Surgery
of the Knee

SECTION EDITORS

W. Norman Scott, MD, FACS
Clinical Professor
Department of Orthopaedic Surgery
Albert Einstein College of Medicine
Associate Orthopaedic Attending
Lenox Hill Hospital
Director
Insall Scott Kelly Institute for Orthopaedics and Sports
  Medicine
New York, New York

Henry D. Clarke, MD
Assistant Professor of Orthopaedics
Mayo Clinic College of Medicine
Rochester, Minnesota
Senior Associate Consultant
Department of Orthopaedics
Mayo Clinic
Scottsdale, Arizona

Fred D. Cushner, MD
Assistant Clinical Professor
Department of Surgery
Division of Orthopaedic Surgery
Albert Einstein College of Medicine
Attending Orthopaedic Surgeon
Lenox Hill Hospital
Beth Israel Medical Center
Director
Insall Scott Kelly Institute for Orthopaedics and Sports
  Medicine
New York, New York

A. Seth Greenwald, DPhil (Oxon)
Director
Orthopaedic Research and Education
Orthopaedic Research Laboratories
Lutheran Hospital
Cleveland Clinic Health System
Cleveland, Ohio

George J. Haidukewych, MD
Orthopaedic Trauma and Adult Reconstruction
Florida Orthopaedic Institute
Temple Terrace, Florida

Mary I. O'Connor, MD
Chair
Department of Orthopaedic Surgery
Associate Professor
Mayo Clinic College of Medicine
Jacksonville, Florida

Susan Craig Scott, MD
Surgeon
Hand Surgery Service
Hospital for Joint Diseases
New York, New York

Giles R. Scuderi, MD
Assistant Clinical Professor of Orthopaedic Surgery
Albert Einstein College of Medicine
Orthopaedic Surgeon
Lenox Hill Hospital
Director
Insall Scott Kelly Institute for Orthopaedics and Sports
  Medicine
New York, New York

Carl L. Stanitski, MD
Professor of Orthopaedic Surgery and Pediatrics
Medical University of South Carolina
Charleston, South Carolina

INSALL & SCOTT

Surgery
of the Knee

Fourth Edition
VOLUME 1

W. Norman Scott, MD, FACS
Clinical Professor
Department of Orthopaedic Surgery
Albert Einstein College of Medicine
Associate Orthopaedic Attending
Lenox Hill Hospital
Director
Insall Scott Kelly Institute for Orthopaedics and Sports Medicine
New York, New York

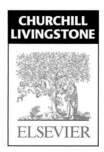

CHURCHILL
LIVINGSTONE

ELSEVIER

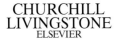

CHURCHILL
LIVINGSTONE
ELSEVIER

1600 John F. Kennedy Blvd.
Ste 1800
Philadelphia, PA 19103-2899

INSALL & SCOTT SURGERY OF THE KNEE

Copyright © 2006, 2001, 1993, 1984 by Elsevier Inc.

E-dition ISBN-13: 978-0443-06961-1
E-dition ISBN-10:   0443-06961-1
ISBN-13: 978-0-443-6671-1
ISBN-10:   0-443-6671-X
Volume 1: PN 9996000389
Volume 2: PN 9996001342

NOTICE

Knowledge and best practice in orthopaedic surgery are constantly changing. As new research and experience broaden our knowledge, changes in practice, treatment, and drug therapy may become necessary or appropriate. Readers are advised to check the most current information provided (i) on procedures featured or (ii) by the manufacturer of each product to be administered, to verify the recommended dose or formula, the method and duration of administration, and contraindications. It is the responsibility of the practitioner, relying on his or her own experience and knowledge of the patient, to make diagnoses, to determine dosages and the best treatment for each individual patient, and to take all appropriate safety precautions. To the fullest extent of the law, neither the publisher nor the editors assume any liability for any injury and/or damage to persons or property arising out of or related to any use of the material contained in this book.

The Publisher

Library of Congress Control Number 2005054901

ISBN-13: 978-0-443-06671-1
ISBN-10:   0-443-06671-X

Publishing Director: Kim Murphy
Developmental Editor: Janice Gaillard
Publishing Services Manager: Tina Rebane
Project Manager: Norm Stellander
Interior Design: Steven Stave
Cover Design: Louis Forgione

Printed in the United States of America

Last digit is the print number: 9 8 7 6 5 4 3 2 1

Dedication

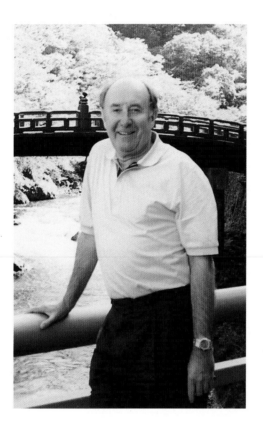

To John N. Insall (1930–2000)

*He is greatly missed by all his students and friends,
whose lives have been enriched by his many contributions.*

Contributors

Paolo Aglietti, MD
Professor of Orthopaedics and Traumatology, and
    Director, First Orthopaedic Clinic, University of
    Florence, Florence, Italy

J. Winslow Alford, MD
Staff Orthopaedic Surgeon, West Bay Orthopaedics,
    Shoulder and Sports Medicine Division, Warwick,
    Rhode Island

Annunziato Amendola, MD
Professor, Department of Orthopaedics and
    Rehabilitation, University of Iowa; Director, University
    of Iowa Sports Medicine Center, Department of
    Orthopaedic Surgery, University of Iowa Hospitals and
    Clinics, Iowa City, Iowa

Jean-Noël A. Argenson, MD
Professor and Chairman of Orthopaedic Surgery, Aix-
    Marseille University; Service de Chirurgie
    Orthopedique et de Traumatologie, Hôpitaux de
    Marseille, Marseille, France

Steven P. Arnoczky, DVM
Professor of Orthopaedic Surgery, College of Human
    Medicine and College of Orthopaedic Medicine,
    Michigan State University; Director, Laboratory for
    Comparative Orthopaedic Research, College of
    Veterinary Medicine, Michigan State University, East
    Lansing, Michigan

Bernard R. Bach, Jr., MD
The Claude N. Lambert, MD—Helen S. Thomson
    Professor, and Director, Division of Sports Medicine,
    Department of Orthopedic Surgery, Rush University
    Medical Center, Chicago, Illinois

David Backstein, MD, MEd, FRSC(C)
Assistant Professor of Surgery, and Director of
    Undergraduate Education, Department of Surgery,
    University of Toronto, Toronto, Ontario, Canada

Scott A. Banks, PhD
Assistant Professor, Mechanical and Aerospace
    Engineering, University of Florida, Gainesville;
    Technical Director, The BioMotion Foundation, West
    Palm Beach, Florida

Sanjiv Bansal, MD
Attending Orthopedic Surgeon, New York Westchester
    Square Medical Center and Our Lady of Mercy
    Medical Center, Bronx, and North Shore University
    Hospital, Queens, New York

Scott A. Barbour, MD
Founder, Comprehensive Orthopaedic Group, Northside
    Forsyth Hospital, Cumming, Georgia

Michael Battaglia, MD
Associate Clinical Professor, University of Washington,
    Seattle, Washington; Associate Clinical Professor,
    University of California, San Diego, La Jolla,
    California; Bethesda National Naval Medical Center,
    Bethesda, Maryland

Todd C. Battaglia, MD, MS
Fellow in Sports Medicine, Department of Orthopaedic
    Surgery, University of Virginia, Charlottesville,
    Virginia

Joshua Baumfeld, MD
Orthopaedic Surgery Resident, Mayo Clinic, Rochester,
    Minnesota; Sports Medicine/Orthopaedic Fellowship,
    University of Virginia, Charlottesville, Virginia

Christopher P. Beauchamp, MD
Associate Professor, Mayo Clinic Graduate School of
    Medicine; Chair, Department of Orthopaedics, Mayo
    Clinic Scottsdale, Scottsdale, Arizona

John A. Bergfeld, MD
Director of Medical Affairs, Cleveland Clinic Sports
    Health, Department of Orthopaedics, The Cleveland
    Clinic Foundation, Cleveland, Ohio

Thomas Bernasek, MD
Adult Reconstruction, Florida Orthopaedic Institute,
    Temple Terrace, Florida

J. David Blaha, MD
Professor, Department of Orthopaedic Surgery,
    University of Michigan, Ann Arbor, Michigan

Robert B. Bourne, MD, FRCSC
Professor and Chairman, Division of Orthopaedic
    Surgery, University of Western Ontario; Chief of
    Orthopaedics, London Health Sciences Centre,
    London, Ontario, Canada

Marc F. Brassard, MD, MS
Anne Arundel Medical Center, Annapolis, Maryland

K. K. Briggs, MPH
Director of Clinical Research, Steadman Hawkins
    Research Foundation, Vail, Colorado

Thomas E. Brown, MD
Assistant Professor, Department of Orthopaedic Surgery, and Co-Director, Orthopaedic Surgery Residency Program, University of Virginia, Charlottesville, Virginia

Richard Brull, MD, FRCPC
Lecturer, Department of Anesthesia, University of Toronto; Staff Anesthesiologist, Toronto Western Hospital, University Health Network, Toronto, Ontario, Canada

Joseph A. Buckwalter, MD
Professor and Head, Orthopaedic Surgery and Rehabilitation, Department of Orthopaedics, University of Iowa Hospitals, Iowa City, Iowa

William D. Bugbee, MD
Associate Professor, Department of Orthopaedic Surgery, University of California, San Diego, La Jolla, California

Michael T. Busch, MD
Orthopaedic Surgeon, Department of Pediatric Orthopaedics, Children's Healthcare of Atlanta at Scottish Rite; Surgical Director, Sports Medicine Program, Children's Healthcare of Atlanta, Atlanta, Georgia

David N. M. Caborn, MB, ChB
Professor, Orthopaedic Surgery, University of Louisville; Chief of Sports Medicine, Jewish Hospital, Louisville, Kentucky

John J. Callaghan, MD
The Lawrence and Marilyn Dorr Chair and Professor, University of Iowa Health Care, Iowa City, Iowa

Anikar Chhabra, MD, MS
Canyon Orthopaedic Surgeons, Ltd., Scottsdale, Arizona

Chang Haw Chong, MBBS, FRCS (Ed), FAMS
Consultant, Department of Orthopedic Surgery, Changi General Hospital, Singapore

Charles R. Clark, MD
Dr. Michael Bonfiglio Professor of Orthopaedics and Rehabilitation, and Professor of BioMedical Engineering, University of Iowa; Staff Physician, Department of Orthopaedics, University of Iowa Hospital and Clinics, Iowa City, Iowa

Henry D. Clarke, MD
Assistant Professor of Orthopaedics, Mayo Clinic College of Medicine, Rochester, Minnesota; Senior Associate Consultant, Department of Orthopaedics, Mayo Clinic, Scottsdale, Arizona

Brian J. Cole, MD, MBA
Associate Professor, Departments of Orthopedics and Anatomy and Cell Biology, Rush University; Director, Rush Cartilage Restoration Center, Rush University Medical Center, Chicago, Illinois

John P. Collier, DE
Myron Tribus Professor of Engineering, Senior Lecturer, and Director, Dartmouth Biomedical Engineering Center, Thayer School of Engineering, Dartmouth College, Hanover, New Hampshire

Matthew J. Crawford, DO, PhD
Clinical Instructor, Michigan State University, East Lansing, Michigan

R. Alexander Creighton, MD
Assistant Professor, Department of Orthopaedic Surgery, University of North Carolina at Chapel Hill, Chapel Hill, North Carolina

Pierluigi Cuomo, MD
First Orthopaedic Clinic, and PhD Candidate, University of Florence, Florence, Italy

Fred D. Cushner, MD
Assistant Clinical Professor, Department of Surgery, Division of Orthopaedic Surgery, Albert Einstein College of Medicine, Bronx; Attending Orthopaedic Surgeon, Lenox Hill Hospital and Beth Israel Medical Center; Director, Insall Scott Kelly Institute for Orthopaedics and Sports Medicine, New York, New York

Diane L. Dahm, MD
Assistant Professor of Orthopaedic Surgery, Mayo Clinic College of Medicine; Orthopaedic Surgeon, Mayo Clinic, Rochester, Minnesota

Timothy A. Damron, MD
David G. Murray Professor of Orthopedics, State University of New York Upstate Medical University; Adjunct Professor, Department of Bioengineering and Neuroscience, Syracuse University, and Department of Neuroscience and Physiology, State University of New York Upstate Medical University, Syracuse, New York

A. Lee Dellon, MD, FACS
Professor, Department of Plastic Surgery—Neurosurgery, Johns Hopkins University, Baltimore, Maryland; Professor of Plastic Surgery, Neurosurgery, and Anatomy, University of Arizona; and Director, Dellon Institute for Peripheral Nerve Surgery, Baltimore, Maryland

Douglas A. Dennis, MD
Adjunct Professor, Department of Biomedical
Engineering, University of Tennessee, Knoxville;
Medical Director, Center for Musculoskeletal
Research, Oak Ridge National Laboratory, Oak Ridge,
Tennessee

Ian D. Dickey, MD
Adjunct Professor of Orthopaedics, University of Maine;
Eastern Maine Medical Center, Cancer Care of Maine,
and Eastern Orthopaedic Oncologist, Bangor, Maine

Todd B. Dietrick, MD
Orthopaedic Surgeon, Congress Medical Associates, Inc.,
Pasadena, California

Anthony M. DiGioia III, MD
Senior Research Scientist and Co-Director, Center for
Medical Robotics and Computer Assisted Surgery,
Carnegie Mellon University; Director, Institute for
Computer Assisted Orthopaedic Surgery, The Western
Pennsylvania Hospital; Orthopaedic Surgeon,
Renaissance Orthopaedics, PC, Pittsburgh,
Pennsylvania

Thomas DiPasquale, DO
Affiliate Assistant Professor, University of South Florida,
Tampa; Associate Director of Orthopaedic Trauma
Service, Tampa General Hospital, Tampa, and Florida
Orthopaedic Institute, Temple Terrace, Florida

Julie A. Dodds, MD
Associate Professor, Michigan State University, East
Lansing, Michigan

Jeffrey B. Driban, MEd, ATC, CSCS
Kinesiology, Temple University, Philadelphia,
Pennsylvania

Zsófia Duska
Physiotherapist, Department of Orthopaedics, Uzsoki
Hospital, Budapest, Hungary

Mark E. Easley, MD
Assistant Professor, Duke University Medical Center;
Consultant, Veterans Administration Medical Center
and Durham Regional Medical Center, Durham, North
Carolina

Thomas H. Eickmann, MD
Orthopedic Surgeon, Centura Avista Adventist Hospital,
Louisville, Colorado

Gregory C. Fanelli, MD
Chief, Arthroscopic Surgery and Sports Medicine,
Geisinger Medical Center, Danville, Pennsylvania

Philip M. Faris, MD
Orthopaedic Surgeon, St. Frances Hospital, Mooresville,
Mooresville, Indiana

Christopher M. Farrell, MD
Fellow, Insall Scott Kelly Institute for Orthopaedics and
Sports Medicine, New York, New York

Thomas K. Fehring, MD
Attending Surgeon, OrthoCarolina Hip and Knee Center,
Charlotte, North Carolina

John M. Flynn, MD
Associate Chief of Orthopaedic Surgery and Associate
Professor of Orthopaedic Surgery, University of
Pennsylvania School of Medicine; Associate Chief of
Orthopaedic Surgery and Associate Orthopaedic
Surgeon, Children's Hospital of Philadelphia,
Philadelphia, Pennsylvania

Lynanne J. Foster, MD
Assistant Professor, Department of Orthopaedics,
University of Texas Health Sciences Center at Houston
Medical School, Houston, Texas

Andrew G. Franks, Jr., MD, FACP
Clinical Professor, New York University School of
Medicine; Attending Physician, Tisch Hospital, The
University Hospital of New York University, New
York, New York

Marc J. Friedman, MD
Assistant Clinical Professor, University of California, Los
Angeles, School of Medicine, Los Angeles; Attending
Surgeon, Southern California Orthopedic Institute,
Van Nuys, California

Richard J. Friedman, MD, FRCSC
Clinical Professor of Orthopaedic Surgery, Medical
University of South Carolina; Medical Director,
Charleston Orthopaedic Associates, Charleston, South
Carolina

Wolfgang Fitz, MD
Clinical Instructor, Orthopaedic Surgery, Harvard
Medical School; Associate Surgeon, Department of
Orthopaedic Surgery, Brigham and Women's Hospital,
Falkner Hospital, and New England Baptist Hospital,
Boston, Massachusetts

Freddie H. Fu, MD
David Silver Professor and Chairman of Orthopaedic
Surgery, University of Pittsburgh School of Medicine
and University of Pittsburgh Medical Center,
Pittsburgh, Pennsylvania

John P. Fulkerson, MD
Clinical Professor of Orthopedic Surgery, and Sports
Medicine Fellowship Director, University of
Connecticut, Farmington, Connecticut

John A. Gallagher, MBBS, FAACS
Fellow, University of Western Ontario, and London
Health Sciences Centre, London, Ontario, Canada

Theodore J. Ganley, MD
Assistant Professor of Orthopaedic Surgery, University of
 Pennsylvania; Attending Surgeon, and Orthopaedic
 Director of Sports Medicine, Department of
 Orthopaedic Surgery, Children's Hospital of
 Philadelphia, Philadelphia, Pennsylvania

Francesco Giron, MD, PhD
Lecturer, University of Florence, and Attending, First
 Orthopaedic Clinic, University of Florence, Florence,
 Italy

Vipool K. Goradia, MD
President, Goradia Orthopedics and Sports Medicine,
 Chester, Virginia

Robert S. Gotlin, DO
Assistant Professor, Rehabilitation Medicine, Albert
 Einstein College of Medicine, Bronx; Director,
 Orthopaedic and Sports Rehabilitation, Beth Israel
 Medical Center, New York, New York

A. Seth Greenwald, DPhil (Oxon)
Director, Orthopaedic Research and Education,
 Orthopaedic Research Laboratories, Lutheran
 Hospital, Cleveland Clinic Health System, Cleveland,
 Ohio

Allan Gross, MD, FRCSC
Bernard I. Ghert Foundation Chair, Lower Extremity
 Reconstruction Surgery, and Professor of Surgery,
 Faculty of Medicine, University of Toronto, Toronto,
 Ontario, Canada

Mahmoud A. Hafez, MD, FRCS Ed
Clinical Research Fellow, Institute for Computer
 Assisted Orthopaedic Surgery, The Western
 Pennsylvania Hospital, Pittsburgh, Pennsylvania

George J. Haidukewych, MD
Orthopaedic Trauma and Adult Reconstruction, Florida
 Orthopaedic Institute, Temple Terrace, Florida

Lázsló Hangody, MD, PhD, DSc
Head, Department of Orthopaedics, Uzsoki Hospital,
 Budapest, Hungary

Arlen D. Hanssen, MD
Professor of Orthopaedic Surgery, Mayo Clinic College
 of Medicine; Consultant in Orthopaedic Surgery, Mayo
 Clinic, Rochester, Minnesota

Melinda K. Harman, DPhil, MSc
Director of Research, The BioMotion Foundation, Palm
 Beach, Florida

Christopher D. Harner, MD
Professor, Department of Orthopedic Surgery, University
 of Pittsburgh School of Medicine; UPMC Center for
 Sports Medicine, Pittsburgh, Pennsylvania

David E. Haynes, MD
Orthopaedic Surgeon, Southwest Sports Medicine and
 Orthopaedics, Waco, Texas

William L. Healy, MD
Professor of Orthopaedic Surgery, Boston University
 School of Medicine, Boston; Chairman and
 Orthopaedic Surgeon, Lahey Clinic, Burlington,
 Massachusetts

Joseph E. Herrera, DO
Fellow, Orthopaedic Sports and Spine Rehabilitation,
 Beth Israel Medical Center, New York, New York

Richard Y. Hinton, MD, MPH
Attending, Union Memorial Hospital, Baltimore,
 Maryland

Aaron A. Hofmann, MD
Professor, Department of Orthopedic Surgery,
 University of Utah School of Medicine, Salt Lake City,
 Utah

Ginger E. Holt, MD
Assistant Professor, Division of Musculoskeletal
 Oncology, Department of Orthopaedic Surgery,
 Vanderbilt Medical Center, Nashville, Tennessee

Johnny Huard, PhD
Henry J. Mankin Associate Professor, Department of
 Orthopaedic Surgery, and Associate Professor,
 Molecular Genetics and Biochemistry and
 Bioengineering, University of Pittsburgh, School of
 Medicine; Director, Growth and Development
 Laboratory, Children's Hospital of Pittsburgh,
 Pittsburgh, Pennsylvania

David S. Hungerford, MD
Professor of Orthopaedic Surgery, Johns Hopkins
 University School of Medicine; Attending, Good
 Samaritan Hospital, Baltimore, Maryland

Marc W. Hungerford, MD
Johns Hopkins University School of Medicine, and
 Chief, Johns Hopkins Orthopedics at Good Samaritan
 Hospital, Baltimore, Maryland

Anthony Infante, DO
Clinical Faculty, Michigan State University, East
 Lansing, Michigan; Orthopaedic Traumatologist,
 General Orthopaedic Surgery, Tampa General
 Hospital, Brandon Regional Hospital, Tampa,
 Florida

John N. Insall, MD*
Formerly Clinical Professor of Orthopaedic Surgery,
   Albert Einstein College of Medicine, Bronx; Director,
   Insall Scott Kelly Institute for Orthopaedics and
   Sports Medicine, Beth Israel Medical Center, New
   York, New York

Richard Iorio, MD
Assistant Professor of Orthopaedic Surgery, Boston
   University School of Medicine, Boston; Active Staff,
   Department of Orthopaedic Surgery, Lahey Clinic,
   Burlington, Massachusetts

David J. Jacofsky, MD
Chairman, The CORE Institute, The Center for
   Orthopedic Research and Education, Sun City West,
   Arizona

Branislav Jaramaz, PhD
Associate Professor, Robotics Institute, Carnegie Mellon
   University; Scientific Director, Institute for Computer
   Assisted Orthopaedic Surgery, The Western
   Pennsylvania Hospital, Pittsburgh, Pennsylvania

James G. Jarvis, MD, FRCS(C)
Associate Professor of Surgery, University of Ottawa;
   Chief, Division of Pediatric Orthopaedics, Children's
   Hospital of Eastern Ontario, Ottawa, Ontario, Canada

Charles E. Johnston II, MD
Professor, Department of Orthopaedic Surgery,
   University of Texas Southwestern Medical School;
   Assistant Chief of Staff, Texas Scottish Rite Hospital
   for Children, Dallas, Texas

Novák Pál Kaposi, MD
National Institute of Rheumatology and Physiotherapy,
   Musculoskeletal Diagnostic Center, Budapest,
   Hungary

Anastassios Karistinos, MD
Sports Medicine Fellow, Advanced Orthopaedics and
   Sports Medicine, Salt Lake City, Utah; Attending
   Physician, Department of Orthopaedic Surgery, Athens
   Naval Hospital, Athens, Greece

Craig M. Kessler, MD
Professor of Medicine, Georgetown University Medical
   Center, Washington, DC

Harpal S. Khanuja, MD
Assistant Professor, Department of Orthopaedic Surgery,
   The Johns Hopkins University School of Medicine;
   Attending, Good Samaritan Hospital, Baltimore,
   Maryland

Warren King, MD
Team Physician, Oakland Raiders; USA Rugby Partner;
   Fellowship Director, Sports Medicine, Palo Alto
   Medical Clinic, Palo Alto, California

*Deceased.

John J. Klimkiewicz, MD
Assistant Professor, Department of Orthopaedic Surgery,
   Georgetown University Hospital, Washington, DC

Kevin Klingele, MD
Attending Orthopaedic Surgeon, Columbus Children's
   Hospital, Columbus, Ohio

Donald M. Knapke, MD
Attending Orthopedic Surgeon, Adult Reconstruction,
   William Beaumont Hospital, Royal Oak, Michigan

Mininder S. Kocher, MD, MPH
Assistant Professor of Orthopaedic Surgery, Harvard
   Medical School; Associate Director, Division of Sports
   Medicine, Children's Hospital, Boston, Massachusetts

Richard D. Komistek, PhD
Professor, Biomedical Engineering, University of
   Tennessee, Knoxville; Director, Center for
   Musculoskeletal Research, Oak Ridge National
   Laboratory, Oak Ridge, Tennessee

Kenneth A. Krackow, MD
Professor and Vice Chairman, Department of
   Orthopaedic Surgery, State University of New York at
   Buffalo; Clinical Director, Department of Orthopaedic
   Surgery, Kaleida Health—Buffalo General Hospital,
   Buffalo, New York

John E. Kuhn, MD
Associate Professor, Division of Sports Medicine,
   Department of Orthopaedics and Rehabilitation,
   Vanderbilt University Medical Center, Nashville,
   Tennessee

Amit Lahav, MD
Fellow, Department of Orthopedic Surgery, University of
   Utah School of Medicine, Salt Lake City, Utah

Jason E. Lang, MD
Chief Resident, Division of Orthopaedic Surgery, Duke
   University Medical Center, Durham, North Carolina

James M. Leone, MD, FRCSC
Instructor of Orthopaedic Surgery, Mayo College of
   Medicine, Rochester, Minnesota

Scott M. Lephart, PhD, ATC
Acting Chair, and Associate Professor, Department of
   Sports Medicine and Nutrition, University of
   Pittsburgh, Pittsburgh, Pennsylvania

Randall J. Lewis, MD
Clinical Professor, Department of Orthopaedic Surgery,
   George Washington University Medical Center;
   Director, Washington Center for Hip and Knee
   Surgery, Washington, DC

Eric M. Lindvall, DO, MS
Orthopaedic Traumatologist, Tampa General Hospital, Tampa, Florida

David R. Lionberger, MD
Clinical Assistant Professor, Department of Orthopedic Surgery, Baylor College of Medicine, Houston; Active Staff, The Methodist Hospital and Twelve Oaks Hospital, Houston; and Active Staff, Bellville General Hospital, Bellville, Texas

Frank Liporace, MD
Attending Physician, Department of Orthopaedics, University of Medicine and Dentistry of New Jersey, Newark, New Jersey

Steve S. Liu, MD
Research Assistant, University of Iowa Health Care, Iowa City, Iowa

T. Thomas Liu, MD, PhD
Orthopaedic Surgery Resident, University of Pittsburgh Medical Center, Pittsburgh, Pennsylvania

Jess H. Lonner, MD
Director, Joint Arthroplasty Fellowship, and Director, Knee Replacement Surgery, Booth Bartolozzi Balderston Orthopaedics, Pennsylvania Hospital, Philadelphia, Pennsylvania

Paul A. Lotke, MD
Professor of Orthopaedic Surgery, University of Pennsylvania School of Medicine; Chief of Implant Service, Hospital of the University of Pennsylvania, Philadelphia, Pennsylvania

Steven Lyons, MD
Adult Reconstruction, Florida Orthopaedic Institute, Temple Terrace, Florida

Mohamed R. Mahfouz, PhD
Co-Director, Center for Musculoskeletal Research, University of Tennessee, Knoxville; Oak Ridge National Laboratory, Oak Ridge, Tennessee

Stephen G. Manifold, MD
Orthopaedic Surgeon, Bayhealth Medical Center, Dover, Delaware

J. Bohannon Mason, MD
Adjunct Professor, Department of Mechanical Engineering, University of North Carolina at Charlotte; Attending Surgeon, OrthoCarolina Hip and Knee Center, Charlotte, North Carolina

Henry Masur, MD
Clinical Professor of Medicine, George Washington University School of Medicine, Washington, DC; Chief, Critical Care Medicine, National Institutes of Health, Bethesda, Maryland

Kevin R. Math, MD
Associate Professor of Clinical Radiology, Albert Einstein College of Medicine, Bronx; Chief of Musculoskeletal Radiology, Beth Israel Medical Center, New York, New York

Leslie S. Matthews, MD, MBA
Assistant Clinical Professor, Johns Hopkins Hospital, and Chief of Orthopaedic Surgery, Union Memorial Hospital, Baltimore, Maryland

James P. McAuley, MD, FRCSC
Associate Clinical Professor, University of Maryland, Baltimore, Maryland; Consultant; Anderson Orthopaedic Clinic and Research Institute, Alexandria, Virginia

David A. McGuire, MD
Clinical Instructor, University of Washington, Seattle, Washington; Affiliate Professor, University of Alaska, Anchorage, Alaska

Nathan M. Melton, DO
Resident, Grandview Hospital, Dayton, Ohio

R. Michael Meneghini, MD
St. Vincent Center for Joint Replacement, Joint Replacement Surgeons of Indiana, Indianapolis, Indiana

Theodore T. Miller, MD
Associate Professor of Radiology, New York University School of Medicine, New York; Chief, Division of Musculoskeletal Imaging, Department of Radiology, North Shore University Hospital–Long Island Jewish Medical Center, Great Neck, New York

Tom Minas, MD, MS
Associate Professor, Harvard Medical School, Boston; Director, Cartilage Repair Center, Brigham and Women's Hospital, Chestnut Hill, Massachusetts

Timothy S. Mologne, MD
Sports Medicine Center, Appleton, Wisconsin

Michael A. Mont, MD
Director, Center for Joint Preservation and Reconstruction, Sinai Hospital of Baltimore, Rubin Institute for Advanced Orthopedics, Baltimore, Maryland

Adam Mor, MD
Research Fellow in Rheumatology, New York University School of Medicine, New York, New York

Edward A. Morra, MSME
Manager, Computational Testing Services, Orthopaedic Research Laboratories, Lutheran Hospital, Cleveland Clinic Health System, Cleveland, Ohio

Kevin J. Mulhall, MD, MCh, FRCSI(TR and Orth)
Fellow, Adult Reconstructive Surgery, Department of Orthopaedic Surgery, University of Virginia, Charlottesville, Virginia

Sandeep Munjal, MCh (Orth), MD
Orthopaedic Attending, Department of Orthopaedics, Physicians' Clinic of Iowa, Cedar Rapids, Iowa

Cass Nakasone, MD
Fellow, University of Southern California, Los Angeles, California

Michael D. Neel, MD
Clinical Assistant Professor in Orthopaedics, University of Tennessee; Adjunct Faculty, Department of Orthopaedics, St. Jude Children's Research Hospital, Memphis, Tennessee

Mary I. O'Connor, MD
Chair, Department of Orthopaedic Surgery, and Associate Professor, Mayo Clinic College of Medicine, Jacksonville, Florida

Mark W. Pagnano, MD
Associate Professor of Orthopaedic Surgery, Mayo College of Medicine; Consultant, Division of Adult Reconstruction, Department of Orthopaedic Surgery, Mayo Clinic, Rochester, Minnesota

Richard D. Parker, MD
Education and Fellowship Director, Cleveland Clinic Sports Health, Department of Orthopaedics, The Cleveland Clinic Foundation, Cleveland, Ohio

Todd A. Parker, MD
Senior Medical Officer, USS Gunston Hall

Lonnie E. Paulos, MD
Partner, Advanced Orthopedics and Sports Medicine, Salt Lake City, Utah

Henrik B. Pedersen, MD
Director of Medical Multimedia, Insall Scott Kelly Institute for Orthopaedics and Sports Medicine, New York, New York

Catherine Petchprapa, MD
Assistant Professor, Department of Radiology, Beth Israel Hospital, New York, New York

Lars Peterson, MD, PhD
Professor, Department of Orthopaedics, University of Goteborg; Clinical Director, Gothenburg Medical Center, Frolunda, Sweden

Russell S. Petrie, MD
Clinical Instructor, Western University Physician Assistant Program, Pomona; Chairman, Department of Orthopedic Surgery, Hoag Memorial Hospital Presbyterian, Newport Beach, California

Pascal Poilvache, MD
Associate Professor, Catholic University of Louvain; Chief, Hip and Knee Reconstruction, Saint-Luc University Hospital, Brussels, Belgium

W.R. Post, MD
Associate Professor, Vice-Chairman, Chief, Section of Sports Medicine and Shoulder Surgery, Department of Orthopedics, West Virginia University School of Medicine, Morgantown, West Virginia

Anthony H. Presutti, MD
Active Staff, Department of Surgery (Privileges in Orthopaedics), Cheshire Medical Center, Dartmouth-Hitchcock Keene, Keene, New Hampshire

Lisa A. Pruitt, PhD
Professor, Department of Mechanical Engineering, University of California, Berkeley, Berkeley, California

Craig S. Radnay, MD, MPH
Orthopaedic Fellow, Insall Scott Kelly Institute for Orthopaedics and Sports Medicine, New York, New York; Fellow, Florida Orthopaedic Institute, Tampa, Florida

Phillip S. Ragland, MD
Center for Joint Preservation and Reconstruction, Rubin Institute for Advanced Orthopedics, Sinai Hospital of Baltimore, Baltimore, Maryland

Robert Lor Randall, MD, FACS
Associate Professor, Department of Orthopaedics, and Director, Sarcoma Services, Huntsman Cancer Institute at the University of Utah and Primary Children's Medical Center, Salt Lake City, Utah

Robert Siskind Reiffel, MD
Attending and Chief Emeritus of Plastic Surgery, and Secretary/Treasurer, Medical Staff, White Plains Hospital, White Plains, New York

Michael D. Ries, MD
Professor of Orthopedic Surgery, Department of Orthopaedic Surgery, and Chief of Arthroplasty, University of California, San Francisco, San Francisco; Professor of Mechanical Engineering, Department of Mechanical Engineering, University of California, Berkeley, Berkeley, California

William G. Rodkey, DVM, Dip ACVS
Director, Basic Science Research and Assistant
Fellowship Director, Steadman–Hawkins Research
Foundation; Vice President, Scientific Affairs, ReGen
Biologics, Inc., Vail, Colorado

Juan J. Rodrigo, MD
Adjunct Professor of Biomedical Engineering, Clemson
University; Emeritus Professor of Orthopaedics,
Department of Orthopaedics, University of California,
Davis, Sacramento, California; Steadman-Hawkins
Clinic of the Carolinas, Spartanburg, South Carolina

Cecil H. Rorabeck, MD, FRCSC
Professor, University of Western Ontario; Attending
Orthopaedic Surgeon, Department of Orthopaedic
Surgery, London Health Sciences Center, London,
Ontario, Canada

Aaron G. Rosenberg, MD
Professor of Surgery and Director of Adult
Reconstructive Orthopaedics, Rush University Medical
Center, Chicago, Illinois

Oleg Safir, MD
Clinical Fellow, University of Toronto and Mount Sinai
Hospital, Toronto, Ontario, Canada

**Khaled J. Saleh, MD, MSc (Epid),
FRCS(C), FACS**
Division Head and Fellowship Director, Adult
Reconstruction; Associate Professor, Department of
Orthopaedic Surgery; and Associate Professor, Health
Evaluation Sciences, University of Virginia,
Charlottesville, Virginia

Roy Sanders, MD
Clinical Professor of Orthopaedics, Department of
Orthopaedic Surgery, University of South Florida;
Chief, Department of Orthopaedics, Tampa General
Hospital, Tampa, Florida

Richard D. Scott, MD
Professor of Orthopaedic Surgery, Harvard Medical
School; Senior Surgeon, Brigham and Women's
Hospital and New England Baptist Hospital, Boston,
Massachusetts

Susan Craig Scott, MD
Surgeon, Hand Surgery Service, Hospital for Joint
Diseases, New York, New York

W. Norman Scott, MD, FACS
Clinical Professor, Department of Orthopaedic
Surgery, Albert Einstein College of Medicine;
Associate Orthopaedic Attending, Lenox Hill
Hospital; Director, Insall Scott Kelly Institute for
Orthopaedics and Sports Medicine, New York, New
York

Giles R. Scuderi, MD
Assistant Clinical Professor of Orthopaedic Surgery,
Albert Einstein College of Medicine, Bronx;
Orthopaedic Surgeon, Lenox Hill Hospital, and
Director, Insall Scott Kelly Institute for Orthopaedics
and Sports Medicine, New York, New York

Jon K. Sekiya, MD
Assistant Professor, Center for Sports Medicine,
University of Pittsburgh Medical Center, Pittsburgh,
Pennsylvania

Alison Selleck, MD
Clinic Physician, National Institute of Allergy and
Infectious Disease, Warren G. Magnuson Clinical
Center, National Institutes of Health Critical Care
Medicine Department, Bethesda, Maryland

Krishn M. Sharma, MD
Resident, Orthopaedics, Union Memorial Hospital,
Baltimore, Maryland

Nigel E. Sharrock, MB, ChB
Clinical Professor, Weill Medical College of Cornell
University; Senior Scientist and Attending
Anesthesiologist, Department of Anesthesiology, The
Hospital for Special Surgery, New York, New York

Stephen G. Silver, MD
Attending, Lenox Hill Hospital, New York, New York;
Attending, Hackensack Medical Center, Hackensack,
New Jersey

Carl L. Stanitski, MD
Professor of Orthopaedic Surgery and Pediatrics, Medical
University of South Carolina, Charleston, South
Carolina

J. Richard Steadman, MD
Clinical Professor, University of Texas Southwestern
Medical School, Dallas, Texas; Orthopaedic Surgeon
and Chairman of the Board, Steadman-Hawkins Clinic
and Research Foundation, Vail, Colorado

James B. Stiehl, MD
Clinical Associate Professor, Department of Orthopaedic
Surgery, Medical College of Wisconsin; Staff
Physician, Columbia St. Mary's Hospital, Milwaukee,
Wisconsin

Michael J. Stuart, MD
Professor of Orthopaedics, Mayo Clinic College of
Medicine; Co-Director, Sports Medicine Center, and
Vice-Chairman, Department of Orthopaedics, Mayo
Clinic, Rochester, Minnesota

S. David Stulberg, MD
Professor, Clinical Orthopaedic Surgery, Northwestern
University Feinberg School of Medicine; Director,
Section of Joint Reconstruction and Implant Surgery,
Northwestern Memorial Hospital, Northwestern
Orthopaedic Institute, Chicago, Illinois

Charles Buz Swanik, PhD, ATC
University of Delaware, Department of Health,
Nutrition, and Exercise Sciences, Human Performance
Laboratory, Newark, Delaware

Imre Szerb, MD
Assistant Leader of the Department of Orthopaedics,
Uzsoki Hospital, Budapest, Hungary

Kimberly Templeton, MD
Associate Professor of Orthopaedic Surgery and McCann
Professor of Women in Medicine and Science,
University of Kansas School of Medicine, Kansas City,
Kansas

Alfred J. Tria, Jr., MD
Clinical Professor of Orthopaedic Surgery, and Director
of Orthopaedic Fellowship Training, Robert Wood
Johnson Medical School, New Brunswick, New Jersey

Hans K. Uhthoff
Professor Emeritus, Research Associate, Ottawa Hospital,
Ottawa, Ontario, Canada

Anthony S. Unger, MD
Associate Professor, Department of Orthopaedic Surgery,
George Washington University Medical Center;
Director, Washington Center for Hip and Knee
Surgery, Washington, DC

Thomas Parker Vail, MD
Professor of Orthopaedic Surgery and Director of Adult
Reconstructive Surgery, Duke University Medical
Center, Durham, North Carolina

Douglas W. Van Citters, MS
PhD Candidate, Thayer School of Engineering,
Dartmouth College, Hanover, New Hampshire

Nikhil Verma, MD
Assistant Professor, Rush University Medical Center,
Chicago, Illinois

Vincent J. Vigorita, MD
Professor of Pathology and Orthopaedic Surgery,
Department of Pathology and Orthopaedic Surgery,
State University of New York Health Sciences Center
at Brooklyn/Downstate Medical Center, Brooklyn;
Director of Orthopaedic Research, St. Vincent's
Medical Center, New York, New York

Kelly G. Vince, MD
Associate Professor, University of Southern California
Center for Arthritis, Los Angeles, California

James A. Walker, PhD
Sports Science Director, The Orthopaedic Specialty
Hospital, Salt Lake City, Utah

Kurt R. Weiss, MD
Orthopaedic Surgery Resident, University of Pittsburgh
Medical Center, Pittsburgh, Pennsylvania

David R. Whiddon, MD
Bone and Joint/Sports Medicine Institute, Department of
Orthopaedic Surgery, Naval Medical Center,
Portsmouth, Virginia

Leo A. Whiteside, MD
Clinical Professor of Orthopaedic Surgery, St. Louis
University; Orthopaedic Surgeon, St. Joseph Hospital
of Kirkwood, and Director, Biomechanical Research
Foundation, Missouri Bone and Joint Center, St.
Louis, Missouri

Thomas L. Wickiewicz, MD
Professor, Weill Medical College of Cornell University,
and Chief, Sports Medicine and Shoulder Service,
Hospital for Special Surgery, New York, New York

William M. Wind, MD
University Sports Medicine, Buffalo Sports Medicine,
Buffalo, New York

Edward M. Wojtys, MD
Professor, Department of Orthopaedic Surgery, and
Director of Sports Medicine, University of Michigan
Health System, Ann Arbor, Michigan

Syed Furqan Zaidi, MD
Chief Resident of Diagnostic Radiology, Beth Israel
Medical Center, New York, New York

Foreword

In the past two decades knee surgery has progressed from a small specialty in its infancy, with a limited basic science foundation, crude imaging and diagnostic modalities, and rudimentary treatment methods, to a huge field that encompasses many subspecialties, each with its own core of knowledge and literature. The field has been dynamic, and much has been learned over a relatively short time period.

A field that has come into its own deserves a textbook that reflects this arrival: *Insall & Scott Surgery of the Knee* is a comprehensive textbook that fulfills this important role. The scope of this text is broad. The book covers basic science of knee disorders, ligament and tendon disorders and reconstruction, fractures about the knee, pediatric knee disorders, and the practice and biomechanics of knee replacement and its alternatives.

The quality of an undertaking of this magnitude is dependent on the individual contributions of each author. A review of chapter authorship reveals this text is written by masters—and in many cases the fathers—of each topic. Authors provide their best work when the subject is their passion and when the book in which their work is to appear is the standard-bearer for a profession. *Insall & Scott Surgery of the Knee* fulfills both criteria, which helps to explain the exceptional quality of the material.

Textbook editors are challenged to produce a text that stays current in the face of a rapidly evolving specialty.

The editors of this book address this dilemma with an innovative idea: a companion electronic version, to include cutting-edge monthly content updates to complement the book. Illustrating surgical technique in a manner that is useful to the surgeon also is a challenge for textbook editors. The editors of this text surmount the challenge with modern technology: an accompanying digital video disk augments the text and illustrates key operative techniques.

A textbook derives its content, organization, and style from its editors and section editors. This text already has a rich heritage. The late John Insall is widely acknowledged as the father of modern reconstructive knee surgery. Norman Scott has been one of the foremost practitioners and educators in the combined fields of sports medicine of the knee and reconstructive knee surgery for the past two decades. This book, their brainchild, now in its fourth edition, provides a comprehensive, authoritative, dynamic, and innovative text that will be the standard on the subject for today's knee surgeons.

Daniel J. Berry, MD
Professor and Chairman
Department of Orthopaedic Surgery
Mayo Clinic
Rochester, Minnesota

Preface

In 1984, John Insall almost single-handedly wrote the first edition of *Surgery of the Knee*. There were only 24 contributors to that single volume. In 1993, the second edition had 40 contributors and four associate editors and consisted of two volumes. In 2001, we combined efforts (*The Knee*, Mosby, 1994) to enhance the third edition (159 contributors) of *Surgery of the Knee*. Thus in 17 years three editions were published, and now the fourth edition has published less than five years later. This shortened publication time reflects our interest in being current and in using the latest technology and leading experts to inform our readers. In this fourth edition of *Surgery of the Knee*, we have updated basic chapters and introduced new information utilizing text and visual aids (DVDs), and we are inaugurating a new feature, a companion online e-dition: www.scottkneesurgery.com. The e-dition website will include full text search, hyperlinks to PubMed, an image library, and monthly content updates, to minimize the customary complaint of the "perpetual lag" inherent with textbooks in general. Our goal is to create an interactive current environment for all of us students of the diagnosis and treatment of knee disorders.

The fourth edition of *Surgery of the Knee* has 12 sections, 112 chapters, and 191 international contributors. The DVD sections include (1) a classic video recorded in 1994 (Drs. Insall and Scott) detailing "Exposures, Approaches and Soft Tissue Balancing in Knee Arthroplasty"; (2) interactive anatomical and physical examination recordings, which enhance the material presented in Chapters 1, 2, 3, 5, 6, and 7; and (3) three commonly used minimally invasive surgical techniques for knee arthroplasty.

In Section I, Basic Science, Chapters 1 to 5, the core information presented in the third edition is updated. The DVD of the Anatomy Section is interactive with the imaging in Section II, so the reader can see the normal and abnormal findings side by side. Chapter 3, Clinical Examination of the Knee, now, as mentioned, has the added feature of an actual examination on the DVD to enhance the text.

Section III, Biomechanics, has been expanded under the guidance of A. Seth Greenwald, DPhil (Oxon), to include soft issue and implant considerations that are essential to executing surgical decisions.

With the plethora of Internet information available to patients today, it behooves the knee physician to be absolutely familiar with the various nonoperative and operative alternatives for the treatment of articular cartilage and meniscal disorders (Section IV). Dr. Henry Clarke has done a magnificent job in assembling the innovators in the field. The 18 chapters in this section truly capture the basic science, including the potential of gene therapy, biomechanics, and various treatment options, presented in great detail with the most current results. The section is further highlighted by Dr. Clarke's algorithm for clinical management of articular cartilage injuries.

The advances in the treatment of knee ligament injuries since 1984 are, needless to say, overwhelming. The success achieved today in the treatment of ligament injuries would have been unimaginable 25 years ago. As Section Editor of Section V, Ligament Injuries, Dr. Fred Cushner has assembled most of the people associated with these improvements. The foundations for treatments, controversies, and specific techniques are well chronicled throughout this section. Similarly, Section VI, Patellar and Extensor Mechanism Disorders, represents an updated comprehensive review by Dr. Aglietti and surgical chapters by Drs. Fulkerson and Scuderi.

Sections VII and VIII are "must reads" for all knee clinicians. In addition to discussing the normal and abnormal synovium, we have recruited distinguished authors to discuss the application of current topics of concern to both the patient and clinician, e.g., HIV and hepatitis (Chapter 59), anesthesia for knee surgery (Chapter 60), and an understanding of reflex sympathetic dystrophy (Chapter 61). The orthopaedic knee surgeon must have an absolute awareness of the potential problems inherent in the skin about the knee. In Chapter 63, Soft-Tissue Healing, Drs. Susan Scott and Robert Reiffel give us a foundation for avoiding and treating these potential problems.

Section IX focuses on fractures about the knee and has been organized by Dr. George Haidukewych. These fracture experts have covered all the fractures that occur, including the difficult periprosthetic fractures. Treatment modalities are detailed and reflect the current options with the latest equipment.

Section X, Pediatric Knee, has been reinvigorated with the help of Carl Stanitski. We decided to present the orthopaedic pediatric approach, rather than the sole viewpoint of the knee physician who treats pediatric injuries. The section is well organized, comprehensive, and, I believe, an improvement over the third edition of *Surgery of the Knee*.

The largest section in this two-volume edition is Section XI, Joint Replacement and Its Alternatives. Dr. Gil Scuderi has organized this section of the surgical treatment of the arthritic knee, including osteotomy, unicompartment replacement, patellofemoral arthroplasty, total knee replacement, and the more challenging revision surgery. While establishing the indications and contraindications for techniques, he has been careful to include the identification and management of difficult complications, such as infection, bone defects, extensor mechanism disruption, blood management, and thrombophlebitis. The tremendous success achieved in knee arthroplasty has paralleled the improvements in surgical instrumentation. In this section several authors have detailed the current concepts of computer and navigation surgery, a truly exciting recent development. In the aforementioned e-dition version of *Surgery of the Knee*, the first several streaming videos will focus on specific techniques. Thus, these chapters provide an excellent foundation for interpreting the subsequent e-version techniques.

Dr. Mary O'Connor has developed Section XII, Tumors about the Knee, in a concise, clinically rational framework for those physicians who do not necessarily treat many of these difficult problems. Chapters 106 to 112 are well written and are truly outstanding contributions to this text.

Surgery of the Knee is a text that includes audiovisual teaching aids and now a monthly means of communicating current information in a timely audiovisual manner. To me, it's very exciting, and I look forward to integrating the contributions of these authors into a rapidly current technology for the benefit of all our patients.

W. Norman Scott, MD

Acknowledgments

I would like to express my appreciation to Dr. Henrik Pedersen, without whom the DVDs and e-version addition would not have been possible; to Kathleen Lenhardt for doing everything imaginable during the transition; and to Ruth O'Sullivan for being a reservoir of dependability.

Contents

Contents

Surgery
of the Knee

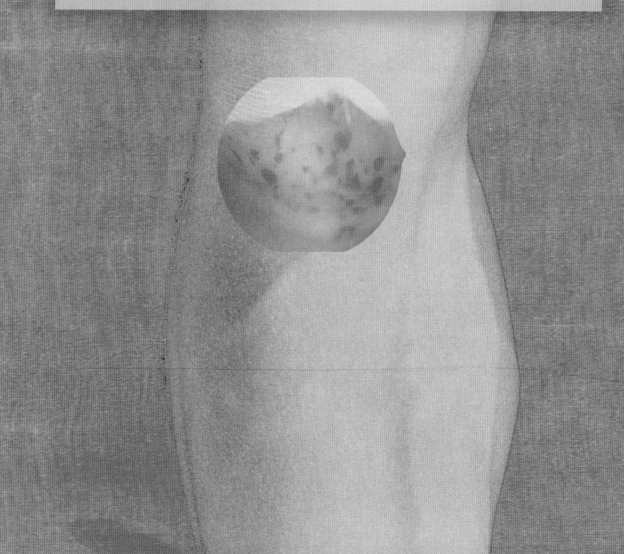

SECTION I

Basic Science

Anatomy

Henry D. Clarke • W. Norman Scott • John N. Insall
Henrik B. Pedersen • Kevin R. Math • Vincent J. Vigorita
Fred D. Cushner

The anatomy of the knee can be examined on a number of levels from the microscopic to the gross and with a variety of techniques, including physical examination, anatomic dissection, radiographic and cross-sectional imaging, and arthroscopic examination. Any practitioner interested in diagnosing and treating disorders of the knee requires a detailed understanding of both normal and abnormal regional anatomy. Furthermore, the ability to interpret and correlate information obtained from different sources is highly beneficial. However, it is also paramount that the clinician gain the knowledge that is required to be able to interpret the significance of an identifiable anatomic abnormality within the context of a patient's complaints. It is the goal of this chapter to present a thorough review of knee anatomy to help the reader more successfully assimilate the material presented in subsequent chapters. To provide a comprehensive description of pertinent anatomic details, text, illustrations, arthroscopic photographs, radiographs, and pictures from cross-sectional imaging studies are used. In addition, in many situations the same structures are presented from different perspectives. Rather than being redundant, we hope that this approach will facilitate the development of a more complete appreciation of the anatomy about the knee. The descriptions that follow are partly taken from standard anatomic texts.[3,8,61,97]

NORMAL SKELETAL STRUCTURES

Bone Physiology

Bone is composed of mineral crystals embedded in an organic matrix. Of the dry weight of bone (about 10% of the actual weight in situ), approximately 70% is due to the mineral content and 30% is organic matter. The mineral is primarily calcium and phosphorus in a ratio of 2:1. The organic matter is composed of collagen, noncollagenized matrix, and proteins. Collagen is the major extracellular component of bone and is composed of fibrils. Collagen fibrils, which form a parallel, highly organized arrangement, are known as *intrinsic fibers*, whereas those that tend to anchor ligaments and tendons at attachment sites and often insert in a perpendicular manner are *extrinsic fibers*. The matrix is populated by mesenchymal cells, which differentiate into osteocytes, osteoblasts, and osteoclasts. These cells perform key functions in the turnover and

remodeling of bone in response to both physical and metabolic stimuli. Osteoblasts are cuboid in nature and have abundant cytoplasm. The main function of osteoblasts is to produce osteoid, a collagenized protein that mineralizes at the tidemark zone as hydroxyapatite crystals are incorporated (Fig. 1–1). As the matrix becomes mineralized bone, these cells become embedded and transform into osteocytes. The osteocyte is in contact with the osteoblast through the cannular system. Osteoclasts are multinucleated macrophage-like cells that perform bone resorption at mineralized bone surfaces (Fig. 1–2). Other associated tissues such as periosteum (Fig. 1–3), fatty and hematopoietic marrow elements, and tendon and ligament attachments create a complex system with mechanical, metabolic, and hematopoietic functions.

Bony Architecture

The knee joint consists of three bony structures—the femur, tibia, and patella—that form three distinct and partially separated compartments: the medial, lateral, and patellofemoral compartments.

PATELLA

The patella is the largest sesamoid bone in the body and sits in the femoral trochlea. It is an asymmetric oval in shape with its apex directed distally. The fibers of the quadriceps tendon envelop it anteriorly and blend with the patella ligament distally. The articulation between the patella and femoral trochlea forms the anterior or patellofemoral compartment (Fig. 1–4).

The posterior aspect of the patella is described as possessing seven facets. Both the medial and lateral facets are divided vertically into approximately equal thirds, whereas the seventh or odd facet lies along the extreme medial border of the patella. Overall, the medial facet is smaller and slightly convex; the lateral facet, which consists of roughly two-thirds of the patella, has both a sagittal convexity and coronal concavity (Fig. 1–5). Six morphological variants of the patella have been described (Fig. 1–6). Types I and II are stable, whereas the other variants are more likely to give rise to lateral subluxation as a result of unbalanced forces.[10,96] The facets are covered by the thickest hyaline cartilage in the body, which may

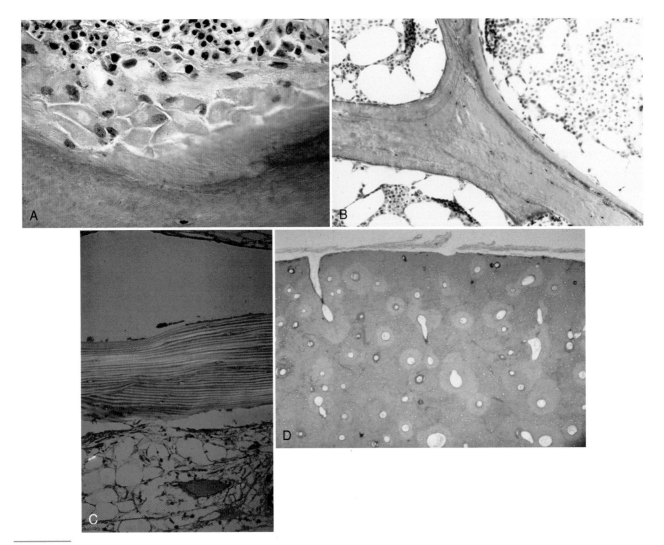

Figure 1–1. **A,** Osteoblasts. Plump, cytoplasmic-rich osteoblasts actively making osteoid, the type I collagen that in the normal sequence of events becomes the fibrous matrix of mineralized bone. **B,** Normal cancellous (trabecular, spongy) bone bathed in normal hematopoietic marrow. Bone surfaces are smooth. Osteoid deposition (light pink surface) is interfaced with mature bone by the basophilic mineralization front. **C,** Normal cancellous bone. With the use of polarized light microscopy, the organized lamellar or pleated deposition of the collagen matrix of mineralized bone is appreciated. **D,** Cross-section of cortical bone showing numerous haversian systems of varying age. The cortical bone is surrounded on its surface by periosteum. The cortical bone itself is composed of haversian bone systems, which represent interwoven longitudinal, circumferential, and concentric bone-forming units (osteons) characterized by central haversian canals of various size and shape. Remodeling is ongoing throughout life; most of it occurs in an axial direction down the shaft.

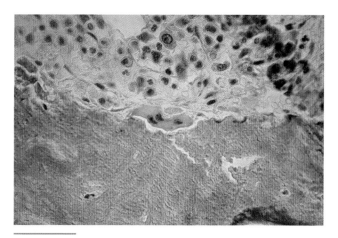

Figure 1–2. Osteoclast. A multinucleated osteoclast is resorbing bone at a crenated surface, Howship's lacuna.

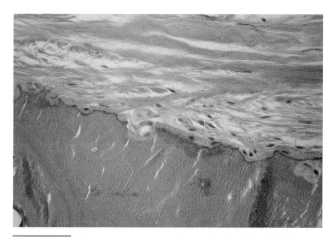

Figure 1–3. Periosteum. The often inconspicuous spindle-shaped fibroblast-like cells of the periosteum belie their remarkable capacity to become activated as bone-forming cells.

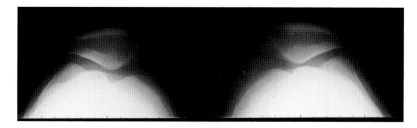

Figure 1–4. Merchant view radiograph of a normal patellofemoral joint. The tibial tubercle is superimposed over the apex of the femoral trochlea.

measure up to 6.5 mm in thickness.[96] The relationship between surface degeneration of this articular surface, or chondromalacia, seen arthroscopically in adolescents and young adults, and pain is unclear.

The femoral trochlea is separated from the medial and lateral femoral condyles by indistinct ridges; the lateral ridge is more prominent. The patella fits in the trochlea of the femur imperfectly, and the contact patch between the patella and femur varies with position as the patella sweeps across the femoral surface. The contact patch has been investigated by dye[32] and casting techniques.[2] Both methods produce very similar results and indicate that the area of contact never exceeds about one-third of the total patellar articular surface. At 10 to 20 degrees of flexion, the distal pole of the patella first contacts the trochlea in a narrow band across both the medial and lateral facets (Fig. 1–7).[32,44] As flexion increases, the contact area moves proximally and laterally. The most extensive contact is made at approximately 45 degrees, where the contact area is an ellipse in continuity across the central portion of the medial and lateral facets. By 90 degrees, the contact area has shifted to the upper part of the medial and lateral patellar facets. With further flexion, the contact area separates into distinct medial and lateral patches.[2,32,44] Because the odd facet makes contact with the femur only in extreme flexion (such as in the act of squatting), this facet is habitually a noncontact zone in humans in Western cultures, a fact that is thought to have some pathological significance.

The main biomechanical function of the patella is to increase the moment arm of the quadriceps mechanism.[52] The load across the joint rises as flexion increases, but because the contact area also increases, the higher force is dissipated over a larger area. However, if extension against resistance is performed, the force increases while the contact area shrinks, which may exacerbate pain from the patellofemoral region. Straight-leg raises eliminate force transmission across the patellofemoral joint because in full extension, the patella has not yet engaged the trochlea.[44]

FEMUR

The architecture of the distal end of the femur is complex. Furthermore, this area serves as the attachment site of numerous ligaments and tendons (Fig. 1–8). In shape and dimensions, the femoral condyles are asymmetric; the larger medial condyle has a more symmetric curvature. The lateral condyle viewed from the side has a sharply increasing radius of curvature posteriorly. The femoral condyles viewed from the surface, articulating with the tibia, show that the lateral condyle is slightly shorter than the medial. The long axis of the lateral condyle is slightly longer and is placed in a more sagittal plane than the long axis of the medial condyle, which is oriented at a mean angle of about 22 degrees and opened posteriorly.[51] The lateral condyle is slightly wider than the medial condyle at the center of the intercondylar notch. Anteriorly, the condyles are separated by a groove: the femoral trochlea

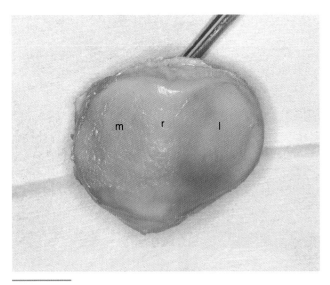

Figure 1–5. Articular surface of the patella. The median ridge (r) divides the smaller medial facet (m) from the larger lateral facet (l).

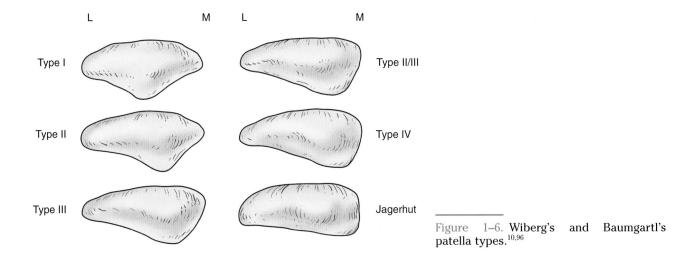

Figure 1–6. Wiberg's and Baumgartl's patella types.[10,96]

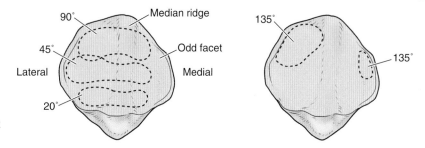

Figure 1–7. Patellofemoral contact areas at different degrees of flexion.

(Fig. 1–9). The sulcus represents the deepest point in the trochlea. Relative to the midplane between the condyles, the sulcus lies slightly laterally.[23] Reproducing this anatomic relationship is important for accurate patellofemoral mechanics after total knee replacement.

The intercondylar notch separates the two condyles distally and posteriorly. The lateral wall of the notch has a flat impression where the proximal origin of the anterior cruciate ligament (ACL) arises. On the medial wall of the notch is a larger site where the posterior cruciate ligament (PCL) originates. The mean width of the notch is narrowest at the distal end and widens proximally (1.8 to 2.3 cm); in contrast, the height of the notch is greatest at the midportion (2.4 cm) and decreases proximally (1.3 cm) and distally (1.8 cm).[57] The dimensions of the notch have become an important topic because of the association between narrow notch width and an increased risk for ACL tear. This risk does not seem to be related to the intrinsic characteristics of the ACL because normal-size ligaments have been identified in specimens with narrow notches.[69] Therefore, the increased risk of ACL failure is probably due to impingement on the ligament.[31,58,69] Notchplasty or sculpting of the intercondylar notch to increase the dimensions has become an integral part of ACL reconstruction.

The lateral condyle has a short groove just proximal to the articular margin, in which lies the tendinous origin of the popliteus muscle. This groove separates the lateral epicondyle from the joint line. The lateral epicondyle is a small but distinct prominence to which attaches the lateral (fibular) collateral ligament (LCL). On the medial condyle the prominent adductor tubercle is the insertion site of the adductor magnus. The medial epicondyle lies anterior and distal to the adductor tubercle and is a C-shaped ridge with a central depression or sulcus (Fig. 1–10). Rather than originating from the ridge, the medial collateral ligament (MCL) originates from the sulcus. The epicondylar axis passes through the center of the sulcus of the medial epicondyle and the prominence of the lateral epicondyle (Fig. 1–11). This line serves as an important reference line in total knee replacement. In relation to a line tangent to the posterior femoral condyles, the epicondylar axis is externally rotated about 3.5 degrees in males and 1 degree in females with normal knees.[11] In patients with osteoarthritis and valgus knee alignment, the transepicondylar axis has been shown to be externally rotated up to 10 degrees relative to the posterior condylar line.[33] Recent studies have also identified that racial differences probably exist in the rotational anatomy of the distal femur, with more natural external rotation of the transepicondylar axis in Asian populations.[99] Measurements of the width of the distal femur along the transepicondylar axis suggest that women have narrower femurs than males relative to the anteroposterior dimension.[16,38,78] These racial and gender differences have significant implications for both prosthesis development and surgical technique in total knee arthroplasty.[74]

TIBIA

In a macerated skeleton, inspection of the tibial plateau suggests that the femoral and tibial surfaces do not conform at all. The larger medial tibial plateau is nearly flat and has a squared-off posterior aspect that is quite distinct on a lateral radiograph.[20] In distinction, the articular surface of the narrower lateral plateau borders on convexity. Both have a posterior inclination of approximately 10 degrees with respect to the shaft of the tibia. However, the lack of conformity between the femoral and tibial articular surfaces is more apparent than real. In an intact knee, the menisci enlarge the contact area considerably and increase the conformity of the joint surfaces. The median portion of the tibia between the plateau is occupied by an eminence: the spine of the tibia. Anteriorly there is a depression, the anterior intercondylar fossa, to which, from anterior to posterior, the anterior horn of the medial meniscus, the ACL, and the anterior horn of the lateral meniscus are attached. Behind this region are two elevations: the medial and lateral tubercles. They are divided by a gutter-like depression: the intertubercular sulcus. On an anteroposterior radiograph, the medial tubercle usually projects more superiorly than the lateral tubercle; on a lateral radiograph, the medial tubercle is located anterior to the lateral tubercle (Fig. 1–12). The tubercles do not function as attachment sites for the cruciate ligaments or menisci but may act as side-to-side stabilizers by projecting toward the inner sides of the femoral condyles. In concert with the menisci, the tibial spine enhances the impression of cupping seen in intact specimens. In the posterior intercondylar fossa, behind the tubercles, the lateral and then the medial menisci are attached anteriorly to posteriorly. Most posteriorly, the PCL inserts on the margin of the tibia between the condyles. On the anterior aspect of the tibia, the tuberosity is the most prominent feature and is the attachment site of the patellar tendon. Approximately 2 to 3 cm lateral to the tibial tubercles is Gerdy's tubercle, which is the insertion site of the iliotibial band (ITB).

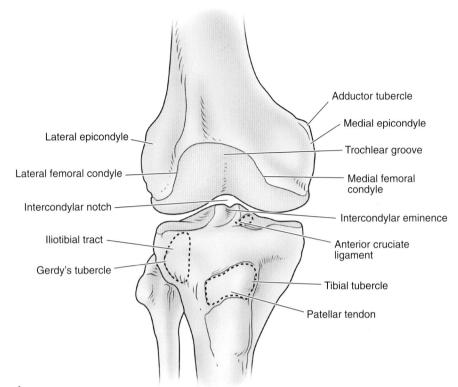

Adductor tubercle

Medial epicondyle

Lateral epicondyle

Trochlear groove

Lateral femoral condyle

Medial femoral condyle

Intercondylar notch

Intercondylar eminence

Iliotibial tract

Anterior cruciate ligament

Gerdy's tubercle

Tibial tubercle

Patellar tendon

A

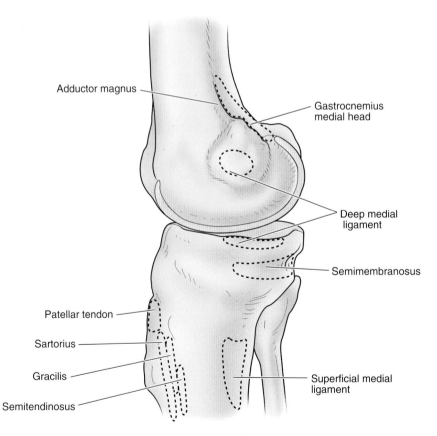

Adductor magnus

Gastrocnemius medial head

Deep medial ligament

Semimembranosus

Patellar tendon

Sartorius

Gracilis

Superficial medial ligament

Semitendinosus

B

Figure 1–8. Bony landmarks with ligament and tendon attachment sites on the anterior (**A**), and medial (**B**).

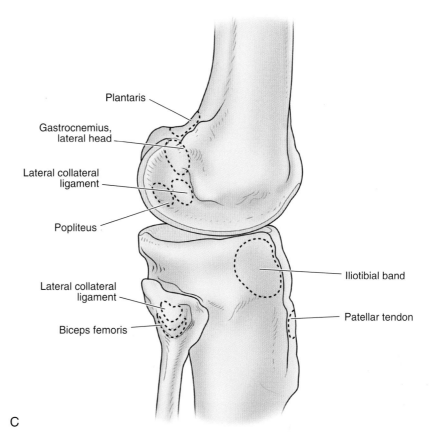

C

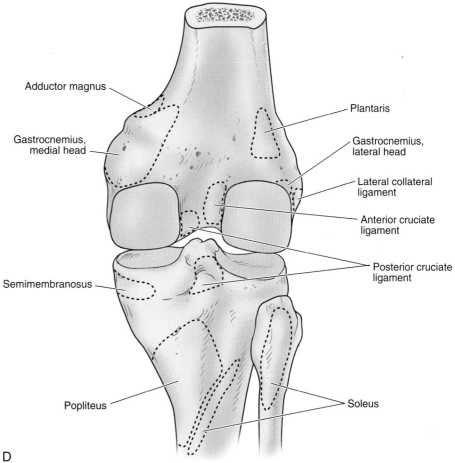

Figure 1–8, cont'd. Medial (**C**), and posterior (**D**) aspects of the knee.

D

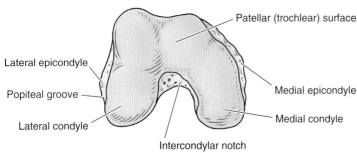

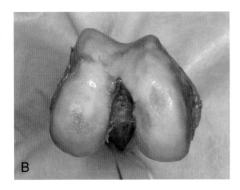

A

B

Figure 1–9. **A,** Bony architecture of the distal femur. **B,** Anatomic specimen of the distal femur. The femoral trochlea separates the lateral and medial femoral condyles. The deepest point lies slightly offset to the lateral side. The anterior aspect of the lateral condyle is more prominent than the medial side.

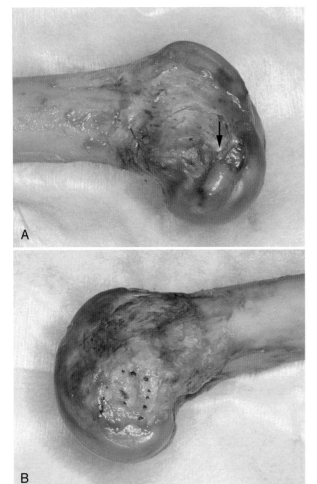

A

B

Figure 1–10. **A,** Bony landmarks of the lateral aspect of the distal femur. The characteristic groove for the popliteus tendon lies just proximal to the articular surface of the lateral condyle. The prominence of the lateral epicondyle (*arrow*) is located posterior to this groove. **B,** Bony landmarks of the medial aspect of the distal femur. The center of the sulcus of the C-shaped, ridge-like medial epicondyle (both marked) represents the center of attachment of the medial collateral ligament.

TIBIOFIBULAR JOINT

In an embryo, both the fibula and tibia are in contact with the femur. However, because the tibia grows at a faster rate than the fibula does, the distance from the femorotibial articulation to the fibula increases. A portion of the capsule that initially surrounds the knee is retained by the fibula and forms the superior tibiofibular joint. The articular surface of the head of the fibula is directed superiorly and slightly anteromedially to articulate with the postero-lateral portion of the tibial metaphysis. The styloid process projects superiorly from the posterolateral aspect of the fibula and is the insertion site for the LCL, biceps femoris tendon, fabellofibular ligament, and arcuate ligament.

The superior tibiofibular joint is lined with synovial membrane and possesses a capsular ligament that is strengthened by anterior and posterior ligaments. In contrast, the inferior tibiofibular joint is a syndesmosis, and the bones are joined by a strong intraosseous ligament. The intraosseous membrane originates from the intraosseous border of the fibula, and the fibers run distally and medially to attach to the intraosseous border of the tibia. A large opening is present superiorly that allows passage of the anterior tibial vessels.

The anterior aspect of the superior tibiofibular joint and the adjoining portions of the tibia and fibula give rise to the origins of the tibialis anterior, extensor digitorum longus, and peroneus longus muscles. The posterior aspect of the same region gives rise to a portion of the soleus muscle. The anterior tibial artery, the terminal branch of the popliteal artery, enters the anterior compartment of the leg through the opening in the intraosseous membrane, two fingerbreadths below the superior tibiofibular joint. A recurrent branch contributes to the anastomosis around the knee. The anterior tibial nerve and a terminal branch of the common peroneal nerve also pierce the anterior intermuscular septum between the extensor digitorum longus and the fibula and come to lie at the lateral side of the artery. The superficial peroneal nerve arises from the common peroneal nerve on the lateral side of the neck of the fibula and runs distally and forward in the substance of the peroneus longus muscle.

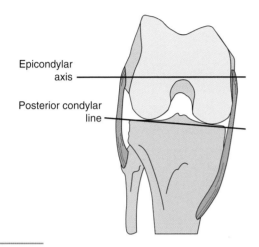

Figure 1–11. The epicondylar axis, which connects the prominence of the lateral epicondyle and the sulcus of the medial epicondyle, is externally rotated relative to the posterior condylar line.

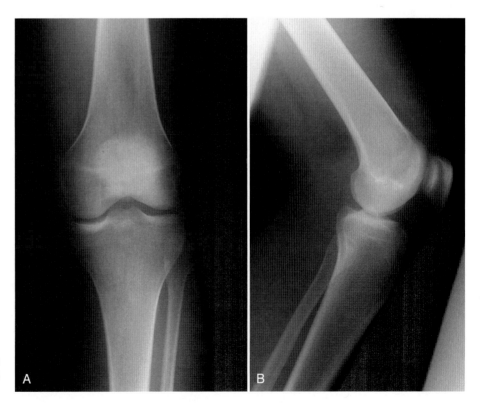

Figure 1–12. Anteroposterior (**A**) and lateral (**B**) radiographs of a normal knee.

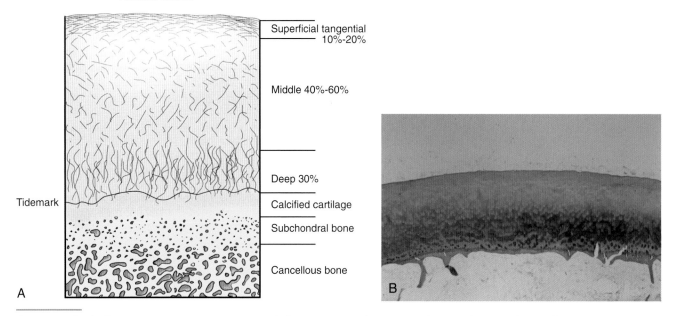

Figure 1–13. **A,** Diagrammatic representation of the transition from articular cartilage to bone. **B,** Normal articular (hyaline) cartilage composed of water, collagen, and proteoglycan. The sparsely cellular, smooth superficial zone becomes increasingly cellular in deeper layers. A distinct basophilic line, the mineralization front, can be seen where cartilage becomes calcified.

HYALINE/ARTICULAR CARTILAGE

Articular cartilage is a specialized connective tissue composed of hydrated proteoglycans within a matrix of collagen fibrils. Proteoglycans are complex glycoproteins consisting of a central protein core to which are attached glycosaminoglycan chains. The structure of hyaline cartilage is not uniform, but rather can be divided into distinct zones based on the arrangement of the collagen fibrils and the distribution of chondrocytes. The density of chondrocytes is highest close to subchondral bone and decreases toward the articular surface (Fig. 1–13). Calcification occurs in a distinct basophilic zone at the deepest level of chondrocyte proliferation termed the *tidemark*. Beneath this region is a zone of calcified cartilage that anchors the cartilage to the subchondral plate. Cartilage is avascular, and chondrocytes in the superficial zones are believed to derive nutrition from synovial fluid. Deeper zones probably obtain nutrition from subchondral bone.

Examination of gross specimens or arthroscopic visualization reveals normal cartilage to be a white, smooth, firm material. Articular cartilage damage or degeneration, termed chondromalacia, can be quite readily identified (Fig. 1–14). These characteristic changes seen during arthroscopic examination have been classified by Outerbridge[71]: grade 0 is normal, white-appearing cartilage; grade I is swelling or softening of an intact cartilage surface; grade II is represented by fissuring and fibrillation over a small area (<0.5 inch); grade III is the same pathological changes over a larger area (>0.5 inch); and grade IV changes represent erosion to subchondral bone and are indistinguishable from osteoarthritis. Chondral flap tears

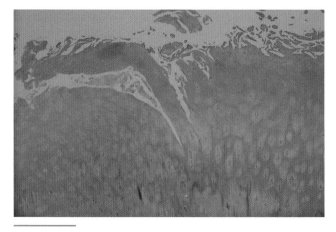

Figure 1–14. Degenerative or chondromalacic articular cartilage. Irregular thickness, surface fibrillation, longitudinal slits, increased chondrocyte cellularity, and altered matrix staining are evident.

caused by delamination of the articular cartilage may also be encountered (Fig. 1–15). These changes in articular cartilage cannot be directly visualized on conventional radiographs but may be seen on magnetic resonance imaging (MRI) studies. However, even MRI is unreliable for detecting early stages of chondromalacia, which may appear as foci or areas of diffuse abnormal signal with a normal surface. Grade III or IV chondromalacia is visible as thinning, irregularity, and fissuring of cartilage (Fig. 1–16).

Damage to the articular cartilage and joint surface may result indirectly from pathological changes in subchondral

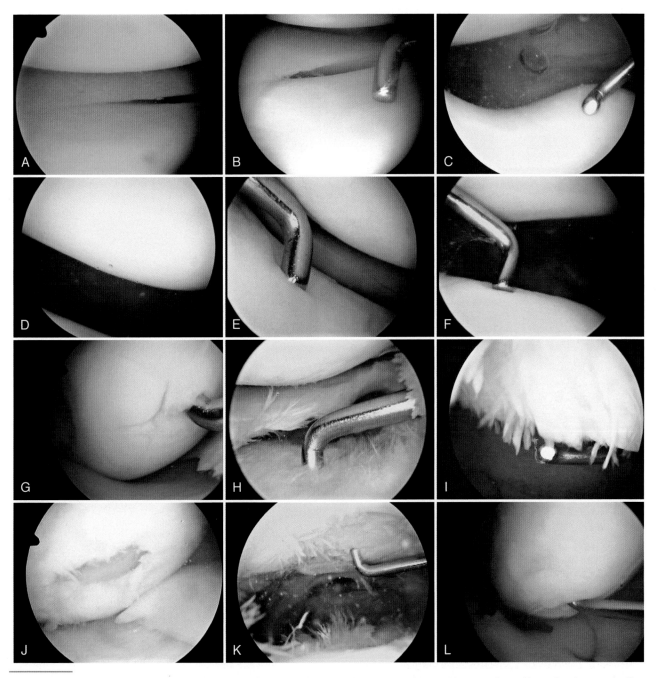

Figure 1–15. Arthroscopic views of articular cartilage. Normal white, smooth articular cartilage (Outerbridge grade 0) in the medial (**A**), lateral (**B**), and patellofemoral compartments (**C** and **D**). Softening of the articular surface of the lateral tibial plateau (**E**) and patellofemoral articulation (**F**) with indentation at the probe tip (Outerbridge grade I) is noted. **G,** A small fissure and fibrillation of the medial femoral condyle (Outerbridge grade II). Extensive fibrillation of the articular cartilage involving the tibial plateau (**H**) and patella (**I**) (Outerbridge grade III). Erosion of articular cartilage to subchondral bone involving the medial femoral condyle (**J**) and patella (**K**) (Outerbridge grade IV). Arthroscopic view of a chondral flap tear (**L**); the probe tip is deep to a flap of delaminated articular cartilage on the medial femoral condyle.

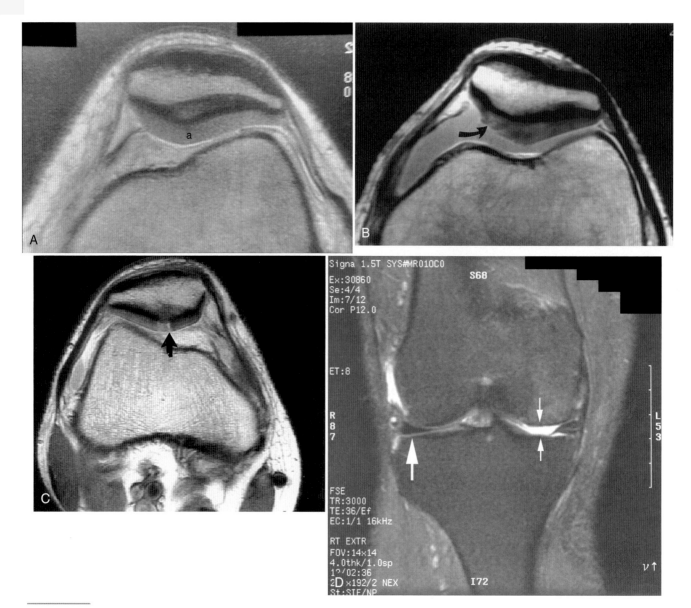

Figure 1–16. **A,** Axial magnetic resonance image (MRI) showing normal articular cartilage (a) on the patellar facets. The cartilage has a uniform signal thickness and appearance. **B,** Axial MRI revealing fissuring and fibrillation of articular cartilage on the medial facet of the patella (*arrow*). **C,** Axial MRI with advanced chondromalacia of the patella. The signal irregularity extends to subchondral bone, and a deep fissure is identified (*arrow*). **D,** Coronal MRI demonstrating complete loss of the articular cartilage of the medial compartment (*thin arrows*). For comparison, the gray band of articular cartilage on the lateral tibial plateau is also identified (*thick arrow*).

bone. Both osteonecrosis and osteochondritis dissecans (OCD) may lead to destruction of the articular surface. In the knee, OCD tends to occur on the intercondylar aspect of the medial femoral condyle in young people. These lesions may separate from the surface and form a loose body. The base of these lesions will reveal vascular subchondral bone if débrided (Fig. 1–17). Classic radiographic findings include a lucent osseous defect that may have a fragmented or corticated osseous density within the lucency (Fig. 1–18). On MRI studies, increased signal about the defect on T2-weighted images represents joint fluid surrounding the lesion; irregularity of the articular surface may also be noted (Fig. 1–19). Osteonecrosis

results in a similar osteochondral fragment but tends to occur in elderly patients on the weightbearing aspect of the medial femoral condyle (Fig. 1–20). In distinction to the lesions in OCD, fragments in osteonecrosis separate from a bed of avascular bone (Fig. 1–21). Again, radiographs may reveal a lucent defect at the involved site, but MRI is more reliable for the evaluation of these defects (Fig. 1–22). A curvilinear area of low signal with variable bone edema is characteristic. Although the articular cartilage is initially normal, both processes may lead to detachment of osteochondral loose bodies, fragmentation, and collapse of the articular surface with resultant degenerative changes.

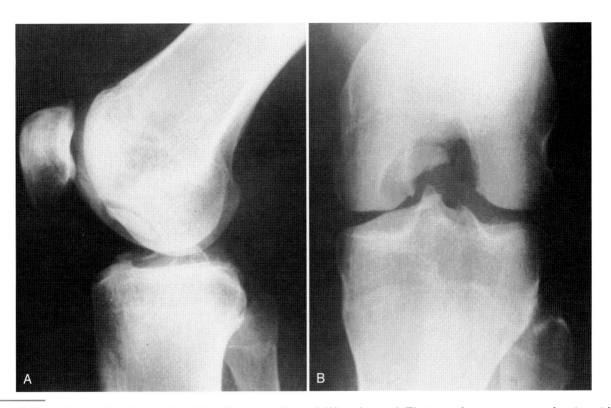

Figure 1–17. Arthroscopic view of osteochondritis of the femoral condyle. **A,** Osteochondral fragment of the articular surface of the femoral condyle. **B,** Punctate bleeding from the base of vascular subchondral bone with the osteochondral fragment mobilized.

Figure 1–18. Radiographs of osteochondritis dissecans. Lateral (**A**) and tunnel (**B**) views show an osseous density within a lucent defect on the medial femoral condyle.

MENISCI

The menisci are two crescentic fibrocartilage structures that serve to deepen the articular surfaces of the tibia for reception of the femoral condyles (Fig. 1–23). The most abundant components of the menisci include collagen (75%) and noncollagenized proteins (8% to 13%). Glycosaminoglycans and glycoproteins are also key constituents. Although there are four main types of collagen in the menisci, type I collagen is the predominant component and accounts for about 90% of the total collagen. Histological examination reveals a population of fibroblasts and fibrocartilaginous cells dispersed in an organized matrix of eosinophilic collagen fibrils. The collagen

bundles are arranged in a circumferential pattern that is optimal for absorption of compressive loads (Fig. 1–24). Radial fibers found at the surface and in the midsubstance parallel to the plateau may act to increase structural rigidity and help prevent longitudinal splitting.[76] Elastin fibers, which constitute approximately 0.6% of the dry weight of the meniscus, seem to help in recoil to the original shape after deformation.[90] In degenerative menisci, metaplasia of the cell population occurs with a trend toward chondroid cell appearance (Fig. 1–25).

Each meniscus covers approximately the peripheral two-thirds of the corresponding articular surface of the tibia. The peripheral border of each meniscus is thick, convex, and attached to the capsule of the joint; the opposite border tapers to a thin, free edge. The proximal sur-

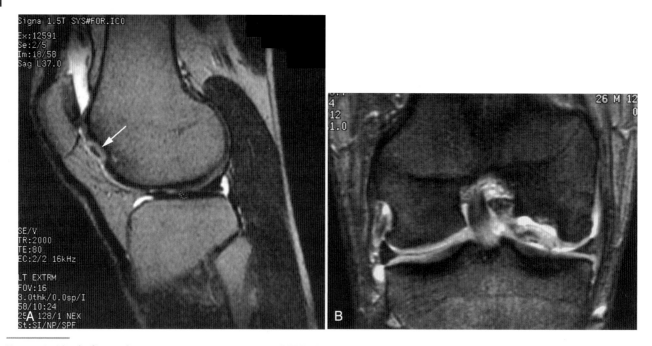

Figure 1–19. **A,** Sagittal magnetic resonance image (MRI) demonstrating a well-demarcated osteochondral lesion (*arrow*) in the anterior aspect of the lateral femoral condyle. **B,** Coronal MRI showing high-signal fluid about a loose osteochondral fragment of the medial femoral condyle. (Courtesy of Martin Broker, M.D.)

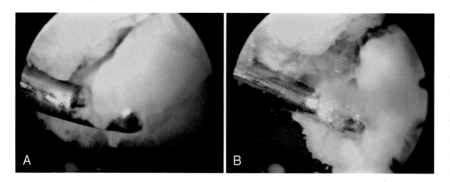

Figure 1–20. Arthroscopic views of osteonecrosis of the femoral condyle. **A,** Disruption of the articular surface by a detached osteochondral fragment. **B,** A probe elevates the loose fragment to reveal a base of almost completely avascular, dead subchondral bone.

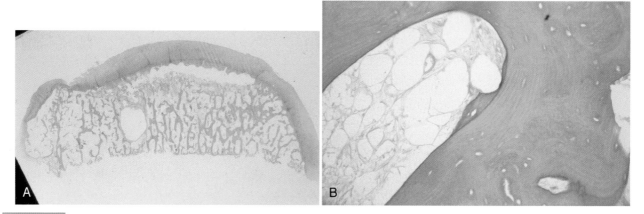

Figure 1–21. **A,** Osteonecrosis. A subchondral lucent zone is surrounded by intact articular cartilage and a thin plate of subchondral bone superficially with collapsed necrotic bone and granulation tissue inferiorly. **B,** Osteonecrosis (high power). Dead bone is characterized by marrow fat necrosis imparting a foggy, acellular appearance and bone devoid of osteocytes (empty lacunar spaces) and bone-lining cells.

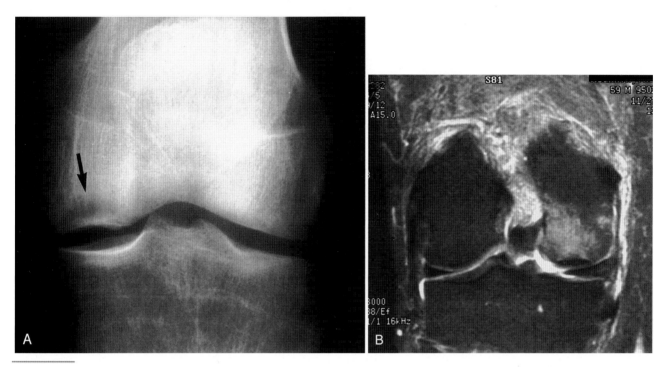

Figure 1–22. Osteonecrosis. **A,** Anteroposterior radiograph of the knee with a focal lucency and flattening of the articular surface of the medial femoral condyle (*arrow*). **B,** Fat-suppressed proton density coronal magnetic resonance image with a curvilinear area of low signal in the necrotic bone and surrounding marrow edema.

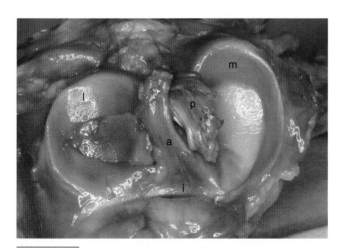

Figure 1–23. Anatomic dissection of the tibial plateau. The menisci act to increase the conformity of the articular surface of the tibial plateau. The medial meniscus (m) is C shaped, whereas the lateral meniscus (l) is more circular. The remnants of the anterior cruciate ligament (a) and posterior cruciate ligament (p) are also marked, as is the transverse intermeniscal ligament (i).

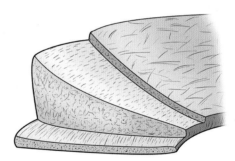

Figure 1–24. Trilaminar cross-sectional area of the meniscus.

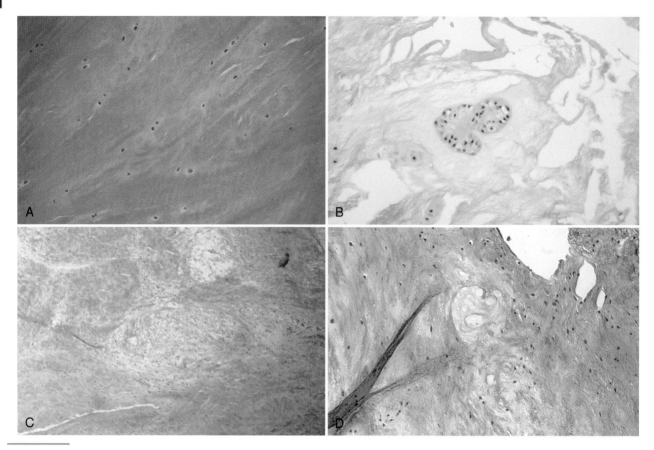

Figure 1–25. Cross-section of the medial meniscus (fibrocartilage) demonstrating the eosinophilic collagen matrix in interwoven bands within which can be seen the nuclei of fibroblasts, here more prominent than seen in tendons and ligaments with occasional perinuclear spaces, often similar to immature cartilaginous cells (**A**). With trauma or degeneration, chondroid metaplasia (**B**), loss of matrix (**C**), and cystic changes (**D**) take place.

faces of the menisci are concave and in contact with the femoral condyles; the distal surfaces are flat and rest on the tibial plateau. On MRI studies, normal menisci are best seen on sagittal views and have low-signal characteristics with no or little internal signal. The posterior horn of the medial meniscus is larger than the anterior horn, whereas the anterior and posterior horns of the lateral menisci are typically of similar size (Fig. 1–26). Increased signal within the menisci may be noted and classified on a scale ranging from I to III. Patchy areas of increased signal that do not touch the inferior and superior borders of the menisci represent grade I changes. Grade II changes typically have a linear configuration, but again they do not touch the superior and inferior surfaces. These signal changes probably represent the normal aging process in the menisci. Increased signal with a linear appearance that contacts one of the articular surfaces of the menisci is classified as grade III change and represents a true meniscal tear (Fig. 1–27).[64,84] A variety of meniscal tears may be identified on MRI but are best delineated by arthroscopic examination (Fig. 1–28). Patterns include vertical and horizontal cleavage tears, radial tears, bucket handle tears (detachment of the body of the menisci at the periphery with intact anterior and posterior horn attachments), and complex degenerative tears (Fig. 1–29). The technique of arthroscopic repair and partial meniscectomy has super-

seded open meniscectomy; therefore, examination of intact resected specimens is rarely possible (Fig. 1–30).

Calcification may occur within the fibrocartilage of the menisci and is referred to as *chondrocalcinosis*. This abnormality has classically been described in association with calcium pyrophosphate dihydrate deposition disease. However, chondrocalcinosis may be noted incidentally on radiographs or during arthroscopic examination (Fig. 1–31).

The menisci perform several important functions, including (1) load transmission across the joint, (2) enhancement of articular conformity, (3) distribution of synovial fluid across the articular surface, and (4) prevention of soft-tissue impingement during joint motion. The medial meniscus also confers some stability to the joint in the presence of ACL insufficiency in that the posterior horn acts as a wedge to help reduce anterior tibial translation.[63] However, the lateral meniscus does not perform a similar function.[62] The rapid progression of degenerative changes, first observed by Fairbank, that occur as a result of complete meniscectomy have been well documented.[24] These changes include (1) osteophyte formation on the femoral condyle projecting over the site of meniscectomy, (2) flattening of the femoral condyle, and (3) narrowing of the joint space on the involved compartment.

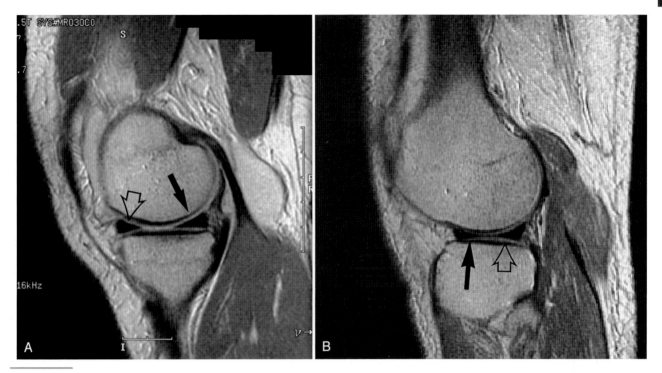

Figure 1–26. **A,** Sagittal magnetic resonance image (MRI) of the medial compartment with a normal medial meniscus. The posterior horn (*thin arrow*) is larger than the anterior horn (*thick arrow*). **B,** Sagittal MRI of the lateral compartment of the knee. The low-signal anterior and posterior horns of the lateral meniscus (*solid arrow* and *open arrow*, respectively) have a uniform appearance and a triangular shape.

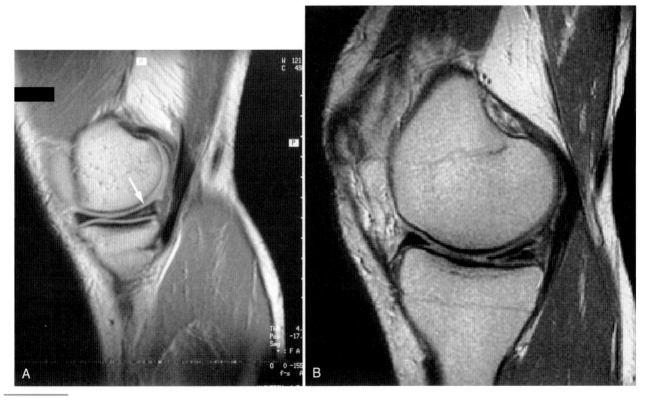

Figure 1–27. Sagittal magnetic resonance images. **A,** Linear intrameniscal signal (*arrow*) in the posterior horn that does not contact the meniscal surface (grade II). **B,** Obliquely oriented linear signal in the posterior horn of the medial meniscus. The signal abnormality touches the inferior surface and is consistent with a meniscal tear (grade III).

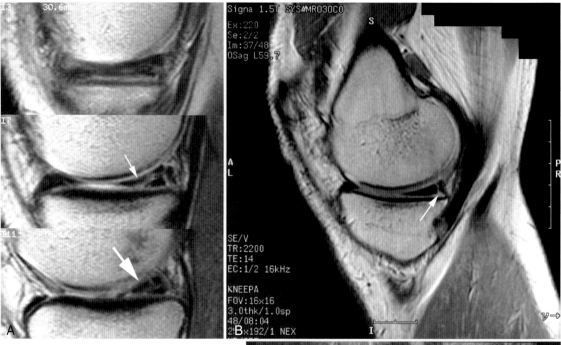

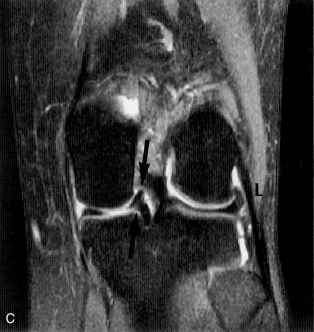

Figure 1–28. **A,** Three sagittal magnetic resonance imaging (MRI) views ("meniscal windows") with multiple linear intrameniscal signals that contact the superior (*thick arrow*) and inferior meniscal surfaces (*thin arrow*) representing a complex degenerative tear. **B,** Sagittal MRI showing a peripheral vertical cleavage tear (*arrow*) of the posterior horn of the medial meniscus. **C,** Coronal MRI demonstrating a displaced bucket handle meniscal tear with the fragment displaced into the notch (*arrows*). The lateral collateral ligament (L) is also well visualized.

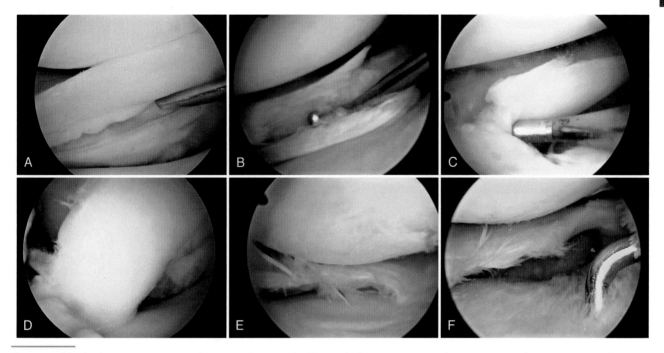

Figure 1–29. Arthroscopic views of meniscal tears. **A,** Vertical cleavage tear with separation of the meniscus from the peripheral attachment. **B,** Horizontal cleavage meniscal tear. **C,** Radial tear in the midbody of the meniscus. **D,** Detached meniscal bucket handle tear with a fragment displaced into the intercondylar notch. **E,** Complex degenerative tear of the posterior body and horn of the medial meniscus. **F,** Degenerative fraying of the meniscus without a gross tear.

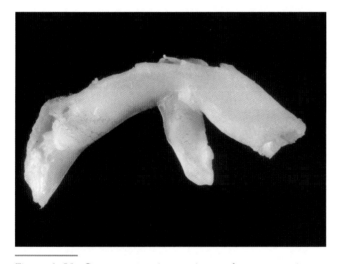

Figure 1–30. Gross anatomic specimen of a torn meniscus.

Medial Meniscus

The medial meniscus is nearly semicircular in form and about 3.5 cm in length. It has a triangular cross-section and is asymmetric, with a considerably wider posterior horn than anterior horn. It is firmly attached to the posterior intercondylar fossa of the tibia directly anterior to the PCL insertion (Fig. 1–32). The anterior attachment is more variable; usually, it is firmly attached to the anterior intercondylar fossa approximately 7 mm anterior to the anterior margin of the ACL insertion in line with the medial tibial tubercle, but this attachment can be quite flimsy.[46] There is also a fibrous band of variable thickness,

the transverse intermeniscal ligament, that connects the anterior horn of the medial meniscus with the lateral meniscus (Fig. 1–33). Peripherally, the medial meniscus is continuously attached to the capsule of the knee. The midpoint of the medial meniscus is more firmly attached to the femur via a condensation in the capsule known as the deep medial ligament (Fig. 1–34). The tibial attachment of the meniscus, sometimes known as the coronary ligament, attaches to the tibial margin a few millimeters distal to the articular surface, where it gives rise to a synovial recess. Posteromedially, according to Kaplan,[51] the meniscus receives a portion of the insertion of the semimembranosus via the capsule.

Lateral Meniscus

In contrast to the C-shaped medial meniscus, the lateral meniscus is nearly circular and covers a larger portion of the articular surface than the medial meniscus does (see Fig. 1–32). The anterior horn is attached to the intercondylar fossa, directly anterior to the lateral tibial tubercle and adjacent to the ACL. The posterior horn is attached to the intercondylar fossa directly posterior to the lateral tibial tubercle and adjacent and anterior to the posterior horn of the medial meniscus.[46] Somewhat variable fibrous bands, the meniscofemoral ligaments, connect the posterior horn of the lateral meniscus to the intercondylar wall of the medial femoral condyle. These meniscofemoral ligaments, which embrace the PCL, are also known by the eponyms Humphry and Wrisberg (Fig. 1–35). The ligament of Humphry passes anterior to the PCL, whereas the ligament of Wrisberg passes poste-

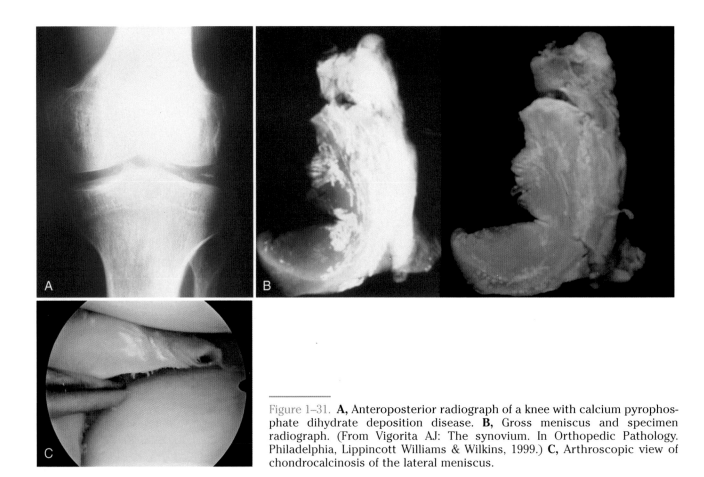

Figure 1–31. **A,** Anteroposterior radiograph of a knee with calcium pyrophosphate dihydrate deposition disease. **B,** Gross meniscus and specimen radiograph. (From Vigorita AJ: The synovium. In Orthopedic Pathology. Philadelphia, Lippincott Williams & Wilkins, 1999.) **C,** Arthroscopic view of chondrocalcinosis of the lateral meniscus.

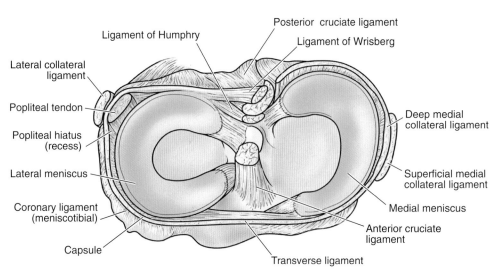

Figure 1–32. Superior aspect of the tibial plateau.

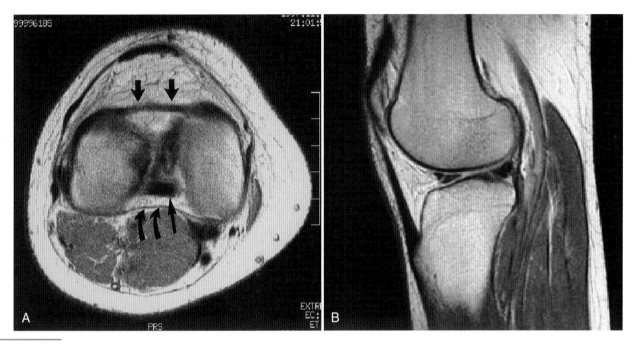

Figure 1–33. **A,** Axial magnetic resonance image (MRI) with the low-signal transverse intermeniscal ligament (*short arrows*) connecting the anterior horns of the medial and lateral menisci. The posterior capsule (*curved arrows*) and posterior cruciate ligament (*long arrow*) are also identified. **B,** Sagittal MRI through the lateral compartment of the knee shows the interface between the transverse intermeniscal ligament and the anterior horn of the meniscus. This may be misidentified as a meniscal tear.

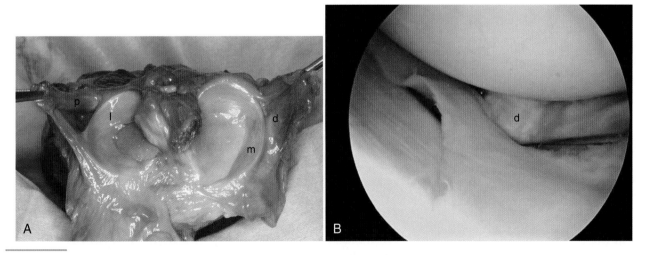

Figure 1–34. **A,** Tibial plateau. The C-shaped medial meniscus has a continuous attachment to the capsule. The deep medial collateral ligament (MCL) (d, retracted in the forceps) is directly attached to the periphery of the midbody of the medial meniscus (m). Laterally, the popliteus tendon (p, retracted in the forceps) enters the joint via the popliteal hiatus. In this location the capsular attachment of the lateral meniscus (l) is interrupted. **B,** Arthroscopic view of the deep MCL. The fibers of the deep MCL (d), which represents a thickening in the medial capsule, can be seen at the tip of the probe.

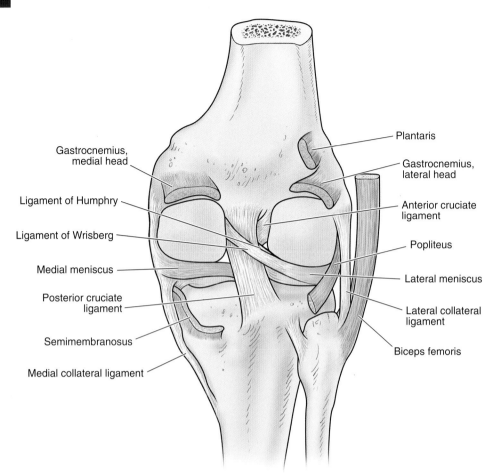

Figure 1–35. Posterior aspect
of the knee. The ligaments
of Humphry and Wrisberg,
which attach the posterior
horn of the lateral meniscus
to the medial femoral condyle, embrace the posterior
cruciate ligament. The popliteal tendon partially inserts
into the posterola-teral aspect of the lateral meniscus.

rior to the PCL (Fig. 1–36). One or the other of these
meniscofemoral ligaments has been identified in between
71% and 100% of cadaver knees; the ligament of Wrisberg
is a more constant finding, and both ligaments together
are found in only a small percentage of specimens.[76,89,91]
Meniscofemoral ligaments running from the anterior
horns of the medial and lateral menisci to the intercondylar notch anterior to the ACL have also been identified. Wan and Felle[91] reported a 15% incidence of both
of these structures in 60 cadaver knees, and one or the
other was present in 25% of the specimens. In general, the
ligaments of Wrisberg and Humphry were much more
robust structures than either of the meniscofemoral ligaments originating from the anterior horns.

The peripheral capsular attachment of the medial
meniscus is continuous, but the attachment of the lateral
meniscus is interrupted by the popliteal hiatus through
which passes the popliteal tendon (Fig. 1–37). In addition,
unlike the anatomy on the medial side, the lateral meniscus does not have a direct attachment to the collateral ligament. Posterolaterally at the popliteal hiatus the lateral
meniscus is grooved by the popliteal tendon. Some fibers
of the tendon insert into the periphery and superior
border of the meniscus at this site.[52,53] Because the lateral
meniscus is not as extensively attached to the capsule
as the medial meniscus is, it is more mobile and may displace up to 1 cm. The controlled mobility of the lateral

meniscus, which is guided by the popliteal tendon and
meniscofemoral ligament attachments, may explain why
meniscal injuries occur less frequently on the lateral
side.[59,60] Although the meniscofemoral ligaments appear to
perform an important function, little is known about the
significance of injuries to these structures.

CAPSULE

The capsule is a fibrous membrane containing areas of
thickening that may be referred to as discrete ligaments.
The anterior capsule is thin, and directly anteriorly it is
replaced by the patellar ligament. Proximally, the capsule
of the knee joint attaches to the femur approximately
three to four fingerbreadths above the patella. Distally, it
attaches circumferentially to the tibial margin except
where the popliteal tendon enters the joint through the
hiatus. Posteriorly, the capsule consists of vertical fibers
that arise from the condyles and the walls of the intercondylar fossa of the femur. In this region, the capsule is
augmented by the fibers of the oblique popliteal ligament,
which is derived from the semimembranosus tendon. This
broad, flat band is attached proximally to the margin of
the intercondylar fossa and posterior surface of the femur
close to the articular margins of the condyles. The fasci-

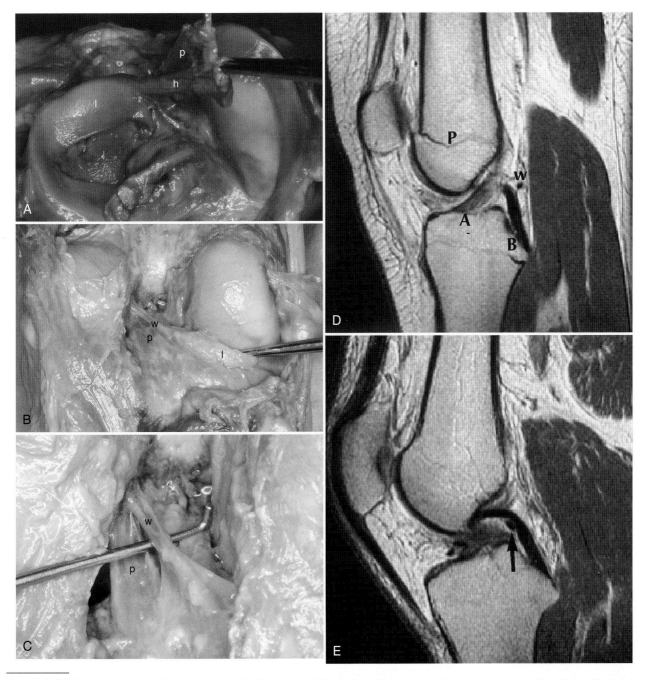

Figure 1–36. Meniscofemoral ligaments. **A,** The ligament of Humphry (h, retracted in the forceps) arises from the posterior horn of the lateral meniscus (l) and passes anterior to the posterior cruciate ligament (PCL) (p). **B,** Posterior view of the knee with the capsule removed laterally revealing the ligament of Wrisberg (w), which originates from the lateral meniscus (l, tip of the forceps) and then passes posterior to the PCL (p). **C,** Close-up view of an anatomic dissection of the posterior aspect of the knee with the capsule removed from the intercondylar notch. The ligament of Wrisberg (w) lies posterior to the PCL fibers (p). **D,** Sagittal magnetic resonance image (MRI) showing the ligament of Wrisberg (w) posterior to the PCL (B). Also identified are the anterior cruciate ligament (A) and physeal scar (P). **E,** Sagittal MRI with the small oval ligament of Humphry identified anterior to the PCL (*arrow*).

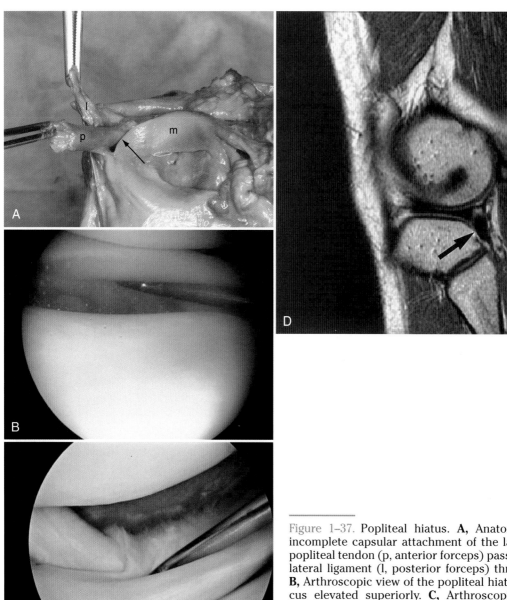

Figure 1–37. Popliteal hiatus. **A,** Anatomic dissection revealing incomplete capsular attachment of the lateral meniscus (m). The popliteal tendon (p, anterior forceps) passes deep to the lateral collateral ligament (l, posterior forceps) through the hiatus (*arrow*). **B,** Arthroscopic view of the popliteal hiatus with the lateral meniscus elevated superiorly. **C,** Arthroscopic view of the popliteal tendon passing between the periphery of the lateral meniscus and the capsule. **D,** Sagittal magnetic resonance image with the popliteus tendon (*arrow*) traversing the popliteal hiatus posterior to the lateral meniscus.

cles are separated by apertures for the passage of vessels and nerves. The oblique popliteal ligament forms part of the floor of the popliteal fossa, and the popliteal artery rests on it. At the site of the popliteal hiatus, the capsule is displaced inferiorly toward the fibula head, forming the arcuate ligament between the lateral meniscus and fibular styloid.

SYNOVIAL CAVITY

Synovium is normally a smooth, translucent pink tissue. Histologically, a thin layer of synovial cells, or synoviocytes, is found at the surface (Fig. 1–38). The synoviocytes consist of two cell populations, broadly classified into those that have macrophage-type function and those with a synthetic function. Type 1 cells contain numerous mitochondria, lysosomes, phagosomes, and surface undulations indicative of their macrophage function. Type 2 cells have rough endoplasmic reticulum and free ribosomes characteristic of secretory cells. This layer of cells, the intimal layer, lies above a fibrovascular zone, the subintimal layer, that contains arterioles, fat, and a variety of con-

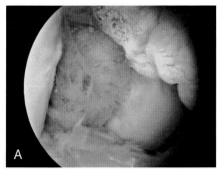

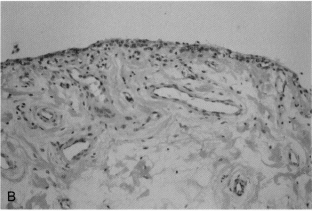

Figure 1–38. **A,** Arthroscopic view of normal synovium. Normal synovium is a fine pink layer that covers the intra-articular surfaces of the knee. **B,** Section of essentially normal synovium demonstrating the synovial intimal layer consisting of synoviocytes, one to two cells thick, beneath which rests the highly vascular subintimal layer, usually sparsely cellular, but containing fibroblasts, histiocytes, fat cells, and occasional mast cells.

nective tissue cells, including fibroblasts and histiocytes. The fibrovascular zone gradually becomes more fibrous at capsular insertions. In specific disease processes, including rheumatoid arthritis, the synovium becomes hypertrophic and inflamed and contributes to intra-articular destruction (Fig. 1–39).

Synovium invests the interior of the knee joint and extends proximally into the suprapatellar pouch above the patella. The suprapatellar pouch is separated from the anterior surface of the femur by a layer of fat (Fig. 1–40). The uppermost limit of the pouch is attached to a small muscle, the articularis genus, that originates from the anterior surface of the femoral shaft. The articularis genus serves to prevent invagination of the suprapatellar pouch beneath the patella.

Intra-articularly, the synovium invests the cruciate ligaments and the popliteal tendon. A synovial recess or sleeve extends around the popliteal tendon for a variable distance beyond the posterolateral capsule. The synovium also lines the coronal recesses beneath the menisci and anteriorly invests the fat pad, which lies posterior to the patellar ligament and capsule. Although the synovium approximates the capsule, it is much more redundant. Synovial folds occur quite frequently, particularly in the suprapatellar pouch. Plicae probably represent remnants of synovial septa normally absorbed during embryonic development. The infrapatellar (ligamentum mucosum), suprapatellar, and medial patellar plicae are the three most common plicae (Fig. 1–41). Visualization of plicae on MRI studies can be difficult without an associated intra-articular effusion. In most cases, sagittal and axial images provide the best detail (Fig. 1–42). Rarely, plicae, especially medial patellar plicae, can become inflamed and painful; in these circumstances, arthroscopic resection may be considered.

The posterior synovial cavity communicates with a popliteal bursa that is found between the semimembranosus tendon and the medial head of the gastrocnemius in about 50% of people (Fig. 1–43).[98] This bursa may be distended when dye is injected into the knee; the bursa can also become enlarged by an intra-articular effusion and result in a popliteal or Baker's cyst. With this exception, the synovial cavity does not normally communicate with any of the other bursae around the knee.

BURSAE

Of the numerous bursae about the knee, those with the most clinical significance include the prepatellar, infrapatellar, and anserine bursae (Fig. 1–44). The prepatellar bursa is large and lies subcutaneously anterior to the patella. The infrapatellar bursa lies posterior to the patellar ligament and separates the ligament from the tibia and lower portion of the fat pad. The pes anserinus bursa lies between the sartorius, gracilis, and semitendinosus tendons and the tibia; another bursa separates the superficial medial ligament from the pes tendons. These bursae may become inflamed as a result of trauma or overuse. The significance of the semimembranosus bursa has previously been discussed.

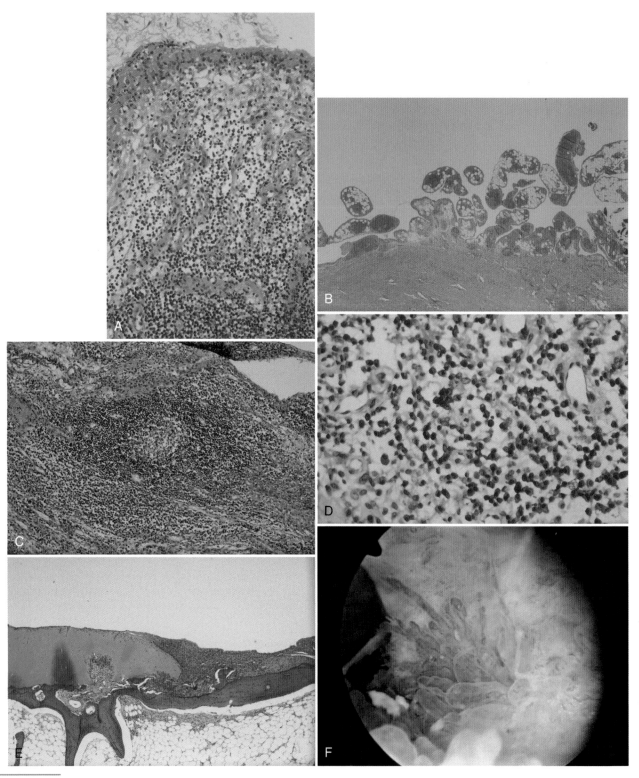

Figure 1–39. Rheumatoid synovium. In rheumatoid arthritis the synovium becomes thickened, edematous, fibrinous, and inflamed (**A**). There is marked lymphocytosis (**B,** low power) with germinal center formation (**C**) and plasma cell prolif-eration (**D**). The inflamed synovium or pannus (**E**) causes chondrolysis and invades the cartilage and bone. **F,** Arthro-scopic view of inflamed synovium with hypertrophic, red villi.

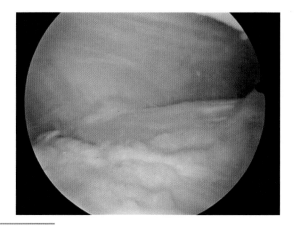

Figure 1–40. Arthroscopic view of the suprapatellar pouch. A thin layer of translucent synovium covers the interior surfaces.

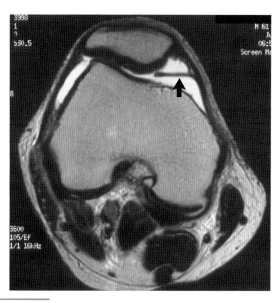

Figure 1–42. Axial magnetic resonance image with a low-signal, thick medial plica (*arrow*) that is highlighted by the large effusion.

Figure 1–41. Arthroscopic views of intra-articular plicae. **A,** The infrapatellar plica (ligamentum mucosum) passes between the intercondylar notch and anterior fat pad. **B,** A large medial patellar plica is seen interposed between the anterior surface of the medial femoral condyle and the patella. **C,** Thickening along the margin of a large medial patellar plica caused by irritation and abrasion on the femoral condyle. **D,** A suprapatellar plica may occlude the opening to the suprapatellar pouch. In some cases, this plica may be continuous with a medial patellar plica.

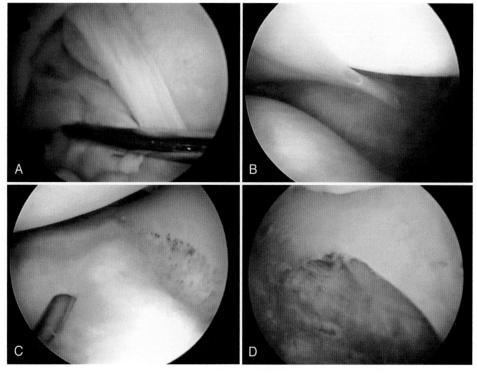

CRUCIATE LIGAMENTS

The cruciate ligaments consist of a highly organized collagen matrix, which accounts for approximately three-fourths of their dry weight. The majority of the collagen is type I (90%), and the remainder is type III (10%).[22] In the ACL this collagen is organized into multiple fiber

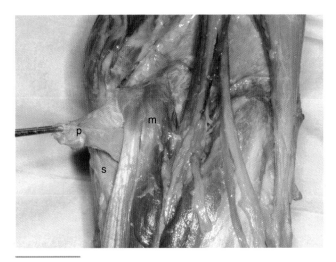

Figure 1–43. Popliteal bursa. Anatomic dissection of the popliteal fossa with a popliteal bursa (p, forceps) originating between the medial head of the gastrocnemius (m) and the semimembranosus tendon (s).

bundles 20 μm wide that are grouped into fascicles 20 to 400 μm in diameter.[18] Occasional fibroblasts and other substances, such as elastin (<5%) and proteoglycans (1%), make up the remainder of the dry weight.[22] Water constitutes 60% of the net weight under physiological conditions. At the microscopic level, ligament and tendon insertions into bone have a characteristic structure consisting of collagen fibrils directly continuous with fibrils within the bone. A calcified front, similar to that seen between osteoid and mineralized bone, can be distinguished (Fig. 1–45).

The cruciate ligaments are named for their attachments on the tibia and are essential to function of the knee joint.[37,56,59,95] The cruciate ligaments act to stabilize the knee joint and prevent anteroposterior displacement of the tibia on the femur. The presence of numerous sensory endings also implies a proprioceptive function. These ligaments are intra-articular but, because they are covered by synovium, are considered extrasynovial. They receive their blood supply from branches of the middle genicular and both inferior genicular arteries. The anatomy of the cruciate ligaments has been studied by Girgis et al[29] (Fig. 1–46).

Anterior Cruciate Ligament

The ACL originates from the medial surface of the lateral femoral condyle posteriorly in the intercondylar notch in the form of a segment of a circle (Fig. 1–47). The anterior side of the attachment is almost straight and the posterior

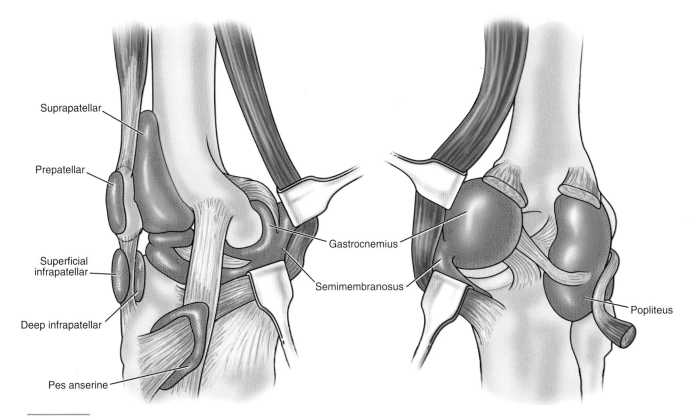

Suprapatellar

Prepatellar

Superficial infrapatellar

Deep infrapatellar

Pes anserine

Gastrocnemius

Semimembranosus

Popliteus

Figure 1–44. Bursae around the knee.

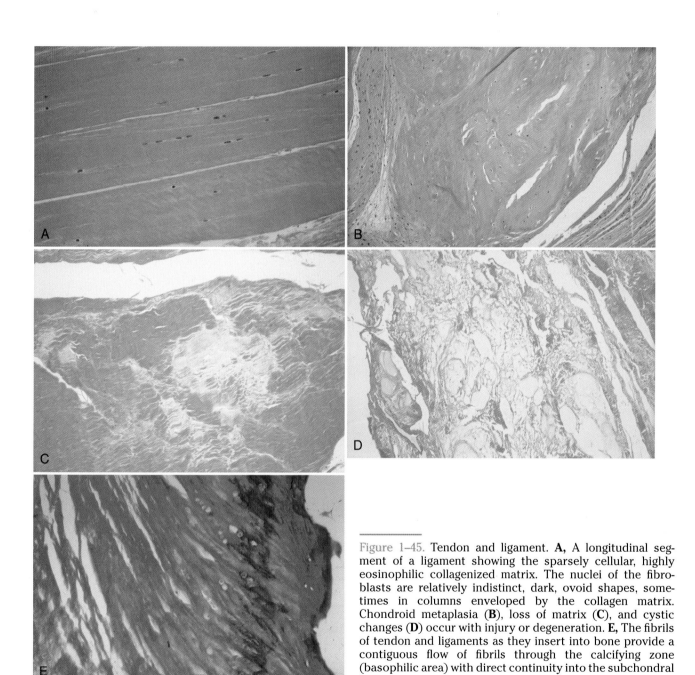

Figure 1–45. Tendon and ligament. **A,** A longitudinal segment of a ligament showing the sparsely cellular, highly eosinophilic collagenized matrix. The nuclei of the fibroblasts are relatively indistinct, dark, ovoid shapes, sometimes in columns enveloped by the collagen matrix. Chondroid metaplasia (**B**), loss of matrix (**C**), and cystic changes (**D**) occur with injury or degeneration. **E,** The fibrils of tendon and ligaments as they insert into bone provide a contiguous flow of fibrils through the calcifying zone (basophilic area) with direct continuity into the subchondral plate.

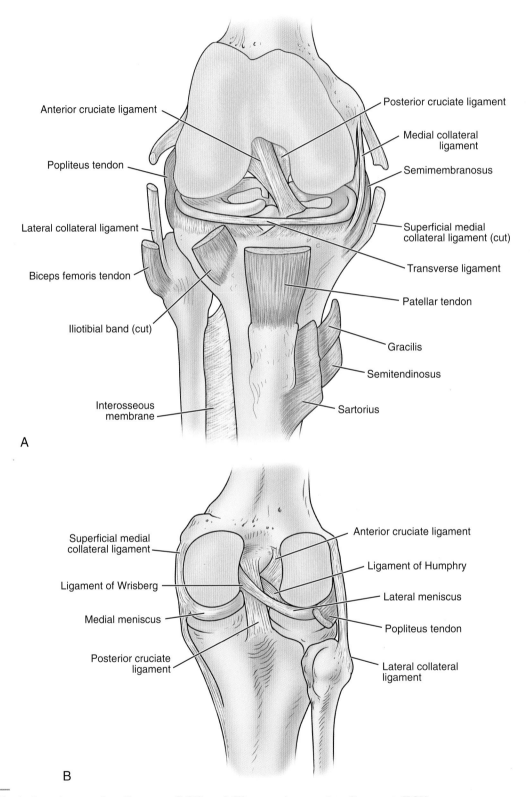

Anterior cruciate ligament

Popliteus tendon

Lateral collateral ligament

Biceps femoris tendon

Iliotibial band (cut)

Interosseous membrane

Posterior cruciate ligament

Medial collateral ligament

Semimembranosus

Superficial medial collateral ligament (cut)

Transverse ligament

Patellar tendon

Gracilis

Semitendinosus

Sartorius

A

Superficial medial collateral ligament

Ligament of Wrisberg

Medial meniscus

Posterior cruciate ligament

Anterior cruciate ligament

Ligament of Humphry

Lateral meniscus

Popliteus tendon

Lateral collateral ligament

B

Figure 1–46. **A,** Anterior cruciate ligament (ACL) and (**B**) posterior cruciate ligament (PCL).

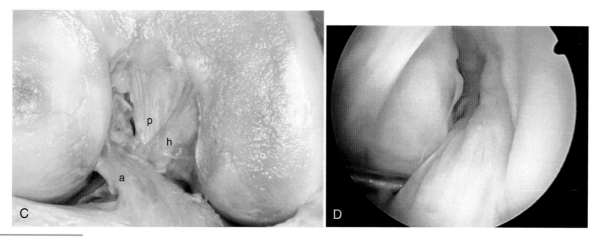

Figure 1–46, cont'd. **C,** Close-up of an anatomic specimen seen from the anterior aspect demonstrating the relationship of the ACL (a), ligament of Humphry (h), and PCL (p) from anterior to posterior in the intercondylar notch. **D,** Arthroscopic view of the contents of the intercondylar notch showing, from left to right, the ligamentum mucosum, PCL, and ACL (probe posterior to the ACL).

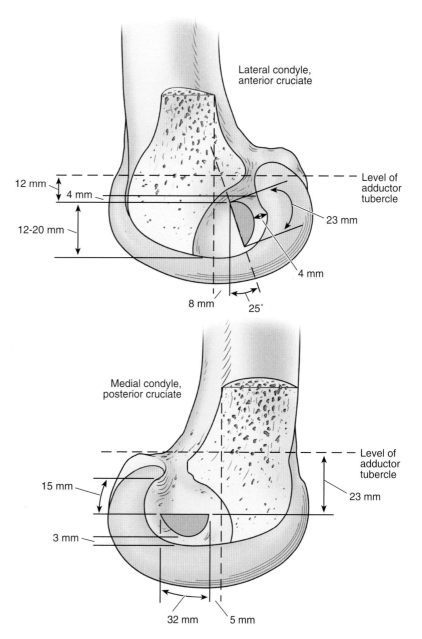

Figure 1–47. Attachments of the anterior and posterior cruciate ligaments to the femur. (From Girgis FG, Marshall JL, Al Monajem ARS: The cruciate ligaments of the knee joint. Clin Orthop 106:216, 1975.)

side convex. The ligament courses anteriorly, distally, and medially toward the tibia (Fig. 1–48). Over the length of its course, the fibers of the ligament undergo slight external rotation. The average length of the ligament is 38 mm and the average width 11 mm.[29] About 10 mm below the femoral attachment, the ligament stands out as it proceeds distally to the tibial attachment, which is a wide, depressed area anterior and lateral to the medial tibial tubercle in the intercondylar fossa (Fig. 1–49). The tibial attachment is oriented in an oblique direction and is more robust than the femoral attachment. There is a well-marked slip to the anterior horn of the lateral meniscus.[29]

On MRI the ACL is best visualized on sagittal images. Because of its oblique course the ACL should routinely be evaluated on two or three sagittal sections. A normal ACL has a relatively low signal, but toward the distal insertion the ACL may appear striated (Fig. 1–50). A discontinuity in the fibers or a soft-tissue mass in the notch with high-signal characteristics resulting from edema and hemorrhage indicates an ACL tear. Partial ACL tears may be suggested by increased signal, thickening, or redundancy in the ligament. However, accurate diagnosis of partial injuries remains challenging (Fig. 1–51). Arthroscopic evaluation of the ACL remains the gold standard for evaluating suspected partial and complete tears (Fig. 1–52).

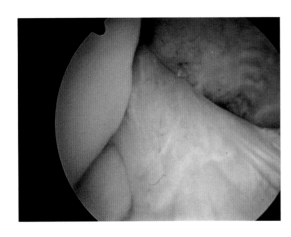

Figure 1–48. Arthroscopic view of a normal anterior cruciate ligament (ACL). The fibers of the ACL fan out distally, anteriorly, and medially to insert on the tibia. The origin of the posterior cruciate ligament can be visualized posterior to the ACL.

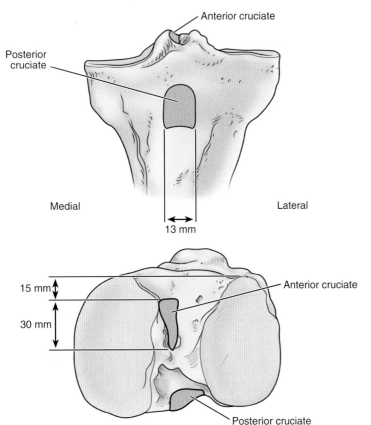

Figure 1–49. Attachments of the anterior and posterior cruciate ligaments to the tibia. (From Girgis FG, Marshall JL, Al Monajem ARS: The cruciate ligaments of the knee joint. Clin Orthop 106:216, 1975.)

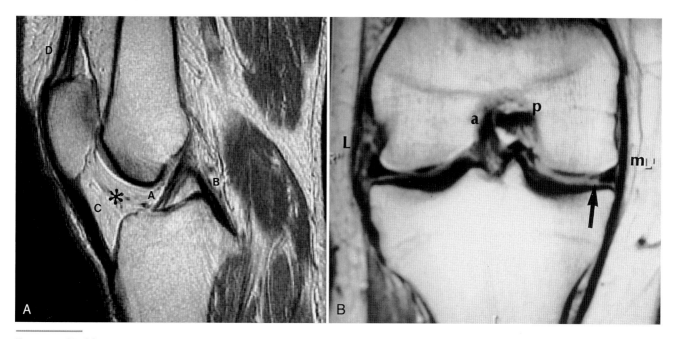

Figure 1–50. Magnetic resonance imaging of the knee. **A,** Sagittal view demonstrating a normal anterior cruciate ligament (ACL) (A) and posterior cruciate ligament (PCL) (B). The low-signal patellar (C) and quadriceps (D) tendons and high-signal fat pad (*asterisk*) can be identified anteriorly. **B,** Coronal view with the ACL (a) lateral to the PCL (p) in the inter-condylar notch. The low-signal medial collateral ligament (m) runs from the femur, with the superficial fibers extending distally onto the medial aspect of the tibia. The lateral collateral ligament (L) and a small tear in the medial meniscus (*arrow*) can be seen.

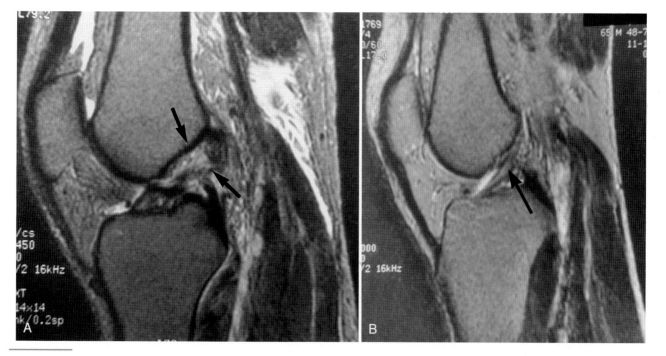

Figure 1–51. **A,** Sagittal magnetic resonance image (MRI) of a torn anterior cruciate ligament (ACL) with disruption at the femoral origin (*arrows*) and an abnormal wavy contour. **B,** Sagittal MRI showing hemorrhage about the ACL and intra-substance signal (*arrow*) consistent with a partial ACL tear, later confirmed by arthroscopic examination.

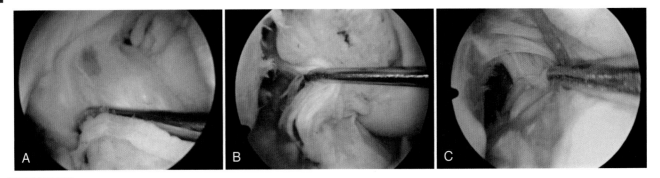

Figure 1–52. Arthroscopic views of anterior cruciate ligament (ACL) tears. **A,** A significant partial proximal ACL tear with a small number of intact fibers inferiorly. **B,** Complete ACL tear with the remaining stump of ruptured fibers at the tibial insertion retracted medially. The bare intercondylar wall (empty wall sign) of the lateral condyle is evident. **C,** Close-up view of the empty wall sign. The stump of the ACL is retracted medially to reveal that the intercondylar wall of the lateral femoral condyle is devoid of the normal ACL origin.

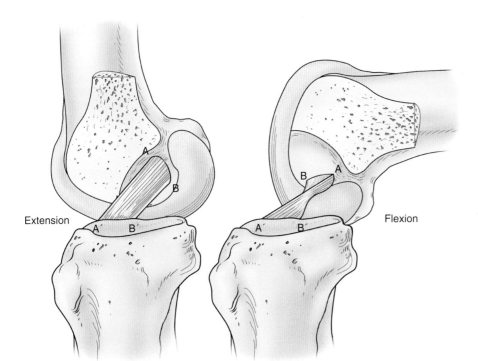

Extension

Flexion

Figure 1–53. Diagram of the anterior cruciate ligament in extension and flexion. Note that in extension the posterolateral bulk is taut whereas in flexion, the anteromedial band is tight and the posterolateral bulk is relatively relaxed. (From Girgis FG, Marshall JL, Al Monajem ARS: The cruciate ligaments of the knee joint. Clin Orthop 106:216, 1975.)

The ACL is the prime static stabilizer against anterior translation of the tibia on the femur and accounts for up to 86% of the total force resisting anterior draw.[14,27,39,54] At different stages of knee motion distinct portions of the ACL appear to act to stabilize the knee joint. Anatomic examination has failed to reveal distinct bundles; therefore, the bundles seem to represent functional, rather than anatomic, structures. An anteromedial bundle becomes taut at 90 degrees of flexion, and a posterolateral bundle becomes tight as full extension is approached (Fig. 1–53).[27,29,95] The ACL also plays a lesser role in resisting internal and external rotation. The maximum tensile strength of the ACL is approximately 1725 ± 270 N,[70] which is less than the peak force that occurs in vigorous athletic activities. Stability is enhanced by dynamic stabilizers, such as the muscles that exert a force across the knee joint. For the muscles to aid in protective stabilization of the knee, effective proprioceptive feedback regarding joint position is crucial. It appears that the ACL plays an important proprioceptive function because a variety of mechanoreceptors and free nerve endings have been identified.[7,22,53,79,80] In humans with ACL-deficient knees, a significantly higher threshold for detecting passive motion of the involved knee has been reported.[7] The afferent and efferent signals involving the ACL are carried by branches of the posterior tibial nerve.

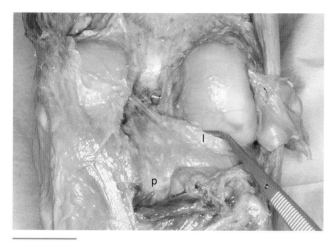

Figure 1–54. Anatomic dissection of the posterior aspect of the knee. The posterior cruciate ligament (p) originates on the lateral aspect of the medial femoral condyle and inserts on the posterior aspect of the tibia distal to the articular surface (l, probe on the superior aspect of the lateral meniscus).

Posterior Cruciate Ligament

The PCL originates from the posterior part of the lateral surface of the medial femoral condyle in the intercondylar notch (see Fig. 1–47). As with the ACL, the origin is in the form of a segment of a circle and is oriented horizontally. The superior boundary of the attachment is straight and the inferior boundary convex. The PCL has an average length of 38 mm and an average width of 13 mm.[29,89] It is narrowest in its midportion and fans out to a greater extent superiorly than it does inferiorly. The fibers are attached to the tibial insertion in a lateromedial direction, whereas in the femur they arise in an anteroposterior direction. The tibial attachment occurs in a depression posterior to the intra-articular upper surface of the tibia (see Fig. 1–49). The attachment extends for up to 1 cm distally onto the adjoining posterior surface of the tibia (Fig. 1–54). Immediately proximal to the tibial attachment, the PCL sends a slip to blend with the posterior horn of the lateral meniscus.[29,89]

A normal PCL has a uniformly low signal intensity on MRI studies with a hockey stick shape. The PCL can be well visualized in both the sagittal and coronal planes (see Fig. 1–50A and B). In addition, the meniscofemoral ligaments of Humphry and Wrisberg may be identified close to the anterior and posterior aspects of the PCL. Tears of the ligament appear as bright signal intensity within the tendon substance, indicative of discontinuity of the fibers (Fig. 1–55). Chronic tears may appear as thinning or an abnormal contour of the ligament.

The PCL is considered to be the primary stabilizer of the knee because it is located close to the central axis of rotation of the joint and is almost twice as strong as the ACL.[17,41,55,89,95] The PCL has been shown to provide approximately 95% of the total restraint to posterior translation of the tibia on the femur.[14] It is maximally taut at full flexion and also becomes tighter with internal rotation

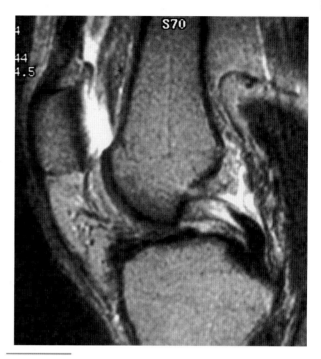

Figure 1–55. Sagittal magnetic resonance image showing increased signal within the femoral half of the posterior cruciate ligament, consistent with a partial tear.

(Fig. 1–56). Two inseparable components of the PCL have been identified. Anterior fibers form the bulk of the ligament and are believed to be taut in flexion and lax in extension. The opposite applies to the thinner posterior portion. The PCL appears to function in concert with the LCL and popliteus tendon to stabilize the knee. Cutting studies have demonstrated that posterior translation in flexion significantly increases when only the PCL is cut, but if the LCL and popliteus are also transected, the translation is significantly greater.[30,89]

Injuries to the PCL are less common than injuries to the ACL and usually result from hyperextension or anterior blows to a flexed knee. Rarely do these injuries result in symptomatic instability, but they may be associated with chronic pain. Significant degenerative changes that involve the medial compartment in 90% of cases have been associated with chronic PCL injuries.[17]

The nature of the superior attachment of the cruciate ligaments results in the bands being twisted around their longitudinal axes on flexion. The ACL and PCL are twisted in opposite directions because they are attached to opposing surfaces. From the front, the direction of torsion will appear to be toward the center of the joint.

ANTERIOR ASPECT

The quadriceps muscle group consists of four distinct parts that share a common tendon of insertion (Fig. 1–57). The rectus femoris arises as two heads, direct and indirect, from the ilium that unite and form a muscle belly running

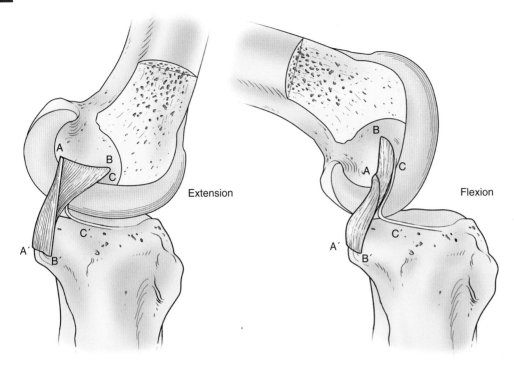

Extension

Flexion

Figure 1–56. Posterior cruciate ligament. In flexion the bulk of the ligament becomes tight, whereas in extension it is relaxed. (From Girgis FG, Marshall JL, Al Monajem ARS: The cruciate ligaments of the knee joint. Clin Orthop 106: 216, 1975.)

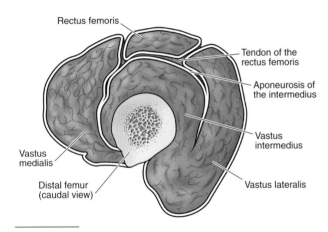

Rectus femoris

Tendon of the rectus femoris

Aponeurosis of the intermedius

Vastus intermedius

Vastus lateralis

Vastus medialis

Distal femur (caudal view)

Figure 1–57. Four components of the quadriceps muscle shown through a cross-section at the junction of middle and distal thirds of the femur. The four components then fuse to form the trilaminar tendon of the quadriceps muscle.

distally in the anterior aspect of the thigh. It narrows to a tendon 5 to 8 cm proximal to the superior pole of the patella.[75] The rectus femoris accounts for about 15% of the cross-section of the quadriceps group. The vastus lateralis arises from a broad linear strip, beginning at the proximal end of the trochanteric line and extending halfway down the linea aspera. It also arises from the lateral intermuscular septum. A fibrous expansion from the distal margin of the vastus lateralis blends with the lateral patellar retinaculum through which there is a direct attachment to the tibia. The vastus medialis originates from the distal part of the trochanteric line and follows the spiral line to the medial lip of the linea aspera. The most distal fibers of the muscle arise from the tendon of the adductor magnus and pass almost horizontally anterior to the insertion into the common tendon and the medial border of the patella. This part of the muscle is sometimes described as the vastus medialis obliquus (VMO). Like the vastus lateralis, the vastus medialis has a distal fibrous expansion that blends with the medial patellar retinaculum. The vastus intermedius arises from the anterior and lateral aspects of the shaft of the femur; medially, it partly blends with the vastus medialis. The four muscles become confluent distally and form the quadriceps tendon, which extends anteriorly about the patella and becomes the patellar tendon (ligament) (Fig. 1–58). The fibers of the rectus femoris and vastus intermedius insert almost perpendicularly into the superior pole of the patella, whereas the fibers of the vastus medialis and lateralis insert obliquely at mean angles of approximately 55 degrees (range, 28 to 70 degrees) and 14 degrees (range, 6 to 45 degrees), respectively.[40,75] The quadriceps tendon is often depicted as a trilaminar structure; the anterior layer is formed by the rectus femoris, the intermediate layer by the vastus medialis and lateralis, and the deep layer by the tendon of the vastus intermedius.[59,75] In reality, the organization is more complex and variable.[75] On MRI the multilaminar nature of the tendon may produce a striated appearance on sagittal views rather than a uniformly low-signal structure (see Fig. 1–50A). A discontinuity or increased signal intensity within the tendon substance and in the surrounding tissues on T2-weighted images is suggestive of quadriceps rupture (Fig. 1–59). Distally, the quadriceps tendon inserts into the patella via an expansion that passes anterior to the patella. In most cases, only fibers from the rectus femoris portion of the tendon continue in the distal

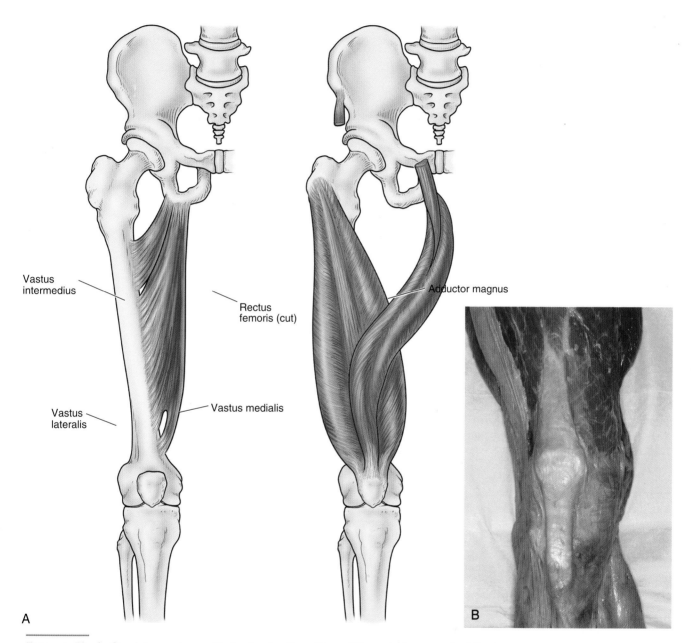

Vastus
intermedius

Rectus
femoris (cut)

Vastus
lateralis

Vastus medialis

Adductor magnus

A

B

Figure 1–58. **A,** Quadriceps group. **B,** Anatomic dissection of the anterior aspect of the knee.

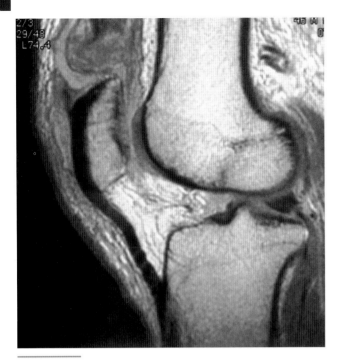

Figure 1–59. Sagittal magnetic resonance image of a complete quadriceps tendon tear with a discontinuity in the fibers at the attachment site on the superior pole of the patella.

expansion over the patella. However, in some cases, fibers from the vastus lateralis can also directly insert distally. In addition, extensions from the medial and lateral vasti insert into the tibia via the patellar retinaculum.

The patellar tendon runs from the lower border of the patella to the tubercle of the tibia. Because the shaft of the femur has an inclination, the quadriceps muscle does not pull in a direct line with the patellar tendon. The angle formed is always valgus, and the average is 14 degrees in males and 17 degrees in females.[1] This angle, the quadriceps (Q) angle, is accentuated by internal rotation of the femur (Fig. 1–60). The resulting tendency toward lateral patellar displacement is resisted by the lateral lip of the femoral trochlea, the horizontal fibers of the VMO, and the medial patellar retinaculum. Selective strengthening of the VMO has been proposed as treatment of patellofemoral pain and subluxation. Although the quadriceps group's most visible function is to extend the knee (with a secondary function to flex the hip), the primary physiological action is to decelerate flexion of the knee during the early stance phase of gait by contracting in an eccentric manner. The four segments of the quadriceps femoris are supplied by the femoral nerve.

The patellar tendon is a strong, flat ligamentous band about 5 cm in length. Proximally, it originates from the apex and adjoining margins of the patella and the rough depression on the posterior surface. Distally, the patellar tendon inserts into the tuberosity of the tibia; superficial fibers are continuous over the front of the patella with those of the tendon of the quadriceps femoris.[75] Medial and lateral portions of the quadriceps tendon pass down on either side of the patella and insert into the proximal

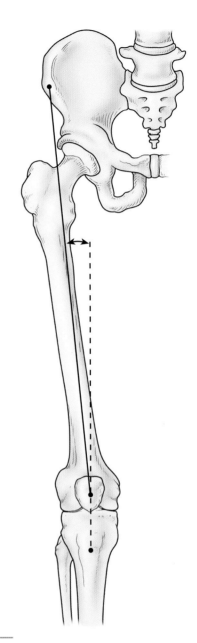

Figure 1–60. Quadriceps (Q) angle.

end of the tibia on either side of the tuberosity. These expansions merge into the capsule and form the medial and lateral patellar retinacula. The patellar tendon normally has low signal intensity on MRI, but it is not uncommon for it to contain intermediate signal at the patella or tibial attachments. As elsewhere, focal discontinuity or high signal intensity in and about the tendon is indicative of a disruption or tear (Fig. 1–61).

The posterior surface of the patellar tendon is separated from the synovial membrane of the joint by a large infrapatellar pad of fat and from the tibia by a bursa. The fat pad fills the space between the femoral condyles and the patellar tendon and adjusts its shape as the size of this potential cavity varies with movement. The fat pad is pierced by numerous blood vessels derived from the genicular arteries. The patellar tendon forms an incomplete

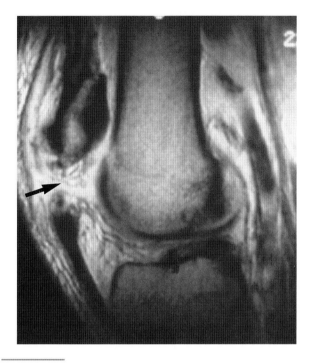

Figure 1–61. Sagittal magnetic resonance image of a patellar tendon tear at the inferior pole of the patella (*arrow*).

septum between the anterior intercondylar notch of the femur and the fat pad.

MEDIAL ASPECT

According to Warren and Marshall,[92] the supporting structures on the medial side of the knee can be divided into three layers. Layer 1 is the most superficial, being the first fascial plane encountered after a skin incision is made on the medial side of the knee. The plane is defined by the fascia that invests the sartorius muscle (Fig. 1–62). The sartorius inserts into this network of fascial fibers and does not have a distinct insertion distally on the tibia. Posteriorly, a layer of fatty tissue lies between layer 1 and the deeper structures. The gracilis and semitendinosus tendons lie in the plane between layers 1 and 2 (Fig. 1–63). Further posteriorly, layer 1 is a fascial sheet that overlies the two heads of the gastrocnemius and the structures of the popliteal fossa. This layer serves as a support for the muscle bellies and the neurovascular structures in the popliteal region. Layer 1 can always be separated from the underlying parallel and oblique portions of the superficial MCL. If a vertical incision is made posterior to the parallel fibers of the ligament, the anterior

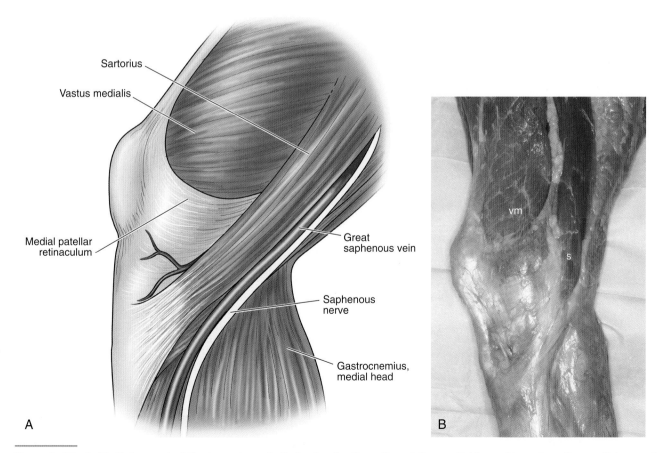

Figure 1–62. **A,** Medial aspect of the knee, layer 1. **B,** Anatomic dissection of the medial knee. Layer 1 on the medial aspect of the knee is defined by the fascial layer, which invests the sartorius muscle (s) (vm, vastus medialis).

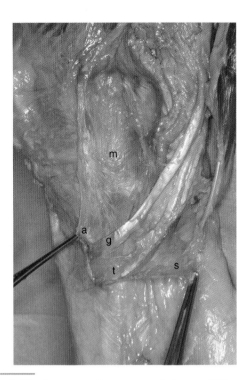

Figure 1–63. Anatomic dissection of the medial aspect of the knee. The tendons of the gracilis (g) and the semitendinosus (t) lie between layer 1 (the fascia investing the sartorius) and layer 2 (m, the superficial medial collateral ligament). In this specimen, layer 1 has been divided, and the sartorius insertion and fascia are retracted posteriorly (s, inferior forceps) and the anterior fascial margin retracted anteriorly (a, superior forceps).

portion of layer 1 can be reflected anteriorly to expose the superficial MCL. Approximately 1 cm anterior to the superficial MCL, layer 1 blends with the anterior portion of layer 2 and the medial patellar retinaculum derived from the vastus medialis. Anteriorly and distally, layer 1 joins the periosteum of the tibia.

Layer 2 is the plane of the superficial MCL. The superficial MCL, as described by Brantigan and Voshell,[13] consists of parallel and oblique portions (Fig. 1–64). The anterior or parallel fibers arise from the sulcus of the medial epicondyle of the femur and consist of heavy, vertically oriented fibers running distally to an insertion on the medial surface of the tibia. This insertion is on average 4.6 cm inferior to the tibial articular surface and is immediately posterior to the insertion of the pes anserinus. The posterior oblique fibers run from the medial epicondyle and blend with layer 3 to form the posteromedial joint capsule.

Anteriorly, according to Warren and Marshall,[92] layer 2 splits vertically. The fibers anterior to the split proceed cephalad to the vastus medialis and join the plane of layer 1 to form the parapatellar retinaculum. The fibers posterior to the split run cephalad to the femoral condyle, from which transverse fibers run forward in the plane of layer 2 to the patella and form the medial patellofemoral ligament. This medial patellofemoral ligament connects the patella to the medial femoral condyle and passively limits

lateral patellar excursion. At the inferior border of the medial patella is the medial meniscopatellar ligament, which connects the patella to the anterior horn of the medial meniscus. The medial retinaculum can be visualized well on routine MRI. Disruptions or tears with the surrounding edema and hemorrhage that occur in association with patella dislocations can also be seen (Fig. 1–65).

Layer 3, the capsule of the knee joint, can be separated from layer 2 except toward the margin of the patella, where it becomes very thin (Fig. 1–66). Deep to the superficial MCL, layer 3 becomes thicker and forms a vertically oriented band of short fibers known as the deep MCL. The deep MCL extends from the femur to the midportion of the peripheral margin of the meniscus and tibia (Fig. 1–67). Anteriorly, the deep MCL is clearly separated from the superficial MCL, with a bursa interposed, but posteriorly the layers blend because the meniscofemoral portion of the deep ligament tends to merge with the overlying superficial ligament near its cephalad attachment. The meniscotibial portion of the deep MCL, however, is readily separated from the overlying superficial ligament and is referred to as the coronary ligament. The components of the MCL are well seen on MRI studies. Coronal images provide clear visualization, but axial images can provide complementary information. Normal ligament fibers have low signal intensity (see Fig. 1–50B). With partial and complete tears, the fibers become less distinct, and increased signal on T2-weighted images can be identified in the ligament as a result of edema and bleeding (Fig. 1–68).

The posteromedial region formed by the merging of layers 2 and 3 is reinforced by five insertions of the semimembranosus tendon and tendon sheath. The semimembranosus has a direct tendinous insertion on the posteromedial corner of the tibia and a second tibial insertion deep to the superficial MCL (see Fig. 1–66). A third tract blends with the oblique fibers of the superficial MCL, and a fourth doubles back to insert proximally in the capsule over the medial meniscus. The fifth tract runs proximally and laterally across the posterior capsule and forms the oblique popliteal ligament (of Winslow) (Fig. 1–69).[92]

On the medial side, the three layers are most obviously separated in the region of the superficial MCL. Anteriorly, the superficial layer and a portion of the middle layer blend and merge with the overlying retinacular expansion from the quadriceps. The other cephalad portion of the middle layer, formed where it splits anterior to the superficial medial ligament, persists as a separate layer forming the patellofemoral ligament. Anteriorly, the deep layer, though separate, becomes extremely thin and difficult to define. Posteriorly, layer 1 becomes the deep fascia, and layers 2 and 3 blend to form the joint capsule.

The superficial MCL functions as the primary restraint against valgus stress, a restraint to external rotation of the tibia, and a weak restraint to anterior tibial translation in ACL-deficient knees.[85,93] The parallel fibers of the superficial MCL are under tension from full extension to 90 degrees of flexion but become maximally taut at 45 to 90 degrees of flexion.[93] The oblique fibers seem to play a minimal role in overall function of the superficial MCL.

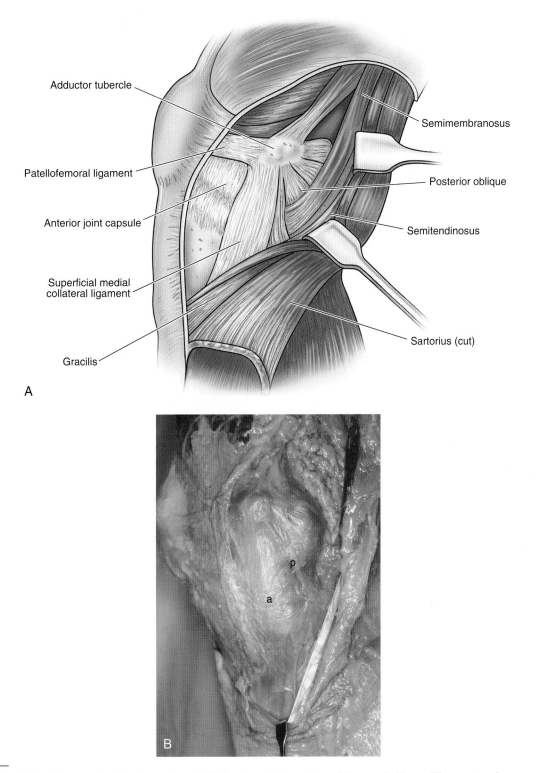

Figure 1–64. **A,** Medial aspect of the knee, layer 2. **B,** Anatomic dissection of the medial knee. The pes tendons are retracted distally and posteriorly to reveal the anterior parallel fibers (a) and the posterior oblique fibers (p) of the superficial medial collateral ligament (layer 2).

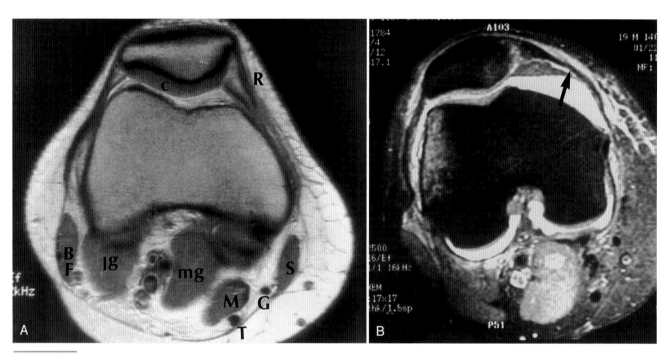

Figure 1–65. **A,** High-resolution axial magnetic resonance image (MRI) of the knee. The popliteal vessels and tibial nerve can be identified between the two heads of the gastrocnemius. The other following structures are marked: patella articular cartilage (c), medial patellar retinaculum (R), sartorius muscle (S), gracilis muscle (G), semimembranosus muscle (M), semitendinosus tendon (T), medial head of the gastrocnemius (mg), lateral head of the gastrocnemius (lg), and biceps femoris (BF). **B,** Axial MRI demonstrating a partial tear of the medial retinaculum (*arrow*) with increased signal on either side secondary to acute lateral patella dislocation.

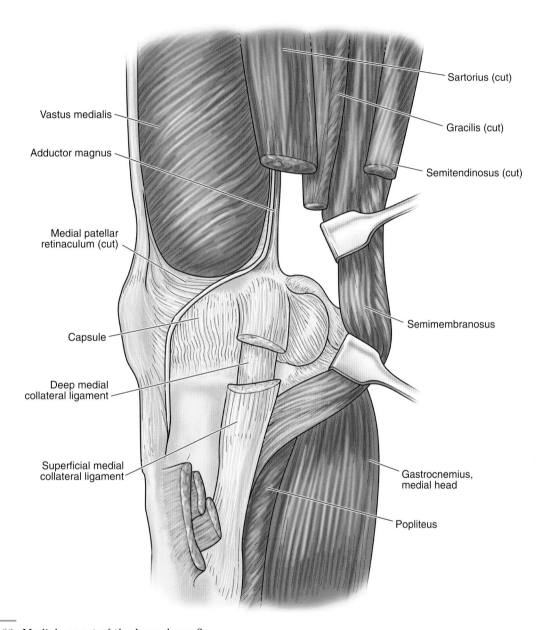

Vastus medialis

Adductor magnus

Medial patellar
retinaculum (cut)

Capsule

Deep medial
collateral ligament

Superficial medial
collateral ligament

Sartorius (cut)

Gracilis (cut)

Semitendinosus (cut)

Semimembranosus

Gastrocnemius,
medial head

Popliteus

Figure 1–66. Medial aspect of the knee, layer 3.

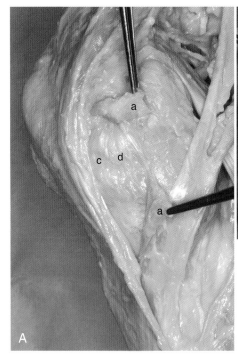

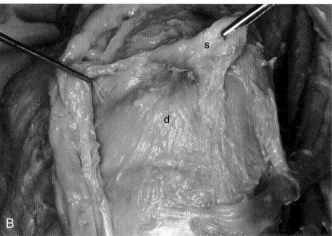

Figure 1–67. Anatomic dissections of the medial aspect of the knee. **A,** The anterior parallel fibers (a) of the superficial medial collateral ligament (MCL) (layer 2) have been sectioned transversely through the middle of the ligament and retracted posteriorly (both forceps) to reveal the fibers of the deep MCL (d) and capsule (c, layer 3). **B,** Close-up view of the fibers of the deep MCL (d) from the femur to the periphery of the meniscus attachment on the tibia. The superficial MCL (s) has been sectioned and the proximal portion retracted proximally (forceps).

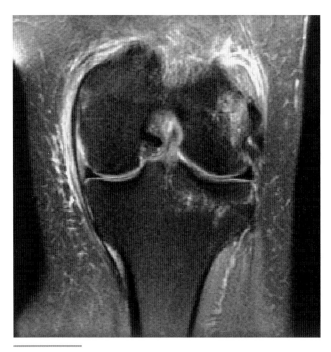

Figure 1–68. Coronal magnetic resonance image with increased fluid signal about the medial collateral ligament consistent with a sprain.

The deep MCL also performs only a weak secondary role as a stabilizer against valgus stress.

LATERAL ASPECT

The supporting structures on the lateral side of the knee have also been described as consisting of three layers.[81]

Layer 1 contains the superficial fascia (fascia lata), the iliotibial tract, and the biceps femoris with its expansion posteriorly (Fig. 1–70). Layer 2 is formed by the quadriceps retinaculum anteriorly and is incomplete posteriorly, where it consists of two patellofemoral ligaments. Layer 3 is composed of the lateral capsule (Fig. 1–71). Posterior to the overlying iliotibial tract, the posterior capsule is divided into two laminae. The deep lamina is composed of the coronary ligament and the arcuate ligament and is newer phylogenetically. The superficial lamina represents the original capsule and consists of the LCL and the fabellofibular ligament. The inferior lateral geniculate artery passes between the two lamina (Fig. 1–72).

The ITB is a longitudinal thickening in the fascia lata that runs along the lateral side of the knee and inserts into Gerdy's tubercle on the tibia. Some of the fibers proceed across Gerdy's tubercle to the tibial tuberosity. Proximally, the fascia lata is adherent to the lateral intermuscular septum, where it is attached to the femur. Posteriorly, the fascia lata merges into the biceps fascia.[49] The biceps femoris muscle is formed from two heads; the long head arises in common with the semitendinosus from the ischial tuberosity, whereas the short head arises from the lateral lip of the linea aspera, the lateral supracondylar line, and the lateral intermuscular septum. The nerve supply of both heads is derived from the sciatic nerve, but from different branches; the long head is innervated by the tibial branch and the short head by the common popliteal nerve. The two heads unite above the knee joint in a common tendon that folds around the LCL insertion on the fibular styloid and then divides into three layers.[67] The superficial layer spreads out and inserts as a wide expansion over the adjoining part of the proximal tibia. The middle layer is a thin, poorly defined layer that envelopes the LCL and is separated from the ligament by a bursa.

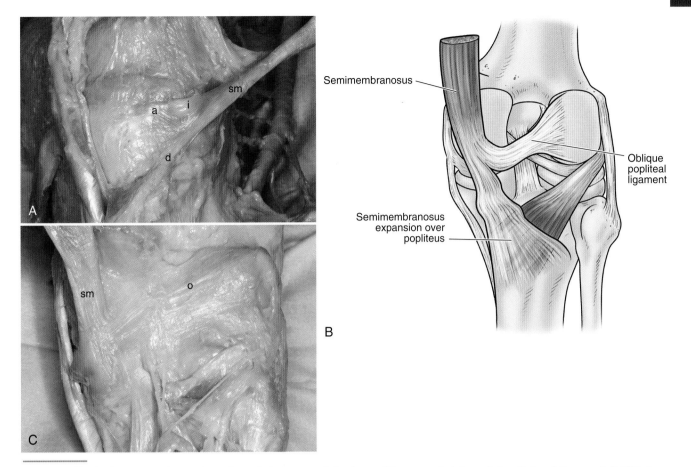

Figure 1–69. **A,** Anatomic dissection of medial aspect of the knee. The superficial medial collateral ligament (MCL) has been sectioned and retracted to reveal the direct insertion (i) of the semimembranosus (sm) on the posteromedial tibia and the anterior extension (a) deep to the superficial MCL. A band of fibers (d) also runs distally to insert into the retracted superficial MCL. **B,** Relationship of the oblique popliteal ligament (o) to the semimembranosus muscle. **C,** Anatomic dissection of the posterior aspect of the knee demonstrating the oblique popliteal ligament (o), which passes obliquely across the posterior capsule to insert on the lateral femoral condyle.

The deep layer bifurcates and inserts on the fibular styloid and on the tibia at Gerdy's tubercle. The biceps functions mainly as a knee flexor but additionally acts as a weaker hip extensor and external rotator of the tibia. The biceps is also believed to be an important static and dynamic stabilizer of the lateral aspect of the knee, especially as the knee flexes beyond 30 degrees.[67,87]

The lateral knee retinaculum has been described by Fulkerson and Gossling[26] (Fig. 1–73). The lateral patellar retinaculum is composed of two major components: the superficial oblique retinaculum and the deep transverse retinaculum. The superficial oblique retinaculum runs superficially from the ITB to the patella (Fig. 1–74). The deep transverse retinaculum is more dense and consists of three major components. The epicondylopatellar band, also known as the transverse patellofemoral ligament, provides superolateral patellar support. The transverse retinaculum courses directly from the ITB to the midpatella and provides the primary support for the lateral patella. The patellotibial band, the third component, runs between the patella and the tibia inferiorly (Fig. 1–75). Overall, the lateral retinaculum provides stronger support to the patella than its medial counterpart does.

In layer 3, the lateral joint capsule is a thin, fibrous layer that is circumferentially attached to the femur and tibia at the proximal and distal margins of the knee joint. The attachment at the margin of the inferior border of the lateral meniscus, which runs to the edge of the articular margin of the tibia, has been termed the coronary ligament.[60,81] The LCL originates on the lateral epicondyle of the femur anterior to the origin of the gastrocnemius. It runs beneath the lateral retinaculum to insert into the head of the fibula, where it blends with the insertion of the biceps femoris. On MRI studies the LCL is best seen on coronal images and appears as a thin band of low signal intensity (see Fig. 1–50B). Two to three sequential images are usually required to visualize the entire structure because of the oblique course of the ligament. A tear appears as a disruption in the fibers, thickening, or increased signal on T2-weighted images in and about the ligament as a result of edema.

The fabellofibular ligament is a condensation of fibers lying between the LCL and arcuate ligaments that runs from the fabella, a sesamoid bone found in the lateral head of gastrocnemius, to the fibular styloid.[50] The arcuate ligament has been variously described; according to Last,[60]

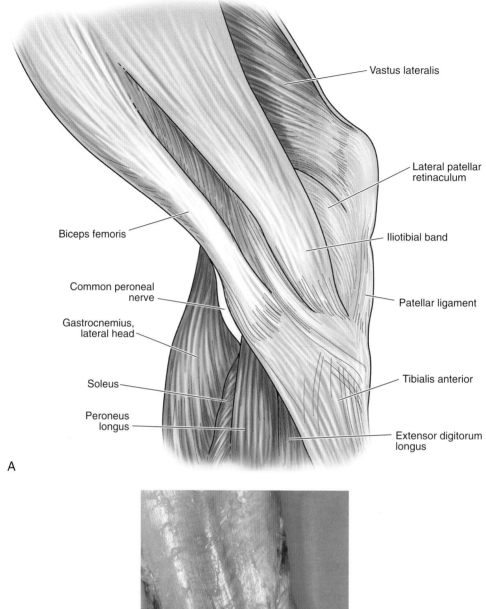

A

B

Figure 1–70. **A,** Lateral aspect of the knee, layer 1. **B,** Anatomic dissection of the lateral knee. Layer 1 on the lateral side of the knee with a prominent iliotibial band (i) insertion on Gerdy tubercle (g).

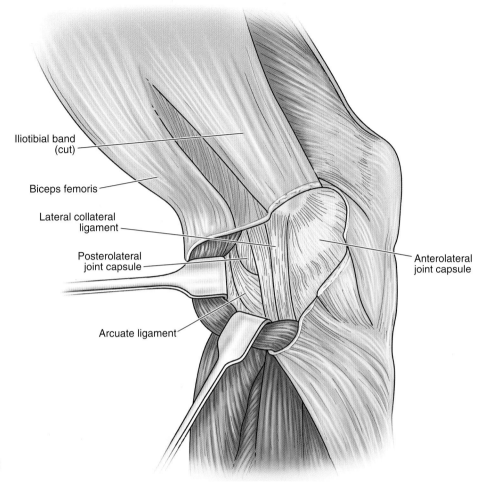

Iliotibial band
(cut)

Biceps femoris

Lateral collateral
ligament

Posterolateral
joint capsule

Anterolateral
joint capsule

Arcuate ligament

Figure 1–71. Lateral aspect of
the knee, layer 3.

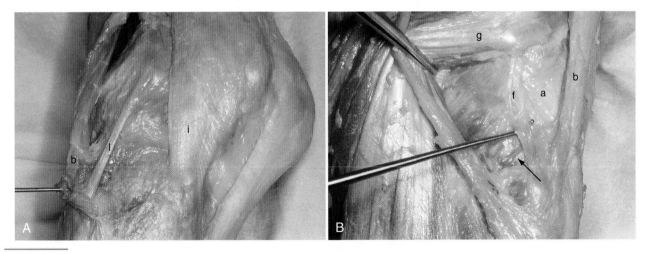

Figure 1–72. Anatomic dissections of the posterolateral aspect of the knee. **A,** The superficial layers along the posterior margin of the iliotibial band (i) have been incised and retracted posteriorly to reveal layer 3 of the lateral aspect of the knee. The prominent lateral collateral ligament (l) inserts deep to the biceps (b, retracted by the probe) on the fibular head. **B,** The lateral head of the gastrocnemius (g) has been retracted medially (forceps) to expose the fabellofibular (f) and arcuate ligaments (a). The inferior lateral geniculate artery (*arrow*) passes between the fabellofibular ligament (superficial lamina of layer 3) and the arcuate ligament (deep lamina of layer 3) just distal to the probe placed between the two laminae (b, biceps femoris).

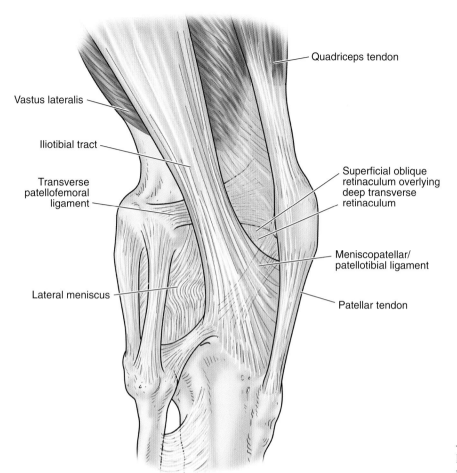

Quadriceps tendon

Vastus lateralis

Iliotibial tract

Transverse
patellofemoral
ligament

Superficial oblique
retinaculum overlying
deep transverse
retinaculum

Meniscopatellar/
patellotibial ligament

Lateral meniscus

Patellar tendon

Figure 1–73. Structures of the lateral retinaculum.

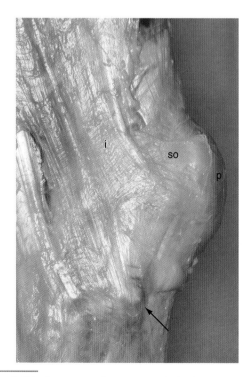

Figure 1–74. Anatomic dissection of the lateral aspect of the knee. The superficial oblique (so) fibers of the lateral retinaculum run between the anterior margin of the iliotibial band (i) and the lateral aspect of the patella (p) (*arrow*, Gerdy's tubercle).

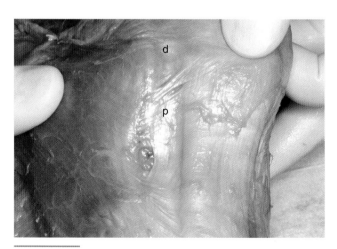

Figure 1–75. Close-up of an anatomic dissection of the lateral retinaculum. With the superficial oblique retinaculum removed, the patellotibial band (p) and transverse fibers (d) of the deep retinaculum can be identified.

"In truth, there is at this part of the capsule such a complexity of fibers running in many directions that, by artful dissection, almost any pattern desired by the dissector could be made." Some fibers extend from the lateral condyle of the femur to the posterior part of the capsule. The strongest and most consistent fibers of the arcuate ligament, however, form a triangular sheet that diverges upward from the fibular styloid. The lateral limb of this mass is dense and strong and is attached to the femur and the popliteal tendon. The weaker medial limb curves over the popliteal muscle and blends with the fibers of the oblique popliteal ligament. The free edge of this medial limb is crescentic, and the lateral or femoral part of the popliteus emerges beneath it to approach its tibial attachment. Three common variations in the fabellofibular and arcuate ligaments have been described. In most knees (67%), both the fabellofibular and arcuate ligaments are present, but in the case of a large fabella, the fabellofibular ligament dominates and the arcuate ligament is absent (20%); however, in the absence of a fabella, only the arcuate ligament is present (13%).[81] Watanabe et al[94] further divided these categories into a total of seven types based on the presence or absence of a fibular insertion of a portion of the popliteal tendon.

The popliteal muscle arises by a strong tendon about 2.5 cm long from a depression at the anterior part of the groove on the lateral condyle of the femur. The tendon, which is invested in synovial membrane, passes beneath the medial limb of the arcuate ligament and forms a thin, flat, triangular muscle that inserts into the medial two-thirds of the triangular surface proximal to the popliteal line on the posterior surface of the tibia. A direct attachment to the fibular head has also been redefined.[68,94] The tendon is also attached to the arcuate ligament, and according to Last,[60] up to half of its fibers are attached to the lateral meniscus. The synovial membrane below the meniscus herniates deep to the muscle as the popliteal bursa. The function of the popliteus is controversial, but it may act in conjunction with the meniscofemoral ligaments to control motion of the meniscus as the knee flexes.[9,47,60,88] However, its primary role appears to be unlocking the knee to allow flexion by producing external rotation of the femur in the loaded position.[9,60,65] The nerve to the popliteus arises from the tibial nerve and runs distally across the popliteal vessels to reach the lower border of the muscle, where it enters the deep surface.

The LCL, PCL, and popliteal-arcuate complex act in concert to stabilize the posterolateral corner of the knee against varus stress, external tibial rotation, and posterior flexion. Damage to these structures results in posterolateral rotatory instability.[6,42,43]

POSTERIOR ASPECT

The popliteal fossa is bounded laterally by the biceps femoris and medially by the semimembranosus and tendons of the pes anserine. Distally, the space is closed by the two heads of the gastrocnemius. The roof of the fossa is formed by the deep fascia; the floor consists of the popliteal surface of the femur, the posterior capsule of the knee joint, and the popliteus muscle with its fascial covering (Fig. 1–76).

The biceps femoris lies posterior to the ITB and forms the lateral wall of the popliteal fossa; it has previously been described. The semitendinosus arises from the ischial tuberosity and runs distally and medially on the surface of the semimembranosus. The semimembranosus arises from the upper and lateral impressions on the ischial tuberosity. It passes distally and medially deep to the origin of the biceps and semitendinosus (Fig. 1–77). Its tendon forms the proximal and medial boundaries of the popliteal fossa and inserts into a groove on the posteromedial aspect of the tibia. Multiple expansions reinforce the posteromedial capsule as previously described. Directly posteriorly, a robust expansion called the oblique popliteal ligament passes proximally and laterally and blends with the posterior capsule and arcuate ligament from the lateral side. The nerve supply to the hamstring muscles is derived from the tibial branch of the sciatic nerve. The gracilis muscle arises from the inferior pubic ramus and runs distally along the medial side of the thigh. In the lower third of the thigh, the fibers end in a long tendon that lies medial to the tendon of the semitendinosus. It is innervated by the obturator nerve. The sartorius muscle arises from the anterior superior iliac spine and runs distally and medially across the front of the thigh, where it forms the roof of the subsartorial canal. Its nerve supply is derived from the femoral nerve. Distally, the sartorius tendon is wider and less well defined than the gracilis and semitendinosus nerves. Rather than inserting directly into the tibia, the diffuse tendinous fibers blend with layer 1 of the medial aspect of the knee. Together, the tendons of the sartorius, gracilis, and semitendinosus form the pes anserinus (see Fig. 1–77). The sartorius tendon expansion lies superficially and covers the insertions of the gracilis and semitendinosus. The semitendinosus inserts into the tibia just distal to the gracilis and forms a conjoint structure with a mean width of 20 mm; the proximal-most point of the insertion begins a mean of 19 mm distal and 22.5 mm medial to the apex of the tibial tubercle.[72] The muscles, which insert at the pes, act to flex and internally rotate the knee.

When the knee is flexed, the biceps tendon can be felt subcutaneously on the lateral side. Medially, two tendons are prominent, the gracilis lying medial to the semitendinosus.

The ischial fibers of the adductor magnus are a derivative of the hamstring group. The fibers run distally and end in a short tendon that inserts into the prominent adductor tubercle on the medial condyle of the femur. Through a gap in the insertion of this muscle, the femoral vessels enter the popliteal fossa. Like the hamstrings, this portion of the adductor magnus is supplied by the sciatic nerve.

The gastrocnemius muscle arises as a lateral head from the lateral aspect of the lateral femoral condyle and as a larger medial head from the popliteal surface of the femur and medial aspect of the medial femoral condyle (Fig. 1–78). The lateral head has a largely fleshy origin, but the portion of the medial head that arises from the medial condyle adjoining the attachment of the medial collateral ligament is tendinous. The two heads merge and form a

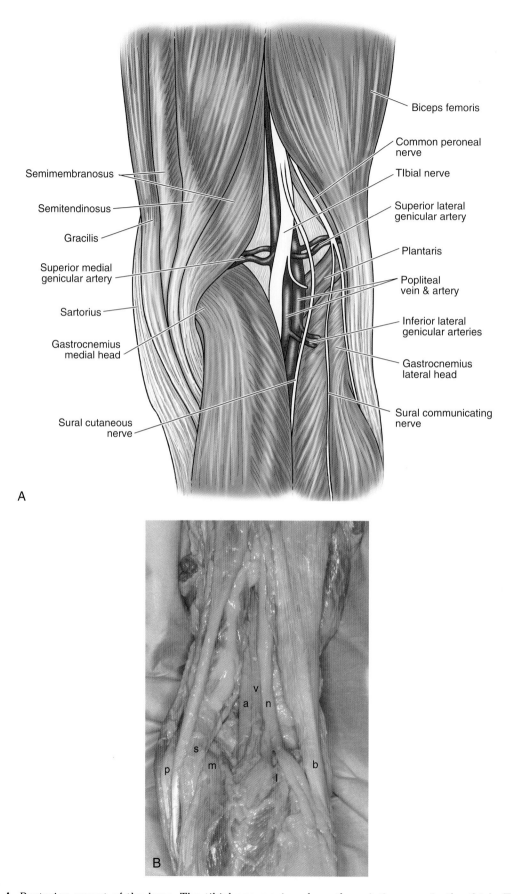

Figure 1–76. **A,** Posterior aspect of the knee. The tibial nerve arises from the sciatic nerve in the thigh. The popliteal artery and vein are in close proximity. **B,** Anatomic dissection of the popliteal fossa. From left to right (medial to lateral), the identified structures at the level of the joint line are the pes tendons (p); semimembranosus (s); medial head of the gastrocnemius (m); popliteal artery (a), vein (v), and nerve (n); lateral head of the gastrocnemius (l); and biceps femoris tendon (b).

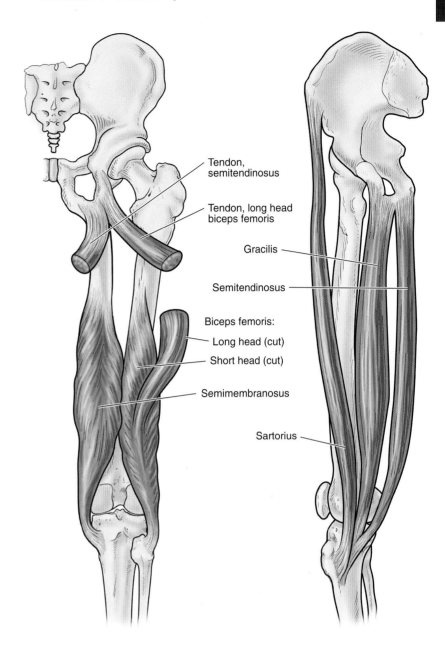

Figure 1–77. **Posterior musculature.**

common tendon with the soleus, which narrows distally and inserts into the tendo calcaneus.

The plantaris muscle has a small, fleshy belly that arises from the lateral supracondylar line of the femur deep to the lateral head of the gastrocnemius. It gives rise to a very long, narrow tendon that runs distally deep to the medial head of the gastrocnemius. The plantaris is absent in about 7% of individuals and is believed to represent a vestigial structure in humans.[21]

The soleus arises from multiple origins, including the upper fourth of the posterior surface of the shaft and head of the fibula, the tendinous arch crossing the posterior tibial vessels and nerve, and the soleal line of the posterior surface of the tibia. Its tendon joins the deep surface of the tendo Achilles. The gastrocnemius, plantaris, and soleus are supplied by the tibial nerve.

NERVES

Although considerable individual variation exists, predominant patterns of innervation about the knee have been identified.[28,53] Two distinct groups of afferent nerves have been differentiated. The first, a posterior group, includes the posterior articular branch of the tibial nerve and obturator nerves. The second group is anterior and includes the articular branches of the femoral, common peroneal, and saphenous nerves.

The tibial nerve (medial or internal popliteal nerve) arises from the sciatic nerve halfway down the thigh. It runs distally through the popliteal fossa, lying at first in the fat beneath the deep fascia. More distally, it is found deeper in the interval between the two heads of the gas-

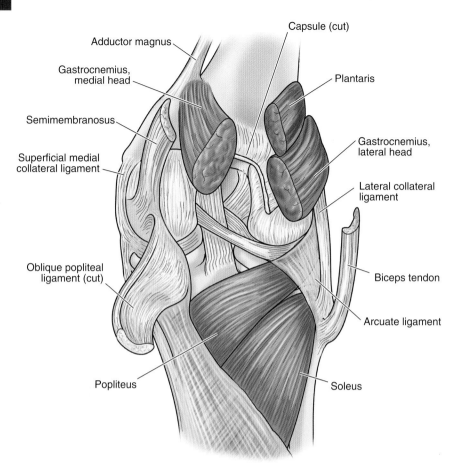

Figure 1–78. Popliteal fossa.

trocnemius. A cutaneous branch, the sural nerve, descends on the surface of the gastrocnemius (see Fig. 1–76). Muscular branches are given off to both heads of the gastrocnemius, plantaris, soleus, and popliteal muscles. In addition, there are several articular branches. The largest and most consistent branch, the posterior articular nerve, has a variable origin but often arises within the popliteal fossa. In other circumstances, it may arise from the tibial portion of the sciatic nerve in the thigh.[28] It courses laterally and wraps around the popliteal vessels before passing deep to join the popliteal plexus. Fibers from the plexus penetrate through the oblique popliteal ligament to innervate the posterior and perimeniscal capsule and synovial covering of the cruciates. The extent of the innervation of the menisci is controversial; evidence supports both nerve fibers penetrating into the outer third of the menisci and innervation limited to only the perimeniscal capsule.[53] The terminal branch of the posterior division of the obturator nerve, which follows the course of the femoral artery into the popliteal fossa, also contributes to the popliteal plexus and thus to the innervation of the capsule and menisci.

The capsule and ligaments on the anteromedial and anterolateral areas of the knee are innervated by the anterior afferent group, in particular, the articular branches of the nerves, which supply the quadriceps muscles. The largest branch arises from the nerve supplying the vastus medialis and supplies a portion of the anteromedial capsule. Laterally, a branch from the nerve to the vastus

lateralis innervates the superolateral capsule, and anteriorly, afferent fibers from the suprapatellar pouch join nerves to the vastus intermedius. The saphenous nerve arises from the posterior division of the femoral nerve. At the lower end of the subsartorial canal, the nerve pierces the deep fascia on the medial side of the knee between the sartorius and gracilis tendons. The infrapatellar branch traverses the sartorius muscle and joins the patellar plexus; it provides innervation to the anteromedial capsule, patellar tendon, and skin anteromedially (Fig. 1–79).[45] Distally, the sartorial branch of the saphenous nerve is joined by the long saphenous vein and runs along the medial aspect of the leg (Fig. 1–80). The patellar plexus lies in front of the patella and patellar tendon. It is formed by the numerous communications between the terminal branches of the lateral, intermediate, and medial cutaneous nerves of the thigh and the infrapatellar branch of the saphenous nerve.

The common peroneal nerve (lateral or external popliteal nerve) enters the popliteal fossa on the lateral side of the tibial nerve and runs distally along the medial side of the biceps tendon (Fig. 1–81). The common peroneal nerve passes between the biceps femoris tendon and the lateral head of the gastrocnemius and runs distally posterior to the fibula head (Fig. 1–82). It next winds superficially across the lateral aspect of the neck of the fibula before piercing the peroneus longus through a fibrous tunnel and dividing into the superficial peroneal (musculocutaneous) and deep peroneal (anterior tibial)

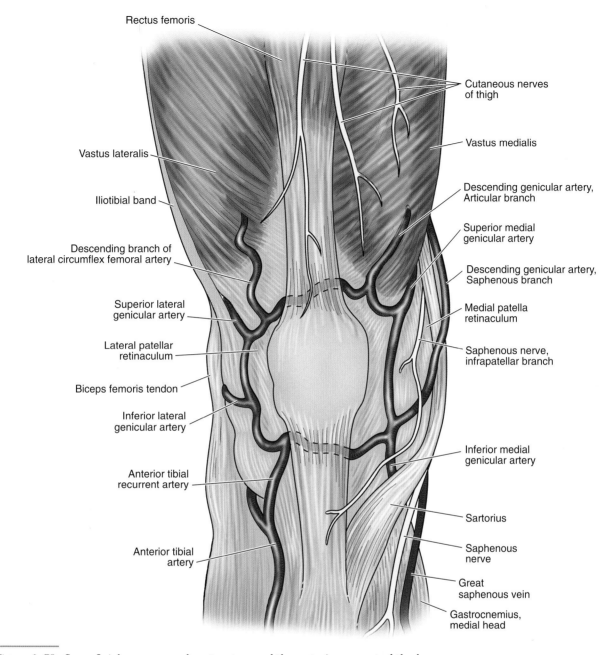

Figure 1–79. Superficial neurovascular structures of the anterior aspect of the knee.

nerves. The cutaneous branches are the sural communicating nerve, which joins the sural nerve, and a small branch to the skin over the upper anterolateral aspect of the leg. Two articular branches of the common peroneal nerve are the lateral articular nerve, which arises at the level of the joint line and innervates the inferior lateral capsule and LCL, and the recurrent peroneal nerve, which ascends the anterior surface of the tibia in the peroneus longus and enters the joint anterolaterally.[53]

The individual structures involved in specific functions such as pain sensation and proprioception in the knee are controversial. Kennedy et al[53] indicated that deep fibrous structures such as the ligaments and menisci rarely contain nerve fibers whereas both pain and specialized

mechanoreceptors are found in the surrounding connective tissues of the capsule and synovium. Stretching of the capsule causes pain, and effusions greater than 60 mL have been shown to cause reflex quadriceps inhibition.[53,83] Because of the numerous mechanoreceptors, the capsule also probably plays a significant role in proprioception.

BLOOD SUPPLY

Before passing through the adductor hiatus, the femoral artery gives off the descending genicular artery. This vessel, in turn, gives off the saphenous branch, an articu-

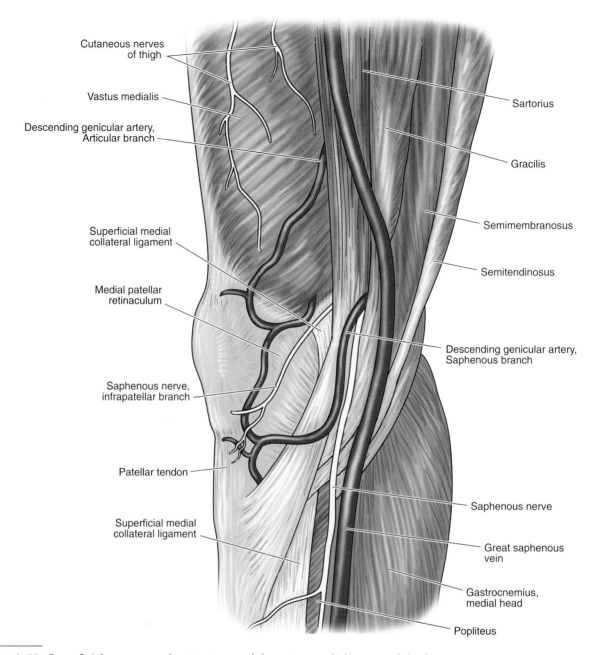

Figure 1–80. Superficial neurovascular structures of the anteromedial aspect of the knee.

lar branch, and the deep oblique branch. The saphenous branch travels distally with the saphenous nerve and passes between the sartorius before anastomosing with the medial inferior genicular artery. The articular branch extends distally within the vastus medialis and anastomoses with the lateral superior genicular artery to contribute to the peripatellar network. The deep oblique branch courses along the medial aspect of the femur and gives off branches to the supracondylar femur as well as collateral muscular branches. The popliteal artery exits from Hunter's canal and enters the popliteal fossa at the junction of the middle and lower thirds of the femur (Fig. 1–83). Proximally, it is separated from the femur by a thick

pad of fat, but distally in the region of the posterior joint line it lies in direct contact with the oblique posterior ligament. Further distally, the artery runs superficial to the popliteus fascia and ends at the lower border of the popliteus by dividing into the anterior and posterior tibial arteries. The popliteal artery gives off numerous muscular branches and five articular branches (Fig. 1–84). The middle genicular artery arises from the anterior aspect of the popliteal artery and pierces the posterior oblique ligament to supply the posterior capsule and intracapsular structures, including the posterior horns of the menisci (Fig. 1–85).[78] Ligamentous branches of this artery traverse the synovium and form a plexus of vessels that cover both

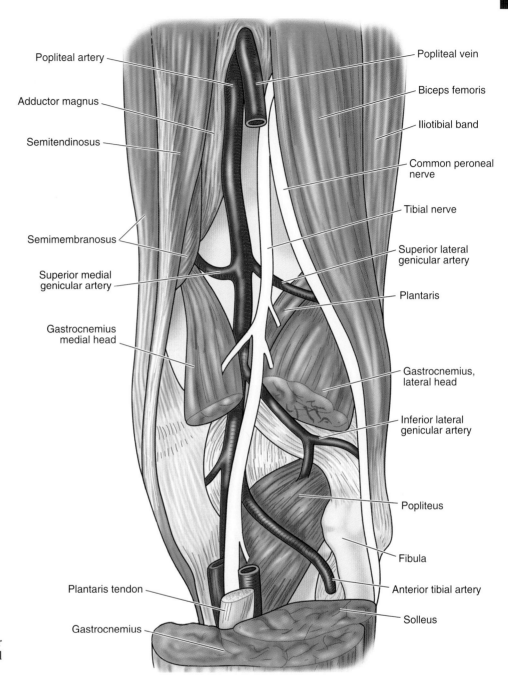

Popliteal artery

Adductor magnus

Semitendinosus

Semimembranosus

Superior medial
genicular artery

Gastrocnemius
medial head

Plantaris tendon

Gastrocnemius

Popliteal vein

Biceps femoris

Iliotibial band

Common peroneal
nerve

Tibial nerve

Superior lateral
genicular artery

Plantaris

Gastrocnemius,
lateral head

Inferior lateral
genicular artery

Popliteus

Fibula

Anterior tibial artery

Solleus

Figure 1–81. Neurovascular
structures of the popliteal
fossa.

the ACL and PCL and perforate the ligaments to anasto-mose with small vessels, which run parallel to the colla-gen fibrils.[78] The cruciates may also receive terminal branches from the inferior genicular arteries. The ACL receives essentially no blood supply from the ligament-bone insertion sites.[4] The medial and lateral superior genicular arteries originate from the posterior aspect of the artery and then wind around the lower end of the femur immediately proximal to the condyles. The lateral supe-rior genicular artery passes deep to the biceps femoris tendon and then anastomoses with the descending branch of the lateral femoral circumflex artery. The medial supe-rior genicular branch courses anteriorly deep to the semi-

membranosus and semitendinosus and proximal to the origin of the medial head of the gastrocnemius. Arising more distally at a level below the joint line from either side of the popliteal artery are the medial and lateral inferior genicular arteries. The inferior lateral genicular artery lies immediately adjacent to the lateral joint line. It passes deep to the LCL, proximal to the fibular head, as it trav-erses anterolaterally to join the anterior anastomosis. The inferior medial genicular artery passes two fingerbreadths distal to the medial joint line, deep to the MCL, and also joins the anterior anastomosis. Branches from the inferior genicular arteries form a complex capillary network in the anterior fat pad and provide abundant supply to the

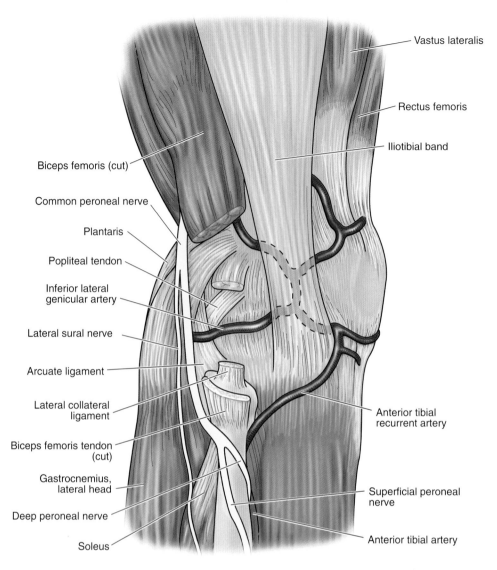

Figure 1–82. Superficial neurovascular structures of the lateral aspect of the knee.

fat pad, synovial cavity, and patellar tendon. Terminal branches of all four medial and lateral genicular arteries also extend into the menisci, but Arnoczky and Warren[5] have shown that the predominant vascular supply comes from the superior and inferior lateral genicular arteries. Rather than providing uniform supply to the entire menisci, only the peripheral 30% receives these vascular branches (Fig. 1–86). Tears that occur in this peripheral vascular zone are considered to be the best candidates for repair.

The anterior anastomosis around the knee is formed by the four inferior and superior genicular arteries, branches of the descending genicular artery, the descending branch of the lateral circumflex femoral artery, and recurrent branches of the anterior tibial artery. The anastomosis thus connects the femoral artery at the origin of its profundus branch with the popliteal and anterior tibial arteries (Fig. 1–87). Anteriorly, the anastomosis forms a vascular circle around the patella from which, according to Scapinelli,[77] 9 to 12 nutrient arteries arise at the lower pole of the patella and run proximally on the anterior surface of the bone in a series of furrows (Fig. 1–88). These vessels penetrate the anterior surface of the patella in the middle third. Additional polar vessels penetrate the patella in the apical region. The patellar retinaculum on the medial side is supplied by the anastomosis, with the main contribution coming from the descending genicular artery. The lateral retinaculum receives almost all of its supply from the lateral anastomosis formed by the superior and inferior lateral genicular arteries.[19] The arterial supply to the patellar tendon appears to be derived from two anastomotic arches that are fed by medial and lateral pedicles.[82] The descending and inferior medial genicular arteries appear to be important contributors to the medial pedicles, whereas on the lateral side, the lateral genicular arteries and recurrent tibial anterior arteries provide the greatest contributions.[82] Perforating collateral vessels from the superior (retropatellar) and inferior (supratubercular) anastomotic arches create two distinct vascular zones that anastomose in the middle third of the tendon.[82]

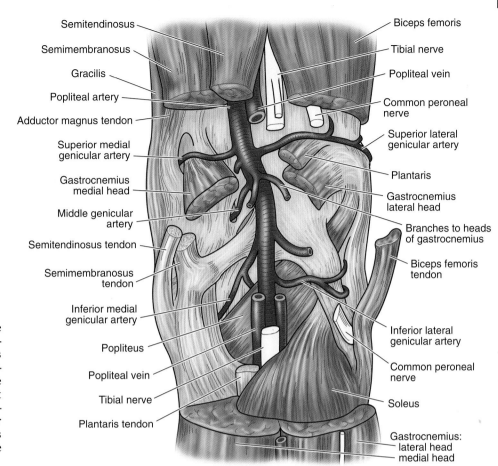

Semitendinosus
Semimembranosus
Gracilis
Popliteal artery
Adductor magnus tendon
Superior medial genicular artery
Gastrocnemius medial head
Middle genicular artery
Semitendinosus tendon
Semimembranosus tendon
Inferior medial genicular artery
Popliteus
Popliteal vein
Tibial nerve
Plantaris tendon

Biceps femoris
Tibial nerve
Popliteal vein
Common peroneal nerve
Superior lateral genicular artery
Plantaris
Gastrocnemius lateral head
Branches to heads of gastrocnemius
Biceps femoris tendon
Inferior lateral genicular artery
Common peroneal nerve
Soleus
Gastrocnemius: lateral head, medial head

Figure 1–83. Branches of the popliteal artery in the popliteal space. The artery lies on the oblique posterior ligament at the level of the joint line. More proximally, it is separated from the posterior of the femur by a layer of fat. The femoral vein is interposed between the artery and the tibial nerve.

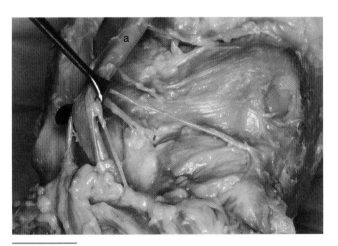

Figure 1–84. Anatomic dissection of the popliteal artery. The popliteal artery (a) has been elevated (probe) to reveal, from proximal to distal, the superior lateral genicular, middle genicular (passing through the posterior oblique ligament), inferior lateral and medial genicular, and two sural branches.

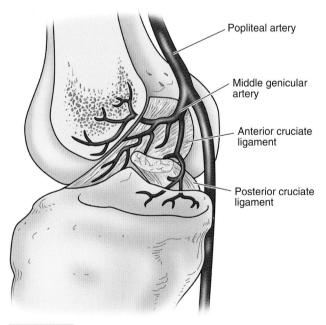

Popliteal artery
Middle genicular artery
Anterior cruciate ligament
Posterior cruciate ligament

Figure 1–85. Middle genicular artery with supply to the cruciate ligaments.

The skin overlying the anterior aspect of the knee receives its blood supply via three routes: direct cutaneous, musculocutaneous, and septocutaneous (intermuscular) vessels.[15,35,36] These vessels provide arterial inflow in both random perforating and axial-type distributions. Perforating vessels include terminal branches

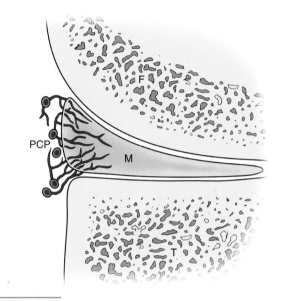

Figure 1–86. Diagrammatic representation of the peripheral blood supply to the medial meniscus (M). F, femur; PCP, perimeniscal capillary plexus; T, tibia.

from the anterior anastomosis, as well as additional musculocutaneous terminal branches from the rectus femoris and vastus muscle group. Once they have perforated through the deep fascia, these vessels run parallel to the skin surface for a considerable distance in the loose areolar layer that separates the deep fascia from subcutaneous fat. In this layer these vessels form an interconnecting fascial plexus.[35,86] Branches from this fascial plexus traverse the subcutaneous tissue and anastomose with other branches to create a subdermal plexus.[34,86] Because the skin relies on the distribution from the fascial plexus just superficial to the deep fascia, the true surgical plane of the anterior knee is beneath the deep fascia; consequently, undermining of the skin in a manner that creates elevated skin and subcutaneous flaps should be minimized.[34] Furthermore, although the skin receives arterial inflow from both the medial and lateral contributions to the anterior anastomosis, the principal vascular supply is from the medial side.[19,35] In particular, the saphenous artery, which arises in a common trunk with the descending genicular vessel from the superficial femoral artery, provides a major contribution to the fascial plexus.[19,35]

Surgical exposure of the knee interrupts flow into variable portions of this network of perforating terminal branches. In a healthy individual, a single midline anterior incision presents little problem for wound healing, but multiple previous incisions or ischemic disease can lead to wound complications or skin necrosis. In general, a previous transverse incision may be crossed perpendicularly. If multiple longitudinal incisions are present, the most lateral midline incision should be selected in the majority of circumstances to avoid creating large laterally

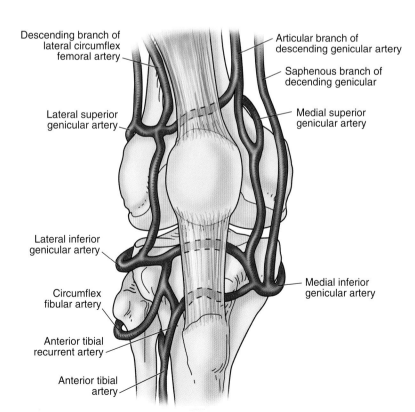

Figure 1–87. Genicular artery circulation and anterior artery anastomosis of the knee.

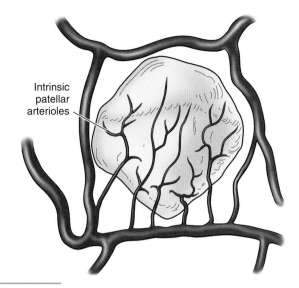

Intrinsic
patellar
arterioles

Figure 1–88. Vascular circle around the patella, which, according to Scapinelli,[77] supplies the patella via nutrient arteries that enter predominantly at the inferior pole. The genicular arteries and their branches lie in the most superficial layer of the deep fascia.

based flaps as a result of the medially biased arterial inflow.[19]

The popliteal vein enters the popliteal fossa on the lateral side of the artery; it crosses superficial to the artery and lies on the medial side in the lower part of the fossa. Throughout the popliteal fossa, it is interposed between the artery and the tibial nerve (see Fig. 1–65A).

MOTION AND FUNCTION

The knee joint is a modified hinge that possesses limited inherent stability from the bony architecture. The lack of conformity between the bony surfaces allows 6 degrees of freedom of motion about the knee, including translation in three planes (medial-lateral, anterior-posterior, proximal-distal) and rotation in three planes (flexion-extension, internal-external, and varus-valgus). Motion and stability of the joint are controlled by additional intra-articular static stabilizers, including the menisci and cruciate ligaments, as well as extra-articular static and dynamic stabilizers, such as the collateral ligaments and muscles.[39,48,66,95] In full extension, both the collateral and cruciate ligaments are taut, and the anterior aspects of both menisci are snugly held between the condyles of the tibia and the femur. At the beginning of flexion, the knee "unlocks" and external rotation of the femur on the tibia occurs, which according to Last,[60] is brought about by contraction of the popliteus muscle. During the first 30 degrees of flexion, rollback of the femur on the tibia occurs and is more pronounced laterally. After 30 degrees, the femoral condyles spin at one point on the tibial condyles.[12,73] New evidence from dynamic MRI studies demonstrates that the medial condyle essentially remains static on the tibia as flexion occurs, with rollback basically

limited to the lateral condyle.[25] The menisci, which are squeezed between the joint surfaces in extension, move posteriorly with the femur in flexion, the lateral more so than the medial. The articular surface of the medial femoral condyle is larger than that of the lateral femoral condyle; when the direction of motion is reversed, the lateral compartment reaches a position of full extension first before the medial compartment is fully extended. Terminal extension is achieved and the knee is "locked" by the femur rotating internally on the tibia—the so-called screw home mechanism—until the medial compartment also reaches the limits of extension (Fig. 1–89).

Some portion of the superficial MCL remains taut throughout flexion, whereas the LCL is taut only in extension and relaxes as soon as the knee is flexed, thereby permitting greater excursion of the lateral tibial condyle.

The superficial MCL is the most important medial stabilizer.[93] The parallel fibers move in a posterior direction as the knee is flexed. The attachments to the femoral condyle are such that with the knee in extension, the posterior fibers are taut and the anterior fibers relax and are drawn in under the posterior part of the ligament (Fig. 1–90). With flexion of the knee, the anterior fibers move proximally and become tight and are then subjected to increasing tension as the joint is flexed (Fig. 1–91). This action, according to Palmer,[73] is attributable to the oval shape of the femoral origin, which changes its orientation in flexion such that the attachments of the most anterior fibers are elevated. As the anterior border becomes tight, the posterior fibers slacken as the knee flexes and remain relaxed throughout flexion. The posterior oblique fibers are relaxed in extension and lie partially beneath the parallel fibers. In flexion, the fibers are drawn out (Fig. 1–92); according to Palmer, because of their attachment to the capsule and periphery of the medial meniscus, they check the backward sliding of the meniscus that occurs in flexion. In the presence of intact parallel fibers, there is approximately 1 to 2 mm of medial opening to valgus stress. The joint is slightly tighter in full extension; the greatest degree of medial opening occurs at 45 degrees.[93] The parallel fibers of the superficial MCL also control rotation, and sectioning these fibers not only increases the amount of medial opening to valgus stress but also causes a significant increase in external rotation. In distinction, sectioning the capsule, deep MCL, or oblique fibers of the superficial MCL causes little or no increase in rotation.[93]

Lateral stability is provided by several structures.[42] In extension, the fibers of the iliotibial tract are crucial, and because these fibers attach proximally to the femur and distally to the tibia, they may be regarded as a true ligament. However, Kaplan[49] demonstrated, through electrical stimulation of the tensor fascia lata and traction on the iliotibial tract in cadavers, that contractions of the tensor fascia lata and gluteus maximus are not transmitted to the tibia and, therefore, the iliotibial tract does not represent a tendon. As the knee flexes, the iliotibial tract moves posteriorly and becomes somewhat relaxed; beyond approximately 30 degrees of flexion the tendon of the biceps femoris may become an important lateral stabilizer.[67]

The lateral ligament is also taut in extension but relaxed throughout flexion. The same is also true of the arcuate

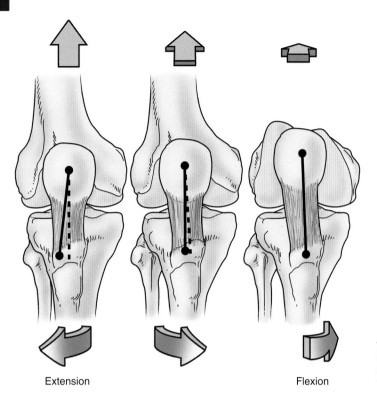

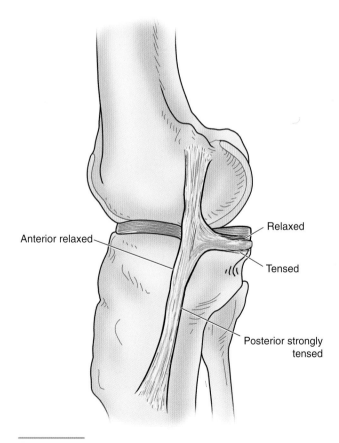

Extension   Flexion

Figure 1–89. Screw home mechanism. At full extension, the tibial tubercle lies lateral to the midpoint of the patella.

Anterior relaxed

Relaxed

Tensed

Posterior strongly tensed

Figure 1–90. In extension, the posterior margin of the medial collateral ligament is tense and the anterior border relatively relaxed. Proximal anterior fibers are drawn underneath the posterior fibers.

ligament. Thus, in flexion, a much greater degree of rotation is possible laterally than medially. This rotation is permitted by the attachments of the lateral meniscus and by relaxation of the supporting ligaments in flexion. There is also a greater degree of rolling of the femur on the tibia, whereas medially this motion is only slight. The attachment of the popliteal tendon to the lateral meniscus draws the meniscus posteriorly and prevents entrapment as the knee is flexed.[60]

The ACL consists of two functional bands: an anteromedial band and a stronger, thicker posterolateral part. In extension, the ligament appears as a flat band, and the posterolateral bulk of the ligament is taut (see Fig. 1–53). Almost immediately after flexion begins, the smaller anteromedial band becomes tight, and the bulk of the ligament slackens. In flexion, it is the anteromedial band that provides the primary restraint against anterior displacement of the tibia.[29]

The PCL consists of two inseparable parts. An anterior portion forms the bulk of the ligament, and a smaller posterior part runs obliquely to the back of the tibia. In extension, the bulk of the ligament is relaxed and only the posterior band is tight. In flexion, the major portion of the ligament becomes tight and the small posterior band is loose (see Fig. 1–56).[28,89]

The ACL is a check against both hyperextension and internal and external rotation. The PCL is a check against posterior instability in the flexed knee but not against hyperextension, provided that the anterior cruciate is intact.

According to Palmer,[73] the tightening of the anterior cruciate in extension fixes the lateral femoral condyle anteriorly; thus, continuation of the movement into

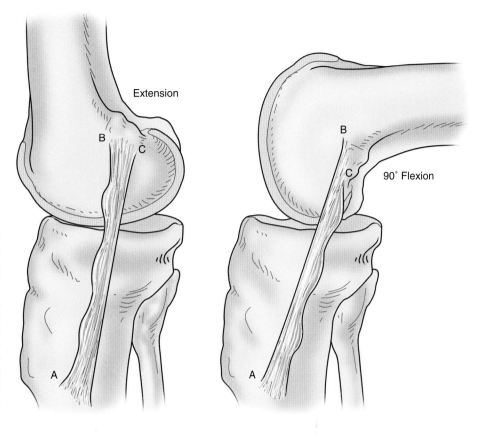

Figure 1–91. Diagram of the superficial medial ligament with flexion and extension of the knee. Because point B moves superiorly, the anterior border is tightened in flexion. Conversely, in extension, point C moves proximally and tightens the posterior margin of the ligament. (From Warren LF, Marshall JL, Girgis FG: The prime static stabilizer of the medial side of the knee. J Bone Joint Surg Am 56:665, 1974.)

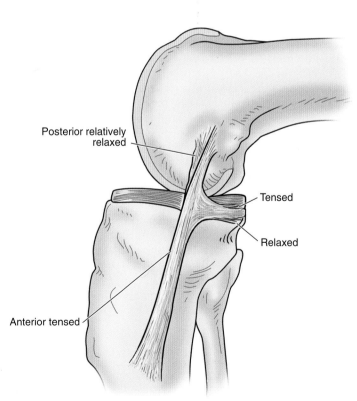

Figure 1–92. The posterior oblique fibers become more tense in flexion. (From Palmer I: On the injuries to ligaments of the knee joint: A clinical study. Acta Chir Scand 81[Suppl 53]:3, 1938.)

hyperextension is only possible where there is simultaneous inward rotation of the femur.

Rotation occurs around an axis through the center of the medial femoral condyle as a result of the tighter anchorage of this condyle by the superficial MCL. If this ligament is ruptured, the axis shifts laterally. According to Palmer, because of the medially shifted axis of rotation, external rotation of the tibia relaxes the ACL through the forward travel of the lateral femoral condyle, at the same time stretching the PCL.[73] Internal rotation reverses this sequence, tensing the anterior cruciate and relaxing the posterior cruciate.

A fibrous band connects the posterior cruciate with the posterior margin of the lateral meniscus (the tibiomeniscal ligament of Kaplan). This band probably restricts the forward sliding motion of the lateral meniscus in internal rotation.

Girgis et al[29] have shown that rotary movements of the tibia on the femur occur in all ranges of motion. Their studies indicate that the anterior cruciate is a check against external rotation in flexion but does not significantly limit internal rotation. In extension, the ACL is a check against external rotation and to a lesser degree against internal rotation. Thus, there is some disagreement about the precise function of the cruciate ligaments with regard to rotation.

Action of the Muscles

The movements of the knee are flexion, extension, and rotation. Flexion is performed by the hamstrings and biceps femoris and, to a lesser extent, by the gastrocnemius and popliteus. Flexion is limited by the soft tissues at the back of the knee. Extension is performed by the quadriceps, and because of the shape of the articulation and the ligament attachments, the femur rotates medially on the tibia in terminal extension, the screw home mechanism that locks the joint. This movement is purely passive, as are other rotary movements occurring during activity, and is due to the articular geometry and static stabilizers as previously described. The exception is the lateral rotation of the femur that precedes flexion by unlocking the joint. This movement is performed by the popliteus. The sartorius, gracilis, and hamstrings are weak rotators of the knee but probably do not act as such. The sartorius, gracilis, and semitendinosus medially and the iliotibial tract laterally mostly act as "guy ropes" to stabilize the pelvis.

References

1. Aglietti P, Insall JN, Cerulli G, et al: Patella pain and incongruence. I: Measurements of incongruence. Clin Orthop 176:217, 1983.
2. Aglietti P, Insall JN, Walker PS, et al: A new patella prosthesis: Design and application. Clin Orthop 107:175, 1975.
3. Anderson JE: Grant's Atlas of Anatomy, 7th ed. Baltimore, Williams & Wilkins, 1978.
4. Arnoczky SP, Dipl AC: Blood supply to the anterior cruciate ligament and supporting structures. Orthop Clin North Am 16:15, 1985.
5. Arnoczky SP, Warren RF: Microvasculature of the human meniscus. Am J Sports Med 10:90, 1982.
6. Baker CL, Norwood LA, Hughston JC: Acute posterolateral rotatory instability of the knee. J Bone Joint Surg Am 65:614, 1983.
7. Barrack RL, Skinner HB, Buckley SL: Proprioception in the anterior cruciate deficient knee. Am J Sports Med 17:1, 1989.
8. Basmajian JV: Grant's Method of Anatomy, 10th ed. Baltimore, Williams & Wilkins, 1980.
9. Basmajian JV, Lovejoy JF Jr: Functions of the popliteus muscle in man: A multifactorial electromyographic study. J Bone Joint Surg Am 53:557, 1971.
10. Baumgartl F: Das Kniegelenk. Berlin, Springer-Verlag, 1944.
11. Berger RA, Rubash HE, Seel MJ, et al: Determining the rotational alignment of the femoral component in total knee arthroplasty using the epicondylar axis. Clin Orthop 286:40, 1993.
12. Brantigan OC, Voshell AF: The mechanics of the ligaments and menisci of the knee joint. J Bone Joint Surg 23:44, 1941.
13. Brantigan OC, Voshell AF: The tibial collateral ligament: Its function, its bursae, and its relation to the medial meniscus. J Bone Joint Surg 25:121, 1943.
14. Butler DL, Noyes FR, Grood ES: Ligamentous restraints to anterior-posterior drawer in the human knee: A biomechanical study. J Bone Joint Surg Am 62:259, 1980.
15. Carriquiry C, Costa MA, Vasconez LO: An anatomic study of the septocutaneous vessels of the leg. Plast Reconstr Surg 76:354, 1985.
16. Chin KR, Dalury DF, Zurakowski D, Scott RD: Intraoperative measurements of male and female distal femurs during primary total knee arthroplasty. J Knee Surg 15:213, 2002.
17. Clancy WG, Shelbourne KD, Zoellner GB, et al: Treatment of knee joint instability secondary to rupture of the posterior cruciate ligament: Report of a new procedure. J Bone Joint Surg Am 65:310, 1983.
18. Clark JM, Sidles JA: The interrelation of fiber bundles in the anterior cruciate ligament. J Orthop Res 8:180, 1990.
19. Colombel M, Mariz Y, Dahhan P, et al: Arterial and lymphatic supply of the knee integuments. Surg Radiol Anat 20:35, 1998.
20. Danzig LA, Newell JD, Guerra J Jr, et al: Osseous landmarks of the normal knee. Clin Orthop 156:201, 1981.
21. Daseler EH, Anson BJ: The plantaris muscle: An anatomical study of 750 specimens. J Bone Joint Surg 25:822, 1943.
22. Dodds JA, Arnoczky SP: Anatomy of the anterior cruciate ligament: A blueprint for repair and reconstruction. Arthroscopy 10:132, 1994.
23. Eckhoff DG, Burke BJ, Dwyer TF, et al: Sulcus morphology of the distal femur. Clin Orthop 331:23, 1996.
24. Fairbank TJ: Knee joint changes after meniscectomy. J Bone Joint Surg Br 30:664, 1948.
25. Freeman MA, Pinskerova V: The movement of the knee studied by magnetic resonance imaging. Clini Orthop 410:35, 2003.
26. Fulkerson JP, Gossling HR: Anatomy of the knee joint lateral retinaculum. Clin Orthop 153:183, 1980.
27. Furman W, Marshall JL, Girgis FG: The anterior cruciate ligament: A functional analysis based on postmortem studies. J Bone Joint Surg Am 58:179, 1976.
28. Gardner E: The innervation of the knee joint. Anat Rec 101:109, 1948.
29. Girgis FG, Marshall JL, Al Monajem ARS: The cruciate ligaments of the knee joint. Clin Orthop 106:216, 1975.
30. Gollehon DL, Torzilli PA, Warren RF: The role of the posterolateral and cruciate ligaments in the stability of the human knee: A biomechanical study. J Bone Joint Surg Am 69:233, 1987.
31. Good L, Odensten M, Gillquist J: Intercondylar notch measurements with special reference to anterior cruciate ligament surgery. Clin Orthop 263:185, 1991.
32. Goodfellow J, Hungerford DS, Zindel M: Patello-femoral mechanics and pathology. I. Functional anatomy of the patello-femoral joint. J Bone Joint Surg Br 58:287, 1976.
33. Griffin FM, Insall JN, Scuderi GR: The posterior condylar angle in osteoarthritic knees. J Arthroplasty 13:812, 1998.
34. Haertsch P: The surgical plane in the leg. Br J Plast Surg 34:464, 1981.
35. Haertsch P: The blood supply to the skin of the leg: A post-mortem investigation. Br J Plast Surg 34:470, 1981.
36. Hallock GG: Salvage of total knee arthroplasty with local fasciocutaneous flaps. J Bone Joint Surg Br 76:1236, 1990.
37. Hey Groves EW: Operation for repair of the cruciate ligaments. Clin Orthop 147:4, 1980.

38. Hitt K, Shurman JR 2nd, Greene K, et al: Anthropometric measurements of the human knee: Correlation to the sizing of current knee arthroplasty systems. J Bone Joint Surg Am 85(Suppl 4):115, 2003.

39. Hsieh H-H, Walker PS: Stabilizing mechanisms of the loaded and unloaded knee joint. J Bone Joint Surg Am 58:87, 1976.

40. Hubbard JK, Sampson HW, Elledge JR: Prevalence and morphology of the vastus medialis oblique muscle in human cadavers. Anat Rec 249:135, 1997.

41. Hughston JC, Andrews JR, Cross MJ, et al: Classification of knee ligament instabilities: Part I. The medial compartment and cruciate ligaments. J Bone Joint Surg Am 58:159, 1976.

42. Hughston JC, Andrews JR, Cross MJ, et al: Classification of knee ligament instabilities: Part II. The lateral compartment. J Bone Joint Surg Am 58:173, 1976.

43. Hughston JC, Norwood LA Jr: The posterolateral drawer test and external rotational recurvatum test for posterolateral rotatory instability of the knee. Clin Orthop 147:82, 1980.

44. Hungerford DS, Barry M: Biomechanics of the patellofemoral joint. Clin Orthop 144:9, 1979.

45. Hunter LY, Louis DS, Ricciardi JR, et al: The saphenous nerve: Its course and importance in medial arthrotomy. Am J Sports Med 7:227, 1979.

46. Johnson DL, Swenson TM, Livesay MS, et al: Insertion site anatomy of the human menisci: Gross, arthroscopic, and topographical anatomy as a basis for meniscal transplantation. Arthroscopy 11:386, 1995.

47. Jones CDS, Keene GCR, Christie AD: The popliteus as a retractor of the lateral meniscus of the knee. Arthroscopy 11:270, 1995.

48. Kaplan EB: Factors responsible for the stability of the knee joint. Bull Hosp Jt Dis 18:51, 1957.

49. Kaplan EB: The iliotibial tract: Clinical and morphological significance. J Bone Joint Surg Am 40:817, 1958.

50. Kaplan EB: The fabellofibular and short lateral ligaments of the knee joint. J Bone Joint Surg Am 43:169, 1961.

51. Kaplan EB: Some aspects of functional anatomy of the human knee joint. Clin Orthop 23:18, 1962.

52. Kaufer H: Mechanical function of the patella. J Bone Joint Surg Am 53:1551, 1971.

53. Kennedy JC, Alexander IJ, Hayes KC: Nerve supply of the knee and its functional importance. Am J Sports Med 10:329, 1982.

54. Kennedy JC, Fowler PJ: Medial and anterior instability of the knee: An anatomical and clinical study using stress machines. J Bone Joint Surg Am 53:1257, 1971.

55. Kennedy JC, Hawkins RJ, Willis RB, et al: Tension studies of human knee ligaments: Yield point, ultimate failure, and disruption of the cruciate and tibial collateral ligaments. J Bone Joint Surg Am 58:350, 1976.

56. Kennedy JC, Weinberg HW, Wilson AS: The anatomy and function of the anterior cruciate ligament as determined by clinical and morphological studies. J Bone Joint Surg Am 56:223, 1974.

57. Koukoubis TD, Glisson RR, Bolognesi M, et al: Dimensions of the intercondylar notch of the knee. Am J Knee Surg 10:83, 1997.

58. Laprade RF, Burnett QM II: Femoral intercondylar notch stenosis and correlation to anterior cruciate ligament injuries. Am J Sports Med 22:198, 1994.

59. Last RJ: Some anatomical details of the knee joint. J Bone Joint Surg Br 30:683, 1948.

60. Last RJ: The popliteus muscle and the lateral meniscus. J Bone Joint Surg Br 32:93, 1950.

61. Last RJ: Anatomy: Regional and Applied, 6th ed. Edinburgh, Churchill Livingstone, 1978.

62. Levy IM, Torzilli PA, Gould JD, et al: The effect of lateral meniscectomy on motion of the knee. J Bone Joint Surg Am 71:401, 1989.

63. Levy IM, Torzilli PA, Warren RF: The effect of medial meniscectomy on anterior-posterior motion of the knee. J Bone Joint Surg Am 64:883, 1982.

64. Lotysch M, Mink J, Crues JV, et al: Magnetic resonance in the detection of meniscal injuries. Magn Reson Imaging 4:185, 1986.

65. Mann RA, Hagy JL: The popliteus muscle. J Bone Joint Surg Am 59:924, 1977.

66. Markolf KL, Mensch JS, Amstutz HC: Stiffness and laxity of the knee: The contributions of the supporting structures: A quantitative in vitro study. J Bone Joint Surg Am 58:583, 1976.

67. Marshall JL, Girgis FG, Zelko RR: The biceps femoris tendon and its functional significance. J Bone Joint Surg Am 54:1444, 1972.

68. Maynard MJ, Deng X, Wickiewicz TL, et al: The popliteofibular ligament: Rediscovery of a key element in posterolateral stability. Am J Sports Med 24:311, 1996.

69. Muneta T, Takakuda K, Yamamoto H: Intercondylar notch width and its relation to the configuration and cross-sectional area of the anterior cruciate ligament. Am J Sports Med 25:69, 1997.

70. Noyes FR, Butler DL, Grood ES, et al: Biomechanical analysis of human ligament grafts used in knee-ligament repairs and reconstructions. J Bone Joint Surg Am 66:344, 1984.

71. Outerbridge R: The etiology of chondromalacia patellae. J Bone Joint Surg Br 43:752, 1961.

72. Pagnani MJ, Warner JJP, O'Brien SJ, et al: Anatomic considerations in harvesting the semitendinous and gracilis tendons and a technique of harvest. Am J Sports Med 21:565, 1993.

73. Palmer I: On the injuries to the ligaments of the knee joint: A clinical study. Acta Chir Scand 53(Suppl), 1938.

74. Poilvache PL, Insall JN, Scuderi GR, et al: Rotational landmarks and sizing of the distal femur in total knee arthroplasty. Clin Orthop 331:35, 1996.

75. Reider B, Marshall JL, Koslin B, et al: The anterior aspect of the knee joint: An anatomical study. J Bone Joint Surg Am 63:351, 1981.

76. Renstrom P, Johnson RJ: Anatomy and biomechanics of the menisci. Clin Sports Med 9:523, 1990.

77. Scapinelli R: Blood supply of the human patella: Its relation to ischaemic necrosis after fracture. J Bone Joint Surg Br 49:563, 1967.

78. Scapinelli R: Vascular anatomy of the human cruciate ligaments and surrounding structures. Clin Anat 10:151, 1997.

79. Schultz RA, Miller DC, Kerr CS, et al: Mechanoreceptors in human cruciate ligaments: A histological study. J Bone Joint Surg Am 66:1072, 1984.

80. Schutte MJ, Dabezies EJ, Zimny ML, et al: Neural anatomy of the human anterior cruciate ligament. J Bone Joint Surg Am 69:243, 1987.

81. Seebacher JR, Inglis AE, Marshall JL, et al: The structure of the posterolateral aspect of the knee. J Bone Joint Surg Am 64:536, 1982.

82. Soldado F, Reina F, Yuguero M, Rodriguez-Baeza A: Clinical anatomy of the arterial supply of the human patellar ligament. Surg Radiol Anat 24:177, 2002.

83. Spencer JD, Hayes KC, Alexander IJ: Knee joint effusion and quadriceps reflex inhibition in man. Arch Phys Med Rehabil 65:171, 1984.

84. Stoller DW, Martin C, Crues JV III, et al: Meniscal tears: Pathologic correlation with MR imaging. Radiology 163:731, 1987.

85. Sullivan D, Levy IM, Sheskier S, et al: Medial restraints to anterior-posterior motion of the knee. J Bone Joint Surg Am 66:930, 1984.

86. Taylor GI, Palmer JH: The vascular territories (angiosomes) of the body: Experimental study and clinical applications. Br J Plast Surg 40:113, 1987.

87. Terry GC, LaPrade RF: The biceps femoris muscle complex at the knee: Its anatomy and injury patterns associated with acute anterolateral-anteromedial rotatory instability. Am J Sports Med 24:2, 1996.

88. Tria AJ Jr, Johnson CD, Zawadsky JP: The popliteus tendon. J Bone Joint Surg Am 71:714, 1989.

89. VanDommelen BA, Fowler PJ: Anatomy of the posterior cruciate ligament: A review. Am J Sports Med 17:24, 1989.

90. Walker PS, Erkman MJ: The role of the menisci in force transmission across the knee. Clin Orthop 109:184, 1975.

91. Wan ACT, Felle P: The menisco-femoral ligaments. Clin Anat 8:323, 1995.

92. Warren LF, Marshall JL: The supporting structures and layers on the medial side of the knee: An anatomical analysis. J Bone Joint Surg Am 61:56, 1979.

93. Warren LF, Marshall JL, Girgis FG: The prime static stabilizer of the medial side of the knee. J Bone Joint Surg Am 56:665, 1974.

94. Watanabe Y, Moriya H, Takahashi K, et al: Functional anatomy of the posterolateral structures of the knee. Arthroscopy 9:57, 1993.

95. Welsh PR: Knee joint structure and function. Clin Orthop 147:7, 1980.

96. Wiberg G: Roentgenographic and anatomic studies on the femoropatellar joint: With special reference to chondromalacia patellae. Acta Orthop Scand 12:319, 1941.

97. Williams PL, Warwick R: Gray's Anatomy, 36th British ed. Philadelphia, WB Saunders, 1980.

98. Wilson PD, Eyre-Brook AL, Francis JD: A clinical and anatomical study of the semimembranosus bursa in relation to popliteal cyst. J Bone Joint Surg 20:963, 1938.

99. Yip DK, Zhu YH, Chiu KY, Ng TP: Distal rotational alignment of the Chinese femur and its relevance in total knee arthroplasty. J Arthroplasty 19:613, 2004.

CHAPTER 2

Anatomic Aberrations

Henry D. Clarke • W. Norman Scott • John N. Insall

Variations of normal anatomy and frankly abnormal structures are occasionally encountered by the practitioner. Without a fundamental understanding of the more common abnormalities, it may be difficult to identify and interpret the significance of these structures. The goal of this chapter is to provide an overview of some of the reported structural anomalies and information regarding their clinical relevance. It is not our intent to review anatomic abnormalities resulting from traumatic or degenerative causes. In addition, developmental phenomena occurring as a result of disordered maturation in the pediatric population are reviewed elsewhere.

SKELETAL ABNORMALITIES

A number of major skeletal dysplasias, including proximal femoral focal deficiencies, tibial dysplasia, fibular aplasia, amelia, and phocomelia, involve the bones of the knee joint to varying degrees but are beyond the scope of this chapter. Here we emphasize abnormalities that may represent incidental findings in some patients but can have significant clinical implications.

Femur

TROCHLEAR DYSPLASIA

Trochlear dysplasia may be relatively subtle or more marked. Clinical manifestations depend not only on the extent of the dysplasia but also on other anatomic factors such as soft-tissue tension. Symptoms may relate to chronic maltracking or frank dislocation. Pain related to the patellofemoral joint resulting from chronic patellar malalignment is typically manifested as an anterior knee ache when sitting with the knee flexed and as acute exacerbations during squatting, kneeling, and stair-climbing activities. On physical examination, crepitus from the patellofemoral joint, pain with patellar compression, and peripatellar tenderness may be noted. Specific radiological criteria have been reported that define normal trochlear anatomy.[8] The sulcus angle is defined on the Merchant view by the intersection of lines connecting the highest point of the femoral condyles to the deepest point of the femoral trochlea; the mean angle in normal knees is 130 to 137 degrees (range, 112 to 151 degrees).[1,40] Significant differences in this angle have been reported in patients with recurrent patellar dislocation and chondro-malacia patellae (Fig. 2–1).[1] The lateral-medial trochlear ratio is the ratio between the segments joining the highest point of the femoral condyles to the deepest point of the trochlea. A ratio greater than 1.7 indicates trochlear dysplasia.[8] If nonoperative treatment such as activity modification and physical therapy fail to relieve symptoms, lateral release and proximal realignment may be considered in patients with disabling symptoms and documented anatomic abnormalities. In carefully selected patients, 91% excellent and good results have been achieved at intermediate-term follow-up by Insall et al.[54] In a small group of pediatric patients with a severely dysplastic trochlea, successful results have been reported after a sulcus-creating procedure in conjunction with soft-tissue realignment.[9]

Patella

CONGENITAL ABSENCE AND HYPOPLASIA

Congenital absence of the patella and hypoplasia are extremely rare anomalies, especially as isolated findings.[12,100] An association with other abnormalities has been reported, including ischiopubic malformations and as part of the nail-patella syndrome (nail and patellar dysplasia, radial head subluxation and elbow malformation, renal abnormalities, and iliac horns).[100,103] Other patellar dysplasias include duplication in both the coronal and sagittal plane; in some cases these abnormalities have been associated with multiple epiphyseal dysplasia.[41,48,84,118]

BIPARTITE PATELLA

Anomalies of patellar development are relatively common, especially failure of accessory ossification centers to fuse, which can lead to bipartite, tripartite, and multipartite patellae (Fig. 2–2). Fragmentation of the patella has been noted in about 2% to 5% of knees. The bipartite type accounts for the majority of cases; approximately 50% of cases occur bilaterally.[16,101,118] The Saupe classification describes three types of patellar fragmentation based on the location of the accessory ossification center: type 1 (5%) is located at the inferior pole, type 2 (20%) at the lateral margin, and type 3, the most frequent (75%), at the superolateral pole.[16,101]

Most bipartite patellae represent incidental findings; only 13% are associated with symptoms. When pain devel-

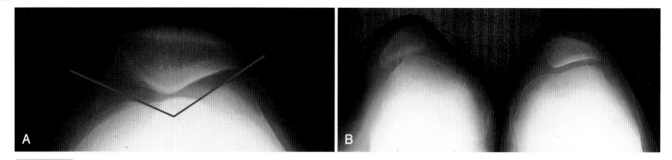

Figure 2–1. Radiographs of the patellofemoral joint. **A,** Merchant view with a normal sulcus angle of the femoral trochlea marked. **B,** Bilateral Merchant view showing a severely dysplastic femoral trochlea with almost flat sulcus angles and patellar dislocation.

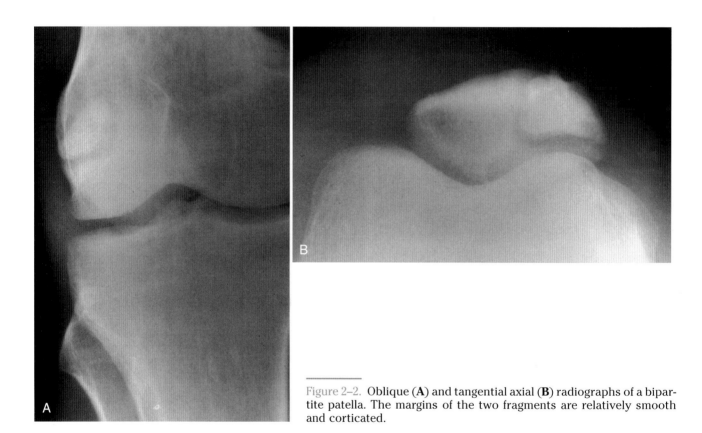

Figure 2–2. Oblique (**A**) and tangential axial (**B**) radiographs of a bipartite patella. The margins of the two fragments are relatively smooth and corticated.

ops, it may occur acutely after trauma or gradually.[16,20,43,101,117] In the acute setting, a traumatic fracture must be ruled out. In such cases, the margins of the fracture fragments usually appear more ragged on plane radiographs, whereas the accessory fragments noted in atraumatic fragmentation tend to have sclerotic smooth margins. Magnetic resonance imaging (MRI) may be helpful in distinguishing incidental fragmentation because in these cases the accessory piece demonstrates low signal intensity without surrounding marrow edema (Fig. 2–3).[101] Initial treatment may include activity modification, anti-inflammatory medication, and immobilization. In patients with persistent symptoms, successful excision of symptomatic fragments has been reported.[16,43,101,117]

LIGAMENT ABNORMALITIES

Anterior Cruciate Ligament

CONGENITAL ABSENCE

Congenital absence of the anterior cruciate ligament (ACL) is a rare anomaly that has been reported, in most circumstances, to occur in association with other knee abnormalities, including congenital knee dislocation, tibial dysplasia, congenital dislocation of the patella, femoral dysplasia, ring meniscus, discoid meniscus,

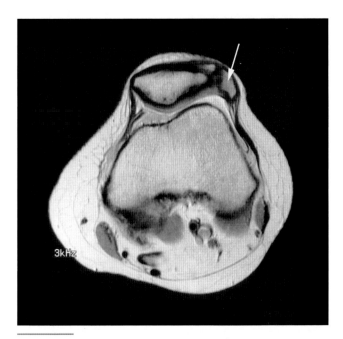

Figure 2–3. Axial magnetic resonance image demonstrating a bipartite patella with a small lateral fragment (*arrow*). The lack of surrounding marrow edema and hemorrhage is consistent with a bipartite patella rather than an acute patellar fracture.

absence of the meniscus, absence of the posterior cruciate ligament (PCL), and congenital leg length discrepancy.[3,60,76,111] An association with other musculoskeletal abnormalities not limited to the knee has also been reported, with at least one other significant anomaly noted in each patient in one series.[111] However, rare cases of isolated absence of the ACL have been reported in otherwise normal individuals.[7] On physical examination, a positive anterior draw test and 3+ Lachman test are common findings. Complex instability may also be noted; in one study, 25% of patients demonstrated medial and lateral translational instability.[111] Therefore, it is evident that this patient population is not entirely analogous to the group that experiences traumatic ACL rupture. Radiographic features that have been associated with congenital absence of the ACL include hypoplasia of the lateral aspect of the tibial spine, hypoplasia of the lateral femoral condyle, a narrow or tight A-frame intercondylar notch, and hypoplasia of the medial part of the tibial plateau.[60,111] Many patients with this anomaly are asymptomatic as children and do not complain of instability.[60] Because the long-term consequences of this type of deficiency are unknown, the need for ligament reconstruction has not been clearly defined. In several series, asymptomatic patients have been treated by observation only with good short-term results.[7,57,111]

OTHER ABNORMALITIES

An abnormal origin of the ACL has been described. Rather than the usual discrete origin, an origin extending completely between the anterior and posterior margins of the intercondylar notch was observed in a young child. Symptoms developed in this patient as a result of impingement of the abnormal ACL against the anterior portion of a discoid lateral meniscus at approximately 100 degrees of flexion.[49]

Posterior Cruciate Ligament

Abnormalities of the PCL are extremely rare. Congenital absence of the PCL has been reported in association with other congenital anomalies, including absence of the ACL, leg length discrepancies, and Larsen's syndrome (multiple congenital dislocations of the elbows, knees, and hips and unusual facies).[36,57,60] The multiple anomalies present in these patients typically result in positive anterior and posterior draw tests and posterolateral rotatory instability. In one patient, an anomaly of the PCL has also been reported in association with congenital absence of the ACL. An anterior insertion of the PCL on the tibia was noted to compensate for the aplastic ACL.[3]

MENISCAL ABNORMALITIES

Anomalous Attachments

A variety of anomalous attachments of the medial meniscus have been described, including insertion of the anterior horn into the ACL, intercondylar notch, and infrapatellar fold and insertion of the posterior horn into the ACL.[13,59,64,78,97,102] Between 10.6% and 22.6% of all Asian patients undergoing arthroscopy were found to have anomalies of the anterior horn of the medial meniscus.[78] In a large study of 953 arthroscopies, 103 (10.8%) of the knees did not demonstrate the normal attachment of the anterior horn of the medial meniscus onto the tibia. Four variants of the anterior horn were observed in this study: 51 (49.5%) had only an attachment to the lateral meniscus via the transverse intermeniscal ligament, 39 (37.9%) inserted into the ACL, 11 (10.7%) inserted into the coronary ligament, and 2 (1.9%) inserted into the infrapatellar synovial fold. In these patients, the abnormal anterior horn attachment rendered the anterior portion of the meniscus hypermobile while the posterior body remained firmly attached. This aberration predisposed the patients to symptomatic tears at the junction of the midbody and posterior body as a result of accumulated stress.[78] Successful arthroscopic resection of symptomatic anomalous insertions has been reported.[97,102] In these cases, a stable, normal-appearing anterior horn was fashioned, which relieved the preoperative knee pain. In one case, symptoms appeared to be related to subluxation of the abnormal bundle under the femoral condyle with flexion.[97] Nonetheless, other authors have reported good results after observation of incidentally discovered anomalies.[13,59]

Hypoplasia and Congenital Absence

The incidence of hypoplasia and congenital absence of the medial and lateral menisci is unknown. An association with other ipsilateral knee and generalized musculoskeletal anomalies, including congenital absence of the ACL, discoid lateral meniscus, thrombocytopenia–absent radius syndrome, and anomalous insertions of the popliteus tendon, has been reported in several cases.[37,77,112,113] The association of simultaneous intra-articular anomalies in some cases is probably due to the common mesenchymal origin of several structures.[13] Condensation of the menisci takes place at approximately 7 to 8 weeks of embryological development and occurs in concert with the intra-articular cruciate ligaments.[13,24,102]

Discoid Meniscus

The first discoid meniscus was reported by Young in 1889.[2,28,58,99] In an early report, Smillie[104] described three variants: primitive, intermediate, and infantile. This classification reflected the belief that the menisci are discoid in a normal fetus and gradually assume an adult form through resorption of the central part; however, anatomic studies have suggested that this supposition is incorrect because discoid menisci do not occur during any part of routine development.[24,58,62,93] Kaplan[62] suggested that abnormal motion of the lateral menisci resulting from deficient peripheral attachments may cause a meniscus that is normal at birth to become discoid during development.[14] However, this explanation does not satisfactorily account for the occurrence of discoid medial menisci. Rather than representing an arrest in normal development, discoid menisci are believed to be congenital anomalies.[14,28]

MEDIAL

Discoid medial menisci are very rare phenomena. The first undisputed case was reported by Cave and Staples[22] in 1941. Its incidence in the general population is reported to be approximately 0.06% to 0.3%.[14,25,28,99] Discoid medial menisci may be asymptomatic, especially in children and adolescents. Meta-analysis has revealed that 65% of all patients with symptomatic discoid medial menisci were older than 18 years.[28] The most common symptoms associated with a discoid medial meniscus are the same as those for a medial meniscal tear and include aching medial joint line pain, intermittent swelling, locking, weakness, instability, and an inability to extend the knee fully.[14,28,58] On physical examination, a block to full extension, effusion, joint line tenderness, and a positive McMurray test may be noted.[28]

Radiographs of the involved knee are usually unremarkable; abnormalities are identified in less than 10% of patients with a discoid medial meniscus.[28] Occasionally, medial joint space widening or deepening of the medial tibial hemiplateau has been observed but may be quite subtle.[14,28] MRI is the best test for identifying discoid menisci. On sagittal views, the menisci should be monitored on serial images. Rather than observing the usual central tapering between the anterior and posterior horns as the image plane moves laterally toward the intercondy-

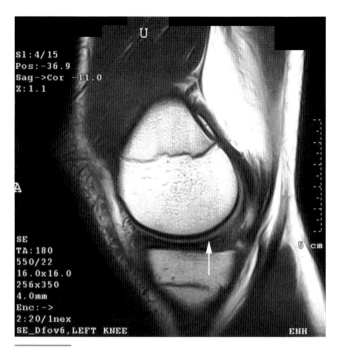

Figure 2–4. Sagittal magnetic resonance image of a discoid medial meniscus showing a block-like appearance that was present on most sagittal cuts through the medial compartment. Intrameniscal signal was considered highly suggestive of a meniscal tear (*arrow*).

lar notch, the horns remain in continuity (Fig. 2–4). Visualization of a continuous band of meniscus on more than three peripheral sagittal images indicates a discoid meniscus. In addition, on coronal images, an abnormally thick meniscus, which can extend into the notch, may be visualized.[14]

Because of the rarity of this phenomenon, its treatment has not been extensively reported. Several authors have suggested that incidentally discovered intact discoid menisci may be left intact.[14,64] However, in these cases, the presence of central and inferior surface cleavage tears, which may be difficult to observe, should be excluded.[25,99] In patients with intra-articular symptoms and no other abnormalities, discoid menisci should be very carefully examined for incomplete inferior or cleavage tears because they may be missed if only the superior surface is examined (Fig. 2–5).

Successful short-term results of arthroscopic débridement with partial meniscectomy and contouring of discoid medial menisci have been reported.[14,64] Because many symptomatic patients are initially seen as young adults, we attempt to fashion as nearly normal a functional meniscus as possible to, it is hoped, minimize the long-term degenerative changes associated with meniscectomy.[34]

LATERAL

Discoid lateral menisci occur more frequently than on the medial side of the knee (Fig. 2–6). In the general population the incidence has been reported to be approximately 1.4% to 15.5%, but certain races appear to have a higher

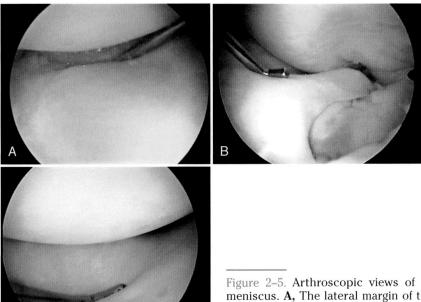

Figure 2–5. Arthroscopic views of the same patient with a discoid medial meniscus. **A,** The lateral margin of the discoid medial meniscus has been elevated to reveal an intact inferior surface. **B** and **C,** The superior surface was also intact.

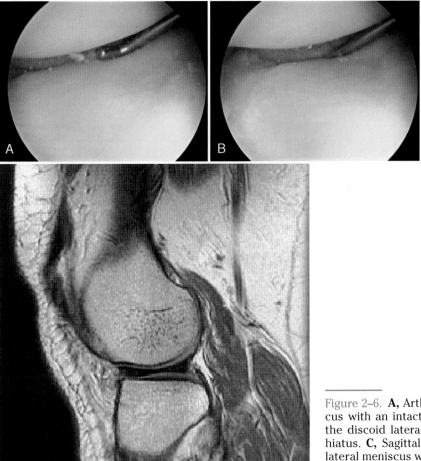

Figure 2–6. **A,** Arthroscopic view of a discoid lateral meniscus with an intact superior surface. **B,** Superior surface of the discoid lateral meniscus with a probe in the popliteal hiatus. **C,** Sagittal magnetic resonance image of a discoid lateral meniscus with a characteristic block-like appearance that was present on the majority of sagittal views through the lateral compartment.

incidence.[29] Whereas a discoid lateral meniscus is thought to occur in less than 5% of white individuals, it has been identified in up to 16.6% of Asians.[21,53] Washington et al identified three types of discoid lateral menisci based on the degree of coverage of the tibial plateau and the presence or absence of normal posterior attachments,[116] including incomplete and complete discoid menisci, which have normal posterior tibial attachments via the coronary ligament, and the Wrisberg type, which lacks the usual posterior tibial attachment, with only one attachment posteriorly via the posterior meniscofemoral ligament (ligament of Wrisberg). Because the Wrisberg type is often not associated with a true discoid appearance, Neuschwander et al[75] suggested that this anomaly be classified as a separate entity, the lateral meniscal variant with absence of the posterior coronary ligament. Though somewhat rare, discoid lateral menisci have been noted to occur in association with a number of other anomalies, including hypoplasia of the lateral femoral condyle, hypoplasia of the lateral tibial spine, a high fibular head, abnormal ACL attachment, and anomalous insertions of the medial meniscus.[49,64]

Patients may have symptoms related to a discoid lateral meniscus in childhood or middle age. The classic complaint of patients with a discoid meniscus is a snapping or popping knee.[2,116] However, in one large series of 62 symptomatic patients, knee pain was the most common problem (89%); other frequent complaints at initial evaluation included the classic clunk or click (58%), swelling (48%), locking (27%), and giving way (19%).[2] On physical examination, the pathognomonic clunk related to abnormal motion of the meniscus as the knee is brought into full extension was elicited in 39% of the patients in the same study; other frequent findings were joint line tenderness (35%), effusion (19%), and locking (11%).[2] Radiographic findings, including widening of the lateral joint line (8%), cupping of the lateral tibial plateau (5%), and sclerosis of the lateral tibial plateau (3%), were identified in a minority of patients.[2] MRI can predictably identify discoid menisci and associated meniscal tears (Fig. 2–7). Treatment of incidentally identified intact complete and incomplete discoid lateral menisci is not thought to be necessary. However, as with medial discoid menisci, tears may be difficult to see and could be missed.[45] In particular, inferior surface cleavage tears should be carefully excluded, especially in patients with intra-articular symptoms and no other identifiable lesions. Treatment of symptomatic tears in the complete and incomplete types is somewhat controversial. Some authors reported successful results after compete meniscectomy, and in some studies the results appear to surpass those achieved after partial meniscectomy and saucerization.[53,116] Radiographic changes consistent with significant degenerative alterations in the lateral compartment after complete meniscectomy in children for discoid menisci have rarely been noted; this is believed to reflect possible adaptive changes of the knee and mechanical alignment.[2,116] However, in one study, early degenerative changes were noted in three of eight patients at 17 years' follow-up.[116] Moreover, significant long-term consequences of meniscectomy have been documented in other circumstances as well.[70] Concern regarding the potential for early degenerative

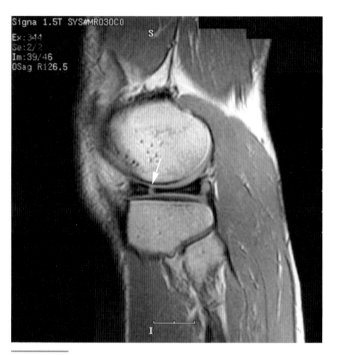

Figure 2–7. Sagittal magnetic resonance image revealing a discoid lateral meniscus with an associated radial tear (*arrow*) at the junction of the anterior horn and body.

disease has prompted many authors to advocate arthroscopic partial meniscectomy with salvage of the most functional remnant possible.[11,29,30,45] Excellent short-term results have been reported with this strategy.[11,29,30,83] We believe that even though the long-term outcome is not clear, the potential consequences associated with early degenerative arthritis in this young patient population make arthroscopic partial meniscectomy and saucerization with resection to a stable, well-contoured remnant the preferred treatment of symptomatic tears of complete- and incomplete-type discoid menisci.

Treatment of a Wrisberg-type discoid meniscus, which is inherently unstable because of a lack of posterior tibial attachments, has traditionally involved complete meniscectomy. However, successful reattachment by suturing the posterior horn to the capsule has been reported, and in a small series of six patients treated in this manner no clinical retears were noted at a mean of 32 months.[75,92] If the long-term results are also successful, this treatment is again theoretically more appealing than complete meniscectomy when the long-term incidence of degenerative changes is not clear.

Other Structural Meniscal Anomalies

Extremely rare structural abnormalities have been reported, including ring-shaped lateral menisci and accessory lateral menisci that appear as a double-layered meniscus.[4,32,65,76,109] When symptoms were believed to be related to these abnormalities, arthroscopic resection of the abnormal portion of the meniscus has proved successful.

Meniscofemoral Ligaments

The anterior and posterior meniscofemoral ligaments (of Humphry and Wrisberg, respectively) run between the posterior horn of the lateral meniscus and the intercondylar notch (Fig. 2–8). They embrace the PCL and are named for their location relative to the ligament. The presence of the anterior meniscofemoral ligament (of Humphry) is less consistent, with an incidence of 33% to 83% in anatomic studies; the posterior meniscofemoral ligament (of Wrisberg) is a more constant structure and is noted in 90% to 93% of the same specimens.[87,115] Overall, 100% of the specimens had at least one of these ligaments. In other studies, one or the other of these meniscofemoral ligaments was identified in 71% to 94% of specimens.[46,90,114] In general, the ligament of Wrisberg is more robust than the ligament of Humphry.

The presence of meniscofemoral ligaments running between the anterior horns of the medial and lateral menisci and the intercondylar notch has also been observed. In Wan and Felle's study,[115] an anterior medial meniscofemoral ligament running between the anterior horn of the medial meniscus and the intercondylar notch, just anterior to the ACL, was observed in 15% of specimens. A similar number of specimens (15%) demonstrated an anterolateral meniscofemoral ligament running between the anterior horn of the lateral meniscus and the intercondylar notch. At least one of these ligaments was present in 25% of specimens; however, both were present in only 5% of knees.[115] The anteromedial meniscofemoral ligament was never more than half the thickness of the ACL, whereas the anterior lateral ligament was never more than the a third the size of the ACL. In all cases, the ligaments of Humphry and Wrisberg were more robust than the anteromedial and anterolateral meniscofemoral ligaments.[115]

Oblique Intermeniscal Ligaments

Oblique intermeniscal (meniscomeniscal) ligaments have been identified in 1% to 4% of specimens.[27,121] These ligaments derive their name from their anterior meniscal point of origin. The medial oblique intermeniscal ligament arises from the central part of the anterior horn of the medial meniscus and passes obliquely posteriorly to the posterior horn of the lateral meniscus. The lateral intermeniscal ligament runs between the anterior horn of the lateral meniscus and the posterior horn of the medial meniscus, passing between the cruciates (Fig. 2–9).[27] The functional significance of these ligaments has not been clearly defined.

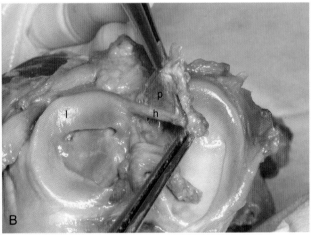

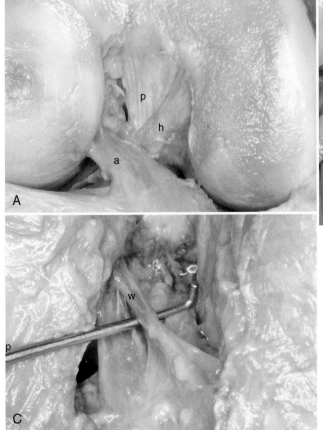

Figure 2–8. Meniscofemoral ligaments. **A,** Anterior view of the intercondylar notch with the ligament of Humphry (h) passing obliquely between the anterior cruciate ligament (ACL) (a) and posterior cruciate ligament (PCL) (p). **B,** The ligament of Humphry (h, inferior forceps) originates from the lateral meniscus (l) and embraces the anterior aspect of the PCL (p). **C,** Posterior view of the intercondylar notch with the ligament of Wrisberg (w) directly posterior to the PCL (p, probe deep to the ligament of Wrisberg).

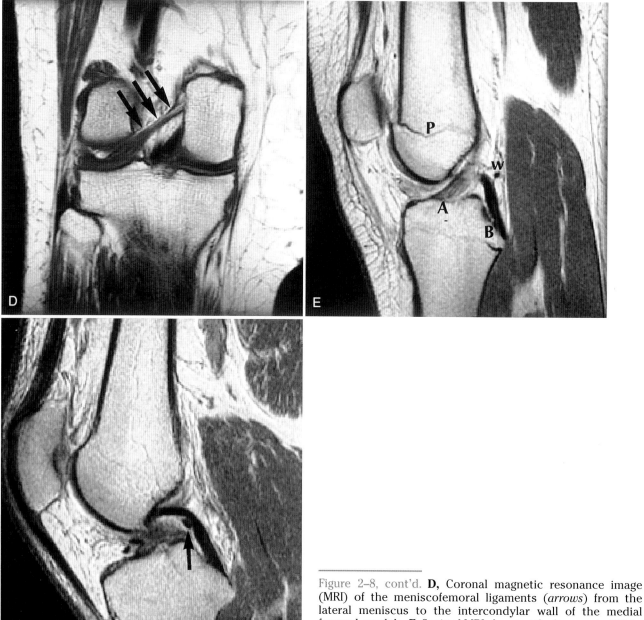

Figure 2–8, cont'd. **D,** Coronal magnetic resonance image (MRI) of the meniscofemoral ligaments (*arrows*) from the lateral meniscus to the intercondylar wall of the medial femoral condyle. **E,** Sagittal MRI showing the ligament of Wrisberg (w) posterior to the PCL (B). Also identified are the ACL (A) and a physeal scar (P). **F,** Sagittal MRI with the small oval ligament of Humphry identified anterior to the PCL (*arrow*).

MUSCLE ABNORMALITIES

Anomalous Attachments

A number of variations in the muscle attachments about the popliteal fossa have been described and are clinically significant in circumstances associated with popliteal artery compression, as described subsequently. The most commonly reported anomalies include lateral and more proximal origins of the medial head of the gastrocnemius.

Anomalous attachments of the pes muscles and hamstrings have also been observed. In one case report, an abnormal attachment of the biceps femoris was noted to be the cause of painful snapping; the biceps inserted entirely on the proximal end of the tibia rather than onto the normal insertion site on the fibula.[47] During extension, subluxation of the tendon over the fibular head was noted. Transposition of the biceps insertion successfully relieved the pain and snapping.

Variations in the pes tendon insertions are quite common; half the specimens in one cadaver study demonstrated one of seven variations ranging from fascial loops connecting the sartorius tendon with the medial collateral ligament to separate tendon slips from each of the three tendons inserting separately into the tibia.[55] These anatomic variations can be clinically important when har-

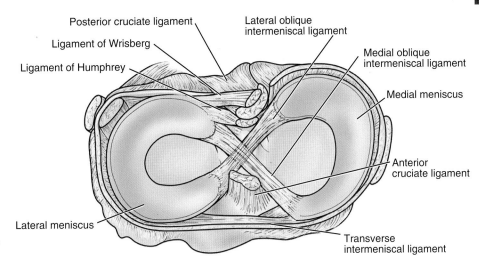

Figure 2–9. Oblique intermeniscal ligaments.

Accessory or Hypertrophic Muscles

Anomalous muscles in the popliteal fossa and posterior aspect of the knee are rare. In a report of 300 anatomic dissections over a 15-year period, the authors observed only a single anomalous muscle.[105]

The popliteus muscle normally flattens and forms a tendon before passing deep to the fibular collateral ligament. In a small number of specimens (≈14%), a more robust muscle with an abnormally short tendon that intruded into the joint was observed.[19] In theory, the extra bulk of this anomalous structure may impinge posteriorly and require recession during total knee replacement.

A third head of the gastrocnemius originating from the posterior and inferior aspects of the femur and joining either the medial or lateral head has been noted in 2% to 5% of individuals and appears to be more common in the Japanese population.[56] Another reported anomaly is an accessory or hypertrophied semimembranosus that lies more laterally in the fossa than normal and rests superficial to the neurovascular bundle.[15,107] A hypertrophied plantaris muscle with a large and more distal origin from the medial aspect of the lateral head of the gastrocnemius has also been observed. This anomalous muscle runs distally and medially and passes under the neurovascular bundle.[15] All these anomalies may lead to symptomatic compression of the popliteal vessels. However, the true incidence of these variations is unknown because many are asymptomatic.

Hypoplasia

Hypoplasia of the vastus medialis muscle may contribute to patellofemoral pathomechanics. The vastus medialis is the last muscle of the quadriceps group to form, and in some individuals this muscle develops poorly, with result-

ant lateral and superior displacement of the patella. This hereditary or congenital anomaly has been identified to some degree in up to 40% of individuals but is frequently asymptomatic.[39] However, in some individuals, such hypoplasia may contribute to abnormal patellar tracking and result in subluxation, dislocation, or patellofemoral pain syndromes. Clinical findings may include observation of a poorly developed vastus medialis relative to the vastus lateralis, lateral hypermobility of the patella, pain with patellar compression, and peripatellar tenderness. Physical therapy with selective strengthening of the vastus medialis may be successful in patients with patellofemoral pain. However, in cases of dislocation or subluxation, identification of all abnormalities in the patellofemoral joint is required, with appropriate surgical intervention, which may include lateral release and proximal soft-tissue realignment.

ARTERIAL ANOMALIES

Persistent Sciatic Artery

The sciatic artery represents a persistence of the embryonic axial artery that is the predominant vascular supply to the lower limb bud during early development (Fig. 2–10). The incidence of this structural anomaly has been reported to be approximately 0.01% to 0.05%.[17] In the early embryo, the axial artery is a continuation of the internal iliac artery. During normal development, it involutes by the 22-mm embryo stage, and the femoral artery provides the major vascular supply to the lower extremity. The only normal remnants of the axial artery are the proximal portions of the anterior and superior gluteal vessels and the popliteal and peroneal vessels. When normal development fails and a persistent sciatic artery occurs, it may be either complete or incomplete. In patients with a complete persistent sciatic artery, it is the predominant arterial supply to the limb. However, in incomplete cases, the sciatic artery is hypoplastic and the femoral artery predominates. In some patients, a persistent sciatic vein may accompany the arterial abnormality.

vesting tendon autografts for reconstructive procedures on the knee ligaments.

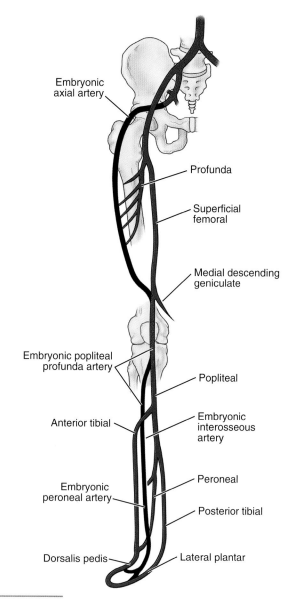

Figure 2–10. Embryonic and adult artery distribution in the lower extremity. The *black* portions regress during normal development, whereas the *red* portions form part of the adult vascular supply. (Redrawn from Mandell VS, Jaques PF, Delany DJ, et al: Persistent sciatic artery: Clinical, embryologic, and angiographic features. AJR Am J Roentgenol 144:245, 1985.)

A persistent sciatic artery follows a characteristic course in which it initially passes through the greater sciatic foramen below the piriform. Next, it passes inferior to the gluteus maximus muscle and posterior to the greater trochanter; it then runs distally along the posterior margin of the adductor magnus muscle to the popliteal fossa.[17,69] On physical examination, the presence of a persistent sciatic artery may be suspected if a pulsatile mass is found in the buttock. In addition, the presence of palpable popliteal and pedal pulses without a femoral pulse may be noted. However, in most cases the femoral artery is developed enough proximally to produce a normal pulse. Sciatic arteries have a high incidence of aneurysm forma-

tion (up to 44%), which may require revascularization procedures.[17] Visualization of this anomalous vessel along its entire course can be difficult and it may be misinterpreted on routine angiograms as atherosclerotic occlusion of the superficial femoral vessel. If this anomaly is suspected, selective internal iliac artery injection or additional delayed-timing injections can assist in correct angiographic identification.[69]

Persistent Deep Popliteal Artery

During embryonic development, the deep popliteal artery represents the distal continuation of the sciatic artery. The deep popliteal artery, which passes between the popliteal and the posterior aspect of the tibia, is normally replaced at the 18-mm crown-rump embryonic stage by the superficial popliteal artery, which runs posterior to the popliteus.[94] Persistence of the earlier embryonic artery has been reported to be a rare cause of popliteal artery entrapment syndrome, which is discussed in more detail next.[10,94]

Popliteal Artery Entrapment Syndrome

Compression of the popliteal artery may be caused by a number of anomalous structures in the popliteal fossa, including deviation of the artery anterior and medial to the origin of the medial head of the gastrocnemius, passage of the artery through the medial head of the gastrocnemius, a high origin of the medial head of the gastrocnemius, a fibrous band running from the medial head of the gastrocnemius to the lateral condyle, hypertrophy of the plantaris muscle, an accessory head of the gastrocnemius, and hypertrophy or an accessory portion of the semimembranosus (Fig. 2–11).[10,15,44,56,94] The incidence of this syndrome was noted to be 0.165% in one large series of 20,000 patients and it appears to be more frequent in young adult males.[15,44,94] Most cases are thought to be due to abnormalities in embryonic muscle development, but as previously noted, rare cases may result from persistence of embryonic arterial structures.[10,94]

Patients most frequently complain of activity-related claudication (54%) but can have acute signs of ischemia (5%) when arterial thrombosis occurs.[10,94] Other symptoms may include swelling, limping, or muscle cramps. On physical examination, absence of a pedal pulse or diminishment with dynamic maneuvers, including active plantar flexion and passive dorsiflexion of the foot with the knee in active extension, may be noted. Lower extremity edema or severe varicosities may be observed if compression of the popliteal vein also occurs. Diagnostic tests such as arteriograms, ultrasonograms, and MRI can be helpful in evaluating young people with complaints of claudication. An arteriogram may show local compression or medial deviation of the popliteal artery in patients with an abnormal origin or path of the medial head of the gastrocnemius. In patients with an acute onset, complete obstruction caused by thrombosis may be observed.[44,94] Dynamic maneuvers performed during arteriography or

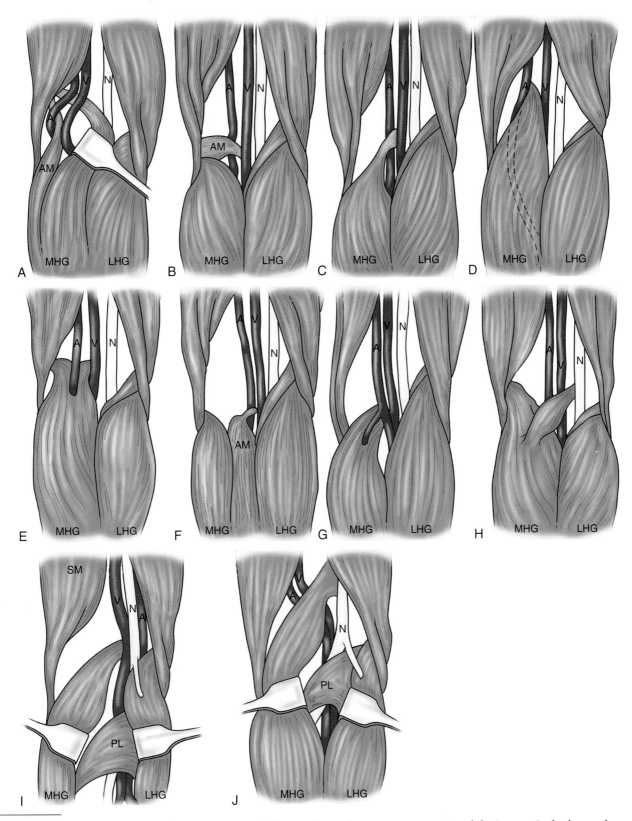

Figure 2–11. **A-J,** Diagrammatic representations of abnormal muscle anatomy encountered during surgical release of symptomatic popliteal artery entrapment. Popliteal artery entrapment may be due to the presence of a variety of anomalous muscle bodies and tendons, deviation of normal muscle attachments (particularly the medial gastrocnemius), and abnormal muscle hypertrophy. A and V, popliteal artery and vein; AM, anomalous muscle; MHG and LHG, medial and lateral heads of the gastrocnemius; N, tibial nerve; PL, abnormal plantaris; SM, hypertrophied semimembranosus. (Redrawn from Bouhoutsos J, Daskalakis E: Muscular abnormalities affecting the popliteal vessels. Br J Surg 68:501, 1981.)

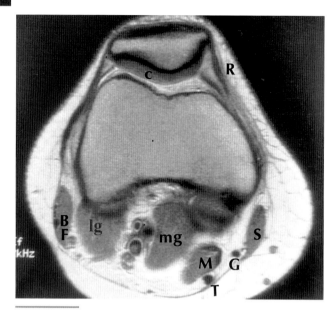

Figure 2–12. Axial magnetic resonance image of the knee. The contents of the popliteal fossa and location of the neurovascular structures between the two heads of the gastrocnemius can be readily identified. BF, biceps femoris; c, patella cartilage; G, gracilis; M, semimembranosus muscle; mg and lg, medial and lateral gastrocnemius; R, medial retinaculum; S, sartorius muscle; T, semitendinosus tendon.

duplex ultrasonography may also demonstrate active compression. MRI can be quite helpful in identifying anomalous structures that compress the artery and has become the gold standard for evaluating the anatomy of the popliteal fossa (Fig. 2–12).[35,94]

In patients with documented symptomatic compression, simple release of anomalous bands or resection or transposition of abnormal or accessory muscles may be performed. However, in those with chronic scarring of the artery or acute thrombosis, revascularization procedures may be required.[10,15,94]

NERVE ABNORMALITIES

Sensory Distribution Variations

Sensation to the anterior and medial aspect of the knee is supplied by the infrapatellar branch of the saphenous nerve. In the majority of patients, the infrapatellar branch originates after the saphenous nerve emerges through the deep fascia between the sartorius and gracilis in the distal part of the thigh. It then traverses through the sartorius muscle and joins the patellar plexus, curving distal and medial to the patella.[52] Anterior and medial surgical approaches to the knee place these branches at risk and have been associated with neuroma formation postoperatively if transected.[23] Frequent variations in anatomy, including more proximal origins of the saphenous nerve and infrapatellar branches, which result in a more anterior course of the infrapatellar branch, make it difficult to

avoid the cutaneous nerves reliably, and we do not routinely attempt to preserve them. Multiple patterns of the cutaneous innervation to the lateral aspect of the knee have also been described.[50]

CYSTS

Ganglion Cysts

Ganglion or synovial cysts have been reported to originate from numerous structures in and around the knee joint, including the ACL, PCL, popliteal tendon, and menisci. In most cases, these cysts are believed to be related to either cystic degeneration of the structure or herniation of synovial fluid and cells through a defect into surrounding tissue; however, in some cases they may represent congenital anomalies.[61,68,80,95,98,106] Symptoms related to these cysts may include palpable masses, recurrent effusions, aching pain, and locking or catching. Successful open excision and arthroscopic débridement of these cysts have been reported in a limited number of cases.[61,68,80,91,98] However, if the underlying disease is not addressed, the risk of recurrence is a concern.

Meniscal Cysts

Meniscal cysts represent a subgroup of ganglion cysts that occur in association with meniscal tears. Originally, the cause of these lesions was controversial; possibilities included myxoid generation, trauma, and synovial rests. However, a link with meniscal tears has now been documented.[80,95] Cysts involve the lateral aspect of the knee more often than the medial. The most common site of occurrence is along the lateral joint line anterior to the lateral collateral ligament. Patients may note a palpable mass that disappears in flexion (Pisani's sign), aching knee pain, or an effusion.[95]

MRI is the test of choice for both evaluating a suspected cyst and detecting associated meniscal tears (Fig. 2–13). Lateral cysts commonly occur at the junction of the anterior and middle third of the body, whereas medial cysts are most frequently located in the posterior horn.[95,110] A horizontal cleavage or transverse tear is typically identified at this site in each case.[42,80,95]

Nonoperative treatment, including aspiration and injection of cortisone into the cyst, has been used successfully, but an approximately 25% short-term recurrence rate has been reported.[72] We do not favor this approach because of the association with intra-articular disease. Surgical intervention previously consisted of open cyst excision, complete meniscectomy, or both.[67] However, arthroscopic partial meniscectomy of the involved torn meniscus with intra-articular cyst drainage has become the accepted intervention.[42,80,81,95] If initial attempts at cyst decompression by the application of external pressure are unsuccessful, an 18-gauge needle can be percutaneously passed through the cyst and accompanying meniscal defect to facilitate intra-articular decompression of the loculated fluid.[81] Alternatively, an arthroscopic punch or shaver may be passed through the meniscal defect into the cyst.[42,80] With these techniques, good and excellent clinical results have been reported in approximately 90% of patients, with no recurrences observed in several series.[80,81,95]

Popliteal Cysts

The posterior synovial cavity communicates with a popliteal bursa that is found between the semimembranosus tendon and the medial head of the gastrocnemius

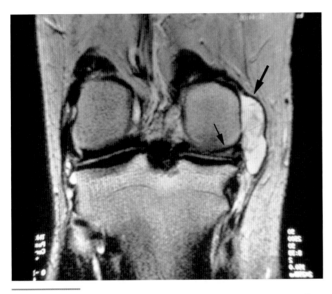

Figure 2–13. Coronal magnetic resonance image of a medial meniscal cyst (*thick arrow*) with high-signal fluid contents in association with a meniscal tear (*thin arrow*).

in about 50% of people (Fig. 2–14).[119] This bursa may be distended when dye is injected into the knee; the bursa can also become enlarged by an intra-articular effusion and result in a popliteal or Baker cyst.[5] Once trapped in the bursa, fluid is unable to return to the joint because of a functional one-way valve. In two large series of patients who underwent MRI of the knee, a 5% to 19% incidence of popliteal cysts was identified.[26,38,71] A higher incidence in older patients was noted.[71] In adult patients, popliteal cysts commonly occur in association with intra-articular abnormalities, including meniscal tears, ACL tears, and degenerative or inflammatory arthritis, which results in increased joint fluid.[26,38,71,108] Fielding et al[38] reported an 82% incidence of posterior horn medial meniscus tears in patients with documented popliteal cysts. Histological examination has revealed that popliteal cysts are generally lined with flattened mesothelium-like cells surrounded by fibroblasts and lymphocysts and contain a viscous, fibrin-rich fluid.[26] Burleson et al[18] identified three types of popliteal cysts. Type 1 cysts have a thin, 1- to 2-mm fibrous wall with flat endothelial-like cells; type 2 cysts have thicker walls that are poorly defined and lined with cuboid-type cells; and type 3 cysts have walls up to 8 mm thick with more lymphocytes, plasma cells, and histiocytes. A small number of cysts could not be adequately classified and were termed transitional types.[18]

In pediatric patients, an asymptomatic swelling in the popliteal fossa is the most common manifestation, but in adult patients, vague posterior aches or symptoms related to the intra-articular disease are commonly present. A pseudothrombophlebitis syndrome with severe calf swelling and pain related to rupture of a cyst has been described.[26,63] On examination, the cyst can often be palpated in the medial aspect of the popliteal fossa as a firm mass that is best appreciated with the knee in extension.

Plain radiographs are rarely helpful in diagnosis except to identify associated arthritic changes. Both MRI and

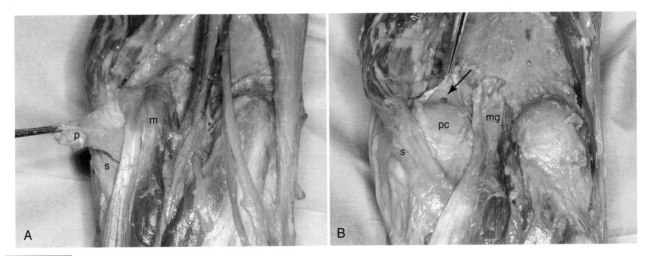

Figure 2–14. Anatomic dissections of a popliteal cyst (semimembranosus bursa). **A,** An evacuated popliteal cyst (p, forceps) originates between the semimembranosus (s) and the medial head of the gastrocnemius (m). **B,** The wall of the cyst has been removed and the medial head of the gastrocnemius (mg) has been detached from its origin on the posterior aspect of the medial femoral condyle and transposed medially to reveal the posterior capsule (pc). A small hole in the capsule (*arrow*, inferior to the tip of the forceps) in the base of the cyst communicates with the intra-articular cavity (s, semimembranosus).

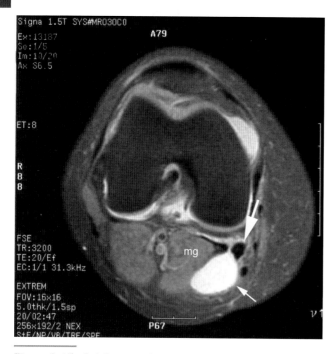

Figure 2–15. Axial magnetic resonance image of a popliteal cyst with the high signal of a fluid-filled cyst (*thin arrow*) dissecting into the popliteal fossa from its origin between the semimembranosus (*thick arrow*) and the medial head of the gastrocnemius (mg).

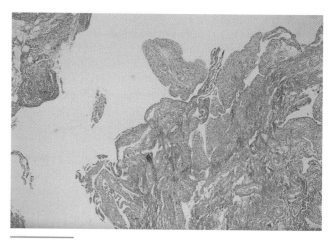

Figure 2–16. Histology of a synovial plica. A bland fibrous membrane is lined with rather indistinct synovial-like lining cells. (From Vigorita VJ: The synovium. In Vigorita VJ, Ghelman B: Orthopaedic Pathology. Philadelphia, Lippincott Williams & Wilkins, 1999.)

ultrasonography can be used to distinguish between cystic and solid masses in the popliteal fossa.[26,79] However, MRI is also excellent at demonstrating associated meniscal tears and other intra-articular disease. Because of the fluid content, popliteal cysts appear bright on T2-weighted images and have low signal intensity on T1-weighted images (Fig. 2–15). The best visualization of these cysts appears to be obtained with axial fat-suppressed fast T2-weighted images.[71]

In the pediatric population, popliteal cysts rarely require operative intervention; in the majority of patients treated by observation, the cysts spontaneously resolve within 1 to 2 years.[31] In symptomatic adults, treatment can include nonsteroidal anti-inflammatory medications, compression, and physical therapy. However, if symptoms persist or are disabling, arthroscopic examination and débridement of the associated intra-articular disease should be considered. We do not favor aspiration or injection of corticosteroids because these solutions are rarely definitive. Open excision is rarely required, but if attempted after failure of arthroscopic management, complete excision of the cyst and stalk with simple closure of the capsular defect may be considered.[51] Transposition of a portion of the medial gastrocnemius tendon over the capsular repair has been reported to decrease the rate of cyst recurrence.[26,88]

PLICAE

During fetal development, the knee is separated into three compartments by synovial membranes. At about 4 to 5 months of embryonic development, these partitions resorb to form a single cavity; incomplete or partial resorption results in incomplete synovial folds or plicae.[33,120] Three plicae are most commonly described: suprapatellar, infrapatellar, and medial patellar. Histological examination reveals a bland fibrous membrane (Fig. 2–16). Visualization of these plicae on MRI is difficult without an associated intra-articular effusion, but it is possible, particularly on sagittal and axial views. Rarely, these plicae become inflamed and fibrotic and may become symptomatic. Arthroscopic resection has proved successful in relieving symptoms in carefully selected patients.[33,66,73,82,89]

Medial Patellar Plica

A medial patellar plica has its origin on the medial wall of the knee joint and runs obliquely distally toward and inserts into the synovium, covering the medial infrapatellar fat pad. It may occur in association with or in continuity with a suprapatellar plica. A medial patellar plica has been noted in 5% to 55% of all individuals but becomes symptomatic in only a small number of patients.[6,66,73,82,96] A fenestrated plica is less common but is more likely to be symptomatic.[6]

A previously asymptomatic plica may become symptomatic after a knee injury. It is postulated that the effusion and synovitis related to the original injury may cause the plica to become edematous, which in turn produces a fibrotic reaction leading to tightening, bowstringing, and impingement of the plica against the medial femoral condyle or medial patellar facet. This irritation leads to further thickening and contraction of the fibrous band.[73,82] Patients complain of dull, aching medial knee pain that may be exacerbated by activity or prolonged sitting. Patients may also have mechanical symptoms such as crepitus or pseudolocking. In one study, the most frequent symptoms were pain (92%), snapping (80%), swelling (67%), and pseudolocking (35%).[73] Physical examination consistently reveals tenderness over the medial condyle, and a painful band may be palpated approximately one fingerbreadth away from the medial border of the patella.[82] A snap or catching may also be elicited.[73]

Koshino and Okamoto[66] described two provocation tests that they found helpful in diagnosing symptomatic plicae. The first, the rotation valgus test, involves flexing the knee and applying a valgus force with internal and then external rotation of the tibia while simultaneously attempting to displace the patella medially. The second, the holding test, involves attempting to flex the knee against active resistance. If either test elicits pain, with or without a click, it is positive.

MRI is the most appropriate imaging modality and has been reported to be quite reliable for detection of medial patellar plicae, with a sensitivity of 93% and a specificity of 81%.[74] These plicae have low signal intensity on both T1- and T2-weighted images, which is believed to be due to recurrent synovitis and fibrosis of the plica (Fig. 2–17).[74]

Arthroscopic examination may reveal a thickened plica that impinges on the femur or patella. Sakakibara and Watanabe[96] described a classification of medial patellar plicae based on the arthroscopic appearance. Type A is a cord-like elevation in the medial wall; type B has a shelf-like appearance, but it does not arthroscopically cover the anterior surface of the medial condyle; type C has a large shelf-like appearance that covers the anterior surface of the medial femoral condyle; and type D is a special variation in which double insertions in the medial wall are seen.[96] Chondromalacia or groove formation may be noted at the site of impingement on the medial femoral condyle or medial patellar facet (Fig. 2–18).[82]

Nonoperative treatment includes a reduction in activity, nonsteroidal anti-inflammatory medications, and physical therapy. These modalities are all aimed at reducing the inflammation and breaking the cycle of irritation and edema within the plica. If nonoperative measures are ineffective, arthroscopic examination and plica excision may be considered. Arthroscopic débridement of symptomatic medial patellar plicae has been moderately successful in carefully selected patients, with 66% to 90% experiencing complete pain relief; however, overdiagnosis and resection of incidental plicae have been cautioned against.[6,66,73,82]

Suprapatellar Plica

A suprapatellar plica is a crescent-shaped septum that may be found between the suprapatellar pouch and the knee joint. It is attached to both the medial and lateral walls of the knee joint, as well as the undersurface of the quadriceps tendon (Fig. 2–19). In a large cadaver study, the presence of a persistent plica was observed in 17% of specimens. In 95 of these specimens, the plica was complete and divided the suprapatellar pouch into two parts, and in 8% the plica was incomplete.[120] A large suprapatellar plica may shield loose bodies and, if in continuity with a medial patellar plica, can contribute to symptomatic impingement against the femoral condyle or patella.[33,82] Symptoms may also occur in patients with division of the pouch by a complete plica.[33]

Patients have symptoms similar to those associated with patellofemoral pain syndrome; pain is aggravated by stair climbing and knee flexion. Swelling in the suprapatellar region may be noted after activity. When the pouch is completely isolated from the knee joint, it has been postulated that distention of the bursae related to activity with occasional dissection between the planes of the quadriceps mechanism leads to pain.[33,85,86] In other cases, pain is probably related to impingement and entrapment of the plica. Again, MRI is the best imaging modality for identifying these plicae (Fig. 2–20). Successful arthroscopic resection of a symptomatic suprapatellar plica has also been reported, although the number of cases is small.[33,73]

Infrapatellar Plica

An infrapatellar plica, commonly known as the ligamentum mucosum, traverses from the intercondylar notch to the infrapatellar fat pad. It widens from its origin in the notch and fans out as it inserts distally in the fat pad. It is the most common plica and is not considered pathological.[73] Rarely, this plica is very large and thickened; in such cases it is referred to as a persistent vertical septum (Fig. 2–21).[89] The only clinical significance of this plica relates to the problems caused by the membrane during arthroscopy or arthrography. During arthroscopic examination, a large infrapatellar plica or a persistent vertical septum can be an obstacle to easy passage of the arthroscope and instruments.[73,89] Resection of these membranes when encountered facilitates easy maneuvering inside the anterior knee joint.

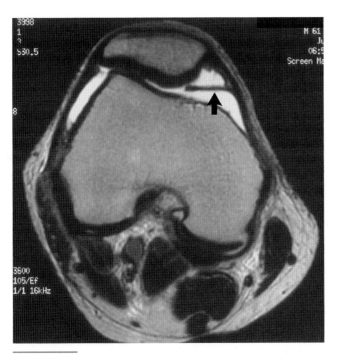

Figure 2–17. Axial magnetic resonance image with a low-signal, thick medial patellar plica (*arrow*) that is highlighted by the large effusion.

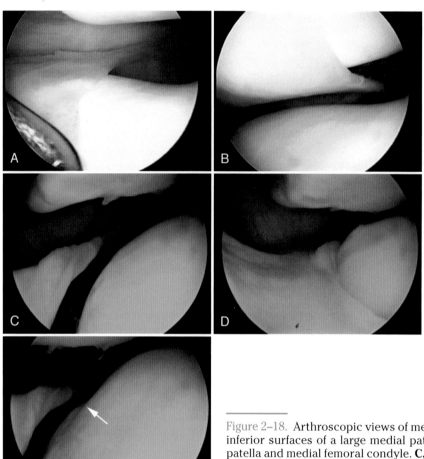

Figure 2–18. Arthroscopic views of medial patellar plicae. **A** and **B,** Superior and inferior surfaces of a large medial patellar plica that is impinging between the patella and medial femoral condyle. **C,** Thickened edge of a fibrotic medial plica. **D,** Impingement by a thickened plica on the medial femoral condyle. **E,** Erosion in the medial femoral condyle articular cartilage as a result of chronic impingement (*arrow*).

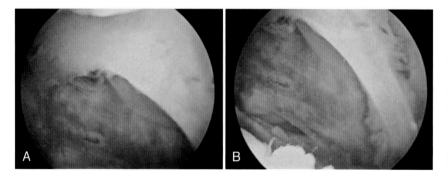

Figure 2–19. Arthroscopic views of a suprapatellar plica. **A,** Incomplete crescent-shaped suprapatellar plica with an opening to the suprapatellar pouch. **B,** Extension of the same suprapatellar plica distally and posteriorly along the intra-articular surface of the medial capsule.

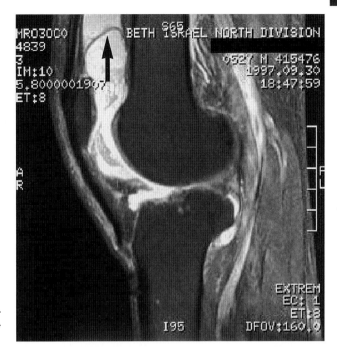

Figure 2–20. Sagittal magnetic resonance image with a curvilinear suprapatellar plica (*arrow*) outlined by an intra-articular effusion.

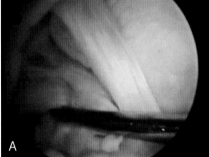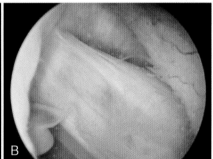

Figure 2–21. **A,** Arthroscopic view of an infrapatellar plica (ligamentum mucosum seen anterior to the anterior cruciate ligament (ACL) (probe tip posterior to the ACL). **B,** Arthroscopic view of a persistent vertical septum with almost complete division of the medial and lateral compartments anteriorly.

SUMMARY

A large number of anatomic variations have been reported and in many cases represent incidental findings. However, in certain circumstances, such as trauma or degeneration, these structures may become symptomatic. To interpret the significance of these findings and render suitable treatment, the first step is correct identification.

References

1. Aglietti P, Insall JN, Cerulli G: Patellar pain and incongruence: I. Measurements of incongruence. Clin Orthop 176:217, 1983.
2. Aichroth PM, Patel DV, Marx CL: Congenital discoid lateral meniscus in children: A follow-up study and evolution of management. J Bone Joint Surg Br 73:932, 1991.
3. Andersson AP, Ellitsgaard N: Aplasia of the anterior cruciate ligament with a compensating posterior cruciate ligament. Acta Orthop Belg 58:240, 1992.
4. Bailey WH, Blundell GE: An unusual abnormality affecting both knee joints in a child: Case report. J Bone Joint Surg Am 56:814, 1974.
5. Baker WM: The classic. On the formation of synovial cysts in the leg in connection with disease of the knee-joint. Clin Orthop 299:2, 1994.
6. Barber FA: Fenestrated medial patella plica. Arthroscopy 3:253, 1987.
7. Barrett GR, Tomasin JD: Bilateral congenital absence of the anterior cruciate ligament. Orthopedics 11:431, 1988.
8. Beaconsfield T, Pintore E, Maffulli N, et al: Radiological measurements in patellofemoral disorders: A review. Clin Orthop 308:18, 1994.
9. Beals RK, Buehler K: Treatment of patellofemoral instability in childhood with creation of a femoral sulcus. J Pediatr Orthop 17:516, 1997.
10. Becquemin J-P, Melliere D, Lamour A, et al: The popliteal entrapment syndrome. Anat Clin 6:203, 1984.
11. Bellier G, Dupont J-Y, Larrain M, et al: Lateral discoid menisci in children. Arthroscopy 5:52, 1989.
12. Bernhang AM, Levine SA: Familial absence of the patella. J Bone Joint Surg Am 55:1088, 1973.
13. Bhargava A, Ferrari DA: Posterior medial meniscus-femoral insertion into the anterior cruciate ligament: A case report. Clin Orthop 348:176, 1998.
14. Blacksin MF, Greene B, Botelho G: Bilateral discoid medial menisci diagnosed by magnetic resonance imaging: A case report. Clin Orthop 285:214, 1992.
15. Bouhoutsos J, Daskalakis E: Muscular abnormalities affecting the popliteal vessels. Br J Surg 68:501, 1981.
16. Bourne MH, Bianco AJ Jr: Bipartite patella in the adolescent: Results of surgical excision. J Pediatr Orthop 10:69, 1990.

17. Brantley SK, Rigdon EE, Raju S: Persistent sciatic artery: Embryology, pathology, and treatment. J Vasc Surg 18:242, 1993.

18. Burleson RJ, Bickel WH, Dahlin DC: Popliteal cyst: A clinicopathological survey. J Bone Joint Surg Am 38:1265, 1956.

19. Burman M: The high-bellied popliteus muscle: An anomaly of the popliteus muscle. J Bone Joint Surg Am 50:761, 1968.

20. Carter SR: Traumatic separation of a bipartite patella. Injury 20:244, 1989.

21. Casscells SW: Gross pathological changes in the knee joint of the aged individual: A study of 300 cases. Clin Orthop 132:225, 1978.

22. Cave EF, Staples OS: Congenital discoid meniscus: A cause of internal derangement of the knee. Am J Surg 54:371, 1941.

23. Chambers GH: The prepatellar nerve: A cause of suboptimal results in knee arthrotomy. Clin Orthop 82:157, 1972.

24. Clark CR, Ogden JA: Development of the menisci of the human knee joint: Morphological changes and their potential role in childhood meniscal injury. J Bone Joint Surg Am 65:538, 1983.

25. Comba D, Quaglia F, Magliano G: Massive discoid medial meniscus: A case report. Acta Orthop Scand 56:340, 1985.

26. Curl WW: Popliteal cysts: Historical background and current knowledge. J Am Acad Orthop Surg 4(3):129, 1996.

27. Dervin GF, Paterson RS: Case report. Oblique meniscomeniscal ligament of the knee. Arthroscopy 13:363, 1997.

28. Dickason JM, Del Pizzo W, Blazina ME, et al: A series of ten discoid medial menisci. Clin Orthop 168:75, 1982.

29. Dickhaut SC, DeLee JC: The discoid lateral-meniscus syndrome. J Bone Joint Surg Am 64:1068, 1982.

30. Dimakopoulos P, Patel D: Partial excision of discoid meniscus: Arthroscopic operation of 10 patients. Acta Orthop Scand 61:40, 1990.

31. Dinham JM: Popliteal cysts in children: The case against surgery. J Bone Joint Surg Br 57:69, 1975.

32. D'Lima DD, Copp SN, Colwell CW Jr: Isolated lateral ring meniscus: Case report. Am J Knee Surg 8(3):117, 1995.

33. Elmer RM: Case report. Persistent congenital isolation of the suprapatellar pouch mimicking patellofemoral disease. J Pediatr Orthop 4:623, 1984.

34. Fairbank TJ: Knee joint changes after meniscectomy. J Bone Joint Surg Br 30:664, 1948.

35. Fermand M, Houlle D, Fiessinger JN, et al: Entrapment of the popliteal artery: MR findings. AJR Am J Roentgenol 154:425, 1990.

36. Ferrone JD Jr: Congenital deformities about the knee. Orthop Clin North Am 7:323, 1976.

37. Fetto JF, Marshall JL, Ghelman B: An anomalous attachment of the popliteus tendon to the lateral meniscus. J Bone Joint Surg Am 59:548, 1977.

38. Fielding JR, Franklin PD, Kustan J: Popliteal cysts: A reassessment using magnetic resonance imaging. Skeletal Radiol 20:433, 1991.

39. Fox TA: Dysplasia of the quadriceps mechanism: Hypoplasia of the vastus medialis muscle as related to the hypermobile patella syndrome. Surg Clin North Am 55:199, 1975.

40. Galland O, Walch G, Dejour H, et al: An anatomical and radiological study of the femoropatellar articulation. Surg Radiol Anat 12:119, 1990.

41. Gasco J, Del Pino JM, Gomar-Sancho F: Double patella: A case of duplication in the coronal plane. J Bone Joint Surg Br 69:602, 1987.

42. Glasgow MMS, Allen PW, Blakeway C: Arthroscopic treatment of cysts of the lateral meniscus. J Bone Joint Surg Br 75:299, 1993.

43. Green WT: Painful bipartite patellae: A report of three cases. Clin Orthop 110:197, 1975.

44. Harris JD, Jepson RP: Entrapment of the popliteal artery. Surgery 69:246, 1971.

45. Hayashi LK, Yamaga H, Ida K, et al: Arthroscopic meniscectomy for discoid lateral meniscus in children. J Bone Joint Surg Am 70:1495, 1988.

46. Heller L, Langman J: The meniscofemoral ligaments of the human knee. J Bone Joint Surg Br 46:307, 1964.

47. Hernandez JA, Rius M, Noonan KJ: Snapping knee from anomalous biceps femoris tendon insertion: A case report. Iowa Orthop J 16:161, 1996.

48. Hodkinson HM: Double patellae in multiple epiphysial dysplasia. J Bone Joint Surg Br 44:569, 1962.

49. Hoffmann FF: Case report. Abnormal femoral origin of the anterior cruciate ligament combined with a discoid lateral meniscus. Arthroscopy 13:254, 1997.

50. Horiguchi M, Yamada TK, Koizumi M: Aberrant cutaneous nerve of the thigh arising from the sciatic nerve in the human. Acta Anat 133:118, 1988.

51. Hughston JC, Baker CL, Mello W: Operative technique—popliteal cyst: A surgical approach. Orthopedics 14:147, 1991.

52. Hunter LY, Louis DS, Ricciardi JR, et al: The saphenous nerve: Its course and importance in medial arthrotomy. Am J Sports Med 7:227, 1979.

53. Ikeuchi H: Arthroscopic treatment of the discoid lateral meniscus: Technique and long-term results. Clin Orthop 167:19, 1982.

54. Insall JN, Aglietti P, Tria AJ Jr: Patellar pain and incongruence: II. Clinical application. Clin Orthop 176:225, 1983.

55. Ivey M, Prud'homme J: Anatomic variations of the pes anserinus: A cadaver study. Orthopedics 16:601, 1993.

56. Iwai T, Sato S, Yamada T, et al: Popliteal vein entrapment caused by the third head of the gastrocnemius muscle. Br J Surg 74:1006, 1987.

57. Johansson E, Aparisi T: Congenital absence of the cruciate ligaments: A case report and review of the literature. Clin Orthop 162:108, 1982.

58. Johnson RG, Simmons EH: Discoid medial meniscus. Clin Orthop 167:176, 1982.

59. Jung YB, Yum JK, Bae YJ, et al: Case report: Anomalous insertion of the medial menisci. Arthroscopy 14:505, 1998.

60. Kaelin A, Hulin PH, Carlioz H: Congenital aplasia of the cruciate ligaments: A report of six cases. J Bone Joint Surg Br 68:827, 1986.

61. Kang C-N, Lee S-B, Kim S-W: Case report. Symptomatic ganglion cyst within the substance of the anterior cruciate ligament. Arthroscopy 11:612, 1995.

62. Kaplan EB: Discoid lateral meniscus of the knee joint: Nature, mechanism, and operative treatment. J Bone Joint Surg Am 39:77, 1957.

63. Katz RS, Zizic TM, Arnold WP, et al: The pseudothrombophlebitis syndrome. Medicine (Baltimore) 56:151, 1977.

64. Kim S-J, Choi C-H: Case report. Bilateral complete discoid medial menisci combined with anomalous insertion and cyst formation. Arthroscopy 12:112, 1996.

65. Kim S-J, Jeon C-H, Koh C-H: Case report. A ring-shaped lateral meniscus. Arthroscopy 11:738, 1995.

66. Koshino T, Okamoto R: Resection of painful shelf (plica synovialis mediopatellaris) under arthroscopy. Arthroscopy 1:136, 1985.

67. Lantz B, Singer KM: Meniscal cysts. Clin Sports Med 9:707, 1990.

68. Liu SH, Osti L, Mirzayan R: Ganglion cysts of the anterior cruciate ligament: A case report and review of the literature. Arthroscopy 10:110, 1994.

69. Mandell VS, Jaques PF, Delany DJ, et al: Persistent sciatic artery: Clinical, embryologic, and angiographic features. AJR Am J Roentgenol 144:245, 1985.

70. Manzione M, Pizzutillo PD, Peoples AB, et al: Meniscectomy in children: A long-term follow-up study. Am J Sports Med 11:111, 1983.

71. Miller TT, Staron RB, Koenigsberg T, et al: MR imaging of Baker cysts: Association with internal derangement, effusion, and degenerative arthropathy. Radiology 201:247, 1996.

72. Muddu BN, Barrie JL, Morris MA: Aspiration and injection for meniscal cysts. J Bone Joint Surg Br 74:627, 1992.

73. Muse GL, Grana WA, Hollingsworth S: Arthroscopic treatment of medial shelf syndrome. Arthroscopy 1:63, 1985.

74. Nakanishi K, Inoue M, Ishida T, et al: MR evaluation of mediopatellar plica. Acta Radiol 37:567, 1996.

75. Neuschwander DC, Drez D Jr, Finney TP: Lateral meniscal variant with absence of posterior coronary ligament. J Bone Joint Surg Am 74:1186, 1992.

76. Noble J: Congenital absence of the anterior cruciate ligament associated with a ring meniscus. J Bone Joint Surg Am 57:1165, 1975.

77. Ohana N, Plotquin D, Atar D: Case report. Bilateral hypoplastic lateral meniscus. Arthroscopy 11:740, 1995.

78. Ohkoshi Y, Takeuchi T, Inoue C, et al: Arthroscopic studies of variants of the anterior horn of the medial meniscus. Arthroscopy 13:725, 1997.

79. Ostergaard M, Court-Payen M, Gideon P, et al: Ultrasonography in arthritis of the knee: A comparison with MR imaging. Acta Radiol 36:19, 1995.

80. Parisien JS: Arthroscopic treatment of cysts of the menisci. Clin Orthop 257:154, 1990.

81. Passler JM, Hofer HP, Peicha G, et al: Arthroscopic treatment of meniscal cysts. J Bone Joint Surg Br 75:303, 1993.
82. Patel D: Plica as a cause of anterior knee pain. Orthop Clin North Am 17:273, 1986.
83. Pellacci F, Montanari G, Prosperi P, et al: Lateral discoid meniscus: Treatment and results. Arthroscopy 8:526, 1992.
84. Petty MJ: Two cases of abnormal patellae. Br J Surg 12:799, 1924.
85. Pipkin G: Lesions of the suprapatellar plica. J Bone Joint Surg Am 32:363, 1950.
86. Pipkin G: Knee injuries: The role of the suprapatellar plica and suprapatellar bursa in simulating internal derangements. Clin Orthop 74:161, 1971.
87. Poynton AR, Javadpour SM, Finegan PJ, et al: The meniscofemoral ligaments of the knee. J Bone Joint Surg Br 79:327, 1997.
88. Rauschning W: Popliteal cysts (Baker's cysts) in adults: II. Capsuloplasty with and without a pedicle graft. Acta Orthop Scand 51:547, 1980.
89. Reider B, Marshall JL, Warren RF: Brief note. Persistent vertical septum in the human knee joint. J Bone Joint Surg Am 63:1185, 1981.
90. Renstrom P, Johnson RJ: Anatomy and biomechanics of the menisci. Clin Sports Med 9:523, 1990.
91. Roeser WM, Tsai E: Case report. Ganglion cysts of the anterior cruciate ligament. Arthroscopy 10:574, 1994.
92. Rosenberg TD, Paulos LE, Parker RD, et al: Discoid lateral meniscus: Case report of arthroscopic attachment of a symptomatic Wrisberg-ligament type. Arthroscopy 3:277, 1987.
93. Ross JA, Tough ICK, English TA: Congenital discoid cartilage: Report of a case of discoid medial cartilage, with an embryological note. J Bone Joint Surg Br 40:262, 1958.
94. Rosset E, Hartung O, Brunet C, et al: Popliteal artery entrapment syndrome. Anatomic and embryologic bases, diagnostic and therapeutic considerations following a series of 15 cases with a review of the literature. Surg Radiol Anat 17:161, 1995.
95. Ryu RKN, Ting AJ: Arthroscopic treatment of meniscal cysts. Arthroscopy 9:591, 1993.
96. Sakakibara J, Watanabe M: Arthroscopic study on Iino's band (plica synovialis mediopatellaris). J Jpn Orthop Assoc 50:513, 1976.
97. Santi MD, Richardson AB: Case report. Bilaterally painful anomalous insertion of the medial meniscus in a volleyball player with marfanoid features. Arthroscopy 9:217, 1993.
98. Scapinelli R: A synovial ganglion of the popliteus tendon simulating a parameniscal cyst: Two case reports. J Bone Joint Surg Am 70:1085, 1988.
99. Schonholtz GJ, Koenig TM, Prince A: Bilateral discoid medial menisci: A case report and literature review. Arthroscopy 9:315, 1993.
100. Scott JE, Taor WS: The "small patella" syndrome. J Bone Joint Surg Br 61:172, 1979.
101. Scuderi GR, Scuderi DM: Patellar fragmentation. Am J Knee Surg 7:125, 1994.
102. Shea KG, Westin C, West J: Anomalous insertion of the medial meniscus of the knee. J Bone Joint Surg Am 77:1894, 1995.
103. Silverman ME, Goodman RM, Cuppage FE: The nail-patella syndrome: Clinical findings and ultrastructural observations in the kidney. Arch Intern Med 120:68, 1967.
104. Smillie IS: The congenital discoid meniscus. J Bone Joint Surg Br 30:671, 1948.
105. Somayaji SN, Vincent R, Bairy KL: An anomalous muscle in the region of the popliteal fossa: Case report. J Anat 192:307, 1998.
106. Stener B: Unusual ganglion cysts in the neighbourhood of the knee joint: A report of six cases—three with involvement of the peroneal nerve. Acta Orthop Scand 40:392, 1969.
107. Stoane JM, Gordon DH: MRI of an accessory semimembranosus muscle. J Comput Assist Tomogr 19:161, 1995.
108. Stone KR, Stoller D, De Carli A, et al: The frequency of Baker's cysts associated with meniscal tears. Am J Sports Med 24:670, 1996.
109. Suzuki S, Mita F, Ogishima H: Double-layered lateral meniscus: A newly found anomaly. Arthroscopy 7:267, 1991.
110. Tasker AD, Ostlere SJ: Relative incidence and morphology of lateral and medial meniscal cysts detected by magnetic resonance imaging. Clin Radiol 50:778, 1995.
111. Thomas NP, Jackson AM, Aichroth PM: Congenital absence of the anterior cruciate ligament: A common component of knee dysplasia. J Bone Joint Surg Br 67:572, 1985.
112. Tolo VT: Congenital absence of the menisci and cruciate ligaments of the knee: A case report. J Bone Joint Surg Am 63:1022, 1981.
113. Twyman RS, Ferris BD: Congenital hypoplasia of the medial meniscus: A report of two cases. Arthroscopy 7:148, 1991.
114. Van Dommelen BA, Fowler PJ: Anatomy of the posterior cruciate ligament: A review. Am J Sports Med 17:24, 1989.
115. Wan ACT, Felle P: The menisco-femoral ligaments. Clin Anat 8:323, 1995.
116. Washington ER III, Root L, Liener UC: Discoid lateral meniscus in children: Long-term follow-up after excision. J Bone Joint Surg Am 77:1357, 1995.
117. Weaver JK: Bipartite patellae as a cause of disability in the athlete. Am J Sports Med 5:137, 1977.
118. Weinberg S: Case report 177: Duplication of the patella ("double" patella). Skeletal Radiol 7:223, 1981.
119. Wilson PD, Eyre-Brook AL, Francis JD: A clinical and anatomical study of the semimembranosus bursa in relation to popliteal cyst. J Bone Joint Surg 20:963, 1938.
120. Zidorn T, Tillmann B: Morphological variants of the suprapatellar bursa. Ann Anat 174:287, 1992.
121. Zivanovic S: Menisco-meniscal ligaments of the human knee joint. Anat Anz 135(Suppl):35, 1974.

CHAPTER 3

Clinical Examination of the Knee

Alfred J. Tria, Jr.

HISTORY

Clinical examination of the knee should begin with a complete history of the symptoms and/or a full description of the mechanism of injury. Often, the history will direct the examiner to the area of knee involvement and help sharpen the physical examination.

OBSERVATION AND INSPECTION

The examination should begin with evaluation of the gait pattern and the stance position of the lower limb. A shortened stance phase of gait (antalgic gait) will confirm the side of involvement. A short leg gait requires confirmation of limb length and may be accompanied by a significant varus or valgus deformity at the knee. Varus or valgus alignment should be noted, as well as any medial or lateral thrust in the stance phase of gait (Fig. 3–1) The clinical alignment of the lower part of the leg (anatomic axis) measures the femorotibial angle (Fig. 3–2) and is different from the mechanical axis of the limb (Fig. 3–3), as measured from the femoral head through the knee into the ankle on a standing roentgenogram. With a goniometer applied to the anterior aspect of the thigh and lower part of the leg and centered on the patella, the examiner can report the clinical varus or valgus alignment. This measurement can be used along with the roentgenographic measurements.

Patellar alignment is influenced by femoral neck anteversion, tibial torsion, the anatomy of the individual patellar facets, and the depth and angle of the femoral sulcus (Fig. 3–4). The Q angle is drawn from the middle of the tibial tubercle to the middle of the patella and then to the anterior superior iliac spine of the pelvis. The normal angle is 10 to 20 degrees and combines the effects of femoral neck anteversion and tibial torsion. The angle should be measured with the patient supine and the hip and knee in full extension. If the knee is allowed to flex slightly, the Q angle decreases with internal rotation of the tibia on the femur (Fig. 3–5).

Clinical effusion may be apparent visually. Active range of motion should be recorded along with any limitations to full extension or flexion so that active range of motion can be further evaluated with palpation and passive range of motion of the knee (Fig. 3–6). It is customary that full extension be considered 0 degrees, and flexion is recorded as an increasing number or as the distance of the heel of the foot from the buttocks. An inability to fully extend may represent lag, a locked knee, or a flexion contracture. An inability to fully flex may be due to an effusion, pain, or extension contracture.

Quadriceps atrophy is sometimes apparent visually and can help confirm the involved side. The appearance should lead to circumferential measurement during the palpation phase of the physical examination.

PALPATION

All the bony landmarks should be palpated and identified. The Q angle, Gerdy's tubercle, the fibular head, the epicondyles of the femur, the patellar margins, and the tibiofemoral joint lines should be identified.

Effusions can be graded in size by compressing the suprapatellar pouch and then noting any fluid (grade 1), slight lift-off of the patella (grade 2), a ballotable patella (grade 3), or a tense effusion with no ability to compress the patella against the femoral sulcus (grade 4) (Fig. 3–7).

The muscle atrophy noted on observation can now be measured. The circumference of the thigh should be measured at a set distance above the patella with the knee in full extension and then compared with the opposite side.

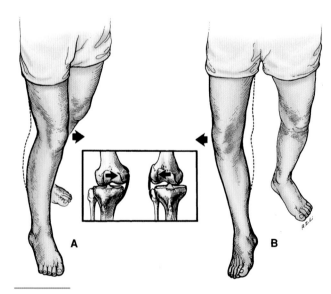

Figure 3–1. Medial thrust of the femur indicates shift of the femur medially on the tibia through the stance phase of gait in the coronal plane (**A**). Lateral thrust indicates lateral shift of the femur in the coronal plane (**B**). (From Tria AJ Jr, Klein KS: An Illustrated Guide to the Knee. New York, Churchill Livingstone, 1992.)

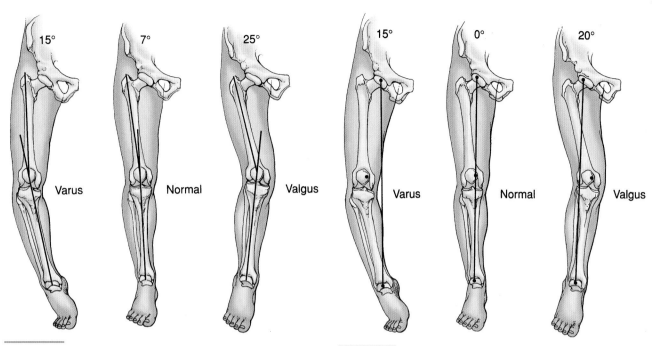

Figure 3–2. The anatomic axis is measured by drawing lines parallel to the long axis of the femur and the tibia and measuring the intercepting angle. (From Tria AJ Jr, Klein KS: An Illustrated Guide to the Knee. New York, Churchill Livingstone, 1992.)

Figure 3–3. The mechanical axis of the leg is measured in the standing position with an imaginary "plumb line" dropped from the femoral head to the ground. This angular measurement gives the best functional evaluation of lower extremity alignment. (From Tria AJ Jr, Klein KS: An Illustrated Guide to the Knee. New York, Churchill Livingstone, 1992.)

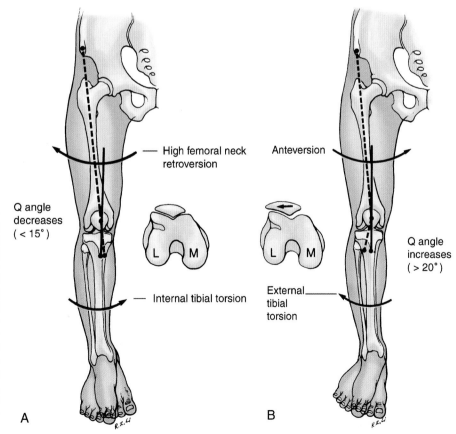

Figure 3–4. High femoral neck retroversion rotates the distal end of the femur externally. In combination with internal tibial torsion, the Q angle is decreased. Patellar tracking is improved, and patellofemoral sulcus alignment is normal. High femoral neck anteversion rotates the distal end of the femur internally. In combination with external tibial torsion, the Q angle is increased. Patellar tracking is compromised, and the patella tends to track laterally. (From Tria AJ Jr, Klein KS: An Illustrated Guide to the Knee. New York, Churchill Livingstone, 1992.)

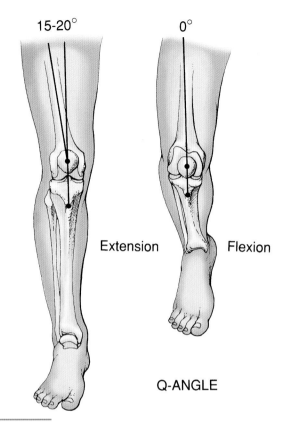

Q-ANGLE

Figure 3–5. Flexion of the knee decreases the Q angle because of the internal tibial rotation. (From Tria AJ Jr, Klein KS: An Illustrated Guide to the Knee. New York, Churchill Livingstone, 1992.)

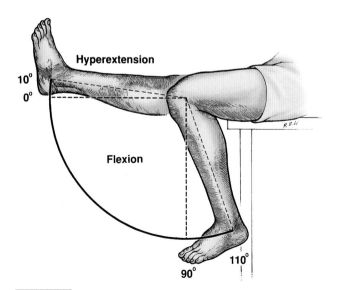

Figure 3–6. Full extension of the knee is the zero or neutral point. (From Tria AJ Jr, Klein KS: An Illustrated Guide to the Knee. New York, Churchill Livingstone, 1992.)

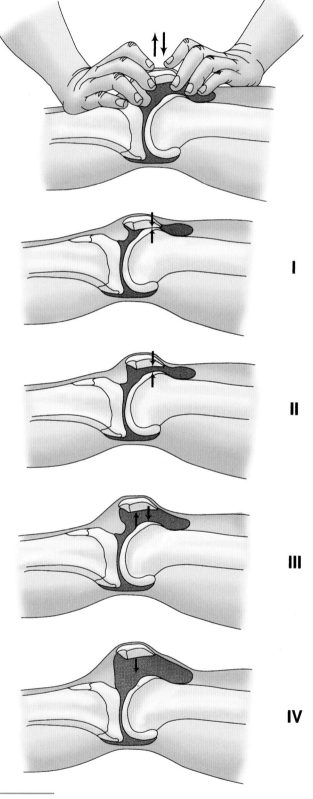

Figure 3–7. Effusions of the knee are graded from 1 to 4. (From Tria AJ Jr, Klein KS: An Illustrated Guide to the Knee. New York, Churchill Livingstone, 1992.)

The calf should be measured at its greatest circumference in the lower part of the leg.

Crepitation in and of itself may or may not represent evidence of a disorder. The location should be recorded for future reference. It may involve the medial or lateral patellofemoral articulation, the medial tibiofemoral articulation, or the lateral tibiofemoral articulation.

The Patellofemoral Joint

Examination of the patellofemoral joint includes both static and dynamic evaluation. Tracking of the patella from full extension into flexion should be recorded visually. In full extension, the patella begins with contact of the median ridge and the lateral facet with the lateral side of the sulcus. The patella moves more centrally and the facets increase their contact with the femoral condyles as flexion increases (Fig. 3–8).

Because the patellar facets do not begin to contact the femoral sulcus until the knee is flexed 30 degrees, the medial and lateral patellofemoral articulation should be palpated in this degree of flexion. One should evaluate tenderness of either the medial or lateral side of the patella, apprehension with either medial or lateral compression, and evidence of crepitation.

The Tibiofemoral Joint

Examination of the tibiofemoral joint should note the presence of any cystic mass (ganglion) along the joint line, localized tenderness, crepitation, snapping, or clicking.

Meniscal tears occur as a result of injury to or degeneration of fibrocartilage. Physical examination of a knee with a torn meniscus reveals joint line tenderness with a palpable click or snap. Range of motion may be limited

Table 3–1. Meniscal Tests

PALPATION	ROTATION
Bragard	Apley
McMurray	Apley grind
Steinmann second	Bohler
	Duck walking
	Helfet
	Merke
	Pavr
	Steinmann first

secondary to displacement of a meniscal tear. A block to full extension may be indicative of a locked knee.

Tests for meniscal tears can be divided into two groups: those that depend on palpation to elicit tenderness or clicks and those that depend on symptoms of joint line pain with rotation (Table 3–1).[1]

The primary palpation tests are the Bragard, McMurray, and Steinmann second tests. With palpation of the joint line, the Bragard test demonstrates that external tibial rotation and knee extension increase tenderness along the joint line. The test brings the meniscus more anterior and closer to the examining finger. Internal rotation and flexion cause less tenderness. If an articular surface irregularity of either the femur or the tibia leads to tenderness, there will be no difference between the two positions. The joint line will remain tender in the same location throughout the range of motion.

The McMurray test elicits a palpable click on the joint line.[15] Medially, it is demonstrated by external tibial rotation and passive motion from flexion to extension. Laterally, it is demonstrated with the tibia in internal rotation and passive motion from flexion to extension. If the click is palpable within the initial few degrees from full flexion, some examiners believe that the tear is more pos-

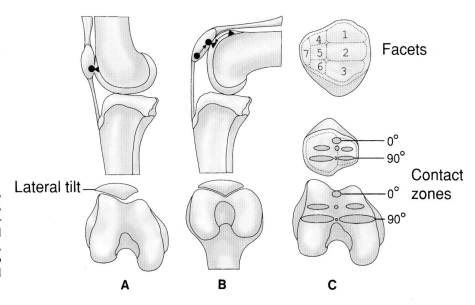

Figure 3–8. As flexion increases, the patella moves more medially, and the contact zones shift proximally and to the medial and lateral facets. (From Tria AJ Jr, Klein KS: An Illustrated Guide to the Knee. New York, Churchill Livingstone, 1992.)

Facets

Contact zones

Lateral tilt

A   B   C

terior. If the click is palpated later as the knee is brought into more extension, the tear is believed to be more anterior.

The Steinmann second test demonstrates joint line tenderness that moves posteriorly with knee flexion and anteriorly with knee extension. This finding is consistent with a meniscal tear that moves with range of motion of the knee and not with a joint line disorder, in which it should remain stationary throughout the range of motion (Fig. 3–9).

Other tests depend on pain with rotation. The Apley grind test forces the tibiofemoral surfaces together to elicit pain. A positive finding is believed to confirm a meniscal tear. The Apley test is also performed with the knee surfaces distracted. If this test elicits less discomfort than the compression test does, the finding of a meniscal tear is favored over a fixed joint line disorder. If the distraction test is equally painful as compression, an articular surface disorder is favored (such as an irregular surface secondary to osteoarthritic erosion).

The Bohler test is performed with varus stress to demonstrate a medial tear with compression (a lateral tear is diagnosed with valgus stress and compression). Duck

walking increases the compressive force on the posterior horns of the torn menisci, thus causing pain.

The Helfet test is appropriate when the knee is locked. Because there is a mechanical block to normal motion, the tibial tubercle cannot rotate externally with extension, and the Q angle cannot increase to normal with extension of the knee. Failure of the knee to externally rotate normally with extension is a positive test result.

The Merke test is the first Steinmann test and is performed with the patient in the weightbearing position. Pain with internal rotation of the body produces external rotation of the tibia and medial joint line pain when the medial meniscus is torn. The opposite occurs when the lateral meniscus is torn.

The Payr test is performed with the patient in the "Turkish sitting position" and downward force applied to the knee. A torn medial meniscus results in medial pain.

In the Steinmann first test, the knee is flexed to 90 degrees, and the tibia is suddenly externally rotated to assess for possible medial meniscal tears. A positive result produces pain along the medial joint line. The internal tibial rotation is used to confirm lateral meniscal tears (Fig. 3–10).

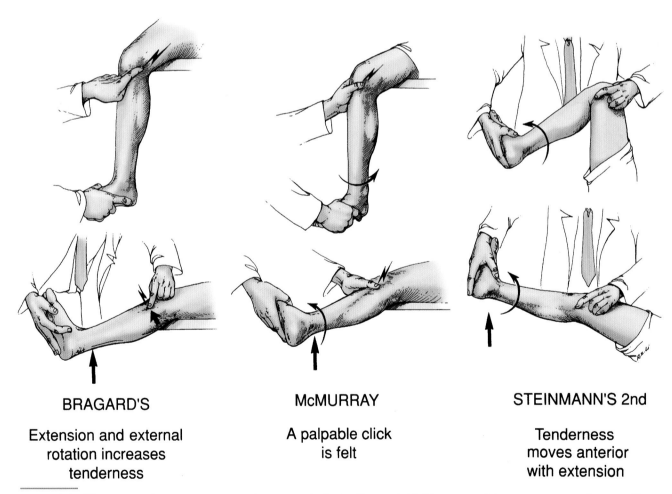

BRAGARD'S

Extension and external
rotation increases
tenderness

McMURRAY

A palpable click
is felt

STEINMANN'S 2nd

Tenderness
moves anterior
with extension

Figure 3–9. The meniscal tests requiring palpation include the Bragard, McMurray, and Steinmann second tests. (From Tria AJ Jr, Klein KS: An Illustrated Guide to the Knee. New York, Churchill Livingstone, 1992.)

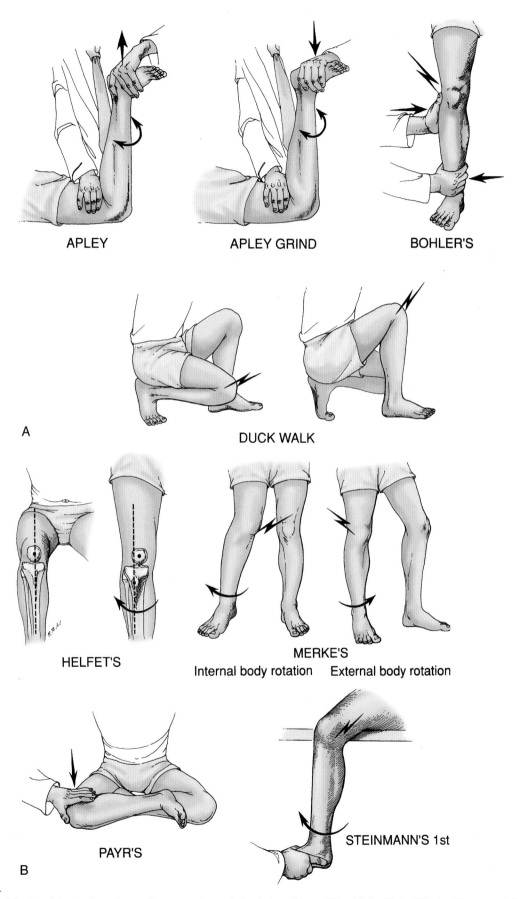

APLEY

APLEY GRIND

BOHLER'S

A

DUCK WALK

HELFET'S

MERKE'S
Internal body rotation   External body rotation

PAYR'S

STEINMANN'S 1st

B

Figure 3–10. Meniscal tests that depend on rotation of the knee. (From Tria AJ Jr, Klein KS: An Illustrated Guide to the Knee. New York, Churchill Livingstone, 1992.)

EXAMINATION OF THE LIGAMENTS AND ASSOCIATED CAPSULAR STRUCTURES

Stress examination can evaluate the status of the two collateral ligaments, the cruciate ligaments, and the posteromedial and posterolateral capsular structures.[8,9,14] Valgus stress in full extension is used to assess the medial collateral ligament and the associated posteromedial capsule. In 30 degrees of flexion, the same stress isolates the collateral ligament by relaxing the capsule (Fig. 3–11). Thus, full extension evaluates the ligament and capsule; flexion evaluates the ligament alone. In similar fashion, varus stress examination is performed in full extension and 30 degrees of flexion to evaluate the lateral collateral ligament and the posterolateral capsule (Fig. 3–12). During stress testing, the examiner should record the quality of the endpoint of the stress force. It can be graded from I to III or by the number of millimeters that the joint opens as determined by the examiner.[3] Neither approach is very objective; therefore, the author prefers to use the grading system. A grade I tear corresponds to a stress examination that allows minimal to no opening with the stress, but the manipulation causes pain along the line of the collateral ligament, most especially at the site of the tear. A grade II tear corresponds to a physical examination that shows some opening of the joint but with a distinct endpoint. A grade III tear shows no distinct endpoint to the evaluation, with the knee opening almost an unlimited degree.

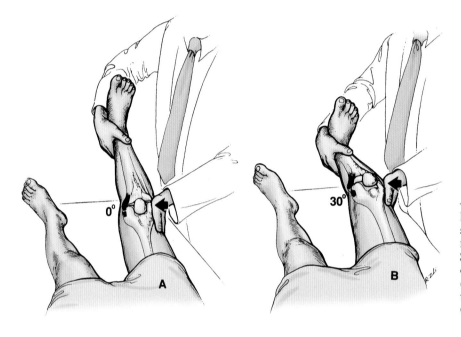

Figure 3–11. Valgus stress in extension tests the medial collateral ligament and the posteromedial capsule. Stress in 30 degrees of flexion tests only the medial collateral ligament. (From Tria AJ Jr, Klein KS: An Illustrated Guide to the Knee. New York, Churchill Livingstone, 1992.)

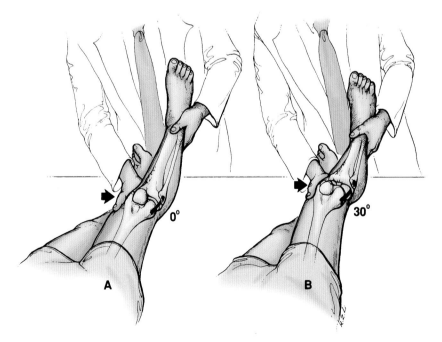

Figure 3–12. Varus stress in extension tests the lateral collateral ligament and the posterolateral capsule. Stress in 30 degrees of flexion tests only the lateral collateral ligament. (From Tria AJ Jr, Klein KS: An Illustrated Guide to the Knee. New York, Churchill Livingstone, 1992.)

A multitude of examinations can be used to determine the integrity of the anterior cruciate ligament. The Lachman (Fig. 3–13) and anterior drawer (Fig. 3–14) tests apply anterior stress to the tibia at 30 and 90 degrees of flexion, respectively.[18] The Lachman test is thought to be more sensitive for the posterolateral bundle of the cruciate and the anterior drawer test more sensitive for the anteromedial bundle. If the knee is held at 30 degrees of flexion and the patient is asked to contract the quadriceps muscle, an anterior cruciate–deficient knee will pull the tibia slightly forward before the lower part of the leg begins to extend (quadriceps active test for the anterior cruciate ligament) (Fig. 3–15).[4]

The flexion rotation drawer test builds on the Lachman test and notes tibial motion and femoral rotation from 15 to 30 degrees of flexion (Fig. 3–16).[16] Anterior force is applied to the tibia, starting at 15 degrees of flexion. This maneuver leads to anterior subluxation, much as in the Lachman test. With further knee flexion, the tibia reduces beneath the femur with a noticeable "clunk" and internal rotation of the femur.

The jerk, pivot-shift, and Losee tests emphasize anterolateral motion of the tibia beneath the femur. The Lachman, drawer, and flexion rotation drawer tests can be applied to the knee with the patient completely awake and unmedicated. The anterolateral tests produce more discomfort for the patient and are difficult to perform on a knee that has been recently injured; however, in a knee with chronic instability, the anterolateral tests are easier to perform than the Lachman, drawer, and flexion rotation drawer tests. In the chronic setting, the patient will often allow the examiner to perform the test and will comment that the motion and discomfort in the knee are similar to the instability experienced when the knee is actually symptomatic.

The jerk test is initiated in flexion with associated internal tibial rotation, forward pressure on the fibular head, and valgus stress (Fig. 3–17). This combination subluxes the lateral tibial condyle anteriorly. As the knee is brought into extension, the tibia reduces with a palpable clunk that is sometimes visible.

The pivot-shift test begins with the knee in full extension.[5-7] Valgus stress is applied along with internal tibial rotation and forward pressure on the fibular head. As flexion is commenced, the lateral aspect of the tibia again comes forward and then reduces on further flexion with a palpable clunk (Fig. 3–18). On occasion, this test may cause medial joint line pain indicative of an associated medial meniscal tear.

The Losee test is similar to the jerk test.[11-13] It also begins with the knee in flexion and valgus stress. The tibia, however, is initially held in external rotation. As the knee is gradually extended, the tibia is rotated internally, and the clunk of the reduction is again felt as in the jerk

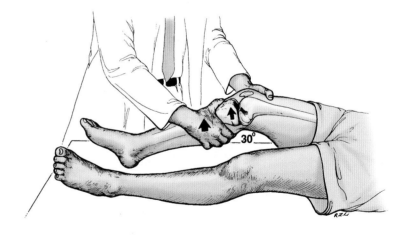

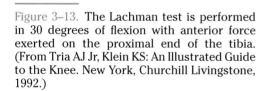

Figure 3–13. The Lachman test is performed in 30 degrees of flexion with anterior force exerted on the proximal end of the tibia. (From Tria AJ Jr, Klein KS: An Illustrated Guide to the Knee. New York, Churchill Livingstone, 1992.)

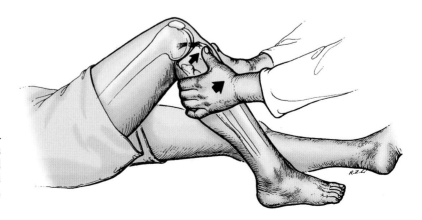

Figure 3–14. The anterior drawer test is performed with the knee flexed to 90 degrees and anterior force applied to the proximal end of the tibia. (From Tria AJ Jr, Klein KS: An Illustrated Guide to the Knee. New York, Churchill Livingstone, 1992.)

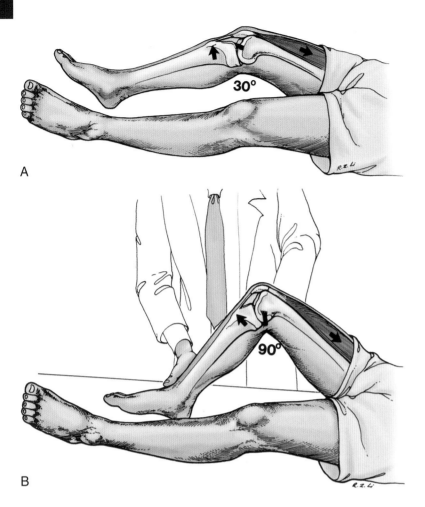

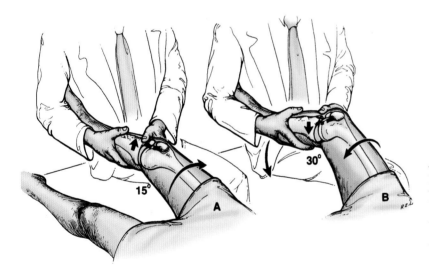

Figure 3–15. Quadriceps active test for the anterior cruciate ligament in 30 degrees of flexion (**A**) and for the posterior cruciate ligament in 90 degrees of flexion (**B**). (From Scott WN [ed]: The Knee. St Louis, CV Mosby, 1994.)

Figure 3–16. In the flexion rotation drawer test, the tibia is cradled in the examiner's hands while the knee is flexed to demonstrate tibial reduction and internal femoral rotation. (From Tria AJ Jr, Klein KS: An Illustrated Guide to the Knee. New York, Churchill Livingstone, 1992.)

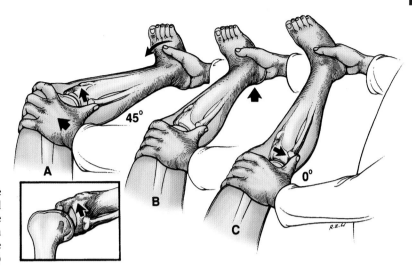

Figure 3–17. The jerk test begins with the knee in flexion, and internal rotation and valgus stress are applied to demonstrate anterolateral subluxation of the tibia. (From Tria AJ Jr, Klein KS: An Illustrated Guide to the Knee. New York, Churchill Livingstone, 1992.)

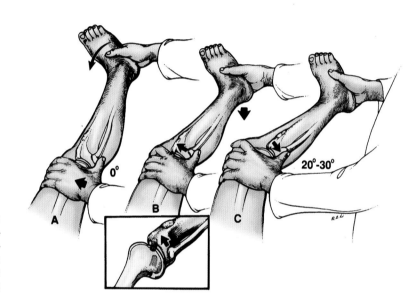

Figure 3–18. The pivot-shift test begins with the knee in full extension, and internal rotation and valgus stress are applied to demonstrate anterolateral subluxation. (From Tria AJ Jr, Klein KS: An Illustrated Guide to the Knee. New York, Churchill Livingstone, 1992.)

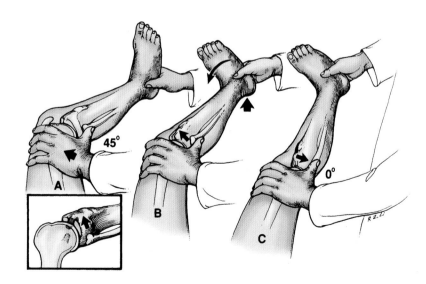

Figure 3–19. The Losee test begins with the knee in flexion, but the foot is externally rotated. Valgus stress is applied, and the tibia is internally rotated as the knee is extended. (From Tria AJ Jr, Klein KS: An Illustrated Guide to the Knee. New York, Churchill Livingstone, 1992.)

test. The test attempts to accentuate the subluxation with external tibial rotation (Fig. 3–19).

The posterior cruciate ligament can be evaluated with two primary tests and one secondary test. The "posterior" Lachman test is performed in 30 degrees of flexion, and the tibia is forced posteriorly (Fig. 3–20). In the posterior drawer test (Fig. 3–21), the knee is positioned in 90 degrees of flexion, and posterior force is then applied. The varus stress examination in full extension is said to include the posterior cruciate ligament. If the lateral aspect of the knee opens with varus stress in full extension, from the discussion earlier, the lateral collateral ligament and the posterolateral capsular structures are included. Some examiners believe that this opening cannot occur without posterior cruciate disruption. The author disagrees with this statement and believes that the varus stress examination can have a positive result with an intact posterior cruciate ligament. Grading of the degree of opening will sometimes help in determining the total amount of injury. A grade I or II laxity test is more likely to include a lateral collateral ligament and a posterolateral capsule tear with an intact posterior cruciate ligament, whereas grade III laxity with a completely indistinct endpoint may indeed include a posterior cruciate ligament tear.

A knee with chronic posterior cruciate ligament laxity will often have a posterior sag. If the patient attempts to contract the quadriceps muscle with the knee in 90 degrees of flexion, the tibia will come forward before the lower part of the leg begins to extend (quadriceps active test for the posterior cruciate ligament) (see Fig. 3–15).

The posteromedial capsule is evaluated with the Slocum test (anterior drawer test at 90 degrees of flexion with external rotation of the lower part of the leg).[2,17] When the tibia is rotated externally, the posteromedial capsule should tighten and allow less anterior excursion than with the drawer test in neutral rotation. When the posteromedial capsule is torn, the Slocum test demonstrates an increase in anterior motion of the tibia versus the drawer test in neutral, and the tibia tends to "roll out" (Fig. 3–22).

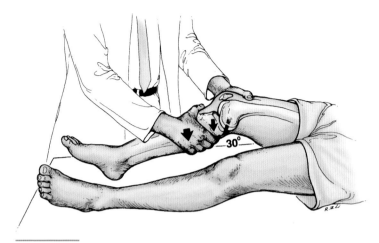

Figure 3–20. The "posterior" Lachman test applies posterior force to the proximal end of the tibia with the knee flexed 30 degrees. (From Tria AJ Jr, Klein KS: An Illustrated Guide to the Knee. New York, Churchill Livingstone, 1992.)

The posterolateral capsule is tested with the anterior drawer test at 90 degrees of flexion and internal tibial rotation. If the posterolateral capsule is torn, the drawer test with internal rotation will show an increase in anterior motion versus the drawer test in neutral, and the tibia will tend to "roll in" (Fig. 3–23). The hyperextension recurvatum sign correlates with injury to the posterolateral capsule. If the leg is held in full extension, the knee hyperextends and the tibia rotates externally because of absence of the posterolateral capsule and its supporting structures (Fig. 3–24). The reverse pivot-shift test is performed with

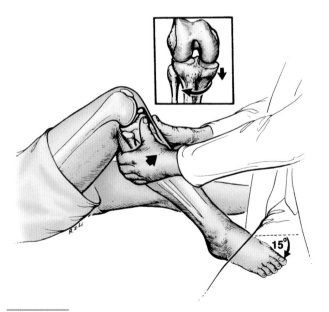

Figure 3–22. The Slocum test is performed in 90 degrees of flexion with the foot externally rotated and anterior proximal tibial force applied to test the posteromedial capsule. (From Tria AJ Jr, Klein KS: An Illustrated Guide to the Knee. New York, Churchill Livingstone, 1992.)

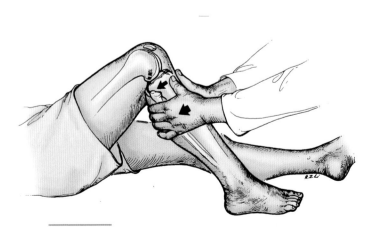

Figure 3–21. The posterior drawer test is performed in 90 degrees of flexion with posterior force on the proximal end of the tibia. (From Tria AJ Jr, Klein KS: An Illustrated Guide to the Knee. New York, Churchill Livingstone, 1992.)

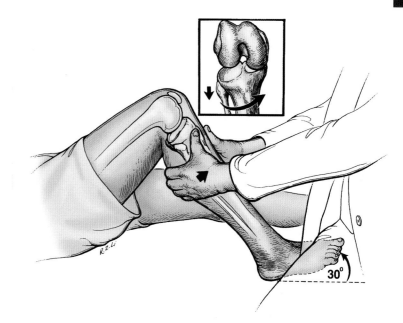

Figure 3–23. The posterolateral capsule is tested with the knee flexed to 90 degrees and anterior proximal tibial force applied with the tibia rotated internally. (From Tria AJ Jr, Klein KS: An Illustrated Guide to the Knee. New York, Churchill Livingstone, 1992.)

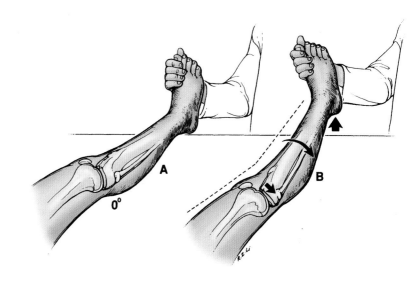

Figure 3–24. The hyperextension recurvatum test demonstrates increased extension of the knee along with the external tibial rotation and drop-back. (From Tria AJ Jr, Klein KS: An Illustrated Guide to the Knee. New York, Churchill Livingstone, 1992.)

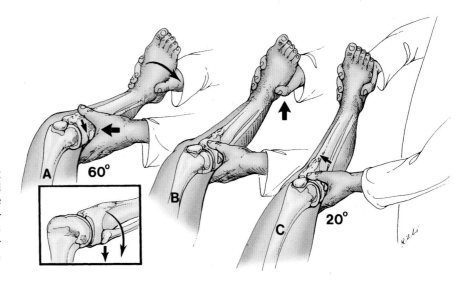

Figure 3–25. The reverse pivot-shift test begins with the knee flexed, and the tibia is externally rotated. The knee is then extended to demonstrate posterolateral capsular laxity. (From Tria AJ Jr, Klein KS: An Illustrated Guide to the Knee. New York, Churchill Livingstone, 1992.)

Table 3–2. Stress Examination (in Order
of Sensitivity)

LIGAMENT	TEST
MCL	Valgus stress (30 degrees flexion)
LCL	Varus stress (30 degrees flexion)
ACL	Lachman, flexion-rotation-drawer, anterior drawer, jerk, pivot, Losee
PCL	Posterior Lachman, posterior drawer, sag (late), (? varus laxity in full extension)
Posteromedial capsule	Valgus in full extension, Slocum
Posterolateral capsule	Varus in full extension, drawer in internal rotation, hyperextension recurvatum test

ACL, anterior cruciate ligament; LCL, lateral collateral ligament; MCL, medial collateral ligament; PCL, posterior cruciate ligament.

the tibia rotated externally and the knee flexed. As the knee is extended, the tibia reduces with a palpable clunk, indicative of a deficient posterolateral capsule (Fig. 3–25).[10]

During examination of each ligament and capsular structure, all the tests should be applied to each area as indicated. Despite sophisticated computers and measurement devices, physical examination of the knee remains the most reliable tool for diagnostic evaluation of the supporting structures. On occasion, diagnostic evaluation of the knee may not be complete despite physical examination, magnetic resonance imaging, and local anesthetic infiltration. Some of the stress tests are more sensitive than others (Table 3–2), and the examiner may rely on that sensitivity, or it may be necessary to perform an examination under anesthesia along with arthroscopy to completely confirm the anatomy of the injury. Diagnostic accuracy is the key to appropriate therapeutic intervention.

References

1. Apley AC: The diagnosis of meniscal injuries. J Bone Joint Surg 29:78, 1947.
2. Bargar WL, Moreland JR, Markolf KL, et al: The effect of tibia-foot rotatory position on the anterior drawer test. Clin Orthop 173:200, 1983.
3. Committee on the Medical Aspects of Sports, American Medical Association: Standard Nomenclature of Athletic Injuries. Chicago, American Medical Association, 1968, pp 99-101.
4. Daniel DM, Stone ML, Barnett P, et al: Use of the quadriceps active test to diagnose posterior cruciate ligament disruption and measure posterior laxity of the knee. J Bone Joint Surg Am 70:386, 1988.
5. Feagin JA, Cooke TD: Prone examination for anterior cruciate ligament insufficiency. J Bone Joint Surg Br 71:863, 1989.
6. Fetto JF, Marshall JL: Injury to the anterior cruciate ligament producing the pivot-shift sign. J Bone Joint Surg Am 61:710, 1979.
7. Galway RD, Beaupre A, MacIntosh DL: Pivot shift: A clinical sign of symptomatic anterior cruciate insufficiency. J Bone Joint Surg Br 54:763, 1972.
8. Hughston JC, Andrews JR, Cross MJ, et al: Classification of knee ligament instabilities. Part I. The medial compartment and cruciate ligaments. J Bone Joint Surg Am 58:159, 1976.
9. Hughston JC, Andrews JR, Cross MJ, et al: Classification of knee ligament instabilities. Part II. The lateral compartment. J Bone Joint Surg Am 58:173, 1976.
10. Jakob RP, Hassler H, Staeubli HU: Observations on rotatory instability of the lateral compartment of the knee: Experimental studies on the functional anatomy and pathomechanics of the true and the reversed pivot shift sign. Acta Orthop Scand 52:1, 1981.
11. Larson RL: Physical examination in the diagnosis of rotatory instability. Clin Orthop 172:38, 1983.
12. Losee RE: Diagnosis of chronic injury to the anterior cruciate ligament. Orthop Clin North Am 16:83, 1985.
13. Losee RE, Johnson TR, Southwick WO: Anterior subluxation of the lateral tibial plateau. J Bone Joint Surg Am 60:1015, 1978.
14. Marshall JL, Baugher WH: Stability examination of the knee: A simple anatomic approach. Clin Orthop 146:78, 1980.
15. McMurray TP: The semilunar cartilages. J Bone Joint Surg 29:407, 1942.
16. Noyes FR, Butler D, Grood E, et al: Clinical paradoxes of anterior cruciate instability and a new test to detect its instability. Orthop Trans 2:36, 1978.
17. Slocum DB, Larson RL: Rotatory instability of the knee: Its pathogenesis and a clinical test to demonstrate its presence. J Bone Joint Surg Am 50:211, 1968.
18. Torg JS, Conrad W, Kalen V: Clinical diagnosis of anterior cruciate ligament instability in the athlete. Am J Sports Med 4:84, 1976.

CHAPTER 4

Neurophysiology of the Knee

Charles Buz Swanik • Christopher D. Harner • Scott M. Lephart • Jeffrey B. Driban

Contemporary research regarding the preservation and restoration of knee function now recognizes the significant neurosensory role of capsuloligamentous and tenomuscular structures, as well as their contribution to neuromuscular coordination and the dynamic restraint mechanism. The clinical relevance can be appreciated by noting the strong correlations established between knee dysfunction and aberrations in the sensorimotor system that compromise joint homeostasis.[11,93] The following will review knee neurophysiology, discuss the sensorimotor system in normal and pathological joints, and outline considerations for surgical management and rehabilitation.

TERMINOLOGY

The recent abundance of clinical research investigating sensorimotor function has led to some confusion related to proper nomenclature that should be addressed. The foundation of somatosensory awareness depends on populations of specialized nerve endings called mechanoreceptors that innervate cutaneous, capsuloligamentous, and tenomuscular tissue. The sensory information from mechanoreceptors that provides conscious and unconscious appreciation of joint position is termed *proprioception*, whereas *kinesthesia* refers to the sensation of joint motion or acceleration.[111] Mechanoreceptors are also capable of providing a *sense of force* that allows the body to differentiate between various loads.[24,74] Proprioceptive and kinesthetic signals are transmitted via *afferent* (sensory) pathways, and the motor responses propagate along *efferent* pathways.[46] In general, the "transformation of neural information [motor commands] back into physical energy" via muscle activation is referred to as *neuromuscular control*.[75,76] Three mechanisms for motor control are involved in interpreting afferent information and coordinating efferent responses.[39,76] The first is *feed-forward* neuromuscular control and involves planning movements and preprogramming muscle activation based on past experience.[86] The second is a *feedback* process that continuously modifies muscle activity through numerous reflex pathways.[106] The dynamic systems model, the third theory, incorporates the previous two mechanisms and proposes that variability in motion is unavoidable and necessary to develop the unique movement patterns that account for environmental, task-specific, and anatomic variations.[37] The level of muscle activation and the elastic properties of the tenomuscular unit determine total muscle stiffness.[109,112,119] From a mechanical perspective,

muscle stiffness is the degree to which a muscle resists length changes.[105] Bach et al[3] suggested that the neuromuscular control apparatus modifies muscle stiffness, depending on the requirements of a task, to optimize these properties. Therefore, neural regulation of muscle stiffness appears to be an important component in the selection and performance of movement strategies and dynamic restraint capabilities.[3,150] Dynamic restraint, the active contribution to joint stability, is dictated by several neuromuscular characteristics, including preparatory and reactive muscle activation, muscle stiffness, flexibility, and muscle force production.[141]

SENSORIMOTOR SYSTEM

Histology and Structural Anatomy

CAPSULOLIGAMENTOUS MECHANORECEPTORS

Cognitive appreciation of joint load, position, movement, speed, and direction is mediated by peripheral mechanoreceptors.[52] Mechanoreceptors are capable of detecting the deformation of adjacent tissue and encoding sensory signals that provide information concerning intrinsic and extrinsic joint forces. Capsuloligamentous structures appear to contain significant volumes of neuronal tissue (1.0% to 2.5% in the anterior cruciate ligament [ACL]), and a large portion of the afferent fibers entering the spinal cord originate from joint mechanoreceptors.[72,156,159] Freeman and Wyke[44] classified the capsuloligamentous mechanoreceptors identified in the knee by morphology. Their four categories include type I (Ruffini endings and Mazzoni endings), type II (pacinian corpuscles and Meissner corpuscles), type III (Golgi endings), and type IV (free nerve endings; Fig. 4–1).[44] Each type of mechanoreceptor can be distinguished by its location, adaptation to stimulation, and perceived sensation (Table 4–1). When mechanical energy is applied to the receptor, deformation-responsive ion channels are disrupted, and the resting membrane potential is altered. If the membrane potential exceeds the generator threshold for that mechanoreceptor, an action potential is transmitted along the peripheral afferent fiber (Fig. 4–2).[55,76] Greater mechanical deformation can be coded by both an increase in the rate of discharge (temporal summation) and an increase in the quantity of mechanoreceptors stimulated.[44,55] Direct recordings from joint afferent fibers via microneurography

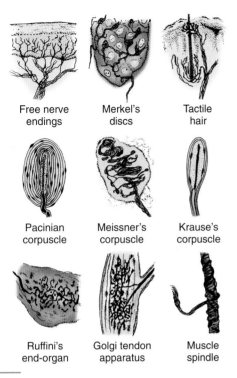

Figure 4–1. Capsuloligamentous, tenomuscular, and cutaneous mechanoreceptors found in the periphery. (From Guyton AC: Human Physiology and Mechanisms of Disease, 6th ed. Philadelphia, WB Saunders, 1997, p 377.)

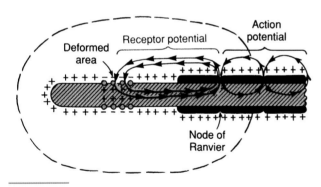

Figure 4–2. Mechanoreceptor nerve ending. Mechanical energy applied to the receptor produces a receptor potential. If the receptor potential exceeds the generator threshold, an action potential is transmitted along peripheral afferent fibers. (Modified from Loëwenstein WR: Excitation and inactivation in a receptor membrane. Ann N Y Acad Sci 94:510, 1961.)

have demonstrated that small loads (1.8 to 5 g) applied to the knee ligaments are sufficient to elicit neural responses.[1,55,109] However, significant motor recruitment is produced only at forces that would be nearly capable of tearing the ligament.[137]

Mechanoreceptors are classified by their morphology and response/adaptation to a sustained stimulus. Quick-adapting (QA) mechanoreceptors cease discharging within milliseconds after the onset of a stimulus, whereas the action potentials of slow-adapting (SA) mechanoreceptors persist in the presence of a continued stimulus (Fig. 4–3).[30] Therefore, QA mechanoreceptors can provide conscious and unconscious kinesthetic sensations of joint motion or acceleration, and SA mechanoreceptors provide continuous proprioceptive feedback relative to joint position.[2,133,134]

TENOMUSCULAR RECEPTORS

In addition to capsuloligamentous receptors, muscle spindles and Golgi tendon organs provide sensory feedback through changes in the length and tension of tenomuscular structures. Muscle spindles are completely encapsulated organs embedded in series with skeletal muscle.[5,31,55] The capsules contain intrafusal fibers and, on each end, extrafusal fibers (Fig. 4–4). Intrafusal fibers are the sensory organs innervated by afferent nerves, whereas extrafusal fibers have contractile properties and are innervated by small gamma motor (efferent) nerves. Gamma efferents are anatomically independent of the large alpha motor fibers innervating skeletal muscle, but they often work in harmony.[5,89] Gamma motor nerves can be directly stimulated by afferent signals from cutaneous, muscular,

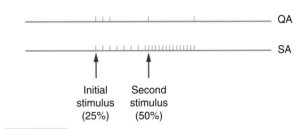

Figure 4–3. Characteristics of slow-adapting (SA) and quick-adapting (QA) mechanoreceptors at two intensity levels.

Table 4–1. Capsuloligamentous Mechanoreceptors

TYPE	RECEPTORS	LOCATION	ADAPTATION	SENSATION
I	Ruffini endings Mazzoni endings	Capsule and extrinsic ligaments	SA	Proprioception
II	Pacinian corpuscles Meissner corpuscles	Deep capsule and fat pads	QA	Kinesthesia
III	Golgi endings	Intrinsic/extrinsic ligaments	SA	Proprioception
IV	Free nerve endings	Capsule, ligaments, fat pads, synovium, and blood vessels	SA	Pain

QA, quick adapting, SA, slow adapting.

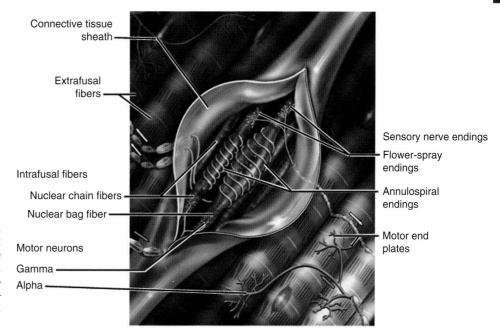

Connective tissue
sheath

Extrafusal
fibers

Sensory nerve endings

Flower-spray
endings

Intrafusal fibers

Nuclear chain fibers

Annulospiral
endings

Nuclear bag fiber

Motor neurons

Motor end
plates

Gamma

Alpha

Figure 4–4. Muscle spindles. (Reprinted from Saladin KS: Anatomy & Physiology: The Unity of Form and Function, 2nd ed. New York, McGraw-Hill, 2001, p 564, with permission from The McGraw-Hill Companies.)

and articular receptors. The excitation level of gamma motor nerves regulates the contraction of extrafusal fibers, but only to modify the length or maintain tension of the intrafusal fibers. The independent function of gamma motor nerves regulates the sensitivity of muscle spindles to muscle length/velocity and accommodates for muscle shortening while continuously transmitting afferent signals.[5] The concentration of muscle spindles in a specific muscle correlates with the sensitivity to changes in muscle length.[120] Therefore, the musculature of the neck (46 to 107 muscle spindles per gram of muscle) would be more sensitive to small perturbations/movements than the leg musculature would (13 to 19 muscle spindles per gram).[120] Afferent signals from muscle spindles provide sensory information but also project directly on skeletal motor nerves through very fast monosynaptic pathways.[154] This is the mechanism (stretch reflexes) whereby muscle spindles have a profound effect on muscle activity.[106,154] If the gamma loop becomes disrupted (i.e., ACL rupture), maximal voluntary activation can be hindered because the muscle spindles are not able to optimally stimulate the Ia afferents needed to recruit high-threshold motor units.[82]

The second type of mechanoreceptor, the Golgi tendon organ (GTO), populates the musculotendinous junction and is responsible for monitoring muscle tension.[55] Because changes in muscle length also alter muscle tension, GTOs protect the tenomuscular unit by reflexively inhibiting agonist and exciting antagonist muscles.[67] GTOs therefore have the opposite effect of muscle spindles. When stimulated by high muscle tension, they elicit reflexive inhibition (relaxation) in the agonist muscle being loaded (Fig. 4–5).[55,67] An additional function of GTOs is to provide feedback along with supplemental signals from cutaneous, articular, and other muscle receptors; these signals can be processed to generate a perception of force and weight.[26] The sense of force and weight discrimination represents a peripherally driven sense of

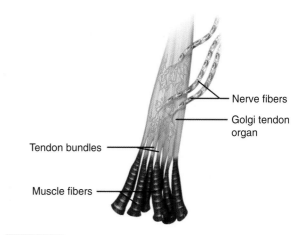

Nerve fibers

Golgi tendon
organ

Tendon bundles

Muscle fibers

Figure 4–5. Golgi tendon organs (GTOs). (Reprinted from Saladin KS: Anatomy & Physiology: The Unity of Form and Function, 2nd ed. New York, McGraw-Hill, 2001, p 567, with permission from The McGraw-Hill Companies.)

force and a centrally incorporated sense of effort, which together allow an individual to determine the "just noticeable difference" between loads.[24,74]

Speculation on how sensory information from peripheral mechanoreceptors is transmitted to the central nervous system (CNS) was originally based on the labeled line theorem.[19] This model suggests that individual mechanoreceptors have private pathways to convey sensory information.[19] However, recent experiments support more complex patterns of afferent information transmitted by populations (ensembles) of mechanoreceptors, referred to as *ensemble coding*.[19] Research has established that a given ensemble contains mechanoreceptors with varying response profiles and sensitivities to different types of mechanical stimuli. The combination of these properties gives ensemble-coded signals the capacity to furnish more discrete information concerning peripheral sensations.

NEURAL PATHWAYS

Decoding and utilization of the sensory information from articular and tenomuscular structures require analysis of the pathways engaged by peripheral afferents and their influence on motor control at three distinct levels: spinal, brainstem, and cerebral cortex. Sherrington[127] first outlined the conceptual role of peripheral receptors as a source of signals for joint sensations and for mediating reflexes of the neuromuscular control system. Encoded signals concerning joint load, motion, and position are transmitted from peripheral receptors via afferent pathways to the CNS.[44,46,127] The conduction velocity of afferent pathways is determined by their diameter (0.2 to 70 μm) and covering (myelinated or unmyelinated). At velocities ranging from 0.3 to 120 m/s, the fastest peripheral sensation could travel from the foot to the brain in 15 ms.[55] However, signals in the nervous systems become

delayed (0.5 ms) as synapses are encountered (synaptic delay); therefore, monosynaptic pathways represent the most efficient signals.[125]

Levels of Motor Control

At the spinal level, peripheral afferents enter the CNS through the dorsal root ganglion.[76] Within the spinal cord, monosynaptic reflex pathways directly link muscle spindle afferents with alpha motor nerves in the agonist muscle. Interneurons also form polysynaptic junctions linking the peripheral afferent fibers with additional alpha and gamma motor nerves (Fig. 4–6). The afferent signal from one extremity is capable of influencing the kinematics bilaterally through spinal interneurons, thereby leading to complex involuntary motor patterns, such as the stepping response in gait.[76] These observations emphasize the important reflexive contribution of articular mechanoreceptors in the regulation of muscle stiffness/recruitment, joint protection, postural control, and coordination of movement. Although articular afferent

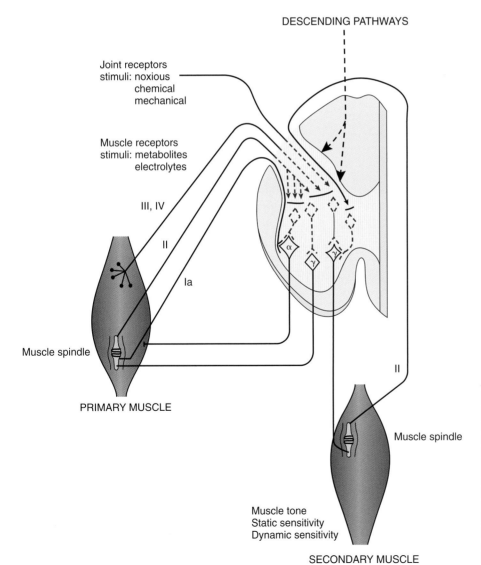

Figure 4–6. Monosynaptic and polysynaptic pathways linking afferent (sensory) mechanoreceptors with alpha and gamma efferent (motor) nerves. (Redrawn from Johansson H, Sojka P: Pathophysiological mechanisms involved in genesis and spread on muscular tension in occupational muscle pain and in chronic musculoskeletal pain syndromes: A hypothesis. Med Hypotheses 35:196, 1991.)

pathways do not exert as much influence directly on skeletal motoneurons as previously reported, they do have frequent and potent effects on muscle spindles via gamma motor nerves.[73,76] Muscle spindles in turn regulate muscle activation through the monosynaptic stretch reflex. This sophisticated articular-tenomuscular link is described as the "final common input."[1,73] The final common input suggests that muscle spindles integrate peripheral afferent information and transmit a final modified signal to the CNS.[2,71] This feedback loop is responsible for continuously modifying muscle activity during locomotion via the muscle spindle's stretch reflex arc.[64,112] However, disruption of afferent feedback as a result of soft-tissue injury can have a profound effect on motor control.[11,21,29,35,90,141]

The network of synapses in the spinal cord also propagates afferent signals through the dorsal columns and spinocerebellar ascending tracts.[55,76] Long-loop reflexes in the brainstem are responsible for postural stability and the maintenance of balance. Postural control is regulated by the same peripheral afferent mechanism that mediates somatosensory input and is partially dependent on the inherent ability to integrate joint sensations with neuromuscular control. The highest level of motor control occurs at the cerebral cortex, where joint load, motion, and position are perceived in the somesthetic area.[55] The sensory feedback from errors and success in movement patterns can be retained and used as a reference for preprogramming muscle activation strategies (Fig. 4–7).

Presynaptic Inhibition

Presynaptic inhibition at the interneuron (in the spinal cord) refers to a decrease in the release of neurotransmitters from the presynaptic terminal. This suppression is continuously mediating normal reflexes, which if left unregulated, would often produce exaggerated responses to the applied demands. The reduction in neurotransmitters leads to an inhibitory effect on the interneuron that directly influences the excitability of the motoneuron pool (a collection of neurons transmitting signals to the muscles).[65] Presynaptic inhibition may play a critical role in balance. It has been reported that younger patients in a standing position suppress their reflexes, whereas older patients fail to restrict the release of neurotransmitters, which leads to greater postural sway.[145] The Jendrassik

maneuver, a contraction of the muscles in the upper part of the body (particularly the forearm and jaw muscles), is a common clinical means of minimizing presynaptic inhibition.[158] The reduction in presynaptic inhibition is due to a decrease in tonic descending input, which leads to a greater contraction in response to a rapid stretch (tendon tap).[158] During rehabilitation, presynaptic inhibition presents a challenge in the presence of joint effusion as a main component of autogenic muscle inhibition. Autogenic muscle inhibition is a protective mechanism leading to a decrease in the ability to actively recruit the surrounding musculature even though it has not been directly traumatized.[65]

Reflex Reversal

During normal gait, group 1 (large diameter, myelinated) afferents may result in different responses during the swing and stance phases.[78,100] Stimulation of the common peroneal nerve during the swing phase induces suppression (autogenic inhibition) of the biceps femoris, but during the early stance phase, such stimulation facilitates contraction.[100] This reflex reversal is caused by a reduction in the inhibitory pathway and selective facilitation of the excitatory pathways. Reflex reversal is a key mechanism that helps stabilize the knee during the stance phase of gait. As reflexes facilitate contraction of the biceps femoris during the early stance phase, a reflexive burst in the quadriceps leads to a cocontraction that increases the stability of the knee when body weight is introduced.[100]

Feed-Forward and Feedback Neuromuscular Control

Traditional beliefs on the processing of afferent signals into efferent responses for dynamic stabilization were based on reactive or feedback neuromuscular control pathways.[89] More contemporary theories emphasize feed-forward control and the significance of preparatory muscle tension in anticipation of movements and joint loads. Feed-forward motor control uses advance information about a task, usually from experience, to preprogram muscle activity.[39,86] This requires building an internal

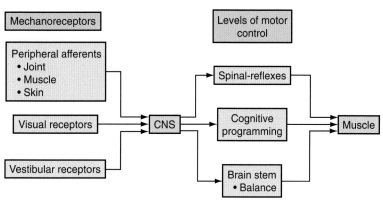

Figure 4–7. Schematic diagram depicting the neural pathways and three levels of motor control governing muscle activation strategies. CNS, central nervous system. (Adapted, by permission, from Lephart S, Henry T: The physiological basis for open and closed kinetic chain rehabilitation for the upper extremity. J Sport Rehabil 5:78, 1996.)

model depicting the expected conditions with all of the known parameters of a task.[39,76] These centrally generated motor commands are responsible for preparatory muscle activity and high-velocity movements.[76] The feed-forward mechanism is not dependent on reflex pathways and, once initiated, executes motor commands very quickly.[76] Furthermore, preparatory excitation of the alpha motor nerves is frequently accompanied by activation of the gamma motor nerves, referred to as alpha-gamma coactivation.[31,38,71,89,106] Alpha-gamma coactivation, which helps couple muscle and muscle spindle length changes, increases the sensitivity of the muscle spindles to stretch, referred to as gain, thereby heightening the awareness of joint motion and position.[33,53] In addition, the heightened sensitivity of spindles evokes more vigorous stretch reflexes that are superimposed on descending motor commands.[38,112] Sensory information in feed-forward motor control is used to evaluate the results after a task and help preprogram future muscle activation strategies to improve coordination. Preactivated muscles may also identify unexpected joint loads more quickly and decrease the electromechanical delay influencing feedback neuromuscular control.[33,38,53]

The feedback mechanism of motor control is characterized by numerous reflex pathways that continuously adjust ongoing muscle activity.[23,39,89,106] Information from joint and muscle receptors reflexively coordinates muscle activity toward the completion of a task. This feedback process is responsible for regulating muscle tone, but polysynaptic and cortical pathways result in long conduction delays. Feedback neuromuscular control is best equipped for regulating slow movements and maintaining posture.[76] The efficacy of reflex-mediated dynamic joint stabilization has been questioned and appears to require much quicker responses (30 to 70 ms) if it is to be effective in protecting the joint.[14,151,152] It is likely that the presence of preparatory muscle activity enhances the reactive properties of muscle so that unexpected joint perturbations are more quickly detected by the muscle spindles.[38,40] The stretch reflex then facilitates reactive muscle activity in already pretensioned muscle, thereby increasing the reactive capability of muscle.

Adaptations to feed-forward and feedback neuromuscular control can refine motor coordination if the sensory and motor pathways are habitually stimulated through practice. Furthermore, as the body performs a specific task, it repeats the pattern with a certain degree of variability (Fig. 4–8). Based on a dynamic systems approach, this variability allows the body to adjust to unique constraints (personal, task, and environmental) and is critical for the neuromuscular system to remain flexible enough to adapt to future complex environments.[37] Each time a signal passes through a sequence of synapses, the synapses become more capable of transmitting the same signal.[55] When these pathways are "facilitated" regularly, memory of that signal is created and can be recalled to program future movement patterns.[55] Frequent facilitation therefore enhances both the memory of tasks for preprogrammed motor control and the reflex pathways for reactive neuromuscular control. Injuries are also capable of altering the activation patterns, as demonstrated by females with an ACL-deficient knee. After

an ACL injury, it has been reported that preparatory activity, the feed-forward response, is increased and provides the injured knee with greater stability; however, it is still debated whether the reflex characteristics change.[14-16,70,87,123,141,151,152]

Static and Dynamic Restraint Mechanism

The soft-tissue structures of the knee provide static support, govern knee kinematics, and restrict excessive motion. Thus their primary roles are to support, stabilize, and guide skeletal segments.[155] This requires all elements to possess complex biomechanical characteristics contingent on their responsibilities as primary and secondary restraints. The orientation and contractile and elastic properties of muscles and tendons also assist in joint stability and enable skeletal muscle to impart or absorb joint forces while restricting excessive motion.[149] By transmitting, absorbing, and storing energy, the contractile and elastic components function much like a spring; however, the musculotendinous tissues dissipate energy with time and are less efficient.[149,150] The mechanical properties of tenomuscular structures can assist in joint stability because of their dampening qualities, which are velocity dependent and will resist faster length changes with more force.

Recently, the interaction between static and dynamic restraint mechanisms has received even greater appreciation in the restoration of functional joint stability. Injury to the static restraints results in not only mechanical disturbance but also loss of joint sensation because of partial deafferentation of peripheral mechanoreceptors.[7,8,94,95] This disrupts the sensory feedback mediating neuromuscular control at the spinal, brainstem, and cortical levels. Substantial evidence suggests that the aberration in muscle activity subsequent to a knee injury is a result of disrupted afferent pathways.[15,21,29,90,123,135,140,141,151] Therefore, injury to the static structures not only reduces the joint's mechanical stability but also often diminishes the capability of the dynamic restraint mechanism and thus renders the knee functionally unstable (Fig. 4–9). When excessive or repetitive loads are placed on the joint, the dynamic restraint mechanism must compensate for mechanical instability to avoid reinjury.[9,95,152]

Previous research suggests that several neuromuscular characteristics contribute to the dynamic restraint mechanism.[12,15,22,27,91,105,137,141,151] The individual expression and interaction of these characteristics in the thigh muscles and the gastrocnemius govern dynamic restraint and the restoration of functional stability. Clinical research quantifying these characteristics has provided insight in improving the quality of injury prevention, management, and rehabilitation.

Sensorimotor Testing Models

Clinically based research on neuromuscular control has focused on questions regarding the sensory role of capsuloligamentous structures and the pathoetiology of joint

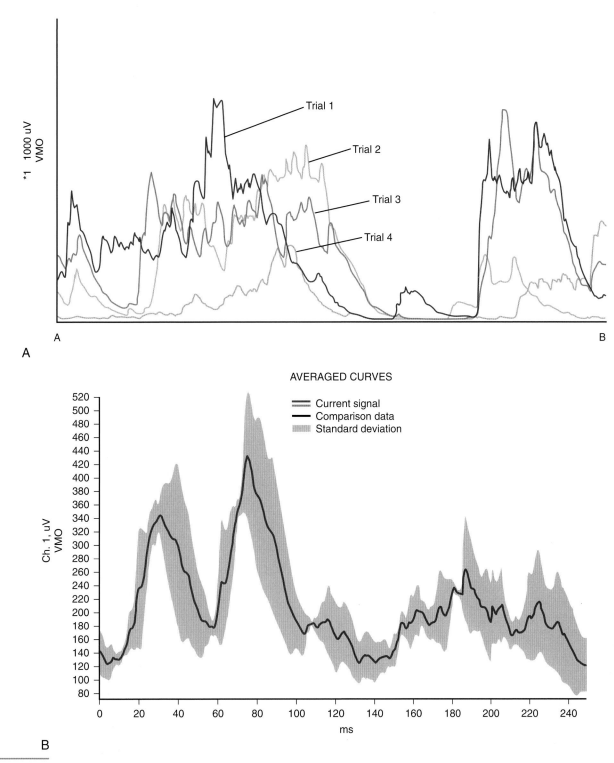

Figure 4–8. **A** and **B**, Vastus medialis activity over four consecutive cycles of motion demonstrating the variability in reactive muscle activity (Reprinted, by permission, from Swanik CB, Lephart SM, Giraldo JL, et al: Reactive muscle firing of anterior cruciate ligament–injured females during functional activities. J Athl Training 34:127, 1999.)

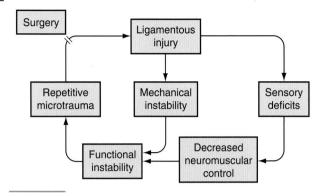

Figure 4–9. Paradigm suggesting a cyclic pattern beginning with injury to the static restraints (ligaments, joint capsule). Joint deafferentation diminishes sensory feedback, thereby inhibiting the normal motor response and decreasing neuromuscular control. The combination of decreased neuromuscular control and mechanical instability results in functional joint instability and contributes to an insidious pattern of repetitive injury. (Reprinted, by permission, from Lephart S, Henry T: The physiological basis for open and closed kinetic chain rehabilitation for the upper extremity. J Sport Rehabil 5:80, 1996.)

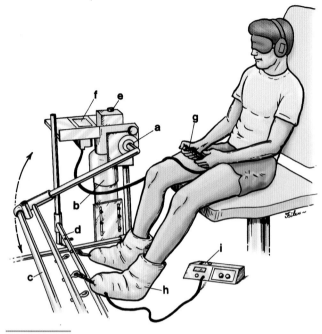

Figure 4–10. Proprioception testing device. a, Rotational transducer; b, motor; c, moving adapter; d, stationary arm; e, control panel; f, digital microprocessor; g, hand-held on/off switch; h, compression sleeve; i, pneumatic compression device. (Reprinted, by permission, from Lephart SM, Kocher MS, Fu FH, et al: Proprioception following anterior cruciate ligament reconstruction. J Sport Rehabil 1:191, 1992.)

injury. The objectives of this research have been to establish neuromuscular profiles by evaluating both the sensory and the motor characteristics specific to several clinical conditions, including the effects of injury, surgery, rehabilitation, prevention programs, and strength and conditioning routines. These sensorimotor characteristics include proprioception and kinesthesia, sense of force, muscle activation strategies and reflex latencies, strength, balance or postural stability, and muscle stiffness. The test models used to assess these characteristics include proprioception testing devices, dynamic electromyography (EMG), somatosensory evoked potentials, joint perturbation devices, isokinetic dynamometers, force platforms, and balance stabilometry units. These characteristics in the knee govern dynamic restraint and the restoration of functional stability.

PROPRIOCEPTION AND KINESTHESIA

Assessment of joint position and motion sense in the knee provides some insight into the afferent pathways contributing to neuromuscular control in normal, pathological, and surgically reconstructed joints. Testing usually involves the construction of a device (Fig. 4–10) that measures active and passive joint rotation, but it can be accomplished with goniometers and/or motion analysis equipment (Fig. 4–11). To assess proprioception, subjects are required to reproduce joint position, either active or passive, and the error between an angle presented to the subject and the reproduced angle is recorded.[18,60,121] A larger error implies diminished proprioception. Kinesthesia is assessed by passively rotating the knee (0.5 to 2.0 degrees/s) until the subject indicates that motion is

perceived. This measurement is referred to as the threshold to detection of passive motion, with a larger score indicating decreased joint motion sense.[121,122]

FORCE PERCEPTION

The sense of force is centrally derived but receives peripheral input from cutaneous, joint, and muscle receptors (primarily GTOs).[24,26] Several methods have been developed to evaluate a patient's ability to determine loads. The contralateral limb–matching approach involves the participant using one extremity to produce a given force (typically percent maximal voluntary contraction) while receiving feedback. On completion, subjects are then asked to use the opposite extremity to reproduce that degree of force without feedback. Another method, weight discrimination (a just noticeable difference), involves asking an individual to feel two weights and notify the tester which weight was heavier. Force perception has been found to be altered by fatigue and numerous neurological disorders.[26,74]

DYNAMIC ELECTROMYOGRAPHY

The study of EMG is concerned with measuring the efferent response of muscles to descending and reflexive motor commands. Descending commands are associated with

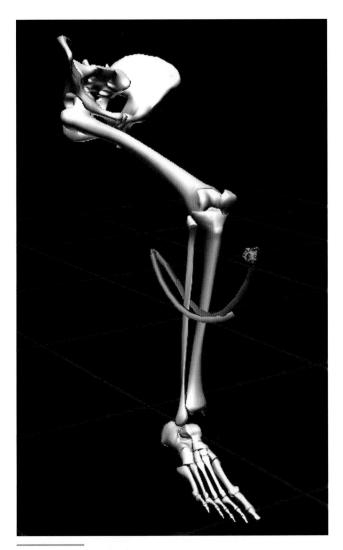

Figure 4–11. Motion analysis systems can be used to evaluate variation between movements.

preparatory muscle activity and feed-forward neuromuscular control, and reflexive commands mediate reactive muscle activity through the feedback process of motor control. Preparatory muscle activity is necessary to position the knee and anticipate joint loads, whereas reactive muscle activation compensates for unexpected events. Surface or indwelling electrodes adjacent to muscle tissue can detect the action potentials of many muscle fibers (ranging between a few microvolts to a few millivolts) as they pass the electrode.[13] Surface electrodes offer a gross observation of the muscle activity in a region, whereas a fine indwelling wire offers data limited to a small sphere around the end of the wire. Both techniques have many advantages: indwelling electrodes are optimal for measuring small or deep muscles (popliteus), and surface electrodes can provide a more encompassing data set on the activity of a larger region/muscle (i.e., medial hamstrings). The data acquired from EMG can be used to determine the onset, sequence, pattern, and magnitude of muscle activity. Frequency spectral analysis is occasionally performed to monitor muscle fatigue, which is characterized by a decrease in the mean frequency.[36] To interpret EMG data,

it is often necessary to synchronize the muscle activity with physical events. Markers are used to denote the time of physical events such as joint movement or ground contact. The magnitude of muscle activity is then quantified relative to a resting or maximum activation level, referred to as amplitude normalization.[156] When assessing muscle activation strategies during functional activities (running), repetitive cycles of motion can be recorded and normalized for time so that muscle activity is described relative to the phases of motion such as stance and swing.[156] EMG instrumentation is valuable for describing conscious and unconscious muscle activity in response to feed-forward and feedback motor commands; however, inference to muscle tension or force based on EMG data requires discretion (Fig. 4–12).

MICRONEUROGRAPHY

Microneurography involves the use of a concentric or tungsten needle percutaneously inserted into a nerve while the participant is conscious. The needle can be used to record neural activity or apply a stimulus to specific sites in the nerve (Fig. 4–13). This has enabled researchers to gain data on isolated muscle spindles and other mechanoreceptors relative to controlled ligamentous and musculotendinous stretching.[57,58]

REFLEXIVE MUSCLE ACTIVATION

The time of onset of muscle activity in response to joint perturbation is a critical factor if feedback neuromuscular control is to provide dynamic restraint. The reflex pathways involve fast monosynaptic stretch reflexes (M1 response), polysynaptic reflexes from ligaments (M2 response), and longer cortical pathways through the brainstem and cerebral cortex (M3 response).[73,76] Knee perturbation devices are designed to impart variable force on the knee while the amount of displacement and onset of muscle activity are recorded. The delay between joint displacement and muscle activity is termed reflex latency (Fig. 4–14).

Reflexive muscle activation can also be observed by eliciting a deep tendon reflex via a tendon tap (rapid stretch stimulating muscle spindles). Tendon reflexes, quantified by various scales, have high intra-rater reliability but often weaker inter-rater reliability because of varying tapping forces or discrepancies in the perception of response. The National Institute of Neurological Disorders and Stroke/American Academy of Neurology scale is a five-point rating commonly used to describe the reflexive response (Table 4–2).

HOFFMANN REFLEX TESTING

The Hoffmann reflex (H-reflex) is an electrically induced monosynaptic reflex similar to a stretch reflex (i.e., deep tendon reflex). However, it bypasses the effects of the gamma motoneuron and muscle spindle discharge. The

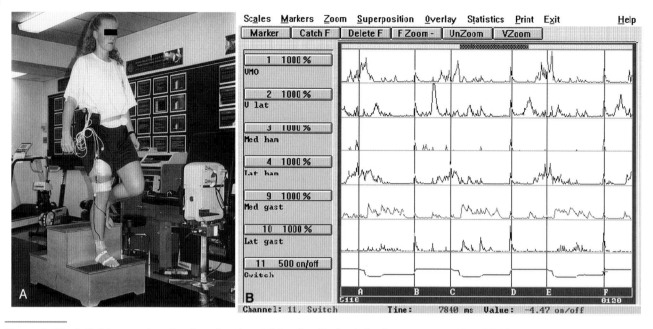

Figure 4–12. **A,** Subject performing functional activities (landing) while electromyographic (EMG) recording of muscle activation patterns is synchronized with landing phases. **B,** EMG activity in the lower extremity with markers identifying the stance and swing phases.

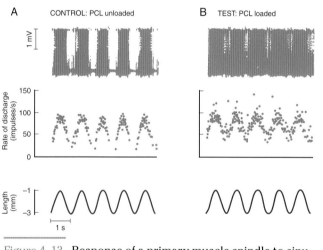

Figure 4–13. Response of a primary muscle spindle to sinusoidal stretching without stretch and during ongoing stretch of the posterior cruciate ligament (PCL) as recorded via microneurography. (From Sojka P, Johansson H, Sjölander P, et al: Fusimotor neurons can be reflexly influenced by activity in receptor afferents from the posterior cruciate ligament. Brain Res 483:177-183, 1989.)

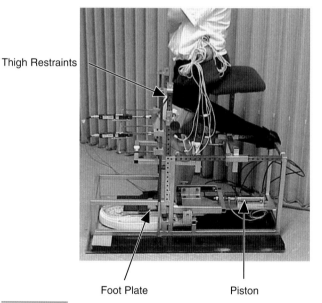

Figure 4–14. Joint perturbation device for the knee. A pneumatic piston initiates tibial translation, which is synchronized with electromyographic equipment measuring reflexive muscle activity.

Table 4–2. NINDS/AAN Myotatic Reflex Scale

GRADE	DESCRIPTION
0	Reflex absent
1	Reflex small, less than normal; includes trace response or response brought out only with reinforcement
2	Reflex in lower half of normal range
3	Reflex in upper half of normal range
4	Reflex enhanced, more than normal; includes clonus if present, which can optionally be noted by an added verbal description of reflex

AAN, American Academy of Neurology; NINDS, National Institute of Neurological Diseases and Stroke.

electrical impulse generates two unique signals (M-wave and H-reflex) that are measured via EMG of the muscle receiving its innervations from the peripheral nerve (Fig. 4–15). A common method of evaluation of the H-reflex is to report the maximum peak values of each signal as the H-reflex–M-wave ratio. Changes in the H-reflex can be indicative of alterations in the excitability of the motoneurons, variations in the amount of neurotransmitters released by the afferent terminals, and/or variations in the intrinsic properties of the motoneurons.[107,157]

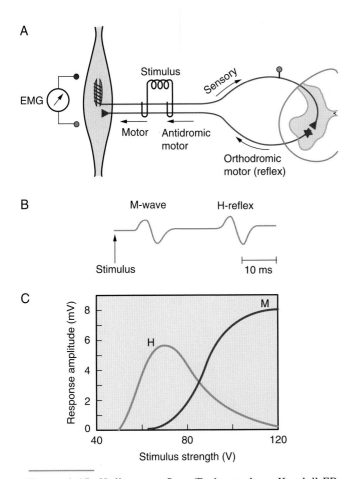

Figure 4–15. Hoffmann reflex. (Redrawn from Kandell ER, Schwartz JH, Jessell TM: Principles of Neural Science, 3rd ed. Norwalk, CT, Appleton & Lange, 1996, p 731, with permission from The McGraw-Hill Companies.)

SOMATOSENSORY EVOKED POTENTIALS

Somatosensory evoked potentials test the integrity of the afferent pathways to the cerebral cortex.[113,114,121] Electroencephalographic and neurological measures are monitored while an external stimulus is introduced to the body (electrical stimulation or joint motion). When the tibial nerve is electrically stimulated, measures, including amplitude changes, wavelength changes, and latencies, can be recorded at the level of the sciatic nerve, at the spinal cord, or at the higher centers. Somatosensory evoked potentials have been used to help determine the afferent contribution from repopulated ACL grafts.[113,114]

ISOKINETIC RESEARCH

The contractile ability and joint movements of various muscle groups are assessed through the use of isokinetic dynamometry by providing reciprocal muscle and bilateral limb profiles in pathological and rehabilitative models. If muscles are to provide dynamic restraint, there must be a significant force produced in a timely fashion.[151,152] A prolonged period of force development or an insufficient amount of force may jeopardize static structures during excessive loads. To assess muscle performance, researchers can quantify peak torque, peak torque normalized to body weight, time to peak torque, and the rate of torque production. Typically, isokinetic strength testing is performed at low velocities (i.e., 60 degrees/s); however, higher velocities (i.e., 240 degrees/s) may be used to evaluate isokinetic endurance. The relationship between isokinetic torque parameters and isolated EMG activity can be evaluated to examine neuromuscular activation and coactivation patterns at various levels of muscle contraction (Fig. 4–16).[137] In addition, analysis of the signal frequency and power spectrum can provide supplementary information

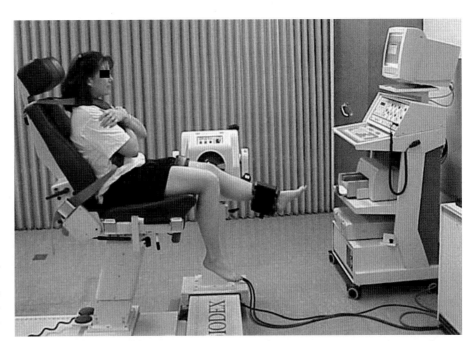

Figure 4–16. Biodex System 2 Dynamometer (Biodex, Inc., Shirley, NY) used to assess isometric and isokinetic strength. When interfaced with electromyography, muscle recruitment, fatigue, synchronization, and coactivation can be measured.

concerning motor unit recruitment during fatiguing contractions.[66,83,84,110]

TWITCH INTERPOLATION AND BURST SUPERIMPOSITION

Twitch interpolation and burst superimposition are two methods of detecting failure of voluntary muscle activation. Both techniques require the application of an electrical stimulus while the patient attempts a voluntary contraction. During the contraction the patient is unable to engage all of the muscle fibers; however, the electrical stimulus is capable of recruiting the additional motor units. Optimally, the difference in force production between the voluntary contraction and the electrically stimulated contraction would be zero, thus indicating that the patient was capable of full recruitment. The two techniques differ in the type of stimulation used to promote additional force production. The twitch interpolation technique superimposes a single pulse on various levels of muscle contraction (including a resting state). The burst superimposition procedure requires a train of pulses (100 Hz) only during maximal volitional effort.[96]

BALANCE AND POSTUROGRAPHY

The ability to maintain upright balance and posture requires that one be able to integrate somatosensory information with vestibular and visual cues, and it is mediated by motor control pathways at the brainstem level of the CNS.[76] Assessment of postural control from an orthopedic perspective can include both static and dynamic testing methods under various visual and stance conditions. During static stance, postural sway can be quantified with the use of a forceplate posturographic system, whereas multiaxial platforms allow for assessment of dynamic balance. Collectively, both these methods (static and dynamic) provide a means to determine the effect of joint pathology, surgery, and rehabilitation on postural control (Fig. 4–17).

STIFFNESS

The level of muscle activation, whether it be preparatory or reactive, largely determines the stiffness properties of the muscle. The stiffness of a muscle is primarily dependent on autogenic and heterogenic input from the muscle spindles to the motoneurons.[72,73] From a mechanical perspective, muscle stiffness is the ratio of the change in force to the change in length. Forces that act to displace the bony segments of a joint must also impart length changes to the surrounding musculature. As muscle stiffness increases, joint stiffness is enhanced because stiffer muscles will resist sudden joint movement. Cocontraction of the antagonist may further stiffen the involved joint and promote stability.[99,101] Increased levels of joint stiffness also lead to an increase in the load delivered to muscle

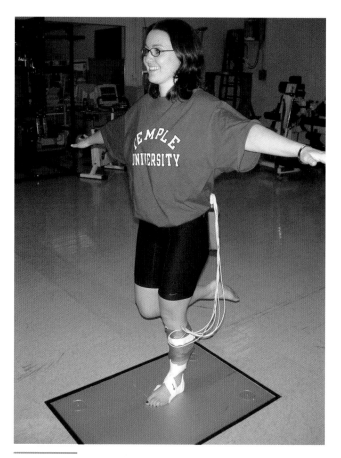

Figure 4–17. **Kistler Force Plate** (Kistler Instrument Corp., Amherst, NY) used to measure postural control.

spindles and thereby decrease the response time to joint perturbations.[105,121] During functional tasks (e.g., landing and cutting), the ability of patients to increase muscle stiffness appropriately is critical to knee stability and the efficiency of motion. Recent research has investigated the landing patterns of female athletes, who typically land with less stiffness than male athletes do, thus possibly revealing one reason for their predisposition to ACL injuries.[51] However, after an ACL injury, female ACL-deficient patients demonstrate less muscle stiffness at rest than their healthy counterparts do, but greater dynamic stability because of an increase in preparatory activity and an increase in the ability to rapidly produce greater force.[141] The capacity of the muscle to resist or absorb excessive force is therefore beneficial to dynamic restraint because joint congruity can be preserved. In vivo measurements of tenomuscular and joint stiffness are performed by modeling the viscoelastic properties of muscles after a single degree of freedom, a mass-spring system. Inverse kinematics from forceplate landings and sinusoid changes in limb velocity detected by accelerometers or motion analysis systems are used to calculate stiffness values. These objective measures of stiffness do not, however, correlate with patients' complaints of stiffness.[61,62] Muscle stiffness has been correlated with muscle performance in healthy populations and with the level of function in ACL-deficient individuals.[3,105,149]

PATHOLOGY

Pain and Effusion

The influence of proprioception on injury varies in the acute and chronic setting. Acutely, proprioception may play a protective role in an injured knee through reflexive muscular splinting. The protective reflex arc initiated by mechanoreceptors and muscular spindle receptors occurs much more quickly than the reflex arc initiated by nociceptors (70 to 100 m/s versus 1 m/s).[7] Pope and colleagues[117] calculated the average time between ligament loading and rupture to be approximately 34 msec. Thus, proprioception appears to play a more significant role than pain sensation in preventing injury in the acute setting. In the chronic setting, proprioceptive deficits contribute more to the etiology of cumulative trauma and reinjury. Initial knee injury can result in partial deafferentation and a sensory deficit, which can predispose one to further injury.[77] The direct effects of residual joint injury on proprioception have been studied by Glencross and Thornton[49] at 8 months after joint injury. When compared with normal controls, there was a decreased ability to reproduce passive positioning that seemed more pronounced at the extremes of motion.[49] This decrease in proprioception places the injured joint at increased risk for reinjury. However, several studies have indicated that chronic pain alone is not responsible for decreases in proprioception.[18,60]

The presence of joint effusion is common, both after injury and after surgical intervention. It has clearly been established that capsular distention contributes to decreased mechanoreceptor afferents and thereby results in the inhibition of muscular contractions. In the knee, this inhibition is mediated by SA mechanoreceptors and appears to provide long-term quadriceps shutdown, particularly in the vastus medialis.[77,138] A 30% to 50% inhibition of reflex-evoked quadriceps contraction can be observed with 60 cm^3 of intra-articular effusion, and decreases in the threshold of the vastus medialis occur with as little as 20 cm^3 of effusion.[138] This muscular inhibition severely disrupts neuromuscular training during rehabilitation and provides fundamental evidence for the wisdom of relieving joint effusion, if only from a neurological point of view.

The direct effects of knee joint effusion on proprioception have not been fully established. The effect of knee joint effusions on articular mechanoreceptors and normal neuromuscular reflexes has been demonstrated to be less influential in the acute setting. McNair and associates[103] found that 90 cm^3 of fluid injected into the knee acutely did not affect the ability of the patient to dynamically track the contralateral limb when compared with control subjects. Contrary to this finding, in the chronic setting it appears as though proprioceptive measures are affected by prolonged capsular distention through the presence of an effusion.[54] Furthermore, this proprioceptive deficit resulting from chronic joint effusion may contribute to the inability to provide neuromuscular joint control and could potentially contribute to continued joint degeneration and/or increased risk of reinjury.[94]

From these studies it is clear that injury and effusion affect joint position sense by several mechanisms. It is difficult to determine whether this loss of joint position sense is secondary to deficits in the joint mechanoreceptors, muscular receptors, or some combination of these proprioceptive afferent inputs. Appreciation of these mechanisms is crucial in returning the joint to its preinjury status. A residual proprioceptive deficit may detract from the functional result of knee surgery, may inhibit complete rehabilitation, and may predispose the patient to reinjury. Therefore, it is clear that any treatment algorithm designed to return patients to their normal preinjury level of function should include a comprehensive rehabilitation program that includes an extensive proprioceptive component.

Anterior Cruciate Ligament–Deficient Knee

PROPRIOCEPTION AND KINESTHESIA

Injury to the ACL results in some level of deafferentation to ligamentous and probably capsular mechanoreceptors as evidenced by deficits in proprioception and kinesthesia.[7,8,11,35,45] In the acute phase of healing, joint inflammation and pain compound the sensory deficits.[12,103] However, inflammation and pain cannot account for the chronic deficits in proprioception and kinesthesia associated with ACL-deficient knees.[11,35] These proprioceptive and kinesthetic deficits may result directly from loss of the ACL afferents or from their reflexive influence on the muscle spindles. Because the neuromuscular control system is mediated by this sensory information, aberrations in the dynamic restraint mechanism can be expected. Compensatory strategies for dynamic restraint must be developed if joint function is to be restored. The neuromuscular characteristics exhibited in ACL-injured subjects are presumably attempts to regain functional stability. If compensatory strategies are not acquired, functional stability is compromised and activity level is limited.

ELECTROMYOGRAPHIC PATTERNS

Functionally stable ACL-deficient subjects exhibit similar patterns of EMG activity while walking and landing. Several profiles have demonstrated increased lateral hamstring activity during the stance phase of walking and cutting maneuvers.[21,29,90,141] When performing landing tasks, the preparatory hamstring activity is greater than that in healthy controls and can be observed approximately 128 ms before contact.[102,141] The increased hamstring activation compensates for ACL insufficiency by inhibiting anterior tibial translation and rotation. Furthermore, during "the swing to strike" transition phase of the gait, quadriceps activity has been shown to decrease (Fig. 4–18).[90] Preprogrammed quadriceps inhibition, before heel strike, may prevent excessive anterior shearing forces at ground contact. The feed-forward process of

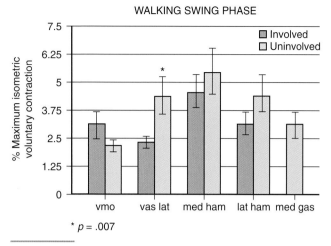

WALKING SWING PHASE

Figure 4–18. A significant decrease in the vastus lateralis of anterior cruciate ligament–deficient subjects demonstrates preprogrammed quadriceps inhibition before heel strike, thereby preventing excessive anterior shearing forces at ground contact. (Redrawn from Lephart SM: EMG profile of the functional ACL-deficient patient during dynamic activities. Presented at a meeting of the American Orthopaedic Society for Sports Medicine, 1997, San Francisco.)

motor control is responsible for compensatory preactivation and inhibition of the dynamic stabilizers during ambulation. Therefore, hamstring activation and quadriceps inhibition reflect preparatory mechanisms to anticipated joint loads. The net effect preserves joint equilibrium and stability through dynamic restraint.[137]

These functionally stable ACL-deficient patients are occasionally termed "copers," whereas their unstable counterparts are categorized as "non-copers" in some research.[28,123] Copers are characterized as individuals who are capable of returning to a high level of activities without episodes of giving way. Non-copers demonstrate altered kinematics and a delayed onset to peak activity in the lateral hamstrings and medial gastrocnemius, thus resulting in a less effective means of stabilizing the knee from anterior shearing.[28,123]

REFLEX LATENCY

Assessment of the reactive characteristics of dynamic restraint in ACL-deficient subjects has included observation of muscle activity in response to joint loads during landing tasks and evaluation of reflex latency with experimentally reproduced joint perturbation. McNair and Marshall[102] demonstrated that ACL-deficient subjects with greater hamstring muscle activation were capable of reducing loads on the knee during landing tasks. However, not all subjects automatically adopted this strategy, and it is unclear whether these subjects were also more or less functional. Simulating episodes of knee perturbation by inducing anterior tibial translation elicits hamstring activation via feedback from the ACL and probably also from muscle spindle receptors.[11,16,25,152] The first experimentally

reproduced latency in the muscle activation of ACL-deficient subjects was published by Beard et al.[15] The hamstring latency in the involved leg (99 ms) was nearly twice that of uninvolved (53 ms) and control limbs (43 ms). It was concluded that the delay was due to proprioceptive deficits and may impair joint function. Wojtys and colleagues,[152] with a similar model, were able to substantiate differences in the timing of muscle firing in the ACL-deficient limb. Jennings and Seedhom,[70] however, were not able to reproduce these results (uninvolved limb, 41 ms; ACL-deficient limb, 32 ms). Swanik et al[141] recently reported findings similar to those of Jennings and Seedhom (ACL-deficient limb, 42.54 ms; control limb, 39.80 ms). These discrepancies may result from the peripheral site where sensory feedback originates. Afferent signals originating in muscle spindles are monosynaptic and therefore project directly on motoneurons within the CNS. Sensory information from other mechanoreceptors must pass through a series of synapses (polysynaptic) before stimulating a motor response.[44,72] The onset times recorded by joint perturbation tests appear to coincide with the stretch reflex mechanism and may therefore be unaffected by ACL injury.

HAMSTRING STIFFNESS

Numerous intrinsic and extrinsic factors are involved in the regulation of total muscle stiffness, including preparatory and reactive muscle activation patterns, muscle fiber type, and flexibility.[79,97,105,149,150] The complex interaction between these components mediates muscle stiffness and the mechanical properties of the tenomuscular unit. For example, research has shown that the stretch reflex can increase muscle stiffness 1 to 3 times and that muscle activation increases joint stiffness 10-fold.[56,81,97] These mechanical properties are believed to be incorporated into the neuromuscular control strategy best suited to provide dynamic restraint and functional performance in normal and ACL-deficient individuals.[3,149] Although McNair and associates[105] did not observe significant differences in hamstring stiffness between the involved and uninvolved limbs of ACL-deficient subjects, a strong correlation ($r = .73$) existed between stiffness and functional ability. The results of a second study by McNair and Marshall[102] showed that ACL-deficient subjects with lower ground reaction forces (soft landings) had greater hamstring muscle activity, but also exhibited lower hamstring muscle stiffness. This finding suggests that there is a relationship or interaction between muscle activation strategies, muscle stiffness, and function in the ACL-deficient population. However, further research is needed before concluding that low muscle stiffness is beneficial to dynamic restraint in ACL-deficient subjects. Recently, Swanik et al[141] reported that ACL-deficient patients have increased preparatory activity and decreased hamstring stiffness, which allows them to produce greater force in a shorter period, thereby promoting dynamic stability. However, it is still unclear whether these neuromuscular characteristics are preexisting traits or a compensatory effect from the injury.

BALANCE AND POSTURAL SWAY

Research investigating the influence of ACL injury on balance and postural sway is conflicting, possibly the result of a variety of testing instrumentation and methodology. In addition, several measurement variables such as the center of pressure, platform deviation, and speed of platform oscillations make comparisons among subject populations and instruments difficult. Evaluations of involved and uninvolved limbs have demonstrated both symmetry and deficits with ACL injury.[41,47,69] However, group comparisons of functionally stable and unstable ACL-deficient subjects reveal significant deficits in postural sway, speed, and the number of frontal plane oscillations.[47,69,108] These results may illustrate disturbances in the sensorimotor system resulting from ACL injury and emphasize the importance of brainstem activity for restoring knee joint function. It is important to note that these objective scores fail to describe the individual strategies (increased hip/ankle activity) that have been observed in patients when trying to promote postural stability.[124]

The Effects of Aging and Osteoarthritis

With changes in the articular surface, the surrounding capsuloligamentous supporting structures, and alignment, the effects of aging and osteoarthritis on the knee from a mechanical perspective are well documented.[34] The effect of these processes on joint position sense and how they might contribute to clinical performance and further deterioration of the knee joint have also been studied. These reports uniformly agree that aging results in overall decreased proprioception of the knee.[10,12,132,133] This has been demonstrated by both a decrease in the reproduction of passive positioning and a decrease in the threshold to passive motion with aging. Furthermore, this overall decrease in position sense is more profound in patients with osteoarthritis than in age-matched controls (Fig. 4–19).[10] What is less certain is the cause of this decrease in position sense. Are these changes in proprioception the result of the arthritic change in the joint surface and surrounding structures, or are they a contributing cause to their formation?

SURGICAL MANAGEMENT

Anterior Cruciate Ligament Reconstruction

Surgical ACL reconstruction may restore its mechanical function in the knee, but the issue of graft reinnervation and its effect on muscle activity remain undetermined.[6] However, recent evidence has indicated that ACL reconstructions may resume their role as afferent transducers. Shimizu et al[128] demonstrated that the concentration of mechanoreceptors in bone-patellar-bone autografts drops during the first 2 weeks after surgery but is comparable to that of the contralateral ACL by the eighth week in white

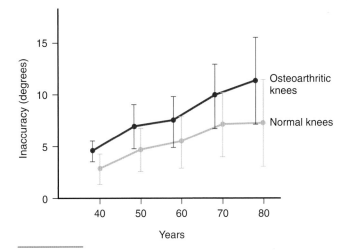

Figure 4–19. Greater inaccuracy while reproducing joint position demonstrated by subjects with osteoarthritis than by age-matched controls. (Reproduced with permission and copyright of the British Editorial Society of Bone and Joint Surgery: Barrett DS, Cobb AG, Bentley G: Joint proprioception in normal, osteoarthritic, and replaced knees. J Bone Joint Surg Br 73:53, 1991.)

rabbits. Additional human studies (bone-patellar-bone and semitendinosus-gracilis) have demonstrated re-emergence of the ACL-hamstring reflex arc and somatosensory evoked potentials and an improvement in position sense, thus indicating that these new mechanoreceptors are providing afferent feedback.[113,144] Clinical research assessing proprioception and kinesthesia in ACL-reconstructed populations is encouraging. Barrack and Skinner[7] measured the threshold to detection of passive motion and observed that kinesthesia is partially restored through the midrange of motion (45 degrees) in ACL-reconstructed subjects. Similar studies assessing this threshold in ACL-reconstructed subjects have demonstrated that kinesthetic deficits persist when comparisons are made to the uninvolved limb.[93] Likewise, ACL reconstruction combined with rehabilitation appears to restore some proprioceptive abilities when assessed by reproducing joint positions. The proprioceptive measures of ACL-reconstructed subjects are more normalized than those of ACL-deficient subjects and occasionally do not differ significantly from the uninvolved extremities (Fig. 4–20).[11,32,59] These results are most likely explained by a combination of factors, including the restoration of joint mechanics and capsuloligamentous tension, compensatory sensory feedback from various mechanoreceptor populations, and peripheral adaptations induced by rehabilitation exercises.[9,32,59,68,91,92,152]

Total Knee Arthroplasty

Because proprioceptive decline is part of the normal aging process, this phenomenon has been found to be further exacerbated in the osteoarthritic knee.[12,132,133] Capsuloligamentous laxity, loss of the cartilaginous surface, and malalignment as a result of this pathological process are each thought to contribute to the loss of "position sense"

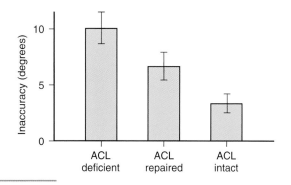

Figure 4–20. Greater inaccuracy while reproducing joint position demonstrated by anterior cruciate ligament (ACL)-deficient and ACL-repaired subjects. (Reproduced with permission and copyright of the British Editorial Society of Bone and Joint Surgery: Barrett DS, Cobb AG, Bentley G: Joint proprioception in normal, osteoarthritic, and replaced knees. J Bone Joint Surg Br 73:53, 1991.)

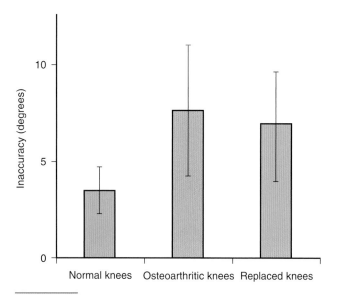

Figure 4–21. Partial restoration of the ability to reproduce joint position demonstrated by subjects with total knee arthroplasties. (Reproduced with permission and copyright of the British Editorial Society of Bone and Joint Surgery: Barrett DS, Cobb AG, Bentley G: Joint proprioception in normal, osteoarthritic, and replaced knees. J Bone Joint Surg Br 73:53, 1991.)

in affected patients. Although conservative treatment of this condition may lead to compensatory efforts in gait to combat this change in proprioception, operative resurfacing of the knee with either a unicondylar or total knee replacement has been found to enhance the proprioceptive "feel" of the knee. Through replacement of the diseased articular surface, in combination with restoration of alignment and soft-tissue balancing, proprioception and postural stability are restored to a level somewhere between its diseased state and normal levels for age-matched controls (Fig. 4–21).[12,140] This improvement, but not complete restoration of knee proprioception, may be one contributing factor why gait patterns after knee

replacement do not return to normal despite the relief of pain and correction of the deformity. In fact, return of normal gait parameters after total knee replacement seems to be most closely related to preoperative proprioceptive function.[20,134]

Analysis of the different designs of knee replacement systems has been performed to determine their different effects on restoration of proprioception. More specifically, it has been hypothesized that maintenance of the proprioceptive input of the posterior cruciate ligament (PCL) in PCL-retaining knee systems may enhance overall proprioception. Several studies have examined the difference in perceived proprioception between PCL-sacrificing and PCL-retaining total knee systems and have come to different conclusions. Warren and colleagues[147] reported enhanced proprioception with PCL-retaining total knee systems, whereas Faris and associates[42] reported equal proprioception in these two groups. Swanik et al[140] tested the reproduction of passive positioning, detection of passive motion, and balance and found the two designs equivalent except when the patient was asked to reproduce a joint position when the knee was extended from a flexed position. Simmons and associates[130] reported no significant difference in postoperative proprioceptive ability between the two designs, but found improved results with PCL-sacrificing knee systems in a subset of patients with severe preoperative degenerative changes. The rationale for this finding was that although the cruciate ligaments' proprioceptive contributions are well established, their role in the degenerative knee is less clear. As the ligaments age, the actual number of mechanoreceptors appears to decline, and in these instances the capsular contributions to proprioception become more important.[126,129] Thus, designs that most effectively restore soft-tissue balancing and tension appear to perform better under these parameters.[43]

Similarly, it has been theorized that maintenance of both cruciate ligaments may provide enhanced proprioceptive feedback in unicondylar knee replacements, and this has resulted in knee replacements that more closely resemble the "normal knee." Laurencin et al[88] analyzed 23 patients with a unicondylar knee replacement and total knee replacement on contralateral sides to determine whether clinically there was a difference in "feel" or performance. In this group of patients, the unicondylar replacements more frequently provided a subjectively "better" knee than the tricompartmental knee replacement did.[88] Simmons et al,[129] using more objective measurements of proprioception, likewise examined these two knee designs. Maintenance of the cruciate ligaments in this patient cohort provided no enhanced proprioception in that the two groups performed equally well in proprioceptive testing.

From these studies that have compared different total knee designs and unicondylar replacements, conflicting reports regarding proprioception emerge. A benefit of retaining the PCL or ACL in these different designs to improve proprioception has not been consistently demonstrated from these studies. Although retaining these structures may improve the kinematics of the replaced knee, it appears that their role in providing proprioceptive feedback to the osteoarthritic knee is less important. This may be related to the decrease in mechanoreceptor population that occurs with normal aging and that is accelerated in the osteoarthritic joint.[126]

REHABILITATION

Damage to the articular structures, whether traumatic or arthritic, appears to cause distinctive proprioceptive, kinesthetic, and neuromuscular deficits.[9,14,21,25,91,92,146] Developing or reestablishing the sensory characteristics and motor function in injured patients will minimize the risk of reinjury and enhance function. Capsuloligamentous retensioning and reconstruction, coupled with traditional rehabilitation, provide one option that appears to normalize some of these deficits, though not always equal to noninvolved limbs.[68,93]

The objective of neuromuscular rehabilitation is to develop or reestablish the afferent and efferent characteristics that enhance function of the sensorimotor system. Four basic elements that are crucial to reestablishing neuromuscular control and functional stability are proprioceptive and kinesthetic sensation, dynamic joint stabilization, reactive neuromuscular control, and functional motor patterns.[85,94,139] In a pathological joint, these elements require compensatory adaptations to dynamic mechanisms because the static restraints have been disrupted, and such adaptations can result in a functionally stable joint.

Several afferent and efferent characteristics contribute to the maintenance of neuromuscular control, including the sensitivity of peripheral receptors and facilitation of afferent pathways, the onset of reflex muscle activation, the magnitude of muscle activity, agonist/antagonist coactivation, muscle stiffness, and discriminatory muscle activation. By using specific rehabilitation techniques these characteristics can be modified to significantly improve dynamic restraint and function.[14,68,94,139,151]

Several exercise techniques appear to facilitate beneficial adaptations to sensory characteristics, whereas plasticity of the neuromuscular system permits modifications that enhance preparatory and reactive muscle activity.[14,63,67,90,146,152] These techniques include closed kinetic chain activities, balance training, eccentric loading, high-repetition exercises, reflex facilitation, stretch-shortening activities, and biofeedback training.[13,48,50,80,81,118,148] A proper active and passive warm-up is also an important component of the patient's program because it facilitates nerve conduction and neurotransmitter release. Traditional rehabilitation, supplemented with these specific techniques, results in beneficial adaptations to the sensorimotor system responsible for dynamic restraint and will ultimately enhance the efficiency of movement and functional stability. Prevention programs attempt to incorporate some of these therapeutic exercises in an effort to promote optimal dynamic restraint strategies. Many of these programs have demonstrated a reduction in the injury rate in comparison to control groups, but kinetic and kinematic studies have thus far failed to demonstrate the mechanism of action in healthy, physically active individuals.[17,136] Recent research, however, has indicated that preventive/plyometric training programs may lead to neuromuscular adaptations as demonstrated by improvements in postural stability, proprioception, kinesthesia, and muscular performance.[115,142]

To restore the preparatory and reactive muscle activation strategies necessary for functional stability, one must use simulated positions of vulnerability that necessitate dynamic muscle stabilization. Despite an inherent risk to placing the knee in positions of vulnerability, if performed in a controlled and progressive fashion, neuromuscular adaptations will result and permit the athlete to return to competitive situations with confidence that the dynamic mechanisms will protect the joint from subluxation and reinjury.[139] Appreciation of the afferent and efferent characteristics that contribute to the sensorimotor system and dynamic restraint mechanism will assist in the development of a comprehensive rehabilitation protocol (Table 4–3).

KNEE BRACING

The use of braces, either prophylactically or in response to ligamentous injury of the knee to prevent future injury,

Table 4–3. Restoration of Proprioception and Neuromuscular Control

ELEMENTS	REHABILITATION TECHNIQUES	AFFERENT/EFFERENT CHARACTERISTICS
Proprioception and kinesthesia	Joint repositioning Functional range of motion Axial loading Closed kinetic chain exercises	Peripheral receptor sensitivity Facilitate afferent pathways
Dynamic restraint	Closed kinetic chain exercises and translatory forces High repetition/low resistance Eccentric loading Stretch-shortening exercises Balance training	Agonist/antagonist coactivation Muscle activation rate and amplitude Peripheral receptor sensitivity Muscle stiffness
Reactive neuromuscular control	Reaction to joint perturbation Stretch-shortening, plyometrics Balance reacquisition	Reflex facilitation Muscle activation rate and amplitude
Functional motor patterns	Biofeedback Sport-specific drills Control-progressive participation	Discriminatory muscle activation Arthrokinematics Coordinated locomotion

has been the subject of many investigations that both support and refute the use of these devices as a means of reducing the number of knee injuries.[4,21,22,131,143] Clinical and laboratory studies of functional braces have demonstrated that some functional knee braces can limit motion and protect ligaments from strain under conditions of low-load application. However, these loads are well below the physiological loads experienced by the knee in vivo.[4,21,22,153] Biomechanical cadaveric studies only approximate the actual effect of these braces in clinical applications. Additionally, poor brace fit has been reported as a large limitation in interpreting these studies purely on biomechanics.[98] Many have proposed that braces produce their effect by increasing knee proprioception and that biomechanical testing evaluates the static and not the dynamic contributions of a specific knee brace. Branch and colleagues studied the effects of an ACL functional brace on dynamic stability of the knee, as measured by EMG patterns of the hamstrings and quadriceps activity during a side-step cutting maneuver. Although this study demonstrated increased hamstring activity in both the stance and swing phases of gait for ACL-deficient patients without a brace as compared with controls, there was no difference in EMG activity in the braced versus unbraced group of ACL-deficient patients. Based on the similar patterns of muscle activity between these two groups, the authors concluded that functional braces do not provide the increased proprioceptive feedback that contributes to increased dynamic knee stability.[21,22]

In contrast to the findings just presented, others have found an increase in proprioception with a "knee sleeve" type of brace. McNair and associates[104] demonstrated an increased ability to reproduce normal passive positioning by about 11% in patients when the knee sleeve was worn. Perlau and colleagues[116] found approximately 25% improvement in similar tasks when an elastic bandage was worn by uninjured subjects. Much larger improvements in proprioception were demonstrated by a subgroup of patients with a lower level of baseline proprioception (up to 66% improvement).[116] This finding was also reported by Barrett and associates,[12] who noted up to a 40% increase in proprioceptive function in osteoarthritic knees, and by Lephart and colleagues[93] in ACL-deficient knees after reconstruction.

Therefore, the benefits of knee bracing from a proprioceptive standpoint are beginning to be uncovered slowly. What types of braces and under what conditions these braces seem warranted have yet to be fully elucidated. It does appear, however, that patients with different levels of baseline proprioception respond differently to this intervention. More study is required to determine who will benefit most from knee bracing. In answering this question, many variables should be considered that include, but are not limited to, patient selection (including associated instability and activity level) and the static and dynamic properties of the brace chosen.

References

1. Andrew BL, Dodt E: The development of sensory endings at the knee joint of the cat. Acta Physiol Scand 28:287, 1953.
2. Appleburg B, Hulliger M, Johansson H, et al: Excitation of dynamic fusimotor neurones of the cat triceps surae by contralateral joint afferents. Brain Res 160:529, 1979.
3. Bach TM, Chapman AE, Calvert TW: Mechanical resonance of the human body during voluntary oscillations about the ankle. J Biomech 16:85, 1983.
4. Baker BE, Bogosian S, Werner FW, et al: A biomechanical study of the static stabilizing effect of knee braces on medial instability. Am J Sports Med 15:566, 1987.
5. Barker D: The morphology of muscle receptors. In Hunt CC (ed): Handbook of Sensory Physiology. Berlin, Springer-Verlag, 1974, pp 191-234.
6. Barrack RL, Lind PJ, Munn BG, et al: Evidence of reinnervation of free patellar tendon autograft used for anterior cruciate ligament reconstruction. Am J Sports Med 25:196, 1997.
7. Barrack RL, Skinner HB: The sensory function of knee ligaments. In Daniel DM, Akeson WH, O'Connor JJ (eds): Knee Ligaments: Structure, Function, Injury. New York, Raven Press, 1990.
8. Barrack RL, Skinner HB, Brunet ME, et al: Joint laxity and proprioception in the knee. Phys Sports Med 11:130, 1983.
9. Barrack RL, Skinner, HB, Brunet ME, et al: Joint kinesthesia in the highly trained knee. J Sports Med 24:18, 1984.
10. Barrack RL, Skinner HB, Cook SD, et al: Effect of articular disease and total arthroplasty on knee joint-position sense. J Neurophysiol 50:684, 1983.
11. Barrett DS: Proprioception and function after anterior cruciate reconstruction. J Bone Joint Surg Br 73:83, 1991.
12. Barrett DS, Cobb AG, Bentley G: Joint proprioception in normal, osteoarthritic, and replaced knees. J Bone Joint Surg Br 73:53, 1991.
13. Basmajian JV (ed): Biofeedback: Principles and Practice for Clinicians. Baltimore, Williams & Wilkins, 1979, pp 17-20.
14. Beard DJ, Dodd CAF, Trundle HR, et al: Proprioception enhancement for anterior cruciate ligament deficiency. J Bone Joint Surg Br 76:654, 1994.
15. Beard DJ, Kyberd PJ, Fergusson CM, et al: Proprioception after rupture of the anterior cruciate ligament. J Bone Joint Surg Br 75:311, 1993.
16. Beard DJ, Kyberd PJ, O'Connor JJ, et al: Reflex hamstring contraction latency in anterior cruciate ligament deficiency. J Orthop Res 12:219, 1994.
17. Bencke J, Nasborg H, Simonsen EB, et al: Motor pattern of the knee joint muscles during side-step cutting in European team handball. Influence on muscular co-ordination after an intervention study. Scand J Med Sci Sports 10:68, 2000.
18. Bennell KL, Hinman RS, Metcalf BR, et al: Relationship of knee joint proprioception to pain and disability in individuals with knee osteoarthritis. J Orthop Res 21:792, 2003.
19. Bergenheim M, Johansson H, Pedersen J, et al: Ensemble coding of muscle stretches in afferent populations containing different types of muscle afferents. Brain Res 734:157, 1996.
20. Berman AT, Bosacco SJ, Israelit C: Quantitative gait analysis after unilateral or bilateral total knee replacement. J Bone Joint Surg Am 69:1340, 1987.
21. Branch TP, Hunter R: Functional analysis of anterior cruciate ligament braces. Clin Sports Med 9:771, 1990.
22. Branch T, Hunter R, Donath M: Dynamic EMG analysis of the anterior cruciate ligament–deficient legs with and without bracing during cutting. Am J Sports Med 17:35, 1989.
23. Brener J: Sensory and perceptual determinants of voluntary visceral control. In Schwartz GE, Beatty J (eds): Biofeedback: Theory and Research. New York, Academic Press, 1977, pp 29-66.
24. Brockett C, Warren N, Gregory JE, et al: A comparison of the effects of concentric versus eccentric exercise on force and position sense at the human elbow joint. Brain Res 771:251, 1997.
25. Caraffa A, Cerulli G, Proietti M, et al: Prevention of anterior cruciate ligament injuries in soccer. A prospective controlled study of proprioceptive training. Knee Surg Sports Traumatol Arthrosc 4:19, 1995.
26. Carson RG, Riek S, Shahbazpour N: Central and peripheral mediation of human force sensation following eccentric and concentric contraction. J Physiol 539:913, 2002.
27. Chimera NJ, Swanik KA, Swanik CB, et al: Effects of plyometric training on muscle-activation strategies and performance in female athletes. J Athl Train 39:24, 2004.

28. Chmielewski TL, Rudolph KS, Snyder-Mackler L: Development of dynamic knee stability after acute ACL injury. J Electromyogr Kinesiol 12:267, 2002.

29. Ciccotti M, Kerlain R, Perry J, et al: An electromyographic analysis of the knee during functional activities. II. The anterior cruciate ligament–deficient knee and reconstructed profiles. Am J Sports Med 22:651, 1994.

30. Clark FJ, Burgess PR: Slowly adapting receptors in cat knee joint: Can they signal joint angle? J Neurophysiol 38:1448, 1975.

31. Clark FJ, Burgess RC, Chapin JW, et al: Role of intramuscular receptors in the awareness of limb position. J Neurophysiol 54:1529, 1985.

32. Co FH, Skinner HB, Cannon WD: Effect of reconstruction of the anterior cruciate ligament on proprioception of the knee and the heel strike transient. J Orthop Res 11:696, 1993.

33. Colebatch JG, McClosky DI: Maintenance of constant arm position or force: Reflex and volitional components in man. J Physiol 386:247, 1987.

34. Cooke TD, Bryant JT, Scudamore RA: Biomechanical factors in alignment and arthritic disorders of the knee. In Fu FH, Warner CD (eds): Knee Surgery. Baltimore, Williams & Wilkins, 1994, pp 1061-1079.

35. Corrigan JP, Cashmen WF, Brady MP: Proprioception in the cruciate deficient knee. J Bone Joint Surg Br 74:247, 1992.

36. Cram JR, Kasman GS: Introduction to Surface Electromyography. Gaithersburg, MD, Aspen Publishers, 1998, pp 52-53.

37. Davids K, Glazier P, Araujo D, et al: Movement systems as dynamical systems: The functional role of variability and its implications for sports medicine. Sports Med 33:245, 2003.

38. Dietz V, Noth J, Schmidtbleicher D: Interaction between pre-activity and stretch reflex in human triceps brachii during landing from forward falls. J Physiol 311:113, 1981.

39. Dunn TG, Gillig SE, Ponser SE, et al: The learning process in biofeedback: Is it feed-forward or feedback? Biofeedback Self Regul 11:143, 1986.

40. Dyhre-Poulsen P, Simonsen B, Voigt M: Dynamic control of muscle stiffness and H reflex modulation during hopping and jumping in man. J Physiol 437:287, 1991.

41. Faculjak PF, Firoozbakhshsh KK, Wausher D, et al: Balance characteristics of normal and anterior cruciate ligament deficient knees. Phys Ther 73(Suppl): S22, 1993.

42. Faris PM, Otis JC, Manouel M: Proprioceptive input of the posterior cruciate ligament in total knee prostheses. Trans Orthop Res Soc 13:358, 1988.

43. Ferrell WR, Crighton A, Sturrock RD: Position sense at the proximal interphalangeal joint is distorted in patients with rheumatoid arthritis of finger joints. Exp Physiol 77:675, 1992.

44. Freeman MAR, Wyke B: Articular contributions to limb reflexes. Br J Surg 53:61, 1966.

45. Friden T, Zatterstrom R, Lindstand A, et al: Disability in anterior cruciate ligament insufficiency: An analysis of 19 untreated patients. Acta Orthop Scand 61:131, 1990.

46. Gardner E, Latimer F, Stiwell D: Central connections for afferent fibers from the knee joint of a cat. Am J Physiol 159:195, 1949.

47. Gauffin H, Tropp H: Altered movement and muscular activation patterns during the one-legged jump in patients with old anterior cruciate ligament rupture. Am J Sports Med 20:182, 1992.

48. Glaros AG, Hanson K: EMG biofeedback and discriminative muscle control. Biofeedback Self Regul 15:135, 1990.

49. Glencross D, Thornton E: Position sense following joint injury. J Sports Med Phys Fitness 21:23, 1981.

50. Gollhofer A, Kyrolaninen H: Neuromuscular control of the human leg extensor muscles in jump exercises under various stretch-load conditions. Int J Sports Med 12:34, 1991.

51. Granata KP, Padua DA, Wilson SE: Gender differences in active musculoskeletal stiffness. Part II. Quantification of leg stiffness during functional hopping tasks. J Electromyogr Kinesiol 12:127, 2002.

52. Grigg P: Peripheral neural mechanisms in proprioception. J Sports Rehabil 3:1, 1994.

53. Griller S: A role for muscle stiffness in meeting the changing postural and locomotor requirements for force development by ankle extensors. Acta Physiol Scand 86:92, 1972.

54. Guido J, Blackburn TA, Kidder JD, et al: The effects of chronic effusion on knee joint proprioception: A case study. J Orthop Sports Phys Ther 25:208, 1997.

55. Guyton AC: Textbook of Medical Physiology, 6th ed. Philadelphia, WB Saunders, 1981, pp 534-536, 562-564, 588-595.

56. Hagood S, Solomonow M, Baratta R, et al: The effect of joint velocity on the contribution of the antagonist musculature to knee stiffness and laxity. Am J Sports Med 18:182, 1990.

57. Hallin RG, Wu G: Protocol for microneurography with concentric needle electrodes. Brain Res Brain Res Protoc 2:120, 1998.

58. Hallin RG, Wu G: Fitting pieces in the peripheral nerve puzzle. Exp Neurol 172:482, 2001.

59. Harter RA, Osternig LR, Singer KM, et al: Long-term evaluation of knee stability and function following surgical reconstruction for anterior cruciate ligament insufficiency. Am J Sports Med 16:434, 1988.

60. Hassan BS, Doherty SA, Mockett S, et al: Effect of pain reduction on postural sway, proprioception, and quadriceps strength in subjects with knee osteoarthritis. Ann Rheum Dis 61:422, 2002.

61. Helliwell PS: Normal vibration perception thresholds in rheumatoid arthritis—evidence against the neurogenic theory of articular stiffness. Clin Rheumatol 13:51, 1994.

62. Helliwell PS, Howe A, Wright V: Lack of objective evidence of stiffness in rheumatoid arthritis. Ann Rheum Dis 47:754, 1988.

63. Hodgson JA, Roy RR, DeLeon R, et al: Can the mammalian lumbar spinal cord learn a motor task? Med Sci Sports Exerc 26:1491, 1994.

64. Hoffer JA, Andreassen S: Regulation of soleus muscle stiffness in premammillary cats: Intrinsic and reflex components. J Neurophysiol 45:267, 1981.

65. Hopkins JT, Ingersoll CD, Krause BA, et al: Effect of knee joint effusion on quadriceps and soleus motoneuron pool excitability. Med Sci Sports Exerc 33:123, 2001.

66. Horita T, Ishiko T: Relationships between muscle lactate accumulation and surface EMG activities during isokinetic contractions in men. J Appl Physiol Occup Physiol 56:18, 1987.

67. Hutton RS, Atwater SW: Acute and chronic adaptations of muscle proprioceptors in response to increased use. Sports Med 14:406, 1992.

68. Ihara H, Nakayama A: Dynamic joint control training for knee ligament injuries. Am J Sports Med 14:309, 1986.

69. Irrgang JJ, Whitney SL, Cox ED: Balance and proprioceptive training for rehabilitation of the lower extremity. J Sports Rehabil 3:68, 1994.

70. Jennings AG, Seedhom BB: Proprioception in the knee and reflex hamstring contraction latency. J Bone Joint Surg Br 76:491, 1994.

71. Johansson H, Sjolander P, Sojka P: Actions on γ-motoneurones elicited by electrical stimulation of joint afferent fibers in the hind limb of the cat. J Physiol (Lond) 375:137, 1986.

72. Johansson H, Sjolander P, Sojka P: A sensory role for the cruciate ligaments. Clin Orthop 268:161, 1991.

73. Johansson H, Sjolander P, Sojka P: Receptors in the knee joint ligaments and their role in the biomechanics of the joint. Crit Rev Biomed Eng 18:341, 1991.

74. Jones LA: Perception of force and weight: Theory and research. Psychol Bull 100:29, 1986.

75. Jonsson H, Karrholm J, Elmquist LG: Kinematics of active knee extension after tear of the anterior cruciate ligament. Am J Sports Med 17:796, 1989.

76. Kandell ER, Schwartz JH, Jessell TM: Principles of Neural Science, 3rd ed. Norwalk, CT, Appleton & Lange, 1996, pp 535-537, 619.

77. Kennedy JC, Alexander IJ, Hayes KC: Nerve supply of the human knee and its functional importance. Am J Sports Med 103:329, 1982.

78. Knop G, Denzer L, Buschges A: A central pattern-generating network contributes to "reflex reversal"–like leg motoneuron activity in locust. J Neurophysiol 86:3065, 2001.

79. Koceja DM, Burke JR, Kamen G: Organization of segmental reflexes in trained dancers. Int J Sports Med 12:285, 1991.

80. Koceja DM, Kamen G: Conditioned patellar tendon reflexes in sprint- and endurance-trained athletes. Med Sci Sports Exerc 20:172, 1988.

81. Kochner MS, Fu FH, Harner CD: Neuropathophysiology. In Fu FH, Harner CD (eds): Knee Surgery, vol 1. Baltimore, Williams & Wilkins, 1994, pp 231-249.

82. Konishi Y, Konishi H, Fukubayashi T: Gamma loop dysfunction in quadriceps on the contralateral side in patients with ruptured ACL. Med Sci Sports Exerc 35:897, 2003.

83. Krivickas LS, Nadler SF, Davies MR, et al: Spectral analysis during fatigue. Surface and fine wire electrode comparison. Am J Phys Med Rehabil 75:15, 1996.

84. Krivickas LS, Taylor A, Maniar RM, et al: Is spectral analysis of the surface electromyographic signal a clinically useful tool for evaluation of skeletal muscle fatigue. J Clin Neurophysiol 15:138, 1998.

85. Kyrolaninen H, Komi PV: The function of neuromuscular system in maximal stretch-shortening cycle exercises: Comparison between power- and endurance-trained athletes. J Electromyogr Kinesiol 5:15, 1995.

86. La Croix JM: The acquisition of autonomic control through biofeedback: The case against an afferent process and a two process alternative. Psychophysiology 18:573, 1981.

87. Lass P, Kaalund S, LeFevre S et al: Muscle coordination following rupture of the anterior cruciate ligament. Electromyographic studies of 14 patients. Acta Orthrop Scand 62:9, 1991.

88. Laurencin CT, Scott RD, Ewald FC: Unicompartmental versus total knee arthroplasty in the same patient: A comparative study. Clin Orthop 273:151, 1991.

89. Leksell L: The action potential and excitatory effects of the small ventral root fibers to skeletal muscle. Acta Physiol Scand 10:1, 1945.

90. Lephart SM: EMG profile of the functional ACL-deficient patient during dynamic activities. Presented at a meeting of the American Orthopaedic Society for Sports Medicine, February 1997, San Francisco.

91. Lephart SM, Giraldo JL, Borsa PA, et al: Knee joint proprioception: A comparison between female intercollegiate gymnasts and controls. Knee Surg Sports Traumatol Arthrosc 4:121, 1996.

92. Lephart SM, Henry TJ: The physiological basis for open and closed kinetic chain rehabilitation for the upper extremity. J Sports Rehabil 5:71, 1996.

93. Lephart SM, Kocher MS, Fu FH, et al: Proprioception following ACL reconstruction. J Sports Rehabil 1:188, 1992.

94. Lephart SM, Pincivero DM, Giraldo JL, et al: The role of proprioception in the management and rehabilitation of athletic injuries. Am J Sports Med 25:130, 1997.

95. Lephart SM, Warner JJP, Borsa PA, et al: Proprioception of the shoulder joint in healthy, unstable, and surgically repaired shoulders. J Shoulder Elbow Surg 3:37, 1994.

96. Lewek MD, Rudolph KS, Snyder-Mackler L: Quadriceps femoris muscle weakness and activation failure in patients with symptomatic knee osteoarthritis. J Orthop Res 22:110, 2004.

97. Lieber RL, Friden J: Neuromuscular stabilization of the shoulder girdle. In Matsen FA (ed): The Shoulder: A Balance of Mobility and Stability. Rosemont, IL, American Academy of Orthopaedic Surgeons, 1992, pp 91-106.

98. Liu SH: Current review: Functional knee bracing. Clin Orthop 317:273, 1995.

99. Louie JK, Mote CD Jr: Contribution of the musculature to rotatory laxity and torsional stiffness at the knee. J Biomech 20:281, 1987.

100. Marchand-Pauvert V, Nielson JB: Modulation of heteronymous reflexes from ankle dorsiflexors to hamstring muscles during human walking. Exp Brain Res 142:402, 2002.

101. Markolf KL, Graff-Radford A, Amstutz MD: In vivo knee stability: A quantitative assessment using an instrumented clinical testing apparatus. J Bone Joint Surg Am 60:664, 1978.

102. McNair PJ, Marshall RN: Landing characteristics in subjects with normal and anterior cruciate ligament–deficient knee joints. Arch Phys Med Rehabil 75:584, 1994.

103. McNair PJ, Marshall RN, Maguire K, et al: Knee joint effusion and proprioception. Arch Phys Med Rehabil 76:566, 1995.

104. McNair PJ, Stanley SN, Strauss GR: Knee bracing: Effects on proprioception. Arch Phys Med Rehabil 77:287, 1996.

105. McNair PJ, Wood GA, Marshall RN: Stiffness of the hamstring muscles and its relationship to function in anterior cruciate–deficient individuals. Clin Biomech 7:131, 1992.

106. Merton PA: Speculations on the servo-control of movement. In Wolstenholme GEW (ed): The Spinal Cord. London, Churchill, 1953, pp 247-255.

107. Misiaszek JE: The H-reflex as a tool in neurophysiology: Its limitations and uses in understanding nervous system function. Muscle Nerve 28:144, 2003.

108. Mizuta H, Shiraishi M, Kubota K, et al: A stabilometric technique for evaluation of functional instability in the anterior cruciate ligament–deficient knee. Clin J Sports Med 2:235, 1992.

109. Morgan DL: Separation of active and passive components of short-range stiffness of muscle. Am J Physiol 32:45, 1977.

110. Moritani T, Nagata A, Muro M: Electromyographic manifestations of muscular fatigue. Med Sci Sports Exerc 14:198, 1982.

111. Mountcastle VS: Medical Physiology, 14th ed. St Louis, CV Mosby, 1980.

112. Nichols TR, Houk JC: Improvements in linearity and regulation of stiffness that results from actions of stretch reflex. J Neurophysiol 39:119, 1976.

113. Ochi M, Iwasa J, Uchio Y, et al: The regeneration of sensory neurones in the reconstruction of the anterior cruciate ligament. J Bone Joint Surg Br 81:902, 1999.

114. Ochi M, Iwasa J, Uchio Y, et al: Induction of somatosensory evoked potentials by mechanical stimulation in reconstructed anterior cruciate ligaments. J Bone Joint Surg Br 84:761, 2002.

115. Paterno MV, Myer GD, Ford KR, et al: Neuromuscular training improves single-limb stability in young female athletes. J Orthop Sports Phys Ther 34:305, 2004.

116. Perlau R, Frank C, Fick G: The effects of elastic bandages on human knee proprioception in the uninjured population. Am J Sports Med 23:251, 1995.

117. Pope MH, Johnson RJ, Brown DW, et al: The role of the musculature in injuries to the medial collateral ligament. J Bone Joint Surg Am 61:398, 1972.

118. Pousson M, Hoecke JV, Goubel F: Changes in elastic characteristics of human muscle induced by eccentric exercise. J Biomech 23:343, 1990.

119. Rack PMH, Westbury DR: The short range stiffness of active mammalian muscle and its effect on mechanical properties. J Physiol 240:331, 1974.

120. Richmond FJ, Bakker DA: Anatomical organization and sensory receptor content of soft tissues surrounding upper cervical vertebrae in the cat. J Neurophysiol 48:49, 1982.

121. Riemann BL, Myers JB, Lephart SM: Sensorimotor system measurement techniques. J Athl Train 37:85, 2003.

122. Risberg MA, Beynnon BD, Peura GD, et al: Proprioception after anterior cruciate ligament reconstruction with and without bracing. Knee Surg Sports Traumatol Arthrosc 7:303, 1999.

123. Rudolph KS, Axe MJ, Buchanan TS, et al: Dynamic stability in the anterior cruciate ligament deficient knee. Knee Surg Sports Traumatol Arthrosc 9:62, 2001.

124. Runge CF, Shupert CL, Horak FB, et al: Ankle and hip postural strategies defined by joint torques. Gait Posture 10:161, 1999.

125. Saladin KS: Anatomy & Physiology: The Unity of Form and Function, 2nd ed. New York, McGraw-Hill, 2001, p 476.

126. Schultz RA, Miller DC, Kerr CS, et al: Mechanoreceptors in human cruciate ligaments. J Bone Joint Surg Am 66:1072, 1984.

127. Sherrington CS: The Integrative Action of the Nervous System. New Haven, CT, Yale University Press, 1911.

128. Shimizu T, Takahashi T, Wada Y, et al: Regeneration process of mechanoreceptors in the reconstructed anterior cruciate ligament. Arch Orthop Trauma Surg 119:405, 1999.

129. Simmons S, Lephart S, Rubash H, et al: Proprioception after unicondylar knee arthroplasty versus total knee arthroplasty. Clin Orthop 331:179, 1996.

130. Simmons S, Lephart S, Rubash H, et al: Proprioception following total knee arthroplasty with and without the posterior cruciate ligament. J Arthroplasty 11:763, 1996.

131. Sitler M, Hopkinson W, Wheeler J, et al: The efficacy of a prophylactic knee brace to reduce injuries in football: A prospective, randomized study at West Point. Am J Sports Med 18:310, 1990.

132. Skinner HB, Barrack RL: Joint position sense in the normal and pathologic knee joint. J Electromyogr Kinesiol 1:180, 1991.

133. Skinner HB, Barrack RL, Cook SD: Age-related decline in proprioception. Clin Orthop 184:208, 1984.

134. Skinner HB, Barrack RL, Cook SD, et al: Joint position sense in total knee arthroplasty. J Orthop Res 1:276, 1984.

135. Snyder-Mackler L, DeLuca PF, Williams PR, et al: Reflex inhibition of the quadriceps femoris muscle after injury or reconstruction of the anterior cruciate ligament. J Bone Joint Surg Am 76:555, 1994.

136. Soderman K, Werner S, Pietila T, et al: Balance board training: Prevention of traumatic injuries of the lower extremities in female soccer players? A prospective randomized intervention study. Knee Surg Sports Traumatol Arthrosc 8:356, 2000.

137. Solomonow M, Baratta R, Zhou BH, et al: The synergistic action of the anterior cruciate ligament and thigh muscles in maintaining joint stability. Am J Sports Med 15:207, 1987.

138. Spencer JD, Alexander IJ: Knee joint effusion and quadriceps reflex inhibition in man. Arch Phys Med Rehabil 65:171, 1984.

139. Swanik CB, Lephart SM, Giannantonio FP, et al: Reestablishing proprioception and neuromuscular control in the ACL-injured athlete. J Sports Rehabil 6:182, 1997.

140. Swanik CB, Lephart SM, Rubash HE: Proprioception, kinesthesia, and balance after total knee arthroplasty with cruciate-retaining and posterior stabilized prostheses. J Bone Joint Surg Am 86:328, 2004.

141. Swanik CB, Lephart SM, Swanik KA, et al: Neuromuscular dynamic restraint in women with anterior cruciate ligament injuries. Clin Orthop 425:189, 2004.

142. Swanik KA, Lephart SM, Swanik CB, et al: The effects of shoulder plyometric training on proprioception and selected muscle performance characteristics. J Shoulder Elbow Surg 1:579, 2002.

143. Tietz CC, Hermanson BK, Kronmal RA, Diehr PH: Evaluation of the use of braces to prevent injury to the knee in collegiate football players. J Bone Joint Surg Am 69:2, 1987.

144. Tsuda E, Ishibashi Y, Okamura Y, et al: Restoration of anterior cruciate ligament–hamstring reflex arc after anterior cruciate ligament reconstruction. Knee Surg Sports Traumatol Arthrosc 11:63, 2003.

145. Tsuruike M, Koceja DM, Yabe K, et al: Age comparison of H-reflex modulation with the Jendrassik maneuver and postural complexity. Clin Neurophysiol 114:945, 2003.

146. Walla DJ, Albright JP, McAuley E, et al: Hamstring control and the unstable anterior cruciate ligament–deficient knee. Am J Sports Med 13:34, 1985.

147. Warren PJ, Cobb AG, Bentley G: Proprioception after knee arthroplasty: The influence of prosthetic design. Clin Orthop 297:182, 1993.

148. Wilk KE, Escamilla RF, Fleisig GS, et al: A comparison of tibiofemoral joint forces and electromyographic activity during open and closed kinetic chain exercises. Am J Sports Med 24:518, 1996.

149. Wilson GJ, Wood GA, Elliott BC: The relationship between stiffness of the musculature and static flexibility: An alternative explanation for the occurrence of muscular injury. Int J Sports Med 12:403, 1991.

150. Wilson GJ, Wood GA, Elliott BC: Optimal stiffness of series elastic component in a stretch-shorten cycle. J Appl Physiol 70:825, 1991.

151. Wojtys E, Huston L: Neuromuscular performance in normal and anterior cruciate ligament–deficient lower extremities. Am J Sports Med 22:89, 1994.

152. Wojtys E, Huston L, Taylor PD, et al: Neuromuscular adaptations in isokinetic, isotonic, and agility training programs. Am J Sports Med 24:187, 1996.

153. Wojtys EM, Goldstein SA, Redfern M, et al: A biomechanical evaluation of the Lennox Hill knee brace. Clin Orthop 220:179, 1987.

154. Wolf SL, Segal RL: Conditioning of the spinal stretch reflex: Implications for rehabilitation. Phys Ther 70:652, 1990.

155. Woo SL, Sofranko RAZ, Jamison JP: Biomechanics of knee ligaments relating to sports medicine. In Fu FF, Stone DA (eds): Sports Injuries: Mechanism, Prevention, Treatment. Baltimore, Williams & Wilkins, 1994, pp 67-80.

156. Yang JF, Winter DA: Electromyographic amplitude normalization methods: Improving their sensitivity as diagnostic tools in gait analysis. Arch Phys Med Rehabil 65:517, 1984.

157. Zehr PE: Considerations for use of the Hoffman reflex in exercise studies. Eur J Appl Physiol 86:455, 2002.

158. Zehr PE, Stein RB: Interaction of the Jendrassik maneuver with segmental presynaptic inhibition. Exp Brain Res 124:474, 1999.

159. Zimmy ML, Shutte M, Dibezies E: Mechanoreceptors in the human anterior cruciate ligament. Anat Rec 214:204, 1986.

CHAPTER 5

Surgical Approaches to the Knee*

Giles R. Scuderi

Critical to exposing the knee surgically is a complete understanding of the local anatomy, which is described in Chapter 1. With such knowledge, the pathological condition, anatomy, and planned surgery can be correlated. Although well-defined soft-tissue layers provide reproducible planes of dissection,[25,30,40] the blood supply to the skin should be respected, especially when previous incisions are present or multiple incisions are planned. Most of the blood supply to the skin arises from the saphenous artery and the descending geniculate artery on the medial side of the knee (Fig. 5–1).[11,43] The vessels perforate the deep fascia and form an anastomosis superficial to the deep fascia. Continuing through the subcutaneous fat to supply the epidermis, there is little communication in the superficial layer. Therefore, dissection should be deep to the fascia to maintain the blood supply to the skin.[42] The blood supply to the skin should not be confused with the blood supply to the patella.

Many of the incisions and approaches to the knee joint were originally designed for open meniscectomy and reconstructive procedures before the advent of arthroscopy.[1] The intent of this chapter is to provide these approaches for historical review because they still have current applications. Some approaches are extensile, and only a portion of the incision may be necessary for the planned surgery.[13] It is usually preferable to perform a single incision rather than multiple smaller incisions because it may not be the last operation performed on the involved knee and multiple scars may cause later skin problems.

A straight anterior skin incision is extensile and can be extended proximally and distally to expose the distal end of the femur, the patella, and the proximal end of the tibia. This anterior incision also allows exposure of the medial and lateral supporting structures and can be reopened if a reoperation is necessary. Through this skin incision a medial parapatellar arthrotomy can be performed, which is the most versatile approach in that it allows the broadest exposure to the knee joint. Historically, meniscectomy incisions were transverse or curvilinear along the medial or lateral joint line. These incisions are limited and are not extensile. The approach to the posteromedial or posterolateral corner can be through a longitudinal or gentle curvilinear incision. Lazy S incisions in this area have no value. Posteriorly, an S incision is the exception to the straight incision rule and provides extensile exposure.

*Adapted from Scott WN: The Knee, vol 1. St Louis, Mosby–Year Book, 1994, pp 55-71.

ANTERIOR APPROACHES

Skin Incisions

The anterior midline skin incision has been a utilitarian extensile approach to the knee (Fig. 5–2). With proximal and distal extension of the skin incision, large flaps can be developed to expose the anterior, medial, and lateral supporting structures.[20] If the midline skin incision is moved medially, it will be parallel to Langer's cleavage lines and subject to less tension and disrupting force than would an anterior midline incision.[38] Incisions parallel to the cleavage lines heal faster, gain strength quicker, and result in a neater scar.[22] There is no evidence that this position creates any more hypoxia in the lateral skin margin than an anterior midline incision does.

The anterior Kocher U incision[23] and the Putti inverted U incision[30] have become obsolete, primarily because of complications associated with vascular compromise to the surrounding skin. The anterior transverse incision may be cosmetically pleasing, but it does not allow extensile exposure (see Fig. 5–2).[38]

Arthrotomy

The medial parapatellar arthrotomy, or anteromedial approach, has been the most used approach for exposure of the knee joint. It provides extensive exposure and is useful for open anterior cruciate ligament reconstruction, total knee replacement, and fixation of intra-articular fractures. Because this approach has been implicated in compromise of the patellar circulation (see Fig. 5–1C),[33,34] some authors have advocated the subvastus, midvastus, and trivector approaches for exposure of the knee joint. Whereas these approaches expose the knee from the medial side, the anterolateral approach exposes the knee joint from the lateral side. With careful planning and arthrotomy selection, the anterior aspect of the joint can be fully exposed with these arthrotomies.

MEDIAL PARAPATELLAR ARTHROTOMY

A medial parapatellar arthrotomy allows excellent exposure to most structures of the knee joint (Fig. 5–3). von Langenbeck[38] originally described dissection of the vastus medialis from the quadriceps tendon with distal extension through the medial patella retinaculum and along the

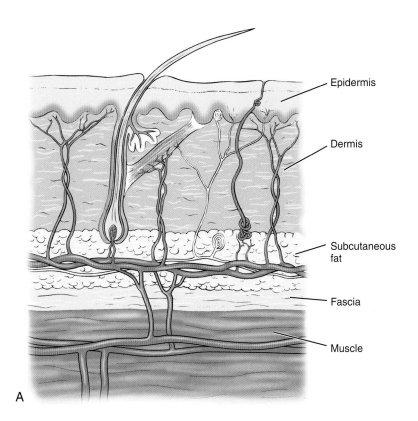

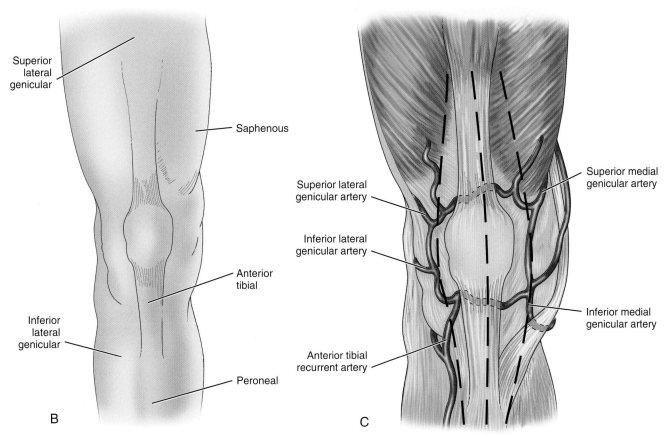

Figure 5–1. Blood supply to the knee. **A,** Microcirculation to the skin. **B,** Vessels contributing to the blood supply to the skin. **C,** Patella blood supply. (**A** and **B,** Redrawn from Younger AS, Duncan CP, Masri BA: Surgical exposures in revision total knee arthroplasty. J Am Acad Orthop Surg 6:55, 1998. **C,** Redrawn from Scott WN: The Knee, vol 1. St Louis, Mosby–Year Book, 1994, p 56.)

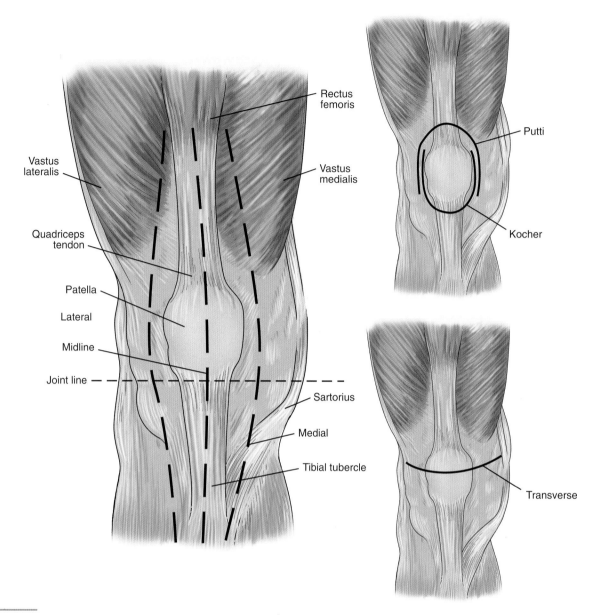

Figure 5–2. Anterior approaches to the knee. (Redrawn from Scott WN: The Knee, vol 1. St Louis, Mosby–Year Book, 1994, p 56.)

patellar ligament. The synovium is divided in line with the capsular incision, and the fat pad is retracted or incised. As dissection continues to the joint line, one must be aware of the anterior horn of the medial meniscus, as well as the transverse ligament between the medial and lateral meniscus. Completion of this arthrotomy permits the patella to be everted and dislocated laterally. When the patella is dislocated and the knee is flexed, care should be taken to not avulse the patellar tendon from the tibial tubercle. If there is difficulty dislocating the patella laterally, the proximal quadriceps tendon incision should be extended superiorly or the patellar tendon carefully reflected subperiosteally along the medial border of the tibial tubercle to its crest. Do not detach the patellar tendon from the tibial tubercle.

Insall[17] modified the split patella approach, as described by Sir Robert Jones, because of damage to the patellar articular surface (Fig. 5–4). The extensor mechanism is exposed through a midline skin incision, the quadriceps tendon is divided 8 to 10 cm above the patella, and the incision is continued distally in a straight line over the patella and along the medial border of the patellar tendon. The quadriceps expansion is peeled from the anterior surface of the patella by sharp dissection until the medial border of the patella is visualized. The synovium is divided, and the fat pad is split along the midline. The patella is then dislocated laterally. There is no internervous plane with this approach; however, both the rectus femoris and the vastus medialis are supplied by the femoral nerve proximal to this incision.

When the anteromedial approach is performed, the infrapatellar branch of the saphenous nerve comes into view (see Fig. 5–4B). The saphenous nerve travels posterior to the sartorius muscle and pierces the fascia between the tendons of the sartorius and gracilis muscles, where it becomes superficial to the medial aspect of the knee. At this level the infrapatellar branch of the saphenous nerve arises to supply the skin over the anteromedial aspect of the knee. Kummel and Zazanis,[24] as well as Chambers,[7] noted variation of this infrapatellar branch and recommended protecting it at the time of surgery to avoid painful neuromas. Insall[18] believes that neuroma formation is more related to the patient's temperament than to an actual pathological condition (see Chapter 92, "Minimally Invasive Total Knee Arthroplasty").

SUBVASTUS APPROACH

The subvastus approach, which allows direct access to the anterior knee joint, has been heralded as being more anatomic than the medial parapatellar arthrotomy (Fig. 5–5).[14,26] The subvastus approach is applicable to most reconstructive procedures of the knee, with the exception of lateral unicompartmental replacement.

This approach uses a straight midline skin incision that is extended above and below the patella. After development of a medial subcutaneous flap, the lower border of the vastus medialis is visualized. Because the vastus medialis inserts into the superior medial corner of the patella, the fascial sheath along the inferior border of the vastus medialis is incised from the patella down to the inter-

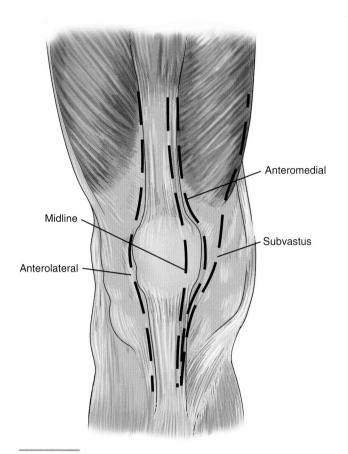

Figure 5–3. Preferred anterior approaches to the knee. (Redrawn from Scott WN: The Knee, vol 1. St Louis, Mosby–Year Book, 1994, p 57.)

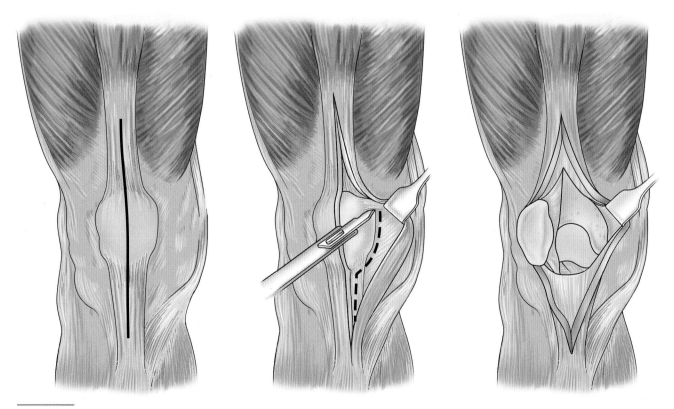

Figure 5–4. Insall's anterior approach. (Redrawn from Scott WN: The Knee, vol 1. St Louis, Mosby–Year Book, 1994, p 57.)

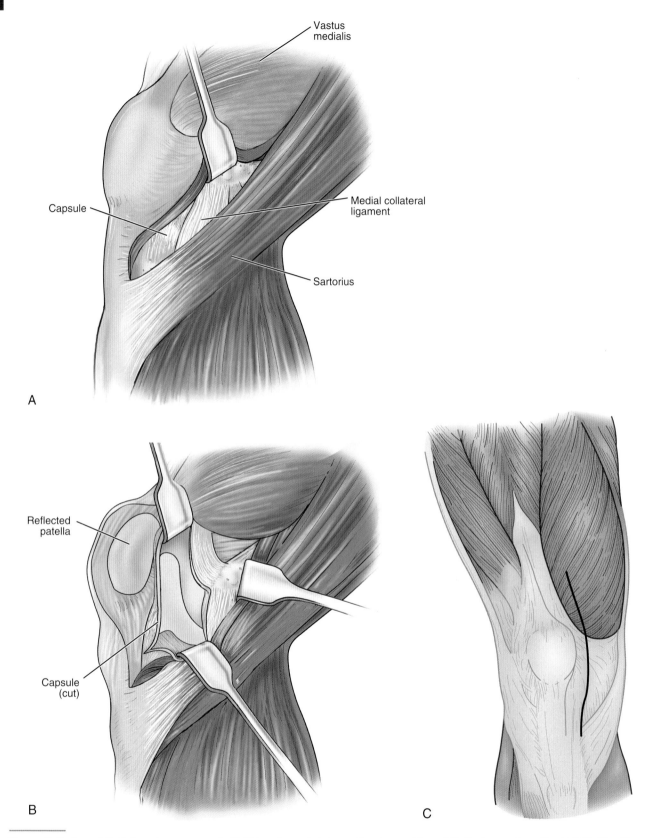

Figure 5–5. **A** and **B,** Subvastus approach. **C,** Trivector-retaining arthrotomy. (**A** and **B,** Redrawn from Scott WN: The Knee, vol 1. St Louis, Mosby–Year Book, 1994, p 58. **C,** Redrawn from Scuderi GR, Tria AJ: Surgical Techniques in Total Knee Arthroplasty. New York, Springer Verlag, 2002.)

muscular septum. This incision separates the vastus medialis from the intermuscular septum. The arthrotomy then continues distally along the medial margin of the patella, with the medial retinaculum incised along the medial border of the patellar tendon and down onto the tibia. The vastus medialis is then peeled proximally, with blunt dissection, from the intermuscular septum. Care should be taken at this point to avoid injury to the neurovascular contents of Hunter's canal. To gain access to the joint, the capsule of the suprapatellar pouch should be divided to release the patella, which is everted and dislocated laterally as the knee is flexed (see Chapter 92).

MIDVASTUS APPROACH

The midvastus muscle-splitting approach is performed through a standard anterior midline skin incision. The incision is carried down through subcutaneous tissue and deep fascia to expose the quadriceps musculature. The vastus medialis is identified and split full thickness, parallel to its muscle fibers. The quadriceps tendon is not incised. The incision is extended to the superior medial corner of the patella and then continued distally along the medial patella and patellar tendon to the level of the tibial tubercle. As in the subvastus approach, the capsule of the suprapatellar pouch is divided so that the patella can be everted and dislocated laterally. Advocates of this approach believe that it is easier to evert the patella with the midvastus approach than with the subvastus approach because of the reduced bulk of the vastus medialis. In addition, this approach splits the muscle well away from its neurovascular supply.[9]

TRIVECTOR-RETAINING ARTHROTOMY

The quadriceps musculature is exposed through an anterior midline skin incision. The trivector-retaining arthrotomy begins with transection of the vastus medialis obliquus muscle fibers 1.5 to 2 cm medial to the quadriceps tendon. Because the quadriceps tendon is not incised with this approach, the incision is extended distally 1 cm medial to the patella and the patellar tendon to the level of the tibial tubercle. It is recommended that this approach be performed with the knee flexed 90 to 110 degrees so that the quadriceps musculature is under maximal tension during the incision. To evert the patella and dislocate it laterally, the capsule of the suprapatellar pouch must be divided.[2]

ANTEROLATERAL APPROACH

The anterolateral approach, as described by Kocher,[22] consists of a lateral capsular incision that begins approximately 8 cm proximal to the patella at the insertion of the vastus lateralis muscle into the quadriceps tendon and continues distally along the lateral retinaculum (see Fig. 5–3). The incision can be extended distally through the fat pad for visualization of the lateral compartment and

ends just distal to the tibial tuberosity. This approach is less favorable than the anteromedial approach because it is more difficult to dislocate the patella medially than laterally.

LATERAL PARAPATELLAR APPROACH

The lateral parapatellar approach may be considered in total knee arthroplasty for fixed valgus deformities that are isolated or combined with flexion contracture or external tibial rotation. Fixed varus deformity represents the only relative contraindication.

In performing this approach, a curvilinear midline skin incision or a laterally placed anterior skin incision is made and extended distally over the lateral border of the tibial tubercle. The joint is entered through a lateral parapatellar incision that extends from the lateral border of the quadriceps tendon, over the lateral margin of the patella, and continues distally into the anterior compartment fascia, 1.5 cm from the tibial tubercle and for a distance of 3 cm from the tibial tubercle. To dislocate the patella medially and expose the joint, a thin segment of the tubercle is osteotomized with the attached patellar tendon. A medial periosteal hinge is maintained along with the infrapatellar fat pad, which is used for later closure of the lateral retinacular defect.[5,21]

LATERAL APPROACHES

Lateral approaches are limited in their exposure but are ideal for lateral meniscectomy and excision of meniscal cysts.[35] Bruser[4] recommended that the horizontal lateral skin incision be made at the level of the joint line with the knee in a fully flexed position (Fig. 5–6). The skin incision begins at the joint line and extends posteriorly from the patellar tendon to an imaginary line between the fibular head and the lateral femoral epicondyle. The iliotibial tract is identified and incised in line with its fibers, and the capsule is opened transversely, anterior to the lateral collateral ligament and superior to the lateral meniscus. Brown[3] modified the Bruser approach by making a vertical incision anterior to the iliotibial tract. O'Donoghue suggested positioning the knee in flexion, with the skin incision having a horizontal component that starts along the lateral edge of the patella and then courses vertically along the patellar tendon to the tibial tubercle.[37] The iliotibial tract is then split along its length. Smillie[36] described positioning the knee in flexion, with a skin incision starting near the lower pole of the patella and sloping downward and posteriorly to end just below the joint line. The capsule is incised in the interval between the patellar tendon and the iliotibial tract. Pogrund,[28] in an effort to obviate the difficulties associated with a large fat pad in the lateral compartment, described a skin incision that begins close to the inferior lateral aspect of the patella and curves gently downward and posteriorly (Fig. 5–7). The anterior capsule is incised in line with the skin incision.

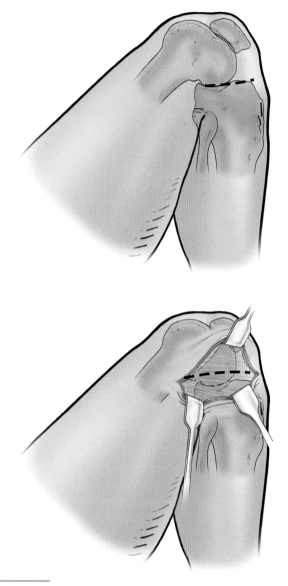

Figure 5–6. Bruser's approach. (Redrawn from Scott WN: The Knee, vol 1. St Louis, Mosby–Year Book, 1994, p 59.)

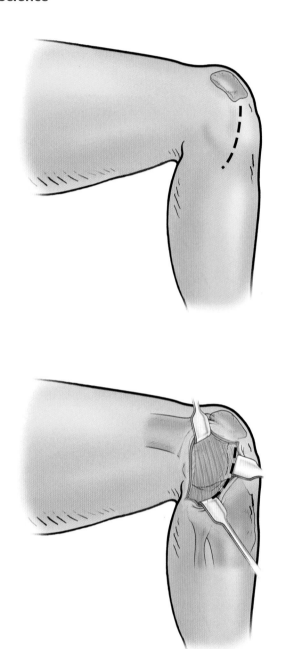

Figure 5–7. Pogrund's approach. (Redrawn from Scott WN: The Knee, vol 1. St Louis, Mosby–Year Book, 1994, p 59.)

For exposing the lateral aspect of the joint, Cave[6] described a curved skin incision that begins posterior to the lateral femoral epicondyle and curves downward and forward to the patellar tendon. The anterior capsule incision is made anterior to the lateral collateral ligament, and the posterior incision is made behind and in line with the lateral collateral ligament. This approach allows full exposure of the lateral meniscus.

MEDIAL APPROACHES

Like lateral incisions, medial approaches are limited and indicated for medial meniscectomy and excision of meniscal cysts. Hoppenfeld and Deboer[15] prefer an incision that begins at the inferomedial corner of the patella and curves anteriorly and posteriorly to end just below the joint line

(Fig. 5–8). The capsule is incised in line with the skin incision. Henderson[12] described a vertical posteromedial incision behind the medial collateral ligament, which allows the best exposure to the posteromedial corner. Both capsular incisions provide complete exposure of the medial meniscus. A transverse skin incision is made along the medial joint line. The capsule is then incised obliquely, anterior to the medial collateral ligament and vertically posterior to the ligament.

Cave[6] described an approach to the medial aspect of the joint that involves the use of a hockey stick skin incision (Fig. 5–9). The knee is flexed to 90 degrees, and the incision begins posterior to the medial epicondyle, is carried downward and gradually curves anteriorly just below the

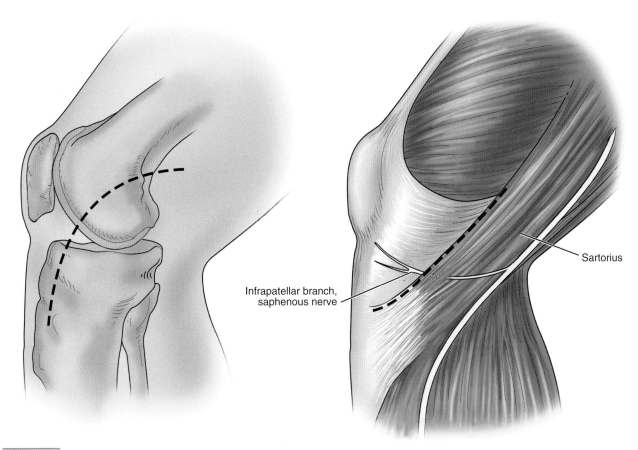

Sartorius

Infrapatellar branch,
saphenous nerve

Figure 5–8. Hoppenfeld's medial approach. (Redrawn from Scott WN: The Knee, vol 1. St Louis, Mosby–Year Book, 1994, p 60.)

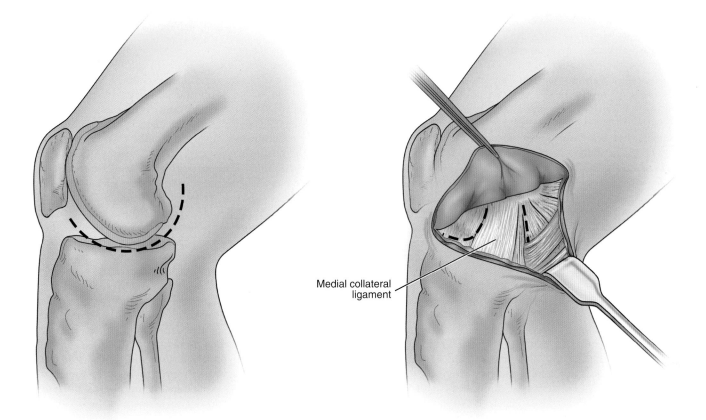

Medial collateral
ligament

Figure 5–9. Cave's approach. (Redrawn from Scott WN: The Knee, vol 1. St Louis, Mosby–Year Book, 1994, p 61.)

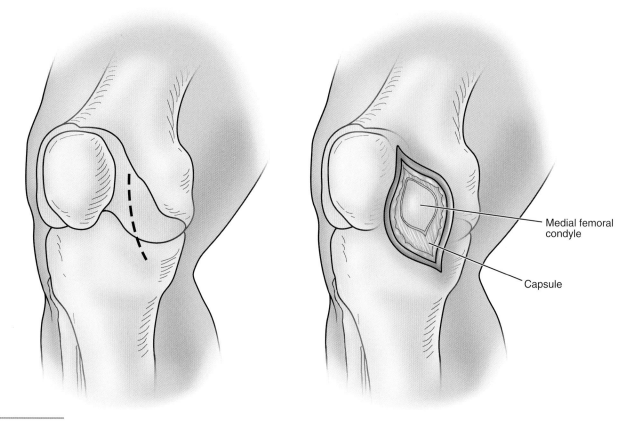

Figure 5–10. The oblique anteromedial incision is short and provides limited exposure. (Redrawn from Scott WN: The Knee, vol 1. St Louis, Mosby–Year Book, 1994, p 61.)

joint line, and is then carried forward to the medial border of the patellar tendon. The joint is entered through two separate incisions, one anterior and the other posterior to the medial collateral ligament. Both capsular incisions allow complete excision of the medial meniscus.

The oblique anteromedial incision is short and provides limited exposure (Fig. 5–10). The skin incision begins midway between the patella and medial femoral epicondyle and extends toward the tibial tubercle. The capsule and synovium are divided in line with the skin incision. The incision cannot be extended without dividing the medial retinaculum.[13]

To approach the medial supporting structures, a curvilinear incision is made 2 cm proximal to the adductor tubercle with the knee flexed 60 degrees; the incision curves over the medial collateral ligament and extends distally past the knee joint to the anteromedial aspect of the tibia (Fig. 5–11).[16] The fascia along the superior border of the sartorius is incised, and with further knee flexion, the sartorius retracts posteriorly to expose the semitendinosus and the gracilis. All three tendons are retracted to expose the tibial attachment of the medial collateral ligament. A medial parapatellar arthrotomy will expose the anterior aspect of the joint. To expose the posterior joint structures, the medial head of the gastrocnemius is separated from the joint capsule and retracted posteriorly with the tendons of the pes anserinus. A longitudinal incision is made in the posterior capsule, posterior to the medial collateral ligament.

POSTEROMEDIAL APPROACH

With the knee flexed 90 degrees, the adductor tubercle is palpated, and a curvilinear skin incision is made convex anteriorly, extending from the adductor tubercle along the medial collateral ligament and ending at the level of the pes anserinus tendons. The dissection continues in the interval between the vastus medialis and sartorius to expose the posteromedial capsule and the medial head of the gastrocnemius. The posteromedial aspect of the joint can be visualized through a longitudinal incision in the posteromedial capsule, posterior to the medial collateral ligament (see Fig. 5–11E). Distally, the insertions of the sartorius, gracilis, and semitendinosus are seen. The semimembranosus resides in the posterior portion of the incision. The saphenous nerve within Hunter's canal is anterior to the tendon of the adductor magnus and deep to the sartorius. The sartorius covers the adductor, or Hunter's, canal, and retraction of the sartorius exposes the contents of Hunter's canal, including the superficial femoral artery and vein, the saphenous nerve, and the motor nerve to the vastus medialis proximally. Proximal extension leads to the popliteal fossa and exposes the roof of Hunter's canal. Exposure of the medial aspect of the femur is achieved by displacing the vastus medialis anteriorly and subperiosteally and elevating the adductor musculature.

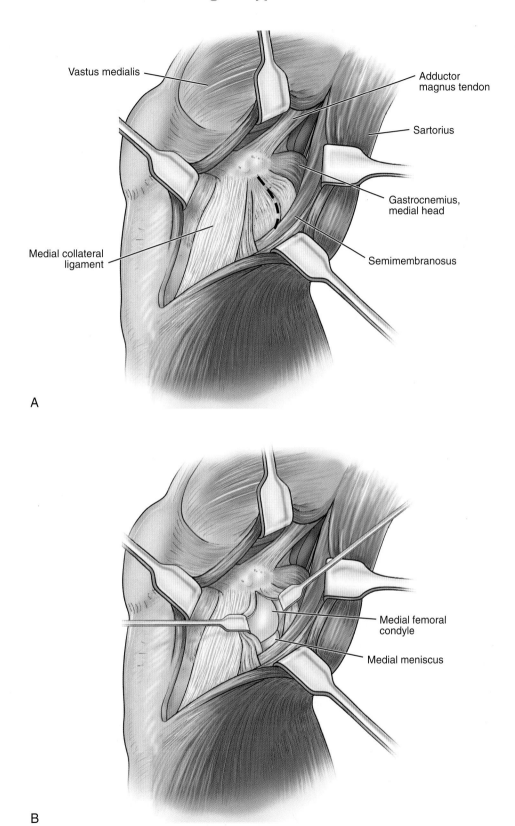

Figure 5–11. Medial approach. A medial parapatellar arthrotomy will expose the anterior aspect of the joint, and the posteromedial surface of the joint can be visualized through a longitudinal incision in the posteromedial capsule, posterior to the medial collateral ligament. (Redrawn from Scott WN: The Knee, vol 1. St Louis, Mosby–Year Book, 1994, p 62).

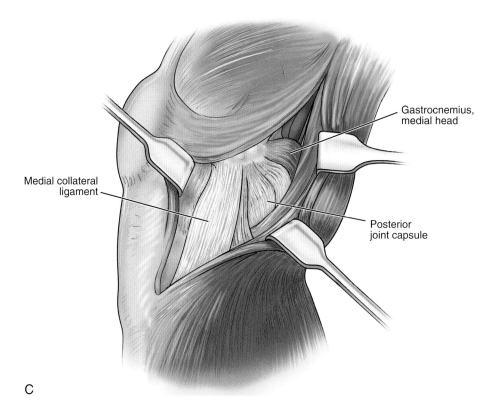

C

Figure 5–11, cont'd.

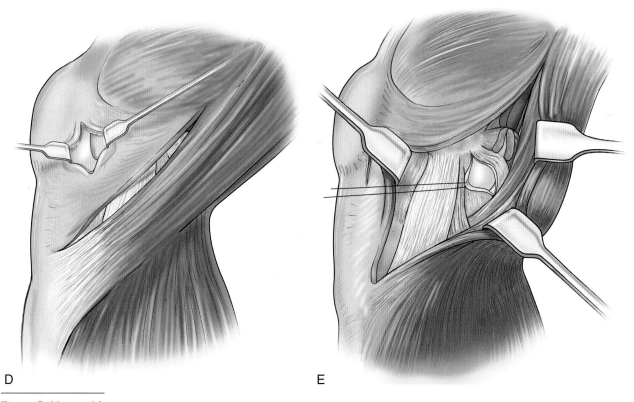

D

E

POSTEROLATERAL APPROACH

With the knee flexed, a curvilinear incision is made anterior to the tendon of the biceps femoris and the head of the fibula. The incision is placed at the interval between the posterior margin of the iliotibial tract and the anterior margin of the biceps femoris, thereby avoiding the common peroneal nerve (Fig. 5–12). The plantaris and lateral head of the gastrocnemius are retracted posteriorly to allow visualization of the posterolateral capsule and the lateral collateral ligament. Alternatively, Insall[17] has

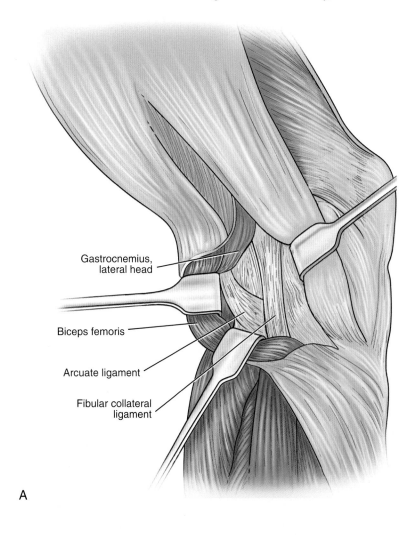

Gastrocnemius, lateral head

Biceps femoris

Arcuate ligament

Fibular collateral ligament

A

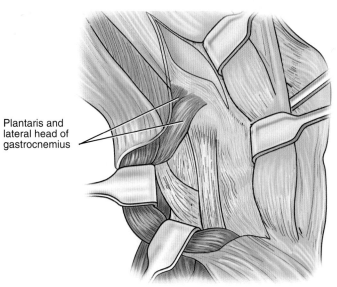

Plantaris and lateral head of gastrocnemius

B

Figure 5–12. Approaching the posterolateral structures. (Redrawn from Scott WN: The Knee, vol 1. St Louis, Mosby–Year Book, 1994, p 63.)

described subperiosteal dissection approximately 3 to 4 cm superior to the lateral femoral condyle (see Fig. 5–12B). The posterior capsule is thereby elevated from its attachment to the femur anterior to the lateral head of the gastrocnemius. This initiates the "over-the-top" approach. Proximal extension exposes the lateral femoral shaft, including the vastus lateralis and intermuscular septum. Distal extension exposes the head of the fibula and the peroneal nerve posterior to the biceps femoris.

POSTERIOR APPROACHES

A posterior approach permits visualization of the popliteal fossa with its neurovascular structures, including the posterior capsule of the knee joint, the posterior attachments of the menisci, the posterior compartments of the knee, the posterior aspect of the femoral and tibial condyles, and the origin of the posterior cruciate ligament. Because the popliteal fossa is a flexion crease, it should not be crossed with a longitudinal incision. An S-shaped skin incision is preferred and can begin on either the medial or lateral side (Fig. 5–13). When starting laterally, the incision begins longitudinally over the biceps femoris; it crosses the popliteal fossa obliquely and turns distally over the medial

head of the gastrocnemius. Medially, the skin incision begins over the tendon of the semitendinosus, crosses the popliteal fossa, and extends distally over the lateral head of the gastrocnemius. The skin flaps are retracted. Lying on the deep fascia is the small saphenous vein, which passes at the midline of the calf. Lateral to the vein is the medial sural cutaneous nerve. The fascia is excised, and the medial sural cutaneous nerve is followed to its origin, the tibial nerve. The popliteal fossa is diamond shaped (Fig. 5–14A). Proximally, the apex is bordered by the semimembranosus on the medial side and by the biceps femoris on the lateral side. Distally, the apex is bordered by the two heads of the gastrocnemius. The common peroneal nerve runs along the posterior border of the biceps femoris. Motor branches of the medial popliteal nerve to the gastrocnemius, popliteus, sartorius, and plantaris can be seen. The popliteal artery and vein lie deep and medial to the tibial nerve. The artery has five branches: the superior lateral geniculate, superior medial geniculate, middle, inferior lateral geniculate, and inferior medial geniculate. The vessels approach the nerve from the medial side proximally and cross anterior to the nerve to lie lateral distally.

The posterior medial joint capsule can be reached by detaching the tendinous origin of the medial head of the gastrocnemius muscle. The popliteal vessel and nerve are

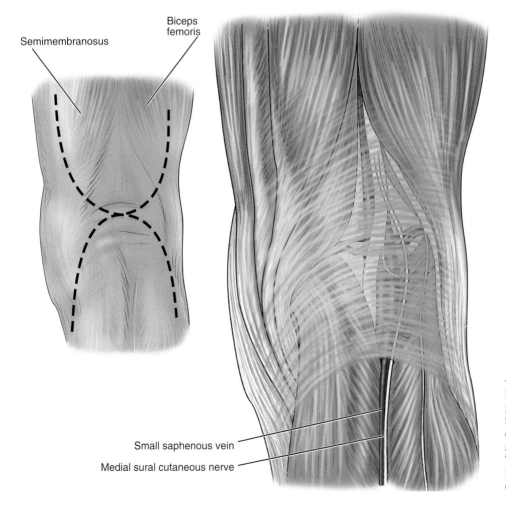

Semimembranosus

Biceps femoris

Small saphenous vein

Medial sural cutaneous nerve

Figure 5–13. An S-shaped posterior incision is preferred and can begin on either the medial or lateral side. (Redrawn from Scott WN: The Knee, vol 1. St Louis, Mosby–Year Book, 1994, p 64.)

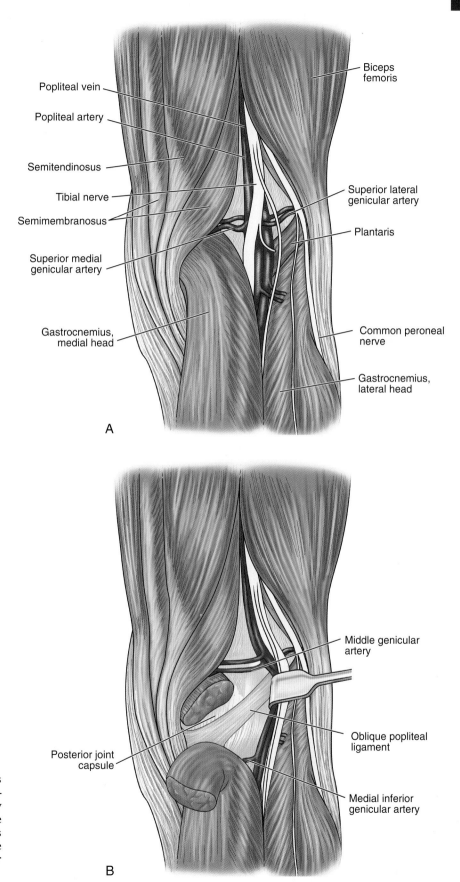

Figure 5–14. **A,** The popliteal fossa is diamond shaped. **B,** The posteromedial joint capsule can be reached by detaching the tendinous origin of the medial head of the gastrocnemius muscle. (Redrawn from Scott WN: The Knee, vol 1. St Louis, Mosby–Year Book, 1994, p 64.)

retracted laterally (Fig. 5–14B). The posterolateral capsule can be approached by detaching the tendinous origin of the lateral head of the gastrocnemius muscle. The nerve and vessels are then retracted medially.

LATERAL APPROACH TO THE DISTAL FEMUR

The lateral approach to the distal end of the femur exposes the posterior aspect of the lateral femoral condyle and the supporting structures (Fig. 5–15). It also allows exposure of the posterior intercondylar notch for the over-the-top approach. With the knee flexed 90 degrees, a curvilinear skin incision is made along the lateral aspect of the distal end of the femur and extended distally over Gerdy's tubercle; it ends about 5 cm distal to the joint line. The interval between the iliotibial band and the biceps femoris is developed. The iliotibial band is retracted anteriorly and the biceps femoris is retracted posteriorly to expose the lateral collateral ligament and the posterolateral corner. The anterior horn of the lateral meniscus can be visualized through a lateral parapatellar incision in the joint capsule. To avoid cutting the lateral meniscus, the arthrotomy should begin 2 cm above the joint line. To expose the posterior horn of the lateral meniscus, the lateral head of the gastrocnemius is retracted posteriorly, and a longitudinal incision is made in the capsule posterior to the lateral collateral ligament and proximal to the joint line. For the over-the-top approach, the vastus lateralis is identified and retracted anteriorly. The lateral superior geniculate artery can now be seen below the vastus lateralis and should be ligated. Subperiosteal dissection of the lateral head of the gastrocnemius and the intermuscular septum is carried medially to the linea aspera and distally over the lateral femoral condyle and into the posterior intercondylar notch.

PATELLAR TURNDOWN APPROACHES

Coonse and Adams[8] originally described a quadriceps turndown. They used a paramedian skin incision that begins at the lower end of the quadriceps tendon along the patella and extends along the medial border of the patellar tendon. Skin flaps are developed, the quadriceps tendon is split down the middle, and about 1 cm above the patella the incision is swung both medially and laterally and continues along the patella and the patellar tendon. The patella and patellar tendon can be turned down to allow complete exposure of the joint (Fig. 5–16).

Further modification of the patellar turndown approach[18] involves the use of an anterior midline incision. A medial parapatellar arthrotomy is performed, and a second incision is made at an inclination of 45 degrees from the apex of the quadriceps tendon and extended laterally through the vastus lateralis and the upper portion of the iliotibial tract. This lateral incision stops short of the inferior lateral geniculate artery to preserve the blood supply (Fig. 5–17). The full patellar turndown is now rarely necessary because cutting the quadriceps tendon

proximally yields excellent soft-tissue exposure, and functional reconstruction is possible (Fig. 5–18). This technique has been called the "quadriceps snip" by Insall.[18]

ANTERIOR APPROACH TO THE KNEE WITH OSTEOTOMY OF THE TIBIAL TUBERCLE

An anterior midline incision is made that extends 8 to 10 cm below the tibial tubercle. The medial parapatellar arthrotomy extends from 6 cm above the patella and distally along the tibial tubercle and anterior crest (Fig. 5–19). Whiteside and Ohl[40] used this exposure for difficult total knee arthroplasty, and they recommend using an oscillating saw to transect the tibial crest 8 to 10 cm below the tibial tubercle and elevating the tibial crest from the tibia. The lateral periosteum and musculature structures are left attached, as well as the lateral aspect of the quadriceps mechanism. Fernandez[10] recommends tibial tubercle osteotomy for bicondylar tibial fractures. He uses a straight anterolateral parapatellar incision. Large medial and lateral subcutaneous flaps are developed. The osteotomy of the tibial tubercle is performed with an oscillating saw and osteotomes. The osteotomy is trapezoidal, 5 cm long, 2 cm wide, and 1.5 cm wide distally. Once the tibial tubercle and the anterior tibial crest are freed, the entire extensor mechanism is elevated proximally and the retropatellar fat pad is divided to expose the entire joint.

TRANSVERSE LATERAL APPROACH TO THE PROXIMAL TIBIA

With the knee flexed 90 degrees, a transverse skin incision is made proximally 1 to 2 cm superior to the tibial tubercle and extended posteriorly along the lateral aspect of the tibia to the head of the fibula (Fig. 5–20). The fibular head, iliotibial band, lateral collateral ligament, and biceps femoris tendon are identified. The peroneal nerve need not be visualized because it lies beneath the biceps tendon. A vertical incision is made along the lateral border of the patellar tendon, and a horizontal incision is made along the anterolateral metaphyseal flare of the tibia and extended to the superior tibiofibular synovial joint. The iliotibial band is elevated subperiosteally from Gerdy's tubercle. The anterolateral musculature, the anterior tibialis, and the proximal portion of the extensor digitorum longus are elevated subperiosteally from the tibia. The superior tibiofibular joint is divided at the posterolateral corner of the proximal end of the tibia, and the popliteus is elevated from the posterior surface of the tibia to expose the entire proximal lateral aspect of the tibia. The anterior tibial recurrent artery arises from the anterior tibial artery at the interosseous membrane and tracks posterolaterally to an anastomosis with the lateral inferior geniculate artery at the lateral tibial condyle. This vessel should be protected or coagulated to avoid a postoperative hematoma. This approach is useful for a high tibial osteotomy.

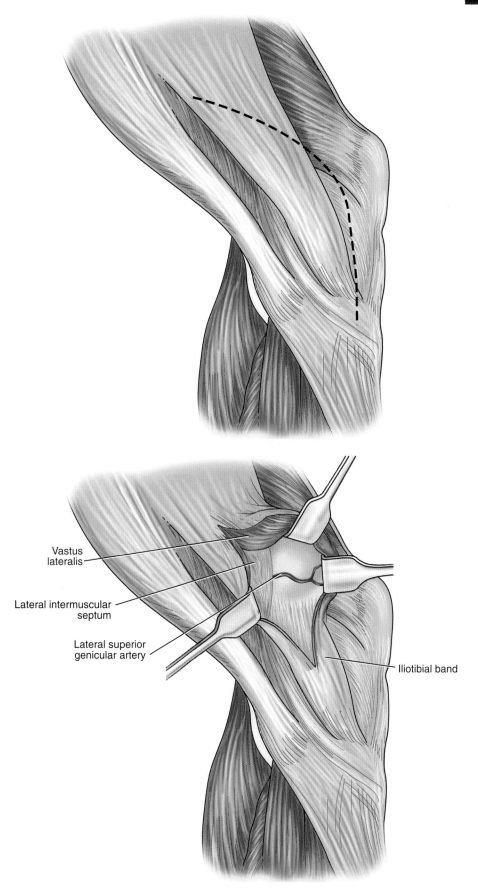

Figure 5–15. Lateral approach to the distal end of the femur. (Redrawn from Scott WN: The Knee, vol 1. St Louis, Mosby–Year Book, 1994, p 65.)

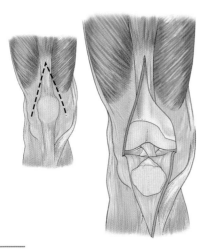

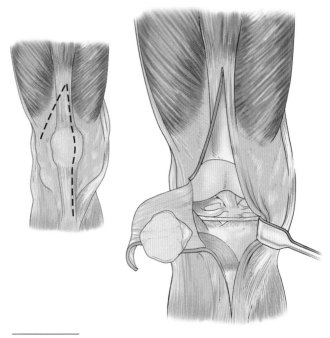

Figure 5–16. Coonse-Adams quadriceps turndown. (Redrawn from Scott WN: The Knee, vol 1. St. Louis, Mosby-Year Book, 1994, p 66.)

Figure 5–17. Modified Coonse-Adams quadriceps turndown. (Redrawn from Scott WN: The Knee, vol 1. St Louis, Mosby–Year Book, 1994, p 66.)

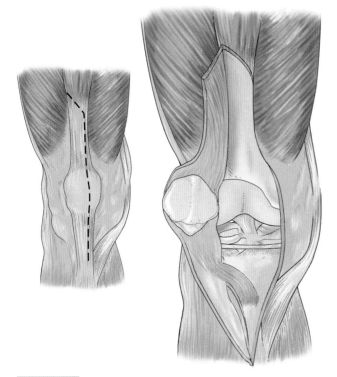

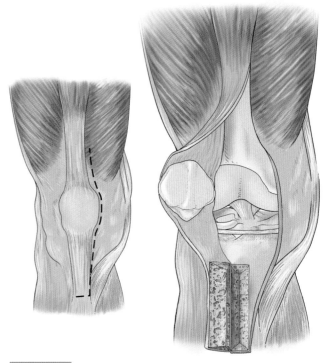

Figure 5–18. Insall's quadriceps snip. (Redrawn from Scott WN: The Knee, vol 1. St Louis, Mosby–Year Book, 1994, p 67.)

Figure 5–19. Anterior approach to the knee with osteotomy of the tibial tubercle. (Redrawn from Scott WN: The Knee, vol 1. St Louis, Mosby–Year Book, 1994, p 67.)

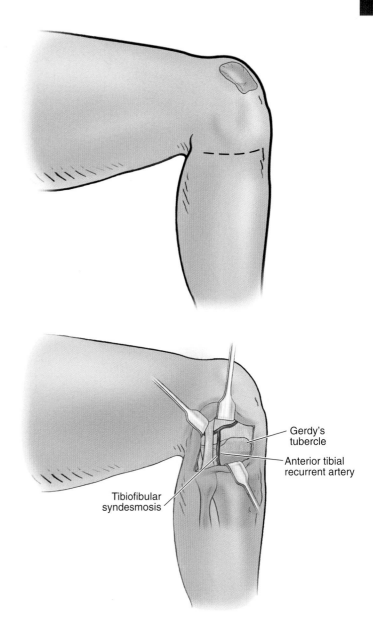

Gerdy's
tubercle

Anterior tibial
recurrent artery

Tibiofibular
syndesmosis

Figure 5–20. Transverse lateral approach to the proximal end of the tibia. (Redrawn from Scott WN: The Knee, vol 1. St Louis, Mosby–Year Book, 1994, p 68.)

ARTHROSCOPIC APPROACHES

Arthroscopy has become a valuable tool in the treatment of many ailments about the knee.[32] Numerous arthroscopic portals have been described (Fig. 5–21) whose utilization has made many arthrotomies less favorable.[27,39]

The superior medial portal is made through a skin puncture site approximately 3 to 4 cm superior to the patella and in line with the medial border of the patella. This portal is generally used for an inflow cannula or for viewing patellar tracking from above.

The superior lateral portal is made through a skin puncture site approximately 3 to 4 cm superior to the patella along its lateral margin. This portal is useful for visualization of patellofemoral tracking or placement of an inflow cannula.

For the anteromedial portal, the knee is flexed. The skin puncture site is approximately 2 cm above the anterior joint line and either at the medial edge of the patellar tendon or 1 cm farther medial to avoid the fat pad. The capsule and synovium are pierced with the arthroscopic sheath and trocar. The anteromedial portal allows visualization of both the medial and lateral compartments. However, it is occasionally difficult to visualize the posterior horn of the medial meniscus from this portal.

For the anterolateral portal the skin puncture site is approximately 2 cm superior to the anterior joint line at the lateral edge of the patellar tendon. The arthroscopic sheath and trocar then pierce the capsule and synovium. This portal is versatile for viewing both the medial and lateral compartments, as well as the patellofemoral joint.

The medial auxiliary portal is made immediately above the medial meniscus and 2 to 3 cm more medial than the anteromedial portal. The scalpel blade should be inserted parallel to the medial meniscus to avoid cutting the meniscus. The portal is posterior to the convexity of the medial femoral condyle and permits more direct access to

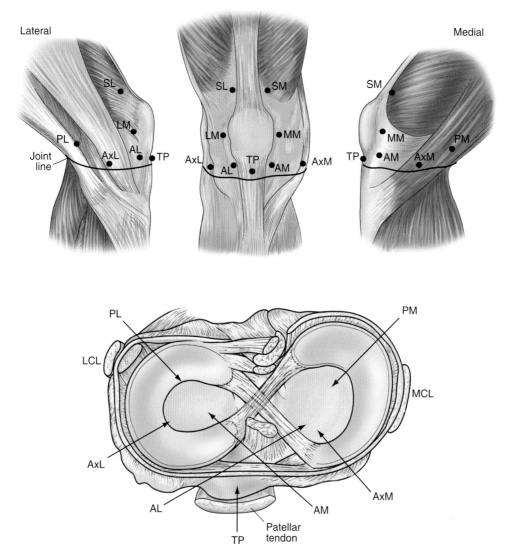

Figure 5–21. Arthroscopic approaches to the knee joint. AL, anterolateral; AM, anteromedial; AxL, lateral auxiliary; AxM, medial auxiliary; LCL, lateral collateral ligament; LM, lateral midpatellar; MCL, medial collateral ligament; MM, medial midpatellar; PL, posterolateral; PM, posteromedial; SL, superior lateral; SM, superior medial; TP, transpatellar. (Redrawn from Scott WN: The Knee, vol 1. St Louis, Mosby–Year Book, 1994, p 69.)

the posterior horn of the medial meniscus. This portal is useful if two instruments are needed in the medial compartment.

The lateral auxiliary portal is made immediately above the lateral meniscus and 2 to 3 cm further lateral than the anterolateral portal. The scalpel blade should be inserted parallel to the lateral meniscus to avoid cutting the meniscus. The portal is posterior to the convexity of the lateral femoral condyle and permits direct access to the posterior horn of the lateral meniscus. This portal is useful if two instruments are needed in the lateral compartment.

The medial and lateral midpatellar portals are more superior to the joint line at about the waist of the patella. The portal is made 5 cm from the medial or lateral margin of the patella. The arthroscope is placed in the anterior portion of the desired compartment and allows viewing of the contralateral meniscus.

The transpatellar portal is made distal to the inferior angle of the patella directly through the patellar tendon. The incision should be made parallel to the fibers of the patellar tendon to avoid cutting it. This portal allows visualization of the medial and lateral compartments and is useful for the three-portal technique of arthroscopic surgery.

For the posteromedial approach the knee is flexed, and the skin puncture site is approximately 2 to 3 cm above the medial joint line and posterior to the medial collateral ligament, usually in the soft spot of the posteromedial corner. It has been suggested that transillumination of the posteromedial compartment, done by placing the arthroscope in the anterolateral portal and passing it through the intercondylar notch, will assist with placement of this portal.[41] Before insertion of the scalpel blade, placement may be confirmed with a spinal needle. The scalpel should

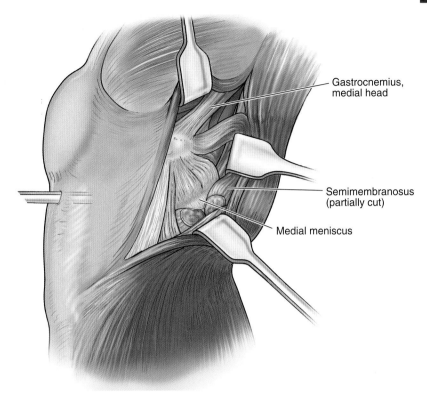

Figure 5–22. Posteromedial incision for arthroscopic repair of the medial meniscus. (Redrawn from Scott WN: The Knee, vol 1. St Louis, Mosby–Year Book, 1994, p 70.)

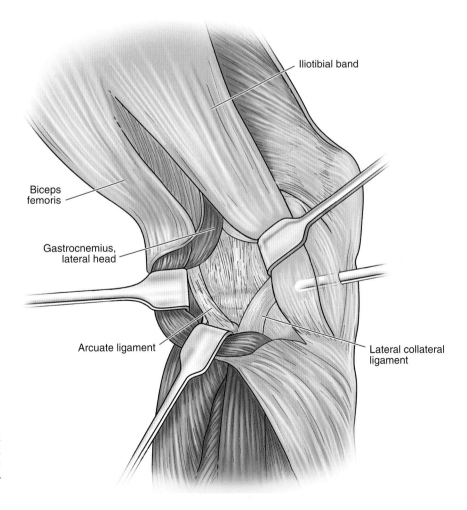

Figure 5–23. Posterolateral incision for arthroscopic repair of the lateral meniscus. (Redrawn from Scott WN: The Knee, vol 1. St Louis, Mosby–Year Book, 1994, p 70.)

pierce the skin and capsule, whereas the synovium is pierced with a cannula and blunt trocar.

The posterolateral portal is made with the knee flexed, and the soft spot posterior to the lateral collateral ligament and above the biceps femoris tendon is palpated. A spinal needle is passed at this point posterior to the lateral femoral condyle. The skin portal is made at this site, and a cannula with a blunt trocar is inserted into the joint.

COMBINED POSTERIOR INCISION AND ARTHROSCOPIC INTRA-ARTICULAR MENISCAL REPAIR

With the advent of meniscal repair,[19] Scott et al[31] described a combined posterior incision and arthroscopic repair to avoid neurovascular injury. For medial repair, a 5-cm longitudinal posteromedial skin incision is made. The sartorius and sartorial branches of the saphenous nerve are retracted posteriorly. The gracilis and semitendinosus are visualized and also retracted posteriorly. Occasionally, 2 to 3 mm of the direct head of the semimembranosus must be divided, and the medial half of the medial head of the gastrocnemius is elevated. The retractor is placed at this level to protect the neurovascular structures, including the tibial nerve and the popliteal artery and vein (Fig. 5–22). After this dissection, suturing of the medial meniscus may be performed with arthroscopic techniques.

For the lateral repair, a 6-cm longitudinal posterolateral incision is made posterior to the lateral collateral ligament. Blunt dissection is carried between the posterior margin of the iliotibial tract and the anterior aspect of the biceps femoris. Dissection is carried further between the lateral half of the gastrocnemius tendon and the posterolateral corner and includes the arcuate ligament complex. The retractor is placed at this level to protect the neurovascular structures. The dissection is not done more medially than the midportion of the lateral head of the gastrocnemius to avoid neurovascular injury. The peroneal nerve is protected by the tendon of the biceps femoris (Fig. 5–23). Once this incision is made, a tear of the lateral meniscus may be repaired with arthroscopic techniques.

References

1. Abbott LC, Carpenter WF: Surgical approaches to the knee joint. J Bone Joint Surg 27:277, 1945.
2. Bramlett KW: The Trivector Arthrotomy Approach. AAOS Instructional Videotape, June 1994.
3. Brown CW: A simplified operative approach for the lateral meniscus. J Sports Med 3:265, 1975.
4. Bruser DM: A direct lateral approach to the lateral compartment of the knee joint. J Bone Joint Surg Br 45:348, 1960.
5. Buechel FF: Lateral approach. In Lotke PA (ed): Master Technique in Orthopedic Surgery: Knee Arthroplasty. New York, Raven Press, 1995, pp 25-39.
6. Cave EF: Combined anterior-posterior approach to the knee joint. J Bone Joint Surg 17:427, 1935.
7. Chambers GH: The prepatellar nerve: The cause of suboptimal results in knee arthrotomy. Clin Orthop 82:157, 1972.
8. Coonse KD, Adams JD: A new operative approach to the knee joint. Surg Gynecol Obstet 77:344, 1943.
9. Engh GA, Holt BT, Parks NL: A midvastus muscle splitting approach for total knee arthroplasty. J Arthroplasty 12:322, 1997.
10. Fernandez DL: Anterior approach to the knee with osteotomy of the tibial tubercle for bicondylar tibial fractures. J Bone Joint Surg Am 70:208, 1988.
11. Haertsch PA: The blood supply to the skin of the leg: A post-mortem investigation. Br J Plast Surg 34:470, 1981.
12. Henderson MS: Posterolateral incision for the removal of loose bodies from the posterior compartment of the knee joint. Surg Gynecol Obstet 33:698, 1921.
13. Henry AK: Extensile Exposure, 2nd ed. Baltimore, Williams & Wilkins, 1970.
14. Hofman AA, Plaster RI, Murdock LE: Subvastus (southern) approach for primary total knee arthroplasty. Clin Orthop 269:70, 1991.
15. Hoppenfeld S, Deboer P: Surgical Exposures in Orthopedics: The Anatomic Approach. Philadelphia, JP Lippincott, 1984.
16. Hughston JC: A surgical approach to the medial and posterior ligaments of the knee. Clin Orthop 91:29, 1973.
17. Insall J: A midline approach to the knee. J Bone Joint Surg Am 53:1584, 1971.
18. Insall JN (ed): Surgery of the Knee. New York, Churchill Livingstone, 1984, pp 41-54.
19. Jakob RP: The arthroscopic meniscal repair: Techniques and clinical experience. Am J Sports Med 16:137, 1988.
20. Johnson DP, Houghton TA, Radford P: Anterior midline or medial parapatellar incision for arthroplasty of the knee: A comparative study. J Bone Joint Surg Br 68:812, 1986.
21. Keblish PA: Valgus deformity in total knee arthroplasty: The lateral retinacular approach. Orthop Trans 9:28, 1985.
22. Kocher T: Textbook of Operative Surgery, 3rd ed, Stiles HJ, Paul CB (trans). London, Adam & Charles Black, 1911.
23. Ksander GA, Vistnes LM, Rose EH: Excisional wound biomechanics, skin tension lines and elastic contraction. Plast Reconstr Surg 59:398, 1977.
24. Kummel BM, Zazanis GA: Preservation of intrapatellar branch of saphenous nerve during knee surgery. Orthop Rev 3:32, 1974.
25. Langer K: On the anatomy and physiology of the skin. I. The cleavability cutis. Br J Plast Surg 31:3, 1978.
26. Mullen M: The subvastus approach for total knee arthroplasty. Tech Orthop 6:64, 1991.
27. Patel D: Proximal approaches to arthroscopic surgery of the knee. Am J Sports Med 9:296, 1981.
28. Pogrund H: A practical approach for a lateral meniscectomy. J Trauma 16:365, 1976.
29. Putti V: Arthroplasty of the knee joint. J Orthop Surg 2:530, 1920.
30. Reider B, Marshall JL, Koslin B, et al: The anterior aspect of the knee joint: An anatomical study. J Bone Joint Surg Am 63:351, 1981.
31. Scott GA, Jolly BE, Henning CE: Combined posterior incision in arthroscopic intraarticular repair of the meniscus. J Bone Joint Surg Am 63:847, 1986.
32. Scuderi GR, Alexiades M: The evolution of arthroscopy. In Scott WN (ed): Arthroscopy of the Knee. Philadelphia, WB Saunders, 1990, pp 1-10.
33. Scuderi G, Scharf SC, Meltzer L, et al: The relationship of lateral releases to patella viability in total knee arthroplasty. J Arthroplasty 2:209, 1987.
34. Scuderi G, Scharf SC, Meltzer L, et al: Evaluation of patella viability after disruption of the arterial circulation. Am J Sports Med 15:490, 1987.
35. Seebacher JR, Inglis AE, Marshall JL, et al: The structure of the posterolateral aspect of the knee. J Bone Joint Surg Am 64:536, 1982.
36. Smillie IS: Injuries of the Knee Joint. New York, Churchill Livingstone, 1928.
37. Tria AJ, Klein KS: Illustrated Guide to the Knee. New York, Churchill Livingstone, 1991.
38. von Langenbeck B: Über die Schussverietzungen des Hüftgelenks. Arch Klin Chir 16:263, 1874.
39. Warren RF, Marshall JL: The supporting structures and layers on the medial side of the knee: An anatomical analysis. J Bone Joint Surg Am 61:56, 1979.

40. Whiteside LA, Ohl MD: Tibial tubercle osteotomy for exposure of the difficult total knee arthroplasty. Clin Orthop 206:6, 1990.

41. Wilson RM, Fowler P: Arthroscopic anatomy. In Scott WN (ed): Arthroscopy of the Knee. Philadelphia, WB Saunders, 1990, pp 49-66.

42. Younger ASE, Duncan CP, Masri BA: Surgical exposures in revision total knee arthroplasty. J Am Acad Orthop Surg 6:55, 1998.

43. Younger ASE, Masri BA: Surgical exposures in revision TKA. J Am Acad Orthop Surg 6:55, 1998.

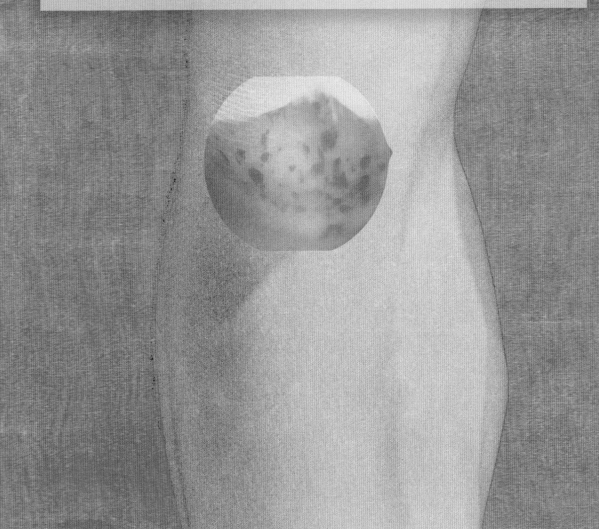

SECTION II

Imaging of the Knee

CHAPTER 6

Imaging in Evaluation of the Knee

Kevin R. Math

ROUTINE RADIOGRAPHIC EXAMINATION OF THE KNEE

Routine radiographic examination of the knee consists of standard anteroposterior (AP) and lateral and tangential axial ("sunrise") views. Other supplemental views include the tunnel view and the flexed, weightbearing posteroanterior (PA) view. The AP view is obtained with the knee extended, the cassette behind the knee, and the central x-ray beam perpendicular to the cassette. A standing (weightbearing) AP view provides more accurate assessment of joint space width than one taken from the supine position[1,2,68,82] and should be routinely obtained if tolerated by the patient (Fig. 6–1). This view depicts the medial and lateral joint compartments and soft tissues; provides images of the weightbearing aspects of the femoral condyles, tibial plateau, patella, and proximal end of the fibula; and gives a rough assessment of femorotibial alignment (Fig. 6–2A).

The lateral view of the knee is obtained with the knee flexed 30 degrees and the patient lying on the affected limb. The cassette is positioned under the lateral side of the knee and the x-ray beam is directed perpendicular to the cassette. This view depicts the patella and patellar height, the quadriceps and patellar tendons, the suprapatellar pouch, the distal end of the femur, and the proximal ends of the tibia and fibula (see Fig. 6–2B).

The tangential axial view of choice is the Merchant view.[40,75,80] The patient is placed in the supine position on the radiography table, the knees are flexed 45 degrees (using a fixed or adjustable platform), and the cassette is placed on the proximal part of the shins. Both knees are exposed simultaneously, with the x-ray beam directed toward the feet, inclined 30 degrees from the horizontal (Fig. 6–3A). This view provides an excellent assessment of patellofemoral alignment and is ideal for assessing the osseous patellofemoral articular surfaces and morphological features (see Fig. 6–3B). Other tangential axial views include the Laurin view,[40,67] which is obtained with the knees flexed 20 degrees, the cassette resting on the midthigh, and the x-ray beam directed from the feet toward the patient. The skyline view, obtained with the knee in maximum flexion, also demonstrates the posterior surface of the patella and the anterior surface of the femur, but the imaged femoral surface is not at the patellofemoral joint. Furthermore, accurate assessment of patellofemoral alignment is limited when the knee is flexed excessively.[15,40]

The tunnel view is a frontal view obtained with the knee flexed 60 degrees; it can be obtained as either AP, with the patient in the supine position, or PA, with the patient prone or kneeling on the cassette (central x-ray beam directed perpendicular to the tibia). This view demonstrates the posterior aspect of the intercondylar notch, the inner posterior aspects of the medial and lateral femoral condyles, and the tibial spines and tibial plateau (Fig. 6–4A). It is ideal for evaluating patients with suspected osteochondritis dissecans (OCD), which tends to occur more posteriorly in the intercondylar notch (see Fig. 6–4B and C).

The flexed, weightbearing PA view of the knee is obtained with the patient standing and flexing the knee 45 degrees. Both patellae touch the film cassette, and the x-ray beam is centered at the level of the inferior pole of the patella and directed 10 degrees caudad. This view is excellent for detecting cartilage loss and resultant joint space narrowing that may be unappreciated or underestimated on the conventional AP weightbearing view (Fig. 6–5).[16,17,53,110,112] With the knee flexed, it reflects the joint space width of the more posterior aspect of the femorotibial joint and also serves as a modified tunnel view. Comparison of intraoperatively observed cartilage loss with the narrowing observed on the radiographs demonstrates that the flexed PA weightbearing view has higher accuracy, sensitivity, and specificity than the conventional extension weightbearing radiograph does.[112]

Oblique views of the knee are not a necessary part of routine knee examination, except to further evaluate a radiographic finding identified on routine views. For the two oblique views, one at 45 degrees of external rotation and the other at 45 degrees of internal rotation, the patient is supine, lying on the cassette with the knee extended. These views show the posterior articular surfaces of the medial and lateral femoral condyles and the patella.

NORMAL RADIOGRAPHIC FINDINGS

Soft Tissues

The soft tissues of the knee are optimally demonstrated with low kilovoltage. On the lateral view, one can see the quadriceps, patellar tendons, and suprapatellar pouch. The collapsed suprapatellar pouch is a vertical radiodensity measuring 2 to 3 mm within the lucent triangular area between the distal end of the femur and the quadriceps

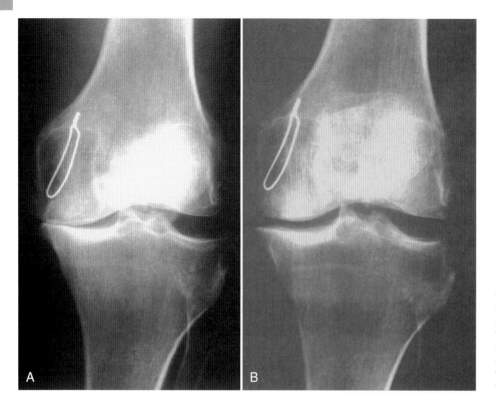

Figure   6–1. Anteroposterior
supine versus weightbearing
views. The severe medial joint
space narrowing is much more
apparent on the weightbearing
view (**A**) than on the supine
view (**B**).

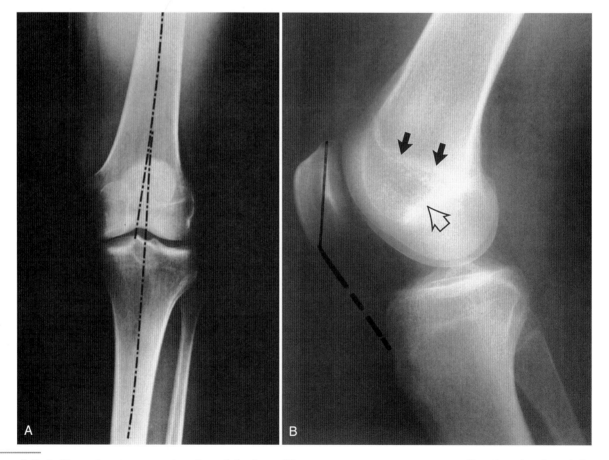

Figure 6–2. **A,** Normal anteroposterior view of the knee. The osseous structures are normally mineralized, and the articular cortices are smooth. Femoral-tibial alignment is in 7 degrees of valgus. The lateral compartment is normally slightly wider than the medial compartment. **B,** Lateral view of the knee. Blumensaat's line (*open arrow*) represents the roof of the intercondylar notch. The physeal scar is indicated by the *solid arrows*. The patella is commonly located between these two lines, with the lower pole approximately at the level of Blumensaat's line. The Insall-Salvati ratio is a more accurate method of assessing patellar height: the length of the patellar tendon (*dotted line*) divided by the greatest diagonal length of the patella (*solid line*) should be approximately 1 (0.8 to 1.2).

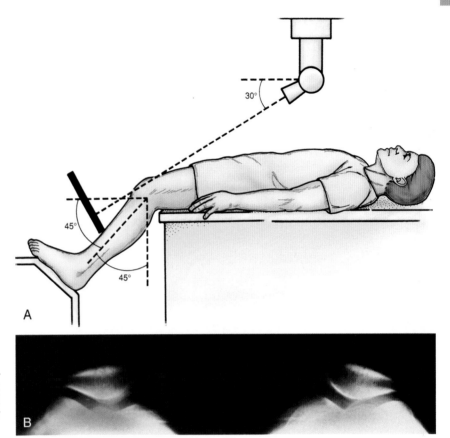

Figure 6–3. Merchant's view. **A,** Technique. **B,** Normal Merchant's view. Patellofemoral alignment is normal bilaterally, and the osseous articular cortices are normal.

tendon. The quadriceps tendon inserts on the superior aspect of the patella, and the patellar tendon extends from the lower pole of the patella to the tibial tubercle. Both these soft-tissue structures are normally straight, are of uniform thickness, and are sharply demarcated posteriorly by fat.

The soft tissues demonstrated on the AP view are the medial and lateral supporting ligaments; however, they have no distinguishing radiographic characteristics unless they are calcified.

Osseous Structures

The osseous structures of the knee include the bones and their articulations. Radiographically, the mineralization, alignment, integrity, and articulation of the bones are examined. The bones of the knee are the distal femur, proximal tibia and fibula, patella, and, on occasion, a fabella and/or cyamella. The fabella is a sesamoid bone in the lateral head of the gastrocnemius and is identified on the lateral view posterior to the distal femur; on the AP view it is superimposed on the lateral femoral condyle (Fig. 6–6A and B). The cyamella is a sesamoid bone in the popliteus tendon and is identified on the AP and oblique views in the groove in the lateral aspect of the lateral femoral condyle (see Fig. 6–6C).

ALIGNMENT

The knee joint consists of three joint compartments: the medial and lateral femorotibial compartments and the patellofemoral compartment. Alignment and joint space width of the medial and lateral compartments are best assessed on the AP view, whereas the patellofemoral compartment is most optimally assessed on the Merchant view.[80] The lateral joint compartment is normally wider than the medial compartment (see Fig. 6–2A); this asymmetry should not be misinterpreted as cartilage loss.

The angle formed by a line drawn through the long axis of the femur and a line through the long axis of the tibia depicts the *anatomic axis* of the knee (see Fig. 6–2A); on a standing AP view, there is normally approximately 7 degrees of valgus alignment at the knee. Standing AP long-leg radiographs (hip to ankle) are often obtained to assess the *mechanical axis* of the lower limb.[22,94-96,98,121] This axis is the angular measurement formed by one line extending from the center of the femoral head to the intercondylar notch of the femur and a second line drawn from the center of the tibial eminence to the center of the tibial plafond. Assessment of the anatomic and mechanical axes on long-length films is important for surgical planning before total knee arthroplasty.

On the tangential axial view of the knee, the patella should be centered directly over the femoral trochlear

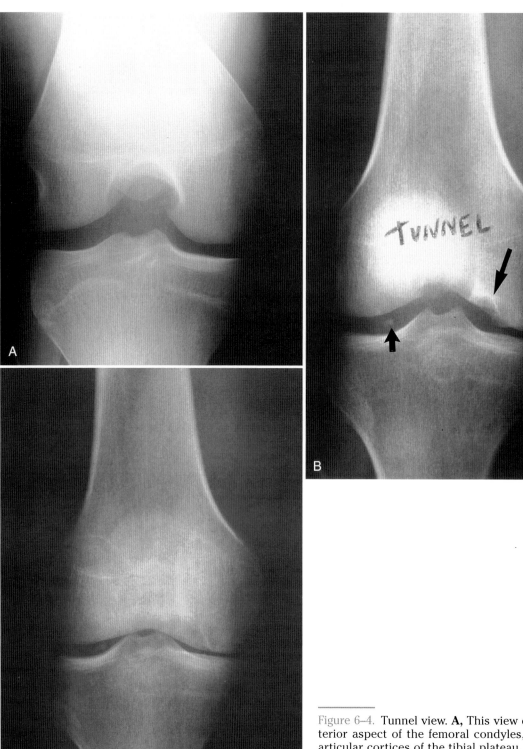

Figure 6–4. Tunnel view. **A,** This view demonstrates the posterior aspect of the femoral condyles, the tibial spines, the articular cortices of the tibial plateau, and the intercondylar notch. **B** and **C,** Osteochondritis dissecans. **B,** This tunnel view of the knee demonstrates an osteochondral defect at the inner aspect of the medial femoral condyle (*long arrow*) and a loose body overlying the lateral joint compartment (*short arrow*). **C,** These findings are extremely subtle on the routine anteroposterior view.

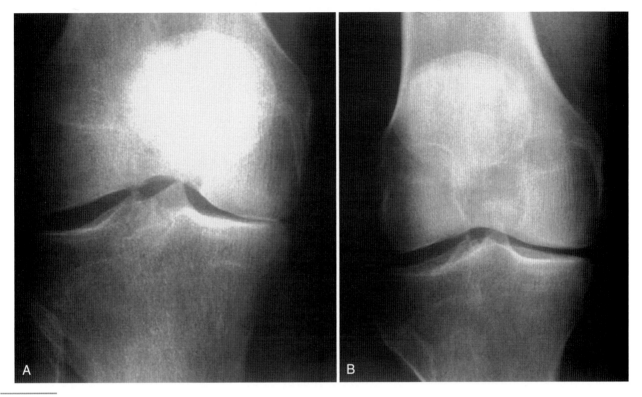

Figure 6–5. The flexed weightbearing tunnel view (**A**) demonstrates significant narrowing of the medial joint compartment, which is not present on the routine standing film (**B**).

articular surface. Calculation of the *congruence angle* provides an objective assessment of axial patellar alignment; the mean normal congruence angle is −6 degrees (standard deviation, 11 degrees) (Fig. 6–7).[80] Routine Merchant views of the knees can usually detect patients with significant patellofemoral malalignment. However, because abnormal tracking of the patella is maximal in the earlier degrees of flexion and the Merchant view is obtained at 45 degrees of knee flexion, other imaging techniques are sometimes necessary to detect patients with transient lateral patellar subluxation. A computed tomography (CT) scan with static axial images through the patellofemoral joints obtained at varying degrees of flexion can be helpful in evaluating patients with suspected patellar maltracking and normal radiographic studies (Fig. 6–8).[40,75] Contiguous images 5 mm thick are obtained through the patellofemoral joints at 0, 15, 30, 45, and 60 degrees of flexion. In addition to detecting patients with transient subluxation, CT provides excellent anatomic assessment of femoral trochlear and patellar morphological features. CT accurately depicts patients with a dysplastic trochlea or a hypoplastic lateral femoral condyle. Other modalities for dynamic assessment of patellar tracking during active flexion are kinematic CT and magnetic resonance imaging (MRI)[15,122]; however, the necessary equipment and software for these techniques are not widely available.

Although several methods of assessing vertical patellar height have been described,[75] the Insall-Salvati ratio remains the most widely used.[56] On the lateral view, the length of the patellar tendon (LT), measured from the lower pole of the patella to the tibial tubercle, should be roughly equal to the greatest diagonal length of the patella (LP) (see Fig. 6–2B). Patella alta exists when the LT/LP ratio exceeds 1.2; a ratio less than 0.8 is termed patella baja or patella infra. Causes of patella alta include patella tendon rupture[104] and spastic neuromuscular diseases (e.g., cerebral palsy). Patella baja is most commonly seen in association with quadriceps tendon rupture but can also occur with flaccid neuromuscular diseases (e.g., polio) and achondroplasia, as well as postoperatively (e.g., after total knee arthroplasty).

ANATOMIC VARIANTS

Normal developmental variations exist in the immature skeleton that can be confused with an abnormality.[7,33,129] These skeletal variants are usually incidental findings and asymptomatic. The most common variations are found at the following locations:

1. Posterior articular cortical surface of the medial and/or lateral femoral condyles. The irregularity on the posterior aspect of the femoral condyles is best visualized on the tunnel and oblique views (Fig. 6–9). The cartilage covering the osseous area of irregularity is intact.
2. Distal metaphysis of the medial femoral condyle. There can be a metaphyseal defect at the insertion site of the adductor muscles on the medial aspect of the distal end of the femur, best visualized on the

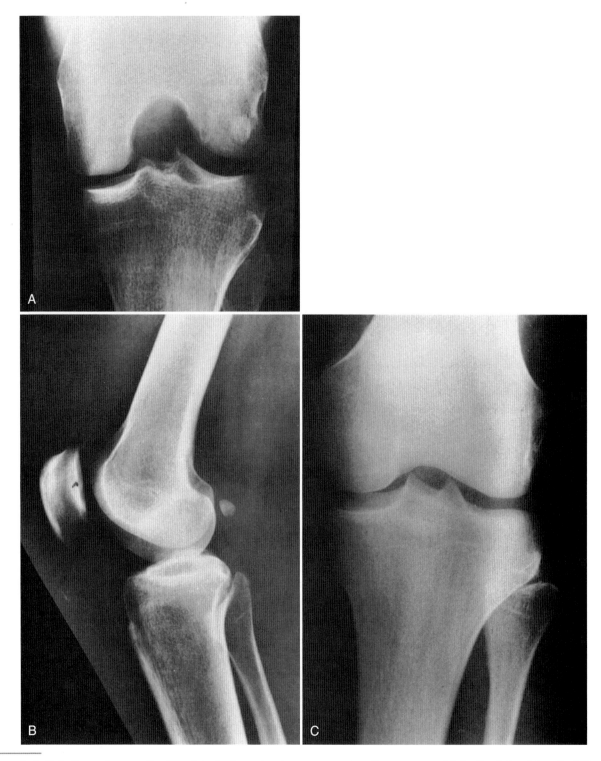

Figure 6–6. Fabella and cyamella. The fabella is a circular osseous density, a sesamoid, in the lateral head of the gastrocnemius muscle. **A,** On the anteroposterior view it is superimposed on the lateral femoral condyle. **B,** On the lateral view, the fabella is posterior to the femoral condyles. **C,** A cyamella is a circular osseous density, a sesamoid, in the popliteus tendon. On the anteroposterior view the cyamella is seen within the notch at the lateral aspect of the lateral femoral condyle.

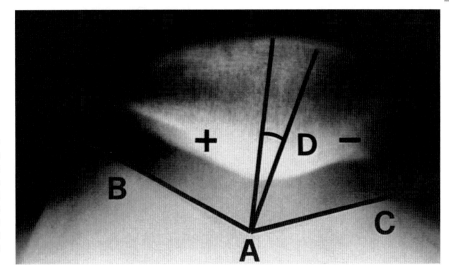

Figure 6–7. Merchant's view; measurement of the sulcus and congruence angles. The sulcus angle (BAC) is bisected by the reference line. A second line (AD) is then drawn from the sulcus to the patellar ridge. If the apex of the patellar apex is lateral to the reference line, the value of the angle is positive; if it is medial, the value of the angle is negative.

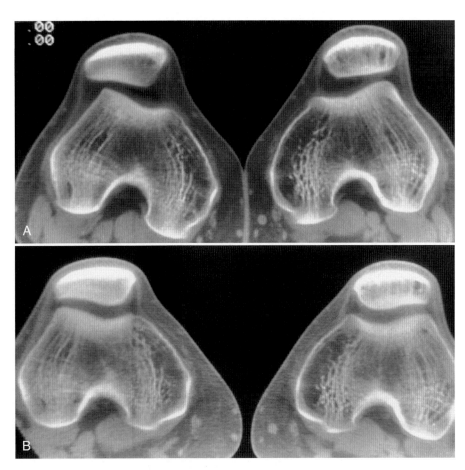

Figure 6–8. Computed tomography (CT) assessment of patellar tracking. Axial CT images obtained at 30 degrees (A) and 45 degrees (B) of flexion demonstrate transient bilateral lateral patellar subluxation. The patellar subluxation present at 30 degrees reduces at 45 degrees of flexion, thus explaining the normal Merchant view in this symptomatic patient.

oblique view (Fig. 6–10). It may represent a benign cortical defect or a reaction to microtrauma; it must be recognized as a normal variant to avoid unnecessary biopsy.

3. Tibial tubercle. The size and shape of the tubercle vary; it may be fragmented and/or separate from the tibia. Normal fragmentation of the tibial tubercle ossification center should not be mistaken for the pathological changes seen in Osgood-Schlatter disease.[92,93]

4. Patella. The patella can have two or more osseous centers, referred to as a bipartite or multipartite patella (Fig. 6–11). A bipartite patella is the most common variant, is seen in 1% of the population, and is bilateral 50% of the time.[75] Bipartite patellae are rarely symptomatic and must be distinguished from patellar fracture.

Accurate differentiation between a bipartite patella and a fracture is usually possible by considering the following features[75]:

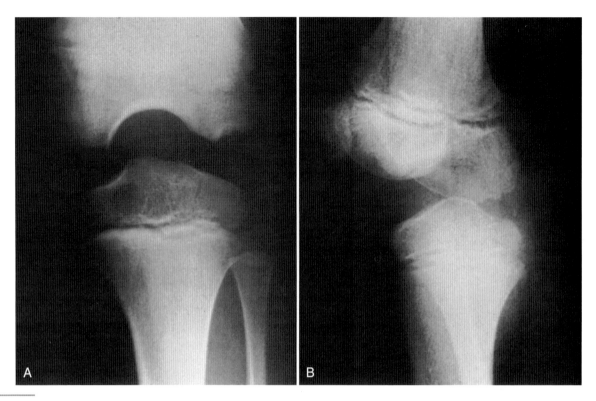

Figure 6–9. Anteroposterior (**A**) and oblique (**B**) views of a child's knee demonstrate irregularity and fragmentation of the posterior articular surface of the lateral femoral condyle. This is a normal variation, and the articular cartilage over the defect is intact.

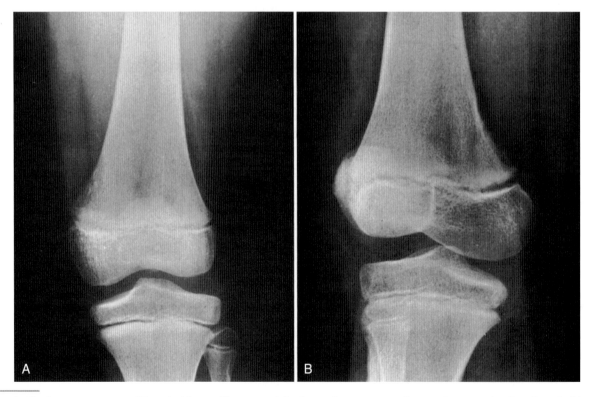

Figure 6–10. Anteroposterior (**A**) and oblique (**B**) views of the knee show a cortical irregularity in the distal medial femoral metaphysis. This cortical defect is an incidental finding that should not be subjected to biopsy.

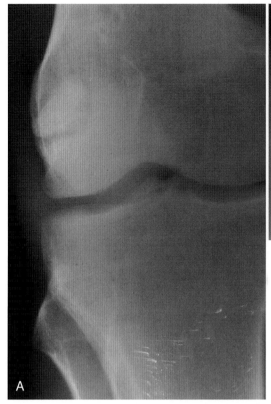

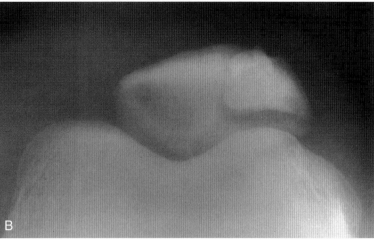

Figure 6–11. Bipartite patella. Oblique (**A**) and tangential axial (**B**) views of the patella demonstrate a crescentic radiolucency traversing the superolateral aspect of the patella. This lucency forms the interface between the two osseous centers of the bipartite patella. The superolateral location is typical of this entity.

Location—The cleavage plane in a bipartite patella is generally at the superolateral aspect of the patella.

Interface—Fracture fragments normally fit evenly together like pieces of a jigsaw puzzle, whereas the interface margins of a bipartite patella do not appear congruent.

Width—The coronal width of a bipartite patella, assessed on a tangential axial view, is usually greater than that of the contralateral patella.

Cartilage integrity—The cartilage overlying a bipartite patella, as depicted on MRI, is intact, unlike fractures, in which osteochondral integrity is disrupted.

A dorsal defect of the patella is another anatomic variant[43,58] that is manifested as a lytic-appearing area at the superolateral patella and is usually detected as an incidental finding (Fig. 6–12). Pathologically, the lesion is composed of fibrous tissue and spicules of bone. This uncommon entity is seen in children and typically fills in with normal or sclerotic bone in adulthood.

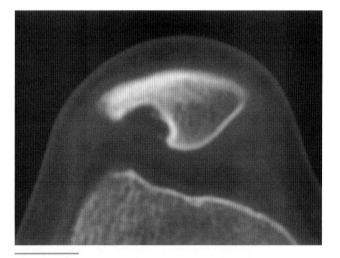

Figure 6–12. Dorsal defect of the patella. This axial computed tomography scan demonstrates a large lucent dorsal defect involving the majority of the lateral facet of the patella. The patient had a smaller, similar lesion in the contralateral patella. This finding is bilateral in approximately one-third of individuals.

SOFT TISSUE

Radiographically, the most common abnormality in the knee is an oval, soft-tissue density posterior to the quadriceps tendon (Fig. 6–13A). It indicates abnormal distention of the suprapatellar pouch by either joint effusion or synovial hypertrophic tissue. A joint effusion may consist of synovial fluid, blood, or pus.

When a joint effusion is present in a patient with a clinically suspected occult fracture, a "cross-table" lateral view is often helpful. This view is obtained with the patient

supine, the cassette perpendicular to the table top, and the central x-ray beam perpendicular to the cassette. A fracture that involves an articular surface bleeds into the joint; this blood contains bone marrow fat. Because fat has lower specific gravity than blood does, it separates from the blood and layers on top of it, analogous to oil floating on water. The sharp interface between the low density of fat

Figure 6–13. Joint effusion. **A,** A lateral view demonstrates an oval soft-tissue density representing a joint effusion within the suprapatellar pouch posterior to the quadriceps tendon. **B,** A cross-table lateral view shows a fat-fluid level (*arrows*) indicating an intra-articular fracture with lipohemarthrosis. (From Torg JS, Pavlov H, Morris VB: Salter-Harris type III fracture of the medial femoral condyle occurring in the adolescent athlete. J Bone Joint Surg Am 63:586, 1981.) **C,** A sagittal T1-weighted magnetic resonance image obtained with the patient supine demonstrates high-signal fat (*asterisk*) floating on top of intra-articular hemorrhage. An acute supracondylar fracture is also noted (*arrows*).

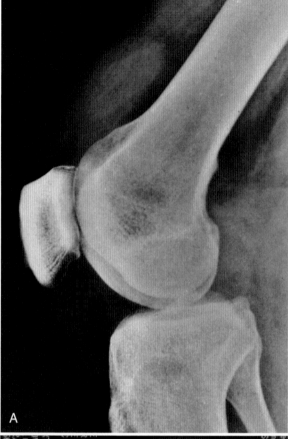

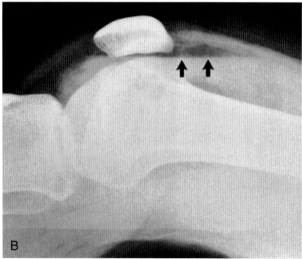

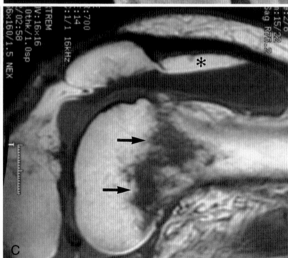

and the soft-tissue density of blood, the so-called fat-fluid level, can be distinguished radiographically on this view (see Fig. 6–13B and C).

Popliteal (Baker's) cysts are often visualized as a soft-tissue mass in the popliteal fossa. They are almost always accompanied by a joint effusion and represent communication of the synovial cavity with a bursa/recess at the posteromedial aspect of the knee. The communication between the joint and this recess exists between the tendon of the medial head of the gastrocnemius and the semimembranosus. Plain films are insensitive in diagnosing popliteal cysts because the soft-tissue density of the gastrocnemius muscle obscures visualization of them. The cyst and communication with the joint can be accurately diagnosed most cost-effectively by ultrasonography (Fig. 6–14A) but can also be clearly delineated with MRI (see Fig. 6–14B).

Calcifications

Calcifications at the knee can be extra-articular or intra-articular, and the cause of these calcifications

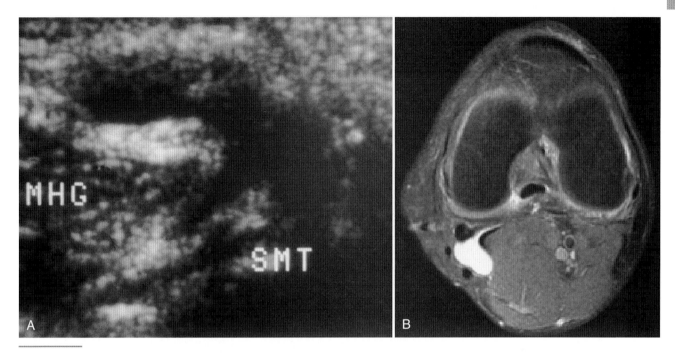

Figure 6–14. Popliteal (Baker's) cyst. Cross-sectional images from ultrasonography (**A**) and magnetic resonance imaging (**B**) show the cystic mass extending into the medial popliteal region. The cyst communicates with the joint through a channel between the medial head of the gastrocnemius (muscle and tendon) located laterally and the semimembranosus tendon located medially.

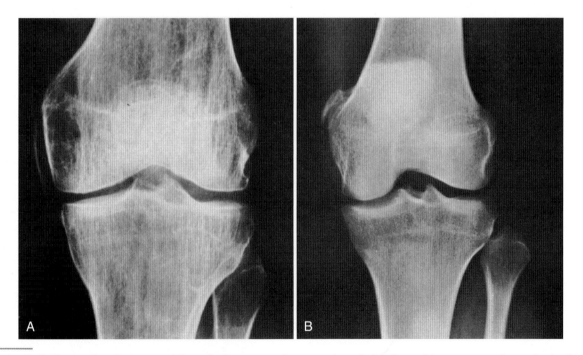

Figure 6–15. Pellegrini-Stieda disease. The calcification in the injured medial collateral ligament can be in the body of the ligament (**A**) or at its proximal attachment (**B**). (From Pavlov H: Radiology for the orthopaedic surgeon. Contemp Orthop 6:85, 1983.)

can often be determined by fairly specific distinguishing characteristics.

Causes of extra-articular calcifications include normal anatomic structures (fabella, cyamella), tendon and ligament calcification, calcific bursitis, calcified neoplasm, aneurysm, tumoral calcinosis, and myositis ossificans.

TENDON AND LIGAMENT CALCIFICATION

Pellegrini-Stieda disease is linear calcification or ossification within and around the medial collateral ligament (MCL) secondary to previous injury (Fig. 6–15).

Calcification/fragmentation at the tibial tubercle insertion of the patellar tendon is the hallmark of *Osgood-Schlatter* disease (Fig. 6–16A). Unlike the normal fragmentation that occurs at this ossification center, there is also localized soft-tissue swelling and soft-tissue infiltration of the infrapatellar fat pad.[92,93,120] The same findings occur at the patellar attachment of the patellar tendon in Sinding-Larsen-Johansson disease[124] (see Fig. 6–16B and C) and in patients with chronic tensile stress on the patellar tendon ("jumper's knee").

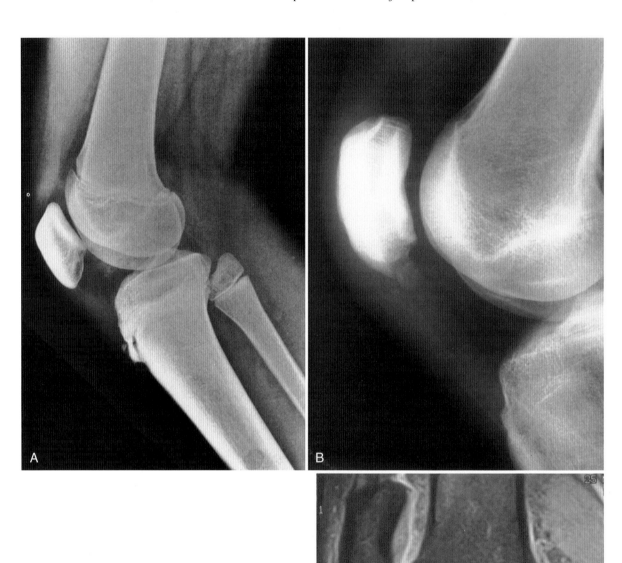

Figure 6–16. **A,** Osgood-Schlatter disease. This lateral radiograph shows the typical findings of a thickened distal patellar tendon, fragmentation of the tibial tubercle, and soft-tissue swelling anterior to the tubercle. In Sinding-Larsen-Johansson disease, there is ossification at the proximal patellar tendon insertion on the lower pole of the patella with soft-tissue swelling (**B**). A sagittal fat-suppressed proton density magnetic resonance image in the same patient (**C**) reveals high-signal soft-tissue edema surrounding the rectangular ossification (*straight arrow*). Note the concomitant injury of the more distal patellar tendon at its tibial tubercle attachment (*curved arrow*).

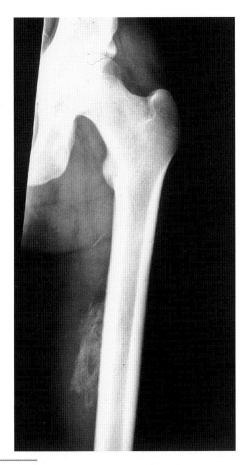

Figure 6–17. Myositis ossificans, medial aspect of the thigh. Soft-tissue ossification consistent with myositis ossificans is seen in the medial aspect of the thigh. Note the characteristic pattern of denser ossification more peripherally than centrally.

Myositis ossificans is marked by ossification in the soft tissues, usually as a result of direct trauma. Patients have a soft-tissue mass that starts to ossify at the periphery in about 2 to 3 weeks. It has a characteristic pattern of ossification in a centripetal fashion and starts "filling in" from the periphery over the next 4 to 6 weeks[90] (Fig. 6–17). This "zonal maturation phenomenon" is the typical pattern of ossification in this condition and distinguishes it from other, more ominous calcifying processes, such as a sarcoma arising from bone or soft tissue. Equivocal cases should be further evaluated with CT, which optimally depicts the peripheral ossification. These lesions often have an aggressive appearance on MRI and can mimic osteosarcoma on biopsy.

BURSAL CALCIFICATION

Aside from the suprapatellar pouch/bursa, there are three bursae located at the anterior aspect of the knee: the prepatellar bursa, the superficial infrapatellar bursa, and the deep infrapatellar bursa. These bursae can become distended with fluid in acute bursitis and can calcify in the chronic setting.

Prepatellar bursitis is distention/inflammation of the prepatellar bursa that extends from the midpatella to the midpatellar tendon. Also known as "housemaid's knee,"[10] chronic disease results in coarse, speckled calcifications anterior to the patella and upper patellar tendon (Fig. 6–18A to C).

"Preacher's knee" is bursitis of the superficial infrapatellar bursa, which is located superficial to the distal patellar tendon and anterior to the tibial tubercle (see Fig. 6–18D). The coarse calcifications in chronic bursitis reflect the typical location of this bursa.

CALCIFIED SOFT-TISSUE NEOPLASMS

In a patient with a calcified soft-tissue tumor near a joint, the diagnosis of synovial sarcoma should be considered. This type of tumor occurs most commonly in young adults and can have associated calcifications. Despite its name, synovial sarcoma is typically extra-articular and not uncommonly located distant from the joint.

Causes of intra-articular calcifications include calcification within the articular (hyaline) cartilage or meniscal (fibro-) cartilage (chondrocalcinosis), calcified loose bodies, and calcification in the infrapatellar fat pad (Hoffa's disease).

Hoffa's disease is an obscure condition characterized by necrosis of the infrapatellar fat pad. Radiographically, patients have irregular calcific flecks or dense clumps of calcification inferior to the patella in the fat pad (Fig. 6–19).

Chondrocalcinosis is deposition of calcium pyrophosphate dihydrate crystals within the articular cartilage or menisci (Fig. 6–20); it occurs equally in men and women in the middle-aged to older population.[54,77,109] Asymptomatic chondrocalcinosis is seen in association with aging, hyperparathyroidism, hemochromatosis, and gout. Different terminologies are used when the cartilage calcification is associated with clinical findings. Pseudogout is the term used when there is cartilage calcification in association with acute arthritic symptoms and joint effusion, with aspiration of weakly positive birefringent crystals (calcium pyrophosphate dihydrate). Pyrophosphate arthropathy is the term used for severe degenerative joint disease (DJD), most pronounced at unusual locations such as the patellofemoral joint. The term calcium pyrophosphate deposition disease encompasses numerous clinical manifestations of arthritis associated with chondrocalcinosis.

Loose Bodies

Circular, coarse calcifications are typical of intra-articular osteocartilaginous bodies (Fig. 6–21A). Intra-articular loose bodies result from cartilaginous fragments that grow by nourishment from synovial fluid. Loose bodies commonly rest within the intercondylar notch, the suprapatellar pouch, a popliteal cyst, or the popliteus bursa. They can be a result or source of degenerative changes. Posterior loose bodies can be overlooked or misinterpreted as

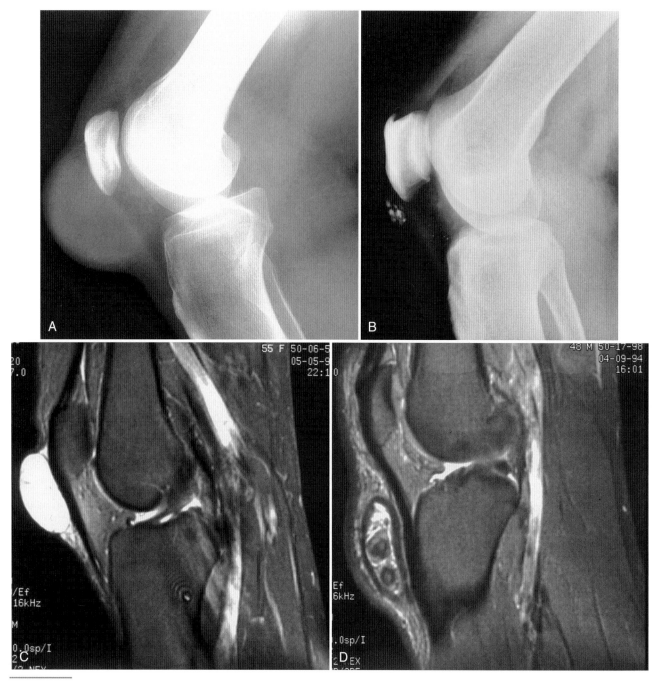

Figure 6–18. Prepatellar bursitis ("housemaid's knee"). **A,** A lateral radiograph shows the massively distended bursa seen in acute bursitis. **B,** Coarse calcifications in the prepatellar region indicate chronic calcific prepatellar bursitis. **C,** Sagittal fat-suppressed proton density magnetic resonance imaging (MRI) shows a large oval distended prepatellar bursa in this patient with acute bursitis. **D,** Sagittal fat-suppressed proton density MRI shows a thick-walled, distended, superficial infrapatellar bursa in this patient with prepatellar bursitis ("preacher's knee"). The rounded low-signal structures within the bursa are calcifications present in chronic calcific bursitis.

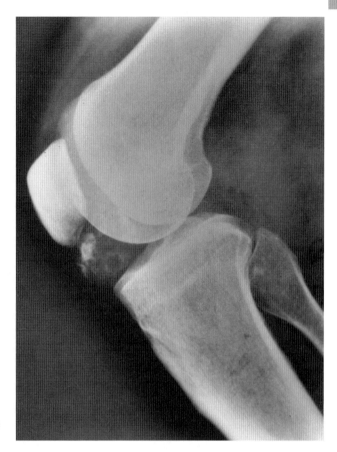

Figure 6–19. Hoffa's disease. Coarse calcifications in the infrapatellar fat pad are characteristic of this condition.

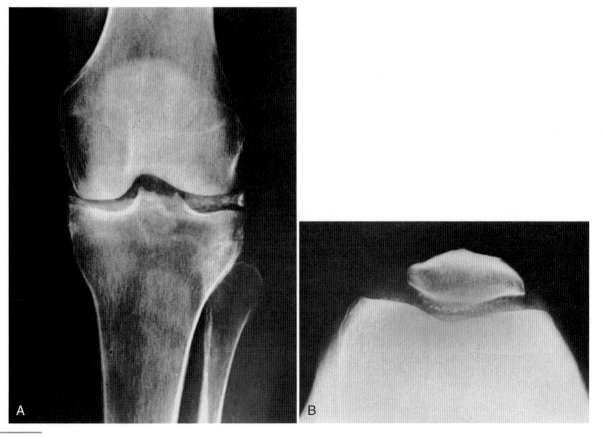

A

B

Figure 6–20. Chondrocalcinosis involves the medial and lateral menisci (fibrocartilage) on the anteroposterior view (**A**) and hyaline articular cartilage at the patellofemoral joint on the tangential axial view (**B**).

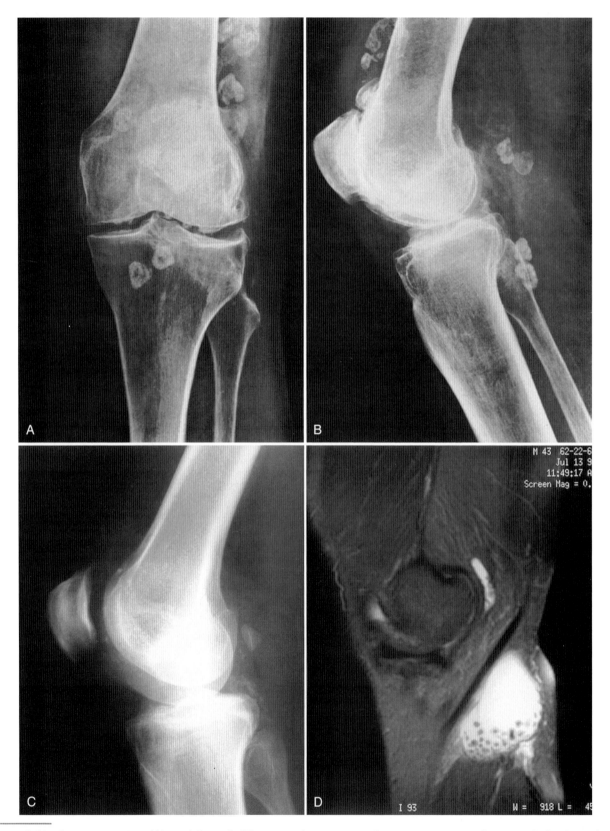

Figure 6–21. Anteroposterior (**A**) and lateral (**B**) views demonstrate degenerative joint disease of the lateral and patellofemoral joint compartments with multiple osteochondral loose bodies (secondary synovial chondromatosis). **C,** Lateral view of the knee in a patient with primary synovial chondromatosis. There are multiple, small, uniformly sized intra-articular calcifications posterior to the tibial plateau in the region of the popliteal hiatus. Faint calcified bodies are also present in the retropatellar and suprapatellar regions. **D,** A sagittal fat-suppressed proton density magnetic resonance image (different patient) shows multiple loose bodies layering within a popliteal cyst. The patient had primary synovial chondromatosis, and conventional radiographs revealed only a joint effusion.

a normal fabella or cyamella (see Fig. 6–21B). Single or multiple osteochondromatous loose bodies are a common finding in degenerative arthritis and can also arise in osteonecrosis and OCD. In the less common primary form of *synovial osteochondromatosis*, chondroid metaplasia of the subsynovial connective tissue occurs and results in innumerable chondral or osteochondral bodies within the synovial cavity (see Fig. 6–21C and D). Synovial osteochondromatosis most commonly affects the knee, and the loose bodies calcify about two-thirds of the time. Noncalcified loose bodies can be detected with arthrography or MRI.

MAGNETIC RESONANCE IMAGING

After conventional radiography, MRI has emerged as the imaging modality of choice for evaluation of the musculoskeletal system. MRI provides a noninvasive multiplanar assessment of bones and joints with exquisite anatomic detail and superior spatial resolution, without exposing the patient to ionizing radiation.

MRI detects very subtle changes and differences in tissue characteristics, thereby allowing earlier and more specific diagnosis of pathological processes than with any other imaging modality.

Tissue Characterization

Different tissues in the body behave in a reproducible manner on specific pulse sequences, and knowledge of these characteristics is helpful for detection of pathological processes. For example, adipose tissue is bright (hyperintense) on T1-weighted images and slightly less intense on T2-weighted images; hematopoietic bone marrow is lower in signal intensity on T1- and T2-weighted images than fatty marrow is because of its lower fat content (Fig. 6–22). Water is bright on T2-weighted images and dark on T1-weighted images. Because pathological processes (tumor, infection, contusion) are typically associated with increased water content, abnormalities usually appear hyperintense to the adjacent tissues on T2-weighted images and lower in signal intensity on T1-weighted images.

The signal intensity of hemorrhage is time dependent and variable, but generally a hematoma tends to get brighter on both T1- and T2-weighted images until it is chronic, at which point hemosiderin deposition will give rise to a low signal on these sequences. The low signal characteristics of hemosiderin in chronic hemorrhage (especially on T2-weighted images) are clearly evident in pigmented villonodular synovitis and hemophilic arthropathy (Fig. 6–23).[57] Mature fibrotic tissue, ligaments, and tendons tend to be low in signal intensity on T1- and T2-weighted images. Calcifications produce signal voids on all sequences, and cortical bone, which has relatively immobile protons, will similarly appear dark on all pulse sequences. Tissues that are bright on T1-weighted images are few; they include fat, subacute

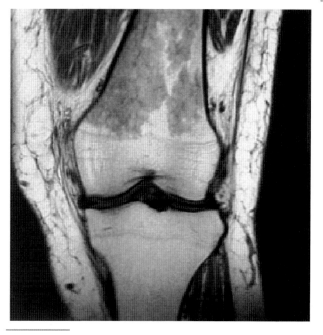

Figure 6–22. Magnetic resonance imaging; marrow signal. A coronal T1-weighted image shows bright marrow signal in the tibia and at the end of the femur, which represents fatty (yellow) marrow. The dark signal in the metaphysis and distal shaft of the femur represents hematopoietic (red) marrow hyperplasia. Note that the red marrow almost never crosses the growth plate scar.

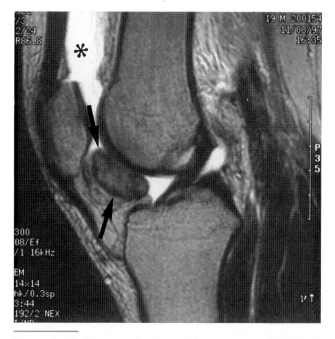

Figure 6–23. Pigmented villonodular synovitis (PVNS). A sagittal T2-weighted magnetic resonance image demonstrates an oval low-signal mass in the infrapatellar fat pad (*arrows*). This is typical of the localized form of PVNS. A calcified loose body would also be considered; however, it was not present on routine plain films of the knee. A large joint effusion (*asterisk*) is also present.

hemorrhage (methemoglobin), proteinaceous fluid collections, and melanin.

In musculoskeletal imaging, in which it is important to detect disorders in subcutaneous fat and bone marrow, the normal high signal intensity of fat on T2-weighted images can inhibit the detection of hyperintense signal abnormalities. An MRI technique known as fat suppression can preferentially suppress the hyperintense signal imparted by fat protons while preserving the normal signal characteristics of water protons. This suppression serves to make the presence and extent of pathological processes more conspicuous on T2-weighted and proton density sequences. Fat suppression can be accomplished either by preferentially saturating the fat protons (chemical saturation) or by a technique known as short tau inversion recovery imaging. The former technique is more commonly used.

Contrast Agents

The primary contrast agent used in MRI is gadopentetate dimeglumine (gadolinium), which is a heavy metal that causes a decrease in T1 and T2 relaxation times in areas in which increased blood flow exists. A decrease in the T1 relaxation time results in relatively increased signal on T1-weighted images. Pathological processes such as infection and tumor will demonstrate enhancement after intravenous contrast injection and will be easier to visualize on T1-weighted images. The relative blood flow to an abnormality is reflected by the degree of contrast enhancement. Intravenous contrast is also helpful for delineating the enhancing margins of fluid collections and for differentiating solid tissue from cystic or necrotic tissue. Intravenous contrast, though helpful in imaging patients with suspected infection or tumor, has no specific role in imaging patients with suspected internal derangement of the knee.

MR-arthrography is MRI of a joint after intra-articular injection of a dilute mixture of gadolinium or, less commonly, saline.[41] This procedure converts the noninvasive MRI study to an invasive study and has much greater clinical utility in shoulder imaging than knee imaging. MR-arthrography can help in determining whether a cystic lesion around the knee joint communicates with the synovial cavity (e.g., differentiating a ganglion cyst from a meniscal cyst) (Fig. 6–24). In addition, MR-arthrography can potentially improve the MRI evaluation of patients with a history of meniscal repair.[5,14,30,35] Patients with an adequately healed meniscus may exhibit linear signal at the site of the repair as a result of granulation tissue and/or fibrosis, which can simulate a persistent tear. Demonstration of gadolinium extension into the site of a previous meniscal repair on MRI signifies a persistent cleavage plane at the site of the tear.

Contraindications to MRI

Although MRI is considered safe for most individuals and uses no ionizing radiation, there are specific contraindications. These contraindications are directly related to implanted internal devices or metallic clips, which can either cease functioning or move when exposed to a

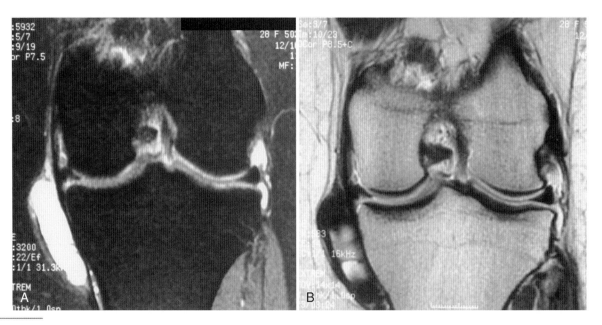

Figure 6–24. Meniscal cyst. **A,** Coronal fat-suppressed fast spin-echo proton density MRI reveals a cystic lesion at the medial aspect of the proximal end of the tibia. The differential diagnosis includes meniscal cyst, ganglion cyst, and pes anserinus bursitis. **B,** MR arthrograph. Coronal T1-weighted MRI, obtained after the administration of intra-articular gadolinium, shows areas of bright signal (gadolinium) within the lesion, indicative of communication with the joint and confirming the suspected diagnosis of meniscal cyst. Note the blunting of the free edge of the medial meniscus and abnormal peripheral signal indicative of a tear.

powerful magnetic field. Devices that can malfunction in the MRI suite and for which MRI is contraindicated include cardiac pacemakers, external defibrillators, cochlear implants, implantable neurostimulators (transcutaneous electrical nerve stimulation unit), and bone growth stimulators. A shift in position of cerebral aneurysm clips and certain prosthetic heart valves can have devastating consequences, and the radiologist, before performing MRI, must know the exact type of clips or valves used for these procedures to ensure that they are not paramagnetic. Sheet metal workers or individuals at risk for metallic foreign bodies near the cornea or orbits must first have conventional radiographs of the orbit to check for metal fragments, which can potentially cause corneal abrasion or blindness. Patients with metallic joint prostheses or spinal instrumentation rods can safely be imaged. Imaging of the tissues near a prosthesis or rod can be challenging or impossible because of the magnetic susceptibility artifact of the implant.

Normal MRI Anatomy

Figure 6–25 demonstrates normal anatomic structures of the knee on sagittal, coronal, and axial images.

MENISCI

The menisci are fibrocartilaginous structures that are arbitrarily divided into an anterior horn, a body, and a posterior horn. They are best seen on sagittal images and have a bowtie configuration peripherally and a triangular configuration more centrally. The base of the triangle represents the peripheral portion of the meniscus where it attaches to the capsule, and the other two sides form the superior and inferior articulating surfaces. The apex of the meniscus should be sharply pointed; it represents the meniscal free edge. The medial meniscus, which has a larger radius than the lateral meniscus does, is more firmly attached to the joint capsule, and its posterior horn is larger than the anterior horn. The more mobile lateral meniscus has a smaller radius and a looser capsular attachment near the junction of the body and posterior horn. The popliteus tendon passes through the capsular attachment of the posterior horn of the lateral meniscus at the popliteal hiatus (Fig. 6–26). Unlike the medial meniscus, the anterior and posterior horns of the lateral meniscus are equivalent in size.

The menisci are normally low-signal (black) structures with little or no internal signal because of their lack of mobile protons. Meniscal tears appear on MRI as abnormal signal intensity within the meniscus that touches an articulating surface of the meniscus or as abnormal meniscal morphological features (Fig. 6–27).[9,23,28,37,85,100,101,130] Not all intrameniscal signal is pathological[66]; a grading system that classifies meniscal signal as grade I, II, or III has been established and correlated with histological findings.[85,130] Grade I changes appear as a spherical or globular area of increased signal that does not reach an articulating surface. Grade II changes are linear areas of

increased signal within the meniscus that do not touch an articulating surface. These signal changes correlate with mucoid degeneration or microscopic clefts within the meniscus and do not represent tears. After the fifth decade, intrameniscal signal is more the rule than the exception, and grade I and II changes probably represent a normal aging phenomenon. Intrameniscal signal is a fairly common finding in children and young adults and is believed to represent normal perforating vascular channels.[132]

Grade III changes are characterized by abnormal signal intensity that reaches the superior or inferior articular surface or free edge of the meniscus, and they represent true meniscal tears. In other words, grade III signal is a meniscal tear; there is no such thing as a grade I or II tear. In the great majority of cases it is possible to discern whether intrameniscal signal touches an articular surface. Occasionally, it is difficult to differentiate between extensive grade II signal and grade III signal (tear); as a rule, if extension of signal to the articular surface is equivocal, it is unlikely to represent a tear.[28,60] Often, coronal images can be helpful in questionable cases. Tears can be classified as horizontal, vertical, or oblique, based on the orientation of the abnormal signal.

The majority of meniscal tears are visualized to best advantage on sagittal images and, because of their orientation, may not be seen clearly in the coronal plane. Tears may uncommonly be seen best in the coronal plane (see Fig. 6–27B),[28] thus underscoring the importance of close evaluation in more than one imaging plane. Tears involving the free edge of the meniscus (e.g., "flap tears") are usually manifested as blunting of the normally pointed free edge of the meniscus, a finding that is often subtle. This blunting can also be seen with bucket handle tears and as a result of previous partial meniscectomy.

Because the normal meniscus is C shaped, one can usually see a continuous band of meniscus on the most peripheral two to three sagittal images. Absence of this continuous meniscus and blunting of the free edge are findings seen in bucket handle tears of the meniscus.[51] The displaced bucket handle fragment is well visualized on coronal images and is usually located in the intercondylar notch (Fig. 6–28A).[140] On sagittal images, the displaced fragment is often situated as an elongated structure beneath the posterior cruciate ligament (PCL) (see Fig. 6–28B), a finding described as the "double-PCL sign."[125] Visualization of a continuous band of meniscus on more than three contiguous peripheral sagittal images indicates a discoid meniscus (Fig. 6–29).[123] This abnormally shaped meniscus is typically seen laterally and is prone to tearing.

Routine inspection of knee MRI studies should include evaluation of the meniscocapsular junction. Detachment of the peripheral meniscus from its capsular attachment can be subtle and evidenced only by the slightly increased distance between the periphery of the meniscus and the capsule or by increased T2 signal at the outer margin of the meniscus.[30,85,114] The periphery of the meniscus normally extends to the outer cortex of the tibial plateau, a helpful relationship when assessing for meniscocapsular injuries. MRI signs of meniscocapsular separation have been shown to have very low positive predictive value and

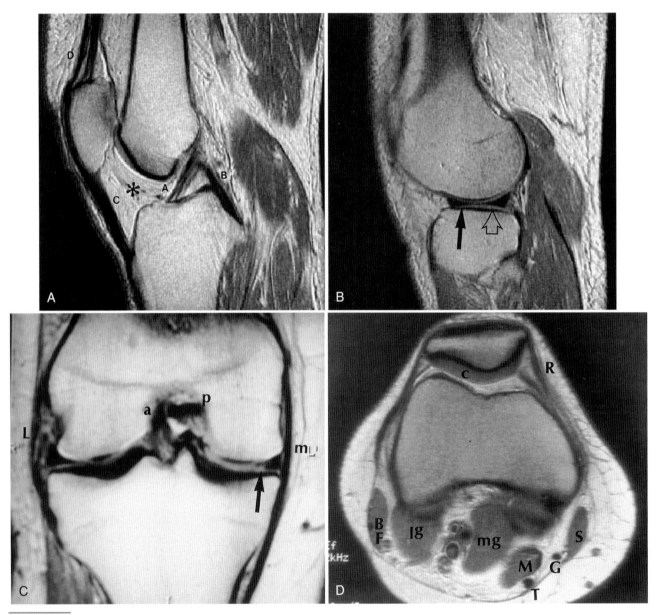

Figure 6–25. Normal magnetic resonance anatomy. A proton density midsagittal image (**A**) reveals the normal anterior (A) and posterior (B) cruciate ligaments. The low-signal patellar (C) and quadriceps (D) tendons are seen anteriorly. The infrapatellar fat pad (*asterisk*) has high signal intensity. A more lateral parasagittal image (**B**) shows the normal triangular/bow tie configuration of the lateral meniscus. The low-signal anterior and posterior horns are indicated by *solid* and *open arrows*, respectively. **C,** A coronal T1-weighted image shows the low-signal medial collateral ligament (m) extending from the upper aspect of the medial femoral condyle. The superficial fibers continue distally to insert on the medial aspect of the proximal tibial metaphysis. The lateral collateral ligament (L) is seen on the same image. Within the intercondylar notch, the anterior cruciate ligament (a) is located lateral to the posterior cruciate ligament (p). Note the tear at the free edge of the body of the medial meniscus (*arrow*). **D,** Axial high-resolution proton density image. BF, biceps femoris muscle; c, patellar articular cartilage; G, gracilis tendon; lg, lateral gastrocnemius; M, semimembranosus muscle; mg, medial head of the gastrocnemius muscle; R, medial patellar retinaculum; S, sartorius muscle; T, semitendinosus tendon. The popliteal vessels are situated between the lateral and medial heads of the gastrocnemius muscles.

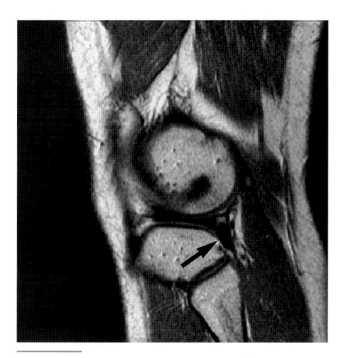

Figure 6–26. Popliteal hiatus. This sagittal image shows the oval low-signal popliteus tendon (*arrow*) passing through the popliteal hiatus, posterior to the lateral meniscus.

poor sensitivity, thus suggesting that MRI is not reliable for making this diagnosis.[114]

The most common pitfall in MRI evaluation of the meniscus is interpreting grade II signal as a tear, which results in a false-positive study.[59] Four other pitfalls involve misinterpreting normal structures, closely contiguous with the meniscus, as meniscal tears[52]:

1. The transverse meniscal ligament connects the anterior horns of the medial and lateral menisci. On sagittal images, the interface of this structure with the anterior horn of the lateral meniscus often simulates a tear (Fig. 6–30).[37,52] Following this "pseudotear" over several images is helpful in identifying it as a normal structure.

2. As the popliteus tendon passes through the popliteal hiatus, it is closely adjacent to the posterior horn of the lateral meniscus, often having linear signal at the interface. This linear signal can be misinterpreted as a peripheral vertical meniscal tear.

3. In the medial compartment, a normal linear area of increased signal is visualized between the periphery of the body of the meniscus and the MCL. This bursa or fat plane should not be mistaken for a tear.

4. The meniscofemoral ligament attaches the posterior horn of the lateral meniscus to the medial femoral condyle (Fig. 6–31). The interface of this ligament with the posterior horn of the lateral meniscus can simulate a meniscal tear.[18]

In the presence of a meniscal tear, the periphery of the meniscus should be evaluated carefully for an associated meniscal cyst. These cysts are more commonly associated with lateral meniscal tears (horizontal cleavage type) and

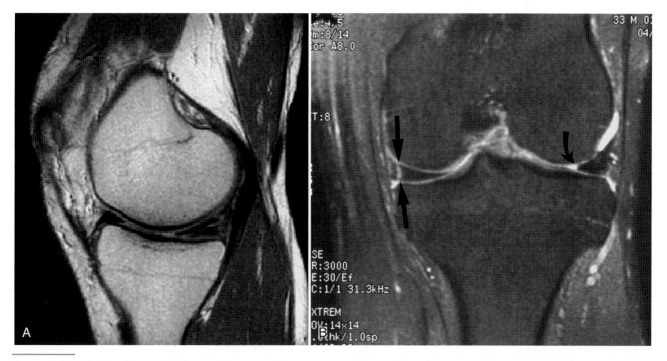

Figure 6–27. Meniscal tears. **A,** A sagittal proton density image shows obliquely oriented linear signal traversing the posterior horn of the medial meniscus and touching its inferior articular surface. This is a classic meniscal tear. **B,** A coronal fat-suppressed proton density image shows two meniscal tears. There is a vertical peripheral tear of the body of the medial meniscus (*straight arrows*) and a flap tear at the free edge of the lateral meniscus manifested as blunting (*curved arrow*).

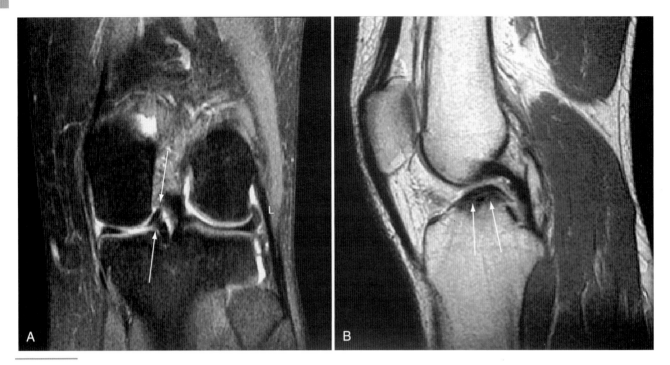

Figure 6–28. Bucket-handle tear, medial meniscus. **A,** A coronal fat-suppressed T2-weighted image shows a large displaced bucket-handle meniscal fragment displaced into the medial aspect of the intercondylar notch (*arrows*). Note the normal-appearing lateral collateral ligament (L). **B,** A sagittal proton density image shows the "double–posterior cruciate ligament (PCL) sign" of a bucket-handle tear. The curved low-signal bucket-handle fragment (*arrows*) parallels the normal low-signal PCL.

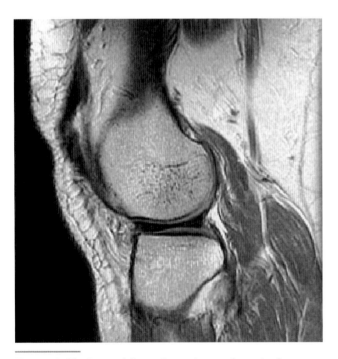

Figure 6–29. Discoid lateral meniscus. A sagittal proton density magnetic resonance image shows a "block-like" continuous band of meniscus; the lateral meniscus had this configuration through it on nearly all sagittal images. A normal meniscus has this appearance on the more peripheral images and assumes the appearance of two separate triangles (anterior and posterior horns) as one approaches the intercondylar notch.

can be manifested as a mass at the joint line. They have the appearance of a rounded cystic mass at the peripheral edge of the meniscus (see Fig. 6–24) and tend to be larger when associated with medial meniscal tears.

MRI has proved to be an effective technique for evaluation of the menisci; a summary of the sensitivity, specificity, and accuracy for detection of meniscal tears follows (averages in parentheses)[12,25,38,59,66,85,100]:

1. Medial meniscal tears: sensitivity, 90% to 98% (95%); specificity, 82% to 95% (88%); accuracy, 89% to 95% (92%)
2. Lateral meniscal tears: sensitivity, 71% to 92% (81%); specificity, 91% to 99% (96%); accuracy, 86% to 97% (92%)

Notably, in the presence of anterior cruciate ligament (ACL) tears, the sensitivity of MRI for detection of meniscal tears has been shown to be lower. DeSmet and Graf[25] reported that the sensitivity for medial meniscal tears dropped from 97% to 88% when an ACL tear was present and dropped from 94% to 69% for lateral meniscal tears. This decrease in sensitivity is multifactorial, but it is largely the result of the fact that, in posterior and peripheral tears of the lateral meniscus when the ACL is torn, the relatively higher frequency is more difficult to detect.

CRUCIATE LIGAMENTS

Anterior Cruciate Ligament

The ACL originates from the medial side of the lateral femoral condyle and inserts on the anterior tibial spines,

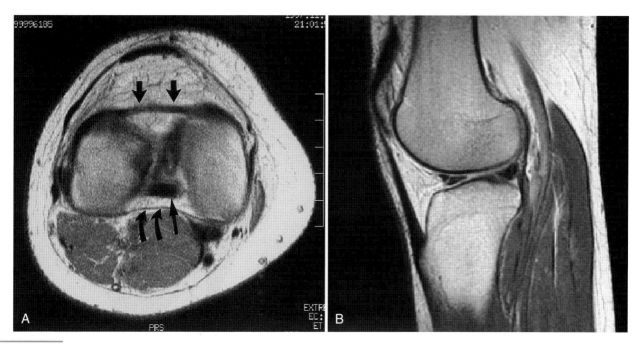

Figure 6–30. Transverse meniscal ligament. **A,** An axial proton density magnetic resonance image shows the low-signal transverse meniscal ligament (TML) (*short arrows*) connecting the anterior horns of the lateral and medial menisci. Also seen on this image are the posterior cruciate ligament (*long arrow*) and the posterior joint capsule (*curved arrows*). **B,** A sagittal proton density image through the lateral meniscus shows a linear interface between the anterior margin of the anterior horn of the lateral meniscus and the TML. The TML can be mistaken for a portion of the lateral meniscus, and the interface can therefore simulate a tear.

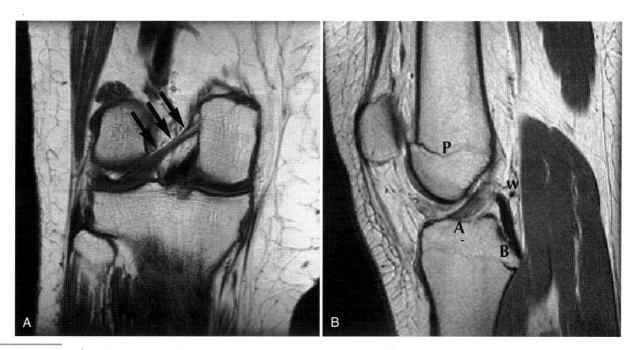

Figure 6–31. Meniscofemoral ligament. **A,** A coronal T1-weighted image shows the meniscofemoral ligament (*arrows*) coursing from the inner aspect of the lateral meniscus to the notch of the medial femoral condyle. **B,** A sagittal proton density image shows the ligament of Wrisberg (w) and part of the meniscofemoral ligament coursing posterior to the posterior cruciate ligament (B). The anterior cruciate ligament (A) and physeal scar of the distal end of the femur (P) are also indicated.

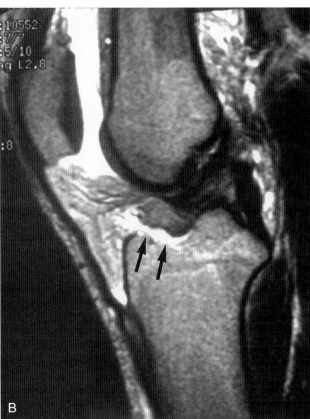
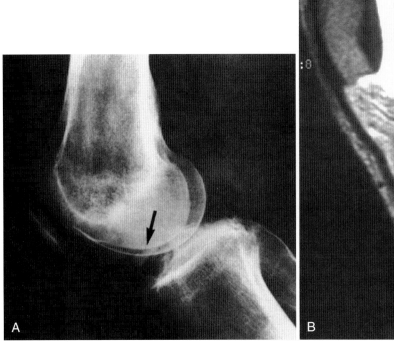

Figure 6–32. Anterior cruciate ligament avulsion fracture. **A,** A lateral radiograph shows the avulsed bony attachment of the anterior cruciate ligament (*arrow*). **B,** A sagittal T2-weighted magnetic resonance image (different patient) demonstrates the triangular bony avulsion fragment with hyperintense fluid seen at its interface with the tibia (*arrows*).

about 10 mm behind the anterior articular surface of the tibia. It is usually 11 to 13 mm thick and is enveloped by a thin sheath.[62] Because the ACL courses at a shallow angle in a lateral-to-medial direction, it is often not imaged in its entirety on a single sagittal image and must be evaluated on two to three contiguous images. Occasionally, it is necessary to obtain oblique sagittal images, tangential to the course of the ACL, for optimal visualization. Although the ACL is best visualized on sagittal images, coronal and axial images are often helpful for thorough assessment of the integrity of this structure, especially when there is a question of a subtle tear.

A normal ACL is relatively low in signal intensity, primarily at its femoral attachment. However, a striated appearance of the distal portion of the ACL on sagittal images (representing fat, connective tissue, and synovium separating the fascicles of the ligament) is a common finding and should not be mistaken for a tear.

Two avulsion fractures that occur at the knee are associated with injury to the ACL or its attachment. Tibial avulsion fractures at the ACL insertion have a characteristic radiographic appearance consisting of an osseous fragment anterior and superior to the tibial spines (Fig. 6–32). These injuries tend to occur in a younger patient population, and the ACL remains intact. Segond's fracture is an avulsion injury at the bony insertion of the meniscal capsular component of the lateral capsular ligament. It is characterized by a small linear fracture fragment adjacent

to the lateral aspect of the lateral tibial plateau (Fig. 6–33). This injury carries a high association with ACL tears and with meniscal injury.[44,139]

MRI is highly accurate for detection of ACL tears, with a sensitivity ranging from 92% to 100% and a specificity of 89% to 97%.* The primary signs of an acute ACL tear include the following:

1. A heterogeneous "pseudomass" (hematoma) in the intercondylar notch with increased signal on T2-weighted images (Fig. 6–34A). This pseudomass is the result of hemorrhage and edema associated with the injury.
2. Discontinuity or disruption of ligament fibers (see Fig. 6–34B).

Findings associated with a chronic ACL tear include nonvisualization of the ligament (as a result of atrophy of its fibers) and an abnormal horizontal orientation of the ACL[136] (see Fig. 6–34C). The abnormally oriented ACL maintains low signal in chronic tears and commonly scars down to the PCL.

Acute ACL tears are typically associated with a large joint effusion (hemarthrosis). Numerous secondary MRI findings of ACL tears have been described[40,80,111,126,134] and can be helpful supportive evidence of an ACL injury, especially when the primary findings of ACL tears are equiv-

*See references 12, 25, 38, 59, 69, 85, 100, 108, 134, 137.

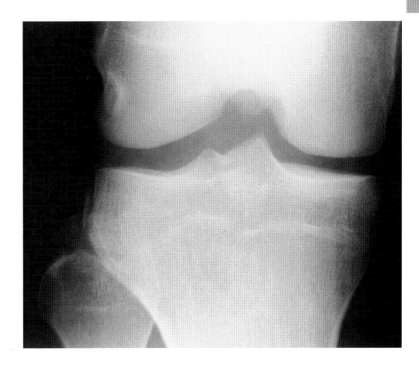

Figure 6–33. Segond's fracture. There is a linear bony fragment at the lateral margin of the tibial plateau representing an avulsion at the attachment of the lateral capsular ligament.

ocal. Bone contusions at the anterior aspect of the lateral femoral condyle and the posterior aspect of the tibial plateau (Fig. 6–35A) occur as a result of impaction injury from anterior translation of the tibia relative to the femur; the location of these contusions is highly specific for ACL injury.[42,79,111,126] This type of force can give rise to an osteochondral injury of the lateral femoral condyle and occasional depression of the articular surface; this depression can sometimes be appreciated on the lateral radiograph (see Fig. 6–35B and C).[20,138] Other secondary signs of ACL tear include "buckling" of the PCL and hanging of the posterior horn of the lateral meniscus over the posterior margin of the lateral femoral condyle (both secondary to anterior translation of the tibia).

Partial tears of the ACL are more difficult to detect, and the sensitivity and specificity ranges for detection of these injuries are approximately 40% to 75% and 62% to 89%, respectively.[135] The MRI findings of focal ligamentous thickening, increased signal, and waviness of ligament fibers are often subtle.

Patients with a history of ACL reconstructive surgery can be effectively imaged with MRI despite the presence of local artifact from metallic screws.[6,76,86,103,106,117] The ACL graft is generally low in signal when imaged more than 6 months after surgery; increased signal in and around the graft before 6 months is not uncommon and is the result of synovial tissue, residual edema, and postoperative changes. Torn ACL grafts demonstrate abnormal signal, abnormal morphological features, or frank disruption or discontinuity.

Posterior Cruciate Ligament

The PCL arises from the posterolateral aspect of the medial femoral condyle and inserts into the posterior intercondylar portion of the tibia. The PCL is thicker than the ACL, varying from 12 to 20 mm in thickness. The PCL

is diffusely low in signal intensity and has a hockey stick configuration. The ligament is clearly visualized on sagittal and coronal images of the knee. One can often see the ligament of Humphry or that of Wrisberg associated with the anterior or posterior aspect of the PCL, respectively (Fig. 6–36A).

PCL tears appear on MRI as a bright signal within the substance of the ligament or as a disruption of ligament fibers (see Fig. 6–36B).[47,128] Chronic tears of the PCL can result in thinning or nonvisualization of the ligament or abnormal angulation (buckling) of this structure. MRI is not a reliable predictor of the integrity of the PCL in patients with chronic PCL insufficiency; fibrosis bridging the tear can result in a normal-appearing ligament on MRI.[133] Avulsion fractures at the tibial attachment are less common than ACL avulsions but have a characteristic radiographic appearance (see Fig. 6–36C).

COLLATERAL LIGAMENTS

Medial Collateral Ligament

The MCL provides support to the medial aspect of the knee. It is divided anatomically into superficial and deep fibers. The superficial fibers, or the tibial collateral ligament, extend from the medial femoral condyle to the medial aspect of the tibia, about 5 cm below the joint line. The deep fibers arise from the joint capsule and the medial meniscus and attach to the tibia and femur close to the joint line. The superficial and deep fibers are separated from each other by a bursa.

The MCL is clearly visualized and well evaluated on coronal MRI (see Fig. 6–25). The ligament fibers are low in signal intensity and can be followed in their entirety from their origin on the femur to their insertion on the tibia. Axial images provide complementary information and are also helpful in assessing the integrity of the MCL.

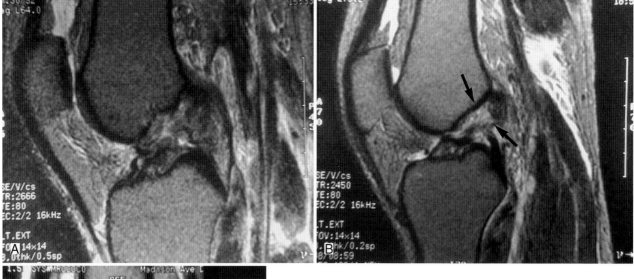

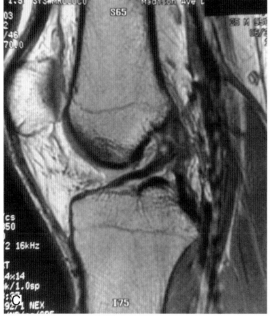

Figure 6–34. Anterior cruciate ligament (ACL) tear, magnetic resonance image. **A,** A sagittal T2-weighted image demonstrates a heterogeneous hematoma involving the majority of the ACL with relative sparing of its tibial attachment fibers. There is an associated large joint effusion in this patient with an acute ACL tear. **B,** Disruption of ACL fibers at its femoral attachment (*arrows*) with waviness in contour of the middle third of the ligament and a large joint effusion. The patient sustained a complete acute ACL tear in a ski accident. **C,** Sagittal proton density magnetic resonance image showing a chronically torn ACL. The dark ligament is nearly horizontally oriented and scarred down to the posterior cruciate ligament. Note the lack of increased signal at the site of the tear and the lack of joint effusion, indicative of a chronic injury.

MCL tears result in partial or complete disruption in continuity of the normally dark bands of ligament fibers; these bands become less distinct and demonstrate increased internal signal intensity.[119] The torn ligament commonly has a wavy configuration rather than the normally seen straight, band-like configuration. Mild sprains of the MCL (grade I) are typically associated with increased T2 signal surrounding the normal-appearing ligament fibers, whereas partial and complete tears of the ligament (grades II and III) have bright signal within the substance of the ligament (Fig. 6–37); this high signal intensity results from the edema and hemorrhage associated with the injury.

Lateral Collateral Ligament

The lateral collateral ligament (LCL) complex comprises the iliotibial band anteriorly, the tendon of the biceps femoris posteriorly, and the fibular collateral ligament situated between these two structures. The fibular collateral ligament arises from the lateral aspect of the lateral femoral condyle (at the lateral epicondyle) and inserts on the styloid process of the fibular head. The LCL joins the biceps femoris tendon to form the conjoined tendon, which inserts on the head of the fibula. The LCL is superficial to the popliteal tendon, which passes through the popliteal hiatus posterior to the posterior horn of the lateral meniscus. The LCL complex, along with the lateral patellar retinaculum, arcuate ligament, lateral capsular ligament, and fabellofibular ligament, contributes to support of the lateral aspect of the knee. Injury to the LCL is considerably less frequent than injury to its medial counterpart.

Like the MCL, the LCL is best evaluated in the coronal plane, and axial images are helpful to corroborate any equivocal findings. The LCL normally has the appearance of a thin band of low signal intensity (see Fig. 6–25); because it courses obliquely posteroinferiorly, it must

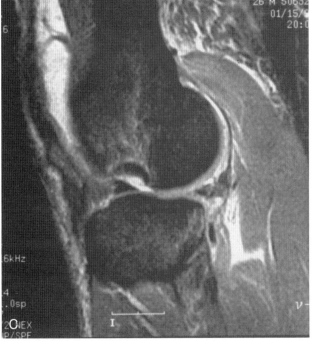
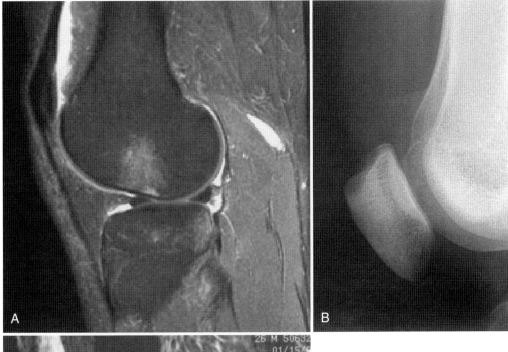

Figure 6–35. Anterior cruciate ligament (ACL) tear—bone contusions. **A,** A sagittal fat-suppressed proton density magnetic resonance image shows bright signal at the anterior aspect of the lateral femoral condyle and posterior aspect of the lateral tibial plateau, typical locations of bone contusions associated with an ACL tear. **B,** A lateral radiograph demonstrates focal depression of the anterior aspect of the lateral femoral condyle (*arrow*) as a result of translational osteochondral impaction injury associated with an ACL tear. **C,** A sagittal fat-suppressed magnetic resonance image (same patient as in **B**) reveals marrow edema underlying the osteochondral depression and a large joint effusion.

usually be assessed on two or three contiguous coronal images. A tear of the LCL will result in loss of continuity of the bands of the ligament, ligamentous thickening, or increased signal in or around this structure (indicating hemorrhage and/or edema).

Extensor Mechanism Injuries

The extensor mechanism of the knee comprises the quadriceps and patellar tendons and the patella. These structures are most optimally assessed in the sagittal

plane. The quadriceps and patellar tendons are normally dark structures; however, knowledge of certain normal MRI variations will avoid overdiagnosis of tendon disorders. Because the quadriceps tendon is made up of contributions from four separate tendons, it commonly has a striated (usually trilaminar) appearance on sagittal images, with longitudinal linear intermediate signal seen within its substance. In addition, it is not uncommon for the normal patellar tendon to have intermediate internal signal at its patellar or tibial tubercle attachments.

Severe disruption of the quadriceps tendon leads to quadriceps insufficiency and resultant patella baja.[89] Quadriceps tears are more commonly seen in an older

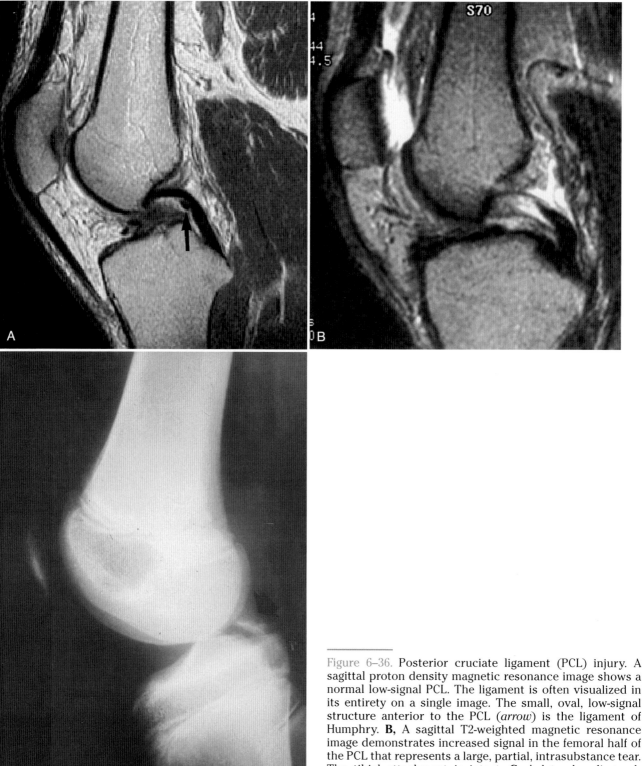

Figure 6–36. Posterior cruciate ligament (PCL) injury. A sagittal proton density magnetic resonance image shows a normal low-signal PCL. The ligament is often visualized in its entirety on a single image. The small, oval, low-signal structure anterior to the PCL (*arrow*) is the ligament of Humphry. **B**, A sagittal T2-weighted magnetic resonance image demonstrates increased signal in the femoral half of the PCL that represents a large, partial, intrasubstance tear. The tibial attachment is intact. **C**, A lateral radiograph shows a well-corticated avulsion fragment at the tibial attachment of the PCL (*arrow*), indicative of a chronic PCL avulsion fracture.

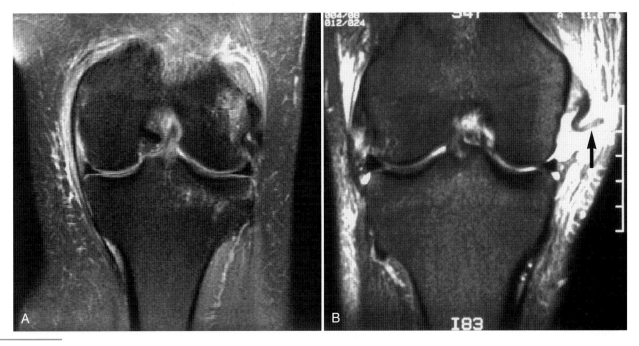

Figure 6–37. Medial collateral ligament (MCL) tear. **A,** A coronal fat-suppressed magnetic resonance image demonstrates increased signal around the MCL fibers, representing a mild ligament sprain. **B,** A coronal magnetic resonance image shows complete disruption of the midportion of the MCL. The torn proximal end of the MCL (*arrow*) is surrounded by extensive soft-tissue edema. (Courtesy of Hollis G. Potter, M.D.)

patient population than patellar tendon tears are and their increases incidence in patients receiving steroid therapy and those with chronic renal disease.[88] Patellar tendon tears are usually partial injuries and tend to occur in younger, more athletic individuals. Conventional radiographs may reveal focal or fusiform thickening of the involved segment and surrounding soft-tissue swelling; complete patellar tendon disruption can result in patella alta.

MRI can clearly define the exact site of the tear and the extent of injury and can determine whether the tear is partial or complete. Tendon tears result in disruption in continuity of the normally low-signal tendon and bright T2 signal at the site of the tear, usually in the surrounding soft tissues (Fig. 6–38).[125] Retracted tendons associated with complete tears tend to be thickened with heterogeneous increased internal signal. The MRI findings of quadriceps or patellar tendinitis and a partial tendon tear are identical, thus suggesting that these two conditions are one and the same.[142] The most commonly seen abnormality of the patellar tendon on MRI is "jumper's knee." Jumper's knee is tendinitis or a partial tear of the patellar tendon at its patellar attachment and results in wedge-shaped hyperintense T2 signal within the tendon, typically involving its more posterior fibers.[34,63]

Patellar disruption and quadriceps tendon disruption are uncommon complications after total knee arthroplasty.[70] Because of the pronounced regional artifact caused by the metallic implants, these relatively superficial structures are best visualized with ultrasonography.

THE PATELLOFEMORAL JOINT

Normal Anatomy
The patella is the largest sesamoid in the body and normally ossifies between 3 and 5 years of age. It has multiple facets, only three of which can be reliably imaged; the lateral facet and the shorter, more steeply angled medial facet articulate with the patella at the patellofemoral joint. The nonarticular odd facet forms the medial margin of the patella and is not covered by articular cartilage. The convex peak separating the medial and lateral facets is the patellar apex.

Chondromalacia Patellae
Articular cartilage cannot be visualized on conventional radiographs, except in pathological states such as chondrocalcinosis. Plain films are very insensitive for detecting symptomatic chondral abnormalities such as injury, chondromalacia, or early DJD[19,36]; plain film findings of cartilage loss will be detected only if the chondral disease is so advanced that it causes joint space narrowing and/or subchondral bony changes. CT-arthrography and MRI can provide visualization of the surface of the patellar articular cartilage, and the latter modality can detect earlier internal chondral disorders.[13,32,49,74,78,99] The sensitivity, specificity, and accuracy ranges for detection of patellar cartilage abnormalities have been reported as 48% to 100%, 50% to 97%, and 52% to 91%, respectively.[32,41,48,78,105] Joint fluid can aid in evaluating the artic-

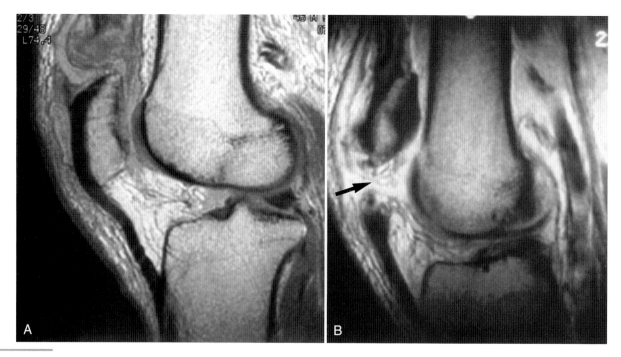

Figure 6–38. Extensor mechanism injury—magnetic resonance image. **A,** A sagittal magnetic resonance image shows complete disruption of the quadriceps tendon at its attachment on the superior pole of the patella. Note the heterogeneous thickened tendon, with discontinuity at the superior aspect of the patella. The patellar tendon is normal in signal and is continuous. **B,** A sagittal magnetic resonance image reveals a complete tear of the patellar tendon at the lower pole of the patella (*arrow*). The quadriceps tendon is intact.

ular cartilage by serving as a natural contrast medium and separating the cartilage of the femur and patella.

The articular cartilage of the patella is the thickest in the body and should have uniform thickness and signal intensity on MRI (see Fig. 6–25). The MRI findings of chondromalacia parallel the morphological changes seen at arthroscopy. Early stages of chondromalacia will demonstrate focal or diffuse abnormal signal within the cartilage, with a normal-appearing surface. As the condition progresses, one can visualize thinning, irregularity, and fissuring of cartilage on MRI (Fig. 6–39A and B), which may progress to subchondral cystic changes. The findings of chondromalacia on CT-arthrography are surface irregularity, chondral thinning, and extension of contrast into chondral fissures, known as imbibition (see Fig. 6–39C). MRI and CT-arthrography are highly sensitive for detecting grade III and IV pathological changes of articular cartilage; however, the sensitivity for detection of early chondral disorder is not optimal,[41,143] and newer techniques that will provide more accurate and sensitive assessment of articular cartilage are currently under investigation.[32,78,99,105,107]

Synovial Plicae

Synovial plicae are remnants of septa present in the embryologically developing knee that can persist into adulthood. They consist of the suprapatellar, infrapatellar, and medial patellar plicae; however, it is the thickened medial plica that has been implicated as a cause of anterior knee pain (plica or "shelf" syndrome).[8,31] The suprapatellar and medial patellar plicae are best visualized in the sagittal and axial planes, respectively (Fig. 6–40). These embryological remnants are commonly encountered as incidental findings on routine MRI of the knee. They are rarely significant clinically, unless they become thickened and inflamed. Without a joint effusion, synovial plicae are difficult to visualize; CT-arthrography is another technique that provides visualization of these bands, particularly the medial plica.

Lateral Patellar Dislocation

Imaging findings of lateral patellar dislocation have been well-documented in the radiology literature,[39,64,65,71,102] particularly because of the characteristic findings on MRI and plain films and the relative difficulty of making a clinical diagnosis. The patella is typically completely or partially reduced at initial evaluation, thus making the diagnosis more challenging. Not uncommonly, these patients have a telltale bony fragment at the medial margin of the patella, strongly indicative of this type of injury (Fig. 6–41A).[39] MRI findings of lateral patellar dislocation include medial patellar retinacular disruption and bone contusion or osteochondral injury at the medial margin of the patella and the lateral margin of the lateral femoral condyle (see Fig. 6–41B).[64,65,102] These classic sites of osteochondral injury result from impaction of the medial patella and the lateral condyle during relocation of the patella. Acute lateral dislocation of the patella is typically associated with a large hemarthrosis secondary to medial retinacular injury and/or osteochondral fracture.

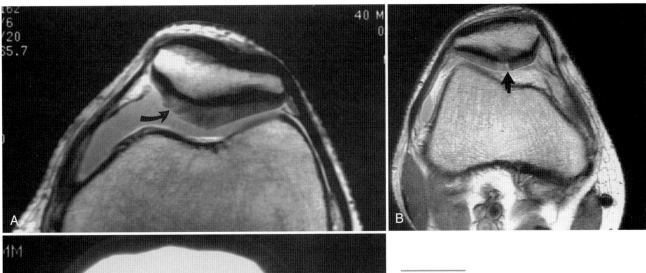

Figure 6–39. Chondromalacia patellae. **A,** An axial high-resolution magnetic resonance image reveals fibrillation and fissuring of the surface of the medial facet articular cartilage (*curved arrow*). Note the normal homogeneous cartilage over the lateral facet and its sharply defined articular surface. **B,** An axial high-resolution magnetic resonance image shows more advanced chondromalacia. The signal abnormality extends down to subchondral bone with a deep fissure at the patellar apex (*arrow*). **C,** A CT-arthrogram shows extension of contrast into the lateral facet articular cartilage with focal cartilage ulceration (*arrow*) in patient with severe chondromalacia.

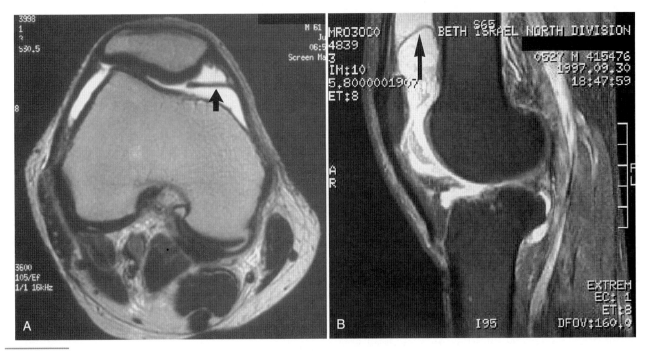

Figure 6–40. Synovial plicae. **A,** An axial magnetic resonance image shows a low-signal thickened medial patellar plica (*arrow*). Visualization of this structure is facilitated by the high-signal joint effusion. **B,** A sagittal fat-suppressed proton density magnetic resonance image shows a curvilinear suprapatellar plica (*arrow*) outlined by a large joint effusion in the suprapatellar pouch.

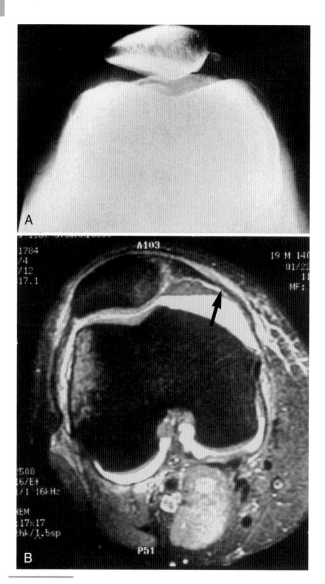

Figure 6–41. Lateral patellar dislocation. **A,** A tangential view of the patella demonstrates an osseous fragment at the medial margin of the patella, consistent with previous lateral patellar dislocation. **B,** An axial fat-suppressed magnetic resonance image shows a partial tear of the medial patellar retinaculum manifested as increased signal on either side of it (*arrow*). There is increased signal in the medial aspect of the patella and at the lateral margin of the lateral femoral condyle, indicative of bone contusions, and there is a large joint effusion. This constellation of findings is characteristic of a recent lateral patellar dislocation.

SKELETAL TRAUMA

Imaging of patients with knee trauma should always start with routine conventional radiographs, which will detect the majority of skeletal injuries. More sophisticated imaging modalities, such as a radionuclide bone scan or MRI, should be reserved for specific clinical instances such as suspected occult bony injury or cartilage or soft-tissue disorders.

Fractures may be complete, partial, impacted, epiphyseal, avulsion, or osteochondral. A complete fracture involves both cortices and can be simple or comminuted. It can be horizontal, oblique, spiral, or vertical. A fracture is radiographically described according to the displacement or angulation of the distal fragment relative to the proximal fragment.

Growth Plate Injuries

The growth plate is the weakest site in the immature skeleton and is even more susceptible to injury than the more elastic and resilient supporting ligaments. As such, growth plate injuries are relatively common fractures in children and result from severe force on a joint. These fractures are described according to the Salter-Harris classification.[115] There are five types of Salter fractures (Fig. 6–42). A Salter fracture should be suspected when the physis is wider than usual; a type V injury is suspected if the physis is narrower than usual, especially if only part of the growth plate is affected. In the setting of trauma, patients with joint effusion, particularly children, should undergo a cross-table lateral view to seek a fat-fluid level occurring with occult fracture. Children with nondisplaced Salter I fractures may have only focal soft-tissue swelling over a growth plate; follow-up films reveal the periosteal new bone seen with fracture healing. Occult growth plate injury and premature growth plate fusion after physeal injury can be reliably detected on MRI.

Tibial Plateau Fracture

Tibial plateau fractures are usually visualized on routine conventional radiographs as cortical disruption and/or depression at the tibial articular surface (Fig. 6–43A). (Lipo)hemarthrosis commonly accompanies these injuries because of blood and marrow fat bleeding into the joint from the fracture. CT is ideal for demonstrating the degree of comminution, fragmentation, and articular depression and the extent of bony involvement associated with these fractures. Once the raw data are obtained on thin (3 mm or less) axial images, sagittal and coronal reconstructed two-dimensional and three-dimensional images can easily be displayed with widely available CT software (see Fig. 6–43B and C).

Patients with equivocal fractures or suspected occult bony injury are best evaluated with MRI (see Fig. 6–43D and E)[84,141]; not only can the presence of a fracture be confirmed or excluded, but other clinically significant disorders such as meniscal or ligament injury can also be detected.

Stress Fracture

Stress fractures are separated into two categories: fatigue fractures, which occur from excessive stress applied to

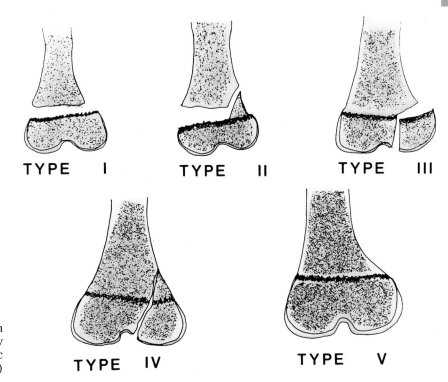

TYPE I   TYPE II   TYPE III

TYPE IV   TYPE V

Figure 6–42. Salter-Harris classification of growth plate injuries. (From Pavlov H: Radiology for the orthopaedic surgeon. Contemp Orthop 4:515, 1982.)

normal bone, and insufficiency fractures, which result from normal stress applied to abnormal bone. The latter tend to occur in individuals who are osteoporotic as a result of advanced age, metabolic bone disease, or steroid therapy.[118] The locations of stress fractures are predictable. These fractures can be cortical or cancellous. In the femur, stress fractures are supracondylar and involve the anterior and posterior cortex. In the proximal end of the tibia, cortical stress fractures occur in the posterior cortex at the junction of the proximal and middle thirds; cancellous fractures occur inferior to the medial or lateral plateau.[72] Cortical stress fractures are lucent and linear and are generally within an area of localized cortical thickening or hyperostosis. Cancellous stress fractures are dense because of impaction of the fractured trabeculae, osteoblastic activity, or endosteal callus.[116] Follow-up radiographs demonstrate a horizontal area of increased density in the proximal end of the tibia below the articular surface fracture that represents healing of the fracture (Fig. 6–44A). Cortical and cancellous stress fractures may be difficult to identify radiographically, so a radionuclide bone scan or MRI should be performed whenever a fracture is clinically suspected and radiographs are normal or equivocal (Figs. 6–44B, 6–45, and 6–46).[69,97]

Osteochondritis Dissecans

OCD is a focal injury to articular cartilage and/or subchondral bone that occurs at characteristic locations in the knee and less commonly at the convex articular surfaces of other joints. The most common site of OCD in the knee

is the intercondylar aspect of the medial femoral condyle,[55] which accounts for about 85% of cases. Other sites of chondral and osteochondral fractures include the posterior aspect of the medial and lateral femoral condyles, the superior and anterior aspect of the lateral femoral condyle, and, uncommonly, the patella. When the patella is involved, the lesion most commonly occurs in the region of the convex articular surface of the patellar apex and the medial facet. When injuries are acute or confined completely to cartilage, conventional radiographs appear normal. Injuries that also involve subchondral bone demonstrate classic radiographic findings with any of the following manifestations:

1. A lucent osseous defect (see Fig. 6–4)
2. A fragmented osseous density within a lucent defect (Fig. 6–47A)
3. A corticated osseous density within a lucent defect (see Fig. 6–47B and C)

The diagnosis of OCD is usually readily apparent on conventional radiographs. Unfortunately, plain films provide little information regarding the stability of these lesions and no information about the presence of a chondral flap. Before MRI, arthrography and radionuclide bone scan were the best imaging studies for determining whether the cartilage overlying an osseous defect was intact or whether a loose osteochondral fragment was present.[81,83] Currently, MRI is the most useful imaging study for this purpose. MRI has proved to be highly accurate in predicting the stability of an osteochondral lesion.[24,26,27,29,81] DeSmet et al[26,27,29] have described four MRI criteria that correlate with instability of a chondral or osteochondral lesion:

Text continued on p. 183

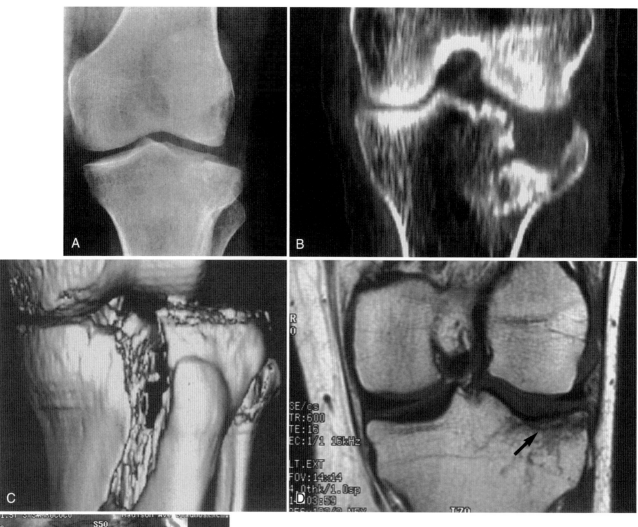

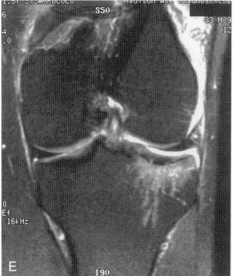

Figure 6–43. Tibial plateau fracture. **A,** An anteroposterior view demonstrates an impacted fracture of the lateral tibial plateau. The articular cortical border of the plateau is interrupted, and the lateral fragment is depressed. **B,** A two-dimensional coronal reconstructed computed tomography (CT) scan shows a comminuted, depressed fracture of the lateral tibial plateau. **C,** Three-dimensional CT image of a displaced oblique fracture of the medial tibial plateau. There is also a fracture of the fibular head and neck. The fracture can be viewed from any angle. Coronal T1-weighted (**D**) and fat-suppressed proton density (**E**) images of a patient with a skiing injury and a normal plain film (except for joint effusion) show minimal depression of the lateral tibial plateau, indicative of a fracture. A subcortical fracture line is seen in **D** (*arrow*), and marrow edema is seen in **E**. The high-signal marrow edema indicates that the fracture is acute.

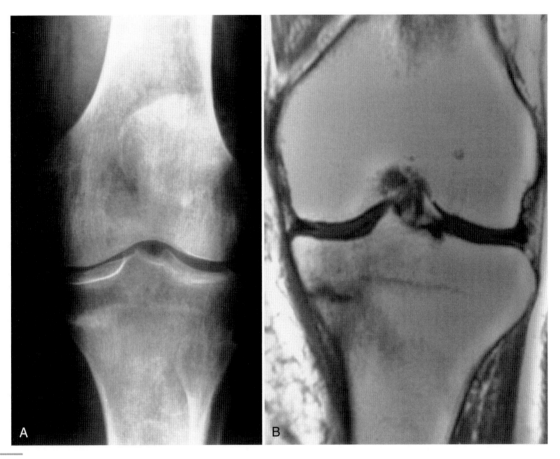

Figure 6–44. Stress fracture. **A,** An anteroposterior view demonstrates a cancellous stress fracture in the medial tibial plateau, represented as a horizontal linear density at the level of the growth plate scar. **B,** A coronal T1-weighted magnetic resonance image shows a linear fracture line corresponding to the fracture seen in **A.** The decreased signal surrounding the fracture represents bone marrow edema.

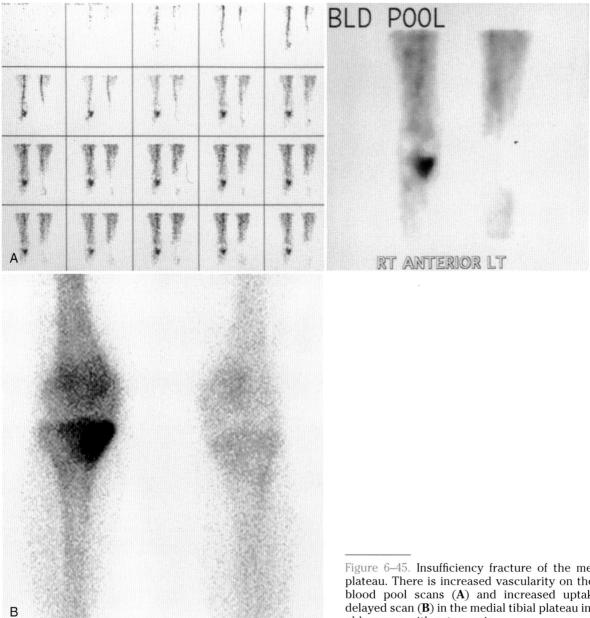

Figure 6–45. Insufficiency fracture of the medial tibial plateau. There is increased vascularity on the flow and blood pool scans (**A**) and increased uptake on the delayed scan (**B**) in the medial tibial plateau in a 70-year-old woman with osteopenia.

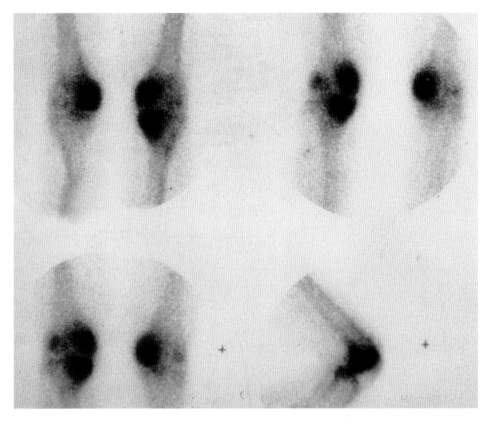

Figure 6–46. Osteomalacia. The patient complained of knee pain. There is increased uptake in the femoral condyles and tibial plateaus bilaterally representing insufficiency fractures. This diagnosis was confirmed with magnetic resonance imaging.

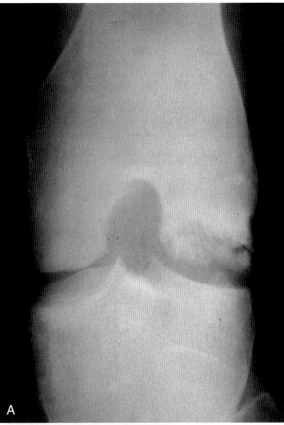

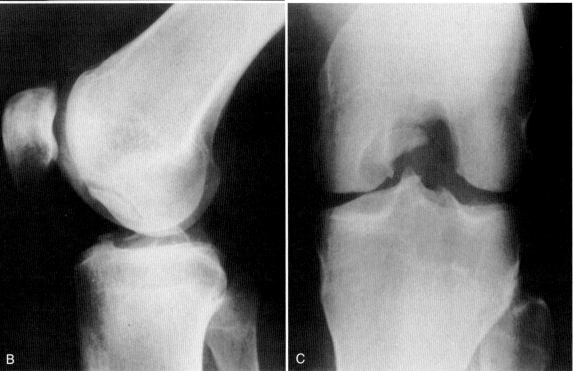

Figure 6–47. Osteochondritis dissecans. A tunnel view (**A**) shows a large fragmented osteochondral lesion of the medial femoral condyle. Lateral (**B**) and tunnel (**C**) views of another patient demonstrate a corticated osseous density within a lucent defect in the intercondylar aspect of the medial femoral condyle.

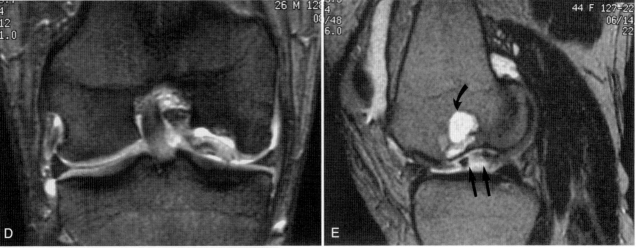

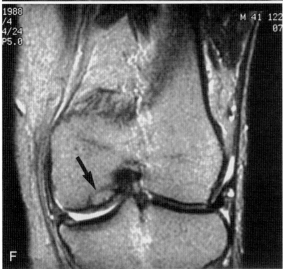

Figure 6–47, cont'd. **D,** A coronal gradient-echo magnetic resonance image shows high-signal fluid surrounding a loose osteochondral fragment at the medial femoral condyle. (Courtesy of Martin Broker, M.D.) **E,** A sagittal T2-weighted image (different patient) shows marked high-signal cystic changes (*curved arrow*) underlying a fragmented loose osteochondral lesion (*straight arrows*). **F,** A coronal T2-weighted magnetic resonance image shows a healed osteochondral lesion of the medial femoral condyle (*arrow*). Note the lack of fluid extending around the lesion and the intact overlying articular cartilage.

1. Fluid signal surrounding an osteochondral fragment on T2-weighted images (Fig. 6–47D)
2. Hyperintense signal underlying the lesion, indicative of granulation tissue
3. Cystic changes underlying the fragment (Fig. 6–47E)
4. Irregularity of articular cartilage overlying the lesion, indicative of a chondral flap

MRI can also be used to monitor lesions that are managed conservatively and can document healing of osteochondral fractures (Fig. 6–47F).

OSTEONECROSIS

Spontaneous osteonecrosis of the knee (SONK) is typically manifested as sudden-onset severe medial knee pain, most common in elderly women. Patients generally have fairly normal-appearing radiographs, and plain film findings of SONK often take 2 to 3 months to develop. Plain film findings of SONK include a focal radiolucency at the weightbearing surface of the medial femoral condyle, often with surrounding sclerosis.[113] Advanced cases progress to collapse/flattening of the articular surface (Fig. 6–48A).[73,113] A triple-phase radionuclide bone scan may reveal focal intense increased uptake at the medial femoral condyle on all three phases, which supports this diagnosis (Fig. 6–49).[3,46,87,113] However, nuclear medicine findings of increased uptake are notoriously nonspecific, and similar findings can occur with medial compartment osteoarthritis, fracture, or bone contusion (Fig. 6–50).

MRI can establish the diagnosis of SONK with a high degree of accuracy and specificity.[11,21,50] Furthermore, unlike plain films, which are usually normal at initial evaluation, both the bone scan and MRI have high sensitivity for detecting SONK at the stage when it becomes symptomatic. Patients with SONK typically have a curvilinear area of low signal near the articular surface of the medial condyle and often have variable degrees of surrounding bone marrow edema (see Fig. 6–48B and C). Whereas

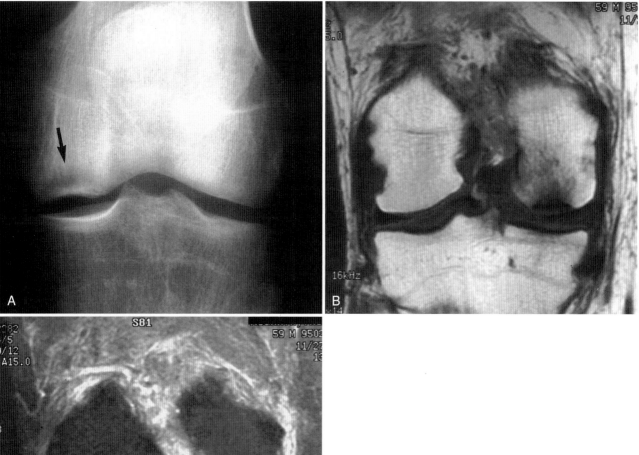

Figure 6–48. Spontaneous osteonecrosis. **A,** An anteroposterior view shows a focal radiolucency at the weight-bearing surface of the medial femoral condyle with mild surrounding sclerosis. There is also mild flattening of the articular surface in this patient with advanced osteonecrosis. Coronal T1-weighted **(B)** and fat-suppressed proton density **(C)** images in a patient with osteonecrosis of the medial femoral condyle and normal radiographs show a curvilinear band of low signal in the subcortical necrotic bone and surrounding marrow edema, best appreciated in **C.**

osteonecrosis involves the ends of bones, medullary bone infarctions typically occur in the diametaphysis of long bones. On conventional radiographs they have a characteristic appearance of peripheral serpiginous calcification in the medullary cavity of the diametaphysis.

ARTHRITIS

The primary signs of DJD are joint space narrowing, articular sclerosis, subchondral cysts, and hypertrophic osteo-

phytic spurring involving any or all of the three joint compartments (Fig. 6–51).[4,45] The medial joint compartment is affected most commonly, followed by the patellofemoral joint and the lateral compartment. Severe DJD of the lateral or medial joint compartment results in genu valgus or genu varus deformities, respectively. Isolated patellofemoral DJD suggests the presence of pyrophosphate arthropathy or chronic abnormal patellofemoral tracking.

Inflammatory arthritides are marked by pannus formation and secondary chondral and bony erosive changes. All inflammatory arthritides, including septic arthritis, rheumatoid arthritis, and the seronegative spondy-

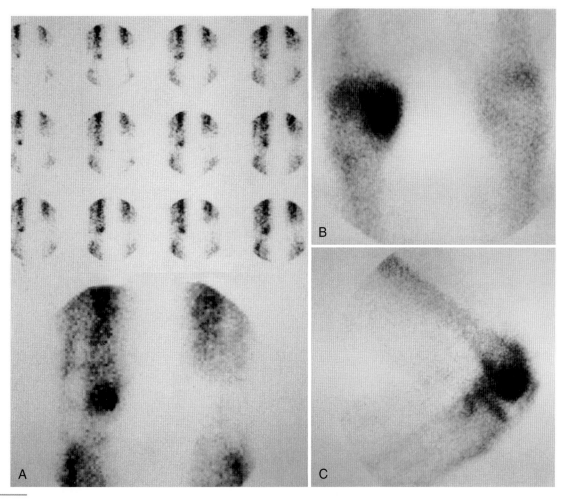

Figure 6–49. Spontaneous osteonecrosis. There is increased vascularity on the flow and blood pool scans (**A**) and increased uptake on the delayed anterior (**B**) and lateral (**C**) views localized to the right medial femoral condyle on a three-phase bone scan.

loarthropathies, are associated with the following radiographic findings (Fig. 6–52):
1. Periarticular osteoporosis secondary to hyperemia associated with inflammation
2. Uniform narrowing of the joint compartments
3. Articular cortical erosions; initially, they are marginal, at the "bare areas" of the bone, and later progress to involve the articular surface
4. Lack of signs of repair: little or no sclerosis and/or hypertrophic spurring

Rheumatoid arthritis is usually polyarticular, and septic arthritis is usually monarticular.

Neuropathic arthropathy is the severe articular disease that occurs as a result of neurological disease or neuropathy. There are numerous causes of neuropathic arthropathy; however, diabetes and syphilis are the ones that most commonly affect the knee. Other causes of neuropathic joints include leprosy, congenital insensitivity to pain, and syringomyelia (most commonly affecting the upper extremity). The hallmark of a neuropathic joint is bony fragmentation, sclerosis, and dislocation or subluxation (Fig. 6–53).[61] The atrophic form occurs much less often than the hypertrophic form, and the two are readily dis-

tinguished on the basis of bone mineralization. The main differential considerations are trauma and infection.

NEOPLASTIC DISEASE

Bone Tumors

The knee is the most common joint affected by primary bone neoplasms such as osteogenic sarcoma and giant cell tumor. In adults, the majority (more than 90%) of bone tumors are metastases or multiple myeloma. Osseous metastatic disease and myeloma most commonly involve the axial skeleton and proximal appendicular skeleton; involvement at the level of or distal to the knees and elbows is uncommon.

An osseous neoplasm is evident by a localized alteration in density, expansion, or destruction of the cortex and/or medullary cavity. Conventional radiographs are the study of choice for assessment of the aggressiveness of a bone tumor. Radiographic signs of a nonaggressive lesion include a narrow zone of transition between normal and

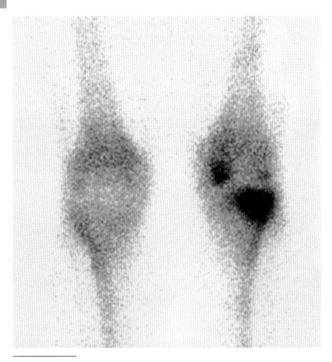

Figure 6–50. Bone bruise. Increased uptake is seen in the medial femoral condyle and lateral tibial plateau after trauma.

abnormal bone, a sclerotic rim, and the lack of periosteal reaction or a soft-tissue mass (Fig. 6–54A). Malignant bone tumors have an ill-defined line of demarcation and a wide zone of transition, and they may have an irregular or interrupted periosteal reaction and/or a soft-tissue mass (see Fig. 6–54B). Tumors should be inspected for internal matrix, which may be chondroid (coarse calcifications: "rings and broken rings") or osteoid (coalescent, cloudy).

After evaluation of bone tumors with plain films, MRI is the study of choice for assessing the extent of marrow involvement, cortical destruction, and involvement of adjacent soft tissues such as nerves and vessels.[131] MRI is ideal for evaluation of patients with suspected bone tumors and normal or equivocal radiographs (see Fig. 6–54C to E). Osteoid osteoma is virtually the only bone tumor for which CT is favored over MRI for further evaluation; the lucent nidus present in these tumors is seen to much better advantage on CT than on MRI (see Fig. 6–54F).

Soft-Tissue Tumors

Imaging evaluation of all soft-tissue tumors should begin with conventional radiographs, which will detect any

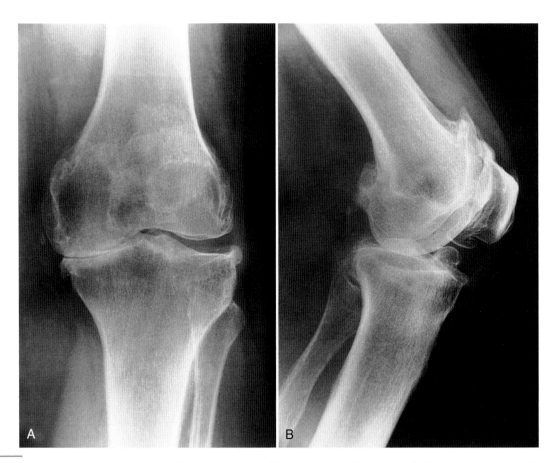

Figure 6–51. Degenerative joint disease. Anteroposterior (A) and lateral (B) views of the knee show the characteristic finding of osteoarthritis. There is joint space narrowing and osteophyte formation at the medial and patellofemoral compartments with varus alignment at the knee. A large suprapatellar joint effusion is also apparent.

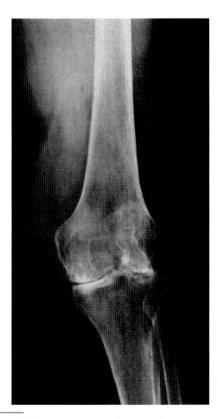

Figure 6–52. Rheumatoid arthritis. An anteroposterior view shows uniform narrowing of the medial and lateral compartments, periarticular osteopenia, and genu valgus deformity.

internal calcification or ossification and confirm that such is arising from the soft tissues rather than bone. After plain films, MRI is the study of choice for evaluation of all soft-tissue tumors[131]; it demonstrates the exact location and extent of the lesion in all three planes and any involvement of neurovascular structures. The MRI appearance of most soft-tissue tumors is notoriously nonspecific. Unlike the case with bone tumors, where plain film findings can determine the aggressiveness of the lesion, the MRI appearance of soft-tissue tumors can be misleading. Specifically, malignant soft-tissue tumors can have a relatively "benign" appearance on MRI; they may be small, well marginated, and homogeneous in signal intensity. Conversely, benign soft-tissue tumors may exhibit "malignant" MRI features such as extensive soft-tissue edema, ill-defined margins, and heterogeneous signal intensity. Myositis ossificans is the most notable soft-tissue tumor that can have an aggressive appearance on MRI as well as histopathologically. The diagnosis of myositis ossificans can be much more readily made on plain films than on MRI (see Fig. 6–17).[90]

Some soft-tissue tumors such as lipoma and plantar fibroma can be accurately diagnosed with MRI (Fig. 6–55); however, the majority of lesions are nonspecific, and biopsy of these tumors is often necessary.

CONCLUSION

In summary, conventional radiographs are the standard method of evaluating the bones and soft tissues of the

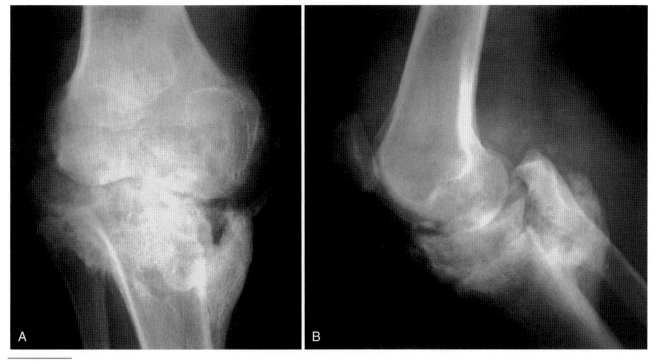

Figure 6–53. Neuropathic arthropathy of the knee. Anteroposterior (**A**) and lateral (**B**) views of the knee show marked deformity, fragmentation, and collapse of the tibial plateau, with surrounding heterotopic ossification and sclerotic changes. This patient has severe neuropathic changes of the knees secondary to long-standing syphilis (tabes dorsalis).

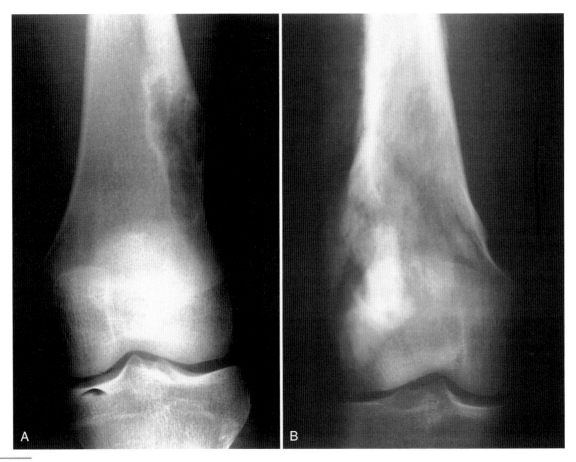

Figure 6–54. Bone tumors. **A,** Benign fibrous lesion. An anteroposterior view demonstrates a lucent lesion involving the cortical and medullary bone of the lateral aspect of the distal femoral diametaphysis. The sharp margins and sclerotic border of the lesion indicate that it is nonaggressive. **B,** Osteogenic sarcoma. An anteroposterior view demonstrates a mixed lytic and sclerotic lesion involving a large segment of the distal femoral shaft and metaphysis. The irregular periosteal reaction at the femoral shaft, combined with the infiltrative, poorly defined nature of the lesion, indicates that it is aggressive.

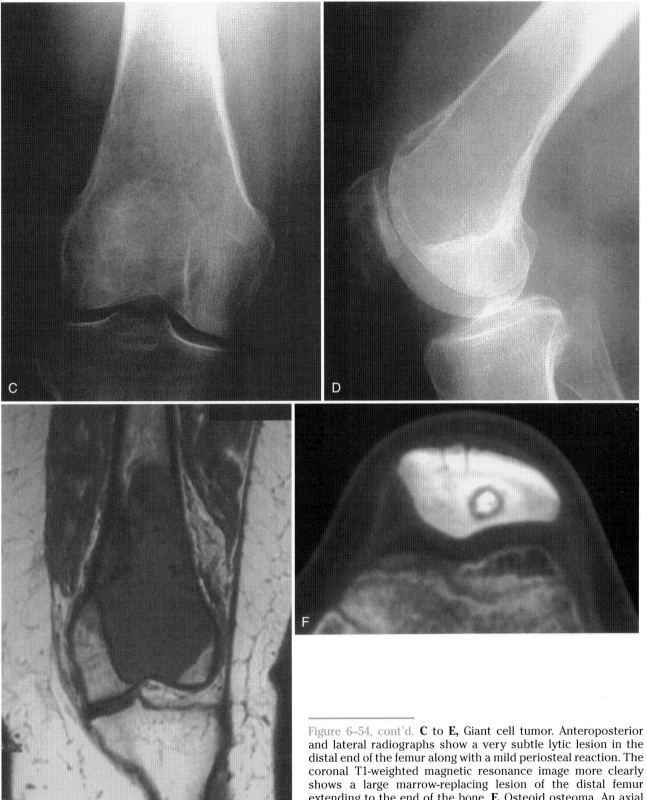

Figure 6–54, cont'd. **C** to **E,** Giant cell tumor. Anteroposterior and lateral radiographs show a very subtle lytic lesion in the distal end of the femur along with a mild periosteal reaction. The coronal T1-weighted magnetic resonance image more clearly shows a large marrow-replacing lesion of the distal femur extending to the end of the bone. **F,** Osteoid osteoma. An axial computed tomography scan of the patella shows a focal lytic lesion in the lateral facet representing the lucent nidus. There is central calcification within the lesion.

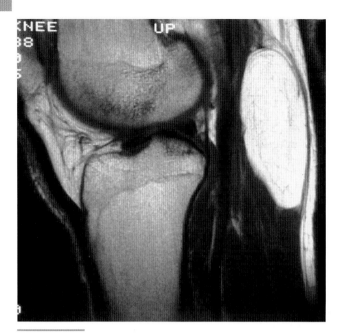

Figure 6–55. Soft-tissue lipoma. A sagittal T1-weighted magnetic resonance image shows a large, oval, high-signal mass in the popliteal soft tissues. The mass has fatty signal and is encapsulated (note the superior margin), thus indicating that it is a lipoma.

knee and assessing osseous integrity and bony alignment. More sophisticated imaging modalities, such as nuclear scanning, CT, and MRI, are used for addressing specific clinical questions. MRI has effectively replaced arthrography for evaluation of intra-articular knee pathology, and its range of clinical applications continues to grow at a rapid rate.

A focused imaging approach tailored for cost-effective evaluation of suspected clinical problems by using an appropriate combination of imaging modalities will generally permit the orthopedist to arrive at a prompt, accurate diagnosis and subsequent treatment plan.

References

1. Adams ME, Wallace CJ: Quantitative imaging of osteoarthritis. Semin Arthritis Rheum 20:26, 1991.
2. Ahlback S: Osteoarthritis of the knee: A radiographic investigation. Acta Radiol Suppl (Stockh) 277:7, 1968.
3. Al-Rowaih A, Wingstrand H, Lindstrand A, et al: Three-phase scintimetry in osteonecrosis of the knee. Acta Orthop Scand 61:120, 1990.
4. Altman RD, Fries JF, Bloch DA, et al: Radiographic assessment of progression of osteoarthritis. Arthritis Rheum 30:1214, 1987.
5. Applegate GR, Flannigan BD, Tolin BS, et al: MR diagnosis of recurrent tears in the knee: Value of intraarticular contrast material. AJR Am J Roentgenol 161:821, 1993.
6. Autz G, Goodwin C, Singson R: Magnetic resonance evaluation of anterior cruciate ligament repair using the patellar tendon double bone block technique. Skeletal Radiol 20:585, 1991.
7. Barnes GR, Gwin JL: Distal irregularities of the femur simulating malignancy. AJR Am J Roentgenol 122:180, 1974.
8. Barton J: Appearance of medial plica of the knee on MR images: Retrospective review. Radiology 173:233, 1989.
9. Bellon EM, Keith MW, Coleman PE, et al: Magnetic resonance imaging of internal derangements of the knee. Radiographics 8:95, 1988.
10. Bellon EM, Sacco DC, Steiger DA, et al: Magnetic resonance imaging in "housemaid's knee" (prepatellar bursitis). Magn Reson Imaging 5:175, 1987.
11. Bjorkengren AG: Spontaneous osteonecrosis of the knee: Value of MR imaging in determining prognosis. AJR Am J Roentgenol 154:331, 1990.
12. Bonamo JJ, Saperstein AL: Contemporary magnetic resonance imaging of the knee: The orthopedic surgeon's perspective. MRI Clin North Am 2:481, 1994.
13. Broderick LS, Turner DA, Renfrew DL, et al: Severity of articular cartilage abnormality in patients with osteoarthritis: Evaluation with fast spin-echo MR vs arthroscopy. AJR Am J Roentgenol 162:99, 1994.
14. Bronstein R, Kirk P, Hurley J: The usefulness of MRI in evaluating menisci after meniscus repair. Orthopedics 15:149, 1992.
15. Brossman J, Muhle C, Bull CC, et al: Evaluation of patellar tracking in patients with suspected patellar malalignment: Cine MR imaging vs arthroscopy. AJR Am J Roentgenol 162:361, 1994.
16. Buckland-Wright JC, Macfarlane DG, Jasani MK, et al: Quantitative microfocal radiographic assessment of osteoarthritis of the knee from weightbearing tunnel and semiflexed standing views. J Rheumatol 21:1734, 1994.
17. Camp JD, Coventry MB: The use of special views in roentgenography of the knee joint. US Nav Med Bull 44:56, 1944.
18. Carpenter WA: Meniscofemoral ligament simulating tear of the lateral meniscus: MR features. J Comput Assist Tomogr 14:1033, 1990.
19. Chan WP, Lang P, Stevens MP, et al: Osteoarthritis of the knee: Comparison of radiography, CT and MR imaging to assess extent and severity. AJR Am J Roentgenol 157:799, 1991.
20. Cobby MJ, Schweitzer ME, Resnick D: The deep lateral femoral notch: An indirect sign of a torn anterior cruciate ligament. Radiology 184:855, 1992.
21. Coleman BC, Kressel HY, Dalinka MK, et al: Radiographically negative avascular necrosis: Detection with MR imaging. Radiology 168:525, 1988.
22. Cooke TDV, Li J, Scudamore RA: Radiographic assessment of bony contributions to knee deformity. Orthop Clin North Am 25:387, 1994.
23. Crues JV III, Mink JH, Levy LT, et al: Meniscal tears of the knee: Accuracy of MR imaging. Radiology 164:445, 1987.
24. DeSmet AA, Fisher DR, Graf BK, et al: Osteochondritis dissecans of the knee: Value of MR imaging in determining lesion stability and the presence of articular cartilage defects. AJR Am J Roentgenol 155:549, 1990.
25. DeSmet AA, Graf BK: Meniscal tears missed on MR imaging: Relationship to meniscal tear patterns and anterior cruciate ligament tears. AJR Am J Roentgenol 162:905, 1994.
26. DeSmet AA, Ilahi OA, Graf BK: Reassessment of the MR criteria for stability of osteochondritis dissecans in the knee and ankle. Skeletal Radiol 25:159, 1996.
27. DeSmet AA, Ilahi OA, Graf BK: Untreated osteochondritis dissecans of the femoral condyles: Prediction of patient outcome using radiographic and MR findings. Skeletal Radiol 26:463, 1997.
28. DeSmet AA, Norris MA, Yandow DR, et al: MR diagnosis of meniscal tears of the knee: Importance of high signal in the meniscus that extends to the surface. AJR Am J Roentgenol 161:101, 1993.
29. DeSmet A, Sapega AA, Banakdarpour A, et al: Osteochondritis dissecans of the knee: Value of MR imaging in determining lesion stability and the presence of articular cartilage defects. AJR Am J Roentgenol 155:549, 1990.
30. Deutsch AL, Mink JH, Fox JM, et al: Peripheral meniscal tears: MR findings after conservative treatment or arthroscopic repair. Radiology 176:485, 1990.
31. Deutsch AL, Resnick D, Dalinka MK: Synovial plicae of the knee. Radiology 141:627, 1981.
32. Disler DG, Peters TL, Muscoreil SJ, et al: Fat-suppressed spoiled GRASS imaging of knee hyaline cartilage: Technique optimization with conventional MR imaging. AJR Am J Roentgenol 163:887, 1994.
33. Dunham WK, Marcus NW, Enneking WF, et al: Developmental defects of the distal femoral metaphysis. J Bone Joint Surg Am 62:801, 1980.

34. El-Khoury GY, Wira RL, Berbaum KS, et al: MR imaging of patellar tendinitis. Radiology 184:849, 1992.

35. Farley TE, Howell SM, Love KF, et al: Meniscal tears: MR and arthroscopic findings after meniscal repair. Radiology 180:517, 1991.

36. Fife RS, Brandt KD, Braunstein EM, et al: Relationship between arthroscopic evidence of cartilage damage and radiographic evidence of joint space narrowing in early osteoarthritis of the knee. Arthritis Rheum 34:377, 1991.

37. Firooznia H, Golimbu C, Rafii M: MR imaging of the menisci: Fundamentals of anatomy and pathology. MRI Clin North Am 2:325, 1994.

38. Fischer SP, Fox JM, Del Pizzo W, et al: Accuracy of diagnoses from magnetic resonance imaging of the knee. J Bone Joint Surg Am 73:2, 1991.

39. Freiberger RH, Kotzen LM: Fracture of the medial margin of the patella: A finding diagnostic of lateral dislocation. Radiology 88:902, 1967.

40. Fulkerson JP: Imaging the patellofemoral joint. In Fulkerson JP: Disorders of the Patellofemoral Joint. Baltimore, Williams & Wilkins, 1997, pp 73-104.

41. Gagliardi JA, Chung EM, Chandnani VP, et al: Detection and staging of chondromalacia patellae: Relative efficacies of conventional MR imaging, MR arthrography and CT arthrography. AJR Am J Roentgenol 163:629, 1994.

42. Gentili A, Seeger LL, Yao L, et al: Anterior cruciate ligament tear: Indirect signs at MR imaging. Radiology 193:835, 1994.

43. Goergen TG, Resnick D, Greenway G, et al: Dorsal defect of the patella: A characteristic radiographic lesion. Radiology 130:333, 1979.

44. Goldman AB, Pavlov H, Rubenstein D: The Segond fracture of the proximal tibia: A small avulsion that reflects major ligamentous damage. AJR Am J Roentgenol 151:1163, 1988.

45. Gresham GE, Rathey UK: Osteoarthritis in knees of aged persons: Relationship between roentgenographic and clinical manifestations. JAMA 233:168, 1975.

46. Greyson ND, Lotem MM, Gross AE, et al: Radionuclide evaluation of spontaneous femoral osteonecrosis. Radiology 142:729, 1982.

47. Grover JS, Bassett LW, Gross ML, et al: Posterior cruciate ligament: MR imaging. Radiology 174:527, 1990.

48. Handelberg F, Shahabpour M, Casteleyn PP: Chondral lesions of the patella evaluated with computed tomography, magnetic resonance imaging and arthroscopy. Arthroscopy 6:24, 1990.

49. Hayes C, Sawyer RW, Conway WF: Patellar cartilage lesions: In vitro detection and staging with MR imaging and pathologic correlation. Radiology 176:479, 1990.

50. Healy WL: Osteonecrosis of the knee detected only by MRI. Orthopedics 14:703, 1991.

51. Helms CA, Laorr A, Cannon DW Jr: The absent bow tie sign in bucket-handle tears of the menisci in the knee. AJR Am J Roentgenol 170:57, 1998.

52. Herman LJ, Beltran J: Pitfalls in MR imaging of the knee. Radiology 167:775, 1988.

53. Holmsblad EC: Postero-anterior x-ray of the knee in flexion. JAMA 109:1196, 1937.

54. Hosking GE, Clennar G: Calcifications in articular cartilage. J Bone Joint Surg Br 42:530, 1960.

55. Hughston JC, Hergenroeder PT, Courtney BG: Osteochondritis dissecans of the femoral condyle. J Bone Joint Surg Am 66:1340, 1984.

56. Insall J, Salvati E: Patella position in the normal knee joint. Radiology 101:101, 1971.

57. Jelinek JS, Kransdorf MJ, Utz JA, et al: Imaging of pigmented villonodular synovitis with emphasis on MR imaging. AJR Am J Roentgenol 152:337, 1989.

58. Johnson JF, Brogdon BG: Dorsal defect of the patella: Incidence and distribution. AJR Am J Roentgenol 138:339, 1982.

59. Justice WW, Quinn SF: Error patterns in the MR imaging evaluation of menisci of the knee. Radiology 196:617, 1995.

60. Kaplan PA, Nelson NL, Garvin KL, et al: MR of the knee: The significance of high signal in the meniscus that does not clearly extend to the surface. AJR Am J Roentgenol 156:333, 1991.

61. Katz I, Rabinowitz JG, Dzaidiw R: Early changes in Charcot's joints. AJR Am J Roentgenol 86:965, 1961.

62. Kennedy JC, Weinberg HW, Wilson AS: The anatomy and function of the anterior cruciate ligament. J Bone Joint Surg Am 56:223, 1974.

63. Khan KM, Bonar F, Desmond PM, et al: Patellar tendinosis (jumper's knee): Findings at histopathologic examination, US and MR imaging. Radiology 200:821, 1996.

64. Kirsch MD, Fitzgerald SW, Friedman H, et al: Transient lateral patellar dislocation: Diagnosis with MR imaging. AJR Am J Roentgenol 161:109, 1993.

65. Lance E, Deutsch AL, Mink JH: Prior lateral patellar dislocation: MR imaging findings. Radiology 189:905, 1993.

66. LaPrade RF, Burnett QM, Veenstra MA, et al: The prevalence of abnormal magnetic resonance imaging findings in asymptomatic knees: With correlation of magnetic resonance imaging to arthroscopic findings in symptomatic knees. Am J Sports Med 22:739, 1994.

67. Laurin CA, Levesque HP, Dussault R, et al: The abnormal lateral patellofemoral angle: A diagnostic roentgenographic sign of recurrent patellar subluxation. J Bone Joint Surg Am 60:55, 1978.

68. Leach RE, Gregg T, Siber FJ: Weight-bearing radiography in osteoarthritis of the knee. Radiology 97:265, 1970.

69. Lee JK, Yao L, Phelps CT, et al: Anterior cruciate ligament tears: MR imaging compared with arthroscopy and clinical tests. Radiology 166:861, 1988.

70. Lynch AF, Rorabeck CH, Bourne RB: Extensor mechanism complications following total knee arthroplasty. J Arthroplasty 2:135, 1987.

71. Macnab I: Recurrent dislocation of the patella. J Bone Joint Surg Am 34:957, 1952.

72. Manco LG, Schneider R, Pavlov H: Insufficiency fractures of the tibial plateau. AJR Am J Roentgenol 140:1211, 1983.

73. Mankin JH: Nontraumatic necrosis of bone (osteonecrosis). N Engl J Med 326:1473, 1992.

74. Martel W, Adler RS, Chan K, et al: Overview: New methods in imaging osteoarthritis. J Rheumatol 1:889, 1991.

75. Math KR, Ghelman B, Potter HG: Imaging of the patellofemoral joint. In Scuderi BR (ed): The Patella. New York, Springer-Verlag, 1995, pp 83-125.

76. Maywood RM, Murphy BJ, Uribe JW, et al: Evaluation of arthroscopic anterior cruciate ligament reconstruction using magnetic resonance imaging. Am J Sports Med 21:523, 1993.

77. McCarty DJ Jr, Haskin ME: The roentgenographic aspects of pseudogout: An analysis of 20 cases. AJR Am J Roentgenol 90:1248, 1963.

78. McCauley TR, Disler DG: MR imaging of articular cartilage. Radiology 209:629, 1998.

79. McCauley TR, Moses M, Kier R, et al: MR diagnosis of tears of the anterior cruciate ligament of the knee: Importance of ancillary findings. AJR Am J Roentgenol 162:115, 1994.

80. Merchant AC, Mercer RL, Jacobsen RH, et al: Roentgenographic analysis of patellofemoral congruence. J Bone Joint Surg Am 56:1391, 1974.

81. Mesgarzedeh M, Sapega AA, Bondakdarpour A, et al: Osteochondritis dissecans: Analysis of mechanical stability with radiography, scintigraphy and MR imaging. Radiology 165:775, 1987.

82. Messiah SS, Fowler PJ, Munro T: Anteroposterior radiographs of the osteoarthritic knee. J Bone Joint Surg Br 72:639, 1990.

83. Milligram JW, Rodgers LS, Miller JW: Osteochondral fractures: Mechanism of injury and fate of fragments. AJR Am J Roentgenol 130:651, 1978.

84. Mink JH, Deutsch AL: Occult cartilage and bone injuries of the knee: Detection, classification and assessment with MR imaging. Radiology 170:823, 1989.

85. Mink JH, Levy T, Crues JV III: Tears of the anterior cruciate ligament and menisci of the knee: MR imaging evaluation. Radiology 167:769, 1988.

86. Moeser P, Brechtold RE, Clark T, et al: MR imaging of anterior cruciate ligament repair. J Comput Assist Tomogr 13:105, 1989.

87. Murray IPC, Dixon J, Kohan L: SPECT for acute knee pain. Clin Nucl Med 15:828, 1990.

88. Nance EP Jr, Kaye JJ: Injuries of the quadriceps mechanism. Radiology 142:301, 1982.

89. Newberg A, Wales L: Radiographic diagnosis of quadriceps tendon rupture. Radiology 125:367, 1977.

90. Norman A, Dorfman HD: Juxtacortical circumscribed myositis ossificans: Evolution and radiographic features. AJR Am J Roentgenol 96:301, 1970.

91. O'Brien SJ, Ngeow J, Gibney MA, et al: Reflex sympathetic dystrophy of the knee: Causes, diagnosis and treatment. Am J Sports Med 23:655, 1995.

92. Ogden JA, Southwick WO: Osgood Schlatter's disease and tibial tuberosity development. Clin Orthop 116:180, 1976.

93. Osgood RB: Lesions of the tibial tubercle occurring during adolescence. Boston Med Surg J 148:114, 1903.

94. Paley D, Herzenberg JE, Tetsworth K, et al: Deformity planning for frontal and sagittal plane corrective osteotomies. Orthop Clin North Am 25:425, 1994.

95. Paley D, Tetsworth K: Mechanical axis deviation of the lower limbs: Preoperative planning of uniapical deformities of the tibia or femur. Clin Orthop 280:48, 1992.

96. Patel DV, Ferris BD, Aichroft PM: Radiologic study of alignment after total knee replacement: Short radiographs or long radiographs? Int Orthop 15:209, 1991.

97. Pentecost RL, Murray RA, Brindley HH: Fatigue, insufficiency and pathologic fractures. JAMA 187:1001, 1964.

98. Petersen TL, Engh GA: Radiographic assessment of knee alignment after total knee arthroplasty. J Arthroplasty 3:67, 1988.

99. Potter HG, Linklater JM, Allen AA, et al: Magnetic resonance imaging of articular cartilage in the knee: An evaluation with use of fast spin-echo imaging. J Bone Joint Surg Am 80:1276, 1998.

100. Quinn SF, Brown SF, Szumoswski J: Menisci of the knee: Radial MR imaging correlated with arthroscopy in 259 patients. Radiology 185:577, 1992.

101. Quinn SF, Muus C, Sara A, et al: Meniscal tears: Pathologic correlation with MR imaging. Radiology 166:580, 1988.

102. Quinn SF, Rose PM, Brown TR, et al: MR imaging of the patellofemoral compartment. MRI Clin North Am 2:425, 1994.

103. Rak KM, Gillogly SD, Schaefer RA, et al: Anterior cruciate ligament reconstruction: Evaluation with MR imaging. Radiology 178:553, 1991.

104. Rand JA, Morrey BF, Bryan AS: Patellar tendon rupture after total knee arthroplasty. Clin Orthop 244:233, 1989.

105. Recht MP, Kramer J, Marcelis S, et al: Abnormalities of articular cartilage of the knee: Analysis of available MR techniques. Radiology 187:473, 1993.

106. Recht MP, Piraino DW, Cohen MAH, et al: Localized anterior arthrofibrosis (Cyclops lesion) after reconstruction of the anterior cruciate ligament: MR imaging findings. AJR Am J Roentgenol 165:383, 1995.

107. Recht MP, Resnick D: MR imaging of articular cartilage: Current status and future directions. AJR Am J Roentgenol 163:283, 1994.

108. Remer EM, Fitzgerald SW, Friedman H, et al: Anterior cruciate ligament injury: MR imaging diagnosis and patterns of injury. Radiographics 12:901, 1992.

109. Resnick D, Niwayama G, Goergen TG, et al: Clinical, radiographic and pathologic abnormalities in calcium pyrophosphate dihydrate deposition disease (CPPD): Pseudogout. Radiology 122:1, 1977.

110. Resnick D, Vint V: The "tunnel" view in assessment of cartilage loss in osteoarthritis of the knee. Radiology 97:265, 1970.

111. Robertson PL, Schweitzer ME, Bartolozzi AR, et al: Anterior cruciate ligament tears: Evaluation of multiple signs with MR imaging. Radiology 193:829, 1994.

112. Rosenberg TD, Paulos LE, Parker RD, et al: The forty-five degree posterior anterior flexion weightbearing radiograph of the knee. J Bone Joint Surg Am 70:1479, 1988.

113. Rozing PM, Insall J, Bohne WJ: Spontaneous osteonecrosis of the knee. J Bone Joint Surg Am 62:2, 1980.

114. Rubin DA, Britton CA, Towers JD, et al: Are MR imaging signs of meniscocapsular separation valid? Radiology 201:829, 1996.

115. Salter RB, Harris R: Injuries involving epiphyseal plate. J Bone Joint Surg Am 45:587, 1963.

116. Savoca CL: Stress fractures: A classification of the earliest radiographic signs. Radiology 100:519, 1971.

117. Schatz JA, Potter HG, Rodeo SA, et al: MR imaging of anterior cruciate ligament reconstruction. AJR Am J Roentgenol 169:223, 1997.

118. Schneider R, Kaye JJ: Insufficiency and stress fractures of the long bones occurring in patients with rheumatoid arthritis. Radiology 116:595, 1975.

119. Schweitzer ME, Tran D, Deely DM, et al: Medial collateral ligament injuries: Evaluation of multiple signs, prevalence and location of associated bone bruises, and assessment with MR imaging. Radiology 194:825, 1995.

120. Scotti DM, Sadhu VK, Heimgerg F, et al: Osgood-Schlatter's disease: An emphasis on soft tissue changes in roentgen diagnosis. Skeletal Radiol 4:21, 1979.

121. Shearman CM, Brandser EA, Kathol MH, et al: An easy linear estimation of the mechanical axis on long-leg radiographs. AJR Am J Roentgenol 170:1220, 1998.

122. Shellock FG, Mink JH, Deutsch AL, et al: Patellar tracking abnormalities: Clinical experience with kinematic MR imaging in 130 patients. Radiology 172:799, 1989.

123. Silverman JM, Mink JH, Deutsch AL: Discoid menisci of the knee: MR imaging experience. Radiology 173:351, 1989.

124. Sinding-Larsen C: A hitherto unknown affliction of the patella in children. Acta Radiol 1:171, 1921.

125. Singson RD: MR imaging of bucket-handle tear of the medial meniscus. AJR Am J Roentgenol 156:121, 1991.

126. Snearly WN, Kaplan PA, Dussault RG: Lateral-compartment bone contusions in adolescents with intact anterior cruciate ligaments. Radiology 198:205, 1996.

127. Sonin AH: Magnetic resonance imaging of the extensor mechanism. MRI Clin North Am 2:401, 1994.

128. Sonin AH, Fitzgerald SW, Friedman H, et al: Posterior cruciate ligament injury: MR imaging diagnosis and patterns of injury. Radiology 190:455, 1994.

129. Sontag LW, Pyle SI: The appearance and nature of cyst-like areas in the distal femoral metaphysis of children. AJR Am J Roentgenol 46:185, 1941.

130. Stoller DW: Meniscal tears: Pathologic correlation with MR imaging. Radiology 163:731, 1987.

131. Sundaram M, McLeod RA: MR imaging of tumor and tumor-like lesions of bone and soft tissue. AJR Am J Roentgenol 155:817, 1990.

132. Takeda Y, Ikata T, Yoshida S, et al: MRI high-signal intensity in the menisci of asymptomatic children. J Bone Joint Surg Br 80:463, 1998.

133. Tewes DP, Fritts HM, Fields RD, et al: Chronically injured posterior cruciate ligament: Magnetic resonance imaging. Clin Orthop 335:224, 1997.

134. Tung GA, Davis LM, Wiggins ME, et al: Tears of the anterior cruciate ligament: Primary and secondary signs at MR imaging. Radiology 188:661, 1993.

135. Umans H, Wimpfheimer O, Haramati N, et al: Diagnosis of partial tears of the anterior cruciate ligament of the knee: Value of MR imaging. AJR Am J Roentgenol 165:893, 1995.

136. Vahey TN, Broome DR, Kayes KJ, et al: Acute and chronic tears of the anterior cruciate ligament: Differential features at MR imaging. Radiology 181:251, 1991.

137. Vahey TN, Meyer SF, Shelbourne KD, et al: MR imaging of anterior cruciate ligament injuries. MRI Clin North Am 2:365, 1994.

138. Warren RF, Kaplan N, Bach BR: The lateral femoral notch sign of anterior cruciate ligament insufficiency. Am J Knee Surg 1:119, 1988.

139. Woods GW, Stanley RF Jr, Tullos HS: Lateral capsular sign: X-ray clue to a significant knee instability. Am J Sports Med 7:27, 1979.

140. Wright DH, DeSmet AA, Norris M: Bucket-handle tears of the medial and lateral menisci of the knee: Value of MR imaging in detecting displaced fragments. AJR Am J Roentgenol 165:621, 1995.

141. Yao L, Lee JK: Occult intraosseous fracture: Detection with MR imaging. Radiology 167:749, 1988.

142. Yu JS, Popp JE, Kaeding CC, et al: Correlation of MR imaging and pathologic findings in athletes undergoing surgery for chronic patellar tendinitis. AJR Am J Roentgenol 165:115, 1995.

143. Yulish BS, Montanez J, Goodfellow DB, et al: Chondromalacia patellae: Assessment with MR imaging. Radiology 164:763, 1987.

CHAPTER 7

Imaging of the Painful Total Knee Arthroplasty

Kevin R. Math • Syed Furqan Zaidi • Catherine Petchprapa

The most common causes of revision total knee replacement (TKR) include prosthetic loosening, infection, and instability.[31,32] Although the cause of a painful TKR can often be determined from routine radiographs[36] combined with a thorough clinical and laboratory evaluation, additional studies such as computed tomography (CT), arthrography, and radionuclide imaging are often helpful in establishing a diagnosis in more challenging cases.

LOOSENING

The radiographic signs of prosthetic loosening include any or all of the following[1,10]:

1. Periprosthetic radiolucency. Such lucency can be seen at the prosthesis-cement interface or the cement-bone interface. Normally, there is no lucency at the metal-cement interface and less than 2 mm at the cement-bone interface. Periprosthetic lucency in an asymptomatic knee arthroplasty is not uncommon, and comparison with previous radiographs is essential to confirm stability or document progression. The Knee Society has developed a scoring system that assists in serial assessment of radiographic findings.[8] A wide or progressive zone of lucency is suggestive of loosening in the appropriate clinical setting (Fig. 7–1A). Occasionally, a fluoroscopically obtained frontal view of the knee may be necessary to detect clinically significant periprosthetic lucency that is not evident on standard radiographs.[20]
2. Shift in position of a component or components on serial radiographic examinations. A loose tibial component tends to shift into varus alignment (best seen on the anteroposterior view) (see Fig. 7–1B), whereas a loose femoral component tends to shift into flexion (best seen on the lateral view).
3. Cement fracture.

INFECTION

Radiographic signs of an infected joint replacement may be subtle or absent. Any or all of the following signs may be present:

1. Loosening. Differentiation of mechanical loosening from septic loosening is not usually possible on plain films, unless signs of osteomyelitis are present.
2. Periosteal reaction. Immature periosteal reaction suggests osteomyelitis and is fairly specific for infection. Periosteal reaction is rare in aseptic loosening (Fig. 7–2A and B).
3. Soft-tissue gas. Gas can be seen within abscess cavities associated with gas-forming organisms. This is the most specific radiographic sign of infection but is rarely seen (see Fig. 7–2C).

MECHANICAL LOOSENING VERSUS SEPTIC LOOSENING

A *radionuclide bone scan* can be very helpful in detecting prosthetic loosening before the appearance of suspicious radiographic findings. It can also be used to confirm equivocal or suspicious findings seen on plain films. There is increased vascularity and uptake for about a year after surgery, which limits the use of bone scanning in this postoperative period. The increased uptake around well-fixed components can persist for many years after surgery (in contrast to total hip replacement, where uptake usually returns to normal within 1 year),[7,28,29,35] thus making evaluation for loosening more challenging.

Loosening can be detected on a radionuclide bone scan as disproportionate increased uptake surrounding the loose component (Fig. 7–3). The characteristic scintigraphic finding of loosening is increased uptake around the prosthetic component; greater degrees of uptake, more extensive uptake, or a relative increase in uptake on serial examinations carry an even higher probability of loosening. The characteristic findings of an infected TKR are increased uptake at the affected knee on all three phases of the study (Fig. 7–4).[26] This sign has high sensitivity, but its specificity is limited by the fact that aseptic loosening can result in identical findings. Supplemental inflammation-specific studies are often necessary to increase the accuracy and improve the specificity of the diagnosis of infection.[30]

GALLIUM 67 CITRATE OR INDIUM 111 LEUKOCYTE SCANNING

For joint replacements, indium 111–labeled leukocyte scanning is more accurate and sensitive and is much more widely used than gallium. A normal indium-labeled white blood cell (WBC) scan strongly mitigates against the diag-

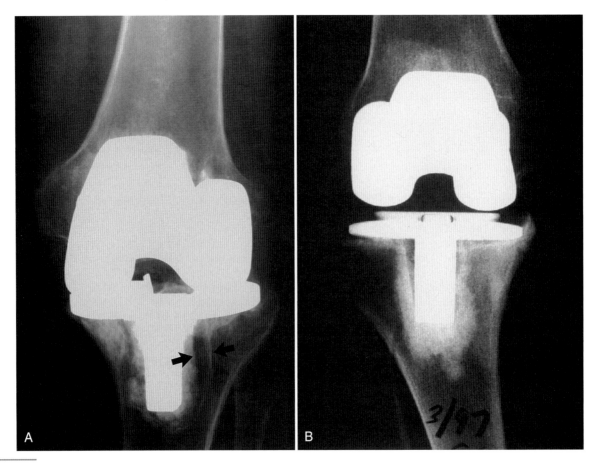

Figure 7–1. Loose total knee replacement. **A,** Anteroposterior view of the knee demonstrating a wide zone of lucency at the lateral aspect of the tibial stem (*arrows*) in this loose tibial prosthesis. **B,** Anteroposterior view showing that the loose tibial component has shifted into varus alignment. There is lucency around the tibial stem, more apparent laterally.

nosis of infection. An infected TKR will have increased uptake at the knee on an indium WBC scan.[15,17,18] After joint replacement surgery, there is a known redistribution of marrow elements around joint replacement components that can cause spuriously increased periprosthetic indium uptake[33] and can decrease the specificity to the 50% range. Although a "hot" indium scan by itself lacks specificity, a normal indium WBC scan strongly mitigates against the diagnosis of infection.

To improve accuracy, specificity, and sensitivity for diagnosis of an infected TKR, it is ideal to perform the three-phase bone scan and indium-labeled WBC scan together for all cases and comparatively assess findings on both studies.[11,13,14,19,29,38] This strategy will help arrive at a more accurate diagnosis than possible for each study alone. If there is abnormal indium activity that is normal on the bone scan or a comparatively greater degree or different distribution of uptake on the indium scan, the results are interpreted as "incongruent" or mismatched. This finding correlates with a high incidence of infection, with sensitivity and specificity reported in the 85% range (Fig. 7–5). Conversely, if the indium uptake completely matches the bone scan uptake, these findings are "congruent" and correlate with a low likelihood of infection.

TECHNETIUM SULFUR COLLOID BONE MARROW SCAN

Sulfur colloid is taken up by cells of the reticuloendothelial system (liver, spleen, and bone marrow). Uptake will be uniform and homogeneous in areas of normal cellular marrow, and it will be inhibited or decreased in infected marrow.[9] This study may be useful in the assessment of a suspected infected TKR,[6,21,22] especially if the mismatched findings on the dual bone scan/indium scan are thought to be falsely positive. If indium uptake around the components is spurious as a result of aberrant cellular marrow elements around the prosthesis, the increased indium uptake will be completely matched by uptake on the marrow scan. If the incongruent findings are secondary to an infected TKR, the areas of increased uptake on the indium scan will be "cold" on the sulfur colloid marrow scan; a mismatch using dual scanning with indium-labeled WBCs and Tc sulfur colloid correlates with a high likelihood of infection.

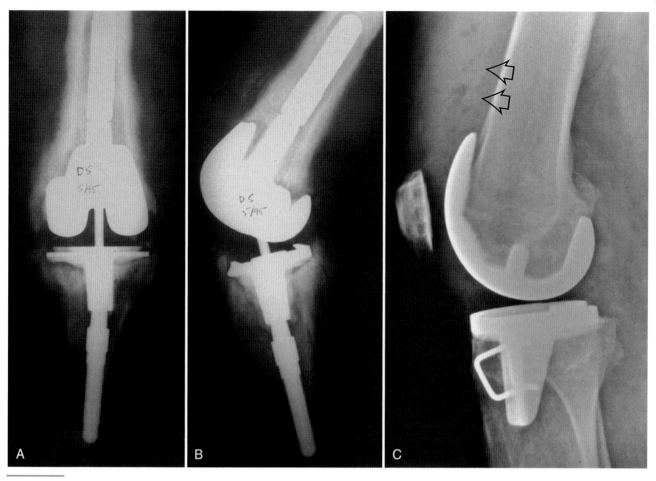

Figure 7–2. Infected total knee replacement (TKR). Anteroposterior (**A**) and lateral (**B**) views of the knee show a loose, infected TKR. There is periosteal reaction at the distal end of the femur, lucency surrounding the tibial and femoral stems, and subsidence of the tibial component. **C,** Lateral view showing multiple gas bubbles (*arrows*) in the suprapatellar region representing an abscess associated with an infected TKR.

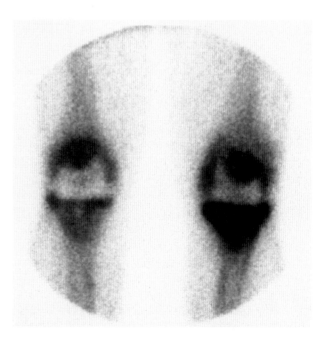

Figure 7–3. Loose tibial component—radionuclide bone scan. There is disproportionately increased uptake surrounding the loose left tibial component. Note the normal uptake around the right total knee replacement components.

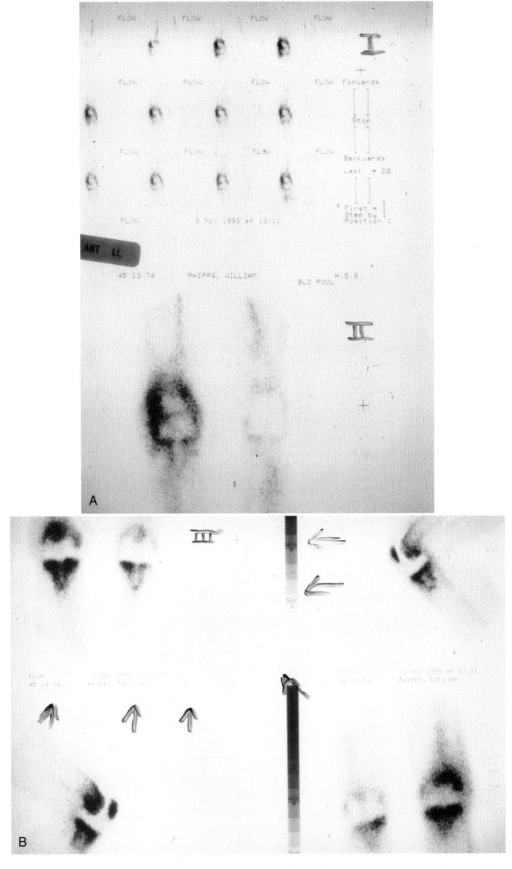

Figure 7–4. Infected total knee replacement (TKR)—triple-phase radionuclide bone scan. Early (**A**) and delayed (**B**) images of the knees demonstrate increased uptake at the right TKR on all three phases. There is hyperemia (I), increased soft-tissue uptake (II), and increased uptake around all components (III).

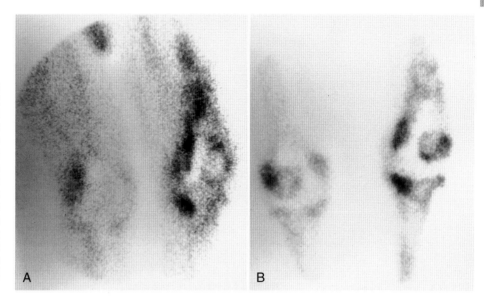

Figure 7–5. Infected total knee replacement (TKR)—nuclear imaging. **A,** There is significant increased indium activity at the mid and distal aspects of the femur and, to a lesser degree, at the medial tibial plateau. The uptake is greater in degree and differs in distribution when compared with the third phase of the bone scan (**B**). This mismatch is consistent with an infected TKR, and the patient proved to have septic arthritis and osteomyelitis of the distal end of the femur.

POLYETHYLENE COMPLICATIONS

Complications of polyethylene implants include dissociation, wear, osteolysis, and metallosis. Dissociation of the polyethylene implant in TKRs most often involves the patellar component (Fig. 7–6A). Polyethylene wear can be detected on conventional radiographs by observing an interval decrease or asymmetry in the joint spaces. Polyethylene wear debris results in an enormous number of particles within the joint (wear debris) that can incite a foreign-body granulomatous reaction. This reaction can subsequently give rise to bone resorption (osteolysis) at the margins of the joint and then around the components. This indolent process often progresses to pathological fracture or prosthetic loosening (see Fig. 7–6B).[12,23,34] CT can be used to define the location and extent of periprosthetic osteolytic lesions (see Fig. 7–6C). Severe polyethylene wear can progress to metal-on-metal contact, especially in TKRs with metal-backed patellar components, and friction between the components can eventually cause metal wear debris (see Fig. 7–6D).[24,37]

COMPONENT MALALIGNMENT

Varus/valgus malalignment is normally readily appreciated on frontal knee radiographs or long-length standing films. However, rotational malalignment, primarily of the femoral component, can result in pain and patellofemoral symptoms[2-4,25,27] and is difficult to detect on standard radiographs. Many surgeons attempt to align the femoral component parallel to a line drawn across the medial and lateral femoral epicondyles (the transepicondylar axis). Rotational malalignment can be assessed on axial CT scanning despite the presence of metal artifact.[5] The epicondylar axis is drawn from the peak of the lateral femoral condyle to the base of the sulcus of the medial epicondyle (which has a shallow W configuration). The angle between this line and a second line extending across the posterior margin of the femoral prosthesis is measured and represents the rotational alignment of the femoral component.[3,16,27] If the lines diverge medially, the component is externally rotated. If they diverge laterally, the femoral component is internally rotated. Symptomatic internal rotation of the femoral component and secondary patellar malalignment (Fig. 7–7) can be readily detected on a CT scan.

ULTRASOUND

Musculoskeletal ultrasound has widespread applications in the diagnosis and guided treatment of orthopedic injuries and diseases and can be particularly useful in the setting of total knee arthroplasty (TKA), where the metal components may be associated with significant artifact on CT or magnetic resonance imaging (MRI) that may preclude their evaluation on these modalities.

Regarding TKA, ultrasound is most useful for assessing the integrity of the quadriceps and patellar tendons or for detecting the presence of effusion or abscess. Ultrasound has also been investigated as a means of evaluating the tibial polyethylene insert for wear.[34]

MAGNETIC RESONANCE IMAGING

The role of MRI in evaluating TKRs is not yet clearly defined. Although MRI is recognized as the imaging "gold standard" for evaluating musculoskeletal diseases, the magnetic susceptibility artifact associated with metal prostheses has limited the role of this modality in this patient population. In the last several years, major advancements have been made in the protocols used for scanning patients with metal implants and minimizing metal artifact. Specifically, techniques such as increasing the imaging bandwidth, reducing TE, using a fast spin-echo technique with a longer imaging train, and avoiding chem-

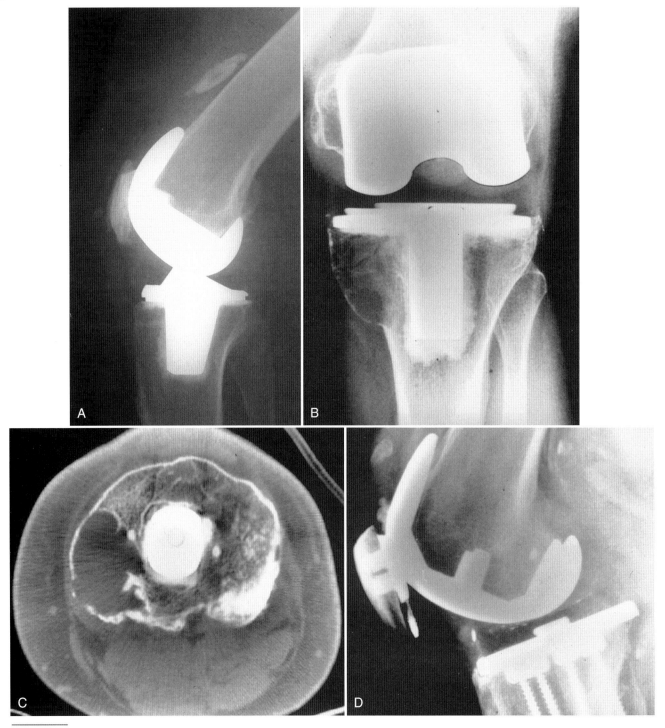

Figure 7–6. Polyethylene complications. **A,** Lateral view of the knee showing dissociation of the patellar implant and migration into the suprapatellar pouch. **B,** Anteroposterior view of the knee demonstrating a large osteolytic lesion of the medial tibial plateau secondary to polyethylene wear debris. There is relative narrowing of the medial joint compartment and a pathological fracture through the lytic lesion. **C,** Axial computed tomography through the proximal end of the tibia clearly defines the size and extent of an area of tibial osteolysis, as well as its proximity to the tibial prosthesis. Thinning and disruption of the medial cortex are present. **D,** Lateral view showing intra-articular metal debris secondary to severe polyethylene wear and metal-on-metal contact at the patellofemoral joint. The metal debris coats the polyethylene surfaces at the lower aspect of the patella and tibial implant, thereby giving an "arthrogram effect."

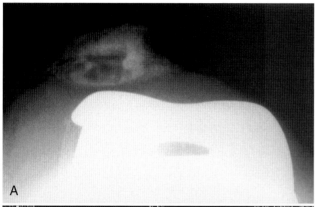

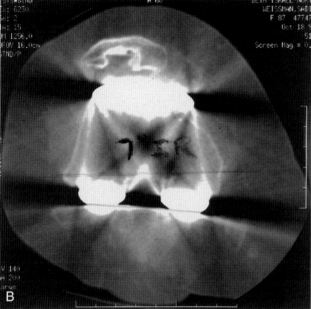

Figure 7–7. Rotational alignment of the femoral component. **A,** Merchant view of a patient with a total knee replacement; the anterior knee pain was caused by lateral patellar subluxation. **B,** Axial computed tomographic assessment of the femoral component at the level of the epicondyles shows that the component is internally rotated by 7 degrees, thus accounting for the patellar malalignment.

ical fat saturation and gradient echo imaging have been shown to improve image quality in joint replacement patients, and as some of the more recent technological advancements are made more widely available, the role of MRI will certainly increase.

CONCLUSION

Patients with a painful TKA represent a challenging population for the general orthopedic surgeon and joint reconstruction specialist alike. Diagnostic imaging using a range of imaging modalities, including plain films, nuclear scanning, CT, and ultrasound or MRI, can be extremely helpful in establishing a diagnosis in patients who have unclear clinical findings. Consultation between the ortho-

pedist and radiologist with appropriate clinical correlation is essential in this challenging patient population for selection of the optimal imaging approach and interpretation of the results based on the individual clinical setting.

References

1. Allen AM, Ward WG, Pope TL Jr: Imaging of total knee arthroplasty. Radiol Clin North Am 33:289, 1995.
2. Anouchi YS, Whiteside LA, Kaiser AD, et al: The effects of axial rotational alignment of the femoral component on knee stability and patellar tracking in total knee arthroplasty demonstrated on autopsy specimens. Clin Orthop 287:170, 1993.
3. Berger RA, Seel MJ, Rubash HE, et al: Determining the rotational alignment of the femoral component in total knee arthroplasty using the epicondylar axis. Clin Orthop 286:40, 1992.
4. Chao EYS, Neluheni EVD, Hsu RWW, et al: Biomechanics of malalignment. Orthop Clin North Am 25:379, 1994.
5. Crossett LS, Rubash HE, Berger R: Computerized tomography in total knee arthroplasty. In Insall JN, Scott WN, Scuderi GR (eds): Current Concepts in Primary and Revision Total Knee Arthroplasty. Philadelphia, Lippincott-Raven, 1996, pp 235-248.
6. Datz FL, Taylor A Jr: The clinical use of radionuclide bone marrow imaging. Semin Nucl Med 15:239, 1985.
7. Duus BR, Boeckstyns M, Kjaer L, et al: Radionuclide scanning after total knee replacement: Correlation with pain and radiolucent lines—a prospective study. Invest Radiol 22:891, 1987.
8. Ewald FC: The Knee Society total knee arthroplasty roentgenographic evaluation and scoring system. Clin Orthop 248:9, 1989.
9. Feigin DS, Strauss HW, James AW: The bone marrow scan in experimental osteomyelitis. Skeletal Radiol 1:103, 1976.
10. Gelman MI, Dunn HK: Radiology of knee joint replacement. AJR Am J Roentgenol 127:447, 1976.
11. Johnson JA, Christie MJ, Sandler C, et al: Detection of occult infection following total joint arthroplasty using sequential technetium 99m HDP bone scintigraphy and indium-111 WBC imaging. J Nucl Med 29:1347, 1988.
12. Knezevich S, Vaughn BK, Lombardi AW, et al: Failure of the polyethylene tibial component of a total knee replacement associated with asymptomatic loosening secondary to polyethylene and metallic wear debris. Orthopedics 16:1136, 1993.
13. LaManna MM, Garbarino JL, Berman AT, et al: An assessment of technetium and gallium scanning in the patient with painful total joint arthroplasty. Orthopedics 6:580, 1983.
14. Lisbona R, Roenthall L: Observations on the sequential use of 99m Tc-phosphate complex and 67-Ga imaging in osteomyelitis, cellulitis and septic arthritis. Radiology 123:123, 1977.
15. Magnuson JE, Brown ML, Hauser MF, et al: In-111–labeled leukocyte scintigraphy in suspected orthopedic prosthesis infection: Comparison with other imaging modalities. Radiology 168:235, 1988.
16. Math KR, Griffin F, Scuderi GR, et al: Imaging of the epicondylar axis of the distal femur: Utility in the evaluation of the painful total knee arthroplasty. Presented at the Radiological Society of North America Scientific Assembly, December 1997, Chicago.
17. McKillop JH, McKay I, Cuthbert GF, et al: Scintigraphic evaluation of the painful prosthetic joint: A comparison of gallium-67 citrate and indium-111–labeled leukocyte imaging. Clin Radiol 35:239, 1984.
18. Merkel KD, Brown ML, Dewanjee MK, et al: Comparison of indium-labeled leukocyte imaging with sequential technetium-gallium scanning in the diagnosis of low-grade musculoskeletal sepsis. J Bone Joint Surg Am 67:465, 1985.
19. Merkel KD, Brown ML, Fitzgerald RH Jr: Sequential technetium-99m HMDP–gallium-67 citrate imaging for the evaluation of infection in the painful prosthesis. J Nucl Med 27:1413, 1986.
20. Mintz AD, Pilkington CAJ, Howie DW: A comparison of plain and fluoroscopically guided radiographs in the assessment of arthroplasty of the knee. J Bone Joint Surg Am 9:1343, 1989.
21. Palestro CJ, Kim CK, Swyer AJ, et al: Total hip arthroplasty: Periprosthetic indium-111–labeled leukocyte activity and complementary technetium-99m sulfur colloid imaging in suspected infection. J Nucl Med 31:1950, 1990.

22. Palestro CJ, Swyer AJ, Kim CK, et al: Infected knee prosthesis: Diagnosis with In-111 leukocyte, Tc-99m sulfur colloid, and Tc-99m MDP imaging. Radiology 179:645, 1991.
23. Peters PC, Engh GA, Dwyer KA, et al: Osteolysis after total knee arthroplasty without cement. J Bone Joint Surg Am 74:864, 1992.
24. Quale JL, Murphey MD, Huntrakoon B, et al: Titanium-induced arthropathy associated with polyethylene-metal separation after total joint replacement. Radiology 182:855, 1992.
25. Ranawat CS, Rodriguez JA: Malalignment and malrotation in total knee arthroplasty. In Insall JN, Scott WN, Scuderi GR (eds): Current Concepts in Primary and Revision Total Knee Arthroplasty. Philadelphia, Lippincott-Raven, 1996, pp 115-122.
26. Reing CM, Richin PF, Kenmore PI: Differential bone scanning in the evaluation of a painful total joint replacement. J Bone Joint Surg Am 61:933, 1979.
27. Rhoades DD, Noble PC, Reuben JD, et al: The effect of femoral component positioning on patellar tracking after total knee arthroplasty. Clin Orthop 260:43, 1990.
28. Rosenthal L, Lepanto L, Raymond F: Radiophosphate uptake in asymptomatic knee arthroplasty. J Nucl Med 28:1546, 1987.
29. Rosenthal L, Lisbona R, Hernandez M, et al: Tc-99m-PP and Ga-67 imaging following insertion of orthopedic devices. Radiology 133:717, 1979.
30. Schauwecker DS: The role of nuclear medicine in osteomyelitis. In Collier BD Jr, Fogelman I, Rosenthall L (eds): Skeletal Nuclear Medicine. St Louis, Mosby–Year Book, 1996, pp 182-203.
31. Schneider R, Hood RW, Ranawat CS: Radiographic evaluation of knee arthroplasty. Orthop Clin North Am 13:225, 1982.
32. Schneider R, Soudry M: Radiographic and scintigraphic evaluation of total knee arthroplasty. Clin Orthop 205:108, 1986.
33. Seabold JE, Nepola JV, Marsh JL, et al: Postoperative bone marrow alterations: Potential pitfalls in the diagnosis of osteomyelitis with In-11–labeled leukocyte scintigraphy. Radiology 180:741, 1991.
34. Sofka CM, Adler RS, Laskin R: Sonography of polyethylene liners used in total knee arthroplasty Am J Roentgenol 180:1437-1441, 2003.
35. Tucker WF Jr, Rosenberg AF: Osteolysis following total knee arthroplasty. In Insall JN, Scott WN, Scuderi GR (eds): Current Concepts in Primary and Revision Total Knee Arthroplasty. Philadelphia, Lippincott-Raven, 1996, pp 131-146.
36. Utz JA, Lull RJ, Galvin EG: Asymptomatic total hip prosthesis: Natural history determined using Tc-99m MDP bone scans. Radiology 61:509, 1986.
37. Weissman BN: Radiographic evaluation of total joint replacement. In Sledge CB, Ruddy S, Harris ED Jr, et al (eds): Arthritis Surgery. Philadelphia, WB Saunders, 1994, pp 846-907.
38. Weissman BN, Scott RD, Brick GW, et al: Radiographic detection of metal-induced synovitis as a complication of arthroplasty of the knee. J Bone Joint Surg Am 73:1002, 1991.

CHAPTER 8

Magnetic Resonance Imaging of the Knee

Theodore T. Miller

Physical examination is the basis of diagnostic evaluation of a painful or injured knee, supplemented with magnetic resonance (MR) imaging when thought necessary by the examining physician. Careful physical examination is as accurate as MR imaging for tears of the menisci and rupture of the anterior cruciate ligament (ACL),[54,80,141] but a survey of members of the ACL study group showed that 44% of respondents routinely order preoperative MR examinations for patients with suspected ACL injury and 51% order MR examinations for patients with suspected posterior cruciate ligament (PCL) injury.[20] In cases in which the physical examination is equivocal or multiple injuries are present, MR imaging does have a significant effect on surgical decision making,[2,117,166,168] and 63% of the respondents of the ACL study group order MR examinations for patients with multiple ligament injuries.[20] Discerning use of MR imaging by orthopedic surgeons was described by Sherman et al,[154] who found that patients referred by nonorthopedic surgeons had a statistically significant higher rate of normal MR examinations than did patients referred by orthopedic surgeons.

One should keep in mind that there is wide variation in the field strengths of clinical magnets (ranging from 0.2 to 3 T), the configuration of the magnets (open or closed), the sequences (e.g., T1, T2, proton density, conventional spin echo, fast spin echo, gradient echo), and slice thicknesses used to image the knee, in addition to wide variation in the skill of the radiologist interpreting the images. All of these factors have bearing on the accuracy of the MR examination,[47] as well as the anecdotal usefulness of the modality to the referring physician.

MENISCAL TEAR

The two imaging criteria that should be used for determining a meniscal tear are (1) the presence of linear signal intensity within the meniscus that convincingly reaches either the superior or the inferior articular surface and (2) abnormal meniscal morphology. The abnormal signal should convincingly reach the articular surface on two or more consecutive slices to have a 90% likelihood of truly being a tear; if the signal reaches the surface on only one image slice, the likelihood of a tear is 55% for the medial meniscus and only 30% for the lateral meniscus.[37] Early descriptions of abnormal signal within the meniscus used a grading system in which grade I was globular signal within the meniscus, grade II was linear signal within the meniscus that did not reach an articular surface, and grade III was linear signal in the meniscus that did reach an

articular surface.[29,161] Grades I and II represent intrasubstance degeneration and grade III is a tear, but most musculoskeletal radiologists do not use this system anymore and, instead, just report that the meniscus is either normal, has intrasubstance degeneration, or is torn. Some tears can be diagnosed only by recognizing the abnormal morphology of the meniscus, such as a truncated or abnormal shape, and not by visualizing abnormal signal intensity within the meniscus.

The sensitivity and specificity of MR imaging for the detection of meniscal tears generally range from 77% to 100%,[3,95,134] but a wide variety of results can be found in both the radiology and orthopedic literature. In the presence of an acute ACL tear, the sensitivity for meniscal tears decreases, especially for tears of the posterior horn of the lateral meniscus; DeSmet and Graf[35] reported a sensitivity of 94% for lateral meniscus tears without ACL injury, but it dropped to 69% in the presence of an ACL tear, and Jee et al[69] reported only 57% sensitivity for lateral meniscus tears in the presence of a torn ACL.

Specific types of tears and their MR imaging appearances are as follows:

1. Radial tear—the tear is perpendicular to the free edge of the meniscus. The normal wedge-shaped meniscus may appear truncated, blunted, or even absent when the image slice is directly in the plane of the tear, and high signal intensity is present in the tear on T2-weighted images (Fig. 8–1).[94] Magee et al[94] found a 32% incidence of these tears in patients with new knee pain after previous partial meniscal resection.

2. Parrot beak tear—this tear is similar to a radial tear except that the plane of the tear is curved.

3. Bucket handle tear—the tear runs longitudinally along the length of the meniscus, and the inner rim flips into the intercondylar notch while remaining attached to the anterior and posterior horns. The flipped fragment lies inferior and anterior to the PCL on a midline sagittal image,[41,182] thus giving the so-called "double-PCL" sign (Fig. 8–2).[156]

4. Flap tear—this tear is similar to a bucket handle tear except that the meniscal fragment is detached from the outer rim at one end.

5. Meniscocapsular separation—vertically oriented high signal intensity is present on T2-weighted images at the periphery of the meniscus.[33]

Sometimes a tear of the meniscus will allow joint fluid to be expressed through the tear and into the soft tissues adjacent to the meniscus, thereby forming a meniscal cyst.

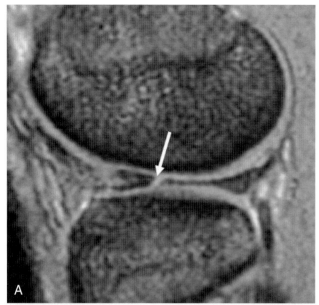

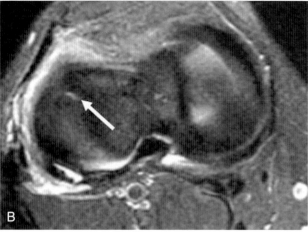

Figure 8–1. Radial tear. **A**, A sagittal gradient-echo T2-weighted sequence shows focal high signal intensity (*arrow*) at the junction of the body and anterior horn of the lateral meniscus with blunting of the anterior horn. **B**, An axial fat-suppressed T2-weighted sequence shows the linear radial tear (*arrow*) involving the inner rim of the lateral meniscus.

One large study found an 8% incidence of cysts with meniscal tears,[21] with two-thirds of the cysts occurring in the medial compartment. These cysts can be either intrameniscal or parameniscal[102] and can be large and multiloculated (Fig. 8–3), but in the series of Campbell et al,[21] only 15% were palpable. The most common type of tear associated with cysts is a horizontal cleavage tear,[169] although occasionally the original tear responsible for the cyst cannot be demonstrated because it has healed, with only the cyst remaining. The cysts may dissect into the surrounding soft tissues, and erosion of adjacent bone by the cyst has been reported.[13] The cysts may occasionally be heterogeneous in appearance because of septations and hemorrhage; however, Mountney and Thomas[115] caution that a heterogeneous mass adjacent to the meniscus

without a demonstrable meniscal tear must be viewed with suspicion for a soft-tissue neoplasm.

For patients with contraindications to MR imaging, such as pacemakers or cerebral aneurysm clips, computed tomography (CT)-arthrography and sonography provide alternative means of evaluation of meniscal tears. CT-arthrography should be considered the second-line modality after MR imaging. Conventional knee arthrography has been replaced by the advent of helical CT and powerful computer processors that can reconstruct and reformat the large volume of CT data. After intra-articular injection of 20 to 40 mL of iodinated contrast, thin slices are imaged in a helical fashion through the knee in the axial plane, with the data reformatted into the coronal and sagittal planes, thus resembling the planes of an MR examination. The normal low-density (dark) meniscus will be outlined by the high-density (bright) contrast, and contrast will insinuate itself into a tear. Accordingly, on the reformatted sagittal and coronal CT images, the high-density linear tear will look similar to the high–signal intensity tear on MR imaging (Fig. 8–4). Reported sensitivities and specificities of this technique are 92% to 100% and 88% to 98%, respectively, even in the presence of ACL tears.[89,173,174]

Sonographically, a meniscal tear can be visualized either as blunting or truncation of the normal meniscal wedge or as a hypoechoic line in the normally homogeneously echogenic meniscus. The published performance of sonography for meniscal tears is 82% to 89% sensitivity and 78% to 88% specificity,[22,49] but sonographic examination of a suspected torn meniscus requires extensive operator experience. A meniscal cyst typically appears as an anechoic mass adjacent to the meniscus, although it may also have a misleading hyperechoic heterogeneous appearance.[151] Sonography can also guide percutaneous decompression of the cyst.

A challenging aspect of meniscal imaging is evaluation of a postoperative meniscus. Even though repaired, the abnormal linear signal intensity that was formerly the tear may persist for years because of granulation tissue and may mimic a retear on postoperative MR imaging.[38,46,74] Similarly, after the meniscus is trimmed and reshaped, intrasubstance degenerative signal intensity, which formerly did not reach an articular surface, may now abut the reshaped surface and mimic a new tear. Thus, the overall accuracy of conventional MR imaging for evaluation of a postoperative meniscus is 66% to 82%.[4,92,150] MR- and CT-arthrography have been advocated for evaluation in these scenarios; a tear is present if contrast insinuates itself into the meniscus. MR-arthrography has an accuracy of 88% to 92% for all postoperative menisci,[4,150] but it is most useful for patients who have undergone meniscal resection of more than 25% or in whom meniscal repair has been performed.[4,93] Magee et al[93] found that conventional MR imaging had only 52% sensitivity for meniscal tears in patients with greater than 25% resection, but MR-arthrography had 100% sensitivity for this subgroup and was necessary to correctly evaluate all patients after meniscal repair who had persistent linear signal on conventional MR images. CT-arthrography has similar reported results.[120] Indirect MR-arthrography (a technique in which gadolinium contrast is injected intravenously

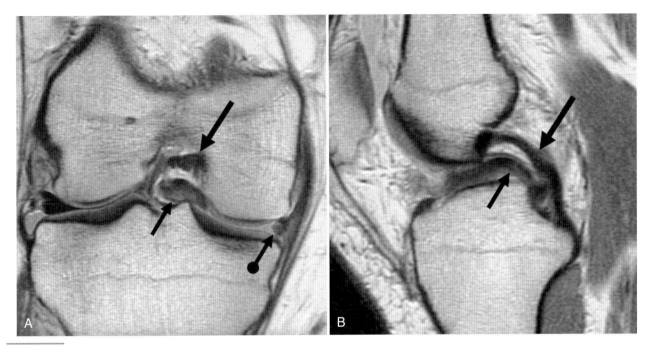

Figure 8–2. Bucket handle tear of the medial meniscus. **A,** A coronal proton-density image shows the meniscal fragment displaced into the intercondylar notch (*small arrow*). The posterior cruciate ligament (PCL) (*large arrow*) is present in the notch above the meniscal fragment. The remainder of the periphery of the medial meniscus stays attached to the joint capsule (*round-tailed arrow*). **B,** The displaced meniscal fragment (*small arrow*) has a configuration paralleling the overlying PCL (*large arrow*), thus forming the "double-PCL" sign.

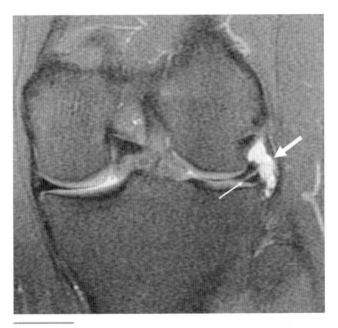

Figure 8–3. Meniscal cyst. A fat-suppressed coronal T2-weighted sequence shows a high–signal intensity meniscal cyst (*large white arrow*) with an associated oblique tear (*small white arrow*) in the body of the lateral meniscus.

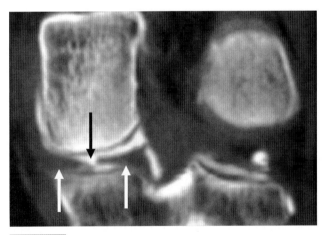

Figure 8–4. CT-arthrography of a meniscal tear. A coronally reformatted CT image after intra-articular injection of contrast shows high-density contrast (*black arrow*) outlining a tear in the posterior horn of the medial meniscus (*white arrows*).

and diffuses into the joint) has reported sensitivities of 83% to 91% and specificities of 78% to 100%,[176,183] but evaluation can be confounded by the fact that healing tears will enhance.[59] Having the preoperative MR imaging examination available for comparison to see the original

tear configuration can also be helpful, regardless of the postoperative imaging technique used.

A "discoid" meniscus, which occurs in 4.5% to 13% of the population,[51,140] is a developmental abnormality of unknown cause in which the meniscus is a large slab of fibrocartilage instead of being a crescent-shaped wedge. It is far more common on the lateral side[155] and is easily recognizable on both sagittal and coronal MR images as a

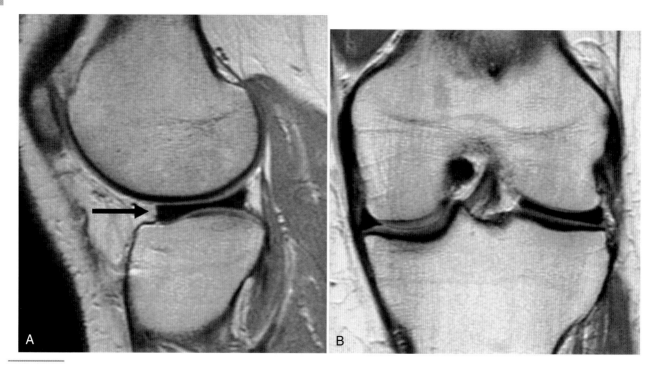

Figure 8–5. Discoid meniscus. **A,** A sagittal proton-density image shows the slab-like lateral meniscus (*arrow*). This appearance was present on every sagittal slice. **B,** A coronal proton-density image shows the large slab-like meniscus and the wedge shape of the contralateral normal medial meniscus.

rectangular block on every slice (Fig..8–5), whereas a normal meniscus should appear as a wedge in the majority of slices. One cannot use the number of imaging slices in which the slab appears as the diagnostic criterion because there is no standard slice thickness used by all imaging facilities. If the lateral meniscus has a wedge shape but the wedges are larger than the corresponding portions of the medial meniscus, the lateral meniscus is considered an incomplete discoid. The literature is controversial on whether the complete[6,79] or the incomplete[12,159] form is more common. A discoid meniscus has a higher incidence of tearing than a normal meniscus does,[5] most often as a result of horizontal tears,[12,144] and tearing occurred in 71% of discoid menisci in one large series.[140] Klingele et al[79] found that instability was more common in complete discoid menisci than in incomplete ones and usually occurred at the anterior peripheral aspect.

MR imaging of meniscal allografts can demonstrate intrasubstance signal abnormality, tears, shrinkage, mild displacement and frank extrusion, and high signal intensity along the transplant-capsular junction,[123,124,127,172] but van Arkel et al[172] reported that MR imaging performed worse than both clinical examination and arthroscopy in evaluation of the status of the transplanted meniscus in their 16 patients. They suggested, however, that such poor performance could be attributed to their MR technique, which used a low–field strength magnet combined with a large interslice gap. Wirth et al[185] had better correlation between the MR appearance and clinical outcome.

LIGAMENT INJURY

Anterior Cruciate Ligament

The normal ACL has a straight course paralleling or slightly steeper than the intercondylar roof (Blumensaat's line), and on sagittal T2-weighted images it has a linear striated appearance with intermediate signal intensity (Fig. 8–6). The anterior margin may occasionally have a darker and thicker appearance than the rest of the ligament, but this does not necessarily correspond anatomically to the anterior bundle. An acutely ruptured ACL will appear on MR imaging as either replacement of the normal linear striated appearance by an amorphous cloud-like appearance of high signal intensity or as a discrete discontinuity of the ligament with fibers that do not course parallel to the intercondylar roof (Fig. 8–7); such findings have 92% to 96% sensitivity and 89% to 99% specificity.[9,80,141] Using quantitative measurement of the ACL angle, Mellado et al[107] and Murao et al[118] found that an ACL angle of 45 degrees or less had 93% to 100% sensitivity and 84% to 100% specificity. Other authors have reported that the use of an oblique coronal sequence, oriented along the plane of the ACL, can also increase the diagnostic accuracy of MR imaging.[62,73] The distal stump may become displaced anteriorly and cause locking or a block to full extension; it appears either as a nodular mass in the anterior aspect of the intercondylar notch or as a tongue-like free edge folded on itself.[65] A large hemarthro-

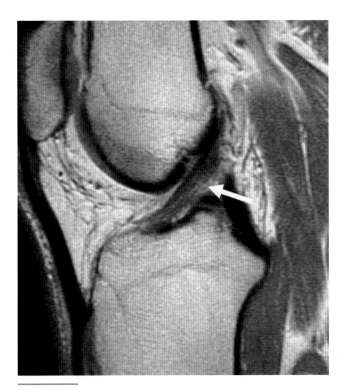

Figure 8–6. Normal anterior cruciate ligament (ACL). A sagittal proton-density image shows a normal ACL (*arrow*). The ACL is striated, has intermediate signal intensity, and is straight, paralleling Blumensaat's line. The anterior margin of the ACL has lower signal intensity than the rest of it does.

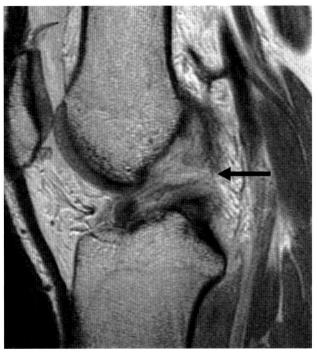

Figure 8–7. Acute anterior cruciate ligament (ACL) rupture. A sagittal proton-density image shows disruption and discontinuity of the ACL (*arrow*). Notice also that its proximal and distal fibers are no longer parallel to Blumensaat's line.

sis usually accompanies an acute ACL rupture because of the well-vascularized nature of this ligament. Partial tears of the ACL may appear as focal loss of the normal striated appearance that does not affect the entire diameter of this ligament, thus leaving some intact fibers on at least one imaging slice, or as increased signal intensity on T2-weighted images with mild swelling of the ligament,[24] but the reported sensitivity and specificity for distinguishing partial tears from ruptures are only 40% to 75% and 62% to 89%, respectively.[170] Pitfalls in the interpretation of ACL injury are cruciate ganglion cysts[52,83,132] and mucoid degeneration of the ACL,[106,122] both of which are not usually associated with a traumatic episode but can cause swelling and abnormal signal intensity within an otherwise intact ACL.

In a patient who cannot undergo MR imaging, CT-arthrography should be considered the next reasonable imaging modality, with Vande Berg et al[173] reporting 90% sensitivity and 96% specificity. Sonographic evaluation of ruptured ACLs has been described but relies on indirect signs of injury, such as hematoma in the notch and a sonographic drawer sign, because the ACL cannot be visualized directly.[49,53]

Other knee injuries often accompany an ACL tear, such as "O'Donoghue's triad," which consists of ACL rupture, medial collateral ligament (MCL) injury, and tear of the medial meniscus. As previously mentioned, however, the sensitivity of MR imaging for detecting a meniscal tear in the setting of acute ACL rupture is diminished. The

Segond fracture is a small vertically oriented fracture caused by avulsion of the lateral joint capsule from the anterolateral aspect of the proximal end of the tibia, just distal to the plateau, and is always associated with ACL rupture and often with a tear of either the medial or lateral meniscus (Fig. 8–8).[30,57,181]

In addition to a Segond fracture, other types of bone injury are often associated with ACL rupture. The most common involves the combination of bone bruises in the weightbearing portion of the lateral femoral condyle and the posterior aspect of the lateral tibial plateau (Fig. 8–9). This offset pattern of lateral bone bruises occurs as a result of internal rotation of the tibia and valgus angulation of the knee, which allows the posterolateral aspect of the tibial plateau to impact the weightbearing portion of the lateral side of the lateral femoral condyle.[135] However, it should be noted that in children, this pattern of offset lateral bone bruises may not have an associated ACL tear because of normal pediatric ligamentous laxity.[88,157] Bone bruises represent trabecular microfracture, but the overlying hyaline cartilage may also be injured, with histological evidence of chondrocyte degeneration[70] and follow-up MR studies showing cartilage thinning over the site even after the bone bruise has resolved.[27,175] "Kissing" bone bruises may occur in the anterior aspect of the tibial plateau and anterior aspects of the femoral condyles as a result of a hyperextension injury when the anterior aspects of the tibia and femoral condyles impact each other. A less common site of bone injury is the posterior aspect of the medial tibial plateau, consisting of a bone

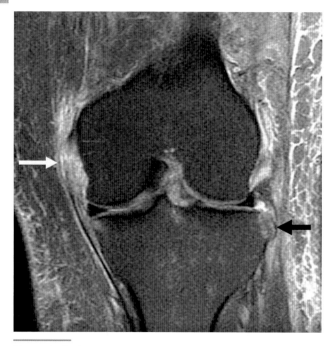

Figure 8–8. Segond fracture. A coronal fat-suppressed T2-weighted sequence shows a small avulsed piece of bone representing a Segond fracture (*black arrow*). The patient also has a rupture of the proximal aspect of the medial collateral ligament (*white arrow*).

bruise, impaction fracture, or a small chip fracture due to avulsion of the semimembranosus tendon,[23] and this site of bone injury is almost always accompanied by tear of the periphery or meniscocapsular junction of the posterior horn of the medial meniscus.[72]

These bony injuries are not only clues to the existence of an ACL tear but are also comorbid causes of pain. Other secondary signs of ACL injury, though not injuries themselves, are anterior subluxation of the tibia relative to the femur, with resultant uncovering of the posterior horn of the lateral meniscus (Fig. 8–10), and buckling of the PCL (Box 8–1).[55,139,167]

In skeletally immature patients, the tibial attachment of the ACL is weaker than the ligament itself, so ACL injuries may occur as tibial avulsions of the ACL rather than rupture of the ligament. The avulsed fracture fragment, immediately anterior to the anterior tibial spine and sometimes involving it, can often be appreciated on radiographs, but CT scanning with sagittally reformatted images can better evaluate the amount of bony distraction.

A chronically ruptured ACL will be manifested as nonvisualization of the ligament or as angulation of the ligament (instead of a straight course) because of scarring and tethering, or it will have a shallow orientation instead of paralleling the intercondylar roof (Fig. 8–11).[9,40,171]

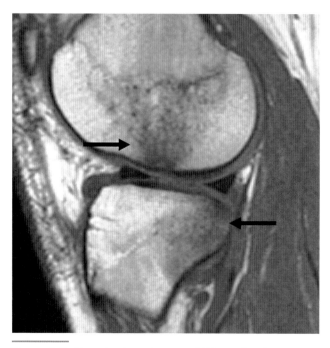

Figure 8–9. Bone bruises. A sagittal T1-weighted sequence shows offset bone bruises in the weightbearing portion of the lateral femoral condyle and the posterior aspect of the lateral tibial plateau (*arrows*) that were due to acute rupture of the anterior cruciate ligament.

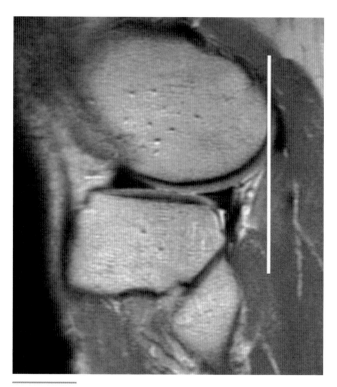

Figure 8–10. Tibial subluxation. A sagittal proton-density image shows anterior subluxation of the tibia relative to the lateral femoral condyle. A vertical line (*white line*) drawn tangential to the posterior aspect of the lateral femoral condyle is more than 7 mm from the posterior cortex of the lateral side of the tibia. Also notice that the posterior horn of the lateral meniscus seems to be sliding off the articular surface of the lateral tibial plateau, called "an uncovered" meniscus. These findings result from anterior cruciate ligament insufficiency.

Box 8-1. Secondary Signs of ACL Tear

Offset bone bruises in the weightbearing portion of the lateral femoral condyle and posterior aspect of the lateral tibial plateau

Anterior "kissing" bone bruises in the anterior aspect of the tibial plateau and anterior aspects of the femoral condyles

Bone bruise or fracture in the posterior aspect of the medial tibial plateau

Deepened condylopatellar sulcus of the lateral femoral condyle

Buckling of the PCL

PCL line sign—a line drawn along the curve of the PCL on sagittal images does not intersect the femur within 5 cm of the distal aspect of the femur

Anterior subluxation of the tibia—a line drawn vertically along the posterior aspects of the femoral condyles is more than 7 mm from the posterior cortex of the tibial plateau

Uncovering of the posterior horn of the lateral meniscus—a line drawn vertically along the posterior cortex of the tibial plateau intersects the posterior horn of the lateral meniscus

Horizontal shearing tear of Hoffa's fat pad

Occasionally, scarred remnants may mimic an intact ligament.[171] The associated findings of acute ACL injury, such as a large hemarthrosis and bone bruises, are typically not present with a chronic ACL tear, although there may be anterior subluxation of the tibia and buckling of the PCL because of residual joint laxity. A deepened condylopatellar sulcus on the lateral femoral condyle, called the "deep lateral femoral notch sign," is also an indication of chronic ACL insufficiency, but it may likewise be seen in acute ACL injury as a result of traumatic impaction (Fig. 8–12).[26,121]

A surgically reconstructed ACL is well visualized with MR imaging. Bioabsorbable interference screws have a lower MR artifact profile than metal ones do,[85,180] but even the dephasing artifact from the metal interference screws is not usually severe enough to preclude MR imaging of either the reconstructed ligament or the menisci. A reactive inflammatory edema pattern has been noted in the marrow around lactide-glycolide screws, but not around polylactic acid screws.[180] The intact, functionally competent neoligament can have variable signal intensity, depending in part on the type of donor tendon used and imaging time after placement,[103] and it usually has a straight course but may occasionally be mildly bowed.[63] On sagittal images, the entrance of the femoral tunnel should be at the intersection of a line drawn along the posterior femoral cortex and a line drawn along the roof of the intercondylar notch, and the anterior margin of the tibial tunnel should be posterior to the intersection of the tibia and a line drawn along the roof of the intercondylar

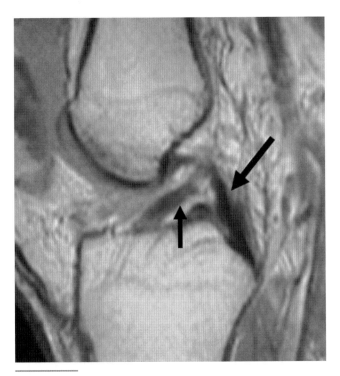

Figure 8–11. Chronic anterior cruciate ligament (ACL) tear. A sagittal proton-density image shows an ACL (*small arrow*) that has scarred onto the posterior cruciate ligament (*large arrow*). Notice that the course of the ACL is more shallow than that of Blumensaat's line and that no femoral attachment of the ACL is present.

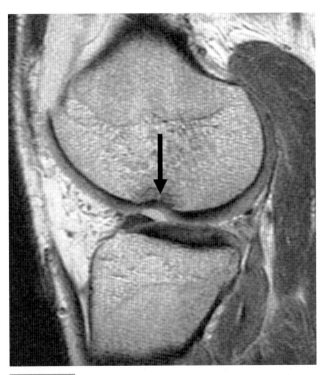

Figure 8–12. Deep lateral femoral notch sign. A sagittal proton-density image shows a deep condyle-patellar sulcus (*arrow*) resulting from impaction during acute anterior cruciate ligament rupture.

notch.[103,165] The course of the reconstructed ligament is thus more steep than that of the native ACL, averaging approximately 67 degrees from the plane of the tibial plateau versus 51 degrees, respectively.[8] Fujimoto et al[50] stress that attention must also be paid to the course of the ACL graft in the coronal plane. In their study, the average angle of the native ACL in the coronal plane relative to the tibial plateau was 67 degrees, that of asymptomatic ACL grafts was 72 degrees, and that of ACL grafts that impinged the PCL was 79.5 degrees. This latter group also had no intervening space between the graft and the PCL on coronal images (Fig. 8–13).

Both normal neovascularization of the graft, especially within the first 2 years of placement,[160,177] and notch impingement[64] can cause high T2-weighted signal intensity, thus decreasing the usefulness of high signal intensity for diagnosing tears. Using conventional MR imaging and evaluating the graft in both the coronal and sagittal plane with such criteria as diffuse or focal signal intensity changes, graft orientation, discontinuity, and focal graft thinning, Horton et al[63] achieved only 50% sensitivity, 100% specificity, and 87.5% accuracy for rupture of the graft and 0% sensitivity, 67% specificity, and 37.5% accuracy for a partial tear. Using MR-arthrography, McCauley et al[104] improved both the sensitivity and specificity for graft rupture to 100%.

Notch impingement of the graft may occur if the tibial bone tunnel is too anterior or the notch is too small. Even though tibial tunnel placement is well depicted on MR imaging, interpretation of the images as impingement is quite variable, with a sensitivity of 32% to 83%, specificity of 52% to 100%, and poor interobserver agreement.[104] Moreover, May et al[101] reported recortication of the notchplasty site and an overlying layer of fibrocartilage within 6 months of the ACL reconstruction that caused narrowing of the initially adequate notchplasty. The "Cyclops" lesion can be detected with 85% accuracy[16] and appears as a nodular soft-tissue mass of intermediate signal intensity on proton-density and T2-weighted imaging anterior to the entrance of the tibial tunnel (Fig. 8–14).[16,133] Cyclops lesions have a histological spectrum of fibrosis and fibrocartilage, but they may not be caused by graft impingement inasmuch as Bradley et al[16] found no difference in tunnel placement or notch size between patients with and without these lesions.

In reconstructions using a hamstring and EndoButton technique, Jansson et al[68] reported that the diameter of the femoral and tibial bone tunnels increased by up to 33% over a period of 2 years even though the knees were clinically stable and asymptomatic, whereas no such change occurred with a bone–patellar tendon–bone graft. In addition, regeneration of the hamstring tendon at the harvest site has been documented clinically[136] and experimentally.[90] In cases involving bone–patellar tendon–bone grafts, the patellar tendon harvest site may show postop-

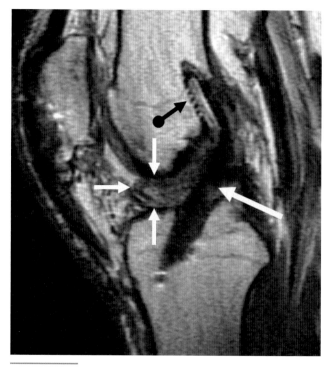

Figure 8–14. Cyclops lesion. A sagittal proton-density image shows a large globular mass of fibrous scar tissue (*small white arrows*) in the anterior aspect of the intercondylar notch after anterior cruciate ligament reconstruction. The graft itself has a normal appearance, with a straight course and uniform low signal intensity (*large white arrow*). The femoral interference screw (*round-tailed arrow*) is well seen because it is bioabsorbable and has a lower dephasing profile than metal interference screws do. It is appropriately positioned at the junction of the posterior femoral cortex and Blumensaat's line.

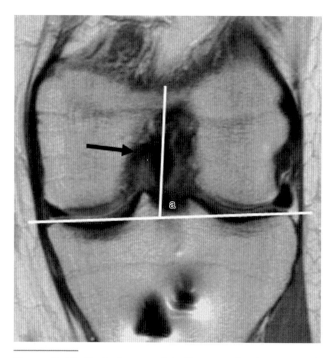

Figure 8–13. Posterior cruciate ligament impingement. A coronal proton-density image after anterior cruciate ligament (ACL) reconstruction shows that the course of the ACL graft has an angle (a) of 84 degrees with a line drawn along the tibial plateau. This steeply oriented graft is impinging on the posterior cruciate ligament (*arrow*).

erative changes consisting of a persistent defect in the central third and increased width for as long as 6 years after surgery.[162]

Posterior Cruciate Ligament

A normal PCL has uniform low signal intensity on all MR pulse sequences and a gentle curve on sagittal images (Fig. 8–15). The meniscofemoral ligaments of Humphrey and Wrisberg can occasionally be seen in cross-section, anterior and posterior, respectively, to the PCL on sagittal images. Injury of the PCL does not look the same as injury of the ACL. PCL ruptures tend to appear as generalized thickening of the ligament on MR imaging, with intermediate signal intensity on T1-weighted sequences and heterogeneous high signal intensity on T2-weighted MR sequences (Fig. 8–16).[158] Occasionally there may be focal ligamentous discontinuity. Because the force necessary to injure the PCL is greater than that needed to injure other ligaments of the knee, it is important to look for associated injuries of the ACL and the posterolateral stabilizers, such as the fibular collateral ligament and popliteus tendon. The incidence of bone bruises associated with PCL tear is similar to that of ACL injury, but their pattern is more diverse and widespread than with ACL injury.[96] In addition, avulsion of the medial tibial plateau by the deep fibers of the MCL has been described in association with PCL tears and has been termed a "reverse Segond" fracture.[45]

Healed PCLs regain their normal low signal intensity and continuity,[152] corresponding to functional competence, whereas nonhealed, functionally incompetent ligaments remain high signal intensity.[1] Similarly, Mariani et al[99] reported the serial MR imaging appearance of PCL reconstructions with bone–patellar tendon–bone graft and found heterogeneous signal intensity lasting up to at least 1 year and no correlation between the MR appearance of the graft and the clinical status of the knee during this period. After 1 year, however, signal intensity changes did correlate with changes in clinical stability. In addition, MR imaging of PCL reconstructions may demonstrate poor femoral tunnel location in patients with persistent instability.[98]

Medial Collateral Ligament

The MCL is injured as a result of valgus stress on the knee and may therefore be associated with injury to the menisci and ACL. Injury is best appreciated on coronal fat-suppressed T2-weighted MR images. A grade I sprain, representing mild partial interstitial tearing, appears as edema along the superficial aspect of this structure. A grade II sprain, representing more extensive interstitial partial tearing, is manifested as thickening of the ligament with internal signal abnormality or even frank thinning of the ligament as a result of more extensive partial tearing. A grade III sprain, or complete rupture of the ligament, can occur from either the proximal or distal attachments and

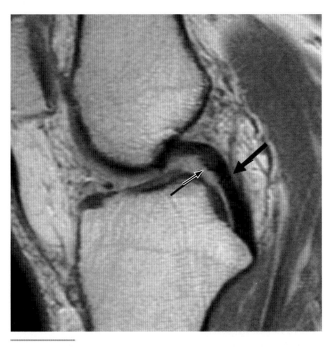

Figure 8–15. Normal posterior cruciate ligament (PCL). A sagittal proton-density image shows the uniformly low signal intensity and gentle curve of a normal PCL (*thick arrow*). The meniscofemoral ligament of Humphrey is present in the concavity of the curve (*thin arrow*).

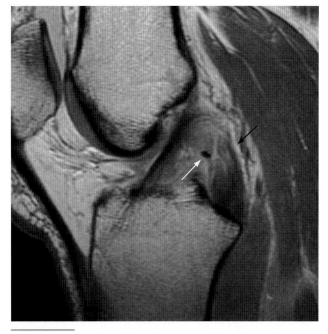

Figure 8–16. Acute posterior cruciate ligament rupture. A sagittal proton-density image shows a swollen, ill-defined, and intermediate–signal intensity ligament (*black arrow*). The meniscofemoral ligament of Humphrey (*white arrow*) maintains its normal low signal intensity.

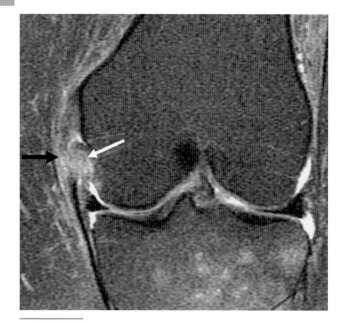

Figure 8–17. Medial collateral ligament rupture. A coronal fat-suppressed T2-weighted image shows high–signal intensity edema in and around the medial collateral ligament. The proximal aspect itself is wavy and discontinuous (*black arrow*). The femoral attachment of the medial joint capsule is also injured (*white arrow*), as manifested by swelling and high signal intensity as a result of edema and hemorrhage.

will appear as focal discontinuity on MR imaging (Fig. 8–17).[149] The ligament sometimes heals with heterotopic ossification, which is radiographically visible and is referred to as "Pellegrini-Stieda" disease.

POSTEROLATERAL LIGAMENT INJURY

Clinically unrecognized instability of the posterolateral corner of the knee can lead to failure of cruciate ligament reconstruction. Injury is best assessed on fat-suppressed T2-weighted MR images by looking for soft-tissue edema around the arcuate complex or frank disruption of these structures (Fig. 8–18).[108] The coronal imaging may be optimized by obliquing the coronal plane along the course of the fibular collateral ligament.[86,188] Avulsion of the conjoined ligament of the distal biceps tendon and the fibular collateral ligament from the fibular head may produce a displaced bony fragment.[86]

ILIOTIBIAL BAND INJURY

Injury to the iliotibial band is usually an overuse phenomenon that typically occurs in runners and bicyclists. The iliotibial band rubs against the lateral femoral condyle and becomes inflamed and painful, a condition called the "iliotibial band friction syndrome." On coronal fat-suppressed T2-weighted MR images one should look for high–signal intensity edema surrounding the iliotibial band (Fig. 8–19).[116,119]

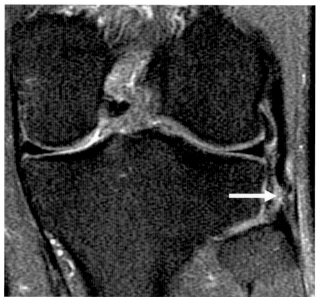

Figure 8–18. Fibular collateral ligament rupture. A coronal fat-suppressed T2-weighted image shows the wavy and discontinuous distal aspect of the fibular collateral ligament (*arrow*). There is a mild amount of surrounding high–signal intensity edema indicative of a subacute injury.

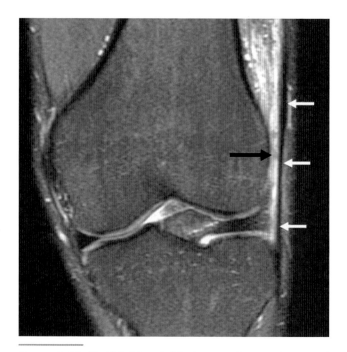

Figure 8–19. Iliotibial band friction syndrome. A coronal fat-suppressed T2-weighted image shows high–signal intensity edema (*black arrow*) surrounding the distal aspect of the iliotibial band (*white arrows*).

EXTENSOR MECHANISM INJURY

The quadriceps and patellar tendons are subject to both rupture and chronic degeneration secondary to overuse. The quadriceps tendon is more prone to tearing, whereas the patellar tendon is more prone to overuse injury.

Rupture is usually seen in unconditioned "weekend" athletes, in people with systemic disease such as diabetes or rheumatoid arthritis, or in individuals with chronic steroid use. The mechanism of injury can be trivial, such as walking up or down stairs, but it is usually due to stumbling in which there is an eccentric contraction of the extensor mechanism as the flexing knee tries to extend against the weight of the stumbling person. Although the diagnosis is usually made clinically, it is not always easy to differentiate a partial tear, which can be treated conservatively, from a complete rupture, which may be treated surgically. Both sagittal T2-weighted MR images and longitudinal sonographic images can be used to assess the degree of tendon rupture and retraction. Rupture typically appears as a balled-up and mildly retracted tendon edge with surrounding soft-tissue edema and edema/hemorrhage in the tendon gap (Fig. 8–20). Some cases of nonretracted quadriceps tendon rupture can be difficult to distinguish from a partial tear of the tendon; sonography can be helpful in such cases by imaging the patient in both the extended and flexed positions and looking for separation or retraction of the torn tendon edge in the flexed position.[11,84]

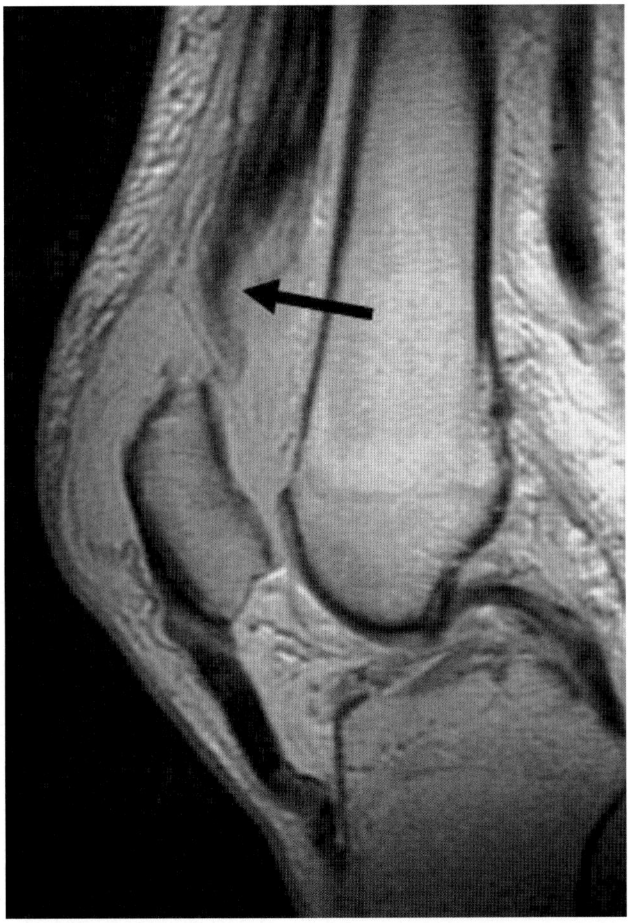

"Jumper's knee," or "patellar tendinitis," is an overuse injury of the proximal aspect of the patellar tendon[147] that is characterized by degeneration of the collagen fibers of the tendon and subsequent partial tearing, which can be painful,[75,91] but may also be asymptomatic.[97] "Jumper's knee" gets its name because it is commonly seen in basketball and volleyball players, although other athletes are likewise susceptible.[91] The term "tendinitis" is a misnomer because there is mucoid degeneration rather than acute inflammation histologically.[75] Sagittal and axial T2-weighted MR images demonstrate swelling of the proximal aspect of the patellar tendon with focal internal high signal intensity (Fig. 8–21). In some cases of chronic degeneration of the proximal patellar tendon, radiographically visible areas of heterotopic ossification may form near the patellar attachment, called Sinding-Larsen-Johansson syndrome.

"Osgood-Schlatter" disease is degeneration of the distal aspect of the patellar tendon near its insertion on the tibial tubercle[142] and consists of the triad of pain, soft-tissue swelling, and radiographically visible ossification in the distal aspect of the patellar tendon. On sagittal MR images the distal aspect of the patellar tendon may be enlarged with low–signal intensity foci of heterotopic ossification. There may be distention of the deep infrapatellar bursa manifested as fluid located between the anterior cortex of the tibia and the deep surface of the patellar tendon (Fig. 8–22).

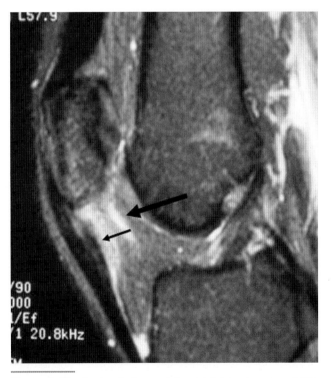

Figure 8–20. Rupture of the quadriceps tendon. A sagittal proton-density image shows discontinuity of the distal aspect of the quadriceps tendon (*arrow*). The tendon is mildly retracted. Incidentally, notice the areas of tendinosis in the proximal and distal aspects of the patellar tendon manifested by intermediate to high signal intensity.

Figure 8–21. Jumper's knee. A sagittal fat-suppressed T2-weighted image shows fusiform swelling of the proximal aspect of the patellar tendon (*small arrow*) with internal signal heterogeneity and marked surrounding high–signal intensity edema (*large arrow*) in Hoffa's fat pad.

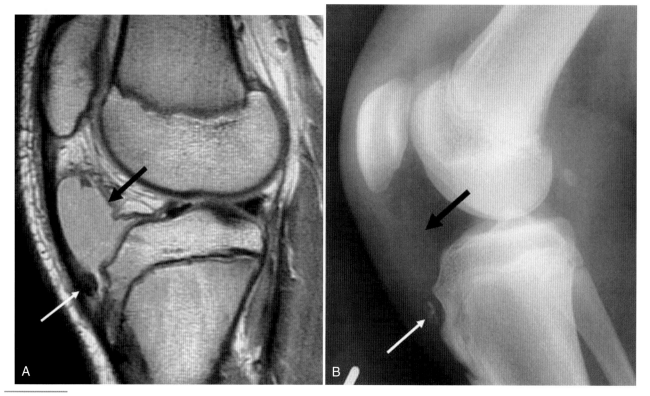

Figure 8–22. Osgood-Schlatter disease. **A**, A sagittal proton-density image shows a thickened distal aspect of the patellar tendon with internal round low signal intensity (*white arrow*) as a result of heterotopic ossification. There is also marked distention of the deep infrapatellar bursa (*black arrow*). **B**, A lateral radiograph of the same patient shows the heterotopic ossification in the distal patellar tendon (*white arrow*). The outline of the deep surface of the patellar tendon is ill defined because of the adjacent distended deep infrapatellar bursa (*black arrow*).

The patellar tendon can exhibit other manifestations of chronic degeneration on sagittal MR images, most commonly focal areas of intermediate signal intensity on T1- and T2-weighted images without focal tendon thickening. The tendon may also appear somewhat wrinkled or may be diffusely thickened.[43,148] A patellar tendon that is as thick as the quadriceps tendon is abnormal.

Lateral dislocation of the patella with spontaneous reduction can also be a cause of anterior knee pain. MR imaging in the axial plane shows bone bruises in the medial aspect of the patella and the lateral aspect of the lateral femoral condyle that occur as the patella spontaneously reduces. There may be associated tearing of the medial retinaculum manifested as thickening and internal high signal intensity on T2-weighted images, as well as associated tearing of the distal aspect of the vastus medialis oblique muscle manifested as feathery high signal intensity within this muscle on T2-weighted sequences (Fig. 8–23).[42,125]

Patellar maltracking and abnormal contact stress can occur if the patella is too high ("patella alta") or too low ("patella infera") within the femoral trochlear groove. Miller et al[109] have shown that the Insall-Salvati[66] ratio can be applied to sagittal MR images by using an image with the longest patellar length and an image through the middle of the patellar tendon.

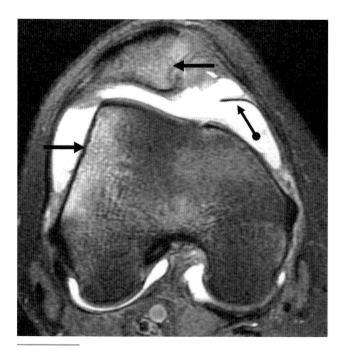

Figure 8–23. Lateral dislocation of the patella. An axial, fat-suppressed T2-weighted image shows offset bone bruises in the medial aspect of the patella and lateral aspect of the lateral femoral condyle (*straight arrows*). Incidentally noted is an incomplete medial plica (*round-tailed arrow*).

BURSITIS

Numerous bursae occur around the knee joint, and any one of them can become distended or inflamed and thereby symptomatic. Some bursae, such as the suprapatellar bursa and deep infrapatellar bursa, are actually extensions of the knee joint itself, and therefore the term "bursa," though commonly used, is actually a misnomer.

Other than a joint effusion in the suprapatellar recess, the most commonly seen fluid collection around the knee is the semimembranosus–medial gastrocnemius bursa, also called a Baker cyst. This cavity is a potential space located between the semimembranosus tendon and the medial head of the gastrocnemius muscle.[179] It has a communication with the posterior aspect of the joint capsule of the knee in adults that allows fluid to be squeezed from the joint into the bursa. Although the prevalence of these cysts is higher in people who have rheumatoid arthritis, degenerative arthritis, joint effusion, or internal derangement of the knee,[100] there is a baseline level of prevalence in the general population.[110] This distended bursa is best appreciated on axial MR images, on which it appears comma shaped, with its neck extending between the tendon of the medial gastrocnemius and the semimembranosus tendon (Fig. 8–24). When large, the patient may complain of pain or tightness in the back of the knee, and the cysts may track superiorly into the posterior aspect of the thigh or inferiorly into the calf, especially in patients with rheumatoid arthritis. The cysts may leak or rupture, best appreciated on axial fat-suppressed T2-weighted images as ill-defined soft-tissue edema adjacent to the distal aspect of the cyst, thus exposing the surrounding tissue to irritative synovial fluid, which can cause severe pain and swelling and mimic deep venous thrombosis. These cysts can also actually cause deep venous thrombosis as a result of either frank compression of the popliteal vein or rupture or leakage because the irritative synovial fluid can cause a reactive thrombophlebitis. In children, cysts in the semimembranosus–medial gastrocnemius bursa do not communicate with the knee joint,[32,110] are not associated with internal derangements, and are more appropriately called popliteal cysts rather than Baker cysts.

Bursae that occur posteromedially are the pes anserinus and the semimembranosus–tibial collateral ligament bursae. The pes anserinus bursa is located between the tendons of the pes anserinus and the distal aspect of the medial collateral ligament (Fig. 8–25).[48] The semimembranosus–tibial collateral ligament bursa is located along the medial side of the distal aspect of the semimembranosus tendon and should be distinguished from a Baker cyst by the fact that it is medial to the semimembranosus tendon whereas a Baker cyst is lateral to the semimembranosus tendon; it should also be distinguished from the pes anserinus bursa by the fact that the semimembranosus–tibial collateral ligament bursa is deep to the MCL (see Fig. 8–24).[48,143] The Baker cyst, pes anserinus bursa, and semimembranosus–tibial collateral ligament bursa do not communicate with each other. The tibial collateral ligament bursa, located within the MCL, is rarely seen but may mimic a meniscocapsular separation on coronal T2-weighted images if it is distended.

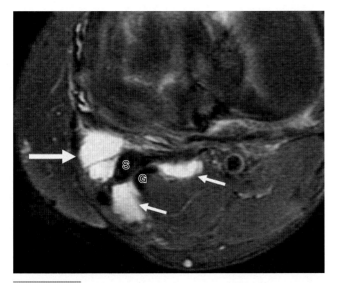

Figure 8–24. Baker's cyst and semimembranosus–tibial collateral ligament (STCL) bursitis. A Baker cyst (*small white arrows*) is a C-shaped or bilobed collection of fluid with a thin neck running between the semimembranosus tendon (S) and the tendon of the medial gastrocnemius muscle (G). The STCL bursa (*large white arrow*) is located medial to the semimembranosus tendon and does not communicate with the Baker cyst. The STCL bursa in this case has a thin septation within it.

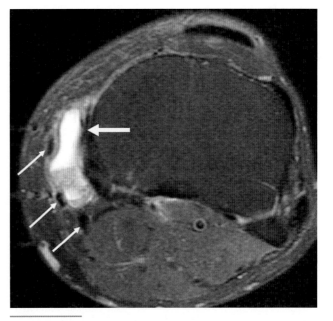

Figure 8–25. Pes anserinus bursitis. An axial fat-suppressed T2-weighted image shows a high–signal intensity fluid-filled bursa with low–signal intensity internal debris located between the pes anserinus tendons (*small white arrows*) and the medial collateral ligament (*large white arrow*).

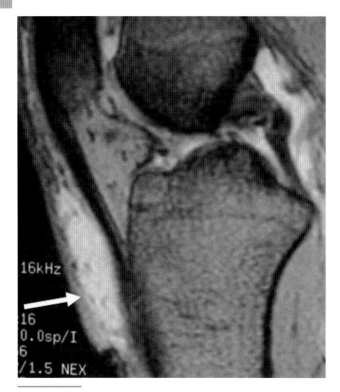

16 kHz
16
0.0sp/I
6
/1.5 NEX

Figure 8–26. Preacher's knee. A sagittal gradient-echo T2-weighted image shows distention of the superficial infrapatellar bursa (*arrow*).

Two bursae of clinical concern in the anterior aspect of the knee are the prepatellar bursa and the superficial infrapatellar bursa.[102] The prepatellar bursa is located anterior to the patella, and the superficial infrapatellar bursa is located anterior to the tibial tubercle and the distal aspect of the patellar tendon. MR imaging demonstrates these two structures as low signal intensity on T1-weighted sequences and high signal intensity on T2-weighted sequences (Fig. 8–26). Prepatellar bursitis is also called "housemaid's knee" because in the days when housemaids used to scrub a floor on their hands and knees, the irritation of the patella rubbing against the hard surface of the floor would cause inflammation and distention of this bursa. A symptomatic superficial infrapatellar bursa is called "preacher's knee" because this bursa is compressed between the tibial tubercle and the wooden bench on which a preacher kneels.

CARTILAGE AND OSTEOCHONDRAL INJURY

Because of the ubiquity of degenerative arthritis, extensive research has been focused on imaging of articular cartilage. Numerous types of MR imaging sequences and techniques have been described both for gross detection of defects and for detection of the earliest chemical changes.[17,56,58,81,114,126,163,182,187] Most of these efforts have been performed with 1.5-T magnets, but as 3-T and higher–field strength units become more widespread,

efforts to evaluate ultrastructure will continue. A trilaminar appearance of hyaline articular cartilage has been described on MR imaging, although it does not perfectly correspond histologically to the true anatomic layers of articular cartilage.[112] There is no single standard cartilage imaging sequence, and many musculoskeletal radiologists have their own particular sequences that they routinely use, but the Articular Cartilage Imaging Committee of the International Cartilage Repair Society advocates proton-density or T2-weighted fast spin-echo sequences (with or without fat suppression) and T1-weighted three-dimensional spoiled gradient-echo sequences (with fat suppression or water excitation).[131] If metal instrumentation or metal debris is present from previous knee surgery, the fast spin-echo technique is preferable because it is not as susceptible to dephasing as the gradient-echo technique is.

Chondromalacia represents a spectrum of cartilage degeneration ranging from proteoglycan breakdown and release of free water to frank full-thickness loss of cartilage (Fig. 8–27).[19,105] The early stages of this condition are seen on MR imaging as signal heterogeneity within the cartilage and surface blistering, but these findings have poor correlation with arthroscopic observations because of the fact that the arthroscopist cannot see the inside of the cartilage and may fail to appreciate focal early softening of the surface. The higher grades of this process, with frank cartilage defects, have better correlation between the MR appearance and arthroscopy.

Osteochondral injury runs the gamut from focal cartilage contusion to a loose osteochondral fragment. The imaging challenge with an osteochondral fragment is to determine its stability. Appearances suggestive of instability on conventional MR imaging are T2-weighted fluid signal intensity in the interface between the fragment and donor pit and cystic change adjacent to the donor pit (Fig. 8–28).[34,36,61] Occasionally, MR-arthrography or CT-arthrography may be needed to clarify the integrity of the cartilage surface and the nature of the fragment-donor interface.[18]

With the advent of cartilage transplant procedures, such as autologous osteochondral transplantation (mosaicplasty), autologous chondrocyte implantation, and allograft osteochondral transplantation, MR imaging has been used to noninvasively monitor the healing process and incorporation of the graft material. Sanders et al[146] and Recht et al[131] have described the serial MR appearance of the autologous osteochondral transplantation process: within the first 4 weeks of implantation, the bony plugs have fatty signal intensity; at 4 to 6 weeks after implantation, the plugs will demonstrate an edema-like signal intensity and will enhance with intravenous gadolinium, all of which suggests revascularization of the plugs; and by 1 year the signal intensity of the plugs should return to normal, even though small foci of edema-like signal intensity may remain. The signal intensity of the articular cartilage of the plugs should remain normal, although high signal intensity may occasionally occur (Fig. 8–29).[146] The signal intensity of the fibrocartilage that develops to fill in the gaps between the hyaline cartilage surfaces of the plugs may give the entire graft a mildly heterogenous signal intensity.[131] In the series of Koulalis

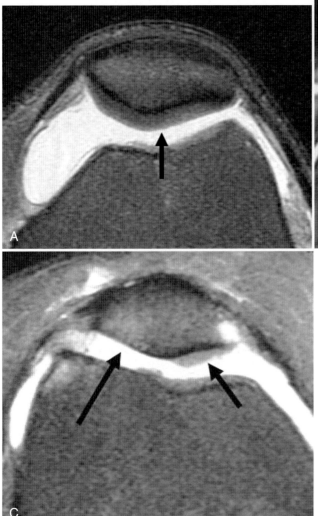

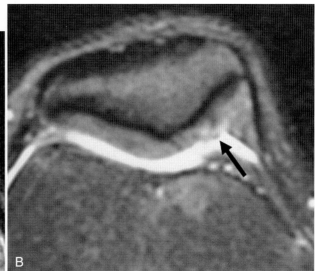

Figure 8–27. Chondromalacia. **A**, An axial fat-suppressed T2-weighted image shows the uniform thickness and uniform low signal intensity of normal patellar articular cartilage (*arrow*). It is well outlined in this case by the small high–signal intensity effusion. The *thin dark line* deep to the articular cartilage is the cortex of the patella. **B**, An axial fat-suppressed T2-weighted image of a different patient shows grade II chondromalacia manifested as blistering (*arrow*). **C**, An axial fat-suppressed T2-weighted image in a different patient shows grade IV chondromalacia manifested as complete denudation of cartilage overlying the lateral patellar facet (*large arrow*). Cartilage remains over the medial patellar facet (*small arrow*) but is thinned, has surface irregularity, and is associated with a focus of high–signal intensity subchondral fibrocystic change.

et al,[82] almost 40% of patients had a joint effusion on MR imaging for an average of 5 months after the procedure. The development of cystic change adjacent to the implant can be a sign of plug instability or loosening.[131]

The MR appearance of autologous chondrocyte implantation is more varied than that of autologous osteochondral transplantation. Both Tins et al[164] and Recht et al[131] reported that the repair tissue generally has signal intensity lower than that of fluid or adjacent normal cartilage, but Henderson et al[60] reported normal or nearly normal signal intensity in 93% of their patients at 1 year, as did Wada et al.[178] Roberts et al[138] found a correlation between the MR appearance of the autologous chondrocyte implantation graft and histology, whereas Tins et al[164] found no relationship between the signal intensity, thickness, surface smoothness, or bony integration of the graft and its histological appearance 1 year after implantation. Similarly, the presence of underlying marrow edema is variable at 1 year, with 56% of 41 patients in Tins and colleagues' series[164] having edema but only 9% of Henderson and associates' 57 patients[60] demonstrating it.

Linear fluid-like signal intensity occurring at the junction of a mature graft and underlying bone suggests poor integration or delamination.[131] Partial or complete delamination of the graft is well evaluated with MR imaging, but periosteal delamination can be difficult to distinguish from periosteal hypertrophy.[131]

ARTHRITIS AND ARTHROPATHY

MR imaging, because of its tomographic nature, is able to demonstrate osteophytes more readily than radiographs can, and because of its capability of demonstrating soft tissue, MR imaging can reveal degenerative cartilage thinning or inflammatory synovitis that radiographs cannot.

The MR imaging features of degenerative arthritis are thinning or loss of articular cartilage, osteophytes, and subchondral signal intensity changes such as sclerosis, edema, or fibrocysts. MR imaging signs of inflammatory arthritis are synovial thickening and enhancement, effu-

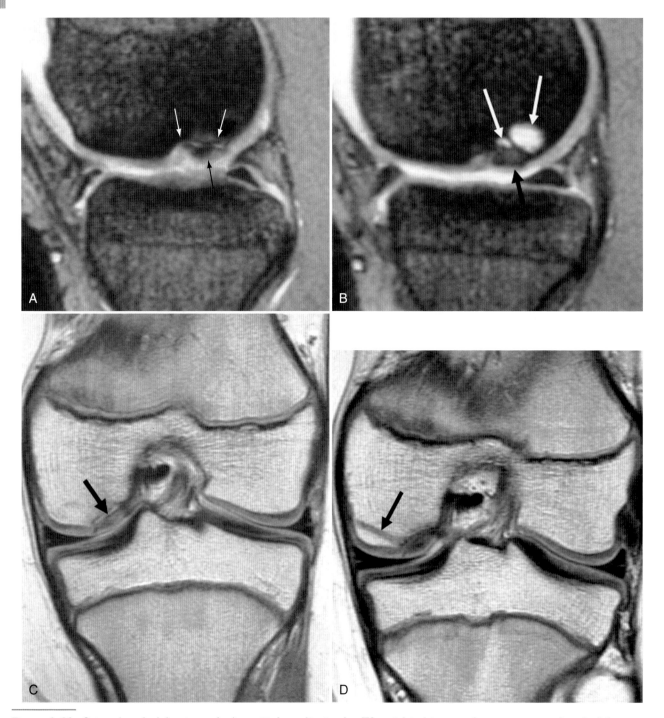

Figure 8–28. Osteochondral fracture. **A**, A sagittal gradient-echo T2-weighted image shows an osteochondral fragment (*black arrow*) in situ, with high–signal intensity fluid (*white arrows*) between the fragment and the parent bone, indicative of instability. **B**, A sagittal gradient-echo T2-weighted image of the same patient at a slightly different level shows the osteochondral fragment (*black arrow*) with two areas of fibrocystic change (*white arrows*), which also indicates instability. **C**, A preoperative coronal proton-density image of a different patient shows an in situ osteochondral fragment with linear high signal intensity (*arrow*) at the interface with the parent bone, indicative of instability. **D**, Postoperative coronal proton-density image of the same patient as in **C**. The track of a bioabsorbable "smart nail" is visible (*arrow*). The high–signal intensity fluid at the fragment-parent interface is no longer present, thus indicating healing.

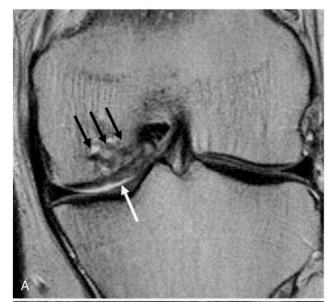

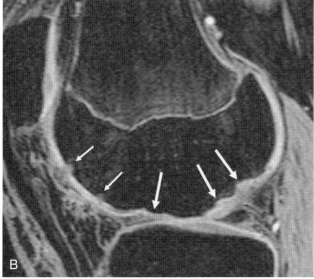

Figure 8–29. Autologous osteochondral transplant (AOT). **A**, A coronal proton-density image after an AOT procedure shows healing of the bone plugs (*black arrows*). The surface of the bone plugs is flush with the cortex of the condyle. The overlying articular cartilage is mildly heterogeneous but has the same signal intensity as the adjacent native cartilage. Mild irregularity is present in the articular cartilaginous surface (*white arrow*). **B**, A sagittal fat-suppressed gradient-echo image in a different patient shows subsidence of the osteochondral plugs (*large white arrows*). Mild signal heterogeneity is present in the overlying articular cartilage as a result of fibrocartilaginous ingrowth. There is also thinning of cartilage over the anterior plug. The faint outlines of the donor sites (*small arrows*) are still visible. (Courtesy of Dr. Michael Recht.)

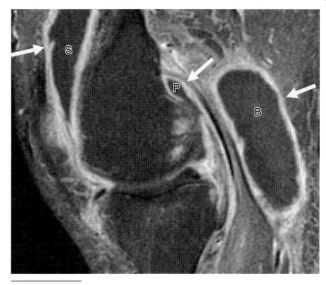

Figure 8–30. Synovitis. A sagittal fat-suppressed T1-weighted image after intravenous contrast injection shows marked enhancement of thickened synovium (*white arrows*) around the suprapatellar recess (S), posterior recess of the joint (P), and a large Baker cyst (B). This appearance can be seen in any inflammatory synovitis such as a septic joint or rheumatoid arthritis.

sion, and occasionally erosions (depending on the chronicity of the process), but MR imaging cannot distinguish septic inflammation from noninfectious inflammation such as rheumatoid arthritis (Fig. 8–30).

There are numerous diseases and abnormalities of the infrapatellar fat pad, all of which can be causes of pain or locking. As outlined by Jacobson et al[67] and Saddik et al,[145] the abnormalities can be grouped according to intrinsic processes, such as impingement (Hoffa's disease), focal nodular synovitis, and postarthroscopy/postsurgical fibrosis, and extrinsic causes, which encompass any abnormality that involves the knee joint, such as meniscal cysts and synovitis.

Plicae, or remnants of fetal synovial tissue, are common, but usually asymptomatic incidental findings on MR imaging. They may be suprapatellar,[10,78] medial parapatellar,[14] or infrapatellar (the so-called ligamentum mucosum).[15,28] All three types can become symptomatic and cause anterior knee pain with or without snapping, but it is the medial type that is most often symptomatic. A medial plica can be symptomatic if it is complete and forms a shelf from the medial side of the joint capsule to the infrapatellar fat pad; in such cases it can rub against the anterior aspect of the medial femoral condyle and become thickened, inflamed, and painful. This is typically an overuse injury associated with such sports as running and bicycling. It is best appreciated on axial T2-weighted MR images, which show the thickened low–signal intensity plica extending across the medial aspect of the knee joint (Fig. 8–31). A symptomatic infrapatellar plica will display linear edema-like signal intensity in Hoffa's fat pad.[28] Very rarely a suprapatellar plica is imperforate, and thus fluid in the suprapatellar recess can become trapped and mimic a mass clinically.

Two common arthropathies of the knee are pigmented villonodular synovitis and synovial chondromatosis. Pigmented villonodular synovitis is an idiopathic hemorrhagic proliferative synovitis and has both diffuse and focal forms.[5,7,77] The MR imaging hallmark of the disease is thick linear or globular foci of marked low signal inten-

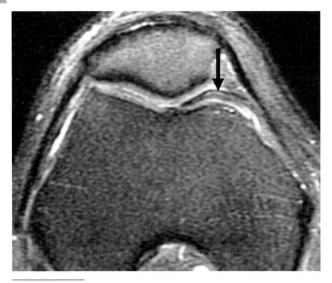

Figure 8–31. Complete medial plica. An axial fat-suppressed T2-weighted image shows a thickened complete medial plica (*arrow*).

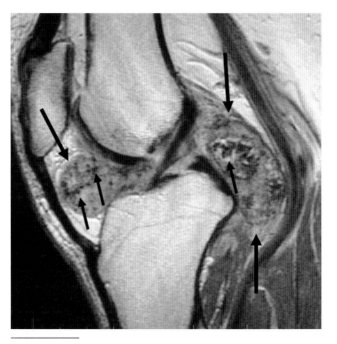

Figure 8–32. Synovial osteochondromatosis. A sagittal proton-density image shows large masses of metaplastic synovium (*large black arrows*) with numerous areas of punctate signal void (*small arrows*) indicating mineralization.

sity within the joint as a result of hemosiderin deposition, but in the early phase of the disease only synovial thickening may be present.[25] Moreover, hemosiderin deposition and synovial thickening are also features of hemophiliac arthropathy. Synovial chondromatosis is an idiopathic chondroid metaplasia of the synovium that yields masses of globular or punctate synovium with high signal intensity on T2-weighted images.[137] If the metaplastic synovium mineralizes (synovial osteochondromatosis), the masses will have a punctate, low–signal intensity appearance (Fig. 8–32).

ABNORMALITIES OF BONE

Abnormalities of the bones themselves, in addition to osteochondral injury, can also cause knee pain. Bone ischemia has a spectrum of pathology and MR appearances. Initially, ischemia produces a large area of ill-defined marrow edema, usually involving a single condyle. If the ischemic event is transient and without frank osteonecrosis, the edema will resolve over a period of approximately 2 months and leave a normal-appearing condyle.[87] If osteonecrosis occurs during the ischemic event, the demarcated zone of necrosis will become evident as the marrow edema subsides (Fig. 8–33). Zones of necrosis occurring in the subchondral portions of bone are referred to as "avascular necrosis," whereas those occurring elsewhere are referred to as "infarcts." The zone of necrosis may have a single or double rim of demarcation and may have the appearance of fat, edema, blood, or sclerosis.[111] Occasionally, the ischemic region of marrow

edema will migrate intra-articularly, indicating intra-articular regional migratory osteoporosis.[113] Avascular necrosis is a rare complication of arthroscopic menisectomy[31,44,71,129] and is perhaps caused by altered weight-bearing forces, although some cases may actually represent insufficiency fractures.

The entity known as spontaneous osteonecrosis of the knee (SONK) has been reclassified since the previous edition of this book and is now considered a subchondral insufficiency fracture of the knee (SIFK).[76,130,186] Radiographic and histological examination of the affected areas shows a subchondral fracture as the primary event, with osteonecrosis occurring as part of the fracture process.[186] MR imaging demonstrates the subchondral linear component, which represents the fracture itself, with surrounding marrow edema (Fig. 8–34).[130]

Physiological red marrow hyperplasia is often seen on MR imaging of the knee and may occur as a result of anemia, chronic disease, smoking, aerobic conditioning, and obesity.[39,128,153,184] It has signal intensity similar to that of muscle on T1-weighted images and becomes mildly high signal intensity on T2-weighted images (Fig. 8–35). Red marrow hyperplasia is usually of no clinical significance and can be distinguished from an infiltrative neoplastic process such as myeloma or lymphoma by the fact that it does not extend across the physeal scar into the end of the bone.

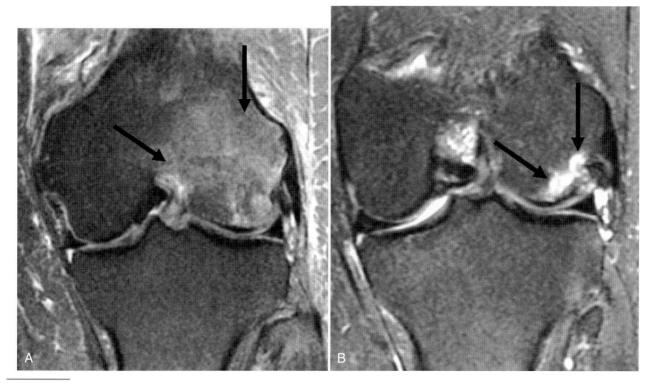

Figure 8–33. Evolving avascular necrosis. **A**, A coronal fat-suppressed T2-weighted MR image at the time of the patient's initial evaluation for pain shows ill-defined marrow edema (*arrows*) without a focal demarcated zone of necrosis. **B**, A corresponding coronal fat-suppressed T2-weighted MR image 8 months later shows resolution of the generalized edema and appearance of a demarcated zone of avascular necrosis (*arrows*).

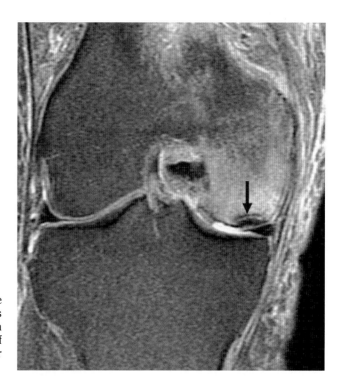

Figure 8–34. Subchondral insufficiency fracture of the knee (SIFK). A coronal fat-suppressed T2-weighted image shows a thin linear low–signal intensity fracture (*arrow*) with surrounding high–signal intensity edema and collapse of the weightbearing portion of the medial femoral condylar cortex.

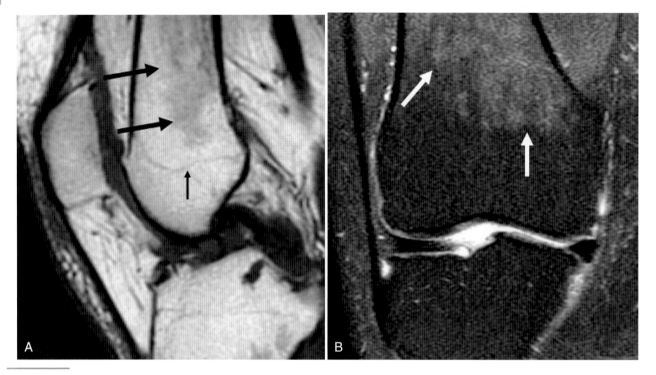

Figure 8–35. Red marrow hyperplasia. **A**, A sagittal T1-weighted image shows ill-defined intermediate–signal intensity red marrow (*large arrows*) in the distal shaft of the femur. It does not extend across the physeal scar (*small arrow*). **B**, A corresponding fat-suppressed coronal T2-weighted sequence shows the mildly high signal intensity of the red marrow (*arrows*).

References

1. Akisue T, Kurosaka M, Yoshiya S, et al: Evaluation of healing of the injured posterior cruciate ligament: Analysis of instability and magnetic resonance imaging. Arthroscopy 17:264, 2001.
2. Alioto RJ, Browne JE, Barnthouse CD, et al: The influence of MRI on treatment decisions regarding knee injuries. Am J Knee Surg 12:9, 1999.
3. Anderson MW, Raghavan N, Seidenwurm DJ, et al: Evaluation of meniscal tears: Fast spin-echo versus conventional spin-echo magnetic resonance imaging. Acad Radiol 2:209, 1995.
4. Applegate GR, Flannigan BD, Tolin BS, et al: MR diagnosis of recurrent tears in the knee: Value of intraarticular contrast material. AJR Am J Roentgenol 161:821, 1993.
5. Araki Y, Ashikaga R, Fujii K, et al: MR imaging of meniscal tears with discoid lateral meniscus. Eur J Radiol 27:153, 1998.
6. Araki Y, Tanaka H, Yamamoto H, et al: MR imaging of pigmented villonodular synovitis of the knee. Radiat Med 12:11, 1994.
7. Asik M, Erlap L, Altinel L, et al: Localized pigmented villonodular synovitis of the knee. Arthroscopy 17:e23, 2001.
8. Ayerza MA, Muscolo L, Costa-Paz M, et al: Comparison of sagittal obliquity of the reconstructed anterior cruciate ligament with native anterior cruciate ligament using magnetic resonance imaging. Arthroscopy 19:19, 2003.
9. Barry KP, Mesgarzadeh M, Triolo R, et al: Accuracy of MRI patterns in evaluating anterior cruciate ligament tears. Skeletal Radiol 25:365, 1996.
10. Base DK, Nam GU, Sun SD, et al: The clinical significance of the complete type of suprapatellar membrane. Arthroscopy 14:830, 1998.
11. Bianchi S, Zwass A, Abdelwahab IF, et al: Diagnosis of tears of the quadriceps tendon of the knee: Value of sonography. AJR Am J Roentgenol 162:1137, 1994.
12. Bin SI, Kim JC, Kim JM, et al: Correlation between type of discoid lateral menisci and tear pattern. Knee Surg Sports Traumatol Arthrosc 10:218, 2002.
13. Blair TR, Schweitzer M, Resnick D: Meniscal cysts causing bone erosion: Retrospective analysis of seven cases. Clin Imaging 23:134, 1999.
14. Boles CA, Butler J, Lee JA, et al: Magnetic resonance characteristics of medial plica of the knee: Correlation with arthroscopic resection. J Comput Assist Tomogr 28:397, 2004.
15. Boyd CR, Eakin C, Matheson GO: Infrapatellar plica as a cause of anterior knee pain. Clin J Sports Med 15:98, 2005.
16. Bradley DM, Bergman AG, Dillingham MF: MR imaging of Cyclops lesions. AJR Am J Roentgenol 174:719, 2000.
17. Bredella MA, Tirman PF, Peterfy CG, et al: Accuracy of T2-weighted fast spin-echo MR imaging with fat saturation in detecting cartilage defects in the knee: Comparison with arthroscopy in 130 patients. AJR Am J Roentgenol 172:1073, 1999.
18. Brossmann J, Preidler KW, Daenen B, et al: Imaging of osseous and cartilaginous intraarticular bodies in the knee: Comparison of MR imaging and MR arthrography with CT and CT arthrography in cadavers. Radiology 200:509, 1996.
19. Brown T, Quinn SF: Evaluation of chondromalacia of the patellofemoral compartment with axial magnetic resonance imaging. Skeletal Radiol 22:325, 1993.
20. Campbell JD: The evolution and current treatment trends with anterior cruciate, posterior cruciate, and medial collateral ligament injuries. Am J Knee Surg 11:128, 1998.
21. Campbell SE, Sanders TG, Morrison WB: MR imaging of meniscal cysts: Incidence, location, and clinical significance. AJR Am J Roentgenol 177:409, 2001.
22. Casser HR, Sohn C, Kiekenbeck A: Current evaluation of sonography of the meniscus. Results of a comparative study of sonographic and arthroscopic findings. Arch Orthop Trauma Surg 109:150, 1990.
23. Chan KK, Resnick D, Goodwin D, et al: Posteromedial tibial plateau injury including avulsion fracture of the semimembranosus tendon insertion site: Ancillary sign of anterior cruciate ligament tear at MR imaging. Radiology 211:754, 1999.
24. Chen WT, Shih TT, Tu HY, et al: Partial and complete tear of the anterior cruciate ligament. Acta Radiol 43:511, 2002.

25. Cheng XG, You YH, Liu W, et al: MRI features of pigmented villonodular synovitis (PVNS). Clin Rheumatol 23:31, 2004.

26. Cobby MJ, Schweitzer ME, Resnick D: The deep lateral femoral notch: An indirect sign of a torn anterior cruciate ligament. Radiology 184:855, 1992.

27. Costa-Paz M, Muscolo DL, Ayerza MA, et al: Magnetic resonance imaging follow-up study of bone bruises associated with anterior cruciate ligament ruptures. Arthroscopy 17:445, 2001.

28. Cothran RL, McGuire PM, Helms CA, et al: MR imaging of infrapatellar plica injury. AJR Am J Roentgenol 180:1443, 2003.

29. Crues JV 3rd, Mink J, Levy TL, et al: Meniscal tears of the knee: Accuracy of MR imaging. Radiology 164:445, 1987.

30. Davis DS, Post WR: Segond fractures: Lateral capsular ligament avulsion. J Orthop Sports Phys Ther 25:103, 1997.

31. De Falco RA, Ricci AR, Balduini FC: Osteonecrosis of the knee after arthroscopic meniscectomy and chondroplasty: A case report and literature review. Am J Sports Med 31:1013, 2003.

32. De Maeseneer M, Debaere C, Desprechins B, et al: Popliteal cysts in children: Prevalence, appearance, and associated findings at MR imaging. Pediatr Radiol 29:605, 1999.

33. De Maeseneer M, Shahabpour M, Vanderdood K, et al: Medial meniscocapsular separation: MR imaging criteria and diagnostic pitfalls. Eur J Radiol 41:242, 2002.

34. De Smet AA, Fisher DR, Graf BK, et al: Osteochondritis dissecans of the knee: Value of MR imaging in determining lesion stability and the presence of articular cartilage defects. AJR Am J Roentgenol 155:549, 1990.

35. De Smet AA, Graf BK: Meniscal tears missed on MR imaging: Relationship to meniscal tear patterns and anterior cruciate ligament tears. AJR Am J Roentgenol 162:905, 1994.

36. De Smet AA, Ilahi OA, Graf BK: Reassessment of the MR criteria for stability of osteochondritis dissecans in the knee and ankle. Skeletal Radiol 25:159, 1996.

37. De Smet AA, Norris MA, Yandow DR, et al: MR diagnosis of meniscal tears of the knee: Importance of high signal in the meniscus that extends to the surface. AJR Am J Roentgenol 161:101, 1993.

38. Deutsch AL, Mink JH, Fox JM, et al: Peripheral meniscal tears: MR findings after conservative treatment or arthroscopic repair. Radiology 176:485, 1990.

39. Deutsch AL, Mink JH, Rosenfelt FP, et al: Incidental detection of hematopoietic hyperplasia on routine knee MR imaging. AJR Am J Roentgenol 152:333, 1989.

40. Dimond PM, Fadale PD, Hulstyn MJ, et al: A comparison of MRI findings in patients with acute and chronic ACL tears. Am J Knee Surg 11:153, 1998.

41. Dorsay TA, Helms CA: Bucket-handle meniscal tears of the knee: Sensitivity and specificity of MRI signs. Skeletal Radiol 32:266, 2003.

42. Elias DA, White LM, Fithian DC: Acute lateral patellar dislocation at MR imaging: Injury patterns of medial patellar soft-tissue restraints and osteochondral injuries of the inferomedial patella. Radiology 225:736, 2002.

43. El-Khoury GY, Wira RL, Berbaum KS, et al: MR imaging of patellar tendinitis. Radiology 184:849, 1992.

44. Encalada I, Richmond JC: Osteonecrosis after arthroscopic meniscectomy using radiofrequency. Arthroscopy 20:632, 2004.

45. Escobedo EM, Mills WJ, Hunter JC: The "reverse Segond" fracture: Association with a tear of the posterior cruciate ligament. AJR Am J Roentgenol 178:979, 2002.

46. Farley TE, Howell SM, Love KF, et al: Meniscal tears: MR and arthrographic findings after arthroscopic repair. Radiology 180:517, 1991.

47. Fischer SP, Fox JM, Del Pizzo W, et al: Accuracy of diagnosis from magnetic resonance imaging of the knee. A multi-center analysis of one thousand and fourteen patients. J Bone Joint Surg Am 73:2, 1991.

48. Forbes JR, Helms CA, Janzen DL: Acute pes anserine bursitis: MR imaging. Radiology 194:252, 1995.

49. Friedl W, Glaser F: Dynamic sonography in the diagnosis of ligament and meniscal injuries of the knee. Arch Orthop Trauma Surg 110:132, 1991.

50. Fujimoto E, Sumen Y, Deie M, et el: Anterior cruciate ligament graft impingement against the posterior cruciate ligament: Diagnosis using MRI plus three-dimensional reconstruction software. Magn Reson Imaging 22:1125, 2004.

51. Fukuta S, Masaki K, Korai F: Prevalence of abnormal findings in magnetic resonance images of asymptomatic knees. J Orthop Sci 7:287, 2002.

52. Garcia-Alvarez F, Garcia-Pequerul JM, Avila JL, et al: Ganglion cysts associated with cruciate ligaments of the knee: A possible cause of recurrent knee pain. Acta Orthop Belg 66:490, 2000.

53. Gebhard F, Authenrieth M, Strecker W, et al: Ultrasound evaluation of gravity induced anterior drawer following anterior cruciate ligament lesion. Knee Surg Sports Traumatol Arthrosc 7:166, 1999.

54. Gelb JH, Glasgow SG, Sapega AA, et al: Magnetic resonance imaging of knee disorders. Clinical value and cost-effectiveness in a sports medicine practice. Am J Sports Med 24:9, 1996.

55. Gentili A, Seeger LL, Yao L, et al: Anterior cruciate ligament tear: Indirect signs at MR imaging. Radiology 193:835, 1994.

56. Gold GE, Fuller SE, Hargreaves BA, et al: Driven equilibrium magnetic resonance imaging of articular cartilage: Initial clinical experience. J Magn Reson Imaging 21:476, 2005.

57. Goldman AB, Pavlov H, Rubenstein D: The Segond fracture of the proximal tibia: A small avulsion that reflects major ligamentous damage. AJR Am J Roentgenol 151:1163, 1988.

58. Graichen H, Al-Shamari D, Hinterwimmer S, et al: Accuracy of quantitative MRI in the detection of ex vivo focal cartilage defects. Ann Rheum Dis Epub Jan 7, 2005.

59. Hantes ME, Zachos VC, Zibis AH, et al: Evaluation of meniscal repair with serial magnetic resonance imaging: A comparative study between conventional MRI and indirect MR arthrography. Eur J Radiol 50:231, 2004.

60. Henderson IJ, Tuy B, Connell D, et al: Prospective clinical study of autologous chondrocyte implantation and correlation with MRI at three and 12 months. J Bone Joint Surg Br 85:1060, 2003.

61. Hinshaw MH, Tuite MJ, De Smet AA: "Dem bones": Osteochondral injuries of the knee. Magn Reson Imaging Clin North Am 8:335, 2000.

62. Hong SH, Choi JY, Lee GK, et al: Grading of anterior cruciate ligament injury. Diagnostic efficacy of oblique coronal magnetic resonance imaging of the knee. J Comput Assist Tomogr 27:814, 2003.

63. Horton KL, Jacobson JA, Lin J, et al: MR imaging of anterior cruciate ligament reconstruction graft. AJR Am J Roentgenol 175:1091, 2000.

64. Howell SM, Berns GS, Farley TE: Unimpinged and impinged anterior cruciate ligament grafts: MR signal intensity measurements. Radiology 179:639, 1991.

65. Huang GS, Chain-Her K, Chan WP, et al: Acute anterior cruciate ligament stump entrapment in anterior cruciate ligament tears: MR imaging appearance. Radiology 225:537, 2002.

66. Insall J, Salvati E: Patella position in the normal knee joint. Radiology 101:101, 1971.

67. Jacobson JA, Lenchik L, Ruhoy MK, et al: MR imaging of the infrapatellar fat pad of Hoffa. Radiographics 17:675, 1997.

68. Jansson KA, Harilainen A, Sandelin J, et al: Bone tunnel enlargement after anterior cruciate ligament reconstruction with the hamstring autograft and endobutton fixation technique. A clinical, radiographic and magnetic resonance imaging study with 2 years follow-up. Knee Surg Sports Traumatol Arthrosc 7:290, 1999.

69. Jee WH, McCauley TR, Kim JM: Magnetic resonance diagnosis of meniscal tears in patients with acute anterior cruciate ligament tears. J Comput Assist Tomogr 28:402, 2004.

70. Johnson DL, Urban WP Jr, Caborn DN, et al: Articular cartilage changes seen with magnetic resonance imaging–detected bone bruises associated with acute anterior cruciate ligament rupture. Am J Sports Med 26:409, 1998.

71. Johnson TC, Evans JA, Gilley JA, et al: Osteonecrosis of the knee after arthroscopic surgery for meniscal tears and chondral lesions. Arthroscopy 16:254, 2000.

72. Kaplan PA, Gehl RH, Dussault RG, et al: Bone contusions of the posterior lip of the medial tibial plateau (countrecoup injury) and associated internal derangements of the knee at MR imaging. Radiology 211:747, 1999.

73. Katahira K, Yamashita Y, Takahashi M, et al: MR imaging of the anterior cruciate ligament: Value of thin slice direct oblique coronal technique. Radiat Med 19:1, 2001.

74. Kent RH, Pope CF, Lynch JK, et al: Magnetic resonance imaging of the surgically repaired meniscus: Six-month follow-up. Magn Reson Imaging 9:335, 1991.

75. Khan KM, Bonar F, Desmond PM, et al: Patellar tendinosis (jumper's knee): Findings at histopathologic examination, US, and

MR imaging. Victorian Institute of Sports Tendon Study Group. Radiology 200:821, 1996.

76. Kidwai AS, Hemphill SD, Griffiths HJ: Radiologic case study: Spontaneous osteonecrosis of the knee reclassified as insufficiency fracture. Orthopedics 28:333, 2005.

77. Kim RS, Lee JY, Lee KY: Localized pigmented villonodular synovitis attached to the posterior cruciate ligament of the knee. Arthroscopy 19:e37, 2003.

78. Kim SJ, Shin SJ, Koo TY: Arch type pathologic suprapatellar plica. Arthroscopy 17:536, 2001.

79. Klingele KE, Kocher MS, Hresko MT, et al: Discoid lateral meniscus: Prevalence of peripheral rim instability. Pediatr Orthop 24:79, 2004.

80. Kocabey Y, Tetik O, Isbell WM, et al: The value of clinical examination versus magnetic resonance imaging in the diagnosis of meniscal tears and anterior cruciate ligament rupture. Arthroscopy 20:696, 2004.

81. Kornaat PR, Doornbos J, van der Molen AJ, et al: Magnetic resonance imaging of knee cartilage using a water selective balanced steady-state free precession sequence. J Magn Reson Imaging 20:850, 2004.

82. Koulalis D, Schultz W, Heyden M, et al: Autologous osteochondral grafts in the treatment of cartilage defects of the knee joint. Knee Surg Sports Traumatol Arthrosc 12:329, 2004.

83. Krudwig WK, Schulte KK, Heinemann C: Intra-articular ganglion cysts of the knee joint: A report of 85 cases and review of the literature. Knee Surg Sports Traumatol Arthrosc 12:123, 2004.

84. La S, Fessell DP, Femino JE, et al: Sonography of partial-thickness quadriceps tendon tears with surgical correlation. J Ultrasound Med 22:1323, 2003.

85. Lajtai G, Noszian I, Humer K, et al: Serial magnetic resonance imaging evaluation of operative site after fixation of patellar tendon graft with bioabsorbable interference screws in anterior cruciate ligament reconstruction. Arthroscopy 15:709, 1999.

86. La Prade RF, Gilbert TJ, Bollom TS, et al: The magnetic resonance imaging appearance of individual structures of the posterolateral knee. Am J Sports Med 28:191, 2000.

87. Lecouvet FE, Van de Berg BC, Maldague BE, et al: Early irreversible osteonecrosis versus transient lesions of the femoral condyles: Prognostic value of subchondral bone and marrow changes on MR imaging. AJR Am J Roentgenol 170:71, 1998.

88. Lee K, Siegel MJ, Lau DM, et al: Anterior cruciate ligament tears: MR imaging–based diagnosis in a pediatric population. Radiology 213:697, 1999.

89. Lee W, Kim HS, Kim SJ, et al: CT arthrography and virtual arthroscopy in the diagnosis of the anterior cruciate ligament and meniscal abnormalities of the knee joint. Korean J Radiol 5:47, 2004.

90. Leis HT, Sanders TG, Larsen KM, et al: Hamstring regrowth following harvesting for ACL reconstruction: The lizard tail phenomenon. J Knee Surg 16:159, 2003.

91. Lian OB, Engebretsen L, Bahr R: Prevalence of jumper's knee among elite athletes from different sports: A cross-sectional study. Am J Sports Med 33:561, 2005.

92. Lim PS, Schweitzer ME, Bhatia M, et al: Repeat tear of postoperative meniscus: Potential MR imaging signs. Radiology 210:183, 1999.

93. Magee T, Shapiro M, Rodriguez J, et al: MR arthrography of postoperative knee: For which patients is it useful? Radiology 229:159, 2003.

94. Magee T, Shapiro M, Williams D: Prevalence of meniscal radial tears of the knee revealed by MRI after surgery. AJR Am J Roentgenol 182:931, 2004.

95. Magee T, Shapiro M, Williams D: Usefulness of simultaneous acquisition of spatial harmonics technique for MRI of the knee. AJR Am J Roentgenol 182:1411, 2004.

96. Mair SD, Schlegel TF, Gill TJ, et al: Incidence and location of bone bruises after acute posterior cruciate ligament injury. Am J Sports Med 32:1681, 2004.

97. Major NM, Helms CA: MR imaging of the knee: Findings in asymptomatic collegiate basketball players. AJR Am J Roentgenol 179:641, 2002.

98. Mariani PP, Adriano E, Bellelli A, et al: Magnetic resonance imaging of tunnel placement in posterior cruciate ligament reconstruction. Arthroscopy 15:733, 1999.

99. Mariani PP, Margheritini F, Camillieri G, et al: Serial magnetic resonance imaging evaluation of the patellar tendon after posterior cruciate ligament reconstruction. Arthroscopy 18:38, 2002.

100. Marti-Bonmati L, Molla E, Dosda E, et al: MR imaging of Baker cysts—prevalence and relation to internal derangements of the knee. MAGMA 10:205, 2000.

101. May DA, Snearly WN, Bents R, et al: MR imaging findings in anterior cruciate ligament reconstruction: Evaluation of notchplasty. AJR Am J Roentgenol 169:217, 1997.

102. McCarthy CL, McNally EG: The MRI appearance of cystic lesions around the knee. Skeletal Radiol 33:187, 2004.

103. McCauley TR: MR imaging evaluation of the postoperative knee. Radiology 234:53, 2005.

104. McCauley TR, Elfar A, Moore A, et al: MR arthrography of anterior cruciate ligament reconstruction grafts. AJR Am J Roentgenol 181:1217, 2003.

105. McCauley TR, Kier R, Lynch KJ, et al: Chondromalacia patellae: Diagnosis with MR imaging. AJR Am J Roentgenol 158:101, 1992.

106. McIntyre J, Moelleken S, Tirman S: Mucoid degeneration of the anterior cruciate ligament mistaken for ligamentous tears. Skeletal Radiol 30:312, 2001.

107. Mellado JM, Calmet J, Olona M, et al: Magnetic resonance imaging of anterior cruciate ligament tears: Reevaluation of quantitative parameters and imaging findings including simplified method for measuring the anterior cruciate ligament angle. Knee Surg Sports Traumatol Arthrosc 12:217, 2004.

108. Miller TT, Gladden P, Staron RB, et al: Posterolateral stabilizers of the knee: Anatomy and injuries with MR imaging. AJR Am J Roentgenol 169:1641, 1997.

109. Miller TT, Staron RB, Feldman F: Patellar height on sagittal MR imaging of the knee. AJR Am J Roentgenol 167:339, 1996.

110. Miller TT, Staron RB, Koenigsberg T, et al: MR imaging of Baker cysts: Association with internal derangement, effusion, and degenerative arthropathy. Radiology 201:247, 1996.

111. Mitchell DG, Steinberg ME, Dalinka MK, et al: Magnetic resonance imaging of the ischemic hip. Alterations within osteonecrotic, viable, and reactive zones. Clin Orthop 244:60, 1989.

112. Modl JM, Sether LA, Haughton VM, et al: Articular cartilage: Correlation of histologic zones with signal intensity at MR imaging. Radiology 181:853, 1991.

113. Moosikasuwan JB, Miller TT, Math K, et al: Shifting bone marrow edema of the knee. Skeletal Radiol 33:380, 2004.

114. Mosher TJ, Dardzinski BJ: Cartilage MRI T2 relaxation time mapping: Overview and applications. Semin Musculoskel Radiol 8:355, 2004.

115. Mountney J, Thomas NP: When is a meniscal cyst not a meniscal cyst? Knee 11:133, 2004.

116. Muhle C, Ahn JM, Yeh L, et al: Iliotibial band friction syndrome: MR imaging findings in 16 patients and MR arthrographic study of six cadaveric knees. Radiology 212:103, 1999.

117. Munshi M, Davidson M, MacDonald PB, et al: The efficacy of magnetic resonance imaging in acute knee injuries. Clin J Sports Med 10:34, 2000.

118. Murao H, Morishita S, Nakajima M, et al: Magnetic resonance imaging of the anterior cruciate ligament (ACL) tears: Diagnostic value of ACL–tibial plateau angle. J Orthop Sci 3:10, 1998.

119. Murphy BJ, Hechtman KS, Uribe JW, et al: Iliotibial band friction syndrome: MR imaging findings. Radiology 185:569, 1992.

120. Mutschler C, Vande Berg BC, Lecouvet FE, et al: Postoperative meniscus: Assessment at dual–detector row spiral CT arthrography of the knee. Radiology 228:635, 2003.

121. Nakauchi M, Kurosawa H, Kawakami A: Abnormal lateral notch in knees with anterior cruciate ligament injury. J Orthop Sci 5:92, 2000.

122. Narvekar A, Gajjar S: Mucoid degeneration of the anterior cruciate ligament. Arthroscopy 20:141, 2004.

123. Noyes FR, Westin-Barber SD, Rankin M: Meniscal transplantation in symptomatic patients less than fifty years old. J Bone Joint Surg Am 86:1392, 2004.

124. Patten RM, Rolfe BA: MRI of meniscal allografts. J Comput Assist Tomogr 19:243, 1995.

125. Pope TL Jr: MR imaging of patellar dislocation and relocation. Semin Ultrasound CT MR 22:371, 2001.

126. Potter HG, Linklater JM, Allen AA, et al: Magnetic resonance imaging of articular cartilage in the knee. An evaluation with use of fast spin-echo imaging. J Bone Joint Surg Am 80:1276, 1998.
127. Potter HG, Rodeo SA, Wickiewicz TL, et al: MR imaging of meniscal allografts: Correlation with clinical and arthroscopic outcomes. Radiology 198:509, 1996.
128. Poulton TB, Murphy WD, Duerk JL, et al: Bone marrow reconversion in adults who are smokers: MR imaging findings. AJR Am J Roentgenol 161:1217, 1993.
129. Prues-Latour V, Bonvin JC, Fritschy D: Nine cases of osteonecrosis in elderly patients following arthroscopic meniscectomy. Knee Surg Sports Traumatol Arthrosc 6:142, 1998.
130. Ramnath RR, Kattapuram SV: MR appearance of SONK-like subchondral abnormalities in the adult knee: SONK redefined. Skeletal Radiol 33:575, 2004.
131. Recht M, White LM, Winalski CS, et al: MR imaging of cartilage repair procedures. Skeletal Radiol 32:185, 2003.
132. Recht MP, Applegate G, Kaplan P, et al: The MR appearance of cruciate ganglion cysts: A report of 16 cases. Skeletal Radiol 23:597, 1994.
133. Recht MP, Piraino DW, Cohen MA, et al: Localized anterior arthrofibrosis (Cyclops lesion) after reconstruction of the anterior cruciate ligament: MR imaging findings. AJR Am J Roentgenol 165:383, 1995.
134. Reeder JD, Matz SO, Becker L, et al: MR imaging of the knee in the sagittal projection: Comparison of three-dimensional gradient-echo and spin-echo sequences. AJR Am J Roentgenol 153:537, 1989.
135. Remer EM, Fitzgerald SW, Friedman H, et al: Anterior cruciate ligament injury: MR imaging diagnosis and patterns of injury. Radiographics 12:901, 1992.
136. Rispoli DM, Sanders TG, Miller MD, et al: Magnetic resonance imaging at different time periods following hamstring harvest for anterior cruciate ligament reconstruction. Arthroscopy 17:2, 2001.
137. Roberts D, Miller TT, Erlanger SM: Sonographic appearance of primary synovial chondromatosis of the knee. J Ultrasound Med 23:707, 2004.
138. Roberts S, McCall IW, Darby AJ, et al: Autologous chondrocyte implantation for cartilage repair: Monitoring its success by magnetic resonance imaging and histology. Arthritis Res Ther 5:R60, 2003.
139. Robertson PL, Schweitzer ME, Bartolozzi AR, et al: Anterior cruciate ligament tears: Evaluation of multiple signs with MR imaging. Radiology 193:829, 1994.
140. Rohren EM, Kosarek FJ, Helms CA: Discoid lateral meniscus and the frequency of meniscal tears. Skeletal Radiol 30:316, 2001.
141. Rose NE, Gold SM: A comparison of accuracy between clinical examination and magnetic resonance imaging in the diagnosis of meniscal and anterior cruciate ligament tears. Arthroscopy 12:398, 1996.
142. Rosenberg ZS, Kawelbaum M, Cheung YY, et al: Osgood-Schlatter lesion: Fracture or tendinitis? Scintigraphic, CT, and MR imaging features. Radiology 185:853, 1992.
143. Rothstein CP, Laorr A, Helms CA, et al: Semimembranosus–tibial collateral ligament bursitis: MR imaging findings. AJR Am J Roentgenol 166:875, 1996.
144. Ryu KN, Kim IS, Kim EJ, et al: MR imaging of tears of discoid lateral menisci. AJR Am J Roentgenol 171:963, 1998.
145. Saddik D, McNally EG, Richardson M: MRI of Hoffa's fat pad. Skeletal Radiol 33:433, 2004.
146. Sanders TG, Mentzer KD, Miller MD, et al: Autogenous osteochondral "plug" transfer for the treatment of focal chondral defects: Postoperative MR appearance with clinical correlation. Skeletal Radiol 30:570, 2001.
147. Schmid MR, Hodler J, Cathrein P, et al: Is impingement the cause of jumper's knee? Dynamic and static magnetic resonance imaging of patellar tendinitis in an open-configuration system. Am J Sports Med 30:388, 2002.
148. Schweitzer ME, Mitchell DG, Ehrlich SM: The patellar tendon: Thickening, internal signal, buckling, and other MR variants. Skeletal Radiol 22:411, 1993.
149. Schweitzer ME, Tran D, Deely DM, et al: Medial collateral ligament injuries: Evaluation of multiple signs, prevalence and location of associated bone bruises, and assessment with MR imaging. Radiology 194:825, 1995.
150. Sciulli RL, Boutin RD, Brown RR, et al: Evaluation of the postoperative meniscus of the knee: A study comparing conventional arthrography, conventional MR imaging, MR arthrography with iodinated contrast material, and MR arthrography with gadolinium-based contrast material. Skeletal Radiol 28:508, 1999.
151. Seymour R, Lloyd DC: Sonographic appearances of meniscal cysts. J Clin Ultrasound 26:15, 1998.
152. Shelbourne KD, Jennings RW, Vahey TN: Magnetic resonance imaging of posterior cruciate ligament injuries: Assessment of healing. Am J Knee Surg 12:209, 1999.
153. Shellock FG, Morris E, Deutsch AL, et al: Hematopoietic bone marrow hyperplasia: High prevalence on MR images of the knee in asymptomatic marathon runners. AJR Am J Roentgenol 158:335, 1992.
154. Sherman PM, Penrod BJ, Lane MJ, et al: Comparison of knee magnetic resonance imaging findings in patients referred by orthopaedic surgeons versus nonorthopaedic practitioners. Arthroscopy 18:201, 2002.
155. Silverman JM, Mink JH, Deutsch AL: Discoid menisci of the knee: MR imaging appearance. Radiology 173:351, 1989.
156. Singson RD, Feldman F, Staron R, et al: MR imaging of displaced bucket-handle tear of the medial meniscus. AJR Am J Roentgenol 156:121, 1991.
157. Snearly WN, Kaplan PA, Dussault RG: Lateral-compartment bone contusions in adolescents with intact anterior cruciate ligaments. Radiology 198:205, 1996.
158. Sonin AH, Fitzgerald SW, Hoff FL, et al: MR imaging of the posterior cruciate ligament: Normal, abnormal, and associated injury patterns. Radiographics 15:51, 1995.
159. Stark JE, Siegel MJ, Weinberger E, et al: Discoid menisci in children: MR features. J Comput Assist Tomogr 19:608, 1995.
160. Stockle U, Hoffmann R, Schwedke J, et al: Anterior cruciate ligament reconstruction: The diagnostic value of MRI. Int Orthop 22:288, 1998.
161. Stoller DW, Martin C, Crues JV, et al: Meniscal tears: Pathologic correlation with MR imaging. Radiology 163:731, 1987.
162. Svensson M, Kartus J, Ejerhed L, et al: Does the patellar tendon normalize after harvesting its central third? Am J Sports Med 32:34, 2004.
163. Tiderius CJ, Tjornstrand J, Akeson P, et al: Delayed gadolinium-enhanced MRI of cartilage (dGEMRIC): Intra- and interobserver variability in standardized drawing of regions of interest. Acta Radiol 45:628, 2004.
164. Tins BJ, McCall IW, Takahashi T, et al: Autologous chondrocyte implantation in knee joint: MR imaging and histologic features at 1-year follow-up. Radiology 234:501, 2005.
165. Tomczak RJ, Hehl G, Mergo PJ, et al: Tunnel placement in anterior cruciate ligament reconstruction: MRI analysis as an important factor in the radiological report. Skeletal Radiol 26:409, 1997.
166. Treishmann HW Jr, Mosure JC: The impact of magnetic resonance imaging of the knee on surgical decision making. Arthroscopy 12:550, 1996.
167. Tung GA, Davis LM, Wiggins ME, et al: Tears of the anterior cruciate ligament: Primary and secondary signs at MR imaging. Radiology 188:661, 1993.
168. Twaddle BC, Hunter JC, Chapman JR, et al: MRI in acute knee dislocation. J Bone Joint Surg Br 78:573, 1996.
169. Tyson LL, Daughters TC Jr, Ryu RK, et al: MRI appearance of meniscal cysts. Skeletal Radiol 24:421, 1995.
170. Umans H, Wimpfheimer O, Haramati N, et al: Diagnosis of partial tears of the anterior cruciate ligament of the knee: Value of MR imaging. AJR Am J Roentgenol 165:893, 1995.
171. Vahey TN, Broome DR, Kayes KJ, et al: Acute and chronic tears of the anterior cruciate ligament: Differential features at MR imaging. Radiology 181:251, 1991.
172. van Arkel ER, Goei R, de Ploeg I, et al: Meniscal allografts: Evaluation with magnetic resonance imaging and correlation with arthroscopy. Arthroscopy 16:517, 2000.
173. Vande Berg BC, Lecouvet FE, Poilvache P, et al: Dual-detector spiral CT arthrography of the knee: Accuracy for detection of meniscal abnormalities and unstable meniscal tears. Radiology 216:851, 2000.
174. Vande Berg BC, Lecouvet FE, Poilvache P, et al: Anterior cruciate ligament tears and associated meniscal lesions: Assessment at dual-detector spiral CT arthrography. Radiology 223:403, 2002.

175. Vellet AD, Marks PH, Fowler PJ, et al: Occult posttraumatic osteochondral lesions of the knee: Prevalence, classification, and short-term sequelae evaluated with MR imaging. Radiology 178:271, 1991.

176. Vives MJ, Homesley D, Ciccotti MG, et al: Evaluation of recurring meniscal tears with gadolinium-enhanced magnetic resonance imaging: A randomized, prospective study. Am J Sports Med 31:868, 2003.

177. Vogl TJ, Schmitt J, Lubrich J, et al: Reconstructed anterior cruciate ligaments using patellar tendon ligament grafts: Diagnostic value of contrast-enhanced MRI in a 2-year follow-up regimen. Eur Radiol 11:1450, 2001.

178. Wada Y, Watanabe A, Yamashita T, et al: Evaluation of articular cartilage with 3D-SPGR MRI after autologous chondrocyte implantation. J Orthop Sci 8:514, 2003.

179. Ward EE, Jacobson JA, Fassell DP, et al: Sonographic detection of Baker's cysts: Comparison with MR imaging. AJR Am J Roentgenol 176:373, 2001.

180. Warden WH, Friedman R, Teresi LM, et al: Magnetic resonance imaging of bioabsorbable polylactic acid interference screws during the first 2 years after anterior cruciate ligament reconstruction. Arthroscopy 15:474, 1999.

181. Weber WN, Neumann CH, Barakos JA, et al: Lateral tibial rim (Segond) fractures: MR imaging characteristics. Radiology 180:731, 1991.

182. Weiss KL, Morehouse HT, Levy IM: Sagittal MR images of the knee: A low-signal band parallel to the posterior cruciate ligament caused by a displaced bucket-handle tear. AJR Am J Roentgenol 156:117, 1991.

183. White LM, Schweitzer ME, Weishaupt D, et al: Diagnosis of recurrent meniscal tears: Prospective evaluation of conventional MR imaging, indirect MR arthrography, and direct MR arthrography. Radiology 222:421, 2002.

184. Wilson AJ, Hodge JC, Pilgram TK, et al: Prevalence of red marrow around the knee joint in adults demonstrated on magnetic resonance imaging. Acad Radiol 3:550, 1996.

185. Wirth CJ, Peters G, Milachowski KA, et al: Long-term results of meniscal allograft transplantation. Am J Sports Med 30:174, 2002.

186. Yamamoto T, Bullough PG: Spontaneous osteonecrosis of the knee: The result of subchondral insufficiency fracture. J Bone Joint Surg Am 82:858, 2000.

187. Yoshioka H, Stevens K, Hargreaves BA, et al: Magnetic resonance imaging of articular cartilage of the knee: Comparison between fat-suppressed three-dimensional SPGR imaging, fat-suppressed FSE imaging, and fat-suppressed three-dimensional DEFT imaging, and correlation with arthroscopy. J Magn Reson Imaging 20:857, 2004.

188. Yu JS, Salonen DC, Hodler J, et al: Posterolateral aspect of the knee: Improved MR imaging with a coronal oblique technique. Radiology 198:199, 1996.

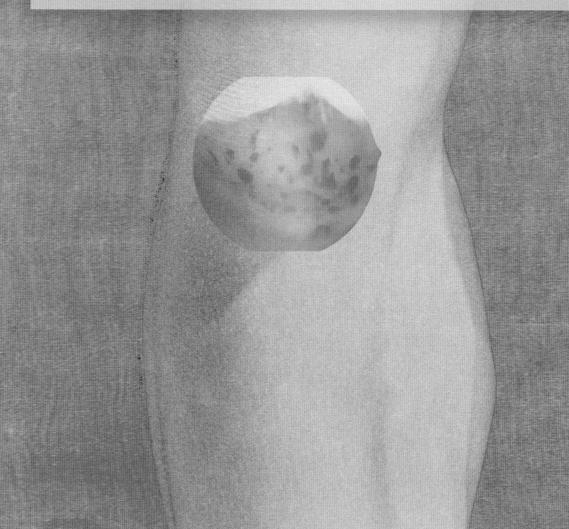

SECTION III

Biomechanics

CHAPTER 9

Motion and Stability of the Normal Knee

J. David Blaha and Edward Wojtys

Surgery on the knee is based on the presumption that the surgical procedure we choose will improve the patient's function. With the possible exception of a case in which tissue will be resected for tumor, operative interventions for repair or reconstruction are predicated on alteration of existing structures to improve the patient's ability to use the joint in tasks ranging from activities of daily living to high-level athletic competition. As a general principle, the closer the knee can be made to "normal," the better the patient's function will be. The literature is replete with complex mechanical and biomechanical descriptions of the motion of the human knee, often seeming to contradict one another. This chapter describes a simple model of tibiofemoral joint motion (excluding the patellofemoral joint) that can serve as a basis for understanding the function of the knee.

RANGE OF MOTION OF THE KNEE

Knee motion occurs in 6 degrees of freedom (Fig. 9–1). Three rotations and three translations can occur, with all motion limited by the fact that the tibia and the femur cannot occupy the same space at the same time. For the sake of explanation, if one considers the femur as fixed and the tibia as moving relative to the femur, the clinically apparent rotations are flexion-extension, internal-external rotation and abduction-adduction (also known as varus-valgus motion). Again, considering the femur fixed and the tibia moving relative to the femur, the tibia can translate medial-lateral, anterior-posterior, and distal-proximal.

The conformity of the articular surfaces of the femur and tibia in concert with the soft tissues around the knee constrains motion so that the knee has limits beyond which it cannot move. The limits define both the range of motion and stability of the normal knee. Evaluations of the knee in the laboratory with cadaveric specimens, in controlled laboratory environments with living subjects, and in clinical practice are used to define "normal" ranges of motion. In essentially all evaluations the knee moves easily in the midrange, becomes less compliant as the extreme is approached, and finally cannot be forced further without failure of some anatomic element. Establishment of the extremes of motion, either actively or passively, is one way to define normal. Yet another measure of normal is determination of the range of motion necessary for a given activity. Still another is to define the path taken by the tibia and femur relative to one another during knee motion.

KINEMATICS OF THE KNEE

Techniques for accurately measuring small displacements and accelerations have been greatly improved with advances in technology and use of computers to process large amounts of data. These techniques have been applied to the human knee to establish the path taken by one bone in relation to the other as the knee moves. Measurement of this relative motion of the tibia to the femur establishes the "kinematics" of the knee.

When presenting data from kinematic experiments, usually one of the bodies is considered fixed and establishes the frame of reference (i.e., the coordinate system) that allows motion of the other body to be characterized (Fig. 9–2). The motion of a moving body can be expressed as Euler angles with a sequence of translations and rotations about three orthogonal axes giving 6 degrees of freedom. Alternatively, the motion can be represented by a single axis along which and around which the moving body travels in progressing from a first point to a second. The single axis is the *helical axis* or the *screw axis*. (If a curve representing every position of the moving object can be drawn, the axis at every instant—the *instantaneous axis*—can be calculated. If only discrete points are known, the axis calculated is a *finite axis*.) Since the axis is the point around which a body is moving, it represents the *line of zero velocity*. If the problem is considered in two dimensions, the point where the axis pierces the plane is the *point of zero velocity*, or the *center of rotation*. While both eularian values (rotation and translation) and the helical axis have been used to define knee motion, the model presented here is better understood with the latter.

Kinematic Terms: Roll, Spin, Countertranslation, and Concordant Translation

Many terms have been used to describe the kinematics of knee motion. Terms such as slip, slide, translate, glide, and others are used in the literature, but kinematically the terms are ambiguous enough that further specific terms are necessary. Five terms that can be applied to any knee

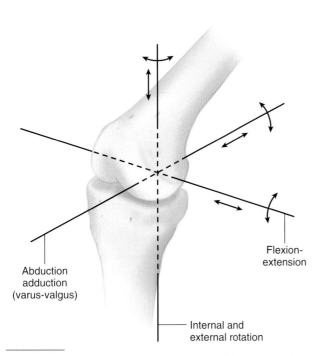

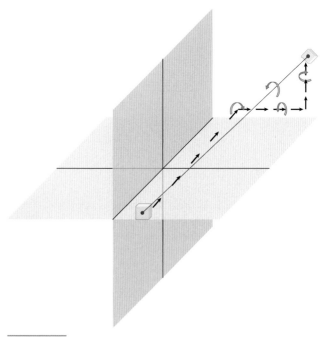

Figure 9–1. The knee has six degrees of freedom—three rotations and three translations about the three orthogonal axes. As the coordinate system is shown, the axes cross in the middle of the medial condyle. For the sake of explanation, if one considers the femur fixed and the tibia as moving relative to the femur, the clinically apparent rotations are flexion-extension, internal-external rotation, and abduction-adduction (also known as varus-valgus motion). Again, considering the femur fixed and the tibia moving relative to the femur, the tibia can translate medial-lateral, anterior-posterior, and distal-proximal.

Figure 9–2. Instead of three rotations and three translations, motion can be characterized as a single axis around which and along which an object moves in getting from a starting position to an ending position. The single axis is the *helical* axis or the *screw* axis. In considering rotation, the axis represents the *line of zero velocity.*

motion (normal or pathologic) can be defined relative to a simplified "disk on a flat surface" model. The terms are presented here first in two dimensions and then in three dimensions and are based on the point of zero velocity (2-D, center of rotation) or a line of zero velocity (3-D, axis of rotation).

Consider first the two-dimensional situation of a disk in contact with a surface (Fig. 9–3A). If the disk turns with the center of rotation at the contact point between the disk and the surface, the kinematic condition is called *rolling.* The disk progresses across the surface for a distance equal to its circumference through as many degrees as the disk turned.

Consider the same disk in contact with the same surface, again turning but in this condition the center of rotation is at the center of the disk (Fig. 9–3B). The condition is called *spinning.* The disk does not progress across the surface but rather stays in the same relative position.

If the center of rotation of the disk falls between its center and its surface, some combination of rolling and spinning occurs (Fig. 9–3C). This condition has been described in the literature with the term "slip ratio" to denote the amount of progression of the disk across the surface relative to the amount that would take place in pure rolling.[29] In these definitions the term would be "spin-roll" ratio. Note that in this case the direction of pro-

gression is always the same as would have taken place with pure rolling.

The center of rotation may fall outside the zone of spinning and rolling. If the center falls above the center of the disk, the contact point will move in one direction while the disk turns in the other. This motion is termed *countertranslation* (Fig. 9–3D). Finally, the center of rotation may fall below the contact point. In this case the contact point will move in the same direction as the turning of the disk. This motion is termed *concordant translation* (Fig. 9–3E). The further the point of zero velocity is away from the center of the disk, the greater will be the progression across the surface for an angular change. When the zero point is located at the extreme, the motion is pure translation.

To begin to apply these concepts to the knee, consider two disks separated but firmly held together with an axle (Fig. 9–4A). (It is generally agreed that the medial condyle is bigger than the lateral condyle, so this model uses one disk larger than the other.) It is possible for both disks to spin, roll, or translate identically, or one disk can exhibit one type of motion and the other a different type of motion. If, for example, one disk is spinning while the other is rolling, the center of rotation will be at the center for the spinning disk and at the contact point for the rolling disk (Fig. 9–4B). The screw axis will pass through the centers of rotation (Fig. 9–4C). The motion will be progression of the rolling disk across the surface while the spinning disk stays in the same place, and the combined disks will appear to turn on the surface (Fig. 9–4D). The turning motion is fully characterized by the screw axis that passes through the center of rotation of each disk.

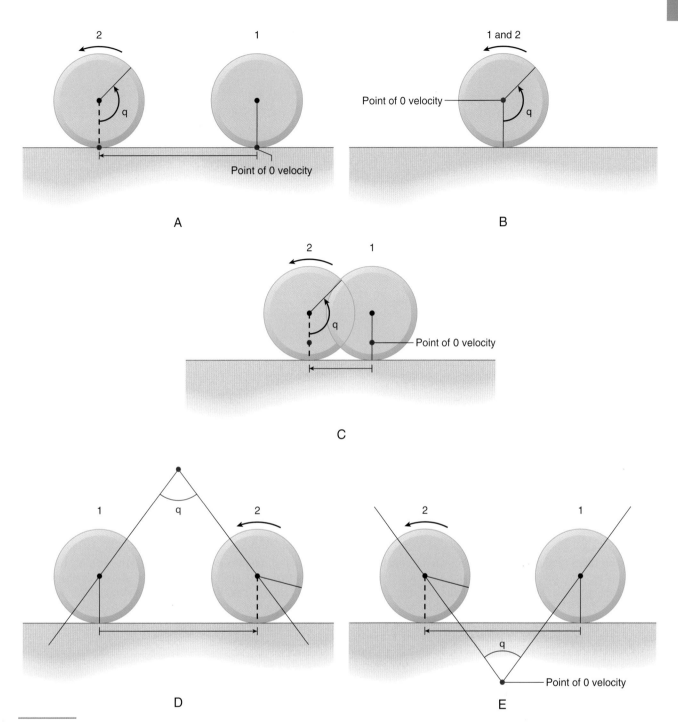

Figure 9–3. Nonambiguous kinematic terms, *roll, spin, combined roll-spin, concordant translation,* and *countertranslation,* can be defined by considering a disk on a flat surface. **A,** Roll. The disk turns such that the point of zero velocity is at the contact point between the disk and the surface as the disk turns through an angle θ°. The disk progresses across the surface for a distance equal to its circumference through θ°. **B,** Spin. The disk turns such that the point of zero velocity is at the center of the disk as the disk turns through an angle of θ°. In this case, the disk does not progress across the surface. **C,** Combined roll and spin. The disk turns such that the point of zero velocity is between the contact point and the center of the disk as the disk turns through an angle of θ°. The disk progresses across the surface less than it would have in pure rolling as a function of the ratio of spinning to rolling. This equivalent to what has been termed the "slip-ratio." **D,** Countertranslation. The disk turns such that the point of zero velocity is above the disk as the disk moves through an angle of θ°. The turning of the disk is in one direction while the disk moves across the surface in the opposite direction. The further the point of zero velocity is above the center of the disk, the greater will be the countertranslation. **E,** Concordant translation. The disk turns such that the point of zero velocity is below the contact point of the disk on the surface while the disk moves through an angle of θ°. The turning of the disk is in the same direction as the translation. The further the point of zero velocity is below the contact surface, the greater will be the concordant translation.

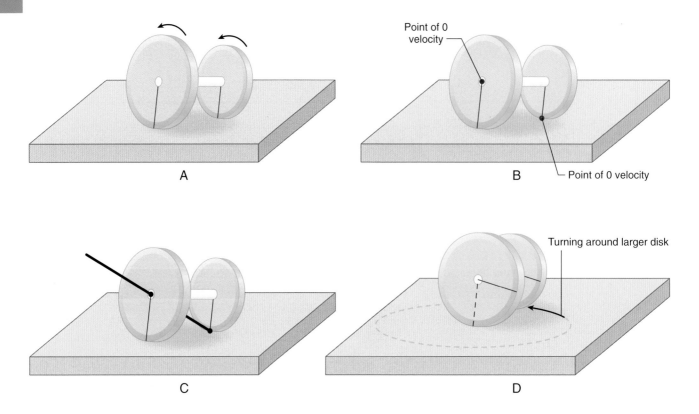

Figure 9–4. The knee can be modeled as two disks, with the medial disk being larger than the lateral. If the axis of rotation is calculated for a given motion, the place that it pierces each disk will define the motion of that disk. **A,** The model of two disks sits on the surface. **B,** The disks turn in such a way that the point of zero velocity is at the center of the larger disk and at the contact point between the smaller disk and the surface. The larger disk will spin, the smaller will roll. **C,** The points of zero velocity for the disks lie on the helical axis. Thus, if the helical axis is known, the motion of the object is fully characterized. **D,** In this case, the larger disk stays in the same place on the surface while the smaller progresses across the surface. The object turns on the surface.

As a simplified model the human knee can be considered as two disks (the medial and lateral condyles) that are connected (through the intercondylar region of the femur).[5,10,17,21,27,28,31,40] Motions of the tibia around the femur can be calculated as a screw axis, and these can be related to the centers of the condyles to determine the individual kinematics of the medial and lateral sides of the joint. Under experimental conditions simulating an "open-chain" exercise on cadaver knees, the kinematics of the medial and lateral sides of the knee are markedly different.[1,20]

The helical axis calculated in the open-chain model stays close to the center of the medial condyle throughout flexion-extension motion. Thus, the medial side moves through the majority of the range in largely spinning kinematics. That is, the center of the femur stays in very nearly the same place relative to the femur. The helical axis calculated in the open-chain model on the lateral side is more variable and pierces the condyle in different locations, sometimes at the contact point, the center, in between, above the center, and below the contact point. Thus, the lateral side of the joint is markedly more variable and demonstrates countertranslation, spinning, rolling, and concordant translation (Fig. 9–5A-F).

The kinematics in this open-chain model has been found in multiple studies of the knee in both cadaver specimens and in vivo experiments.[4,7,8,11,13,16,25,35] Although

details and magnitudes differ among the studies reported, the picture that emerges is one that shows asymmetry of the kinematics of the medial and lateral sides, with the femoral condyle on the medial side having much less anterior-posterior change in position than on the lateral side.

THE CLASSIC MODEL OF KNEE KINEMATICS: THE CROSSED FOUR-BAR LINK

The findings of a relatively stable medial side and a more mobile lateral side call into question the more traditional model of knee joint motion known as the "four-bar link" model or, more correctly, the "crossed four-bar link" model.

The four-bar link model was probably first introduced near the beginning of the 20th century (Fig. 9–6A and B).[6,29,47] As was initially proposed, in the four-bar link model the cruciate ligaments are presumed to be tense at all times and to act as ropes or checkreins linking the femur and tibia. If the theoretic motion of the tibia around the femur under the conditions of the classic four-bar link is plotted, a path of motion for the joint is produced that shows the femur moving progressively backward on the

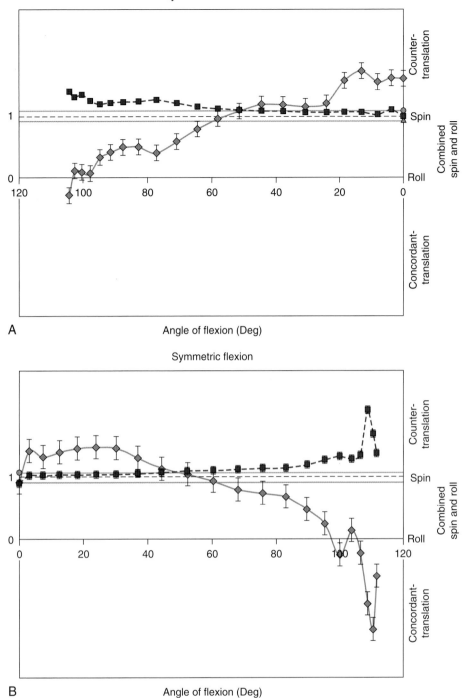

Symmetric extension

A   Angle of flexion (Deg)

Symmetric flexion

B   Angle of flexion (Deg)

Figure 9–5. Cadaveric human knees were moved in an open-chain model using physiologic extension loads through the quadriceps tendon and variable hamstring loads. Using video-motion analysis equipment, the position of the tibia as it moved about the fixed femur was determined and the helical axis was calculated. That axis was related to a CT scan of the specimen. The piercing point of the axis was determined for the mid-sagittal outline of the medial and lateral condyles, which were prepared as the circle representing the bony outline of the condyle. The position of the piercing point relative to the center of the circle and contact point was used to calculate β. The calculated β for each condyle at various angles of flexion in the extending knee and the flexing knee with symmetric and asymmetric hamstring loads is plotted as the mean value with standard error for seven specimens. The band encompassing the β value of 1 represents the 95% confidence interval. Each curve represents the data from seven knees, each of which had two trials. Therefore, 14 data points combine for each point (with the standard error) on each curve. There is some variation in the graphs of the β value based on the direction of motion (flexion or extension) and the type of hamstring loading. However, the results are remarkably similar and show the spinning kinematics on the medial side contrasted to the lateral side, which shows elements of rolling, spinning, combined spinning and rolling, countertranslation, and concordant translation. **A,** For the extending knee with symmetric hamstring loads, the medial side starts with slight countertranslation that moves to spinning by 60°. The lateral side starts in concordant translation, progresses to spinning by 60°, and then to countertranslation. **B,** For the symmetrically loaded flexing knee, the data show qualitatively the same motion as the extending knee except for some spikes of translation at full flexion. The spikes are probably artifact from the sudden deceleration of the knee at full flexion.

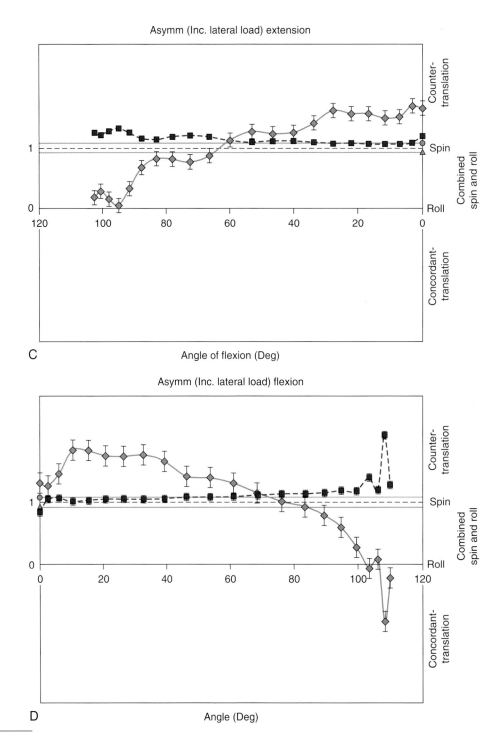

Figure 9–5, cont'd. **C,** With lateral asymmetric load in the extending trials, the kinematics of the medial side are nearly the same countertranslation then spinning motion as in the symmetric loading case. The lateral side also behaves very much like the symmetrically loaded case, starting with concordant translation, progressing to spinning, and then to countertranslation. **D,** With lateral asymmetric load in the flexing trials, again the kinematics of each side show qualitatively the same motion as the extending case. Again, the spikes of translation at full flexion are artifact from the rapid deceleration of the knees at full flexion.

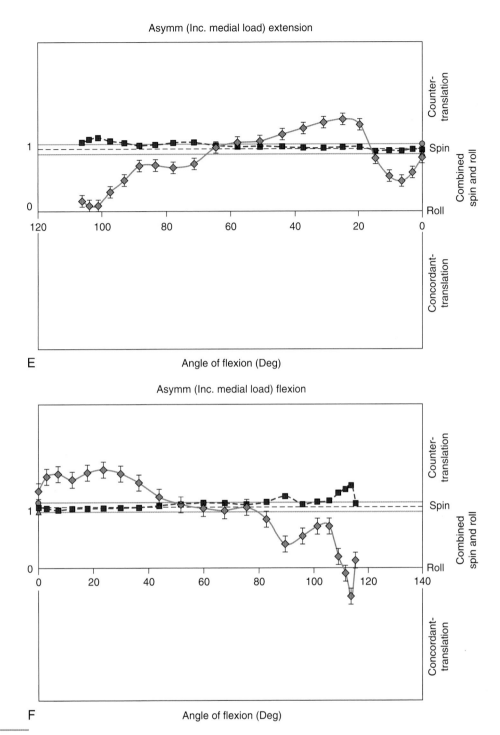

Figure 9–5, cont'd. **E,** With medial asymmetric load in the extending trials, the graphs for each condyle's motion are qualitatively the same but there is less deviation from the β = 1 (spinning) value. **F,** With medial asymmetric load, the flexing trials show marked similarity to the extending trials and again show the translation spikes, although considerably damped compared with the other conditions. (From Blaha JD, Mancinelli CA, Simons WH, et al: Kinematics of the human knee using an open chain cadaver model. Clin Orthop 410:25-32, 2003.)

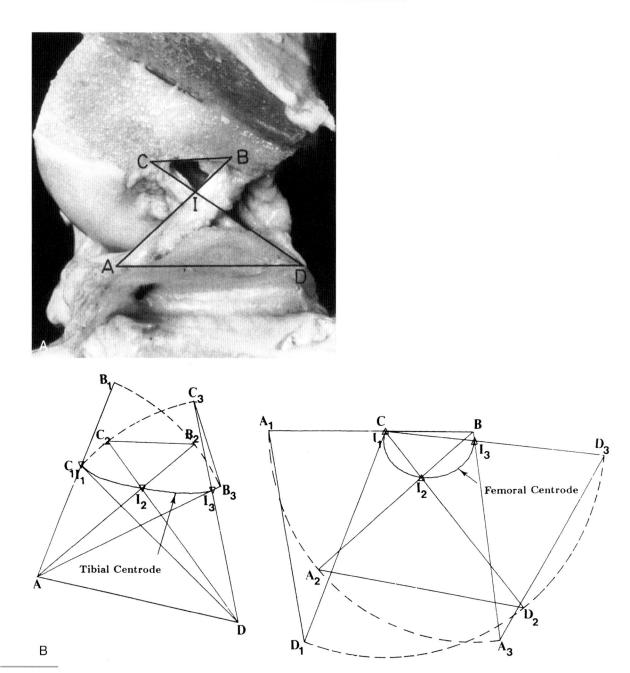

Figure 9–6. The classic description of the crossed four-bar link model demonstrates the anatomic location of the links and the proposed kinematics based on rigid elements. **A,** The elements of the four-bar link are the femur (CB), the tibia (AD), the anterior cruciate ligament (AB), and the posterior cruciate ligament (CD). **B,** If all of the elements remain rigid (i.e., inelastic and always under equal tension), then the point of zero velocity must always be at the crossing point of the cruciate ligaments. Since the crossing point is anterior in extension and posterior in flexion this model predicts that there will be posterior movement of the femur in the tibia with flexion and the reverse with extension. (From Pedowitz RA, O'Connor JJ, Akeson WH (eds): *In* Daniels: Knee Injuries, 2nd ed. Philadelphia, Lippincott-Williams & Wilkins, 2003, pp 67-68.)

tibia with increasing flexion. This backward motion with flexion has been called *rollback*. (The term is certainly a misnomer. Although the four-bar link model predicts backward motion with flexion, it is most certainly not rolling. Nonetheless, the term is ubiquitous in the orthopedic literature.) Using the terminology proposed earlier, the motion is combined spin and roll.

The four-bar link model exhibits its motion characteristics because of two critical elements of its structure. The

links must all be rigid and two of the elements must cross. The mechanics of the four-bar link is such that the point of zero velocity is always at the intersection point of the two crossed segments. If all the elements of the model were rigid, both condyles should move backward with flexion (i.e., roll back) equally.

The model has been modified to add elasticity to the ligaments and to add differing bundles to the ligaments based on anatomic dissections with differing mechanical properties of the ligament bundles and their attachments to the femur and tibia.[29,30] These changes in the model have yielded motion characteristics much closer to those observed in cadaver and living subject experiments with asymmetry between the medial and lateral sides of the knee. As the models are refined, it is clear that the initial idea of the cruciate ligaments acting as ropes to guide motion has been replaced with more complicated models that divide the ligaments into separate elements and integrate their function with the shape of the articular surfaces.

ROLE OF THE CRUCIATE LIGAMENTS

Most studies of the cruciate ligaments can be classified into three broad categories (Fig. 9–7A and B). The first category is "rupture" studies.[26,39,45] In this type of experiment the ultimate force required to cause failure of the ligament at various angles of knee flexion and various loading rates is determined. The second category is "knee compliance" studies.[22,30] At various degrees of knee flexion with various loading, the tibia or the femur is translated

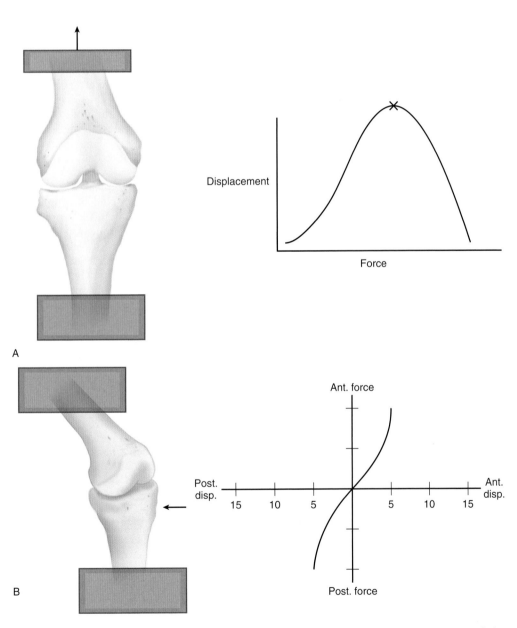

Figure 9–7. Mechanical studies of the cruciate ligaments can be categorized into two main groups: failure studies and compliance studies. **A,** Failure studies apply load to a ligament until it fails. The angle of the joint, loading rate, and other experimental conditions have given a good picture of the mechanical properties of the cruciate ligaments. **B,** Compliance studies generally fix one of the bones of the knee (either femur or tibia) and move the other in various combinations of the 6 degrees of freedom of the joint. The angle of the joint, loading rate, and other experimental conditions have given a good picture of the contributions of various structures to the stability of the knee. The force displacement curves generated show a relatively compliant joint in mid-range and an increasingly noncompliant joint at the extremes.

and/or angulated to measure force versus displacement. By sectioning either the anterior or the posterior cruciate ligament, or both, the contribution of each ligament to knee compliance is calculated. The third category is ultrastructural or neurophysiologic studies.[9,14,15,33,37,38]

Taken as a whole, these studies suggest that the cruciate ligaments cannot be functioning in the classic four-bar link model because they are not entirely rigid, and thus it is appropriate that the more recent modifications of that model have been introduced. In the studies of ultimate strength and in the compliance studies, some translation and/or angulation (within the elasticity of the ligament) is demonstrated before the ligaments prevent further motion, and thus no part of either ligament is actually rigid unless some displacement is induced. The amount of displacement allowed by the ligament compliance exceeds that demonstrated in the normal human knee during activity. At the extreme of motion, stiffness (rigidity) increases rapidly, and clearly the ligaments can be ruptured by the application of further force. Ultrastructural studies have demonstrated that there are distinct bundles of fibers in the ligaments and that there are mechanoreceptors in the ligaments. Taken together, these findings suggest that there is a dual function for the cruciate ligaments.

The cruciate ligaments are first "strain gauges" used as input for control of the limb. The external loads caused by activity tend to perturb the relative position of the femur and tibia; the cruciate ligaments provide a measure of that perturbation so that muscular contraction can stiffen the joint and restrain the relative motion of the femur and tibia within an acceptable range. Only at the extreme do they function as a "checkrein" to fully limit motion.   Anterior cruciate ligament grafts return the checkrein function of the ligament but probably do not restore the sensory function, and this has led to the suggestion that degeneration of the knee can occur despite an apparently well-functioning graft (to clinical examination) because of neuromuscular instability.[3,12,18,24,34,36,41,42,44]

A MODEL OF KNEE KINEMATICS WITH THREE ENVELOPES OF MOTION

Knee joint motion is clearly asymmetric when considering the medial and lateral compartments. That is, the medial and lateral sides behave kinematically differently.[1,4,7,8,11,13,16,20,25,35] The medial side of the joint behaves overall like a ball in a shallow socket (Fig. 9–8A). Without perturbation, the medial condyle stays in nearly the same position relative to the tibia throughout motion (as in the open-chain model experiment). There is some posterior movement of the contact point of the femur on the tibia that can be explained at least in part by the shape of the medial femoral condyle. There are two radii to the medial condyle, with the distal radius (the extension radius) frequently being larger than the more posterior radius (termed the flexion radius).[2,11,34,43] The extension radius is, however, markedly variable, with some specimens demonstrating a nearly flat surface in the sagittal plane (i.e., a large radius) and others having a radius the same

as the flexion radius (i.e., a single radius to the condyle).[2] When there is a significant difference in the radii, motion of the joint shows a change in contact position of the medial femur with the tibia as the joint is flexed. This "rocking" type of motion can give the appearance that the condyle is moving backward when in fact it simply moved from one part of the medial condyle to the other. After the flexion radius contacts the tibia, the femur stays reasonably steady with little further progression in the posterior direction.

The anatomy of the medial side of the tibia is consistent with this kinematic model.[19] The overall shape of the tibia is concave, with the depth of the concavity being roughly in the center of the plateau. The medial meniscus is firmly applied to the tibia and deepens the concavity. The medial collateral ligament is stout and holds the medial condyle in the concavity of the medial tibial plateau. With valgus stress there is limited opening of the medial side throughout the range of motion.

The lateral joint behaves like two disks (Fig. 9–8B). The femur is free to move into an anterior or posterior position while the tibia rotates around the center of the concavity on the medial side. Left to itself with no external perturbation, the tibia internally rotates with knee flexion, and this action moves the contact point to the posterior part of the tibia. This has been termed "lateral rollback," but because of the specific meaning in the context of the four-bar link that should be applied to the term rollback, it has led to confusion in interpreting knee kinematics.

The anatomy of the lateral side of the tibia is consistent with this kinematic model.[19] The overall shape of the tibia is convex with no central concavity. The meniscus is more loosely applied and can translate front to back to accommodate the position of the femur on the tibia. The lateral collateral ligament is a much less substantial structure than is the medial collateral ligament. Lateral stability is enhanced by the iliotibial band and the popliteus muscle, which individually and combined provide muscular restraint to opening of the lateral side of the joint but allow considerably more laxity (as demonstrated by the opening of the joint in the "figure 4" position) than the medial.

This model, which seems to encompass most of the available experimental data, is one that has three "envelopes" of motion at the knee (Fig. 9–9). The most central envelope is that motion demonstrated in the open-chain cadaver kinematic model in which no external forces are applied. This motion is characterized as medial ball-in-socket and lateral two-disk motion as described earlier. The second envelope of motion is a neuromuscular control range. In this range external loads perturb the open-chain kinematics and the ligaments provide input to the musculature to restrain motion to an acceptable amount. The final envelope is at the extreme of perturbation when the ligaments must act as the restraint to further motion. This range is a "danger zone" because further displacement can lead to ligament rupture.

The knee is like a universal joint connecting the upper (thigh) and lower (leg and foot) part of the lower extremity. A universal joint is "a shaft coupling capable of transmitting rotation from one shaft to another not coliner with

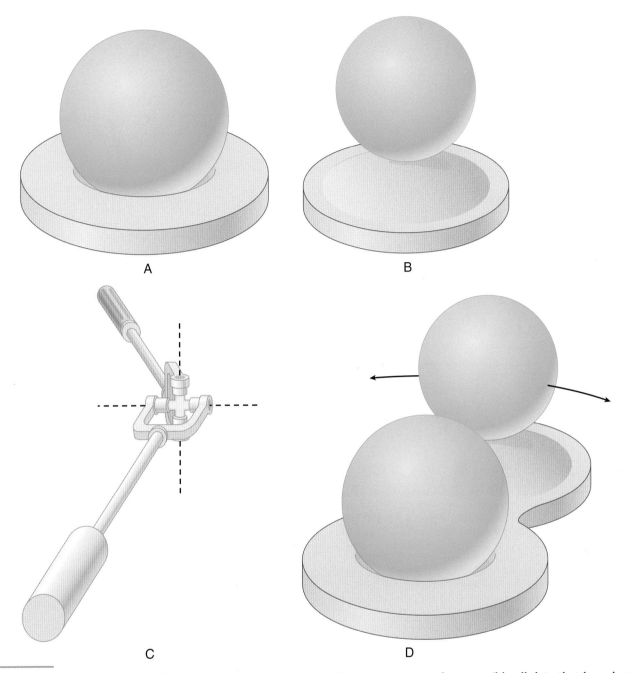

Figure 9–8. This proposed model of the knee joint attempts to incorporate as much as possible all data that have been generated about the kinematics of the human knee joint. **A,** The medial side of the joint acts like a ball in a shallow socket. Under most conditions, the condyle remains at or near the center of the concavity on the top of the tibia. **B,** The lateral side of the joint acts like two disks. The two disks can contact anteriorly on the tibia (tibial external rotation) or posteriorly (tibial internal rotation) to accommodate the function of the limb. **C,** Taken together, the joint is like a universal joint. A universal joint can transmit torque in multiple positions. **D,** The medial side of the knee remains stable while the lateral side rotates around it to accommodate the rotational position required for a given function. The positioning occurs in the mid-section of the compliance curves of the knee where there is the least stability provided by the cruciate ligaments. External forces can disturb the stability afforded by the articular surfaces and menisci and can displace the medial side out of its concavity. The cruciate ligaments are then in perfect position to serve as "strain gauges" to act as input for neuromuscular control that can set muscle tone and provide stability.

it"[23] (Fig. 9–8C). By remaining stable in ball-in-shallow-socket motion on the medial side, a large area for carriage of compressive load is maintained. The two disks' motion on the lateral side permits the knee joint to rotate to a limited degree in internal and external rotation to allow the foot and ankle to find a firm position (Fig. 9–8D and E). The quadriceps can then contract against a stable knee to accelerate the body.

The knee has an added safety factor, however, to prevent the damage that might result from being too rigid. Because

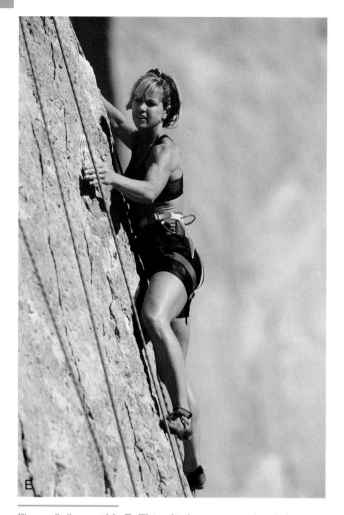

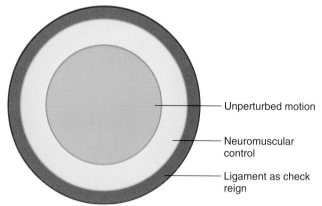

Unperturbed motion

Neuromuscular control

Ligament as check reign

Figure 9–9. There are three "envelopes of motion" for the knee. As diagrammed here the most central envelope represents medial ball-in-socket and lateral two-disk kinematics. If the knee is moved in the open-chain model, the motion will remain in this envelope. With the application of external forces, the knee can move in the next envelope, which represents neuromuscular control. The two sides of the joint can, within limits, spin, roll, or translate (in countertranslation or concordant translation) to accommodate the motion of the limb, but the envelope is limited by neuromuscular control, with the cruciate ligaments acting as an important part of the control mechanism. At the limit of the neuromuscular control envelope, the cruciate ligaments become checkreins to limit further motion. At this range, further application of load can lead to rupture of the ligaments. Patients sense the most central envelope as a normal knee and the next as a knee that requires muscular effort to maintain a feeling of stability. The final envelope is sensed as a knee that is at risk and is actively avoided.

Figure 9–8., cont'd. **E,** This climber is using her left lower extremity to ascend the rock face. She has flexed and fully externally rotated the knee to allow her foot to find a crevasse in the rock. Activation of her quadriceps will extend her knee, using it as a universal joint to transmit the torque necessary to push her up the wall. The cruciates, acting as strain gauges, will help maintain the tone around the knee to maintain acceptable kinematics.

the socket is shallow, the medial condyle can translate out of the concavity for a limited distance. If it were not able to do so because of the rigidity of the ligaments, those ligaments would be in danger of rupture from any external force that translated the femur and tibia. When functioning within the design specifications the joint remains stable. If pushed beyond the specifications, limited slipping is possible. With immediate feedback from the cruciate ligaments, the neuromuscular system is capable of altering load to within the specified limits.

SUMMARY

Operative intervention on the knee is done to return a patient to the highest level of function possible. It is reasonable to assume that the closer the knee is to "normal," the better the functional result will be. Thus, it is imper-

ative to consider the motion and stability of the normal knee when designing and performing knee surgery. The four-bar link has long been the model of knee joint kinematics and stability. Recent kinematic studies have confirmed information that was published in the 1800s. A model of knee kinematics that has three envelopes of motion explains more of the experimental data derived from kinematic and stability studies of the knee. In this model the cruciate ligaments are first displacement transducers that provide input to the neuromuscular control system. Only in the extreme are they "checkreins" that directly constrain motion.

References

1. Blaha JD, Mancinelli CA, Simons WH, et al: Kinematics of the human knee using an open chain cadaver model. Clin Orthop 410:25, 2003.
2. Blaha JD, Mancinelli CA, Simons WH: Using the transepicondylar axis to define the sagittal morphology of the distal part of the femur. J Bone Joint Surg [Am] 84(Suppl 2):48, 2002.
3. Dye SF, Wojtys EM, Fu FH, et al: Factors contributing to function of the knee joint after injury or reconstruction of the anterior cruciate ligament. J Bone Joint Surg [Am] 80:1380, 1998.
4. Dye SF: An evolutionary perspective of the knee. J Bone Joint Surg [Am] 69:976, 1987.
5. Elias SG, Freeman MA, Gokcay EI: A correlative study of the geometry and the anatomy of the distal femur. Clin Orthop 260:98, 1990.

6. Goodfellow J, O'Connor J: The mechanics of the knee and prosthesis design. J Bone Joint Surg [Br] 60:358, 1978.

7. Hefzy MS, Kelly BP, Cooke TD, et al: Knee kinematics in-vivo of kneeling in deep flexion examined by bi-planar radiographs. Biomed Sci In strum 33:453, 1997.

8. Hill PF, Vedi V, Williams A, et al: Tibiofemoral movement 2: The loaded and unloaded living knee studied by MRI. J Bone Joint Surg [Br] 82:1196, 2001.

9. Hogervorst T, Brand RA: Joint mechanoreceptors and knee function. In Pedowitz RA, O'Connor JJ, Akeson WH (eds): Daniel's Knee Injuries. Philadelphia, Lippincott Williams and Wilkins, 2003, pp 127-148.

10. Hollister AM, Jatana S, Singh A, et al: The axes of rotation of the knee. Clin Orthop 290:259, 1993.

11. Iwaki H, Pinskerova V, Freeman, MA: Tibiofemoral movement 1: The shapes and relative movements of the femur and tibia in the unloaded cadaver knee. J Bone Joint Surg [Br] 82:1189, 2001.

12. Jomha NM, Pinczewski LA, Clingeleffer A, et al: Arthroscopic reconstruction of the anterior cruciate ligament with patellar-tendon autograft and interference screw fixation. The results at seven years. J Bone Joint Surg [Br] 81:775, 1999.

13. Karrholm J, Brandsson S, Freeman MA: Tibiofemoral movement 4: Changes in axial rotation caused by forced rotation of the weight bearing knee studied by RSA. J Bone Joint Surg [Br] 82:1201, 2000.

14. Kennedy JC, Alexander IJ, Hayes KC: Nerve supply of the human knee and its functional importance. Am J Sports Med 10:329, 1982.

15. Kennedy JC, Weinberg HW, Wilson AS: The anatomy and functions of the anterior cruciate ligament. J Bone Joint Surg [Am] 56:223, 1974.

16. Komistek RD, Denis DA, Mahfouz M: In vivo fluoroscopic analysis of the normal human knee. Clin Orthop 410:69, 2003.

17. Kurosawa H, Walker P, Abe S, Hunter T: Geometry and motion of the knee for implant for implant and orthotic design. J Biomech 18:487, 1985.

18. Larsen E, Jensen PK, Jensen PR: Long-term outcome of knee and ankle injuries in elite football. Scand J Med Sci Sports 9:285, 1999.

19. Levangie PK, Norkin CC: The knee in joint structure and function: A comprehensive analysis. In Levangie PK, Norkin CC (eds): Joint Structure and Function: A Comprehensive Analysis, 4th ed. Philadelphia, FA Davis, 2005, p 395.

20. Mancinelli CA: The instantaneous axis of rotation of the human knee joint. Dissertation for the degree of PhD. West Virginia University, 1994.

21. Martelli S, Pinskerova V: The shapes of the tibial and femoral articular surfaces in relation to tibio-femoral movement. J Bone Joint Surg [Br] 89:607, 2002.

22. McCarty EC, Ibarra C, Torzilli PA, Warren R: Ligament cutting studies. In Pedowitz RA, O'Connor JJ, Akeson WH (eds): Daniel's Knee Injuries. Philadelphia, Lippincott Williams & Wilkins, 2003, pp 81-96.

23. Merriam-Webster's Collegiate Dictionary, 10th ed. Springfield, MA, Merriam-Webster.

24. Myklebust G, Holm I, Mæhlum S, et al: Clinical, functional, and radiologic outcome in team handball players 6 to 11 years after anterior cruciate ligament injury: A follow-up study. Am J Sports Med 31:981, 2003.

25. Nakagawa SMD, Kadoya Y, Todo S, et al: Tibiofemoral movement 3: Full flexion in the living knee studied by MRI. J Bone Joint Surg [Br] 82:1199, 2000.

26. Noyes FR, Grood ES: The strength of the anterior cruciate ligament in humans and Rhesus monkeys. J Bone Joint Surg [Am] 58:1074, 1976.

27. Nuno, A, Ahmed M: Sagittal profile of the femoral condyles and its application to femorotibial contact analysis. J Biomech Eng 123:18, 2001.

28. Nuno A, Ahmed M: Three-dimensional morphometry of the femoral condyles. Clin Biomech (Bristol Avon) 18:924, 2003.

29. O'Connor JJ, Feikes J, Gill RHS, Zavatsky AB: Mobility of the knee. In Pedowitz RA, O'Connor JJ, Akeson WH (eds): Daniel's Knee Injuries. Philadelphia, Lippincott Williams & Wilkins, 2003, pp 49-79.

30. O'Connor JJ, Zavatsky AB, Gill RHS: Stability of the knee. In Pedowitz RA, O'Connor JJ, Akeson WH (eds): Daniel's Knee Injuries. Philadelphia, Lippincott Williams & Wilkins, 2003, pp 149-184.

31. O'Connor JJ, Shercliff TL, Biden E, et al: The geometry of the knee in the sagittal plane. J Eng Med Proc Inst Mech Eng (Part H) 203:223, 1989.

32. O'Connor JJ, Zavatsky AB, Gill RHS: Stability of the knee. In Pedowitz RA, O'Connor JJ, Akeson WH (eds): Daniel's Knee Injuries. Philadelphia, Lippincott Williams & Wilkins, 2003, pp 149-184.

33. Palmer I: Plastic surgery of the ligaments of the knee. Acta Chir Scand 91:37, 1944.

34. Pinczewski LA, Deehan DJ, Salmon LJ, et al: A five-year comparison of patellar tendon versus four-strand hamstring tendon autograft for arthroscopic reconstruction of the anterior cruciate ligament. Am J Sports Med 30:523, 2002.

35. Pinskerova V, Maquet P, Freeman MAR: Annotation: Writings on the knee between 1836 and 1917. J Bone Joint Surg [Br] 82:1100, 2000.

36. Roos H, Mrnell M, Gardsell P, et al: Soccer after anterior cruciate ligament injury—an incompatible combination? A national survey of incidence and risk factors and a 7-year follow-up of 310 players. Acta Orthop Scand 66:107, 1995.

37. Schultz RA, Miller DC, Kerr CS, et al: Mechanoreceptors in human cruciate ligaments. J Bone Joint Surg [Am] 66:1072, 1984.

38. Schutte MJ, Dabzies EJ, Zimmy MI: Neural anatomy of the human anterior cruciate ligament. J Bone Joint Surg [Am] 69:243, 1987.

39. Shrive NG, Thornton GM, Hart DA, Frank CB: Ligament mechanics, structural behavior, and material properties of normal and injured ligaments. In Pedowitz RA, O'Connor JJ, Akeson WH (eds): Daniel's Knee Injuries. Philadelphia, Lippincott Williams & Wilkins, 2003, pp 97-112.

40. Siu D, Rudan J, Weaver HW, Griffith P: Femoral articular shape and geometry. A three dimensional computerized analysis of the knee. J Arthroplasty 11:166, 1996.

41. Snyder-Mackler L, Fitzgerald GK, Bartolozzi AR III, Ciccotti MG: The relationship between passive joint laxity and functional outcome after anterior cruciate ligament injury. Am J Sports Med 25:191, 1997.

42. Sommerlath K, Lysholm J, Gillquist J: The long-term course after treatment of acute anterior cruciate ligament ruptures. A 9-16 year followup. Am J Sports Med 19:156, 1991.

43. Weber WE, Weber EFM: Mechanik der menschlichen Gehwerkseuge. Göttingen, Dietrichschen Buchhandlung, 1836.

44. Wojtys EM, Huston LJ: Neuromuscular performance in normal and anterior cruciate ligament-deficient lower extremities. Am J Sports Med 22:89, 1994.

45. Woo SLY, Young EP, Kwan MK: Fundamental studies in knee ligament mechanics. In Daniel DM, Akeson WH, O'Connor JJ (eds): Knee Ligaments: Structure, Function, Injury, Repair. New York, Raven Press, 1990, pp 115-134.

46. Yagi T, Sasaki T: Tibial torsion in patients with medial-type osteoarthritic knee. Clin Orthop 213:177, 1986.

47. Zuppinger H: Die aktive Flexion in unbelasteten Kniegelenk: Züricher Hab il Schr Wiesbaden, Bergmann, 1904, p 703.

CHAPTER 10

Soft-Tissue Reconstruction and Fixation in the Knee

David E. Haynes • *John A. Bergfeld*
William M. Wind • *Richard D. Parker*

This chapter is the second of seven in the section "Biomechanics." As authors in this section, we have been asked to focus our chapter on soft-tissue mechanics, kinematics, implant design and selection, materials, and component retrieval, where appropriate. Emphasis is directed at clinical appreciation of clinical dilemmas. Therefore, this chapter deals with the biomechanical assessment of both posterior cruciate ligament (PCL) and anterior cruciate ligament (ACL) reconstruction through a variety of techniques. Emphasis has been placed on the biomechanical rationale for selection of a surgical procedure, from graft choice to tunnel placement and fixation.

POSTERIOR CRUCIATE LIGAMENT

This section reviews the pertinent anatomy/biomechanics, epidemiology/classification, clinical evaluation, natural history, nonoperative treatment, and operative treatment of the PCL with a focus on discussion of the tibial tunnel versus the tibial inlay and the one-bundle versus the two-bundle (tunnel) femoral techniques.

Anatomy and Biomechanics

Anatomic studies have shown the PCL to average between 32 and 38 mm in length from origin to insertion.[46] It has a cross-sectional area of 31.2 mm^2 at its midsubstance, which is 1.5 times greater than that of the ACL.[46,62,64] The PCL femoral and tibial insertion sites are approximately three times larger in cross-section than its midsubstance, which makes anatomic reconstruction difficult.[58,64]

The PCL is divided functionally into an anterolateral (AL) and a posteromedial (PM) bundle. This standard nomenclature refers to the anatomic location of the femoral insertion to the tibial insertion.[46] Each bundle exhibits different tensioning patterns depending on the degree of knee flexion. The AL bundle tightens in knee flexion and loosens in knee extension. The PM bundle tightens in knee extension and is lax in knee flexion.[46,157] Division of the PCL into distinct bundles may be an oversimplification according to some authors, with three- and four-bundle divisions being described, as well as a continuum of fibers of different length and attachment characteristics.[93,99]

The femoral insertion site characteristics of the PCL were recently mapped and found to have a broad attachment with an angle of 88 ± 5.5 degrees to the roof.[99] The anterior portion inserts in a more vertical orientation than the posterior portion, which inserts on the flat intercondylar surface (Fig. 10–1). The midpoint of the femoral PCL attachment is 1 cm proximal to the articular cartilage of the medial femoral condyle.[29] The tibial insertion of the PCL is 1.0 to 1.5 cm inferior to the posterior rim of the tibia in a defined PCL facet.

The recommendations for reconstruction of the AL bundle via the single-bundle technique are due to its superior structural properties (ultimate strength, stiffness) and its size, which is twice the cross-sectional area of the PM bundle.[64,125] In addition, the AL bundle is the preferred bundle for reconstruction because it tightens in flexion, where PCL function is most important. Harner et al[64] have shown that the AL bundle is 2.1 times stiffer and has an ultimate load 2.7 times greater than the PM bundle does. The complex fiber anatomy and nonisometric nature of the PCL make reconstruction to restore its normal anatomy and function difficult.[67]

In addition to the AL and PM bands of the PCL, there are also two variable meniscofemoral ligaments (MFLs). The anterior ligament of Humphrey and the posterior ligament of Wrisberg originate from the posterior horn of the lateral meniscus and insert anterior and posterior to the PCL on the medial femoral condyle, respectively.[87] These anatomic ligaments can cause confusion in the normal demarcation of the PCL; however, the MFLs can be identified by tracing their origin to the posterior horn of the lateral meniscus. Although the presence of these ligaments is believed to be variable, a recent anatomic study found that 93% of 84 knees had at least one MFL (ligament of Humphrey in 74%; ligament of Wrisberg in 69%).[53]

Biomechanical studies have demonstrated the importance of the MFLs.[64,87] The MFLs have a stiffness and ultimate load that is slightly greater than that of the PM bundle of the PCL.[64,87] They represent 30% of the anatomic femoral attachment (footprint) and provide 30% to 60% of the resistance to posterior stress with the knee at 90 degrees of flexion.[64] Further studies are needed to fully characterize the biomechanics of these ligaments. The MFLs are important in the overall strength of the PCL, and we attempt to preserve them during PCL reconstruction.

The primary function of the PCL complex (PCL and MFLs) is to restrict posterior tibial translation. It acts as a

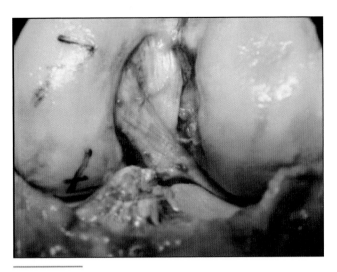

Figure 10–1. Vertical orientation of the anterolateral bundle of the posterior cruciate ligament in a left knee.

secondary restraint to tibial varus, valgus, and external rotation.[21,47,51,159] When compared with the ACL, the PCL has slightly higher stiffness and ultimate tensile load.[124] Cutting studies have shown that isolated sectioning of the PCL complex results in increased posterior translation, most pronounced at 90 degrees of flexion.[47,51,61,159] The posterolateral corner (PLC) also plays a role in limiting posterior tibial translation, but its primary role is to resist varus and external rotation force with the knee at 30 to 45 degrees of flexion.[47,108,109] When both the PCL and PLC are cut, posterior translation is significantly greater than when either structure is cut alone.[47,51] Varus and external rotation are also increased at both 30 and 90 degrees.[47,51]

Epidemiology and Classification

There is considerable variability in the reported incidence of PCL injuries, which varies from 1% to 44% of all acute knee injuries.[139] The incidence reported in the general population (3%) is much lower than in the traumatic setting, where 37% of all hemarthroses have an associated PCL injury.[34,35,105] Traumatic high-velocity knee injuries often result in PCL tears in conjunction with other ligamentous injuries. The incidence of these combined injuries in the emergency department setting can be as high as 95%.[35]

The incidence of PCL injuries in the athletic population is sport specific, with injuries occurring more frequently in contact sports. Parolie and Bergfeld[119] found a 2% incidence of PCL injury in asymptomatic college football players at National Football League predraft examinations. Data from other studies have shown a relatively low incidence of PCL injuries in other sports, with injuries occurring more frequently in sports involving high contact force.[7,27,40,82,89,107,142]

Motor vehicle accidents are a more common cause of PCL injuries.[1,35,88] A dashboard injury occurs with the knee in a flexed position as a posteriorly directed force is applied to the tibia. When this force is combined with a varus or rotational component, the lateral or posterolateral structures may also be injured.

The most common mechanism of PCL injury in an athlete is a fall on a flexed knee with a plantar-flexed foot or hyperflexion of the knee.[33,122] The PCL and posterior capsule can also be torn by a hyperextension mechanism.

Clinical Evaluation

Clinical evaluation begins with a careful history of the mechanism of injury, which may help identify potential injury to associated structures. The mechanism dictates the severity of injury in the wide spectrum of potential injury. When eliciting a history from a patient with an acute isolated PCL tear, unlike an ACL tear, the patient will often not report feeling a "pop" or "tear." With acute tears resulting from low force (sports injury), patients typically have mild to moderate knee effusion, a slight limp, pain in the back of the knee, and a 10- to 20-degree deficit in flexion. More instability is experienced in combined injuries than in isolated tears. Patients with chronic PCL tears may complain more of disability than instability.[25] Frequently, patients with a chronic PCL tear have difficulty walking up or down inclines such as a ramp.

The most accurate test to assess the integrity of the PCL is the posterior drawer test.[25,30] This test is performed with the knee at 90 degrees of flexion and the tibia in neutral and in external and internal rotation. In isolated PCL tears, there is a decrease in posterior tibial translation with internal tibial rotation. Bergfeld et al showed that the medial collateral ligament (MCL) and posterior oblique ligament contribute to this secondary restraint.[12,128]

Classification of PCL injuries can be based on the time interval from injury (acute versus chronic) and the presence or absence of associated injuries (isolated versus combined). Grading of PCL tears is typically based on the position of the medial tibial plateau relative to the medial femoral condyle at 90 degrees of flexion. It is important to recognize that the tibia normally lies approximately 1 cm anterior to the femoral condyles in its resting position. In grade I injuries, the tibia continues to lie anterior to the femoral condyles, but it is slightly diminished (0- to 5-mm patholaxity). Grade II injuries represent a tibia that is flush with the femoral condyles (5- to 10-mm patholaxity). When the tibia no longer has a medial step-off and can be pushed beyond the medial femoral condyle (>10-mm patholaxity), it is classified as a grade III injury. Grade III injuries often represent combined injuries, and involvement of the capsular ligaments must be ruled out.

It is important to distinguish isolated PCL injuries from combined PCL, PLC, and posteromedial corner (PMC) injuries. All structures need to be addressed at the time of surgery when involved. Injury to the PCL and PLC can be distinguished with the tibial external rotation (dial) test with the knee in both 30 and 90 degrees of flexion (Fig. 10–2).[47,51,160] The test is performed by passively rotating both feet externally at 30 and 90 degrees of flexion with the patient either prone or supine. The thigh-foot angle is then measured, with more than 10 to 15 degrees of external rotation versus the uninjured side being considered pathological. Asymmetry with the knee at 30 degrees of flexion is associated with a PLC injury, whereas asymmetry at both 30 and 90 degrees of flexion represents an injury to both the PCL and PLC.

The integrity of the PMC can be tested with the posteromedial pivot test.[116] This test evaluates the integrity of the PCL, MCL, and posterior oblique ligament. A positive test results when the knee shifts anteriorly as it is extended to approximately 20 degrees while applying a varus, compression, and internal rotation stress to the tibia.

In addition to examining the knee for PCL, PMC, and PLC laxity, it is important to test the function of the other ligamentous structures of the knee for their integrity. Associated meniscal as well as chondral injury should be evaluated. The overall alignment of the knee should be assessed. A primary varus knee will be more susceptible to difficulty with a posterolateral injury and is the cause

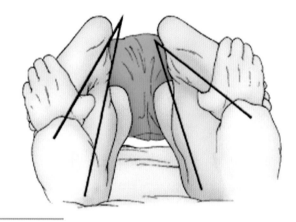

Figure 10–2. Dial test. An increase of 10 to 15 degrees in the tibiofemoral angle versus the normal side represents a significant injury.

of the chronic medial joint problems seen in 15% of isolated PCL injuries. Gait should be assessed with the patient both standing and walking to observe for genu varum or a varus thrust. These findings are more common in patients with chronic PCL deficiencies.

A neurovascular examination is essential, especially when combined injuries are detected. Pulses (dorsalis pedis, posterior tibial) should be documented, as well as motor/sensory function (particularly the peroneal nerve). Any concern regarding the vascular status of the limb should be evaluated with an arteriogram. Caution should be exercised in the situation in which pulses are intact, but diminished because of the probable presence of an intimal tear. An arteriogram is recommended in this setting and when the ankle-brachial index is less than 0.8 in comparison to the unaffected extremity.

Plain radiographs are the next step in the evaluation of PCL injuries. Standard series consist of bilateral standing anteroposterior, 45-degree posteroanterior flexion weight-bearing, Merchant patellar views, and a lateral view of the affected extremity. Plain radiographs will document evidence of arthritis (especially the flexion weightbearing views), avulsion fractures, posterior sag on the lateral view, and lateral joint space widening. The lateral radiograph also provides a measurement of proximal tibia slope.

Stress radiographs (Telos) are an important adjunct to routine knee radiographs (Fig. 10–3) and have several advantages over physical examination and arthrometric testing. They allow a noninvasive and objective comparison of sagittal translation between the injured and intact knee. They also eliminates errors from compliance of soft tissues by measuring skeletal displacement alone. Stress radiographs may even be more accurate than KT-1000 arthrometry or clinical testing, with greater than 8 mm of posterior translation being indicative of a complete PCL rupture.[71]

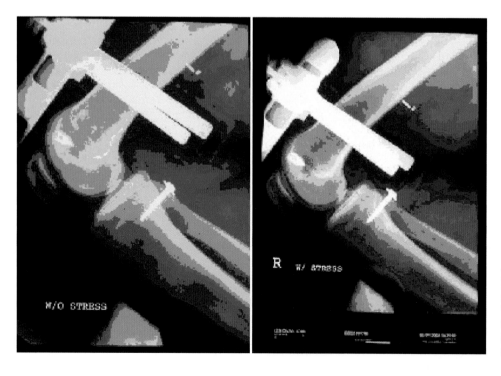

W/O STRESS

R W/ STRESS

Figure 10–3. Plain radiographic Telos stress views. The degree of posterior translation of the tibia is measured with both stress and nonstress views.

Magnetic resonance imaging (MRI) is now the preferred imaging technique for evaluating PCL injuries. It has been reported to have an accuracy in the range of 96% to 100%.[39,52,70,123,156] MRI can determine the location of the PCL injury, in addition to other ligament, meniscal, and cartilage injury in the knee. Moreover, it can determine whether the injured PCL is in continuity, which may then heal clinically. A normal PCL appears dark on T1- and T2-weighted images and is curvilinear in appearance. However, the shape of the ligament should not be used as a criterion for normal PCL function because its shape may vary.

With chronic PCL injuries, MRI may appear normal in grade I and II injuries. Therefore, as for acute injuries, the history and physical examination become important in the diagnosis of PCL tears. Bone scans are also a valuable tool in patients with symptomatic, chronic PCL tears. A bone scan may show early arthritic changes in the knee joint before radiographs or MRI does. Such patients have a higher risk for the development of articular cartilage degenerative changes (increased uptake) in the patellofemoral and medial compartments. Some authors advocate reconstruction in this setting to decrease knee patholaxity; however, no study has proved this or that PCL reconstruction can prevent the progression of arthritis.[36,122]

pendent of the grade of PCL laxity. In addition, half the patients returned to the same sport at the same or higher level and half were not able to return at the same level.

The incidence of meniscal and chondral injury associated with PCL tears has not been as extensively studied as the incidence of these injuries with ACL tears. The incidence of meniscus tears ranges from 16% to 28% in the literature,[40,45,55] with longitudinal tears of the anterior horn of the lateral meniscus being the most common location.[55] There is also a high incidence of radial tears in the middle or posterior lateral meniscus.[55]

Articular cartilage injury may also occur with PCL tears; however, its incidence is more varied because of different criteria/grading of the lesions. Fowler and Messiah[40] reported a 31% incidence, whereas Geissler and Whipple[45] found that 12% of knees had articular cartilage lesions requiring arthroscopic surgery. A more recent study, which included milder lesions, noted a 52% incidence, with grade III or higher lesions found in only 16%.[55] The medial femoral condyle was the most common site of severe cartilaginous lesions.

Long-term outcome studies have shown that chronic, isolated PCL-deficient knees may deteriorate over time.[16,25,31,84] In some patients, articular cartilage degenerative changes eventually develop in the medial and patellofemoral compartment.[25,30,145]

Natural History

Natural history studies allow for a comparison of the results of operative and nonoperative treatment. Some authors believe that isolated PCL tears will typically follow a benign short-term course when treated nonoperatively[40,119,135,155] whereas the prognosis is guarded with combined injuries[139] and those at long-term follow-up.[16] In addition, most studies have shown that patients with acute, isolated PCL tears treated nonoperatively achieve a level of knee function that is independent of the grade of laxity.[16,119,155]

Fowler and Messiah[40] prospectively monitored 13 athletes treated nonoperatively for PCL tears for a mean of 2.6 years and found that 3 had good objective results but all 13 had good subjective results. Parolie and Bergfeld[119] concluded in a population of 25 athletes at a mean of 6.2 years after injury that regaining quadriceps strength was an important factor in return to sports without surgery. Twenty patients (80%) were satisfied with their overall knee function. Torg et al[155] monitored 14 patients with isolated PCL instability and found 5 (36%) to have an excellent result and 7 a good result. They advocated nonsurgical treatment of isolated PCL tears.

Shelbourne et al[139] evaluated 133 patients with acute, isolated grade I/II PCL tears at a mean follow-up of 5.4 years. Sixty-eight returned for a long-term follow-up examination. The authors concluded that the objective grade of PCL laxity did not increase with time from injury or correlate with the amount of radiographic joint space narrowing. Overall, they found that patients with acute, isolated PCL tears, when treated nonoperatively, achieved a level of objective and subjective function that was inde-

Nonoperative Treatment

Nonoperative treatment is indicated for patients with acute, isolated grade I or II PCL tears.[40,84,119] Physical examination is crucial for determining whether the injury is restricted to the PCL because a knee with an isolated injury to the PCL is a candidate for nonoperative treatment. For operative treatment, the physical examination may be outside this envelope of isolated PCL examination. MRI continuity of the PCL also leads to a favorable prognosis for nonoperative treatment. The integrity of secondary restraints and the healing capacity of the PCL result in a more favorable prognosis for these low-grade injuries. Our approach is a 2-week period of relative immobilization and protected weightbearing with crutches, followed by early range-of-motion exercises and a quadriceps-strengthening rehabilitation program. Quadriceps strengthening is emphasized to counteract posterior tibial subluxation.[73,126] Return to sport typically takes 4 to 6 weeks.

Treatment of patients with acute grade III injuries is more controversial. These patients have generally also injured the PLC or PMC, and thus a period of 2 to 4 weeks of relative immobilization in full extension is considered.[59] Weightbearing is also limited. Exercises emphasizing the quadriceps, such as quad sets and straight-leg raises, are encouraged, with antagonistic hamstring exercises not initiated until later. Return to sport is delayed for 3 to 4 months in patients with higher-grade injuries.

Nonoperative treatment of chronic PCL injuries consisting of physical therapy and rehabilitation is usually adequate. A brace is fitted to protect the terminal 15 degrees of extension initially. The brace is opened to full extension when the posterior knee pain has resolved. If symptoms develop, patients typically report pain and recurrent swelling. With negative radiographs, a bone scan and MRI are performed. If the bone scan is positive in patients with grade I/II PCL tears who are unable to modify their activities or in patients with a grade III PCL injury, we recommend surgical intervention. The PLC or PMC will usually need to be addressed in grade III injuries at the time of PCL reconstruction.

Consideration must be given to bone alignment, as well as the slope of the tibial plateau. Osteotomy procedures that increase the posterior slope of the tibia and result in decreased posterior translation have recently been tested in the laboratory. In addition, biplanar osteotomies to correct varus alignment and posterior slope have been proposed for salvage of difficult chronic PCL deficiency, particularly in patients who have medial pain.

Operative Treatment

Current surgical indications for PCL injuries include combined ligament injuries involving the PCL, symptomatic grade III laxity, and bony avulsion fractures.[100,127,131,135,144] However, some natural history studies,[16,25,31,84] which have shown deterioration in knee function over time, as well as improvement in surgical techniques for correcting knee laxity, may lead to expansion of these indications in the future.

The timing of PCL reconstruction depends on the severity of the injury and the associated ligamentous structures involved. Knees with multiligament injuries should be addressed within the first 2 to 3 weeks[112] to provide the best opportunity for anatomic ligament repair if possible and decrease capsular scarring.

A number of graft options are available for PCL reconstruction and should be discussed preoperatively with the patient. Autologous tissues that are available include bone–patellar tendon–bone (BPTB) and the hamstring (HS) and quadriceps tendons, of which the BPTB is the most frequently used. BPTB grafts allow for superior fixation; however, problems of harvest site morbidity, graft-tunnel mismatch, and incomplete filling of tunnels with collagen may make this graft less desirable. In addition, the quadriceps mechanism is compromised, and it is imperative that the quadriceps have maximal strength and endurance for a successful outcome. Quadruple HS grafts have decreased surgical morbidity but inferior graft fixation methods require healing within the tunnel to be successful. Staubli et al believe that use of the quadriceps tendon is arguably associated with less donor site morbidity than use of the BPTB is and has demonstrated biomechanical properties comparable to those of the BPTB.[148]

We currently prefer allograft Achilles tendon as our graft of choice for PCL reconstruction. The use of allografts decreases harvest site morbidity and surgical time.[18,36,111] Achilles tendon allografts contain an abundance of collagen for reconstruction of the AL band of the PCL. They may also facilitate double-bundle reconstruction by splitting the soft-tissue aspect of the graft for each bundle. The osseous portion of the graft can provide excel-

lent bony fixation on the tibia with a cancellous screw via the inlay technique. We use a soft-tissue screw and staple technique to fix the soft-tissue portion of the graft on the femur.

The indications for PCL reconstruction have been outline earlier, and a number of different surgical techniques have been described. Current popular techniques include single- and double-bundle reconstructions using the tibial inlay or tunnel method.

Our rationale for use of the tibial inlay technique has stemmed from basic science research. The tibial inlay technique involves open, anatomic placement of the tibial graft by creating a trough at the PCL tibial insertion. This method of tibial fixation avoids the so-called killer turn commonly seen with the tunnel technique. Bergfeld et al[12] have shown that at time zero, both posterior tibial inlay reconstruction and the tibial tunnel method produce stable knees. Cyclic loading of cadaveric knees resulted in increased laxity in the tibial tunnel reconstruction in comparison to the inlay reconstruction. Transillumination of these grafts showed thinning and fraying at 30, 60, and 90 degrees at the site of maximal graft curvature around the proximal posterior aspect of the tibia (Fig. 10–4).

Markolf et al compared inlay versus tibial tunnel PCL reconstruction and showed that 10 of 31 grafts passed through a tibial tunnel failed at the acute angle before 2000 cycles whereas 31 of 31 inlay grafts survived the testing intact. Tibial tunnel grafts also had increased graft elongation and thinning, especially at the "killer turn."[96] Other studies comparing the two techniques, however, have shown no difference in the generation of graft force.[98,115] Avoiding the killer curve and more closely duplicating the normal PCL anatomy are reasons for preferring the PCL tibial inlay technique.

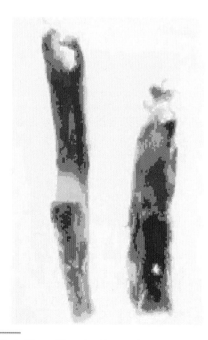

Figure 10–4. Transillumination of reconstructed grafts showed thinning at the bone plug–graft junction in the area of the "killer turn" with the tibial tunnel reconstruction technique versus the tibial inlay technique.

Before surgical reconstruction, an examination of both knees under anesthesia is performed. If evidence of injury to the posterolateral or posteromedial structures is detected, these secondary restraints must be addressed at the time of PCL reconstruction. Any malalignment, especially varus, should also be taken into consideration.

TIBIAL INLAY TECHNIQUE

The surgical procedure begins with diagnostic arthroscopy. The PCL injury is documented, and any associated internal derangements of the knee are addressed. The PCL remnant is then débrided while attempting to preserve any of the remaining MFLs. The normal femoral PCL anatomic attachment is identified and marked with a sharp curet. The femoral tunnel is then established with an outside-in technique such that the femoral insertion of the PCL/MFL complex is closely duplicated and the tunnel is aimed in the direction of the native ligament. The anterior aspect of the tunnel should be 1 to 2 mm from the articular margin. The MFLs are looked for and, if intact, are preserved. Although it is not unusual to find one or the other MFL intact, we have never found both to be present in the event of a PCL complex injury. A commercial graft passer or 18-gauge wire is placed through the femoral tunnel and directed toward the back of the knee to facilitate passage of the graft once it is secured to the tibia.

The entire leg is placed in a sterile Mayo stand cover and wrapped circumferentially. The patient is then turned to the prone position on another operating room table. The leg is reprepared and draped for the posterior exposure. We have found that turning the patient to the prone position, though cumbersome, requires only an additional 15 minutes of operating room time.

A modified Burks posterior approach to the tibia is then performed without a tourniquet, thus ensuring hemostasis. This approach has been shown to be safe with respect to the popliteal artery.[103] The interval between the medial head of the gastrocnemius and the semitendinosus is bluntly dissected (Fig. 10–5). A broad, low-profile blunt retractor works well to retract the medial head of the gastrocnemius and the neurovascular bundle. The posterior capsule is then visualized and incised longitudinally to expose the PCL stump. The graft passer is often palpable underneath the capsule.

During the exposure, an assistant can prepare the Achilles tendon allograft, which again, is our graft of choice. A Krackow stitch with No. 5 nonabsorbable suture is placed in the soft-tissue end, and the bone plug is sized to 10 mm in width by 20 mm in length. A 35-mm-long, 6.5-mm-diameter, partially threaded cancellous screw with a washer is placed in the bone plug and oriented in a slightly distal direction. The screw is placed so that the cancellous side of the plug will be facing the cancellous trough.

A trough the size of the bone plug is created with sharp osteotomes at the native PCL footprint (Fig. 10–6). The graft is placed into the graft passer and passed through the femoral tunnel. The bone plug is then recessed into the tibia and the screw advanced (Fig. 10–7). The poste-

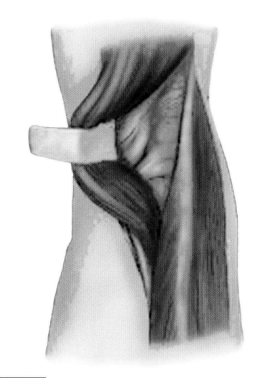

Figure 10–5. Modified Burks posterior tibial approach for the inlay technique. Dissection in the interval between the medial head of the gastrocnemius and the semitendinosus reveals the posterior capsule.

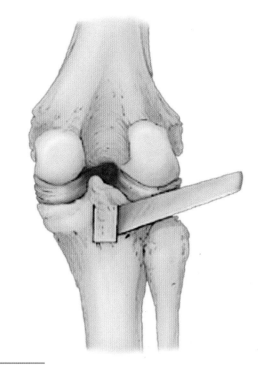

Figure 10–6. A trough is created with sharp osteotomes at the site of the native posterior cruciate ligament footprint.

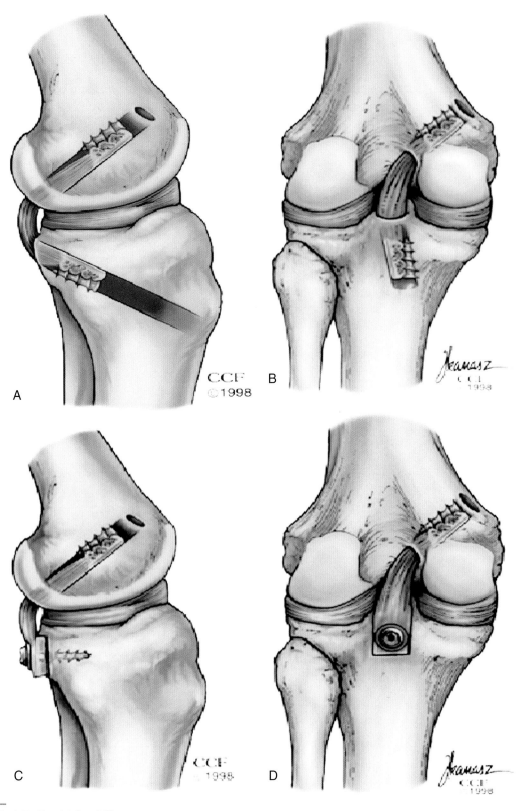

Figure 10–7. **A-D,** Final inlay PCL reconstruction.

rior capsule and the surgical incisions are closed, and the patient is turned back to the supine position.

After repreparing and draping the patient, the soft-tissue graft is fixed in the femoral tunnel with a soft-tissue interference screw and reinforced to the femur with staples. The graft is tensioned with a force of 20 N in 70 to 90 degrees of flexion while performing an anterior drawer test before fixation. We routinely require an overnight stay in the hospital for vascular monitoring and pain management.

Postoperatively, a locked knee brace in full extension is applied. Exercises include straight-leg raises, quad sets, and calf pumps. The brace may be unlocked for patient-assisted tibial lifts in flexion limited to 60 degrees. At 4 weeks the brace is unlocked as the patient increases weightbearing and range of motion to 90 degrees. Exercises include resisted cycling, straight-leg raises, eccentric quadriceps contraction, open-chain quadriceps progressive resistive exercises, Theraband leg presses, and quad sets at 90 degrees of knee flexion. A PCL functional brace is fitted at 4 to 6 weeks, at which time the crutches are discontinued. Progressive quadriceps exercises are emphasized; however, HS progressive resistive exercises are not performed until 3 to 6 months postoperatively. A slide board may be used at 4 months, with jogging and sport-specific exercises beginning at 6 months. Full return to sport may vary from 8 to 12 months, depending on the individual and the demands of their sport.

TIBIAL TUNNEL TECHNIQUE

The tibial tunnel method of PCL reconstruction addresses the tibial PCL attachment site arthroscopically as opposed to the open approach. Visualization of the PCL stump is enhanced with a 70-degree scope and by establishing a PM portal. After débridement of the PCL stump, a PCL guide is used to drill a guide pin from a point just distal and medial to the tibial tubercle and aimed at the distal and lateral aspect of the PCL footprint. An intraoperative radiograph or C-arm is helpful to confirm correct placement of the guide wire. A tunnel is then created with a reamer over the guide wire, with care taken to protect the posterior neurovascular structures.

The femoral tunnel can be created with either an inside-out or an outside-in approach. The outside-in approach may be technically easier and more properly restores the native orientation of the PCL. In single-bundle reconstructions, for reasons previously mentioned, most surgeons attempt to reproduce the AL component of the PCL. The femoral tunnel should be placed just under the subchondral bone, with sufficient bone maintained on the medial femoral condyle to reduce the risk of osteonecrosis.[24,101,102]

One of the most difficult steps of the arthroscopic reconstruction is passage of the graft around the abrupt turn at the back of the tibial plateau. The direction of graft passage often depends on the type of graft used. The tibial inlay technique avoids this difficult step with an open exposure. The graft is then pretensioned and fixed at 70 and 90 degrees of flexion while an anterior drawer test is performed.

The other option for femoral-sided reconstruction is the double-bundle technique, in which both the AL and PM bundles are reconstructed. In a recent biomechanical analysis, Harner et al[60] showed that double-bundle reconstruction more effectively restores normal knee kinematics than single-bundle reconstruction does throughout the full range of flexion. In addition, posterior tibial translation was decreased by up to 3.5 mm with this technique when compared with single-bundle reconstruction.

The double-bundle reconstruction technique, though conceptually attractive, is technically more challenging. Two tunnels are created; a larger tunnel is drilled for the AL component and a smaller tunnel for the PM bundle. An Achilles tendon allograft is a commonly used graft for the AL bundle and a double semitendinosus autograft for the smaller PM bundle. The AL graft is tensioned and fixed at 90 degrees of knee flexion and the PM bundle at 30 degrees. Long-term outcome data are needed to determine whether this technique offers any advantages over single-bundle reconstruction.

Conclusion

Continued interest in PCL injuries has resulted in numerous recent anatomic and biomechanical studies. Although most would agree on the indications for PCL reconstruction, debate centers on the technique that will most accurately restore normal knee kinematics. Long-term outcome studies are needed to determine the best method of treatment of these injuries. Present outcome studies in the literature are a cacophony of index patient injuries, reconstructive techniques, and standard reporting systems.

ANTERIOR CRUCIATE LIGAMENT

Current techniques for ACL reconstruction provide improved knee stability and outcomes.[6,20] The evolution of these techniques has been based on attempts to reestablish normal ligament function as described in Chapter 1. Techniques such as aperture fixation and double-bundle reconstruction are examples of these attempts. Recent data obtained by open-access MRI evaluation of ACL-reconstructed knees suggest that the knee is stabilized in the sagittal plane but that the relationship between the femur and the tibia is different in the reconstructed knee than in the normal knee.[91] Tashman and associates used stereoradiographic evaluation to show significant differences in reconstructed and uninjured knees. Reconstructed knees were more adducted and externally rotated.[153] These studies suggest that although current techniques improve stability and most patients are satisfied with the results of surgery, the normal kinematics of the knee is not completely restored. Outcome studies of newer techniques, as well as research on normal biomechanics of the knee, will influence the future direction of progress. However, until these outcome studies are available, clinicians must carefully weigh their choice of surgical procedure and not abandon a reasonably successful procedure for an unproven, popular postulate.

Biomechanics

Understanding the rationale behind reconstructive techniques requires knowledge of the native anatomy and biomechanics of the ACL. Chapter 1 describes in detail the properties and functions of the native ACL. Its role as a primary restraint to anterior translation and a secondary restraint to internal rotation is well described. The ACL is responsible for 82% to 89% of restraint to an applied load at 30 degrees of flexion. This percentage decreases slightly with increasing flexion. Reconstruction has focused on restoring the primary function of the ACL, that is, anterior translation of the tibia on the femur.[32,43,151]

Traditionally, the ACL, in conjunction with the PCL, has been described as part of a "crossed four-bar linkage." This two-dimensional description requires the cruciates to function isometrically and remain static in length. Recent data have shown that the native ACL is not literally isometric and that changes in length do occur throughout a range of motion.[32,75] Multiple studies have also demonstrated the ACL to have a role in rotational stability of the knee. Anderson and Dyhre-Poulsen showed a statistically significant increase in total arc of internal/external rotation at 10 and 30 degrees of knee flexion after sectioning of the ACL.[5,44] These recent biomechanical studies support the complex role of the ACL.

Consideration must also be given to the environment in which the ACL exists. It functions within a system that includes the synovium, articular surfaces, menisci, PCL, collateral ligaments, joint capsule, and surrounding musculature. Papageorgiou and associates demonstrated that the force in the medial meniscus doubles as a result of ACL deficiency and that in situ force in the ACL increases 33% to 50% after medial meniscectomy.[117] Sakane et al also confirmed that significant load sharing occurs among the ACL, PCL, MCL, posterolateral structures, and articular surface contact.[134] Knowledge of the biomechanics and anatomy of the ACL is the basis for current reconstruction techniques and will continue to be the impetus for improvement.

Single-Bundle Reconstruction

Multiple studies have shown greater than 90% successful clinical results with single-bundle ACL reconstruction.[6,9,20] Although it has enjoyed long-term success, the procedure has continued to evolve to incorporate principles of appropriate tunnel positions, graft types, and methods of fixation that are based on basic science. Research has provided data about the characteristics of the native ACL. Girgis et al divided the ACL into two functional parts: the anteromedial (AM) bundle and the posterolateral (PL) bundle.[46] The names refer to the position of insertion on the tibia. The AM bundle attaches to the femur on the most proximal and posterior aspect of the "footprint" and the PL bundle on the distal aspect.

ISOMETRY

Single-bundle ACL reconstruction simulates the AM bundle of the ACL. The rationale behind this approach is that the AM bundle, though not completely isometric, experiences less change in length and more constant in situ force at various degrees of knee flexion.[75,133,151] Furia et al described central fibers originating from the poste-

rior and inferior femoral "footprint" that change less than 1 mm in length throughout a range of motion. The authors in this study also suggest that "physiologic isometry," in which intraoperative changes in length throughout a range of motion are less than 2 to 3 mm and mimic the native ACL, can be achieved.[44] Others have also confirmed that the most isometric attachment sites on the femur are near the posterior end of Blumensaat's line.[172] These studies have typically used a tibial attachment site in the central portion of the footprint. Changes in the tibial insertion have proved to have less effect on isometry.[66]

TUNNEL POSITION

The goal of proper placement of the graft in ACL reconstruction has led to investigation of appropriate tunnel placement. Multiple authors have advocated placement of the tibial tunnel in a central or posterior position within the native tibial insertion site. This position decreases the likelihood of impingement on the roof of the intercondylar notch in full extension.[43] As stated earlier, the position of the tibial tunnel has less impact on in situ force and thus less potential for causing degeneration and/or early failure of the graft.

Placement of the femoral tunnel is critical to successful ACL reconstruction. Improper anterior placement of the femoral tunnel seen radiographically correlates with decreasing clinical outcomes[146] (Fig. 10–8). Multiple studies have contributed data to predict this correlation.[4,66,68] Anterior femoral tunnel placement is the most common error and results in a shorter graft and increased tension in flexion. Such graft placement may result in lim-

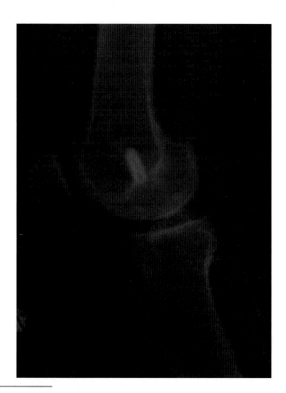

Figure 10–8. Incorrect femoral tunnel placement.

itation of flexion or early failure as a result of increased tension. This clinical scenario is known as a "captured knee." In addition to considerable data on the problems with anterior graft placement in the sagittal plane, recent studies have addressed biomechanical issues related to changes in the coronal plane. Scopp et al showed that more oblique placement of the femoral tunnel in the coronal plane restores internal rotation stability at 30 degrees of knee flexion whereas more vertical femoral tunnel placement does not. This oblique placement did not have a significant effect on external rotation stability or internal rotation stability at a flexion angle other than 30 degrees.[137] A separate study determined that oblique placement of femoral tunnels, lower on the lateral wall of the intercondylar notch, decreases graft tension at 120 degrees of knee flexion and reduces the pretensioning force required to restore anterior laxity comparable to that of an intact ligament. Positions tested were 80 degrees, or 10 degrees off vertical, 70 degrees, and 60 degrees. They found that a 60-degree femoral tunnel provided the lowest graft tension. They also found that with placement of more vertical tunnels, the increased tension was due to impingement on the PCL.[143] These findings are consistent with other studies that have supported oblique placement of the tibial and femoral tunnels[76] (Fig. 10–9). One must remember that the individual graft fascicles, like the native ACL, are subject to different tension, stress, and strain at different angles of motion.

NOTCHPLASTY

The development of arthroscopic techniques for ACL reconstruction has introduced different sources of error in the placement of femoral and tibial tunnels. Anterior placement of the femoral tunnel is the most common technical error associated with failure of reconstruction.[56,146] Notchplasty evolved to improve visualization, prevent impingement of the graft on the lateral wall and roof of the intercondylar notch, and facilitate graft passage during arthroscopic ACL reconstruction. The effects of notchplasty on in situ force and excursion of the graft were largely unknown before some recent data on these issues. Markolf et al described excursion, anterior-posterior laxity, and in situ graft force before and after a 2- and 4-mm notchplasty. The results showed increased excursion of the graft, increased pretensioning force required to restore anterior laxity, and increased force in the graft after notchplasty.[95] Hame et al showed that these detrimental effects of notchplasty persisted with variations in femoral tunnel position.[56] The opinion of secondary author JAB is that notchplasty of the roof or lateral wall is rarely necessary in a well-done ACL reconstruction. Notchplasty can be helpful in the occasional A-frame, tight notch. This subset represents approximately 10% of reconstructions.

GRAFT TENSION

Animal studies, cadaveric studies, and clinical studies have all attempted to characterize the appropriate magnitude and knee flexion angle at which initial tensioning should occur. Undertensioning risks increased laxity and overtensioning risks decreased range of motion and increased force in the graft, thereby potentially leading to failure. No consensus has been reached, but several studies have supported tensioning as an important element in successful ACL reconstruction.[15,169] In a cadaveric study, Burks and Leland found that the tensioning required to restore anterior-posterior laxity was tissue specific, with BPTB grafts requiring less tension (16 N) and semitendinosus and iliotibial band grafts requiring more tension (38 and 61 N, respectively). Therefore, it is likely that appropriate tensioning is tissue specific.[19] Boylan et al studied tension degradation with cyclic loading at different levels of initial graft tension. This cadaveric study used a quadruple HS graft fixed on the tibia with suture and post. Three separate levels of tensioning were examined, 23 N (5 lb), 45 N (10 lb), and 68 N (15 lb). This study revealed that 68 N was required to most closely restore anterior-posterior laxity after 1000 cycles. It was noted that in all groups an approximately 50% degradation took place after cyclic loading.[15] Clinical studies have shown no significant differences in symptoms, but do confirm subjective increased laxity with lower levels of tensioning and overconstraint and loss of range of motion at higher levels of tensioning with short-term follow-up.[69,169]

Recommendations for the knee flexion angle at the time of tensioning vary. Biomechanical data showing excursion of the ligament in full extension and higher flexion angles are in agreement with data on reconstruction that show increased force on the graft at full extension and higher flexion angles. These findings have led some to tension the graft with the knee at 30 degrees of flexion in an attempt to minimize force and excursion at extreme flexion and extension.[15,32] Some have proposed that with an appropriately placed graft, the flexion angle at the time of tensioning has no effect on kinematics.[15,32,69] Graft tensioning should be tailored to the graft type and

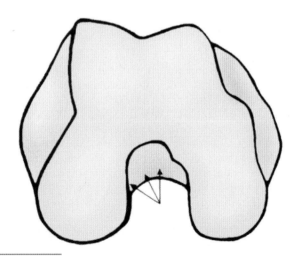

Figure 10–9. Coronal plane anatomy for femoral tunnel placement in a right knee. (From Hame SL, Markolf KL, Hunter DM, et al: Effects of notchplasty and femoral tunnel position on excursion patterns of an anterior cruciate ligament graft. Arthroscopy 19:340-345, 2003.)

intraoperative evaluation of excursion. After femoral fixation, if the graft has significant excursion, it should be tensioned in extension to avoid overconstraining the knee while realizing the trade-off that exists with anterior-posterior laxity.

Double-Bundle Reconstruction

Double-bundle or "anatomic" reconstruction is based on the description of the AM and PL bundles of the ACL.[46] It is likely that these "bundles" described in the literature are different fascicles of the ACL experiencing different strain at different flexion angles. Some authors have divided the ACL into three bundles, whereas others have proposed that no distinct bundles exist. However, the functions of the AM and PL bundles have been well described.[43] The AM bundle tightens with knee flexion, whereas the PL bundle is relatively loose. In extension, the PL bundle tightens and the AM bundle remains tight, but not as tight as the PL bundle (Fig. 10–10). Biomechanical evaluation of double-bundle reconstruction is ongoing. In a cadaveric study, Yagi et al compared the intact ACL with single-bundle reconstruction and double-bundle reconstruction. Performance when subjected to an anterior tibial load and combined rotatory and valgus load was evaluated. The double-bundle reconstruction had significantly less anterior tibial translation and more closely duplicated the in situ force of the intact ACL when subjected to anterior tibial load. Under a combined rotatory and valgus load, the double-bundle reconstruction again more closely reproduced the kinematics of the intact ACL.[168] In a clinical study, Muneta et al showed a trend toward improved

stability when compared with previous results of single-bundle reconstruction and a similar rehabilitation protocol.[106] Conversely, a prospective, double-blind study with a 32-month average follow-up showed no significant difference in anterior laxity or joint position sense when comparing double-bundle with single-bundle reconstruction.[2] This study agrees with the results of Hamada et al, which showed no significant difference in anterior stability.[54] Despite the theoretic and apparent biomechanical advantages of double-bundle reconstruction, clear clinical advantages have not been shown.

Graft Selection

Biological grafts are used extensively for ACL reconstruction, the most common choices being BPTB and quadruple semitendinosus/gracilis (HS) tendon autografts or an allograft.[43,104] Each of these graft types has been extensively studied, and graft choice is based on patient preference, the availability of tissue, and surgeon experience and philosophy. Recent studies have shown no statistically significant difference with regard to pain, instability, arthrometric measurement, and graft failure.[22,63,121,140] The advantages of an autograft include essentially no risk of disease transmission, rejection, or pathological inflammatory reaction. The advantages of an allograft include no donor site morbidity and decreased postoperative pain.[43] Synthetic grafts are rarely used because of high failure rates, and tissue-engineered ligaments and ligament scaffolds are in their infancy.[41,43,141] The characteristics of the graft material should be considered when evaluating graft choices. Mechanical properties, the biology of incorporation, and donor site morbidity are important issues when matching the graft with the clinical situation. The surgeon should be familiar with BPTB and quadrupled semitendinosus/gracilis and quadriceps tendon autografts. Common allografts include Achilles' tendon, BPTB, posterior tibialis, and anterior tibialis.

AUTOGRAFTS

The ideal autograft for ACL reconstruction would have the biomechanical properties of the native ligament after healing and minimal donor site morbidity. Biomechanical parameters of different grafts have been reported in the literature. Interpretation of these data is difficult because of the fact that much of it is from cadaveric studies with different methods. These studies do not take into account the changes that occur in vivo after ACL reconstruction. Rougraff et al described stages of ligamentization in postoperative biopsy specimens harvested from BPTB autografts. Repopulation with fibroblasts occurs in the first 2 months. Remodeling occurs in the first postoperative year and includes degeneration of mature collagen fibrils, neovascularization, and increased numbers of active fibroblasts. Maturation of the graft occurs 1 to 3 years postoperatively, and after 3 years the process of ligamentization is complete.[132] The histological changes that occur in HS autografts and allografts have been studied

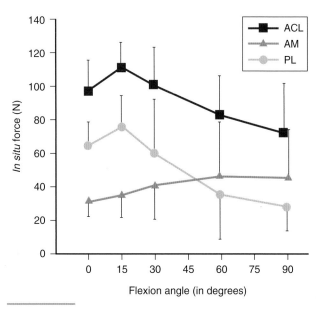

Figure 10–10. In situ force in the anterior cruciate ligament (ACL) with a 134-N anterior displacement load at various knee flexion angles. AM, anteromedial; PL, posterolateral. (From Sakane M, Fox RJ, Woo SL, et al: In situ forces in the anterior cruciate ligament and its bundles in response to anterior tibial loads. J Orthop Res 15:285-293, 1997.)

in animal models and are similar to those described earlier.[49,79] These biological changes have biomechanical consequences that have been documented in humans and animals. Animal studies have shown a decrease in the load to failure in the first 3 months to 53% of the contralateral donor tissue. This value increased to 81% at 9 months.[10] Beynnon et al reported a case in which an ACL graft was evaluated 8 months postoperatively and showed a load to failure that was 87% of the normal ACL.[14] Further studies are needed to determine the differences, if any, in the biomechanical characteristics of different types of healed ACL grafts.

Bone–Patella Tendon–Bone

The BPTB autograft has been referred to as the gold standard for ACL reconstruction.[104,141] Several studies have quantified the biomechanical properties of the native ACL. Noyes et al found the ultimate tensile strength and stiffness to be 1725 N and 182 N/mm.[113] Woo et al tested similar properties and took into account the knee flexion angle and anatomic position of the ligament. The results were an ultimate tensile strength of 2160 N and stiffness of 242 N/mm.[166] Given the properties of the native ACL and the previously described changes that occur with healing of a graft, a suitable graft would have an initial strength greater than that of the native ACL. Noyes et al found BPTB grafts to have 168% of the strength of the native ACL.[113] Woo et al found the strength and stiffness of BPTB grafts to be 2376 N and 812 N/mm, respectively.[166] These authors measured the strength of the native ACL, as stated previously, and the strength of grafts, thus minimizing the difficulty of interpreting nominal values from different studies. Other studies have also found the initial strength and stiffness of BPTB grafts to be adequate.[28,136]

Potential complications include anterior knee pain, pain with kneeling, patellar fracture, quadriceps weakness, and numbness as a result of transection of the infrapatellar branch of the saphenous nerve.[141] The most often cited problems are anterior knee pain and pain with kneeling. Recent studies have reported patellofemoral pain in 5% to 55% of patients.[104] Feller and Webster and others have shown a significantly higher incidence of anterior knee pain and pain on kneeling with BPTB than with HS autografts.[37,141] However, in a prospective, randomized clinical trial in 2004, Aglietti and associates reported a 22% incidence of patellofemoral crepitation in the BPTB group and a 23% incidence in the HS group.[3] Similarly, Shelbourne et al studied 602 patients with a BPTB autograft and found a similar anterior knee pain score as an age-matched control group.[139] Several studies have correlated patellofemoral pain with quadriceps circumference and weakness.[104] With multiple studies on both sides of the issue, it is unlikely that anterior knee pain is related solely to graft harvest in ACL reconstruction with a BPTB autograft.

Hamstring

The perception of donor site morbidity in BPTB autografts in conjunction with increasing data on the properties of HS autografts has produced renewed interest in the later.

The reported biomechanical properties of HS autografts have seemed to improve over the past 2 decades. However, the changes responsible for this apparent improvement include the use of quadrupled grafts instead of single and double grafts, as well as improved fixation techniques. Recent studies have shown the ultimate tensile strength and stiffness of HS grafts to be 4108 N and 776 N/mm, respectively.[57] Wilson et al, in a cadaveric study, documented the load to failure, stiffness, and size of both BPTB and HS grafts. For 15 matched pairs, the mean load to failure was 1784 ± 580 N for BPTB and 2422 ± 538 N for HS. The mean cross-sectional area for BPTB autografts was 45 mm^2, and that for HS autografts was 57 mm^2. No significant difference in stiffness was found.[165] These studies suggest that the biomechanical properties of HS autografts are adequate for ACL reconstruction.

Donor site morbidity in ACL reconstruction with an HS autograft consists mainly of potentially decreased knee flexion strength. Several studies with at least 2-year follow-up that have compared BPTB and HS autografts have shown decreased knee flexion strength in the HS group.[8,13,152] Viola et al and Segawa et al have shown a persistent decrease in internal tibial rotation strength.[138,162] Some of the same authors and others have failed to demonstrate significant functional differences in the two groups of patients, and one study[8] showed higher patient satisfaction in the HS group despite decreased knee flexion strength.[3,8,37] Therefore, the significance of the quantitative findings is uncertain.

Bone–Patellar Tendon–Bone versus Hamstring Autografts

The increasing number of studies comparing BPTB and HS autografts has prompted the performance of two meta-analyses. Freedman et al evaluated 1976 patients and found significantly lower rates of graft failure, less laxity, higher patient satisfaction, but a higher incidence of anterior knee pain in the BPTB group.[42,141] Yunes et al reported on four studies that included 411 patients and found that BPTB grafts were associated with less laxity and higher rates of "return to preinjury level of activity."[141,170] Interpretation of these meta-analyses is difficult because of variability in the studies included. Differences in methods among studies introduce confounding variables that affect the conclusions.[50] It should be noted that a recent randomized, prospective clinical trial with a 2-year follow-up showed no significant differences in visual analog scale, International Knee Documentation Committee scores, KT-1000 arthrometer measurements, anterior knee pain, muscle strength recovery, and return to sports activities.[3] This contrast illustrates that the data are not conclusively in support of one graft over the other.

Quadriceps

The quadriceps tendon is a less often used graft for ACL reconstruction. Staubli et al have advocated its use and shown the initial mechanical properties to be adequate. The ultimate tensile strength of a 10-mm-wide graft is 2352 N and its stiffness is 326 N/mm. The cross-sectional area was shown to be 64.4 mm^2.[148] However, few studies have shown long-term results, and quadriceps muscle weakness is a concern. The graft can be used in revision surgery when other graft options are unavailable and does appear to have appropriate initial biomechanical properties.

ALLOGRAFT

Traditionally, ACL reconstruction with allografts has been performed for revision cases, multiple-ligament injuries, and lower-demand patients.[77] The continued search for the ideal ACL reconstruction graft, together with improved screening for potentially transmittable diseases, has stimulated continued investigation of allograft tissues. Continued debate over donor site morbidity with autografts has also contributed. Advantages include decreased surgical time, no harvest site morbidity, and improved cosmesis. Disadvantages include potential disease transmission or immune reaction, slower incorporation and remodeling, higher cost, and potential negative effects of processing and sterilization.[104]

Numerous allograft options are available. The Achilles tendon and BPTB are the most common and have been demonstrated to have appropriate biomechanical properties for ACL reconstruction.[77,167] Recent reports have shown the biomechanical properties of doubled anterior tibialis, doubled posterior tibialis, and doubled peroneus longus tendons to also be adequate for ACL reconstruction.[120]

The greatest advantage of allografts is the absence of graft harvest morbidity. Without the aforementioned potential problems, as well as less postoperative pain, the patient could theoretically recover quicker from surgery. However, such difference in postoperative recovery between allograft and autograft ACL reconstruction has not been shown in the literature.[104] No graft harvest is necessary; therefore, surgical time is reduced and the incision used to perform the reconstruction can be more cosmetic.

Disadvantages of allograft tissue have been extensively studied in the literature. The risk of transmission of human immunodeficiency virus (HIV) in a screened allograft is approximately 1 in 1,500,000. Allograft tissue is also screened for hepatitis B, hepatitis C, and syphilis. Contamination is also an issue, and in 2001 a patient died of *Clostridium sordelli* septic shock after receiving an infected graft.[141] Before using any allograft tissue, the surgeon should be familiar with the vender from which the tissue was obtained and the processing techniques used.

In the past, allografts have been sterilized with radiation and ethylene oxide. Ethylene oxide sterilization has resulted in persistent synovitis, cystic changes in the bone tunnels, and graft failure and is therefore no longer used.[80,104,129] Gamma irradiation is still used to sterilize allograft tissue, and several studies have addressed its effects on mechanical properties. A dose greater than 2.0 Mrad has been shown to affect the biomechanical properties of the graft, and the dose required to reduce HIV to undetectable levels has been shown to be 3.0 Mrad.[38,158] Because of the potential effects of these sterilization tech-

niques, the allografts currently used in ACL reconstruction are most commonly fresh frozen and cryopreserved. Tissue screening and aseptic harvest techniques are used to prevent disease transmission.[141]

Allografts and autografts undergo similar stages of ligamentization.[142] However, Jackson et al showed delayed incorporation of patellar tendon allografts versus autografts in a goat model. The differences were observed at 6 months postoperatively.[79] Other studies have supported this conclusion as well.[78,94] In contrast, Nikolaou et al showed allografts and autografts to have similar biomechanical properties at 36 weeks.[110] A higher rerupture rate has also been shown in allograft ACL reconstruction. This rate ranges from 7% to 13%; by comparison, the BPTB autograft rerupture rate ranges from 0% to 5%.[22] Of note, one recent series of 50 ACL reconstructions using cryopreserved grafts had no reruptures at 3- to 5-year follow-up.[77] No cause-and-effect relationship has been established between slower incorporation and higher rerupture rates.

A local immunological response to allograft tissue has been reported after ACL reconstruction.[65] Both humans and animals have displayed this immunological reaction, but no clinical significance has been shown. Widening of the tibial bone tunnel has also been reported, particularly with allografts sterilized with ethylene oxide and with allografts in general.[65] Hoher et al stated that possible causes of tibial tunnel widening were shielding, improper tunnel placement, and aggressive rehabilitation.[74] A recent series showed tibial tunnel widening that was radiographically stable 6 weeks postoperatively, which is similar to the findings of Linn et al, who showed stabilization of tunnel widening.[77,90] Many causes have been proposed, both mechanical and biological, but after a review of the literature, Wilson et al concluded that the etiology remains unknown and is most likely multifactorial.[164] The tunnel widening seen in these studies has not been associated with graft failure or increased laxity, and thus its clinical significance is unclear.

A significant number of allograft ACL reconstructions are being performed and thus several published studies have compared allograft with BPTB autograft. Any conclusions from these comparisons are clouded by the variability in allograft, technique, fixation, and sterilization processes. However, trends may be discernible. At least three separate series have found no significant differences between allograft and autograft.[22,121,140] Harner et al compared 64 allografts with 26 autografts at a 3- to 5-year follow-up and found a trend toward limited knee extension in the autograft patients, but no significant differences.[63] Victor et al found no significant decrease in morbidity at a 2-year follow-up when compared with autograft. However, this study and a series by Stringham et al showed an increased number of reruptured grafts in the allograft group.[150,161]

Allografts provide a viable alternative to autografts, and the aforementioned review shows that comparable results have been achieved with both grafts. The surgeon should be aware of the clinical and basic science literature regarding both grafts. An individual approach to each patient and clinical situation will allow the patient and surgeon to make the most appropriate graft choice.

Fixation

Many types of fixation are available for the femoral as well as the tibial side of an ACL reconstruction. The surgeon must realize that the femur–ACL graft–tibia construct is only as strong as its weakest portion. With advances in the study of properties of the graft and thus the selection of grafts with appropriate biomechanical properties, tibial fixation is now the weakest element.[72,97] Issues to consider when choosing a fixation device include the strength and stiffness that the device provides to the construct, as well as the type of graft being used. The device must provide adequate strength to prevent failure of the construct during the early postoperative period, before biological incorporation of the graft. Adequate stiffness will theoretically prevent excessive motion between the graft and the one tunnel. Finally, the bone-to-bone integration that occurs in BPTB grafts has different fixation requirements than free tendon-to-bone integration does, and this difference between grafts should be considered when choosing a fixation device.

The evolution of BPTB autografts for ACL reconstruction began with Jones' report of using the central third of the patellar tendon in 1963.[83] Investigation of the healing of a bone block in a bone tunnel has progressed, and it has been shown to be reliable in animal studies.[118,154] In a goat model, complete incorporation of the bone block was seen at 6 weeks.[118] Clinical studies have also shown ACL reconstruction with an BPTB autograft to be highly successful.[8,81]

As discussed earlier in the chapter, free tendon grafts, most prominently HS, have gained popularity recently. The healing of free tendons in a bone tunnel is the subject of intense research.[48,118,130] Rodeo et al reported collagen bone connections at 12 weeks postoperatively in a canine model, and Goradia et al examined histology and biomechanical properties and concluded that graft incorporation occurred by 24 weeks. Despite this reportedly longer time to integration in animal models, clinical studies have shown the results of HS autografts to be equivalent to those of BPTB autografts.[3]

FEMUR

Rigid fixation of a bone block in the femoral tunnel is most commonly achieved with interference screws. Kurosaka et al found superior fixation characteristics with the use of an interference screw in a BPTB graft as compared with staples or suture over a button.[86] The screw is typically inserted to the junction of the tendon and bone block, thereby preventing abrasion of the graft by the screw and providing aperture fixation of the graft. The most common diameters are 7 and 8 mm.[97] The angle of insertion of the screw with the bone block has been studied, and greater than 20 degrees of divergence is biomechanically detrimental; however, clinical studies have shown no significant increase in laxity or graft failure.[17] The discussion of interference screws must include biodegradable implants. Biodegradable interference screws are being advocated for fixation of HS grafts and have shown acceptable outcomes.[97] Multiple studies have reported fixation characteristics similar to those of metal implants; therefore, the selection of one over the other should be based on potential complications. Metal screws can distort MRI scans and can be more problematic in the revision setting. A higher incidence of graft laceration has been reported, but some attribute this problem to early screw design.[17] Disadvantages of biodegradable screws include a risk of implant fracture on insertion and unknown biomechanics of fixation as the material degrades.[17,163]

The EndoButton is a suspension-type, extracortical femoral fixation device for HS or BPTB grafts. The metal device is placed on the outer surface of the distal end of the femur and suspends the graft in the bone tunnel via suture or a polyester loop. It can be used for primary ACL reconstruction, or it can address potential complications such as fracture of the posterior femoral tunnel. Disadvantages include lower stiffness and increased graft tunnel motion.[97]

Transfemoral or cross-pin fixation is achieved by insertion of a metal or biodegradable implant into the lateral distal aspect of the femur. Typically a soft-tissue ACL graft is then secured in a suspension-type fixation; however, biodegradable pins have been shown to have adequate biomechanical characteristics when used with BPTB grafts.[171] An example of cross-pin fixation is the TransFix (Arthrex Corp., Naples, FL) device, which is a 3-mm pin secured to the lateral femoral cortex with a 7-mm-wide head. This implant has been shown to have the highest strength and stiffness of any HS femoral fixation device.[11,97]

TIBIA

Interference screw fixation has been advocated in tibial BPTB and soft-tissue grafts and has shown appropriate properties in vitro and good functional results in clinical studies.[23,26] Bone mineral density and insertion torque have been correlated with the ultimate tensile strength of fixation with biodegradable interference screws.[114] This biomechanical finding is supported by clinical data from Hill et al, who found significantly increased laxity in women with biodegradable screws alone versus biodegradable screws and staples for tibial fixation in ACL reconstruction with an HS autograft. The authors concluded that the lower average bone mineral density of females contributed to the findings.[72]

Other tibial fixation systems include a screw and soft-tissue spiked washer, a screw as a post, and four-quadrant tibial graft fasteners. The WasherLoc system (Artrotek, Warsaw, IN), which is a bicortical screw and spiked washer system, has performed well in multiple studies.[26,85,92] Magen et al showed that suture tied to a screw as a post had significantly greater slippage, as did double staples.[92] The four-quadrant tibial fastener (Intrafix, Mitek Products, Norwood, MA) consists of a plastic four-quadrant sheath that is placed in the tibial tunnel with one strand of the HS graft in each quadrant. The central plastic screw is then inserted. This device depends on friction between the plastic sheath and the surrounding cancellous bone for fixation. It was shown to have less slippage and greater strength than a metal interference screw in two separate studies.[85,147]

Conclusion

ACL reconstruction continues to evolve with recent studies in each of the areas of biomechanics, graft type, and fixation methods. The most important step is translating new data into better clinical outcomes for patients. Reliable outcomes measures will be important in future studies to ensure actual improvement in ACL reconstruction.

References

1. Abbott LC, Saunders JB, Bost FC: Injuries to ligaments of the knee joint. J Bone Joint Surg Am 26:503-521, 1944.
2. Adachi N, Ochi M, Uchio Y, et al: Reconstruction of the anterior cruciate ligament. Single- versus double-bundle multistranded hamstring tendons. J Bone Joint Surg Br 86:515-520, 2004.
3. Aglietti P, Giron F, Buzzi R, et al: Anterior cruciate ligament reconstruction: Bone–patellar tendon–bone compared with double semitendinosus and gracilis tendon grafts. A prospective, randomized clinical trial. J Bone Joint Surg Am 86:2143-2155, 2004.
4. Amis AA, Jakob RP: Anterior cruciate ligament graft positioning, tensioning and twisting. Knee Surg Sports Traumatol Arthrosc 6(Suppl 1):S2-S12, 1998.
5. Andersen HN, Dyhre-Poulsen P: The anterior cruciate ligament does play a role in controlling axial rotation in the knee. Knee Surg Sports Traumatol Arthrosc 5:145-149, 1997.
6. Arciero RA, Scoville CR, Snyder RJ, et al: Single versus two-incision arthroscopic anterior cruciate ligament reconstruction. Arthroscopy 12:462-469, 1996.
7. Arendt E, Dick R: Knee injury patterns among men and women in collegiate basketball and soccer. NCAA data and review of literature. Am J Sports Med 23:694-701, 1995.
8. Aune AK, Holm I, Risberg MA, et al: Four-strand hamstring tendon autograft compared with patellar tendon–bone autograft for anterior cruciate ligament reconstruction. A randomized study with two-year follow-up. Am J Sports Med 29:722-728, 2001.
9. Bach BR Jr, Tradonsky S, Bojchuk J, et al: Arthroscopically assisted anterior cruciate ligament reconstruction using patellar tendon autograft. Five- to nine-year follow-up evaluation. Am J Sports Med 26:20-29, 1998.
10. Bartlett RJ, Clatworthy MG, Nguyen TN: Graft selection in reconstruction of the anterior cruciate ligament. J Bone Joint Surg Br 83:625-634, 2001.
11. Becker R, Voigt D, Starke C, et al: Biomechanical properties of quadruple tendon and patellar tendon femoral fixation techniques. Knee Surg Sports Traumatol Arthrosc 9:337-342, 2001.
12. Bergfeld JA, McAllister DR, Parker RD, et al: The effects of tibial rotation on posterior translation in knees in which the posterior cruciate ligament has been cut. J Bone Joint Surg Am 83:1339-1343, 2001.
13. Beynnon BD, Johnson RJ, Fleming BC, et al: Anterior cruciate ligament replacement: Comparison of bone–patellar tendon–bone grafts with two-strand hamstring grafts. A prospective, randomized study. J Bone Joint Surg Am 84:1503-1513, 2002.
14. Beynnon BD, Risberg MA, Tjomsland O, et al: Evaluation of knee joint laxity and the structural properties of the anterior cruciate ligament graft in the human. A case report. Am J Sports Med 25:203-206, 1997.
15. Boylan D, Greis PE, West JR, et al: Effects of initial graft tension on knee stability after anterior cruciate ligament reconstruction using hamstring tendons: A cadaver study. Arthroscopy 19:700-705, 2003.
16. Boynton MD, Tietjens BR: Long-term followup of the untreated isolated posterior cruciate ligament–deficient knee. Am J Sports Med 24:306-310, 1996.
17. Brand J Jr, Weiler A, Caborn DN, et al: Graft fixation in cruciate ligament reconstruction. Am J Sports Med 28:761-774, 2000.
18. Bullis DW, Paulos LE: Reconstruction of the posterior cruciate ligament with allograft. Clin Sports Med 13:581-597, 1994.
19. Burks RT, Leland R: Determination of graft tension before fixation in anterior cruciate ligament reconstruction. Arthroscopy 4:260-266, 1988.
20. Buss DD, Warren RF, Wickiewicz TL, et al: Arthroscopically assisted reconstruction of the anterior cruciate ligament with use of autogenous patellar-ligament grafts. Results after twenty-four to forty-two months. J Bone Joint Surg Am 75:1346-1355, 1993.
21. Butler DL, Noyes FR, Grood ES: Ligamentous restraints to anterior-posterior drawer in the human knee. A biomechanical study. J Bone Joint Surg Am 62:259-270, 1980.
22. Chang SK, Egami DK, Shaieb MD, et al: Anterior cruciate ligament reconstruction: Allograft versus autograft. Arthroscopy 19:453-462, 2003.
23. Charlton WP, Randolph DA Jr, Lemos S, Shields CL Jr: Clinical outcome of anterior cruciate ligament reconstruction with quadrupled hamstring tendon graft and bioabsorbable interference screw fixation. Am J Sports Med 31:518-521, 2003.
24. Clancy WG, Bisson LJ: Double tunnel technique for reconstruction of the posterior cruciate ligament. Op Tech Sports Med 7:110-117, 1999.
25. Clancy WG Jr, Shelbourne KD, Zoellner GB, et al: Treatment of knee joint instability secondary to rupture of the posterior cruciate ligament. Report of a new procedure. J Bone Joint Surg Am 65:310-322, 1983.
26. Coleridge SD, Amis AA: A comparison of five tibial-fixation systems in hamstring-graft anterior cruciate ligament reconstruction. Knee Surg Sports Traumatol Arthrosc 12:391-397, 2004.
27. Cooper DE: Clinical evaluation of posterior cruciate ligament injuries. Sports Med Arthrosc Rev 7:248-252, 1999.
28. Cooper DE, Deng XH, Burstein AL, Warren RF: The strength of the central third patellar tendon graft. A biomechanical study. Am J Sports Med 21:818-823, discussion 823-824, 1993.
29. Cosgarea AJ, Jay PR: Posterior cruciate ligament injuries: Evaluation and management. J Am Acad Orthop Surg 9:297-307, 2001.
30. Covey CD, Sapega AA: Injuries of the posterior cruciate ligament. J Bone Joint Surg Am 75:1376-1386, 1993.
31. Dejour H, Walch G, Peyrot J, Eberhard P: [The natural history of rupture of the posterior cruciate ligament.] Rev Chir Orthop Reparatrice Appar Mot 74:35-43, 1988.
32. Dienst M, Burks RT, Greis PE: Anatomy and biomechanics of the anterior cruciate ligament. Orthop Clin North Am 33:605-620, v, 2002.
33. Eakin CL, Cannon WD Jr: Arthrometric evaluation of posterior cruciate ligament injuries. Am J Sports Med 26:96-102, 1998.
34. Fanelli GC: Posterior cruciate ligament injuries in trauma patients. Arthroscopy 9:291-294, 1993.
35. Fanelli GC, Edson CJ: Posterior cruciate ligament injuries in trauma patients: Part II. Arthroscopy 11:526-529, 1995.
36. Fanelli GC, Giannotti BF, Edson CJ: Arthroscopically assisted combined posterior cruciate ligament/posterior lateral complex reconstruction. Arthroscopy 12:521-530, 1996.
37. Feller JA, Webster KE: A randomized comparison of patellar tendon and hamstring tendon anterior cruciate ligament reconstruction. Am J Sports Med 31:564-573, 2003.
38. Fideler BM, Vangsness CT Jr, Moore T, et al: Effects of gamma irradiation on the human immunodeficiency virus. A study in frozen human bone–patellar ligament–bone grafts obtained from infected cadavera. J Bone Joint Surg Am 76:1032-1035, 1994.
39. Fischer SP, Fox JM, Del Pizzo W, et al: Accuracy of diagnoses from magnetic resonance imaging of the knee. A multi-center analysis of one thousand and fourteen patients. J Bone Joint Surg Am 73:2-10, 1991.
40. Fowler PJ, Messieh SS: Isolated posterior cruciate ligament injuries in athletes. Am J Sports Med 15:553-557, 1987.
41. Frank CB, Jackson DW: The science of reconstruction of the anterior cruciate ligament. J Bone Joint Surg Am 79:1556-1576, 1997.
42. Freedman KB, D'Amato MJ, Nedeff DD, et al: Arthroscopic anterior cruciate ligament reconstruction: A metaanalysis comparing

patellar tendon and hamstring tendon autografts. Am J Sports Med 31:2-11, 2003.

43. Fu FH, Bennett CH, Lattermann C, Ma CB: Current trends in anterior cruciate ligament reconstruction. Part 1: Biology and biomechanics of reconstruction. Am J Sports Med 27:821-830, 1999.

44. Furia JP, Lintner DM, Saiz P, et al: Isometry measurements in the knee with the anterior cruciate ligament intact, sectioned, and reconstructed. Am J Sports Med 25:346-352, 1997.

45. Geissler WB, Whipple TL: Intraarticular abnormalities in association with posterior cruciate ligament injuries. Am J Sports Med 21:846-849, 1993.

46. Girgis FG, Marshall JL, Monajem A: The cruciate ligaments of the knee joint. Anatomical, functional and experimental analysis. Clin Orthop 106:216-231, 1975.

47. Gollehon DL, Torzilli PA, Warren RF: The role of the posterolateral and cruciate ligaments in the stability of the human knee. A biomechanical study. J Bone Joint Surg Am 69:233-242, 1987.

48. Goradia VK, Rochat MC, Grana WA, et al: Tendon-to-bone healing of a semitendinosus tendon autograft used for ACL reconstruction in a sheep model. Am J Knee Surg 13:143-151, 2000.

49. Goradia VK, Rochat MC, Kida M, Grana WA: Natural history of a hamstring tendon autograft used for anterior cruciate ligament reconstruction in a sheep model. Am J Sports Med 28:40-46, 2000.

50. Graham SM, Parker RD: Anterior cruciate ligament reconstruction using hamstring tendon grafts. Clin Orthop 402:64-75, 2002.

51. Grood ES, Stowers SF, Noyes FR: Limits of movement in the human knee. Effect of sectioning the posterior cruciate ligament and posterolateral structures. J Bone Joint Surg Am 70:88-97, 1988.

52. Grover JS, Bassett LW, Gross ML, et al: Posterior cruciate ligament: MR imaging. Radiology 174:527-530, 1990.

53. Gupte CM, Smith A, McDermott ID, et al: Meniscofemoral ligaments revisited. Anatomical study, age correlation and clinical implications. J Bone Joint Surg Br 84:846-851, 2002.

54. Hamada M, Shino K, Horibe S, et al: Single- versus bi-socket anterior cruciate ligament reconstruction using autogenous multiple-stranded hamstring tendons with EndoButton femoral fixation: A prospective study. Arthroscopy 17:801-807, 2001.

55. Hamada M, Shino K, Mitsuoka T, et al: Chondral injury associated with acute isolated posterior cruciate ligament injury. Arthroscopy 16:59-63, 2000.

56. Hame SL, Markolf KL, Hunter DM, et al: Effects of notchplasty and femoral tunnel position on excursion patterns of an anterior cruciate ligament graft. Arthroscopy 19:340-345, 2003.

57. Hamner DL, Brown CH Jr, Steiner ME, et al: Hamstring tendon grafts for reconstruction of the anterior cruciate ligament: Biomechanical evaluation of the use of multiple strands and tensioning techniques. J Bone Joint Surg Am 81:549-557, 1999.

58. Harner CD, Baek GH, Vogrin TM, et al: Quantitative analysis of human cruciate ligament insertions. Arthroscopy 15:741-749, 1999.

59. Harner CD, Hoher J: Evaluation and treatment of posterior cruciate ligament injuries. Am J Sports Med 26:471-482, 1998.

60. Harner CD, Janaushek MA, Kanamori A, et al: Biomechanical analysis of a double-bundle posterior cruciate ligament reconstruction. Am J Sports Med 28:144-151, 2000.

61. Harner CD, Janaushek MA, Ma CB, et al: The effect of knee flexion angle and application of an anterior tibial load at the time of graft fixation on the biomechanics of a posterior cruciate ligament–reconstructed knee. Am J Sports Med 28:460-465, 2000.

62. Harner CD, Livesay GA, Kashiwaguchi S, et al: Comparative study of the size and shape of human anterior and posterior cruciate ligaments. J Orthop Res 13:429-434, 1995.

63. Harner CD, Olson E, Irrgang JJ, et al: Allograft versus autograft anterior cruciate ligament reconstruction: 3- to 5-year outcome. Clin Orthop 324:134-144, 1996.

64. Harner CD, Xerogeanes JW, Livesay GA, et al: The human posterior cruciate ligament complex:. An interdisciplinary study. Ligament morphology and biomechanical evaluation. Am J Sports Med 23:736-745, 1995.

65. Harris NL, Indelicato PA, Bloomberg MS, et al: Radiographic and histologic analysis of the tibial tunnel after allograft anterior cruciate ligament reconstruction in goats. Am J Sports Med 30:368-373, 2002.

66. Hefzy MS, Grood ES: Sensitivity of insertion locations on length patterns of anterior cruciate ligament fibers. J Biomech Eng 108:73-82, 1986.

67. Hefzy MS, Grood ES, Lindenfeld TL: The posterior cruciate ligament: A new look at length patterns. Trans Orthop Res Soc 11:128, 1986.

68. Hefzy MS, Grood ES, Noyes FR: Factors affecting the region of most isometric femoral attachments. Part II: The anterior cruciate ligament. Am J Sports Med 17:208-216, 1989.

69. Heis FT, Paulos LE: Tensioning of the anterior cruciate ligament graft. Orthop Clin North Am 33:697-700, 2002.

70. Heron CW, Calvert PT: Three-dimensional gradient-echo MR imaging of the knee: Comparison with arthroscopy in 100 patients. Radiology 183:839-844, 1992.

71. Hewett TE, Noyes FR, Lee MD: Diagnosis of complete and partial posterior cruciate ligament ruptures. Stress radiography compared with KT-1000 arthrometer and posterior drawer testing. Am J Sports Med 25:648-655, 1997.

72. Hill PF, Russell VJ, Salmon LJ, Pinczewski LA: The influence of supplementary tibial fixation on laxity measurements after anterior cruciate ligament reconstruction with hamstring tendons in female patients. Am J Sports Med 33:94-101, 2005.

73. Hoher J, Harner CD, Vogrin TM, et al: Hamstring loading increases in situ forces in the PCL. Trans Orthop Res Soc 23:48, 1998.

74. Hoher J, Moller HD, Fu FH: Bone tunnel enlargement after anterior cruciate ligament reconstruction: Fact or fiction? Knee Surg Sports Traumatol Arthrosc 6:231-240, 1998.

75. Hollis JM, Takai S, Adams DJ, et al: The effects of knee motion and external loading on the length of the anterior cruciate ligament (ACL): A kinematic study. J Biomech Eng 113:208-214, 1991.

76. Howell SM, Gittins ME, Gottlieb JE, et al: The relationship between the angle of the tibial tunnel in the coronal plane and loss of flexion and anterior laxity after anterior cruciate ligament reconstruction. Am J Sports Med 29:567-574, 2001.

77. Indelli PF, Dillingham MF, Fanton GS, Schurman DJ: Anterior cruciate ligament reconstruction using cryopreserved allografts. Clin Orthop 420:268-275, 2004.

78. Jackson DW, Corsetti J, Simon TM: Biologic incorporation of allograft anterior cruciate ligament replacements. Clin Orthop 324:126-133, 1996.

79. Jackson DW, Grood ES, Goldstein JD, et al: A comparison of patellar tendon autograft and allograft used for anterior cruciate ligament reconstruction in the goat model. Am J Sports Med 21:176-185, 1993.

80. Jackson DW, Windler GE, Simon TM: Intraarticular reaction associated with the use of freeze-dried, ethylene oxide–sterilized bone–patella tendon–bone allografts in the reconstruction of the anterior cruciate ligament. Am J Sports Med 18:1-10, discussion 10-11, 1990.

81. Jansson KA, Linko E, Sandelin J, Harilainen A: A prospective randomized study of patellar versus hamstring tendon autografts for anterior cruciate ligament reconstruction. Am J Sports Med 31:12-18, 2003.

82. Jarrett GJ, Orwin JF, Dick RW: Injuries in collegiate wrestling. Am J Sports Med 26:674-680, 1998.

83. Jones KG: Reconstruction of the anterior cruciate ligament. A technique using the central one-third of the patellar ligament. J Bone Joint Surg Am 45:925-932, 1963.

84. Keller PM, Shelbourne KD, McCarroll JR, Rettig AC: Nonoperatively treated isolated posterior cruciate ligament injuries. Am J Sports Med 21:132-136, 1993.

85. Kousa P, Jarvinen TL, Vihavainen M, et al: The fixation strength of six hamstring tendon graft fixation devices in anterior cruciate ligament reconstruction. Part II: Tibial site. Am J Sports Med 31:182-188, 2003.

86. Kurosaka M, Yoshiya S, Andrish JT: A biomechanical comparison of different surgical techniques of graft fixation in anterior cruciate ligament reconstruction. Am J Sports Med 15:225-229, 1987.

87. Kusayama T, Harner CD, Carlin GJ, et al: Anatomical and biomechanical characteristics of human meniscofemoral ligaments. Knee Surg Sports Traumatol Arthrosc 2:234-237, 1994.

88. Lee HG: Avulsion fracture of the tibial attachment of the cruciate ligaments. J Bone Joint Surg Am 19:460-468, 1937.

89. Levy AS, Wetzler MJ, Lewars M, Laughlin W: Knee injuries in women collegiate rugby players. Am J Sports Med 25:360-362, 1997.

90. Linn RM, Fischer DA, Smith JP, et al: Achilles tendon allograft reconstruction of the anterior cruciate ligament–deficient knee. Am J Sports Med 21:825-831, 1993.

91. Logan M, Dunstan E, Robinson J, et al: Tibiofemoral kinematics of the anterior cruciate ligament (ACL)-deficient weightbearing, living knee employing vertical access open "interventional" multiple resonance imaging. Am J Sports Med 32:720-726, 2004.

92. Magen HE, Howell SM, Hull ML: Structural properties of six tibial fixation methods for anterior cruciate ligament soft tissue grafts. Am J Sports Med 27:35-43, 1999.

93. Makris CA, Georgoulis AD, Papageorgiou CD, et al: Posterior cruciate ligament architecture: Evaluation under microsurgical dissection. Arthroscopy 16:627-632, 2000.

94. Malinin TI, Levitt RL, Bashore C, et al: A study of retrieved allografts used to replace anterior cruciate ligaments. Arthroscopy 18:163-170, 2002.

95. Markolf KL, Hame SL, Hunter DM, et al: Biomechanical effects of femoral notchplasty in anterior cruciate ligament reconstruction. Am J Sports Med 30:83-89, 2002.

96. Markolf KL, Zemanovic JR, McAllister DR: Cyclic loading of posterior cruciate ligament replacements fixed with tibial tunnel and tibial inlay methods. J Bone Joint Surg Am 84:518-524, 2002.

97. Martin SD, Martin TL, Brown CH: Anterior cruciate ligament graft fixation. Orthop Clin North Am 33:685-696, 2002.

98. McAllister DR, Markolf KL, Oakes DA, et al: A biomechanical comparison of tibial inlay and tibial tunnel posterior cruciate ligament reconstruction techniques: Graft pretension and knee laxity. Am J Sports Med 30:312-317, 2002.

99. Mejia EA, Noyes FR, Grood ES: Posterior cruciate ligament femoral insertion site characteristics. Importance for reconstructive procedures. Am J Sports Med 30:643-651, 2002.

100. Meyers MH: Isolated avulsion of the tibial attachment of the posterior cruciate ligament of the knee. J Bone Joint Surg Am 57:669-672, 1975.

101. Miller MD, Gordon WT: Posterior cruciate ligament reconstruction: Tibial inlay technique—principles and procedures. Op Tech Sports Med 7:127-133, 1999.

102. Miller MD, Harner CD, Koshiwaguchi S: Acute posterior cruciate ligament injuries. In Fu FH, Harner CD, Vince KJ (eds): Knee Surgery, vol 1. Baltimore, Williams & Wilkins, 1994, pp 749-767.

103. Miller MD, Kline AJ, Gonzales J, Beach WR: Vascular risk associated with a posterior approach for posterior cruciate ligament reconstruction using the tibial inlay technique. J Knee Surg 15:137-140, 2002.

104. Miller SL, Gladstone JN: Graft selection in anterior cruciate ligament reconstruction. Orthop Clin North Am 33:675-683, 2002.

105. Miyasaka KC, Daniel DM: The incidence of knee ligament injuries in the general population. Am J Knee Surg 4:3-8, 1991.

106. Muneta T, Sekiya I, Yagishita K, et al: Two-bundle reconstruction of the anterior cruciate ligament using semitendinosus tendon with endobuttons: Operative technique and preliminary results. Arthroscopy 15:618-624, 1999.

107. Mykleburst G, Maehlum S, Engebretsen L, et al: Registration of cruciate ligament injuries in Norwegian top level team handball: A prospective study covering two seasons. Scand J Med Sci Sports 7:289-292, 1997.

108. Nielson S, Helmig P: The static stabilizing function of the popliteal tendon in the knee. Arch Orthop Trauma Surg 103:165-169, 1984.

109. Nielson S, Ovesen J, Rasmussen O: The posterior cruciate ligament and rotatory knee instability. Arch Orthop Trauma Surg 104:53-56, 1985.

110. Nikolaou PK, Seaber AV, Glisson RR, et al: Anterior cruciate ligament allograft transplantation. Long-term function, histology, revascularization, and operative technique. Am J Sports Med 14:348-360, 1986.

111. Noyes FR, Barber-Westin SD: Posterior cruciate ligament allograft reconstruction with and without a ligament augmentation device. Arthroscopy 10:371-382, 1994.

112. Noyes FR, Barber-Westin SD: Treatment of complex injuries involving the posterior cruciate and posterolateral ligaments of the knee. Am J Knee Surg 9:200-214, 1996.

113. Noyes FR, Butler DL, Grood ES, et al: Biomechanical analysis of human ligament grafts used in knee-ligament repairs and reconstructions. J Bone Joint Surg Am 66:344-352, 1984.

114. Nyland J, Kocabey Y, Caborn DN: Insertion torque pullout strength relationship of soft tissue tendon graft tibia tunnel fixation with a bioabsorbable interference screw. Arthroscopy 20:379-384, 2004.

115. Oakes DA, Markolf KL, McWilliams J, et al: Biomechanical comparison of tibial inlay and tibial tunnel techniques for reconstruction of the posterior cruciate ligament. Analysis of graft forces. J Bone Joint Surg Am 84:938-944, 2002.

116. Owens TC: Posteromedial pivot shift of the knee: A new test for rupture of the posterior cruciate ligament. A demonstration in six patients and a study of anatomical specimens. J Bone Joint Surg Am 76:532-539, 1994.

117. Papageorgiou CD, Gil JE, Kanamori A, et al: The biomechanical interdependence between the anterior cruciate ligament replacement graft and the medial meniscus. Am J Sports Med 29:226-231, 2001.

118. Papageorgiou CD, Ma CB, Abramowitch SD, et al: A multidisciplinary study of the healing of an intraarticular anterior cruciate ligament graft in a goat model. Am J Sports Med 29:620-626, 2001.

119. Parolie JM, Bergfeld JA: Long-term results of nonoperative treatment of isolated posterior cruciate ligament injuries in the athlete. Am J Sports Med 14:35-38, 1986.

120. Pearsall AW 4th, Hollis JM, Russell GV Jr, Scheer Z: A biomechanical comparison of three lower extremity tendons for ligamentous reconstruction about the knee. Arthroscopy 19:1091-1096, 2003.

121. Peterson RK, Shelton WR, Bomboy AL: Allograft versus autograft patellar tendon anterior cruciate ligament reconstruction: A 5-year follow-up. Arthroscopy 17:9-13, 2001.

122. Petrie RS, Harner CD: Evaluation and management of the posterior cruciate injured knee. Op Tech Sports Med 7:93-103, 1999.

123. Polly DW Jr, Callaghan JJ, Sikes RA, et al: The accuracy of selective magnetic resonance imaging compared with the findings of arthroscopy of the knee. J Bone Joint Surg Am 70:192-198, 1988.

124. Prietto MP, Bain J, Stonebrook S, et al: Tensile strength of the human posterior cruciate ligament. Trans Orthop Res Soc 13:195, 1988.

125. Race A, Amis AA: The mechanical properties of the two bundles of the human posterior cruciate ligament. J Biomech 27:13-24, 1994.

126. Renstrom P, Arms SW, Stanwyck TS, et al: Strain within the anterior cruciate ligament during hamstring and quadriceps activity. Am J Sports Med 14:83-87, 1986.

127. Richter M, Kiefer H, Hehl G, Kinzl L: Primary repair for posterior cruciate ligament injuries. An eight-year followup of fifty-three patients. Am J Sports Med 24:298-305, 1996.

128. Ritchie JR, Bergfeld JA, Kambic H, Manning, T: Isolated sectioning of the medial and posteromedial capsular ligaments in the posterior cruciate ligament–deficient knee. Influence on posterior tibial translation. Am J Sports Med 26:389-394, 1998.

129. Roberts TS, Drez D Jr, McCarthy W, Paine R: Anterior cruciate ligament reconstruction using freeze-dried, ethylene oxide–sterilized, bone–patellar tendon–bone allografts. Two year results in thirty-six patients. Am J Sports Med 19:35-41, 1991.

130. Rodeo SA, Arnoczky SP, Torzilli PA, et al: Tendon-healing in a bone tunnel. A biomechanical and histological study in the dog. J Bone Joint Surg Am 75:1795-1803, 1993.

131. Roman PD, Hopson CN, Zenni EJ Jr: Traumatic dislocation of the knee: A report of 30 cases and literature review. Orthop Rev 16:917-924, 1987.

132. Rougraff B, Shelbourne KD, Gerth PK, Warner J: Arthroscopic and histologic analysis of human patellar tendon autografts used for anterior cruciate ligament reconstruction. Am J Sports Med 21:277-284, 1993.

133. Sakane M, Fox RJ, Woo SL, et al: In situ forces in the anterior cruciate ligament and its bundles in response to anterior tibial loads. J Orthop Res 15:285-293, 1997.

134. Sakane M, Livesay GA, Fox RJ, et al: Relative contribution of the ACL, MCL, and bony contact to the anterior stability of the knee. Knee Surg Sports Traumatol Arthrosc 7:93-97, 1999.

135. Satku K, Chew CN, Seow H: Posterior cruciate ligament injuries. Acta Orthop Scand 55:26-29, 1984.

136. Schatzmann L, Brunner P, Staubli HU: Effect of cyclic preconditioning on the tensile properties of human quadriceps tendons and patellar ligaments. Knee Surg Sports Traumatol Arthrosc 6(Suppl 1):S56-S61, 1998.
137. Scopp JM, Jasper LE, Belkoff SM, Moorman CT 3rd: The effect of oblique femoral tunnel placement on rotational constraint of the knee reconstructed using patellar tendon autografts. Arthroscopy 20:294-299, 2004.
138. Segawa H, Omori G, Koga Y, et al: Rotational muscle strength of the limb after anterior cruciate ligament reconstruction using semitendinosus and gracilis tendon. Arthroscopy 18:177-182, 2002.
139. Shelbourne KD, Davis TJ, Patel DV: The natural history of acute, isolated, nonoperatively treated posterior cruciate ligament injuries. A prospective study. Am J Sports Med 27:276-283, 1999.
140. Shelton WR, Papendick L, Dukes AD: Autograft versus allograft anterior cruciate ligament reconstruction. Arthroscopy 13:446-449, 1997.
141. Sherman OH, Banffy MB: Anterior cruciate ligament reconstruction: Which graft is best? Arthroscopy 20:974-980, 2004.
142. Shino K, Oakes BW, Horibe S, et al: Collagen fibril populations in human anterior cruciate ligament allografts. Electron microscopic analysis. Am J Sports Med 23:203-208, discussion 209, 1995.
143. Simmons R, Howell SM, Hull ML: Effect of the angle of the femoral and tibial tunnels in the coronal plane and incremental excision of the posterior cruciate ligament on tension of an anterior cruciate ligament graft: An in vitro study. J Bone Joint Surg Am 85:1018-1029, 2003.
144. Sisto DJ, Warren RF: Complete knee dislocation. A follow-up study of operative treatment. Clin Orthop 198:94-101, 1985.
145. Skyhar MJ, Warren RF, Ortiz GJ, et al: The effects of sectioning of the posterior cruciate ligament and the posterolateral complex on the articular contact pressures within the knee. J Bone Joint Surg Am 75:694-699, 1993.
146. Sommer C, Friederich NF, Muller W: Improperly placed anterior cruciate ligament grafts: Correlation between radiological parameters and clinical results. Knee Surg Sports Traumatol Arthrosc 8:207-213, 2000.
147. Starch DW, Alexander JW, Noble PC, et al: Multistranded hamstring tendon graft fixation with a central four-quadrant or a standard tibial interference screw for anterior cruciate ligament reconstruction. Am J Sports Med 31:338-344, 2003.
148. Staubli HU, Schatzmann L, Brunner P, et al: Quadriceps tendon and patellar ligament: Cryosectional anatomy and structural properties in young adults. Knee Surg Sports Traumatol Arthrosc 4:100-110, 1996.
149. Staubli HU, Schatzmann L, Brunner P, et al: Mechanical tensile properties of the quadriceps tendon and patellar ligament in young adults. Am J Sports Med 27:27-34, 1999.
150. Stringham DR, Pelmas CJ, Burks RT, et al: Comparison of anterior cruciate ligament reconstructions using patellar tendon autograft or allograft. Arthroscopy 12:414-421, 1996.
151. Takai S, Woo SL, Livesay GA, et al: Determination of the in situ loads on the human anterior cruciate ligament. J Orthop Res 11:686-695, 1993.
152. Tashiro T, Kurosawa H, Kawakami A, et al: Influence of medial hamstring tendon harvest on knee flexor strength after anterior cruciate ligament reconstruction. A detailed evaluation with comparison of single- and double-tendon harvest. Am J Sports Med 31:522-529, 2003.
153. Tashman S, Collon D, Anderson K, et al: Abnormal rotational knee motion during running after anterior cruciate ligament reconstruction. Am J Sports Med 32:975-983, 2004.
154. Tomita F, Yasuda K, Mikami S, et al: Comparisons of intraosseous graft healing between the doubled flexor tendon graft and the bone–patellar tendon–bone graft in anterior cruciate ligament reconstruction. Arthroscopy 17:461-476, 2001.
155. Torg JS, Barton TM, Pavlov H, Stine R: Natural history of the posterior cruciate ligament–deficient knee. Clin Orthop 246: 208-216, 1989.
156. Turner DA, Prodromos CC, Petasnick JP, Clark JW: Acute injury of the ligaments of the knee: Magnetic resonance evaluation. Radiology 154:717-722, 1985.
157. Van Dommelen BA, Fowler PJ: Anatomy of the posterior cruciate ligament. A review. Am J Sports Med 17:24-29, 1989.
158. Vangsness CT Jr, Garcia IA, Mills CR, et al: Allograft transplantation in the knee: Tissue regulation, procurement, processing, and sterilization. Am J Sports Med 31:474-481, 2003.
159. Veltri DM, Deng XH, Torzilli PA, et al: The role of the cruciate and posterolateral ligaments in stability of the knee. A biomechanical study. Am J Sports Med 23:436-443, 1995.
160. Veltri DM, Warren RF: Isolated and combined posterior cruciate ligament injuries. J Am Acad Orthop Surg 1:67-75, 1993.
161. Victor J, Bellemans J, Witvrouw E, et al: Graft selection in anterior cruciate ligament reconstruction—prospective analysis of patellar tendon autografts compared with allografts. Int Orthop 21:93-97, 1997.
162. Viola RW, Sterett WI, Newfield D, et al: Internal and external tibial rotation strength after anterior cruciate ligament reconstruction using ipsilateral semitendinosus and gracilis tendon autografts. Am J Sports Med 28:552-555, 2000.
163. Weiler A, Windhagen HJ, Raschke MJ, et al: Biodegradable interference screw fixation exhibits pull-out force and stiffness similar to titanium screws. Am J Sports Med 26:119-126, 1998.
164. Wilson TC, Kantaras A, Atay A, Johnson DL: Tunnel enlargement after anterior cruciate ligament surgery. Am J Sports Med 32:543-549, 2004.
165. Wilson TW, Zafuta MP, Zobitz M: A biomechanical analysis of matched bone–patellar tendon–bone and double-looped semitendinosus and gracilis tendon grafts. Am J Sports Med 27:202-207, 1999.
166. Woo SL, Hollis JM, Adams DJ, et al: Tensile properties of the human femur–anterior cruciate ligament–tibia complex. The effects of specimen age and orientation. Am J Sports Med 19:217-225, 1991.
167. Wren TA, Yerby SA, Beaupre GS, Carter DR: Mechanical properties of the human Achilles tendon. Clin Biomech (Bristol, Avon) 16:245-251, 2001.
168. Yagi M, Wong EK, Kanamori A, et al: Biomechanical analysis of an anatomic anterior cruciate ligament reconstruction. Am J Sports Med 30:660-666, 2002.
169. Yasuda K, Tsujino J, Tanabe Y, Kaneda K: Effects of initial graft tension on clinical outcome after anterior cruciate ligament reconstruction. Autogenous doubled hamstring tendons connected in series with polyester tapes. Am J Sports Med 25:99-106, 1997.
170. Yunes M, Richmond JC, Engels EA, Pinczewski LA: Patellar versus hamstring tendons in anterior cruciate ligament reconstruction: A meta-analysis. Arthroscopy 17:248-257, 2001.
171. Zantop T, Welbers B, Weimann A, et al: Biomechanical evaluation of a new cross-pin technique for the fixation of different sized bone–patellar tendon–bone grafts. Knee Surg Sports Traumatol Arthrosc 12:520-527, 2004.
172. Zavras TD, Race A, Bull AM, Amis AA: A comparative study of "isometric" points for anterior cruciate ligament graft attachment. Knee Surg Sports Traumatol Arthrosc 9:28-33, 2001.

CHAPTER 11

Understanding Knee Arthroplasty Kinematics: News You Can Use

Scott A. Banks

Radiographic imaging and shape-matching techniques have been used since the late 1980s to quantify the motions of knee replacements in vivo. These studies have shown how knee implants move in vivo, how implant design affects knee kinematics, and how different surgical and design factors influence knee mechanics and patient function. In general, knee implants that definitively control the anteroposterior (AP) position of the femur with respect to the tibia achieve greater weightbearing flexion and exhibit kinematics that are more likely to result in better patient function and implant longevity.

THREE-DIMENSIONAL KINEMATICS FROM TWO-DIMENSIONAL IMAGES

By the late 1980s, total knee arthroplasty (TKA) had become a fairly routine procedure for the treatment of severe knee arthritis. A wide variety of implant designs were being used with predictable success and reasonable durability. The focus of designers was shifting from basic knee function and implant fixation to improvement in knee performance and implant longevity. In part, what was needed to continue evolving knee replacements was more precise information on how knee replacements moved once implanted. Unfortunately, the gait laboratories and computed tomography (CT) scanners of the day could not provide accurate three-dimensional kinematic information of knee replacement motion during weightbearing dynamic activities.

In 1988, my surgeon colleague W. Andrew Hodge and I set out to develop a better method for measuring knee arthroplasty kinematics. Having failed to use the gait laboratory motion capture system to accurately measure implant motion, Hodge suggested that we should directly image the joint with x-ray fluoroscopy and develop an image-based measurement technique. I developed a "shape-matching"–based measurement approach that worked well,[1,3] and this technique and evolved forms have been used since to provide a better understanding of knee replacement function.

The details of shape-matching–based motion measurement are beyond the scope of this volume, but the process follows logically: radiographic images are produced when x-rays pass through space and are attenuated by the patient's anatomy before striking a sensitive medium and causing a chemical or electrical reaction. The x-ray beam emanates from a single point in space with rays diverging in all directions to create a perspective projection of the object—in essence a shadow (Fig. 11–1). The location of the x-ray source with respect to the image plane can be measured so that the same projection can be reproduced on a computer. Computer-aided design information is available for knee implant components, and bone surfaces can be reconstructed from CT or magnetic resonance imaging (Fig. 11–2), thus making it a simple process to synthesize on the computer images of implants at any possible position. These synthetic views can be iteratively modified until they match the views obtained from patients. Once matched, the positions and orientations of the models represent the physical position and orientation of the patients' implants that created the radiographic projection.

Many groups the world over have used shape-matching techniques for determining implant motion from single-plane radiographic views and have studied a range of activities, including gait,[12] stair climbing,[13] and deep knee bends.[19] Although details of the methods vary, measurement precision for each moving segment is typically 0.5 to 1.0 mm for implant motions parallel to the image plane and 0.5 to 1.0 degree for rotations. Importantly, this is monocular vision, not stereo or binocular, and all these techniques have much reduced accuracy for determining translation perpendicular to the image plane, where precision is typically 3.0 to 6.0 mm. Propagating these measurement errors to the articular surfaces, one can typically expect measurement uncertainties of greater than 1.2 mm for single observations of condylar contact or separation.

POSITIONAL FINDINGS

Findings from image-based TKA studies can be organized into positional and dynamic observations. Positional observations relate closely to how implant design and surgical alignment influence articular contact and knee function at the extreme ranges of motion.

Knee implants are typically designed to maximize the tibiofemoral contact area with the knee in extension and to accommodate 10 to 15 degrees of hyperextension. Implant wear testing is performed such that the implants reach 0 degrees relative flexion at simulated early stance. Yet neither context takes into account the fact that surgical alignment may place the implants in positions that differ from 0 degrees relative flexion. Femoral components implanted with intramedullary rods or extramedullary

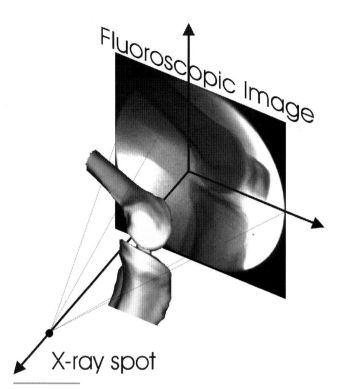

Figure 11–1. Fluoroscopic and radiographic projections are created by a spot source of rays so that the image is a "perspective" projection, or shadow, that is a three-dimensional function of the projection geometry and the position and orientation of the bones. This geometry allows three-dimensional kinematics to be derived from sequences of two-dimensional radiographic images.

techniques are aligned to the distal femur. The anterior bow of the femoral shaft results in the femoral implant component being flexed forward in the sagittal plane by 5 to 7 degrees. Similarly, tibial implant techniques range from alignment perpendicular to the long axis of the tibia to alignment matching the normal posterior slope of the tibial plateau. The net result of typical surgical placement is that the implants are in 5 to 12 degrees of relative hyperextension. Simultaneous measurements of skeletal flexion using goniometry or motion capture (Fig. 11–3) and implant flexion using fluoroscopy have shown an average

of 9.5 degrees implant hyperextension when compared with the skeletal flexion angle.[2]

This simple and intuitive observation has at least three important ramifications. First, implants that have hyperextension stops will probably experience much greater contact and possible wear than the designers anticipated.[2,11] Posterior-stabilized designs with tibial posts and some posterior cruciate ligament (PCL)-retaining designs accommodate limited hyperextension, often 5 to 15 degrees. With the implants routinely placed in almost 10 degrees of hyperextension at 0 degrees knee flexion, many of these designs will experience anterior impingement during routine activity. Second, standard evaluations of TKA designs, whether by computer or machine, do not account for implant alignment. The evaluations assume that the straight leg corresponds to 0 degrees of implant flexion. Given that many designs have surfaces with changing curvatures in early flexion, it is possible that these tests will predict performance differing from the clinical experience. Third, implant features designed to guide implant motions at particular flexion angles will engage later in the flexion arc. Post and cam mechanisms in posterior-stabilized knees will engage at approximately 10 degrees greater anatomic flexion than anticipated by the design. In very deep flexion, there is some concern that the proximal "edge" of the femoral condyles (where the articular and bone-cut surfaces meet) will dig into the tibial articular surface. Normal implant alignment means that this phenomenon will occur 10 degrees later in the flexion arc, if at all.

Fluoroscopic evaluations have elucidated the mechanics of TKAs in deeply flexed postures. It has long been assumed that greater posterior femoral translation on the tibia permits greater knee flexion.[29] In a study of 16 different TKA designs in patients with excellent clinical outcomes, there was a significant linear relationship between the amount of posterior femoral translation and maximum weightbearing flexion.[9] This relationship, 1.4 degrees greater flexion for each additional millimeter of posterior femoral translation, held true for all types of TKA design (Fig. 11–4). Implant designs that definitively controlled tibiofemoral position in flexion achieved greater femoral "rollback" and demonstrated greater weightbearing flexion than did designs that required the

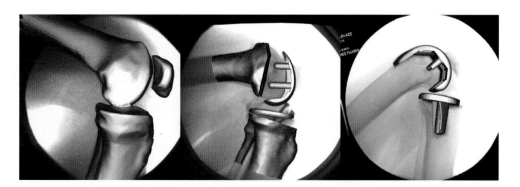

Figure 11–2. Three-dimensional measurement of dynamic knee motion using fluoroscopy and shape-matching techniques has been performed for natural knees *(left)*, knees with partial arthroplasty *(middle)*, and knees with total arthroplasty *(right)*. The bone surface models can be created from computed tomographic and magnetic resonance imaging scans, and the implant models are obtained from the manufacturer or three-dimensional laser scans.

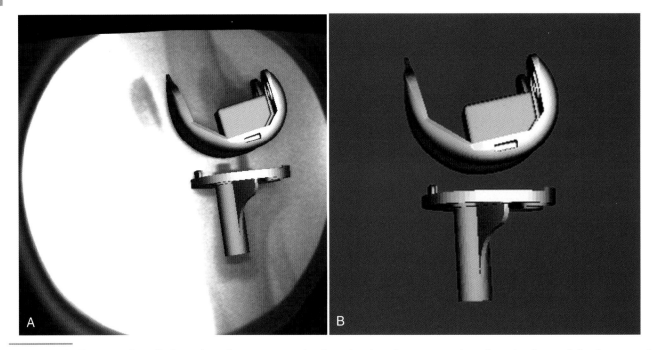

Figure 11–3. Knees with well-aligned implants commonly show implant hyperextension. Anterior bow of the femur and posterior slope of the tibial plateau bias implant alignment by an average of 10 degrees hyperextension. Thus, when the knee is fully extended at toe-off during gait (**A**), the implants are in hyperextension (**B**).

soft tissues and muscles to control tibiofemoral position. These findings suggest that the flexion space, particularly in PCL-retaining TKA, ought not to be made too loose because the additional laxity may allow unwanted anterior translation of the femur and a concomitant decrease in maximum weightbearing flexion.

Similar analyses have demonstrated the importance of posterior condylar geometry on knee flexion range. Bellemans et al[10] showed a significant linear relationship between changes in the posterior condylar offset, or the maximum AP distance from the femoral shaft to the most posterior point on the condyles, and changes in passive range of motion. They found that reducing the posterior condylar offset by 1 mm from its anatomic value decreased passive range of motion by 6 degrees (Fig. 11–5). This finding is particularly relevant for surgeons using anterior referencing instrumentation: when a knee measures

in-between component sizes, common practice argues for selecting the smaller component. This will typically reduce the anatomic posterior condylar offset by several millimeters and thus potentially reduce the flexion range by 10 degrees or more! Using the larger femoral component, when possible, or adjusting the position of the smaller femoral component can reduce the effect on the posterior condylar offset and provide the patient with the best possible range of motion.

DYNAMIC CHARACTERISTICS

Early fluoroscopic studies of TKA kinematics demonstrated that dynamic motions could differ markedly from those of a normal knee.[8] These and subsequent studies

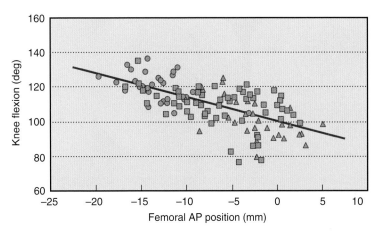

Figure 11–4. Maximum weightbearing knee flexion as a function of femoral anteroposterior (AP) position for 121 knees. Femoral posterior positions are negative, anterior is positive, and zero represents the AP midpoint of the tibial component. *Circles* represent posterior-stabilized knees; *asterisks* represent posterior cruciate–retaining, fixed-bearing knees; and *triangles* represent mobile-bearing knees. The *solid line* shows the linear regression with a slope of 1.4 degrees more flexion per millimeter femoral posterior translation ($r = 0.64$, $p < 0.001$). (From Banks SA, Bellemans J, Nozaki H, et al: Tibio-femoral translation and maximum weight-bearing flexion in fixed and mobile bearing knee arthroplasties. Clin Orthop 410:131-138, 2003.)

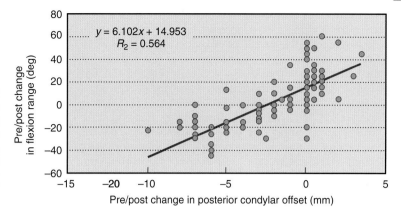

Figure 11–5. Correlation of restoration of posterior condylar offset (postoperative minus preoperative) with postoperative flexion gain (+)/loss (−) for 150 consecutive knees. Overlapping points are not shown. (From Bellemans J, Banks SA, Victor J, et al: Fluoroscopic analysis of deep flexion kinematics in total knee arthroplasty: The influence of posterior condylar offset. J Bone Joint Surg Br 84:50-53, 2002.)

showed that in knees lacking the anterior cruciate ligament and menisci, there is a tendency for the femur to slide forward on the tibia with flexion and backward with extension. However, tibial rotations were normal, with the tibia rotating inward with flexion. A simple method to quantify these translations and rotations is to consider the average center of rotation: in a healthy knee, posterior translation of the femur and internal rotation of the tibia with flexion result in a medial center of rotation. The lateral condyle moves posterior with flexion about a relatively stationary medial condylar position. In unconstrained TKA, the medial condyle is observed to slide forward with flexion about a relatively stationary lateral condylar position. Thus, a lateral center of rotation has been observed in unconstrained TKA designs. An analysis of stair-climbing motions in 25 different TKA designs showed a significant relationship between the intrinsic constraints of the implant and the average center of rota-

tion (Fig. 11–6): designs with greater intrinsic control had central or medial centers of rotation, whereas up to 86% of unconstrained devices had lateral centers of rotation.[4] This analysis included only patients with high satisfaction and excellent clinical scores and showed that a wide range of knee motion patterns are compatible with good clinical results. Hence, implant designers and surgeons may have wide latitude to modulate knee motion patterns to achieve further improvement in patient strength, range of motion, and implant longevity.

Fluoroscopic studies of TKA kinematics comparing different activities have shown that TKA motions can vary dramatically depending on the activity and implant design.[5] Many implant designs have articular surfaces with varying curvatures or mechanisms that engage at different parts of the flexion arc. Intuitively, these changing constraints might result in different kinematic patterns depending on the flexion range of the activity. Conversely,

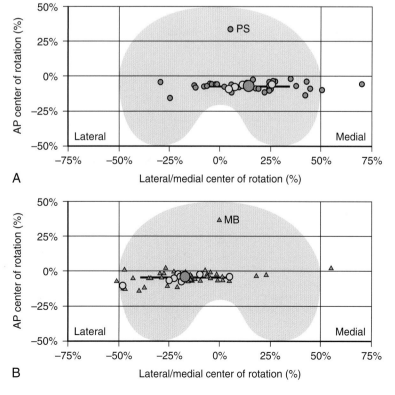

Figure 11–6. The average center of rotation is strongly influenced by the intrinsic constraints of the implant design for stair step activities. Posterior-stabilized knees, which force the femur posterior on the tibia with flexion, mostly show medial centers of rotation (A). Gait-congruent, mobile-bearing knee designs allow relatively free anteroposterior translation of the femur in flexion, with most knees showing a lateral center of rotation (B). Each red circle and red triangle represents the center of rotation in one knee; the blue circles represent the average center of rotation for a specific implant design, and the large purple circle represents the average center of rotation for all knees of that type. (From Banks SA, Hodge WA: Implant design affects knee arthroplasty kinematics during stair-stepping. Clin Orthop 426:187-193, 2004.)

implant designs with consistent intrinsic constraint over the flexion arc might be expected to show similar motion patterns across the range of activities. Comparison of TKA motions during the stance phase of gait and during stair activities confirms these concepts (Fig. 11–7). For example, posterior-stabilized, fixed-bearing TKA designs consistently showed more medial centers of rotation during stair activities than during gait (Fig. 11–7A). During stair climbing, the post-cam mechanism controls motion and forces posterior femoral translation with flexion. During gait, the post-cam mechanism is not engaged and the femur tends to slide posterior with *exten-*sion, more so on the medial side. The opposite situation is observed in rotating platform, mobile-bearing knees with gait-congruent articulations (Fig. 11–7B). During gait, the tibiofemoral articulation is fully conforming and allows only axial rotation with flexion/extension. Stair climbing flexes the knee beyond the range of tibiofemoral congruency, and the femur slides forward on the tibia with flexion, more on the medial side. Implants with condyles that have the same sagittal radius from 0 to 75 degrees flexion and correspondingly consistent tibiofemoral constraint did exhibit similar motion for the gait and stair activities (Fig. 11–7C).

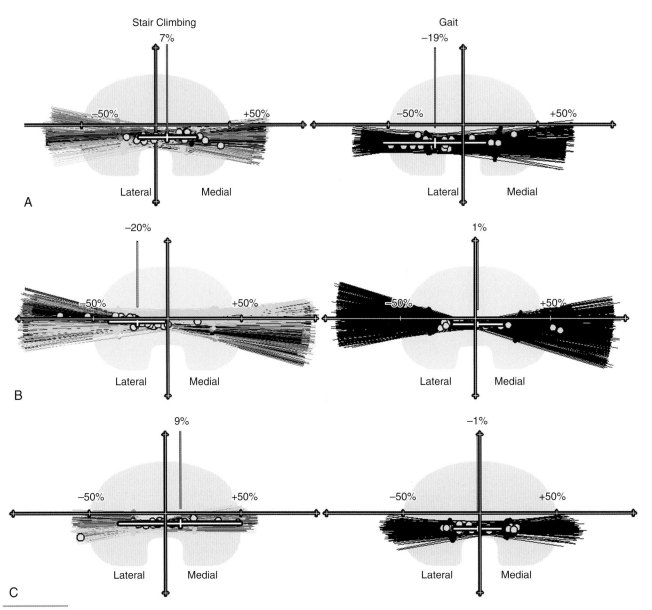

Figure 11–7. Patterns of knee motion vary with activity and implant design. **A**, Sagittally unconstrained, posterior-stabilized knees show a medial center of rotation during stair-climbing activities *(left)*, but greater femoral sliding and a lateral center of rotation during the stance phase of gait. **B**, Gait-congruent, rotating platform mobile-bearing knees show anterior sliding of the femur in flexion during stair activities and a lateral center of rotation, but they are constrained to pure internal/external tibial rotation with flexion during the stance phase of gait *(right)*. **C**, Knees that maintain similar conformity over the flexion range show more similar knee motion patterns for the gait and stair activities. Each *line* represents the location and orientation of the femoral condyles with respect to the tibial plateau for all frames of data for a group of subjects. The *gray dots* indicate the average center of rotation for a single motion trial, and the *white cross* indicates the mean and standard deviation for the group average center of rotation.

OTHER APPLICATIONS FOR IN VIVO DATA

In vivo kinematic data are unquestionably useful for understanding the interplay of implant design and surgical factors in TKA performance. In addition, these data provide important corroboration or guidance for other studies. For example, interpretation of wear patterns on retrieved tibial inserts is greatly enhanced with knowledge of that particular implant's in vivo kinematics.[18] In vivo kinematics can be used to implement increasingly realistic and more powerfully predictive mechanical wear tests. With advanced computer codes, it is now possible to input in vivo kinematics and make reasonably accurate predictions of that implant's wear performance over its service life.[14]

CONCLUSION

Fluoroscopy has provided a unique window for direct observation and measurement of dynamic knee replacement motions. Shape-matching–based measurements are a powerful tool for accurately quantifying knee motions, and they provide informative characterization of implant design and surgical factors that influence patient outcomes. In addition to providing an enhanced understanding of implant design and surgical issues, these in vivo data are a useful complement to retrieval studies, gait laboratory analyses, and computer simulations.

NEWS YOU CAN USE

1. *Surgical technique matters.* Surgical balancing of the ligaments and soft tissues can have a significant effect on weightbearing knee kinematics, particularly in unconstrained arthroplasty designs.[23] When using unconstrained tibiofemoral articulations, the surgeon has the opportunity to restore near-physiological knee motion. However, many kinematic studies of unconstrained devices demonstrate abnormal knee motions wherein the femur slides forward with flexion instead of moving backward with flexion.[2,6,7,10,25-28]

2. *Axial rotation range is maintained in healthy, reconstructed, unicondylar, and total knee arthroplasties of many types.* The total amount of tibial internal/external rotation appears to be maintained after ligament reconstruction or arthroplasty. However, the specific pattern of rotation can change with reconstruction. Knees generally exhibit tibial internal rotation with early flexion, approximately 5 degrees in the stance phase of gait and 8 degrees during stair climbing.[5] These ranges of rotation are similar for healthy and reconstructed knees.[20] At a minimum, new surgical techniques or knee replacements ought to provide for these ranges of axial rotation.

3. *Axial rotation is activity dependent, not obligatory, with total knee replacements in deep flexion postures.* With TKA, early tibial rotation with flexion does not necessarily continue into deeply flexed postures, and achieving high flexion is not correlated to the amount of axial rotation. Different high-flexion postures, such as squatting, kneeling, or lunging, show rotations more closely related to the body position than to the degree of flexion achieved.[9,19] This situation may differ considerably from an intact normal knee.

4. *Restoring normal posterior condylar geometry permits greater maximum knee flexion.* Normal posterior condylar geometry elevates the femoral cortex with respect to the tibia to allow deep flexion without impingement. When this posterior condylar offset is diminished during arthroplasty, posterior impingement can occur earlier in the flexion arc and block full flexion potential.[10] Reduced condylar offset can also provide greater laxity in flexion and allow the femur to translate forward in flexion—likewise reducing flexion potential.

5. *A posterior femoral position enhances maximum weightbearing flexion.* Knee arthroplasties that achieve a relatively posterior position of the femur on the tibia exhibit greater maximum weightbearing flexion.[9] Arthroplasty designs with definitive control of tibiofemoral translation, through either conforming tibial surfaces or PCL substitution, maintain a more posterior position of the femur on the tibia in flexion. For patients desiring lifestyles involving deeply flexed postures, the surgeon might consider arthroplasty designs or modular tibial inserts that provide enhanced control of the tibiofemoral position in flexion.

6. *With normal surgical alignment, implant components are biased toward hyperextension.* Anterior bowing of the femur and posterior slope of the tibial plateau cause arthroplasty components to have approximately 10 degrees of hyperextension with neutral surgical alignment.[2] This often places components close to the design limit for allowable hyperextension and thus accounts for the very common observation of anterior impingement damage on many types of retrieved knee arthroplasty components.[2,11,15,16,18,21,22,24] Posterior translation of the femur with knee extension exacerbates anterior impingement. Anterior impingement damage is commonly observed in retrieved posterior-stabilized knees with post/cam stabilization. Surgeons using this type of arthroplasty should know and take into account the allowable hyperextension range during component alignment.

7. *The center of rotation in the knee can be changed by varying articular constraints.* Kinematic studies of clinically successful knee arthroplasties during a variety of activities demonstrate a wide range of motion patterns. Unconstrained arthroplasties with either translating, mobile-bearing or flat, fixed-bearing tibial inserts show a lateral center of rotation wherein the medial condyle moves forward with flexion. This center of rotation, or the AP movement of the femur, can be modulated by changing

tibiofemoral conformity or the AP constraints in the knee.[5,17,27,28] By knowing how tibiofemoral motions are modulated throughout the functional range of motion, one can develop better expectations for patient and device performance.

References

1. Banks SA: Model Based 3D Kinematic Estimation from 2D Perspective Silhouettes: Application with Total Knee Prostheses [doctoral dissertation]. Cambridge, MA, Massachusetts Institute of Technology, 1992.
2. Banks SA, Harman MK, Hodge WA: The mechanism of anterior impingement damage in total knee replacement. J Bone Joint Surg Am 84(Suppl 2):37-42, 2002.
3. Banks SA, Hodge WA: Accurate measurement of three-dimensional knee replacement kinematics using single-plane fluoroscopy. IEEE Trans Biomed Eng 43:638-649, 1996.
4. Banks SA, Hodge WA: Implant design affects knee arthroplasty kinematics during stair-stepping. Clin Orthop 426:187-193, 2004.
5. Banks SA, Hodge WA: Design and activity dependence of kinematics in fixed and mobile bearing knee arthroplasties—the Hap Paul Award Paper. J Arthroplasty 19:809-816, 2004.
6. Banks SA, Markovich GD, Hodge WA: The mechanics of knee replacements during gait. In vivo fluoroscopic analysis of two designs. Am J Knee Surg 10:261-267, 1997.
7. Banks SA, Markovich GD, Hodge WA: In vivo kinematics of cruciate-retaining and -substituting knee arthroplasties. J Arthroplasty 12:297-304, 1997.
8. Banks SA, Riley PO, Spector C, et al: In vivo bearing motion with meniscal bearing TKR. Orthop Trans 15:544, 1991.
9. Banks SA, Bellemans J, Nozaki H, et al: Tibio-femoral translation and maximum weight-bearing flexion in fixed and mobile bearing knee arthroplasties. Clin Orthop 410:131-138, 2003.
10. Bellemans J, Banks S, Victor J, et al: Fluoroscopic analysis of the kinematics of deep flexion in total knee arthroplasty. Influence of posterior condylar offset. J Bone Joint Surg Br 84:50-53, 2002.
11. Callaghan JJ, O'Rourke MR, Goetz DD, et al: Tibial post impingement in posterior-stabilized total knee arthroplasty. Clin Orthop 404:83-88, 2002.
12. Dennis DA, Komistek RD, Mahfouz MR: In vivo fluoroscopic analysis of fixed-bearing total knee replacements. Clin Orthop 410:114-130, 2003.
13. Fantozzi S, Benedetti MG, Leardini A, et al: Fluoroscopic and gait analysis of the functional performance in stair ascent of two total knee replacement designs. Gait Posture 17:225-234, 2003.
14. Fregly BJ, Sawyer WG, Harman MK, Banks SA: Computational wear prediction of a total knee replacement from in vivo kinematics. J Biomech 38:305-314, 2005.
15. Furman BD, Gillis AM, Schmieg JJ, et al: Wear and damage to the post in posterior stabilized total knee replacements: An unexpected source of polyethylene debris. Trans Soc Biomaterials 22:476, 1999.
16. Gillis AM, Furman B, Schmieg J, et al: The effect of post impingement in posterior stabilized total knee replacements on femoral rotation and damaged area as determined from analysis of retrieved tibial inserts. Trans Orthop Res Soc 26:1098, 2001.
17. Haas BD, Komistek RD, Stiehl JB, et al: Kinematic comparison of posterior cruciate sacrifice versus substitution in a mobile bearing total knee arthroplasty. J Arthroplasty 17:685-692, 2002.
18. Harman MK, Banks SA, Hodge WA: Polyethylene damage and knee kinematics after total knee arthroplasty. Clin Orthop 392:383-393, 2001.
19. Kanekasu K, Banks SA, Honjo S, et al: Fluoroscopic analysis of knee arthroplasty kinematics during deep flexion kneeling. J Arthroplasty 19:998-1003, 2004.
20. Kanisawa I, Banks AZ, Banks SA, et al: Weight bearing knee kinematics in subjects with two types of anterior cruciate ligament reconstructions. Knee Surg Sports Traumatol Arthrosc 11:16-22, 2003.
21. Landy MM, Walker PS: Wear of ultra-high molecular-weight polyethylene components of 90 retrieved knee prostheses. J Arthroplasty 3(Supp):S73-S85, 1988.
22. Noble P, Vagner G, Conditt M, et al: The role of the cam mechanism in posterior stabilized TKR: An analysis of 75 retrieved components. Trans Orthop Res Soc 26:1102, 2001.
23. Nozaki H, Banks SA, Suguro T, Hodge WA: Observations of femoral rollback in cruciate-retaining knee arthroplasty. Clin Orthop 404:308-314, 2002.
24. Puloski SK, McCalden RW, MacDonald SJ, et al: Tibial post wear in posterior stabilized total knee arthroplasty. An unrecognized source of polyethylene debris. J Bone Joint Surg Am 83:390-397, 2001.
25. Stiehl JB, Komistek RD, Dennis DA: Fluoroscopic analysis of kinematics after posterior-cruciate-retaining knee arthroplasty. J Bone Joint Surg Br 77:884-889, 1995.
26. Stiehl JB, Komistek RD, Dennis DA: Detrimental kinematics of a flat on flat total condylar knee arthroplasty. Clin Orthop 365:139-148, 1999.
27. Uvehammer J, Karrholm J, Brandsson S: In vivo kinematics of total knee arthroplasty. Concave versus posterior-stabilised tibial joint surface. J Bone Joint Surg Br 82:499-505, 2000.
28. Uvehammer J, Karrholm J, Brandsson S, et al: In vivo kinematics of total knee arthroplasty: Flat compared with concave tibial joint surface. J Orthop Res 18:856-864, 2000.
29. Walker PS, Garg A: Range of motion in total knee arthroplasty. A computer analysis. Clin Orthop 262:227-235, 1991.

CHAPTER 12

Alternative Bearings for Knee Articulation: Hopes and Realities

Lisa A. Pruitt • Michael D. Ries

This chapter reviews contemporary experience with conventional metal-polyethylene resurfacing and delves into the evolving, highly cross-linked polyethylene and alternative femoral component finishing in total knee arthroplasty (TKA).

In TKA, the tibial and patellar components that typically articulate against a cobalt-chrome (CoCr) or ceramic femoral counter bearing are composed of ultrahigh molecular weight polyethylene (UHMWPE). Sliding and rolling of the counterface in TKA lead to the imposition of cyclic stress on components that can range as high as 10 MPa in tension to 40 MPa in compression as the articulating surface sweeps from flexion to extension.[5] These components are subjected to a large assortment of damage modes such as catastrophic failure, fatigue damage, and delamination wear, as well as scratching, pitting, and burnishing.[38,63] Particulate wear can also occur in knee components, although the particle size is generally larger than that observed in hip replacements because of greater contact stress in the patellofemoral and tibial components than in the acetabular component.[6,34,43]

UHMWPE serves as a gold standard for total joint arthroplasty because it has exceptional mechanical integrity as a result of its chain entanglements, high tie molecule density, crystallinity, and very high molecular weight. The degree of crystallinity of UHMWPE is a very important morphologic parameter. Higher-crystallinity UHMWPEs generally have a larger modulus of elasticity, superior yield strength, improved resistance to creep deformation, and enhanced fatigue strength. Fatigue strength is very important because it relates to the ability of UHMWPE to resist cyclic damage modes, which are prevalent in knee components. Factors that affect the performance of UHMWPE include its sterilization method, its processing conditions, and molecular factors such as the degree of cross-linking. Additionally, UHMWPE performance is affected by the properties of the counter bearing material. These factors are discussed in the text that follows.

FACTORS AFFECTING WEAR IN TOTAL JOINT ARTHROPLASTY

Sterilization of UHMWPE

Sterilization of UHMWPE components is an important variable in device longevity because it is known that ionizing radiation degrades the mechanical and wear properties of UHMWPE.[7,19,52] Until the mid to late 1990s, UHMWPE components of total joint replacements were packaged in air and subsequently sterilized with a 25- to 37-kGy dose of gamma radiation. It is well known that radiation causes cross-linking, chain scission, and long-term oxidative degradation of polyethylene. The effects of ionizing radiation on postirradiation aging of several types of polyethylene, including pressure-crystallized UHMWPE, were studied in detail by Bhateja et al.[8,9] Costa and coworkers have shown that oxidation can also occur in ethylene oxide–sterilized UHMWPE, albeit to a much smaller extent than in gamma radiation–sterilized UHMWPE.[11,18] It is now well established that long-term postirradiation aging can have detrimental effects on the morphology and mechanical properties of UHMWPE.[10,53] The effects of postirradiation aging have been well documented in analyses of TKA retrievals. Recent reviews summarize various issues related to sterilization, its chemistry, and effects on UHMWPE for total joint arthroplasty prostheses.[18,37]

Orthopedic manufacturers now recognize the harmful effects of long-term oxidation. In response, many manufacturers sterilize UHMWPE with nonradiation methods, such as ethylene oxide or gas plasma sterilization. Some orthopedic manufacturers have resorted to packaging of components in low-oxygen environments, such as vacuum foil packaging and packaging in nitrogen or argon gas. These methods slow down the rate of oxidation during storage. However, it is not yet known whether in vivo oxidation rates would eventually affect the clinical performance of conventional UHMWPE that is packaged in low-oxygen environments and then sterilized with 25- to 37-kGy doses of gamma radiation.

Alternative Forms of UHMWPE

Contact stress of UHMWPE components in TKAs can be reduced by a design approach that increases the conformity of the metal and UHMWPE components. However, such an approach can limit the range of motion for a patient. In addition, more constraint imparts greater stress on fixation interfaces. A preferred approach is to improve the material and tribologic properties of UHMWPE to enable greater flexibility in implant design. One approach that was attempted more than 2 decades ago was to blend UHMWPE with carbon fibers to fabricate total joint replacement components.[62] However, although carbon fiber–reinforced polyethylene showed excellent resistance to creep and improved compressive strength in in vitro tests, there was a large decrease in fatigue resistance. More importantly, no improvement in resistance to wear was observed, and black-colored debris caused by the presence of carbon fibers was found in retrieved components. The material fared poorly in a clinical setting, and within a short time after implantation many devices failed as a result of elevated wear.

High-pressure crystallization was used in the early 1990s to produce UHMWPE components. This bulk material with enhanced crystallinity was known as Hylamer (DePuy-Dupont Orthopaedics, Inc.). High crystallinity in UHMWPE results in an increase in mechanical properties such as yield stress, Young's modulus, resistance to creep deformation, and resistance to fatigue crack propagation.[13,14] Although it seems that this form of UHMWPE would be advantageous for use in joint replacement applications, clinical results revealed early failures because of excessive wear.[14,41] It is now well recognized that Hylamer is more susceptible to oxidative degradation associated with gamma radiation sterilization, which leads to early failure as a result of high wear rates.[15] Even though this form of polyethylene is no longer manufactured, a significant number of Hylamer acetabular cups remain in use today.

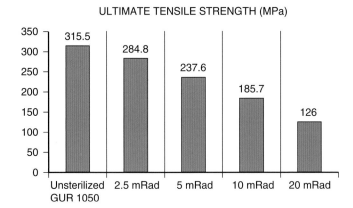

ULTIMATE TENSILE STRENGTH (MPa)

Figure 12–2. Plot of true ultimate tensile strengths for a range of cross-link densities in UHMWPE. Note that tensile strength decreases with radiation dosage (cross-link density).

particulate wear because of cross-linking would outweigh the risk of fatigue failure of UHMWPE components in these devices. Regardless, radiation cross-linked UHMWPE acetabular cups are now in clinical use for total hip replacements, and it is yet to be determined whether they will lead to higher survivorship than cups with conventional, non–cross-linked UHMWPE.

Cross-linked UHMWPE

Over the last several years, cross-linking has been shown to improve the wear performance of UHMWPE.[46,50,51] Laboratory tests have shown a significant decrease in the wear rate with increased cross-linking of UHMWPE.[46] However, a concern associated with cross-linking of UHMWPE is that it causes a reduction in fatigue crack propagation resistance, a reduction in ultimate tensile strength, and a decrease in fracture toughness.[3,4,36] Figure 12–1 shows the reduction in fatigue crack inception in UHMWPE for a range of cross-link dosages. Figure 12–2 shows the concomitant reduction in ultimate tensile strength. Because these are important mechanical properties of UHMWPE for application in total knee replacement components, it is not yet clear that the benefits of resistance to

UHMWPE: Future Directions

In the near future, radiation cross-linking processes may be optimized to improve the resistance to particulate wear without a large decrease in mechanical properties such as resistance to fatigue crack propagation, ultimate tensile strength, and J integral fracture toughness. One complication with most of the radiation cross-linking methods that involve complete melting to initiate cross-linking is that melting of UHMWPE erases the thermal history induced by ram extrusion and compression molding. Because cooling or recrystallization after melting is carried out without any application of pressure, it generally decreases the overall degree of crystallinity of radiation cross-linked UHMWPE. This reduced crystallinity in turn leads to a low Young modulus in radiation cross-linked

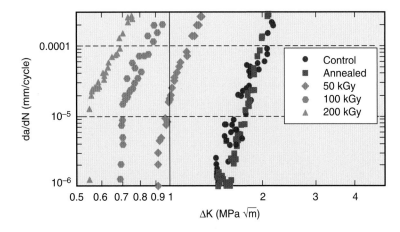

Figure 12–1. Plot of fatigue crack propagation resistance for a range of cross-link densities in UHMWPE. Note that fatigue crack inception decreases with radiation dosage (cross-link density).

UHMWPE, which is generally associated with lower resistance to creep deformation. A recent study by Simis et al[57] investigated the coupled effects of cross-linking and enhanced crystallinity via high-pressure methods to improve the mechanical properties of UHMWPE. This tailored microstructure provided a material with good wear resistance as a result of the cross-linking and improved fatigue resistance because of higher crystallinity and larger lamellae. These material developments are especially important for TKAs, where high cyclic stress can lead to fatigue wear mechanisms.

Effect of Counterface Roughening on Wear

Both abrasive and fatigue wear occur in TKAs. Whereas fatigue wear typically occurs in knees as a result of cyclic contact stress, the abrasive wear component is significantly influenced by the roughness of the counterface.[21,25] The roughness of a metal bearing surface can be increased by oxidative wear and scratching. The wear rate of UHMWPE is proportional to the counterface roughness, and a single scratch can increase the wear rate by a factor of 10.[24,56] The metal bearing surfaces used in total joint replacements have an oxide surface film that forms spontaneously on exposure to the environment. If this film is worn or scratched, the underlying metal substrate may be released into solution by a corrosion reaction as the passive film reforms. This process causes a net loss of metal or surface material displacement and an increase in surface roughness.

When a metallic bearing surface is scratched, a trough is created with a pileup of metal adjacent to both sides of the trough. The pileup of material that lies above the main bearing surface causes an increase in wear by plowing or cutting into the corresponding bearing surface material. Indentations in the bearing surface without an associated pileup above the surface have little effect on wear.[24,25] Wear is also influenced by the direction of scratches. A scratch transverse to the direction of motion causes greater wear than more longitudinally oriented scratches do.[24,25]

Particles of bone cement containing barium sulfate have been found embedded in the surfaces of clinically retrieved UHMWPE implants.[56] Barium sulfate or zirconium used as a radiopacifying agent in polymethylmethacrylate (PMMA) has sufficient hardness to scratch CoCr alloys.[32]

In vitro wear tests demonstrate an increase in wear when a roughened CoCr femoral component is articulated against UHMWPE. The method used to roughen the component should ideally reproduce roughness values similar to those of in vivo retrieved components to accurately predict the effect of in vivo counterface roughening on wear. Widding et al[61] described a method of counterface roughening in which total knee femoral components were tumbled in alumina particles before testing to create surface roughness values similar to those of in vivo retrieved femoral components. Wear of both conventional and highly cross-linked UHMWPE in TKA was increased after counterface roughening. Muratoglu et al[47] implanted on a knee simulator clinically retrieved total knee femoral components that had been roughened in vivo. When compared with unimplanted control components, wear was increased in both conventional and highly cross-linked polyethylene with the in vivo roughened components.

Counterface Hardness

Third-body abrasives such as particles of bone, PMMA, or porous coatings have been implicated as a cause of in vivo scratching of metal bearing surfaces.[16,20,33,42] The resultant increase in surface roughness is associated with an increase in UHMWPE wear. When compared with CoCr alloys, titanium alloys are more susceptible to articular roughening because of their inferior hardness and their poor resistance to shear of the surface oxide from sliding wear.[21] Figure 12–3 shows an example of this scratching in a titanium alloy used in total knee replacement. Severe in vivo wear of titanium bearing surfaces in total hip replacements has also been observed.[1,48] Therefore, CoCr alloys are the preferred metallic counterfaces for total joint prostheses.

The CoCr femoral heads used in total hip replacements are forged alloys with greater hardness and scratch resistance than cast cobalt chrome. However, the CoCr femoral components used in total knee replacements are typically cast alloys, which may leave them more susceptible to surface roughening. Scratches on the femoral condyles are frequently observed on clinically retrieved CoCr total knee femoral components.[40]

Ceramics such as zirconia and alumina have been used successfully in total hip arthroplasty, and they maintain a certain nearly pristine bearing surface finish even in the presence of third-body abrasives such as bone or PMMA.[16,17,20,21] Because these ceramics are metal oxides, oxidative wear cannot occur. However, ceramics have

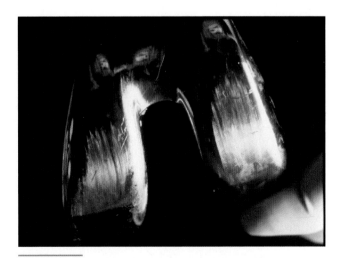

Figure 12–3. Retrieved titanium femoral component with marked abrasion of both condyles after 2 years of in vivo use. No third-body abrasive particles such as bone, cement, or metallic debris were found in the joint.

lower fracture toughness than metals do, which makes them more brittle.

Fracture of ceramic components has been reported in total hip arthroplasty and has been linked to improper design or fabrication procedures.[12,26,31,32,35,44,54] This experience has limited the application of ceramics for femoral components in TKA, where the loading conditions and implant geometry are more complex.

Methods to Improve Counterface Hardness

Numerous approaches have been proposed for enhancing the abrasion resistance of CoCr and titanium alloy counterfaces.[20,22] Nitrogen ion implantation increases their surface hardness and wettability. Though more wear resistant than nontreated surfaces, the submicron-thick ion-implanted surface layer is still subject to scratching and oxidative wear and, in several wear studies, has been found to have worn away.[21,45,59] Thermally driven diffusion hardening of the metallic surface can produce a thicker surface layer than ion implantation can, but scratching and oxidative wear are still possible.[22,39] Vapor deposition of a microns-thick titanium nitride oxide coating increases the surface hardness and prevents oxidative wear, but there have been reports of coating breakthrough possibly caused by homogeneities inherent in the coating process.[29]

A thick (approximately 5 μm) uniform zirconium oxide surface can be formed on zirconium alloys by diffusion of oxygen.[21,45] Laboratory testing has shown that oxidized Zr-2.5Nb alloy combines the wear resistance of a ceramic with the fracture toughness of a metal. The oxide also remains adherent to the substrate metal if damaged. This combination of material and mechanical properties may be advantageous for a femoral component used in TKA.

IN VITRO WEAR TESTING WITH A CERAMIC COUNTERFACE

Knee simulator tests have been used to compare the wear behavior of OxZr and CoCr counterfaces under a number of conditions. The first study of this type was conducted with a simulator that mimics the rolling and plowing motions of knee prosthesis kinematics.[60] Early OxZr prototypes made from castings were used in this study, and the oxide was relatively thin. In addition, the tibial polyethylene inserts were gamma-irradiated in air. Despite these material limitations, the OxZr components produced significantly fewer wear features and none of the macroscopic polyethylene delamination observed in tests with the CoCr components. It was also noted that the CoCr surfaces roughened during testing, whereas the OxZr surfaces were not affected.

A later study was conducted with a four-axis, displacement-controlled, physiologic knee simulator.[58] Components were tested for 6 million cycles of 90% walking gait and 10% stair-climbing activity, and polyethylene wear was measured periodically during the test by weight loss and by wear particle characterization. In comparison to CoCr, OxZr produced an aggregate wear rate of polyethylene that was 85% less. It was noted that all of the OxZr components generated lower polyethylene wear rates and produced less burnishing of the inserts. In contrast to the OxZr surfaces, the CoCr surfaces were found to have roughened during testing even though the lubricant was filtered before testing.

A separate study was conducted on a different component design in the same type of simulator, but the test parameters were modified to produce greater wear rates and less measurement variability with just a walking-gait motion.[30] In comparison to CoCr, OxZr produced a mean wear rate that was 42% less when measured either gravimetrically or volumetrically. This reduction is substantial, though less than the 85% reduction of the previous study. The later study may be more representative of the "normal" performance advantage of OxZr knees because it achieved a 95% confidence limit and the relative performance is similar to that found with hip simulators.[28] This study continued on, however, to show that the knee wear rates were sensitive to test conditions. The wear rate using OxZr was 62% less than that using CoCr under conditions of greater rotation and an additional varus moment. This finding indicated that the performance advantage for OxZr might increase for conditions associated with "more demanding" patient kinematics or implant malposition.

To assess the effect of in vivo conditions on wear with CoCr and OxZr components with simulated roughening, CoCr femoral components were tumbled in an abrasive alumina powder before wear testing.[55] The resulting femoral component roughness values were within the clinically relevant range. The components were tested for 5 million cycles with a displacement-controlled simulator. OxZr components were tumbled via the same procedure, but they roughened less and produced an aggregate polyethylene wear rate that was 89% less ($p < .05$). A separate test using preroughened components was conducted for 5 million cycles with a force-controlled simulator.[23] When compared with CoCr in this test, OxZr produced an average wear rate that was 82% less ($p < .001$).

Collectively, these knee simulator tests indicate that OxZr components can reduce wear of the polyethylene counterface by 40% to 90%, depending on test conditions. Similar wear reductions have been found for monolithic ceramic femoral components in knee simulator tests.[2,49]

References

1. Agins HJ, Alcock NW, Bansal M, et al: Metallic wear in failed titanium-alloy total hip replacements. A histological and quantitative analysis. J Bone Joint Surg Am 71:347-356, 1988.
2. Alberts LR, Neff JR, Webb JD: Wear simulation comparison of a zirconia and a cobalt chrome femoral knee implant. Trans Orthop Res Soc 26:1101, 2001.
3. Baker DA, Bellare A, Pruitt L: The effects of degree of crosslinking on the fatigue crack initiation and propagation resistance of orthopedic-grade polyethylene. J Biomed Mater Res A 66: 146-154, 2003.

4. Baker DA, Hastings RS, Pruitt L: Study of fatigue resistance of chemical and radiation cross-linked medical grade ultrahigh molecular weight polyethylene. J Biomed Mater Res 46:573-581, 1999.

5. Bartel DL, Bicknell VL, Wright TM: The effect of conformity, thickness, and material on stresses in ultra-high molecular weight components for total joint replacement. J Bone Joint Surg Am 68:1041-1051, 1986.

6. Bartel DL, Rawlinson JJ, Burstein AH, et al: Stresses in polyethylene components of contemporary total knee replacements. Clin Orthop 317:76-82, 1995.

7. Bhateja SK: Changes in the crystalline content of irradiated linear polyethylenes upon ageing. 23:654-655, 1982.

8. Bhateja SK, Andrews EH: Radiation-induced crystallinity changes in polyethylene blends. J Mater Sci 20:2839-2845, 1985.

9. Bhateja SK, Andrews EH, Yarbrough SM: Radiation induced crystallinity changes in linear polyethylenes: Long term aging effects. Polymer J 21:739-750, 1989.

10. Birkinshaw C, Buggy M, Daly S: The effect of gamma radiation on the physical structure and mechanical properties of ultrahigh molecular weight polyethylene. J Appl Polymer Sci 38:1967-1973, 1989.

11. Brach del Prever E, Crova M, Costa L, et al: Unacceptable biodegradation of polyethylene in vivo. Biomaterials 17:873-878, 1996.

12. Callaway GH, Flynn W, Ranawat CS, Sculco TP: Fracture of the femoral head after ceramic-on-polyethylene total hip arthroplasty. J Arthroplasty 10:855-859, 1995.

13. Champion AR, Li S, Saum K, et al: The effect of crystallinity on the physical properties of UHMWPE. Presented at the 40th Annual Meeting of the Orthopaedic Research Society, 1994.

14. Chmell MJ, Poss R, Thomas WH, Sledge CB: Early failure of Hylamer acetabular inserts due to eccentric wear. J Arthroplasty 11:351-353, 1996.

15. Collier JP, Bargmann LS, Currier BH, et al: An analysis of Hylamer and polyethylene bearings from retrieved acetabular components. Orthopedics 21:865-871, 1998.

16. Cooke FW: Ceramics in orthopedic surgery. Clin Orthop 276:135-146, 1992.

17. Cooper JR, Dowson D, Fisher J, Jobbins B: Ceramic bearing surfaces in total artificial joints: Resistance to third body wear damage from bone cement particles. J Med Eng Tech 15:63-67, 1991.

18. Costa L, Brach del Prever E (eds): UHMWPE for Arthroplasty: Characterisation, Sterilisation and Degradation. Torino, Italy, Edizioni Minerva Medica, 2000.

19. Costa L, Luda MP, Trossarelli L, et al: In vivo UHMWPE biodegradation of retrieved prosthesis. Biomaterials 19:1371-1385, 1998.

20. Davidson JA: Characteristics of metal and ceramic total hip bearing surfaces and their effect on long-term ultra high molecular weight polyethylene wear. Clin Orthop 294:361-378, 1993.

21. Davidson JA, Asyian CM, Mishra AK, Kovacs P: Zirconium (ZrO$_2$) coated zirconium–2.5 Nb alloy for prosthetic knee bearing applications. In Bioceramics 5. Kyoto, Japan, Kobunski Kankokai, 1992, pp 389-401.

22. Dearnley PA: A review of metallic, ceramic and surface-treated metals used for bearing surfaces in human joint replacements. Proc Inst Mech Eng 213:107-135, 1999.

23. DesJardins JD, LaBerge M: UHMWPE in-vitro wear performance under roughened oxidized zirconium and CoCr femoral knee components. Trans Soc Biomaterials 26:364, 2003.

24. Dowson D, Diab M, Gillis B, Atkinson JR: Influence of counterface topography on the wear of UHMWPE under wet or dry conditions. In Polymer Wear and Its Control. New York, American Chemical Society, 1985, pp 171-187.

25. Dowson D, Thaheri S, Wallbridge NC: The role of counterface imperfections in the wear of polyethylene. Wear 119:227-293, 1987.

26. Fritsch EW, Gleitz M: Ceramic femoral head fractures in total hip arthroplasty. Clin Orthop 328:129-136, 1996.

27. Gomoll A, Wanich T, Bellare A: J-integral fracture toughness and tearing modulus measurement of radiation cross-linked UHMWPE. J Orthop Res 20:1152-1156, 2002.

28. Good V, Ries M, Barrack RL, et al: Reduced wear with oxidized zirconium femoral heads. J Bone Joint Surg Am 85(Suppl 4):105-110, 2003.

29. Harman MK, Banks SA, Hodge WA: Wear analysis of a retrieved hip implant with titanium nitride coating. J Arthroplasty 12:938-945, 1997.

30. Hermida JC, Patil S, D'Lima DD, et al: Polyethylene wear against metal-ceramic composite femoral components. Am Acad Orthop Surg Ann Mtg Proc 5:449, 2004.

31. Higuchi F, Shiba N, Inoue A, Wakebe I: Fracture of an alumina ceramic head in total hip arthroplasty. J Arthroplasty 10:851-854, 1995.

32. Hummer CD III, Rothman RH, Hozack WJ: Catastrophic failure of modular zirconium-ceramic femoral head components after total hip arthroplasty. J Arthroplasty 10:848-850, 1995.

33. Jasty M, Bragdon CR, Lee K, et al: Surface damage to cobalt-chrome femoral head prostheses. J Bone Joint Surg Br 76:73-77, 1994.

34. Jin ZM, Dowson D, Fisher J: A parametric analysis of the contact stress in ultra-high molecular weight polyethylene acetabular cups. Med Eng Phys 16:398-405, 1994.

35. Krikler S, Schatzker J: Ceramic head failure. J Arthroplasty 10:860-862, 1995.

36. Krzypow D, Bensusan J, Sevo K, et al: The fatigue crack propagation resistance of gamma radiation or peroxide cross-linked UHMW polyethylene. Presented at the 6th World Biomaterials Congress, 2000.

37. Kurtz SM, Muratoglu OK, Evans M, Edidin AA: Advances in the processing, sterilization, and crosslinking of ultra-high molecular weight polyethylene for total joint arthroplasty. Biomaterials 20:1659-1688, 1999.

38. Landy MM, Walker PS: Wear of ultra-high-molecular-weight polyethylene components of 90 retrieved knee prostheses. J Arthroplasty 3(Suppl):S73-S85, 1988.

39. Laurent M, Shetty R: Wear and surface characterization of nitrided Co-Cr-Mo alloy knees. Trans Orthop Res Soc 24: 895, 1999.

40. Levesque M, Livingstone BJ, Jones WM, Spector M: Scratches on condyles in normal functioning total knee arthroplasty. Trans Orthop Res Soc 23:247, 1998.

41. Livingston BJ, Chmell MJ, Spector M, Poss R: Complications of total hip arthroplasty associated with the use of an acetabular component with a Hylamer liner. J Bone Joint Surg Am 79:1529-1538, 1997.

42. Lombardi AV Jr, Mallory TH, Vaughn BK, Drouillard P: Aseptic loosening in total hip arthroplasty secondary to osteolysis induced by wear debris from titanium-alloy modular femoral heads. J Bone Joint Surg Am 71:1337-1342, 1989.

43. McNamara JL, Collier JP, Mayor MB, Jensen RE: A comparison of contact pressures in tibial and patellar total knee components before and after service in vivo. Clin Orthop 299:104-113, 1994.

44. Michand RJ, Rashad SY: Spontaneous fracture of the ceramic ball in a ceramic-polyethylene total hip arthroplasty. J Arthroplasty 10:863-867, 1995.

45. Mishra AK, Davidson JA: Zirconium/zirconium: A new abrasion resistant material for orthopaedic applications. Mater Tech 8:1621, 1993.

46. Muratoglu OK, Bragdon CR, O'Connor DO, et al: A novel method of cross-linking ultra-high-molecular-weight polyethylene to improve wear, reduce oxidation, and retain mechanical properties. Recipient of the 1999 HAP Paul Award. J Arthroplasty 16:149-160, 2001.

47. Muratoglu O, Burroughs B, Christensen S, et al: In vitro wear of highly cross-linked tibias articulating with explanted rough femoral components. Trans Orthop Res Soc 29:297, 2004.

48. Nasser S, Campbell PA, Kilgus D, et al: Cementless total joint arthroplasty prostheses with titanium-alloy articular surfaces. A human retrieval analysis. Clin Orthop 261:171-185, 1990.

49. Oonishi H, Hanatate Y, Tsuji E, Yunoki H: Comparisons of wear of UHMW polyethylene sliding against metal and alumina in total knee prostheses. In Oonishi H, Aoki H, Sawai K (eds): Bioceramics, vol 1. Tokyo, Ishiyaku EuroAmerica, 1989, pp 219-224.

50. Oonishi H, Ishimaru H, Kato A: Effect of cross-linkage by gamma radiation in heavy doses to low wear polyethylene in total hip prostheses. J Mater Sci Mater Med 7:753-763, 1996.

51. Oonishi H, Kadoya Y: Wear of high-dose gamma-irradiated polyethylene in total hip replacements. J Orthop Sci 5:223-228, 2000.

52. Premnath V, Harris WH, Jasty M, Merrill EW: Gamma sterilization of UHMWPE articular implants: An analysis of the oxidation problem. Ultra High Molecular Weight Poly Ethylene. Biomaterials 17:1741-1753, 1996.

53. Pruitt L, Ranganathan R: Effect of sterilization on the structure and fatigue resistance of medical grade UHMWPE. c3:91-93, 1995.

54. Pulliam IT, Trousdale RT: Fracture of a ceramic femoral head after a revision operation. A case report. J Bone Joint Surg Am 79:118-121, 1997.

55. Ries MD, Salehi A, Widding K, Hunter G: Polyethylene wear performance of oxidized zirconium and cobalt-chromium knee components under abrasive conditions. J Bone Joint Surg Am 84(Suppl 2):129-135, 2002.

56. Rose RM, Crugnola A, Ries M, et al: On the origins of high in vivo wear rates in polyethylene components of total joint prostheses. Clin Orthop 145:277-286, 1979.

57. Simis K, Bellare A, Pruitt L: The effect of high pressure crystallisation and crosslinking on the fatigue crack inception behaviour of medical grade ultra high molecular weight polyethylene. Presented at 12th International Conference on the Deformation, Yield and Fracture of Polymers, Cambridge, UK, April 2003, pp 69-72.

58. Spector M, Ries MD, Bourne RB, et al: Wear performance of ultra-high molecular weight polyethylene on oxidized zirconium total knee femoral components. J Bone Joint Surg Am 83(Suppl 2):80-86, 2001.

59. Weightman B, Light D: The effect of surface finish of alumina and stainless steel on the wear rate of UHMWPE. Biomaterials 7:20-24, 1986.

60. White SE, Whiteside LA, McCarthy DS, et al: Simulated knee wear with cobalt chromium and oxidized zirconium knee femoral components. Clin Orthop 309:176-184, 1994.

61. Widding K, Scott M, Jani S, Good V: Cross-linked UHMWPE in knees: Clean versus abrasive conditions. Trans Orthop Res Soc 28:1427, 2003.

62. Wright TM, Fukubayashi T, Burstein AH: The effect of carbon fiber reinforcement on contact area, contact pressure, and time-dependent deformation in polyethylene tibial components. J Biomed Mater Res 15:719-730, 1981.

63. Wright TM, Rimnac CM, Stulberg SD, et al: Wear of polyethylene in total joint replacements. Observations from retrieved PCA knee implants. Clin Orthop 276:126-134, 1992.

CHAPTER 13

Computational Models Can Predict Polymer Insert Damage in Total Knee Replacements

Edward A. Morra • Melinda K. Harman • A. Seth Greenwald

A computational model that successfully predicts clinically observed damage occurring in the polymer insert component of a total knee arthroplasty (TKA) prosthesis is a powerful predictive tool. This chapter demonstrates use of the finite element method to visualize the magnitude and location of stress on and within the polymer insert associated with wear for a wide range of contemporary knee replacement designs. Such models increase the orthopedic surgeon's visualization of the mechanisms leading to material wear of polymer inserts. The effect of any innovative component design changes on long-term polymer insert wear can also be readily explored. The results presented herein suggest that the best-performing TKA designs are the ones that achieve low stress on and within the tibial insert without being overly conforming.

Successful TKA is dependent on many factors. A surgeon's experience with accurate component placement, ligamentous balance, and optimization of limb alignment contributes significantly to a good to excellent outcome. Patient variables such as the extent of deformity, weight, and joint kinematics also influence success. The choice of materials used in implant design coupled with manufacturing processes that accurately create the desired component conformities completes the orthopedic triad of factors influencing the long-term outcome of this surgical procedure.

Primary to the longevity of total joint replacement is the long-term efficacy of the joint bearing surface. In contemporary knee designs, this is directly related to the durability of the ultrahigh-molecular-weight polyethylene (UHMWPE) tibial insert component. Sharkey et al[29] found that UHMWPE wear was the primary reason for 25% of revision TKA surgeries. UHMWPE components contribute to the failure of joint arthroplasty through component creep, generation of debris, "wear through," delamination, and fracture.[5,15] UHMWPE debris has been linked to a biological response leading to osteolysis, loosening, and pain.[6,9,31]

Many researchers[2,24,25] have associated the accumulated damage observed in UHMWPE to specific states of cyclic stress that arise when a femoral component articulates with a tibial insert. Abrasive wear is related to the magnitude and distribution of compressive normal (contact) stress on the surface of the tibial insert and relative tangential velocities between components. Delamination cracks that propagate parallel to but just below the articulating surface are associated with von Mises stress.

Pitting (cracks that develop in a direction perpendicular to the articulating surface) is a function of the range of maximum principal stress that any given point in the polymer experiences in a gait cycle.

FINITE ELEMENT METHOD

Material science can predict the mechanical response of a material with a very simple geometry, such as a cube, with a single equation when a load is applied. If a cube of stainless steel resting on a table has a force applied equally across its topmost face, the decrease in height and increase in width can be readily calculated. The finite element method allows the mechanical response of a material with a complex geometry such as a tibial insert to be calculated by breaking the shape down into a large number of finite elements of a simpler shape, such as a cube. The same simple equation can be used for each finite element, but the response of one element affects all the elements around it. A large number of equations arise that are mathematically coupled to their neighbors' equations, and the use of a powerful computer is needed to determine the overall response of the complex geometry.

A three-dimensional, finite element model (Fig. 13–1) was created for each total knee design by measuring the articular surfaces of implantable quality parts with a coordinate-measuring machine and laser profilometer.[19] The resulting cloud of data points represented the actual manufactured surfaces (Fig. 13–2) and was imported into the finite element software to define the geometries of both the femoral and tibial insert components. The modeled tibial insert was positioned in the computer according to the specified surgical procedure from each manufacturer; for instance, many designs prescribed a 3-degree posteriorly sloped tibial bone cut.

The femoral surface was treated as a rigid body and was articulated with the modeled tibial insert by using the average values for the heel strike portion of the level walking cycle[20,21,23] (1950 N) and flexion angle[1,14,22] (0-degree flexion). To aid in comparison, all polymer inserts were characterized by the same gamma-irradiated, nonlinear material[30] 10 mm in thickness and maintained at 37° C. The virtual components were allowed to settle into their preferred alignments without consideration of friction or soft-tissue constraints. The resulting stress distributions on and within the polymer insert were then photorealistically imaged to allow visual comparison of the different implant designs.

FINITE ELEMENT RESULTS

The results for heel strike loading are broken into two groups, mobile-bearing designs (Figs 13–3 to 13–9) and fixed-bearing designs (Figs. 13–10 to 13–13), and ranked in order from the largest contact area to the smallest. Three images are presented for each design and represent stress associated with polymer damage in the tibial insert: (A)

proximal contact stress, (B) subsurface delamination stress, and (C) subsurface pitting stress. All designs are appreciated from a superior posterior view of the left knee. Tabulated numeric data for contact area, peak contact stress, peak delamination stress, and compressive and tensile subsurface peak pitting stress and their range are available for mobile bearings in Table 13–1 and for fixed bearings in Table 13–2.

The distribution of proximal compressive contact stress in the first-row images (A) gives an indication of areas where surface abrasion caused by contact with the femoral component can occur during heel strike. The higher the contact stress, the greater the propensity for abrasive damage. The proximal contact areas are determined by using a 1-MPa threshold. The minimum and maximum contact areas for mobile bearings as a group were 381 mm^3 and 875 mm^2, respectively. Peak contact stress for mobile bearings ranged from 8.5 to 15.0 MPa. The minimum and maximum contact areas for fixed bearings as a group were

Text continued on p. 6

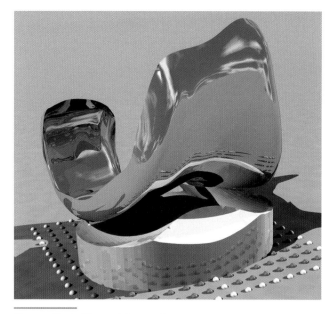

Figure 13–1. Typical finite element model used in the protocol. The tibial insert is free to slide and rotate on a bed of frictionless spring-loaded elements to achieve optimal component alignment with equal loads applied in the medial and lateral compartments.

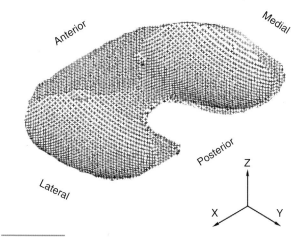

Figure 13–2. "Cloud of points" measurement data used in building a finite element model that represents actual manufactured component geometries.

Table 13–1. Mobile-Bearing Results

TOTAL KNEE ARTHROPLASTY DESIGN NAME	MANUFACTURER OF RECORD	YEAR OF COMPONENT MANUFACTURE	PROXIMAL CONTACT AREA (mm^2)	PEAK PROXIMAL CONTACT STRESS (MPa)	VON MISES DELAMINATION, PEAK STRESS (MPa)	COMPRESSIVE MAXIMUM PRINCIPAL PEAK PITTING STRESS (MPa)	TENSILE MAXIMUM PRINCIPAL PEAK PITTING STRESS (MPa)	MAXIMUM PRINCIPAL PITTING STRESS RANGE (MPa)
LCS Rotating Platform	DePuy	1996	875	10.4	15.4	−5.9	9.5	15.4
e.motion	Aesculap	2003	666	8.5	11.8	−3.8	6.2	10.0
Dual Bearing Knee	Finsbury	2003	595	15.0	21.2	−4.7	6.4	11.1
Interax	Howmedica	1997	530	10.9	12.5	−6.8	9.7	16.5
Profix MBK	Smith & Nephew	1998	507	13.9	16.4	−6.4	9.0	15.4
MBK	Zimmer	1998	429	11.4	15.0	−5.2	9.5	14.7
PFC Sigma Rotating Platform	DePuy	2001	381	14.1	9.3	−7.4	2.9	10.3

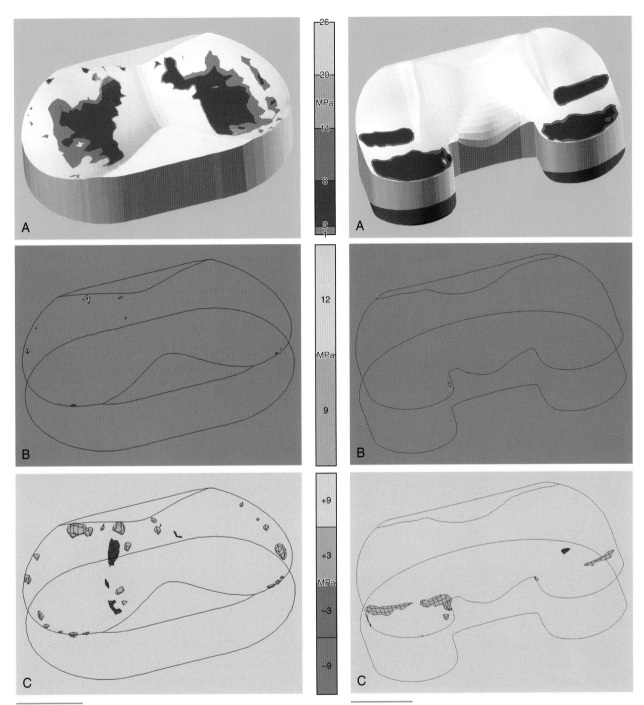

Figure 13–3. Product name: LCS Rotating Platform; manufacturer of record: DePuy; component manufacture year: circa 1996. **A,** Contact area (mm²): 875; peak proximal contact stress (MPa): 10.4. **B,** Peak delamination stress (MPa): 15.4. **C,** Peak maximum principal stress (MPa): tensile, 9.5; compressive, –5.9; range, 15.4.

Figure 13–4. Product name: e.motion; manufacturer of record: Aesculap; component manufacture year: circa 2003. **A,** Contact area (mm²): 666; peak proximal contact stress (MPa): 8.5. **B,** Peak delamination stress (MPa): 15.4. **C,** Peak maximum principal stress (MPa): tensile, 6.2; compressive, –3.8; range, 10.0.

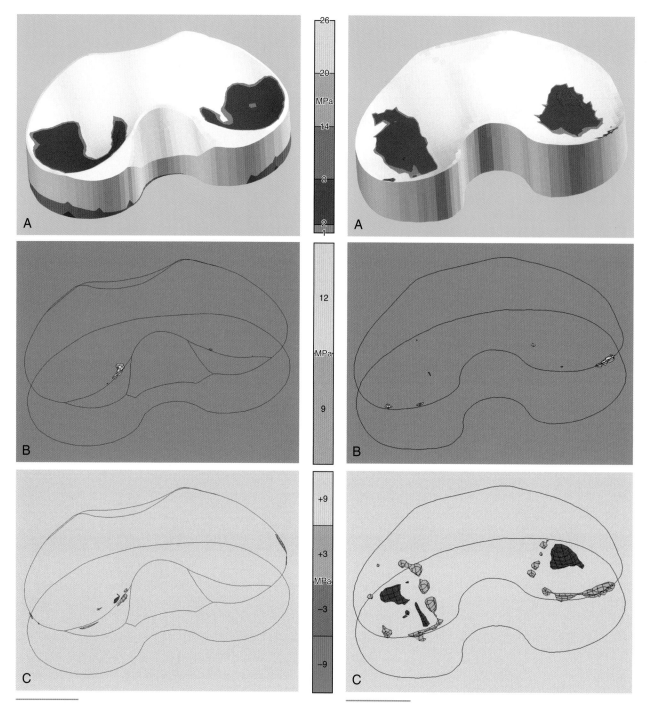

Figure 13–5. Product name: Dual Bearing Knee; manufacturer of record: Finsbury; component manufacture year: circa 2003. **A,** Contact area (mm²): 595; peak proximal contact stress (MPa): 15.0. **B,** Peak delamination stress (MPa): 21.2. **C,** Peak maximum principal stress (MPa): tensile, 6.4; compressive, –4.7; range, 11.1.

Figure 13–6. Product name: Interax; manufacturer of record: Howmedica; component manufacture year: circa 1997. **A,** Contact area (mm²): 530; peak proximal contact stress (MPa): 10.9. **B,** Peak delamination stress (MPa): 12.5. **C,** Peak maximum principal stress (MPa): tensile, 9.7; compressive, –6.8; range, 16.5.

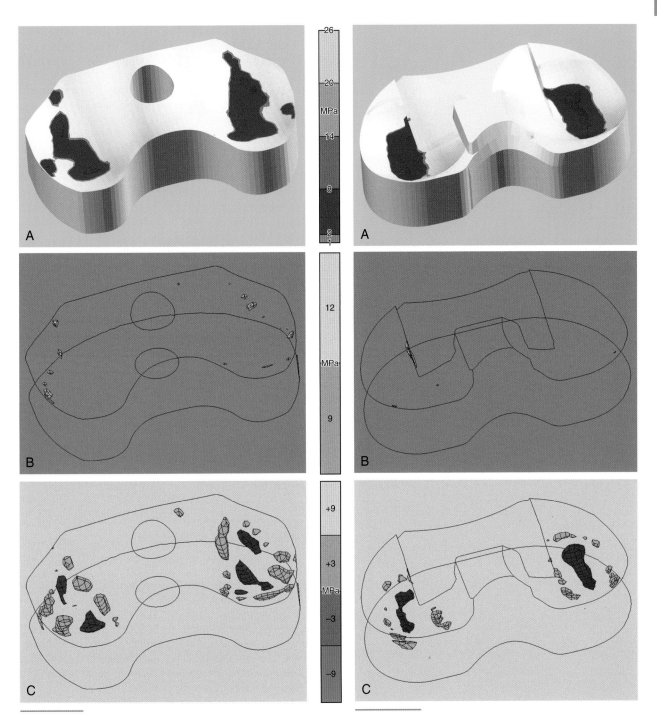

Figure 13–7. Product name: Profix MBK; manufacturer of record: Smith & Nephew; component manufacture year: circa 1998. **A,** Contact area (mm²): 507; peak proximal contact stress (MPa): 13.9. **B,** Peak delamination stress (MPa): 13.1. **C,** Peak maximum principal stress (MPa): tensile, 9.0; compressive, –6.4; range, 15.4.

Figure 13–8. Product name: MBK; manufacturer of record: Zimmer; component manufacture year: circa 1998. **A,** Contact area (mm²): 429; peak proximal contact stress (MPa): 11.4. **B,** Peak delamination stress (MPa): 15.0. **C,** Peak maximum principal stress (MPa): tensile, 9.5; compressive, –5.2; range, 14.7.

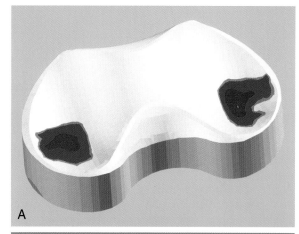

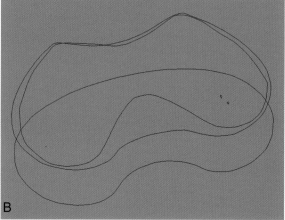

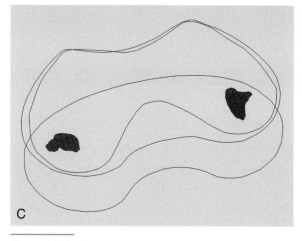

Figure 13–9. Product name: PFC Sigma Rotating Platform; manufacturer of record: DePuy; component manufacture year: circa 2001. **A,** Contact area (mm²): 381; peak proximal contact stress (MPa): 14.1. **B,** Peak delamination stress (MPa): 9.3. **C,** Peak maximum principal stress (MPa): tensile, 2.9; compressive, –7.4; range, 10.3.

212 mm² and 313 mm², respectively. Peak contact stress for fixed bearings ranged from 11.5 to 30.7 MPa.

The second-row images (B) depict three-dimensional isosurfaces of Von Mises (delamination) stress and indicate locations where shear cracks may propagate parallel to, but just below the articulating surface. Isosurfaces are defined by points of identical stress magnitude. Peak stress occurs at isolated points within the volume bounded by an isosurface and located near the articulating surface. In Figure 13–13 the peak stress is located directly below the center of contact and occurs approximately 2.5 mm beneath the articulating surface. In general, the stress in more conforming systems is lower in magnitude and its location shifted to a ring outside the edge of contact and closer to the surface. Peak Von Mises stress ranged from 9.3 to 21.2 MPa for mobile bearings and from 9.7 to 21.8 MPa for fixed bearings.

The third-row images (C) depict three-dimensional isosurfaces of maximum principal (pitting) stress and indicate locations where cracks may form perpendicular to the articulating surface. Peak stress occurs at isolated points within the volume bounded by an isosurface. Compressive (negative) maximum principal stress occurs directly beneath the center of contact. Tensile (positive) maximum principal stress occur outside the edge of contact, generally distributed in a ring. The opposition of compressive and tensile maximum principal stress is conducive to opening vertical cracks in the articulating surface. The larger the range between the values, the greater the propensity for pitting. The range of maximum principal stress was between 10.0 and 16.5 MPa for mobile bearings and between 16.2 and 31.0 MPa for fixed bearings.

FINITE ELEMENT DISCUSSION

The mobile-bearing results in Figures 13–3 through 13–9 demonstrate contact patterns indicating good component fit at full extension. This leads to low contact stress and large contact areas. Although the visualized delamination stresses are above a damage threshold, all involve a small volume of polymer. Pitting stress is distributed widely across most of the available compartment area for most mobile bearings; the ones with the lowest range of stress involve a small amount of polymer.

The fixed-bearing results in Figures 13–10 through 13–12 are mostly similar to the mobile-bearing results. Their good component fit allows low contact stress, and damaging delamination stress involves a small volume of polymer. However, the range of pitting stress is more intense and the distribution more tightly focused. The results of the least conforming design presented in Figure 13–13 are typical of a classic fixed-bearing design with low-contact areas, high contact stress, sphere-like delamination stress involving large volumes of polymer directly below the contact locations, and intense, tightly focused distributions of pitting stress. To scale these results to clinical reality, it should be noted that despite the large stress that this design manifests, it is generally considered a clinical success.[8]

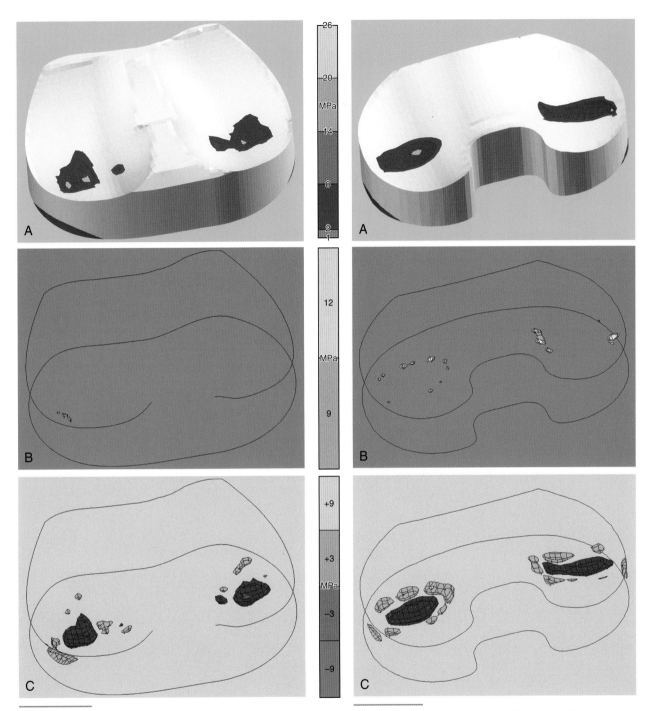

Figure 13–10. Product name: NK II Ultracongruent; manufacturer of record: Intermedics; component manufacture year: circa 1995. **A,** Contact area (mm^2): 313; peak proximal contact stress (MPa): 15.4. **B,** Peak delamination stress (MPa): 9.7. **C,** Peak maximum principal stress (MPa): tensile, 6.2; compressive, −10.0; range, 16.2.

Figure 13–11. Product name: Genesis II CR; manufacturer of record: Smith & Nephew; component manufacture year: circa 1995. **A,** Contact area (mm^2): 293; peak proximal contact stress (MPa): 11.5. **B,** Peak delamination stress (MPa): 20.0. **C,** Peak maximum principal stress (MPa): tensile, 16.6; compressive, −7.8; range, 24.4.

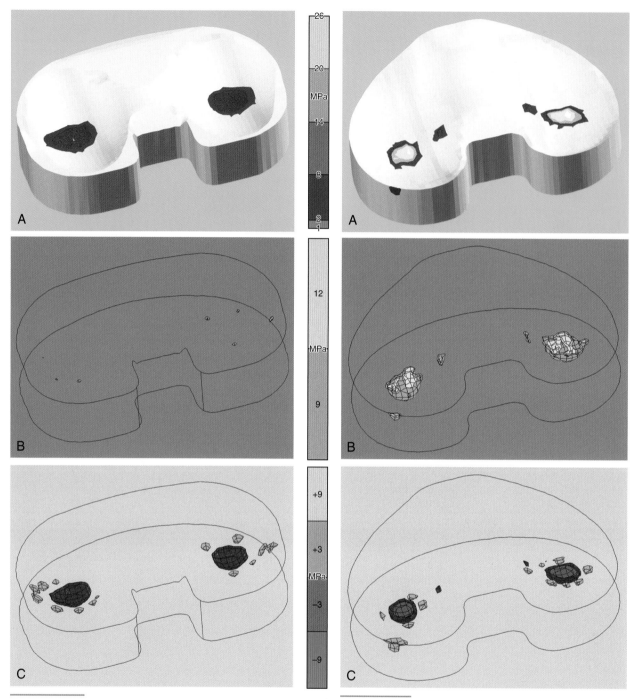

Figure 13–12. Product name: PFC Sigma Curved; manufacturer of record: Johnson & Johnson; component manufacture year: circa 1997. **A,** Contact area (mm²): 247; peak proximal contact stress (MPa): 14.3. **B,** Peak delamination stress (MPa): 14.3. **C,** Peak maximum principal stress (MPa): tensile, 6.9; compressive, −11.3; range, 18.2.

Figure 13–13. Product name: Duracon; manufacturer of record: Howmedica; component manufacture year: circa 1995. **A,** Contact area (mm²): 212; peak proximal contact stress (MPa): 30.7. **B,** Peak delamination stress (MPa): 21.8. **C,** Peak maximum principal stress (MPa): tensile, 13.8; compressive, −17.2; range, 31.0.

Table 13–2. Fixed-Bearing Results

TOTAL KNEE ARTHROPLASTY DESIGN NAME	MANUFACTURER OF RECORD	YEAR OF COMPONENT MANUFACTURE	PROXIMAL CONTACT AREA (mm²)	PEAK PROXIMAL CONTACT STRESS (MPa)	VON MISES DELAMINATION, PEAK STRESS (MPa)	COMPRESSIVE MAXIMUM PRINCIPAL PEAK PITTING STRESS (MPa)	TENSILE MAXIMUM PRINCIPAL PEAK PITTING STRESS (MPa)	MAXIMUM PRINCIPAL PITTING STRESS RANGE (MPa)
NK II Ultracongruent	Intermedics	1995	313	15.4	9.7	−10.0	6.2	16.2
Genesis II CR	Smith & Nephew	1995	293	11.5	20.0	−7.8	16.6	24.4
PFC Sigma Curved	Johnson & Johnson	1997	247	14.3	14.3	−11.3	6.9	18.2
Duracon	Howmedica	1995	212	30.7	21.8	−17.2	13.8	31.0

Model Caveats

The finite element protocol focuses on the effect of articulating geometry on the stress associated with the long-term wear response of the tibial insert. Design features known to affect stress magnitude and distribution, including polymer thickness, polymer material response, and tibial tray fixation, were modeled for each design in the same manner. By holding these aspects of all designs constant, direct comparison of results is possible.

The results represent best-case scenarios because of average heel strike loads being applied to optimally aligned components. The effect of soft tissues is not considered in this model; only the intrinsic curvatures of the components guide their optimal alignment. The results also serve as a detailed spot check of manufacturing processes because models were built from measurements of actual manufactured components and not perfect geometries contained in computer-aided design files.

UHMWPE wear is a function of polymer stress and the kinematics of articulation. Although the model results presented in this chapter convey detailed maps of surface and subsurface stress associated with clinically observed damage, it is only for one moment during the walking gait cycle. The kinematics of component articulation during cyclic activities such as walking gait and stair climbing will propel the visualized stress patterns about the tibial insert, and they will change in shape and intensity. Phenomena such as rollback, internal/external rotation, and anterior/posterior sliding were not captured in these models because of the "settling" methods used to position the femoral and tibial components together in a repeatable and consistent manner for all designs.

Material Damage Thresholds

Material failure theories for polymers[32] suggest that pitting and delamination in a UHMWPE tibial insert are unlikely to develop when cycled through a stress range less than 9 MPa. As stress associated with these damage modes exceeds this threshold, there is a higher potential for crack development. This threshold applies to stress that occurs within the material only, not contact stress occurring on the surface of a tibial insert.

In contrast, the minimum contact stress value that initiates in vivo abrasive damage under cyclic loading is not universal for UHMWPE[24,25] and is likely to vary with the choice of resin, material processing, design characteristics, and articular kinematics. Therefore, a general threshold is unavailable and inappropriate for analyzing the nonlinear contact stress used to predict abrasive wear of UHMWPE tibial inserts.

Peak Stress Values

Peak stress values are reported for comparison to the results of other researchers. These values are easily determined from output data and convenient to report; however, they are not very meaningful by themselves when describing wear phenomena. The scalar value of peak stress is not enough information for drawing conclusions concerning wear; the spatial location of that peak stress value must also be considered.

When determining the potential for polymer damage, it is important to consider both the magnitude of the stress and the material volume involved. A very high peak stress involving a very small volume of polymer is less significant than a large volume of polymer at a lower, but potentially damaging stress level. Reporting only peak values tends to obfuscate their significance in terms of their potential for actual polymer damage.

Range of Pitting Stress

The scalar range of maximum principal stress within a tibial insert has been reported to be associated with the propensity for a crack to form perpendicular to the articulating surface.[2] This is not a precise statement. The range of maximum principal stress that *a given point* within a tibial insert experiences defines the propensity for a crack to form *at that point*. Because the cyclic nature of patient kinematics repeatedly moves the areas of contact around on a tibial insert, a given point of polymer may at one moment be under great tension followed by a moment of large compression, thereby fatiguing the material. Fixed-bearing designs tend to have a higher range of pitting stress than mobile-bearing designs do, and their less conforming geometries may allow for greater excursions of contact during ambulation, thus making them more susceptible to pitting damage.

Confluence of Stress

When the locations of pitting stress are spatially coincident with the locations of abrasive and delamination stress, there is a potential for pitting to exacerbate both the abrasion and delamination modes of wear. Bulk degradation of tibial inserts is clinically associated with synovitis and is visualized on retrievals as component fracture or gross scarring of the articular surface. These failures are caused by large subsurface stress in the polymer component. Pitting damage is not sufficient to independently cause gross malfunction of tibial components. However, vertical cracks can create defects on the articulating surface and propagate distally to intersect a horizontal delamination crack, thereby leading to gross scarring.

Effect of Conformity

Large contact area (conformity) is often a major design goal because it is assumed that increasing contact area always leads to lower stress, which in turn leads to less abrasion, pitting, and delamination of the tibial insert. However, the finite element results presented in this chapter demonstrate a wide range of conformities for both mobile- and fixed-bearing designs, all leading to generally very good results. The components were well manufactured and fit together well, thus creating low contact stress and subsequently small volumes of polymer that sustained damaging subsurface stress levels.

However, other investigations in this laboratory[17,18] have discovered several conforming systems with large contact areas that suffer from poorly fitting components leading to damaging stress levels. The fit of more conforming design components is much less forgiving of small variations in dimension than a less conforming design is. Recent tribological evidence[16,26,28] suggests that higher-contact *areas* are associated with increases in the volume of wear debris, thus implying an upper limit to the amount of conformity that may be advantageous.

Although contact area is a simple and often used performance benchmark, it is a poor predictor of wear performance, especially in an ill-fitting design. Contact stress and its distribution on the articulating surface are directly related to abrasion, pitting, and delamination of the tibial insert and are far more reliable predictors of long-term wear performance than contact area is.

MODEL VALIDATION

A feature common to analytic and computational models is the inclusion of simplifying assumptions meant to reduce a complex problem to one that is more easily understood. It is very important to check the effect of a model's simplifying assumptions against a set of relevant benchmarks to ensure that an oversimplification does not lead to errant conclusions. A model is also more valuable if it can be validated to several extreme cases. This provides more confidence that the model can be exercised in a range of circumstances and still yield accurate and useful results. When modeling wear in TKA components, comparison with damage patterns observed on UHMWPE inserts retrieved after in vivo function is a widely accepted standard benchmark. Comparing computational results with physical models such as implanted cadaver motion studies, fluoroscopy, mechanical wear testing, and laboratory contact studies can also be valuable.

Similarity between a model result and a benchmark increases confidence in the validity of the model. Figure 13–14A is a proximal view of the heel strike contact areas predicted by the finite element model in the least-conforming design presented in Figure 13–13. These contact locations serve as a "paintbrush" that distributes damage across the tibial insert when propelled by patient kinematics. The image in Figure 13–14B is an overlay plot that visualizes all damage pattern measurements from a series of 17 retrieved UHMWPE tibial inserts of the same design as presented in Figure 13–14A. The darker areas on this plot indicate that a greater number of inserts had damage in these locations, with black consistent with all inserts having damage. It is apparent that if the predicted contact areas in Figure 13–14A were swept by typical patient kinematics, a similar wear pattern as visualized in Figure 13–14B would be predicted. Comparison of these images indicates that the finite element model predicted the real-world component fit well because the contact areas coincide with locations of wear damage in clinical retrievals.

Figure 13–15A is a proximal view of the locations of pitting predicted by the finite element model in the most-conforming design presented in Figure 13–3. Figure 13–15B is an overlay plot that is limited to only displaying pitting damage on 11 retrievals of the same design as presented in Figure 13–15A. Light amounts of pitting damage can be seen distributed broadly around the periphery of each compartment. Comparison of these images indicates that the finite element model accurately predicted the light, peripheral pitting damage found in clinical retrievals.

Mobile-bearing implant designs allow motion between both the femoral and tibial tray components and the polymer insert in an effort to distribute the kinematic requirements of knee joint function between the proximal and distal surfaces of the tibial insert. This allows more conforming geometries between the components to be used in mobile-bearing designs. In theory, higher conformity leads to a reduction in damaging polymer stress and should improve component longevity. However, in

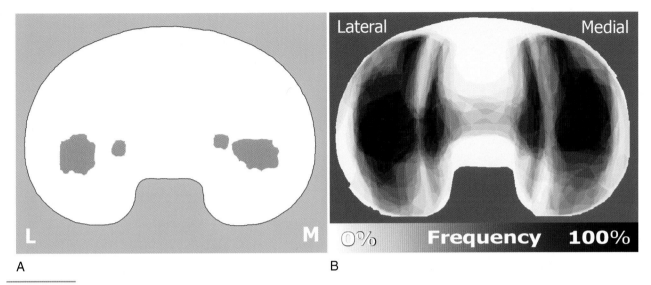

Figure 13–14. **A,** Proximal view of contact locations predicted by the finite element model at heel strike for the least conforming system presented in Figure 13–13. These locations serve as a "paintbrush" that distributes damage across the tibial insert when propelled by patient kinematics. **B,** Proximal view of an overlay damage plot for 17 clinical retrievals[12] of the same design as presented in **A.** Darker areas indicate that a greater number of inserts had damage in those locations.

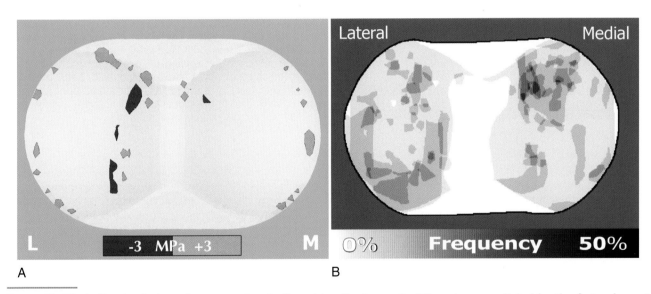

Figure 13–15. **A,** Proximal view of compressive (red) and tensile (orange) pitting stress predicted by the finite element model at heel strike for the most conforming system presented in Figure 13–3. **B,** Proximal view of an overlay pitting damage plot on seven clinical retrievals[13] of the same design as presented in **A.** Light pitting damage is noted in the periphery of each compartment.

practice, achieving the desired conformity through precision manufacturing can be a difficult proposition.

An example of the consequence of a poor fit between the femoral component and the proximal surface of a mobile bearing is seen in Figure 13–16A. The poor fit propagates to the distal interface and creates contact patterns along the edge of the distal surface (Fig. 13–16B). The amplifying effect of prescribed kinematics in a laboratory mechanical wear specimen[3] can be appreciated in a photograph of the distal surface of the same design (Fig. 13–16C). Comparison of Figure 13–16B and C indicates

that the finite element model is capable of accurately predicting locations of abrasion in laboratory wear specimens, even in an extreme case in which component fit was poor.

CONCLUSIONS

The finite element computational models herein have successfully predicted clinical wear observed in a wide range

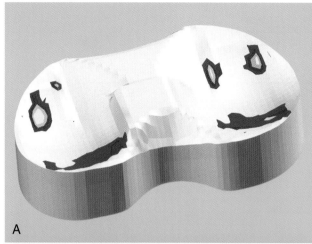

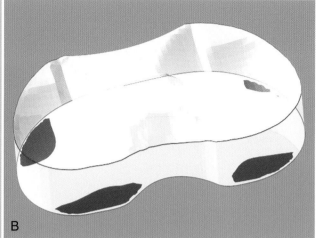

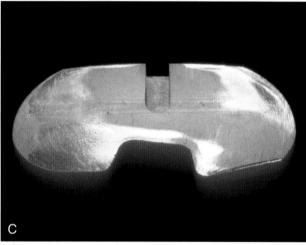

Figure 13–16. **A,** Proximal contact stress on a poorly fitting mobile bearing circa 1998. **B,** Distal contact stress on the backside interface between the tibial insert and the tibial tray of the same design as presented in **A. C,** Backside wear at 2 million cycles of walking gait wear simulation[3] for comparison to **B**. The applied walking gait motions amplify the effect of the peripheral contact locations.

of retrievals and, as such, may prove to be a valuable tool for extending the clinician's vision by determining a priori the wear performance of new implant designs. These models may also prove useful in the manufacturer's design stage to vet product concepts computationally before investing the time and expense required for physical laboratory wear testing and clinical trials.

The finite element model results in this chapter illustrate that a wide range of well-manufactured conformities can lead to a successful outcome. Highly conforming mobile-bearing designs with more than three times the contact area of a fixed design demonstrate only marginal improvement in stress performance. Coupled with evidence that good component fit is often not achieved in the manufacture of highly conforming designs and that large contact areas may be associated with an increase in volumetric wear, a case can be made for a happy medium when designing component conformity.

FUTURE WORK

Knee kinematics must be considered in any model with the goal of predicting the distribution of wear damage observed in clinical retrievals of TKA polyethylene inserts.

Femoral contact location, measured experimentally by fluoroscopy during dynamic activities, is a significant predictor of the damage location on polyethylene tibial inserts retrieved after in vivo function.[11] Finite element models have recently been extended to consider kinematics using an explicit analysis[10] and cyclic damage accumulation in the tibial insert.[27] These modeling techniques can be combined to produce a very powerful computational wear simulator.

Unlike finite element models that can calculate subsurface stress associated with delamination and pitting, another approach is dynamic contact (DC) models[7] that address surface deformation caused by compressive creep and material removal as a result of mild wear. Mild wear is consistent with adhesive-abrasive damage modes, such as the scratching, burnishing, and tractive striations that commonly occur on inserts retrieved for reasons other than mechanical failure.[11] DC models consider tibiofemoral motion along with design geometry, polymer material properties, and joint load to predict surface creep and abrasion wear damage depths on the polymer insert. DC models can also accommodate the variations in tibiofemoral kinematics and contact area locations that occur over the full range of knee flexion[4] when comparing different prostheses.

CODA

Orthopaedic Research Laboratories of Cleveland, Ohio, has analyzed more than 40 knee implants over the last decade with this finite element protocol to create a compendium of directly comparable performance results for a variety of contemporary designs, of which a subset is presented in this chapter. A searchable database of other results using this methodology, including unicompartmental designs, can be found at our website *http://orl-inc.com* for various activities such as high flexion, walking gait, and external torque.

The BioMotion Foundation's Orthopaedic Research Laboratory of West Palm Beach, Florida, has operated an implant retrieval program since 1992. Hundreds of different knee components have been retrieved after revision surgery and at autopsy. Quantitative assessment of surface wear modes, damage area, and surface deformation is available for model validation for a variety of designs from different manufacturers.

References

1. Apkarian J, Naumann S, Cairns B: A three-dimensional kinematic and dynamic model of the lower limb. J Biomech 22:143-155, 1989.
2. Bartel DL, Bicknell MS, Wright TM: The effect of conformity, thickness, and material on stresses in UHMWPE components for total joint replacement. J Bone Joint Surg Am 68:1041-1051, 1986.
3. Bell CJ, Walker PS, Saathasivam S, et al: Differences in wear between fixed bearing and mobile bearing knees. Trans Orthop Res Soc 24:962, 1999.
4. Bourne RB, Masonis J, Anthony M: An analysis of rotating-platform total knee replacements. Clin Orthop 410:173-180, 2003.
5. Collier JP, Mayor MB, McNamara JL, et al: Analysis of the failure of 122 polyethylene inserts from uncemented tibial knee components. Clin Orthop 273:232-242, 1991.
6. Dannenmaier WC, Haynes DW, Nelson CL: Granulomatous reaction and cystic bony destruction associated with high wear rate in a total knee prosthesis. Clin Orthop 198:224-230, 1985.
7. Fregly B, Sawyer W, Harman M, et al: Computational wear prediction of a total knee replacement from in vivo kinematics. J Biomech 38:305-314, 2005.
8. Furnes O, Espehaug B, Lie SA, et al: Early failures among 7,174 primary total knee replacements: A follow-up study from the Norwegian Arthroplasty Register 1994-2000. Acta Orthop Scand 73:117-129, 2002.
9. Goodman SB, Chin RC, Chiou SS, et al: A clinical-pathologic-biochemical study of the membrane surrounding loosened and nonloosened total hip arthroplasties. Clin Orthop 244:182-187, 1989.
10. Halloran JP, Petrella AJ, Rullkoetter PJ: Explicit finite element modeling of total knee replacement mechanics. J Biomech 38:323-331, 2005.
11. Harman M, Banks S, Hodge W: Polyethylene damage and knee kinematics after total knee arthroplasty. Clin Orthop 392:383-393, 2001.
12. Harman MK, Banks SA, Schmitt S, et al: Total knee replacement performance beyond 5 years: Can in vivo fluoroscopy and retrieved implant analysis lead the way? Presented at the 69th Annual Meeting of the American Academy of Orthopaedic Surgeons, Dallas, 3:738, 2002.
13. Harman MK, Markovich GD, Banks SA, et al: Cementless LCS total knee arthroplasty after 9 years in-situ: Articular and backside wear on retrieved meniscal and rotating platform polyethylene bearings. Presented at the 71st Annual Meeting of the American Academy of Orthopaedic Surgeons, San Francisco, 5:462, 2004.
14. LaFortune MA, Cavanaugh PR, Sommer HJ, et al: Three-dimensional kinematics of the human knee during walking. J Biomech 25:347-357, 1992.
15. Landy MM, Walker PS: Wear of ultra-high molecular-weight polyethylene components of 90 retrieved knee prostheses. J Arthroplasty 3:S73-S85, 1988.
16. Mazzucco D, Spector M: Effects of contact area and stress on the volumetric wear of ultrahigh molecular weight polyethylene. Wear 254:514-522, 2003.
17. Morra EA, Postak PD, Greenwald AS: The influence of mobile bearing knee geometry on the wear of UHMWPE tibial inserts III: A finite element study. Presented at the 67th Annual Meeting of the American Academy of Orthopaedic Surgeons, Orlando, 1:617, 2000.
18. Morra EA, Postak PD, Greenwald AS: Tibial plateau abrasion in mobile bearing knee systems during walking gait: A finite element study. Presented at the 71st Annual Meeting of the American Academy of Orthopaedic Surgeons, San Francisco, 5:462, 2004.
19. Morra EA, Postak PD, Plaxton MS, et al: The effects of external torque on polyethylene tibial insert damage patterns. Clin Orthop 410:90-100, 2003.
20. Morrison JB: Function of the knee joint in various activities. Biomed Eng 4:573-580, 1969.
21. Morrison JB: The mechanics of the knee joint in relation to normal walking. J Biomech 3:51-61, 1970.
22. Murray MP, Drought AB, Kory RC: Walking patterns in normal men. J Bone Joint Surg Am 46:335-360, 1964.
23. Paul JP: Forces transmitted by joints in the human body. Proc Inst Mech Eng 181:358, 1967.
24. Rose RM, Goldfarb HV: On the pressure dependence of the wear of ultrahigh molecular weight polyethylene. Wear 92:99-111, 1983.
25. Rostoker W, Galante JO: Contact pressure dependence of wear rates of ultra high molecular weight polyethylene. J Biomed Mater Res 13:957-964, 1979.
26. Saikko V, Ahlroos T: Wear simulation of UHMWPE for total hip replacement with a multidirectional motion pin-on-disk device: Effects of counterface material, contact area, and lubricant. J Biomed Mater Res 49:147-154, 2000.
27. Sathasivam S, Walker PS: The conflicting requirements of laxity and conformity in total knee replacement. J Biomech 32:239-247, 1999.
28. Sathasivam S, Walker PS, Campbell PA, et al: The effect of contact area on wear in relation to fixed bearing and mobile bearing knee replacements. J Biomed Mater Res 58:282-290, 2001.
29. Sharkey PF, Hozack WJ, Rothman RH, et al: Why are total knee arthroplasties failing today? Clin Orthop 404:7-13, 2002.
30. Waldman SD, Bryant JT: Compressive stress relaxation behavior of irradiated ultra-high molecular weight polyethylene at 37° C. J Appl Biomater 5:333-338, 1994.
31. Willert HG, Bertram H, Buchhorn GH: Osteolysis in alloarthroplasty of the hip: The role of ultra-high molecular weight polyethylene wear particles. Clin Orthop 258:95-107, 1990.
32. Williams JG: Stress Analysis of Polymers. John Wiley & Sons, Halstead Press, 1984.

CHAPTER 14

Choosing Your Implant

James McAuley • Tom Eickmann

With many implant designs and levels of constraint, selecting the optimum implant can be a difficult process. The advantage of increasing the level of constraint is added stability. However, added constraint of the components will increase stress on the implant and bone interface.[36] In principle, the lowest level of constraint that provides adequate stability should be used.[31,36] Posterior cruciate–retaining and posterior cruciate–substituting knees are used in the vast majority of primary knee arthroplasties. In some cases, however, varus/valgus-constrained or hinged components are required.[18] It is important to recognize the potential need for additional constraint preoperatively so the appropriate implants are available in the operating room.

PREOPERATIVE PLANNING

In deciding on the appropriate level of constraint, preoperative clinical and radiographic examination is critical. The knee should be examined for signs of posterior cruciate ligament (PCL) instability, including the posterior sag sign and the posterior drawer and quadriceps active tests. Assessing the knee for an effusion is also important because it can be an indication of underlying instability, such as the triad of anterior knee pain, swelling, and giving way found in PCL-deficient knees.[34] The knee should be examined with varus and valgus stress to delineate collateral ligamentous laxity and whether any deformity is fixed or correctable. It is important to recognize the difference between laxity (which implies pathologic stretching of the ligament on the convex side of the deformity) and pseudolaxity (which is simply the sensation of instability produced by an underlying bony deficiency). Evaluation of the gait pattern will also reveal varus or valgus thrust, which can be an indicator of collateral ligamentous laxity and subsequent tibiofemoral subluxation.

Radiographic examination is an essential part of the preoperative examination. We routinely perform anteroposterior (AP) weightbearing and 90-degree lateral views. Twenty-degree flexion and notch views are performed if needed to document the extent of degenerative changes. Sunrise views are used to assess the patellofemoral joint. In addition to confirming proper indications for surgery, the amount of deformity can be quantified. The flexion view demonstrates rollback of the femur on the tibia and gives an indication of the functional status of the PCL: Excessive rollback is seen in PCL contracture, whereas the posterior sag sign occurs with PCL insufficiency.

Bone deficiency should be noted because defects may necessitate metal augmentation or allograft reconstruction.

CRUCIATE-RETAINING IMPLANTS

Cruciate-retaining implants represent the lowest level of component constraint, but no knee components are truly "unconstrained" (Fig. 14–1).[22] For example, in one manufacturer's cruciate-retaining design, no varus-valgus stability is provided by the implant, but rotation is limited to 15 degrees internally and externally.[37] Indications for cruciate retention versus cruciate substitution are controversial. It does make sense that optimal results will be obtained in a sound biomechanical environment. Severe deformity, large bone defects, or significant soft-tissue deficiency can compromise knee kinematics and thus may not be ideal situations for cruciate-retaining designs. For a knee replacement to be cruciate retaining, there must be a functional PCL. If a surgeon is considering the use of a cruciate-retaining design, the status of the PCL must be specifically addressed and optimized by recession if needed to avoid the limitations to full flexion that result from an excessively tight PCL. In some cases the PCL may be contracted, and different techniques can then be used to balance the knee.[5]

In some patients, release of a contracted PCL can result in posterior sag and AP laxity in flexion, and thus a posterior-stabilized implant may be preferred.

Cruciate-retaining knees have historically been used predominantly for varus osteoarthritis, but Krackow and colleagues reported successful use of cruciate-retaining implants in valgus knees despite the need for soft-tissue release.[17] Our experience of repair of 159 valgus knees at the Anderson Orthopaedic Research Institute (AORI) has revealed that the cruciate could be retained in 150 cases without excessive rollback and with good correction of the deformity. Survivorship was 93% at 8 years postoperatively. These data suggest that cruciate-retaining designs can be used successfully in valgus knees and are a reasonable alternative to using posterior-stabilized implants in knees with valgus deformities.[9]

Cruciate-retaining designs are rarely indicated in the revision scenario. Prerequisites include good bone stock, a healthy surrounding soft-tissue envelope, and a functional PCL. Unicondylar arthroplasty revisions, early failure of fixation, and polyethylene insert wear are conditions that may lend themselves to cruciate-retaining revision knees. However, cruciate-retaining knees would

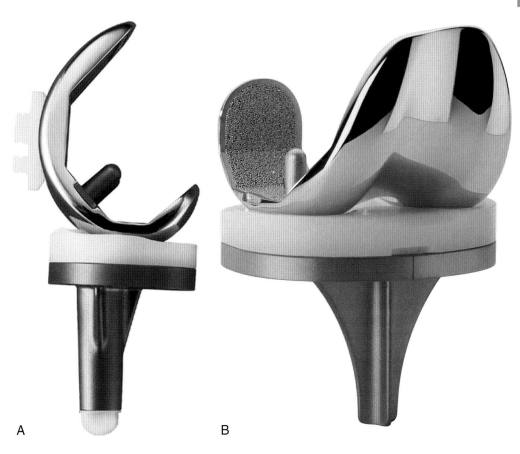

Figure 14–1. **A** and **B**, Cruciate-retaining implant. (Courtesy of DePuy, Warsaw, IN.)

A

B

not be indicated in most revision circumstances. Attempts at using cruciate-retaining designs in knees with PCL insufficiency and a loose flexion space have produced disappointing results.[28,34] Augments, wedges, and stems are not available in many cruciate-retaining designs, which limits their usefulness in a revision scenario (Figs. 14–2 and 14–3).

POSTERIOR-STABILIZED IMPLANTS

Posterior-stabilized or cruciate-substituting implants are the next level of constraint in knee arthroplasty (Fig. 14–4). The PCL is routinely resected in the posterior-stabilized technique, thus eliminating the subjective aspects of PCL evaluation and balancing. However, more bone stock is lost by making a box cut, and in osteoporotic bone, such loss of bone stock may increase the risk for supracondylar periprosthetic fracture.[21] The box in the femoral component may also come in contact with the quadriceps tendon in extreme flexion, which can lead to fibrous thickening of the tendon. The fibrous thickening may become symptomatic and is manifested as a painful patellar clunk when the knee is actively extended from extreme flexion.[10]

With the PCL resected, there is no anatomic structure to encourage rollback in flexion. In most cases, PCL function is substituted in posterior-stabilized designs by a post on the polyethylene that engages in the box of the femoral

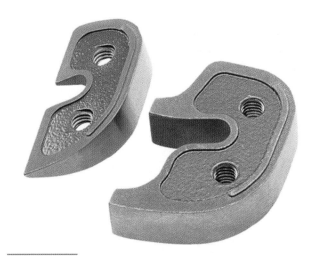

Figure 14–2. Metal augments. (Courtesy of Zimmer, Warsaw, IN.)

component at around 75 degrees; engagement of the post produces obligatory rollback and prevents posterior sag of the tibia under the femur.[37] Rollback is important in allowing extreme flexion. Addition of the post does add stability, but it also introduces the potential problems of post wear and impingement.

The design of a posterior-stabilized component may allow better contact area between components and subse-

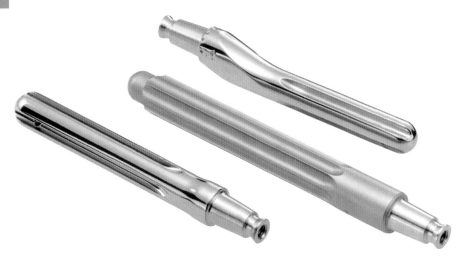

Figure 14–3. Stems. (Courtesy of Zimmer, Warsaw, IN.)

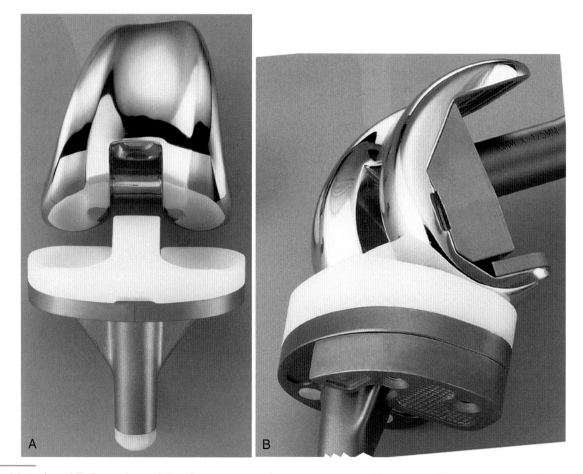

A

B

Figure 14–4. **A** and **B**, Posterior-stabilized or cruciate-substituting implant. (Courtesy of DePuy, Warsaw, IN.)

quently be a more favorable environment for the tibial polyethylene. The contact area of one manufacturer's posterior-stabilized design is 289 mm^2 in extension and 154 mm^2 in flexion.[37] Cruciate-retaining designs tend to have less contact area. For example, one manufacturer's cruciate-retaining knee, depending on the style of polyethylene, would have 148 to 270 mm^2 contact area in extension and 120 to 169 mm^2 in flexion.[3] Increasing the contact area theoretically reduces contact stress on the polyethylene and thus reduces wear.

Posterior-stabilized implants offer no improvement in varus/valgus stability over cruciate-retaining designs.[15] It is important to realize that the polyethylene becomes more conforming in posterior-stabilized designs and additional rotational constraint is introduced. One manufacturer's design allows 12 degrees of internal and external rotation.[37] Another's design offers 7.5 degrees of internal and external rotation in its posterior-stabilized knee.[3] It is very important to ensure optimum rotational match of the femoral and tibial components in fixed-bearing posterior-stabilized designs. Producing equal flexion and extension spaces is an essential aspect of the posterior-stabilized implant technique to optimize knee function. Producing a relatively loose flexion space can be disastrous because of the potential for post dislocation posteriorly from the femoral box.[8] An alternative to the traditional posted cruciate-substituting designs is the use of an ultracongruent polyethylene insert with anterior buildup, which also limits posterior subluxation. The downside of a more rounded or constrained insert is the potential for transmitting higher stress to the prosthesis, which may contribute to aseptic loosening or backside wear in modular inserts.[2]

Posterior-stabilized implants may be used in uncomplicated varus knees, are commonly used in valgus knees, and are recommended in cases of previous patellectomy, PCL deficiency, complex primary arthroplasty, and most revision arthroplasties. A posterior-stabilized level of constraint is all that is required to obtain a full complement of augments, wedges, and stems to address cases of severe bone loss.[12]

VARUS-VALGUS–CONSTRAINED IMPLANTS

The next level of constraint is varus-valgus constraint (Fig. 14–5). These implants inherently produce varus-valgus stability, but they also result in further rotational limitation. One manufacturer's design allows 2.2 degrees of varus and valgus motion and 4.3 degrees of internal and external rotation.[3] Another's design allows 1.25 degrees of varus and valgus motion and 2 degrees of rotation.[37]

Constrained implants can succeed only if the deforming forces are corrected.[33] For long-term durability in cases of severe varus-valgus instability, adjunctive soft-tissue reconstruction is often needed to provide long-term stability. Inadequate correction of deformity can predispose soft-tissue reconstructions to failure.[16] If a patient has perfect alignment, it is possible for medial instability to be asymptomatic.[15] Residual collateral ligamentous deficiency is much better tolerated on the lateral side of the knee than on the medial side, but only if valgus alignment of the knee is restored. Conversely, lateral collateral deficiency will be poorly tolerated if the leg is in varus alignment.[24]

The AORI experience with varus-valgus–constrained implant designs as the sole treatment of varus-valgus instability has been very disappointing, with success

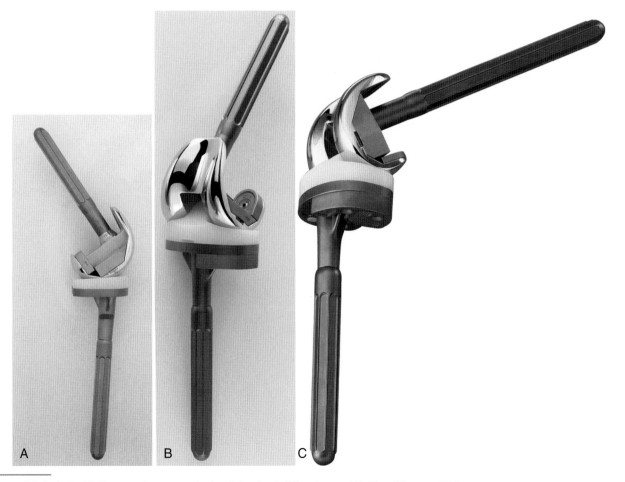

Figure 14–5. **A** to **C**, Varus-valgus–constrained implant. (Courtesy of DePuy, Warsaw, IN.)

achieved in only 20%. The mode of failure was late recurrence of the instability.[23]

Varus-valgus–constrained implants transmit higher stress to the prosthesis-bone interface, and the long-term outcome may be adversely affected by this higher stress.[35] Stems can be used in varus-valgus–constrained knees to help distribute the stress and transfer it to the diaphyseal segment of the bone.[6] Stems are commonly used at this level of constraint, although the indications for using them remain controversial.[19,27]

To provide increased varus-valgus stability, tibial post height is greater than in posterior-stabilized designs. It is critical to remember that posterior dislocation is still a potential problem with a loose flexion space. The odds of a dislocation occurring, however, are lower than with posterior-stabilized designs, which have a much shorter post.

Varus-valgus–constrained implant designs are rarely indicated in a primary arthroplasty setting; an example of the need for this level of constraint would be an incompetent collateral on the convex side of a severe deformity that cannot be corrected by standard ligament-balancing techniques.[7] Significant collateral ligament laxity in primary knee arthroplasty can still be addressed many times by using a less constrained design, but only if the soft-tissue envelope has the potential to provide long-term stability in the knee.[4] In the case of iatrogenic injury to the medial collateral ligament, good results may be obtained with primary repair or reattachment and postoperative bracing.[20] In the revision setting, it is more common to require varus-valgus constraint because of frequent compromise of the soft-tissue envelope from previous surgery. In principle, the minimal level of constraint that restores mechanical stability should be used.[26]

HINGED DESIGNS

Hinged or linked designs represent the ultimate level of constraint (Fig. 14–6). As our experience has shown, constrained designs have severe limitations in patients with collateral ligamentous deficiency or flexion instability. Unfortunately, along with increasing levels of constraint, the forces transmitted to the bone-prosthesis interface become greater.[1,32,36] This has historically resulted in disappointing results with frequent and early loosening.[11,13,29]

Despite the reduced rotational constraint with rotating hinges, early results were disappointing.[30] Newer designs of rotating hinges have produced more encouraging early results.[1,35] However, in some cases there is no good alternative to a linked design.

The indications for a hinged implant have continued to evolve. The strongest indications for this level of constraint are global instability, complete absence of collateral ligamentous support, and severe flexion instability.[1,24] Relative indications include neuropathic joints and elderly

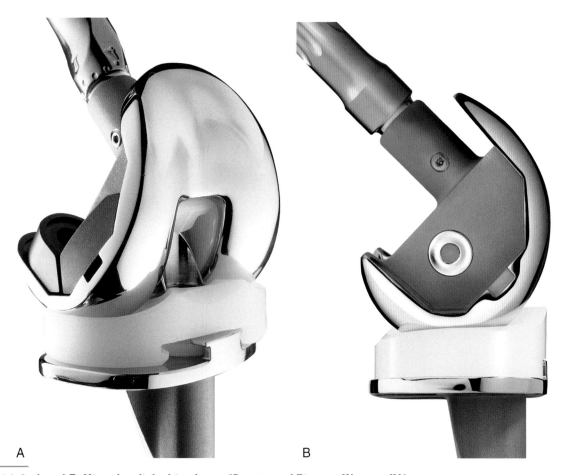

A   B

Figure 14–6. **A** and **B**, Hinged or linked implants. (Courtesy of Zimmer, Warsaw, IN.)

patients with distal femoral fractures.[1] Another potential indication would be a case in which greater than 1 inch of leg lengthening is required to achieve stability.[14] In our opinion, the progression to a linked component design is determined by the soft-tissue envelope, not by bone deficiencies, which can be successfully handled with modern graft or augmentation techniques.

Hinged implants are rarely indicated in primary knee arthroplasty. The primary cause of instability in primary knee arthroplasty is malalignment.[24,25] Complex cases involving a severe deformity have an increased probability of soft-tissue compromise, which may warrant having a hinged prosthesis available. In patients with severe flexion-extension mismatch or deficient medial soft tissues, a rotating hinge should be considered.[18] This clinical scenario is more common in revision knee arthroplasty.

To obtain optimal long-term clinical results, careful preoperative planning and having the necessary implants available at the time of surgery are important. Careful attention at the time of surgery to the soft-tissue envelope and gap balancing is essential for optimal long-term results. If this cannot be accomplished, increasing the level of constraint is essential to provide acceptable results beyond the short term.

References

1. Barrack R: Evolution of the rotating hinge for complex total knee arthroplasty. Clin Orthop 392:292, 2001.
2. Callaghan J, O'Rourke M, Goetz D, et al: Tibial post impingement in posterior-stabilized total knee arthroplasty. Clin Orthop 404:83, 2002.
3. DePuy Design Rationale.
4. Edwards E, Miller J, Chan K: The effect of postoperative collateral ligament laxity in total knee arthroplasty. Clin Orthop 236:44, 1988.
5. Engh G: The difficult knee. Clin Orthop 416:58, 2003.
6. Engh G, Ammeen D: Bone loss with revision total knee arthroplasty: Defect classification and alternatives for reconstruction. Instr Course Lect 48:167, 1999.
7. Fehring T, Valadie A: Knee instability after total knee arthroplasty. Clin Orthop 229:157, 1994.
8. Gebhard J, Kilgus D: Dislocation of a posterior stabilized total knee prosthesis. Clin Orthop 254:225, 1990.
9. Hamilton W, Collier M, McAuley J, Engh G: Total knee arthroplasty with posterior cruciate retention for treatment of valgus osteoarthritis. Unpublished data, Anderson Orthopaedic Research Institute.
10. Hozack W, Rothman R, Booth R, et al: The patellar clunk syndrome. A complication of posterior stabilized total knee arthroplasty. Clin Orthop 241:203, 1989.
11. Inglis A, Walker P: Revision of failed knee replacement using fixed-axis hinges. J Bone Joint Surg Br 73:757, 1991.
12. Insall J: Revision of total knee replacement. Instr Course Lect 35:290, 1986.
13. Karpinski M, Grimer R: Hinged knee replacement in revision arthroplasty. Clin Orthop 220:185, 1987.
14. Kaufer H, Matthews L: Revision total knee arthroplasty: Indications and contraindications. Instr Course Lect 35:297, 1986.
15. Krackow K: Revision total knee replacement ligament balancing for deformity. Clin Orthop 404:152, 2002.
16. Krackow K: Instability in total knee arthroplasty. J Arthroplasty 18:45, 2003.
17. Krackow K, Jones M, Teeny S, et al: Primary total knee arthroplasty in patients with fixed valgus deformity. Clin Orthop 273:9, 1991.
18. Kumar J, Dorr L: Severe malalignment and soft-tissue imbalance in total knee arthroplasty. Am J Knee Surg 10:1, 1997.
19. Lachiewicz P, Falatyn S: Clinical and radiographic results of the total condylar III and constrained condylar total knee arthroplasty. J Arthroplasty 11:916, 1996.
20. Leopold S, McStay C, Klafeta K, et al: Primary repair of intraoperative disruption of the medial collateral ligament during total knee arthroplasty. J Bone Joint Surg Am 83:86, 2001.
21. Lombardi A, Mallory T, Waterman R, et al: Intercondylar distal femoral fracture. J Arthroplasty 10:643, 1995.
22. McAuley J, Engh G: Constraint in total knee arthroplasty. J Arthroplasty 18:51, 2003.
23. McAuley J, Engh G, Ammeen D: Treatment of the unstable total knee arthroplasty. Instr Course Lect 53:237, 2004.
24. Moore M, McAuley J: Instability after total knee arthroplasty. In Callaghan JJ, Rosenburg AG, Rubash HE, Simonian PT, Wickiewicz TL, (eds): The Adult Knee. Philadelphia, Lippincott Williams & Wilkins, 2003, p 1377.
25. Moreland J: Mechanisms of failure in total knee arthroplasty. Clin Orthop 226:49, 1988.
26. Naudie D, Rorabeck C: Managing instability in total knee arthroplasty with constrained and linked implants. Instr Course Lect 53:207, 2004.
27. Nazarian D, Mehta S, Booth R: A comparison of stemmed and unstemmed components in revision knee arthroplasty. Clin Orthop 404:256, 2002.
28. Pagnano M, Hanssen A, Lewallen D, Stuart M: Flexion instability after primary posterior cruciate retaining total knee arthroplasty. Clin Orthop 356:39, 1998.
29. Pritsch M, Fitzgerald R, Bryan R: Surgical treatment of ligamentous instability after total knee arthroplasty. Arch Orthop Trauma Surg 102:154, 1984.
30. Rand J, Chao E, Stauffer R: Kinematic rotating-hinge total knee arthroplasty. J Bone Joint Surg Am 69:489, 1987.
31. Scuderi G: Revision total knee arthroplasty. Clin Orthop 392:300, 2001.
32. Shaw J, Balcom W, Greer R: Total knee arthroplasty using the kinematic rotating hinge prosthesis. Orthopedics 12:647, 1989.
33. Vince K: Why knees fail. J Arthroplasty 18:39, 2003.
34. Waslewski G, Marson B, Benjamin J: Early incapacitating instability of posterior cruciate ligament–retaining total knee arthroplasty. J Arthroplasty 13:763, 1998.
35. Westrich G, Mollano A, Sculco T, et al: Rotating hinge total knee arthroplasty in severely affected knees. Clin Orthop 379:195, 2000.
36. Whiteside L, Kasselt M, Haynes D: Varus-valgus and rotational stability in rotationally unconstrained total knee arthroplasty. Clin Orthop 219:147, 1987.
37. Zimmer Design Rationale.

CHAPTER 15

The Retrieval Laboratory: Making Sense of Knee Implant Revisions

Douglas W. Van Citters • John P. Collier

Over 30,000 total knee arthroplasty revision surgeries are performed each year, a figure that represents nearly 10% of all total knee replacements performed.[35,45] These surgeries include revisions for pain, infection, trauma, malposition, loosening, and osteolysis. Given the range of reasons for revision, it is natural for all the parties involved in the surgery to be curious about the root causes of the failure. More importantly, the surgeon, patient, and manufacturer would all like to identify ways in which a process, material, or design can be improved to reduce the likelihood of failure in the future. It is therefore important to investigate every aspect of the system, including the failed device (Fig. 15–1). These failure analyses are some of the most valuable tools in promoting future success.

Retrieval analysis, though currently performed by a very small number of laboratories and scientists, is a significant component of any orthopedic quality improvement program. The importance of knee prosthesis retrieval has been recognized since the early 1980s, when Hood et al began examining long-term outcomes of total condylar knees.[29] Over the past 20 years, hundreds of publications related to retrieval analysis have been produced, and in 2000 the National Institutes of Health (NIH) released a state-of-the-science statement recognizing the importance and need for a national retrieval program.[46]

Unfortunately, the orthopedic specialty is a long way from developing a standardized national retrieval program. Although some surgeons and their research teams analyze devices that they have revised and a very few independent retrieval centers exist, the vast majority of knee implants removed during revision surgery are not evaluated. Furthermore, postmortem analysis during autopsy is rarely performed, thus denying the cohort of "successful" components from inclusion in most scientific studies.

Despite the lack of a national system, retrieval studies have nonetheless been instrumental in changing the way that implants are designed and manufactured. After identifying factors that can lead to implant failure, some of the techniques and limitations of retrieval analysis will be described. The time and complexity that are often associated with solving an industry-wide problem will be illustrated through the example of the ultrahigh-molecular-weight polyethylene (UHMWPE) oxidation problem. The historical example will be followed by a description of some of the questions that retrieval programs are currently trying to answer. Finally, the continued need for retrieval studies will be presented in the context of the current orthopedic market.

FAILURE TYPES

Orthopedic implant failures can be broadly classified according to the root causes of malfunction. Although different researchers create various categories to best suit their particular line of investigation, perhaps the simplest and most elegant failure classification was presented by Morrey in 1993.[43] He separates implant failures into three categories based on the major factor: the patient, the procedure, and the device.[43]

Patient Factors

Patient factors such as activity levels or adverse physiological reactions are difficult to control and, in some cases, impossible to avoid. For instance, revision surgery and component retrieval may be necessary for a patient who was in a vehicle accident (Fig. 15–2). In such a case, the joint has failed, but there is nothing that the orthopedic surgeon or the manufacturer of the orthopedic device could have done. Likewise, a patient who subjects the device to unusual duty cycles during a game of full-contact football or marathon running may also be solely responsible for failure of the device.

Figure 15–3 illustrates one of the more common types of failure associated with patient factors. The patient weighed 250 lb and led an active lifestyle. The cause of failure was determined to be fatigue fracture of the material as a result of patient weight and activity level. Recent studies have estimated that over 60% of the U.S. population is overweight or obese.[27] Because of the high stress placed on their joints, overweight patients have a higher incidence of knee and hip problems than do patients within a healthy weight range.[22] Although joint replacement may provide at least a temporary solution to joint pain or instability, patient weight will continue to have deleterious effects on the joint. Total knee prostheses are designed to operate within a set of parameters associated with normal activity for the majority of the population. However, the high stress associated with obesity, combined with an unusual stress environment, may result in catastrophic failure of the device.[7]

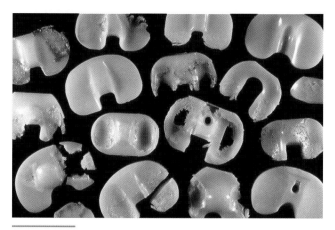

Figure 15–1. Panorama of failed total knee devices.

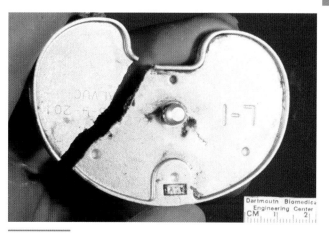

Figure 15–3. Tibial tray failure attributed to patient weight.

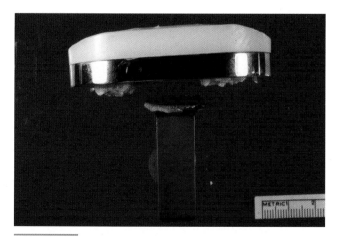

Figure 15–2. Tibial component failure caused by a single, high-stress event, in this case a vehicle accident.

Procedure Factors

The second set of factors leading to failure is related to the surgical procedure. Though possibly preventable, these failures may be somewhat more difficult to analyze because the retrieval scientist is rarely present during the primary surgery. Determining whether additional surgical guides or training could have prevented the failure is hence difficult and requires a complete set of radiographs or case notes to analyze. Unfortunately, complete details are seldom submitted with the retrieved devices, and concrete indications regarding surgical technique during the original implantation are often not provided.

Occasionally, egregious errors during primary surgery lead to device failure and subsequent revision surgery. For instance, wrong-site surgeries could result in left knee devices being inserted in right knees or vice versa. Simple solutions such as the American Academy of Orthopaedic Surgeons "Sign Your Site" campaign have been introduced to eliminate such errors. Although it is still too early to determine results in the United States, a similar campaign in Canada has proved successful in reducing the incidence of wrong-site surgery.[23]

More commonly, procedure factors lead to less severe and more difficult to identify conditions such as a mal-aligned device or a poorly cemented component. For instance, Silva et al noted that poor alignment during the initial surgery led to eventual tibial loosening.[54] Likewise, Moreland et al identified alignment as a critical factor in stability and fixation.[42] These alignment problems, in turn, can produce mechanical loading for which an implant was not designed. When coupled with cyclic loading, these factors can lead to material fatigue or wear and eventual failure.

Device Factors

Although procedural and patient factors can lead to joint revision, many factors that lead to joint failure are related to the device itself. Morrey further differentiates device factors into three categories based on manufacturing and design changes that can be implemented to avoid this type of failure. These categories include inadequate design, poor material selection, and inappropriate manufacturing process.[43] Figures 15–4 to 15–6 show examples of each type of failure.

In reality, failure factors often do not occur independent of one another. As an example, wear of a poorly selected material, a design factor, may result in particulate debris that causes bone loss in a person with a predisposition to osteolysis. Osteolysis, in turn, may be responsible for implant loosening and eventual failure of the implant to perform its intended function. Although the patient factor is ultimately responsible for the revision, it is the device that can be more readily addressed through a design or material change.

RETRIEVAL LABORATORY TOOLS

Although device failures can often be identified visually, the possible scenarios leading to failure are best identified with a well-equipped testing facility. Rather than just an archive, a retrieval laboratory can be thought of as a pathology laboratory for mechanical devices. Even though the methods and materials may differ between the two, failure analysis and problem solving are performed at each site. Furthermore, in both cases the results of an investigation are based on observations and analysis of the samples provided by the surgeon.

Figure 15–7 presents a copy of the retrieval form used by the Dartmouth Biomedical Engineering Center for Orthopaedics. At first glance, it may seem unusual to include surgical interpretations in a mechanical or materials study, but an understanding of the failure environment is incomplete without clues regarding patient history and diagnoses. This critical information allows for a detailed and accurate report that provides more complete causal relationships.

Whereas a surgeon's judgment is influenced by patient-related observations such as device position, pain, tissue condition, and patient activity, the retrieval scientist focuses on mechanical performance of the device. This is approached both destructively and nondestructively by using a host of material testing techniques. Nondestructive tests provide information related to the dimensional, morphological, or appearance changes sustained in vivo.

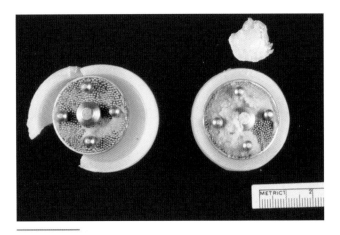

Figure 15–4. Design failure: patellar failure caused by high stress in thin polyethylene.

Destructive tests explore the mechanical and chemical changes occurring in vivo.

The most common nondestructive test is optical analysis. Components can be viewed with the naked eye or with a stereomicroscope to determine color, surface appearance and texture, wear scarring, or other damage. If necessary, higher-resolution images can be obtained with the aid of an environmental scanning electron microscope. Individual characteristics can be quantified with either method, although it is often more efficient to assign a qualitative rating to each type of damage. For instance, burnishing, pitting, scratching, delamination, abrasion, creep, and cracking can all be evaluated on a 0 through 3 scale per the scoring system of Hood et al.[29] Many of these same attributes could be counted, mapped, and measured, but there is questionable value in investing extra time to gain the additional information. The reader is nonetheless cautioned that sorting such observations into larger qualitative bins still relies heavily on interobserver repeatability. This can be overcome through training and use of a well-defined scale.

Results less subject to interobserver variation can be obtained through other nondestructive tests. Measurements using calipers or a micrometer can determine postimplantation dimensions to quantify abrasion or creep. If it is necessary to take dimensional and textural measurements on an even smaller scale, coordinate measurement, laser profiling, and surface metrology can be used.

Conditt et al published two related papers showing the utility of quantification and qualification in knee bearing analysis. The first study reported on the severity of signs of wear across a large collection of knee retrievals.[16] The focus of the study was whether wear is of universal concern to the industry, and hence a quantified review was unnecessary. Their second article, however, focused on a single design and investigated a possible correlation between micromotion and wear in a modular prosthesis.[15] The study design necessitated quantification of wear, locking mechanism clearance, and range of movement between the tibial components for each device.

In some cases, even chemical measurements can be determined nondestructively. Energy-dispersive x-ray

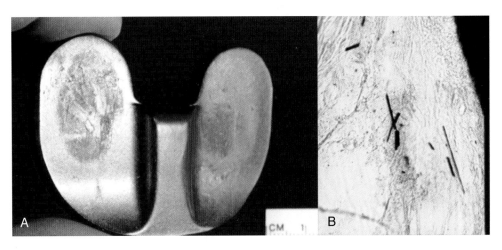

Figure 15–5. Material selection. Carbon fiber–reinforced polyethylene wore in vivo (**A**) and left shards of carbon in the surrounding tissue (**B**).

analysis and Raman spectrometry can be used to determine the atomic and molecular composition of a device without damage. For instance, McDonald and Bloebaum used backscattered electron imaging and elemental analysis to better visualize third-body debris embedded in poly-ethylene inserts.[40] Such a technique can prove useful to determine the cause of wear when the third body is difficult to detect by optical means.

After nondestructive tests are complete, destructive tests may provide additional insight into the reason that dimensional changes and unexpected visible damage have occurred. Chemical analysis is often used to determine whether the device's initial character has changed over time as a result of in vivo chemical processes. Some of the most common techniques available for chemical analysis include Fourier transform infrared spectrometry, differential scanning calorimetry, Raman spectrometry, and electron spin resonance.

Beyond the atomic and molecular level, grain and crystal scale measurements can be performed with metallurgic techniques. Such studies can determine grain sizes, impurity contents, and phase distribution in a retrieved device. In addition, x-ray diffraction can be used to determine crystal structure and composition.

Figure 15–6 shows a device in which the porous coating separated from the tibial tray. In this laboratory and others, metallurgy performed on similar devices showed that the strength of the bead/substrate bond was insufficient to perform as designed.[17,34,47] These results led to new

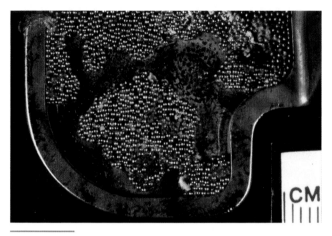

Figure 15–6. Process failure. Poor metallurgy allowed the porous coating to break away from the tibial component.

IMPLANT RETRIEVAL FORM   DBEC Number:_____
See reverse for shipping procedure   For Laboratory Use Only

SURGEON INFORMATION: Retrieval Surgeon:_____
Address:_____
Telephone:_____   FAX #:_____   E-mail address:_____
Did you implant the retrieved prosthesis? *yes*   *no*   If not, who did?_____

PATIENT INFORMATION: Name:_____   M   F   Age:_____   Wt:_____lbs Ht:_____in
Patient activity level prior to the onset of symptoms: *very active   active   ambulatory w/aids   nonambulatory*
Patient activity level immediately prior to surgery: *very active   active   ambulatory w/aids   nonambulatory*
Description of pain (prior to surgery):   1) severity: *none   mild   moderate   severe*
                                           2) location: *groin   buttock   thigh   knee   other:_____*
                                           3) duration:_____*months*
What was the primary diagnosis for which this prosthesis was implanted?_____
Were there any additional significant diagnoses prior to surgery?   *yes   no*
If so, please describe:_____

IMPLANT INFORMATION: *Left / Right*   Manufacturer:_____   Model:_____
Implant LOT #'s (high priority for LOT #'s of polyethylene components): _____
(if possible, please enclose photocopies of the ***retrieved*** implants' identification stickers from the patient file)
Date of Implantation: /   /   Date of Retrieval: /   /
Was this implant inserted as a Primary or a Revision?   *P   R   unknown*
Why was this prosthesis removed? *loose   subsidence   painful   position   instability   dislocation   lysis*
     wear of: poly – metal   fracture of: poly – implant – bone   sepsis   postmortem   other:_____
     Which component?_____
Pertinent history:_____
Did the poly insert disassociate in vivo?   *yes   no   loosely attached*
Was this implant Hydroxyapatite (HA) coated?   *yes   no*
What was the quality of bone at the time of revision?   *poor   fair   good   excellent*
Was there evidence of significant debris?   *no   poly   metal   cement   other:_____*
                                lytic activity at revision?   *none   mild   moderate   severe*
                                loosening?   *none   mild   moderate   severe*
                                stress shielding?   *none   mild   moderate   severe*
                                osteoporosis?   *yes   no*   If so, was it: *clinical   radiographic   both*
What was the removal difficulty?   *none   mild   moderate   severe*
What surgical instruments were used?_____
What is the replacement prosthesis?   Manufacturer:_____   Model:_____

CLINICAL DETAIL: If you implanted this retrieved prosthesis,
Were you initially satisfied with its size?   *yes   no*   its orientation?   *yes   no*
Were there any complications?_____
What was the post-operative management?   bed rest_____days   protection_____days/weeks
Additional comments:_____

Please Enclose All Retrieved Items including metal shells, stems, heads, screws, pegs, clips, etc.

Enclosed_____Under Separate Cover_____

Figure 15–7. Sample DBEC retrieval form.

fabrication methods and, in many devices, elimination of beads in favor of cemented fixation.

If the chemical or structural character of the device has changed, it is useful to know what effect this has on mechanical properties such as tensile strength, ductility, modulus, and toughness. Likewise, inferior performance may be a function of poor material selection or quality assurance, both of which can result in unacceptable mechanical properties. Several mechanical tests are routinely used to determine these properties, including tensile and compressive tests and, more recently, the small-punch test. All three tests are standardized by the American Society for Testing of Materials (ASTM International) and hence provide data that are easily compared between laboratories.[1-4,13,19,36]

Despite the wealth of tools and methods available in a well-equipped laboratory, the most important asset is the experience and ingenuity of its employees. In reality, the most important job of the retrieval scientist is to act as the lead detective. No matter how much data are collected, synthesis and subsequent development of a story about the life of an implant are the most critical components of retrieval analysis. It is this fusion of information that leads to industry-wide process and material improvement.

EVOLUTION OF A PROBLEM

With an understanding of the factors leading to failure and the tools available to analyze them, an example can be presented that shows the evolution of a solution to the worldwide problem of irradiation-induced oxidation. This case in point highlights the time and volume of retrievals necessary to generate evidence sufficiently compelling to cause an industry-wide change. The resulting reduction in specific implant failure modes demonstrates the efficacy and importance of a retrieval laboratory.

The first knee retrieval was received by our laboratory in March 1980. Rather than demonstrating a mode of failure from patient factors such as sepsis, aseptic loosening, or subluxation, the polyethylene tibial component had catastrophically failed after 36 months through contact fatigue and subsequent delamination. At the time, oxidation of polyethylene was not recognized as a problem in orthopedic devices, and the polyethylene tested by manufacturers and independent laboratories showed remarkable toughness and fatigue fracture properties. Because product testing and development used nonsterile or recently sterilized components, there was no reason to believe that polyethylene would suffer degraded mechanical properties by the time of implantation or during in vivo service.

As more devices arrived at our facility, it became apparent that a significant percentage of polyethylene components exhibited cracking and delamination. In fact, the first paper on the topic published by this laboratory reported a fatigue failure rate of 61% in 122 knee retrievals.[12] At the time, the limited series of knees showed a strong correlation between material loss on the articular surface of the component and consolidation defects in the bulk. All available evidence pointed to inconsistencies and

consolidation problems in the original manufacturing of the polyethylene. These findings led to multiple studies and processing changes to improve the homogeneity of the bulk material.

Although these findings did not reveal the ultimate cause of failure, the discovery of consolidation defects led to important improvements in material quality control. The defects indeed existed and reduced the mechanical properties of UHMWPE tibial components by up to 20%.[62] However, the introduction of better consolidation processes did not eliminate the problem of delamination and fatigue.

At the same time that the consolidation studies were performed, research was also focused on the correlation between failure and high contact stress in particular component designs.[5,12,21,59,60] Contact stress was shown to be higher in some designs than others, and many failures were observed in high–contact stress regions. Thin polyethylene tibial components were also found to correlate with failure in a number of designs. The majority of the published studies analyzed only single designs or, at best, designs by single manufacturers. Thus, although early studies provided good information leading to designs incorporating thicker polyethylene components or more tolerable uniform stress distributions, a comprehensive study of components across designs and manufacturers revealed that some fatigue failures could not be attributed to high contact stress.[61] This was particularly true for components with a short in vivo duration. As with process improvements to minimize consolidation defects, stress analysis and component redesign were necessary advances in the orthopedic specialty, but they did not completely solve the fatigue failure problem.

It was not until the mid-1990s that a sufficiently large series of retrieved components spanning multiple years, multiple manufacturers, and multiple designs were assembled for study. The overwhelming finding, and the clue that chemical kinetics was involved in the degradation of components, was that the number of failed components was related to the time that the components had spent on the shelf or in vivo after irradiation.

In 1995 the (then) radical concept of irradiation-induced oxidation of UHMWPE orthopedic components was presented. The initial scientific publication on the subject explained the phenomenon in the context of explanted hips obtained through a retrieval program.[56] The discovery showed that oxidation increased as a function of time and that mechanical properties decreased as a function of oxidation. In particular, it was shown that elongation at failure (ductility) and ultimate tensile strength both decrease to well below ASTM specifications at oxidation levels reached after only a few years on the shelf. The combined losses in these two properties lead to a significant drop in fracture toughness and, hence, a decrease in overall fatigue strength.

An article showing the same effect in knees was subsequently published,[13] followed by one focusing on a large series of unicompartmental knees.[58] The knees had been explanted for various reasons, but half showed neither cracking nor delamination after a long in vivo duration. The only major difference between these inserts and those that had failed catastrophically was the sterilization method. Ethylene oxide was correlated with longevity,

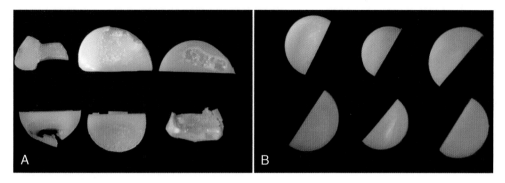

Figure 15–8. **A,** Unicompartmental knees failed because of irradiation-induced oxidation. **B,** The components show no failure and were sterilized with ethylene oxide.

whereas gamma irradiation resulted in eventual revision after fatigue failure or wear-through (Fig. 15–8).

Further studies published by this laboratory and others eventually led to sweeping changes in the orthopedic industry. UHMWPE components are no longer irradiation-sterilized in the presence of oxygen; they are either barrier-packaged or sterilized by a nonirradiation technique. Furthermore, the components are stored in oxygen-impermeable packages to eliminate oxidation during storage.

In retrospect, the solution to the problem may now seem obvious, but this case study provides a good example of how large numbers of components were required to uncover the cause-and-effect relationship underlying component failures. Despite a single process leading to industry-wide failure, there existed multiple overlying reasons for failure. These design-specific variables were eliminated as global problems through large-scale data collection across different types and brands of devices.

The magnitude of such studies also allowed for grouping of components beyond the manufacturer or design. Instead, groups could be established for all treatments through the life cycle of the device. Of critical importance was the cooperation of all stakeholders, including the resin manufacturer, the polyethylene consolidator, the orthopedic companies, the surgeons, and the researchers.

This success notwithstanding, the solution may have been less elusive had certain basic quality control measures been taken during the early 1980s. Before medical device tracking laws and the Safe Medical Devices Act, no tibial components were marked with serial numbers or other identification indicating the date of manufacture and sterilization. Without this information, all time-related data analysis had to be based purely on in vivo duration. Unfortunately, this method did not take shelf time into account, thus allowing for significant oxidation variation between components of similar implantation time but different dates of sterilization.

Looking back, the identification of irradiation-related oxidation is perhaps the best available example to demonstrate the importance of impartiality, large sample size, and good laboratory-surgeon-manufacturer relationships. The problem was identified through a large retrieval population that controlled for and looked beyond the range of design, patient, surgical, and manufacturing variables.

Through industry-wide cooperation, manufacturing and sterilization processes have improved dramatically, thereby enhancing the overall quality of care for the patient.

RETRIEVAL STUDIES CAN CONTRADICT INDUSTRY MOMENTUM

The orthopedic industry relies on input from surgeons, engineers, and academic scientists to drive orthopedic device changes. In addition, indirect design input is derived from sources such as marketing departments, the government (Medicare), the economy, and patient perception. Change in industry is not always driven by results from retrieval studies.

This collective input has led to discontinuation of a variety of knee devices over the years. Although changes are usually in the patients' best interests, components of a given type from all manufacturers are sometimes discontinued because of faulty understanding of cause and effect. In many cases, retrieval analysis contradicts the perception that drives market changes. Examples include a misunderstanding of polyethylene failure in unicompartmental knees, heat-polished components, and metal-backed patellae and fixation failure in cementless tibial components.

Although metal-backed patellae, heat polishing, and porous coatings are rarely used today, they may see a rebirth if the performance of their replacements does not live up to expectations.

Unicompartmental Knees

Historically, the polyethylene in unicompartmental knee designs was intentionally left thin to minimize bone resection. Furthermore, most geometries were "curved-on-flat" designs to ease implantation and alignment. The thin polyethylene combined with the high contact stress inherent in the design was thought to be the source of numerous polyethylene bearing failures.[15] Hence, this component style largely fell out of favor during the 1990s.

As previously mentioned, in vivo unicompartmental knee performance varied widely as a function of the sterilization method. A comprehensive analysis of retrievals demonstrated that the actual source of failure was oxidation of the polyethylene secondary to gamma irradiation in air.[58] No fatigue damage was observed in a series of ethylene oxide–sterilized polyethylene unicompartmental knees of similar design.

This knowledge has allowed the unicompartmental knee to make a slow return to the market as a viable alternative to total knee arthroplasty.

Metal-Backed Patellae

Metal-backed patellae were developed as part of the effort to market a completely cementless total knee system. A porous-coated metal backing was added to the button-style patellae to provide a surface for bone ingrowth. After a short in vivo duration, many of these components failed because of fatigue of the polyethylene and/or separation of the bearing from the metal backing. High contact stress and thin polyethylene were identified in the literature as the primary causes of failure, although many cemented patellae of identical geometry had survived over long periods.[31,41,52]

Once again, gamma-in-air sterilization was a contributor to many of the failures. Nonetheless, metal-backed patellae were largely abandoned because of apparently conflicting design requirements: a thick polyethylene component to reduce stress, a metal backing to permit ingrowth, and an overall thin component to provide proper geometry. Interestingly, one design that combined a thin polyethylene bearing with a porous-coated metal backing performed very satisfactorily despite being sterilized by gamma radiation in air. This very congruent, self-aligning, mobile-bearing patellar component was introduced in the early 1980s and has remained essentially unchanged for more than 20 years.

Heat Surfacing

In the 1980s, heat pressing was applied to machined components to attain the same glossy articular surface texture as found on molded components. Early failure of these devices was attributed to this heat-polishing process, as well as thin polyethylene and high contact stress. Later examination of the components revealed high oxidation levels after gamma sterilization in air.

Although heat processing was the focus of criticism, there was no series of heat-processed, non–gamma-sterilized components to provide a comparison set. Instead, heat polishing was discontinued without a critical determination of its role in the failure process. It is now known that many tibial components of similar thickness and contact stress failed at similar durations without having been heat-polished. In these cases, oxidation related to gamma sterilization in air has been identified as the primary contributor to failure.

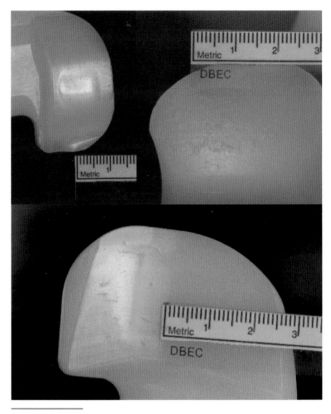

Figure 15–9. Three commonly found articular features: wear (**A**), pitting (**B**), and burnishing (**C**).

Porous Coating

Cementless fixation of knee components was inspired by the success of cementless hip arthroplasty and the failure of many cemented knees. Reliable ingrowth of the femoral and patellar components was generally achieved, but ingrowth of the tibial trays was far less frequently observed in retrievals.[14] Examination of many different types of designs made it clear that secure initial fixation was the key to ingrowth. The addition of porous-coated pegs and the use of screws dramatically improved the likelihood of well-fixed tibial components.

Paradoxically, as the problems with these systems were identified and solved, improvements in cemented fixation were leading many clinicians back to cemented designs. There were advances in cement-mixing techniques and increased consistency and quality between batches.[26,33,39] Furthermore, these less technically demanding installations used devices that were less expensive than porous-coated components.

CURRENT CHALLENGES FACING RETRIEVAL LABORATORIES

The need for retrieval laboratories has not disappeared. In fact, it appears that device failures have remained constant at about 1% to 3% of the total installed base for the past 25 years. There are few metal-backed patellae on the market, polyethylene bearings are thicker, and fewer beads from porous coatings are coming off. In addition, we have been receiving fewer delaminated devices because of abandonment of gamma-in-air sterilization. However, the proportion of devices that we evaluate after revision for osteolysis or looseness has been steadily increasing.

The oxidation problem of the mid-1990s highlights the importance of examining each incoming device not just as an individual case or design study, but also as it relates to industry-wide trends. Some trends have been present since the very first retrievals were analyzed. For instance, the articular surfaces of many tibial inserts show pitting, burnishing, and wear (Fig. 15–9). Although they may have low or no oxidation, the components have characteristics indicative of third-body debris, generation of polyethylene debris, and material failure. Despite identification in the first modern retrieval study,[29] several decades of material testing and refinement have failed to provide an appropriate solution to the problem.

Most recently, trends have been identified regarding wear, unintended articulation, and third-body debris.

Rotational Motion, Micromotion, and Wear

Historically, spalling, delamination, and fatigue failure of polyethylene knee bearings have been responsible for the generation of large particles of polyethylene in the joint space. Though painful for the patient and associated with failure of the implant, these millimeter- to centimeter-sized particles do not cause an undesirable physiological response. In comparison, in specific circumstances, adhesive and abrasive wear of conventional polyethylene can produce millions of submicron-sized particles, which have a higher potential to elicit a lytic response.[30,53]

The wear problem is not solely a process at the intended articulation. Studies have shown that at revision, many tibial components exhibit more wear on the backside than on the articular surface.[15,18,38] It has been suggested that micromotion of the polyethylene tibial component in the tray might be responsible for a significant proportion of this wear. Furthermore, several factors have the potential to exacerbate this process.[16] For instance, most titanium tibial trays are left with a matte finish. The surface roughness of this finish is much greater than that of a polished surface and hence could be responsible for greater wear of the polyethylene.

It is difficult to reproduce backside wear in vitro, thus making determination of the direct cause more difficult. However, many retrieved tibial inserts show indications of motion within the tray. For instance, one might find multiple marks on the nonarticular surfaces that are several hundred microns in length (Fig. 15–10). These "stippling" marks assume a circumferential shape around a common center of rotation, indicative of relative motion between the tibial tray and the insert. Occasionally, the motion can be quantified by assembling the tibial components and applying a small torque to exact movement between the two.

As previously mentioned, wear volume can be estimated through precision measuring techniques such as coordinate measurement and laser profiling. However, qualitative indicators of wear are also discernible on components and are equally useful in device analysis. For instance, asymmetric thinning between different portions of tibial components can be observed as a missing "wedge" of material that can be graded on a qualitative scale. However, to make such an observation, a substantial amount of material must be missing.

Smaller material loss can nonetheless be identified. For example, machining marks or the manufacturer's identification numbers can be worn away during in vivo use. Figure 15–11 shows several examples of this phenomenon. In each case, the only machining marks that remain are found in areas that do not contact the tibial tray. This

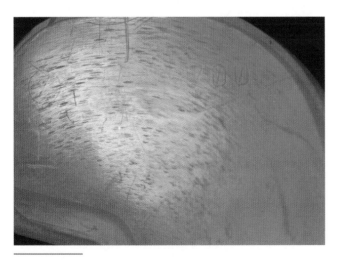

Figure 15–10. Backside markings showing polyethylene micromotion.

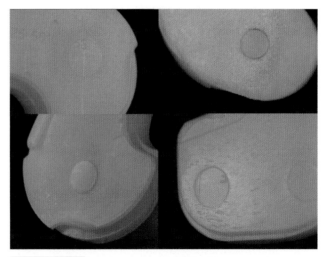

Figure 15–11. Tibial insert backsides. The machining marks remain only over the screw holes. Most of the manufacturers' identification marks are worn away, and there is evidence of micromotion.

is most often an area above a screw hole or access point to a modular peg. Furthermore, the linear wear distance can be estimated by the relative difference in elevation between the unworn surface above the hole and the adjacent worn surface.

Tibial Tray Marks

Rotational motion is also evident on the nonarticulating side of retrieved tibial trays (Fig. 15–12). Most currently manufactured tibial trays are cast from a titanium-aluminum-vanadium alloy with a hardness and toughness much greater than that of polyethylene. Therefore, any marks created on the tibial tray are indicative of a third body acting as an abrasive between the insert and the tray. No one has documented the source or composition of this debris, but possibilities include bone cement, stainless steel from surgical tooling, abrasive compounds from the manufacturing and polishing process, metallic beads from porous coating, and bone chips.

Although titanium scratching in the knee has not in itself been shown to be harmful, it is nonetheless of great interest. Because the knee is a synovial joint, the metal debris generated during a micromotion process is not immediately carried away in the bloodstream. A finite length of time is required for it to break down into ions and diffuse out of the joint space. Therefore, the overall process leads to two debris-related questions. First, one must ask whether the metallic particles are exacerbating the wear process through persistence in the interface as a third body. After the metal breaks down, it is equally important to know the effects of the elevated ion concentration in the joint space. Elevated ion concentrations manifest themselves in blood and urine samples and are currently being studied in the context of metal-on-metal total hip replacements. However, further research is needed to identify whether metal ions, in the concentration found in the synovial space, are harmful.

Anterior Impingement

Many retrieved posterior-stabilized devices from various manufacturers demonstrate significant removal of material on the anterior portion of the tibial posts (Fig. 15–13). In some cases, burnishing and removal of material are also apparent at the top of the post. Because neither of these two locations is an intended point of articulation, current investigations are aimed at determining the design or procedural changes that must occur to prevent such events.

Anterior impingement suggests one or more possible conditions:
1. A highly unstable knee
2. A hyperextended knee. Reasons for hyperextension include
   a. Anatomic anomaly or instability of the knee joint
   b. Progressive laxity of the knee joint
   c. Surgical placement of the components, including
      i. Tibial component too far anterior
      ii. Too much posterior tilt of the tibial component
      iii. Posterior placement of the femoral component and/or
      iv. Femoral component placed in flexion

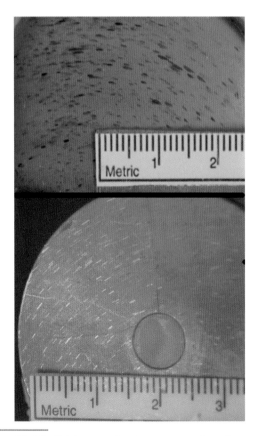

Figure 15–12. **Evidence of micromotion found on tibial trays.**

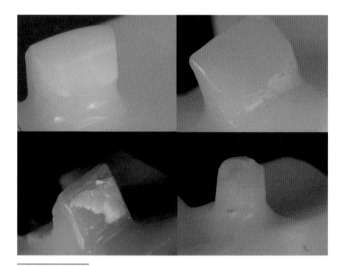

Figure 15–13. **Anterior impingement has been found on several different styles of stabilized knees.**

Note that procedure and patient factors account for the large number of conditions that could lead to impingement. Furthermore, though not specifically identified, device factors can also play a part. If a design does not allow for flexibility in the surgical procedure or accommodate inherent variations between patients, the likelihood of impingement and eventual failure is much higher.

It should be noted that few of the previously mentioned factors account for wear and burnishing on other areas of the tibial posts. However, in the event that anterior impingement changes the geometry of the tibial post through wear or creep, the top of the post might contact the top of the femoral box during hyperextension of the leg. Such contact will also occur if the tibial condyles wear during the course of normal articulation, thereby decreasing the distance between the femur and the tibia. Burnishing marks at the tops of some posts suggest that one of these two scenarios is occurring.

Both anterior impingement and unintended articulation at the top of the post indicate debris generation and failure of the device to perform as designed. Moreover, because a stress concentrator is created, fatigue or extreme stress conditions could be responsible for separation of the tibial post from the insert. Though uncommon, this phenomenon has been documented in other laboratories.[10]

IN VITRO COMPARISONS

Although the primary goal of retrieval analysis is to establish causal relationships, the previous sections related to in vivo wear also point to an important, but often overlooked application. Organizations such as ASTM and the International Organization for Standardization (ISO) have published standards for testing new orthopedic materials and designs that involve conventional materials evaluation techniques and equipment.[1] Additional guidelines exist for testing with specialized devices such as knee simulators or the aforementioned small-punch test.[4,32] Regardless of the experiment, the outcomes are intended to predict in vivo performance. Therefore, benchmarks and reliability studies should always be established. Although the example of UHMWPE is used here, similar examples can be found for titanium and cobalt-chrome components.

Even though UHMWPE has been shown to have reliable mechanical properties in its virgin and recently sterilized state, the long-term behavior of medical implants is a crucial decision factor in the design process. The most common method for in vitro component analysis is the knee simulator. Commercially available machines can simulate the motion of the human knee in all six axes. When a component is mounted on the machine, the operator can program an infinite number of gait patterns, including flexion extremes and load variations. The machines are useful for testing component design and performance under prescribed gait cycles, but they do little to analyze the root causes of material failure. Indeed, the varying stress and motion imposed during a standard human gait are very complex and do not lend themselves to analysis by standard contact mechanics and fatigue theory.

Despite the complexities associated with operating a knee simulator, in vitro failures of oxidized polyethylene components appear similar to failed retrievals and are hence of value in the design and permitting process. Comparing device failures produced by using a simulator with failures of retrieved components allows for validation of the machine and possible redesign of tests to more closely mimic the in vivo environment. A machine can be trusted to realistically test novel components only after in vitro failures of currently marketed components match in vivo failures. It is critical to note that this condition is necessary, but not sufficient to ensure a reliable in vitro test. The machines work by using either load control or displacement control, but they are not adaptive to motion or stress in the same way that the physiological system is.

In addition, researchers have devoted time to testing materials with various accepted tribotesters in an effort to better control stress or motion conditions. These tests include disk-on-disk, pin-on-disk, pin-on-flat, flat-on-disk, and flat-on-flat contact.[6,7,20,25,48-51,55,57] Tribotesting methods such as these do a very good job of quantifying wear and fatigue behavior of UHMWPE in contact with a counterface such as CoCrMo or Ti6Al4V. Although many of these methods use sample geometries quite different from the final implant shape, all tests must somehow be validated against an in vivo model, which necessitates a large collection of knee retrievals that exhibit failure under different environmental conditions. An example of a comparison between an explanted knee and a tribotester result is shown in Figure 15–14. Although the specimen geometry is quite different from the explanted component, the oxidation, stress conditions, time to failure, and failure mode are all similar.[57]

RETRIEVAL STUDY LIMITATIONS

No chapter written about a retrieval study is complete without a discussion of the limitations inherent in retrieval analysis. The implants that retrieval scientists have the opportunity to analyze are not representative of the overall population. By their nature, retrievals are generally failed devices.

The installed implant base has been estimated at over 1 million components, and more than 30,000 total knee revisions are performed every year.[35,45] The largest influx of retrievals to our laboratory was only 300 knees annually, which equates to 1% of the total number of revised knees and 0.03% of the installed base. It is impossible to accurately extrapolate on the basis of this small and potentially biased sample; one can only identify phenomena.

The gross disparity between the number of retrieved components and the number of revised knees leads to the first limitation of retrieval studies. All numbers reported must be viewed in the greater context of the orthopedic market. Whereas a study may report on 40 retrievals, 4 of which display a remarkable trait, the 10% finding may or may not be statistically relevant. There can be a large bias in a retrieval study because surgeons often will not consider sending a device for analysis unless it has a visible

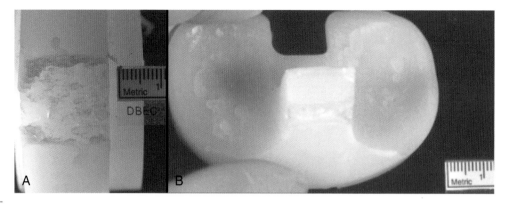

Figure 15–14. Polyethylene failure induced by a rolling, sliding tribotester (**A**) versus failure experienced in vivo (**B**).

defect or unusual clinical performance. It follows that the surgeon may, in fact, retrieve a large number of components over a certain time frame and send only a very small fraction to the retrieval laboratory. The laboratory then finds additional information or interest in just a fraction of these components. Through this selection by the surgeon and the laboratory, publications and reports will show a failure rate that may be artificially high or low when compared with the actual number failed and the actual number of revisions.

This problem of identifying the denominator is not likely to see a solution in the near term. Without a joint registry, the total number of knees installed in the United States is only an estimate that must be determined by scrutinizing closely guarded sales statistics, Medicare reimbursement records, and hospital discharge surveys. Furthermore, it can be overwhelming and perhaps impractical for a busy practice to package all the retrieved knees, document the patient and surgery information, and send them to a retrieval laboratory.

Statistical significance is also hard to assign to some retrievals in which a catastrophic failure is identified, but only one or two cases are presented. Because of patient, surgeon, and manufacturing variations, it may not be reasonable to change an otherwise proven design based on isolated failures from such a narrow sample.

Finally, independent of the surgeons, manufacturers, and laboratories, the patient factor is always a significant variable. Individual response to an implant can be predicted to a certain extent, but it may still vary greatly in a population. Each patient will treat the implant differently. Despite cautions by surgeons and manufacturers, it is well known that some patients will impose a much more demanding duty cycle on their implant. Even if all the recommendations are followed, patients who are more active and mobile will subject their device to a greater number of annual cycles than will patients who have reduced mobility for other health or lifestyle reasons.

Likewise, patient reaction to implant materials and wear debris will vary greatly within a population. Although we can proactively identify certain metal allergies, host response might also be affected by the particular drugs that a patient is taking. Or, it is possible that someone might be a "responder" to polyethylene particles or metal

ions. In either case, the implant or its byproducts may then elicit a host response that necessitates revision. Without detailed information related to the patient history and propensity to respond, drawing correlations between design or material and device failure may be difficult, if not impossible.

The aforementioned limitations deal solely with the statistics and variables inherent in a retrieval study. Numerous external barriers also exist to the establishment of retrieval programs and joint registries, but they are beyond the scope of this section. The reader is referred to the NIH consensus statement for an in-depth review of these barriers, including legal, religious, and economic issues.[46]

THE FUTURE NEED FOR RETRIEVAL LABORATORIES

While studies of existing devices are ongoing, new designs and materials are constantly being introduced, often with little knowledge of their long-term in vivo behavior. These changes can be small, such as tighter fits in the tray-insert assembly, lower roughness values, or more sophisticated instrumentation. Conversely, the changes can be major, such as the introduction of a new material, a change in the kinematic behavior of a device, or a move to an alternative fixation method.

New innovations in orthopedic component design, manufacture, and implantation will require continued studies at retrieval laboratories to determine efficacy and the prognosis for long-term outcomes. Examples of recent innovations requiring further analysis include barrier-packaged components, cross-linked polymers, and international designs.

Barrier-Packaged Components

It is recognized that shelf storage after irradiation in air can lead to high oxidation, reduced mechanical properties, and loss of longevity. As a result, manufacturers have moved to alternative sterilization and storage methods.

One of the leading techniques is irradiation in a vacuum or inert gas and subsequent storage in an oxygen-free package. The favorable wear properties of irradiated polyethylene can be realized, and aside from the brief exposure to atmospheric oxygen in the operating room, a tibial insert theoretically has no time to oxidize. Nonetheless, there exists concern that oxidation can occur in vivo, and the resulting decrease in mechanical properties would limit long-term implant survivorship. Retrieval study results are well suited to show whether this phenomenon occurs and, if so, to what effect.

Cross-linked Polymers

The most recent change in the knee industry has been the introduction of cross-linked polymers into tibial bearings. Although gamma irradiation raises the potential for harmful oxidation, subsequent quenching using heat is believed to eliminate the free radicals through carbon chain cross-linking and recombination. Furthermore, many researchers have concluded that cross-linked materials are superior to conventional UHMWPE in their wear properties.[8,9,20,24,37,44] This decrease in particle generation and material breakdown may lower the risk of osteolysis, and thus the new material could be a reasonable replacement for the conventional material. However, it is also well known that cross-linking reduces the ability of a polymer to withstand fatigue.[28] Despite this knowledge, few tests have been published that address in vivo fatigue of medical-grade cross-linked UHMWPE. It is quite possible that despite wear reduction and a decrease in revisions because of UHMWPE-related osteolysis, the number of mechanical failures of cross-linked UHMWPE components could rise.

A recent study has identified the mechanical properties of several currently marketed cross-linked polyethylenes.[11] As the radiation dose received by the material increases, the ultimate tensile strength drops. The study further finds that materials with the highest doses have ultimate tensile strengths of around 30 MPa. Because some knee designs are subjected to cyclic contact stress approaching 20 MPa during regular walking and can be subjected to compressive stress of more than 30 MPa during stair climbing or jumping, a higher potential for fatigue failure exists with these materials.

The first cross-linked and quenched knee components have been in use for less than 5 years, thus implying that their duty life is on the order of 10 million cycles or less. Because high-cycle fatigue failure could be a catastrophic event, surgeons will need to continue sending explanted components to retrieval laboratories to determine whether fatigue is responsible for product failure. Likewise, there is an ever-present need for postmortem retrievals, particularly from more active patients with high-longevity total knee devices. As previously mentioned, these "success stories" are critical in establishing a baseline for performance. Postmortem analyses may also reveal potential long-term problems before they manifest themselves in patients.

International Designs

New materials represent only one portion of the interesting components being delivered to today's retrieval laboratories. The U.S. regulatory environment makes it increasingly difficult and expensive to perform investigational and trial surgeries. This necessary and appropriate concern for patient safety often results in a large amount of time between the invention of a device and its availability on the market. Understandably, surgeons, patients, and manufacturers all wish to realize the benefits of a new device sooner rather than later. It is for this reason that many experimental components are placed into service in foreign countries with less restrictive rules regarding patient safety and long-term results.

Because of the frequency and popularity of international travel, it has become increasingly common for our laboratory to receive components that were originally marketed and installed in foreign countries, but explanted in the United States. Examination of these components gives a sneak preview into the future results of domestic clinical trials and in some cases can speed or slow the permitting process. Components that represent the U.S. outlook in materials and design may already have seen several years of use in foreign countries.

CONCLUSION

It has been nearly 2 decades since the first publication related to a total knee retrieval. In those years, device designs have come and gone, different materials have been introduced and eliminated, and surgical techniques have been continuously improved. Although in vitro testing has accomplished much and lent insight into the nature of material and implant system behavior, the true test of performance is always borne by the patient. Perfect in vivo results are the ultimate goal in any medical discipline, and although this may never be realized, it is our belief that continuous improvement through retrieval analysis will allow the orthopedic industry to eliminate most, if not all, device-related failures.

ACKNOWLEDGMENTS

The authors wish to thank the researchers of the Dartmouth Biomedical Engineering Center for their valuable assistance in preparing this chapter. Moreover, the authors would like to acknowledge the more than 700 surgeons who have supplied retrieved orthopedic components to our laboratory.

References

1. American Society for Testing of Materials: ASTM F648-00e1: Standard Specification for Ultra-High-Molecular-Weight Polyethylene Powder and Fabricated Form for Surgical Implants. Philadelphia, ASTM, 2000.

2. American Society for Testing of Materials: ASTM D882-02: Standard Test Method for Tensile Properties of Thin Plastic Sheeting. Philadelphia, ASTM, 2002.

3. American Society for Testing of Materials: ASTM D2990-01: Standard Test Methods for Tensile, Compressive, and Flexural Creep and Creep-Rupture of Plastics. Philadelphia, ASTM, 2002.

4. American Society for Testing of Materials: ASTM F2183-02: Standard Test Method for Small Punch Testing of Ultra-High Molecular Weight Polyethylene Used in Surgical Implants. Philadelphia, ASTM, 2002.

5. Bartley RE, Stulberg SD, Robb WJ 3rd, Sweeney HJ: Polyethylene wear in unicompartmental knee arthroplasty. Clin Orthop 299:18-24, 1994.

6. Blanchet TA, Kennedy FE: The development of transfer films in ultra-high molecular weight polyethylene/stainless steel oscillatory sliding. Tribol Trans 32:371-379, 1989.

7. Bragdon CR, O'Connor DO, Lowenstein JD, et al: A new pin-on-disk wear testing method for simulating wear of polyethylene on cobalt-chrome alloy in total hip arthroplasty. J Arthroplasty 16:658-665, 2001.

8. Burroughs BR, Blanchet TA: Factors affecting the wear of irradiated UHMWPE. Tribol Trans 44:215-223, 2001.

9. Chiesa R, Tanzi MC, Alfonsi S, et al: Enhanced wear performance of highly crosslinked UHMWPE for artificial joints. J Biomed Mater Res 50:381-387, 2000.

10. Clarke HD, Math KR, Scuderi GR: Polyethylene post failure in posterior stabilized total knee arthroplasty. J Arthroplasty 19:652-657, 2004.

11. Collier JP, Currier BH, Kennedy FE, et al: Comparison of crosslinked polyethylene materials for orthopaedic applications. Clin Orthop 414:289-304, 2003.

12. Collier JP, Mayor MB, McNamara JL, et al: Analysis of the failure of 122 polyethylene inserts from uncemented tibial knee components. Clin Orthop 273:232-242, 1991.

13. Collier JP, Sperling DK, Currier JH, et al: Impact of gamma sterilization on clinical performance of polyethylene in the knee. J Arthroplasty 11:377-389, 1996.

14. Collier JP, Mayor MB, Surprenant VA, et al: Biological ingrowth of porous-coated knee prostheses. In Goldberg VM (ed): Controversies of Total Knee Arthroplasty. New York, Raven Press, 1991, pp 95-104.

15. Conditt MA, Ismaily SK, Alexander JW, Nobel PC: Backside wear of modular ultra-high molecular weight polyethylene tibial inserts. J Bone Joint Surg Am 86:1031-1037, 2004.

16. Conditt MA, Stein JA, Noble PC: Factors affecting the severity of backside wear of modular tibial inserts. J Bone Joint Surg Am 86:305-311, 2004.

17. Cook SD, Thomas KA: Fatigue failure of noncemented porous-coated implants. A retrieval study. J Bone Joint Surg Br 73:20-24, 1991.

18. Cuckler JM, Lemons J, Tanparapalli JR, Beck P: Polyethylene damage on the nonarticular surface of modular total knee prostheses. Clin Orthop 410:248-253, 2003.

19. Currier BH, Currier JH, Collier JP, et al: Shelf life and in vivo duration. Impacts on performance of tibial bearings. Clin Orthop 342:111-122, 1997.

20. Endo MM, Barbour PS, Barton DC, et al: Comparative wear and wear debris under three different counterface conditions of crosslinked and non-crosslinked ultra high molecular weight polyethylene. Biomed Mater Eng 11:23-35, 2001.

21. Engh GA, Dwyer KA, Hanes CK: Polyethylene wear of metal-backed tibial components in total and unicompartmental knee prostheses. J Bone Joint Surg Br 74:9-17, 1992.

22. Foran JR, Mont MA, Etienne G, et al: The outcome of total knee arthroplasty in obese patients. J Bone Joint Surg Am 86:1609-1615, 2004.

23. Furey A, Stone C, Martin R: Preoperative signing of the incision site in orthopaedic surgery in Canada. J Bone Joint Surg Am 84:1066-1068, 2002.

24. Furman BD, Bhattacharyya S, Hernoux C, et al: Independent evaluation of wear properties of commercially available cross linked UHMWPE. Presented at 27th Annual Meeting of the Society for Biomaterials in conjunction with the 33rd International Biomaterials Symposium, St. Paul, 2001.

25. Gonzalez-Mora V, Hoffmann M, Hampshire J, et al: Wear of ultra high molecular weight polyethylene sliding against a CoCrMo coating applied by physical vapor deposition. Presented at the 14th International Conference on Surface Modification Technologies, 2001, Paris.

26. Grelsamer R: More recent advances in cementing technique . . . cement centrifugation and vacuum mixing have significantly improved the results of cement femoral implants. J Arthroplasty 13:484, 1998.

27. Hedley AA, Ogden CL, Johnson CL, et al: Prevalence of overweight and obesity among US children, adolescents, and adults, 1999-2002. JAMA 291:2847-2850, 2004.

28. Hertzberg RW, Manson J: Fatigue of Engineering Plastics. New York, Academic Press, 1980.

29. Hood RW, Wright TM, Burstein AH: Retrieval analysis of total knee prostheses: A method and its application to 48 total condylar prostheses. J Biomed Mater Res 17:829-842, 1983.

30. Howling GI, Barnett PI, Tipper JL, et al: Quantitative characterization of polyethylene debris isolated from periprosthetic tissue in early failure knee implants and early and late failure Charnley hip implants. J Biomed Mater Res 58:415-420, 2001.

31. Hsu HP, Walker PS: Wear and deformation of patellar components in total knee arthroplasty. Clin Orthop 246:260-265, 1989.

32. International Organization for Standardization: ISO 14243-3:2004: Loading and Displacement Parameters for Wear-Testing Machines with Displacement Control and Corresponding Environmental Conditions for Test. ISO, Geneva, Switzerland, 2004.

33. Jasty M, Mulroy R, Harris WH: Borderline indications for use of cement in total joint replacements. Chir Organi Mov 77:397-404, 1992.

34. Kohn DH, Ducheyne P, Cuckler JM, et al: Fractographic analysis of failed porous and surface-coated cobalt-chromium alloy total joint replacements. Med Prog Technol 20:169-177, 1994.

35. Kozak LJ, Owings MF, Hall MJ: National Hospital Discharge Survey: 2001 annual summary with detailed diagnosis and procedure data. Vital Health Stat 13 156:1-198, 2004.

36. Kurtz SM, Jewett CW, Bergstrom JS, et al: Miniature specimen shear punch test for UHMWPE used in total joint replacements. Biomaterials 23:1907-1919, 2002.

37. Kurtz SM, Muratoglu OK, Evans M, Edidin AA: Advances in the processing, sterilization, and crosslinking of ultra-high molecular weight polyethylene for total joint arthroplasty. Biomaterials 20:1659-1688, 1999.

38. Li S, Scuderi G, Furman BD, et al: Assessment of backside wear from the analysis of 55 retrieved tibial inserts. Clin Orthop 404:75-82, 2002.

39. Linden U: Fatigue properties of bone cement. Comparison of mixing techniques. Acta Orthop Scand 60:431-433, 1989.

40. McDonald MD, Bloebaum RD: Distinguishing wear and creep in clinically retrieved polyethylene inserts. J Biomed Mater Res 29:1-7, 1995.

41. McNamara JL, Collier JP, Mayor MB, Jensen RE: A comparison of contact pressures in tibial and patellar total knee components before and after service in vivo. Clin Orthop 299:104-113, 1994.

42. Moreland JR: Mechanisms of failure in total knee arthroplasty. Clin Orthop 226:49-64, 1988.

43. Morrey BF (ed): Biological, Material, and Mechanical Considerations of Joint Replacement. New York, Raven Press, 1993.

44. Muratoglu OK, Bragdon CR, O'Connor DO, et al: Unified wear model for highly crosslinked ultra-high molecular weight polyethylenes (UHMWPE). Biomaterials 20:1463-1470, 1999.

45. National Center for Health Statistics: National Hospital Discharge Survey. Hyattsville, MD, National Center for Health Statistics, 2001.

46. National Institutes of Health: State of the Science Statement 19: Improving Medical Implant Performance through Retrieval Information: Challenges and Opportunities, http://consensus.nih.gov/ta/019/019_statement.htm, 9/29/2004.

47. Ranawat CS, Johanson NA, Rimnac CM, et al: Retrieval analysis of porous-coated components for total knee arthroplasty. A report of two cases. Clin Orthop 209:244-248, 1986.

48. Saikko V, Ahlroos T, Calonius O: A three-axis knee wear simulator with ball-on-flat contact. Wear 249:310-315, 2001.

49. Saikko V, Ahlroos T, Calonius O, Keranen J: Wear simulation of total hip prostheses with polyethylene against CoCr, alumina and diamond-like carbon. Biomaterials 22:1507-1514, 2001.

50. Saikko V, Keranen J: Wear simulation of alumina-on-alumina pros-thetic hip joints using a multidirectional motion pin-on-disk device. J Am Ceram Soc 85:2785-2791, 2002.

51. Schmidt MB, Hamilton JV, De Grenier C, et al: Comparison of UHMWPE wear produced by pin-on-flat and hip simulator testing. Presented at the 24th Annual Meeting of the Society for Biomaterials, San Diego, 1998.

52. Schwartz O, Aunallah J, Levitin M, Mendes DG: Wear pattern of retrieved patellar implants. Acta Orthop Belg 68:362-369, 2002.

53. Shanbhag AS, Bailey HD, Hwang DS, et al: Quantitative analysis of ultrahigh molecular weight polyethylene (UHMWPE) wear debris associated with total knee replacements. J Biomed Mater Res 53:100-110, 2000.

54. Silva M, Kabbash CA, Tiberi JV 3rd, et al: Surface damage on open box posterior-stabilized polyethylene tibial inserts. Clin Orthop 416:135-144, 2003.

55. Smith SL, Unsworth A: Simplified motion and loading compared to physiological motion and loading in a hip joint simulator. Proc Inst Mech Eng [H] 214:233-238, 2000.

56. Sutula LC, Collier JP, Saum KA, et al: The Otto Aufranc Award. Impact of gamma sterilization on clinical performance of polyethyl-ene in the hip. Clin Orthop 319:28-240, 1995.

57. VanCitters DW, Kennedy FE, Currier JH, et al: A multi-station rolling/sliding tribotester for knee bearing materials. ASME J Tribol 126:380-385, 2004.

58. Williams IR, Mayor MB, Collier JP: The impact of sterilization method on wear in knee arthroplasty. Clin Orthop 356:170-180, 1998.

59. Wright TM, Bartel DL: The problem of surface damage in polyeth-ylene total knee components. Clin Orthop 205:67-74, 1986.

60. Wright TM, Rimnac CM, Stulberg SD, et al: Wear of polyethylene in total joint replacements. Observations from retrieved PCA knee implants. Clin Orthop 276:126-134, 1992.

61. Wrona M, Mayor MB, Collier JP, Jensen RE: The correlation between fusion defects and damage in tibial polyethylene bearings. Clin Orthop 299:92-103, 1994.

62. Wu JJ, Buckley CP, O'Connor JJ: Mechanical integrity of compres-sion-moulded ultra-high molecular weight polyethylene: Effects of varying process conditions. Biomaterials 23:3773-3783, 2002.

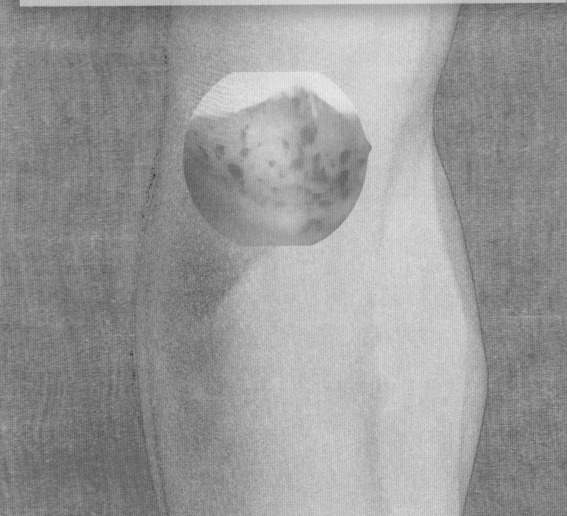

SECTION IV

Articular Cartilage and Meniscal Considerations

CHAPTER 16

Articular Cartilage and Meniscus: Biology, Biomechanics, and Healing Response

Joseph A. Buckwalter • Annunziato Amendola • Charles R. Clark

Articular cartilage and the menisci have very important and specialized biomechanical functions.[46] Articular cartilage provides a lubricated bearing surface and is a deformable shock absorber.[46] The meniscus is a primary knee stabilizer.[17] It has very important load-bearing, shock-absorbing, and load-transmitting functions.[17,23]

Articular cartilage lacks a blood or lymphatic supply. In addition, it has no neurological elements and is sheltered from the immune system. Consequently, there is limited healing potential of articular cartilage because of its poor regenerative capacity.[24,34,38] The inner two-thirds of the meniscus is also avascular and does not heal well, and thus only the periphery of the meniscus has the potential to heal. In fact, the location of a meniscal tear is the most important factor related to the healing response.[37] The major issue with regard to these tissues is whether these problems can be overcome and whether we can enable articular cartilage and the meniscus to heal.

The options for treatment of afflictions involving articular cartilage and the meniscus can be summed up in the four r's: restore, replace, relieve, and resect.[34] Treatment in the past has largely centered on the last modality: resection. Loss of the meniscal load-bearing capacity predictably results in arthrosis.[33] Recent advances in articular cartilage[34] and meniscal transplantation,[33] as well as exciting developments in gene therapy,[24,34,38] suggest that this problem of a lack of healing response will be overcome.[12]

To solve the problems of articular cartilage and meniscal repair, basic science must be integrated into clinical practice.[12] Understanding the basic science of articular cartilage and menisci, including the anatomy, biology, biomechanical function, and healing response, is the basis for developing effective treatment of injuries and afflictions of these tissues.

The purpose of this chapter is to present the basic science of articular cartilage and the menisci, including the biology, biomechanics, and healing response.

ARTICULAR CARTILAGE: INTRODUCTION

Articular cartilage gives synovial joints the ability to provide low-friction, pain-free motion. It varies in thickness, cell density, matrix composition, and mechanical properties within the same joint and among joints. Yet in all synovial joints it consists of the same components, has the same general structure, and performs the same functions. Only a few millimeters thick, it has surprising stiffness to compression, resilience, and an exceptional ability to distribute loads, thereby minimizing peak stress on subchondral bone. Perhaps most impressive, it has great durability—in many people it provides normal joint function for 80 years and more.

Biology

Grossly and microscopically, adult articular cartilage appears to be a simple inert tissue. Opening a synovial joint exposes the smooth, slick, firm articular cartilage surfaces that when probed resist deformation. It consists primarily of extracellular matrix with a sparse population of cells, and it lacks blood vessels, lymphatic vessels, and nerves.[10] Despite its unimpressive appearance, articular cartilage has an elaborate, highly ordered structure.

CHONDROCYTES

Only one type of cell exists within normal articular cartilage: the highly specialized chondrocyte.[14] Chondrocytes from different cartilage zones differ in size, shape, and probably metabolic activity, but all these cells contain the organelles necessary for matrix synthesis, including endoplasmic reticulum and Golgi membranes. Chondrocytes surround themselves with their extracellular matrix and do not form cell-to-cell contact. A spheroidal shape, synthesis of type II collagen, large aggregating proteoglycans, and specific noncollagenous proteins distinguish mature chondrocytes from other cells. To produce a tissue that can provide normal synovial joint function, chondrocytes first synthesize appropriate types and amounts of macromolecules and then assemble and organize them into a highly ordered macromolecular framework. Maintenance of the articular surface requires turnover of the matrix macromolecules, that is, continual replacement of degraded matrix components.[14,15] To accomplish these activities, the cells must sense changes in matrix composition caused by degradation of macromolecules and the mechanical demands placed on the articular surface and respond by synthesizing appropriate types and amounts of macromolecules.

EXTRACELLULAR MATRIX

The articular cartilage matrix consists of two components: tissue fluid and the framework of structural macromolecules that gives the tissue its form and stability.[10,14] Interaction of the tissue fluid and the macromolecular framework gives the tissue its mechanical properties of stiffness and resilience.

TISSUE FLUID

Water contributes up to 80% of the wet weight of articular cartilage, and the interaction of water with the matrix macromolecules significantly influences the mechanical properties of the tissue. This tissue fluid contains gases, small proteins, metabolites, and a high concentration of cations to balance the negatively charged proteoglycans. At least some of the water can move freely in and out of the tissue. Its volume, concentration, and behavior within the tissue depend primarily on its interaction with the structural macromolecules, in particular, the large aggregating proteoglycans that help maintain the fluid within the matrix and the fluid electrolyte concentrations.

STRUCTURAL MACROMOLECULES

The cartilage structural macromolecules—collagens, proteoglycans, and noncollagenous proteins—contribute 20% to 40% of the wet weight of the tissue. The three classes of macromolecules differ in their concentrations within the tissue and in their contributions to tissue properties. Collagens contribute about 60% of the dry weight of cartilage, proteoglycans contribute 25% to 35%, and the noncollagenous proteins and glycoproteins contribute 15% to 20%. Collagens are distributed relatively uniformly throughout the depth of the cartilage, except for the collagen-rich superficial zone. The collagen fibrillar meshwork gives cartilage its form and tensile strength. Proteoglycans and noncollagenous proteins bind to the collagenous meshwork or become mechanically entrapped within it, and water fills this molecular framework. Some noncollagenous proteins help organize and stabilize the matrix macromolecular framework, whereas others help chondrocytes bind to the macromolecules of the matrix.

Collagens

Articular cartilage, like most tissues, contains multiple, genetically distinct collagen types, specifically, collagen types II, VI, IX, X, and XI. Collagen types II, IX, and XI form the cross-banded fibrils seen by electron microscopy. The organization of these fibrils into a tight meshwork that extends throughout the tissue provides the tensile stiffness and strength of articular cartilage and mechanically entraps the large proteoglycans. The principal articular cartilage collagen, type II, accounts for 90% to 95% of the cartilage collagen and forms the primary component of the cross-banded fibrils. The functions of type IX

and type XI collagen remain uncertain, but presumably they help form and stabilize the collagen fibrils assembled primarily from type II collagen. The projecting portions of type IX collagen molecules may also help bind the collagen fibril meshwork together and connect the collagen meshwork with proteoglycans. Type VI collagen appears to form an important part of the matrix immediately surrounding chondrocytes and helps chondrocytes attach to the matrix. The presence of type X collagen only near the cells of the calcified cartilage zone of articular cartilage and the hypertrophic zone of the growth plate (where the longitudinal cartilage septa begin to mineralize) suggests that it has a role in cartilage mineralization.

Proteoglycans

Proteoglycans consist of a protein core and one or more glycosaminoglycan chains (long unbranched polysaccharide chains consisting of repeating disaccharides that contain an amino sugar). Each disaccharide unit has at least one negatively charged carboxylate or sulfate group, so the glycosaminoglycans form long strings of negative charges that repel other negatively charged molecules and attract cations. Glycosaminoglycans found in cartilage include hyaluronic acid, chondroitin sulfate, keratan sulfate, and dermatan sulfate. The concentration of these molecules varies among sites within articular cartilage and also with age, cartilage injury, and disease.

Articular cartilage contains two major classes of proteoglycans: large aggregating molecules, or aggrecans, and smaller proteoglycans, including decorin, biglycan, and fibromodulin. Aggrecans have large numbers of chondroitin sulfate and keratan sulfate chains attached to a protein core filament. Decorin has one dermatan sulfate chain, biglycan has two dermatan sulfate chains, and fibromodulin has several keratan sulfate chains. Aggrecan molecules fill most of the interfibrillar space of the cartilage matrix. They contribute about 90% of the total cartilage matrix proteoglycan mass, whereas large nonaggregating proteoglycans contribute 10% or less and small nonaggregating proteoglycans contribute about 3%. Although the small proteoglycans contribute relatively little to the total mass of proteoglycans when compared with the aggrecans, because of their small size, they may be present in equal or higher molar amounts.

In the articular cartilage matrix, most aggrecans noncovalently associate with hyaluronic acid (hyaluronan) and link proteins, small noncollagenous proteins, to form proteoglycan aggregates. These large molecules have a central hyaluronan backbone that can vary in length from several hundred to more than ten thousand nanometers. Large aggregates may have more than 300 associated aggrecan molecules. Link proteins stabilize the association between monomers and hyaluronic acid and appear to have a role in directing the assembly of aggregates. Aggregate formation helps anchor proteoglycans within the matrix, thereby preventing their displacement during deformation of the tissue, and helps organize and stabilize the relationship between proteoglycans and the collagen meshwork.

The small nonaggregating proteoglycans have shorter protein cores than the aggrecan molecules do, and unlike aggrecans, they do not fill a large volume of the tissue or contribute directly to the mechanical behavior of the tissue. Instead, they bind to other macromolecules and probably influence cell function.

Noncollagenous Proteins and Glycoproteins

A wide variety of noncollagenous proteins and glycoproteins exist within articular cartilage. In general, they consist primarily of protein and a few attached monosaccharides and oligosaccharides. Fibronectin and tenascin, noncollagenous matrix proteins that are found in a variety of tissues, have also been identified within cartilage. Their functions in articular cartilage remain poorly understood, but they may have roles in matrix organization, cell matrix interactions, and responses of the tissue in inflammatory arthritis and osteoarthritis.

STRUCTURE

To form articular cartilage, chondrocytes organize the collagens, proteoglycans, and noncollagenous proteins into a unique, highly ordered structure. The composition, organization, and mechanical properties of the matrix, cell morphology, and probably cell function vary with the depth from the articular surface. Matrix composition, organization, and function also vary with the distance from the cell.

ZONES

The morphological changes in chondrocytes and matrix from the articular surface to subchondral bone make it possible to identify four zones, or layers: the superficial zone, the transitional zone, the radial zone, and the zone of calcified cartilage. The relative size and appearance of these zones vary among joints, and although each zone has different morphological features, the boundaries between zones cannot be sharply defined.

Superficial Zone

The unique structure and composition of the thinnest articular cartilage zone, the superficial zone, give it specialized mechanical and possibly biological properties. It typically consists of two layers. A sheet of fine fibrils with little polysaccharide and no cells covers the joint surface. This portion of the superficial zone presumably corresponds to the clear film, often identified as the "lamina splendens," that can be stripped from the articular surface in some regions. Deep to this acellular sheet of fine fibrils, flattened ellipsoid-shaped chondrocytes arrange themselves so that their major axes are parallel to the articular surface. They synthesize a matrix that has a high collagen concentration and a low proteoglycan concentration relative to the other cartilage zones, and studies of superficial zone cells in culture show that they degrade proteoglycans

more rapidly and synthesize less collagen and proteoglycans than do cells from the deeper zones. Fibronectin and water concentrations are also highest in this zone.

Transitional Zone

As the name "transitional zone" implies, the morphology and matrix composition of the transitional zone is intermediate between that of the superficial zone and the radial zone. It usually has several times the volume of the superficial zone. The cells have a higher concentration of synthetic organelles, endoplasmic reticulum, and Golgi membranes than superficial zone cells do. Transitional zone cells assume a spheroidal shape and synthesize a matrix that has larger-diameter collagen fibrils, a higher proteoglycan concentration, but lower concentrations of water and collagen than present in the superficial zone matrix.

Middle (Radial or Deep) Zone

The chondrocytes in the middle zone are spheroidal in shape, and they tend to align themselves in columns perpendicular to the joint surface. This zone contains the largest-diameter collagen fibrils, the highest concentration of proteoglycans, and the lowest concentration of water. The collagen fibers of this zone pass into the "tidemark," a thin basophilic line seen on light microscopic sections of decalcified articular cartilage that roughly corresponds to the boundary between calcified and uncalcified cartilage.

Calcified Cartilage Zone

A thin zone of calcified cartilage separates the radial zone (uncalcified cartilage) and subchondral bone. The cells of the calcified cartilage zone have a smaller volume than do cells of the radial zone and contain only small amounts of endoplasmic reticulum and Golgi membranes.

MATRIX REGIONS

Variations in the matrix within zones distinguish three regions or compartments: the pericellular region, the territorial region, and the interterritorial region. The pericellular and territorial regions appear to serve the needs of chondrocytes, that is, binding the cell membranes to the matrix macromolecules and protecting the cells from damage during loading and deformation of the tissue. They may also help transmit mechanical signals to the chondrocytes when the matrix deforms during joint loading. The primary function of the interterritorial matrix is to provide the mechanical properties of the tissue.

Pericellular Matrix

Chondrocyte cell membranes appear to attach to the thin rim of the pericellular matrix that covers the cell surface.

This matrix region is rich in proteoglycans and also contains noncollagenous matrix proteins. It has little or no fibrillar collagen.

Territorial Matrix

An envelope of territorial matrix surrounds the pericellular matrix of individual chondrocytes and, in some locations, pairs or clusters of chondrocytes and their pericellular matrices. In the radial zone, a territorial matrix surrounds each chondrocyte column. The thin collagen fibrils of the territorial matrix nearest to the cell appear to adhere to the pericellular matrix. At a distance from the cell they decussate and intersect at various angles to form a fibrillar basket around the cells. An increase in collagen fibril diameter and a transition from the basket-like orientation of the collagen fibrils to a more parallel arrangement mark the boundary between the territorial and interterritorial matrices. However, many collagen fibrils connect the two regions, thus making it difficult to precisely identify the boundary between these regions.

Interterritorial Matrix

The interterritorial matrix makes up most of the volume of mature articular cartilage. It contains the largest-diameter collagen fibrils. Unlike the collagen fibrils of the territorial matrix, these fibrils are not organized to surround the chondrocytes, and they change their orientation relative to the joint surface 90 degrees from the superficial zone to the deep zone. In the superficial zone, the fibril diameters are relatively small and the fibrils generally lie parallel to the articular surface. In the transitional zone, interterritorial matrix collagen fibrils assume more oblique angles relative to the articular surface, and in the radial zone, they usually lie perpendicular (or radial) to the joint surface.

MENISCUS: INTRODUCTION

Injury to the meniscus from both athletic events and activities of daily living is common. As a result, arthroscopic treatment of meniscal injuries has become one of the most common orthopedic surgical procedures, and arthroscopic partial meniscectomy is one of the top 10 orthopedic surgical procedures performed in this country.[2,25] Occurring in isolation or in association with ligamentous injury, meniscal tears can result in abnormal knee joint function, abnormal loading, and subsequent osteoarthritis of the joint.

There has been substantial progress in the management of meniscal tears and deficiency with appreciation of the biomechanical importance of these structures to joint stability and articular preservation. In 1887, Bland-Sutton described the meniscus as "the functionless remains of a leg muscle."[9] Not until 1948 did Fairbank[21] appreciate that "meniscectomy is not wholly innocuous" in his classic report of postmeniscectomy radiographic changes.

In terms of meniscal repair and healing, in November 1883, Thomas Annandale[4] was the first to suture a medial meniscus. Half a century later, in 1936, King[28] showed that degenerative changes would appear in the canine stifle after meniscectomy. He showed that a peripheral meniscal tear has the potential to heal. In the 1950s and 1960s, the menisci were discarded as an unnecessary appendage that can easily be removed. Total meniscectomy was performed for almost any meniscal tear suspected on clinical examination. It took almost a century from Annandale's report until a conservative approach to the management of meniscal tears was applied clinically. In the last 2 decades, understanding of meniscal importance and the development of arthroscopic techniques have improved meniscal preservation and the healing response.

Anatomy

GROSS FEATURES

Various authors have extensively studied meniscal anatomy. In terms of gross anatomy, the menisci are C-shaped or semicircular fibrocartilaginous structures with bony attachments at the anterior and posterior aspects of the tibial plateau (Fig. 16–1). The medial meniscus is C shaped, with the posterior horn larger than the anterior horn in the anteroposterior dimension. The anterior horn attachment of the medial meniscus is variable, an important consideration, particularly for meniscal transplantation. In an anatomic study, Berlet and Fowler[8]

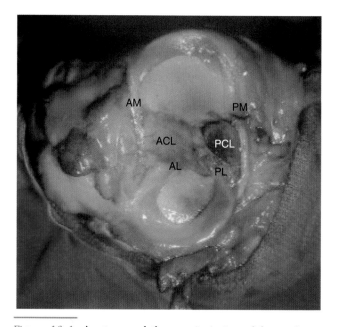

Figure 16–1. Anatomy of the menisci viewed from above. Note the differences in position and shape of the medial and lateral menisci. Meniscus horn insertion sites viewed from above. Note the proximity to the anterior cruciate ligament (ACL). AL, anterior horn lateral meniscus; AM, anterior horn medial meniscus; PCL, posterior cruciate ligament; PL, posterior horn lateral meniscus; PM, posterior horn medial meniscus.

described four types of anterior horn medial meniscus attachments. The type IV variant has no firm bony attachment and is attached to the intermeniscal ligament or the soft tissues at the base of the anterior cruciate ligament (ACL). This variability makes standard bony reattachment difficult, either with replantation or reattachment of an avulsed anterior horn. Nelson and LaPrade[32] found a similar type of attachment in 14% of 47 specimens. In the majority of specimens, however, a firm anterior bony attachment was observed. The posterior root attaches anterior to the insertion of the posterior cruciate ligament and behind the medial tibial eminence. Johnson et al[26] mapped the bony insertion sites of the meniscus in an effort to identify appropriate landmarks for meniscus transplantation. They noted the location of each insertion site (Fig. 16–2) and the insertion site surface area. The anterior horn of the medial meniscus has the largest insertion site surface area (61.4 mm^2), and the posterior horn of the lateral meniscus has the smallest (28.5 mm^2). The remainder of the medial meniscus is firmly attached to the joint capsule and the deep surface of the deep medial capsular ligament. The capsular attachment of the medial meniscus on the tibial side is referred to as the coronary ligament. A thickening of the capsular attachment in the midportion spans from the tibia to the femur and is referred to as the deep medial collateral ligament. The lateral meniscus has an almost semicircular configuration. It covers a larger portion of the tibial articular surface than the medial meniscus does (see Fig. 16–1). Discoid lateral menisci have been reported with a prevalence of 3.5% to 5%, most being the incomplete type.[42] The anterior and posterior horns attach much closer to each other than do those of the medial meniscus, thus making this anatomic area very consistent with a relationship easy to maintain during meniscal transplantation. The anterior horn inserts adjacent to the ACL and can often be used as a landmark

for the drill guide and ACL graft placement. The posterior root is posterior to the lateral tibial eminence. The attachment includes the Wrisberg variation of the discoid lateral meniscus, in which the posterior horn bony attachment is absent and the posterior meniscofemoral ligament of Wrisberg is the only stabilizing structure. This variation can allow excessive motion and result in posterior horn instability, although a hypermobile meniscus may occur without any variant. The anterior meniscofemoral ligament of Humphrey runs from the posterior horn of the lateral meniscus anterior to the posterior cruciate ligament and inserts on the femur. Posterior and lateral to the posterior bony insertion of the lateral meniscus lies the popliteus tendon. The popliteal hiatus identifies the lateral meniscus, and there is no firm peripheral attachment to the femur or tibia in this location, which contributes to the less likely healing of lateral meniscal tears involving this area. Simonian et al[40] have investigated the role that the popliteomeniscal fasciculi play in lateral meniscus stability. Disruption of both these fascicular attachments may increase meniscal motion at the hiatus and be important in causing hypermobility of the posterior horn of the lateral meniscus. In addition, the lateral meniscus is more mobile than the medial meniscus through the knee range of motion, as shown by Thompson et al[41] with three-dimensional magnetic resonance imaging. They demonstrated 11.2 mm of posterior excursion of the lateral meniscus and 5.2 mm of the medial meniscus during knee flexion. The anatomic attachment of the lateral meniscus allows for mobility by less rigorous capsular attachment.

MICROSCOPIC ANATOMY

The fibrocartilaginous structure of the meniscus has been well described and is made of coarse collagen bundles. The orientation of collagen fibers is mainly circumferential, with some radial fibers at the surface and within the midsubstance.[6] This orientation allows compressive loads to be dispersed by the circumferential fibers, whereas the radial fibers act as tie fibers to resist longitudinal tearing (Fig. 16–3). The surface fiber orientation is more of a mesh network or random configuration, which is thought to be important in the distribution of shear stress. The majority of collagen (90%) is type I, and the remainder consists of types II, III, V, and VI. Elastin accounts for approximately 0.6% of the dry weight of the meniscus, and noncollagenous proteins, for 8% to 13%.[30]

The cells of the meniscus have been called fibrochondrocytes because of their appearance and the fact that they synthesize a fibrocartilaginous matrix. The fibrochondrocytes appear to be of two types, with the more superficial cells being oval or fusiform and the deeper cells more rounded. Both types contain abundant endoplasmic reticula and Golgi complexes and few mitochondria.

VASCULARITY

At birth, the entire meniscus is vascular; by 9 months of age, the inner third has become avascular. This decrease

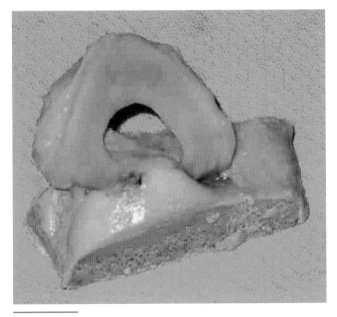

Figure 16–2. Lateral meniscus. Note the proximity of the anterior and posterior horns on either side of the tibial eminence.

in vascularity continues to the age of 10 years, when the meniscus closely resembles the adult meniscus. Arnoczky and Warren[5] studied the adult blood supply and demonstrated that only the outer 10% to 25% of the lateral meniscus and 10% to 30% of the medial meniscus are vascular (Fig. 16–4). This vascularity arises from the superior and inferior branches of the medial and lateral genicular arteries, which form a perimeniscal capillary plexus. A synovial fringe extends a short distance over both the femoral and tibial surfaces of the menisci but does not contribute to the meniscal blood supply. At the popliteal hiatus, the meniscus is relatively avascular, which probably contributes to poorer healing and a higher incidence of retears of the lateral meniscus. Because of the avascular nature of the inner two-thirds of the meniscus, cell nutrition is believed to occur mainly through diffusion of synovial fluid.[31] The neuroanatomy of the meniscus is not totally clear, but the distribution of neural elements has been demonstrated to be in essentially the same anatomic distribution as the vascular supply. The anterior and posterior horns are the most richly innervated, and the body innervation follows the pattern along the periphery. Though not entirely clear, these nerve endings are believed to play a role in sensory feedback and proprioception. It seems that the greatest feedback occurs at the extremes of flexion and extension, when the meniscal horns are compressed and neural elements are stimulated.

Dye et al,[19] who performed neurosensory mapping of the internal structures of the knee, confirmed that probing peripheral tissues is more painful than probing central ones. This finding can be confirmed when performing meniscectomy under local anesthesia only. The innervation of the knee may be important for proprioceptive feedback during motion.

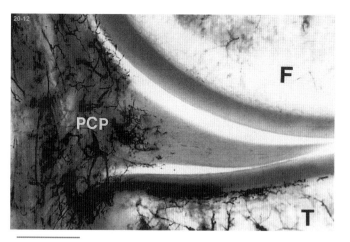

Figure 16–4. The microvasculature of the meniscus. (From Arnockzy SP, Warren RS: Microvasculature of the human meniscus. Am J Sports Med 10:90-95, 1982. Reprinted with permission of Sage Publications, Inc.) F, femur; T, tibia; PCP, perimeniscal capsular periphery.

ARTICULAR CARTILAGE: BIOMECHANICS

Articular cartilage is subjected to a wide range of static and dynamic mechanical loads. The ability of cartilage to withstand physiological compressive, tensile, and shear forces depends on the composition and structural integrity of its extracellular matrix. In turn, maintenance of a functionally intact matrix requires chondrocyte-mediated synthesis, assembly, and degradation of proteoglycans, collagens, noncollagenous proteins and glycoproteins, and other matrix molecules. The collagen fibrils effectively resist tensile and shear deformation forces, whereas the highly charged glycosaminoglycan constituents of aggrecan molecules resist compression and fluid flow within the tissue. Joint loading induces a range of responses in cartilage. Dynamic compression of cartilage results in deformation of cells and extracellular matrix, hydrostatic pressurization of tissue fluid, pressure gradients and the accompanying flow of fluid within the tissue, and streaming potentials and currents induced by tissue fluid flow. The local changes in tissue volume caused by static compression also lead to physiochemical changes within the matrix, including alterations in matrix water content, fixed charge density, mobile ion concentrations, and osmotic pressure. Any of these mechanical, chemical, or electrical phenomena in the environment of the chondrocyte may affect cellular metabolism. Static loading within the physiological range can reversibly inhibit the synthesis of critical components of the cartilage matrix. Such static compressive forces can downregulate the gene expression and production of type II collagen, aggrecan core protein, and link protein, whereas cyclically applied hydrostatic pressure and compressive strain stimulate aggrecan core protein and protein synthesis. Immobilization or reduced loading can decrease the synthesis of proteoglycans and lead to softening of the tissue.

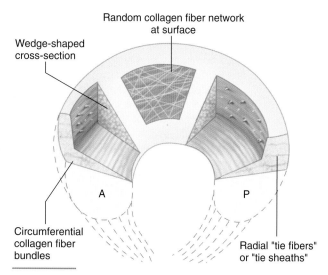

Figure 16–3. Schematic of collagen bundles and their orientation within the meniscus. (Reproduced with permission and copyright © of the British Editorial Society of Bone and Joint Surgery, from Bullough PG, Munuera L, Murphy J, Weinstein AM: The strength of the menisci of the knee as it relates to their fine structure. J Bone Joint Surg Br 52:564-567, 1970.)

MENISCUS: BIOMECHANICS

The menisci are important in many aspects of knee function, including load sharing, shock absorption, reduction in joint contact stress, passive stabilization, increase in congruity and contact area, limitation of extremes of flexion and extension, and proprioception. Many of these functions are achieved through the ability of the menisci to transmit and distribute load over the tibial plateau. The findings of joint space narrowing, osteophyte formation, and squaring of the femoral condyles after total meniscectomy suggested that the meniscus is important in joint protection and led to investigations of the role of the meniscus in joint function. The medial and lateral menisci transmit at least 50% to 70% or more at times of the load when the knee is in extension; it increases to 85% with 90 degrees of knee flexion.[1]

Radin et al[35] demonstrated that these loads were well distributed when the menisci were intact. Removal of the medial meniscus results in a 50% to 70% reduction in femoral condyle contact area and a 100% increase in contact stress.[22,27,44] Total lateral meniscectomy causes a 40% to 50% decrease in contact area and increases contact stress in the lateral compartment to 200% to 300% of normal. In addition, partial removal of the meniscus alters load characteristics, particularly when two-thirds of the posterior horn is removed.[43] With the decrease in contact area within the joint, stress is increased and unevenly distributed. This change results in increased compression and shear across the joint. Along with the biomechanical changes that can occur with meniscectomy, the results of some studies[31] suggest that the biochemical activity of cartilage is also affected. The improved joint congruity, which occurs through meniscus contact, is thought to play a role in joint lubrication and cell nutrition. The meniscus also plays a role in shock absorption. Compression studies using bovine menisci have demonstrated that meniscal tissue is approximately half as stiff as articular cartilage. In one study,[43] the shock absorption capacity of the normal knee was reduced by 20% after meniscectomy. The menisci also play a key role in enhancing joint stability.[29] Medial meniscectomy in an ACL-intact knee has little effect on anteroposterior motion, but in an ACL-deficient knee, it results in an increase in anterior tibial translation of up to 58% at 90 degrees of flexion. Shoemaker and Markolf[39] demonstrated that the posterior horn of the medial meniscus is the most important structure in resisting an applied anterior tibial force in an ACL-deficient knee. Allen et al[2] showed that the resultant force in the medial meniscus of an ACL-deficient knee increases by 52% in full extension and by 197% at 60 degrees of flexion under a 134-N load. Although the inner two-thirds of the meniscus is important in maximizing joint contact area and increasing shock absorption, integrity of the peripheral third is essential for both load transmission and stability.

HEALING RESPONSES: ARTICULAR CARTILAGE

Based on the type of tissue damage, articular surface injuries caused by mechanical forces can be classified into three types (Table 16–1): (1) damage to the cells and matrices of articular cartilage and subchondral bone that is not associated with visible disruption of the joint surface; (2) visible mechanical disruption of articular cartilage limited to articular cartilage that takes the form of chondral fissures, flap tears, or chondral defects; and (3) visible mechanical disruption of articular cartilage and

Table 16–1. Chondral and Osteochondral Injuries

INJURY	EVALUATION	REPAIR RESPONSE	POTENTIAL FOR HEALING
Damage to chondral matrix and/or cells without visible disruption of the articular surface	Inspection of the articular surface and current clinical imaging methods for articular cartilage cannot detect this type of injury MRI of subchondral bone may show edema	Synthesis of new matrix macromolecules Cell proliferation?	If the basic matrix structure is intact and enough viable cells remain, the cells can restore the normal tissue composition If the matrix and/or cell population sustains significant damage or if the tissue sustains further damage, the lesion may progress to cartilage degeneration
Cartilage disruption (chondral fractures or rupture)	CT and MRI imaging can demonstrate these injuries	No fibrin clot formation or inflammation Synthesis of new matrix macromolecules and cell proliferation, but new tissue does not fill the cartilage defect	Depending on the location and size of the lesion and the structural integrity, stability, and alignment of the joint, the lesion may or may not progress to cartilage degeneration
Cartilage and bone disruption (osteochondral fractures)	CT imaging can demonstrate these injuries	Formation of a fibrin clot, inflammation, invasion of new cells, and production of new chondral and osseous tissue	Depending on the location and size of the lesion and the structural integrity, stability, and alignment of the joint, the repair tissue may remodel and serve as a functional joint surface, or it may degenerate

CT, computed tomography; MRI, magnetic resonance imaging.

bone, that is, intra-articular fractures. Each type of tissue damage stimulates a different repair response.[11,13,15,16]

Cell and Matrix Damage

Articular cartilage damage that leaves the overlying articular surface intact occurs with almost every joint injury. The intensity and type of joint loading that can cause chondral and subchondral damage without visible articular surface disruption has not been well defined. Physiological levels of joint loading do not cause this type of joint injury, but impact loading above that generated by normal activities such as walking or lifting light objects but less than that necessary to produce visible cartilage disruption can disrupt the cartilage matrix macromolecular framework, damage or kill chondrocytes, decrease proteoglycan concentration and synthesis, and increase matrix water concentration and permeability.

Experimental evidence suggests that increased degradation or decreased synthesis of aggrecans is the least severe cartilage injury caused by impact loading. However, even this ostensibly minimal injury increases the risk for joint degeneration. Loss of proteoglycans decreases cartilage stiffness and increases its permeability. These alterations may cause greater loading of the remaining macromolecular framework, thus making the tissue more vulnerable to additional damage from loading, including distortion or disruption of the collagen fibril network and collagen-proteoglycan relationships, swelling of the matrix, and chondrocyte injury or death. Impact loading also may cause chondrocyte death directly. Chondrocytes that survive a joint injury may have decreased ability to maintain and repair the tissue as a result of increased mechanical or metabolic stress.

The ability of chondrocytes to sense changes in matrix composition and synthesize new molecules makes it possible for them to repair damage to the macromolecular framework. It is not clear at what point this type of injury becomes irreversible and leads to progressive loss of articular cartilage. Presumably, chondrocytes can restore the matrix if the loss of matrix proteoglycans does not exceed what the cells can produce rapidly, as long as the fibrillar collagen meshwork remains intact and enough chondrocytes remain capable of responding to the matrix damage. When these conditions are not met, the cells cannot restore the matrix, chondrocytes will be exposed to excessive mechanical and metabolic stress, and the tissue will degenerate.

Cartilage Disruption

Chondrocytes respond to injuries that disrupt articular cartilage, but not to those that extend into subchondral bone (see Table 16–1). After this type of injury they proliferate and increase the synthesis of matrix macromolecules near the injury; however, the newly synthesized matrix and proliferating cells do not fill the tissue defect, and soon after injury the increased proliferative and synthetic activity ceases. This leaves a permanent articular surface defect that can alter joint mechanical function and increase the risk for joint degeneration.

Cartilage and Subchondral Bone Disruption (Intra-articular Fractures)

Unlike injuries limited to cartilage, injuries that extend into subchondral bone cause hemorrhage and fibrin clot formation and activate the inflammatory response. As a result, repair and remodeling of intra-articular fractures differ from the events that follow injuries that cause only cell and matrix injury or disruption of the articular surface limited to articular cartilage (see Table 16–1). However, the force required to produce an intra-articular fracture causes cell and matrix damage and chondral disruption. For these reasons, intra-articular fractures include all three types of articular surface injury (see Table 16–1).

The degree of displacement of the fracture and the size of the gaps between fracture fragments influence the extent and outcome of the repair and remodeling responses. Repair of the chondral portions of intra-articular fractures with gaps between the fracture fragments has not been extensively studied, and therefore current understanding of this process is based on studies of osteochondral repair of experimental drill hole defects. These studies show that soon after injury, blood escaping from the damaged bone blood vessels forms a hematoma that temporarily fills the injury site. Fibrin forms within the hematoma and platelets bind to fibrillar collagen. A continuous fibrin clot fills the bone defect and extends for a variable distance into the cartilage defect. Platelets within the clot release vasoactive mediators and growth factors or cytokines (small proteins that influence multiple cell functions, such as migration, proliferation, differentiation, and matrix synthesis), including transforming growth factor β (TGF-β) and platelet-derived growth factor (PDGF). Bone matrix also contains growth factors such as TGF-β, bone morphogenetic proteins (BMPs), PDGF, insulin-like growth factor type I (IGF-I), IGF-II, and possibly others. Release of these growth factors may have an important role in the repair of osteochondral defects. In particular, they probably stimulate vascular invasion and migration of undifferentiated cells into the clot and influence the proliferative and synthetic activities of the cells.

Shortly after entering the tissue defect, the undifferentiated mesenchymal cells proliferate and synthesize a new matrix. Within 2 weeks after injury, some mesenchymal cells assume the rounded form of chondrocytes and begin to synthesize a matrix that contains type II collagen and a relatively high concentration of proteoglycans. These cells produce regions of hyaline-like cartilage in the chondral and bony portions of the defect. Six to 8 weeks after injury, the repair tissue within the chondral region of osteochondral defects contains many chondrocyte-like cells in a matrix consisting of type II collagen, proteoglycans, some type I collagen, and noncollagenous proteins. Unlike the cells in the chondral portion of the defect, the cells in the bony portion of the defect produce immature bone, fibrous tissue, and hyaline-like cartilage. The bony repair tissue is well vascularized, but blood vessels rarely enter the chondral portion of an osteochondral defect. Six to 8 weeks after injury, the chondral repair tissue typically has a composition and structure intermediate between hyaline cartilage and fibrocartilage; it rarely, if ever replicates the elaborate structure of normal articular cartilage.

Repair tissue that fills osteochondral defects is less stiff and more permeable than normal articular cartilage, and the orientation and organization of the collagen fibrils in even the most hyaline-like chondral repair tissue do not follow the pattern seen in normal articular cartilage. In addition, the repair tissue cells may fail to establish the normal relationships between themselves and the matrix and among matrix macromolecules, in particular, the organization of the pericellular, territorial, and interterritorial matrices. The decreased stiffness and increased permeability of repair cartilage matrix may increase loading of the macromolecular framework during joint use and result in progressive structural damage, thereby exposing the repair chondrocytes to excessive loads that additionally compromise their ability to restore the matrix. Experimental studies of osteochondral healing and clinical experience with patients who suffer comminuted displaced intra-articular fractures and regain excellent joint function suggest that chondral repair tissue occasionally progressively remodels to form a functional joint surface. However, in most large osteochondral injuries, the chondral repair tissue does not follow this course. Instead, it begins to show evidence of degeneration, including depletion of matrix proteoglycans, fragmentation and fibrillation, increasing collagen content, and loss of cells with the appearance of chondrocytes within 1 year or less. The remaining cells often assume the appearance of fibroblasts as the surrounding matrix comes to consist primarily of densely packed collagen fibrils. This fibrous tissue usually fragments and often disintegrates, thus leaving areas of exposed bone. The inferior mechanical properties of chondral repair tissue may be responsible for its frequent deterioration.

HEALING RESPONSES: MENISCUS

The key factor in the process of tissue repair is accessibility of cells and inflammatory mediators to the site of injury. The formation of a clot is an initial phase that provides a scaffold for matrix formation and is a chemotactic stimulus for the cellular elements involved in wound healing.[36] In adult menisci, only the peripheral 20% to 30% is vascular.[30] This leaves the injured central 70% to 80% absent of hematoma. Therefore, tears in the vascular zone tend to heal, whereas tears in the avascular central region do not. Because of the vascular anatomy, classification of meniscal tears into red-red, red-white, and white-white zones is common as a means of predicting healing potential. Tears in the red zone are in the vascular region and usually heal, but the most common tears and the dilemma occur in the red-white zone. In this zone a significant portion of the meniscus is usually involved, but healing is also precarious. Therefore, in an attempt to get these tears to heal, every aspect of the process is impor-

tant: technical suturing to provide a stable repair, postoperative cautious rehabilitation and return to activity, and stimulation of the repair site by hematoma. Webber et al[45] showed in tissue culture that meniscal cells can proliferate and synthesize an extracellular matrix when exposed to factors that are normally present in wound hematoma. To promote healing, many have investigated the use of a fibrin clot, fibrin glue, cell growth factors, and creation of traumatic vascular access channels and adjacent synovial bleeding by various methods. Currently, many investigators are looking at the effect and function of extrinsic mediators and growth factors that may affect healing. At this point, abrading the synovium adjacent to the tear and "freshening up" the tear site by rasps or shavers is the common method of providing a hematoma at the tear site.[36] However, this naturally occurring clot may be ineffective if it is dissolved by synovial fluid. Nonetheless, we do know that clinically, the healing rate of meniscal tears is higher in knees with concurrent ACL reconstruction versus isolated meniscal tears, thus indicating that a significant hematoma may help healing, obviously in addition to other factors. Besides stability of the joint, other factors that seem to positively affect healing include the acuity of the tear and younger age of the patient. The presence of degeneration within the meniscal tear (probably correlated with age) has a negative impact on the ability of the tear to heal.[7,20] In terms of rehabilitation and healing response, the meniscus and tear site probably respond to normal physiological stress. Immobilization of the knee joint seems to decrease collagen content in the meniscus, and knee motion tends to prevent collagen loss.[18] With advancing age a normal degenerative process occurs within the meniscus, and therefore its ability to withstand stress is reduced. Consequently, isolated degenerative meniscal tears occur less traumatically and in the older population, that is, usually those older than 30 years. In contrast, younger patients tend to have more traumatic knee injuries and are more likely to sustain combined meniscal and ligamentous injury.

In summary, the menisci are important structures with substantial joint-protective properties. Accordingly, the current approach is to preserve meniscal tissue as much as possible. A clear understanding of the function, biology, and healing capacity of the meniscus is important to allow proper decision making in the clinical setting.

References

1. Ahmed AM, Burke DL: In-vitro measurement of static pressure distribution in synovial joints. Part I: Tibial surface of the knee. J Biomech Eng 105:216-225, 1983.
2. Allen CR, Wong EK, Livesay GA, et al: Importance of the medial meniscus in the anterior cruciate ligament–deficient knee. J Orthop Res 18:109-115, 2000.
3. American Board of Orthopaedic Surgeons, Part II, 2002.
4. Annandale T: An operation for displaced semilunar cartilage. 1885. Clin Orthop 260:3-5, 1990.
5. Arnoczky SP, Warren RF: Microvasculature of the human meniscus. Am J Sports Med 10:90-95, 1982.
6. Beaupre A, Choukroun R, Guidouin R, et al: Knee menisci: Correlation between microstructure and biomechanics. Clin Orthop 208:72-75, 1986.

7. Belzer JP, Cannon WD Jr: Meniscus tears: Treatment in the stable and unstable knee. J Am Acad Orthop Surg 1:41-47, 1993.

8. Berlet GC, Fowler PJ: The anterior horn of the medial meniscus: An anatomic study of its insertion. Am J Sports Med 26:540-543, 1998.

9. Bland-Sutton J (ed): Ligaments: Their Nature and Morphology, 2nd ed. London, JK Lewis, 1897.

10. Buckwalter JA: Articular cartilage. Instr Course Lect 32:349-370, 1983.

11. Buckwalter JA: Articular cartilage injuries. Clin Orthop 402:21-37, 2002.

12. Buckwalter JA: Integration of science in orthopaedic practice: Implications for solving the problem of articular cartilage repair. J Bone Joint Surg Am 85:1-7, 2003.

13. Buckwalter JA, Brown TD: Joint injury, repair, and remodeling roles in post-traumatic osteoarthritis. Clin Orthop 423:7-16, 2004.

14. Buckwalter JA, Mankin HJ: Articular cartilage: Tissue design and chondrocyte-matrix interactions. Instr Course Lect 47:477-486, 1998.

15. Buckwalter JA, Mankin HJ: Articular cartilage: Degeneration and osteoarthritis, repair, regeneration, and transplantation. Instr Course Lect 47:487-504, 1998.

16. Buckwalter JA, Martin JA, Olmstead M, et al: Osteochondral repair of primate knee femoral and patellar articular surfaces: Implications for preventing post-traumatic osteoarthritis. Iowa Orthop J 23:66-74, 2003.

17. Clark CR, Ogden JA: Development of the menisci of the human knee joint: Morphological changes and their potential role in childhood meniscal injury. J Bone Joint Surg Am 65:538-547, 1983.

18. Dowdy PA, Miniaci A, Arnoczky SP, et al: The effect of cast immobilization on meniscal healing. An experimental study in the dog. Am J Sports Med 23:721-728, 1995.

19. Dye SF, Vaupel GL, Dye CC: Conscious neurosensory mapping of the internal structures of the human knee without intraarticular anesthesia. Am J Sports Med 26:773-777, 1998.

20. Eggli S, Wegmuller H, Kosina J, et al: Long-term results of arthroscopic meniscal repair. An analysis of isolated tears. Am J Sports Med 23:715-720, 1995.

21. Fairbank TJ: Knee joint changes after meniscectomy. J Bone Joint Surg Br 30:664-670, 1948.

22. Fukubayashi T, Kurosawa H: The contact area and pressure distribution pattern of the knee: A study of normal and osteoarthritic knee joints. Acta Orthop Scand 51:871-879, 1980.

23. Goto H, Shuller FD, Lamsan C, et al: Transfer LacZ marker gene to the meniscus. J Bone Joint Surg Am 81:915-918, 1995.

24. Hannallah D, Peterson B, Lieberman J, et al: Gene therapy in orthopaedic surgery. Instr Course Lect 52:753-768, 2003.

25. Harner CD: The use of allografts in sports medicine. Presented at the Annual Meeting of the American Orthopaedic Society for Sports Medicine, 2004, Quebec City, Canada.

26. Johnson DL, Swenson TM, Livesay GA, et al: Insertion-site anatomy of the human menisci: Gross, arthroscopic, and topographical anatomy as a basis for meniscal transplantation. Arthroscopy 11:386-394, 1995.

27. Kettelkamp DB, Jacobs AW: Tibiofemoral contact area: Determination and implications. J Bone Joint Surg Am 54:349-356, 1972.

28. King D: The healing of semilunar cartilages. J Bone Joint Surg 18:333-342, 1936.

29. Levy IM, Torzilli PA, Warren RF: The effect of medial meniscectomy on anterior-posterior motion of the knee. J Bone Joint Surg Am 64:883-888, 1982.

30. McDevitt CA, Webber RJ: The ultra-structure and biochemistry of meniscal cartilage. Clin Orthop 252:8-18, 1990.

31. Mow VC, Fithian DC, Kelly MA: Fundamentals of articular cartilage and meniscus biomechanics. In Ewing JW (ed): Articular Cartilage and Knee Joint Function: Basic Science and Arthroscopy. New York, Raven Press, 1990, pp 1-18.

32. Nelson EW, LaPrade RF: The anterior intermeniscal ligament of the knee: An anatomic study. Am J Sports Med 28:74-76, 2000.

33. Noyes FR, Barber-Westin SD, Rankin M: Meniscal transplantation in symptomatic patients less than fifty years old. J Bone Joint Surg Am 86:1392-1404, 2004.

34. O'Driscoll SW: Current concepts review: The healing and regeneration of articular cartilage. J Bone Joint Surg Am 80:1795-1812, 1998.

35. Radin EL, de Lamotte F, Maquet P: Role of the menisci in the distribution of stress in the knee. Clin Orthop 185:290-294, 1984.

36. Ritchie JR, Miller MD, Bents RT, Smith DK: Meniscal repair in the goat model. The use of healing adjuncts on central tears and the role of magnetic resonance arthrography in repair evaluation. Am J Sports Med 26:278-284, 1998.

37. Rodeo SA: Arthroscopic meniscal repair with use of the outside-in technique. Instr Course Lect 49:195-206, 2000.

38. Sellars RS, Peluso D, Morris EA: The effect of recombinant human bone morphogenetic protein-2 (rhBMP-2) on the healing of full-thickness defects of articular cartilage. J Bone Joint Surg Am 79:1452-1463, 1997.

39. Shoemaker SC, Markolf KL: The role of the meniscus in the anterior-posterior stability of the loaded anterior cruciate–deficient knee: Effects of partial versus total excision. J Bone Joint Surg Am 68:71-79, 1986.

40. Simonian PT, Sussmann PS, van Trommel M, et al: Popliteomeniscal fasciculi and lateral meniscal stability. Am J Sports Med 25:849-853, 1997.

41. Thompson WO, Thaete FL, Fu FH, Dye SF: Tibial meniscal dynamics using three-dimensional reconstruction of magnetic resonance images. Am J Sports Med 19:210-216, 1991.

42. Vandermeer RD, Cunningham FK: Arthroscopic treatment of the discoid lateral meniscus: Results of long-term follow-up. Arthroscopy 5:101-109, 1989.

43. Voloshin AS, Wosk J: Shock absorption of meniscectomized and painful knees: A comparative in-vivo study. J Biomed Eng 5:157-161, 1983.

44. Watanabe Y, Scyoc AV, Tsuda E, et al: Biomechanical function of the posterior horn of the medial meniscus: A human cadaveric study. J Orthop Sci 9:280-284, 2004.

45. Webber RJ, Harris MG, Hough AJ: Cell culture of rabbit meniscal fibrochondrocytes: Proliferative synthetic response to growth factors and ascorbate. J Orthop Res 3: 36-42, 1985.

46. Wong M, Hunziker EB: Articular cartilage biology and biomechanics. In Insall JN, Scott WN (eds): Surgery of the Knee, 3rd ed. Philadelphia, Churchill Livingstone, 2000, pp 317-325.

CHAPTER 17

Gene Therapy in the Treatment of Knee Disorders

Kurt R. Weiss • T. Thomas Liu • Freddie H. Fu • Johnny Huard

Impressive advances in the treatment of knee disorders have occurred in the past several years. New instruments, materials, and technology are being tested and improved continually through clinical experience. Incisions have become increasingly smaller, and minimally invasive techniques have exploded in popularity. The limits of early rehabilitation are constantly being challenged, returning patients to sports and activities of daily life faster than ever before. Meniscus that previously was removed and discarded is now being repaired. Patients with arthritis have a wide variety of therapeutic options besides joint replacement. Computers aid clinicians in perfect placement of anterior cruciate ligament (ACL) replacement tunnels. Novel medications keep patients active later into life.

Despite these significant strides in operative techniques, technology, imaging, rehabilitation, and pharmacology, we are still confounded by seemingly immobile truths of nature. Articular cartilage and meniscus do not heal. Ligamentization of ACL graft is painfully slow. Healed tendon never fully regains its preinjury strength and may rupture again. Rheumatoid arthritis (RA) is relentlessly debilitating. The desire to break through these barriers and fundamentally alter the natural history of disease provides the motivation to develop novel treatment options for knee disorders.

DEFINITION AND STRATEGIES

Gene therapy is the process by which cells are genetically modified to change their expression profiles with the intent of exerting a therapeutic effect. Three basic strategies have emerged as to how this might be accomplished. First, one could deliver the cell-altering material or altered cells themselves systemically through the bloodstream. This approach has merit in systemic diseases, where the goal is to modify several cell types throughout the entire body. This systemic approach is probably not logical, however, in the treatment of knee disorders because only a small percentage of the body's cells in a discrete anatomic area are of interest. A second strategy is the direct or in vivo method of gene therapy. In this method, the cell-transforming material is introduced directly into the environment to be modified. In terms of gene therapy for knee disorders, an in vivo approach probably would involve intra-articular injection of the vector. This strategy is technically simple, but what is gained in simplicity is lost in control. With the direct, in vivo method, there is no way to predict which knee cells or structures would be altered by the vector. Also, there is no way to test how successful the genetic manipulation was unless cells are harvested from the joint and analyzed for transgene expression. Finally, the third strategy, the indirect or ex vivo method, uses a stepwise approach. Target cells of interest are maintained under laboratory conditions. When a suitable number of cells have been grown, they are exposed to the cell-altering vector. At this point, the modified cells can be assayed to discern if the manipulation was successful. A set number of modified cells is injected into the knee or implanted into specific tissues within the knee. The ex vivo method offers the highest degree of control at all stages of experimental manipulation. It is, however, much more cumbersome and time-consuming than the in vivo method. Because most gene therapy to the knee is intended for specific tissues, the ex vivo method is the one most often employed (Fig. 17–1).

VECTORS

A vector is simply the vehicle by which DNA encoding the therapeutic gene of interest is presented to the cell. Traditionally, vectors have been divided broadly into viral vectors and nonviral vectors.

Because nonviral vectors are conceptually simpler, they are discussed first. Proven nonviral vectors include naked plasmid DNA and DNA complexed with liposomes or polycations.[34,91,92] Cells endocytose naked plasmid DNA, but their transfection efficiency is poor and tends to be short-lived. Attempts have been made to package the DNA in ways that foster more efficient uptake by the cell. Combining the DNA with liposomes or polycations increases the transfection efficiency and expression of the transgene. The "gene gun" is a process by which microprojectiles of gold or tungsten are coated with the DNA of interest and accelerated by high-pressure helium or high-voltage electrical discharge and essentially shot through the cell membrane.[51,92,95] Finally, exposure of cells or tissue to pulsed electric fields (a process called *electroporation*) transiently increases the permeability of the cell membrane and encourages the transit of more DNA. The advantages of nonviral vectors are their low cost and nearly complete lack of immunogenicity. The major disadvantage of nonviral vectors, as alluded to, is their poor and transient transduction efficiency.

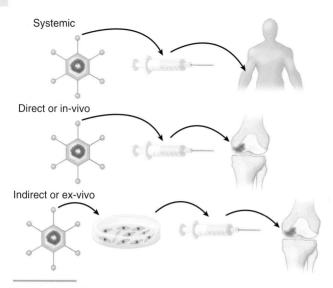

Figure 17–1. Strategies of gene therapy.

Examples of viral vectors include adenovirus, adeno-associated virus (AAV), herpes simplex virus (HSV), retrovirus, and lentivirus. Adenoviruses do not integrate their DNA into the host genome. Their DNA remains in the nucleus as an episome after host cell infection. The main advantage of adenoviruses is their ability to efficiently transduce dividing and nondividing cells, and they have been used extensively for in vitro and animal models of gene therapy. Adenoviruses have several disadvantages, however. First, because their DNA remains episomal and does not integrate, it is subject to degradation and dilution during cell division. Additionally, adenoviral proteins are extremely immunogenic and cytotoxic. As a result of these attributes, the duration of adenoviral transgene expression is only on the order of weeks. Attempts to reduce adenoviral immunogenicity led to the creation of second-generation adenoviruses and "gutless" adenoviruses. The latter require a "helper virus" such as HSV for replication.[23,72,92,94,96] Adenoviral-mediated human gene therapy for ornithine transcarbamoylase deficiency resulted in the death of one of the study patients. This event was not anticipated based on the preclinical animal studies, and it has raised serious concerns regarding the safety of this vector in human subjects.[78]

HSV is a DNA virus similar in many respects to adenovirus. Similar to adenovirus, HSV can efficiently transduce dividing and nondividing cells. This and the ability to transfer very large DNA cassettes are the major advantages of HSV. HSV also shares the penchant of adenovirus for immunogenicity. The virus's complex lifestyle poses specific challenges because it may enter a lytic or latent state. Major ongoing efforts seek to create replication-deficient HSVs that are kept in a pseudolatent state and avoid lysing host cells.[72,92]

Retroviruses also are used extensively in gene therapy. They are RNA viruses and can infect only dividing cells.[21,72,79,92] Retroviruses integrate their genetic material into the host genome and as such provide stable transduction of genes whose expression is not lost through cell division. This ability to impart long-term gene expression without significant immunologic response is the main advantage of retroviruses. A disadvantage of retroviruses is that cells must undergo active division to be transduced. Another theoretical concern of retroviruses, which incorporate randomly into the host genome, is termed *insertional mutagenesis*. Conceivably the introduced genetic material could integrate into a deleterious or disruptive position along the host genome.[91] Finally, the major advantage of retroviruses also could be a potential disadvantage: Retroviruses should be used only for applications requiring prolonged transgene expression.

A subset of retroviruses related to human immunodeficiency virus (HIV) is lentivirus. Similar to other retroviruses, lentivirus incorporates its DNA into the host genome. The distinguishing characteristic between this and other retroviruses is the ability of lentivirus to infect dividing and nondividing cells. The limitations of lentiviruses include the difficulties encountered in the production of high-titer virus stocks and safety concerns related to their similarity to HIV.[59] This vector is not yet widely used in orthopedic applications of gene therapy.

AAV, a member of the parvovirus family, is a single-stranded DNA virus that also requires a helper virus for replication.[10,15,16,31,92,93] AAV combines many strengths of the aforementioned viral vectors. AAV transduces dividing and nondividing cells and has low cytotoxic effects (Table 17–1).[91]

REGULATABLE PROMOTERS

Viral and nonviral vectors are tools that the gene therapist must use appropriately, taking into account their individual attributes and drawbacks and choosing the one that best suits its intended application. Another means of controlling the transgene expression is the use of regulatable promoters. The promoter is a genetic sequence, generally upstream of the coding region of a gene, which acts as a controlling element in the gene's expression. It serves as a recognition signal for the cell's transcription machinery. Vectors now can be constructed such that their promoters require the presence or absence of certain chemicals to function. There are "tet-on" and "tet-off" promoters that require the drug tetracycline to initiate or inactivate gene transcription; this is accomplished easily by adding or withholding tetracycline in the experimental animal's drinking water or in the cell culture medium for in vivo and in vitro applications.[30,68] Besides tetracycline, regulatable promoters have been constructed that recognize doxycycline, rapamycin, ecdysone, and streptogramin.[37,88] This strategy has been used successfully in several of the forthcoming examples of gene therapy.

Another elegant method of controlling the timing of gene expression involves use of the *Cre-Lox* system. *Cre* recombinase is an enzyme that cleaves DNA between highly specific sequences called *loxP* sites and recombines the DNA strand around them. Conceptually the gene of interest could be transduced with superfluous DNA upstream to its coding region flanked by loxP sites, rendering the gene silent. When *Cre* recombinase is introduced, the genetic material between the loxP sites is "cut

Table 17–1. Vectors in Gene Therapy

VECTOR	TYPE	ADVANTAGES	DISADVANTAGES
Plasmid DNA	Nonviral	Low cost; non-immunogenic	Low and transient transfection efficiency; can be improved by complexing with liposomes or polycations, gene gun, or electroporation
Adenovirus	Viral	Efficiently transduces dividing and nondividing cells	DNA does not integrate; immunogenicity leads to rapid clearance
Herpes simplex virus	Viral	Efficiently transduces dividing and nondividing cells; can transfer large amounts of DNA	DNA does not integrate; immunogenicity leads to rapid clearance; complex and as yet uncontrollable life cycle
Retrovirus	Viral	DNA integrates into genome yielding stable transduction	Transduces only dividing cells; insertional mutagenesis
Lentivirus	Viral	DNA integrates into genome yielding stable transduction; transduces dividing and nondividing cells	Difficult to produce; safety concerns related to HIV
Adeno-associated virus	Viral	Lower immunogenicity than adenovirus or herpes simplex virus; transduces dividing and nondividing cells	Requires helper virus for proliferation

HIV, human immunodeficiency virus.

out," the DNA assumes its normal sequence, and transgene expression commences.[48]

STEM CELLS

Another important aspect of gene therapy delivery is choosing the correct cell to express the desired gene product. This choice may be as important as the choice of transgene and vector system. An area of research with which we have had considerable experience is the use of stem cells in gene therapy.

By definition, stem cells are characterized by three features: They are self-renewing, pluripotential, long-term progenitor cells. There are two types of stem cells—embryonic, which are from the zygote stage and are totipotent, and adult stem cells, which reside in postnatal tissues and are responsible for their reparative capacity. Adult mesenchymal stem cells (MSCs) reside in mesenchymal tissues and can differentiate into bone, cartilage, fat, muscle, and tendon.[30,55] Our experience has been mainly with the use of postnatal muscle-derived stem cells. We have shown that under the correct conditions, muscle-derived stem cells possess the capacity to differentiate into myogenic, hematopoietic, osteogenic, endothelial, neuronal, adipose, and chondroid lineages (Fig. 17–2).[18] These stem cells are powerful tools for three reasons. First, muscle-derived stem cells may be genetically engineered to deliver growth factors to the site of injury and initiate the creation of new tissue. Second, they may serve as a source of progenitor cells to assist with the repair of injured tissues. Third, stem cells engineered to express growth factors could exert their effects in autocrine and paracrine fashions.

Proof that the choice of cell per se is critical in gene therapy was illustrated by Gazit and associates,[32] who reported that MSCs transduced with a retrovirus encoding bone morphogenetic protein-2 (BMP2) healed an osseous

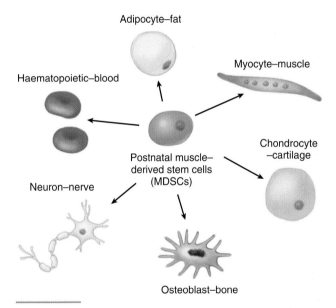

Figure 17–2. Pluripotential/multipotential nature of postnatal muscle-derived stem cells (MDSCs). (Figure provided compliments of B.M. Deasy.)

defect more completely than transduced Chinese hamster ovary cells, despite the fact that the Chinese hamster ovary cells expressed quantitatively more BMP2. This is compelling evidence that, despite a smaller amount of protein, the MSCs were qualitatively better suited to this application.[30,32] Moutsatos and colleagues[68] showed that MSCs expressing BMP2 produced more bone in a mouse radial defect model than did injection of recombinant protein, illustrating that cells contribute more than merely a source of growth factor.[30,68]

The remainder of this chapter is divided by intra-articular tissue. Examples of gene therapy for each tissue since the publication of the previous edition of this book are discussed.

MENISCUS

Damage to the meniscus resulting from trauma or sports-related injury is the leading indication for arthroscopic surgery.[17,43] Meniscectomy is among the most commonly performed procedures in all of orthopedic surgery. Modern research has disclosed that the meniscus, previously routinely removed when injured, has important biomechanical functions, including shock absorption, lubrication, and stabilization of the knee.[3,43,80] Early meniscectomy is associated with articular cartilage damage and degenerative arthritis. After complete meniscectomy, patients can expect the onset of osteoarthritis in 5 to 10 years.[46]

Commensurate with these discoveries, the trend among practicing surgeons has shifted from liberal meniscectomy to reparative procedures that attempt to preserve as much meniscus as possible. Repair techniques have involved the use of sutures, arrows, and staples to attempt stabilization of meniscal injuries.[46] A major anatomic obstacle of this effort mirrors the difficulty experienced with the repair of articular cartilage defects, however: Although injuries to the peripheral vascular zone can heal, the inner two-thirds of the meniscus is avascular and cannot support a regenerative process. For this reason, meniscal allograft procedures are being employed with increasing frequency for injuries that are deemed irreparable.[53] This procedure is technically demanding and carries with it the inherent dangers of allograft use, including disease transmission, immunogenicity, and graft failure. The goal of gene therapy to the meniscus is to heal defects in the central, avascular zone with (1) the use of exogenous cells expressing growth factors that stimulate healing or enhance neovascularization (or both), (2) the recruitment of endogenous cells from the peripheral vascular zone to repair the defect, or (3) a combined approach.

Hidaka and coworkers[43] used functional tissue engineering to illustrate that (1) meniscal cells can populate a bioengineered scaffold, and (2) the cells may be manipulated via gene therapy to improve neoangiogenesis in the artificial meniscal tissue. Bovine meniscal cells were transduced with adenovirus encoding hepatocyte growth factor, an angiogenic growth factor. Transduced cells were seeded onto polyglycolic acid felt scaffolds and placed subcutaneously into nude mice. Scaffolds with hepatocyte growth factor–expressing cells showed dramatically greater blood vessel ingrowth than β-galactosidase-expressing or nontransduced control scaffolds.[43] This study showed the feasibility of using gene therapy and functional tissue engineering to augment meniscal repair. Although encouraging, there is a paucity of research on gene therapy for the meniscus. More innovative studies, such as the one performed by Hidaka and coworkers,[43] are required to generate novel clinical solutions to meniscal injury.

LIGAMENT

The ACL is one of two intra-articular knee ligaments. The ACL resists anterior translation of the tibia and is probably an important rotational stabilizer. It is frequently traumatized, and there are probably more than 100,000 ACL injuries per annum in the United States.[46] The ACL has poor de novo healing capacity, and this characteristic provides the rationale behind ACL replacement surgery. Candidate tissues for replacement include ACL allografts and autologous patellar tendon or hamstring grafts. Disadvantages to these approaches include possible disease transmission and immunogenicity of allograft, donor site morbidity in autologous tissue transfer, and mismatch between the biomechanical properties of transplanted or transferred tissue versus native ACL.

Regardless of the replacement material used, maturation or "ligamentization" of the graft and its bony attachments is the rate-limiting step of functional recovery and may take years to complete. Hastening the ligamentization process would result in faster graft incorporation and return to preinjury activities.[65] To test the ability of genetically engineered cells to populate an ACL and express a transgene, we transduced rabbit ACL-derived fibroblasts and muscle-derived cells with adenovirus encoding the β-galactosidase gene,[65] which then were injected into intact rabbit ACLs. ACL fibroblasts and muscle-derived cells were incorporated into the ligament and expressed the marker protein for 6 weeks. This study offers proof that ACL-derived and muscle-derived cells can be stably transduced and successfully transferred into the ACL.[65] The next logical step would be to introduce cells producing growth factors with the intent of speeding ligamentization or attempting to impart regenerative capacity to the injured ACL.

Another ACL study by Martinek and colleagues[63] examined the effect of BMP2 gene therapy on the ligamentization process. Autologous doubled semitendinosus graft ACL replacements were performed in rabbits. These were injected with adenovirus encoding BMP2, the luciferase marker gene, or nothing. The results showed that treatment with BMP2 gene therapy accelerated the ligamentization process. In BMP2-treated animals, the tendon-bone interface in the osseous tunnel was similar to that of a normal ACL insertion at 6 weeks. In contrast, the luciferase and control groups displayed only dense connective tissue at the interface. These results were mirrored in biomechanical studies that showed statistically higher load-to-failure levels in the BMP2-treated animals compared with luciferase and control groups.[36] This study provides forceful evidence that ACL repair may be enhanced by gene therapy.

In contrast to the ACL, the medial collateral ligament (MCL) possesses some intrinsic healing capacity. This ability is not perfect, however. A rabbit model of MCL injury showed that healed MCLs fail between 30% and 50% of normal values. Additionally, MCL scar tissue has more creep than normal ligament, compromising medial joint stability and predisposing to knee osteoarthritis.[45] One potential reason for the biomechanical inferiority of healed MCL tissue lies in differences of collagen fibril diameter between intact and healing MCL. Decorin is a proteoglycan implicated in collagen fibrillogenesis and associated with small-diameter collagen fibrils. These small-diameter fibrils are disproportionately numerous in injured versus normal MCLs. It was postulated by

Nakamura and associates[69] that blocking decorin expression would lead to better ligament healing with larger diameter collagen fibrils. To test this hypothesis, liposomal antisense decorin complementary DNA (cDNA) was injected into a 4-mm rabbit MCL defect. The antidecorin MCLs showed larger fibril diameter than untreated groups. They also displayed an 85% increase in peak failure stress and a 20% decrease in creep compared with untreated MCLs.[45,69] Although these data are encouraging, the in vivo milieu of healing ligament is extremely complex, and manipulation of one protein is unlikely to restore the preinjury functionality of MCL tissue. The roles of growth factors and collagen type heterogeneity must be investigated more completely if ligament healing is to be optimized.

TENDON

Traumatic and degenerative tendon injuries are extremely common. Tendinopathies represent 50% of all sports injuries.[2,47] Endogenously healed tendons never achieve preinjury strength largely because repair tissue contains a large amount of type III collagen, which has fewer cross-links than type I collagen. Because type I collagen accounts for greater than 90% of the collagen in human tendons, this mismatch translates into reduced tensile strength of healed versus normal tendons.[61] In addition to the formation of biomechanically inferior scar tissue, some healing tendons form adhesions to the surrounding tissue. These adhesions interfere with the normal gliding motion of tendons and compromise proper tendon function, which is of particular concern in the hand where adhesions can have a dramatic effect on range of motion.[45]

Since the publication of the last edition of this text, there has been extraordinary progress in tendon basic science research, which has elucidated the roles of growth factors in tendon. The growth of tenocytes in vitro has been shown to be affected by such diverse mediators as insulin-like growth factor-1 (IGF1), platelet-derived growth factor (PDGF), transforming growth factor (TGF)-β, epidermal growth factor, and fibroblast growth factor (FGF).[22,47,61,90] In uninjured canine flexor tendons, there is a higher baseline level of basic FGF than PDGF. In injured tendon, the inverse relationship occurs.[61] During tendon embryogenesis, BMPs 12 and 13 are expressed, causing increased production of elastin and type I collagen.[61] The BMP-related growth and differentiation factors may be important for tendon healing. Growth and differentiation factors 5, 6, and 7 led to the formation of ectopic tendon tissue when injected into rats.[47] The aforementioned discoveries have provided the rationale behind several applications of gene therapy for tendon.

Jayankura and associates[47] investigated the feasibility of in vivo gene transfer therapy to rat, mouse, and rabbit tendons with plasmid DNA encoding the β-galactosidase reporter gene. Injection of plasmid DNA into the patellar tendon sheath was performed under direct visualization. The reporter gene was transferred successfully in all three models. Additionally, it was discovered that combining injection with the application of a pulsed electric field to the tendon resulted in an approximately 50% increase in the number of transduced cells. It is possible to transfer a therapeutic gene of interest directly into tendon.[47] Proof of this concept also was shown in a canine digital flexor tendon model. Transfection efficiency of 100% was reported by Goomer and colleagues,[35] who delivered the β-galactosidase marker gene via liposomal plasmid DNA.[35,45]

An in vitro study by Wang and coworkers[90] examined the ability of PDGF to augment type I collagen production in cultured cells. Tenocytes from rat flexor digitorum profundus tendon explants were transfected with plasmid cDNA for the PDGF gene. Transfection enhanced type I collagen expression by more than threefold compared with untreated tenocytes. The authors called for further studies to assess the efficacy of PDGF gene therapy in vivo. This challenge was met by Hildebrand and associates,[44] who delivered the PDGF gene to healing rat tendon via liposomal plasmid DNA. The results showed not only the expected increase in collagen type I deposition in the PDGF-treated group, but also enhanced neoangiogenesis. By 8 weeks postinjury, there were no measurable differences between uninjured patellar tendons and experimental tendons treated with PDGF.[44]

Adenovirus expressing BMP13 was injected by Helm and colleagues[42] into the thigh musculature of athymic nude rats and examined with light and electron microscopy at various time points 2 to 100 days after injection. By 100 days after virus injection, the treated tissue displayed the histologic and ultrastructural appearance of ligament or tendon and was demarcated from the adjacent musculature. These data indicate that BMP13-mediated gene therapy may have promise in the treatment of tendon and ligament injuries.[42] Similarly, Lou and associates[57] used BMP12 adenovirus to treat tendon cells in vitro and lacerated chicken tendons in vivo. The in vitro data showed that BMP12 gene transfer caused the tendon cells to increase type I collagen synthesis by 30%. BMP12 transduction in vivo resulted in a twofold increase in strength and stiffness compared with endogenously healed tendons, indicating that BMP12 gene therapy may be beneficial in the tendon healing process.[57] These data are impressive, but there are still numerous factors important to tendon biology whose in vivo effects should be evaluated by themselves and in concert with other mediators.

ARTICULAR CARTILAGE— OSTEOARTHRITIS

In 1743, Hunter observed that "ulcerated cartilage is a troublesome thing, once destroyed is not repaired."[26] Injury to the articular cartilage is a formidable obstacle in orthopedic medicine. Cartilage has extremely limited healing potential because of intrinsic properties of its biology: Adult articular cartilage has neither vascular supply nor innervation. Defects larger than a few millimeters rarely, if ever, heal.[26,53] The healing response is initiated only when full-thickness defects occur that also injure the subchondral bone. When this occurs, the resultant tissue is fibrocartilage, which is histologically dissimilar and biomechanically inferior to normal hyaline cartilage. Fibrocartilage consists predominantly of type I and type III collagen, whereas hyaline cartilage contains mainly type II collagen.[18,41,71] The most common etiology of articular cartilage damage is osteoarthritis.[6]

Epidemiologically the impact of osteoarthritis cannot be overestimated. Osteoarthritis affects 43 million Americans and affects more lives than any other musculoskeletal condition.[12,14,53] Eighty percent of people older than age 75 have this disease, making it the most common pathology of later life. Treatments cost more than $100 billion per annum.[25] These numbers and statistics are expected to increase as the bulging cohort of "baby boomers" grows older and remains active into later life.[12,14,18,26]

Surgical and nonsurgical treatments of osteoarthritis exist. Nonsurgical options include the use of nonsteroidal anti-inflammatory drugs and intra-articular treatments of steroids and hyaluronic acid. Surgical treatments of osteoarthritis pathology include articular surface débridement, mosaicplasty, autologous chondrocyte transplant, and total joint replacement. None of these operative and nonoperative options successfully halts the progression of osteoarthritis, and all have significant intrinsic risks. Novel strategies aimed at the cessation or reversal of osteoarthritis pathology are required.

It is generally held that elevated matrix synthesis is a feature of early osteoarthritis, whereas reduced matrix synthesis occurs in advanced disease. As osteoarthritis progresses, aggrecan (the major proteoglycan of articular cartilage) content decreases dramatically. Although the total amount of collagen does not change significantly, the collagen helices are proteolytically cleaved. There is a higher proportion of type III collagen, an isoform found in scar tissue and basement membrane that is normally absent from articular cartilage. Matrix degradation is mediated by matrix metalloproteinases, free radicals, and perhaps other as yet undiscovered factors. Production of these matrix-degrading enzymes may be driven by cytokines, such as interleukin (IL)-1 and tumor necrosis factor (TNF)-α.[25,76] Because osteoarthritis affects a limited number of weightbearing joints and seems to have no systemic manifestations, it is conceptually well-suited to local, intra-articular gene therapy. The same characteristics of articular cartilage that make it difficult for cells to heal defects (e.g., abundant extracellular matrix and lack of vascularity) pose challenges, however, to the introduction of viral or nonviral vectors. First, the dense matrix essentially immobilizes the chondrocytes, precluding them from migrating and participating in repair processes. Second, the lack of vascularity and lymphatic drainage impedes cell and growth factor traffic to the site of injury. Gene therapy for articular cartilage defects demands four essential elements: (1) An efficient cell type must be selected for tissue repair. (2) The correct growth factors must be chosen to facilitate the repair. (3) An appropriate scaffold must be constructed to deliver the cells and growth factors. (4) The proper biomechanical stimulation must be imparted to the system.[18]

Despite the complexity of osteoarthritis pathology and the difficulties anticipated with articular cartilage gene therapy, significant contributions have been made. The first of these are advances in the understanding of cartilage biology as it relates to growth factors. IGFs, BMPs, TGF-β, and FGFs affect chondrocyte proliferation and extracellular matrix synthesis. In normal cartilage, IGF1 acts as an anabolic growth factor through stimulation of matrix synthesis and inhibition of matrix degradation. IGF1 also serves as a chondrocyte survival factor. Osteoarthritic cartilage fails to respond appropriately to IGF1 because of increased activity of IGF1 binding proteins and inactivation of the IGF1 receptor by free radicals.[25,28,85] These characteristics make IGF1 an attractive candidate for cartilage repair gene therapy. BMP7 is a potent stimulator of human articular chondrocytes, inducing them to synthesize proteoglycan and type II collagen. Stimulation of stem cells with BMP2 and BMP4 induces chondrogenic differentiation. TGF-β regulates chondrocyte homeostasis by stimulating collagen synthesis and inhibiting proteoglycan degradation. TGF-β1, TGF-β2, and TGF-β3 all have displayed the ability to promote chondroid differentiation in bone marrow stromal cells. TGF-β3 in combination with BMP6 has shown additive effects on marrow stromal cell differentiation.[82] FGFs promote mitogenic activity in chondrocytes. FGF2 stimulates chondrocyte proliferation and matrix formation. FGF2 and IGF1 work in concert to promote chondrocyte mitosis and proteoglycan synthesis. Finally, applying mechanical forces to chondrocytes (e.g., shear, compression) increases their production of matrix proteins.[18,29,54,74,85]

Several proof-of-concept research efforts have used nontherapeutic marker genes to test novel vectors, matrices, or other strategies of osteoarthritis gene therapy. Madry and coworkers[60] transfected rabbit chondrocytes with plasmid DNA encoding the luciferase marker gene. Transfected cells were embedded in an alginate gel and placed into rabbit osteochondral defects. Luciferase activity was found to peak at day 5, then decline until day 32, proving the efficacy of this relatively simple strategy.[60]

Another rabbit osteochondral defect model by Pascher and associates[75] compared the use of coagulated bone marrow aspirate versus collagen/glycosaminoglycan matrix as a scaffold for transduced cells. The scaffolds were loaded with adenoviral vectors carrying DNA for the marker genes β-galactosidase, green fluorescent protein, and luciferase and placed into 3 × 8 mm osteochondral defects. Both scaffold groups showed expression of the marker genes for several weeks. Collagen/glycosaminoglycan scaffolds showed significant transgene expression in the surrounding synovium, indicating leakage of the vector from the implanted matrix. Coagulated bone marrow aspirate showed better containment of the vector. It may be concluded from this study that matrix formed from bone marrow aspirate clot is completely natural, native to the host, and a scaffold that should be considered for cell and gene therapy.[75]

A third rabbit study from our laboratory explored the feasibility of using allogeneic muscle-derived cells to treat full-thickness articular cartilage defects and compared them with chondrocytes.[1] Muscle-derived cells and chondrocytes were transduced with retrovirus for the β-galactosidase marker gene. These were placed into collagen gels and grafted into full-thickness rabbit osteochondral defects. Muscle-derived cells and chondrocytes displayed long-term (>1 month) expression of β-galactosidase in essentially equivalent high percentages of the implanted cells. Repair tissues in the chondrocyte and muscle-derived cell groups were histologically superior to control groups, and repair tissue contained mostly type II collagen.[1] This study illustrated that (1) muscle-derived cells may be used successfully to express a transgene long-term in a full-thickness articular cartilage defect, and (2) the cells used to carry a gene of interest also contribute to the healing process and should be chosen carefully.

Other experimental models have applied therapeutic genes of interest. Gelse and coworkers[33] transduced perichondrial mesenchymal cells with adenovirus encoding IGF1 or BMP2. Cells were suspended in fibrin glue and applied to partial-thickness articular cartilage defects in the rat trochlear groove. Control groups, which received nontransduced cells, failed to fill articular cartilage defects or did so with fibrocartilage. Treatment with IGF1-transduced or BMP2-transduced cells healed the partial-thickness defects with hyaline-like cartilage, however, and restored the articular surface.[33] Mi and associates[66] showed that intra-articular injection of adenovirus encoding IGF1 in a rabbit model of osteoarthritis yielded a sufficient amount of IGF production to increase matrix synthesis.

In a rabbit model, Grande and associates[39] transduced periosteal stem cells with either BMP7 or sonic hedgehog (Shh). These cells were loaded onto bioabsorbable polymer scaffolds and placed into full-thickness osteochondral defects. Control defects were filled with fibrocartilage, but the BMP7 and Shh defects were filled with hyaline-like cartilage. The BMP7-treated animals remodeled the osseous portion of the defect much faster than the Shh-treated animals.[39]

Another application of BMP7-mediated gene therapy to articular cartilage was described by Mason and colleagues,[64] who used retrovirus to transduce rabbit MSCs with the BMP7 gene. BMP7-expressing cells were expanded, seeded onto polyglycolic acid scaffolds, and placed into full-thickness osteochondral defects in a rabbit model. The grafts containing BMP7-expressing cells consistently showed complete or nearly complete bone and articular cartilage regeneration, whereas the grafts from the control groups had poor repair by macroscopic, histologic, and immunochemical criteria. This research successfully combined aspects of stem cells, gene therapy, and a scaffold to elicit a therapeutic effect.[64]

The ability of TGF-β1 gene therapy to repair articular cartilage defects was tested by Song and coworkers.[84] NIH 3T3 cells, a well-known fibroblast cell line, were transduced with the gene for TGF-β1, irradiated, and placed into partial-thickness rabbit articular cartilage defects. Animals treated with TGF-β1-expressing cells healed their defects with hyaline-like cartilage. Cells treated with lower doses of radiation (20 Gy) formed histologically superior cartilage compared with cells irradiated at higher levels (40 Gy or 80 Gy). The authors concluded that irradiated heterologous cell–mediated TGF-β1 gene therapy may be a clinically useful and efficient method of regenerating hyaline articular cartilage, but the amount of radiation experienced by transplanted cells is probably an important parameter to be considered.[84]

Guo and associates[40] transfected MSCs with TGF-β1 cDNA via a lipofectamine vector and placed them into rat full-thickness articular cartilage defects. TGF-β1 transgene expression was detectable for 4 weeks after implantation.[40]

Intra-articular injection of adenovirus encoding TGF-β1 in a rabbit model of osteoarthritis illustrated a potential drawback of this approach. TGF-β1 virus administration increased extracellular matrix synthesis, but transduction of other intra-articular structures, such as the synovium, caused massive synovial fibrosis and synovial chondromatosis. Similar experiments in a murine model also displayed these complications.[5,25,67]

Zhang and coworkers[99] sought to use gene therapy for anti-inflammatory cytokines in the treatment of osteoarthritis. They transduced rabbit synoviocytes with retrovirus for the IL-1 receptor-antagonist protein (IL-1Ra) gene and the IL-10 gene. IL-1Ra is a direct inhibitor of IL-1, and IL-10 is an anti-inflammatory cytokine. Their rabbit model of osteoarthritis was established by excision of the MCL plus medial meniscectomy. Five days after this operation, rabbits received IL-1Ra-expressing cells, IL-10-expressing cells, a combination of these two cells, or no cells. Knees receiving the IL-1Ra gene had significantly reduced cartilage breakdown. The IL-10 gene was less effective, showing only modest cartilage protection. Injection of cells expressing both factors showed an additive inhibition of cartilage breakdown. This finding suggested that the simultaneous delivery of several anti-inflammatory factors may be beneficial in the treatment of osteoarthritis.[99]

A novel strategy by Nixon and colleagues[70] designed to promote cartilage repair and inhibit degradation simultaneously employed a combination of IL-1Ra and IGF1 adenoviral gene therapy. Synoviocytes transduced with both factors restored normal proteoglycan levels to equine articular cartilage.[25,70]

In Caron and coworkers'[13] canine model of osteoarthritis, biweekly intra-articular injections of recombinant IL-1Ra inhibited cartilage loss, lowered matrix metalloproteinase expression, and reduced the number and size of osteophytes.[25] Fernandes and associates[27] described a rabbit model of osteoarthritis that yielded similar results with intra-articular injection of liposome-encapsulated IL-1Ra cDNA.[25]

Glutamine:fructose-6-phosphate amidotransferase catalyzes the rate-limiting step of glucosamine synthesis. Gouze and colleagues[38] reported that in vitro, transfection of synovial fibroblasts with glutamine:fructose-6-phosphate amidotransferase cDNA protected them and adjacent chondrocytes from challenge with high doses of IL-1.[25]

Many ambitious efforts have been made in the field of osteoarthritis gene therapy. Some investigators believe that the applicability of these animal models is limited, however, and that investigators ought to strive for even more clinically meaningful research. Evans and colleagues[25] advocate introducing candidate genes into human joints scheduled for replacement so that human studies could be conducted "in a safe and responsible manner."

ARTICULAR CARTILAGE—RHEUMATOID ARTHRITIS

RA is a common disease affecting 0.5% to 1% of the population. It is a chronic inflammatory disease that is thought to be autoimmune in etiology. RA involves mainly diarthroidal joints such as the knee and is characterized by inflammatory cell infiltration and hyperplasia of the synovium, pannus formation, and erosion of articular cartilage and bone. The etiology of RA is unknown, but the inflammatory cytokines IL-1 and TNF-α are thought to be pivotal in the pathogenesis of this condition.[37,53] The disease is relentlessly progressive and characterized by periodic exacerbations or "flare-ups" of the symptoms.[12] The mainstays of pharmacological treatment include chronic systemic glucocorticoids, cytotoxic agents such as methotrexate and leflunomide, and the new TNF-α antagonists infliximab and etanercept.[53] Current treatments for RA do not provide prolonged symptomatic relief, and they do not halt disease progression.[10] Surgery often is required to replace joints that have been damaged to the point that they are deformed, ankylosed, and nonfunctional. Commensurate with the clinical features of the disease, gene therapy for RA falls into three main categories: anti-inflammatory gene therapy, cartilage-repairing gene therapy, and combination gene therapy.

Because IL-1 and TNF-α have been heavily implicated in the pathogenesis of RA, investigations were undertaken to identify the effect of inhibiting these cytokines via gene therapy. Kim and associates[50] used retroviruses encoding IL-1Ra and the soluble tumor necrosis factor receptor (sTNFR-Ig) to transduce autologous rabbit fibroblasts stably. These fibroblasts were then injected into rabbit knees in an antigen-induced arthritis model alone or in combination. Results showed that the delivery of either IL-1Ra-expressing or sTNFR-Ig-expressing fibroblasts decreased arthritis severity in the injected and noninjected joints. Additionally the authors reported that the delivery of both factors resulted in a synergistic amelioration of disease in the treated and nontreated joints.[50] These results not only suggest that blockade of anti-inflammatory cytokines is therapeutic, but also imply that local gene therapy for arthritis could effectively block disease progression in untreated joints.

IL-4 is an anti-inflammatory cytokine that was found to be absent from the joint lavages of patients with RA. Lubberts and coworkers[58] hypothesized that overexpression of IL-4 might protect joints from inflammatory arthritis. They constructed an adenovirus encoding the IL-4 gene and injected it into the knees of mice in a collagen-induced arthritis (CIA) model. Although severe inflammation persisted in mouse knees, IL-4 adenovirus prevented cartilage and bone erosion.[58]

The most successful RA gene therapy trials to date involve blocking the inflammatory effects of IL-1 or TNF-α, but constant blockade of these factors could be deleterious. It is desirable for therapeutic transgenes to become activated in times of disease exacerbations and deactivated when symptoms subside. To create an inflammation-activated gene therapy, Van de Loo and colleagues[87] constructed an adenoviral vector with a novel promoter. The hybrid promoter combined the IL-6 promoter and IL-1 enhancer elements. Using the luciferase marker gene, this IL-1/IL-6 promoter was tested in a murine CIA model. Low basal levels of luciferase were detected. These levels increased threefold to fivefold with experimentally induced disease flares, but returned to baseline levels when the disease stimulus was removed. The IL-1/IL-6 promoter system provides an excellent example of a disease-induced construct that delivers the desired factor at low basal levels and at increased levels with disease flare-up. Ideally the authors will use this exceptionally novel promoter to drive the expression of a therapeutic gene.[87] Bakker and colleagues[4] exhibited an inflammation-induced gene therapy by constructing a hybrid vector that combined the C3 complement promoter with the IL-1Ra gene. This strategy prevented CIA in a mouse model.[10]

A strategy advocated by Gould and coworkers[37] to titrate gene therapy predicated on waxing and waning symptoms involves inducible promoters. Plasmid DNA encoding a dimeric doxycycline-inducible TNF-α receptor was delivered intramuscularly in a murine CIA model. A therapeutic effect was seen only in animals that received doxycycline in their drinking water. This effect disappeared when doxycycline was withdrawn.[37] Tetracycline-inducible promoters also were used successfully by Perez and colleagues[77] to drive an AAV expressing viral IL-10, a potent inhibitor of inflammation.

IL-18 is a proinflammatory cytokine implicated in RA. Smeets and associates[83] developed an adenoviral vector encoding an IL-18 binding protein with the intent of ameliorating the symptoms of inflammatory arthritis in a CIA mouse model. They injected this adenovirus into the knees of arthritic mice and reported less severe arthritis in these animals, as evidenced by decreased inflammation and destruction of bone and cartilage. They also noted that treatment protected against CIA incidence and severity in distal paws. This research lends greater credence to the importance of IL-18 in RA and the therapeutic efficacy of its blockade.[83]

Reactive oxygen species, particularly the free radicals nitric oxide and superoxide, also have been implicated in the pathogenesis of RA. Antioxidant enzymes, such as superoxide dismutase and catalase, block radical-induced events. Dai and colleagues[20] sought to determine if transfer of the genes for superoxide dismutase or catalase by themselves or in concert would alter the progression of rat antigen-induced arthritis. Rat synoviocytes were transfected with plasmids for these respective genes and injected into arthritic rat knees alone or together. Rats treated with cells expressing superoxide dismutase, catalase, or both showed significant suppression of arthritis compared with control groups. No statistically significant difference was found, however, between the groups treated with cells overexpressing superoxide dismutase, catalase, or a combination of both.[20]

The widely held theory among most RA researchers is that autoreactive T lymphocytes are instrumental in driving the pathophysiology of RA. A therapy that could eradicate these autoimmune T cells selectively while sparing normal T cells would be extremely effective. Tumor necrosis factor–related apoptosis-inducing ligand (TRAIL) could provide such a therapy. Dendritic cells expressing TRAIL could be pulsed with the autoantigen responsible for RA. These TRAIL-expressing, primed dendritic cells would recognize autoreactive T cells and cause apoptosis when TRAIL binds with its receptor. Proof of this principle was provided by Liu and coworkers[56] in a murine CIA model, where the autoantigen (type II collagen) is known. Murine dendritic cells were transduced with adenovirus encoding the TRAIL gene under a tetracycline-inducible promoter. These cells were pulsed with type II collagen and delivered systemically to mice. Animals treated with the transduced, primed dendritic cells had a dramatic decrease in disease severity. The culprit autoantigen in human RA is not known. The use of systemic gene therapy for a nonlethal disease should be evaluated carefully in terms of patient safety.[24,56]

TNF-α is a major mediator of disease progression in RA. Zhang and colleagues[98] showed that adenoviral delivery of genes for the type I or type II TNF-α receptor inhibits the progression of disease in murine and lapine models of inflammatory arthritis.[10] Another avenue of inhibiting inflammation is to increase levels of anti-inflammatory cytokines. IL-4, IL-13, IL-10, and viral IL-10 all can inhibit the release of inflammatory cytokines.[10]

Because cartilage and bone destruction are clinical features of RA, growth factors such as TGF-β, BMPs, IGF, FGF, and others may help to repair lesions in affected joints.[7-10] Mi and associates[66] reported that an adenovirus encoding IGF1 resulted in increased proteoglycan synthesis in a rabbit model of antigen-induced arthritis. No chondroprotective or anti-inflammatory effects were appreciated.[88]

Van Beuningen and coworkers[86] compared and contrasted TGF-β and BMP2 gene therapy in a mouse CIA model. TGF-β stimulated proteoglycan synthesis in normal and inflamed mouse knees, but BMP2 stimulated synthesis only in noninflamed knees. A possible mechanism could be that nitric oxide production counteracts the anabolic effects of BMP2 and not TGF-β.[86] TGF-β has been shown to promote fibrosis and osteophyte formation, however. BMP7 and BMP9 have been shown by Majumdar and colleagues[62] to counteract IL-1-mediated proteoglycan loss in vitro, but this finding has not been validated in vivo.[86,88]

Inhibition of matrix-degrading proteolytic enzyme activity is also a logical therapeutic strategy for RA. Theoretically the inhibition of proteolytic destruction ought to shift joint homeostasis toward tissue repair. To this end, Van der Laan and associates[89] used an adenovirus encoding the plasmin inhibitor ATF-BPTI to transduce murine synovium in a mouse model of arthritis. It resulted in a significant reduction of cartilage matrix degradation.[88]

Because RA has inflammatory and destructive aspects, a laudable goal of some gene therapy strategies is to combine anti-inflammatory and anabolic qualities. Receptor activator of NF-κβ (RANK) is highly expressed by osteoclast precursors and is required for their activation. It is activated when its ligand, RANKL, which is expressed by osteoblasts and activated T cells, binds to it and induces osteoclasts to resorb bone. Osteoprotegrin is expressed by osteoblasts and binds RANKL with high affinity, acting as a strong inhibitor of bone resorption. RANKL secretion is enhanced by inflammatory cytokines, such as IL-1 and TNF-α, the two most notorious mediators of RA. IL-4 inhibits RANK-mediated bone destruction.

Saidenberg-Kermanac'h and associates[81] used a mouse CIA model to evaluate the efficacy of IL-4 and osteoprotegrin combination gene therapy. Mouse fibroblasts were transfected with an IL-4 cDNA via a lipofectamine vector system. Mice were injected subcutaneously with IL-4-transfected fibroblasts or osteoprotegrin protein or both. The results suggested that osteoprotegrin inhibited bone loss in CIA mice. The combination of IL-4 and osteoprotegrin showed additive protection from bone loss.[81]

Kim and coworkers[49] hypothesized that because the invasive rheumatoid pannus is hypervascular, perhaps inhibition of angiogenesis would decrease the severity of joint destruction. They transduced NIH 3T3 cells with retrovirus for angiostatin, a potent antiangiogenic factor. Angiostatin-expressing cells were injected into the knee joints of mice in a CIA model. The mouse knees subsequently were evaluated via clinical score and immunostain for angiogenic and inflammatory markers. Pannus formation and cartilage erosion were reduced dramatically in knees treated with angiostatin-expressing cells. The authors also showed amelioration of CIA in ipsilateral paws distal to the injection site. Finally, as expected, angiostatin gene transfer inhibited angiogenesis in treated knees.[49] This research displayed a novel approach to RA gene therapy with antiangiogenic factors.

Gene therapy–mediated synovectomy is possible through a variety of methods. The method described by Goossens and colleagues[36] uses intra-articular thymidine kinase gene therapy via an HSV vector followed by gancyclovir administration, which induces synovial apoptosis. Fas-ligand-mediated gene therapy also can induce synovial cell death. The Fas protein is a receptor whose expression is considerably high in arthritic synoviocytes. When Fas-ligand binds with Fas, a signal transduction cascade is set in motion, which ultimately results in apoptosis, or programmed cell death. Proof of this concept has been provided by Zhang and Okamoto and their colleagues[73,97] with adenoviral vectors in a CIA model. This same cellular mechanism can be exploited by transferring the Fas-associated death domain (FADD) gene into synoviocytes. Introduction of the FADD gene by Kobayashi and associates[52] resulted in programmed cell death in synoviocytes, but not in chondrocytes (Table 17–2).[10,36,52,73,97]

CONCLUSIONS AND FUTURE DIRECTIONS

Gene therapy is a rapidly evolving field that has made significant advances in the years since the last edition of this text. The use of regulatable promoters will become much more common and critical as we better understand the nuances and timing of growth factor expression. Combinations of growth factors will be used to optimize biologic responses and mimic the complex intra-articular milieu.

Table 17–2. Summary of Gene Therapy Studies on Intra-articular Tissues

TISSUE	VECTOR	TRANSFERRED GENE(S)	FIRST AUTHOR, YEAR	REFERENCE NO.
Meniscus	Adenovirus	HGF	Hidaka, 2002	43
Ligament	Adenovirus	β-galactosidase	Menetrey, 1999	65
	Adenovirus	BMP2	Martinek, 2002	63
	Liposomal cDNA	Antisense decorin	Nakamura, 2000	69
Tendon	Plasmid cDNA	β-galactosidase	Jayankura, 2003	47
	Liposomal cDNA	β-galactosidase	Goomer, 2000	35
	Plasmid cDNA	PDGF	Wang, 2004	90
	Liposomal cDNA	PDGF	Hildebrand, 2002	44
	Adenovirus	BMP13	Helm, 2001	42
	Adenovirus	BMP12	Lou, 2001	57
Articular cartilage	Plasmid cDNA	Luciferase	Madry, 2003	60
	Adenovirus	β-galactosidase, luciferase, GFP	Pascher, 2004	75
	Retrovirus	β-galactosidase	Adachi, 2002	1
	Adenovirus	IGF1, BMP2	Gelse, 2003	33
	Adenovirus	IGF1	Mi, 2000	66
	Retrovirus	BMP7, Shh	Grande, 2003	39
	Retrovirus	BMP7	Mason, 2000	64
	Retrovirus	TGF-β1	Song, 2004	84
	Liposomal cDNA	TGF-β1	Guo, 2002	40
	Adenovirus	TGF-β1	Mi, 2003	67
	Adenovirus	TGF-β1	Bakker, 2001	5
	Retrovirus	IL-1Ra, IL-10	Zhang, 2004	99
	Adenovirus	IL-1Ra, IGF1	Nixon, 2003	70
	Recombinant protein	IL-1Ra	Caron, 1996	13
	Liposomal cDNA	IL-1Ra	Fernandes, 1999	27
	Plasmid cDNA	GFAT	Gouze, 2003	38
	Retrovirus	IL-1Ra, sTNFR-Ig	Kim, 2002	50
	Adenovirus	IL-4	Lubberts, 2000	58
	Adenovirus	Luciferase	Van de Loo, 2004	87
	Adenovirus	IL-1Ra	Bakker, 2001	4
	Plasmid cDNA	TNF-αR	Gould, 2004	37
	Adeno-associated virus	Viral IL-10	Perez, 2002	77
	Adenovirus	IL-18 binding protein	Smeets, 2003	83
	Plasmid cDNA	Superoxide dismutase, catalase	Dai, 2003	20
	Adenovirus	TRAIL	Liu, 2003	56
	Adenovirus	TNF-αR I and II	Zhang, 2000	98
	Adenovirus	IGF1	Mi, 2000	66
	Recombinant protein	TGF-β2, BMP2	Van Beuningen, 1998	86
	Recombinant protein	BMP7, BMP9	Majumdar, 2001	62
	Adenovirus	ATF-BPTI	Van der Laan, 2000	89
	Liposomal cDNA	IL-4, osteoprotegrin	Saidenberg-Kermanac'h, 2003	81
	Retrovirus	Angiostatin	Kim, 2002	49
	HSV	Thymidine kinase	Goossens, 1999	36
	Adenovirus	Fas	Zhang, 1997	97
	Adenovirus	Fas	Okamoto, 1998	73
	Adenovirus	FADD	Kobayashi, 2000	52

New vectors will be designed that combine maximum stability, minimal immunogenicity, and the potential for tight regulation. Tissue engineering efforts will optimize the combination of cells, vectors, and scaffolds to elicit the desired biological response. Factors such as age and sex must be investigated and may add increasing complexity to already formidable systems. Finally, the use of human subjects for gene therapy in the treatment of knee disorders will be initiated, ushering in a new era of biologically designed and driven treatment modalities.

References

1. Adachi N, Sato K, Usas A, et al: Muscle derived, cell based ex vivo gene therapy for treatment of full thickness articular cartilage defects. J Rheumatol 29:1920-1930, 2002.

2. Almekinders LC, Temple JD: Etiology, diagnosis, and treatment of tendonitis: An analysis of the literature. Med Sci Sports Exerc 30:1183-1190, 1998.

3. Arnoczky S: Gross and vascular anatomy of the meniscus and its role in medical healing, regeneration, remodeling. In Mow VC, Arnoczky SP, Jackson DW: Knee Meniscus: Basic Clinical Foundations. New York, Raven Press, 1992, pp 1-14.

4. Bakker AC, Van de Loo FA, Beuningen HM, et al: Overexpression of active TGF-beta-1 in the murine knee joint: Evidence for synovial-layer-dependent chondro-osteophyte formation. Osteoarthritis Cartilage 9:128-136, 2001.

5. Bakker AC, Van de Loo FA, Joosten LA, et al: C3-Tat/HIV-regulated intraarticular human interleukin-1 receptor antagonist gene therapy results in efficient inhibition of collagen-induced arthritis superior to cytomegalovirus-regulated expression of the same transgene. Arthritis Rheum 46(6):1661-1670, 2002.

6. Bentley G, Biant LC, Carrington RW, et al: A prospective, randomised comparison of autologous chondrocyte implantation versus mosaicplasty for osteochondral defects in the knee. J Bone Joint Surg Br 85:223-230, 2003.

7. Bessis N, Boissier MC, Ferrara P, et al: Attenuation of collagen-induced arthritis in mice by treatment with vector cells engineered to secrete interleukin-13. Eur J Immunol 26:2399-2403, 1996.

8. Bessis N, Chiocchia G, Kollias G, et al: Modulation of proinflammatory cytokine production in tumour necrosis factor-alpha (TNF-alpha)-transgenic mice by treatment with cells engineered to secrete IL-4, IL-10, or IL-13. Clin Exp Immunol 111:391-396, 1998.

9. Bessis N, Honiger J, Damotte D, et al: Encapsulation in hollow fibres of xenogenic cells engineered to secrete IL-4 or IL-13 ameliorates murine collagen-induced arthritis (CIA). Clin Exp Immunol 117:376-382, 1999.

10. Boissier MC, Bessis N, et al: Therapeutic gene transfer for rheumatoid arthritis. Reumatismo 56:51-61, 2004.

11. Bonadio J: Tissue engineering via local gene delivery: Update and future prospects for enhancing the technology. Advanced Drug Deliv Rev 44:186-194, 2000.

12. Buckwalter JA, Stanish WD, Rosier RN, et al: The increasing need for nonoperative treatment of patients with osteoarthritis. Clin Orthop Rel Res 385:36-45, 2001.

13. Caron JP, Fernandes JC, Martel-Pelletier J: Chondroprotective effect of intraarticular injections of interleukin-1 receptor antagonist in experimental osteoarthritis—an immunohistochemical study. Arthritis Rheum 39:1535-1544, 1996.

14. Centers for Disease Control and Prevention: Impact of arthritis and other rheumatic conditions on the health-care system—United States, 1997. JAMA 281:2177-2178, 1999.

15. Clark KR, Liu X, McGrath JP, Johnson PR: Highly purified recombinant adeno-associated virus vectors are biologically active and free of detectable helper and wild-type viruses. Hum Gene Ther 10:1031-1039, 1999.

16. Collaco RF, Cao X, Trempe JP: A helper virus-free packaging system for recombinant adeno-associated virus vectors. Gene 238:397-405, 1999.

17. Cooper DE, Arnoczky SP, Warren RF: Meniscal repair. Clin Sports Med 10:529, 1991.

18. Corsi K, Li GH, Peng H, Huard J: Muscle-based gene therapy and tissue engineering for cartilage and bone healing. Curr Genomics 5:7-17, 2004.

19. Cuevas P, Burgos J, Baird A: Basic fibroblast growth factor (FGF) promotes cartilage repair in vivo. Biochem Biophys Res Commun 156:611-618, 1988.

20. Dai L, Claxson A, Marklund SL, et al: Amelioration of antigen-induced arthritis in rats by transfer of extracellular superoxide dismutase and catalase genes. Gene Ther 10:550-558, 2003.

21. Danos O, Heard JM: Recombinant retrovirus as tools for gene transfer to somatic cells. Bone Marrow Transplant 9:131-138, 1992.

22. Duffy FJ, Jr., Seiler JG, Gelberman RH, Hergrueter CA: Growth factors and canine flexor tendon healing: Initial studies in uninjured and repair models. J Hand Surg 20:645-649, 1995.

23. Engelhardt JF, Yang Y, Stratford-Perricaudet LD: Direct gene transfer of human CFTR into human bronchial epithelia of xenografts with E-1 depleted adenoviruses. Nat Genet 4:27-34, 1993.

24. Evans CH: On the TRAIL of an arthritis cure. Gene Ther 11:735-736, 2004.

25. Evans CH, Gouze JN, Gouze E, et al: Osteoarthritis gene therapy. Gene Ther 11:379-389, 2004.

26. Felson DT, Lawrence RC, Hochberg MC, et al: Osteoarthritis: New insights. Part 2. Treatment approaches. Ann Intern Med 133:726-737, 2000.

27. Fernandes J, Tardif G, Martel-Pelletier J: In vivo transfer of interleukin-1 receptor antagonist gene in osteoarthritic rabbit knee joints: Prevention of osteoarthritis progression. Am J Pathol 154:1159-1169, 1999.

28. Fernandes JC, Martel-Pelletier J, Pelletier JP: The role of cytokines in osteoarthritis pathophysiology. Biorheology 39:237-246, 2002.

29. Flechtenmacher J, Huch K, Thonar EJ, et al: Recombinant human osteogenic protein 1 is a potent stimulator of cartilage proteoglycans and collagens by human articular chondrocytes. Arthritis Rheum 39:1896-1904, 1996.

30. Gafni Y, Turgeman G, Liebergal M, et al: Stem cells as vehicles for orthopedic gene therapy. Gene Ther 11:417-426, 2004.

31. Gao GP, Qu G, Faust LZ, et al: High-titer adeno-associated viral vectors from a Rep/Cap cell line and hybrid shuttle virus. Hum Gene Ther 9:2353-2362, 1998.

32. Gazit D, Turgeman G, Kelley P, et al: Engineered pluripotent mesenchymal cells integrate and differentiate in regenerating bone: A novel cell-mediated gene therapy. J Gene Med 1:121-133, 1999.

33. Gelse K, von der Mark K, Aigner T, et al: Articular cartilage repair by gene therapy using growth factor-producing mesenchymal cells. Arthritis Rheum 48:430-441, 2003.

34. Goldschmidt TJ, Andersson M, Malmstrom V, Holmdahl R: Activated type II collagen reactive T cells are not eliminated by in vivo anti-CD4 treatment: Implications for therapeutic approaches on autoimmune arthritis. Immunology 184:359-371, 1992.

35. Goomer RS, Maris TM, Gelberman R, et al: Nonviral in vivo gene therapy for tissue engineering of articular cartilage and tendon repair. Clin Orthop 379S:189-200, 2000.

36. Goossens PH, Schouten GJ, Hart BA, et al: Feasibility of adenovirus-mediated nonsurgical synovectomy in collagen-induced arthritis-affected rhesus monkeys. Hum Gene Ther 10:1139-1149, 1999.

37. Gould DJ, Bright C, Chernajovsky Y: Inhibition of established collagen-induced arthritis with a TNF-α inhibitor expressed from a doxycycline regulated plasmid. Arthritis Res Ther 6:R103-R113, 2004.

38. Gouze JN, Gouze E, Palmer GD, et al: Adenovirus-mediated gene transfer to glutamine:fructose-6-phosphate amidotransferase antagonizes the effects of interleukin-1 beta on rat chondrocytes. Osteoarthritis Cartilage 12(3):217-224, 2004.

39. Grande DA, Mason J, Light E, Dines D: Stem cells as platforms for delivery of genes to enhance cartilage repair. J Bone Joint Surg Am 85(Suppl 2):111-116, 2003.

40. Guo X, Du J, Zheng Q, et al: Expression of TGF-β1 in mesenchymal stem cells: Potential utility in molecular tissue engineering for osteochondral repair. J Huazhong Univ Sci Technol Med Sci 22:112-115, 2002.

41. Hangody L, Kish G, Karpati Z, et al: Arthroscopic autogenous osteochondral mosaicplasty for the treatment of femoral condylar articular defects: A preliminary report. Knee Surg Sports Traumatol Arthrosc 5:262-267, 1997.

42. Helm GA, Li JZ, Alden TD, et al: A light and electron microscopic study of ectopic tendon and ligament formation induced by BMP-13 adenoviral gene therapy. J Neurosurg 95:298-307, 2001.

43. Hidaka C, Ibarra C, Hannafin JA, et al: Formation of vascularized meniscal tissue by combining gene therapy with tissue engineering. Tissue Eng 8:93-105, 2002.

44. Hildebrand KA, Jia F, Woo SL: Response of donor and recipient cells after transplantation of cells to the ligament and tendon. Microsc Res Techn 58:34-38, 2002.

45. Hildebrand KA, Frank CB, Hart DA: Gene intervention in ligament and tendon: Current status, challenges, future directions. Gene Ther 11:368-378, 2004.

46. Insall JN, Scott WN (eds): Surgery of the Knee, 3rd ed. Philadelphia, Churchill Livingstone, 2001, pp 1215-1221.

47. Jayankura M, Boggione C, Frisen C, et al: In situ gene transfer into animal tendons by injection of naked DNA and electrotransfer. J Gene Med 5:618-624, 2003.

48. Kaczmarczyk SJ, Green JE: Induction of cre recombinase activity using modified androgen receptor ligand binding domains: A sensitive assay for ligand-receptor interactions. Nucleic Acids Res 31:e86, 2003.

49. Kim JM, Ho SH, Park EJ, et al: Angiostatin gene transfer as an effective treatment strategy in murine collagen-induced arthritis. Arthritis Rheum 46:793-801, 2002.

50. Kim SH, Lechman ER, Kim S, et al: Ex vivo gene delivery of IL-1Ra and soluble TNF receptor confers a distal synergistic therapeutic effect in antigen-induced arthritis. Mol Ther 6:591-600, 2002.

51. Klein RM, Wolf ED, Wu R, Sanford JC: High-velocity micro-projectiles for delivering nucleic acids into living cells. Biotechnology 24:384-386, 1992.

52. Kobayashi T, Okamoto K, Kobata T, et al: Novel gene therapy for rheumatoid arthritis by FADD gene transfer: Induction of apoptosis of rheumatoid synoviocytes but not chondrocytes. Gene Ther 7:527-533, 2000.

53. Koval KJM (ed): Orthopaedic Knowledge Update 7: Home Study Syllabus. Rosemont, IL, American Academy of Orthopaedic Surgeons, 2002.

54. Kramer J, Hegert C, Guan K, et al: Embryonic stem cell-derived chondrogenic differentiation in vitro: Activation by BMP-2 and BMP-4. Mech Dev 92:193-205, 2000.

55. Leichty KW, MacKenzie TC, Shaaban AF, et al: Human mesenchymal stem cells engraft and demonstrate site-specific differentiation after in utero transplantation in sheep. Nat Med 6:1282-1286, 2000.

56. Liu Z, Xu X, Hsu HC, et al: CII-DC-AdTRAIL gene therapy inhibits infiltration of CII-reactive T cells and CII-induced arthritis. J Clin Invest 112:1332-1341, 2003.

57. Lou J, Tu Y, Burns M, et al: BMP-12 gene transfer augmentation of lacerated tendon repair. J Orthop Res 19:1199-1202, 2001.

58. Lubberts E, Joosten LA, Chabaud M, et al: IL-4 gene therapy for collagen arthritis suppresses synovial IL-17 and osteoprotegerin ligand and prevents bone erosion. J Clin Invest 105:1697-1710, 2000.

59. Lundstrom K: Latest development in viral vectors for gene therapy. Trends Biotechnol 21:117-122, 2003.

60. Madry H, Cucchiarini M, Stein U, et al: Sustained transgene expression in cartilage defects in vivo after transplantation of articular chondrocytes modified by lipid-mediated gene transfer in a gel suspension delivery system. J Gene Med 5:502-509, 2003.

61. Maffuli N, Moller HD, Evans CH: Tendon healing: Can it be optimised? Br J Sport Med 36:315-316, 2002.

62. Majumdar MK, Wang E, Morris EA: BMP-2 and BMP-9 promotes chondrogenic differentiation of human multipotential mesenchymal cells and overcomes the inhibitory effect of IL-1. J Cell Physiol 189:275-284, 2001.

63. Martinek V, Latterman C, Usas A, et al: Enhancement of tendon-bone integration of anterior cruciate ligament grafts with bone morphogenetic protein-2 gene transfer: A histological and biomechanical study. J Bone Joint Surg Am 84:1123-1131, 2002.

64. Mason JM, Breitbart AS, Barcia M, et al: Cartilage and bone regeneration using gene-enhanced tissue engineering. Clin Orthop 379(Suppl):S171-S178, 2000.

65. Menetrey J, Kasemkijwattana C, Day CS, et al: Direct-, fibroblast-, and myoblast-mediated gene transfer to the anterior cruciate ligament. Tissue Eng 5:435-442, 1999.

66. Mi Z, Ghivizzani SC, Lechman ER, et al: Adenovirus-mediated gene transfer of insulin-like growth factor 1 stimulates proteoglycan synthesis in rabbit joints. Arthritis Rheum 43:2563-2570, 2000.

67. Mi Z, Ghivizzani SC, Lechman E, Glorioso JC, et al: Adverse effects of adenovirus-mediated gene transfer of human transforming growth factor beta 1 into rabbit knees. Arthritis Res Ther 5:R132-R139, 2003.

68. Moutsatos IK, Turgeman G, Zhou S, et al: Exogenously regulated stem cell mediated gene therapy for bone regeneration. Mol Ther 3:449-461, 2001.

69. Nakamura N, Hart DA, Boorman RS, et al: Decorin antisense gene therapy improves functional healing of early rabbit ligament scar with enhanced collagen fibrillogenesis in vivo. J Orthop Res 18:517-523, 2000.

70. Nixon AJ, Haupt JL, Frisbie DD, et al: Gene mediated restoration of cartilage matrix by combination insulin-like growth factor-1/interleukin-1 receptor antagonist therapy. Gene Ther 12(2):177-186, 2005.

71. O'Driscoll SW: The healing and regeneration of articular cartilage. J Bone Joint Surg Am 80:1795-1812, 1998.

72. Oligino TJ, Yao Q, Ghivizzani SC, Robbins P: Vector systems for gene transfer to joints. Clin Orthop 379:S17-S30, 2000.

73. Okamoto K, Asahara H, Kobayashi T, et al: Induction of apoptosis in the rheumatoid synovium by Fas ligand gene transfer. Gene Ther 5:331-338, 1998.

74. Osborn KD, Trippel SB, Mankin HJ: Growth factor stimulation of adult articular cartilage. J Orthop Res 7:35-42, 1989.

75. Pascher A, Palmer GD, Steinert A, et al: Gene delivery to cartilage defects using coagulated bone marrow aspirate. Gene Ther 11:133-141, 2004.

76. Pelletier JP, Martel-Pelletier J, Abramson SB: Osteoarthritis, an inflammatory disease: Potential implication for the selection of new therapeutic agents. Arthritis Rheum 44:1237-1247, 2001.

77. Perez N, Plence P, Millet V, et al: Tetracycline transcriptional silencer tightly controls transgene expression after in vivo intramuscular electrotransfer: Application to interleukin 10 therapy in experimental arthritis. Hum Gene Ther 13:2161-2172, 2002.

78. Raper SE, Yudkoff M, Chirmule N, et al: A pilot study of in vivo liver-directed gene transfer with an adenoviral vector in partial ornithine transcarbamylase deficiency. Hum Gene Ther 13:163-175, 2002.

79. Robbins PD, Ghivizzani SC: Viral vectors for gene therapy. Pharmacol Ther 80:35-47, 1998.

80. Rodkey WG: Basic biology of the meniscus and response to injury. Instr Course Lect 49:189, 2000.

81. Saidenberg-Kermanac'h N, Bessis N, Lemeiter D, et al: Interleukin-4 cellular gene therapy and osteoprotegerin decrease inflammation-associated bone resorption in collagen-induced arthritis. J Clin Immunol 4:370-378, 2004.

82. Sekiya I, Colter DC, Prockop DJ: BMP-6 enhances chondrogenesis in a subpopulation of human marrow stromal cells. Biochem Biophys Res Commun 284:411-418, 2001.

83. Smeets RL, Van de Loo FA, Arntz OJ, et al: Adenoviral delivery of IL-18 binding protein C ameliorates collagen-induced arthritis in mice. Gene Ther 10:1004-1011, 2003.

84. Song SU, Hong YJ, Oh IS, et al: Regeneration of hyaline articular cartilage with irradiated transforming growth factor beta1-producing fibroblasts. Tissue Eng 10:665-672, 2004.

85. Studer RK, Levicoff E, Georgescu H, et al: Nitric oxide inhibits chondrocyte response to IGF-1: Inhibition of IGF-1Rbeta tyrosine phosphorylation. Am J Cell Physiol 279:C961-C969, 2000.

86. Van Beuningen HM, Glansbeek HL, van der Kraan PM, van den Berg WB: Differential effects of local application of BMP-2 or TGF-β on both articular cartilage composition and osteophyte formation. Osteoarthritis Cartilage 6:306-317, 1998.

87. Van de Loo FA, de Hooge AS, Smeets RL, et al: An inflammation-inducible adenoviral expression system for local treatment of the arthritic joint. Gene Ther 11:581-590, 2004.

88. Van der Kraan PM, van de Loo FA, van den Berg WB: Role of gene therapy in tissue engineering procedures in rheumatology: The use of animal models. Biomaterials 25:1497-1504, 2004.

89. Van der Laan WH, Pap T, Ronday HK, et al: Cartilage degradation and invasion by rheumatoid synovial fibroblasts is inhibited by gene transfer of a cell surface-targeted plasmin inhibitor. Arthritis Rheum 43:1710-1718, 2000.

90. Wang XT, Liu PY, Tang JB: Tendon healing in vitro: Genetic modification of tenocytes with exogenous PDGF gene and promotion of collagen gene expression. J Hand Surg (Am) 29:884-890, 2004.

91. Wooley PH: Immunotherapy in collagen-induced arthritis: Past, present, and future. Am J Med Sci 327:217-226, 2004.

92. Wu D, Razzano P, Grande DA: Gene therapy and tissue engineering in repair of the musculoskeletal system. J Cell Biochem 88:467-481, 2003.

93. Xiao X, Li J, Samulski RJ: Production of high-titer recombinant adeno-associated virus vectors in the absence of helper adenovirus. J Virol 72:2224-2232, 1998.

94. Yang Y, Wilson JM: Clearance of adenovirus-infected hepatocytes by MHC class I-restricted CD4+ CTLs in vivo. J Immunol 155:2564-2570, 1995.

95. Yang NS, Burkholder J, Roberts B, et al: In vivo and in vitro gene transfer to mammalian cells by particle bombardment. Proc Natl Acad Sci U S A 87:9568-9572, 1990.

96. Yang Y, Nunes FA, Berencsi K, et al: Cellular immunity to viral antigens limits E1-depleted adenoviruses for gene therapy. Proc Natl Acad Sci U S A 91:4407-4411, 1994.

97. Zhang H, Yang Y, Horton JL, et al: Amelioration of collagen-induced arthritis by CD95 (Apo-1/Fas)-ligand gene transfer. J Clin Invest 100:1951-1957, 1997.

98. Zhang HG, Xie J, Yang P, et al: Adeno-associated virus production of soluble tumor necrosis factor receptor neutralizes tumor necrosis factor alpha and reduces arthritis. Hum Gene Ther 11:2431-2442, 2000.

99. Zhang X, Mao Z, Yu C: Suppression of early experimental osteoarthritis by gene transfer of interleukin-1 receptor antagonist and interleukin-10. J Orthop Res 22:742-750, 2004.

CHAPTER 18

Nonoperative Treatment of Knee Arthritis

Marc W. Hungerford • Harpal S. Khanuja • David S. Hungerford

Osteoarthritis is one of the most common musculoskeletal ailments,[291] and it is estimated that approximately 15% of Americans (40 million persons) suffer from some form of arthritis.[159] Joints most commonly affected include the cervical and lumbar spine, fingers, knees, and hips,[291] with approximately 6 million Americans suffering from osteoarthritis of the knee.[159] Because it is predominantly an affliction of the elderly, the increasing percentage of the older population of industrialized western countries, including the United States, has provided additional impetus for the prevention and treatment of osteoarthritis. Several new nonsurgical modalities have recently become available, with many other regimens expected in the near future. A more sophisticated understanding of the etiology of osteoarthritis, as well as the biochemical and biomechanical process of the disease, has aided in the development of specifically targeted therapeutic agents. An understanding of the disease process also allows objective monitoring of the effectiveness of these therapies. The aim of this chapter is to provide a general scheme for the nonsurgical treatment of osteoarthritis and review the rationale and indications for currently available nonoperative treatment modalities.

Although the diagnosis may be established with a high degree of sensitivity and specificity in patients with concordant signs and symptoms, the diagnosis is not always straightforward. The typical radiographic changes of subchondral sclerosis, osteophytosis, joint space narrowing, cystic changes, and joint deformity are commonly seen in asymptomatic individuals. Therefore, the presence of arthrosis does not necessarily imply the diagnosis of arthritis. Furthermore, the difficulty in establishing a correct diagnosis and developing a rational treatment plan for patients with joint pain is compounded by the fact that rheumatic disorders are not mutually exclusive. Thus, before embarking on a course of therapy, the question of whether the patient has osteoarthritis and whether the osteoarthritis fully accounts for the symptoms should be carefully considered.

The differential diagnosis for joint pain is huge and covers the spectrum of rheumatological, orthopedic, neurological, and vascular diseases. The differential includes soft-tissue disorders ranging from muscle and ligament strain to pes anserine bursitis or meniscal problems. Inflammatory arthropathies can mimic osteoarthritis and include crystal arthropathy (which has a predilection for the knees and other large joints), rheumatoid arthritis, and systemic lupus erythematosus. Spontaneous osteonecrosis of the knee (SPONK) is not uncommon in patients older than 55 years. Secondary or idiopathic osteonecrosis may occur in younger patients, especially those with relevant risk factors (such as corticosteroid or alcohol abuse). Other causes of knee pain include neurological conditions (radiculopathy, peripheral neuropathy, spinal stenosis), vascular problems (claudication, insufficiency), malignancy, and infection.

Knowledge of the natural history of osteoarthritis should be used to guide the aggressiveness of treatment. Whereas end-stage disease can be extremely painful and debilitating, osteoarthritis in general is not relentlessly progressive. In a survey of 682 elderly people, the prevalence and severity of signs and symptoms of osteoarthritis about the knee remained constant through the seventh, eighth, and ninth decades.[84] In another study documenting radiographic progression in patients older than 54, the percentage of patients with the most severe changes did not increase with age.[158] In some cases radiographic improvement consisting of an increase in joint space has been noted.[258] Therefore, osteoarthritis is a chronic disease with a waxing and waning course. With proper management, many patients should maintain reasonable comfort and function for an indefinite period.

Cartilage is both avascular and aneural. Therefore, the pain of osteoarthritis must come from a different source. Candidates for pain generation in osteoarthritic joints are as plentiful and varied as the physiological changes noted. Muscle strain caused by overuse, microfractures in the subchondral trabeculae, irritation of periosteal nerve endings, ligamentous stress as a result of bone deformity or effusion, and venous congestion caused by remodeling of subchondral bone have all been proposed. In fact, various mechanisms may play a role in different patients. This probability helps explain the variability in patient response to a given treatment regimen. It also highlights the need to more thoroughly define the source of pain so that the most effective treatment modality may be selected.

Synovitis is a prime candidate for the source of pain in osteoarthritis because synovium is richly innervated,[144] but patients with early-stage osteoarthritis may not show much evidence of synovial inflammation.[206] However, in those with more advanced disease, synovial inflammation is common and may be a significant source of pain. Inflammation in osteoarthritis may be induced by proteoglycans[24] or cartilage fragments[74] released by damaged cartilage. Synovial inflammation leads to release of inflammatory mediators, thus sensitizing nociceptive cells and damaging cartilage directly. If synovial inflammation is the predominant source of pain, corticosteroids and anti-inflammatory medications are a rational therapy. However, the inflammation in osteoarthritis is much less intense than that in rheumatoid arthritis, erythema and warmth are uncommon, and morning stiffness is usually brief. In an arthroscopic study of patients with mild or moderate radiographic disease of the knee, nearly 50% of those examined had no appreciable synovitis. No relationship between severity, size, or location of the lesion and synovitis was noted.[206] Although synovitis may cause pain in a large number of patients with osteoarthritis, it would be myopic to view inflammation as the sole target of therapeutic intervention.

PHYSICAL THERAPY

The proven benefit of physical therapy coupled with the absence of side effects argues for a prominent role of these modalities in the treatment of osteoarthritis. The advantageous risk-benefit ratio is further amplified in the elderly, a population that is at greater risk for side effects from pharmacological intervention. The general rehabilitation goals in treating patients with osteoarthritis of the knee are to increase and maintain current function, as well as prevent further joint deterioration. There are multiple modalities that physical therapy uses to achieve these goals, including braces, orthoses, exercise, educational plans, and physical (temperature, electrical stimulation, ultrasound) modalities. In general, a physical therapy program involves the use of heat, cold, or other modalities, followed by an exercise program. This section provides a brief description of these modalities and reviews the literature regarding their efficacy and indications.

Exercise

Exercise programs have been devised with diverse goals, including increasing strength, endurance, and/or range of motion (ROM) in patients with knee arthritis. Most (but not all) of the published and ongoing research is directed at the quadriceps mechanism.* Different types of exercise include passive exercise, in which the joint and thus the muscles are moved by the therapist or by an apparatus (such as a continuous passive motion machine), without active input by the patient. Active or active assisted exercises are performed by active contraction of muscles with assistance by the therapist. Resistive exercises are accomplished by active contraction of muscle by the patient against resistance (mechanical or manual). Isometric, isotonic, and isokinetic contractions may all be used. Stretching exercises to increase joint motion and flexibility are frequently added to the regimen.

RANGE-OF-MOTION AND STRETCHING EXERCISES

ROM and stretching exercises should be a part of every osteoarthritis patient's daily routine. Beneficial effects reported include maintenance of function, decreased

*References 45, 61, 72, 73, 77, 80-82, 126, 135, 153, 179, 180, 193, 194, 201, 212, 233, 237, 249, 252, 267, 276, 282.

edema, stimulation of flexion-extension reflexes, and preparation of the limb for active exercise. Stretching exercises can restore or maintain ROM. Care should be taken with inflamed joints because passive ROM exercise has been shown to increase joint inflammation.

STRENGTHENING EXERCISES

In knee arthritis, loss of strength and function occurs rapidly. A muscle can atrophy up to 30% in 1 week. A muscle at complete rest will lose strength at a rate of 3% per day.[80,82,201] Despite a wealth of published literature, consensus regarding the optimum dosage, modality, and frequency of exercise for strengthening the quadriceps is lacking. In one case study,[179] isometric strengthening of the quadriceps muscles led to improvement in quadriceps torque, clinical status, and pain after walking. This program consisted of exercises performed three times a week for 6 weeks with the knee flexed to 60 degrees. Other studies have demonstrated improvement in function of quadriceps-trained individuals, but most of these studies have failed to compare the results with those in patients who rested. Three randomized, controlled trials[72,77,135] in patients with knee osteoarthritis who underwent quadriceps strengthening with either isometric, isotonic, or resistive exercises showed significant improvement in quadriceps strength, knee pain, and function when compared with controls.

Nevertheless, strengthening exercises must be used with caution. Exercises that involve repetitive joint motion or require full ROM may increase inflammation and pain and thus fail to achieve muscle strengthening. Isometric contraction is less likely to increase joint pain or inflammation. Dynamic (repetitive) exercises using isotonic or isokinetic muscle contraction are appropriate after the pain is controlled. Isokinetic exercises can be performed by patients with ligamentous stability and no internal derangement. Deep knee bends, however, may increase intra-articular pressure and should be avoided.[41]

AEROBIC CONDITIONING

In addition to weakness, patients with osteoarthritis of the knee suffer from decreased cardiovascular endurance.[126] Aerobic exercise can increase the overall vitality, activity, and feeling of well-being in these patients. Suitable endurance exercises include cycling, swimming, and low-impact aerobics. High-impact loading activities, such as jogging, should probably be avoided.

Increased aerobic fitness not only improves overall health but specifically improves arthritic symptoms as well. Kovar and coworkers,[153] in an 8-week supervised fitness walking program involving 102 patients with knee osteoarthritis, reported improvement in 6-minute walking distance and reduction in pain and the use of medications in the exercise group versus controls. In another study, 12 weeks of aerobic walking or aquatic exercise improved overall exercise capacity, and the aerobic gains were maintained at 9 months. In the Fitness, Arthritis, and Seniors

Trial,[73] 439 subjects with radiographically confirmed osteoarthritis of the knee, pain, and disability were randomized to a program of aerobic exercise, resistance exercise, or health education. In this 18-month trial, those in the exercise groups showed improvement in tests of physical performance (climbing and descending stairs, lifting and carrying 10 lb) in comparison to the education group. Pain and disability self-reported scores improved in the exercise groups.

Weight Loss

Weight reduction should also be encouraged on principle. A 1-lb weight loss effects a 3- to 4-lb decrease in load across the joint. A patient who is 33 lb overweight adds more than 100 lb of load on each knee per step. If a patient takes 2000 steps a day, an extra 100 tons is being placed across an already damaged knee per day. A recent study showed that weight loss in middle-aged and older women significantly reduced the incidence of symptomatic osteoarthritis in the knee.[79] Though rational, few controlled data demonstrate a reduction in joint pain or slowed progression of arthrosis with weight loss.[78,79]

Therapy regimens are generally prescribed in a programmatic fashion rather than in isolation. The Arthritis, Diet, and Activity Promotion Trial (ADAPT) recently tried to estimate the relative contribution of each modality. Three hundred sixteen overweight patients with knee osteoarthritis were randomized into four groups: healthy lifestyle (education), diet only, exercise only, and diet plus exercise. At the end of the 18-month trial, the diet-plus-exercise group showed improvement in self-reported function, 6-minute walk distance, stair climb time, and knee pain. The exercise-only group showed improvement in walk distance. The diet-only group was no better than the education group.[191] Whether the benefits persist over the long term remains questionable.[288]

Biomechanical

TAPING

Appliances that alter the biomechanics of the knee joint may be helpful. Cushnaghan and associates[49] found that taping the patella medially was effective in reducing knee pain in patients with patellofemoral arthritis. In this randomized, single-blind, crossover trial with 14 subjects, medial taping was superior to lateral or neutral taping in pain scores, symptomatology, and patient preference. Other authors have used taping before quadriceps exercises for chondromalacia patellae.[189]

KNEE BRACING AND ORTHOTICS

The usefulness of bracing for the treatment of knee osteoarthritis has been controversial.[85,146,249,267] Most clinical and biomechanical studies have shown little or no benefit from these devices. The primary goal of knee brace designs is to assist in restoration of normal mechanical stability. The first step in fitting for a brace is to define the abnormal motion that the brace should control.

A Swedish knee cage or a hinged knee brace may provide support in limiting extension and may help decrease pain.[249] A number of three-point pressure braces are available for control of medial or lateral instability (Donjoy).[267] In selected patients, these devices can be quite effective. In a recent study, Kirkley and coworkers[146] found that valgus-producing functional knee braces were much more effective for the treatment of medial compartment osteoarthritis of the knee than a simple neoprene sleeve was. Furthermore, the quality-of-life (Western Ontario and McMaster University Osteoarthritis Index [WOMAC]) scores of both braced groups exceeded those of a control group receiving standard medical treatment in a prospective, parallel-group, randomized clinical trial.

Immobilization of the knee with a knee immobilizer or posterior splint during periods of increased pain or inflammation may be useful. These modalities support the knee in extension and permit relaxation of the flexor muscles. An elastic bandage may control knee swelling but, strictly speaking, is not a knee orthosis.

ASSISTIVE DEVICES

A cane can successfully unload the knee joint.[21] Assistive devices to unload the knee joint are most effectively used on the side opposite the pathological condition. The use of a crutch or cane will reduce the joint load on the opposite limb by about 50%. A quad cane can be used instead of a straight cane when balance is a problem.

Hydrotherapy

The buoyancy of water is useful for minimizing stress on the knee joint by effectively neutralizing the force of gravity. It is especially helpful when ROM and strengthening exercises are prescribed for an obese patient. The external application of water for therapeutic purposes can provide either heat or cold. Many physiological effects have been reported in patients treated with warm water hydrotherapy, including a rise in body temperature, increased sweating, superficial vasodilatation, increase in peripheral circulation, decrease in blood pressure after immersion, sedative effect on nerve endings, and muscle relaxation. The water temperature should be between 34°C and 37°C. Contraindications to hydrotherapy include skin infections or lesions, open wounds, and cardiovascular disorders.

The efficacy of hydrotherapy has been questioned. One study of hydrotherapy plus home exercise versus home exercise alone found no difference in osteoarthritis of the hip.[113] More research needs to be conducted in patients with knee osteoarthritis to ascertain the efficacy of this modality.

Electrical and Related Energy

HEAT MODALITIES

Therapeutic heat can be applied superficially or to a deep location. Heat is usually applied at temperatures of 41°C to 45°C. Superficial heat is capable of elevating soft-tissue temperature 3°C at a depth of 1 cm without penetrating deeper depths and is thus penetrating the knee joint.[132] Some studies have demonstrated that the threshold for pain can be raised in humans as well as animals by the application of superficial or deep heat.[163] The effect is produced by analgesia of free nerve endings (peripheral nerves and gamma fibers of muscle spindles), and thus muscle relaxation is effected.[163,164] Local heat may also relieve pain by acting on sensory afferents and closing the "pain gate" or by increasing local blood flow and thus washing out the pain-inducing metabolites and inflammatory mediators produced in osteoarthritis.[163,164]

The six general methods that produce superficial heat include diathermy (short waves),[56,237] microwaves,[56] ultrasound,[68] radiation (infrared), conduction (heating pad, water bottle),[214] and convection (sauna, steam room). Moist heat produces a greater temperature elevation than dry heat does and thus may be preferable for clinical applications.[132,214] As in all of these modalities, care must be exercised to avoid burns (especially with uneven application). A towel-wrapped hot water bottle, gel-filled hot pack, or thermostatically controlled electric heating pad provide simple methods for the patient to benefit from superficial heat application at home.

Deep heat can be used as a modality that affects the viscoelastic properties of collagen.[290] Diathermy can use shortwave (11.062-m wavelength at 27.12-MHz frequency) radiation delivered via two electrodes or an induction cable for about 20 minutes.[237] This treatment leads to an increase in skin temperature, blood flow, and pain threshold. These effects are maintained for 15 to 30 minutes after the cessation of treatment.

Diathermy has provided clinical benefit when used in combination with exercise but should not be used indiscriminantly.[237] Shortwave diathermy can exacerbate knee arthritis as a result of heat-induced proliferation of collagenous tissue leading to the development of adhesions and thus decreased ROM. Microwave (12.2-cm wavelength at 2456-, 915-, and 433.9-MHz frequencies) electromagnetic radiation is used less frequently, probably because of safety concerns.[56]

ULTRASOUND

Ultrasound is a well-established deep-heating modality that can induce greater depth of penetration than attainable with shortwave or microwave diathermy.[68,276] Several early studies demonstrated the efficacy of this modality in relieving osteoarthritic pain.[68,163] Its effect is attributed to both thermal and mechanical mechanisms. Ultrasound is absorbed and creates heat in structures with a high protein content. The physiological effects of local tissue heating, as previously described, include an increase in the pain threshold, reduction of muscle spasm, and promotion of the healing process. The nonthermal or mechanical effects include "microstreaming," or small fluid movements around cells that alter cell membrane permeability, promote collagen synthesis, and alter electrical activity in painful nerve afferents.[68]

Ultrasound therapy requires the use of a coupling agent (water or mineral oil) to prevent attenuation of the sound waves in air. Energy exposure of 0.5 to 4.0 W/cm^2 for 5 to 10 minutes is commonly used. The therapist must keep the ultrasound applicator in constant motion to decrease excessive focal heating. The effects of ultrasound have also been found to be additive with nonsteroidal anti-inflammatory treatment.

There is still little documented well-controlled evidence of the effectiveness of ultrasound, as well as its optimal dosage. In fact, two recent meta-analyses concluded that there was little evidence to support the use of ultrasound to treat pain in a variety of musculoskeletal conditions.[92,289] Significant response rates to ultrasound treatment are seen in only approximately 40% of cases.[154]

Ultrasound may be a useful adjunct to other modes of treatment, but it should not be a mainstay of therapy.

SUMMARY OF HEAT TREATMENT MODALITIES

All these heat treatment modalities should be used as adjuncts or precursors to other treatment regimens, such as before exercise, mobilization, or stretching. They should be used cautiously because the application of heat may increase inflammation or joint damage. Use of heat therapy in patients with inadequate thermal sensation is contraindicated.

Acupuncture

Interest in traditional Chinese medicine in general and acupuncture specifically has been increasing steadily since the 1970s. Approximately 1 million patients receive acupuncture treatments in the United States annually, many of them for musculoskeletal ailments. The technique has been applied to a wide variety of conditions, including postoperative pain, arthritis, obesity, and nicotine addiction.

Although interest remains strong, scientific evidence of efficacy is frequently lacking. Studies involving acupuncture frequently suffer significant methodological deficiencies, such as lack of placebo control and lack of blinding. Most of the studies also report small sample sizes.

Birch and coauthors[20] published an overview of systematic reviews and meta-analyses published on acupuncture and separated them by the condition treated. Of the more than 45 such reviews published, those looking at postoperative pain, postoperative nausea, and nausea associated with chemotherapy offered the best evidence of efficacy. Studies of osteoarthritis and many other conditions showed less conclusive support.

Ezzo et al[75] performed a systematic review of studies specific to osteoarthritis of the knee. Of the seven studies identified, there was limited evidence that acupuncture was more effective in improving pain and function than treatment as usual. The authors did find that several of these studies showed significant improvement in pain scores, an effect that lasted more than 1 month after the cessation of treatment. This improvement was not seen in two of three studies in which sham acupuncture was used.

The safety of acupuncture, when practiced by qualified individuals, has been widely documented.

Interferential Therapy

Interferential therapy involves the use of two medium-frequency (approximately 4 KHz) alternating currents applied to the skin through suction cups or adhesive padding. The resultant current has a low frequency, which is the difference between the two original frequencies. This current is usually applied for about 15 minutes for the knee and is experienced as a prickling sensation.

Various pain-relieving mechanisms (blocking of nonmyelinated nociceptive fibers, activation of delta A and C fibers releasing encephalins and endorphins, and activation of the opioid system) have been proposed for the pain relief that this technique provides.[237]

Transcutaneous Electrical Neuromuscular Stimulation

Transcutaneous electrical nerve stimulation (TENS) delivers short–pulse width (50 to 250 microseconds), low-frequency (2 to 150 Hz) waves that are used specifically for pain relief.[116,136] As with interferometry, a prickly sensation is produced. Carbon-rubber electrodes with a coupling gel on the skin or with a self-adhesive substance are used to deliver pulses for 30 to 60 minutes once or twice daily. The finding that large-diameter cutaneous nerve fibers are preferentially stimulated by TENS is thought to account for its efficacy. These fibers inhibit the transmission of painful stimuli to the spinal cord. Double-blind studies using TENS for the control of pain in patients with osteoarthritis of the knee have yielded conflicting results. One study concluded that it provided no greater benefit than placebo did, whereas the other study demonstrated improvement over placebo.[116] More research is needed both to demonstrate the effectiveness of this modality and define optimum parameters for its use.

Cryotherapy

Cold can be used to decrease pain. Joints are cooled by the application of ice packs or commercial gel hydropacks.[214] The pack should be applied for 15 to 20 minutes and should be separated from the skin by a towel to prevent freezing. Decreasing skin and muscle temperature may reduce muscle spasm by reducing muscle spindle activity

and raising the pain threshold.[149,162] Cryotherapy may also provide functional improvement. One study showed that cryotherapy led to improvement in passive ROM and joint stiffness in osteoarthritis.[162]

Cold therapy is contraindicated in patient's with Raynaud's disease and should be used cautiously in those with cardiovascular disease.

Other Methods

MAGNETISM, ELECTRICAL STIMULATION, AND LOW-INTENSITY PULSED ULTRASOUND

Magnetism, electrical stimulation, and low-intensity pulsed ultrasound involve the use of low-energy fields to achieve their effects. The Bionicare device has recently been approved by the Food and Drug Administration (FDA) for the treatment of osteoarthritis of the knee and rheumatoid arthritis of the hand. Zizic et al recently published a short-term clinical study comparing patients with osteoarthritis of the knee treated with this device versus placebo. The treatment group had statistically significant improvement in pain and function scores over the 4-week treatment period.[309] In another recent study, the application of pulsed electromagnetic fields was able to delay the need for total knee arthroplasty when compared with historical controls (Mont, Jones, and Hungerford, unpublished data). There is even some indication that these modalities have a disease-modifying effect. Low-intensity pulsed ultrasound was recently shown to yield more hyaline-like cartilage in a rabbit model than in nontreated controls in a study by Cook and coworkers.[47] Lippiello and colleagues, using the Bionicare device, also reported improved hyaline cartilage repair in a lacerative and bore defect model in rabbits when the animals were treated with electromagnetic stimulation.[169]

EDUCATION

The goals of education are to reduce anxiety, make patients aware of treatment methods, and effect a change in behavior when appropriate. Patients should understand the natural history of the disease and its impact on work and leisure time activities. When patients understand their disease, they can aid in the self-management of their symptoms. It has been shown that regular physician-patient phone contact leads to improvement in pain and functional status and is cost-effective.[299]

A meta-analysis of studies contrasting patient education with ibuprofen therapy concluded that education produced a significant reduction in pain, but not disability. There was some evidence for a synergistic effect of both interventions.[273]

Activities that lead to excessive loading of the knee should be avoided when possible.[167] Loading activities are better performed in short periods; rest periods for 30 minutes between periods of activity may help reduce pain and allow greater overall productivity. Several shorter periods of standing are preferable to a single prolonged period.

ANALGESICS

Acetaminophen is the sole representative of the class of simple, non-narcotic analgesics available in the United States. Nefopam and dipyridone are available elsewhere. Variously classified as a peripheral or central analgesic, its mode of action is poorly understood. Acetaminophen readily penetrates the central nervous system. Its analgesic action may be mediated through the diffuse noxious inhibitory control pathway.[278] Acetaminophen has no significant effect on cyclooxygenase (COX) and thus does not demonstrate the toxicity plaguing nonsteroidal anti-inflammatory drugs (NSAIDs). Acetaminophen can cause interstitial nephritis when consumed in large quantities over a long period. The maximum dose should not exceed 4 g/day. The dosage should be lowered in patients with renal or hepatic impairment.[229,251] Acetaminophen is inexpensive, readily available, well tolerated, and effective and deserves serious consideration as a primary therapeutic agent in osteoarthritis.

NON-STEROIDAL ANTI-INFLAMMATORY AGENTS

NSAIDs are commonly prescribed for arthritis. There are a number of NSAIDs available in the United States today, and more continue to be developed. It is a multibillion dollar industry, yet the rationale for using them as first-line treatment of osteoarthritis remains uncertain.

Mechanism of Action

NSAIDs have a variety of effects on the inflammatory process. They block conversion of arachidonic acid to prostaglandins by binding to the COX enzyme. This is probably the main mechanism for their anti-inflammatory and analgesic effects.[197] The COX-1 isoform is expressed in many normal tissues. Prostaglandins produced by COX-1 play a role in tissue hemostasis, such as mucosal defense and repair in the gastrointestinal system and renal perfusion.[181,253] COX-1 is also found in platelets and plays a role in platelet aggregation.[133,181] COX-2, though found in normal tissue, is also an inducible enzyme and appears in areas of inflammation and injury.[133,140]

Traditional NSAIDs are nonspecific in that they bind to both COX-1 and COX-2 isoforms. COX-2 inhibitors have been developed to avoid the side effects associated with nonspecific COX inhibitors, including gastrointestinal and renal effects.

Mass marketing, together with perceived efficacy of these drugs, and their wide variety of indications have made NSAIDs one of the most popular classes of drugs. They have become the de facto standard of care for the treatment of osteoarthritis. In fact, a survey of practice habits of general practitioners revealed that only 10%

would prescribe a pure nonopioid analgesic for a patient with uncomplicated osteoarthritis. The rest chose either sub-anti-inflammatory or full anti-inflammatory doses of NSAIDs.[183]

NSAIDs versus Analgesics

Although multiple studies have shown that NSAIDs are more effective than placebo, evidence that they are more effective than simple analgesics (such as acetaminophen) in osteoarthritis is not consistent. Several studies have demonstrated a 10% to 20% improvement in scores of pain and stiffness when NSAIDs were compared with placebo.[18,19,283] In a large comparative trial of five different NSAIDs, slightly less than half the patients exhibited a favorable response to treatment. No difference in response rates between drugs was noted.[171]

A 4-week randomized, prospective, and blinded study comparing an anti-inflammatory dose of ibuprofen, an analgesic dose of ibuprofen, and acetaminophen failed to show any significant difference between the three treatment groups.[26] Another study comparing ketoprofen with dextropropoxyphene/acetaminophen (a non-narcotic analgesic) failed to show any difference between the regimens.[65] Consistent with these findings are several studies in which ibuprofen given in an analgesic dose (1200 mg) was equivalent to several other NSAIDs given at anti-inflammatory doses for the treatment of osteoarthritic joint pain.[30,44,54,200,248] Given the evidence, one might consider that the efficacy of NSAIDs lies in their analgesic effect rather than the anti-inflammatory one. A study showing equivalent efficacy of both the R and S enantiomers of flurbiprofen, even though only S-flurbiprofen inhibits prostaglandin synthesis, further supports this hypothesis.[31] Schumacher and coworkers did show that high-dose ibuprofen was superior to acetaminophen in patients with knee arthritis and synovial effusion. Therefore, there may be a subset of patients with osteoarthritis and an inflammatory component who benefit additionally from NSAIDs.[257]

More recent studies do show some potential benefit of NSAIDs over acetaminophen. In a 6-week trial acetaminophen was compared with diclofenac and misoprostol. The latter demonstrated a statistically higher response to treatment in patients with osteoarthritis of the hip and knee.[231] In a multicenter, randomized, double-blind trial, Geba et al compared two different dosages of rofecoxib with celecoxib and the maximal daily dosage of acetaminophen. They concluded that higher-dose rofecoxib (25 mg) was significantly more efficacious than acetaminophen (400 mg), celecoxib (200 mg), and rofecoxib (12.5 mg), as measured by the WOMAC index and patient global assessment of response to therapy.[97]

Efficacy Differences between NSAIDs

NONSPECIFIC COX INHIBITORS

Are there any differences in efficacy between the various nonspecific NSAIDs? Several trials revealed that low-dose ibuprofen was less effective than other NSAIDs, but others show no difference between high-dose ibuprofen and other NSAIDs.[30,34,44,54,119,200] Indomethacin and aspirin are generally believed to be the most toxic.[281] Hedner[119] reviewed nearly 100 comparative trials of NSAIDs in patients with osteoarthritis. Generally, these studies indicated that aspirin was equivalent in efficacy or slightly less effective than other NSAIDs, but patients suffered more side effects. No other consistent differences between nonselective NSAIDs have been found.[18,171,298]

COX-2 Inhibitors versus Nonselective COX Inhibitors

COX-2 inhibitors have been compared with each other and with conventional NSAIDs. There were three oral forms available in the United States: celecoxib, rofecoxib, and valdecoxib. A parenteral form is undergoing clinical trials.

In a multicenter randomized trial involving 1042 patients, 1000 mg of nabumetone was compared with 12.5 mg of rofecoxib. The percentage of patients with a good or excellent response was significantly higher at 6 weeks in those being treated with rofecoxib. In addition, rofecoxib had a significantly quicker onset.[148]

A recent meta-analysis of randomized controlled trials studied the efficacy of valdecoxib versus nonselective NSAIDs.[69] Nine trials with a total of 5726 patients were reviewed. Valdecoxib was significantly better than placebo and as effective as conventional NSAIDs, including naproxen and diclofenac. Valdecoxib also caused fewer adverse events and withdrawals, as well as fewer gastrointestinal ulcers detected by endoscopy.

In a similarly designed meta-analysis of nine randomized controlled trials, Deeks et al reviewed the efficacy of celecoxib in 15,187 patients with rheumatoid arthritis or osteoarthritis. All patients received 12 weeks of therapy, and all trials included comparison to diclofenac, naproxen, or ibuprofen. Five trials included a placebo. For both rheumatoid arthritis and osteoarthritis there was a significant improvement when compared with placebo and no significant differences with the conventional NSAIDs. The number of withdrawals for gastrointestinal events was significantly decreased with celecoxib versus the nonspecific NSAIDs.[55]

Toxicity of NSAIDs

Inhibition of prostaglandin synthesis has detrimental effects. Prostacyclin (PGI_2) and prostaglandin E_2 (PGE_2) are both vasodilators important in maintaining renal perfusion during hypovolemia. Prostaglandin inhibition also leads to sodium retention in the kidney, which may worsen congestive heart failure. Numerous conditions cause dependence on renal prostaglandins to maintain renal profusion, including congestive heart failure, cirrhosis, certain forms of hypertension, and dehydration. In these patients, exposure to NSAIDs will lead to a decline in renal function, even if creatinine clearance was normal before treatment.[46,205,301,302] This decline is usually reversible. NSAIDs may increase the overall risk for chronic renal failure.[178,229] Acute interstitial nephritis has also been noted with most of the NSAIDs, but it is seen most commonly with fenoprofen.[37,178] Sulindac[300,301] and nabumetone[8] are purported to be less likely to cause deterioration in renal function.[38]

The most common toxic side effect of NSAIDs occurs in the gastrointestinal tract. It has been estimated that 15% to 35% of all peptic ulcer complications are attributable to these drugs.[114,115,117,122,123,156] Morbidity includes 41,000 hospitalizations and 3300 deaths annually in the United States alone.[239] Upper gastrointestinal symptoms caused by NSAIDs include dyspepsia, ulceration, hemorrhage, perforation, and death.[91,95,114,115,266] The relative risk of gastrointestinal bleeding is estimated to be increased threefold to fivefold with the use of NSAIDs.[91,122] Risk factors for the development of a bleeding complication with the use of these medications include a history of previous peptic ulcer disease, concomitant use of corticosteroids or anticoagulants, and poor general health.[89,94,117,262,264,265] Because toxicity from NSAIDs is additive, the use of more than one NSAID at a time is contraindicated.[40,192] Moreover, the use of NSAIDs in patients who are also taking systemic corticosteroids should be avoided if at all possible because the incidence of bleeding complications and mortality is significantly elevated.

COX-2 inhibitors do show promise in reducing gastrointestinal adverse events and complications[55,69,252] Two large prospective randomized long-term outcome studies have been performed for celecoxib and rofecoxib. The trials are known by the acronyms CLASS (Celecoxib Long-term Arthritis Safety Study) and VIGOR (Vioxx Gastrointestinal Outcome Research), respectively.[23,263] The CLASS trial compared celecoxib with diclofenac or ibuprofen in 7698 patients. Dosages were 400 mg twice a day for celecoxib, 75 mg twice a day for diclofenac, and 800 mg three times a day for ibuprofen. There was not a significant reduction in the incidence of ulcers between the three regimens at 6 months. There were, however, significantly lower rates of symptomatic and complicated ulcers in the celecoxib group. The design of the study has been called into question.[253] It appears that the concomitant use of aspirin by some patients lessened the gastrointestinal protective effects of celecoxib. When aspirin users were excluded, the incidence of complicated ulcers was significantly lower for Celebrex than for the other NSAIDs.

The VIGOR study compared rofecoxib at a daily dose of 50 mg with naproxen at 1000 mg daily. The median treatment time was 9 months. There was a significant decrease in symptomatic and complicated ulcers with rofecoxib. The efficacy and rate of discontinuation were comparable for both regimens. Both the CLASS and VIGOR studies used doses of COX-2 inhibitors that are twice the dose routinely recommended.

A review was performed of randomized controlled trials and open-label trials that involved valdecoxib and nonselective NSAIDs. As with the other two COX-2 inhibitors, valdecoxib was associated with a significantly lower rate of gastrointestinal ulcer complications.[109]

DETRIMENTAL EFFECTS OF COX-2 INHIBITION

There is much concern about the potential cardiac risk associated with COX-2 inhibitors. This concern has significant merit based on findings in the studies described earlier.

The selectivity of COX-2 inhibitors, though beneficial to the gastrointestinal mucosa, may lead to problems with thrombosis, as well as salt and fluid imbalance.[306] This was borne out in the CLASS and VIGOR studies. Both demonstrated an increase in serious adverse events unrelated to gastrointestinal events. With respect to the VIGOR trial, the incidence of thrombotic cardiovascular events was significantly higher for rofecoxib than for naproxen.[306] The same has not been confirmed for the CLASS trial, although Wright points out that FDA data suggest an increased risk for cardiac events when compared with other NSAIDs.[306]

The hypertensive effects of COX-2 enzymes seem equal to those of conventional NSAIDs. It appears that the COX-2 enzyme is responsible for prostaglandin production, which is important for fluid balance. Blocking its production affects fluid retention and can result in hypertension.[140]

The COX-2 enzyme is also responsible for the production of PGI_2, which is a vasodilator.[83] A number of products of the COX-1 enzyme have vasoconstrictive effects. Therefore, selective inhibition of COX-2 will tip the balance in favor of vasoconstriction. This effect will play a role in both hypertension and heart disease.

The exact mechanism for increased cardiac risk has not been elucidated. In addition to the vasoconstriction that can be associated with COX-2 inhibition, a number of other factors may cause increased cardiac risk. The COX-2 enzyme is expressed in endothelial cells in response to injury.[140] It is also found in atheromatous plaque and may play role in decreasing vascular inflammation.[256] Furthermore, there is no COX-2 expression on platelets. COX-2 inhibitors, unlike their nonselective counterparts, do not block the formation of thromboxane, which plays an important role in platelet aggregation and vasoconstriction.[140]

This increased cardiac risk has been confirmed by the voluntary withdrawal of Vioxx (rofecoxib) from the market. A long-term study of the drug for the use of recurrent colon polyps was halted. Investigators found an increased risk for cardiovascular events, including heart attack and stroke, especially in those taking the medication for more than 18 months (www.fda.gov/cder/drug/ifnopage/vioxx/default.htm). As of this writing, valdecoxib has been withdrawn from the market due to similar concerns.

NSAIDs for Chronic Use

Because osteoarthritis is a chronic disease, the long-term efficacy and tolerability of NSAIDs become relevant questions. Most studies are short term, but several long-term studies have been conducted. Dieppe and associates[58] performed a randomized study in patients receiving chronic NSAID therapy and compared diclofenac with placebo. Patients were also allowed to take up to 4 g of acetaminophen as a rescue medication. At the end of the study period, only 57% had completed the trial. A higher number of the placebo group withdrew in the first 3 months because of lack of efficacy, but a higher number of the treatment group withdrew as a result of side effects and 15% withdrew because of lack of compliance. There was no appreciable difference between the treatment groups with respect to compliance. Outcomes in terms of efficacy at the end of 2 years were similar, with 52% in the diclofenac group reporting improvement versus 45% in the placebo group. The placebo group averaged slightly more acetaminophen intake.[58] Another long-term study by Williams and coworkers[303] in patients with knee osteoarthritis compared naproxen (Naprosyn) with acetaminophen. In this trial only 35% of the patients completed the 2-year study. Similar to the Dieppe study, withdrawal because of lack of efficacy was higher in the acetaminophen group and withdrawal because of side effects was higher with Naprosyn. Again, only a modest percentage of patients showed improvement at the end of the study, and few significant differences between the treatment groups were found.[303] Similar reports indicate that NSAIDs can be discontinued over the long term, at least in elderly patients, without an increase in osteoarthritic symptoms.[138,274] Taken together with the results of the long-term studies,[58,303] these reports seem to indicate that up to two-thirds of patients may do well without NSAID therapy over the long term when other analgesics are available. Therefore, periodic attempts at withdrawal and reassessment of the necessity for NSAID therapy seem warranted.

Does long-term use of NSAIDs accelerate arthritis? There is some evidence to suggest that NSAIDs interfere with synovial blood flow or with repair of microfractures of subchondral bone.[238,271,272] Furthermore, in various animal models it has been observed that the most commonly used NSAID, aspirin, inhibited proteoglycan synthesis and led to enhanced cartilage destruction.[27,29,216,217,219] Early clinical studies implied that NSAIDs were associated with more rapid degeneration of the osteoarthritic joint and earlier performance of surgery. A retrospective analysis of radiographic progression of osteoarthritis of the hip led to the conclusion that indomethacin was associated with greater joint destruction than that seen in control patients.[245] Another study looked at patients with advanced hip osteoarthritis awaiting arthroplasty who were treated with either indomethacin or propozone. The authors concluded that the indomethacin group showed more rapid radiographic deterioration and underwent surgery earlier than did the propozone group.[238] However, the results of this study have been called into question,[63] and in fact, a double-blind study of indomethacin versus placebo showed no increase in disease progression.[127]

Possible Chondroprotective Action of NSAIDs

The traditional view that osteoarthritis is an inevitably progressive disease and results from "wear and tear" of cartilage has been replaced by an understanding of the biochemical and biomechanical factors in the etiology and progression of the disease. Because cartilage is continuously undergoing both degradation and renewal, it appears logical to design a medication that promotes the anabolic activity of cartilage while inhibiting its degradation. The evidence for these beneficial activities of NSAIDs is mixed.[125]

A chondroprotective effect of NSAIDs has been postulated.[62] Proposed mechanisms include improved biomechanics by decreasing arthralgia and inhibition of cartilage catabolism. Cartilage matrix proteoglycans are degraded by enzymes such as metalloproteinases and serine proteases. Some NSAIDs are effective inhibitors of these enzymes.[33,98,165] Release of oxygen free radicals and other inflammatory mediators may also be suppressed by NSAIDs.[124,225,227] Other NSAIDs may actually stimulate glycosaminoglycan production, as indicated by increased sulfate incorporation.

The net effect of NSAIDs on cartilage remains to be determined, and the effect may vary between NSAIDs.[217] In vivo models of surgically induced osteoarthritis and immobilization in dogs showed a detrimental effect of aspirin on the production of articular cartilage proteoglycans when the anterior cruciate ligament was transected and the hind limb immobilized, but a beneficial effect on cartilage proteoglycan maintenance when the anterior cruciate was not transected but the hind limb was immobilized. This finding would seem to indicate that the injured cartilage is predisposed to the harmful effects caused by the inhibition of anabolism with aspirin whereas uninjured and immobilized cartilage may be protected from catabolism by aspirin.[218] Interpretation of animal models is difficult at best because of the extreme variability of results in different species and the fact that the time course and possibly the mechanism of osteoarthritis in animals may differ significantly from that in humans.

The effects of COX-2 inhibitors on articular cartilage have not been studied extensively. The effect of celecoxib and diclofenac on human chondrocyte metabolism was compared in an in vitro model. Celecoxib increased the synthesis of hyaluronan and proteoglycans in these explanted cells, whereas diclofenac did not have such an effect.[71]

There is no concrete evidence for a chondroprotective effect of NSAIDs in humans.

Summary

What, then, should be the strategy for the use of NSAIDs and the treatment of osteoarthritis? If nonpharmacological measures fail, simple analgesics should probably be tried as a first-line measure. In the subset of patients in whom analgesic therapy is not effective, a low dose (less than 1200 mg/day) of ibuprofen often provides effective therapy. Low-dose ibuprofen is not anti-inflammatory and is very inexpensive. In the event that ibuprofen is not effective in an analgesic dose, anti-inflammatory doses of ibuprofen or other nonselective NSAIDs may be tried.

The initial enthusiasm for COX-2 inhibitors has been replaced with caution. COX-2 inhibitors should be considered in younger patients who cannot tolerate nonselective NSAIDs or have a history of gastrointestinal irritation. They should be avoided in patients with hypertension, those with a history of cardiac or renal disease, and the elderly. At this time the overall cardiac risk associated with the COX-2 inhibitors that remain on the market is uncertain. Until further data are obtained, care should be used in prescribing COX-2 inhibitors to individuals.

Once relief is achieved with NSAIDs, periodic withdrawal of therapy plus substitution of a simple analgesic is prudent, especially in the older population. NSAIDs should be avoided in high-risk patients, such as those with a history of ulcer disease, those taking concurrent oral corticosteroids, and those with a history of gastrointestinal bleeding, congestive heart failure, or renal insufficiency. Nonacetylated salicylates, such as Arthropan (choline salicylate), Disalcid/salsalate (salicylsalicylic acid), and Trilisate (choline magnesium trisalicylate), or "renal-sparing" NSAIDs such as sulindac may have a role in the treatment of these patients.

INJECTABLE CORTICOSTEROIDS

Injectable corticosteroids have been part of the therapeutic armamentarium since they were introduced by Hollander and Brown in the 1950s.[131] Despite the frequency of use of these compounds and the length of experience with them, there is little literature to guide the physician in the optimal corticosteroid preparation, frequency of dosage, and length of treatment. In addition, there are few well-controlled studies documenting efficacy. Concern persists about the possible deleterious effects of these medications on cartilage.

Corticosteroids inhibit phospholipase A_2 expression, which blocks both the COX and the lipoxygenase pathways.[76] This is probably their main mechanism of action, although they also affect RNA protein synthesis and cellular metabolism.[16]

A variety of injectable corticosteroids are available. The duration of action appears to be related to the solubility of the compound.[16] Hydrocortisone acetate is absorbed rapidly from the knee (half-life of 1 to 2 hours)[57] and provides only a few days of relief. Triamcinolone hexacetonide is the longest acting, with a half-life of several weeks.[57]

Systemic absorption of these compounds from the joint can occur. Suppression of the hypothalamic-pituitary axis is possible if multiple joints are injected or if injections are given at close intervals.[215] Decreased serum cortisol levels have been noted from even a single intra-articular injection.[160] Suppression of the hypothalamic-pituitary axis does not persist for more than 2 days, and adrenocorticosteroid secretion returns to normal in 3 to 6 days.[150] Systemic absorption is rarely a clinical problem.

Hollander originally reported on 231 patients who received corticosteroid injections over a period of 20 years. Eighty-seven percent of these patients reported complete relief of pain.[128] Another large study by the same author confirmed this favorable view. Sixty percent of nearly 1000 patients treated over a period of 9 years no longer had sufficient symptoms to require injections. Only 20% failed to respond to treatment.[129] The three controlled trials were not quite as enthusiastic.[59,88,307] Patients injected with corticosteroid had a small, but definite improvement in symptoms (but not function) versus placebo at 1 to 2 weeks after injection. By 4 weeks, however, the groups were indistinguishable. As would be expected with an invasive therapy, the response to placebo (saline or vehicle) was high, with 35% to 45% of patients reporting improvement. Contrary to a similar study using NSAIDs, Dieppe and associates found no correlation between therapeutic response and synovial fluid white cell count.[59]

A recent meta-analysis of randomized controlled studies that assessed the efficacy of intra-articular corticosteroid injections was performed.[8] The authors concluded that these studies showed a statistically significant improvement in the short term, at 2 weeks. The few studies reviewed that allowed for evaluation at longer follow-up periods did show significant improvement at 16 to 24 weeks.

Recognized complications from corticosteroid injection include intra-articular infection and inflammatory flair.[110,111] Intra-articular infection is extremely rare, even when rigorous sterile technique is not used. Its incidence is estimated at 0.01% to 0.005%.[255] Postinjection flair is far more common with an incidence of 2% to 5%. Inflammation occurs within hours of injection. It is a neutrophil-dependent inflammatory response most likely caused by the corticosteroid crystals themselves.[186] It is almost always self-limited and resolves within 1 to 3 days.

Dark-skinned individuals may have local discoloration of the skin from subcutaneous injection, and it can be permanent.[210] This cosmetic discoloration is not serious but can lead to considerable consternation on the part of the patient and should therefore be a part of informed consent. Temporary disturbances may include elevated blood sugar, arterial hypertension, and facial flushing.[139,220]

Effects on Cartilage

Evidence for the effects of injected corticosteroids on cartilage metabolism is mixed. Corticosteroids are potent inhibitors of both anabolic and catabolic processes in cartilage. As with NSAIDs, interpretation of animal data is difficult because of the species-specific response to these compounds. Weekly injections into rabbit joints produced histological and macroscopic evidence of cartilage degeneration and depressed synthesis of collagen and proteoglycan.[17,198] Weightbearing joints were more strongly affected. On the other hand, injection of corticosteroid provided significant protection from cartilage breakdown in rabbits with secondary arthritis.[36,199] Similar protective effects have been noted in primates and dogs.[106,224,226,304] A recent in vitro study of human chondrocytes demonstrated that dexamethasone administration decreases proteoglycan concentrations.[270] Whether inhibition of the

anabolic or catabolic effects predominates in humans is unknown.

Anecdotal reports linking intra-articular corticosteroid therapy with accelerated joint destruction have not been borne out either by clinical experience or by historical data. Even in uncontrolled reports it was a rare occurrence.[13,110,143,308] Historical data covering over 330,000 injections put the incidence of this complication at less than 1%, well within the realm of coincidence.[13] Nevertheless, given the possibility of a deleterious effect on the joint, most practitioners are reluctant to inject a joint more frequently than every 4 to 6 weeks.

Theoretically, masking of pain may lead to overuse and subsequent accelerated breakdown. Therefore, some clinicians recommend a period of joint rest after steroid injection.[130,185,209] In rheumatoid arthritis patients, those who had a period of rest after triamcinolone hexacetonide injection experienced a longer period of relief than ambulatory patients did. In animal studies, the articular cartilage damage produced by corticosteroids in menisectomized rabbits seemed to be potentiated by exercise.[198]

Intra-articular corticosteroid therapy is appropriate as a stopgap measure for acute pain in osteoarthritis. It should be considered as long-term treatment only in patients in whom it is effective and other regimens have failed. It appears prudent for patients to rest for a time immediately after injection.

CHONDROPROTECTIVE AGENTS

Recent attention has focused on the development of agents or interventions that could actually slow or reverse the progression of disease. Such proposed agents are called "chondroprotective agents" or disease-modifying osteoarthritis drugs. How could you tell if you had discovered such an agent? Although no consensus definition exists, Ghosh and Brooks proposed that a chondroprotective agent should (1) enhance chondrocyte macromolecule synthesis; (2) enhance the synthesis of hyaluronan; (3) inhibit degradative enzymes; (4) mobilize deposits of thrombin, fibrin, lipids, and cholesterol in vessels surrounding the joint; (5) reduce joint pain; and (6) reduce joint synovitis.[102] With these guidelines in mind, we will examine the evidence for several agents.

Hyaluronic Acid

Hyaluronic acid is a key constituent of both cartilage ground substance and synovial fluid. It is also referred to as hyaluronate or hyaluronan. Early osteoarthritis is characterized by loss and degradation of hyaluronic acid from cartilage and synthesis of lower-molecular-weight hyaluronic acid by synoviocytes. Hyaluronic acid plays a role in both the viscous and elastic properties of synovial fluid. As a pharmacological agent, anti-inflammatory, antinociceptive, and cartilage anabolic effects have been ascribed to hyaluronic acid.[99,100] Hyaluronic acid is a viscous substance with preparations of higher molecular weight exhibiting greater viscosity. Cross-linked molecules have higher molecular weight and viscosity. It is believed that hyaluronate exerts its effect by physical cushioning of the joint.[228] Injection of hyaluronate is thus considered viscosupplementation.

Since Peyron and Balazs reported on the first clinical experience with injected hyaluronate over 30 years ago,[230] numerous clinical and animal studies have been carried out. Despite this lengthy and sustained clinical and laboratory interest in hyaluronate as a possible treatment of osteoarthritis, its use and efficacy remain controversial.[50-52,100,147]

Intra-articular hyaluronic acid has been used in veterinary practice for at least 30 years. Beneficial effects have been noted in several different species, including horses and dogs.[10,35,93,246] Experience in human subjects began in 1974, when Peyron and Balazs reported a beneficial effect of intra-articular hyaluronic acid in a double-blind, placebo-controlled study of 28 patients.[230] Since that time, many clinical studies, including some prospective, randomized, and controlled studies, have lent credence to the assertion that injected hyaluronic acid has a beneficial effect in osteoarthritis.

Dixon and coworkers reported on a multicenter double-blind study involving 63 patients in which sodium hyaluronate was compared with placebo. They found significant differences between groups in the amount of pain at rest after 5 weeks of treatment (hyaluronate better), with the difference widening over time. No difference in activity assessment was found.[60] Another short-term blinded and controlled trial showed similar results.[112] When compared with intra-articular prednisolone, a series of three injections of hyaluronic acid provided similar relief of symptoms after 1 week, with greater improvement thereafter.[161] Several uncontrolled studies confirm these data.[2,175,176,207,300] Investigators generally reported a response rate of 70% to 80% and an improvement of about 30% over placebo.[64,175,176,207]

Leopold et al prospectively studied 100 patients with knee osteoarthritis randomized to receive hylan G-F 20 or corticosteroid. They found modest improvements in both groups, but there was not a significant difference in outcomes between the two groups at 3- and 6-month follow-up.[166]

In addition to the in vitro and in vivo data detailed later, several human studies have tried to investigate the tissue- and disease-modifying properties of injected hyaluronic acid. In a pilot study of 40 patients treated with 20 mg of hyaluronate sodium (Hyalgan) intra-articularly once per week for 5 weeks, Frizziero and coworkers found that 30% had morphological improvement in cartilage and synovial membrane when compared with baseline. Improvements included reconstitution of the superficial amorphous layer, improvement in chondrocyte density and vitality, and reduction of synovial inflammation. However, 60% of patients showed no improvement, 7% worsened, and there was no placebo control group in the study.[90] In a small randomized, but not blinded study of hyaluronan injection versus "standard therapy," Listrat and associates found less deterioration in the structural parameters of cartilage evaluated by arthroscopy in the study group.[172]

Interpretation of human studies is confounded by differing study designs, injection regimens, outcomes evaluation criteria, and importantly, failure to control for concurrent NSAID use. It is well recognized that the placebo effect becomes more pronounced as the therapy becomes more invasive. Indeed, at least two prospective, randomized, and blinded studies showed no difference between injected hyaluronate and placebo.[52,121] Another large, multicenter, controlled study of Hyalgan versus placebo noted no difference between groups as measured by pain, function, motion, or activity scores. When groups were stratified by age and severity, however, there was a significantly greater improvement in patients older than 60 years and those with a higher degree of symptoms when treated with Hyalgan.[173]

In a more recent multicenter, double-blind randomized study of 240 patients, hyaluronate was significantly more effective than saline placebo for the treatment of mild or moderate osteoarthritis.[53]

Injected hyaluronates have been extensively studied in animal and cell culture models. The results generally agree on a therapeutic and "chondroprotective effect." Yet even in these models, not all the evidence supports a therapeutic role. Studies in sheep, horses, dogs, rats, and rabbits have demonstrated a wide variety of beneficial effects. Aihara and associates noted an antinociceptive response in rats.[5] Dose-related inhibition of acute and chronic inflammation in the rat has also been noted.[134] This effect may be due to inhibition of release of arachidonic acid[279] or other inflammatory mediators by synovial fibroblasts.

Hyaluronate injections appeared to prevent early osteoarthritic changes in cartilage and subchondral bone in menisectomized sheep[6,104] and in anterior cruciate ligament–deficient dogs.[254] Studies in horses showed increased weightbearing[11,96] in animals injected with hyaluronate in comparison to those given injections of placebo. This response was dose related, and improvement occurred as rapidly as 1 week.[107] Injected hyaluronan was also effective in preventing loss of proteoglycan from cartilage in the Pond-Nuki model in dogs,[1] as well as in rabbit-derived chondrocyte culture.[260] In opposition to the prevailing view, Smith and coworkers reported no beneficial effect in anterior cruciate ligament–transected mongrel dogs. In fact, these authors reported a slight decrease in proteoglycan content in the cartilage of treated animals and concluded that hyaluronan may inhibit repair.[268]

Because part of the proposed mechanism for hyaluronate efficacy is as a viscous "cushioning" agent, several studies have examined the role of molecular weight on efficacy. Most have concluded that lower-molecular-weight and cross-linked preparations were superior to high-molecular-weight compounds.[9,103,261] However, this conclusion is not universally supported.[145,305]

Intra-articular hyaluronic acid is generally well tolerated, yet infrequent problems may arise. Infection is a small risk and, though not specifically reported, may be assumed to be of the same magnitude as that reported for corticosteroid injection. A local inflammatory reaction is a more frequent occurrence.[3,213] The incidence can be as low as 3%.[175] One author reported local inflammation with 11% of injections, and 27% of patients experienced such inflammation. Occurrence was unpredictable, and symptoms lasted up to 3 weeks.[235]

Despite the wealth of positive clinical and laboratory evidence, the question of efficacy of injected hyaluronates remains to be resolved. No evidence exists to support the use of one commercially available preparation over another, nor have the optimal dosage, injection regimen, and patient selection criteria been determined.

Glucosamine

Recent popular books[277] and media articles have drawn attention to the use of oral glucosamine sulfate as treatment of osteoarthritis. What is surprising is not the spate of new interest in this compound, but rather that its usefulness was not recognized earlier given the wealth of laboratory and clinical support already published. In 1994, McCarty[187] decried the complete lack of interest in glucosamine as a treatment of arthritis in light of the fact that it has been shown in culture studies dating back to the 1950s to enhance secretion of mucopolysaccharides in cartilage-derived fibroblasts. He also cited animal studies that demonstrated a beneficial effect in both prevention and treatment of arthritis, as well as several human studies. Most strikingly, all the human trials demonstrated efficacy of the compound, whereas none showed serious side effects. When these findings are contrasted with the questionable effects of NSAIDs on cartilage,[190] together with the high rate of complications of these compounds, a strong argument emerges for consideration of glucosamine as a first-line agent in the treatment of arthritis.

RATIONALE FOR GLUCOSAMINE

Glucosamine is a simple amino sugar that serves as a substrate for the synthesis of both glycosaminoglycans and hyaluronic acid. Glucosamine is synthesized directly by chondrocytes, but when supplemented, it can be used directly to synthesize larger macromolecules. Most preparations are derived from chitin in crustacean shells.

A wide variety of effects have been documented in in vitro and animal models. They can be broadly classified as substrate, transcriptional, "antireactive," and "antiarthritic" effects.

As far back as 1956, Roden noted increased production of glycosaminoglycans and collagen when glucosamine sulfate was added to cartilage-derived fibroblast cell cultures.[242] Other studies have confirmed this effect.[296,297] Karzel later demonstrated that glucosamine sulfate was efficiently incorporated into mucopolysaccharides. These studies demonstrated a specific effect: N-acetylglucosamine was far less active and glucuronic acid was without effect.[141,155]

Besides functioning as a simple substrate, recent work has shown glucosamine to affect gene transcription within the chondrocyte. Jimenez and Dodge demonstrated a twofold increase in perlecan and aggrecan mRNA levels

and a moderate increase in stromelysine mRNA in chondrocyte cultures incubated with 50 μM of glucosamine.[137] The same authors showed a dose-dependent downregulation of metalloproteinase I and II (enzymes important in degradation of cartilage) mRNA in the same model.[137]

Glucosamine may be more effective in upregulating cartilage metabolism in arthritic or stressed cartilage. Lippiello found an increase in glycosaminoglycan synthesis in arthritic cartilage explants under various types of stress on exposure to glucosamine when compared with young or nonstressed explants.[168] Looking at a biological marker of type II cartilage degradation, Christgau et al determined that patients with higher rates of cartilage turnover (higher levels of CTX-II in urine) benefited the most from glucosamine supplementation.[43]

Glucosamine increases the synovial production of hyaluronic acid, a substance that has itself been shown to have anti-inflammatory effects, induce anabolic activity in chondrocytes, decrease joint pain, and increase mobility in vivo and in clinical studies.[188]

Animal studies have demonstrated an "antireactive effect" of glucosamine by finding that it prevents an inflammatory response to certain irritants known to cause inflammation in rats but has no inhibitory effects on inflammation caused by inflammatory mediators such as bradykinin, serotonin, or histamine.[259] Specifically and importantly, glucosamine did not produce any inhibition of the COX system, thus lending some credibility to the claim of gastrointestinal tolerability. In fact, glucosamine may stimulate the production of protective mucopolysaccharides in the gastric mucosa and therefore may be useful in ulcer therapy.[195]

An "antiarthritic" effect of glucosamine has been demonstrated in animal models of inflammatory arthritis, mechanical arthritis, immunoreactive arthritis, and generalized inflammation. Efficacy in these models was lower than that of indomethacin, but toxicity was significantly lower, so the overall therapeutic margin was much more favorable. Therefore, glucosamine may have a place in the treatment of inflammatory arthritis, in addition to osteoarthritis.[259]

HUMAN STUDIES

Contrary to perception in the United States, glucosamine sulfate has been heavily studied in human arthritis sufferers in the past 25 years. Studies were performed in many countries, including Italy,[48] Germany,[22,67,70,204] Spain,[174] Portugal,[274] China,[236] and the Philippines.[234] Subjects suffered from arthritis of the hand, spine, shoulders, hips, and knees. The results were consistent: all studies showed a beneficial effect of the study drug. Improvement in pain occurred slowly over a period of several weeks. Subjects continued to improve while taking the study drug, in contrast to patients taking placebo, who did not. Subjects also maintained improvement for weeks to months after use of the drug was discontinued. Response to treatment was high, ranging from 56% to over 90%.[234,275] Equally important, no study encountered significant side effects with glucosamine. Early clinical uncontrolled trials performed in Germany beginning in 1969 used an injectable form and a dosage of 400 mg/day. Injections were either intra-articular, intramuscular, or intravenous. All studies reported diminution of pain, some improvement in mobility, and no significant side effects.[22,67,70,204,287] Interest in glucosamine accelerated in Europe with the synthesis of an easily absorbable oral preparation. Since the early 1980s, numerous controlled studies, including 12 double-blind studies,* were carried out. At least five double-blind, single-joint, placebo-controlled studies using a validated outcome tool have been performed.[203,211,221,240,241]

Lopes Vaz studied 40 outpatients with unilateral osteoarthrosis of the knee. Twenty patients who received 1.5 g of glucosamine daily were compared with 20 who received 1.2 g of ibuprofen. Ibuprofen patients noted rapid improvement in the first 2 weeks. Improvement in the glucosamine group was slower, but continued throughout the study and was significantly better by week 8.[174]

Drovanti and associates studied 80 patients for 30 days. Subjects received either 1.5 g of glucosamine or placebo on a randomized, blinded basis. Patients receiving glucosamine experienced greater relief and experienced it faster than those taking placebo did. Very little intolerance was noted. In fact, of the five patients in the study group who had occult gastrointestinal bleeding at the beginning of the study, three were free of occult blood after taking glucosamine.[66]

More recently, Qiu and coauthors studied 178 patients with osteoarthritis of the knee. Randomized cohorts received either 1.5 g of oral glucosamine or 1.2 g of ibuprofen for a period of 4 weeks. Both groups recorded improvement in pain, mobility, and swelling, with an accelerating trend in favor of glucosamine. After discontinuation of treatment, glucosamine demonstrated a greater remnant therapeutic effect, although it was not statistically significant at 2 weeks. Glucosamine was significantly better tolerated than ibuprofen, and the glucosamine group suffered less dropout.[236]

Reichelt and coauthors reported a multicenter, double-blind, placebo-controlled study on the efficacy of intra-muscular glucosamine in patients with osteoarthritis of the knee. One hundred fifty-five patients were treated with 400 mg of glucosamine sulfate twice a week for 6 weeks or with placebo. The glucosamine group had a greater response and a higher rate of responders than the placebo group did.[241]

Criticism of the older literature on glucosamine has centered on the small numbers of patients studied, the short time periods of these studies, and the relative lack of studies independent of corporate sponsorship.[36a] Methodological concerns, specifically the failure of most studies to control for NSAID use, have also been raised.[31a] Recent meta-analyses should help dispel some of the concern over the quality of the clinical evidence. Towheed et al, writing for the Cochrane Database, evaluated 16 randomized controlled trials, 12 comparing glucosamine with placebo and 4 comparing it with an NSAID. The authors concluded that glucosamine was both safe and effective.[280]

McAlindon et al reviewed six studies of glucosamine involving 911 patients. Quality scores for these studies ranged from 12% to 52%. The combined results showed a moderate treatment effect of glucosamine.[184]

Glucosamine may be effective symptomatic treatment of osteoarthritis of the knee, but does it have a chondroprotective effect? Perhaps the most convincing evidence comes from a pair of very similar long-term studies. Reginster and coauthors randomized 212 patients to either glucosamine sulfate (1500 mg/day) or placebo and monitored them for 3 years. Standardized weightbearing knee radiographs were obtained and the minimum medial tibiofemoral joint space measured by digital image analysis. The patients taking placebo showed progressive joint space narrowing of approximately 0.1 mm/yr, whereas those taking glucosamine did not. WOMAC scores worsened slightly in the placebo group versus improvement with glucosamine.[240] Reginster et al allowed the use of several different NSAIDs as rescue medications, and some commentators were concerned that increased knee extension because of symptomatic relief in the glucosamine group could skew the results. To address some of these perceived deficiencies, Pavelka et al performed a very similar study with nearly identical results. In this study 202 patients were randomized to glucosamine sulfate or placebo. Only Tylenol was used for rescue analgesia. The minimum tibiofemoral compartment width at a standard degree of knee flexion and algofunctional scoring were used as endpoints. Progressive joint space narrowing was noted in the placebo group versus joint preservation in the glucosamine group. Lequesne and WOMAC scores also showed statistically significant differences between groups.[221]

Chondroitin

Several other amino sugars or glycosaminoglycans are commercially available for the treatment of osteoarthritis, including chondroitin sulfate, glycosaminoglycan-peptide association complex (Rumalon), glycosaminoglycan polysulfuric acid (GAGPS or Arteparon), and sodium pentosan polysulfate (Cartrofen). Although these compounds enjoy some laboratory and clinical support, they have not gained the popularity nor been as well studied as glucosamine or hyaluronic acid.

Chondroitin sulfate (galactosaminoglycuronoglycan sulfate) is a mucopolysaccharide that together with keratan sulfate and a protein core forms aggrecan. Aggrecan, in turn, associates with hyaluronan to form a hydroscopic macromolecule largely responsible for the physical elasticity of cartilage. During aging, the ratio of keratan sulfate to chondroitin sulfate in aggrecan increases because of a relative loss of chondroitin. In addition, chondroitin sulfate from diseased cartilage is shorter in length than normal.[28]

As a pharmaceutical, chondroitin exhibits anti-inflammatory properties similar to other glycosaminoglycans and glycosaminoglycan precursors.[12] In humans it is well tolerated and has few side effects and reasonable bioavailability.[244] Moreover, like other glycosaminoglycan precursors, stimulatory effects on cartilage have been reported.[142]

---

*References 48, 66, 120, 174, 203, 211, 221, 234, 236, 240, 241, 287.

Chondroitin sulfate has also been shown to neutralize catabolic processes, such as interleukin-1 production and metalloproteinase activation in human osteoarthritic chondrocyte tissue culture.[182]

Several randomized controlled trials demonstrating a beneficial effect of chondroitin sulfate have been published.[25,32,196,247,285,286,292] Morreale and associates, in a rigorous study comparing chondroitin with diclofenac, showed a more rapid response to diclofenac, but a more profound and long-lasting response to chondroitin. The chondroitin group maintained their symptomatic improvement 3 weeks after discontinuation of the drug, whereas symptoms in patients treated with diclofenac returned immediately after cessation of therapy.[196]

There is even some credible evidence that chondroitin alters the course of disease in humans. Studying 120 patients with knee osteoarthritis, Uebelhart and coauthors found that the group given chondroitin sulfate had better functional outcomes and less joint space narrowing on standard radiographs at 1 year than did controls.[284] Verbruggen et al have also reported on two studies in which patients with erosive arthritis of the hand suffered less progression and fewer new lesions when given chondroitin than the control group did.[293]

Glucosamine/Chondroitin Synergy

Looking back to the definition of a "chondroprotective agent" supplied by Ghosh and Brooks, it is clear that neither glucosamine alone nor chondroitin alone satisfies all the criteria. Because they both act through different mechanisms, it is reasonable to suppose they could have a synergistic effect (Table 18–1). Lippiello and coauthors published a dramatic study in a rabbit instability model of knee osteoarthritis. The authors compared glucosamine alone, chondroitin alone, the combination, and the carrier. Although a chondroprotective effect of both glucosamine and chondroitin alone was noted, the combination almost completely prevented the onset of osteoarthritis (Figs. 18–1 to 18–3).[170]

In light of the significant promise that glucosamine and chondroitin seem to hold for the treatment of osteoarthritis, the National Institutes of Health has funded a 4-year trial comparing glucosamine, chondroitin, and the combination with placebo. The results of this study are pending at the time of this writing.

Table 18–1. Postulated Mechanism of Synergy between Glucosamine and Chondroitin Sulfate

CHONDROPROTECTIVE AGENTS	CHARACTERISTICS
Glucosamine	Stimulates chondrocyte and synoviocyte metabolism
Chondroitin sulfate	Inhibits degradative enzymes
	Prevents fibrin thrombi in periarticular tissue

Dangers of "Nutraceuticals"

Most of the studies cited in the previous paragraphs were performed in countries in which glucosamine and chondroitin are considered pharmaceuticals and are regulated accordingly. In the United States, these substances are considered "nutritional supplements" and are therefore not regulated by the FDA. The nutritional supplement

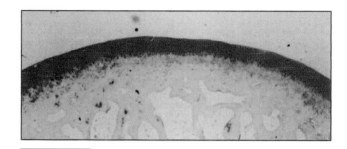

Figure 18–1. Cross-section of normal rabbit femoral condyle stained with safranin O. Cartilage is of normal thickness and shows normal glycosaminoglycan staining.

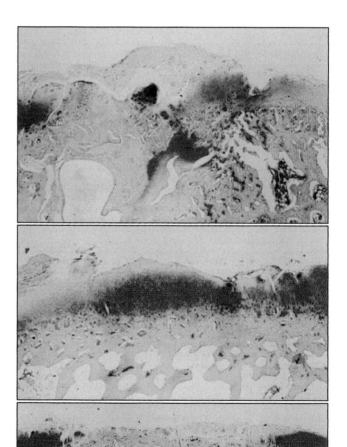

Figure 18–2. Cross-section of an experimental animal treated with placebo. Extensive loss of glycosaminoglycan and cartilage destruction can be noted.

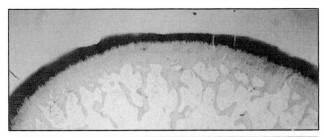
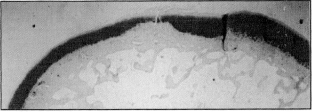
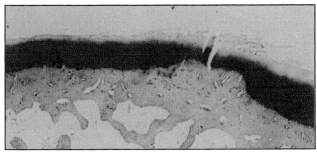

Figure 18–3. Experimental animal treated with a glucosamine/chondroitin combination. Cartilage shows near-perfect preservation.

industry is regulated by the Dietary Supplement Health Education Act, which simply requires that the percentage of active ingredient match the label claim. There is no requirement for safety, efficacy, or bioavailability of the product. Recent investigations have cast doubt that even the percentage of ingredients claimed on the label is accurate.[4] Furthermore, several studies have shown that high-molecular-weight chondroitin sulfate is poorly absorbed and much less permeable in chondrocytes.[4,42] Until the FDA takes a more serious position on these agents, it will be incumbent on the physician to investigate the purity and efficacy of individual formulations before recommending them to patients.

Other agents primarily directed at inhibiting enzymatic or inflammatory cartilage destruction are being investigated. Such agents include orgotein (bovine superoxide dismutase), interleukin-1 receptor antagonist, S-adenosyl-methionine,* and Cartrofen (sodium pentosan polysulfate). Although some encouraging data have been presented,[†] these compounds should be considered investigational at this time.

*References 15, 108, 118, 152, 157, 177, 202, 222, 232, 295.
†References 14, 39, 86, 87, 101, 105, 151, 208, 223, 243, 250, 269, 294.

References

1. Abatangelo G, Botti P, Del Bue M, et al: Intraarticular sodium hyaluronate injections in the Pond-Nuki experimental model of osteoarthritis in dogs. I. Biochemical results. Clin Orthop 241:278-285, 1989.
2. Adams ME: An analysis of clinical studies of the use of crosslinked hyaluronan, hylan, in the treatment of osteoarthritis. J Rheumatol Suppl 39:16-18, 1993.
3. Adams ME: Acute local reactions after intraarticular hylan for osteoarthritis of the knee [letter; comment]. J Rheumatol 23:944-945, discussion 946, 1996.
4. Adebowale A, Cox DS, Zhongming L, Eddington ND: Analysis of glucosamine and chondroitin sulfate content in marketed products and the CaCo-2 permeability of chondroitin sulfate raw materials. JANA 3:37-44, 2000.
5. Aihara S, Murakami N, Ishii R, et al: [Effects of sodium hyaluronate on the nociceptive response of rats with experimentally induced arthritis.] Nippon Yakurigaku Zasshi 100:359-365, 1992.
6. Armstrong S, Read R, Ghosh P: The effects of intraarticular hyaluronan on cartilage and subchondral bone changes in an ovine model of early osteoarthritis. J Rheumatol 21:680-688, 1994.
7. Aronoff GR: Therapeutic implications associated with renal studies of nabumetone. J Rheumatol 19(Suppl 36):25-31, 1992.
8. Arroll B, Goodyear-Smith F: Corticosteroid injections for osteoarthritis of the knee: Meta-analysis. BMJ 328:869, 2004.
9. Asari A, Miyauchi S, Matsuzaka S, et al: Molecular weight–dependent effects of hyaluronate on the arthritic synovium. Arch Histol Cytol 61:125-135, 1998.
10. Asheim A, Lindblad G: Intra-articular treatment of arthritis in race-horses with sodium hyaluronate. Acta Vet Scand 17:379-394, 1976.
11. Auer JA, Fackelman GE, Gingerich DA, Fetter AW: Effect of hyaluronic acid in naturally occurring and experimentally induced osteoarthritis. Am J Vet Res 41:568-574, 1980.
12. Baici A, Bradamante P: Interaction between human leukocyte elastase and chondroitin sulfate. Chem Biol Interact 51:1-11, 1984.
13. Balch HW, Gibson JMC, El-Ghobarey AF, et al: Repeated corticosteroid injections into knee joints. Rheumatol Rehabil 16:137-140, 1977.
14. Baragi VM, Renkiewicz RR, Jordan H, et al: Transplantation of transduced chondrocytes protects articular cartilage from interleukin 1–induced extracellular matrix degradation. J Clin Invest 96:2454-2460, 1995.
15. Barcelo HA, Wiemeyer JC, Sagasta CL, et al: Effect of S-adenosylmethionine on experimental osteoarthritis in rabbits. Am J Med 83(5A):55-59, 1987.
16. Baxter JD, Forsham PH: Tissue effects of glucocorticoids. Am J Med 53:573-589, 1972.
17. Behrens F, Shepard N, Mitchell N: Alterations of rabbit articular cartilage by intra-articular injections of glucocorticoids. J Bone Joint Surg Am 57:70-76, 1975.
18. Bellamy N, Buchanan WW, Chalmers A, et al: A multicenter study of tenoxicam and diclofenac in patients with osteoarthritis of the knee. J Rheumatol 20:999-1004, 1993.
19. Bellamy N, Kean WF, Buchanan WW, et al: Double blind randomized controlled trial of sodium meclofenamate (Meclomen) and diclofenac sodium (Voltaren): Post validation reapplication of the WOMAC Osteoarthritis Index. J Rheumatol 19:153-159, 1992.
20. Birch S, Hesselink JK, Jonkman FA, et al: Clinical research on acupuncture: Part 1. What have reviews of the efficacy and safety of acupuncture told us so far? J Altern Complement Med 10:468-480, 2004.
21. Blount WP: Don't throw away the cane. J Bone Joint Surg Am 38:695-698, 1956.
22. Bohne W: Glokosamine in der donservativen arthosebehandlung. Med Welt 30:1668-1671, 1969.
23. Bombardier C, Laine L, Reicin A, et al: Comparison of upper gastrointestinal toxicity of rofecoxib and naproxen in patients with rheumatoid arthritis. VIGOR Study Group. N Engl J Med 343:1520-1528, 2 p following 1528, 2000.
24. Boniface RJ, Cain PR, Evans CH: Articular responses to purified cartilage proteoglycans. Arthritis Rheum 31:258-266, 1988.
25. Bourgeois P, Chales G, Dehais J, et al: Efficacy and tolerability of chondroitin sulfate 1200 mg/day vs chondroitin sulfate 3 ×

400 mg/day vs placebo. Osteoarthritis Cartilage 6(Suppl A):25-30, 1998.

26. Bradley JD, Brandt KD, Katz BP, et al: Comparison of an antiin-flammatory dose of ibuprofen, an analgesic dose of ibuprofen, and acetaminophen in the treatment of patients with osteoarthritis of the knee. N Engl J Med 325:87-91, 1991.

27. Brandt KD: Effects of nonsteroidal anti-inflammatory drugs on chondrocyte metabolism in vitro and in vivo. Am J Med 83(5A):29-34, 1987.

28. Brandt KD, Palmoski, M: Organization of ground substance pro-teoglycans in normal and osteoarthritic knee cartilage. Arthritis Rheum 19:209-215, 1976.

29. Brandt KD, Palmoski MJ: Effects of salicylates and other nons-teroidal anti-inflammatory drugs on articular cartilage. Am J Med 77(1A):65-69, 1984.

30. Breshnihan B, Hughes G, Essigman WK: Diflunisal in the treatment of osteoarthrosis: A double blind study comparing diflunisal with ibuprofen. Curr Med Res Opin 5:556-561, 1978.

31. Brune K, Beck WS, Geisslinger G, et al: Aspirin-like drugs may block pain independently of prostaglandin synthesis inhibition. Experientia 47:257-261, 1991.

31a. Buckwalter JA, Callaghan JJ, Rosier RN: From oranges and lemons to glucosamine and chondroitin sulfate: Clinical observations stim-ulate basic research. J Bone Joint Surg [Am] 83:1266-1268, 2001.

32. Bucsi L, Poor G: Efficacy and tolerability of oral chondroitin sulfate as a symptomatic slow-acting drug for osteoarthritis (SYSADOA) in the treatment of knee osteoarthritis. Osteoarthritis Cartilage 6(Suppl A):31-36, 1998.

33. Burkhardt D, Ghosh P: Laboratory evaluation of antiarthritic drugs as potential chondroprotective agents. Semin Arthritis Rheum 17(2 Suppl 1):3-34, 1987.

34. Busson M: Update on ibuprofen: Review article. J Int Med Res 14(2):53-62, 1986.

35. Butler J, Rydell NW, Balazs EA: Hyaluronic acid in synovial fluid. VI. Effect of intra-articular injection of hyaluronic acid on the clin-ical symptoms of arthritis in track horses. Acta Vet Scand 11:139-155, 1970.

36. Butler M, Colombo C, Hickman L, et al: A new model of osteoarthrosis in rabbits. III. Evaluation of antiarthritic effects of selected drugs administered intraarticularly. Arthritis Rheum 26:1380-1386, 1983.

36a. Callaghan JJ, Buckwalter JA, Schenck RC Jr: Argument against use of food additives for osteoarthritis of the hip. Clin Orthop Rel Res 381:88-90, 2000.

37. Cameron S: Allergic interstitial nephritis: Clinical features and pathogenesis. Q J Med 250:97-115, 1988.

38. Cangiano JL, Figueroa J, Palmer R: Renal hemodynamic effects of nabumetone, sulindac, and placebo in patients with osteoarthritis. Clin Ther 21:503-512, 1999.

39. Caron JP, Fernandes JC, Martel-Pelletier J, et al: Chondroprotective effect of intraarticular injections of interleukin-1 receptor antago-nist in experimental osteoarthritis. Suppression of collagenase-1 expression. Arthritis Rheum 39:1535-1544, 1996.

40. Caruso I, Biancho Porro G: Gastroscopic evaluation of anti-inflam-matory agents. BMJ 280:75-78, 1980.

41. Chamberlain MA, Care G, Harfield B: Physiotherapy in osteoarthri-tis of the knees: A controlled trial of hospital versus home exer-cises. Int Rehabil Med 4:101-106, 1982.

42. Cho SY, Sim JS, Jeong CS, et al: Effects of low molecular weight chondroitin sulfate on type II collagen–induced arthritis in DBA/1J mice. Biol Pharm Bull 27:47-51, 2004.

43. Christgau S, Henrotin Y, Tanko LB, et al: Osteoarthritic patients with high cartilage turnover show increased responsiveness to the cartilage protecting effects of glucosamine sulphate. Clin Exp Rheumatol 22:36-42, 2004.

44. Cimmino MA, Cutolo M, Samanta, Accardo S: Short term treatment of osteoarthritis: A comparison of sodium meclofenamate and ibuprofen. J Int Med Res 10:46-52, 1982.

45. Clark GR, Willis LA, Steiners L, Nichols PJ: Evaluation of physio-therapy in the treatment of osteoarthritis of the knee. Rheumatol Rehabil 13:190-197, 1974.

46. Clive DM, Stoff JS: Renal syndromes associated with nonsteroidal anti-inflammatory drugs. N Engl J Med 310:563-572, 1984.

47. Cook SD, Salkeld SL, Patron LSP, Ryaby JP: Treatment of osteo-chondral defects with low intensity pulsed ultrasound. Trans Am Acad Orthop Surg 66:175, 1999.

48. Crolle G, D'Este E: Glucosamine sulphate for the management of arthrosis: A controlled clinical investigation. Curr Med Res Opin 7:104-109, 1980.

49. Cushnaghan J, McCarthy C, Dieppe P: Taping the patella medi-ally—a new treatment for osteoarthritis of the knee joint. BMJ 308:753-755, 1994.

50. Dahlberg L: [Intra-articular injection of hyaluronan in the knee. An effective therapy or placebo?] Lakartidningen 91:3406-3408, 1994.

51. Dahlberg L: [Positive discoveries on hyaluronan should be tested in a new trial (letter).] Lakartidningen 91:4244, 1994.

52. Dahlberg L, Lohmander LS, Ryd L: Intraarticular injections of hyaluronan in patients with cartilage abnormalities and knee pain. A one-year double-blind, placebo-controlled study. Arthritis Rheum 37:521-528, 1994.

53. Day R, Brooks P, Conaghan PG, Petersen M: A double blind, ran-domized, multicenter, parallel group study of the effectiveness and tolerance of intraarticular hyaluronan in osteoarthritis of the knee. J Rheumatol 31:775-782, 2004.

54. De Blecourt JJ: A comparative study of ibuprofen ("Brufen") and indomethacin in uncomplicated arthritis. Curr Med Res Opin 3:477, 1975.

55. Deeks JJ, Smith LA, Bradley MD: Efficacy, tolerability, and upper gastrointestinal safety of celecoxib for treatment of osteoarthritis and rheumatoid arthritis: Systematic review of randomised con-trolled trials. BMJ 325:619, 2002.

56. Delpizzo V, Joyner KH: On the safe use of microwave and short-wave diathermy units. Aust J Physiother 33:157-161, 1987.

57. Derendorf H, Möllmann H, Gruner A, et al: Pharmacokinetics and pharmacodynamics of glucocorticoid suspensions after intra-artic-ular administration. Clin Pharmacol Ther 39:313-317, 1986.

58. Dieppe P, Cushnaghan J, Jasani MK, et al: A two-year, placebo-controlled trail of non-steroidal anti-inflammatory therapy in osteoarthritis of the knee joint. Br J Rheumatol 32:595-600, 1993.

59. Dieppe PA, Sathapatayavongs B, Jones HE, et al: Intra-articular steroids in osteoarthritis. Rheumatol Rehabil 19:212-217, 1980.

60. Dixon AS, Jacoby RK, Berry H, Hamilton EB: Clinical trial of intra-articular injection of sodium hyaluronate in patients with osteoarthritis of the knee. Curr Med Res Opin 11:205-213, 1988.

61. Dobson C: A study of the quality and effectiveness of the treatment of knee conditions. Physiotherapy 81:217-221, 1995.

62. Doherty M: "Chondroprotection" by non-steroidal anti-inflammatory drugs. Ann Rheum Dis 48:619-621, 1989.

63. Doherty M, Holt M, MacMillan P, et al: A reappraisal of "analgesic hip." Ann Rheum Dis 45:272-276, 1986.

64. Dougados M, Nguyen M, Listrat V, Amor B: High molecular weight sodium hyaluronate (hyalectin) in osteoarthritis of the knee: A 1 year placebo-controlled trial. Osteoarthritis Cartilage 1:97-103, 1993.

65. Doyle DV, Dieppe PA, Scott J, Huskisson EC: An articular index for the assessment of osteoarthritis. Ann Rheum Dis 40:75-78, 1981.

66. Drovanti A, Bignamini AA, Rovati, AL: Therapeutic activity of oral glucosamine sulfate in osteoarthrosis: A placebo-controlled double-blind investigation. Clin Ther 3:260-272, 1980.

67. Dustmann HO, Puhl W: Die intraartikulaere Injektionstherapie der arthrose—klinissche und tierexperimentell Untersuchungen. Orthop Praxis 14:682-684, 1978.

68. Dyson M: Mechanisms involved in therapeutic ultrasound. Phys-iotherapy 73:116-120, 1987.

69. Edwards JE, McQuay HJ, Moore RA: Efficacy and safety of valde-coxib for treatment of osteoarthritis and rheumatoid arthritis: Sys-tematic review of randomised controlled trials. Pain 111:286-296, 2004.

70. Eichler J, Nöh E: Behandlung der Arthrosis deformans durch Bee-influssung des Knorpelstoffwechsels. Orthop Praxis 6:225-229, 1970.

71. El Hajjaji H, Marcelis A, Devogelaer JP, Manicourt DH: Celecoxib has a positive effect on the overall metabolism of hyaluronan and proteoglycans in human osteoarthritic cartilage. J Rheumatol 30:2444-2451, 2003.

72. Ettinger WH Jr, Afable RF: Physical disability from knee osteoarthritis: The role of exercise as an intervention. Med Sci Sports Exerc 26:1435-1440, 1994.

73. Ettinger WH Jr, Burns R, Messier SP, et al: A randomized trial com-paring aerobic exercise and resistance exercise with a health edu-cation program in older adults with knee osteoarthritis—The

Fitness Arthritis and Seniors Trial (FAST). JAMA 277:25-31, 1997.

74. Evans CH, Mears DC, McKnight JL: A preliminary ferrographic survey of the wear particles in human synovial fluid. Arthritis Rheum 24:912-918, 1981.

75. Ezzo J, Hadhazy V, Birch S, et al: Acupuncture for osteoarthritis of the knee: A systematic review. Arthritis Rheum 44:819-825, 2001.

76. Fadale PD, Wiggins ME: Corticosteroid injections: Their use and abuse. J Am Acad Orthop Surg 2:133-140, 1994.

77. Feinberg J, Marzouk D, Sokolek C, et al: Effects of isometric versus range of motion exercise on joint pain and function in patients with knee osteoarthritis [abstract]. Arthritis Rheum 35:R28, 1992.

78. Felson DT, Anderson JJ, Naimarck A, et al: Obesity and knee osteoarthritis—the Framingham study. Ann Intern Med 109: 18-24, 1988.

79. Felson DT, Zhang Y, Anthony JM, et al: Weight loss reduces the risk of symptomatic knee osteoarthritis in women. Ann Intern Med 116:535-539, 1992.

80. Fisher NM, Gresham GE, Abrams M, et al: Quantitative effects of physical therapy on muscular and functional performance in subjects with osteoarthritis of the knees. Arch Phys Med Rehabil 74:840-847, 1993.

81. Fisher NM, Gresham G, Pendergast DR: Effects of a quantitative progressive rehabilitation program applied unilaterally to the osteoarthritic knee. Arch Phys Med Rehabil 74:1319-1326, 1993.

82. Fisher NM, Pendergast DR, Gresham GE, Calkins E: Muscle rehabilitation its effect on muscular and functional performance of patients with knee osteoarthritis. Arch Phys Med Rehabil 72:367-374, 1991.

83. FitzGerald GA, Patrono C: The coxibs, selective inhibitors of cyclooxygenase-2. N Engl J Med 345:433-442, 2001.

84. Forman MD, Malamet R, Kaplan D: A survey of osteoarthritis of the knee in the elderly. J Rheumatol 10:282-287, 1983.

85. France EP, Paulos LE: Knee bracing. J Am Acad Orthop Surg 2:281-287, 1994.

86. Francis DJ, Forrest MJ, Brooks PM, Ghosh P: Retardation of articular cartilage degradation by glycosaminoglycan polysulfate, pentosan polysulfate, and DH-40J in the rat air pouch model. Arthritis Rheum 32:608-616, 1989.

87. Francis DJ, Hutadilok N, Kongtawelert P, Ghosh P: Pentosan polysulphate and glycosaminoglycan polysulphate stimulate the synthesis of hyaluronan in vivo. Rheumatol Int 13(2):61-64, 1993.

88. Friedman DM, Moore ME: The efficacy of intraarticular steroids in osteoarthritis: A double-blind study. J Rheumatol 7:850-856, 1980.

89. Fries JF, Williams CA, Bloch DA, Michael BA: Nonsteroidal anti-inflammatory drug–associated gastropathy: Incidence and risk factor models. Am J Med 91:213-222, 1991.

90. Frizziero L, Govoni E, Bacchini P: Intra-articular hyaluronic acid in the treatment of osteoarthritis of the knee: Clinical and morphological study. Clin Exp Rheumatol 16:441-449, 1998.

91. Gabriel SE, Jaakkimainen L, Bombardier C: Risk for serious gastrointestinal complications related to use of nonsteroidal anti-inflammatory drugs: A meta-analysis. Ann Intern Med 115:787-796, 1991.

92. Gam AN, Warming S, Larsen LH, et al: Treatment of myofascial trigger-points with ultrasound combined with massage and exercise—a randomised controlled trial. Pain 77:73-79, 1998.

93. Gannon JR: Clinical experiences with intravenous use of sodium hyaluronate in racing greyhounds. Aust Vet J 76:474-475, 1998.

94. Garcia-Rodriguez LA, Jick H: Risk of upper gastrointestinal bleeding and perforation associated with individual non-steroidal anti-inflammatory drugs. Lancet 343:769-772, 1994.

95. Garcia-Rodrigue LA, Walker AM, Gutthann SP: Nonsteroidal anti-inflammatory drugs and gastrointestinal hospitalizations in Saskatchewan: A cohort study. Epidemiology 3:337-342, 1992.

96. Gaustad G, Larsen S: Comparison of polysulphated glycosaminoglycan and sodium hyaluronate with placebo in treatment of traumatic arthritis in horses. Equine Vet J 27:356-362, 1995.

97. Geba GP, Weaver AL, Polis AB, et al: Efficacy of rofecoxib, celecoxib, and acetaminophen in osteoarthritis of the knee: A randomized trial. JAMA 287:64-71, 2002.

98. Ghosh P: Anti-rheumatic drugs and cartilage. Baillieres Clin Rheumatol 2:309-338, 1988.

99. Ghosh P: Osteoarthritis and hyaluronan—palliative or disease-modifying treatment? Semin Arthritis Rheum 22(6 Suppl 1):1-3, 1993.

100. Ghosh P: The role of hyaluronic acid (hyaluronan) in health and disease: Interactions with cells, cartilage and components of synovial fluid. Clin Exp Rheumatol 12:75-82, 1994.

101. Ghosh P, Armstrong S, Read R, et al: Animal models of early osteoarthritis: Their use for the evaluation of potential chondroprotective agents. Agents Actions Suppl 39:195-206, 1993.

102. Ghosh P, Brooks P: Chondroprotection—exploring the concept [editorial]. J Rheumatol 18:161-166, 1991.

103. Ghosh P, Guidolin D: Potential mechanism of action of intra-articular hyaluronan therapy in osteoarthritis: Are the effects molecular weight dependent? Semin Arthritis Rheum 32:10-37, 2002.

104. Ghosh P, Holbert C, Read R, Armstrong S: Hyaluronic acid (hyaluronan) in experimental osteoarthritis. J Rheumatol Suppl 43:155-157, 1995.

105. Ghosh P, Hutadilok N: Interactions of pentosan polysulfate with cartilage matrix proteins and synovial fibroblasts derived from patients with osteoarthritis. Osteoarthritis Cartilage 4:43-53, 1996.

106. Gibson T, Burry HC, Poswillo D, Glass J: Effect of intra-articular corticosteroid injections on primate cartilage. Ann Rheum Dis 36:74-79, 1977.

107. Gingerich DA, Auer JA, Fackelman GE: Effect of exogenous hyaluronic acid on joint function in experimentally induced equine osteoarthritis: Dosage titration studies. Res Vet Sci 30:192-197, 1981.

108. Glorioso S, Todesco S, Mazzi A, et al: Double-blind multicentre study of the activity of S-adenosylmethionine in hip and knee osteoarthritis. Int J Clin Pharmacol Res 5:39-49, 1985.

109. Goldstein JL, Eisen GM, Agrawal N, et al: Reduced incidence of upper gastrointestinal ulcer complications with the COX-2 selective inhibitor, valdecoxib. Aliment Pharmacol Ther 20:527-538, 2004.

110. Gray RG, Gottlieb NL: Intra-articular corticosteroids. An updated assessment. Clin Orthop 177:235-263, 1983.

111. Gray RG, Tenenbaum J, Gottlieb NL: Local corticosteroid injection treatment in rheumatic disorders. Semin Arthritis Rheum 10:231-254, 1981.

112. Grecomoro G, Martorana U, Di Marco C: Intra-articular treatment with sodium hyaluronate in gonarthrosis: A controlled clinical trial versus placebo. Pharmatherapeutica 5:137-141, 1987.

113. Green J, McKenna F, Redfern EJ, Chamberlain MA: Home exercises are as effective as outpatient hydrotherapy for osteoarthritis of the hip. Br J Rheumatol 32:812-815, 1993.

114. Griffin MR, Piper JM, Daugherty JR, et al: Nonsteroidal anti-inflammatory drug use and increased risk for peptic ulcer disease in elderly persons. Ann Intern Med 114:257-263, 1991.

115. Griffin MR, Ray WA, Schaffer W: Nonsteroidal anti-inflammatory drug use and death from peptic ulcer in elderly persons. Ann Intern Med 109:359-363, 1988.

116. Grimmer K: A controlled double blind study comparing the effects of strong burst mode TENS and high rate TENS on painful osteoarthritic knees. Aust J Physiother 38:49-56, 1992.

117. Gutthann SP, Garcia Rodriguez LA, Raiford DS: Individual nonsteroidal anti-inflammatory drugs and the risk of hospitalization for upper gastrointestinal bleeding and perforation in Saskatchewan: A nested case-control study. Pharmacoepidemiol Drug Saf 3:S63, 1994.

118. Harmand MF, Vilamitjana J, Maloche E, et al: Effects of S-adenosylmethionine on human articular chondrocyte differentiation. An in vitro study. Am J Med 83(5A):48-54, 1987.

119. Hedner T: Comparative evaluations of NSAIDs and other analgesics in osteoarthrosis. In Pharmacological Treatment of Osteoarthritis, 2nd ed. Uppsala, Sweden, Almqvist & Wiksell, 1989, pp 173-198.

120. Hehne HJ, Blasius K, Ernst HU: [Therapy of gonarthrosis using chondroprotective substances. Prospective comparative study of glucosamine sulfate and glycosaminoglycan polysulphate.] Fortschr Med 102:676-682, 1984.

121. Henderson EB, Smith EC, Pegley F, Blake DR: Intra-articular injections of 750 kD hyaluronan in the treatment of osteoarthritis: A randomised single centre double-blind placebo-controlled trial of 91 patients demonstrating lack of efficacy. Ann Rheum Dis 53:529-534, 1994.

122. Henry D, Dobson A, Turner C, et al: NSAIDs and risk of upper gastrointestinal bleeding. Lancet 337:730, 1991.

123. Henry D, Lim LLU, Garcia-Rodriguez LA, et al: Variability in risk of major upper gastrointestinal complications with individual NSAIDs. BMJ 312:1563-1566, 1996.

124. Herman JH, Appel AM, Hess EV: Modulation of cartilage destruction by select nonsteroidal antiinflammatory drugs. In vitro effect on the synthesis and activity of catabolism-inducing cytokines produced by osteoarthritic and rheumatoid synovial tissue. Arthritis Rheum 30:257-265, 1987.

125. Herman JH, Appel AM, Khosla RC, Hess EV: The in vitro effect of select classes of nonsteroidal antiinflammatory drugs on normal cartilage metabolism. J Rheumatol 13:1014-1018, 1986.

126. Hochberg MC, Altman RD, Brandt KD, et al: Guidelines for the medical management of osteoarthritis, part II—osteoarthritis of the knee. Arthritis Rheum 38:1541-1546, 1995.

127. Hodgkinson R, Woolf D: A five-year clinical trial of indomethacin in osteoarthrosis of the hip. Practitioner 210:392-396, 1973.

128. Hollander JL: Intraarticular hydrocortisone in arthritis and allied conditions—a summary of two years' clinical experience. J Bone Joint Surg Am 5:983-990, 1953.

129. Hollander JL: Treatment of osteoarthritis of the knees. Arthritis Rheum 3:564, 1960.

130. Hollander JL: Intrasynovial corticosteroid therapy in arthritis. Md State Med J 19:62, 1970.

131. Hollander JL, Brown EM Jr, Jessar RA, Brown CY: Hydrocortisone and cortisone injected into arthritic joints: Comparative effects of and use of hydrocortisone as a local antiarthritic agent. JAMA 147:1629-1635, 1951.

132. Hollander JL, Horvath SM: The influence of physical therapy procedures on the intra-articular temperature of normal and arthritic subjects. Am J Med Sci 218:543-548, 1949.

133. Hutchinson R: COX-2 selective NSAIDs: A review and comparison with non-selective NSAIDs. Am J Nurs 104(3):52-55, 2004.

134. Ialenti A, Di Rosa M: Hyaluronic acid modulates acute and chronic inflammation. Agents Actions 43:44-47, 1994.

135. Jan MH, Lai JS: The effects of physiotherapy on osteoarthritic knees of females. J Formos Med Assoc 90:1008-1013, 1993.

136. Jensen H, Zesler T, Christensen T: Transcutaneous electrical stimulation (TENS) for painful osteoarthrosis of the knee. Int J Rehabil Res 14:356-358, 1991.

137. Jimenez S, Dodge G: The effects of glucosamine sulfate on human chondrocyte gene expression. Osteoarthritis Cartilage 5(SA):72, 1997.

138. Jones AC, Berman P, Doherty, M: Non-steroidal anti-inflammatory drug usage and requirement in elderly acute hospital admissions. Br J Rheumatol 31:45-48, 1992.

139. Jones A, Doherty M: Intra-articular therapies in osteoarthritis. In Brandt KD, Doherty M, Lohmander LS (eds): Osteoarthritis. Oxford, Oxford University Press, 1998, pp 299-306.

140. Justice E, Carruthers DM: Cardiovascular risk and COX-2 inhibition in rheumatological practice. J Hum Hypertens 19:1-5, 2005.

141. Karzel K, Domenjoz R: Effects of hexosamine derivatives and uronic acid derivatives on glycosaminoglycan metabolism of fibroblast cultures. Pharmacology 5:337-345, 1971.

142. Karzel K, Lee KJ: [Effect of hexosamine derivatives on mesenchymal metabolic processes of in vitro cultured fetal bone explants.] Z Rheumatol 41:212-218, 1982.

143. Keagy RD, Keion HA: Intra-articular steroid therapy: Repeated use in patients with chronic arthritis. Am J Med Sci 253:45-51, 1967.

144. Kidd BL, Mapp PI, Blake DR, et al: Neurogenic influences in arthritis. Ann Rheum Dis 49:649-652, 1990.

145. Kikuchi T, Yamada H, Shimmei M: Effect of high molecular weight hyaluronan on cartilage degeneration in a rabbit model of osteoarthritis. Osteoarthritis Cartilage 4:99-110, 1996.

146. Kirkley A, Webster-Bogaert S, Litchfield RB, et al: The effect of bracing on medial compartment osteoarthritis of the knee. Trans Am Acad Orthop Surg 66:51, 1999.

147. Kirwan JR, Rankin E: Intra-articular therapy in osteoarthritis. Baillieres Clin Rheumatol 11:769-794, 1997.

148. Kivitz AJ, Greenwald MW, Cohen SB, et al: Efficacy and safety of rofecoxib 12.5 mg versus nabumetone 1,000 mg in patients with osteoarthritis of the knee: A randomized controlled trial. J Am Geriatr Soc 52:666-674, 2004.

149. Knutsson E, Mattsson E: Effects of local cooling on monosynaptic reflexes in man. Scand J Rehabil Med 1:126-132, 1969.

150. Koehler BE, Urowitz MB, Killinger DW: The systemic effects of intra-articular corticosteroid. J Rheumatol 1:117-125, 1974.

151. Kongtawelert P, Brooks PM, Ghosh P: Pentosan polysulfate (Cartrophen) prevents the hydrocortisone induced loss of hyaluronic acid and proteoglycans from cartilage of rabbit joints as well as normalizes the keratan sulfate levels in their serum. J Rheumatol 16:1454-1459, 1989.

152. Konig B: A long-term (two years) clinical trial with S-adenosylmethionine for the treatment of osteoarthritis. Am J Med 83(5A):89-94, 1987.

153. Kovar PA, Allegrante JP, MacKenzie CR, et al: Supervised fitness walking in patients with osteoarthritis of the knee: A randomized, controlled trial. Ann Intern Med 116:529-534, 1992.

154. Kozanoglu E, Basaran S, Guzel R, Guler-Uysal F: Short term efficacy of ibuprofen phonophoresis versus continuous ultrasound therapy in knee osteoarthritis. Swiss Med Wkly 133(23-24):333-338, 2003.

155. Kutzim H: Über ^{14}C-Markiertes Glukosamin. Report of the Nuclear Medicine Laboratory. Bonn, Germany, University Clinic of Bonn, 1970.

156. Langman MJS, Weil J, Wainwright P, et al: Risks of bleeding peptic ulcer associated with individual non-steroidal anti-inflammatory drugs. Lancet 343:1075-1078, 1994.

157. Laudanno OM: Cytoprotective effect of S-adenosylmethionine compared with that of misoprostol against ethanol-, aspirin-, and stress-induced gastric damage. Am J Med 83(5A):43-47, 1987.

158. Lawrence JS, Bremner JM, Bier F: Osteo-arthrosis. Prevalence in the population and relationship between symptoms and x-ray changes. Ann Rheum Dis 25:1-24, 1966.

159. Lawrence RC, Helmick CG, Arnett FC, et al: Estimates of the prevalence of arthritis and selected musculoskeletal disorders in the United States. Arthritis Rheum 41:778-799, 1998.

160. Lazarevic MB, Skosey JL, Djordjevic-Denic G, et al: Reduction of cortisol levels after single intra-articular and intramuscular steroid injection. Am J Med 99:370-373, 1995.

161. Leardini G, Mattara L, Franceschini M, Perbellini A: Intra-articular treatment of knee osteoarthritis. A comparative study between hyaluronic acid and 6-methyl prednisolone acetate. Clin Exp Rheumatol 9:375-381, 1991.

162. Lee J, Warren M, Mason S: Effects of ice on nerve conduction velocity. Physiotherapy 64:2-6, 1978.

163. Lehmann JF, Brunner GD, Stow RW: Pain threshold measurement after therapeutic application of ultrasound, microwaves, and infrared. Arch Phys Med Rehabil 39:560-565, 1958.

164. Lehmann JF, de Lateur BJ: Therapeutic heat. In Therapeutic Heat and Cold. Baltimore, Williams & Wilkins, 1982, pp 404-562.

165. Lentini A, Ternai B, Ghosh P: Synthetic inhibitors of human granulocyte elastase, Part 4. Inhibition of human granulocyte elastase and cathepsin G by non-steroidal anti-inflammatory drugs (NSAID)s. Biochem Int 15:1069-1078, 1987.

166. Leopold SS, Redd BB, Warme WJ, et al: Corticosteroid compared with hyaluronic acid injections for the treatment of osteoarthritis of the knee. A prospective, randomized trial. J Bone Joint Surg Am 85:1197-1203, 2003.

167. Lindberg H, Montgomery F: Heavy labor and the occurrence of gonarthrosis. Clin Orthop 214:235-236, 1987.

168. Lippiello L: Glucosamine and chondroitin sulfate: Biological response modifiers of chondrocytes under simulated conditions of joint stress. Osteoarthritis Cartilage 11:335-342, 2003.

169. Lippiello L, Chakkalakal D, Connolly JF: Pulsing direct current–induced repair of articular cartilage in rabbit osteochondral defects. J Orthop Res 8:266-275, 1990.

170. Lippiello L, Woodward J, Karpman R, Hammad TA: In vivo chondroprotection and metabolic synergy of glucosamine and chondroitin sulfate. Clin Orthop 381:229-240, 2000.

171. Lister BJ, Poland M, DeLapp RE: Efficacy of nabumetone versus diclofenac, naproxen, ibuprofen, and piroxicam in osteoarthritis and rheumatoid arthritis. Am J Med 95(2A):2S-9S, 1993.

172. Listrat V, Ayral X, Patarnello F, et al: Arthroscopic evaluation of potential structure modifying activity of hyaluronan (Hyalgan) in osteoarthritis of the knee. Osteoarthritis Cartilage 5:153-160, 1997.

173. Lohmander LS, Dalen N, Englund G, et al: Intra-articular hyaluronan injections in the treatment of osteoarthritis of the knee: A randomised, double blind, placebo controlled multicentre trial.

Hyaluronan Multicentre Trial Group. Ann Rheum Dis 55:424-431, 1996.

174. Lopes Vaz A: Double-blind clinical evaluation of the relative efficacy of ibuprofen and glucosamine sulphate in the management of osteoarthrosis of the knee in out-patients. Curr Med Res Opin 8:145-149, 1982.

175. Lussier A, Cividino AA, McFarlane CA, et al: Viscosupplementation with hylan for the treatment of osteoarthritis: Findings from clinical practice in Canada. J Rheumatol 23: 1579-1585, 1996.

176. Luzar MJ, Altawil B: Pseudogout following intraarticular injection of sodium hyaluronate. Arthritis Rheum 41:939-940, 1998.

177. Maccagno A, Di Giorgio EE, Caston OL, Sagasta CL: Double-blind controlled clinical trial of oral S-adenosylmethionine versus piroxicam in knee osteoarthritis. Am J Med 83(5A):72-77, 1987.

178. Marasco WA, Gikas PW, Azziz-Baumgartner R, et al: Ibuprofen-associated renal dysfunction. Arch Intern Med 147:2107-2116, 1987.

179. Marks R: Quadriceps strength training for osteoarthritis of the knee: A literature review and analysis. Physiotherapy 79:13-18, 1993.

180. Marks R: The effects of isometric quadriceps strength training in mid-range for osteoarthritis of the knee. Arthritis Care Res 6:52-56, 1993.

181. Martel-Pelletier J, Pelletier JP, Fahmi H: Cyclooxygenase-2 and prostaglandins in articular tissues. Semin Arthritis Rheum 33:155-167, 2003.

182. Mathieu P: [A new mechanism of action of chondroitin sulfates ACS4-ACS6 in osteoarthritic cartilage.] Presse Med 31:1383-1385, 2002.

183. Mazzuca SA, Brandt KD, Anderson SL, et al: The therapeutic approaches of community based primary care practitioners to osteoarthritis of the hip in an elderly patient. J Rheumatol 18:1593-1600, 1991.

184. McAlindon TE, LaValley MP, Gulin JP, Felson DT: Glucosamine and chondroitin for treatment of osteoarthritis: A systematic quality assessment and meta-analysis. JAMA 283:1469-1475, 2000.

185. McCarty DJ: Intrasynovial therapy with adreno-corticosteroid esters. Wis Med J 77:S75-S76, 1978.

186. McCarty DJ, Hogan JM: Inflammatory reaction after intrasynovial injection of microcrystalline adrenocorticosteroid esters. Arthritis Rheum 7:359-367, 1964.

187. McCarty MF: The neglect of glucosamine as a treatment for osteoarthritis—a personal perspective. Med Hypotheses 42:323-327, 1994.

188. McCarty MF: Enhanced synovial production of hyaluronic acid may explain rapid clinical response to high-dose glucosamine in osteoarthritis. Med Hypotheses 50:507-510, 1998.

189. McConnell JS: The management of chondromalacia patellae: A long term solution. Aust J Physiother 32:215-223, 1986.

190. McKenzie LS, Horsburgh BA, Ghosh P, Taylor TK: Osteoarthrosis: Uncertain rationale for anti-inflammatory drug therapy [letter]. Lancet 1:908-909, 1976.

191. Messier SP, Loeser RF, Miller GD, et al: Exercise and dietary weight loss in overweight and obese older adults with knee osteoarthritis: The Arthritis, Diet, and Activity Promotion Trial. Arthritis Rheum 50:1501-1510, 2004.

192. Miller DR: Combination use of nonsteroidal antiinflammatory drugs. Drug Intell Clin Pharm 15:3-7, 1981.

193. Minor MA: Exercise in the management of osteoarthritis of the knee and hip. Arthritis Care Res 7:198-204, 1994.

194. Minor MA, Hewett JE, Webel RR, et al: Efficacy of physical conditioning exercise in patients with rheumatoid arthritis and osteoarthritis. Arthritis Rheum 32:1396-1405, 1989.

195. Moriga M, Aono M, Murakami M, Uchino H: The activity of N-acetylglucosamine kinase in rat gastric mucosa. Gastroenterol Jpn 15:7-13, 1980.

196. Morreale P, Manopulo R, Galati M, et al: Comparison of the anti-inflammatory efficacy of chondroitin sulfate and diclofenac sodium in patients with knee osteoarthritis. J Rheumatol 23:1385-1391, 1996.

197. Moskowitz RW: Principles of drug therapy.

198. Moskowitz RW, Davis W, Sammarco J, et al: Experimentally induced corticosteroid arthropathy. Arthritis Rheum 13:236-243, 1970.

199. Moskowitz RW, et al: Effects of intraarticular corticosteroids and exercise in experimental models of inflammatory and degenerative arthritis. Arthritis Rheum 18:417, 1975.

200. Moxley TE, Royer GL, Hearron MS, et al: Ibuprofen versus buffered phenylbutazone in the treatment of osteoarthritis: Double-blind trial. J Am Geriatr Soc 23:343-349, 1975.

201. Muller EZ: Influence of training and inactivity on muscle strength. Arch Phys Med 51:449-462, 1970.

202. Muller-Fassbender H: Double-blind clinical trial of S-adenosylmethionine versus ibuprofen in the treatment of osteoarthritis. Am J Med 83(5A):81-83, 1987.

203. Muller-Fassbender H, Bach GL, Haase W, et al: Glucosamine sulfate compared to ibuprofen in osteoarthritis of the knee. Osteoarthritis Cartilage 2:61-69, 1994.

204. Mund-Hoym WD: [The treatment of hip and knee joint arthroses.] ZFA (Stuttgart) 56:2153-2159, 1980.

205. Murray MD, Brater DC: Adverse effects of nonsteroidal anti-inflammatory drugs on renal function. Ann Intern Med 112:559-560, 1990.

206. Myers SL, Brandt KD, Ehlich JW, et al: Synovial inflammation in patients with early osteoarthritis of the knee. J Rheumatol 17:1662-1629, 1990.

207. Namiki O, Toyoshima H, Morisaki N: Therapeutic effect of intra-articular injection of high molecular weight hyaluronic acid on osteoarthritis of the knee. Int J Clin Pharmacol Ther Toxicol 20:501-507, 1982.

208. Nethery A, Giles I, Jenkins K, et al: The chondroprotective drugs, Arteparon and sodium pentosan polysulphate, increase collagenase activity and inhibit stromelysin activity in vitro. Biochem Pharmacol 44:1549-1553, 1992.

209. Neustadt DH: Intra-articular steroid therapy. In Moskowitz RW, Howell DS, Goldberg VM, Mankin HF (eds): Osteoarthritis. Diagnosis and Management. Philadelphia, WB Saunders, 1992, pp 493-510.

210. Newman RJ: Local skin depigmentation due to corticosteroid injection. Br Med J (Clin Res Ed) 288:1725-1726, 1984.

211. Noack W, Fischer M, Forster KK, et al: Glucosamine sulfate in osteoarthritis of the knee. Osteoarthritis Cartilage 2:51-59, 1994.

212. Norden DK, Leventhal LJ, Schumacher, HR: Prescribing exercises for osteoarthritis of the knee. J Musculoskel Med 11:14-21, 1994.

213. O'Hanlon D: Acute local reactions after intraarticular hylan for osteoarthritis of the knee [letter; comment]. J Rheumatol 23:945-946, 1996.

214. Oosterveld FG, Rasker JJ, Jacobs JW, Overmars HJ: The effect of local heat and cold therapy on the intraarticular and skin surface temperature of the knee. Arthritis Rheum 35:146-151, 1992.

215. O'Sullivan MM, Rumfeld WR, Jones MK, Williams BD: Cushing's syndrome with suppression of the hypothalamic-pituitary-adrenal axis after intra-articular steroid injections. Ann Rheum Dis 44:561-563, 1985.

216. Palmoski MJ, Brandt KD: Effect of salicylate on proteoglycan metabolism in normal canine articular cartilage in vitro. Arthritis Rheum 22:746-754, 1979.

217. Palmoski MJ, Brandt KD: Effects of some nonsteroidal anti-inflammatory drugs on proteoglycan metabolism and organization in canine articular cartilage. Arthritis Rheum 23:1010-1020, 1980.

218. Palmoski MJ, Brandt KD: Effects of salicylate and indomethacin on glycosaminoglycan and prostaglandin E_2 synthesis in intact canine knee cartilage ex vivo. Arthritis Rheum 27:398-403, 1984.

219. Palmoski MJ, Colyer RA, Brandt KD: Marked suppression by salicylate of the augmented proteoglycan synthesis in osteoarthritic cartilage. Arthritis Rheum 23:83-91, 1980.

220. Pattrick M, Doherty M: Facial flushing after intra-articular injection of steroid. Br Med J (Clin Res Ed) 295:1380, 1987.

221. Pavelka K, Gatterova J, Olejarova M, et al: Glucosamine sulfate use and delay of progression of knee osteoarthritis: A 3-year, randomized, placebo-controlled, double-blind study. Arch Intern Med 162:2113-2123, 2002.

222. Pellegrini P: [S-adenosylmethionine (SAMe) in osteoarthrosis; a double-blind crossover peroral study.] G Clin Med 61:616-627, 1980.

223. Pelletier JP, Caron JP, Evans C, et al: In vivo suppression of early experimental osteoarthritis by interleukin-1 receptor antagonist using gene therapy. Arthritis Rheum 40:1012-1019, 1997.

224. Pelletier JP, DiBattista JA, Raynauld JP, et al: The in vivo effects of intraarticular corticosteroid injections on cartilage lesions, stromelysin, interleukin-1, and oncogene protein synthesis in experimental osteoarthritis. Lab Invest 72:578-586, 1995.

225. Pelletier JP, Martel-Pelletier J: Evidence for the involvement of interleukin 1 in human osteoarthritic cartilage degradation: Protective effect of NSAID. J Rheumatol Suppl 18:19-27, 1989.

226. Pelletier JP, Martel-Pelletier J: Protective effects of corticosteroids on cartilage lesions and osteophyte formation in the Pond-Nuki dog model of osteoarthritis. Arthritis Rheum 32:181-193, 1989.

227. Pelletier JP, Martel-Pelletier J: The therapeutic effects of NSAID and corticosteroids in osteoarthritis: To be or not to be. J Rheumatol 16:266-269, 1989.

228. Pelletier JP, Martel-Pelletier J: The pathophysiology of osteoarthritis and the implication of the use of hyaluronan and hylan as therapeutic agents in viscosupplementation. J Rheumatol Suppl 39:19-24, 1993.

229. Perneger TV, Whelton PK, Klag MJ: Risk of kidney failure associated with the use of acetaminophen, aspirin, and nonsteroidal anti-inflammatory drugs. N Engl J Med 331:1675-1679, 1994.

230. Peyron JG, Balazs EA: Preliminary clinical assessment of Na-hyaluronate injection into human arthritic joints. Pathol Biol (Paris) 22:731-736, 1974.

231. Pincus T, Koch GG, Sokka T, et al: A randomized, double-blind, crossover clinical trial of diclofenac plus misoprostol versus acetaminophen in patients with osteoarthritis of the hip or knee. Arthritis Rheum 44:1587-1598, 2001.

232. Polli E, Cortellaro M, Parrini L, et al: [Pharmacological and clinical aspects of S-adenosylmethionine (SAMe) in primary degenerative arthropathy (osteoarthrosis).] Minerva Med 66:4443-4459, 1975.

233. Puett DW, Griffin MR: Published trials of nonmedicinal and noninvasive therapies for hip and knee osteoarthritis. Ann Intern Med 121:133-140, 1994.

234. Pujalte JM, Llavore EP, Ylescupidez FR: Double-blind clinical evaluation of oral glucosamine sulphate in the basic treatment of osteoarthrosis. Curr Med Res Opin 7:110-114, 1980.

235. Puttick MP, Wade JP, Chalmers A, et al: Acute local reactions after intraarticular hylan for osteoarthritis of the knee. J Rheumatol 22:1311-1314, 1995.

236. Qiu GX, Gao SN, Giacovelli G, et al: Efficacy and safety of glucosamine sulfate versus ibuprofen in patients with knee osteoarthritis. Arzneimittelforschung 48:469-474, 1998.

237. Quirk A, Newman R, Newman K: An evaluation of interferential therapy, shortwave diathermy and exercise in the treatment of osteoarthritis of the knee. Physiotherapy 71:55-57, 1985.

238. Rashad S, Revell P, Hemingway A, et al: Effect of non-steroidal anti-inflammatory drugs on the course of osteoarthritis. Lancet 2:519-522, 1989.

239. Ray WA, Griffin MR, Shorr RI: Adverse drug reactions and the elderly. Health Affairs (Millwood) 9:114-122, 1990.

240. Reginster JY, Deroisy R, Rovati LC, et al: Long-term effects of glucosamine sulphate on osteoarthritis progression: A randomised, placebo-controlled clinical trial. Lancet 357:251-256, 2001.

241. Reichelt A, Forster KK, Fischer M, et al: Efficacy and safety of intramuscular glucosamine sulfate in osteoarthritis of the knee. A randomised, placebo-controlled, double-blind study. Arzneimittelforschung 44:75-80, 1994.

242. Roden L: Effect of hexosamines on the synthesis of chondroitin sulphuric acid in vitro. Ark Kemi 10:345-352, 1956.

243. Rogachefsky RA, Dean DD, Howell DS, Altman RD: Treatment of canine osteoarthritis with insulin-like growth factor-1 (IGF-1) and sodium pentosan polysulfate. Osteoarthritis Cartilage 1:105-114, 1993.

244. Ronca F, Palmieri L, Panicucci P, Ronca G: Anti-inflammatory activity of chondroitin sulfate. Osteoarthritis Cartilage 6(Suppl A):14-21, 1998.

245. Ronningen H, Langeland N: Indomethacin treatment in osteoarthritis of the hip joint. Does the treatment interfere with the natural course of the disease? Acta Orthop Scand 50:169-174, 1979.

246. Rose RJ: The intra-articular use of sodium hyaluronate for the treatment of osteo-arthrosis in the horse. N Z Vet J 27:5-8, 1979.

247. Rovetta G: Galactosaminoglycuronoglycan sulfate (matrix) in therapy of tibiofibular osteoarthritis of the knee. Drugs Exp Clin Res 17:53-57, 1991.

248. Royer GL Jr, Moxley TE, Hearron MS, et al: A six-month double-blind trial of ibuprofen and indomethacin in osteoarthritis. Curr Ther Res Clin Exp 17:234-248, 1975.

249. Rubin RG, Dixon M, Fanisi M: Prescription procedures for knee orthosis and knee ankle foot orthosis. Orthot Prosthet 31:15, 1977.

250. Sakurai K, Miyazaki K, Kodera Y, et al: Anti-inflammatory activity of superoxide dismutase conjugated with sodium hyaluronate. Glycoconj J 14:723-728, 1997.

251. Sandler DP, Smith JC, Weinberg CR, et al: Analgesic use and chronic renal disease. N Engl J Med 320:1238-1243, 1989.

252. Sasaki T, Yasuda K: Clinical evaluation of the treatment of the osteoarthritic knee with a wedged insole. Clin Orthop 221:181-187, 1987.

253. Scheiman JM: Gastroduodenal safety of cyclooxygenase-2 inhibitors. Curr Pharm Des 9:2197-2206, 2003.

254. Schiavinato A, Lini E, Guidolin D, et al: Intraarticular sodium hyaluronate injections in the Pond-Nuki experimental model of osteoarthritis in dogs. II. Morphological findings. Clin Orthop 241:286-299, 1989.

255. Schnitzer TJ: Management of osteoarthritis. In McCarty DJ, Koopman WJ (eds): Arthritis and Allied Conditions. Philadelphia, Lea & Febiger, 1993, pp 1261-1769.

256. Schonbeck U, Sukhova GK, Graber P, et al: Augmented expression of cyclooxygenase-2 in human atherosclerotic lesions. Am J Pathol 155:1281-1291, 1999.

257. Schumacher HR Jr, Stineman M, Rahman M: The association between synovial fluid and treatment response in osteoarthritis. Intern Med 4:25, 1996.

258. Seifert MH, Whiteside CG, Savage O: A 5-year follow-up of fifty cases of idiopathic osteoarthritis of the hip. Ann Rheum Dis 28:325-326, 1969.

259. Setnikar I, Cereda R, Pacini MA, Revel L: Antireactive properties of glucosamine sulfate. Arzneimittelforschung 41:157-161, 1991.

260. Shimazu A, Jikko A, Iwamoto M, et al: Effects of hyaluronic acid on the release of proteoglycan from the cell matrix in rabbit chondrocyte cultures in the presence and absence of cytokines. Arthritis Rheum 36:247-253, 1993.

261. Shimizu C, Kubo T, Hirasawa Y, et al: Histomorphometric and biochemical effect of various hyaluronans on early osteoarthritis. J Rheumatol 25:1813-1819, 1998.

262. Shorr RI, Ray WA, Daugherty JR, Griffin MR: Concurrent use of nonsteroidal anti-inflammatory drugs and oral anticoagulants places elderly persons at high risk for hemorrhagic peptic ulcer disease. Arch Intern Med 153:1665-1670, 1993.

263. Silverstein FE, Faich G, Goldstein JL:, et al: Gastrointestinal toxicity with celecoxib vs nonsteroidal anti-inflammatory drugs for osteoarthritis and rheumatoid arthritis: The CLASS study: A randomized controlled trial. Celecoxib Long-term Arthritis Safety Study. JAMA 284:1247-1255, 2000.

264. Silverstein FE, Graham DY, Senior JR, et al: Misoprostol reduces serious gastrointestinal complications in patients with rheumatoid arthritis receiving nonsteroidal anti-inflammatory drugs: A randomized, double-blind, placebo-controlled trial. Ann Intern Med 123:241-249, 1995.

265. Singh G: Recent considerations in nonsteroidal anti-inflammatory drug gastropathy. Am J Med 105:(1B):31S-38S, 1998.

266. Smalley WE, Ray WA, Daugherty J, Griffin MR: Nonsteroidal anti-inflammatory drugs and the incidence of hospitalizations for peptic ulcer disease in elderly persons. Am J Epidemiol 141:539-545, 1995.

267. Smith EM, Juvinoll RC, Corell EB, et al: Bracing the unstable arthritic knee. Arch Phys Med Rehabil 51:22-28, 1970.

268. Smith GN Jr, Myers SL, Brandt KD, Mickler EA: Effect of intraarticular hyaluronan injection in experimental canine osteoarthritis. Arthritis Rheum 41:976-985, 1998.

269. Smith MM, Ghosh P, Numata Y, Bansal MK: The effects of orally administered calcium pentosan polysulfate on inflammation and cartilage degradation produced in rabbit joints by intraarticular injection of a hyaluronate-polylysine complex. Arthritis Rheum 37:125-136, 1994.

270. Stove J, Schoniger R, Huch K, et al: Effects of dexamethasone on proteoglycan content and gene expression of IL-1beta–stimulated osteoarthrotic chondrocytes in vitro. Acta Orthop Scand 73:562-567, 2002.

271. Sudmann E, Bang G: Indomethacin-induced inhibition of haversian remodelling in rabbits. Acta Orthop Scand 50:621-627, 1979.

272. Sudmann E, Dregelid E, Bessesen A, Mørland J: Inhibition of fracture healing by indomethacin in rats. Eur J Clin Invest 9:333-339, 1979.

273. Superio-Cabuslay E, Ward MM, Lorig KR: Patient education interventions in osteoarthritis and rheumatoid arthritis: A meta-analytic comparison with nonsteroidal antiinflammatory drug treatment. Arthritis Care Res 9:292-301, 1996.

274. Swift GL, Rhodes J: Are non-steroidal anti-inflammatory drugs always necessary? A general practice survey. Br J Clin Pract 46(2):92-94, 1992.

275. Tapadinhas MJ, Rivera IC, Bignamini AA: Oral glucosamine sulphate in the management of arthrosis: Report on a multi-centre open investigation in Portugal. Pharmatherapeutica 3:157-168, 1982.

276. ter Haar G, Dyson M, Oakley S: The use of ultrasound by physiotherapists in Britain. Ultrasound Med Biol 13:659-664, 1987.

277. Theodosakis JAB, Fox B: The Arthritis Cure. New York, St Martins Press, 1997.

278. Tjølsen A, Lund A, Hole K: Antinociceptive effect of paracetamol in rats is partly dependent on spinal serotonergic systems. Eur J Pharmacol 193:193-201, 1991.

279. Tobetto K, Yasui T, Ando T, et al: Inhibitory effects of hyaluronan on [^{14}C]arachidonic acid release from labeled human synovial fibroblasts. Jpn J Pharmacol 60(2):79-84, 1992.

280. Towheed TE, Anastassiades TP, Shea B, et al: Glucosamine therapy for treating osteoarthritis. Cochrane Database Syst Rev (1):CD002946, 2001.

281. Towheed TE, Hochberg MC: A systematic review of randomized controlled trials of pharmacological therapy in osteoarthritis of the knee, with an emphasis on trial methodology. Semin Arthritis Rheum 26:755-770, 1997.

282. Trock DH, Bollet AJ, Markoll R: The effects of pulsed electromagnetic fields in the treatment of osteoarthritis of the knee and cervical spine: Report of randomized, double blind, placebo trials. J Rheumatol 21:1903-1911, 1994.

283. Tyson VC, Glynne A: A comparative study of benoxaprofen and ibuprofen in osteoarthritis in general practice. J Rheumatol Suppl 6:132-138, 1980.

284. Uebelhart D, Malaise M, Marcolongo R, et al: Intermittent treatment of knee osteoarthritis with oral chondroitin sulfate: A one-year, randomized, double-blind, multicenter study versus placebo. Osteoarthritis Cartilage 12:269-276, 2004.

285. Uebelhart D, Thonar EJ, Delmas PD, et al: Effects of oral chondroitin sulfate on the progression of knee osteoarthritis: A pilot study. Osteoarthritis Cartilage 6(Suppl A):39-46, 1998.

286. Uebelhart D, Thonar EJ, Zhang J, Williams JM: Protective effect of exogenous chondroitin 4,6-sulfate in the acute degradation of articular cartilage in the rabbit. Osteoarthritis Cartilage 6(Suppl A):6-13, 1998.

287. Vajaradul Y: Double-blind clinical evaluation of intra-articular glucosamine in outpatients with gonarthrosis. Clin Ther 3:336-343, 1981.

288. van Baar ME, Dekker J, Oostendorp RA, et al: Effectiveness of exercise in patients with osteoarthritis of hip or knee: Nine months' follow up. Ann Rheum Dis 60:1123-1130, 2001.

289. van der Windt DA, van der Heijden GJ, van den Berg SG, et al: Ultrasound therapy for musculoskeletal disorders: A systematic review. Pain 81:257-271, 1999.

290. Van Laranta H: Effect of shortwave diathermy on mobility and radiological stage of the knee in the development of experimental osteo-arthritis. Am J Phys Med 61:59-65, 1982.

291. van Saase JL, van Romunde LK, Cats A, et al: Epidemiology of osteoarthritis: Zoetermeer survey. Comparison of radiological osteoarthritis in a Dutch population with that in 10 other populations. Ann Rheum Dis 48:271-280, 1989.

292. Verbruggen G, Goemaere S, Veys EM: Chondroitin sulfate: S/DMOAD (structure/disease modifying anti-osteoarthritis drug) in the treatment of finger joint OA. Osteoarthritis Cartilage 6(Suppl A):37-38, 1998.

293. Verbruggen G, Goemaere S, Veys EM: Systems to assess the progression of finger joint osteoarthritis and the effects of disease modifying osteoarthritis drugs. Clin Rheumatol 21:231-243, 2002.

294. Verbruggen G, Veys EM: Intra-articular injection pentosanpolysulphate results in increased hyaluronan molecular weight in joint fluid. Clin Exp Rheumatol 10:249-254, 1992.

295. Vetter G: Double-blind comparative clinical trial with S-adenosylmethionine and indomethacin in the treatment of osteoarthritis. Am J Med 83(5A):78-80, 1987.

296. Vidal y Plana RR, Bizzarri D, Rovati AL: Articular cartilage pharmacology: I. In vitro studies on glucosamine and non steroidal anti-inflammatory drugs. Pharmacol Res Commun 10:557-569, 1978.

297. Vidal y Plana RR, Karzel K: [Glucosamine: Its importance for the metabolism of articular cartilage. 2. Studies on articular cartilage.] Fortschr Med 98:801-806, 1980.

298. Ward DE, Veys EM, Bowdler JM, Roma J: Comparison of aceclofenac with diclofenac in the treatment of osteoarthritis. Clin Rheumatol 14:656-662, 1995.

299. Weinberger M, Tierney WM, Booher P, Katz BP: Can the provision of information to patients with osteoarthritis improve functional status? A randomized, clinical trial. Arthritis Rheum 32:1577-1583, 1989.

300. [What is hyaluronic acid and how does it work?] Orthopade 24(2 Suppl):3-6, 1995.

301. Whelton A, Hamilton CW: Nonsteroidal anti-inflammatory drugs: Effects on kidney function. J Clin Pharmacol 31:588-598, 1991.

302. Whelton A, Stout RL, Spilman PS, Klassen DK: Renal effects of ibuprofen, piroxicam, and sulindac in patients with asymptomatic renal failure. Ann Intern Med 112:568-576, 1990.

303. Williams HJ, Ward JR, Egger MJ, et al: Comparison of naproxen and acetaminophen in a two-year study of treatment of osteoarthritis of the knee. Arthritis Rheum 36:1196-1206, 1993.

304. Williams JM, Brandt KD: Triamcinolone hexacetonide protects against fibrillation and osteophyte formation following chemically induced articular cartilage damage. Arthritis Rheum 28:1267-1274, 1985.

305. Wobig M, Bach G, Beks P, et al: The role of elastoviscosity in the efficacy of viscosupplementation for osteoarthritis of the knee: A comparison of hylan G-F 20 and a lower-molecular-weight hyaluronan. Clin Ther 21:1549-1562, 1999.

306. Wright JM: The double-edged sword of COX-2 selective NSAIDs. CMAJ 167:1131-1137, 2002.

307. Wright V, Chandler GN, Morison RAH, Hartfall SJ: Intra-articular therapy in osteo-arthritis. Comparison of hydrocortisone acetate and hydrocortisone tertiary-butylacetate. Ann Rheum Dis 19:257-259, 1960.

308. Zachariae L: Deleterious effects of corticosteroid administered topically, in particular intra-articularly. Acta Orthop Scand 36:127-136, 1965.

309. Zizic TM, Hoffman KC, Holt PA, et al: The treatment of osteoarthritis of the knee with pulsed electrical stimulation. J Rheumatol 22:1757-1761, 1995.

CHAPTER 19

Arthroscopic Treatment of Degenerative Arthritis of the Knee

Henry D. Clarke • W. Norman Scott

Many treatment options exist for symptomatic osteoarthritis of the knee, including nonsurgical modalities, such as nonsteroidal anti-inflammatory drugs and intra-articular injections, and surgical procedures. Depending on age, activity levels, and patient goals, possible surgical interventions include arthroscopic débridement, osteotomy, and knee arthroplasty. Despite numerous published studies documenting the benefits of arthroscopic intervention, never before has arthroscopic débridement been as controversial as it is now. Part of the confusion in addressing this topic can be attributed to the nonspecific nature of the term *arthroscopic débridement* and the heterogeneous mix of patients and pathology that this technique is used to treat. This confusion makes it difficult to draw comparisons between studies. Many different surgical techniques fall under the umbrella of this chapter. In general, these surgical options can be classified into three broad groups: (1) arthroscopic lavage and débridement, (2) marrow-stimulating cartilage repair techniques, and (3) cartilage transplantation procedures.

CLASSIFICATION OF ARTICULAR CARTILAGE DAMAGE AND ARTHRITIS IN THE KNEE

The comparison of results between series has been difficult, partly as a result of the terminology used to describe the radiographic and intraoperative extent of articular cartilage damage. Because no one radiographic or intraoperative classification system is complete and precise in the description of articular cartilage damage, numerous slightly different systems have been proposed.[1,10,13,20,25,34,36] The most commonly used radiographic classification systems are described by Ahlbach[1] and Kellgren and Lawrence[25] (Table 19–1). These systems are far from comprehensive; in the case of the Kellgren and Lawrence,[25] results are based on a single anteroposterior view of the knee.

The most commonly used intraoperative system, described by Outerbridge[36] in 1961, is based on the arthroscopic appearance of the cartilage and the size of the lesion (Table 19–2 and Fig. 19–1). We use a similar classification system by Insall and colleagues,[20] which is based on the description of the cartilage in simple terms. We have found this system helpful when combined with an assessment of the extent of the articular surface that is involved. The six articular surfaces of the knee (patella, trochlea, medial femoral condyle, lateral femoral condyle, medial tibial plateau, and lateral tibial plateau) are individually graded for the type of damage (based on the worst area) and the percentage of the surface involved; lower grades of damage on the same surface that surround the worst area are ignored.

ARTHROSCOPIC LAVAGE AND DÉBRIDEMENT

Arthroscopic treatment of the arthritic knee is not new, with the first reports dating back to 1931.[9] In 1934, Burman and colleagues[9] reported their results in a subgroup of 12 patients with arthritis in a larger series of 30 patients. The early arthroscopic instruments were crude by today's standards. Despite these limitations, Burman and colleagues[9] noted, "It was in the group of arthritic cases that we had the pleasant surprise of seeing a marked improvement in the joint following arthroscopy. This unlooked for therapeutic effect was so marked in the case of one patient that after his one knee had been examined he begged us to do the same for his other knee." Because the rudimentary instruments allowed little more than a simple joint lavage, Burman and colleagues[9] further commented, "It seems to us that, as already stated, this improvement was due to the withdrawal of the synovial effusion and to the distention and thorough irrigation of the joint." In the modern era, similar benefits have been noted from simple lavage alone. In 1991, Livesley and associates[27] compared physical therapy alone with arthroscopic lavage and physical therapy in a randomized study. Pain with activity was statistically better in the lavage group at 3 and 6 months than in the group receiving therapy alone. Although the exact mechanism of the relief was unknown, Livesley and associates[27] speculated that it was the removal of cartilage debris and other inflammatory agents that resulted in the improved outcomes.

Although there were considerable technical limitations in the early cases, the potential advantages of this minimally invasive technique were clear at the time. During the same era, other surgical alternatives included arthrotomy and joint débridement. Magnuson[29] reported his results of open débridement with removal of all degenerative cartilage to bare bone and excision of the menisci and osteophytes in 1941. Postoperative treatment included Buck's traction and 8 to 10 days of bed rest.[29] Haggart[15] performed a similar procedure on patients with

Table 19–1. Radiographic Classification Systems

SYSTEM	GRADE	CLASSIFICATION OF OSTEOARTHRITIS
Kellgren and Lawrence	0	None
	1	Doubtful
	2	Minimal
	3	Moderate
	4	Severe
Ahlbach	0	Joint space not narrowed
	1	Joint space narrowed
	2	Obliterated, <50%
	3	Obliterated, >50%

arthritic knees, but also included a formal patellectomy. The postoperative course was daunting by today's standards with 5 to 7 days of casting, postoperative manipulation under anesthesia in all patients to break up adhesions, and 3 weeks of hospitalization.[15] Compared with the alternatives, the advantages of arthroscopy performed through stab incisions must have been appealing to the patients and surgeons. Burman and colleagues[9] noted that arthroscopic treatment was particularly valuable in patients who were unwilling to consider an arthrotomy. Despite the potential advantages of arthroscopic débridement, the technical limitations of the instruments restricted the application of this innovative approach, and open débridement remained the main tool available to orthopedic surgeons before the era of modern joint reconstructive techniques and arthroscopy. Despite the protracted postoperative courses noted by Magnuson[29] and Haggart,[15] patients generally responded well to the surgical interventions, providing anecdotal support for the concept of "cleaning out" the degenerative knee. In Magnuson's series,[29] 60 of 62 patients made a complete recovery from their symptoms, and in Haggart's report,[15] at 19 months to 5 years of follow-up, 19 of 20 patients were improved relative to their preoperative condition. With the development of more sophisticated instrumentation in the 1970s, the potential benefits of minimally invasive arthroscopic treatment could be harnessed and quickly supplanted open arthrotomy for the treatment of many forms of intra-articular knee pathology, including torn menisci, loose bodies, and synovitis. Even now, 30 years later, no consensus has yet emerged, however, regarding the role of this operative modality in the management of degenerative arthritis of the knee. Although published results have been inconsistent, independent

centers have reported satisfactory outcomes in approximately one-half to two-thirds of patients who undergo the procedure.[4,5,14,18,35,40,43] The improvements noted in these patients have been hypothesized to result from the removal of mechanical irritants, such as unstable meniscal tears and chondral flaps (Figs. 19–2 and 19–3), and lavage of cartilage debris and destructive enzymes that can provoke the inflammatory cascade. Favorable prognostic indicators include a short duration of mechanical-type symptoms, such as locking and catching; minimal mechanical malalignment of the extremity; absence of flexion contractures; less severe radiographic changes of osteoarthritis; and realistic patient goals and expectations.[4,5,14,18,35,40,43] When these general criteria have been used, statistically significant improvements in objective criteria, such as knee swelling and walking ability, have been achieved.

Sprague,[40] in 1981, was among the first in the modern era to report the advantages of arthroscopic débridement in a group of 78 knees with moderate to extreme arthritis. Intra-articular findings included articular cartilage damage to bone in 61% and meniscal tears in 83% of the knees.[40] At a mean of 13.4 months, 69 of the knees were evaluated, and despite the extensive articular damage identified intraoperatively, 74% of the patients reported good subjective outcomes.[40] In 1990, Baumgaertner et al[4] reported the outcomes of arthroscopic débridement in 49 arthritic knees in patients older than 50 years. Good and excellent results were obtained in 52% of patients at the time of maximal improvement, which occurred at a mean of 15 months; at 33 months postoperatively, only 40% of patients had good or excellent results.[4] Statistically significant correlations with better results were noted in patients with symptoms of less than 1 year duration, mechanical symptoms, mild or moderate radiographic changes, and normal mechanical alignment.[4] The importance of alignment also was noted by Harwin[18] and Ogilvie-Harris and Fitsialos.[35] In a retrospective review of 204 patients at a mean of 7.4 years postoperatively, favorable factors for good outcomes included smaller axial angulation at the time of arthroscopic débridement and the absence of prior surgery.[18] Overall, 63% of the patients were better than preoperatively, but in patients with normal alignment, the success rate was higher, at 84% satisfactory results versus 27% in patients with greater than 5 degrees of axial malalignment on a standing anteroposterior radiograph.[18] The association between better results and normal alignment also was noted by Ogilvie-Harris

Table 19–2. Intraoperative Classification Systems

SYSTEM	GRADE	DESCRIPTION	SIZE
Outerbridge	I	Softening and swelling	—
	II	Fragmentation and fissuring	<0.5 inch
	III	Fragmentation and fissuring	>0.5 inch
	IV	Erosion of cartilage to bone	—
Insall	I	Swelling and softening	—
	II	Deep fissures to subchondral bone	—
	III	Fibrillation	—
	IV	Erosion and exposure of subchondral bone	—

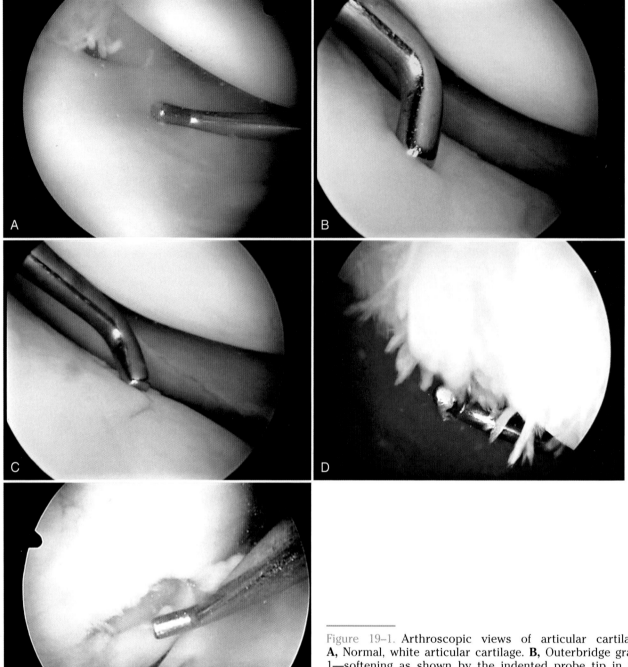

Figure 19-1. Arthroscopic views of articular cartilage. **A,** Normal, white articular cartilage. **B,** Outerbridge grade 1—softening as shown by the indented probe tip in the trochlea. **C,** Outerbridge grade 2—small fissure. **D,** Outerbridge grade 3—extensive fibrillation covering a large area of the patella. **E,** Outerbridge grade 4—erosion to subchondral bone.

and Fitsialos[35] in a study of 551 knees. At a mean of 4.1 years of follow-up, 53% of the patients still had good results.[35] The better results were obtained, however, in patients with normal alignment, unstable meniscal tears identified intraoperatively, and mild arthritis.[35] In addition to angular deformity in the coronal plane, the importance of fixed deformity in the sagittal plane has been noted. In a study by Fond and coworkers,[14] 36 patients with symptomatic knee arthritis that was refractory to nonsurgical

modalities underwent arthroscopic débridement. At 5 years of follow-up, 25 of the 36 patients were satisfied with the results of arthroscopic débridement.[14] Despite these generally favorable outcomes, poor results were correlated with flexion contractures greater than 10 degrees at the time of surgery.[14]

In support of the observation by Baumgaertner and associates,[4] the importance of mechanical symptoms, rather than unremitting pain, has been noted in other

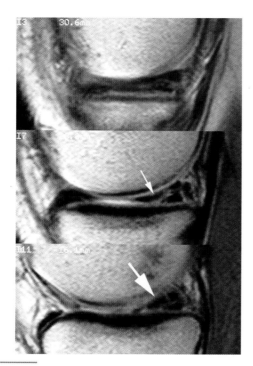

Figure 19–2. Three sagittal MRI "meniscal windows" of a complex, degenerative medial meniscal tear (*arrows*).

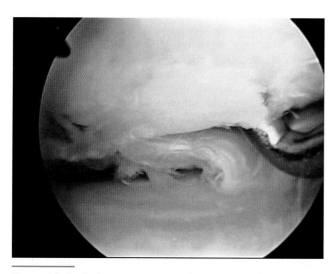

Figure 19–3. Arthroscopic view of a complex, degenerative meniscal tear.

reports. Yang and Nisonson[43] identified the presence of mechanical symptoms and mild articular degeneration as the most important predictors of good outcomes in their study of 105 knees. At a mean of 11.7 months' follow-up, good or excellent outcomes had been achieved in 65% of these knees.[43]

Although the intent of arthroscopic débridement in many of the aforementioned studies was to delay the need for knee replacement, McGinley and coworkers[30] were among the first to address this scenario specifically, where arthroscopic débridement was used selectively as a temporizing procedure in patients with osteoarthritis of

the knee who were apprehensive about undergoing total knee arthroplasty. In this circumstance, arthroscopic débridement should be considered an adjunct to nonsurgical modalities. As with nonsurgical modalities in this patient population, the goal of arthroscopic débridement should be considered symptomatic improvement, rather than complete relief. For successful outcomes to be achieved, when arthroscopic débridement is used in this manner, patient expectations and patient education are crucial.[30] Patients need to understand that lifestyle changes, including activity modification, are important. In their report, McGinley and coworkers[30] noted the results of arthroscopic débridement in a group of 77 patients with knee pain and radiographic changes consistent with significant osteoarthritis (Ahlbach grade 2 or 3), who were considered to be candidates for total knee arthroplasty but elected to undergo arthroscopic débridement as a temporizing procedure. At a mean of 13.2 years postoperatively, 67% had not proceeded to knee replacement; the mean postoperative patient satisfaction score regarding the success of the procedure was 8.6 on a scale of 0 to 10.[30]

Despite many published studies that have supported the use of arthroscopic débridement in the arthritic knee, more recent studies have rekindled the debate about whether this is an effective treatment modality. In a retrospective review of 126 patients, Dervin and associates[12] questioned the accuracy of physicians in predicting which patients would benefit. Only three variables were significantly associated with postoperative improvement: (1) the presence of medial joint line tenderness, (2) a positive Steinman test, and (3) the presence of an unstable meniscal tear identified at the time of the arthroscopy.[12] In 2002, questions also had been raised by another blinded, prospective, randomized study by Moseley and colleagues,[33] which did not show any therapeutic benefit versus the placebo effect seen in the control group. In this study, 180 patients were randomized to three treatment groups: (1) arthroscopic lavage; (2) arthroscopic débridement; and (3) a sham procedure in which the patient was anesthetized, received skin incisions and simulated débridement, but did not undergo any intra-articular intervention.[33] The results of this study suggested that the perceived benefits of arthroscopic débridement were simply due to the placebo effect alone because there were no differences in knee pain between the placebo group and either the lavage group or the débridement group at 1 or 2 years postoperatively.[33] These results challenged the continuing use of arthroscopic débridement in the osteoarthritic knee. Although the results of prospective and randomized studies provide the most convincing experimental data, critics of this study have questioned the validity of the results because of poor study design.[22] In particular, the failure to use previously identified favorable prognostic indicators in the patient selection has been condemned.[22] Rather than applying specific inclusion criteria, any patient younger than 75 years with osteoarthritis of the knee and knee pain, who had been treated with nonsurgical treatments for 6 months but had not undergone arthroscopy of the knee in the prior 2 years, was considered a candidate. Based on prior studies, this broad category of patients would have been considered poor candidates for arthroscopic débridement; it is not surprising that no significant treatment effect was identified in the arthroscopic débridement group versus the placebo group.[22] The radiologic assessment of the extent of the osteoarthritis was criticized because it was based on limited views that were inadequate for disease classification. Other selection bias concerns also were introduced because nearly all of the patients were male and were treated at a Veterans Administration facility. Finally, 44% of the patients who met the selection criteria refused to participate. It is unclear whether these results can be extrapolated to the general population because the motives and expectations of the patients who did consent are unknown.

The importance of applying previously documented favorable selection criteria cannot be underestimated. In 1993, Merchan and Galindo[31] reported the results of a smaller prospective, randomized trial in which tighter selection criteria were used. Inclusion in the study was limited to patients with less than 15 degrees of angular deformity, minimal joint space narrowing and osteophyte formation, pain less than 6 months' duration, and no prior surgery.[31] Comparing the results at final follow-up in the group of patients who underwent arthroscopy versus the patients who were treated without surgery, 75% versus 16% were improved, 14% versus 31% were unchanged, and 11% versus 53% were worse.[31] Although definitive studies have yet to be performed, it seems that a select group of patients with osteoarthritis of the knee are most likely to benefit from arthroscopic débridement. This group includes patients with short duration of mechanical symptoms, good range of motion, less angular deformity, less radiographic evidence of osteoarthritis, and reasonable expectations.[4,5,14,18,35,40,43]

Not only has patient selection been controversial, but also the key elements of the surgical technique have been debated. In general, arthroscopic débridement is now considered to imply arthroscopic joint lavage, excision of torn meniscal fragments, removal of loose bodies, and débridement of fibrillated or loose articular cartilage fragments, while avoiding creation of full-thickness articular cartilage defects. Abrasion arthroplasty, microfracture, and extensive radiofrequency cartilage ablation generally are not considered part of the technique and are discussed under subsequent headings. If the broad patient selection criteria and the general technical principles noted previously are used, it is reasonable to expect symptomatic relief in about one-half to two-thirds of the patients undergoing arthroscopic débridement at short-term to midterm follow-up.[4,5,14,18,35,40,43]

CARTILAGE REPAIR TECHNIQUES

Hyaline cartilage lacks a blood and nerve supply, and as a result partial-thickness and full-thickness injuries have limited healing abilities in adults. In situ repair processes generally require that the subchondral bone be penetrated. This penetration allows mesenchymal cells from the marrow to populate the cartilage defect and produce a fibrocartilage substitute, which is composed primarily of type I collagen, rather than the type II collagen of hyaline cartilage. The mechanical properties of this fibrocartilage substitute are inferior to the original hyaline cartilage. Although the basic biology of cartilage is understood, and a variety of cartilage repair options have proven clinical results in young patients with focal lesions, a durable biological resurfacing for the osteoarthritic knee is not yet a realistic option. Not only is understanding of normal articular cartilage incomplete, but also other pathologic changes that are part of the disease process, including limb malalignment and degenerative and compensatory changes in the ligaments and soft tissues about the knee, confound the problems in treating the diffuse articular cartilage damage of the osteoarthritic knee. In the following sections, the broad categories of cartilage repair techniques that currently exist and the utility of these techniques for treating the osteoarthritic knee are reviewed. In general, although these techniques have achieved good results at midterm follow-up in young patients with isolated articular cartilage defects that are described in detail in other chapters of this text, the indications for use in the osteoarthritic knee are limited.

Marrow-Stimulating Techniques

The concept of drilling through the subchondral bone in an area of cartilage loss, to stimulate reparative cartilage formation, was popularized by Pridie in 1959.[19,37] Successful outcomes were reported in 74% of 62 arthritic knees in which this technique was performed as part of an open débridement.[19] Since that time, a variety of techniques have been used to stimulate the limited fibrocartilage repair mechanism that occurs in the adult knee in vivo, including mechanical abrasion, drilling, and microfracture of the subchondral bone. Each of these techniques is best suited to small, isolated lesions (<1 to 2 cm²) in knees without significant malalignment. The pioneers of these techniques have emphasized the importance of prolonged periods of modified weightbearing postoperatively, with the use of crutches for 6 to 8 weeks and avoidance of pivoting or impact sports for 6 months or more. Although limited success has been reported with the use of these techniques in younger patients, little evidence exists to support the routine use of these procedures in the arthritic knee versus arthroscopic treatment alone, especially considering the significant postoperative restrictions that are recommended.

ABRASION CHONDROPLASTY

Abrasion chondroplasty was one of the first marrow-stimulating techniques described during the 1980s and was first described as a palliative, salvage technique for patients with severe degenerative arthritis who are trying to avoid knee replacement.[23,24] Contraindications include severe malalignment, ligamentous instability, morbid obesity, or unwillingness to comply with 2 months' non-weightbearing requirement.[24] This technique is performed with a mechanical bur, which is used to remove the superficial layer of subchondral bone. The removal of this layer allows the mesenchymal marrow cells that stimulate the fibrocartilage repair process to be released into the lesion. Analysis of biopsy samples, obtained during second-look arthroscopy, has confirmed that the reparative material is fibrocartilage, rather than the original hyaline cartilage.[23] Results of the operation have been mixed. If the success is judged by the avoidance of knee replacement, which is the main goal of the procedure in this patient population, the results have been good. At 5 years' follow-up, Johnson[24] reported that 86% of patients in a cohort of 248 had not required further operations, and only 6% had progressed to total knee replacement. If symptomatic relief is the main criterion, however, results have been more mixed. At a mean follow-up of 3 years, only 24% of the patients did not have complaints of pain, loss of motion, or limp, and 99% had restriction of activity.[24] Results from other centers also have been less good. In 1991, Rand[38] compared the results of arthroscopic débridement alone with débridement and abrasion arthroplasty. At a mean follow-up of 3.8 years, abrasion arthroplasty did not seem to offer any significant advantage over arthroscopic débridement alone, and 50% of the abrasion arthroplasty group had progressed to total knee replacement by 3 years.[38] Similar results had been reported by Bert and Maschka[5] in 1989; at a mean of 60 months' follow-up in 126 patients treated with either arthroscopic débridement alone or arthroscopic débridement and abrasion arthroplasty, the group who had undergone simple débridement had better outcomes. In the arthroscopic débridement group, 66% had good results, 13% had fair results, and 21% had poor results; in distinction, in the group who also had undergone abrasion arthroplasty, only 51% had good to excellent results, 16% had fair results, and 33% had poor results.[5] The unpredictable nature of this technique has limited the general acceptance of this treatment option for patients with arthritic knees.

SUBCHONDRAL DRILLING

Subchondral drilling is another technique for promoting the release of mesenchymal marrow cells to promote the fibrocartilage repair process. In contrast to abrasion arthroplasty, multiple discrete holes are drilled through the denuded areas into the subchondral bone. Few long-term reports have been published, and the results generally fail to show significant advantages versus arthroscopic débridement alone. Richards and Lonergan[39] reported their experience comparing subchondral drilling and arthroscopic débridement with arthroscopic débridement alone; the results were similar for both groups.

MICROFRACTURE

The microfracture technique is a third method that attempts to enhance the native in vivo fibrocartilage repair process.[42] It is indicated for full-thickness loss of articular cartilage in a weightbearing area between the femur and the tibia or an area of contact between the patella and the trochlea; contraindications include patients older than 60 years and mechanical axis alignment greater than 5 degrees varus or valgus on a full-length, standing hip to ankle radiograph.[42] Consequently, many patients with degenerative arthritis are not good candidates for this procedure.

In this technique, the subchondral bone is first denuded of any remaining cartilage with a shaver or curet. Next, an arthroscopic awl is used to create multiple small puncture holes, a few millimeters in diameter. Holes should be about 3 to 4 mm apart and penetrate 2 to 4 mm into the subchondral bone.[42] A significant period of 6 to 8 weeks of crutch-assisted, limited weightbearing is required postoperatively.[42] Theoretical advantages of this technique versus drilling include less thermal damage to the subchondral bone and surrounding cartilage; second, the awls may be contoured, which allows easier access to the entire joint.[42] As with the other marrow-stimulating techniques, inferior fibrocartilage is produced by the repair process, rather than true hyaline cartilage. Although this technique may have some theoretical advantages and may provide some practical advantages for the surgeon, the published clinical results are limited to young patients with focal defects, and little is known about the use in patients with osteoarthritis.[41] Consequently, there can be little support for routine application of this intervention, especially in view of the significant postoperative disability that results from the prolonged recuperation that has been recommended.

Autologous and Allogeneic Cartilage Transplantation

The marrow-stimulating techniques all create a fibrocartilage substitute with inferior mechanical properties to true hyaline cartilage. In contrast, techniques that aim to restore the articular surface with true hyaline cartilage articular surface have been developed. These are generally techniques for transplanting autologous or allogeneic cartilage cells to the damaged area. A wide variety of different techniques fall under this general heading, including transfer of autologous osteochondral plugs of different sizes transplanted from one area of the knee to another; implantation of autologous cells that have been harvested from the patient's knee, cultured in-vivo, and injected in a sterile solution under a watertight perichondral patch; and allogeneic osteochondral plugs or bulk osteochondral grafts. As with the marrow-stimulating techniques, most of these techniques have been developed for use in patients with focal, well-defined traumatic defects, or osteochondritis dissecans, rather than in patients with diffuse degenerative changes and mechanical malalignment. Evidence of reduced healing potential in older patients generally has limited the use of these techniques to patients 50 to 60 years old and younger. Most patients with osteoarthritis of the knee are poor candidates for these techniques. Also as with the marrow-stimulating techniques, these procedures are associated with prolonged periods of activity modification postoperatively. Typically, limited weightbearing for 6 to 12 weeks is required with avoidance of impact activities for a further 6 months or more.

AUTOGENOUS OSTEOCHONDRAL PLUG TRANSFER

Autogenous osteochondral plug transfer involves the harvesting of small plugs of autologous cartilage with the subchondral bone base and transplanting them to an area of chondral damage in the same knee, where the plugs are press-fit into prepared tunnels. The plugs typically are harvested from non-weightbearing areas of the knee, such as adjacent to the intercondylar notch or lateral femoral condyle superior to the sulcus terminalis. This technique may be performed either entirely arthroscopically or in a limited open manner. Alternate methods have been described using a few large plugs, generally 5 to 10 mm in diameter, or multiple smaller plugs 2.7 to 8.5 mm in diameter.[16,17] This latter method, first described by Hangody and associates,[17] has been termed *mosaicplasty*. These multiple small plugs can be used to fill lesions 4 cm^2, but the technique probably is best suited for lesions 1 to 2 cm^2.[16] Smaller lesions usually can be managed entirely arthroscopically, but may require a limited, open arthrotomy. The treatment of larger lesions generally is limited by the availability of donor sites, and in these cases, an open arthrotomy is often required to facilitate harvest of the plugs or transplantation. It is important that the plug harvest, preparation of the recipient tunnel, and implantation of the plug are done perpendicular to the articular surface, to create a uniform articular surface and to avoid damage to the plugs. The small voids between the transplanted plugs become filled with fibrocartilage. In many cases, the microfracture technique can be used to stimulate fibrocartilage between the transplanted plugs. Care should be taken, however, to avoid damaging the area surrounding the plugs that may lead to failure of the press-fit plugs. Using this technique, the resulting composite articular surface has been shown to be composed of approximately 80% transplanted hyaline cartilage and 20% fibrocartilage; typically the donor sites heal with a fibrocartilage cap within approximately 6 to 8 weeks.[16] Favorable postoperative outcomes, based on standardized clinical rating systems, including the modified HSS (Hospital for Special Surgery) score, Lysholm, and Modified Cincinnati scores, have been reported, with good to excellent results in 92% of patients with femoral lesions and 88% of patients with tibial lesions.[16] This technique should be considered only for focal cartilage defects in young patients, however, because the contraindications, including age older than 50 years, malalignment, and instability, preclude most patients with osteoarthritis of the knee. Based on their experience with a group of patients with multiple degenerative lesions who underwent autogenous osteochondral plug transfer, Andres and colleagues[2] in 2003 cautioned against the use of this technique in the arthritic knee. In their experience, better outcomes were not achieved by combining this technique with osteotomy when the limb was malaligned.[2]

AUTOLOGOUS CHONDROCYTE IMPLANTATION

Autologous chondrocyte implantation/transplantation is best suited to larger lesions (typically >2 cm^2) that involve a single condyle of the knee.[6,7,32] The surgical technique is a two-stage process that is separated by weeks to months. In the first operation, chondrocytes from the patient's knee are harvested arthroscopically and cultured in vitro to produce 20 to 50 times the original number of cells. During the culture process, the cells dedifferentiate, and the resulting chondrocytes are similar to mesenchymal cells. At the second operation, which requires a formal open arthrotomy for exposure, these cultured cells are injected in a sterile solution under a watertight periosteal graft patch that is harvested from the proximal tibia and sewn over the damaged articular surface defect. Analysis of cartilage obtained through second-look arthroscopies has shown superior hyaline-like cartilage.[6,7] This is a controversial finding, however. In a report of a randomized, prospective study comparing the results of autologous chondrocyte implantation with microfracture in patients younger than 45 years, Knutsen and coworkers[26] documented that there was no statistically significant histologic difference in the cartilage produced, with hyaline, fibrocartilage, and mixed areas found in both groups. Midterm to long-term follow-up with favorable results have been reported using autologous chondrocyte implantation, but the best results have been obtained in patients with unipolar femoral condyle lesions rather than multifocal or kissing lesions.[7,19,32] In a group of 213 patients at 2 to 10 years' follow-up, 90% of the patients with femoral condyle lesions in the study reported by Brittberg and colleagues[7] had excellent or good results using the Cincinnati rating score versus only 58% with trochlear lesions and 75% with multiple lesions. These favorable results were achieved in young patients with mean ages in the early 30s, however, rather than older patients.[7] Minas[32] reported the results in 71 salvage cases of knees with multiple lesions and early arthritic changes and in knees with bipolar lesions. In this group, in which the mean resurfaced area was a large 11.66 cm^2 per knee, statistically significant improvements in SF36 quality-of-life scores and Cincinnati rating scale were reported at 24 months' follow-up when the patellofemoral joint was not involved.[32] In this group, 80% of the patients reported good or excellent results, and 90% were satisfied with their outcomes; 93% of these patients thought they were better than before the procedure.[32] Approximately 50% of these patients also underwent an osteotomy, however, to correct alignment problems, and it is difficult to determine the relative effects of these individual procedures. In addition, a prospective, randomized study by Knutsen and associates[26] comparing autologous chondrocyte implantation with microfracture failed to show any advantage in the clinical outcomes in the group with the two-stage cartilage implantation; the reoperation rate in the autologous cartilage implantation group was significantly higher. At this time, this technique should be considered experimental for the diffuse cartilage damage that is encountered in the osteoarthritic knee, and use of this technique should be part of a clinical study. The role of this technique in conjunction with simultaneous or staged osteotomy has not been defined clearly and requires further investigation.

ALLOGENEIC OSTEOCHONDRAL TRANSPLANTATION

Transplantation of large osteochondral allografts has been performed, using a variety of techniques, in cases of traumatic articular cartilage injuries and osteochondritis dissecans. These techniques include giant osteochondral plugs ($\geq$2 cm in diameter) that are used in much the same way as the autogenous plugs; resurfacing techniques, in which thin articular sections with the subchondral bone are used; and replacement techniques of an entire hemicondyle. These large grafts are best suited for large areas of cartilage damage more than 3 to 4 cm in diameter, uncontained defects, or lesions with osseous defects more than 1 cm deep that preclude the use of either autologous osteochondral plug transfer or autologous chondrocyte implantation.[3] Although the potential for donor site morbidity is eliminated using these allogeneic grafts, concerns exist about the risks of disease transmission, owing to viral and other submicroscopic vector transmission, and bacterial contamination, owing to improper graft harvest and storage techniques. The immunologic characteristics of the fresh osteochondral allograft have been studied extensively. Although the chondrocytes contain antigens, their location within the cartilage matrix protects them from a significant host response.[8] Although an antibody response can occur, immunologic rejection does not seem to be a clinically significant issue, and no attempt currently is made to match donor and recipient for immunologic parameters.[8]

Long-term results detailing the clinical results of these techniques, used with or without supplemental procedures, such as osteotomy, in patients with osteoarthritis or bipolar cartilage lesions are sparse. In 2001, Aubin and coworkers[3] reported the results of their experience with fresh osteochondral allografts used in 72 patients with post-traumatic cartilage lesions greater than 3 cm in diameter and more than 1 cm deep of the distal femur. In this series, Kaplan-Meier survivorship at 10 years was 85% and at 15 years was 74%; 12 failures had occurred among 60 grafts that were available for long-term follow-up at a mean of 10 years.[3] Because more than physiologic loading was shown on preoperative full-length, weightbearing radiographs, 68% of the patients underwent simultaneous realignment osteotomy.[3] Among the 48 surviving grafts at mean 10-year follow-up, 40 patients (84%) had good or excellent HSS scores.[3] Bugbee and Convery[8] reported their results with large "shell" osteochondral grafts in 1999; at a mean of 2 years postoperatively, the success rate was 86% for patients with monopolar lesions, but in patients with bipolar lesions, who underwent grafting of both lesions, the success rate was only 53%. At a mean of 50 months, 7 of the 30 patients who had undergone bipolar grafting had required further surgery because of treatment failure, with 5 undergoing total knee replacement and 2 electing arthrodesis.[8]

GROWTH FACTORS AND BIOLOGIC AND SYNTHETIC MATRICES

Currently, research is being conducted to identify biologic and synthetic materials that can be used to fill osteochondral defects. These materials may act as simple scaffolds or stimulate extrinsic repair processes through the incorporation of growth factors or even autologous cells. Preformed and injectable materials are being developed. Desirable features of these scaffolds include the ability to provide good initial fixation to the host site, adequate mechanical strength to protect the cells within it, the ability to facilitate cell attachment and growth, and a biodegradable matrix that can be replaced as the new cartilage develops.[11,21] The ultimate goal of tissue engineering is to create histologically and functionally normal tissue via implantation of a scaffold that can serve as a mechanical substrate for cells and bioactive factors to help direct and organize tissue regeneration.[28] Currently, no long-term clinical results of more recent advances in tissue engineering are available, but the potential advantages of these materials for patients with osteoarthritis of the knee and isolated chondral defects continue to stimulate intense research efforts.

CONCLUSIONS

Many treatment options exist for managing patients with symptomatic osteoarthritis, and numerous factors determine how the various modalities should be used, such as age, activity levels, and expectations. Arthroscopic débridement should remain in the armamentarium of orthopedic surgeons for treatment of patients with osteoarthritis of the knee. Key elements of the technique include removal of loose bodies, excision of unstable meniscal fragments and chondral flaps, and avoidance of extensive débridement of fibrillated cartilage. The additional morbidity associated with marrow-stimulating techniques and cartilage transplantation, without correcting limb alignment, precludes the use of these procedures as a routine part of arthroscopic débridement in patients with generalized degenerative cartilage damage. Arthroscopic débridement should be considered complementary to nonsurgical options, including nonsteroidal anti-inflammatory drugs, hyaluronic acid injections, and physical therapy, and other surgical procedures, including osteotomy and knee replacement. Appropriate patient selection is crucial for each of these treatment options. Indications still need to be refined for optimal results with each option, and research will undoubtedly continue. At present, the best prognosis after arthroscopic débridement is for younger patients with mechanical symptoms of short duration, in whom the radiographic changes show mild to moderate osteoarthritis and minimal limb malalignment. In these patients, arthroscopic intervention should be considered palliative and not curative. Above all else, regardless of the treatment option, patient expectations need to be realistic.

References

1. Ahlbach S: Osteoarthrosis of the knee: A radiologic investigation. Acta Radiol 227(Suppl):S7, 1968.

2. Andres BM, Mears SC, Somel DS, et al: Treatment of osteoarthritic cartilage lesions with osteochondral autograft transplantation. Orthopedics 26:1121, 2003.

3. Aubin PP, Cheah HK, Davis AM, Gross AE: Long-term followup of fresh femoral osteochondral allografts for posttraumatic knee defects. Clin Orthop 391(Suppl):S318, 2001.

4. Baumgaertner MR, Cannon WD Jr, Vittori JM, et al: Arthroscopic debridement of the arthritic knee. Clin Orthop 253:197, 1990.

5. Bert JM, Maschka K: The arthroscopic treatment of unicompartmental gonarthrosis: A five-year follow-up study of abrasion arthroplasty plus arthroscopic debridement and arthroscopic debridement alone. Arthroscopy 5:25, 1989.

6. Brittberg M, Lindahl A, Nilsson A, et al: Treatment of deep cartilage defects in the knee with autologous chondrocyte transplantation. N Engl J Med 331:889, 1994.

7. Brittberg M, Tallheden T, Sjogren-Jansson B, et al: Autologous chondrocytes used for articular cartilage repair: An update. Clin Orthop 391(Suppl):S337, 2001.

8. Bugbee WD, Convery FR: Osteochondral allograft transplantation. Clin Sports Med 18:67, 1999.

9. Burman MS, Finkelstein H, Mayer L: Arthroscopy of the knee joint. J Bone Joint Surg Am 16:255, 1934.

10. Casscells SW: Gross pathological changes in the knee joint of the aged individual: A study of 300 cases. Clin Orthop 132:225, 1978.

11. Coutts RD, Healey RM, Ostrander R, et al: Matrices for cartilage repair. Clin Orthop 391(Suppl):S271, 2001.

12. Dervin GF, Stiell IG, Rody K, Grabowski J: Effect of arthroscopic debridement for osteoarthritis of the knee on health-related quality of life. J Bone Joint Surg Am 85:10, 2003.

13. Dougadas M, Ayral X, Listrat V, et al: The SFA system for assessing articular cartilage lesion at arthroscopy of the knee. Arthroscopy 10:69, 1994.

14. Fond J, Rodin D, Ahmad S, Nirschl RP: Arthroscopic debridement for the treatment of osteoarthritis of the knee: 2- and 5-year results. Arthroscopy 18:829, 2002.

15. Haggart GE: Surgical treatment of degenerative arthritis of the knee joint. J Bone Joint Surg Br 22:717, 1940.

16. Hangody L, Feczko P, Bartha L, et al: Mosaicplasty for the treatment of articular defects of the knee and ankle. Clin Orthop 391(Suppl):328, 2001.

17. Hangody L, Kish G, Karpati Z, et al: Mosaicplasty for the treatment of articular cartilage defects: Application in clinical practice. Orthopedics 21:751, 1998.

18. Harwin SF: Arthroscopic debridement for osteoarthritis of the knee: Predictors of patient satisfaction. Arthroscopy 15:142, 1999.

19. Insall J: The Pridie debridement operation for osteoarthritis of the knee. Clin Orthop 101:61, 1974.

20. Insall J, Falvo KA, Wise DW: Chondromalacia patellae: A prospective study. J Bone Joint Surg Am 58:1, 1976.

21. Jackson DW, Scheer MJ, Simon TM: Cartilage substitutes: Overview of basic science and treatment options. J Am Acad Orthop Surg 9:37, 2001.

22. Johnson LJ: Letter to the editor. Arthroscopy 7:683, 2002.

23. Johnson LL: Arthroscopic abrasion arthroplasty: Historical and pathologic status. Arthroscopy 2:54, 1986.

24. Johnson LL: Arthroscopic abrasion arthroplasty: A review. Clin Orthop 391(Suppl):306, 2001.

25. Kellgren JH, Lawrence JS: Radiological assessment of osteo-arthrosis. Ann Rheum Dis 16:494, 1957.

26. Knutsen G, Engebretsen L, Ludvigsen TC, et al: Autologous chondrocyte implantation compared with microfracture in the knee: A randomized trial. J Bone Joint Surg Am 86:455, 2004.

27. Livesley PJ, Doherty M, Needoff M, Moulton A: Arthroscopic lavage of osteoarthritic knees. J Bone Joint Surg Br 73:922, 1991.

28. Lu L, Zhu X, Valenzuela RG, et al: Biodegradable polymer scaffolds for cartilage tissue engineering. Clin Orthop 391(Suppl):S251, 2001.

29. Magnuson PB: Joint debridement: Surgical treatment of degenerative arthritis. Surg Gynecol Obstet 73:1, 1941.

30. McGinley BJ, Cushner FD, Scott WN: Debridement arthroscopy: 10-year follow-up. Clin Orthop 367:190, 1999.

31. Merchan ECR, Galindo E: Arthroscopy-guided surgery versus non-operative treatment for limited degenerative osteoarthritis of the femorotibial joint in patients over 50 years of age: A prospective comparative study. Arthroscopy 9:663, 1993.

32. Minas T: Autologous chondrocyte implantation for focal chondral defects of the knee. Clin Orthop 391(Suppl):S349, 2001.

33. Moseley JB, O'Malley K, Petersen NJ, et al: A controlled trial of arthroscopic surgery for osteoarthritis of the knee. N Engl J Med 347:81, 2002.

34. Noyes FR, Stabler CL: A system for grading articular cartilage lesions at arthroscopy. Am J Sports Med 17:505, 1989.

35. Ogilvie-Harris DJ, Fitsialos DP: Arthroscopic management of the degenerative knee. Arthroscopy 7:151, 1991.

36. Outerbridge RE: The etiology of chondromalacia patellae. J Bone Joint Surg Br 43:752, 1961.

37. Pridie AH: A method of resurfacing osteoarthritic knee joints. J Bone Joint Surg Br 41:617, 1959.

38. Rand JA: Role of arthroscopy in osteoarthritis of the knee. Arthroscopy 7:358, 1991.

39. Richards RN, Lonergan RP: Arthroscopic surgery for relief of pain in the osteoarthritic knee. Orthopedics 7:1705, 1984.

40. Sprague NF III: Arthroscopic debridement for degenerative knee joint disease. Clin Orthop 160:118, 1981.

41. Steadman JR, Briggs KK, Rodrigo JJ, et al: Outcomes of microfracture for traumatic chondral defects of the knee: Average 11-year follow-up. Arthroscopy 19:477-484, 2003.

42. Steadman JR, Rodkey WG, Rodrigo JJ: Microfracture: Surgical technique and rehabilitation to treat chondral defects. Clin Orthop 391(Suppl):S362, 2001.

43. Yang SS, Nisonson B: Arthroscopic surgery of the knee in the geriatric patient. Clin Orthop 316:50, 1995.

CHAPTER 20

Débridement and Microfracture for Full-Thickness Articular Cartilage Defects

J. R. Steadman • W. G. Rodkey • K. K. Briggs • J. J. Rodrigo

Full-thickness articular cartilage defects in the knee are common, and the lesions may occur in a variety of clinical settings and at different ages.[3-6,15,16] A single event, the shearing forces of the femur on the tibia, may result in trauma to the articular cartilage and cause it to fracture, lacerate, and separate from the underlying subchondral bone or separate with a piece of the subchondral bone.[4,15,16] Alternatively, chronic repetitive loading in excess of normal physiological levels may result in fatigue and failure of the articular surface. Single events are usually found in younger groups, whereas chronic degenerative lesions are seen in middle-age and older groups.[4,11,15,16] It has been shown that repetitive impacts can cause cartilage swelling, an increase in collagen fiber diameter, and an alteration in the relationship between collagen and proteoglycans.[15,16] Thus, acute events may not result in full-thickness cartilage loss but rather start a degenerative cascade that can lead to chronic full-thickness loss. The degenerative cascade typically includes early softening and fibrillation (grade I), fissures and cracks in the surface of the cartilage (grade II), severe fissures and cracks with a "crab meat" appearance (grade III), and finally, exposure of subchondral bone (grade IV).[4,11,15,16]

Articular cartilage defects that extend full thickness to subchondral bone rarely heal without intervention.[2-5,19-21,23-28,31,32] Some patients may not experience clinically significant problems from acute full-thickness chondral defects, but most eventually suffer from degenerative changes that can be debilitating.[4,5,21,32] Techniques used to treat chondral defects include abrasion, drilling, osteochondral autografts, osteochondral allografts, and autologous cell transplantation.[2-4,8,11] The senior author (JRS) developed the "microfracture" technique to enhance chondral resurfacing by providing a suitable environment for new tissue formation and taking advantage of the body's own healing potential.[2,7,8,19,21,23-28] The senior author's clinical experience now includes more than 2500 patients in whom microfracture has been performed.

We have found that arthroscopic débridement accompanied by microfracture of subchondral bone is a reliable and repeatable procedure to stimulate biological repair of cartilage defects of the knee in patients in whom nonoperative treatment has failed or in whom acute lesions were encountered during arthroscopy. Thus, more invasive procedures, such as osteotomy, cartilage grafting, or unicompartmental arthroplasty, might be avoided or at least delayed for several years. Specifically, the goals of this procedure are to alleviate the pain and attendant disabilities that result from the chondral lesions and, furthermore, to prevent late degenerative changes in the joint by restoring the joint surface.[21,25]

INDICATIONS FOR MICROFRACTURE

Microfracture was designed initially for patients with post-traumatic articular cartilage lesions of the knee that had progressed to full-thickness chondral defects. Microfracture is still the most commonly indicated technique for full-thickness loss of articular cartilage in either a weight-bearing area between the femur and tibia or an area of contact between the patella and trochlear groove.[19-21,23-28,31] Unstable cartilage that overlies subchondral bone is also an indication for microfracture. If a partial-thickness lesion is probed and the cartilage simply scrapes off down to bone, we consider this to be a full-thickness lesion. Degenerative joint disease in a knee that has proper axial alignment is another common indication for microfracture. These lesions all involve loss of articular cartilage at the bone-cartilage interface.

Patients with acute chondral injuries are treated as soon as practical after the diagnosis is made, especially if the knee is being treated concurrently for meniscus or anterior cruciate ligament pathology. Patients with chronic or degenerative chondral lesions are often treated nonoperatively (conservatively) for at least 12 weeks after a suspected chondral lesion is diagnosed clinically. This treatment regimen includes activity modification, physical therapy, nonsteroidal anti-inflammatory drugs, joint injections, and perhaps dietary supplements that may have cartilage-stimulating properties. If nonoperative treatment is not successful, surgical treatment is considered.[2,19,23-28,31]

No limitations are placed on how large an acute lesion can be and still be considered suitable for microfracture.[23,25] We have observed that even very large acute lesions respond well to microfracture.[21] We have noted empirically that traumatic lesions, acute or chronic, that are less than 400 mm^2 tend to respond better to microfracture than do lesions greater than 400 mm^2, but we have not found this difference to be statistically significant.[17,21] Treatment of chronic degenerative lesions is not specifically limited by size, but more emphasis is placed on proper axial alignment and the presence of global degenerative changes throughout the knee.[17,25]

General considerations for use of the microfracture procedure include patient age, acceptable biomechanical alignment of the knee, the patient's activity level, and the patient's expectations.[17,21,25,26,28] If all these criteria define a patient who could benefit from chondral resurfacing, microfracture is considered.

CONTRAINDICATIONS TO MICROFRACTURE

Specific contraindications to microfracture include axial malalignment (as described later), patients unwilling or unable to follow the required strict and rigorous rehabilitation protocol, partial-thickness defects, and an inability to use the opposite leg for weightbearing during the minimal or non-weightbearing period.[24,25] Other specific contraindications include any systemic immune-mediated disease, disease-induced arthritis, or cartilage disease. A relative contraindication exists for patients older than 65 years because the authors have observed that some patients older than 65 experience difficulty with crutch walking and the required rigorous rehabilitation.[24,25] Other contraindications to microfracture include global degenerative osteoarthrosis and cartilage surrounding the lesion that is too thin to establish a perpendicular rim to hold the marrow clot.[17,24,25] In these advanced degenerative cases, axial malalignment is also a confounding factor.[17]

Two methods for radiographic measurement of the biomechanical alignment of the weightbearing axis of the knee are used in our facility: (1) the angle made between the femur and tibia on anteroposterior views obtained with the patient standing and (2) the weightbearing mechanical axis drawn from the center of the femoral head to the center of the tibiotarsal joint on long, standing (~51 inches/130 cm) radiographs. If the angle drawn between the tibia and femur is greater than 5 degrees of varus or valgus when compared with the normal knee, this amount of axial malalignment would be a relative contraindication to microfracture. Preferably, the mechanical axis weightbearing line should be in the central quarter of the tibial plateau of either the medial or lateral compartment. If the mechanical axis weightbearing line falls outside the central-most quarter of the plateaus, medial or lateral, this weightbearing shift would also be a relative contraindication if left uncorrected. In such cases, a realignment procedure should be included as a part of the overall treatment regimen.[17,25]

PREOPERATIVE PLANNING

Patients with knee joint pain undergo a thorough physical and orthopedic examination. The chondral lesions can be on the joint surfaces of the femur, tibia, and/or patella. At times, the physical diagnosis can be difficult and elusive, especially if only an isolated chondral defect is present. Identification of point tenderness over a femoral condyle or tibial plateau is a useful finding but, in itself, is not diagnostic. If compression of the patella elicits pain, this finding might be indicative of a patellar or trochlear lesion.

For diagnostic imaging, we use long, standing radiographs as described earlier to observe for angular deformity and the joint space narrowing that is often indicative of loss of articular cartilage. We also obtain standard anteroposterior and lateral radiographs of both knees, as well as weightbearing views with the knees flexed to 30 to 45 degrees. Patellar views are also useful to evaluate the patellofemoral joint. Magnetic resonance imaging with newer diagnostic sequences specific for articular cartilage has become a mainstay of our diagnostic workup of patients with suspected chondral lesions.

SURGICAL TECHNIQUE

Three portals are routinely made about the knee for use of the inflow cannula, the arthroscope, and the working instruments. We typically do not use a tourniquet during the microfracture procedure; rather, we vary the arthroscopic fluid pump pressure to control bleeding. An initial thorough diagnostic examination of the knee should be performed. We carefully inspect all geographic areas of the knee, including the suprapatellar pouch, the medial and lateral gutters, the patellofemoral joint, the intercondylar notch and its contents, and the medial and lateral compartments, as well as the posterior horns of both menisci. We do all other intra-articular procedures before performing the microfracture technique, with the exception of ligament reconstruction. This technique helps prevent loss of visualization when the fat droplets and blood enter the knee from the microfracture holes. Importantly, we pay particular attention to soft tissues, such as plicae and the lateral retinaculum, that could potentially produce increased compression between cartilage surfaces.[21,23-26,28]

After carefully assessing the full-thickness articular cartilage lesion, we débride the exposed bone of all remaining unstable cartilage. We use a hand-held curved curet and a full-radius resector to débride the cartilage. It is critical to débride all loose or marginally attached cartilage from the surrounding rim of the lesion. The calcified cartilage layer that remains as a cap to many lesions must be removed, preferably by using a curet. Thorough and complete removal of the calcified cartilage layer is extremely important based on animal studies that we have completed.[7,8] Care should be taken to maintain the integrity of the subchondral plate by not débriding too deeply. This prepared lesion, with a stable perpendicular edge of healthy well-attached viable cartilage surrounding the defect, provides a pool that helps hold the marrow clot, "super clot" as we have termed it, as it forms (Fig. 20-1).[25]

After preparation of the lesion, we use an arthroscopic awl to make multiple holes, or "microfractures," in the exposed subchondral bone plate. We use an awl with an angle that permits the tip to be perpendicular to the bone as it is advanced, typically 30 or 45 degrees. There is also a 90-degree awl that is typically used only on the patella or other soft bone. The 90-degree awl should be advanced only manually, not with a mallet. The holes are made as close together as possible, but not so close that one breaks into another, thus damaging the subchondral plate

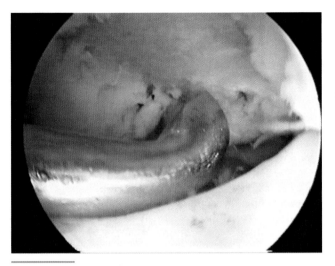

Figure 20–1. A curet is used to remove the calcified cartilage layer of a full-thickness chondral defect. Damaged cartilage has been débrided to form a stable perpendicular edge of healthy cartilage. (From Steadman JR, Rodkey WG, Briggs KK: Microfracture chondroplasty: Indications, techniques, and outcomes. Sports Med Arthrosc Rev 11:236-244, 2003.)

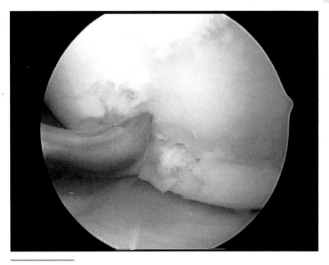

Figure 20–2. A chondral defect has been débrided and is being microfractured. The microfracture holes are started at the periphery of the defect adjacent to the stable cartilage. (From Steadman JR, Rodkey WG, Briggs KK: Microfracture chondroplasty: Indications, techniques, and outcomes. Sports Med Arthrosc Rev 11:236-244, 2003.)

between them. This technique usually results in microfracture holes that are approximately 3 to 4 mm apart. When fat droplets can be seen coming from the marrow cavity, the appropriate depth (approximately 2 to 4 mm) has been reached. The arthroscopic awls probably produce essentially no thermal necrosis of the bone as compared with hand-driven or motorized drills. We make microfracture holes around the periphery of the defect first, immediately adjacent to the healthy stable cartilage rim (Fig. 20–2). Then we complete the process by making the microfracture holes toward the center of the defect (Fig. 20–3). We assess the treated lesion at the conclusion of the microfracture to ensure that a sufficient number of holes have been made before we reduce the arthroscopic irrigation fluid flow (Fig. 20–4). After the arthroscopic irrigation fluid pump pressure is reduced, under direct visualization we are able to observe the release of marrow fat droplets and blood from the microfracture holes into the subchondral bone. We judge the quantity of marrow contents flowing into the joint to be adequate when we observe marrow emanating from all microfracture holes (Fig. 20–5). We then remove all instruments from the knee and evacuate the joint of fluid.[24,25] Intra-articular drains should not be used because the goal is for a surgically induced marrow clot rich in marrow elements to form and stabilize while covering the lesion.[7,8]

Chronic degenerative chondral lesions commonly have extensive eburnated bone and bony sclerosis with thickening of the subchondral plate,[11,17] thus making it difficult to perform an adequate microfracture procedure. In these instances and when the axial alignment and other indications for microfracture are met, we first make a few microfracture holes with the awls in various locations of the lesion to assess the thickness of the subchondral plate. We often use a motorized bur to remove the sclerotic bone until punctate bleeding is seen. After bleeding appears

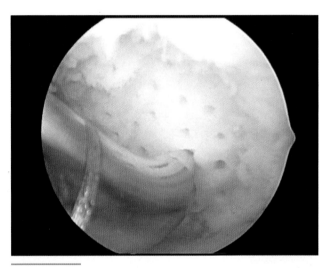

Figure 20–3. Microfracture holes are continued into the central portion of the defect. The microfracture awl is penetrating the subchondral bone approximately 2 to 4 mm in depth. (From Steadman JR, Rodkey WG, Briggs KK: Microfracture chondroplasty: Indications, techniques, and outcomes. Sports Med Arthrosc Rev 11:236-244, 2003.)

uniformly over the surface of the lesion, a microfracture procedure can be performed as previously described.[17,25] We have observed noticeably improved results in patients with chronic chondral lesions since we began using this technique. However, if the surrounding cartilage is too thin to establish a perpendicular rim to hold the marrow clot, we would probably not perform a microfracture procedure in patients with such advanced degenerative lesions.[17,25]

The microfracture awl produces a rough surface in the subchondral bone to which the marrow clot can adhere more easily, yet the integrity of the subchondral plate is

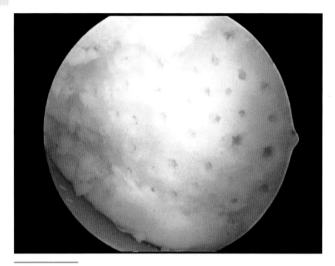

Figure 20–4. The microfracture procedure has been completed. Notice the proximity of the microfracture holes, usually no more than 3 to 4 mm apart. (From Steadman JR, Rodkey WG, Briggs KK: Microfracture chondroplasty: Indications, techniques, and outcomes. Sports Med Arthrosc Rev 11:236-244, 2003.)

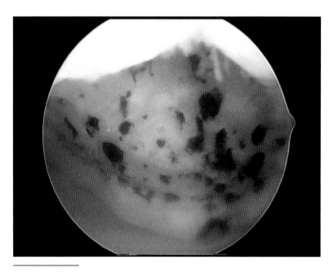

Figure 20–5. Marrow elements, including blood and fat droplets, accessed by the subchondral bone microfracture can be seen coming from essentially all the microfracture holes after the arthroscopic irrigation fluid pressure has been reduced. (From Steadman JR, Rodkey WG, Briggs KK: Microfracture chondroplasty: Indications, techniques, and outcomes. Sports Med Arthrosc Rev 11:236-244, 2003.)

maintained for joint surface shape. The microfracture procedure virtually eliminates thermal necrosis and provides a roughened surface for blood clot adherence, and the different angles of the arthroscopic awls available provide easier access to difficult-to-reach areas of the knee. The awls provide not only perpendicular holes but also improved control of depth penetration when compared with drilling. We believe that the key to the entire procedure is to establish the marrow clot to provide the optimal environment for the body's own pluripotential marrow cells (mesenchymal stem cells or progenitor cells) to differentiate into stable tissue within the lesion.[20,21]

POSTOPERATIVE MANAGEMENT

We have designed the postoperative program to promote the ideal physical environment in which the newly recruited mesenchymal stem cells from the marrow can differentiate into the appropriate articular cartilage–like cell lines.[9,21,24-26] These differentiation and maturation processes must occur slowly, but consistently.[9,10] Our animal studies have confirmed that both cellular and molecular changes are an essential part of the development of durable repair tissue.[7,8]

Our patients are counseled carefully so that they understand that they will probably not start to experience improvement in their knees for at least 6 months after microfracture. Our experience and clinical research data indicate that improvement can be expected to occur slowly and steadily for at least 2 years.[2,19,21,25,26] During this protracted period, the repair tissue matures, pain and swelling resolve, and patients regain confidence and comfort in their knees during increased levels of activity.[21]

REHABILITATION

The rehabilitation program after microfracture for treatment of chondral defects in the knee is crucial to optimize the results of surgery.[9,10,21] Rehabilitation promotes the optimal physical environment for the mesenchymal stem cells to differentiate and produce new extracellular matrix that eventually matures into durable repair tissue. The surgically induced marrow clot provides the basis for the most ideal chemical environment to complement the physical environment.[7,8] This newly proliferated repair cartilage then fills the original defect.

The postoperative rehabilitation program after microfracture necessitates consideration of several factors.[9,21,23-25] The specific protocol recommended depends on both the anatomic location and the size of the defect. These factors are critical to determine the ideal postoperative plan. For example, if other intra-articular procedures are performed concurrently with microfracture, such as anterior cruciate ligament reconstruction, we do not hesitate to alter the rehabilitation program as necessary. All the possible variations of the rehabilitation program are not within the scope of this chapter, but in the following paragraphs we describe two different protocols.

Rehabilitation Protocol for Patients with Lesions on the Femoral Condyle or Tibial Plateau

After microfracture of lesions on the weightbearing surfaces of the femoral condyles or tibial plateaus, we commence immediately with a continuous passive motion

(CPM) machine in the recovery room. The initial range of motion (ROM) is typically 30 to 70 degrees, and then it is increased as tolerated by 10 to 20 degrees until full passive ROM is achieved. The rate of the machine is usually 1 cycle per minute, but the rate can be varied based on patient preference and comfort. Many patients tolerate use of the CPM machine at night. For those who do not, we have observed that intermittent use during the day is probably as beneficial. Regardless of when the CPM machine is used, the goal is to have the patient in the CPM machine for 6 to 8 hours every 24 hours. If the patient is unable to use the CPM machine, instructions are given for passive flexion and extension of the knee with 500 repetitions three times per day. We encourage patients to gain full passive ROM of the injured knee as soon as possible after surgery.

We also prescribe cold therapy for all patients postoperatively. Our experience and observations indicate that cold helps control pain and inflammation, and most patients state that cold therapy provides overall postoperative relief of discomfort. Cold therapy is generally used for 1 to 7 days postoperatively.[18]

We prescribe crutch-assisted touch-down weightbearing ambulation for 6 to 8 weeks, depending on the size of the lesion. For most patients, 6 to 8 weeks seems an adequate time to limit weightbearing. However, for patients with small lesions (<1 cm in diameter), weightbearing may be hastened by a few weeks. Patients with lesions on the femoral condyles or tibial plateaus rarely use a brace during the initial postoperative period. However, we now prescribe an unloading-type brace when the patient becomes more active and the postoperative swelling has resolved.

We begin mobilization immediately after surgery with an emphasis on ROM and patellar and patellar tendon motion. Touch-down weightbearing is started, with 10% of the patient's body weight on the injured leg during weightbearing. Patients begin stationary biking without resistance and a deep water exercise program 1 to 2 weeks after microfracture. The deep water exercises include the use of a flotation vest for deep water running. It is critical and imperative that the foot of the injured leg does not touch the bottom of the pool during this exercise. Patients progress to full weightbearing after about 8 weeks and begin more vigorous biking with increasing resistance. They also begin knee flexion exercises at approximately 8 weeks after microfracture. An elastic resistance cord is added to the exercise regimen at about 12 weeks. A detailed description of use of the cord and the exercises has been published previously.[9] Our observations indicate that the ability to achieve predetermined maximum levels for sets and repetitions of elastic resistance cord exercises is an excellent indicator for progressing to weight training. We permit free or machine weights when the patient has achieved the early goals of the rehabilitation program, but not before 16 weeks after microfracture. We strongly emphasize the importance of proper technique when beginning a weight program. Depending on the clinical examination, size of the patient, the sport, and the size of the lesion, we usually recommend that patients do not return to sports that involve pivoting, cutting, and jumping until at least 4 to 9 months after microfracture.

Rehabilitation Protocol for Patients with Patellofemoral Lesions

All patients treated by microfracture for patellofemoral lesions must use a brace set at 0 to 20 degrees for at least 8 weeks. This brace limits compression of the regenerating surfaces of the trochlea or patella, or both. We allow passive motion with the brace removed, but otherwise the brace must be worn at all times. Patients with patellofemoral lesions are placed in a CPM machine immediately postoperatively. We also use cold therapy as described earlier. With this regimen patients typically obtain pain-free and full passive ROM soon after surgery.

For patients with patellofemoral joint lesions, we carefully observe joint angles at the time of arthroscopy to determine where the defect comes into contact with the patellar facet or the trochlear groove. We make certain to avoid these areas during strength training for approximately 4 months. This avoidance allows for training in the 0- to 20-degree range immediately postoperatively because there is minimal compression of these chondral surfaces with such limited motion.

Patients with lesions of the patellofemoral joint treated by microfracture are allowed weightbearing as tolerated in their brace 2 weeks after surgery. It is essential for patients to use a brace that prevents placing excessive shear force on the maturing marrow clot in the early postoperative period. We routinely lock the brace between 0 and 20 degrees ROM to prevent flexion past the point where the median ridge of the patella engages the trochlear groove. After 8 weeks, we open the knee brace gradually before it is discontinued. When the brace is discontinued, patients are allowed to advance their training progressively. Stationary biking is allowed 2 weeks postoperatively, and increased resistance is added 8 weeks after microfracture. Starting 12 weeks after microfracture, the exercise program is the same as used for femorotibial lesions.

POTENTIAL COMPLICATIONS FROM MICROFRACTURE

Most patients progress through the postoperative period with little or no difficulty.[21,24-26] However, some patients have mild transient pain, most frequently after microfracture in the patellofemoral joint. Small changes in the articular surface of the patellofemoral joint may be detected by a grating or "gritty" sensation of the joint, especially when a patient discontinues use of the knee brace and begins normal weightbearing through a full ROM. Patients rarely complain of pain at this time, and this grating sensation generally resolves spontaneously in a few days or weeks.

Similarly, if a steep perpendicular rim was made in the trochlear groove, patients may notice "catching" or "locking" as the apex of the patella rides over this lesion during joint motion. Some patients may even perceive these symptoms while in the CPM machine. These symptoms usually dissipate within 3 months. If this perceived locking is painful, the patient is advised to limit weightbearing and avoid the symptomatic joint angle for an additional period.[24,25]

Swelling and joint effusion typically resolve within 8 weeks after microfracture.[21] Occasionally, a recurrent effusion develops between 6 and 8 weeks after microfracture, usually when a patient begins to bear weight on the injured leg after microfracture of a defect on the femoral condyle. Although this effusion may mimic the preoperative or immediate postoperative effusion, it is generally painless. We treat this type of painless effusion conservatively. It usually resolves within several weeks after onset. Rarely has a second arthroscopy been required for recurring effusions.

DOCUMENTING OUTCOMES

Database Management

The Steadman Hawkins Research Foundation Clinical Research Database currently has data on over 12,000 knee operative procedures. Of these surgical procedures, 2804 knees underwent microfracture (Table 20–1). Information in this database includes preoperative physician and patient subjective assessment, findings at arthroscopy and treatments, and postoperative physician and patient subjective assessment. At the time of the first examination, the patients are asked to complete a self-administered questionnaire. Patients are then sent the questionnaire yearly for evaluation of symptoms, function, return to sports, activities of daily living, and satisfaction. All patient information is stored anonymously in a relational database. Database files are linked and queried to obtain the desired data. Data analysis is performed with an SPSS (SPSS, Inc., Chicago) software package. All statistics are reviewed by an independent statistician.

Table 20–1. Distribution of Locations of Grade IV Chondral Lesions Treated by Microfracture in the Steadman Hawkins Clinical Research Database ($N = 2804$)

AREA	PATIENTS (%)
MFC	19
LFC	10
MTP	4
LTP	5
TG	13
PAT	4
MFC and MTP	17
LFC and LTP	10
TG and PAT	2
Other	16

LFC, lateral femoral condyle; LTP, lateral tibial plateau; MFC, medial femoral condyle; MTP, medial tibial plateau; PAT, patella; TG, trochlear groove.

Outcome Measures

LYSHOLM SCORE

Knee function in our database is measured by using the Lysholm score. The scale of Lysholm and Gillquist is a condition-specific score that consists of eight domains related to function of the knee: walking with a limp, support, locking, instability, pain, swelling, stair climbing, and squatting.[14] Pain and instability receive the highest point allocation, followed by locking, swelling, and stair climbing. A total score of 95 to 100 points is associated with normal function, 84 to 94 points indicates symptoms related to vigorous activity, and less than 84 points suggests symptoms related to activities of daily living. The Lysholm score has been widely used for various disorders of the knee, and it has recently been validated for use with chondral disorders of the knee.[13]

Kocher et al determined the reliability, validity, and responsiveness of the Lsyholm score.[13] These psychometric properties were analyzed in a group of 1657 patients with chondral disorders of the knee. Test-retest, which entailed the same patient completing the questionnaire twice within 4 weeks, determined the reproducibility of the score between patients, or its reliability. Validity of the score, which included content validity, criterion validity, and construct validity, was also measured. To determine whether the score can assess change, the responsiveness was determined. This study showed that the overall Lsyholm score performed acceptably for the assessment of outcome after treatment of chondral disorders. Some individual domains of the score, however, did not perform as well.[13]

TEGNER ACTIVITY SCALE

Activity level in our database is measured with the use of the Tegner activity scale.[30] In the Tegner scale, a numerical value, 0 to 10, is assigned to specific activities. An activity level of 10 corresponds to competitive sports, including soccer, football, and rugby at the elite level; an activity level of 6 corresponds to recreational sports; and a level of zero corresponds to a person on sick leave or disability pension because of knee problems. Activity levels of 5 to 10 can be achieved only if the patient participates in recreational or competitive sports. The Tegner activity scale is easy to use; however, not all sports are represented in the categories.[30]

WOMAC

In studies documenting the outcomes of patients with osteoarthritis of the knee, we use the WOMAC score in addition to other scores. The Western Ontario and McMaster University Osteoarthritis Index (WOMAC) is a general musculoskeletal instrument for patients who have osteoarthritis of the hip or knee.[1] It has been validated in randomized clinical trials and has been shown to be a responsive tool in measuring outcomes after treatment of osteoarthritis of the knee.[1] WOMAC has three domains:

pain (5 items), stiffness (2 items), and physical functioning (17 items). The questions are ranked on a 5-point Likert scale (0 = none, 1 = slight, 2 = moderate, 3 = severe, 4 = extreme). The score is reported as the sum of the scores for each domain.[1]

PATIENT SATISFACTION

As health care becomes more patient driven, assessing patient satisfaction is a major objective of our data collection. Our goals are to evaluate patient satisfaction with the outcome of treatment and to identify parameters that are related to such satisfaction. With determinants of patient satisfaction from these studies, we can identify elements that are most important to patients after surgery. We assess satisfaction with the outcome of treatment on a scale of 1 to 10, with 10 being very satisfied and 1 being dissatisfied.

RESULTS OF MICROFRACTURE

In 2003, the first long-term outcomes paper was published on the microfracture technique.[21] This study monitored 72 patients for an average of 11 years after microfracture, with the longest follow-up being 17 years. This study included only knees with no joint space narrowing, no degenerative arthritis, and no ligament or meniscus pathology that required treatment. All patients were younger than 45 years. The microfracture technique used on these patients did not include recent improvements to the technique as described in the technique section of this chapter. With a 95% follow-up rate, the results showed improvement in symptoms and function. Patient-reported pain and swelling decreased at postoperative year 1 and continued to decrease at year 2, and the clinical improvements were maintained over the study period. The study identified age as the only independent predictor of Lysholm improvement. Patients older than 35 years improved less than patients younger than 35; however, both groups showed improvement.[21]

Recently, a study compared the outcomes of autologous chondrocyte implantation with microfracture treatment in a randomized trial.[12] Forty patients were treated in each group. At 2 years, both groups showed significant improvement in Lysholm score and pain, with no difference between the groups. However, the microfracture group had more improvement in the SF-36 physical component score. A high physical functioning score corresponds to a person who performs all types of physical activities, including the most vigorous without limitations because of health. The authors theorized that this difference may be due to the fact that microfracture is one arthroscopic procedure, whereas autologous chondrocyte implantation requires one arthroscopic and one open procedure. This study also found age to be a predictor of improvement with microfracture. In addition, it identified activity level and lesion size as predictors of better clinical results. Histological evaluations showed no differences between the groups. Based on these findings, with both techniques resulting in similar outcomes, we believe that microfracture should be the recommended treatment of isolated chondral defects.

Cartilage injuries are common in high-impact sports. We documented the outcome of microfracture in patients who played professional football in the United States.[22] Twenty-five active National Football League players were treated by microfracture between 1986 and 1997. The study found that 76% of players returned to play the next football season. After return to play, those same individuals played an average of 4.6 additional seasons. All players showed decreased symptoms and improvement in function. Of those individuals who did not return to play, most had preexisting degenerative changes in the knee.[22]

Arthroscopic treatment of a degenerative knee is controversial. However, we did document the outcome at 2 years in patients with degenerative chondral lesions treated by microfracture.[17] The goals of this procedure are to alleviate pain, maximize function, and prevent further degenerative changes. With strict patient selection, proper surgical technique, and compliance with a well-defined rehabilitation program, patients showed improvement in function and had decreased symptoms. Pain and swelling significantly decreased, with most patients reporting only mild symptoms. Patients were highly satisfied with their results. Factors that were associated with less Lsyholm improvement included bipolar lesions, lesions larger than 400 mm², and knees with absent menisci. Repeat arthroscopy was reported in 15.5% of these patients. Failures, as defined by revision microfracture or total knee replacement, were documented in 6% of the patients. These results confirm excellent short-term outcomes; however, further studies will be needed to determine how long the results last.[17]

A contraindication to microfracture in a degenerative knee is malalignment of the joint. Medial opening wedge high tibial osteotomy has gained popularity as a means of correcting malalignment in patients with medial compartment arthrosis and varus malalignment who wish to stay active. We recently reported on 39 patients who underwent an opening wedge osteotomy on the medial side of the proximal end of the tibia in conjunction with the microfracture procedure in their degenerative varus knee.[29] Patients showed improvement in function and activity level, as well as decreased symptoms. Most patients had a greater than 20-point increase in their Lysholm score. This study also showed that patients with no previous surgeries had more improvement. Two patients went on to total knee replacement at 3 and 5 years after the high tibial osteotomy. The study concluded that at a minimum of 2 years after surgery, patients with varus alignment and chondral surface lesions of the knee can be treated effectively by high tibial osteotomy and microfracture.[32] These patients returned to an active lifestyle as demonstrated by their high Tegner scores in Table 20–2.

SUMMARY

Based on our extensive experience, we conclude that arthroscopic débridement plus microfracture of subchon-

Table 20–2. Average Functional Scores of All Patients

	PATIENT AGE RANGE	LYSHOLM	TEGNER
Traumatic lesions (Arthroscopy, 2003)	13-45	89	6
Traumatic lesions (J Bone Joint Surg, 2004)	18-45	76	4
NFL players (J Knee Surg, 2003)	22-36	90	9
Degenerative knees (J Knee Surg, 2003)	40-70	83	4.5
High tibial osteotomy and microfracture	34-79	78	5

dral bone is safe and effective in treating full-thickness chondral defects of the knee in clinical patients, both acute and chronic. Microfracture significantly improves functional outcomes and decreases pain in the majority of patients treated. This repair tissue appears tough and durable, yet it is smooth enough to function similar to normal articular cartilage in clinical patients. We believe that microfracture should be considered the initial treatment of choice for full-thickness articular cartilage defects of the knee.

References

1. Bellamy N, Buchanan WW, Goldsmith CH, et al: Validation study of WOMAC: A Health Status Instrument for measuring clinically important patient relevant outcomes to antirheumatic drug therapy in patients with osteoarthritis of the hip or knee. Rheumatology 15:1833-1840, 1988.
2. Blevins FT, Steadman JR, Rodrigo JJ, et al: Treatment of articular cartilage defects in athletes: An analysis of functional outcome and lesion appearance. Orthopedics 21:761-768, 1998.
3. Brittberg M, Lindahl A, Nilsson A, et al: Treatment of deep cartilage defects in the knee with autologous chondrocyte transplantation. N Engl J Med 331:889-895, 1994.
4. Buckwalter JA: Articular cartilage: Injuries and potential for healing. J Orthop Sports Phys Ther 28:192-202, 1998.
5. Cohen NP, Foster RJ, Mow VC: Composition and dynamics of articular cartilage: Structure, function, and maintaining healthy state. J Orthop Sports Phys Ther 28:203-215, 1998.
6. DePalma AF, McKeever CD, Subin DK: Process of repair of articular cartilage demonstrated by histology and autoradiography with tritiated thymidine. Clin Orthop 48:229-242, 1966.
7. Frisbie DD, Oxford JT, Southwood L, et al: Early events in cartilage repair after subchondral bone microfracture. Clin Orthop 407:215-227, 2003.
8. Frisbie DD, Trotter GW, Powers BE, et al: Arthroscopic subchondral bone plate microfracture technique augments healing of large osteochondral defects in the radial carpal bone and medial femoral condyle of horses. J Vet Surg 28:242-255, 1999.
9. Hagerman GR, Atkins JA, Dillman C: Rehabilitation of chondral injuries and chronic degenerative arthritis of the knee in the athlete. Oper Tech Sports Med 3:127-135, 1995.
10. Irrgang JJ, Pezzullo D: Rehabilitation following surgical procedures to address articular cartilage lesions of the knee. J Orthop Sports Phys Ther 28:232-240, 1998.
11. Johnson LL: The sclerotic lesion: Pathology and the clinical response to arthroscopic abrasion arthroplasty. In Ewing JW (ed): Articular Cartilage and Knee Joint Function: Basic Science and Arthroscopy. New York, Raven Press, 1990, pp 319-333.
12. Knutsen G, Engebretsen L, Ludvigsen TC, et al: Autologous chondrocyte implantation compared with microfracture in the knee. J Bone Joint Surg Am 86:455-464, 2004.
13. Kocher MS, Steadman JR, Briggs KK, et al: Reliability, validity, and responsiveness of the Lysholm knee scale for various chondral disorders of the knee. J Bone Joint Surg Am 86:1139-1145, 2004.
14. Lysholm J, Gillquist J: Evaluation of knee ligament surgery with special emphasis on use of a scoring scale. Am J Sports Med 10:150-154, 1982.
15. Mankin HJ: Reaction of articular cartilage to injury and osteoarthritis. N Engl J Med 291:1335-1340, 1974.
16. Mankin HJ: The response of articular cartilage to mechanical injury. J Bone Joint Surg Am 64:460-465, 1982.
17. Miller BS, Steadman JR, Briggs KK, et al: Patient satisfaction and outcome after microfracture of the degenerative knee. J Knee Surg 17:13-17, 2004.
18. Ohkoshi Y, Ohkoshi M, Nagasaki S, et al: The effect of cryotherapy on intraarticular temperature and postoperative care after anterior cruciate ligament reconstruction. Am J Sports Med 27:357-362, 1999.
19. Rodrigo JJ, Steadman JR, Silliman JF, et al: Improvement of full-thickness chondral defect healing in the human knee after débridement and microfracture using continuous passive motion. Am J Knee Surg 7:109-116, 1994.
20. Singleton SB, Silliman JF: Acute chondral injuries of the patellofemoral joint. Oper Tech Sports Med 3:96-103, 1995.
21. Steadman JR, Briggs KK, Rodrigo JJ, et al: Outcomes of microfracture for traumatic chondral defects of the knee: Average 11-year follow-up. Arthroscopy 19:477-484, 2003.
22. Steadman JR, Karas SG, Miller BS, et al: The microfracture technique in the treatment of full-thickness chondral lesions of the knee in National Football League players. J Knee Surg 16:83-86, 2003.
23. Steadman JR, Rodkey WG: Microfracture in the pediatric and adolescent knee. In Micheli LJ, Kocher M (eds): The Pediatric & Adolescent Knee. Philadelphia, WB Saunders, 2004.
24. Steadman JR, Rodkey WG, Briggs KK: Microfracture to treat full-thickness chondral defects. J Knee Surg 15:170-176, 2002.
25. Steadman JR, Rodkey WG, Briggs KK: Microfracture chondroplasty: Indications, techniques, and outcomes. Sports Med Arthrosc Rev 11:236-244, 2003.
26. Steadman JR, Rodkey WG, Rodrigo JJ: "Microfracture": Surgical technique and rehabilitation to treat chondral defects. Clin Orthop 391(Suppl):S362-S369, 2001.
27. Steadman JR, Rodkey WG, Singleton SB, et al: Microfracture technique for full-thickness chondral defects: Technique and clinical results. Oper Tech Orthop 7:300-304, 1997.
28. Steadman JR, Rodkey WG, Singleton SB, et al: Microfracture procedure for treatment of full-thickness chondral defects: Technique, clinical results and current basic science status. In Harner CD, Vince KG, Fu FH (eds): Techniques in Knee Surgery. Media, PA, Williams & Wilkins, 1999, pp 23-31.
29. Sterett WI, Steadman JR: Chondral resurfacing and high tibial osteotomy in the varus knee. Am J Sports Med 32:1243-1249, 2004.
30. Tegner Y, Lysholm J: Rating systems in the evaluation of knee ligament injuries. Clin Orthop 198:43-49, 1985.
31. Urrea LH, Silliman JF: Acute chondral injuries to the femoral condyles. Oper Tech Sports Med 3:104-111, 1995.
32. Walker JM: Pathomechanics and classification of cartilage lesions, facilitation of repair. J Orthop Sports Phys Ther 28:216-231, 1998.

CHAPTER 21

International Experience with Autologous Chondrocyte Transplantation

Lars Peterson

Articular cartilage is a unique tissue with no vascular, nerve, or lymphatic supply. The lack of vascular and lymphatic circulation may be one of the reasons why articular cartilage has such a poor intrinsic capacity to heal. There is no inflammatory response to tissue damage unless there is involvement of subchondral bone in the damaged area. Subsequently, there will be no macrophage invasion to phagocytose and remove the damaged and devitalized tissue and, furthermore, no migration of cells with repair capacity into the damaged area. The chondrocyte itself, encapsulated in its own matrix, is incapable of migrating and repopulating the damaged area.

Chondral injuries that penetrate down to subchondral bone will not heal but may progress to osteoarthritis over time by enzymatic degradation and mechanical wear. Osteochondral injuries that penetrate subchondral bone into trabecular bone with bleeding will result in inflammatory repair tissue filling the lesion with fibrocartilage produced by mesenchymal stem cells or fibroblasts. Unfortunately, the quality of the fibrocartilage repair tissue has been shown to not be able to withstand mechanical wear over time, and the fibrocartilage may degenerate and the lesion progress to osteoarthritis.[4-6,17,21,33]

Excellent results can be achieved with treatment of severe osteoarthritis of the knee by total joint replacement in elderly patients. In young and middle-aged patients, however, there is no optimal treatment. The spectrum of treatment alternatives for articular cartilage defects in young and middle-aged patients can range from simple lavage and débridement, drilling, microfracturing, and abrasion to osteochondral grafting and autologous chondrocyte transplantation.

The optimal healing of an articular cartilage injury should consist of regeneration with tissue identical to hyaline cartilage; however, repair of chondral injury involves filling with tissue not identical to hyaline cartilage (i.e., fibrocartilage). The repair tissue should be able to fill and seal off the defective area with good adhesion to subchondral bone and complete integration to surrounding cartilage. It should be able to withstand mechanical wear over time and gradually be included in the natural turnover of normal cartilage.[5]

The functional unit of articular cartilage includes not only the different layers of cartilage but also subchondral and trabecular bone. Any treatment technique that interferes with subchondral and trabecular bone may not be able to restore the functional unit of cartilage, especially its shock-absorbing function.

Techniques that affect the subchondral bone plate include abrasion, arthroplasty, multiple drilling, and multiple microfracturing. All these techniques may result in stiffening of subchondral and trabecular bone.[3] Osteochondral grafting may affect subchondral and trabecular bone function because the osseous part of the plug has to undergo resorption, revascularization, and remodeling. Periosteal and perichondrial grafting also affect subchondral bone by drilling and abrading the subchondral bone plate.

Chondrocyte transplantation does not violate subchondral or trabecular bone. On the contrary, for success with this technique, bleeding from subchondral bone should be avoided so that fibroblasts or stem cells are not introduced and result in fibroblastic repair tissue.[2]

HISTORICAL BACKGROUND OF AUTOLOGOUS CHONDROCYTE TRANSPLANTATION

In 1965 Smith was successful in isolating and growing chondrocytes in culture for the first time.[10] Epiphysial chondrocytes grown in culture were injected into tibial articular defects in the rabbit knee but did not show any significant repair.

In 1982, experimental work started at the Hospital for Joint Diseases–Orthopedic Institute in New York to design an experimental rabbit model using articular chondrocytes isolated and grown in culture for transplantation into a defect made in the patella and covered with a periosteal flap. The idea was to use articular chondrocytes because they are the only cells committed to form hyaline cartilage.

The initial results of autologous chondrocyte transplantation in this rabbit model were presented in 1984 and showed hyaline-like cartilage filling 80% of the patellar defect. No significant filling was seen in the control side, where the defect was treated with periosteal cover, but no cells.[13,29]

Since 1984, extensive animal studies have been ongoing at the University of Göteborg, Sweden. The results from New York were confirmed and improved.[3]

In 1985, work started on transferring the cell-culturing technique to human chondrocytes, and in 1987 the first autologous chondrocyte transplantation was performed in

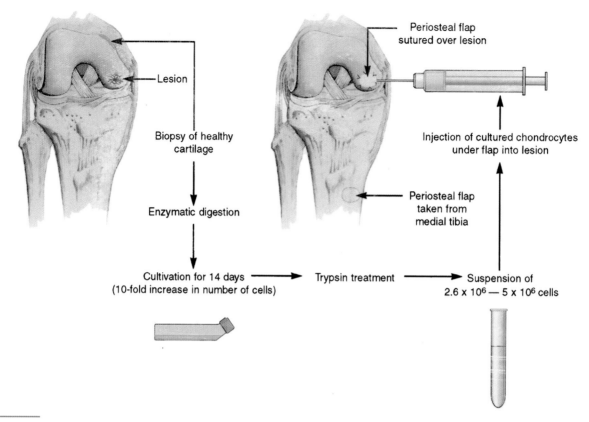

Figure 21-1. Diagram of the autologous chondrocyte transplantation procedure.

the human knee at the Department of Orthopaedics, University of Göteborg, after approval by the Ethical Committee of the Medical Faculty of the University of Göteborg (Fig. 21–1).

A pilot study of 23 patients with 39 months' follow-up reported in the *New England Journal of Medicine* in October 1994 showed that of the 16 patients who underwent femoral condyle procedures, 14 had a good or excellent result. Eleven of 15 biopsy specimens showed hyaline-like cartilage. Of the seven patients who underwent autologous chondrocyte transplantation of the patella, however, only two good or excellent results were achieved, and one biopsy specimen showed hyaline-like cartilage.[2]

Since 1987, more than 1300 patients have been operated on in Gothenburg, Sweden, and since 1995, more than 400 surgeons have performed autologous chondrocyte transplantation on over 20,000 patients outside Sweden.

The clinical results from Sweden have been reported at the American Academy of Orthopaedic Surgeons in 1996, 1997, 1998, 2000, 2001, 2002, 2003, and 2004.[30]

INDICATIONS FOR AUTOLOGOUS CHONDROCYTE TRANSPLANTATION

Autologous chondrocyte transplantation is indicated in patients between 15 and 55 years old with symptomatic, full-thickness, Outerbridge[26] or International Cartilage Repair Society (ICRS)[18] grade III to IV cartilage injuries of the knee with a diameter larger than 10 mm up to an area of 10 to 16 cm^2 (Fig. 21–2). The location of the defect should be on the femoral or patellar articular surface and should be accessible for transplantation via open arthrotomy. Only grade I to II Outerbridge or ICRS classification changes on the reciprocal articular surface should be included.

Osteochondritis dissecans of the medial or lateral femoral condyles with an unstable fragment, separated but attached flap, or empty bed is also an indication for autologous chondrocyte transplantation (Fig. 21–3).[3]

Bipolar chondral injuries (i.e., osteoarthritis) are undergoing investigational studies and are not indicated for this treatment at present. A definite decision regarding the indication is made during arthroscopic evaluation.

CLINICAL EVALUATION

A thorough history of symptoms, trauma, or repetitive loading is important, as well as a careful record of previous surgery. Clinical examination, including signs of local tenderness, swelling, range of motion, and crepitation, is performed.

Varus and valgus deformities are assessed, and patella malalignment, maltracking, or instability is evaluated. Clinical testing of ligament instability is performed.

BACKGROUND FACTORS TO CONSIDER

An understanding of the optimal environment for survival of the repair tissue in the short and long term is of utmost importance. Varus or valgus malalignment should be evaluated on standing x-ray films of the knee in the extended

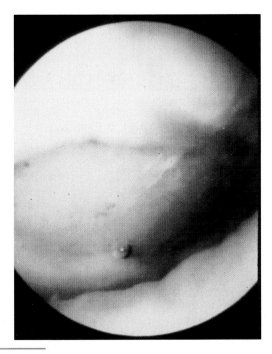

Figure 21–2. Arthroscopic view of a chondral injury down to bone on the medial femoral condyle, an indication for autologous chondrocyte transplantation.

position and 45 degrees of knee flexion. Additional information could be achieved through examining the hip, knee, and ankle axis on long, standing x-ray films. Varus or valgus deformity should be corrected. Magnetic resonance imaging (MRI) could be helpful to evaluate the articular cartilage injury and condition of the subchondral bone in more detail, as well as the status of the menisci. Previous meniscus surgery should be assessed, and after total or subtotal meniscectomy, meniscal transplantation should be considered.

Instability should be evaluated clinically and any instability corrected. Osseous defects deeper than 8 to 10 mm should be considered for autologous bone grafting and chondrocyte transplantation. MRI could be a helpful tool to evaluate any bone pathology.

ARTHROSCOPIC EVALUATION

Under general or spinal anesthesia, complete stability testing of the knee is performed and the results compared with those on the healthy side. A complete examination of the knee joint should be performed, including visualization and probing of the articular cartilage surfaces, synovial lining, menisci, and cruciate ligaments, and the presence of any fragment or loose body should be identified. Undiagnosed pathology may be critical to the outcome of surgery. The cartilage injury is visualized, probed, and assessed for depth, size, and location. The opposing articular surface should be assessed and should be normal or have only fibrillation or superficial fissuring, Outerbridge or ICRS grade I to grade II. The defect should be evaluated regarding containment and shouldering. An uncontained lesion extends into the synovial lining of the joint. It could be unilateral or bilateral, for example,

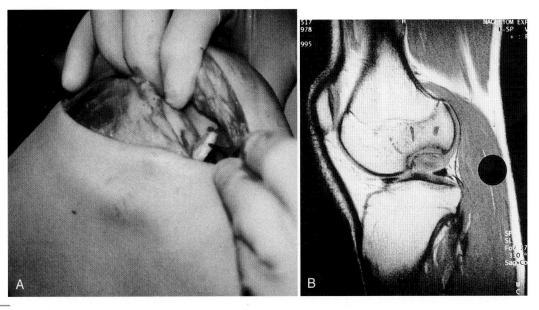

Figure 21–3. **A,** Arthrotomy of a right knee with osteochondritis dissecans of the lateral femoral condyle and an avulsed but attached flap, an indication for autologous chondrocyte transplantation. **B,** Magnetic resonance image showing a deep osseous defect on the lateral femoral condyle.

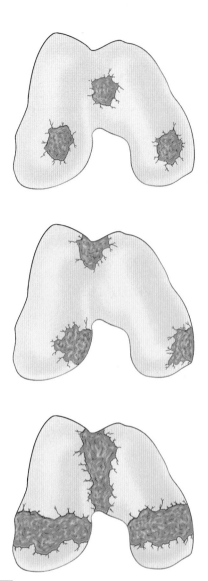

Figure 21–4. Schematic drawing showing containment of defects. The *upper* drawing shows contained defects; the *middle* drawing, unilateral uncontained defects extending to the synovial lining; and the *lower* drawing, bilateral uncontained defects.

extending from the synovial lining of the articular surface of the medial femoral condyle into the synovial lining of the intercondylar notch (Fig. 21–4).[6]

A shouldered defect is a defect surrounded by normal cartilage in which the bone in the center of the defect is not in contact with the opposing articular surface. An unshouldered defect is so large that in a weightbearing position the subchondral bone in the center of the defect is in contact with the opposing articular surface (Fig. 21–5).[4,20] During arthroscopy, the proposed transplantation is evaluated regarding different possibilities of the surgical approach, the intended amount of débridement, the extent of shouldering, containment of the defect, and so on.

Meniscus lesions should be treated at this time, but only after harvesting cartilage for cell culture. Cartilage frag-

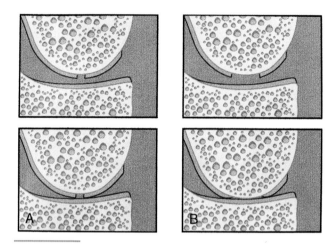

Figure 21–5. **A,** Shouldered defects are usually smaller than 10 mm and are contained. **B,** Unshouldered defects are larger. During weightbearing the center of the defect is in contact with the opposing articular surface.

ments and loose bodies should be removed before harvesting the cartilage.

Only gentle or no débridement of the injury should be performed at this time. When the specifics of the indication have been fulfilled, cartilage is harvested from the upper medial or upper lateral femoral condyle on minor weightbearing areas (Fig. 21–6). It could also be harvested from the intercondylar notch. In 98% of our cases, cartilage is harvested from the upper medial femoral condyle. With a curet, three to four slices of cartilage 3 to 4 mm × 10 mm should be taken down to subchondral bone on the upper medial femoral condyle.[5] Approximately 200 to 300 mg of articular cartilage is required for enzymatic digestion and cell culturing. The harvesting area should extend to the synovial lining to allow fibrous as well as synovial ingrowth for covering the harvest area. In more than 1400 patients who have had cartilage removed for cell culturing, no complications or late symptoms have occurred from the donor site. Optimal harvesting of cartilage is of greatest importance for the success of cell culturing, and optimal cell quality is necessary for the best possible result of this procedure.[3]

SURGICAL PROCEDURE

Chondral Lesions

The patient is placed under general or spinal anesthesia. With a tourniquet-controlled bloodless field, a minor parapatellar incision is made. The joint is opened and the injury assessed. For a good surgical technique it is important to obtain good access to the defect, and the arthrotomy might need to be adjusted accordingly (Fig. 21–7).[3,23] The patella may have to be dislocated in the case of transplantation to multiple femoral or patellar lesions.

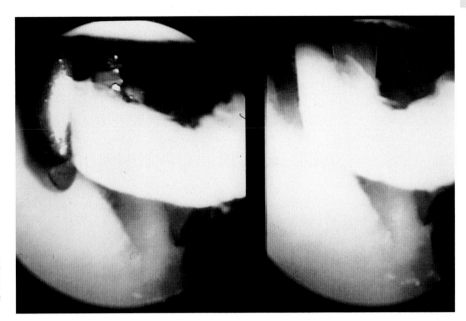

Figure 21–6. Arthroscopic views showing harvesting of articular cartilage from the upper medial femoral condyle with a curette (*right* picture).

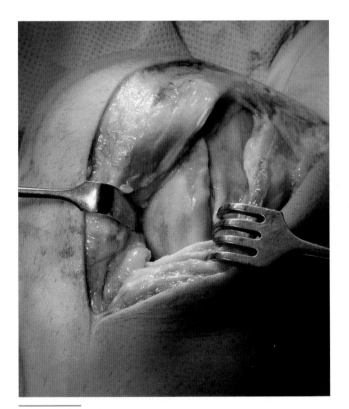

Figure 21–7. The arthrotomy is adjusted for good exposure of the defect.

EXCISION AND DÉBRIDEMENT OF THE LESION

The injured area is excised with vertical edges, including all damaged cartilage. Radical excision is the key to success. The resulting lesions should be as circular or oval as possible. If the lesion is not contained by healthy cartilage, it is better to leave a 3- to 4-mm rim of acceptable cartilage than to have the lesion border bone or synovium. Gentle débridement of the excised area is performed down to subchondral bone without causing any bleeding. If bleeding occurs, an epinephrine sponge or a drop of fibrin glue can stop it. The excised defect is then measured in its longest diameter and longest perpendicular diameter. The defect should be shaped as geometrically as possible. A template of sterile aluminum foil or paper is used to model the exact size of the defect (Fig. 21–8).

HARVESTING OF THE PERIOSTEAL FLAP

Through a separate incision on the upper medial aspect of the tibia, the periosteum is dissected free of fascia, fat, and fibrous tissue. Even passing vessels should be dissected off the flap. Measure the intended periosteal flap, or use the template to create the exact size and form. Oversize the periosteal flap by adding 1 to 2 mm to the periphery of the intended flap. Incise the periosteum and use a sharp elevator to remove the periosteal flap. Use small movements to avoid rifts in the periosteum (Fig. 21–9). Mark the side of the periosteum to be able to identify the cambium layer. Saline is used to keep the periosteal flap moist. The periosteal flap should be as thin as possible and transparent to achieve more volume in the defect and allow the cells to spread and expand. The thinner the periosteal flap, the less risk for hypertrophy, fibrillation, or other complications.

SUTURING OF THE PERIOSTEAL FLAP

Anchor the periosteal flap in four corners with the cambium layer facing the inside of the bone of the defect.

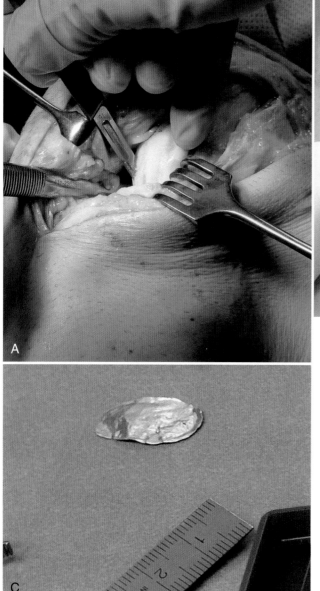

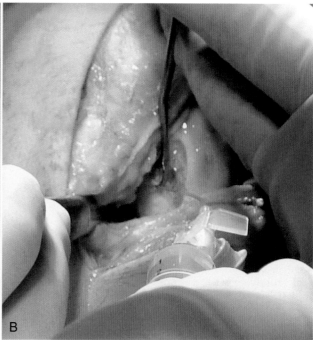

Figure 21–8. All damaged or undermined cartilage is excised (**A**) and carefully débrided (**B**). A template of the defect is made from sterile aluminum foil (**C**).

Then adapt the periosteum to the surrounding cartilage by placing 6-0 resorbable suture at 4- to 6-mm intervals. Insert the suture to a depth of at least 5 to 6 mm to avoid cutting the cartilage. The intervals between the suture are sealed with fibrin glue. An opening in the upper part of the defect is left for injection of the cells.

Before injecting the cells, check that there is no leakage by introducing a soft catheter with a syringe into the defect. Inject saline slowly into the defect and check for any leakage. Then aspirate the saline and inject the cells into the defect, starting distally and withdrawing the syringe proximally as the cells are injected. Close the injection site with suture and fibrin glue (Fig. 21–10).

Osteochondral Lesions (Osteochondritis Dissecans)

When treating osteochondritis dissecans by autologous chondrocyte transplantation, attention must be paid to the depth of the defect. If the bony defect is shallower than 6 to 8 mm, the lesion is treated the same way as a chondral lesion. Gently débride the sclerotic bottom of the defect, but be careful to not cause bleeding. The cartilage is incised and débrided to vertical edges of healthy cartilage. Cover the defect with a periosteal flap, seal, and check for leakage. Then implant the chondrocytes and close the last opening.

If the bony defect is deeper than 6 to 8 mm, autologous chondrocyte transplantation is not enough, and concomitant autologous bone grafting is needed. Start by abrading

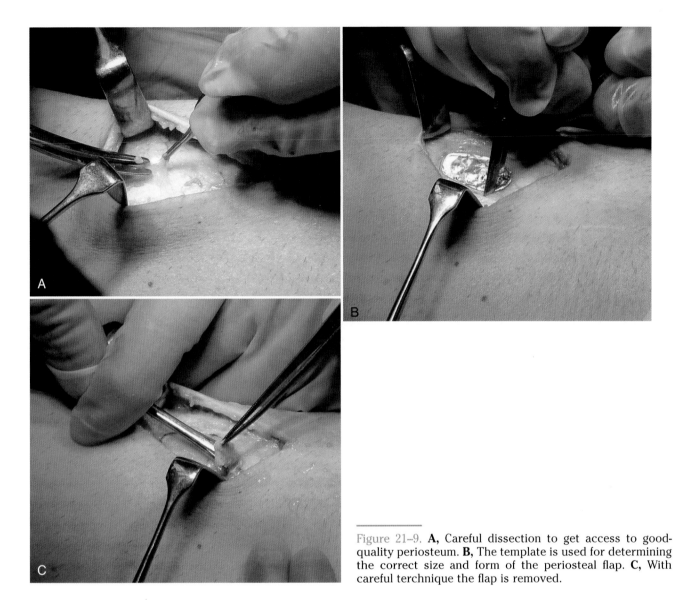

Figure 21–9. **A,** Careful dissection to get access to good-quality periosteum. **B,** The template is used for determining the correct size and form of the periosteal flap. **C,** With careful terchnique the flap is removed.

the sclerotic bottom of the defect to spongy bone and undercut the subchondral bone plate. Use a 2-mm bur and drill multiple holes into the spongy bone. The cartilage is débrided to healthy cartilage with vertical edges. Then harvest cancellous bone for grafting of the bony defect. If the bony defect is small, use bone from the tibial or femoral condyle, but if the defect is larger, bone has to be harvested from the iliac crest. Pack the bone from the bottom up and try to shape the bone graft to the contour of the condyle.

Harvest a periosteal flap to cover the bone graft at the level of subchondral bone, with the cambium layer facing the joint. Anchor it with horizontal or mattress sutures placed into the cartilage or through small drill holes in the subchondral bone plate, and use fibrin glue under the flap for fixation to the bone graft. This technique will avoid bleeding into the cartilage defect. Another periosteal flap is harvested and sutured to the cartilage edges, with the cambium layer facing the defect. Use fibrin glue to seal the intervals between the sutures. Test for a watertight seal with a gentle saline injection. If no leakage is present, aspi-

rate the saline and inject the chondrocytes. Close the last opening and seal with fibrin glue (Fig. 21–11).

THE CONCEPT OF OPTIMAL ENVIRONMENTAL CONDITIONS FOR THE SHORT- AND LONG-TERM SURVIVAL OF REPAIR TISSUE

Over the years it has become obvious when dealing with autologous chondrocyte transplantation and concomitant procedures that it is mandatory to create optimal local environmental conditions for the short- and long-term survival of the repair. Malalignment and instability will need corrective surgery for a good result. Procedures such as anterior cruciate ligament (ACL) reconstruction or high tibial osteotomy may be performed at the same time as the biopsy specimen is harvested. Otherwise, they could be done concomitant with the transplantation. Pathological mechanics in the joint reduces the chance of successful

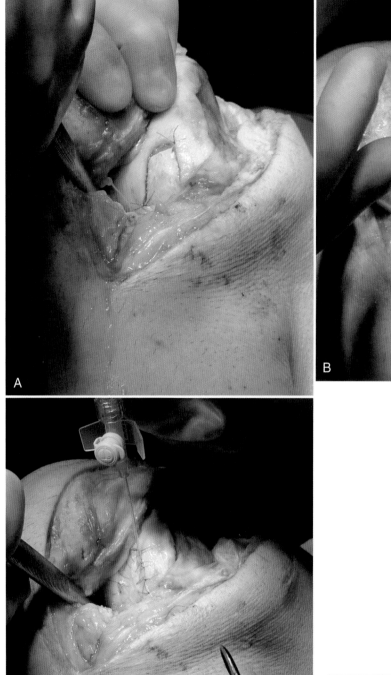

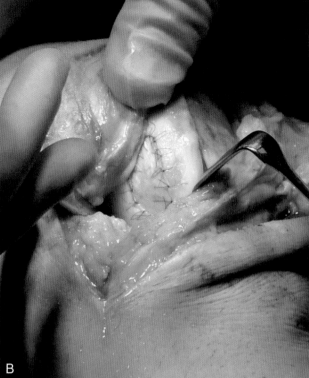

Figure 21–10. **A,** The periosteal flap is first anchored with a suture in each corner. **B,** The flap is then sutured to the cartilage rim. **C,** The integrity of the chamber under the flap is tested with an injection of saline.

repair. Patellar lesions are often related to a maltracking or unstable patella, and the patella must thus be realigned or stabilized for good healing. Stabilizing procedures may include anteromedialization of the tibial tuberosity, lateral release, proximal medial soft-tissue shortening, and trochlear grooveplasty (if it is dysplastic). In patients with trochlear and patellar lesions, especially large and uncontained ones, unloading with ventralization of the tibial tuberosity should be considered. A torn ACL is reconstructed after the cartilage lesion is débrided and covered with periosteum, but before the chondrocytes are injected. To unload the transplanted area when a varus or valgus deformity is present, a high tibial or distal femoral osteotomy is performed. When these corrective surgeries are performed, a brace limiting range of motion to 0 to 60 degrees is used postoperatively for 3 weeks, and for the following 3 weeks, range of motion is limited to 0 to 90 degrees. In patients with previous total or subtotal meniscectomy, meniscus allograft transplantation should be considered.

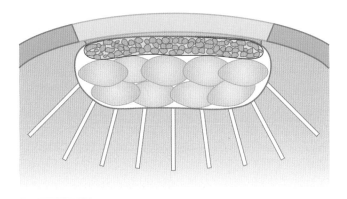

Figure 21–11. Schematic drawing of the sandwich procedure with layers of transplanted bone, periosteal flap, chondrocytes, and periosteal flap.

POSTOPERATIVE TREATMENT

The patient is given antibiotic and thrombotic prophylaxis for 48 hours. Six to 8 hours after surgery, a continuous passive motion machine is used with a range of motion of 0 to 40 degrees. Range of motion is allowed the day after surgery, as well as isometric quadriceps training. Weightbearing is limited during the first weeks. Depending on the size, location, and containment of the lesion and concomitant procedures, weightbearing ranges from loading to the pain threshold for 6 weeks, loading with 30 to 40 lb for 8 weeks, and then gradually increased weightbearing for another 6 weeks. Cycling on a stationary bike with low resistance could be started when the patient has reached 90 to 100 degrees of knee flexion. When full weightbearing is achieved, long-distance walking with increasing distances is encouraged. Swimming is allowed, as well as wet vest training, when the wounds are healed. Cross-country skiing, in-line skating, or outdoor skating if the patient is used to these techniques can be allowed when full weightbearing has been achieved. Running is not allowed until 9 months.

Return to professional sports is permitted after individual assessment, including overall clinical and functional tests and arthroscopic evaluation with the indentation test and probing to determine the hardness and condition of the repair tissue.

It is very important to inform the patient about the healing process, starting with cells in a suspension changing to cotton-like tissue in the first 2 to 3 months and gradually maturing to a rubber-like tissue within 6 months. Continuous maturation with hardening is an ongoing process and is stimulated by gradually increased weightbearing, as well as motion. Such maturation will continue for 12 months or longer.

RESULTS OF AUTOLOGOUS CHONDROCYTE TRANSPLANTATION: LONG-TERM SWEDISH EXPERIENCE

Since October 1987, more than 1300 patients have undergone autologous chondrocyte transplantation in Gothen-burg, Sweden. Two-hundred nineteen of these patients have had a minimum follow-up of 2 years, and 213 have been evaluated 2 to 10 years after surgery. Fifty-seven patients had isolated injury to the femoral condyles, 27 had isolated injury to the femoral condyle and ACL reconstruction, and 32 had osteochondritis dissecans of the femoral condyles. Thirty-two patients had cartilage injury on the patella and 12 on the trochlea of the femur. Fifty-three patients had multiple lesions and could be considered salvage cases.

Patients were evaluated with the use of multiple functional scales, activity scores, clinical examination, and arthroscopic macroscopic assessment. Indentation tests were performed to measure the stiffness of the repair tissue, and biopsy tissue was harvested for analysis of microscopic appearance and biochemistry. The results that are reported mainly concern the injury locations considered an indication for autologous chondrocyte transplantation.[31]

Isolated Injury to the Femoral Condyle

Fifty-seven patients with an average age of 32.9 years had an average follow-up of 4 years. The average size of the defect was 4.2 cm², with the largest being 12 cm². Twenty-nine patients had undergone 58 earlier surgeries for this injury. The results, according to the modified Cincinnati scale, were 2.4 preoperatively and 8.4 postoperatively on a 0 to 10 scale. The overall clinical grading showed excellent results in 58%, good results in 32%, fair results in 7%, and poor results in 3%. Patient self-assessment indicated improvement in 89%.[31]

Isolated Femoral Condyle Injury with Anterior Cruciate Ligament Insufficiency

Twenty-seven patients had an isolated chondral injury on the femur combined with ACL insufficiency. The average follow-up was 4.3 years, and the average age was 30.3 years. The average defect size was 3.9 cm² with a maximum defect of 14 cm². Twenty-seven patients had undergone 55 previous surgeries related to the injury.

The clinical result, graded by the modified Cincinnati rating, was 2.2 preoperatively and 7.0 postoperatively on a 0 to 10 scale. Thirty-three percent had an excellent result, and 41% had a good result. Sixty-three percent considered themselves improved by surgery. If revision ACL patients were excluded, 85% considered themselves improved by the surgery.[31]

Osteochondritis Dissecans of the Femoral Condyle

In a study published in 2003, 58 patients had an average follow-up time of 5.6 years. The average age was 26.4 years, and the average defect size was 5.7 cm² with a maximum defect of 12 cm². Forty-eight patients had

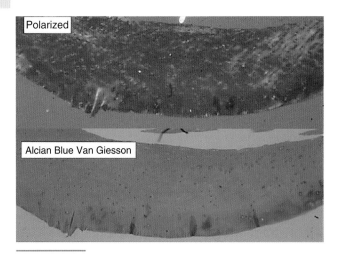

Polarized

Alcian Blue Van Giesson

Figure 21–12. Biopsy specimen from repair tissue 9 years after autologous chondrocyte transplantation.

Table 21–1. Immunohistochemical Analysis Comparing Normal Cartilage with Hyaline and Fibrous Repair Tissue

	NORMAL CARTILAGE	HYALINE REPAIR	FIBROUS REPAIR
Collagen type I	$- \rightarrow +$	$- \rightarrow +$	$+ + \rightarrow + + +$
Collagen type II	$+ + +$	$+ + \rightarrow + + +$	$-$
Cartilage oligomeric matrix protein	$+ + +$	$+ + \rightarrow + + +$	$+ \rightarrow + +$
Aggrecan	$+ + +$	$+ + \rightarrow + + +$	$+ \rightarrow + +$

undergone a mean of 2.1 previous surgeries because of the injury. The score, according to the modified Cincinnati clinical rating, was 2.0 preoperatively and 9.8 postoperatively at follow-up. The overall clinical grading was excellent in 53%, good in 38%, fair in 7%, and poor in 2%. Ninety-three percent of the patients considered themselves improved by self-assessment.[32]

Arthroscopic Assessment and Biopsies

Arthroscopic assessment was performed in 46 patients. Macroscopic evaluation of the defect area showed a maximal defect score of 12 points. Isolated femoral condyle injuries in 20 patients showed an average of 10.3 points. Isolated femoral condyle lesions plus ACL reconstruction had an average score of 10.9 points and, with osteochondritis dissecans, an average score of 10.5 out of 12 maximum, which is complete filling of the defect until total integration to the surrounding cartilage and a normal surface. Biopsy samples were harvested and judged by unbiased scientists, and 80% showed hyaline-like cartilage (Fig. 21–12).[27]

Indentation Test of Repair Tissue

The indentation test with an arthroscopic probe showed no significant difference in stiffness between normal articular cartilage and hyaline-like repair tissue in the transplanted area. Patients with fibrous tissue in the repair area had a significant decrease in stiffness when compared with normal cartilage and the repair tissue of hyaline-like cartilage.[27]

Immunohistochemical Analysis

Twenty-two biopsy specimens were taken from both repair tissue ($n = 19$) and healthy cartilage ($n = 3$). Analysis was

done in blinded fashion and involved the content of type I and II collagen, cartilage oligomeric matrix protein, and aggrecan. Hyaline-like repair tissue had characteristics very similar to those of normal articular cartilage, whereas fibrous repair tissue differed in all analyzed parameters (Table 21–1).

Complications

There were no serious complications, no infections, no chronic synovitis, and no thrombosis. The reoperation rate was 5%. The main complications were periosteal hypertrophy with a clicking or crepitating sensation, sometimes with swelling early in the postoperative period. Most of these symptoms disappeared with time and continued rehabilitation. If symptoms remained, patients were treated arthroscopically by débridement of the hypertrophic periosteum or fibrillation (Fig. 21–13). This complication had no impact on the long-term result. A few patients sustained partial delamination of the grafted area, with or without a new trauma episode. These patients were treated by retransplantation of autologous chondrocytes and achieved good and excellent results.

Long-Term Durability

Fifty of 61 patients with femoral condyle injuries had good or excellent results after 2 years' follow-up. Fifty-one of these patients still had a good or excellent result 5 to 10 years postoperatively, with an average follow-up of 7.4 years. This outcome indicates high durability.[27]

CARTILAGE REGISTRY REPORT

All patients treated by autologous chondrocyte transplantation in the United States and Europe are monitored in a registry outcome study. In a cohort of patients with both single ($n = 28$) and multiple lesions ($n = 11$) on the medial and lateral condyles and the trochlea with a 72-month follow-up, the modified Cincinnati Knee Rating Scale went from 3.15 preoperatively to 6.93 at 72 months.

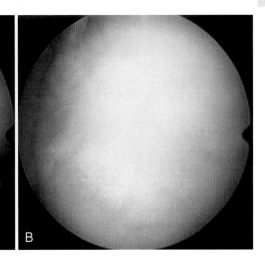

Figure 21–13. **A,** Complication consisting of fibrillation of the periosteal flap 1 year after autologous chondrocyte transplantation of the medial femoral condyle. **B,** After débridement of the superficial fibrillation of the periosteal flap. The fibrillation did not have any impact on the long-term results.

Eighty-two percent of the patients had functional improvement.[9]

A cohort of 15 patients with multiple lesions and a minimum of 60 months' follow-up were evaluated with the modified Cincinnati Knee Rating Scale for overall patient evaluation, pain, and swelling. All parameters increased. The overall patient evaluation category increased from 2.73 to 7.53, pain from 2.80 to 7.33, and swelling from 3.73 to 7.47, and the overall condition was improved in 93% of the patients.[7]

Complications

No infections have been reported since the start of the study in 1995. Adverse events or complications were reported by 5.8% after transplantation, and 2.9% had a complication considered to be at least possibly related to the autologous cultured chondrocytes. The most frequently reported adverse events are hypertrophic tissue at the repair site, intra-articular adhesions, superficial wound infection, hypertrophic synovitis, and postoperative hematoma.[8]

Both the clinical results and the complications were on a level with the Swedish results.

INTERNATIONAL EXPERIENCE WITH AUTOLOGOUS CHONDROCYTE TRANSPLANTATION

Ochi and coworkers have done interesting research with autologous chondrocytes evenly distributed and transplanted in a collagen gel. Twenty-eight knees in 26 patients treated with chondrocytes in collagen gel were monitored for at least 25 months. The treatment resulted in significant improvement in the Lysholm score. Pain and swelling were reduced in all patients, and locking was not present in any patient postoperatively. Arthroscopic

assessment indicated that 26 knees had a good or excellent outcome.[25]

From Australia, Hart and Henderson et al have confirmed the Swedish results in medium-term follow-up.[15,16]

From different centers in Europe, short- to medium-term results of autologous chondrocyte transplantation have been reported.[11,12]

Marcacci et al published promising short-term results on arthroscopic autologous chondrocyte transplantation with the use of Hyalograft, a hyaluronic acid derivative.[22]

Guillen et al reported good to excellent short-term results with type I collagen membranes.[14] Nehrer et al have also shown promising results with matrix-assisted chondrocyte transplantation.[24]

Prospective randomized studies with short-term results have been published by Knutsen et al,[19] with comparison between autologous chondrocyte implantation and microfracture, as well as by Bentley et al,[1] who randomized between autologous chondrocyte implantation and mosaicplasty. Promising clinical results are presented, but the follow-up is too short to draw any conclusions regarding which technique is better suited for the lesions treated.

FUTURE INDICATIONS

In young patients with multiple lesions (two or more in one joint) or bipolar lesion (i.e., bone-to-bone articulation), it is possible to try autologous chondrocyte transplantation. In treating this patient group it is of utmost importance to address background factors such as ligament instability, varus/valgus deformity, total/subtotal meniscectomy, bony defects in osteochondritis dissecans or after fracture, or patella malalignment or instability.

It is very important that the surgeon have optimal access to the defects, especially in the posterior part of the femur and the tibia. For that, you may need to detach the anterior insertion of the meniscus and its capsular insertion to the tibia. If this is not enough to reach the posterior part of the defect, the second step is to incise behind the collateral ligament. If that is not acceptable, do not hesitate to take down the collateral ligament from the femoral epicondyle with a bone block measuring 2×2 cm, and then you can open the joint to achieve excellent access to the posterior part of the tibia and femur.

Postoperative rehabilitation is longer in young early osteoarthritic patients, especially those who undergo concomitant procedures. Usually, we recommend partial weightbearing with 20 kg for 8 weeks and then progressively increased weightbearing up to full weightbearing at 4 months.

Patients with multiple lesions and a minimum of 3 years' follow-up had 84% good or excellent results. Those with bipolar tibial-femoral lesions had 75% good or excellent results, and patients with bipolar patellar-femoral lesions had 75% good or excellent results.

OTHER JOINTS

Autologous chondrocyte transplantation has been used in the ankle joint with osteochondritis dissecans, as well as for cartilage lesions in the shoulder, elbow, and wrist. In principle, this technique can be used in any joint with a localized articular cartilage lesion or osteochondritis dissecans.

The longest follow-up in the talus is now over 8 years, and the results are promising. The approach to medial or lateral localized injuries in the talus usually mandates a medial or sometimes a lateral osteotomy for optimal surgical access to the defect.[28]

The hip has been operated on in six young patients with osteochondritis dissecans or chondral lesions on the caput femoris. The shoulder has been operated on in three cases, in two with lesions of both the glenoid and the head of the humerus. The results seem promising in other joints, but we need more patients and longer follow-up for establishing these indications.

Further data collection and long-term results are needed before indications for these joints can be approved.

SUMMARY

Clinical experience with autologous chondrocyte transplantation is now longer than 17 years. Isolated articular cartilage injuries on the femoral condyles show good to excellent results in 90% of cases. Treatment of osteochondritis dissecans produces good to excellent results in 89% of cases. No serious complications have occurred, and a low number of adverse reactions have been reported. Biopsy specimens have shown hyaline-like cartilage, and indentation tests have not indicated any significant difference between the indentation stiffness of hyaline-like repair tissue and normal surrounding cartilage.

The results from the Swedish study have been confirmed by Cartilage Repair Registry data, with the longest follow-up being 6 years, and by data from Boston and Atlanta, with the longest follow-up being 8 years. In the United States more than 10,000 operations have been performed since 1995.

References

1. Bentley G, Biant LC, Carrington RWJ, et al: A prospective, randomized comparison of autologous chondrocyte implantation versus mosaicplasty for osteochondral defects in the knee. J Bone Joint Surg Br 85:223, 2003.
2. Brittberg M, Lindahl A, Nilsson A, et al: Treatment of deep cartilage defects in the knee with autologous chondrocyte transplantation. N Engl J Med 331:889, 1994.
3. Brittberg M, Nilsson A, Peterson L, et al: Healing of injured rabbit articular cartilage after transplantation with autologously isolated and cultured chondrocytes [abstract]. In Abstracts of the Bat Sheva Seminars on Methods Used in Research on Cartilaginous Tissues, Tel Aviv, Israel, March 16-26, 1989, vol 1. Nof Ginnosar, Israel, Bat Sheva, 1989, pp 28-29.
4. Buckwalter JA: Chondral and osteochondral injuries: Mechanisms of injury and repair responses. Op Tech Orthop 7:263, 1997.
5. Buckwalter JA, Mankin AJ: Articular cartilage II. Degeneration and osteoarthrosis, repair regeneration and transplantation. J Bone Joint Surg Am 54:147, 1997.
6. Buchwalter JA, Rosenberg LC, Hunziker EB: Articular cartilage: Composition, structure, response to injury and methods of facilitating repair. In Ewing JW (ed): Articular Cartilage and Knee Joint Function: Basic Science and Arthroscopy. New York, Raven Press, 1990, pp 19-56.
7. Cartilage Repair Registry Multiple Defect Subanalysis. Registry Report, vol 7. Cambridge, MA, Genzyme Tissue Repair, 2001.
8. Cartilage Repair Registry Periodic Report, vol 4. Cambridge, MA, Genzyme Tissue Repair, 1998.
9. Cartilage Repair Registry Summary Report, vol 8. Cambridge, MA, Genzyme Tissue Repair, 2002.
10. Chesterman PJ, Smith AU: Homotransplantation of articular cartilage and isolated chondrocytes: An experimental study in rabbits. J Bone Joint Surg Br 50:184, 1968.
11. Erggelet C, Steinwachs MR, Reichelt A: The operative treatment of full thickness cartilage defects in the knee joint with autologous chondrocyte transplantation. Saudi Med J 21:715, 2000.
12. Gobbi A, Berruto M, Francisco R: Clinical results in patellofemoral full thickness chondral defects treated with Hyalograft-C: A prospective study at 2-years follow-up [abstract]. Presented at the American Orthopaedic Society for Sports Medicine Specialty Day, February 26, 2005, Washington, DC.
13. Grande DA, Pitman MI, Peterson L, et al: The repair of experimentally produced defects in rabbit articular cartilage by autologous chondrocyte implantation. J Orthop Res 7:208, 1989.
14. Guillen Garcia P, Abelow S, Fernandez Jaen T: Membrane/ matrix autologous chondrocyte implantation. Presented at the University of California at San Francisco Comprehensive Knee Cartilage Symposium: State of the art in 2003. November 8, 2003, San Francisco.
15. Hart J: Arthroscopic evaluation of cartilage repair following autologous chondrocyte implantation (ACI). Presented at the Fourth Biennial ISAKOS Congress, March 8-16, 2003, Auckland, New Zealand.
16. Henderson IJ, Tuy B, Connell D, et al: Prospective clinical study of autologous chondrocyte implantation and correlation with MRI at three and 12 months. J Bone Joint Surg Br 85:1060, 2003.
17. Hubbard MJS: Articular debridement versus washout for degeneration of medial femoral condyle: A five-year study. J Bone Joint Surg Br 78:217, 1996.
18. International Cartilage Repair Society website, www.cartilage.org, downloaded May 2, 2005.
19. Knutsen G, Engebretsen L, Ludvigsen TC, et al: Autologous chondrocyte implantation compared with microfracture in the knee: A randomized trial. J Bone Joint Surg Am 86:455, 2004.
20. Magnusson PB: Technique of debridement of the knee joint for arthritis. Surg Clin North Am 26:226, 1946.
21. Mankin HJ: Current concepts review. The response of articular cartilage to mechanical injury. J Bone Joint Surg Am 64:460, 1982.
22. Marcacci M, Kon E, Zaffagnini S: Tissue engineering of cartilage: 2nd generation autologous chondrocyte transplantation. Presented

at the Fifth Biennial ISAKOS Congress, April 3-7, 2005, Hollywood, FL.

23. Minas T, Peterson L: Chondrocyte transplantation. Op Tech Orthop 7:323, 1997.
24. Nehrer S, Schatz K, Marlovits S, et al: Preliminary results of matrix-assisted chondrocyte transplantation using a hyaluronan matrix. Presented at the International Cartilage Repair Society Symposium, June 15-18, 2002, Toronto.
25. Ochi M, Uchio Y, Kawasaki K, et al: Transplantation of cartilage-like tissue made by tissue engineering in the treatment of cartilage defects of the knee. J Bone Joint Surg Br 84:571, 2002.
26. Outerbridge RE: The etiology of chondromalacia patellae. J Bone Joint Surg Br 43:752, 1961.
27. Peterson L, Brittberg M, Kiviranta I, et al: Autologous chondrocyte transplantation: Biomechanics and long-term durability. Am J Sports Med 30:2, 2002.
28. Peterson L, Brittberg M, Lindahl A: Autologous chondrocyte transplantation of the ankle. Foot Ankle Clin N Am 8:291, 2003.
29. Peterson L, Menche D, Grande D, et al: Chondrocyte transplantation: An experimental model in the rabbit [abstract]. In Transactions from the 30th Annual Orthopaedic Research Society, Atlanta, February 7-9, 1984. Palatine, IL, Orthopaedic Research Society, 1984, p 218.
30. Peterson L, Minas T: Articular cartilage regeneration: Chondrocyte transplantation and other technologies. Presented at the Annual Meeting of the American Academy of Orthopaedic Surgeons, February 12-15, 1997, San Francisco.
31. Peterson L, Minas T, Brittberg M, et al: Two- to 9-year outcome after autologous chondrocyte transplantation of the knee. Clin Orthop 374:212, 2000.
32. Peterson L, Minas T, Brittberg M, et al: Treatment of osteochondritis dissecans of the knee with autologous chondrocyte transplantation: Results at two to ten years. J Bone Joint Surg Am 85(Suppl 2): 17, 2003.
33. Suh J-K, Åören A, Muzzonigro T, et al: Injury and repair of articular cartilage: Related scientific issues. Op Tech Orthop 7:270, 1997.

CHAPTER 22

North American Experience with Autologous Chondrocyte Implantation

Tom Minas

HISTORICAL PERSPECTIVE

Autologous chondrocyte transplantation has been known as autologous chondrocyte implantation (ACI) in North America. The technique as described by Peterson and coworkers[2] has been adapted by the author after several visits to Sweden in the early 1990s. After institutional review board approval, the technique of ACI has been used to manage large acute and chronic focal articular cartilage injuries in the knee since March 1995. To date, over 350 treatments have been performed at our institution, and as of fall 2004, more than 10,000 patients have been treated by ACI in North America.

The use of autologous chondrocytes for patient care in the United States has been carefully regulated by the Food and Drug Administration (FDA, Biologics Division) and has required both good laboratory practices (GLP standards) and good manufacturing practices (GMP standards) since the onset of its introduction in the United States. This has been cost prohibitive to private institutions for patient care and therefore has been performed by industry (Genzyme Bio Surgery, Cambridge, MA). As of August 22nd, 1997, the FDA formally approved ACI (FDA Biologics License 1233) for the management of focal chondral defects of the femoral articular surfaces. Approval was based on the early data of 159 patients evaluated in Sweden as of 1997. Because of early results that were not favorable for management of the patella, tibia, or cases involving early bipolar or arthritic lesions, these defects have been considered "off label." However, before FDA approval, the author had gained considerable experience in the treatment of these "off-label" uses based on patients who were sent for the management of these troublesome lesions.

PRINCIPLES FOR SUCCESSFUL MANAGEMENT OF ARTICULAR CARTILAGE LESIONS

When a full-thickness articular cartilage lesion is discovered by arthroscopy or magnetic resonance imaging (MRI), it is important to identify whether the lesion is symptomatic, as well as the cause of the defect, before pursuing cartilage repair. If one is to undertake cartilage repair without addressing the underlying predisposing factors, the repair technique will probably fail. Common modes of articular failure include anterior cruciate ligament (ACL) disruption in a varus knee, patellofemoral dislocation in the presence of abnormal patellar tracking, a direct impact blow to the knee as a result of a motor vehicle or industrial accident, a repetitive impact injury in the face of varus or valgus malalignment of the axial extremity, a meniscectomized knee, and premature breakdown of articular cartilage as a result of obesity or osteoarthritis at an early age. These factors may be overlooked when they occur in patients with a sports injury, but they are important to address in definitive reconstruction of a knee to achieve successful cartilage repair and clinical resolution of symptoms.

PREOPERATIVE EVALUATION

When evaluating a patient with an articular cartilage injury, the author evaluates patient factors as well as knee factors separately to determine the most appropriate management. Patient factors to consider include age, activity level (whether it be high or low demand), body weight, emotional well-being, and addictive behavior patterns (smoking and narcotic and alcohol use to mention a few). Issues related to the knee include (in order of importance) axial alignment, ligamentous stability, chondral defect size, presence or absence of the meniscus, and cartilage phenotype—other joints that are osteoarthritic, radiographic evidence of osteoarthritis, or a strong family history of osteoarthritis.

In the author's experience, a patient who is highly motivated, realistic about the rehabilitation protocol, a nonsmoker, and not using narcotics for pain management is desirable. A strong social support system and a sense of vitality as measured by the SF-36 Health Survey has proved to be a high statistical predictor of a good physical outcome in a study conducted at our institution and presented at a meeting of the International Cartilage Repair Society in Toronto in 2001.[4] A patient younger than 18 years also has an excellent chance of returning to full activities.[5]

Axial alignment is best measured by long, axial alignment radiographs that include the hip, knee, and ankle on a single cassette; we have used 54-inch cassettes at our institution, which can also be digitized. Radiographs are the only true way to assess the location of the mechanical axis at the level of the knee as opposed to clinical examination. In addition, standing anteroposterior extension, standing 45 degree posteroanterior (Rosenberg), lateral, and patello-femoral tangential (skyline/Merchant) views are taken as a routine baseline assessment in all patients. These films are useful to assess joint space narrowing, as well as axial alignment, in order to rule out bone-on-bone changes, which are not suitable for cartilage repair by any technique. Patellofemoral maltracking is best assessed by clinical evaluation of the quadriceps angle with the patella in the reduced position with the knee in extension to assess patellar subluxation with quadriceps contraction. If there is any question regarding patellar tracking, a computed tomography (CT) scan is performed with the knee in extension to assess patellar location relative to the trochlea when the quadriceps is in both the relaxed and contracted positions. This also is an excellent evaluation tool to assess dysplasia of the trochlea. If a dye arthrogram is performed with the CT scan, we have found it to be an excellent technique to evaluate the articular cartilage surface at the same time.

The author considers ACI for the management of an articular chondral defect when the defect is noted to be symptomatic, it is larger than 2 cm², and other mechanical factors have been identified such as varus alignment or ligamentous instability, which are usually corrected at the time of the cartilage repair procedure. This technique is performed in a highly motivated, compliant, symptomatic patient who requires a high-demand repair. The hyaline-like articular cartilage produced by ACI provides near-normal viscoelastic properties that relieve symptoms, as well as a durable, long-term repair.

TECHNIQUE

The techniques for autologous chondrocyte transplantation have been described in detail in the previous chapter by Lars Peterson, M.D., Ph.D. These techniques have also been described elsewhere.[2,6]

NORTH AMERICAN CLINICAL RESULTS USING AUTOLOGOUS CHONDROCYTE IMPLANTATION

The results to follow include the author's collaborative results of the use of ACI in adolescents and soccer players, as well as personal updated results in treating the patellofemoral joint and the osteoarthritic or salvage group of patients. The North American Cartilage Repair Registry of Genzyme Bio Surgery (Cambridge, MA) completes the chapter.

ACI in Adolescents[5]

Between December 1995 and December 2000, 20 patients with 29 full-thickness articular cartilage lesions in 23 knees were treated by ACI at Boston Children's Hospital and Brigham and Women's Hospital. All patients had failed previous conservative and surgical treatment and had undergone at least one surgical procedure before ACI (mean, 2.5 procedures; range, 1 to 6). The maximum age for inclusion in the study was 18 years. Patient demographics, defect etiology and characteristics, preoperative duration of symptoms, and surgical history were recorded. Injuries were considered chronic if the preoperative duration of symptoms was longer than 12 months. Preoperative radiographs were obtained on every patient and demonstrated open growth plates at the time of ACI in 60% of the adolescent athletes (see Table 22–1).

In two patients the depth of the defect required autologous bone grafting in combination with ACI. Implantation of chondrocytes in these cases was performed by using the "sandwich technique" (see previous chapter). Reconstruction of the ACL was performed in one patient at the time of chondrocyte implantation. One other patient had undergone staged ACL reconstruction before autologous chondrocyte transplantation. Meniscal repair was performed in four patients, at the time of chondrocyte implantation in two and as part of their previous surgical procedures in two. Tibial tubercle osteotomy was performed concomitantly in one patient. Postoperatively, continuous passive motion was initiated within 6 to 12 hours and administered for 2 weeks. Patients remained non-weightbearing for 6 to 8 weeks with gradual progression to full weightbearing by 10 to 12 weeks. Most patients were allowed to return to regular daily activities by 4 months, low-impact pursuits by 6 months, and progression to running at 9 months. Demanding high-impact and pivoting sports were avoided for 12 months.

Table 22–1. Functional Outcome of Knee Articular Cartilage Repair in Adolescent Athletes: Demographic Data and Lesion Characteristics

Gender, M/F (%)	75:25
Age (yr)	15.9 ± 0.3 (12-18)
Previous operations (*n*)	2.5 ± 0.3 (1-6)
Preoperative interval (mo)	21 ± 3.5 (3-60)
≤12 mo	48%
>12 mo	52%
Lesion size (cm²)	6.4 ± 0.7 (2.4-14)
Number of lesions	1.3 ± 0.1 (1-3)
Lesion type	
Traumatic	*n* = 9 (39%)
Osteochondritis dissecans	*n* = 14 (61%)
Single	*n* = 18 (78%)
Multiple	*n* = 5 (22%)
Lesion location (%)*	
Medial femoral condyle	*n* = 14 (61%)
Lateral femoral condyle	*n* = 6 (26%)
Trochlea	*n* = 4 (17%)
Tibial plateau	*n* = 2 (9%)
Patella	*n* = 1 (4%)

*Some patients had multiple lesions.
Data from Tom Minas, MD, Kai Mithöfer, MD, Howard Yeon, MD, and Lyle J. Micheli, MD, Departments of Orthopedic Surgery, Children's Hospital, Cartilage Repair Center, Brigham and Women's Hospital, and Harvard Medical School, Boston.

Patients were evaluated preoperatively and at a mean of 47 ± 4 months postoperatively (range, 23 to 91 months). Functional outcome was determined by using established knee scoring systems, including the Lysholm score and the Tegner activity score. In addition, a questionnaire was used to evaluate the patient's ability to participate in athletics and to provide a subjective rating of knee function, which was graded as either excellent, good, fair, or poor. The level of athletic participation before injury was compared with the athletic ability after chondrocyte transplantation.

Twenty adolescent patients with articular cartilage lesions in 23 knees were treated by autologous chondrocyte transplantation. Seventeen patients had unilateral involvement and 3 had bilateral knee articular cartilage lesions. The mean age at chondrocyte transplantation was 15.9 ± 0.3 years (range, 12 to 18 years). There were 15 male and 5 female adolescent athletes. The average duration of symptoms was 21 months, 12 months or less in 11 knees (48%) and over 12 months in 12 knees (52%). All patients had failed previous conservative and surgical treatment.

Osteochondritis dissecans was the cause of the chondral defect in 14 knees, whereas in the remaining 9 knees the cartilage lesions resulted from acute focal trauma associated with pivoting sports such as basketball, football, and soccer. Two patients had tears of the ACL (10%), and four patients (20%) meniscal injuries. A total of 29 cartilage lesions were observed, the majority being single lesions with an average of 1.3 cartilage defects per knee. The average lesion size was 6.4 cm^2.

At latest follow-up, 96% of patients were able to regularly participate in high-impact, pivoting sports at the recreational level or higher. Sixty percent of the athletes had returned to the same or higher level of athletic activity than before their injury. Tegner activity scores increased in all patients in comparison to preoperative values. Lysholm scores were not available before injury but increased significantly from preoperative values of 64 ± 3 points to 87 ± 7 points at latest follow-up ($p < .01$).

Only 33% of adolescents with chronic preoperative symptoms (>12 months) returned to the same level of athletics, whereas such return was possible in all adolescents with shorter preoperative intervals ($p < .01$). Postoperative Tegner scores (7.2 ± 0.3 points) and Lysholm scores (85 ± 3 points) in adolescents with chronic symptoms were lower than Tegner scores (8.7 ± 0.2 points, $p < .01$) and Lysholm scores (91 ± 2 points) in adolescents with symptoms for 12 months or less. The average preoperative duration of symptoms in adolescents who returned to preinjury athletic levels was 15 ± 4 months and less than in adolescents who failed to return to the same level (31 ± 6 months, $p < .05$). Adolescents with chronic symptoms had undergone an average of 3.2 ± 0.4 previous surgeries as compared with 1.6 ± 0.2 in adolescents with acute symptoms ($p < .05$). The number of previous operations also showed a significant correlation with the ability to return to preinjury athletics ($r = .453$, $p < .05$).

Ninety-six percent of patients rated their results as good or excellent, and only one patient reported a fair outcome. This patient had moderate genu varum and did not consent to primary realignment. He briefly returned to high-impact athletics after autologous chondrocyte transplantation to the medial femoral condyle and trochlea, but recurrent symptoms developed on resumption of athletic activities and graft failure occurred. Secondary high tibial osteotomy was performed. The patient has not yet returned to high-impact activities at the time of last follow-up and awaits revision ACI. Other complications included graft hypertrophy, which was observed in three athletes (15%) and was successfully treated by arthroscopic chondroplasty in all cases.

ACI in adolescent patients is highly successful when used as a first-line treatment strategy for large chondral defects within the first year of injury. Performance of multiple surgeries in an attempt to be less invasive led to chronic dysfunction and a poor clinical outcome in these patients.

ACI in Soccer Players[8]

Between March 1988 and August 2000, 45 soccer players were treated by autologous chondrocyte transplantation at the participating institutions (Table 22–2). All athletes complained of acute or chronic symptoms. Baseline evaluation included a careful history and physical examination and documentation of the type, onset, and duration of symptoms. Demographic data, previous surgical history, and skill level were recorded. Skill level was divided into recreational and high-level competitive sports for athletes who participated in high-school, collegiate, professional, or national team–level soccer.

All patients had full-thickness Outerbridge type IV articular cartilage lesions or osteochondral lesions of the knee demonstrated at arthroscopy. The minimum follow-up duration from the time of implantation was 12 months. At follow-up, the sports activity–based Tegner scale was used to rate the athlete's function. The ability and timing of return to soccer and the skill level after articular cartilage repair were recorded. Successful articular cartilage repair was defined as the ability to return to soccer even if not at the previous skill level. Treatment durability was defined as the percentage of players who returned to soccer and maintained this functional status at subsequent follow-up. Adverse events and complications were carefully documented.

Significant improvement in activity scores was observed in more than 80% of players, thus confirming the overall functional improvements described after ACI in previous studies. Despite the overall increased function, only a third of the players was able to return to soccer. The return rate was significantly higher in competitive than in recreational-level players. An 83% return rate was recorded in competitive soccer players after autologous chondrocyte transplantation in our study. Interestingly, the rate of return to recreational soccer in our study was significantly lower than the return rate at the higher skill level. Significantly prolonged preoperative morbidity was seen in players who failed to return to soccer after autologous chondrocyte transplantation in our study and could also explain the lower return rate of recreational players in the present study. Our data indicate that the longer the time

Table 22–2. Articular Cartilage Repair in High-Demand Athletes by Autologous Chondrocyte Transplantation: Functional Outcome and Return to Competition

DEMOGRAPHIC DATA	ALL PLAYERS	RETURN	NO RETURN
Gender, M/F (%)	72:28	80:20	63:37
Age (yr)	26 ± 1 (14-43)	22.3 ± 1.6*	27.6 ± 1.2
Previous surgeries (*n*)	2.0 ± 0.3 (0-13)	1.5 ± 0.3	2.3 ± 0.5
Skill level (%)			
Recreational	73	16	84
High level	27	83[†]	17
Symptom duration (mo)	26 ± 3.4 (3-96)	16.7 ± 3.8*	30.7 ± 4.5
Lesion size (cm²)	5.7 ± 0.6	5.5 ± 0.8	5.6 ± 0.8
Lesion type (%)			
Single	65	86[†]	14
Multiple	35	30	70
Lesion location (%)			
Femoral condyles	83	75	25
Patellofemoral	24	36	64
Graft failure (%)	13	6	16

*$p < .05$.
[†]$p < .001$.
Data from Kai Mithöfer, MD, and Lars Peterson, MD, PhD, Gothenburg Medical Center, Gothenburg, Sweden; Bert R. Mandelbaum, MD, Santa Monica Orthopedic and Sports Medicine Foundation, Los Angeles; and Tom Minas, MD, Harvard Combined Orthopedic Surgery Program, Boston.

between injury and chondrocyte transplantation, the lower the rate of return to competitive or recreational soccer. In fact, the success rate effectively doubled if autologous chondrocyte transplantation was performed within 1 year after onset of the articular cartilage injury. This finding confirms previous observations in which a significantly better functional outcome was demonstrated if autologous chondrocyte transplantation was performed within 1 year of sustaining the cartilage injury, as in our adolescent patients.

The average time to return to soccer in our study was 18 months, and 87% of returning players were still competing at a mean of 48 months postoperatively. Although initial recovery after chondrocyte transplantation may be more prolonged, our data suggest that this cartilage repair technique provides excellent durability even with very high athletic demand. Some world-class athletes who were treated primarily with autologous chondrocyte transplantation within 4 months of their injury were able to rapidly return to their preinjury level of play and had excellent long-term durability. These excellent results under maximum demand support the use of autologous chondrocyte transplantation as a primary technique for articular cartilage repair in young active patients. In contrast, when autologous chondrocyte transplantation is used as a salvage procedure in older patients with long-standing preoperative symptoms and multiple previous operations, the results are less predictable.

The results with the use of autologous chondrocyte transplantation in soccer athletes are encouraging. An excellent rate of return to demanding athletic activity and long-term function is possible, particularly in young, competitive players with a short duration of symptoms and fewer previous surgical interventions. These results are comparable to those reported for microfracture or

osteochondral mosaicplasty. Long-term evaluation will help determine whether restoration of articular cartilage lesions in the knee in soccer players can effectively reduce the high incidence of osteoarthritis in this population.

ACI in the Patellofemoral Joint[3]

Many factors have been implicated as contributing to abnormal pathomechanics leading to pain in the patellofemoral joint, including patella alta, trochlea dysplasia, an increased quadriceps or Q angle with secondary soft-tissue problems, a weakened or hypoplastic vastus medialis oblique quadriceps muscle with a contracted lateral retinaculum, and/or an absent redundant medial patellofemoral ligament. These pathomechanics lead to abnormal forces across the patella that result in secondary degenerative changes or injury to the articular surfaces of the patellofemoral joint acutely or chronically. Diagnosing as well as correcting these underlying abnormalities when associated with cartilage injury is crucial to a successful outcome when using ACI for repair of these defects. It is for these reasons that the early results of resurfacing of the patella with ACI led to only two good or excellent results in seven patients treated (29%) in the first study in which autologous chondrocyte transplantation was introduced in Sweden in 1994.[2] In later reports,[9,11] as patellar tracking was also addressed by realignment of the extensor mechanism at the time of transplantation, it was noted that the success rate increased at 2 years such that 11 of 17 patients (65%) had good or excellent results,[11] and at 10 years the results had improved to the extent that 13 of 17 patients (76%) had good or excellent results.[9] Two patients who were rated as having a fair result at 2 years had improved to a good results at 3 years; thus the results improved over time. The importance of correcting the underlying cause of the chondral injury cannot be underestimated when attempting surgical correction with cartilage repair techniques.

Anteromedialization (AMZ) of the tibial tubercle has become a useful surgical tool for correcting maltracking and unloading an articular cartilage injury to the patella. Fulkerson and colleagues[12] have demonstrated that a successful clinical outcome of AMZ tibial tubercle osteotomy correlates with the location of the patellar articular lesion (Fig. 22–1). In patients with a type I (inferior patellar pole) or a type II (lateral facet) articular cartilage lesion, unloading of these two locations by an osteotomy yielded 87% good to excellent subjective results, and 100% of these patients said that they would have the procedure done again. Type III (medial facet) lesions had 55% good to excellent results, and with type IV (proximal pole or diffuse) lesions, only 20% had a good or excellent result. Patients with type I or II lesions were significantly more likely to have good or excellent results than were those with type III or IV lesions. Central trochlea lesions were associated with medial patellar lesions, and all patients with central trochlea lesions have poor results. Workers' compensation issues diminish the likelihood of a satisfactory outcome by 19%. They concluded that the location of the articular patellar cartilage lesion was significantly correlated with the success of AMZ tibial tubercle osteotomy.

Localization of the articular cartilage injury at the time of reconstruction is therefore important for determining whether osteotomy surgery alone may achieve a successful outcome. Theoretically, cartilage repair of patellar type III and IV lesions, as well as trochlea lesions, may improve the clinical outcome of these difficult lesions when associated with patellar maltracking or in the absence of abnormal tracking when no other options exist.

ACI is indicated for the management of focal chondral defects in the knee. The author has treated single, multiple, and kissing lesions. However, the cartilage space must be intact on a standard radiograph to indicate that the overall joint space is patent, the margins are well shouldered, and cartilage loss is not diffuse.

Between March 1995 and July 2002, 248 patients had been treated. One hundred seventy patients had a minimum of 2-year follow-up as of July 2002. Of these 170 patients treated, 45 had treatments involving the patella or trochlea, in isolation or combination with other lesions, with a minimum of 2 years of follow-up. These patients were the ones who participated in this study.

Baseline patient demographics were captured, as well as outcomes as assessed by several validated outcomes instruments. In addition, at the time of surgery all patients had their surgeries photographed to assess the appearance of the native chondral injury, the débrided chondral injury, and the surgical site after the completion of suturing of the periosteal patch and injection with autologous cultured chondrocytes. These photographs are maintained on a digital file and were used to classify the patellar defect location as per the Fulkerson classification.[12] Patients filled out questionnaires, including the SF-36, Knee Society Score, Western Ontario McMaster Osteoarthritis Score (WOMAC), the activity-based score of the modified Cincinnati rating scale (0 to 10), and a patient satisfaction survey.

Patients were sent by orthopedists for definitive management of persistent painful knees. There were 27 males and 18 females. The average patient age at surgery was 36.9 years (range, 15 to 54). The average follow-up is 47.5 months (range, 24 to 86 months). The average number of previous surgeries was 2.5 per patient on the affected knee. Twenty-four percent of patients (11/45) had been treated while receiving workers' compensation. There were an average of 2.2 defects per knee, and an average of 2.18 vials times 12 million cells per vial (26.16 million cells) was used to treat each knee. The lesions treated were large with an average surface area per knee joint of 10.45 cm^2.

Technical issues that are specific to the surgical procedure of ACI in the patellofemoral joint include a suture technique that restores the surface articular shape of the patella (Fig. 22–2) and the trochlea (Fig. 22–3), as well as soft-tissue tensioning at the end of the procedure that allows normal medial-to-lateral and proximal-to-distal patellar glide without overconstricting the patellofemoral joint. An AMZ tibial tubercle osteotomy as preferred by the author is demonstrated in Figure 22–4. If patellar instability secondary to a dysplastic trochlea is still present after AMZ tibial tubercle osteotomy and soft-tissue stabilization, trochleoplasty is added to the procedure as described by Peterson et al.[10]

Osteotomy was frequently performed in this series, in 29 of 45 patients (64%) who had tibiofemoral or patellofemoral malalignment, or both. It is thought that a successful cartilage repair includes normal alignment and tracking. Hence, if 2 or more degrees of mechanical malalignment from a neutral mechanical axis is present in the tibiofemoral joint in combination with a large chondral defect, a varus- or valgus-producing osteotomy

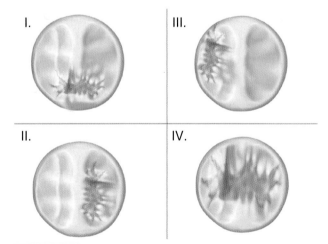

Figure 22–1. Classification of patella articular chondral defects[9]: type 1, inferior patellar pole; type 2, lateral patellar facet; type 3, medial patellar facet; and type 4, global central pan-patellar defect. Type 1 and 2 defects are well managed by an unloading anterior medial tibial tubercle osteotomy. Type 3 and 4 defects do poorly with osteotomy alone.

accompanies the cartilage repair on the weightbearing condyles. If there is evidence of patellar subluxation and tilt with regard to patellar tracking as noted by clinical examination and/or assessment by CT scan, an AMZ tibial tubercle osteotomy is performed in conjunction with resurfacing of the patella or trochlea, or both.

Rehabilitation in the first 6 weeks after surgery has three goals. The first is to restore tibiofemoral range of motion, as well as patellar mobility, to prevent infrapatellar tendon contracture. This is performed by aggressive deep friction, mobilization, stretching, and continuous passive motion for 6 weeks postoperatively and use of a stationary bicycle at 4 weeks. Second, muscle tone must be reestablished with isometric leg lifts, muscle contractions, and stationary bicycling. Finally and most important, the graft must be protected from overloading. The patella and trochlea experience maximal contact force between 40 and 70 degrees of flexion. Therefore, open-chain quadriceps extensions through this range of motion is avoided. If the graft is very large, continuous passive motion is avoided through this range of motion at the early stages of rehabilitation.

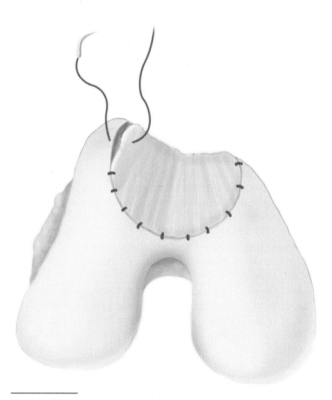

Figure 22–2. The periosteal suturing technique for the trochlea requires microsuturing to restore the concavity of the trochlea.

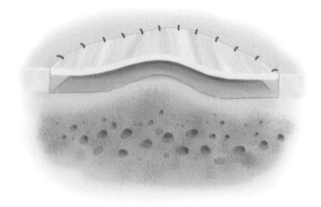

Figure 22–3. The periosteal suturing technique for the patella requires starting at the apex of the median ridge and restoring the "tent" shape to the patella.

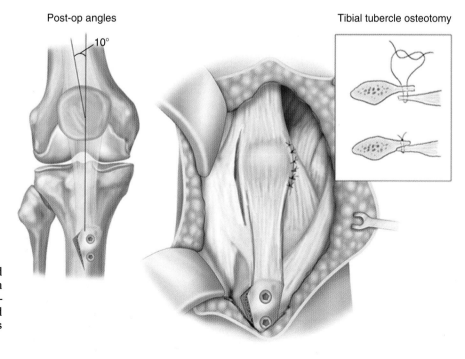

Figure 22–4. The author's preferred technique for anteromedialization tibial tubercle osteotomy accompanied by patella lateral release and vastus medialis oblique–quadriceps advancement.

The principles of therapy involve functional rehabilitation with avoidance of resisted open-chain activities. Stationary followed by outdoor bicycling, treadmill and outdoor walking, and elliptical training devices have all been useful; weight machines have been avoided until at least 6 months after surgery. If the knee becomes painful or swollen or crepitations develop and limit further recovery, the activities are stopped. Clinical evaluation usually followed by MRI with intravenous or intra-articular gadolinium enhancement is performed to evaluate the status of the ACI graft versus periosteal overgrowth, which generally occurs between 3 and 9 months after surgery. MRI evaluation with intravenous gadolinium enhancement to determine the status of the grafts at different time points is the subject of another study and has been very useful in determining graft status.

Typically, patients start to have good pain relief by 4 to 6 months after surgery. Nonimpact sporting activities are commenced at 9 months postoperatively and full impact activities by 18 months. Maximal medical improvement may take as long as 3 years in patients with large areas transplanted to allow for graft maturation and functional strengthening.

Clinical outcome questionnaires were administered by a registered nurse at baseline, 6 months, 1 year, 18 months, 2 years, and annually thereafter. Patient failures were defined as poor clinical outcomes accompanied by evidence of graft failure as a result of delamination from adjacent cartilage and subchondral bone, poor biomechanical properties indicative of fibrous or fibrocartilage repair as evidenced by arthroscopy, or evidence of graft detachment by MRI or arthroscopy despite a good clinical outcome.

The results of ACI in the patellofemoral joint have been successful in this difficult patient population. When assessing the first 45 patients who underwent treatment of the patellofemoral joint by ACI at a minimum of a 2-year follow-up, we have found patient satisfaction to be high. Use of a patient questionnaire regarding overall satisfaction has shown 71% to be satisfied, 16% neutral, and 13% dissatisfied. When compared with the situation before surgery, 76% were better, 18% were the same, and 6% were worse. Eighty-seven percent of patients said that they would choose the surgery again, whereas 13% said that they would not. Overall, patients rated their results as 71% good or excellent, 22% fair, and 7% poor. Marked clinical improvement and statistical significance were achieved with the SF-36, the Knee Society Score, the WOMAC score, and the modified Cincinnati activity score (see Table 22–3).

Our series has shown that the location of the chondral defect on the patella and the trochlea is key to achieving a successful clinical outcome when ACI, in addition to realignment when needed, is used to treat the chondral defect, whereas other series have not.[12] In this series (Table 22–4), 31 of 34 (91%) patellar lesions treated were type III or type IV in location. The location of the other defects was the trochlea ($n = 11$) or a kissing patella and trochlea ($n = 20$). Sixty-four percent of the cases involved osteotomy of the tibial tubercle alone or in combination with a valgus-producing tibial osteotomy. The osteotomy effect alone would not account for the high success rate based on Fulkerson's results[3] because of the size and location of these chondral defects.

Three subgroups in our series—patella plus trochlea ($n = 4$), weightbearing condyles plus patella ($n = 2$), and weightbearing condyles plus trochlea ($n = 2$)—had a small sample size with not very meaningful statistics. However, the groups patella ($n = 8$), trochlea ($n = 9$), and weightbearing condyles plus patella plus trochlea ($n = 20$) demonstrated marked improvement in pain relief and functionality.

The SF-36 Physical Component Summary demonstrated highly significant improvement in physical well-being after ACI. Emotional well-being as measured by the SF-36 Mental Component Summary was also significant for the larger group ($n = 20$), weightbearing condyle plus patella plus trochlea. The WOMAC score, which indicates relief from pain, stiffness, and swelling, was also significant for these three groups, as was the Knee Society Score for the knee rating component of this scoring system. The greatest improvement in sports activity rating, surprisingly, was in the most severely injured knees. This treatment group had the largest surface area of transplantation for the knee, 15.31 cm².

When assessing the overall size of the defects treated, we noted that 35 trochleae with an average surface area of 5.22 cm² and 34 patellae with an average surface area of 4.86 cm² were treated. These were large surfaces that involved the majority of the articular surface. Unlike the weightbearing condyles, however, the average thickness of the articular surface at these sites was 3 to 5 mm versus 2

Table 22–3. Overall Outcome Scores for Autologous Chondrocyte Implantation in the Patellofemoral Joint

OUTCOME MEASURES	PREOPERATIVE	POSTOPERATIVE	P VALUE
SF-36 PCS	35.16	40.25	.0004
SF-36 MCS	47.84	53.39	.0016
WOMAC	37.1	24.4	<.0001
KSS—Knee	53	74	<.0001
KSS—Function	67	78	<.0002
Mod Cincinnati	3.84 (range, 1-8)	5.76 (range, 1-10)	<.0001

KSS, Knee Society Score; MCS, Mental Component Summary; Mod Cincinnati, Modified Cincinnati Rating—Patient; PCS, Physical Component Summary; WOMAC, Western Ontario–McMaster Osteoarthritis Score.

Table 22–4. Autologous Chondrocyte Implantation: Patellofemoral Subgroup Characteristics

SUBGROUP	N	OSTEOTOMY	PATELLAR DEFECT LOCATION	SURFACE AREA TRANSPLANTED (cm²)	AVERAGE AGE
Patella	8	TTO-5	1 Type I 6 Type III 1 Type IV	4.34	35
Trochlea	9	TTO-6	N/A	4.74	37
Patella + trochlea	4	TTO-3	3 Type III 1 Type IV	12.59	50
Weightbearing condyle + patella	2	TTO-1	2 Type IV	6.88	39
Weightbearing condyle + trochlea	2	HTO + TTO-1	N/A	13.05	43
Weightbearing condyle + patella + trochlea	20	TTO-6 HTO-1 HTO + TTO-6	2 Type II 9 Type III 9 Type IV	15.31	38
Total	45	29/45 (64%)	31/34 Type III + IV (91%)	Average, 10.45 cm²/knee	38

All trochlea, $N = 35$; total surface area, 5.22. All patellae, $N = 34$; total surface area, 4.86.
HTO, high tibial osteotomy; N/A, trochlea is not applicable to patellar defect location classification; TTO, tibial tubercle osteotomy.

to 3 mm. We found that pain relief at the weightbearing condyles improved over a period of 6 to 12 months. However, in the patellofemoral joint, continued improvement occurred up to 3 years. This delay may be due to several factors, including the increased cartilage thickness and time required for maturation and growth, the shearing forces across the patellofemoral articulation as opposed to the compressive forces on the weightbearing condyles, and reconditioning of the quadriceps extensor mechanism.

Eleven of 45 (24%) patients were defined as having failed, 3 of whom suffered failure of the weightbearing condyle ACI graft. There were therefore 8 failures (18%) caused by failure of a patella or a trochlea graft. Of the patients treated who received workers' compensation, treatment failed in 5 of 11 (45%). Three patients underwent prosthetic reconstruction: two eventually received a total knee replacement, and one in whom the patella transplant failed received an isolated patellofemoral prosthesis. Three patients who had partial graft failures underwent arthroscopic débridement. Five patients whose grafts failed underwent a revision ACI procedure: two for the trochlea, two for the patella, and one for a medial femoral condyle; they have all had successful revision ACI procedures.

We think that ACI offers a complementary role, not previously available, that can provide symptomatic pain relief and improved function in young patients for whom osteotomy is not successful and prosthetic reconstruction is not desired. Based on the clinical outcomes presented in this study, we have found the following algorithm to be useful in the clinical management of patients with patellofemoral disease.

Successful treatment is based on identification of (1) patellar tilt, (2) patellar subluxation, and (3) the location of the chondrosis.

The arthroscopic lateral release procedure is overused. It is effective for isolated patellar tilt without subluxation of the patella when the lateral retinacular structures of the patella are contracted and mobility of the patella is limited. There may be early grade II Outerbridge chondromalacia associated with a chronically contracted and nonsubluxated patella, which is a relatively rare condition.

If subluxation is associated with patellar tilt, arthroscopic lateral release should not be performed. Persistent subluxation and tilt lead to mechanical overload with subsequent progressive chondral wear. In patients with abnormal mechanics but no chondral changes, medialization of the tibial tubercle performed with a lateral release is highly effective without anterior translation.

When the chondral changes in the patella are Fulkerson type I and type II, an AMZ tibial tubercle osteotomy is highly successful in unloading the damaged articular surface, along with patellar lateral release and possible vastus medialis oblique advancement as needed.

In our series of ACI in the patellofemoral joint, 91% of patients had type III and type IV patellar chondral injuries. Thirty-four patients underwent ACI of the patella with an average defect size of 4.86 cm², and 35 patients underwent ACI of the trochlea with an average defect of 5.22 cm². Overall, the average surface transplanted per knee was 10.45 cm². Patient satisfaction overall was such that 87% would choose the surgery again. Seventy-one percent thought that their clinical outcome was good or excellent, 22% fair, and 7% poor.

Three patients required prosthetic replacement after failure of ACI: two for patellar failure and one for medial femoral condyle failure. When failures occurred, they were readily managed by revision ACI when the source of the failure was robust repair tissue that did not integrate well. If the repair tissue was of poor quality, we would recommend either an osteochondral allograft or prosthetic reconstruction. Hence, despite initial failure, a final good result was usually obtained by biologic means and the patient's function and joint were preserved.

When collapse of the joint space is evident radiographically, as viewed by the Merchant or skyline projection, cartilage repair by ACI is no longer possible. The procedure relies on intact full-thickness cartilage margins to maintain the joint space so that growing cartilage repair tissue can fill the defect. In this situation, we recommend a unicompartmental patellofemoral prosthesis in a middle-aged patient, which has been a useful interim solution.

ACI offers a successful and complementary role in the management of patellofemoral disease. We have achieved successful results when damage to the patella is medial (i.e., Fulkerson type III), proximal pole or pan-patellar (i.e., type IV), or in isolation or combination with disease of the trochlea or weightbearing condyles.

ACI in an Osteoarthritic or Salvage Knee[7]

Perhaps the most gratifying use of ACI is in the management of severely injured young arthritics. This group of patients is outside the realm of sports medicine and too young to undergo prosthetic arthroplasty. They may still obtain successful pain relief, functional improvement, and acceptable quality of life after undergoing ACI. In our most recent follow-up of patients considered to have been treated in our salvage category, an overall satisfaction rate of 75% was achieved.

Between March 1995 and November 2002, 66 patients and 69 knees with early osteoarthritis were treated by ACI. Obscure threat was defined as bipolar focal chondral lesions or generalized grade 2 or greater chondromalacia throughout the joint as assessed arthroscopically. Radiographically, patients demonstrated peripheral osteophyte formation or early joint space narrowing of less than 50%. A total of 152 defects were treated in 69 knees, or an average of 2.2 defects per knee. The average resurfacing area per knee was 11.66 cm^2 with a range per knee of 4.3 to 31.6 cm^2. One to four defects were treated per knee.

These patients were generally older than the average patient treated by ACI. The average age was 38.9 years with a range of 18 to 57. Fifty-seven percent of the patients were male and 43% female.

This heterogeneous group of knee reconstructions consisted of the following:
- High tibial osteotomy plus ACI, $n = 16$
- Tibial tubercle osteotomy plus ACI, $n = 19$
- High tibial osteotomy with tibial tubercle osteotomy plus ACI, $n = 7$
- ACI alone with multiple defects, $n = 20$
- Femoral condyles plus tibial plateau with meniscal allografts, $n = 2$
- Femoral condyles plus tibial plateau, $n = 4$
- Patella plus trochlea, $n = 1$
- Total, 69

These patients were referred by other orthopedists in an attempt to avoid total knee arthroplasty at a young age. They were severely symptomatic, and their baseline scores were poor (see Figs 22–6 and 22–7). The patient satisfaction survey included rating of the results, comparison to the preoperative condition, overall patient satisfaction, and whether the patient would choose the surgery again. Fifty-seven percent of the patients (39/69) rated the results as good or excellent. Seventy-four percent (51/69) thought that they felt better than preoperatively, 81% (56/69) would choose the surgery again, and 75% (52/69) felt that they were better.

The clinical outcomes of these patients varied by the subgroup treated (Figs. 22–5 to 22–7). Those who experienced the highest level of functional improvement as assessed by a sports activity score (overall Cincinnati rating) were those who underwent high tibial valgus osteotomy with ACI to unload a large medial femoral condyle defect in association with varus alignment. These patients were able to return to pivoting sports with only minor modifications in activity. This was followed by the group of patients who underwent high tibial valgus osteotomy with tibial tubercle osteotomy. These patients were also able to return to sporting activities, but with modifications. The other subgroups were also analyzed as noted in Figure 22–7. Pain relief and functional improvement in activities of daily living were also highly significant as noted by the Knee Society and WOMAC scores.

Treatment failure was defined as persistent or worsening symptoms or objective evidence of poor-quality repair tissue arthroscopically or by MRI along with evidence of partial or complete graft delamination despite a good clinical result. Based on this definition, 21 patients (30%)

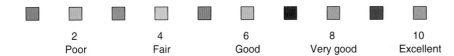

MODIFIED CINCINNATI RATING SCALE
OVERALL CONDITION

Rate overall condition at the present time

2	4	6	8	10
Poor	Fair	Good	Very good	Excellent

2 = Poor	Significant limitations affect activities of daily living
4 = Fair	Moderate limitations affect activities of daily living, no sports
6 = Good	Some limitations with sports but participate; I compensate
8 = Very good	Only a few limitations with sports
10 = Excellent	Able to do whatever I wish (any sport) with no problems

Figure 22–5. Modified Cincinnati overall rating scale.

OVERALL CLINICAL OUTCOME SCORES

	Pre op	Post op	P Value
Modified Cincinnati	3.9	5.7	< 0.0001
WOMAC	35.4	23.1	< 0.0001
KSS-Knee Function	53.7 66.8	72.7 73.1	< 0.0001 0.0192

ACI salvage

Figure 22–6. Overall clinical outcome scores for autologous chondrocyte implantation in an arthritic knee (series, $N = 69$; 2- to 6-year follow-up).

experienced failure. Four patients had evidence of partial or complete delamination, which was not treated because the patients had good symptom relief in comparison to their baseline condition and would choose surgery again. Nine of 21 patients were treated by biologic repair consisting of revision cartilage repair by microfracture, osteochondral grafting, or ACI, depending on the size of the chondral defect that failed. Seven of these nine patients (78%) were better 6 years later. Eight of 21 patients (38%) eventually underwent prosthetic arthroplasty because of either graft failure or progression of arthritic disease in the remainder of the knee joint.

In this series of 69 knees in 66 patients, overall patient satisfaction remained high at 87%. Although patients may have undergone revision cartilage surgery or prosthetic arthroplasty for failed ACI, satisfaction with the final clinical outcome remained high. ACI offers an interim solution that is durable at a midterm average follow-up of 5 years (2- to 6-year follow-up). Further follow-up is needed to determine ongoing durability and improved quality of life in these more severely injured knees. Markers for generalized osteoarthritis would be useful in this population to predict those predisposed to eventual joint failure despite the use of cartilage repair.

U.S. Registry of North American Outcomes[1]

The U.S. Cartilage Repair Registry maintained by Genzyme Bio Surgery is an industry-monitored outcome registry as assessed by the overall Cincinnati rating score system. Multiple national and international registry surgeons monitor these data.

Before 2001, the purpose of the evaluation was to determine the efficacy and safety of ACI for large multiple defects of the distal end of the femur at a minimum of 2 years' follow-up. Multicenter prospective follow-up data consisting of demographics and clinical outcomes as

A   CINCINNATI SCORE (PATIENT)

Group	Pre op	Post op	P Value
HTO + ACI n = 16	4.56	6.94	< 0.002
TTO + ACI n = 19	3.37	4.89	< 0.001
HTO – TTO + ACI n = 7	4.29	5.71	0.118

ACI salvage

B   CINCINNATI SCORES (PATIENT)

Group	Pre op	Post op	P Value
ACI n = 10	3.67	5.00	0.126
MFC + Troch +/– Patella n = 10	3.00	5.20	0.012

ACI salvage

Figure 22–7. **A** and **B**, Cincinnati scores for salvage series subdivided by group.

assessed by the overall Cincinnati rating scale were collected.

A total of 111 patients were treated. Their mean age was 40 years with a range of 15 to 57. Seventy-four percent were male with average body mass index of 28.6 kg/m^2. Sixty-one percent of patients had an acute onset of symptoms and had normal tibiofemoral alignment. Eighty-three percent had normal patellar tracking. Workers' compensation was an issue in 37% of patients. Thirty-five percent of patients underwent previous marrow stimulation techniques for cartilage repair that had failed.

In 111 knees treated, there were 233 defects with a mean total defect size of 9.2 cm^2 per knee and a range of 1 to 36.5 cm^2. Seventy-three percent of the lesions treated were 2 cm^2 or greater. Defect locations included the medial femoral condyles in 47%, lateral femoral condyles in 23%, and the trochlea in 30%. The diagnosis was osteochondritis dissecans in 4%.

Overall, treatment of multiple defects by ACI resulted in improvement in 67% of patients ($p < .0001$, two-sided paired t-test), the same status in 20%, and worsened status in 13%. Thirteen percent met the study definition of treatment failure requiring repeat surgery. The most common complications after surgery were related to adhesions, graft hypertrophy, loose bodies, and patellar maltracking. After ACI in 111 patients, a total of 74 surgeries were performed in 39 patients.

This was a very difficult and complex, challenging group of patients to treat. They frequently had significant functional impairment at baseline with low baseline scores, multiple surgeries, and a large total defect size of 9.2 cm^2. Thirty-seven percent of patients were receiving workers' compensation. Nonetheless, two-thirds of patients improved and have maintained the improvement at final follow-up.

SUMMARY

ACI clearly has achieved outstanding clinical results in juvenile athletes and high-level soccer players when the injury is treated within the first year after injury. Delays in treatment or multiple treatments result in worse clinical outcomes for reasons not yet clear.

ACI in the patellofemoral joint has been successful in treating a difficult management problem when careful attention is paid to patellar tracking. It has been successful in pan-patellar injuries (Fulkerson type IV patella) and medial patellar facet injuries (Fulkerson type III patella). It is effective in managing defects of the trochlea, which has been a problem area until the advent of ACI. It has a complementary role in managing patellofemoral chondral defects in maltracking knees in which realignment osteotomy alone is not successful.

Young arthritic patients pose a particular management dilemma because they are frequently too young to be considered for prosthetic arthroplasty and traditional sports medicine techniques are not effective in alleviating pain by repairing articular cartilage. This group of patients is generally older (40 years old) and requires large areas of surface repair (12 cm^2 on average). Clinical outcomes in this group have been very positive, with a patient satisfaction rate of 87% overall.

U.S. Registry data for multiple femoral defects appear to be similar to that in the author's series of young arthritics or the salvage category of patients. This is not surprising because the average age (40 years old) and the average treatment area (9.3 cm^2) are similar.

The clinical results of ACI in North America appear to be similar to that in Sweden. There is now hope for knees that have large areas of acute and chronic articular cartilage injury since the popularization of ACI. Time will determine whether the durability is also the same.

References

1. Anderson AF, Mandelbaum BR, Browne JE, et al: Treatment outcomes of autologous chondrocyte implantation for multiple defects of the distal femur. Presented at the American Orthopaedic Society for Sports Medicine Specialty Day, March 13, 2004, San Francisco.
2. Brittberg M, Lindahl A, Nilsson A, et al: Treatment of full-thickness cartilage defects in the human knee with cultured autologous chondrocytes. N Engl J Med 331:889-895, 1994.
3. Minas T, Bryant T: ACI in the patellofemoral joint. Presented at a meeting of the Knee Society, September 11, 2004, Jackson Hole, WY.
4. Minas T, Marchie A, Bryant T: SF-36 as a predictor of clinical outcome after autologous chondrocyte implantation in the knee [poster]. Presented at a meeting of the International Cartilage Repair Society, June 2001, Toronto.
5. Minas T, Mithöfer K, Yeon H, Micheli LJ: Functional outcome of knee articular cartilage repair in adolescent athletes. Presented at the American Orthopaedic Society for Sports Medicine Specialty Day, March 13, 2004, San Francisco.
6. Minas T, Peterson L: Advanced techniques in autologous chondrocyte transplantation. Clin Sports Med 18:13-44, 1999.
7. Minas T, Solhpour S, Bryant T: 2-6 Yr prospective clinical follow up for patients with multiple defects treated with ACI. Presented at a meeting of the International Cartilage Repair Society, Session 10c, May 29, 2004, Gent, Belgium.
8. Mithöfer K, Peterson L, Mandelbaum BR, Minas T: Articular cartilage repair in high-demand athletes with autologous chondrocyte transplantation: Functional outcome and return to competition. Presented at a meeting of the American Orthopaedic Sports Medicine Society, June 26, 2004, Quebec City, Canada.
9. Peterson L, Brittberg M, Kiviranta I, et al: Autologous chondrocyte transplantation. Biomechanics and long-term durability. Am J Sports Med 30:2-12, 2002.
10. Peterson L, Karrlson J, Brittberg M, et al: Patellar instability with recurrent dislocation due to patellofemoral dysplasia results after surgical treatment. Bull Hosp Joint Dis 48:130-139, 1988.
11. Peterson L, Minas T, Brittberg M, et al: Two- to 9-year outcome after autologous chondrocyte transplantation of the knee. Clin Orthop 374:212-234, 2000.
12. Pidoriano AJ, Weinstein RN, Buuck DA, Fulkerson JP: Correlation of patellar articular lesions with results from anteromedial tibial tubercle transfer. Am J Sports Med 25:533-537, 1997.

CHAPTER 23

Autologous Osteochondral Transplantation: The "Mosaicplasty" Technique

László Hangody • Imre Szerb • Zsófia Duska • Novák Pál Kaposi

Treatment of full-thickness cartilage damage to the weightbearing articular surfaces of the knee is one of the most frequent problems of orthopedic practice. Localized chondral and osteochondral defects of the weightbearing gliding surfaces can cause numerous problems for the patient (pain, swelling, instability, clicking, etc.) and may well be harbingers of osteoarthritis. Several surgical resurfacing treatment options are available to manage these defects. Subchondral penetration has been shown to have limited value because of the poor biomechanical characteristics of ingrowth reparative fibrocartilage.[6,20] Therefore, in the last 2 decades, several authors have proposed innovative techniques to achieve articular resurfacing with hyaline or hyaline-like tissue. These recently introduced techniques include periosteal and perichondrial grafts, autologous chondrocyte transplantation, morselized autologous osteochondral mixture, osteochondral allografts, biomaterials, and autologous osteochondral transplantation.*

Experience with autogenous osteochondral grafting has shown consistent survival of the transplanted hyaline cartilage. However, two notable problems have been encountered in the process. First, the donor sites must be taken from relatively non-weightbearing surfaces, which limits the procurement field. Additionally, the use of large grafts can cause incongruity at the recipient site and permanently alter the biomechanics of the joint.[7,11,28,31,32]

To solve these two problems, it stood to reason that the use of multiple small grafts would permit more tissue to be transplanted while preserving donor site integrity, and their use in a mosaic implanting pattern would allow progressive contouring of the new surface.[4,16,23]

Initially, the mosaicplasty concept was tested in German Shepherd dog and horse trials supplemented by cadaver application. Macroscopic and histological evaluation of the animal resurfaced areas and the donor sites demonstrated survival of the transplanted hyaline cartilage, formation of a composite cartilage layer consisting of 80% transplanted hyaline cartilage and 20% fibrocartilage, and deep matrix integration at the recipient site. Furthermore, by 8 weeks, the donor sites had filled to the surface with cancellous bone capped by fibrocartilage. Armed with reproducible experimental confirmation of the mosaicplasty concept, clinical application was begun on February 6, 1992. Over the following 6 years, clinical experience matched the animal results, and since 1996 the procedure has been used with equal success at numerous clinics throughout the world.[8,14-18,21]

INDICATIONS

Initially, autologous osteochondral mosaicplasty had been confined to treating small and medium-sized focal chondral and osteochondral defects of the weightbearing surfaces of the femoral condyles and patella. As success was gained through experience, the indications were expanded to include talar, tibial, and recently, femoral head lesions. Theoretic and practical considerations suggest that ideally, the extent of the defect should be between 1.0 and 4.0 cm^2. These limitations are mainly determined by donor site availability and other technical circumstances. Under certain conditions, mosaicplasty can be used for defects up to 8.0 cm^2 as a "salvage procedure." Fifty years of age seems to be the upper age limit for this type of transplantation.

It is very important in patient management, as with any other type of cartilage repair, that resurfacing be recognized as only one element of the therapeutic plan and that in every case it is necessary to treat the underlying cause. Accordingly, treatment of instability, malalignment, and meniscal and ligament tears can be incorporated into the operative and postoperative rehabilitation algorithms. After isolated autologous osteochondral mosaicplasty, patients are permitted immediate full range of motion but require a period of 2 to 3 weeks of non-weightbearing and 2 weeks of partial loading (30- to 40 kg loading). This protocol can easily be modified in accordance with established guidelines for concurrent anterior cruciate ligament reconstruction, high tibial osteotomy, and meniscal reinsertion or resection.

Contraindications to mosaicplasty include infection, tumors, and generalized or rheumatoid arthritis because of the biochemical alterations that they induce in the involved joint's milieu.

---

*References 1-3, 5, 7, 9-13, 19, 20, 22, 24-27, 29, 30.

SURGICAL TECHNIQUE

Procedure Overview

Autologous osteochondral mosaicplasty involves harvesting small cylindrical osteochondral grafts (from 2.7 up to 8.5 mm in diameter) from the less weightbearing periphery of the femoral condyles at the level of the patellofemoral joint and transplanting them to a prepared defect site on the weightbearing surfaces. A combination of different graft sizes allows an 80% filling rate. Fibrocartilage ingrowth and coverage, stimulated by abrasion arthroplasty at the base of the defect, will complete the new surface.

Autologous osteochondral mosaicplasty can be performed as an open procedure (Fig. 23–1), through a miniarthrotomy, or arthroscopically (Fig. 23–2). The technique of these three surgical procedures is similar. Only small technical differences exist at certain steps of each operation.

Operative Preparations

Generally speaking, cartilaginous lesions are defined only at arthroscopy. If the preoperative differential diagnosis includes such a lesion, the patient should be advised of the possibility of mosaicplasty. The patient should be prepared for an open procedure if the site is inaccessible because of posterior location or inability to flex the knee sufficiently. This procedure can lead to an overnight stay and altered weightbearing status for several weeks.

General or regional anesthesia with tourniquet control is recommended for this procedure. Prophylactic antibiotics may support the success of mosaicplasty.

The patient is positioned supine with the knee capable of 120 degrees of flexion. The contralateral extremity is placed in a stirrup.

Steps of the Operation

After the defect is identified, its edges are brought back sharply to a good hyaline cartilage rim with a curet, knife blade, or arthroscopic resector blade. The base of the lesion is abraded or curetted to viable subchondral bone. At this point, the drill guide is used to determine the number of grafts needed.

In the open procedure, both edges of the femoral condyles at the level of the patellofemoral joint can serve as donor sites. In the arthroscopic technique, the medial border of the medial femoral condyle is recommended as a primary donor site because of distention pushing the patella laterally and thus making perpendicular access easiest here. If necessary, the lateral border can be used as a secondary site.

The proper-size tube chisel is introduced perpendicular to the donor site. The harvester is tapped into the donor site. Usually, 15-mm length is recommended for resurfacing cartilage defects and 25-mm length is appropriate for osteochondral defects. After tapping and toggling, the chisel is removed, and with the use of the chisel guards the graft is delivered from the harvester. It is very important to push the grafts out at the bony end to avoid damage to the hyaline cartilage. The necessary grafts are harvested as needed.

Insertion of the grafts is performed though the universal guide. The first step in implantation is to tap the guide into the bony base of the defects. The 3-mm-long cutting edge is introduced into the bony base, and the shoulder of the device will help define a line perpendicular to that part of the defect. With assistance of this universal guide a recipient tunnel is created by the appropriately sized drill bit. A conically shaped dilator is used to create a similarly shaped recipient tunnel for easy insertion of the transplanted graft. Finally, the insertion is performed by using

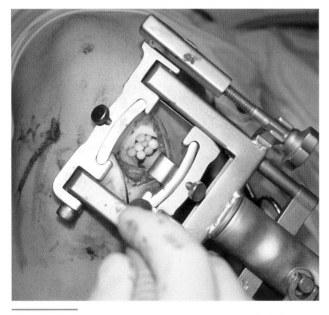

Figure 23–1. Open mosaicplasty on the medial femoral condyle.

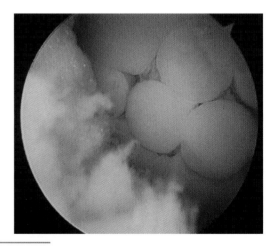

Figure 23–2. Arthroscopic mosaicplasty on the medial femoral condyle.

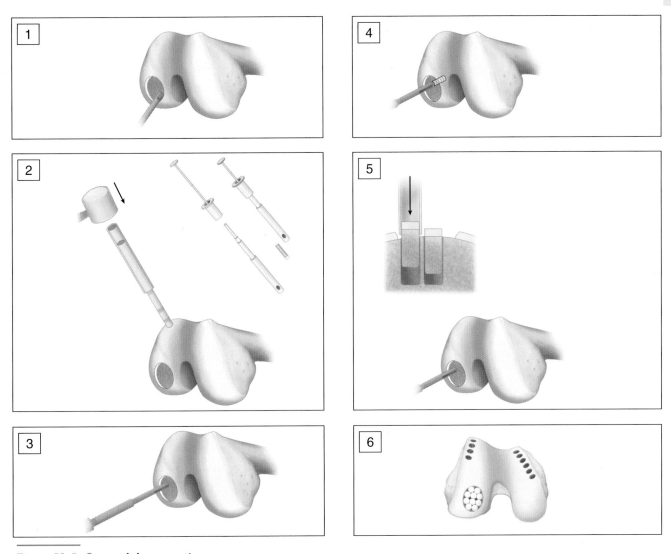

Figure 23–3. **Steps of the operation.**

an adjustable plunger to match the surface of the graft to the surrounding articular surface. With the use of this step-by-step sequence (drilling-dilating-delivering), all the grafts are inserted. When all the holes are filled, the knee is put through a range of motion with varus and valgus stress to fully seat the grafts and ensure their press-fit stability. The portals are closed and the joint drained through the superior portal (Fig. 23–3).

RESULTS

Between February 6, 1992, and February 28, 2002, 831 mosaicplasties have been performed at our institution. Five hundred ninety-seven of the 831 implantations involved the femoral condyles; 118, the patellofemoral joint; 25, the tibia; and 76, the talus. Two-thirds of the patients underwent the operation because of a localized grade III or IV cartilage lesion (Outerbridge classification system), whereas one-third of the implantations were performed because of osteochondral defects. In 85% of the

patients, concomitant surgical interventions also were performed.

The results of these resurfacing procedures have been evaluated at regular intervals by standardized clinical scores and radiographs and, in selected cases, by magnetic resonance imaging, second-look arthroscopy, histological evaluation of biopsy material, and cartilage stiffness measurements. Femoral, tibial, and patellar implantation was evaluated with the modified Hospital for Special Surgery, modified Cincinnati, Lysholm, and International Cartilage Repair Society scoring systems, whereas possible donor site disturbances were evaluated with the Bandi scoring system. The talar patients were subjected to both these knee and ankle Hannover evaluations. During the 10-year period, 83 patients were examined by second-look arthroscopy to assess the quality of the resurfaced area and the morphological features of the donor sites.

The clinical scores demonstrated good to excellent results in 92% of the patients who underwent femoral condylar implantation, 87% of those who underwent tibial resurfacing, 79% of those in whom patellar and/or trochlear mosaicplasty was performed, and 94% of those

TABLE 23–1. Mosaicplasty Rehabilitation Protocol*

General Viewpoints

Immobilization
No immobilization![†]

Ambulation[‡]

Two-crutch ambulation, non-weightbearing	Immediate
Two-crutch ambulation, partial loading (30-40 kg-sec)	2-4 weeks
Discontinue crutches, full weightbearing	4-5 weeks

Functional Exercises

Form walking, gait evaluation	4-5 weeks
Step up	4-5 weeks
Step down	5-6 weeks

Range of Motion

Early range of motion encouraged	Immediate (first week)
Continuous passive motion (in painless range) in case of extended lesions 2-4 cm²	
Full extension, flexion as tolerated	Immediate
Stationary bicycle	3 weeks

Strength Rehabilitation
Quadriceps

Open-chain exercises, leg raises	Immediate
Concentric contraction to full extension	1 week (or earlier if tolerated)
Concentric contraction against resistance	2 weeks
Isometric exercises at different angles	Immediate
Eccentric exercises against resistance	3-4 weeks

Hamstrings

Isometric exercises at different angles	Immediate
Concentric and eccentric strengthening	1-2 weeks
Against resistance	3-4 weeks

Closed-Chain Exercises[§]

Pushing a soft rubber ball with the foot	Immediate
Closed-chain exercises with half weightbearing	2-3 weeks
With full weightbearing	5-6 weeks
Stationary bicycle with resistance	2-4 weeks (if 90-degree knee flexion achieved)
Stairmaster	6-8 weeks

Proprioception Rehabilitation

Balance exercises standing on both feet	5-6 weeks
Standing on one foot (hard ground)	6-8 weeks
Standing on one foot (trampoline or AeroStep)	8-10 weeks

Return to Activity

Jogging	10 weeks
Straight-line running	3 months
Directional changes	4-5 months
Shear forces	5 months[¶]
Sport-specific adaptations	5 months
Sports activity	5-6 months[¶]

*Uzsoki Hospital and Sanitas Private Clinic, Budapest, Hungary.
[†]The main point of the rehabilitation is to ensure early motion of the treated joint to promote appropriate nutrition of transplanted cartilage. Cryotherapy can be used during the first week to avoid postoperative bleeding and decrease postoperative pain. In a case of a concomitant procedure requiring external fixation of the affected joint (e.g., meniscus reinsertion), limitation of range of motion for a short period by bracing can be allowed.
[‡]The extent, type (chondral or osteochondral), and location of the defect may modify weightbearing (see the next section).
[§]Partial loading promotes the transformation of connecting tissue (between transplanted plugs) into fibrocartilage, so these exercises are extremely important, especially in the half-weightbearing period. On the other hand, with some closed-chain exercises (e.g., cycling), it is possible to ensure cyclic loading, which makes fluid and nutrition transport much more efficient between synovial fluid and hyaline cartilage.
[¶]Approximately 4 to 5 months is needed to form a composite hyaline-like surface on the transplanted area that tolerates shear forces.
[¶]Depending on the depth and extent of the defect. If strength, power, endurance, balance, and flexibility are not satisfactory, sports activity is allowed only later.

Special Viewpoints

Weightbearing with Different Defects of the Knee
Femoral or tibial condyle, chondral defect, diameter <15 mm

Non-weightbearing	1 week
Partial weightbearing	1-3 weeks

Femoral or tibial condyle, chondral defect, diameter ≥15 mm

Non-weightbearing	2 weeks
Partial weightbearing	2-4 weeks

Femoral or tibial condyle, osteochondral defect

Non-weightbearing	3 weeks
Partial weightbearing	3-5 weeks

Patellar defect, diameter <15 mm

Partial weightbearing	2 weeks

Patellar defect, diameter ≥15 mm

Partial weightbearing	3 weeks

Quadriceps Strengthening and Patellar Mobilization— Differences at Patellar Defects
Vastus medialis strengthening!

Isometric exercises in extension	Immediate
Patellar mobilization	Immediate!
Isometric exercises at different angles	1 week
Open-chain exercises	2 weeks
Against resistance	3-4 weeks
Eccentric exercises against resistance	4-5 weeks
Closed-chain exercises	2-3 weeks

Treatment of the underlying causes can also modify the rehabilitation program. The most frequent combinations of knee procedures are the following:

Anterior Cruciate Ligament Reconstruction Combined with Mosaicplasty:
2-4 weeks of non-weightbearing (depending on the mosaicplasty)
2 more weeks of partial weightbearing
5-90 degrees range of motion for 4 weeks
Mainly closed-chain exercises for quadriceps strengthening
Hamstring strengthening in open- and closed-chain exercises
Proprioceptive training

Meniscus Reinsertion Combined with Mosaicplasty
4 weeks of non-weightbearing
2 more weeks of partial weightbearing
5-45 degrees range of motion for 4 weeks

Retinaculum Patellae Reconstruction Combined with Mosaicplasty
2-4 weeks of non-weightbearing (depending on the mosaicplasty)
2 more weeks of partial weightbearing
0-45 degrees range of motion for 4 weeks

High Tibial Osteotomy Combined with Mosaicplasty
Weightbearing (for 4 weeks only with crutches and only in extension) depends on the mosaicplasty, pain, and degree of correction of the varus (undercorrection, non-weightbearing; overcorrection, early weightbearing)

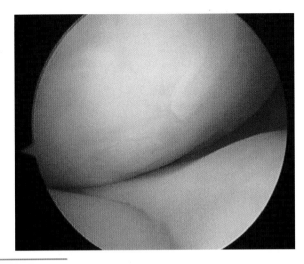

Figure 23–4. Control arthroscopy of mosaicplasty performed 5.5 years earlier for osteochondritis dissecans of a medial femoral condyle. Indication was a second injury.

who underwent a talar procedure. The Bandi score demonstrated slight donor site disturbances in 3%. Sixty-nine of the 83 control arthroscopies have demonstrated good gliding surfaces (Fig. 23–4), histologically proven survival of the transplanted hyaline cartilage, and fibrocartilage covering of the donor sites. Four patients (two with chondral lesions and two with osteochondritis dissecans) have shown degenerative changes at the recipient sites. In the 21 patients who underwent arthroscopic indentation testing, most demonstrated stiffness of the resurfaced area that was similar to that of the surrounding hyaline cartilage. The map of normal human knee articular cartilage, which had been revealed in former studies,[31] enabled us to observe and compare measurements of the resurfaced area.

Patient rehabilitation was carried out according to a special protocol developed at our department (Table 23–1). The rehabilitation process is always carried out on a patient-by-patient basis in line with the principles of the special mosaicplasty rehabilitation protocol. Variances in the rehabilitation program are due to differences in the severity, extent, and site of the resurfaced cartilage defect and the concomitant disorders treated.

During these operations 4 deep infections and 36 post-operative painful hemarthroses have occurred. Infection was treated successfully by arthroscopic or open débridement, whereas hemarthrosis was treated by aspiration, with nine patients undergoing arthroscopic or open débridement. Two patients had thromboembolic complications.

The overall results have been in the good to excellent range. As experience has been gained, the results have improved and the low rate of complications has been further reduced. Consistent with the age limitations of the procedure, it is not surprising that the older segment of this group (>35 years) has faired less well than the young patients.

From these encouraging results it appears that autologous osteochondral mosaicplasty may be a viable alternative treatment of localized full-thickness cartilage damage to the weightbearing surfaces of the knee.

References

1. Aichroth P, Burwell RG, Laurence M: An experimental study of osteoarticular grafts to replace articular surfaces. J Bone Joint Surg Br 53:554, 1971.
2. Bakay A, Csönge L, Papp G, Fekete L: Térdízületi porckárosodások mutéti kezelése osteochondralis allografttal. Magyar Traumat Ortop 39:227, 1996.
3. Brittberg M, Lindahl A, Nilsson A, et al: Treatment of deep cartilage defects in the knee with autologous chondrocyte transplantations. N Engl J Med 331:889, 1994.
4. Bobic V: Arthroscopic osteochondral autogenous graft transplantation in anterior cruciate reconstruction: A preliminary report. Knee Surg Sports Traumatol Arthrosc 3:262, 1996.
5. Bruns J, Kersten P, Lierse W, Silberman M: Autologous rib perichondrial grafts in experimentally induced osteochondral lesions in the sheep-knee joint: Morphological results. Virchows Arch A Pathol Anat Histopathol 421:1, 1992.
6. Buckwalter JA, Mankin HJ: Articular cartilage restoration. Arthritis Rheum 41:1331-1342, 1998.
7. Campanacci M, Cervellati C, Dontiti U: Autogenous patella as replacement for a resected femoral or tibial condyle. A report of 19 cases. J Bone Joint Surg Br 67:557, 1985.
8. Christel P, Versier G, Landreau P, Djian P: Les greffes osteochondrales selon la technique de la mosaicplasty. Maitrise Orthop 76:1, 1998.
9. Convery FR, Akeson WH, Keown GH: The repair of large osteochondral defect. Clin Orthop 82:253, 1972.
10. Coutts RD, Woo SL, Amiel D, et al: Rib perichondrial autografts in full-thickness articular cartilage defects in rabbits. Clin Orthop 275:263, 1992.
11. Fabbricciani C, Schiavone Panni A, Delcogliano A, et al: Osteochondral autograft in the treatment of osteochondritis dissecans of the knee. Presented at the Annual Meeting of the American Orthopaedic Society for Sports Medicine, 1991, Orlando, FL.
12. Garrett JC: Treatment of osteochondritis dissecans of the distal femur with fresh osteochondral allografts: A preliminary report. Arthroscopy 2:222, 1986.
13. Gross AE, Silverstein EA, Falk J, et al: The allotransplantation of partial joints in the treatment of osteochondritis of the knee. Clin Orthop 108:7, 1975.
14. Hangody L, Duska Z, Kárpáti, Z: Osteochondral plug transplantation. In Jackson DW (ed): Master Techniques in Orthopaedic Surgery. Reconstructive Knee Surgery, 2d ed. Philadelphia, Lippincott Williams & Wilkins 2003.
15. Hangody L, Feczkó P, Bartha L, et al: Mosaicplasty for the treatment of articular defects of the knee and ankle. Clin Orthop 391:328, 2001.
16. Hangody L, Kárpáti Z: Súlyos, körülírt térdízületi porckárosodások sebészi kezelésének új lehetosége. Magyar Traumat Ortop 37:237, 1994.
17. Hangody L, Kish G, Szabó ZS: Mosaicplasty for the treatment of osteochondritis dissecans of the talus: Two to seven year results in 36 patients. Foot Ankle Int 7:552, 2001.
18. Hangody L, Ráthonyi G, Duska Z, et al: Autologous osteochondral mosaicplasty. J Bone Joint Surg Am 86(Suppl 1):65, 2004.
19. Homminga GN, Bulstra SK, Bouwmeester PSM, Van der Linden AL: Perichondral grafting for cartilage lesions of the knee. J Bone Joint Surg Br 72:1003, 1990.
20. Insall JN: Intraarticular surgery for degenerative arthritis of the knee: A report of the work of the late K. H. Pridie. J Bone Joint Surg Br 49:211, 1967.
21. Jakob RP, Mainil-Varlet P, Saager C, Gautier E: Mosaicplasty in cartilaginous lesions over 4 square cm and indications outside the knee [abstract]. Presented at the Second Fribourg International Symposium on Cartilage Repair, 1997.
22. Mahomed MN, Beaver RJ, Gross AE: The long-term success of fresh, small fragment osteochondral allografts used for intraarticular post-traumatic defects in the knee joint. Orthopedics 15:1191, 1992.
23. Matsusue Y, Yamamuro T, Hama H: Arthroscopic multiple osteochondral transplantation to the chondral defect in the knee associated with anterior cruciate ligament disruption—case report. Arthroscopy 9:318, 1993.

24. Messner K, Gillquist J: Synthetic implants for the repair of osteo-chondral defects of the medial femoral condyle: A biomechanical and histological evaluation in the rabbit knee. Biomaterials 14:513, 1993.

25. Minns RJ, Muckle DS, Donkin JE: The repair of osteochondral defects in osteoarthritis rabbit knees by the use of carbon fibre. Bio-materials 3:81, 1982.

26. Muckle DS, Minns RJ: Biological response to woven carbon fibre pads in the knee. J Bone Joint Surg Br 82:60, 1990.

27. O'Driscoll SW, Keeley FW, Salter RB, et al: Durability of regenerated cartilage produced by free autogenous periosteal grafts in major full-thickness defects in joint surfaces under the influence of continu-ous passive motion. J Bone Joint Surg Am 70:595, 1988.

28. Outerbridge HK, Outerbridge AR, Outerbridge RE: The use of a lateral patellar autogenous graft for the repair of a large osteochon-dral defect in the knee. J Bone Joint Surg Am 77:65, 1995.

29. Ritsula VA, Santavirts S, Alhopuro S, et al: Periosteal and perichon-drial grafting in reconstructive surgery. Clin Orthop 302:259, 1994.

30. Stone KR, Walgenblach A: Surgical technique and results for articu-lar transplantation to traumatic and arthritic defects in the knee joint. Presented at the Annual Congress of the American Academy of Orthopaedic Surgeons, 1997, San Francisco.

31. Szerb I, Hangody L, Karpati Z: In vivo examination of the biome-chanical characteristics of the hyaline articular cartilage. Osteol Kozl 2:77, 2003.

32. Yamashita F, Sakakida K, Suzu F, Takai S: The transplantation of an autogenic osteochondral fragment for osteochondritis dissecans of the knee. Clin Orthop 201:43, 1985.

CHAPTER 24

Autologous Osteochondral Transplantation: Background, Surgical Indications, and Results

R. Alexander Creighton • Brian J. Cole

The ability to treat symptomatic chondral lesions has improved over the past 10 years. These lesions are difficult because of the requirement of articular cartilage to withstand marked stress and its lack of intrinsic ability to heal. Patients who suffer from this entity are often physically demanding and wish to maintain their active lifestyle. Over 900,000 Americans are affected annually by chondral lesions of the knee and undergo more than 200,000 surgical procedures for high-grade lesions.[5] The treating physician and patient must have realistic goals and understand the complexity of the problem. There is an obvious difference between osteoarthritis and chondral lesions. The former, osteoarthritis, is a diffuse process displaying radiographic changes and disruption on opposing sides of the joint surface and currently represents a contraindication to treatment with many of the available nonarthroplasty solutions. The latter, chondral lesions that are focal with minimal radiographic changes, are often treatable with nonarthroplasty solutions. Even though the natural history of isolated chondral lesions remains unknown, some reports have shown that cartilage injuries have a greater than 50% chance of becoming symptomatic with demonstrable joint space narrowing.[21] The clinical course is multifactorial and related to the size, location, depth, chronicity, patient comorbidity (cruciate deficiency, meniscal damage, limb malalignment, and high body mass index), and previous operative interventions. If a symptomatic lesion does not respond to conservative treatment, surgical intervention is warranted. The treatment goal is to diminish pain and swelling, improve function, and prevent progression with minimal morbidity and at the lowest cost to the health care system. It is reasonable to recommend treatment sooner rather than later. How we deal with these injuries should be critically evaluated because what we do today may be considerably different from what we do in the future.

CHONDRAL LESIONS

The outcome of a cartilage injury is dependent on the size, depth, extent, and location of the damage. Classification of these lesions as modified by the International Cartilage Repair Society (ICRS) is dependent on the extent and depth of the lesion (Table 24–1). The avascularity and high matrix-to-cell ratio of cartilage make healing and repair limited at best. In a horse model, Convery and colleagues[6] assessed the effect of defect size. In the distal end of the femur of horses, they demonstrated that a larger 9-mm-diameter lesion did not heal but a smaller 3-mm lesion did repair in a 3-month period.

The total incidence of these lesions, whether symptomatic or asymptomatic, is unknown. If acute hemarthrosis develops after a sports- or work-related injury, it has been proposed that 5% to 10% of patients have a full-thickness chondral injury.[22] Curl and associates[7] retrospectively reviewed 31,516 knee arthroscopies. Chondral lesions were reported in 19,827 (63%), with over 60% of these lesions being grade III or grade IV chondral lesions. Of the patients with grade IV lesions, 5% were younger than 40 years. Smaller lesions may not be totally asymptomatic either. Levy and colleagues[19] reported on 23 isolated chondral defects in 15 high-caliber soccer players. Thirty-three percent of these lesions were less than 10 mm in diameter, but all players reported knee pain limiting their ability to play soccer.

The clinician must have a high index of suspicion when evaluating patients with focal chondral defects. They can occur in isolation or with other intra-articular pathology. A thorough history and physical examination are a must to decipher symptom-provoking activities, previous injuries, and associated pathology. Symptoms may be subtle but often include localized pain, swelling, catching, and giving way. The symptoms are due to abnormal stress on subchondral bone, debris, and exposed tissue.

Diagnostic imaging is required and helpful in the evaluation of these patients. Our standard protocol begins with standard weightbearing anteroposterior, Merchant, long-leg alignment, and non-weightbearing lateral views. Additionally, a 45-degree flexion weightbearing, posteroanterior radiograph can provide information on subtle joint space narrowing that traditional extension views may underestimate.[25] Magnetic resonance imaging (MRI) may provide extra information in difficult cases. Potter and associates[24] found MRI to be more sensitive than plain radiographs in detecting focal chondral defects, although there are still issues with sensitivity and specificity. MRI techniques, including two-dimensional fast spin-echo and three-dimensional fat suppression, provide the most detail in evaluating articular cartilage.

After diagnosing a focal chondral defect, the magnitude of the patient's symptoms and the extent of the lesion determine the treatment regimen. In highly symptomatic patients, nonsurgical management is largely ineffective and should be reserved for very low-demand patients wishing to avoid or delay surgery. Nonsurgical management includes activity modification, nonsteroidal anti-inflammatory drugs, intermittent corticosteroid injections, braces, oral or injectable chondroprotective agents, and physical therapy.

Table 24–1. Modified International Cartilage Repair Society Chondral Injury Classification System

GRADE OF INJURY	DESCRIPTION
Grade 0	Normal
Grade I	Superficial fissuring
Grade II	Less than half the cartilage depth
Grade III	Greater than the cartilage depth to the subchondral plate
Grade IV	Osteochondral lesion through the plate
Osteochondritis dissecans	Stability, continuity, depth

Once the decision to proceed with surgery has been made, the next decision is the type of surgery to perform. A number of surgical options are available for the treatment of chondral and osteochondral lesions. These interventions all have different success rates that depend on the patient's age, activity level, and the size, location, and depth of the lesion (Fig. 24–1). Options include lavage and débridement (palliative), marrow stimulation technique (reparative), and osteochondral grafting and autologous chondrocyte implantation (restorative). In this chapter we are focusing on the plug technique for autologous osteochondral transplantation.

AUTOLOGOUS OSTEOCHONDRAL GRAFTING

Because chondral lesions are often an expression of damage at the tidemark–subchondral bone interface, it makes intuitive sense to replace the entire cartilage-bone unit when possible. In a goat model, Jackson and

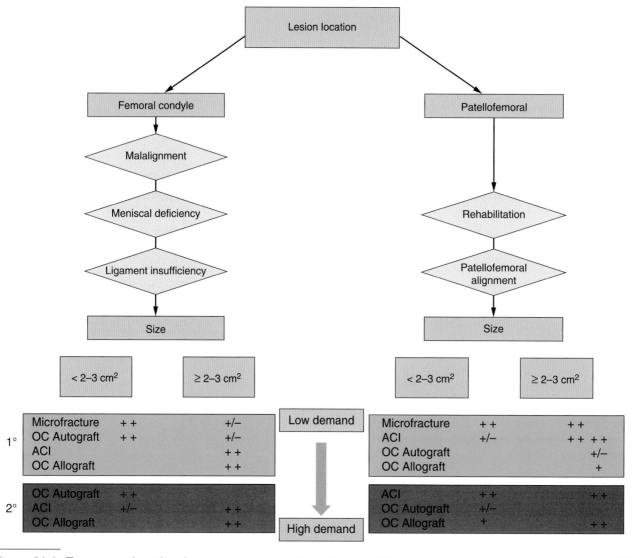

Figure 24–1. Treatment algorithm for symptomatic cartilage lesions. ACI, autologous chondrocyte implantation; OC, osteochondral.

associates[15] found that large, untreated lesions in the weightbearing surface of the medial femoral condyle led to progressive changes in both articular cartilage and bone over time, as well as the surrounding tissues. Osteochondral autograft transplantation is the only surgical technique that restores the height and shape of the articulating surface with composite autologous material. Use of this grafting technique reduces the area of fibrocartilage fill, which has been found to be inferior to true hyaline cartilage. The main disadvantage of the autologous technique is the availability of grafts and the technical demands of the procedure.

We believe that the ideal indication for this technique is a symptomatic patient with a full-thickness femoral chondral defect measuring 10 to 20 mm in diameter with stable surrounding cartilage. These lesions are frequently found in the central weightbearing area of the medial femoral condyle in an anterior cruciate ligament (ACL)-deficient knee, but they are often asymptomatic and observed by us until they become problematic. The upper age limit of the patient is around 50 years, and in general, deep large osteochondral defects are not suitable for an osteochondral autograft transplantation procedure.

TECHNIQUE

After appropriate anesthesia, patient positioning, and examination under anesthesia, diagnostic arthroscopy is performed to critically evaluate the joint for other associated pathology and the lesion itself. Documentation of the size of the lesion and depth, as well as the condition of the surrounding articular cartilage, is paramount to ensure that the lesion is suitable for osteochondral transplantation. The size of the lesion is appropriately measured with the use of color-coded sizers (Arthrex, Inc., Naples, FL) (Fig. 24–2).

Our preferred donor site is along the lateral edge of the lateral femoral condyle, proximal to the sulcus terminalis. This area has three main advantages. First, it is exposed to less contact pressure than other potential donor sites

are.[11,26] Second, it has a convex articular surface that mimics the weightbearing surface of the femoral condyles, where this technique is most often used.[27] Finally, this site is very easy to access with limited morbidity. We prefer to perform a limited arthrotomy to ensure a perpendicular harvest under direct visualization (Fig. 24–3). Alternatively, it may be accessed through a standard lateral portal with the knee in approximately 30 degrees of flexion. Other donor sites are along the superolateral margin of the intercondylar notch. One must thoroughly evaluate this area for fibrocartilage in an ACL-deficient knee, which is inappropriate for transfer. Limitations of this area include an inability to harvest plugs larger than 6 mm in diameter. The surgeon should have already determined whether to transfer a single or multiple osteochondral plugs from evaluation of the defect.

It is paramount that the harvester be perpendicular to ensure a circular graft. The depth markings on the barrel of the harvester should be visible at all times, either directly or arthroscopically. Using a mallet, the harvester is impacted to a depth of approximately 10 to 15 mm. The harvester is removed after the appropriate depth has been attained by abruptly rotating it clockwise 90 degrees and counterclockwise 90 degrees. Gentle rocking superiorly and inferiorly may be necessary to fracture the cancellous bone.

After appropriate sizing, the recipient site is prepared. It is cored to the appropriate depth to match the donor plug and cut at a perpendicular angle similar to the manner in which the donor graft was harvested (Fig. 24–4). The surgeon may need to hyperflex the knee to obtain the appropriate angle. Alternatively, an accessory portal or a limited arthrotomy may be necessary to access the defect. The socket is checked by visualization and the calibrated alignment stick to ensure the correct depth and angle before placing the donor plug (Fig. 24–5).

The donor harvester is placed inside the recipient site, and the donor graft is gently extruded. The collard pin of the harvester is advanced until the pin is flush with the pin calibrator. The pin is designed to advance the graft so that 1 mm of the graft is exposed. A sizer 1 mm larger than

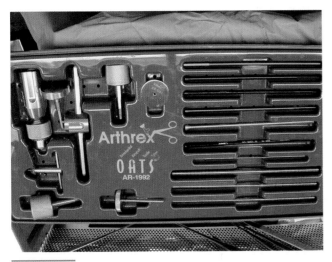

Figure 24–2. OATS set with color-coded sizers by Arthrex, Inc. (Naples, FL).

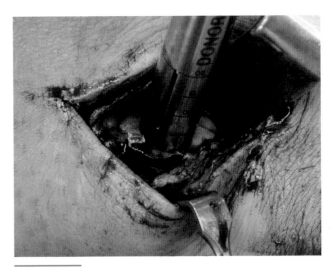

Figure 24–3. Limited arthrotomy for an osteochondral donor plug.

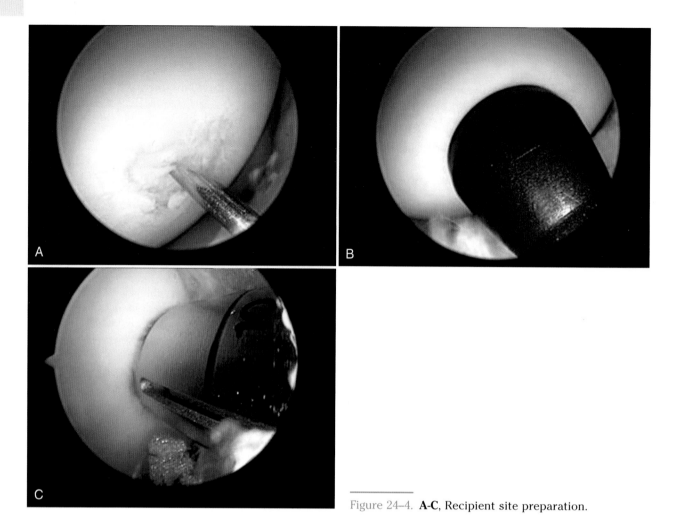

Figure 24–4. **A-C**, Recipient site preparation.

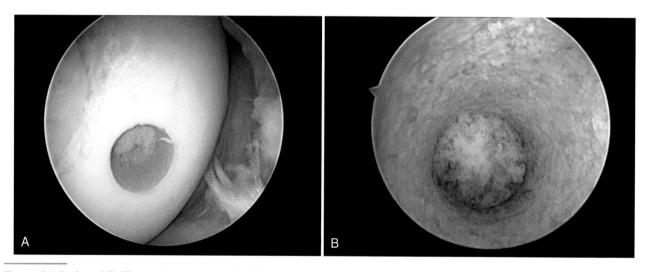

Figure 24–5. **A** and **B**, The recipient site is double-checked.

the graft is used, and gentle tapping fully seats the plug; progress is checked periodically (Fig. 24–6).

If the procedure calls for multiple cores, each transfer should be completed before subsequent creation of the recipient sockets. This technique ensures that the donor sockets are placed appropriately and usually prevents socket wall blowout. It is necessary to fill the defect as completely as possible, usually at least 60% to 80% (Fig. 24–7).

The donor plug holes are usually left unfilled. They fill with a combination of cancellous bone and fibrocartilage at the 12-week mark. It may take up to 1 year for these holes to fill to the level of surrounding articular cartilage. Ongoing research is evaluating different composite materials to fill these defects in an effort to decrease postoperative hematoma formation and to stimulate earlier filling (Fig. 24–8).[10]

Postoperatively, if the procedure is performed appropriately with a well-contained defect, early weightbearing and motion are encouraged. After a multiple-plug technique, full range of motion and protected weightbearing are advised for the first 4 weeks. At 4 weeks, full weightbearing is allowed. Sporting activities are not recommended until 4 to 6 months postoperatively.

The most frequent complication after osteochondral transfer surgery is hemarthrosis. Other complications include pain, donor site morbidity, graft fracture, condylar fracture, and loose bodies. Mosaicplasty has similar complications, but there is higher potential for donor site morbidity and the possibility of avascular necrosis if too many donor grafts are chosen from the same area. In several instances, plug failure has been observed by the senior author when multiple small plugs have been implanted (Fig. 24–9).

RESULTS

The first type of cartilage transfer was performed in 1908 by Judet.[17] He transplanted post-traumatic fragments into their defects and obtained pain relief. A study by Pap[23] found that lesions smaller than 5 mm survived longer than 2 years. Daniel and associates[8] in 1963 showed the importance of bone for survival of the cartilage. Campbell and colleagues[4] also came to this conclusion in a dog model, in which 1- by 2-cm plug survival was related to at least a 5-mm bone plug. The first case report of the

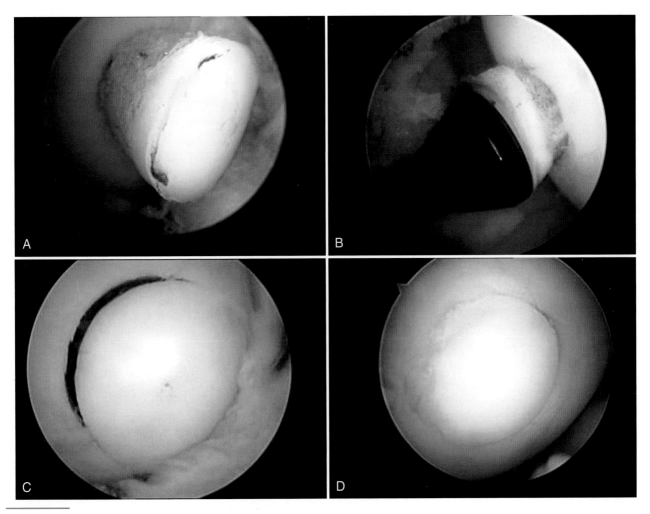

Figure 24–6. **A-D,** The donor graft is placed inside the recipient site.

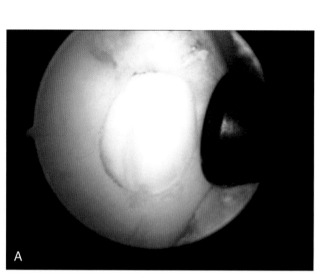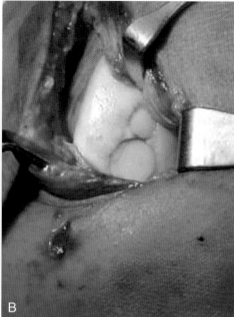

Figure 24–7. **A** and **B**, Multiple plugs.

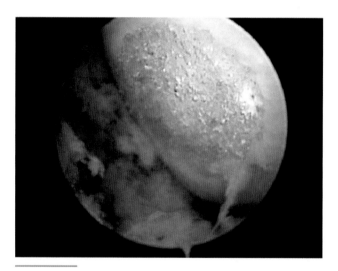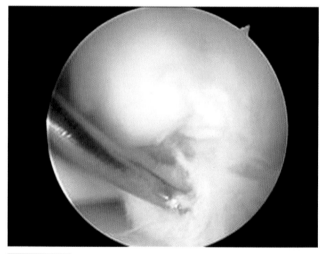

Figure 24–8. Osteochondral defect filled with a 9-mm-diameter OsteoBiologics TruFit BGS Plug. At the time of implantation, the resorbable, porous, backfill scaffold is contoured and tightly fit into the site and has filled with blood and cellular elements. (Courtesy of Wayne Gersoff, M.D., Denver.)

Figure 24–9. Failure of the multiple-plug technique.

arthroscopic technique was published in 1993 and involved a patient with an ACL-deficient knee.[20] Duchow and associates[9] used a porcine model to evaluate the stability of press-fit–implanted osteochondral grafts. They found that failure loads were significantly lower for 10- than for 15-mm-long grafts, as well as for 8- versus 11-mm-diameter grafts. In addition, repeated implantation and levering the graft at harvest reduce primary stability. Koh and colleagues[18] assessed the effect of graft height

mismatch on contact pressure after osteochondral grafting. A plug that was inserted flush normalized the contact pressure. A plug that was left proud, even 0.5 mm, significantly increased peak pressure by 40%. A plug that was countersunk also demonstrated increased contact pressure by about 10%, but not as high as the contact pressure with an empty defect. This study demonstrates the importance of the graft matching the host's articular geometry.

Bobic[3] reported on the treatment of 12 patients with chronic ACL deficiency and full-thickness femoral condyle lesions greater than 10 mm in diameter. He treated the ACL deficiency with a patellar tendon graft and the osteochondral lesion by osteochondral autograft transplantation with modified tubular instruments. The multiple osteochondral cylinders were obtained from the notch area. During second-look arthroscopy at 2 years, 10 of 12 grafts were satisfactory in terms of visual and probed inspection.

Hangody and associates[13] used various techniques to treat 227 patients who had chondral lesions ranging from 1 to 9 cm^2. Superior results were achieved in patients treated with mosaicplasty versus abrasion arthroplasty, microfracture, or Pridie drilling. Treatment of these chondral lesions by penetration of the subchondral bone appeared to deteriorate over time, with improvement ranging from 0% to 34% at 5 years. Mosaicplasty maintained its results at 5 years with an 87% success rate.

Jakob and colleagues[16] treated chondral lesions of the knee in 52 consecutive patients by mosaicplasty with an average follow-up of 37 months. Twenty-three patients were classified as ICRS grade III and 29 as grade IV. Knee function was improved in 92% of patients. Four patients did require surgery for graft failure. They found that patients who required 8 to 12 plugs, 6 to 7 mm in diameter, had more of a problem with donor site morbidity. The authors concluded that autologous osteochondral transplantation is an appropriate option for the treatment of full-thickness osteochondral defects. However, this treatment is limited by the size of the lesion and the number of plugs that can be harvested.

Hangody and Fules[12] reported on their 10-year experience of autologous osteochondral transplantation. Eight hundred thirty-one patients were evaluated over this period. The investigators reported good to excellent results in 92% of femoral condylar implants, 87% of those treated by tibial resurfacing, 79% of patellar or trochlear mosaicplasties, and 94% of talar lesions. Donor site morbidity was assessed by the Bandi score. Long-term morbidity was found in 3% of patients. Other complications included 4 deep infections and 36 painful postoperative hemarthroses. Eighty-three patients were evaluated by second-look arthroscopy. Sixty-nine showed congruent articular gliding surfaces, histological evidence of hyaline cartilage, and fibrocartilage filling of the donor sites.

Andres and associates[1] looked at the effectiveness of osteochondral autograft transplantation in the treatment of osteoarthritic cartilage lesions. Twenty-two transplantations were performed for isolated or multiple degenerative cartilage lesions. At a minimum follow-up of 24 months, the isolated cartilage lesions had significantly better pain relief and functional scores based on the Western Ontario and McMaster Universities Osteoarthritis Index. The authors concluded that osteochondral autograft transplantation is effective in treating isolated arthritic lesions but that it appears to be contraindicated in patients with multiple lesions.

Horas and coworkers[14] performed a prospective, randomized study comparing 40 patients treated by autologous chondrocyte implantation (ACI) with 40 treated by osteochondral cylinder transplantation (OCT) in the knee joint with a 2-year follow-up. Both groups improved their Meyers score and Tegner activity score, but the Lysholm score of the ACI group lagged behind that of the OCT group at 6, 12, and 24 months. Histomorphologic biopsy in a small number of patients demonstrated that the OCT group retained their hyaline cartilage character, whereas the ACI group consisted mainly of fibrocartilage. The authors concluded that both treatments decreased patients' symptoms but that the ACI group lagged behind the OCT group.

Bentley and associates[2] also performed a prospective, randomized comparison of ACI versus mosaicplasty for osteochondral defects of the knee. Fifty-eight patients were treated with ACI and 42 with mosaicplasty, the mean size of the defect was 4.66 cm^2, and the mean followup was 19 months (12 to 26). Using the Cincinnati and Stanmore scores with objective clinical assessment, 88% of the ACI group had excellent or good results, whereas 69% of the mosaicplasty group had excellent or good results. Arthroscopy at 1 year revealed ICRS grades of I or II in 82% of the ACI group but only 34% of the mosaicplasty group. It should be noted that all five of the mosaicplasties performed on the patella failed. The authors concluded that ACI is superior to mosaicplasty in repair of articular defects in the knee.

CONCLUSION

Treatment of symptomatic chondral lesions continues to evolve. Autologous osteochondral transplantation is the only surgical technique that restores the height and shape of the articulating surface with composite autologous material. It has a steep learning curve and is technically dependent. We prefer to perform a limited lateral arthrotomy to ensure a perpendicular donor harvest. In addition, proper preparation of the recipient site is important to ensure flush seating of the plug and limit the possibility of damage to the hyaline cartilage of the plug. We believe that the ideal indication for this technique is a symptomatic patient with a full-thickness femoral chondral defect 10 to 20 mm in diameter and stable surrounding cartilage. The upper age limit of patients is around 50 years, and deep, large osteochondral defects are not suitable for osteochondral autograft transplantation in our opinion. It is always important to individualize any treatment technique toward a particular patient and lesion and to correct any associated ligament laxity, limb malalignment, or significant meniscal deficiency.

References

1. Andres BM, Mears SC, Wenz JF, et al: Treatment of osteoarthritic cartilage lesions with osteochondral autograft transplantation. Orthopedics 26:1121-1126, 2003.
2. Bentley G, Biant LC, Carrington RW, et al: A prospective, randomized comparison of autologous chondrocyte implantation versus mosaicplasty for osteochondral defects in the knee. J Bone Joint Surg Br 85:223-230, 2003.
3. Bobic V: Arthroscopic osteochondral autograft transplantation in anterior cruciate ligament reconstruction: A preliminary clinical study. Knee Surg Sports Traumatol Arthrosc 3:262-264, 1996.
4. Campbell CJ, Ishida H, Takahashi H, Kelly F: The transplantation of articular cartilage. An experimental study in dogs. J Bone Joint Surg Am 45:1579-1592, 1963.
5. Cole B, Frederick R, Levy A, Zaslav K: Management of a 37-year old man with recurrent knee pain. J Clin Outcomes Management 6:46-57, 1999.

6. Convery FR, Akeson WH, Keown GH: The repair of large osteochondral defects: An experimental study in horses. Clin Orthop 82:253-262, 1972.

7. Curl WW, Krome J, Gordon ES, et al: Cartilage injuries: A review of 31,516 knee arthroscopies. Arthroscopy 13:456-460, 1997.

8. Daniel GA, Kahn DS, Entin MA: Experimental autogenous transplantation of hemi-joints in dogs. Surg Forum 14:460-461, 1963.

9. Duchow J, Hess T, Kohn D: Primary stability of press-fit– implanted osteochondral grafts. Am J Sports Med 28:24-27, 2000.

10. Feczko P, Hangody L, Varga J, et al: Experimental results of donor site filling for autologous osteochondral mosaicplasty. Arthroscopy 19:755-761, 2003.

11. Garretson RB III, Katolik LI, Cole BJ, et al: Contact pressure at osteochondral donor sites in the patellofemoral joint. Am J Sports Med 32:967-974, 2004.

12. Hangody L, Fules P: Autologous osteochondral mosaicplasty for the treatment of full-thickness defects of weight-bearing joints. J Bone Joint Surg Am 85:27-32, 2003.

13. Hangody L, Kish G, Karpati Z, et al: Mosaicplasty for the treatment of articular cartilage defects: Application in clinical practice. Orthopedics 21:751-756, 1998.

14. Horas U, Pelinkovic D, Herr G, et al: Autologous chondrocyte implantation and osteochondral cylinder transplantation in cartilage repair of the knee joint. J Bone Joint Surg Am 85:185-192, 2003.

15. Jackson DW, Lalor PA, Aberman HM, Simon TM: Spontaneous repair of full-thickness defects of articular cartilage in a goat model: A preliminary report. J Bone Joint Surg Am 83:53-64, 2001.

16. Jakob RP, Franz T, Gautier E, et al: Autologous osteochondral grafting in the knee: Indications, results, and reflections. Clin Orthop 401:170-184, 2002.

17. Judet H: Essai sur les greffes des tissues articulaires. CR Acad Sci 146:193, 1908.

18. Koh JL, Wirsing K, Lautenschlager E, Zhang LO: The effect of graft height mismatch on contact pressure following osteochondral grafting. Am J Sports Med 32:317-320, 2004.

19. Levy AS, Lohnes J, Sculley S, et al: Chondral delamination of the knee in soccer players. Am J Sports Med 24:634-639, 1996.

20. Matsusue Y, Yamamuro T, Hama H: Arthroscopic multiple osteochondral transplantation to the chondral defect in the knee associated with anterior cruciate ligament disruption. Arthroscopy 9:318-321, 1993.

21. Messner K, Maletius W: The long-term prognosis for severe damage to weight-bearing cartilage in the knee: A 14-year clinical and radiographic follow-up in 28 young athletes. Acta Orthop Scand 67:165-168, 1996.

22. Noyes FR, Bassett RW, Grood ES, Butler DL: Arthroscopy in acute traumatic hemarthrosis of the knee: Incidence of anterior cruciate tears and other injuries. J Bone Joint Surg Am 62:687-695, 1980.

23. Pap K: Reduction and percutaneous fixation of mobile fractures. Acta Med Acad Sci Hung 2:581-618, 1951.

24. Potter H, Linklater L, Allen A, et al: Magnetic resonance imaging of articular cartilage of the knee: An evaluation with use of fast-spin-echo imaging. J Bone Joint Surg Am 80:1276-1284, 1998.

25. Rosenberg T, Paulos L, Oarker R, et al: The 45-degree PA flexion weight-bearing radiograph of the knee. J Bone Joint Surg Am 70:1479-1483, 1988.

26. Simonian PT, Sussmann PS, Wickiewicz TL, et al: Contact pressures at osteochondral donor sites in the knee. Am J Sports Med 26:491-494, 1998.

27. Terukina M, Fujioka H, Yoshiya S, et al: Analysis of the thickness and curvature of articular cartilage of the femoral condyle. Arthroscopy 19:969-973, 2003.

CHAPTER 25

Fresh Osteochondral Allografting

Todd B. Dietrick • William Bugbee

HISTORICAL BACKGROUND

Experience with osteochondral transplantation dates back to 1908, when Lexer first reported a large series of fresh osteochondral allografts.[40] In 1925 he followed this report with an evaluation of the grafts that he had transplanted between 1907 and 1925.[41] His overall assessment was that the results of the operations were "uniformly good."[49] The major long-term problem encountered by Lexer in his series was collapse of the subchondral bone with failure of incorporation. This problem was due in part to slow revascularization of donor bone in the metaphyseal area, which led to fatigue fractures and failure of the structures supporting the cartilage. Initially, he thought that weight-bearing should be avoided for 3 months but later conceded that it should be extended beyond 2 years. He also stated that the cartilage surfaces remained smooth for up to 2 years and then began to deform secondary to "functional demands." Lexer's observations continue to be fundamentally sound, although much of the science and technique of fresh osteochondral allografting has evolved significantly.

Subsequent to the reports of Lexer, Harnach[33] in 1959 published his results using osteochondral "shell" allografts. In 1975, Gross[30,32] reported on nine transplants in eight patients with follow-up of 2 years. His indication for allografting was degenerative disease too severe to be adequately dealt with by osteotomy but insufficient to justify prosthetic replacement. His ideal indication was described as osteoarthritis localized to one compartment of the knee. All grafts were cadaveric in origin and transplanted within 24 hours of death of the donor. They were either medial or lateral tibial plateau and consisted of articular cartilage and a thin shell of underlying bone. At 2 years there were no signs of rejection, with all grafts untied to host bone. This report was followed up in 1985 with a follow-up study that reported long-term results of the first 100 cases of fresh small-fragment osteochondral allografts.[36,44] The best outcomes were reported in patients with traumatic injury, whereas success rates for osteoarthritis were not as encouraging. Gross concluded that the best candidates were patients with post-traumatic injury requiring grafts of only one joint surface. He also pointed out that correction of mechanical alignment was critical to long-term success.

This early clinical experience, along with basic scientific investigation, has provided an understanding for the rationale and support of the current application of fresh osteochondral allografts in the treatment of articular cartilage lesions.[43,58] Fresh osteochondral grafts are used to treat a broad spectrum of articular cartilage pathology, from focal chondral defects to joints with established osteoarthrosis. Most commonly, allografts are used in the treatment of larger traumatic or degenerative chondral lesions, osteochondritis dissecans, osteonecrosis, and post-traumatic reconstruction of the knee. Fresh allografts are also effective primary treatment of smaller chondral femoral condyle lesions, but in our experience they are often used as salvage if other repair procedures such as microfracture, osteochondral autografting, or autologous chondrocyte implantation have failed.

RATIONALE

The fundamental concept governing fresh osteochondral allografting is transplantation of architecturally mature hyaline cartilage, along with living chondrocytes that survive transplantation and are thus capable of supporting the cartilage matrix. Hyaline cartilage possesses many characteristics that make it attractive for transplantation. It is an avascular tissue and therefore does not require a blood supply; it meets its metabolic needs through diffusion from synovial fluid. It is aneural and does not require innervation for function. Third, articular cartilage is relatively immunoprivileged[32,38] because the chondrocytes are embedded within a matrix and are relatively protected from host immune surveillance. The second component of the osteochondral allograft is the osseous portion, which generally functions as support for the cartilage, as well as serving as a vehicle to allow attachment and fixation of the graft to the host. The osseous portion is quite different from hyaline cartilage in that it is vascular tissue and requires a blood supply for survival. The cellular elements of osseous tissue are not thought to survive transplantation; rather, this portion functions as a scaffold for healing to the host by creeping substitution.[31,36] Generally, the osseous portion of the graft is limited to a few millimeters; however, depending on the clinical situation, the allograft may contain more extensive amounts of bone, which is required to restore injured or absent subchondral tissue. This is often the case in osteochondritis dissecans, osteonecrosis, and post-traumatic reconstruction. In addition, the bone is not immunoprivileged like cartilage and tends to elicit an immune response.[23,24,51,57] Thus, a bone and cartilage transplant is treated as two separate components by the host. It is helpful, then, to consider a fresh osteochondral allograft as a composite graft of both bone and cartilage, with a living mature hyaline portion and a nonliving subchondral bone portion. It is also helpful to understand the allografting procedure in the context of tissue or organ transplantation because the graft is essentially transplanted as an intact structural and functional unit replacing a diseased or absent component in the recipient joint. Transplantation of mature hyaline cartilage obviates the need to rely on techniques that induce cells to form cartilage tissue, which are central to other restorative procedures.

In addition to the advantages of mature hyaline cartilage transplantation, fresh osteochondral allografts have their own set of clinical issues, including the following:
1. Complexities of acquisition, processing, and storage of donor tissue
2. Safety concerns with respect to disease transmission from donor tissue to host
3. Immunological behavior of the allograft
4. The allograft-host bone interaction
5. Long-term chondrocyte viability and matrix stability

GRAFT ACQUISITION

The cornerstone of an allografting procedure is the availability of fresh osteochondral tissue. Currently, in fresh osteochondral allografting, the small-fragment allografts are not HLA or blood type matched and are used fresh rather than frozen or processed, as is the case for other bulk allografting or tumor reconstructive procedures. The reason for this is predicated on maximizing the quality of articular cartilage in the graft. Such use is in distinction to cases of large osseous reconstruction, where restoration of the osseous defect is the primary goal and therefore frozen tissue may be more appropriate. Despite numerous efforts at cryopreservation and other freezing protocols that attempt to maintain chondrocyte viability, it has been demonstrated that the freezing process kills chondrocytes.[42,48,52] This process effectively eliminates over 95% of viable chondrocytes in the articular cartilage portion of the osteochondral graft. Furthermore, clinical experience has shown that the articular cartilage matrix of frozen grafts deteriorates over time,[20,21] presumably because there are no cells within the matrix to maintain tissue homeostasis. In 2001, Enneking and Campanacci[20] reported on the retrieval of 28 cryopreserved osteoarticular allografts. Specimens were examined under high-power microscopy after staining with toluidine blue and safranin O solutions. The articular cartilage showed no evidence of viable chondrocytes in all specimens. Five of these specimens retrieved within 1 year of transplantation showed no change in the thickness of articular cartilage; however, specimens retrieved after 1 year demonstrated varying degrees of fibrillation and degeneration on the articular surface. Interestingly, one retrieval was a fresh osteochondral graft at 13 months after transplantation. It demonstrated viable chondrocytes with preserved articular cartilage. It stands to reason, then, that with limited chondrocytes available to support the articular cartilage

matrix, the long-term prognosis for articular cartilage viability is poor.

Chondrocyte viability has been demonstrated in other studies as well.[17,36,45,47] Kandel et al[36] examined the histopathology of 44 failed fresh osteochondral allografts. Specimens were extirpated between 12 and 44 months after transplantation. Each specimen was stained with hematoxylin-eosin and toluidine blue and examined under light and polarized light microscopy. Twenty-seven of 44 grafts showed variable amounts of hyaline articular cartilage along with chondrocytes secreting proteoglycan matrix. Two of the grafts that were 7 years old had viable chondrocytes. Most cases had donor cartilage that was fragmented and showed minor degeneration, whereas areas of severe degeneration were covered by fibrocartilage. In addition, 14 specimens were examined by electron microscopy and demonstrated normal architectural structure. Chondrocytes had increased levels of rough endoplasmic reticulum, thus suggesting increased activity. The osseous portion of the allografts revealed necrotic bone with variable replacement by host bone. Kandel and colleagues concluded that there was no evidence of transplant rejection seen in 44 specimens and that viable cartilage is present as late as 7 years after transplantation. Oakeshott et al[47] reported similar findings in a 1988 retrieval study of 23 fresh osteochondral allografts in 18 patients. The mean time from transplantation to removal was 35 months (range, 3 to 92 months). Of 23 specimens, 17 showed evidence of viable hyaline cartilage. In addition, all grafts older than 44 months demonstrated complete reossification. Interestingly, 15 of 18 failed grafts had increased stress in that compartment as a result of malalignment. Czitrom et al[19] reported the results of cartilage biopsy of four functioning osteochondral allografts. Specimens were stained for both RNA and synthesized proteoglycans. Chondrocyte viability was 96% to 99% at 12 months, 69% to 78% at 24 months, 90% at 41 months, and 37% at 6 years in the four grafts. Recently, Gross et al reported viable chondrocytes in an allograft retrieved 17 years after implantation.[45] These retrieval studies support the use of fresh versus frozen tissue for small osteochondral allografts in the setting of reconstruction of chondral and osteochondral defects.

ALLOGRAFT TESTING AND SAFETY

Understanding the process of tissue recovery, testing, and storage is critically important in the allografting procedure. Historically, the obstacles presented by these fundamental components have led to the development of fresh allograft programs only at specialized centers that not only have a close association with an experienced tissue bank but have also put significant investment of resources into setting up protocols specific for safe and effective transplantation of fresh osteochondral tissue.

Recently, fresh osteochondral allografts have become commercially available and are thus more accessible to the orthopedic community. Procurement, processing, and testing of donor tissue follow the guidelines established by the American Association of Tissue Banks (AATB).[1] The screening process is very extensive and includes a detailed inquiry into the donor's medical, social, and sexual history.[6,35] Current guidelines include serologic testing for human immunodeficiency virus (HIV) I/II antibody, human T-lymphotrophic virus (HTLV) I/II antibody, hepatitis B surface antigen, hepatitis C virus, syphilis, and hepatitis B core antibody. The age criterion for the donor pool of fresh grafts is between 15 and 45 years of age. The joint surface must pass a visual inspection for cartilage quality. These criteria ensure, but do not guarantee acceptable tissue for transplantation.[28] Experienced allograft surgeons will often discuss particular donor characteristics with tissue bank personnel. It is extremely important to acknowledge that fresh human tissue is unique and that no two donors have the same characteristics. Therefore, strict adherence to tissue-banking standards and adherence to protocols and processes in quality control are paramount. Furthermore, an essential part of the informed consent process is a discussion of the risk for bacterial or viral disease transmission.

As with any organ or tissue transplantation, there exists the risk of disease transmission despite extensive donor screening and testing.[16] Advances in serologic testing for HIV, hepatitis, and other entities have improved safety, but a measurable risk still remains.[54] It is imperative that both the surgeon and the patient considering an allografting procedure be aware of the risk for transmission of infectious disease. Unfortunately, this risk is difficult to quantify. Despite more than 5 million allograft transplants performed over the past decade, there are very few documented incidents of disease transmission, especially with fresh osteochondral allografts.[14,35] One death has been reported as a result of transmission of *Clostridium sordellii* by a fresh osteochondral allograft.[13]

In a 20-year experience at our institution we have performed more than 450 fresh osteochondral allografts without a documented case of infectious disease transmission. We believe that strict adherence to the guidelines set forth by the AATB and knowledge of the individual tissue banks that provide the transplanted tissue can minimize the potential risk for disease transmission. Overall, inherent safety of the graft is based on good tissue recovery and processing practices, including donor screening and physical examination and serologic and bacteriologic testing.

ALLOGRAFT STORAGE

Storage of fresh osteochondral grafts before transplantation has recently received attention. Historically, fresh grafts were transplanted within 5 days of donor death, thus obviating the need for prolonged tissue storage. The majority of published clinical studies reflect the situation in which the grafts were recovered, stored in lactated Ringer's solution, and transplanted within 5 days.[2,7,19,59,61] Current tissue bank protocols, however, call for storage of fresh osteochondral allografts while tests for bacterial and viral contamination are carried out. Because some anaerobic organisms require up to 14 days to grow in ideal media solution, the tissue currently recovered is usually transplanted no sooner than 14 days and sometimes as long as 40 days after recovery from the donor. At our institution, we investigated chondrocyte viability and the mechanical properties of human articular cartilage stored in a culture medium.[37,50,60] The superiority of this culture medium over lactated Ringer's solution was demonstrated by Ball et al[3] in a study that compared the effects of storage on fresh human osteochondral allografts in two different solutions, lactated Ringer's and a standard culture medium containing amino acids, glucose, and inorganic salts. Fresh grafts were stored in one of the two solutions. The grafts were then tested for chondrocyte viability and metabolic activity at 7, 14, and 28 days after harvest. After 7 days of storage in lactated Ringer's solution, a significant decline in chondrocyte viability and metabolic activity was seen. Culture media provided significantly better preservation of the cartilage, with viability and metabolic activity remaining essentially unchanged from baseline for as many as 14 days. Chondrocyte viability in lactated Ringer's solution at 14 days was 80% versus 90.5.% in stored culture medium ($p < .05$). Even at 28 days, culture medium provided 83.4% chondrocyte viability versus only 28.9% for lactated Ringer's solution ($p < .001$). In addition, the biochemical and biomechanical properties of the extracellular matrix remained stable with both solutions over time (Table 25–1).

Using this culture medium (which is now standard protocol for storage of fresh osteochondral allografts), Williams et al[60] looked at the effects of prolonged storage on the articular cartilage of fresh human osteochondral allografts. Their experiment examined articular cartilage

Table 25–1. Chondrocyte Viability, Viable Cell Density, Metabolic Activity, and Articular Cartilage Glycosaminoglycan Content after Storage in Modified Culture Media

STORAGE DURATION	1 DAY n = 10	7 DAYS n = 10	14 DAYS n = 10	28 DAYS n = 10
Viability (%)	99.2 ± 1.1	98.3 ± 2.5	97.5 ± 2.2	70.7 ± 11.4
Viable cell density (cells/mm³)	16,297 ± 1919	15,730 ± 2562	16,186 ± 3578	8936 ± 2767
$^{35}SO_4$ uptake (cpm/mg)	395 ± 169	288 ± 152	155 ± 168	49 ± 86
Glycosaminoglycan content (% hexosamine/dry wt)	4.2 ± 0.7	4.1 ± 1.3	4.0 ± 0.5	4.2 ± 0.5

stored in culture medium at 4° C at intervals of 1, 7, 14, and 28 days. The osteochondral plugs were examined at each interval for viability and viable cell density by confocal microscopy, proteoglycan synthesis, glycosaminoglycan content, indentation stiffness, compressive modulus, hydrodynamic permeability, and tensile modulus. The results of the study demonstrated that chondrocyte viability remained unchanged after storage for 7 and 17 days (0.9% and 1.7% decrease) and then declined at 28 days (28% decrease in viability). The marker for proteoglycan synthesis, SO_4 incorporation, showed a decline after 14 days (60.8% decrease) and at 28 days (87.6% decrease). No significant differences were detected in glycosaminoglycan content, indentation stiffness, compressive modulus, permeability, or equilibrium tensile modulus after storage for 28 days. The authors of the study concluded that although the properties of the articular cartilage matrix and chondrocytes remained relatively unchanged over the first 14 days after the death of the donor, a significant decrease in the viability and metabolic activity of this cartilage is seen after this time. In a follow-up study, Robertson et al demonstrated significant changes in gene expression in stored allografts.[50] It is currently unknown whether there is a critical chondrocyte viability threshold that is required to ensure the health of the osteochondral transplant over the long term. Because it is thought that maintenance of the viability of metabolically active chondrocytes is critical for long-term integrity of articular cartilage after transplantation, the findings in this study may have implications for grafts that are transplanted after prolonged storage. Currently, there are no clinical studies of osteochondral allografts that have been stored in culture media and transplanted after 14 days or longer.

IMMUNOLOGY

The immunology of fresh osteochondral allografts bears special consideration. Traditionally, it has been accepted that articular cartilage is relatively immunoprivileged. Evidence for this is largely attributed to a study by Langer and Gross in 1974.[38] They evaluated the immunologic response to articular cartilage and chondrocytes after allotransplantation in both rats and rabbits. They found that although isolated chondrocytes possess transplantation antigens and elicit an immune response from the recipient, when embedded in an intact cartilage matrix, they were protected and a host response was not initiated. In their study the intact articular cartilage surface grafts did not sensitize the recipient animals. Their conclusion was that the articular cartilage component of a fresh osteochondral graft is not susceptible to cell-mediated immunity and that it should survive transplantation.

Despite these experimental findings, it is known and accepted that fresh osteochondral allografts do elicit a variable immune response. A study by Stevenson[57] compared the immune response to transplantation of fresh and frozen leukocyte-matched and leukocyte-unmatched osteochondral allografts in a canine model. The authors reported the greatest immune response in fresh, unmatched osteochondral allografts. Kandel and coauthors[36] reported on the histopathology of 44 failed osteoarticular shell allografts retrieved between 12 and 84 months after insertion. The osseous portion of the grafts showed variable resorption of donor bone with areas of necrosis and variable replacement by viable host bone; this finding was independent of the duration of the graft in situ. The cartilage demonstrated variable areas of degeneration and fibrillation. Pannus formation was present, adjacent to and on top of some specimens, with variable resorption of the articular surface. However, the authors reported no histologic evidence of transplant rejection. Oakeshott et al[47] looked at the histology of 18 failed fresh osteochondral allografts. There was no evidence of rejection, with only mild chronic inflammation in some patients with advanced destruction of the graft.

Despite a lack of clinical or histologic evidence of rejection, a recent study on fresh osteochondral allografts demonstrated that anti-HLA antibodies developed in 50% of recipients after transplantation.[56] In this study, 36 patients who received a fresh osteochondral allograft were analyzed by magnetic resonance imaging (MRI) at 3, 6, 12, 24, and/or 36 months. Additionally, all patients were checked preoperatively and postoperatively for the development of anti-HLA antibodies. The patients who were antibody positive had greater mean edema, a thicker interface, and more abnormal graft marrow, in addition to a higher proportion of surface collapse, than antibody-negative patients did. These results suggest that humoral immunity may play a role in the outcome of fresh allografting. Current clinical practice does not include either HLA or blood type matching of donor and recipient;[11] however, the issue of immune behavior may ultimately become clinically relevant, and it is clearly an area where more knowledge is needed to improve the outcomes of fresh osteochondral allografting.

INDICATIONS FOR FRESH OSTEOCHONDRAL ALLOGRAFTS

Fresh osteochondral allografts possess the ability to restore a wide spectrum of articular and osteoarticular pathology. As a result, the clinical indications cover a broad range of pathology (Table 25–2). As is true for other restorative procedures, careful assessment of the entire

Table 25–2. Indications for Fresh Osteochondral Allografts in the Knee

Traumatic or degenerative lesions of the femoral condyle or trochlea
Osteochondritis dissecans
Osteonecrosis of the femoral condyle
Patellar chondrosis
Failed microfracture, autologous chondrocyte implantation, or osteochondral autologous transfer (OATS), "mosaicplasty"
Unicompartmental or multifocal arthrosis

joint, as well as the individual, is important, in addition to evaluating the particular articular lesion. Many proposed algorithms suggest the use of allografts for large lesions (>2 or 3 cm) or for salvage in difficult reconstructive situations. In our experience, allografts can be considered a primary treatment option for osteochondral lesions larger than 2 cm in diameter, as is typically seen in traumatic or degenerative chondral lesions, osteochondritis dissecans, and osteonecrosis. Additionally, allografts are often used primarily for salvage reconstruction of post-traumatic defects of the tibial plateau or femoral condyle.[3,27] Other indications for allografting of the knee include treatment of patellofemoral chondrosis or arthrosis[34] and select cases of unicompartmental or multifocal tibiofemoral arthrosis.[12] Moreover, allografts are used as a salvage procedure when other cartilage restorative procedures have been unsuccessful, such as microfracture, osteochondral autologous transfer (OATS), or autologous chondrocyte implantation.

CONTRAINDICATIONS

Contraindications to the allografting procedure include joint instability or malalignment of the limb. Creation of a mechanically favorable environment is paramount to successful allograft transplantation. Ligamentous instability and malalignment may be addressed at the time of allografting or as a staged procedure. In general, if an osteotomy is planned at the same site as the allograft (i.e., a distal femoral osteotomy and a lateral femoral condyle allograft), these procedures should be staged to improve the chances of graft healing. If the osteotomy is to be performed opposite the allograft (i.e., proximal tibial osteotomy and medial femoral condyle), it is acceptable to perform both operations at the same procedure. Allografting should not be performed as an alternative procedure in a patient who has an acceptable age and activity level for a prosthetic replacement. In younger individuals, modest success has been achieved with allografting of bipolar and multicompartmental arthrosis; however, the presence of advanced degenerative changes in multiple compartments, regardless of age, is a relative contraindication to the allografting procedure. Other relative contraindications include inflammatory arthropathy, crystal-induced arthropathy, and any unexplained synovitis. The use of fresh osteochondral allografts in patients with altered bone metabolism has not been studied extensively.

TECHNIQUE

Preoperative Planning

As with any surgical procedure, preoperative planning is essential. All patients who elect to undergo an allografting procedure should have long, standing alignment films taken to ensure that the mechanical axis of the limb is not overloading the compartment to be addressed. If so,

consideration should be given to osteotomy. In addition, ligamentous examination should be performed and any instability addressed either before or during the allografting procedure.

MRI is also helpful to evaluate the status of the meniscus and the extent of the osseous defect, especially in cases of osteochondritis dissecans and osteonecrosis (Fig. 25–1A and B). After the mechanical environment has been addressed, correct sizing must be determined for appropriate matching between the donor and recipient. This is performed in the knee by using an anteroposterior radiograph with a 10-cm magnification marker at the level of the joint and measuring the medial-lateral dimension of the proximal end of the tibia (Fig. 25–2). The corrected measurement is used, and the tissue bank makes a direct measurement of the donor tibial plateau. A match is considered acceptable at ±2 to 4 mm; however, anatomy can be quite variable. For example, in treating osteochondritis dissecans, the pathologic condyle is typically larger, wider, and flatter; in these cases a larger donor transplant should generally be used.

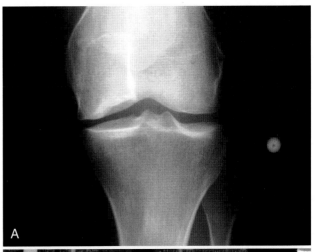
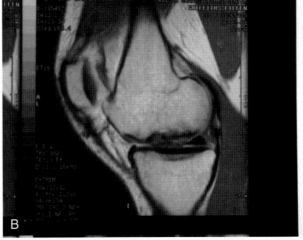

Figure 25–1. **A,** Osteochondritis dissecans of the medial femoral condyle. **B,** T1-weighted magnetic resonance image demonstrating an osteochondritis dissecans lesion.

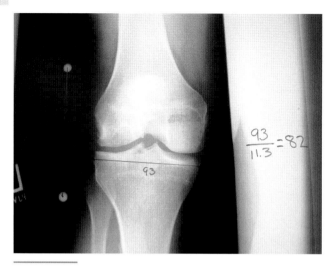

Figure 25–2. Use of a magnification marker on an antero-posterior view of the knee for sizing of the fresh osteochondral allograft.

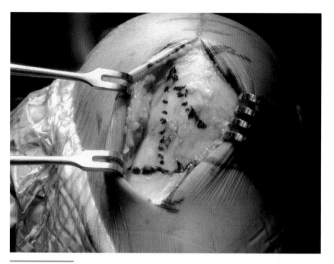

Figure 25–4. Miniarthrotomy with a medial or lateral retinacular incision (*outlined*).

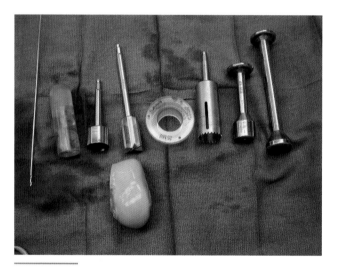

Figure 25–3. Instrument setup for the osteochondral allograft dowel technique.

Surgical Technique

Femoral Condyle

For most femoral condyle lesions, allografting can be performed through a miniarthrotomy, with commercial instruments used to create round or dowel-shaped grafts (Fig. 25–3). Occasionally, a freehand technique using hand tools is necessary to create rectangular or trapezoidal shaped grafts. Arthroscopy has often been performed recently but is not a necessary component of the allografting procedure; however, if there are any unanswered questions regarding meniscal status or the condition of other compartments, diagnostic arthroscopy can be performed before the allografting procedure.

Before making the incision, the fresh graft is inspected to confirm the adequacy of the size match and the quality of the tissue.

The patient is positioned supine with a tourniquet on the thigh. A leg holder is valuable in this procedure to position the leg in 70 to 100 degrees of flexion.

A standard midline incision is made from the center of the patella to the tip of the tibial tubercle. Depending on the location of the lesion (either medial or lateral), a retinacular incision is then made from the superior aspect of the patella inferiorly (Fig. 25–4). Great care is taken to enter the joint and incise the fat pad without disrupting the anterior horn of the meniscus. In some cases in which the lesion is posterior or very large, the meniscus must be taken down; generally, this can be done safely, with a small cuff of tissue left adjacent to the anterior attachment of the meniscus for later repair.

Once the joint capsule and synovium have been incised and the joint entered, retractors are placed medially and laterally to expose the condyle. Care is taken during positioning of the retractor within the notch to protect the cruciate ligaments and articular cartilage. The knee is then flexed and/or extended until the proper degree of flexion is achieved that positions the lesion in the arthrotomy site (Fig. 25–5). Excessive degrees of flexion limit the ability to mobilize the patella. The lesion is then inspected and palpated with a probe to determine the extent, margins, and maximum size. A guide wire is driven into the center of the lesion, perpendicular to the curvature of the articular surface. The size of the proposed graft is then determined by sizing dowels, and a special reamer is used to remove the remaining articular cartilage and 3 to 4 mm of subchondral bone (Fig. 25–6). In deeper lesions, the pathologic bone is removed until healthy, bleeding bone is observed. Generally, the preparation does not exceed 6 to 10 mm, and usually, bone grafting is performed to fill any deeper or more extensive osseous defects. After removal of the guide pin, depth measurements are made in the four quadrants of the prepared recipient site (Fig. 25–7).

The corresponding anatomic location of the recipient site is then identified on the graft. The graft is placed in a graft holder (or alternatively, held with bone-holding forceps). A saw guide is then placed in the appropriate

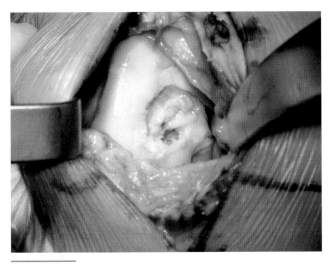

Figure 25–5. Exposure of an osteoarticular defect of the medial femoral condyle.

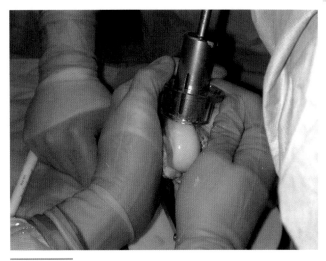

Figure 25–8. Harvesting of an allograft with a hole saw and guide in the appropriate position on the donor condyle.

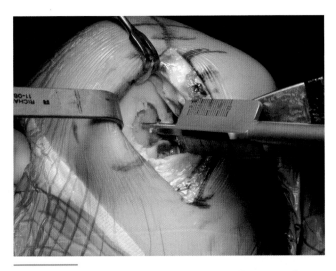

Figure 25–6. Placement of a guide pin and routing device to prepare the lesion for an allograft.

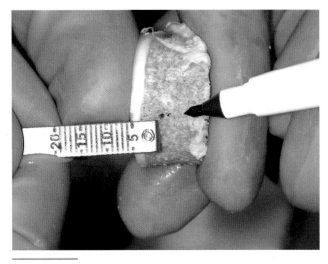

Figure 25–9. The allograft is measured and trimmed to match the recipient site depth.

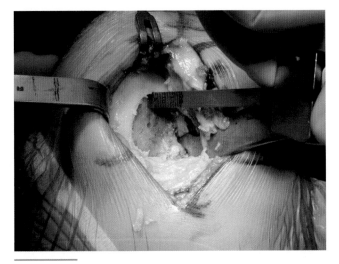

Figure 25–7. Measurement of the recipient site for sizing of an osteoarticular graft.

position, again perpendicular to the articular surface, and an appropriately sized tube saw is used to core out the graft (Fig. 25–8). Once the graft is removed, depth measurements, which were taken from the recipient, are transferred to the graft (Fig. 25–9); the graft is then cut with an oscillating saw and trimmed with a rasp to the appropriate thickness in all four measured quadrants. Often, this process must be done multiple times to ensure precise thickness for matching the prepared defect in the patient. Before implantation, the graft should be irrigated copiously with high-pressure lavage to remove as many marrow elements as possible. The graft is then inserted by hand in the appropriate rotation and gently tamped in place until it is flush (Fig. 25–10). Excessive impacting of the graft can lead to further chondrocyte death. If the graft does not fit, the recipient site can be dilated, or refashioning of either the recipient site or the graft itself should be performed carefully.

Once the graft is seated, a determination is made whether additional fixation is required. Typically,

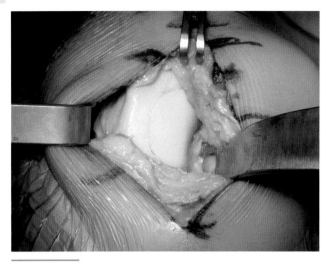

Figure 25–10. Allograft in place with restoration of the original articular contour.

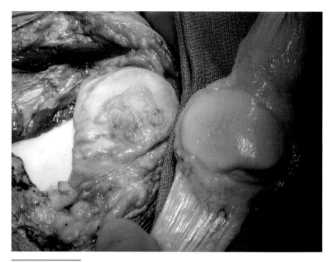

Figure 25–12. Allograft for patellar resurfacing.

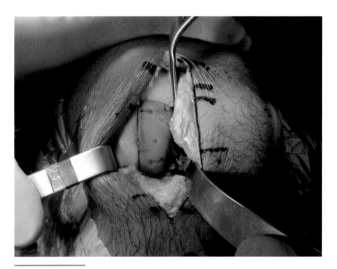

Figure 25–11. Shell allograft used for a large lesion and fixed with absorbable pins.

absorbable pins are used, particularly if the graft is large or has an exposed edge.[55] Frequently, the graft needs to be trimmed in the notch region to prevent impingement. The knee is then brought through a complete range of motion to confirm that the graft is stable and there is no catching or soft-tissue obstruction.

Occasionally, very large or irregularly shaped lesions require either multiple dowel-type grafts or preparation of the graft and host with a freehand "shell" technique to fashion square- or rectangular-shaped grafts (Fig. 25–11). This technique requires the use of small burs, curets, and osteotomes to create matching donor and recipient sites.

TROCHLEAR ALLOGRAFTS

Lesions of the trochlea are approached in a similar manner; however, they are more challenging because the anatomy of the trochlea is much more complex and creation of symmetrically matching recipient sites and donor

grafts can be technically difficult. In this setting, extensive care must be taken to match the anatomic location and the angle of approach because most larger grafts will end up being elliptical as a result of the anatomy of the trochlear groove. Correction of patellofemoral arthrosis, in which the entire trochlea is removed, is performed similar to arthroplasty, with resection of the anterior part of the femur. The graft is resected similarly and fixed in place with interfragmentary screws both medially and laterally. Great care must be taken to not thin the graft in the central portion of the trochlea, which can lead to fracture.

PATELLAR ALLOGRAFTS

The patella is often resurfaced in its entirety when using an osteochondral allograft (Fig. 25–12). In this setting, a technique similar to that for arthroplasty resurfacing is performed. After first measuring patellar thickness, the articular surfaces are resected, with at least 12 to 15 mm of residual patellar bone maintained. The graft is then resected freehand in a similar fashion to ensure minimal thickness in the medial and lateral facets, which generally leads to a maximal thickness of 10 to 12 mm. The graft is seated in appropriate position and rotation, and tracking is noted (Fig. 25–13). The patellar graft can be moved a few millimeters on the recipient surface to optimize patellar tracking. Fixation is typically performed with an interfragmentary screw from the anterior surface of the patella into the median ridge of the graft, which has adequate bone for purchase of a small screw (Fig. 25–14). An extensive lateral release is routinely performed, and proximal or distal patellar realignment is optional. Smaller patellar lesions can be treated with dowel-type grafts in a technique similar to that for the femoral condyle.

TIBIAL PLATEAU ALLOGRAFTS

A tibial plateau allograft is approached similar to the tibial portion of a unicondylar arthroplasty. This technique can

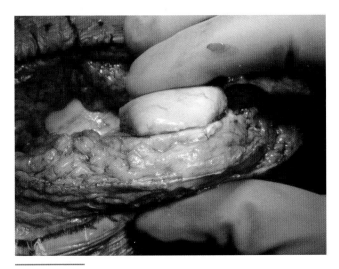

Figure 25–13. Patellar graft in place.

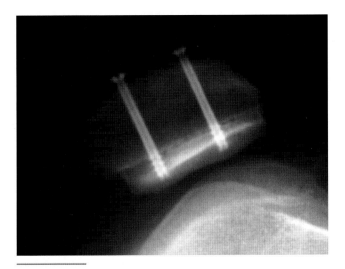

Figure 25–14. Screw fixation of a patellar graft.

typically be performed through a midline arthrotomy without eversion of the patella. Great care must be taken to not damage the cruciate ligaments or meniscal attachments when it is preserved. The proximal tibial resection may be performed with an extramedullary alignment instrument for proximal tibial resection or with a freehand technique under fluoroscopic control. A minimal resection to subchondral bone is made. The vertical portion of the osteotomy should be made parallel to the femoral condyle, with care taken to not resect bone containing the cruciate ligaments. After removal of all diseased tissue, particularly in the back of the joint, the knee is extended and placed in neutral alignment. In this position, the width of the resected compartment and the joint space gap (from the resected surface to the femoral condyle) is measured. Such measurement allows for an estimation of the desired dimensions of the allograft. The tibial allograft is then placed in a graft holder (or secured by assistants), and the desired thickness and width are measured and marked on the graft. Typically, grafts are at least 12 mm thick, with a minimum of 9 mm. A vertical reciprocating

saw cut is then made, and when meniscal transplantation is being performed, the meniscal attachments are included with the graft. An oscillating saw cut is then made by using the guide marks placed on the graft margins. The graft is subsequently remeasured for appropriate width and length and often needs to be thinned in the medial-lateral direction. Trimming is performed as necessary. Before placement of the graft into the recipient, the graft is lavaged to remove all marrow elements. The knee is then brought into flexion and the graft is slid into place, with care taken to not entrap the native meniscus. Once the allograft is seated under the femoral condyle, the knee is brought through a range of motion, and the graft is visualized both clinically and by fluoroscopy for appropriate position, restoration of the joint line, slope, and orientation of the femur relative to the tibial surface. Fine-tuning is performed as necessary. Graft fixation is performed with two 3.0-mm cannulated titanium interfragmentary screws at the anterior and anterolateral edges of the graft. The meniscus is then repaired, or as in the case of an associated meniscal allograft, suturing is performed in the standard fashion. It should be noted that it is vitally important to ensure stability of the tibial graft and prevent mechanical overloading of the graft, either by overstuffing the compartment or by underfilling the compartment, so that increased stress is not placed on the grafted side.

POSTOPERATIVE MANAGEMENT AND REHABILITATION

Rehabilitation of a knee allograft patient in the early postoperative period includes management of pain and swelling and restoration of limb control and range of motion. Assuming rigid graft fixation, patients are allowed touch-down weightbearing for a minimum of 6 to 8 weeks postoperatively, or until bony union is determined by radiographs. Patellofemoral allografts are allowed to bear full weight in extension while locked in a range-of-motion brace and otherwise allowed 0 to 45 degrees of motion for the first 4 weeks and full range thereafter. No bracing is needed for femoral condyle allografts, but if a tibial allograft or an osteotomy is performed, a hinged range-of-motion brace is used for protection until healing is apparent. Tibial grafts associated with a meniscal allograft should be limited to less than 90 degrees of flexion for the initial 6 weeks to allow the soft tissues to heal. Weightbearing is progressed slowly between the second and fourth month, with full weightbearing using a cane or crutch. Sports and recreational activities are not reintroduced until full strength of the limb is complete and radiographic evidence of healing is noted. This generally occurs no sooner than 6 months postoperatively. Continuous passive motion is considered optional. The main objective is restoration of range of motion, strengthening of the quadriceps/hamstrings with isometric exercises, and avoidance of open-chain exercises. We use the stationary bicycle at 4 to 6 weeks in addition to pool therapy if available.

Clinical follow-up includes radiographs at 4 to 6 weeks, 3 months, 6 months, and yearly thereafter. Careful radiographic assessment of the graft-host interface is important. Any concern of delayed healing should lead to a more cautious approach to weightbearing and other high-stress activities.

Patients will typically experience continued improvement over the first postoperative year and often continue to demonstrate functional improvement between years 1 and 2. This often depends on patient motivation, desired activity level, and adherence to a rehabilitation program. Return to sports and recreational activities is individualized in the period between 4 months and 1 year.

RESULTS

The literature has reported on successful results of fresh osteochondral allografting since 1908 with Lexter's reports of fresh allotransplantation.[5,39,40,41] Since that time, the majority of the literature reported has arisen from two centers, the University of Toronto and the University of California at San Diego. Most reports list success and failure based on age group and preoperative diagnosis; this is especially important with regard to fresh osteochondral allografting because of the broad spectrum of disease that this technique addresses.

The experience at the University of California, San Diego, extends over 2 decades. Between 1983 and 2004, 365 fresh allograft procedures have been performed in the knee. Of these, 29% were for complex lesions or salvage situations, 27% for osteochondritis dissecans, 22% for traumatic or degenerative chondral lesions, 14% for patellofemoral conditions, and 8% for steroid-induced osteonecrosis. The anatomic locations of the grafts are outlined in Table 25–3.

In this series, 20% of patients have undergone reoperation, most commonly arthroscopy (6%), revision allografting (5%), and unicompartmental or total knee arthroplasty (TKA) (5%).

In 1985, McDermott et al reported on the long-term results of the first 100 cases of fresh osteochondral allografting performed at the University of Toronto.[44] Of these cases, 95 were available for follow-up. All transplants were performed within 24 hours of donor harvest. The average follow-up in this series was 6 years (range, 5 to 13). The

best results in this series were reported in post-traumatic cases, with 36 of 48 (75%) having a successful result. Results for osteonecrosis and osteoarthritis were not as encouraging in this series, with only 10 of 24 (42%) arthritic cases reporting success and only 3 of 11 (27%) patients with osteonecrosis reporting success. Of interest in this series, 25% of patients had realignment procedures in addition to allografting, but only 38% of this group had a successful result. They concluded that bipolar grafts fared poorly, most likely because of biomechanical considerations.

In 1989, Meyers and coauthors reported on 40 patients available for follow-up at 2 to 10 years after fresh osteochondral allografting of the knee.[46] Of these 40 patients, they reported 31 (77.5%) successes and 9 (22.5%) failures. Patients were rated by using a modified system of Merle d'Aubigne and Postel.[46] An excellent score was given if the patient had complete relief of pain, no limp, and a range of motion of 0 to 130 degrees or more; could perform normal activities; and had returned to work. A good score meant that the patient could return to work and could perform activities of daily living but had occasional pain or swelling, no more than a slight limp, and range of motion of at least 0 to 90 degrees. A fair score meant that the patient had returned to, but had modified work-related activities and those of daily living, might have frequent swelling and less than 90 degrees of motion, and occasionally needed medication for pain. A poor score meant that there was little or no improvement in the patient's complaints or functional capacity. In this system, a successful result was considered excellent, good, or fair, and failure was considered a poor result. Meyers and colleagues reported excellent results in 13, good results in 14, and fair results in 4. On the basis of these results, Meyers et al recommended that fresh osteochondral shell allografts be performed for the treatment of post-traumatic degenerative arthritis of the patella and chondromalacia of the patellofemoral joint, traumatic defects of the tibial plateau and femoral condyle, osteochondritis dissecans, and avascular necrosis. The authors warned against using this technique for unicompartmental degenerative arthritis of both the tibia and the femur (bipolar disease) because the results were successful in only 3 of 10 cases.

Chu et al[15] reported on 55 consecutive knees undergoing osteochondral allografting. This group included patients with diagnoses such as traumatic chondral injury, avascular necrosis, osteochondritis dissecans, and patellofemoral disease. The mean age of this group was 35.6 years, with follow-up averaging 75 months (range, 11 to 147 months). Of the 55 knees, 43 were unipolar replacements and 12 were bipolar resurfacing replacements. On an 18-point scale, 42 of 55 (76%) of these knees were rated good to excellent and 3 of 55 were rated fair, for an overall success rate of 82%. It is important to note that 84% of the knees that underwent unipolar femoral grafts were rated good to excellent and only 50% of the knees with bipolar grafts achieved good or excellent status.

Aubin et al[2] reported on the Toronto experience with fresh osteochondral allografts of the femoral condyle. Sixty knees were reviewed with a mean follow-up of 10 years (range, 58 to 259 months). The cause of the osteochondral lesion was trauma in 36, osteochondritis in 17,

Table 25–3. Anatomic Location of 365 Grafting Procedures

SITE	PERCENTAGE
Bipolar/multifocal femur/tibia	21
Medial femoral condyle	38
Lateral femoral condyle	15
Femoral trochlea	9
Patella	5
Bipolar patellofemoral	5
Isolated lateral tibial plateau	6
Isolated medial tibial plateau	1

osteonecrosis in 6, and arthrosis in 1. Realignment osteotomy was performed in 41 patients and meniscal transplantation in 17. Twelve knees required graft removal or conversion to TKA. The remaining 48 patients averaged a Hospital for Special Surgery (HSS) score of 83 points. The authors reported 85% graft survivorship at 10 years.

Osteochondritis Dissecans

The first report on the results of fresh osteochondral allografting for osteochondritis dissecans was by Garrett.[25] The report included 17 patients with a mean age of 20 years (range, 16 to 46). Success in this study was denoted by an intact articular surface firmly affixed to subchondral bone with flush margins in the remainder of the articular surface. Graft viability was confirmed during hardware removal from 6 months to 6 years after transplantation. At follow-up of 2 to 9 years, 16 of 17 grafts were successful. There was no graft collapse. The one reported failure was a 3 × 4.5-cm graft that demonstrated gross fragmentation on arthroscopy. The author concluded that fresh osteochondral allografting is an effective treatment of large osteochondral defects in the knee.

Similar success with osteochondritis dissecans has been reported by Bugbee and colleagues.[9] The results of fresh osteochondral allografting in 69 knees with osteochondritis dissecans of the femoral condyle were reported in 2003. The mean age at transplantation was 28 years, and the mean allograft size was 7.4 cm². Patients were prospectively evaluated at a mean of 5.2 years (range, 2 to 18) postoperatively. Overall, 53 of 67 (79.1%) knees were rated good/excellent, 10 of 67 (14.9%) were rated fair, and 4 of 67 (6.0%) were rated poor. Two knees were lost to follow-up. Thirteen patients underwent reoperations: 2 were converted to TKA, 5 underwent revision allografting, and 6 patients underwent arthroscopy. Patient satisfaction with the operation was 96%, and 86% reported less pain.

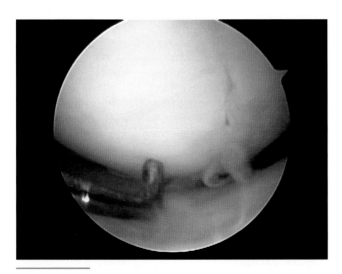

Figure 25–15. Arthroscopic view of a femoral condyle allograft 2 years after implantation for osteochondritis dissecans.

Patellofemoral Disease

In the patellofemoral joint, allografts have been used for the treatment of patellar or trochlear lesions, avascular necrosis, and patellofemoral arthrosis as a result of chronic malalignment. Reports in this group have been limited. Meyers and coworkers reported their results of fresh osteochondral allografting for chondromalacia patellae and patellar arthritis.[46] They reported that at 2 to 8 years of follow-up, five of seven were successful and two had failed.

The largest series to date has been reported by Jamali et al.[34] In this group, 29 knees were evaluated at a mean of 4.5 years. Twenty-two underwent complete patellar resurfacing, 1 underwent trochlear resurfacing, and 7 were treated by combined patellar and trochlear grafting. In this difficult group, 57% were considered to have good or excellent results and 43% were considered fair or poor or underwent reoperation. Reoperations included four revision allografts, three TKAs, and one arthrodesis for sepsis. Four required no further surgery but failed because of a low clinical score.

Osteonecrosis

The use of osteochondral allografts for the treatment of osteonecrosis of the knee has been reported.[4,10,22] In the most recent study of 5.1 years, 19 knees in 15 patients were available for evaluation (3 patients were lost to follow-up). The average age of these patients was 30 years (15 to 68), and all patients had a diagnosis of steroid-induced osteonecrosis of the knee. In these difficult-to-treat patients, 95% reported improved clinical scores. There were 53% good/excellent, 42% fair, and 5% poor results. Notably, 100% of the patients reported satisfaction with the procedure. For younger patients with steroid-induced osteonecrosis, allografting appears to be an effective alternative treatment.

Post-traumatic Arthritis

The results of fresh osteochondral allografting for post-traumatic defects of the knee have been among the most promising.[3,15,27,32,44,46,51] Aubin[2] reported the long-term results of fresh femoral osteochondral allografting for post-traumatic defects in the knee in 2001. This retrospective study focused on 72 patients who received fresh femoral allografts for medial or lateral femoral condyle defects. Sixty of these patients were available for follow-up of at least 10 years. The reported graft survival was 85% at 10 years and 74% at 15 years. The HSS knee score at 10 years averaged 83 points. Patients who underwent simultaneous procedures that included realignment osteotomy or meniscal transplantation had similar scores as those who underwent the allografting procedure alone. Of the 12 reported failures, 3 had their grafts removed and 9 underwent conversion to TKA. The authors concluded that fresh allografting is an effective treatment option in patients with large post-traumatic defects in the distal femoral condyle.

Ghazavi and colleagues[27] reported on the results of fresh osteochondral allografting for post-traumatic defects of the knee. The study included 123 patients with an average age of 35 years. Follow-up averaged 7.5 years (range, 2 to 20 years). All the transplanted grafts in this study were at least 10 mm thick, and in 68 knees osteotomy was performed as part of the procedure. Clinical assessment in this study involved the use of a modified HSS knee-scoring system. Success was defined as an increase in knee score of at least 10 points or maintenance of a score of 75 or more, with no need for further surgery. Using this criteria, 105 of 123 grafts were successful (85%), and 18 (15%) were defined as failures. Survivorship analysis showed 95% graft survival at 5 years, 71% at 10 years, and 66% at 20 years. Failures in this series were associated with age older than 50 years, bipolar defects, malaligned knees, and workers' compensation cases. The authors concluded that young patients with unipolar grafts obtained the best results.

In 2003, Shasha et al[53] reported on the long-term follow-up of fresh tibial osteochondral allografts used for treating failed tibial plateau fractures. There were 65 patients in the study with an average age at surgery of 42.8 years. All patients had a defect in the proximal end of the tibia of at least 3 cm in diameter and 1 cm in depth. The mean follow-up was 12 years. Of 65 patients, 44 had intact grafts at final follow-up. Of these intact grafts, there was an 8.6% prevalence of graft collapse in excess of 3 mm, and 40% demonstrated moderate to severe degenerative changes. The overall survival rate was 95% at 5 years, 80% at 10 years, 65% at 15 years, and 46% at 20 years. There was a reported trend toward increased survivorship for patients who had undergone meniscal transplantation in conjunction with osteochondral allografting, but this trend was not significant. The 21 patients whose grafts failed underwent conversion to TKA. The overall rate of conversion to TKA was 30% at 10 years. The authors concluded that their technique provides a long-lasting and reliable reconstruction in this high-demand population. In addition, this procedure did not make eventual conversion to TKA more difficult.

Tibiofemoral Arthrosis

The results of osteochondral allografting for tibiofemoral arthrosis of the knee have historically been less successful.[30] In 1985 McDermott and associates[44] reported the results of fresh small-fragment osteochondral allografts for the treatment of osteoarthritis. In this group only 10 of 24 (42%) were reported as successful procedures. Bugbee et al[12] reported on the results of fresh allografting for tibiofemoral arthrosis in 41 patients. The average age was 37 years. There were 12 unipolar, 26 bipolar, and 3 multiple-surface allografts. Follow-up in the group averaged 4.5 years, with 21 (54%) successful and 18 (46%) unsuccessful cases. Two patients were lost to follow-up. Of note, the unipolar grafts fared better than arthe bipolar grafts (70% versus 48% success). Of the failures, seven patients

were revised to TKA, five underwent repeat allografting, and one underwent arthrodesis. The author concluded that biologic resurfacing is successful in over half the patients and that failure does not preclude conversion to primary prosthetic arthroplasty.

COMPLICATIONS OF FRESH OSTEOCHONDRAL ALLOGRAFTING

Complications of the allografting procedure can be divided into early and late.

Early Complications

Early complications unique to the allografting procedure are few. There does not appear to be any increased risk for surgical site infection with the use of allografts versus other procedures. The use of a miniarthrotomy in the knee decreases the risk for postoperative stiffness. Occasionally, one sees a persistent effusion, which is typically a sign of overuse but may indicate immune-mediated synovitis. Delayed union or nonunion of the fresh allograft is the most common early finding. This is evidenced by persistent discomfort and/or a visible graft-host interface on serial radiographic evaluation. Delayed union or nonunion is more common in larger grafts, such as those used in the tibial plateau, or in the setting of compromised bone, such as in the treatment of osteonecrosis. In this setting, patience is essential, and complete healing or recovery may take an extended period. Decreasing activities, institution of weightbearing precautions or the use of braces, and possible use of external bone stimulators may be helpful in the early management of delayed healing. Careful evaluation of serial radiographs can provide insight into the healing process, but MRI is rarely helpful, particularly before 6 months postoperatively, because it typically shows extensive signal abnormality that is difficult to interpret.[56] It should be noted that with adequate attention to postoperative weightbearing restrictions and adequate graft fixation, delayed union or nonunion requiring repeat surgical intervention within the first year is extremely uncommon. The natural history of a graft that fails to osseointegrate is unpredictable. Clinical symptoms may be minimal, or there may be progressive clinical deterioration and radiographic evidence of fragmentation, fracture, or collapse. Typical symptoms of this type of graft failure include an increase in pain or sudden onset, often associated with minor trauma. Effusion, crepitus, and localized pain are commonly seen. Careful evaluation of serial radiographs will typically demonstrate collapse, subsidence, fracture, or fragmentation. Computed tomography or MRI can also be used to confirm graft failure, although criteria for failure are lacking.

Treatment of this type of graft failure generally requires either allograft revision or, with more extensive disease, conversion to arthroplasty or arthrodesis in cases in which the graft was used in a salvage procedure.

Late Complications

As previously noted, the requisite event for a successful fresh allograft procedure is healing of the host-graft bony interface and integration of the host bone into the osseous portion of the allograft. This process of so-called creeping substitution is well described in the paradigm of bone graft healing. Revascularization of the allograft bone by the host may take many years and may not be complete.[26] The amount of bone within the allograft may be important in this process, and it is likely that more complete revascularization will be achieved with thinner grafts than with thicker grafts. Retrieval studies[18-20,26] of failed fresh osteochondral allografts have provided tremendous insight into the allograft healing process and have led to the understanding that fresh osteochondral allografts rarely fail because of the cartilage portion of the graft; rather, most failures originate within the osseous portion of the graft or from progression of the host joint disease process (i.e., osteoarthrosis). It is likely that late allograft failure, which has been seen between 2 and 17 years, is the result of graft subsidence, collapse, or fragmentation as a result of fatigue failure, very much like that noted with bulk allografts placed under repetitive loading situations. This clinical finding underscores the need to pay close attention to joint alignment and stability in the initial treatment of the patient. Clinically, the patient will have new pain or mechanical symptoms of either insidious or acute onset. Radiographs will show cysts or sclerosis or perhaps subchondral collapse, typically in the center of the graft, which may be most distant from the revascularization process, or in an area that has been under higher load because of activity of the patient or malalignment. Again, careful review of serial radiographs is important. MRI may also be useful and is generally obtained to confirm the allograft pathology and rule out other sources of pain or sites of pathology in the knee joint. It is important to note that the allografted joint may suffer from the same pathology that is present in any other joint, such as meniscus or ligamentous injury. It should also be noted that radiographic and MRI abnormalities are commonly seen, even in well-functioning allografts,[49] and great care must be taken in interpreting and correlating the imaging studies with clinical findings (Figs. 25–16 and 25–17).

Treatment options for failed allografts include observation if the patient is minimally symptomatic and the joint is thought to be at low risk for further progression of disease. Arthroscopic evaluation and débridement may also be used.[8,9] In many cases, revision allografting is performed and has generally led to a success rate equivalent to that of primary allografting. This appears to be one of the particular advantages of fresh osteochondral allografting in that it does not preclude a revision allograft as a salvage procedure for failure of the initial allograft. In patients with more extensive joint disease, particularly older individuals, conversion to prosthetic arthroplasty is appropriate and can be carried out with little difficulty

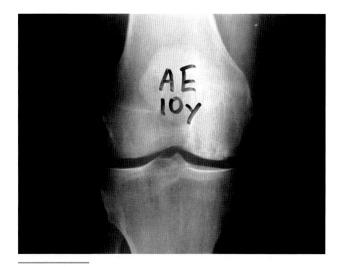

Figure 25–16. Anteroposterior radiograph 10 years after successful medial femoral condyle allograft transplantation. The patient is symptom-free.

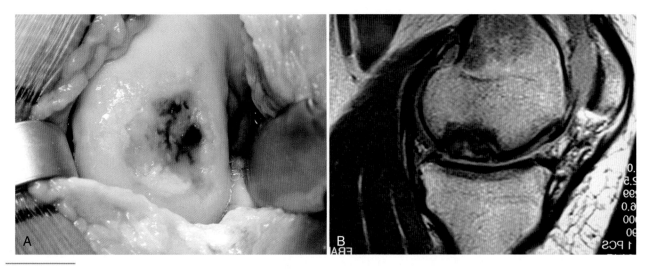

Figure 25–17. **A** and **B**, Clinical and magnetic resonance image of a failed osteochondral allograft.

because significant osseous defects are uncommon with allograft failure.

SUMMARY

Clinical experience with fresh, small-fragment osteochondral allograft transplantation extends nearly 3 decades. The value of this procedure in reconstructing large or difficult chondral and osteochondral lesions is reflected in the increasing use of allografts in cartilage and joint reconstructive procedures. Despite the extensive clinical experience and basic scientific investigation, there are large gaps in our understanding of fresh osteochondral allografts. As with other cartilage restorative procedures, indications for the use of fresh osteochondral allografts are still evolving with respect to the use of allografts in the treatment of focal femoral condyle lesions, as well as more extensive disease states that typify the arthritic joint. One can envision applying allografting techniques to other anatomic locations in special circumstances. The technical aspects of the procedure are evolving rapidly as well, and it is anticipated that improved surgical instrumentation, techniques, and innovations will allow more reproducible results and decrease the number of technical-related early failures. With respect to fresh grafts, we can anticipate further improvements in tissue-banking techniques, not only to improve safety but also to enhance graft quality, and perhaps innovation in the storage of allografts will prolong the storage life of fresh allografts and thus allow more widespread access to this procedure. Further understanding of the immunologic behavior of fresh allografts is clearly needed. Modulating the immunologic response, either by donor-recipient matching or by other therapies, may lead to improvements in the short- and long-term success of allograft procedures. The rapidly emerging field of growth factors and other bioactive substances could provide new methods that would serve to enhance bone healing and improve integration of the allograft bone to the recipient, which is currently the most important event for clinically successful allografting. Processing or manipulation of the osseous portion of the allograft with the addition of growth factors may allow the allograft bone to act more like an autograft and enhance or facilitate the osseointegration so vital to success of the allograft. We may also envision the application of growth factors or other substances to the hyaline cartilage portion of the graft to improve matrix properties or cellular function, effect integrative cartilage repair of the allograft to the host, and limit the detrimental effect of storage on the allografts. When one compares the knowledge and understanding of fresh osteochondral allograft transplantation with the body of knowledge available for the transplantation of other organs and tissues, one recognizes that we are in the very early beginnings of understanding the osteochondral transplant procedure. Nonetheless, osteochondral allograft transplantation is an established and successful technique for treating both simple and complex articular cartilage lesions in the knee.

References

1. American Association of Tissue Banks: Standards for Tissue Banking. Arlington, VA, American Association of Tissue Banks, 1987.
2. Aubin PP, Cheah HK, Davis AM, Gross AE: Long-term followup of fresh femoral osteochondral allografts for posttraumatic knee defects. Clin Orthop 391(Suppl):S318-S327, 2001.
3. Ball ST, Amiel D, Williams SK, et al: The effects of storage on fresh human osteochondral allografts. Clin Orthop 418:246-252, 2004.
4. Bayne O: Osteochondral allografts in the treatment of osteonecrosis of the knee. Orthop Clin North Am 16:727, 1985.
5. Brown KLB, Cruess RL: Bone and cartilage transplantation in orthopaedic surgery. J Bone Joint Surg Am 64:270-279, 1982.
6. Buck BE, Malinin TI: Human bone and tissue allografts: Preparation and safety. Clin Orthop 303:8-17, 1994.
7. Bugbee WD: Fresh osteochondral allografts. J Knee Surg 15:191-195, 2002.
8. Bugbee WD: Fresh osteochondral allografts for the knee. Tech Knee Surg 3:1-9, 2004.
9. Bugbee WD, Emmerson B, Jamali A: Fresh osteochondral allografts in the treatment of osteochondritis dissecans of the femoral condyle [Paper No. 054]. Presented at the 70th Annual Meeting of the American Academy of Orthopaedic Surgeons, February 2003, New Orleans.
10. Bugbee WD, Khadavi B: Fresh osteochondral allografting in the treatment of osteonecrosis of the knee [Paper No. 108]. Presented at the 71st Annual Meeting of the American Academy of Orthopaedic Surgeons, 2004, San Francisco.
11. Bugbee WD, Kwak C, Lebeck L, Bragee M: The effect of ABO blood type on outcome of fresh osteochondral allograft transplantation [Paper No. 110]. Presented at the 71st Annual Meeting of the American Academy of Orthopaedic Surgeons, 2004, San Francisco.
12. Bugbee WD, Rabbani R, Jamali A: Fresh osteochondral allografts for treatment of tibiofemoral arthrosis [Paper No. 027]. Presented at the 69th Annual Meeting of the American Academy of Orthopaedic Surgeons, February 2002, Dallas.
13. Centers for Disease Control and Prevention: Update: Allograft-associated bacterial infections—United States, 2002. MMWR Morb Mortal Wkly Rep 51(10):207-210, 2002.
14. Centers for Disease Control and Prevention: Hepatitis C virus transmission from an antibody-negative organ and tissue donor—United States, 2000-2002. MMWR Morb Mortal Wkly Rep 52(13):273-276, 2003.
15. Chu CR, Convery FR, Akeson WH, et al: Articular cartilage transplantation: Clinical results in the knee. Clin Orthop 360:159-168, 1999.
16. Conrad EU, Gretch DR, Obermeyer KR: Transmission of the hepatitis-C virus by tissue transplantation. J Bone Joint Surg Am 77:214-224, 1995.
17. Convery FR, Akeson WH, Amiel D, et al: Long-term survival of chondrocytes in an osteochondral articular cartilage allograft: A case report. J Bone Joint Surg Am 78:1082-1088, 1996.
18. Czitrom AA, Keating S, Gross AE: The viability of articular cartilage in fresh osteochondral allografts after clinical transplantation. J Bone Joint Surg Am 72:574-581, 1990.
19. Czitrom AA, Langer F, McKee N, Gross AE: Bone and cartilage allotransplantation: A review of 14 years of research and clinical studies. Clin Orthop 208:141-145, 1986.
20. Enneking WF, Campanacci DA: Retrieved human allografts: A clinicopathological study. J Bone Joint Surg Am 83:971-986, 2001.
21. Enneking WF, Mindell ER: Observations on massive retrieved human allografts. J Bone Joint Surg Am 73:1123-1142, 1991.
22. Flynn JM, Springfield DS, Mankin HJ: Osteoarticular allografts to treat distal femoral osteonecrosis. Clin Orthop 303:38-43, 1994.
23. Friedlaender GE: Immune responses to osteochondral allografts: Current knowledge and future directions. Clin Orthop 174:58-68, 1983.
24. Friedlaender GE, Horowitz MC: Immune responses to osteochondral allografts: Nature and significance. Orthopedics 15:1172-1175, 1992.
25. Garrett JC: Fresh osteochondral allografts for treatment of articular defects in osteochondritis dissecans of the lateral femoral condyle in adults. Clin Orthop 303:33-37, 1994.
26. Garrett JC: Osteochondral allografts for reconstruction of articular defects of the knee. Instr Course Lect 47:517-522, 1998.

27. Ghazavi MT, Pritzker KP, Gross AE: Fresh osteochondral allografts for post-traumatic osteochondral defects of the knee. J Bone Joint Surg Br 79:1008-1013, 1997.
28. Glynn SA, Kleinman SH, Wright DJ, Busch MP: International application of the incidence rate/window period model. Transfusion 42:966-972, 2002.
29. Goldberg VM, Heiple KG: Experimental hemijoint and whole-joint transplantation. Clin Orthop 174:43-53, 1983.
30. Gross AE: Reconstruction of skeletal deficits at the knee: A comprehensive osteochondral transplant program. Clin Orthop 174:96-106, 1983.
31. Gross AE: Repair of cartilage defects in the knee. J Knee Surg 15:167-169, 2002.
32. Gross AE, Silverstein EA, Falk J, Langer F: The allotransplantation of partial joints in the treatment of osteoarthritis of the knee. Clin Orthop 108:7-14, 1975.
33. Harnach Z: Prenos kycelniho kloubu u cloveka. Acta Chir Orthop Traumatol Cech 26:276, 1959.
34. Jamali A, Bugbee WD, Chu C, Convery FR: Fresh osteochondral allografting of the patellofemoral joint [Paper No. 177]. Presented at the 68th Annual Meeting of the American Academy of Orthopaedic Surgeons, February 2001, New Orleans.
35. Joyce MJ, Greenwald AS, Mowe J: Musculoskeletal allograft tissue safety. Presented at the 70th Annual Meeting of the American Academy of Orthopaedic Surgeons, 2003, New Orleans.
36. Kandel RA, Gross AE, Ganel A, et al: Histopathology of failed osteoarticular shell allografts. Clin Orthop 197:103-110, 1985.
37. Kwan MK Wayne JS, Woo SL, et al: Histological and biomechanical assessment of articular cartilage from stored osteochondral shell allografts. J Orthop Res 7:637-644, 1989.
38. Langer F, Gross AE: Immunogenicity of allograft articular cartilage. J Bone Joint Surg Am 56:297-304, 1974.
39. Laurence M: Allograft arthroplasty of the knee: Proceedings and reports of councils and associations. J Bone Joint Surg Br 52:781, 1970.
40. Lexer E: Substitution of whole or half joints from freshly amputated extremities by free-plastic operation. Surg Gynecol Obstet 6:601-607, 1908.
41. Lexer E: Joint transplantation and arthroplasty. Surg Gynecol Obstet 40:782-809, 1925.
42. Malinin TI, Mnaymneh W, Lo HK, Hinkle DK: Cryopreservation of articular cartilage. Clin Orthop 303:18-32, 1994.
43. Mankin HJ, Doppelt S, Tomford W: Clinical experience with allograft implantation: The first ten years. Clin Orthop 174:69-86, 1983.
44. McDermott AGP, Langer F, Pritzker KPH, Gross AE: Fresh small-fragment osteochondral allografts: Long term follow-up study on the first 100 cases. Clin Orthop 197:96-102, 1985.
45. McGovern BM, Pritzker KPH, Shasha N, et al: Long-term chondrocyte viability in a fresh osteochondral allograft. J Knee Surg 15:97-100, 2002.
46. Meyers MH, Akeson W, Convery FR: Resurfacing of the knee with fresh osteochondral graft. J Bone Joint Surg Am 71:704-713, 1989.
47. Oakeshott RD, Farine I, Pritzker KPH, et al: A Clinical and histologic analysis of failed fresh osteochondral allografts. Clin Orthop 233:283-294, 1988.
48. Ohlendorf C, Tomford WM, Mankin HJ: Chondrocyte survival in cryopreserved osteochondral articular tissue. J Orthop Res 14:413-416, 1996.
49. Pressman AE, White L, Gross AE: The MRI evaluation of fresh osteochondral allografts: A pilot study. Newsl Clin Res Soc I:217-220, 2002.
50. Robertson CM, Allen RT, Bugbee WD, et al: Gene Expression of Human Fresh Osteochondral Allografts during Prolonged Storage: A Gene Array Analysis. San Diego, CA, UCSD Connective Tissue Biochemistry Laboratory, 2004.
51. Rodrigo JJ, Sakovich L, Travis C, Smith G: Osteocartilaginous allografts as compared with autografts in the treatment of knee joint osteocartilaginous defects in dogs. Clin Orthop 134:342-349, 1978.
52. Rodrigo JJ, Thompson E, Travis C: Deep-freezing versus 4° preservation of avascular osteocartilaginous shell allografts in rats. Clin Orthop 218:268-275, 1987.
53. Shasha N, Krywulak S, Backstein D, et al: Long-term follow-up of fresh tibial osteochondral allografts for failed tibial plateau fractures. J Bone Joint Surg Am 85:33-39, 2003.
54. Shutkin NM: Homologous-serum hepatitis following the use of refrigerated bone-bank bone. J Bone Joint Surg Am 36:160-162, 1954.
55. Sirlin CB, Boutin RD, Brossman J, et al: Polydioxanone biodegradable pins in the knee: MR imaging. AJR Am J Roentgenol 176:83-90, 2001.
56. Sirlin CB, Brossman J, Boutin RD, et al: Shell osteochondral allografts of the knee: Comparison of MR imaging findings and immunologic responses. Radiology 219:35-43, 2001.
57. Stevenson S: The immune response to osteochondral allografts in dogs. J Bone Joint Surg Am 69:573-582, 1987.
58. Tomford WW, Mankin HJ: Investigational approaches to articular cartilage preservation. Clin Orthop 174:22-27, 1983.
59. Tomford WW, Springfield DS, Mankin HJ: Fresh and frozen articular cartilage allografts. Orthopedics 15:1183-1188, 1992.
60. Williams SK, Amiel D, Ball ST, et al: Prolonged storage effects on the articular cartilage of fresh human osteochondral allografts. J Bone Joint Surg Am 85:2111-2120, 2003.
61. Zukor DJ, Oakeshott RD: Osteochondral allograft reconstruction of the knee. Part 2: Experience with successful and failed fresh osteochondral allografts. Am J Knee Surg 2:182-191, 1989.

CHAPTER 26

Allograft Osteochondral Transplantation: Bulk Graft

David Backstein • Oleg Safir • Allan Gross

Full-thickness articular defects of the knee have a poor prognosis as a result of the limited ability of cartilage to conduct repair. Articular defects larger than 2 to 4 mm in diameter rarely heal, even with interventions such as continuous passive motion.[17,21,32,46,47,64,70,74,83,86,92] In the presence of a full-thickness articular cartilage injury, a healing response is initiated with hematoma, stem cell migration, and vascular ingrowth.[14] This healing response produces fibrous cartilage (type I collagen) rather than normal hyaline cartilage.[20] The capacity for fibrocartilage to act as a satisfactory replacement for hyaline cartilage is low because fibrocartilage has inferior resilience, stiffness, and wear characteristics. These differences ultimately may lead to secondary osteoarthritis.

Post-traumatic full-thickness osteochondral injuries in the knee present a particularly challenging situation. These defects are large and deep and predispose to a high incidence of secondary degenerative arthritis (Fig. 26–1). The post-traumatic situation is complicated further by the fact that these patients are often young and have a high physiological demand. The use of prosthetic replacement components (partial knee arthroplasty or total knee arthroplasty [TKA]) in young patients generally is avoided if possible, because of difficulties of early failure. Currently available biological techniques include subchondral drilling; microfracture; autologous chondrocyte transplantation; mosaicplasty; and various cell-mediated, tissue-mediated, or growth factor–mediated processes.

In contrast, fresh osteochondral bulk allografts (FOBAs) have shown chondrocyte viability for 17 years after transplantation.[32,50,69] There is supporting evidence that chondrocytes remain viable in fresh allografts with maintained matrix; however, this is not true of frozen allografts. Gross and colleagues[42,43] have reported extensively on the outcomes after FOBA in numerous patients. Several other long-term follow-up studies have been published from other centers.[15,19,22]

FOBAs provide a potential biological solution to focal and diffuse articular cartilage disease of the knee. This technique is now a well-established management option for the treatment of large cartilage defects of the knee. On the tibial side, survivorship in the range of 95% at 5 years and 80% at 10 years has been reported,[97] and 85% survivorship was found at 10 years on the femoral side.[3,7,22,35,39,59,71,72]

The primary advantage of FOBA is that they provide instantly viable, fully formed, normally contoured articular surfaces and can restore lost subchondral bone stock.[24,93] A further advantage of these grafts is the avail-

ability of large amounts of tissue from each donor, which can manage almost any size lesion.[45] Ultimately, bulk structural grafts provide a complete, congruent articulating surface that heals to host bone by creeping substitution.[80]

Availability and use of allograft materials have increased in recent years. In 1999, more than 20,000 donors provided cadaveric tissue, and in 1999, U.S. tissue banks distributed more than 750,000 allografts.[27] An advantage of autogenous bone and cartilage sources is the lack of immunologic response and risk of transmitting infectious agents. Autogenous sources also seem to have better long-term autograft cell viability.[94] Disadvantages of autologous bone and cartilage include a limited supply of tissue and the morbidity of harvesting graft from healthy areas within the joint (e.g., from the periphery or trochlea). Allograft tissue provides the opportunity to use graft from younger donors than the recipient patient.[79]

One of the most concerning and controversial areas in the use of fresh allograft material is the risk of transmitting infectious organisms, including viral and bacterial disease. In many centers, a significant delay in implantation is needed while awaiting culture results, and graft viability becomes an issue. This delay seems acceptable because allograft storage studies have shown chondrocyte viability for 28 days with a significant decline after 14 days.[81,106] At our institution, grafts typically are used within 48 to 72 hours from procurement to maximize chondrocyte viability.

BASIC SCIENCE

Cartilage is known to have a limited capacity to regenerate. Several factors have been found to influence the ability of cartilage to heal, including the following:

1. *Biological cartilage age.* Chondrocytes from skeletally immature animals have a greater ability to proliferate and synthesize cartilage matrix.[52,77]
2. *Size of defect.* Convery and associates[21] showed that small defects (<3 mm) have a better capacity to heal than larger ones. These authors showed a proportional relationship between increasing size and decreasing healing.
3. *Continuous passive motion.* Continuous passive motion has been reported to enhance the ability of full-thickness defects to heal. Studies have shown accelerated repair rates and formation of tissue

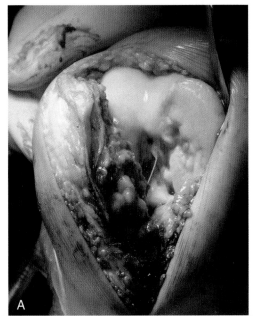

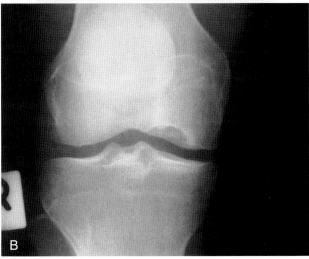

Figure 26–1. **A** and **B,** Large osteochondral defect of the medial femoral condyle in a young man.

closely resembling hyaline cartilage morphologically and histochemically.[75,84-86,90,92] The advantage that fresh bulk osteochondral grafts hold over other forms of grafting lies in the fact that they do not require cartilage repair or regeneration, but instead simply depend on chondrocyte survival and avoidance of rejection in the supporting mature matrix that the graft provides. Host-graft healing occurs via the process of creeping substitution to unite the underlying allograft bone to the host.

Viability of Chondrocytes

Studies on allogeneic cartilage transplantation have shown a high percentage of live transplanted chondrocytes that are able to form matrix without inducing evidence of an immunological or inflammatory reaction.[22,26,54-56,80] At the same time, these live chondrocytes prevent degenerative changes.[24] Retrieval studies of FOBA have shown that live chondrocytes are present in grafts retrieved 17 years post-operatively.[69] It has been shown that even with the most careful cryopreservation techniques and thawing, an acceptable degree of cartilage viability is not possible when frozen grafts are used.[28,29] Tissue matching of FOBA is not required because the matrix that surrounds the chondrocytes isolates them from immunocompetent host cells, and in effect the chondrocytes live in an immuno-protected environment.[54,55]

Allogeneic bone-graft tissues function as a scaffold that is eventually incorporated into the host. Three stages constitute incorporation. Cell death from the donor bone tissue occurs first. This stage is characteristic of fresh tissues only because fresh frozen or freeze-dried preservation methods cause cell death before transplantation. The second stage involves the revascularization of the donor tissue and invasion by host cells.[98] The final phase, remodeling, occurs slowly and may take years to complete.

Gross[38] showed histological viability of chondrocytes in retrieved grafts at 12 years after transplantation and chondrocyte function by radioisotope studies at 6 years. The bony parts of small grafts are replaced by host bone in 2 to 3 years by creeping substitution.[16,32,38,68,80]

Graft Storage

Currently, it is impossible to store articular cartilage for prolonged periods while maintaining a high degree of chondrocyte survival. Cryopreservation techniques have not been successful.[62,87,102,103] The grafts should be transplanted as soon as safely possible. Our policy is to have the transplant procedure completed within 72 hours from the time of donor death.

Immunogenicity

It has been shown that chondrocytes are immunogenic,[55] but when surrounded by matrix, they are isolated from the immunocompetent cells and do not sensitize the host. Articular cartilage is immunologically privileged, meaning that tissue typing is not performed, and no immunosuppression is required for FOBA.[22] In our fresh graft program, no attempt is made to match donor and recipient other than on the basis of size.

In contrast to cartilage, subchondral bone is immunoreactive.[54] It has been shown that the preservation process of freezing decreases the bone immunogenicity, but does not eliminate it completely.[54] Fresh bone is more immunogenic than frozen bone, but there is insufficient difference to affect the clinical behavior or outcome.[54] Bone, whether fresh or preserved, is not viable because of its inability to survive without immediate vascularization, but it remains structurally intact and mechanically strong as it is replaced by host bone via creeping substitution or until it is weakened and absorbed by invasion of granulation tissue.[16,32,80] Freezing kills the cartilage.[99] Even with cryopreservation, the best viability rates that could be achieved have varied from 15% to 50% using glycerol or dimethyl sulfoxide (DMSO) and controlled rates of freezing and thawing.[62,93,102,103]

Fresh corticocancellous bone grafts have been shown to elicit a host immune response,[54] as do articular chondrocytes if they are exposed out of an intact matrix.[55] As long as the articular surface is undamaged, and the matrix surrounds the chondrocytes, articular cartilage is believed to be immunoprivileged.[15,24] This concept has been called into question more recently as Phipatanakul and colleagues[88] compared the sera of 14 fresh osteochondral recipients with that of 14 healthy control subjects. These authors found 8 of 14 allograft recipients displayed reactivity to cartilage-specific protein, whereas only 2 of 14 controls showed a similar response. This study raises the question of what the impact and consequences of host immune responses to such large grafts may be in the long-term.

Viability

It has been well shown that transplanted fresh cadaveric cartilage is viable.[18,22-24,28,50,80,100] Jackson and coworkers[48] found that fresh cartilage allografts contained viable chondrocytes for 1 year after transplantation, but viability decreased after 3 weeks. Live chondrocytes have been observed in grafts retrieved 17 years after transplantation.[69]

In ideal storage conditions, human allograft cartilage viability has been examined at durations of 1, 7, 14, and 28 days after harvest.[106] These data show that after 14 days, chondrocytes undergo a significant decrease in viability, viable cell density, and metabolic activity, with preservation of glycosaminoglycan content and biomechanical properties. Cartilage matrix is preserved during storage for 28 days, but the chondrocytes necessary to maintain the matrix after transplantation decreased over that time period. This research involved storage medium change every 48 to 72 hours, a practice that is not usually employed in clinical situations and that may assist in survivorship of chondrocytes. The consequences and implications of prolonged storage times while awaiting culture results and other investigations must be understood fully by surgeons performing these procedures.

The ability of chondrocytes to survive in frozen allografts has been studied in the presence of cryoprotectants.[29,61,65,94] Delloye and colleagues[25] cultivated frozen cartilage treated with DMSO and observed cell growth with the morphological appearance of living chondrocytes, but did not observe any differences from the control group (allografts frozen without cryoprotectant). Schachar and McGann[94] studied the viability of chondrocytes in vitro and in animal models. These authors showed that the viability of cartilaginous cells was optimized by the use of DMSO as a cryoprotectant and by using slow freezing and rapid thawing of the graft. Only remnants of nucleated chondrocytes with cytomorphological features of via-

bility were found, however, in 4 of 28 osteoarticular specimens. Most human chondrocytes stored by conventional banking techniques do not survive despite the use of cryoprotectants. In contrast, the Schacher study[94] found two fresh specimens had clear histological evidence of chondrocyte survival. This finding confirms the work of Oakeshott and colleagues,[80] which showed that fresh, unfrozen allografts had substantial chondrocyte survival.

INDICATIONS

FOBA is a viable option for physiologically and chronologically young, high-demand patients in whom implants are undesirable, and arthrodesis is not readily acceptable. The primary indications for FOBA of the knee are large post-traumatic defects of the tibial plateaus and femoral condyles. These lesions should involve a minimum of one-third of the condyle or plateau and measure at least 5 mm in depth (Fig. 26–2; see also Fig. 26–1). These indications have been used for approximately 30 years and are well supported by experimental and clinical evidence.[18,23,24,37,50,53,76,80,89,105] A review by Ghazavi and associates[36] of their first 100 cases showed that the best indication for this procedure was a post-traumatic unipolar defect (i.e., a defect on either the femoral or the tibial side but not both). In this study of a relatively young group of patients, the graft provided bone stock and stability, which were able to result in clinically significant

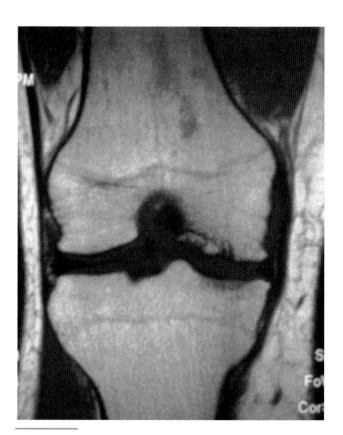

Figure 26–2. Preoperative MRI of a medial femoral condyle lesion.

delay in the need for joint replacement. The failure rate is higher for bipolar grafts than for unipolar grafts, and the results in patients older than age 60 years are inferior to younger candidates.[7] Additional indications mentioned in the literature for FOBA include avascular necrosis of the femoral condyle, patellofemoral disease (including chondrosis and arthrosis), and secondary unicompartmental arthrosis (e.g., postmeniscectomy).[15]

The use of fresh allografts for diseases such as avascular necrosis, focal osteoarthritis, and osteochondritis dissecans has been investigated, but the most favorable results have been found consistently in the post-traumatic defects, in our experience. Other successful outcomes have been achieved, however, in the management of osteochondritis dissecans and avascular necrosis.[7,22,24,36,42,68,71,72] Patients with large osteochondritis dissecans lesions are considered potential candidates for FOBA. Garrett[34] reported a 97% success rate in allografts performed for osteochondritis dissecans with a 1- to 6-year follow-up. Knees with primary osteoarthritis, particularly with multicompartmental disease, are considered to be definite contraindications to FOBA.

Large focal lesions of the tibial plateau resulting from trauma offer fewer management alternatives compared with their femoral condylar counterparts. Femoral-sided lesions are amenable to the alternative treatment modalities of fresh bulk osteochondral allografts, osteochondral plugs, or autologous chondrocyte transplantation, which have not been as successful for tibial plateau lesions.[13,63,78,82] Consequently, osteochondral transplantation is a particularly useful alternative for large tibial plateau lesions.[3,7,36,42,43,58,68,97]

PROCUREMENT, PREPARATION, AND STORAGE

At our institution, FOBAs have been harvested along with other organs on a routine basis since the 1970s. This process has necessitated the development of an organized procurement process and team, which is managed by the Orthopaedic Division in our own institution. This degree of involvement in the procurement process by surgeons is in contrast to many other locations because it has been shown that 65% of surgeons do not know which tissue banks their grafts come from and how the tissue has been processed.[57] In our program, the donors must be younger than 30 years old to provide healthy, viable cartilage. Graft procurement usually is carried out within 24 hours of death, under strict aseptic conditions, with the specimen consisting of the entire joint with the capsule intact (Fig. 26–3).[3,7,36,42,43,58,68,97]

Donors are screened in detail for risk factors of potential exposure to human immunodeficiency virus (HIV), hepatitis B, and hepatitis C.[104] The process includes a detailed medical and social history, serologic tests for HIV antibodies, HIV antigen, polymerase chain reaction HIV, hepatitis B surface antigen, hepatitis B surface antibodies, hepatitis B core antibodies, hepatitis C virus antibodies, and the rapid plasma reagin test for syphilis. A separate study of lymph nodes completes the screening process.

In centers outside of our facility, allograft tissues generally are harvested and processed aseptically. When allograft is harvested by a commercial tissue bank,

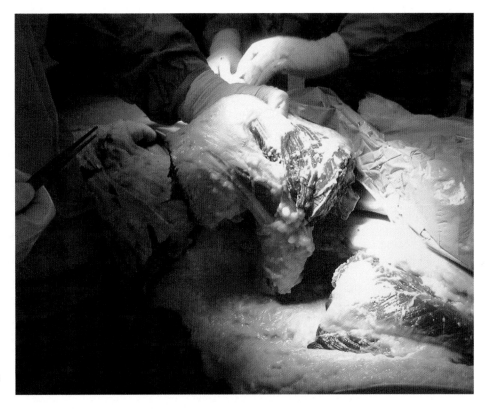

Figure   26–3. Intraoperative photograph of bone harvest.

contamination may occur before the surgeon obtains control of the tissue. This contamination may be the result of an infection in the donor, postmortem infection by bacteria from the gastrointestinal tract, or potential contamination that occurs during the harvesting process. To reduce the chance of infectious disease transmission, some tissue processors use antimicrobial solutions. In our institution, harvested allograft bone is stored in Ringer's lactate with 1 g of cefazolin and 50,000 U of bacitracin at 4°C.

PREOPERATIVE PLANNING

Potential candidates for FOBA are counseled on the risks, benefits, and alternatives to FOBA. These patients usually have been referred after failure of other surgical treatments. They are placed on a waiting list and often given pagers to ensure ease of contact.

As soon as a donor becomes available, the recipients are contacted and instructed to proceed to the hospital for admission. Donors are matched to the recipient by size and bone morphology, using standardized radiographs. Comparison is made in terms of the mediolateral and anteroposterior dimensions on anteroposterior and lateral radiographs. Neither tissue typing nor ABO matching is performed. It is our policy to implement transplantation within 24 to 72 hours from harvest with the understanding that the longer the wait, the greater the death of cartilage cells. Variable durations of storage have been published showing graft viability ranging from 7 to 28 days.[5,81,106]

SURGICAL TECHNIQUE

When the patient and graft are in the hospital, surgery is carried out on an urgent basis. The transplantation is performed in a clean-air operating room. Patients routinely receive preoperative and postoperative prophylactic antibiotics.

The surgical team is composed of two groups. One group prepares the graft, and the other simultaneously prepares the recipient.[96] The favored surgical approach[36,38] is direct midline skin incision and a medial or lateral parapatellar arthrotomy, which allows easy access for the transplant and either proximal tibial or distal femoral osteotomy if indicated. If later salvage to TKA becomes necessary, the same approach is used with little risk of skin complications. The bony defect being addressed is cut down to bleeding cancellous bone, sacrificing little or no healthy bone (Fig. 26–4). On a separate side-table, the donor tissue is cut to appropriate size and shape, often necessitating several fine adjustments (Fig. 26–5). The graft is implanted into the bony defect aiming for a tight fit with accurate reproduction of normal anatomy. All grafts are at least 10 mm thick and are fixed to the prepared defects using 3.5-mm or 4-mm cancellous screws through the bony part of the graft (Fig. 26–6). The use of titanium screws is now advised because of their MRI compatibility. If the host meniscus is significantly damaged or

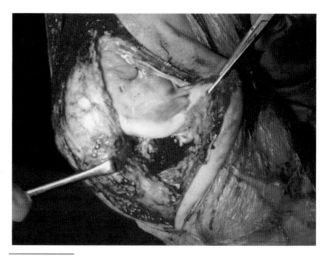

Figure 26–4. Intraoperative photograph after removal of osteochondral defect.

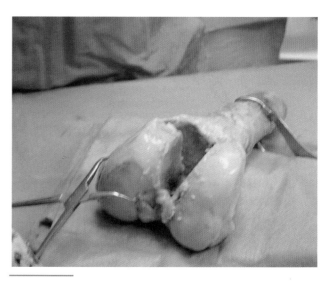

Figure 26–5. Intraoperative photograph of preparation of femoral donor osteochondral graft.

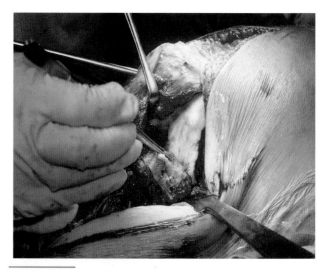

Figure 26–6. Intraoperative photograph of lateral tibial plateau graft fixed in place.

has been excised previously, it is replaced by an allograft meniscus. Dealing with menisci in this way has been reinforced by a review of our results, which showed a trend toward better long-term results when menisci were transplanted.[97] The transplanted meniscus is attached to its own osseous anchors and is implanted further by placement of absorbable sutures to the capsule of the recipient.

The graft itself is never used to correct alignment; this is achieved by osteotomy either before or at the time of allograft implantation. Osteotomy is planned to decrease weightbearing loads on the graft by slightly overcorrecting any malalignment. The preference is to perform either distal femoral varus osteotomy (DFVO) or high tibial valgus osteotomy (HTO) depending on the preoperative deformity. If the realignment procedure involves the same side of the joint as the graft, it may be done several months before transplantation to allow sufficient time for revascularization of host bone, although it is generally our practice to perform the HTO or DFVO concomitant with the graft in most cases (Figs. 26–7 and 26–8).

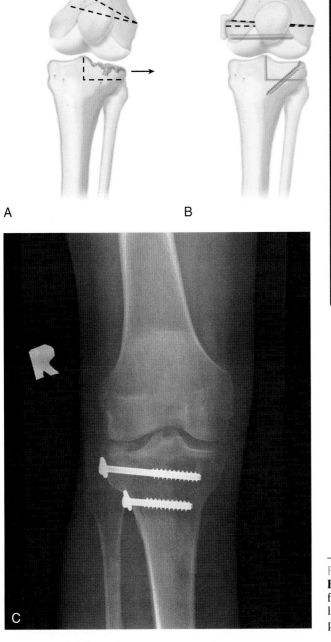

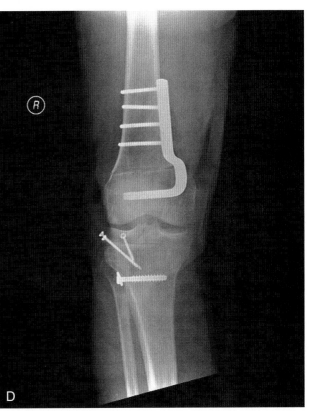

Figure 26–7. **A,** Schematic of lateral tibial plateau defect. **B,** Schematic of postoperative lateral plateau graft and distal femoral varus osteotomy (DFVO). **C,** Preoperative x-ray of lateral plateau defect. **D,** Postoperative x-ray of lateral plateau graft and DFVO.

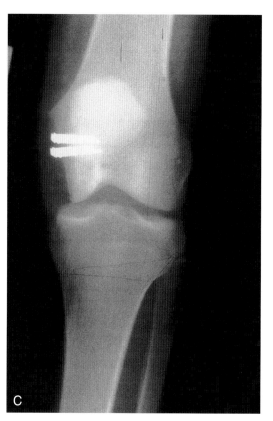

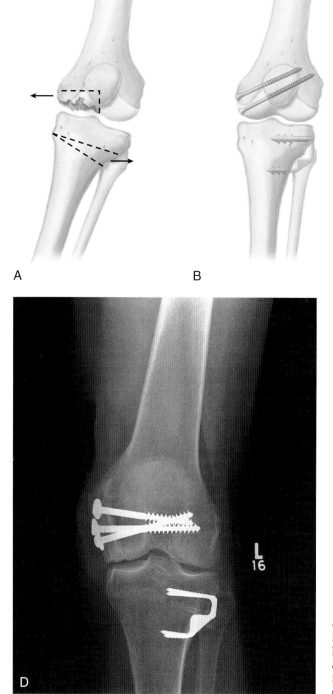

Figure 26–8. **A,** Schematic of medial femoral condyle defect. **B,** Schematic of postoperative medial femoral condyle graft and high tibial valgus osteotomy (HTO). **C,** Preoperative x-ray of medial femoral condyle defect. **D,** Postoperative x-ray of medial femoral condyle graft and HTO.

In a review by Ghazavi and associates,[36] 68 of 126 FOBA procedures had an osteotomy performed. There were 37 osteotomies of the distal femur and 31 of the proximal tibia, performed when the damaged compartment seemed to be under more than a physiological load as seen on long-film standing radiographs. The biomechanical axis of the limb was measured and overcorrected by approximately 2 to 3 degrees. Valgus deformity secondary to fracture of the lateral plateau is managed by a DFVO with an allograft of the lateral tibial plateau. Varus deformity secondary to a medial condylar defect is treated by a HTO and an allograft of the medial femoral condyle.[40,41] Of the 68 osteotomies in one review, 44 were performed at the time of grafting, 19 were done after and 5 before the allograft.

POSTOPERATIVE MANAGEMENT

The senior author's protocol has been to place all patients in a custom-molded ischial bearing brace for 1 year to

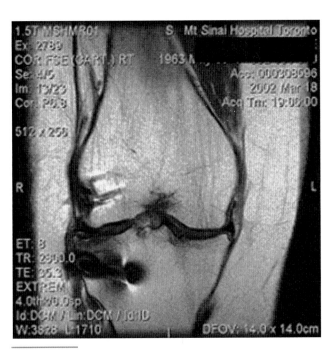

Figure 26–9. Postoperative MRI of lateral tibial plateau graft.

protect the knee from full weightbearing. Patients are allowed to bear weight in the brace when the osteotomy has united, usually at 8 to 12 weeks.[36] At approximately 3 weeks postoperatively, patients are encouraged to begin range-of-motion and muscle-strengthening exercises.

Complete union between the host and graft takes place at about 6 months, and a significant portion of the graft has been replaced at 1 year, although the graft may be subject to collapse for 2 to 3 years.[68,80] Follow-up radiographs are obtained at 6 weeks, 3 months, and 6 months to document union of the allograft to host bone. Magnetic resonance imaging is currently performed for all recipients to assess status of the cartilage, bone, and menisci at least once in the first 5 years postoperatively (Fig. 26–9).

RESULTS

The treatment of post-traumatic defects of femoral condyle and tibial plateau with FOBA has been reported by the senior author with survivorship of 95% at 5 years and 66% at 20 years of follow-up.[7] Similarly positive results have been published by Garrett for the treatment of osteochondritis dissecans.[35] Previous reports have shown little correlation between radiological changes and clinical failures,[58,107,108] but our more recent results have found a highly statistically significant relationship.[3,97] Our survivorship analysis has shown satisfactory results in 95% after 5 years and in 80% after 10 years.[97] We have emphasized previously the importance of patient selection and continue to confirm that young compliant patients with unipolar traumatic defects obtain the best results.[6,7,38,107,108]

Spontaneous osteonecrosis of the knee has not proved to be an ideal indication for this procedure because only

3 patients have obtained successful results out of 11 patients treated for this diagnosis.[7] Results of allografts in the medial and lateral compartments of the knee have been similar to each other. Outcomes have not been found to have any relation to gender. Gross and associates[38] have found that older patients do not tolerate the postoperative bracing as well as younger individuals.

Convery and coworkers[22] reported on nine knees in eight patients with 5 to 6 years of follow-up and found eight of nine (89%) had good or excellent results. Our group[7] followed 92 fresh allografts in 91 patients and found that long-term survival was 76% at 5 years, 69% at 10 years, and 67% at 14 years. The underlying principles that have emerged from almost 3 decades of performing FOBA at our institution include the need for careful patient selection, correction of joint malalignment by osteotomy, and rigid fixation of the graft. Radiographic appearance and clinical result usually correlate.

Garrett[33] reported clinical improvement in 10 patients who were followed for 2 to 4 years after femoral condyle transplants. Our group[36] has reported clinical success in 85% of 126 knees at an average of 7.5 years after the knees had received similar treatment for a post-traumatic osteochondral defect. Analysis revealed a 95% survivorship at 5 years, 71% at 10 years, and 66% at 20 years. Patient factors that were found to be predictive of better outcomes included age younger than 50 years, a unipolar defect (involving only one side of the articulation), and normal alignment or unloading by means of an osteotomy.

Osteotomy

We have performed a realignment osteotomy in more than half of our patients when the weightbearing axis passed through the compartment that was to receive the allograft.[97] Among patients treated with osteotomy, improved results were seen when realignment preceded or was coincident with the allograft surgery. Among patients with intact grafts, improved Hospital for Special Surgery (HSS) scores were associated with early realignment.[97] In patients with failed grafts, conversion to knee arthroplasty was delayed by early osteotomy. Seventy-three percent of the osteotomies were performed at the time of the grafting procedure. Whenever an adjunctive osteotomy is required, we believe it should be performed coincident with the transplantation procedure. Delayed osteotomy should be reserved as a salvage procedure for a deteriorating graft when the mechanical axis passes through the grafted compartment in a very young patient. In patients with intact grafts, the mechanical axis has been overcorrected in 32%, neutral in 55%, and undercorrected in 13%.[97]

Meniscal Transplant

A more recent review by our group[97] has shown that there is a trend toward better survivorship in patients who had meniscal transplantation along with osteochondral allografting. Patients with meniscal allografts who required conversion to total knee replacement underwent arthroplasty at an average of 10.6 years compared with 7.1 years for patients without meniscal allografts. We now believe that increased use of meniscal allografts is warranted.

Functional Outcome

Good to excellent results on the basis of the HSS score were found in 86% of our patients at an average of 12 years (range 5 to 24 years). Only 39% of the knees had moderate to severe degenerative changes at the time of the final follow-up. A correlation between severe degenerative changes and the HSS score was identified. The HSS score did not degrade over time in the absence of degenerative changes.[97] In 1999, in a functional outcome study, we found 93% of FOBA patients had moderately to extremely successful outcomes using SF-36 and Western Ontario and McMaster Universities Osteoarthritis Index as measurement tools.[1]

Femoral-Sided Transplants

At our last review, seventy-two femoral graft transplants had been done in 72 patients with 60 grafts available for follow-up.[3] Average follow-up was 120 months. Sixteen DFVOs and 25 HTOs have been performed in association with the FOBA. Of 60 grafts, 12 have failed, with 3 knees salvaged by having graft removal alone and 9 converted to total knee replacement. Fragmentation and collapse of the graft occurred in four knees at less than 6 years, and osteoarthritis developed in seven patients at more than 5 years postoperatively. Kaplan-Meier survivorship analysis revealed 85% graft survival at 10 years and 74% survival at 15 years. Patients with surviving grafts had good function, with a mean HSS score of 83 points at 10 years' follow-up. Ten patients (17%) underwent concomitant meniscal transplantation, and 41 (68%) required realignment osteotomy done simultaneously with the osteochondral allograft. Patients requiring meniscal transplantation, limb realignment, or both had equally good outcomes at 10 years as patients who underwent osteochondral transplantation alone because osteotomy or meniscal transplants were unnecessary. Likewise, transplantation to the medial or the lateral condyle had no bearing on long-term outcomes.[3]

Tibial-Sided Transplants

Our review of tibial-sided grafts for post-traumatic defects documented 64 FOBAs in 64 patients with an average follow-up of 11.8 years.[97] In total, 59% underwent meniscal allograft and 58% had an osteotomy (25 DFVOs and 12 HTOs). Of 64 grafts, 43 remained in place at most recent follow-up with 21 conversions to TKA. Only 2 of 43 patients had a poor clinical outcome as defined by an HSS score of less than 70. The average HSS score for the 43 remaining grafts was 85. Kaplan-Meier survivorship curves revealed 95% survivorship at 5 years, 85% at 10 years, and 71% at 15 years.

Conversion to Total Knee Arthroplasty

Conversion to a TKA as a salvage procedure for patients with a deteriorating graft was performed for one-third of patients at an average of 10 years after the index allograft surgery. In our opinion, conversion to TKA many years after an allografting procedure does not indicate a failure of the procedure because joint replacement would have been the only option if FOBA had not been performed. In those cases, the FOBA simply bought several additional years of function before finally performing TKA.

Kaplan-Meier survivorship analysis showed an 80% rate of survival at 10 years and a 65% rate of survival at 15 years.[97] This procedure successfully provides an enduring stable, and functional knee in young, high-demand patients. The presence of the tibial allograft did not make TKA technically more difficult. The restoration of bone stock virtually eliminates the need for metal or bony augmentation. Our analysis of TKA in patients with previous FOBA showed that in relatively young patients who have a large tibial defect after a tibial plateau fracture for which conventional treatment has failed, FOBA can delay TKA for a prolonged period while providing functional use of the knee. Any technical complexity of TKA in this context was related to the osteotomy as opposed to the fresh graft.

COMPLICATIONS

Complications from FOBA surgery can be classified as the nonspecific complications inherent to any major knee surgery and the complications specific to this procedure. Nonspecific complications are similar in frequency to other major knee procedures and include infection (1.9%) and knee stiffness (3%) (Gross AE, et al: unpublished data, 2004).

Problems specific to this procedure include approximately a 2% to 4% incidence of failure of the graft to incorporate to host bone.[36] Delayed union or nonunion is more common in extremely large grafts and the treatment of osteonecrosis.[15] Definitive nonunions are treated with autografting and supplemental fixation if indicated. In the study by Ghazavi and coworkers,[36] complications included three stiff knees (as a result of long postoperative immobilization), one wound hematoma, and one patellar tendon rupture. Log-rank analysis revealed a statistically significant relationship of failure to bipolar grafts ($p < .05$) and workers' compensation patients ($p = .0396$), but no significant relationship to other factors, such as osteotomy, meniscus transplant, sex, and medial or lateral side of the knee. In the study by Ghazavi and coworkers,[36] no graft fractures were seen, but 30 of 130 knees showed significant graft collapse or 50% joint space narrowing and early graft degeneration (hypertrophy, delamination, or fragmentation).

Immune Response

The question of what effect large segments of bone and cartilage allograft may have on immune response to a potential future organ transplant has been investigated.[56] Serological data of Kiesau and associates[51] showed that of 72 graft recipients, 25% had sensitization to HLA antigens before transplant, whereas 86% had sensitization after receiving the graft ($p < 0.05$). There was no significant relationship between the immune response and clinical outcome in this study. It may be necessary to consider, however, what implications these serological changes could have on potential future organ transplantation in these patients.

Failure

Ultimate failure of the graft generally presents with new pain or mechanical symptoms and radiographic evidence of collapse or fragmentation.[15] Our center generally has elected to treat late failed grafts with conversion to TKA. Even failed grafts often improve the underlying bone stock to some degree, however, and repeat osteochondral allograft is considered a viable option.

Infection and Contamination

FOBA transplantation is a generally safe procedure, and complications resulting from bacterial or viral transmission are extremely rare. Current tissue banking processing and proper donor screening reduce the risk to very low levels.[2,11,12,101] The risk of infection transmission or contamination is real, however, and must be avoided at all costs. Several standard-setting organizations have been established to help ensure the quality of tissue banks' handling of human tissue. One of the more prominent of these certification agencies is the American Association of Tissue Banks, which offers inspections and accreditation of tissue banks.

The risk of transplanting fresh musculoskeletal tissue that has an undetected viral infection has been quoted to be equal to that of a blood transfusion. The risks from transfusion generally are quantified as 1 in 493,000 for HIV, 1 in 641,000 for human T-lymphotropic virus, 1 in 103,000 for hepatitis C virus, and 1 in 63,000 for hepatitis B virus.[95] The risk of implanting allograft tissue from an undetected HIV carrier actually is probably less than 1 in 1 million when aseptic processing and strict adherence to donor screening and testing are used.[11] We have had zero HIV transmissions out of 270 bulk osteochondal fresh grafts.

With respect to contamination after donor death, Malinin and colleagues[60] examined tissue obtained from 795 consecutive donors of musculoskeletal tissue, and 64 (8.1%) were found to have *Clostridium* contamination, most commonly *C. sordelii*. These authors also found that increased time between death and harvest seems to increase the risk of *Clostridium* contamination. Blood cultures of donors in isolation have been found to be inaccurate predictors of the results of cultured harvested tissue,[67] and it has been recommended that blood and bone marrow cultures be performed. Martinez and associates[66] found that combined marrow and blood cultures are more reliable indicators of tissue contamination than blood cultures alone.

DISCUSSION

The long-term clinical results of large FOBAs have been encouraging. The best indication for this procedure seems to be post-traumatic defects on a single side of the joint (unipolar).[7,58,107] Our early series of grafts did not perform as well as later series because of the early inclusion of bipolar grafts, inadequate deformity correction, and a much wider spectrum of indications. The role of FOBA for post-traumatic joint defects continues to be defined despite positive midterm to long-term results.[4,6,7,15,22,30,31,35,36,42,58,68,72,91] New techniques and technologies for cartilage repair and replacement, such as autologous chondrocyte transplant, likely have restricted osteochondral allografts to treatment of larger defects only.[8-10,13,44,63,73,78] Pure chondral defects less than 3 cm in diameter are better suited to treatment modalities such as microfracture, autologous chondrocyte transplantation, osteochondral autografts (mosaicplasty), or periosteal autografts.[8-10,13,44,63,73,78] The indications for these techniques may include management of defects extending into the subchondral bone (osteochondral defects) when they are less than 3 cm in diameter and 1 cm in depth. Defects larger than these dimensions are better suited to FOBA. Best results from FOBA surgery can be achieved by adhering to principles including correct sizing, realignment, and internal fixation to achieve ideal mechanical conditions along with prompt implantation to maximize cell viability. Mechanical factors seem more important than immunological factors in terms of survival of the graft.

At 10 years of follow-up, we have shown 85% survival on the femoral side and 80% on the tibial side.[3,97] Average survivorship for tibial and femoral bulk grafts is 82.5% at 10 years and 70% at 15 years. For the tibial group, a trend toward increased survivorship ($p = 0.08$) was seen in patients who had undergone meniscal transplantation in conjunction with osteochondral grafting. The longest confirmation of chondrocyte viability at our institution is 17 years after transplantation of a medial femoral condyle graft done for a giant cell tumor.[69]

Allograft tissue has inherent advantages and drawbacks. Among the benefits of allograft tissue is the lack of any donor site morbidity. Tissue is harvested from an organ donor, and no cartilage from the patient's joint must be sacrificed, as is required in autologous osteochondral grafts (mosaicplasty). The donor joint provides large amounts of tissue, which can be used to replace and fill the host's exact size and shape of the osteochondral defect.[80]

Disadvantages of using these large fresh allografts include the potential for infectious disease transmission and the need for a well-organized and resource-intensive transplant program, which is necessary to coordinate the logistics of obtaining tissue and performing the surgery within 48 hours. The surgery generally must be done on an urgent basis and often after-hours because of the erratic nature of donor availability. Disease transmission in fresh allograft tissue remains a concern despite proper screening according to the American Association of Tissue Banks guidelines as reported by Jacobs.[49] Risks are equal to the risks for homologous blood transfusion (HIV risk of 1 in 493,000; hepatitis C virus risk of 1 in 103,000; hepatitis B virus risk of 1 in 63,000), although we believe that the true risk in osteochondral allografts is lower. Finally, there exists a theoretical potential for adverse host immunological consequences in the long-term.[51]

CONCLUSION AND RECOMMENDATIONS

1. Traumatic loss of a joint segment is the best indication for FOBA.
2. Patient selection is a vital consideration.
3. Mechanical conditions seem more important to successful results than immunological factors.
4. Ideal alignment of the extremity to "unload" the graft is an absolute requirement and, if necessary, should be achieved by osteotomy before or simultaneous with allograft implantation.
5. Internal fixation of the allograft should be used.
6. Bipolar allograft should be avoided, if possible.
7. A meniscus should be implanted if the recipient's meniscus is absent or irreparably damaged.

References

1. Agnidis Z, Stimec J, Krajbich J, et al: Health-related quality-of-life following fresh osteochondral allograft of the knee: A minimum five-year follow-up. J Bone Joint Surg Br 81(Suppl I):106, 1999.
2. Asselmeier MA, Caspari RB, Bottenfield S: A review of allograft processing and sterilization techniques and their role in transmission of the human immunodeficiency virus. Am J Sports Med 21:170-175, 1993.
3. Aubin PP, Cheah HK, Davis AM, Gross AE: Long-term followup of fresh femoral osteochondral allografts for posttraumatic knee defects. Clin Orthop 391(Suppl):318-327, 2001.
4. Bakay A, Csonge L, Papp G, et al: Osteochondral resurfacing of the knee joint with allograft: Clinical analysis of 33 cases. Int Orthop 22:277-281, 1998.
5. Ball ST, Amiel D, Williams SK, et al: The effects of storage on fresh human osteochondral allografts. Clin Orthop 418:246-252, 2004.
6. Bayne O, Langer F, Pritzker KP, et al: Osteochondral allografts in the treatment of osteonecrosis of the knee. Orthop Clin North Am 16:727-740, 1985.
7. Beaver RJ, Mahomed M, Backstein D, et al: Fresh osteochondral allografts for post-traumatic defects in the knee: A survivorship analysis. J Bone Joint Surg Br 74:105-110, 1992.
8. Blevins FT, Steadman JR, Rodrigo JJ, et al: Treatment of articular cartilage defects in athletes: An analysis of functional outcome and lesion appearance. Orthopedics 21:761-768, 1998.
9. Bobic V, Carter T: Osteochondral autologous graft transfer. Oper Tech Sports Med 8:168-178, 2000.
10. Brittberg M, Lindahl A, Nilsson A, et al: Treatment of deep cartilage defects in the knee with autologous chondrocyte transplantation. N Engl J Med 331:889-895, 1994.
11. Buck BE, Malinin TI, Brown MD: Bone transplantation and human immunodeficiency virus: An estimate of risk of acquired immunodeficiency syndrome (AIDS). Clin Orthop 240:129-136, 1989.
12. Buck BE, Resnick L, Shah SM, et al: Human immunodeficiency virus cultured from bone: Implications for transplantation. Clin Orthop 251:249-253, 1990.
13. Buckwalter JA, Mankin HJ: Articular cartilage repair and transplantation. Arthritis Rheum 41:1331-1342, 1998.
14. Buckwalter JA, Rosenberg LC, Hunziker EB: Articular cartilage: Composition, structure, response to injury and methods of facilitating repair. In Ewing JW (ed): Articular Cartilage and Knee Joint Function: Basic Science and Arthroscopy. New York, Raven Press, 1990, pp 19-56.
15. Bugbee WD, Convery FR: Osteochondral allograft transplantation. Clin Sports Med 18:67-75, 1999.
16. Burchardt H: The biology of bone graft repair. Clin Orthop 174:28-42, 1983.
17. Calandruccio RA, Gilmer WS Jr: Proliferation, regeneration, and repair of articular cartilage of immature animals. J Bone Joint Surg Am 44:431-455, 1962.
18. Campbell CJ, Ishida H, Takahashi H, Kelly F: The transplantation of articular cartilage: An experimental study in dogs. J Bone Joint Surg Am 45:1579-1592, 1963.
19. Chu CR, Convery FR, Akeson WH, et al: Articular cartilage transplantation: Clinical results in the knee. Clin Orthop 360:159-168, 1999.
20. Convery FR, Akeson WH, Amiel D, et al: Long-term survival of chondrocytes in an osteochondral articular cartilage allograft: A case report. J Bone Joint Surg Am 78:1082-1088, 1996.
21. Convery FR, Akeson WH, Keown GH: The repair of large osteochondral defects: An experimental study in horses. Clin Orthop 82:253-262, 1972.
22. Convery FR, Meyers MH, Akeson WH: Fresh osteochondral allografting of the femoral condyle. Clin Orthop 273:139-145, 1991.
23. Craigmyle MBL: An autoradiographic and histochemical study of long-term cartilage grafts in the rabbit. J Anat 92:467-472, 1958.
24. Czitrom AA, Keating S, Gross AE: The viability of articular cartilage in fresh osteochondral allografts after clinical transplantation. J Bone Joint Surg Am 72:574-581, 1990.
25. Delloye C, De Halleux J, Cornu O, et al: Organizational and investigational aspects of bone banking in Belgium. Acta Orthop Belg 57(Suppl 2):27-34, 1991.
26. Depalma AF, Tsaltas TT, Mauler GG: Viability of osteochondral grafts as determined by uptake of S.35. J Bone Joint Surg Am 45:1565-1578, 1963.
27. Department of Health and Human Services, Office of the Inspector General: Oversight of Tissue Banking. Report No. OEI-01-00-00441. Rockville, MD, DHHS, 2001.
28. Enneking WF, Campanacci DA: Retrieved human allografts: A clinicopathological study. J Bone Joint Surg Am 83:971-986, 2001.
29. Enneking WF, Mindell ER: Observations on massive retrieved human allografts. J Bone Joint Surg Am 73:1123-1142, 1991.
30. Fitzpatrick PL, Morgan DA: Fresh osteochondral allografts: A 6 to 10-year review. Aust N Z J Surg 68:573-579, 1998.
31. Flynn JM, Springfield DS, Mankin HJ: Osteoarticular allografts to treat distal femoral osteonecrosis. Clin Orthop 303:38-43, 1994.
32. Furukawa T, Eyre DR, Koide S, Glimcher MJ: Biochemical studies on repair cartilage resurfacing experimental defects in the rabbit knee. J Bone Joint Surg Am 62:79-89, 1980.
33. Garrett JC: Treatment of osteochondral defects of the distal femur with fresh osteochondral allografts: A preliminary report. Arthroscopy 2:222-226, 1986.
34. Garrett JC: Osteochondral allografts. Instr Course Lect 42:355-358, 1993.
35. Garrett JC: Fresh osteochondral allografts for treatment of articular defects in osteochondritis dissecans of the lateral femoral condyle in adults. Clin Orthop 303:33-37, 1994.
36. Ghazavi MT, Pritzker KP, Davis AM, Gross AE: Fresh osteochondral allografts for post-traumatic osteochondral defects of the knee. J Bone Joint Surg Br 79:1008-1013, 1997.
37. Gibson T, Davis WB, Curran RC: The long-term survival of cartilage homografts in man. Br J Plast Surg 11:177-187, 1958.
38. Gross AE: Use of fresh osteochondral allografts to replace traumatic joint defects. In Czitrom AA, Gross AE (eds): Allografts in Orthopaedic Practice. Baltimore, Williams & Wilkins, 1992, pp 67-82.
39. Gross AE, Beaver RJ, Mohammed MN: Fresh small fragment osteochondral allografts used for posttraumatic defects in the knee joint. In Finerman GAM, Noyes FR (eds): Biology and Biomechanics of the Traumatized Synovial Joint: The Knee as a Model. Rosemont, IL: American Academy of Orthopaedic Surgeons, 1992, pp 123-141.

40. Gross AE, Hutchison CR: Realignment osteotomy of the knee: Part l. Distal femoral varus osteotomy for osteoarthritis of the valgus knee. Oper Tech Sports Med 8:122-126, 2000.

41. Gross AE, Hutchison CR: Realignment osteotomy of the knee: Part 2. Proximal valgus tibial osteotomy for osteoarthritis of the varus knee. Oper Tech Sports Med 8:127-130, 2000.

42. Gross AE, McKee NH, Pritzker KP, Langer F: Reconstruction of skeletal deficits at the knee: A comprehensive osteochondral transplant program. Clin Orthop 174:96-106, 1983.

43. Gross AE, Silverstein EA, Falk J, et al: The allotransplantation of partial joints in the treatment of osteoarthritis of the knee. Clin Orthop 108:7-14, 1975.

44. Hangody LK, Karpati Z: Arthroscopic autogenous osteochondral mosaicplasty for the treatment of femoral condylar articular defects. Knee Surg Sports Traumatol Arthrosc 4:262-269, 1997.

45. Harner CD, Olson E, Irrgang JJ, et al: Allograft versus autograft anterior cruciate ligament reconstruction: 3- to 5-year outcome. Clin Orthop 324:134-144, 1996.

46. Hunter W: The classic of the structure and disease of articulating cartilages. Clin Orthop 317:3-6, 1995.

47. Hurtig MG, Fretz PB, Doige CE, Schnurr DL: Effects of lesion size and location on equine articular cartilage repair. Can J Vet Res 52:137-146, 1988.

48. Jackson DW, Halbrecht J, Proctor C, et al: Assessment of donor cell and matrix survival in fresh articular cartilage allografts in a goat model. J Orthop Res 14:255-264, 1996.

49. Jacobs NJ: Establishing a surgical bone bank. In Fawcett K (ed): Tissue Banking. Arlington, VA, American Association of Blood Banks, 1987, pp 67-96.

50. Kandel RA, Gross AE, Ganel A, et al: Histopathology of failed osteoarticular shell allografts. Clin Orthop 197:103-110, 1985.

51. Kiesau CD, Rapp T, Bruckner J, et al: Poster Presentation P-192. AAOS, San Francisco, CA. March 10-14, 2004.

52. Kreder HJ, Moran M, Keeley FW, et al: Biologic resurfacing of a major joint defect with cryopreserved allogeneic periosteum under the influence of continuous passive motion in a rabbit model. Clin Orthop 300:288-296, 1994.

53. Lane JM, Brighton CT, Ottens HR, Lipton M: Joint resurfacing in the rabbit using an autologous osteochondral graft: A biochemical and metabolic study of cartilage viability. J Bone Joint Surg Am 59:218-222, 1977.

54. Langer F, Czitrom A, Pritzker KP, Gross AE: The immunogenicity of fresh and frozen allogeneic bone. J Bone Joint Surg Am 57:216-220, 1975.

55. Langer F, Gross AE: Immunogenicity of allograft articular cartilage. J Bone Joint Surg Am 56:297-304, 1974.

56. Langer F, Gross AE, West M, Urovitz EP: The immunogenicity of allograft knee joint transplants. Clin Orthop 132:155-162, 1978.

57. Lavernia CJ, Malinin TI, Temple HT, Moreyra CE: Bone and tissue allograft use by orthopaedic surgeons. J Arthroplasty 19:430-435, 2004.

58. Locht RC, Gross AE, Langer F: Late osteochondral allograft resurfacing for tibial plateau fractures. J Bone Joint Surg Am 66:328-335, 1984.

59. Mahomed MN, Beaver RJ, Gross AE: The long-term success of fresh, small fragment osteochondral allografts used for intraarticular post-traumatic defects in the knee joint. Orthopedics 15:1191-1199, 1992.

60. Malinin TI, Buck BE, Temple HT, et al: Incidence of clostridial contamination in donors' musculoskeletal tissue. J Bone Joint Surg 95(7):1051-1054, 2003.

61. Malinin TI, Martinez OV, Brown MD: Banking of massive osteoarticular and intercalary bone allografts—12 years' experience. Clin Orthop 197:44-57, 1985.

62. Malinin TI, Wagner JL, Pita JC, Lo H: Hypothermic storage and cryopreservation of cartilage: An experimental study. Clin Orthop 197:15-26, 1985.

63. Mandelbaum BR, Browne JE, Fu F, et al: Articular cartilage lesions of the knee. Am J Sports Med 26:853-861, 1998.

64. Mankin HJ: Current concepts review: The response of articular cartilage to mechanical injury. J Bone Joint Surg Am 64:460-466, 1982.

65. Mankin HJ, Doppelt S, Tomford W: Clinical experience with allograft transplantation: The first ten years. Clin Orthop 174:69-86, 1983.

66. Martinez OV, Buck BE, Hernandez M, Malinin TI: Blood and marrow cultures as indicators of bone contamination in cadaver donors. Clin Orthop 409:317-324, 2003.

67. Martinez OV, Malinin TI, Valla PH, Flores A: Postmortem bacteriology of cadaver tissue donors: An evaluation of blood cultures as an index of tissue sterility. Diag Microbiol Infect Dis 3:193-200, 1985.

68. McDermott AG, Langer F, Pritzker KP, Gross AE: Fresh small-fragment osteochondral allografts: Long-term follow-up study on first 100 cases. Clin Orthop 197:96-102, 1985.

69. McGoveran BM, Pritzker KP, Shasha N, et al: Long-term chondrocyte viability in a fresh osteochondral allograft. J Knee Surg 15:97-100, 2002.

70. Meachim G, Roberts C: Repair of the joint surface from subarticular tissue in the rabbit knee. J Anat 109:317-327, 1971.

71. Meyers MH: Resurfacing of the femoral head with fresh osteochondral allografts: Long-term results. Clin Orthop 197:111-114, 1985.

72. Meyers MH, Akeson W, Convery FR: Resurfacing of the knee with fresh osteochondral allograft. J Bone Joint Surg Am 71:704-713, 1989.

73. Minas T: Autologous chondrocyte implantation for focal chondral defects of the knee. Clin Orthop 391S:349-361, 2001.

74. Mitchell N, Shepard N: The resurfacing of adult rabbit articular cartilage by multiple perforations through the subchondral bone. J Bone Joint Surg Am 58:230-233, 1976.

75. Moran ME, Kim HK, Salter RB: Biological resurfacing of full-thickness defects in patellar articular cartilage of the rabbit: Investigation of autogenous periosteal grafts subjected to continuous passive motion. J Bone Joint Surg Br 74:659-667, 1992.

76. Mulholland RS, Gross AE: Osteocartilaginous lesions of the talus treated with fresh osteochondral allograft transplantation. Transplantation/Implantation Today 7:15-23, 1990.

77. Nevo Z, Robinson D, Halperin N, et al: Culturing chondrocytes for implantation. In Maroudas A, Kuettner K (eds): Methods in Cartilage Research. London, Academic Press, 1990, pp 98-100.

78. Newman AP: Articular cartilage repair. Am J Sports Med 26:309-324, 1998.

79. Noguchi T, Oka M, Fujino M, et al: Repair of osteochondral defects with grafts of cultured chondrocytes: Comparison of allografts and isografts. Clin Orthop 302:251-258, 1994.

80. Oakeshott RD, Farine I, Pritzker KP, et al: A clinical and histologic analysis of failed fresh osteochondral allografts. Clin Orthop 233:283-294, 1988.

81. Oates KM, Chen AC, Young EP, et al: Effect of tissue culture storage on the in vivo survival of canine osteochondral allografts. J Orthop Res 13:562-569, 1995.

82. O'Driscoll SW: The healing and regeneration of articular cartilage. J Bone Joint Surg Am 80:1795-1812, 1998.

83. O'Driscoll SW, Keeley FW, Salter RB: The chondrogenic potential of free autogenous periosteal grafts for biological resurfacing of major full-thickness defects in joint surfaces under the influence of continuous passive motion: An experimental investigation in the rabbit. J Bone Joint Surg Am 68:1017-1035, 1986.

84. O'Driscoll SW, Keeley FW, Salter RB: Durability of regenerated articular cartilage produced by free autogenous periosteal grafts in major full-thickness defects in joint surfaces under the influence of continuous passive motion: A follow-up report at one year. J Bone Joint Surg Am 70:595-606, 1988.

85. O'Driscoll SW, Salter RB: The induction of neochondrogenesis in free intra-articular periosteal autografts under the influence of continuous passive motion: An experimental investigation in the rabbit. J Bone Joint Surg Am 66:1248-1257, 1984.

86. O'Driscoll SW, Salter RB: The repair of major osteochondral defects in joint surfaces by neochondrogenesis with autogenous osteoperiosteal grafts stimulated by continuous passive motion: An experimental investigation in the rabbit. Clin Orthop 208:131-140, 1986.

87. Ohlendorf C, Tomford WW, Mankin HJ: Chondrocyte survival in cryopreserved osteochondral articular cartilage. J Orthop Res 14:413-416, 1996.

88. Phipatanakul WP, VandeVord PJ, Teitge RA, Wooley PH: Immune response in patients receiving fresh osteochondral allografts. Am J Orthop 33(7):345-348, 2004.

89. Roffman M, Du Toit GT: Osteochondral hemiarthroplasty: An experimental investigation in baboons. Int Orthop 9:69-75, 1985.

90. Rubak JM, Poussa M, Ritsilää V: Effects of joint motion on the repair of articular cartilage defects by free periosteal grafts. Acta Orthop Scand 53:187-191, 1982.

91. Salai M, Ganel A, Horoszowski H: Fresh osteochondral allografts at the knee joint: Good functional results in a followup study of more than 15 years. Arch Orthop Trauma Surg 116:423-425, 1997.

92. Salter RB, Simmonds DF, Malcolm BW, et al: The biological effect of continuous passive motion on the healing of full-thickness defects in articular cartilage: An experimental investigation in the rabbit. J Bone Joint Surg Am 62:1232-1251, 1980.

93. Schachar NS, McAllister D, Stevenson M, et al: Metabolic and biochemical status of articular cartilage following cryopreservation and transplantation: A rabbit model. J Orthop Res 10:603-609, 1992.

94. Schachar NS, McGann LE: Cryopreservation of articular cartilage. In Friedlaender GE, Goldberg VM (eds): Bone and Cartilage Allografts. American Academy of Orthopaedic Surgeons Symposium. 1989, pp 221-230.

95. Schreiber GB, Busch MP, Kleinman SH, et al: The risk of transfusion-transmitted viral infections: The Retrovirus Epidemiology Donor Study. N Engl J Med 334(26):1685-1690, 1996.

96. Shasha N, Gross AE: Allograft transplantation for articular defects of the knee. In Jackson DW (ed): Reconstructive Knee Surgery, 2nd ed. Philadelphia, Lippincott Williams & Wilkins.

97. Shasha N, Krywulak S, Backstein D, et al: Long-term follow-up of fresh tibial osteochondral allografts for failed tibial plateau fractures. J Bone Joint Surg Am 85(Suppl 2):33-39, 2003.

98. Shelton WR, Treacy SH, Dukes AD, et al: Use of allografts in knee reconstruction: I. Basic science aspects and current status. J Am Acad Orthop Surg 6:165-168, 1998.

99. Simon W, Richardson S, Herman W, et al: Long-term effects of chondrocyte death of rabbit articular cartilage in vivo. J Bone Joint Surg Am 58:517-526, 1976.

100. Stevenson S, Dannucci GA, Sharkey NA, Pool RR: The fate of articular cartilage after transplantation of fresh and cryopreserved tissue-antigen-matched and mismatched osteochondral allografts in dogs. J Bone Joint Surg Am 71:1297-1307, 1989.

101. Tomford WW: Current concepts review: Transmission of disease through transplantation of musculoskeletal allografts. J Bone Joint Surg Am 77:1742-1754, 1995.

102. Tomford WM, Duff GP, Mankin HJ: Experimental freeze-preservation of chondrocytes. Clin Orthop 197:11-14, 1985.

103. Tomford WW, Fredericks GR, Mankin HJ: Studies on cryopreservation of articular cartilage chondrocytes. J Bone Joint Surg Am 66:253-259, 1984.

104. U.S. Food and Drug Administration: Guidance for Industry: Screening and Testing of Donors of Human Tissue Intended for Transplantation. Rockville, MD, FDA, 1997.

105. Wakitani S, Kimura T, Hirooka A, et al: Repair of rabbit articular surfaces with allograft chondrocytes embedded in collagen gel. J Bone Joint Surg Br 71:74-80, 1989.

106. Williams SK, Amiel D, Ball ST, et al: Prolonged storage effects on the articular cartilage of fresh human osteochondral allografts. J Bone Joint Surg Am 85:2111-2120, 2003.

107. Zukor DJ, Oakeshott RD, Gross AE: Osteochondral allograft reconstruction of the knee: Part 2. Experience with successful and failed fresh osteochondral allografts. Am J Knee Surg 2:182-191, 1989.

108. Zukor DJ, Paitich B, Oakeshott RD, et al: Reconstruction of post-traumatic articular surface defects using fresh small-fragment osteochondral allografts. In Aebi M, Regazzoni P (eds): Bone Transplantation. Berlin, Springer-Verlag, 1989, pp 293-305.

CHAPTER 27

Clinical Algorithm for Treatment of Chondral Injuries

Henry D. Clarke • Fred D. Cushner • W. Norman Scott

Although the inherent repair mechanisms for chondral injuries remain limited, advances in cell biology and surgical technique have produced a proliferation of cartilage repair procedures. These procedures include a diverse spectrum of techniques based on different rationales, and they have their own distinct potential advantages and limitations. Methods include stimulation of the natural fibrocartilage repair mechanism, transplantation of autologous and allograft osteochondral plugs, and implantation of cultured autologous chondrocytes under a periosteal patch. Elsewhere in this text, each of these methods is thoroughly presented by pioneers and experts in the field of cartilage repair. Therefore, in this chapter we have endeavored to provide a concise and practical approach to managing chondral defects rather than undertake a comprehensive review of each method of cartilage repair. To date, only a few prospective, randomized trials have been undertaken to compare the results of these different techniques.[4,15,17] Therefore, the following material is based on the clinical experience of the two senior authors over the past decade with a wide variety of these techniques, as well as the published and anecdotal results from the pioneers of these procedures, many of whom have contributed to this text. Certainly, few certainties exist in this field, and much of the debate about how to address specific lesions is confused by the diverse types of lesions encountered. Furthermore, the diverse characteristics of the patients in whom these injuries are encountered make it difficult to adhere to a strict algorithm. Concomitant pathology also influences treatment and certainly makes comparison of outcomes between studies difficult. Problems that often must be addressed, either simultaneously or in staged fashion, include ligamentous injuries, meniscal tears and previous meniscectomies, and limb malalignment. In addition, previous surgeries and the response to treatment need to be considered in any evaluation.

Despite the inherent difficulties in creating an algorithm to guide treatment of chondral injuries in the knee, we have attempted to provide a rational approach to these problems (Fig. 27–1). Other authors have also attempted to simplify this difficult decision-making process, and in many ways these algorithms are similar.[1,9-11,21] However, it is also clear from any of these templates that many variables must be considered and the knee surgeon should be familiar with a variety of cartilage repair techniques. Factors that may influence the decision process are discussed next.

PATIENT FACTORS

Age

Although age is a relative indication, data regarding the outcomes of any of these procedures in patients older than 45 to 50 years are limited, and some data have demonstrated better results in patients younger than 30 to 35.[17,23] Therefore, for practical purposes, these techniques are best suited for skeletally mature patients up to approximately 60 years old. Furthermore, age is also a factor in the treatment option that is recommended. In older patients with large lesions, we encourage the use of osteochondral allografts, whereas in younger patients, we may consider autologous chondrocyte implantation (ACI) if the patient is apprehensive about the risk of disease transmission associated with allografts.

Activity Level

Patients with lower activity levels tend to be less symptomatic and therefore may respond to less invasive techniques such as chondroplasty and marrow stimulation. Because there are currently no convincing data that any of these techniques delay or eliminate the development of post-traumatic or degenerative arthritis, the authors generally do not treat asymptomatic lesions. Exceptions include small focal chondral lesions discovered during anterior or posterior cruciate ligament reconstruction where a microfracture technique can be performed with little increased morbidity and no change in postoperative protocols. In such cases we believe that the risk is low and outweighed by the potential gain.

Expectations

Patients must be educated appropriately before any surgical procedure, and avoidance of impact conditioning activities should be emphasized. Expectations regarding the prognosis must be realistic before any reconstructive intervention, and the importance of this concept has been demonstrated.[18,19]

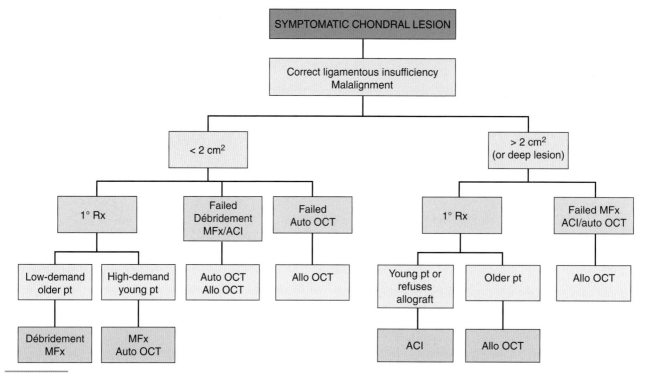

Figure 27–1. Clinical algorithm for the treatment of symptomatic chondral injuries of the femoral condyles. ACI, autologous chondrocyte implantation; Allo OCT, allograft osteochondral transplantation; Auto OCT, autograft osteochondral transplantation; MFx, microfracture.

LESION CHARACTERISTICS

Size

Although there is no true consensus, smaller lesions are generally considered better candidates for the less invasive treatments such as débridement or microfracture. Most authors agree that for treatment purposes, two broad categories of lesions can be defined by their surface area, those less than about 2 to 3 cm^2 and those that are larger.[1,9-11,21]

Location

The best results with virtually all techniques have been reported for isolated femoral condyle lesions; the poorest results have generally been associated with patellar lesions or bipolar lesions.[6,8,13] Only limited data support the use of any technique for chondral defects on the tibial side.[8,13,19,23] Therefore, the clinical algorithm pertains to isolated femoral condyle lesions.

Depth

Deep lesions that involve significant areas of subchondral bone are a distinct problem that significantly influences the appropriate repair technique. Whereas superficial

traumatic chondral injuries can be treated with a number of techniques, we believe that deep lesions, such as encountered with osteochondritis dissecans, are best treated by autologous or allogeneic osteochondral plug transplantation, depending on the diameter of the lesion. If ACI is selected for these deep lesions, the "sandwich technique" is recommended. This technique involves bone-grafting the defect with a periosteal patch followed by a second patch for the chondrocyte injection.

ASSOCIATED PATHOLOGY

The patient should be thoroughly evaluated for associated axial limb malalignment, ligamentous insufficiency, and meniscal tears, which are commonly encountered in this population. In general, we approach these patients by performing ligament reconstruction and meniscal repair or partial meniscectomy as the primary procedure in order to stabilize the knee. At this primary intervention we also use the microfracture technique to address any significant chondral lesions. In these cases we use the standard, accelerated anterior collateral ligament (ACL) rehabilitation protocol and do not specifically protect the microfracture repair. If the patient has persistent symptoms that can be attributed to the known chondral lesion, a secondary reconstructive procedure will be performed 12 months or more after ACL reconstruction. This approach is based on the opposing rehabilitation requirements after ligament reconstruction and cartilage restoration procedures, which we believe potentially limits the results of the ligament reconstruction. In cases in which osteotomy is required to correct limb malalignment to protect the area of cartilage repair, it can be performed simultaneously. It is unclear exactly how much malalignment can be tolerated, but greater than 5 degrees of varus or valgus from normal femorotibial alignment is generally considered unacceptable.[17,25] Sterett and Steadman have reported good results with combined microfracture and high tibial osteotomy.[25] However, in our experience these tend to be chronic cases that have failed previous surgeries, including arthroscopic débridement and microfracture. Therefore, they often represent salvage operations rather than the typical chondral injuries encountered in association with meniscal tears and ligament injuries. In these salvage cases, it is more likely that we would consider the use of allograft osteochondral plug transfer because of the size of the lesions and age of the patients involved.

TREATMENT OPTIONS

Arthroscopic Débridement and Chondroplasty

Arthroscopic débridement plus chondroplasty for unstable flaps is the treatment of choice in older patients, especially those with diffuse areas of involvement. Young patients with isolated lesions smaller than 1 cm^2 and low activity demands may also be treated in this manner. In the setting of diffuse changes in older patients, published results have been inconsistent, but independent centers have reported satisfactory outcomes after about 2- to 10-year follow-up in approximately half to two-thirds of patients who undergo the procedure.[3,5,12,14,18,20,22,26] In their report, McGinley et al noted the results of arthroscopic débridement in a group of 77 patients with knee pain and radiographic changes consistent with significant osteoarthritis (Ahlbach grade 2 or 3 changes) who were considered to be candidates for total knee arthroplasty but elected to undergo arthroscopic débridement as a temporizing procedure.[18] At a mean of 13.2 years postoperatively, 67% had not proceeded to knee replacement; furthermore, the mean postoperative patient satisfaction score regarding the success of the procedure was 8.6 on a scale of 0 to 10.[18]

Marrow-Stimulating Techniques

Each of the marrow-stimulating techniques is best suited to small, isolated lesions in knees without significant malalignment. We favor use of the microfracture technique rather than abrasion arthroplasty or subchondral drilling.[16,24] Microfracture is indicated for full-thickness loss of articular cartilage in a weightbearing area of the femur or trochlea. Lesions between 1 and 2 cm^2 are probably best suited to this technique; however, lesions up to 10 cm^2 have been managed with microfracture.[10,17,23] Contraindications include patients older than 60 years and mechanical axis alignment greater than 5 degrees varus

or valgus on a full-length, standing hip-to-ankle radiograph.[24] In a recent study by Knutsen et al in which patients with femoral lesions were randomized to either ACI or microfracture, there were no statistically significant differences in clinical or histological outcome at 2 years.[17] In distinction, the reoperation rate for recurrent symptoms was significantly higher in the ACI group (25%) than in the microfracture group (10%).[17] Based on these results, as well as our own anecdotal experience, we use microfracture as a primary treatment option for any small, isolated lesion identified during ligament reconstruction and for symptomatic lesions smaller than 2 cm^2 that have not previously been treated. In the latter cases we follow the recommended protocols for protected weightbearing and the use of continuous passive motion for 6 to 12 weeks postoperatively, but in the former cases we do not.[23,24]

Autologous Osteochondral Plug Transfer

Autologous osteochondral plug transfer is indicated for lesions 1 to 4 cm^2 in area.[10,13] However, treatment of lesions up to 8 cm^2 has been reported.[13] Either multiple small plugs a few millimeters in size (the so-called mosaicplasty) or a few 5- to 10-mm plugs can be used. We favor the use of a smaller number of larger plugs and will use a microfracture technique in the small peripheral areas around the central plugs. Smaller lesions can usually be managed entirely arthroscopically, but larger defects may require a limited open arthrotomy. Treatment of larger lesions is generally limited by the availability of donor sites. Because of these considerations, in our practice the best indications for autologous osteochondral plug transfer are lesions smaller than 2 to 3 cm^2 in younger patients in whom previous cartilage repair, such as microfracture, has failed. Small, previously untreated lesions can also be treated with this technique, as long as they are identified preoperatively and the patient has been properly informed of the planned procedure. Favorable postoperative outcomes based on standardized clinical rating systems, including the modified Hospital for Special Surgery (HSS), Lysholm, and Modified Cincinnati scores, have been reported, with 92% good to excellent results in patients with femoral lesions and 88% in patients with tibial lesions.[13] Contraindications include age older than 50 years, malalignment, and instability.

Autologous Chondrocyte Implantation

ACI is best suited to a larger lesion, typically 2 to 10 cm^2, that involves a single condyle of the knee.[6,7,10,19] The surgical technique is a two-stage process that is separated by weeks to months. Favorable midterm to long-term results have been reported with ACI, but the best results have been obtained in patients with unipolar femoral condyle lesions rather than multifocal or kissing lesions.[6,7,19] In a group of 213 patients with 2 to 10 years' follow-up, 90% of patients with femoral condyle lesions in the study reported by Brittberg et al had excellent or good results according to the Cincinnati rating score versus only 58% with trochlear lesions and 75% with multiple lesions.[7] However, these favorable results were achieved in young patients with a mean age in the early 30s rather than older patients.[7] In a recent study Minas reported the results of 71 salvage cases in knees with multiple lesions and early arthritic changes and in knees with bipolar lesions.[19] Even in this group, in which the mean resurfaced area was a very large 11.66 cm^2 per knee, 80% of the patients reported good or excellent results and 90% were satisfied with their outcomes.[19] However, it must also be noted that approximately 50% of these patients also underwent osteotomy to correct alignment problems, and it is therefore difficult to determine the impact of the cartilage repair alone.[19]

A recent prospective, randomized study by Knutsen et al in which ACI was compared with microfracture failed to demonstrate any advantage in clinical or histological outcome in the group that underwent two-stage ACI versus the cheaper single-stage microfracture; furthermore, the reoperation rate in the ACI group was double the rate in the microfracture group.[17] In our anecdotal experience, we have also encountered a significant reoperation rate because of problems such as graft hypertrophy and delamination. Other prospective randomized studies comparing ACI with autologous osteochondral plug transfer have been inconsistent, with Bentley et al reporting superior results with ACI and Horas et al noting the opposite result.[4,15]

As a result of these published reports, our anecdotal experience, the need for two operations, and the significant cost involved, our enthusiasm for the ACI technique has diminished; in many of these situations we now consider the use of allograft osteochondral plug transfer for larger lesions where we may have once considered using ACI. However, in very young patients and those who are concerned about exposure to allograft material, we still use this technique. Because of the anatomy of the trochlea, ACI also remains a good option for large lesions in this area, where it may otherwise be difficult to match the surface contour with other techniques.

Allograft Osteochondral Transplantation

Transplantation of large osteochondral allografts can be performed with a variety of techniques, including giant osteochondral plugs up to 2 cm or more in diameter, which are used in much the same way as autograft plugs; resurfacing techniques in which thin articular sections with subchondral bone are used; and replacement techniques in which an entire hemicondyle is used. These large grafts are best suited for large areas of cartilage damage greater than 3 to 4 cm in diameter and knees with osseous defects deeper than 1 cm that compromise the use of other techniques.[2] However, because of concern about the risk for disease transmission from viral and other submicroscopic vectors and for bacterial contamination from improper graft harvesting and storage, some patients

may not consent to such an option. Cell viability is yet another concern and appears to be related to the period between harvest and implantation.

The long-term clinical results of these techniques, used with or without supplemental procedures such as osteotomy, are limited. In 2001, Aubin et al reported the results of their experience with fresh osteochondral allografts in 72 patients with post-traumatic cartilage lesions of the distal end of the femur greater than 3 cm in diameter and 1 cm in depth.[2] In this series, Kaplan-Meier survivorship was 85% at 10 years and 74% at 15 years; 12 failures had occurred in 60 grafts that were available for long-term follow-up at a mean of 10 years.[2] Sixty-eight percent of the patients underwent simultaneous realignment osteotomy because more than physiological loading was demonstrated on preoperative full-length, weight-bearing radiographs.[2] Among the 48 surviving grafts at a mean 10-year follow-up, 40 patients (83%) had good or excellent HSS scores.[2] Bugbee et al reported their results with large "shell" osteochondral grafts in 1999; at a mean of 2 years postoperatively, the success rate was 86% in patients with monopolar lesions, but in patients with bipolar lesions who underwent grafting of both lesions, the success rate was only 53%.[8]

Although we have experienced favorable anecdotal results with the use of large osteochondral grafts, availability is often limited. Therefore, other options may need to be considered if the patient is not willing to wait or in cases in which the patient is apprehensive about the use of allograft material.

CONCLUSIONS

Many treatment options are available for managing patients with symptomatic chondral injuries. Numerous factors influence the decision on which of the various repair techniques to use, including age, activity level, and patient expectations. Certainly, arthroscopic débridement remains an option for older patients with diffuse changes and young patients with incidental small lesions. Currently, we use microfracture as primary treatment of significant lesions of all sizes on the femur that are noted during ACL reconstruction and for symptomatic lesions of the femur that are less than approximately 1 to 2 cm^2. For lesions that have failed previous treatment, we use autologous osteochondral plug transfer for femoral lesions that are approximately 2 cm^2 or smaller, especially in younger patients and those who are apprehensive about allograft exposure. For larger primary lesions (>2 cm^2) in older patients, deep lesions such as seen in osteochondritis dissecans, and larger lesions that have failed previous microfracture, ACI, or autologous osteochondral plug transfer in any age patient, we favor the use of allograft osteochondral plug transfer. Our use of the ACI technique has declined for the reasons outlined previously; however, this option may be considered in young patients with superficial primary lesions greater than 2 cm^2 and those who are apprehensive about allograft exposure. Combined techniques, such as autogenous grafts in conjunction with biological scaffolds, are another option, but although the early experience has been positive, long-term results from clinical studies remain pending.

References

1. Alford JW, Cole BJ: Cartilage restoration, part 2. Techniques, outcomes, and future directions. Am J Sports Med 33:443, 2005.
2. Aubin PP, Cheah HK, Davis AM, Gross AE: Long-term followup of fresh femoral osteochondral allografts for posttraumatic knee defects. Clin Orthop 391(Suppl):S318, 2001.
3. Baumgaertner MR, Cannon WD Jr, Vittori JM, et al: Arthroscopic débridement of the arthritic knee. Clin Orthop 253:197, 1990.
4. Bentley G, Biant LC, Carrington RWJ, et al: A prospective, randomized comparison of autologous chondrocyte implantation versus mosaicplasty for osteochondral defects in the knee. J Bone Joint Surg Br 85:223, 2003.
5. Bert JM, Maschka K: The arthroscopic treatment of unicompartmental gonarthrosis: A five-year follow-up study of abrasion arthroplasty plus arthroscopic débridement and arthroscopic débridement alone. Arthroscopy 5:25, 1989.
6. Brittberg M, Lindahl A, Nilsson A, et al: Treatment of deep cartilage defects in the knee with autologous chondrocyte transplantation. N Engl J Med 331:889, 1994.
7. Brittberg M, Tallheden T, Sjogren-Jansson B, et al: Autologous chondrocytes used for articular cartilage repair: An update. Clin Orthop 391(Suppl):S337, 2001
8. Bugbee WD, Convery FR: Osteochondral allograft transplantation. Clin Sports Med 18:67, 1999.
9. Cain EL, Clancy WG: Treatment algorithm for osteochondral injuries of the knee. Clin Sports Med 20:321, 2001.
10. Cole BJ, Lee SJ: Complex knee reconstruction: Articular cartilage treatment options. Arthroscopy 19(Suppl 1):1, 2003.
11. Farr J, Lewis P, Cole BJ: Patient evaluation and surgical decision making. J Knee Surg 17:219, 2004.
12. Fond J, Rodin D, Ahmad S, Nirschl RP: Arthroscopic débridement for the treatment of osteoarthritis of the knee: 2- and 5-year results. Arthroscopy 18:829, 2002.
13. Hangody L, Feczko P, Bartha L, et al: Mosaicplasty for the treatment of articular defects of the knee and ankle. Clin Orthop 391(Suppl):S328, 2001.
14. Harwin SF: Arthroscopic débridement for osteoarthritis of the knee: Predictors of patient satisfaction. Arthroscopy 15:142, 1999.
15. Horas U, Pelinkovic D, Herr G, et al: Autologous chondrocyte implantation and osteochondral cylinder transplantation in cartilage repair of the knee joint. J Bone Joint Surg Am 85:185, 2003.
16. Johnson LL: Arthroscopic abrasion arthroplasty: A review. Clin Orthop 391(Suppl):S306, 2001.
17. Knutsen G, Engebretsen L, Ludvigsen TC, et al: Autologous chondrocyte implantation compared with microfracture in the knee. A randomized trial. J Bone Joint Surg Am 86:455, 2004.
18. McGinley BJ, Cushner FD, Scott WN: Débridement arthroscopy: 10-year follow-up. Clin Orthop 367:190, 1999.
19. Minas T: Autologous chondrocyte implantation for focal chondral defects of the knee. Clin Orthop 391(Suppl):S349, 2001.
20. Ogilvie-Harris DJ, Fitsialos DP: Arthroscopic management of the degenerative knee. Arthroscopy 7:151, 1991.
21. Scopp JM, Mandelbaum BR: Cartilage restoration: Overview of treatment options. J Knee Surg 17:229, 2004.
22. Sprague NF III: Arthroscopic débridement for degenerative knee joint disease. Clin Orthop 160:118, 1981.
23. Steadman JR, Briggs KK, Rodrigo JJ, et al: Outcomes of microfracture for traumatic chondral defects of the knee: Average 11-year follow-up. Arthroscopy 19:477, 2003.
24. Steadman JR, Rodkey WG, Rodrigo JJ: Microfracture: Surgical technique and rehabilitation to treat chondral defects. Clin Orthop 391:S362, 2001
25. Sterett WI, Steadman JR: Chondral resurfacing and high tibial osteotomy in the varus knee. Am J Sports Med 32:1243, 2004.
26. Yang SS, Nisonson B: Arthroscopic surgery of the knee in the geriatric patient. Clin Orthop 316:50, 1995.

CHAPTER 28

Spontaneous and Secondary Osteonecrosis of the Knee

Paul A. Lotke • Jess H. Lonner

Two distinct forms of osteonecrosis affect the knee. Spontaneous osteonecrosis involving the medial femoral condyle was described as a distinct entity by Ahlback et al in 1968 (Fig. 28–1).[3] The condition can also occur in the lateral femoral condyle or the tibial plateaus. Spontaneous, idiopathic, or primary osteonecrosis can be distinguished from the more diffuse form, secondary osteonecrosis, which is associated with corticosteroid therapy, excessive alcohol consumption, blood dyscrasias, Gaucher's disease, and caisson disease, among others. This chapter will address the pathology, etiology, clinical course, imaging studies, differential diagnosis, and treatment of these two related but different disorders.

CLINICAL MANIFESTATIONS

Spontaneous osteonecrosis is three times more common in women than in men, and most patients are older than 60 years.[8,12,21,47,65,75,78,80] The usual history is one of a sudden onset of pain about the medial aspect of the knee that may have been precipitated by a specific activity or a minor injury. The pain is frequently worse at night during the acute phase, which may last 6 to 8 weeks after the onset of symptoms. Depending on the size and stage of the lesion, the severe pain of the acute phase may either resolve gradually or become chronic. On clinical examination in the acute phase, the knee may appear locked; that is, the patient cannot fully bend or fully extend the knee because of pain, effusion, and muscle spasm. The examiner can usually find a precise area of severe tenderness on the medial femoral condyle just above the joint line in the flexed knee. As the acute-phase symptoms begin to resolve, the knee continues to remain painful, local tenderness persists, there is variable effusion, ligaments can be shown to be intact, and motion is not limited except by pain and effusion.

Although spontaneous osteonecrosis most commonly involves the medial femoral condyle, it can also occur in the lateral femoral condyle and the tibial plateau.[20,24-25,33,47,52] The area of maximum tenderness alerts the examiner to the involved area. Spontaneous osteonecrosis of the medial tibial plateau is less recognized than osteonecrosis of the medial femoral condyle, but it may be more common, and the initial symptoms are similar.[48,51,54,56] It was first described in 1976 in the French literature by Houpt et al.[33] As is the case with spontaneous osteonecrosis of the medial femoral condyle, most affected persons are women older than 60 years. The most common initial symptom is a sudden onset of pain on the medial side of the knee, often related to minor trauma or increased activity.[26,48,51] A rare case of osteonecrosis in the patella has been reported.[43]

Secondary osteonecrosis is variably referred to as traumatic, ischemic, corticosteroid induced, or idiopathic and is often easily differentiated from spontaneous osteonecrosis. Although the exact incidence of this condition is not well known, it tends to occur in patients younger than 55 years, most commonly in their mid-30s, and involves multiple condyles of the knee. Often, there is polyarticular involvement, The entity tends to be bilateral in more than 80% of cases, and other joints may be involved in as many as 60% to 90% of patients.[60] The knee is affected by spontaneous osteonecrosis less frequently than the hip is, and nonsurgical as well as biological surgical alternatives such as core decompression tend to be less effective than they are for the treatment of secondary osteonecrosis of the hip joint. The exact pathophysiology of the condition is not well understood; however, a number of associated conditions may predispose to the development of osteonecrosis of the knee, including prolonged use of corticosteroids, alcoholism, systemic lupus erythematosus, sickle cell anemia, lipid storage diseases such as Gaucher's disease, and caisson disease.[1,34,36,60]

IMAGING STUDIES

Originally, the diagnosis of osteonecrosis was established by radiographic changes described by Ahlback et al.[3] The diagnosis was confirmed by radionuclide bone scans. The widespread availability of magnetic resonance imaging (MRI) has enhanced the ability to establish a diagnosis and better define the changes in subchondral bone associated with this syndrome.

Radiography

Findings on plain radiographs may be divided into five sequential stages.[2,35,41,82] The process can be arrested at any stage, and only the most severe cases reach stage V.

In stage I, the radiograph is normal. In some patients the symptoms resolve spontaneously and radiographic lesions never develop.[32,53] The diagnosis in this case depends on the radionuclide bone scan and MRI (Fig. 28–2). It is frequently reported as bone edema, best seen

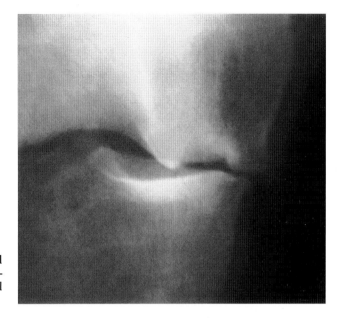

Figure 28–1. Spontaneous osteonecrosis of the medial femoral condyle. This was originally described as a radiolucent lesion surrounded by a sclerotic halo in the medial femoral condyle.

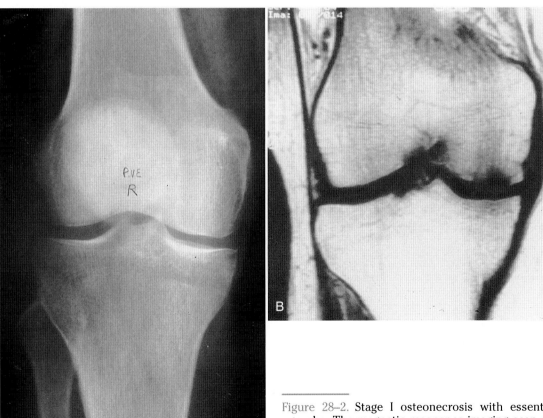

Figure 28–2. Stage I osteonecrosis with essentially normal radiographs. The magnetic resonance imaging scan shows a low-signal defect on the T1-weighted image. The patient's symptoms resolved spontaneously.

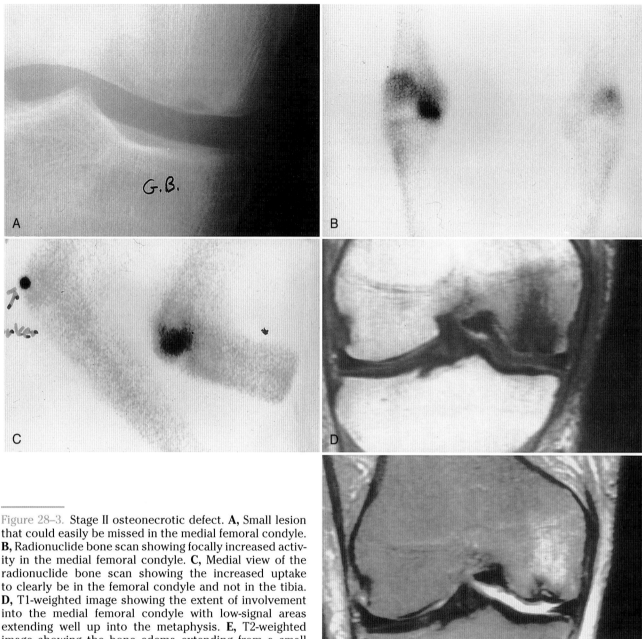

Figure 28–3. Stage II osteonecrotic defect. **A,** Small lesion that could easily be missed in the medial femoral condyle. **B,** Radionuclide bone scan showing focally increased activity in the medial femoral condyle. **C,** Medial view of the radionuclide bone scan showing the increased uptake to clearly be in the femoral condyle and not in the tibia. **D,** T1-weighted image showing the extent of involvement into the medial femoral condyle with low-signal areas extending well up into the metaphysis. **E,** T2-weighted image showing the bone edema extending from a small lesion in the subchondral zone of the medial femoral condyle.

on T2-weighted images. In the case of tibial osteonecrosis, more than half the time the initial radiographs show minor preexisting degenerative changes that are so frequent in elderly patients.

In stage II, there is a subtle flattening of the weight-bearing portion of the affected condyle, which may easily be missed. This finding implies an impending subchondral fracture (Fig. 28–3). In secondary osteonecrosis, the radiographic findings at this stage may include mixed areas of sclerosis and porosis (Fig. 28–3A).

Stage III shows the typical lesion of osteonecrosis. It consists of a radiolucent area of variable size located in subchondral bone and bordered circumferentially by a sclerotic halo. The extent of involvement may be quantified in this stage (Fig. 28–4).

In stage IV, the sclerotic halo thickens, and subchondral bone begins to collapse. There is an increasing sclerotic halo with indefinite borders (Fig. 28–5).

Stage V includes the osseous collapse of stage IV accompanied by secondary degenerative changes in the femoral

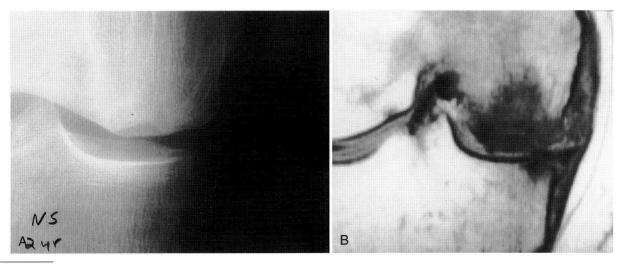

Figure 28–4. Stage III osteonecrotic defect in the medial femoral condyle **A,** Radiograph showing the radiolucent lesion in the medial femoral condyle with minimal collapse. **B,** A magnetic resonance image of the midsized osteonecrotic lesion shows a low-signal area in the condyle with minimal collapse and joint space.

condyle (i.e., osteophyte formation, joint space narrowing, and sclerosis). Secondary degenerative changes can also occur in the corresponding tibial side of the joint. Varus or valgus angulation is present, depending on which condyle is involved (Fig. 28–6).

In stage III, the extent of involvement may be quantified and has prognostic implications. The lesion may be measured as the ratio of the lesion to the size of the condyle[49] or by the area of the lesion (see Fig. 28–5).[65] The area of the lesion was originally used to predict in which knees severe osteoarthritis would eventually develop. Progression to severe degenerative arthritis was unlikely with an average lesion size of 2.5 cm², whereas it was more likely with an average lesion size of 10.4 cm². Nonsurgical treatment was therefore proposed for lesions smaller than 3.5 cm² and surgery only for lesions larger than 5 cm².

The ratio of the width of the lesion to the width of the condyle in the anteroposterior view has also been shown to be a good guide to prognosis.[7,49] The average ratio of knees with a favorable outcome was 0.32, and almost all knees with a ratio less than 0.45 fared well. In contrast, knees with poor outcomes had an average ratio of 0.57, and almost all knees in which the ratio was greater than 0.50 had a poor result (Fig. 28–7). This type of measurement, which is unaffected by errors from varying magnification of the radiograph, is therefore a useful prognostic tool. Al-Rowaih et al have shown that there is no difference between the area and ratio techniques in predicting prognosis.[7,8]

The stage of the lesion is also thought to be important.[41] The earlier the stage of the lesion at the time of diagnosis, the better the prognosis. One problem with staging is that it is done only radiographically and depends on the integrity of subchondral bone. With MRI, we can appreciate widespread involvement into the affected condyle before the lesion is visible radiographically. The prognosis appears to depend on the integrity and size of the lesion

involving the subchondral bone on MRI, but this has not yet been validated.

Radionuclide Bone Scanning

The radionuclide scan is performed with technetium 99m and must be positive to diagnose osteonecrosis.[9,46,53,74] The static-phase image demonstrates a focally intense area of uptake over the affected condyle or tibial plateau. Localization of the increased uptake is easier to see on a lateral view, which clearly demonstrates that the increased uptake is in the femoral condyle as opposed to the tibial plateau (see Fig. 28–3). Increased significant uptake along the condylar contours in both the tibia and femur is more indicative of osteoarthritis than osteonecrosis. Al-Rowaih et al[9] found that the pool phase of a three-phase study did not add useful diagnostic or prognostic information but that persistence of a high flow phase and a static uptake phase for 6 to 12 months correlated directly with poor clinical and radiological outcome.

Magnetic Resonance Imaging

MRI has become the standard for establishing the diagnosis of osteonecrosis. It shows the involvement of the condyle or plateau to be more extensive than can be appreciated on plain radiographs.[15,16,32,44,72,83] On T1-weighted images, the high intensity normally produced by the fat in marrow is replaced by a discrete subchondral area of low signal intensity sometimes surrounded by an area of intermediate signal intensity. A low-signal serpiginous line may differentiate the area of necrotic bone from that involved with edema alone. On T2-weighted images, an area of low signal intensity is surrounded by a variable high-intensity

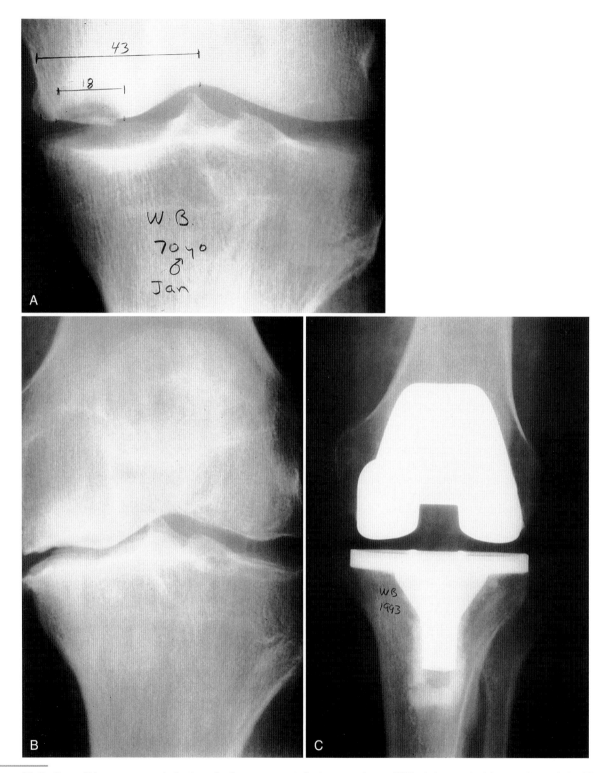

Figure 28–5. Stage IV osteonecrotic lesion. **A,** Osteonecrotic lesion involving 42% of the medial femoral condyle. There is only minimal collapse at this time. **B,** Ten years later, severe osteoarthritis has developed. The saddle-shaped configuration of the osteoarthritic process indicates that this was initially an osteonecrotic lesion with progressive collapse into the medial femoral condyle and tibial plateau. **C,** Total knee replacement for severe secondary degenerative changes.

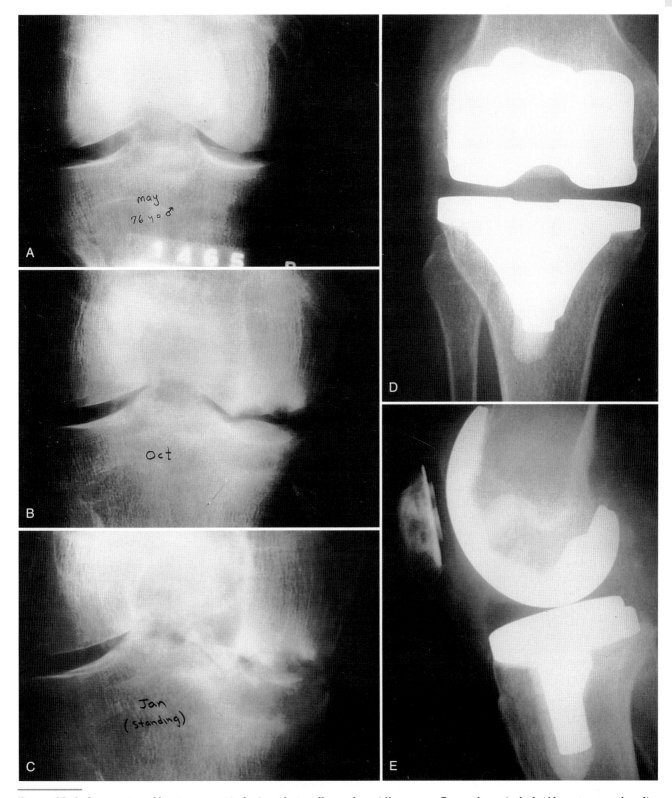

Figure 28–6. Large stage V osteonecrotic lesion that collapsed rapidly over a 7-month period. **A,** Almost normal radiograph, 1 month after the onset of symptoms. **B,** Six months after the onset of symptoms, the entire medial femoral condyle has collapsed. **C,** Eight months after the onset of symptoms, the entire joint, including the tibial side, has collapsed into varus deformity with severe destruction. **D** and **E,** Total knee replacement as the treatment of choice for a severe collapsing osteonecrotic lesion.

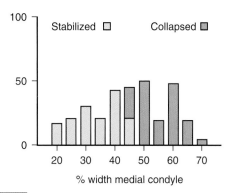

Figure 28–7. The prognosis depends on the size of the lesion as determined by the percentage of the width of the medial femoral condyle that has collapsed from osteonecrosis. Smaller lesions have a better prognosis.

signal that is thought to be caused by edema surrounding the lesion (see Fig. 28–3). In spontaneous osteonecrosis, the lesions are localized to the subchondral regions of the involved condyle or plateau. In the case of secondary osteonecrosis, either or both the medial and lateral femoral condyles or hemiplateaus may be involved, as well as the metaphyseal zones of bone (Fig. 28–8).

MRI is the most common method for recognizing focal tibial osteonecrosis and allows patients to be divided into four distinct types.[54] These types appear to be part of a spectrum of tibial subchondral changes that are associated with this syndrome of sudden onset of pain on the medial side of the knee. The initial symptoms are similar in all patients, and only MRI distinguishes the types.

Type A changes are relatively small, well-localized, low-signal areas in the subchondral zone, best seen on spin-echo T1-weighted images (Fig. 28–9).

Type B changes are low-signal areas also occurring in subchondral bone, but they diffuse down into the tibial metaphysis below the epiphyseal line (Fig. 28–10). They are less focal with a more diffuse area of signal change and are best appreciated on spin-echo TI- and T2-weighted images, as well as fat suppression images.

Type C changes are well-localized changes in subchondral bone in addition to widespread change in the metaphysis. Furthermore, there is a well-marginated low-signal area surrounded by a well-defined serpiginous rim of low signal representing reactive bone circumscribing the lesion in the subchondral collapse that is not visible on standard radiographs. This type C pattern and its serpiginous line are classically associated with osteonecrosis.

Type D is an extension of the type C pattern. The subchondral collapse is large enough to create secondary changes in bone and is therefore able to be seen on standard radiographs (Fig. 28–11).

The MRI classification can be correlated with the prognosis for an individual lesion. Type A and type B lesions, without clearly defined osteonecrotic central segments, generally do well, although patients may have symptoms for 9 to 12 months. The pain is initially acute but then resolves gradually over a long period.

At the end of the year, with conservative management, the symptoms will be minimal and the MRI lesions will also resolve. Only a small subchondral reaction will

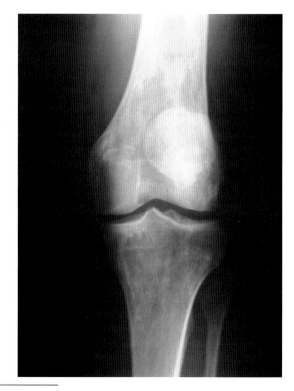

Figure 28–8. Steroid-induced osteonecrosis with diffuse involvement of the condyles and femoral metaphysis. MRI confirmed the diagnosis of osteonecrosis (refer to Figure 28–22).

remain to indicate the original lesion. These symptoms and MRI findings are commonly seen in elderly patients and those who have early degenerative joint disease. The symptoms may recur intermittently, but they are related to the associated arthritis. With time, the arthritis progresses, and the patient has symptoms typical of advancing degenerative arthritis.

Type C lesions also have normal radiographs, but MRI shows the serpiginous low-signal line typically associated with bone necrosis. These patients have a poorer prognosis. At a 2- to 10-year follow-up of patients with this problem, 66% with type C MRI scans had symptoms severe enough to require additional surgery,[54] as compared with only 20% of patients with type A and type B lesions.

Type D changes are marked by plain radiographic evidence of necrosis in addition to MRI changes showing collapse of subchondral bone, a serpiginous lucent line, and metaphyseal involvement (Fig. 28–12). These patients have the worst prognosis. In one report,[26] 84% of patients eventually underwent either total knee or unicompartmental arthroplasty.

The size and depth of the MRI changes noted at the metaphysical area did not appear to offer prognostic information.[54] However, it seems that involvement of the subchondral plate and the size of the subchondral lesion, similar to that seen in osteonecrosis of the femoral condyle, may be more important factors in the ultimate destruction of the joint.

Fat suppression images, which normally have low signal in the marrow, dramatically show high-intensity signal that may extend well into the condylar area (Fig. 28–13).

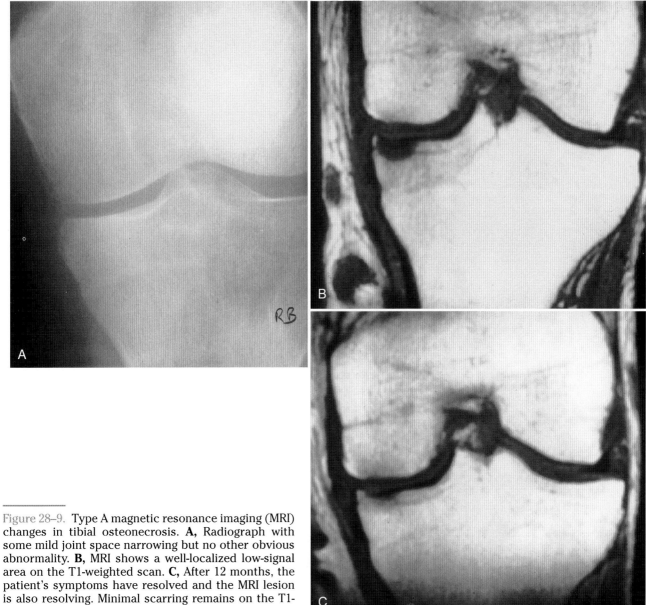

Figure 28–9. Type A magnetic resonance imaging (MRI) changes in tibial osteonecrosis. **A,** Radiograph with some mild joint space narrowing but no other obvious abnormality. **B,** MRI shows a well-localized low-signal area on the T1-weighted scan. **C,** After 12 months, the patient's symptoms have resolved and the MRI lesion is also resolving. Minimal scarring remains on the T1-weighted scan.

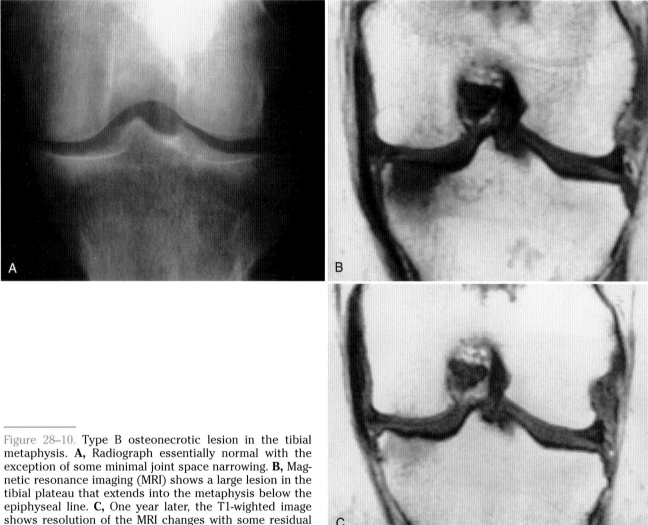

Figure 28–10. Type B osteonecrotic lesion in the tibial metaphysis. **A,** Radiograph essentially normal with the exception of some minimal joint space narrowing. **B,** Magnetic resonance imaging (MRI) shows a large lesion in the tibial plateau that extends into the metaphysis below the epiphyseal line. **C,** One year later, the T1-wighted image shows resolution of the MRI changes with some residual subchondral scarring remaining.

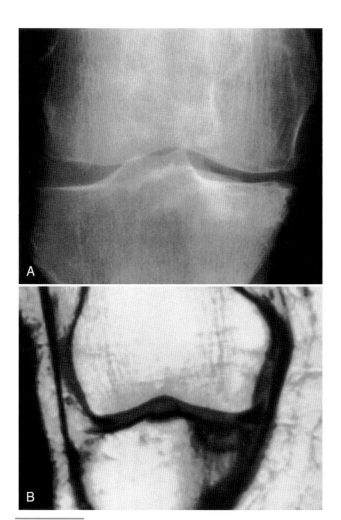

Figure 28–11. Type D tibial osteonecrotic lesion with x-ray evidence of tibial metaphyseal involvement. **A,** Plain radiograph showing an irregular, patchy, sclerotic zone within the subchondral area of the medial tibial metaphysis. **B,** Magnetic resonance imaging showing a typical osteonecrotic lesion with a serpiginous low-signal rim defining the osteonecrotic zone. This lesion will progress to collapse.

The aforementioned MRI changes in patients with osteonecrosis may not be apparent for a variable period from the onset of symptoms. Pollack et al[72] found 10 knees with classic symptoms of osteonecrosis and confirmed with a radionuclide bone scan that 2 knees initially had no evidence of osteonecrosis on MRI. They theorized that the initial small lesion might have been missed because of the thickness of the MRI section. Alternatively, processes other than osteonecrosis might have caused the positive scans. Nakamura et al,[67] using a canine model in the laboratory, noted a delay in histological and MRI changes after surgically induced avascular necrosis in the hip. They found that minimal histological changes could be seen as early as 3 days but that MRI changes did not appear until fibrous tissue developed an interface with normal bone. At 2 weeks, four of seven animals showed MRI changes, but it was not until 4 weeks that all animals demonstrated both histological and MRI evidence of necrosis.

There are several reports of knees with initial MRI examinations negative for osteonecrosis that underwent arthroscopy and then had the typical osteonecrosis lesion eventually develop.[16,66] Brahme et al[16] reported seven cases in which knees that had no evidence of osteonecrosis on the initial MRI scan were treated by arthroscopic partial meniscectomy. Repeat MRI performed because of persistent or recurrent pain showed an area of low signal intensity on a T1-weighted image. None of the patients had undergone radionuclide studies before the arthroscopy. The authors theorized that the diminished bearing capacity of the injured meniscus resulted in microfracture or vascular insufficiency in the contiguous condyle. They did not consider the possibility that the MRI study may have been normal in very early osteonecrosis and that the meniscal tear as seen on MRI may not have been the cause of the initial symptoms.

This alternative hypothesis is suggested by the findings of Bjorkengren et al[15] in a study of 16 patients with spontaneous osteonecrosis and a positive radionuclide study. Two patients had normal T1-weighted images. The MRI studies showed buckling of articular cartilage over the lesion in 12 patients and a tear over the medial meniscus in 9 patients. Four of the knees appeared normal on T2-weighted images, which the authors related to a favorable clinical outcome. The presence of bone marrow edema, without evolving to osteonecrosis, is a finding that is not commonly appreciated. Patients have a classic history of osteonecrosis and MRI findings of edema in subchondral bone. There is no collapse and no evidence of necrosis. Eventually, the symptoms decrease, the marrow edema resolves, and patients return to their baseline activities. This situation is frequently associated with early degenerative joint disease. The significance of the observation is undetermined; however, it should be appreciated or it may lead to unnecessary meniscal surgery.[70,71]

Gadolinium-enhanced MRI may provide useful adjunctive information regarding osseous turnover and activity. Enhanced activity may provide useful prognostic information by suggesting that the lesion may heal; in contrast, lesions without activity may have a poorer prognosis in terms of healing potential.

CLINICAL COURSE

The clinical course of osteonecrosis appears to depend on the size of the lesion. All patients initially have a similar history and examination. The pain will be very intense at first and gradually begin to resolve. Very intense pain may persist for up to 6 weeks. It is not possible to prognosticate at the very onset of symptoms because radiograph and MRI may be negative. Patients suffering from secondary osteonecrosis may often have insidious, but progressive periarticular knee pain. Occasionally, when necrosis has occurred in the metadiaphyseal region of the bone, juxtaarticular pain may be present.

With time, patients can be grouped into those with a poor or those with a satisfactory prognosis. Patients with a satisfactory prognosis usually begin to have diminished symptoms after 6 weeks, with persistence of mild pain for

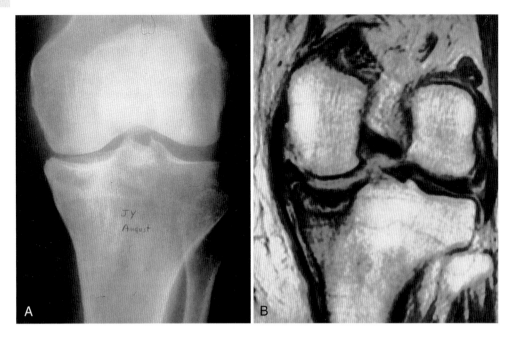

Figure 28–12. Osteonecrotic defect in the tibial metaphysis with collapse. **A,** Plain radiograph showing evidence of sclerosis and radiolucency in the tibial metaphysis; the femoral condyle has not become involved at this point. There is joint space narrowing and early collapse. **B,** Magnetic resonance imaging (MRI) scan showing the zone of collapse and necrosis. There is a serpiginous, low signal intensity area surrounding the necrotic zone on the T1-weighted MRI scan.

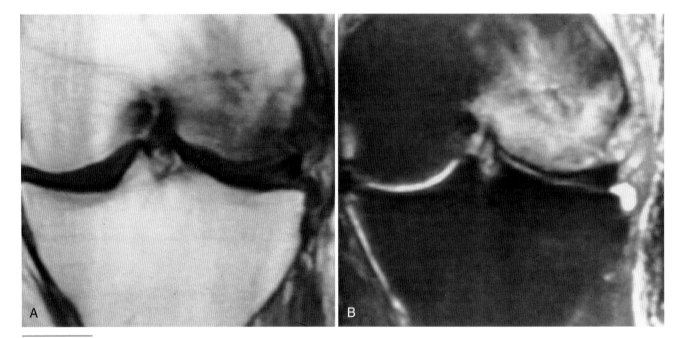

Figure 28–13. Fat suppression T2-weighted images. **A,** T1-weighted image showing only moderate involvement of the condyle with low signal intensity scattered into the femoral condyle. **B,** Effectiveness of fat suppression magnetic resonance images in highlighting the area of involvement in the medial femoral condyle.

12 to 15 months. Either a radiographic lesion will never develop in these patients or they will have small lesions less than 40% of their condylar width. In time, osteoarthritis will develop in most knees with osteonecrosis. The rate of development of the osteoarthritic changes varies with the size of the lesion. Insall et at[35] found that at 2 years almost all patients will have at least grade I osteoarthritis with joint space narrowing (Fig. 28–14).

Patients with a poor prognosis have lesions greater than 50% of their femoral condylar width. These patients never

experience relief of their symptoms and have progressive, unremitting symptoms that never seem to improve. They rapidly progress through stages III, IV, and V with destruction of their knees, sometimes as quickly as within 1 year. In the case of tibial osteonecrosis, the clinical course parallels the radiographic progression. Of patients whose initial radiographs are normal or show only minimal degenerative changes without a collapsing lesion, most will generally do well and gradually become asymptomatic. Later, symptoms related to the associated arthritis

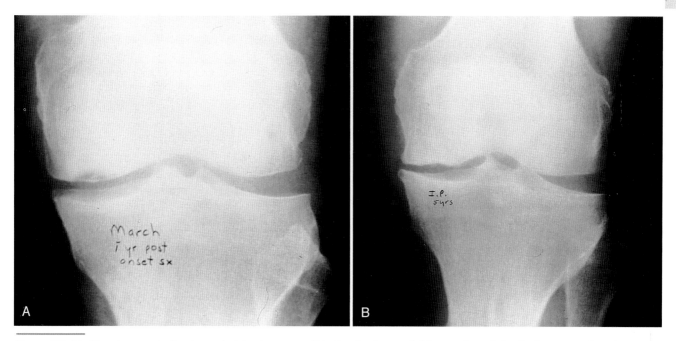

Figure 28–14. Development of osteoarthritis after a small lesion in the medial femoral condyle. **A,** One year after the onset of symptoms, the pain is resolved, but minimal early degenerative changes and joint space narrowing are noted. **B,** Five years later, there is progression of the osteoarthritis with joint space narrowing and increased proliferative changes.

may develop. On the other hand, if collapse is seen on MRI in type C lesions or if the radiographic changes of type D lesions become apparent, the prognosis is much poorer and the patient's initial pain never resolves. Many patients have progressive degenerative changes and require arthroplasty.

It is undetermined whether treatment intervention will alter the prognosis. However, Mont et al[62] suggested that core decompression might improve the prognosis in patients with corticosteroid-induced osteonecrosis. Whether their data would be applicable to spontaneous osteonecrosis is still undetermined but is an attractive option.

PATHOLOGY

Osteonecrosis indicates death of the segment of the weightbearing portion of the condyle with associated subchondral fracture and collapse. Total knee replacement and arthroscopy have allowed physicians to correlate the imaging stage with the macroscopic and histological findings.[4] The histopathology of the lesions of secondary osteonecrosis is identical to that observed with spontaneous osteonecrosis of the knee, but they tend to be more diffuse than in spontaneous osteonecrosis. In the early stages of osteonecrosis, one finds an area of slight flattening or discoloration in the articular cartilage. This is over an area of the condyle and is the size of a Ping-Pong ball indentation. At the edge of the lesion, one might find an irregular line of demarcation on the surface with a ridge of cartilage of altered color.

In later stages, the demarcation can become more pronounced. Gradually, the flap becomes evident. The fragment of cartilage with a thin layer of subchondral bone can easily be freed from its base with forceps. It is usually hinged on a normal cartilage segment (Fig. 28–15). The shape of the lesion is oval with a longer sagittal diameter. In advanced cases, only remnants of the fragments remain and the degenerative process involves the entire compartment. A crater can be found covered by a material varying from dead detritus to regrown fiber cartilage.

In sagittal sections of the distal end of the femur removed for total knee replacement, one can see a cartilage layer of normal thickness and color without any gross fibrillation or fissuring. Just below is a thin layer of whitish yellow necrotic subchondral bone, sometimes in a fragmented state. Proceeding into the depth of the condyle, one encounters a clear, empty space corresponding to the subchondral fracture that has begun at the margins and propagated parallel to the surface. In the bed of the crater above the fractured cleft, one can see necrotic detritus and necrotic trabeculae. The bone around this necrotic area acquires normal growth characteristics with signs of intense perifocal reparative reaction and sometimes sclerosis. In more advanced cases in which degenerative changes have already begun, it might be difficult to find a pathology section of a typical necrotic lesion. Sometimes only after close scrutiny can the pathologist find the remnants of the worn-down crater and fragment. Many believe that osteonecrosis of the knee, like that of the hip, is an important and underestimated cause of osteoarthritis.

In the early stages, the articular cartilage is not only viable histologically but also appears normal or almost normal. The chondrocytes are grouped normally with

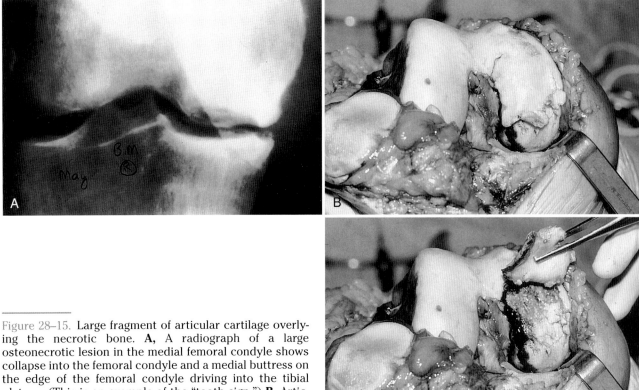

Figure 28–15. Large fragment of articular cartilage overlying the necrotic bone. **A,** A radiograph of a large osteonecrotic lesion in the medial femoral condyle shows collapse into the femoral condyle and a medial buttress on the edge of the femoral condyle driving into the tibial plateau. (This is an example of the "tooth sign.") **B,** Articular cartilage in place, held on an intact hinge. **C,** Raising the cartilage flap on its hinge reveals a bed of necrotic bone.

normal staining matrix around them. Later, if the process has progressed for a while, there might be cloning of the chondrocytes and early fibrillation or erosion in the tidemark layer, which might become wavy and thicker. The subchondral bone has the typical characteristics of necrosis; that is, the marrow exhibits cell lysis, destruction of fat cells, blood vessels in the stroma, and osteolytic lacunae into the trabecular area or has pyknotic nuclei. The marrow in more advanced cases has a typical dusty or smoky appearance.

Signs of reaction are absent. At the base of the crater, in the more superficial layers, one can find some necrotic trabeculae and intense fibrovascular granulation tissue with histiocytes and osteoclasts reabsorbing the necrotic tissue. Islands of fibrocartilage can also be seen. The appearance is very similar to that of fractured callus. Proceeding toward the depth of the condyle, the perifocal reaction gradually shifts toward new bone formation, and one can observe the deposition of new, immature bone around dead trabeculae or thickening of trabeculae and sclerosis. This type of reparative reaction can be very deep in the condyle.

ETIOLOGY

The very term "spontaneous idiopathic osteonecrosis" indicates that the cause of this condition is still unknown.

Two main theories can be identified: the vascular theory and the traumatic theory. Osteonecrosis of the knee has yet to be experimentally reproduced; therefore, etiological hypotheses are borrowed by analogy from those of osteonecrosis of the hip.

The vascular theory remains dominant in osteonecrosis of the hip.[39] Seventy-four percent of patients with avascular necrosis of the hip have been shown to have some underlying coagulopathy or thrombophilia. Glueck et al[31] noted that most cases of osteonecrosis were associated with a coagulation disorder such as hypofibringolysis or thrombophilia, including resistance to activated protein C, low protein C, and low stimulated tissue plasminogen activator activity. They speculated that these coagulopathies cause thrombotic venous occlusion in the head of the femur and consequently lead to venous hypertension and hypoxic death of bone.

Others have proposed that osteonecrosis of the knee may be secondary to some form of trauma.[49] The traumatic theory takes into account that most patients are elderly women in whom osteoporosis is common and therefore minor trauma might cause a microfracture in the weakened subchondral bone. Once the subchondral plate has been violated, fluid may enter the marrow space and thereby increase pressure and cause ischemia and pain (Fig. 28–16). Unfortunately, no confirmatory histological evidence is available to support either of these theories.

The specific cause of secondary osteonecrosis is also not entirely understood, but like spontaneous osteonecrosis,

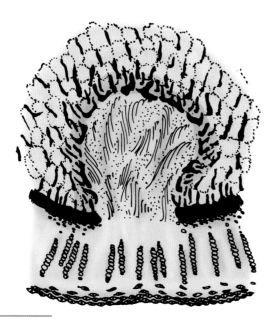

Figure 28–16. With collapse of the subchondral plate, fluid from articular cartilage can be pushed into the subchondral zone and create increased pressure and pain and a reactive sclerotic bone halo.

vascular and traumatic theories have been proposed to explain the initiation and evolution of this process. In the case of corticosteroid use, there may be an increase in the size and volume of fat cells within the bone marrow, and these cells may in turn impede circulation, increase intraosseous pressure, and ultimately cause intraosseous ischemia. Heritable coagulopathies that predispose to thrombophilia or hypofibrinolysis may contribute to the formation of local emboli that can result in bone death.[31]

LABORATORY STUDIES

There are no specific abnormal laboratory findings, with the possible exception of the coagulation abnormalities just mentioned, that can help predict whether a patient is at risk for the development of osteonecrosis or that can be useful objective measures for monitoring the course of the disease or response to treatment of spontaneous or secondary osteonecrosis of the knee.

DIFFERENTIAL DIAGNOSIS

Osteochondritis Dissecans

Historically, the diagnoses of spontaneous osteonecrosis and osteochondritis dissecans have been related since the early descriptions were interpreted as chondritis or osteochondritis of the elderly.[10,22,75,78] However, several differences between these conditions appear to make them separate entities.

The localization of osteochondritis dissecans lesions differs from that of osteonecrosis. In most cases, osteochondritis dissecans lesions are situated on the lateral aspect of the medial femoral condyle toward the inner condylar notch. Sometimes the area extends toward the weightbearing portion of the condyle, but in two-thirds to three-fourths of cases the lesions are located near the notch.[45,84]

The predilection of age and gender is also different. Osteochondritis dissecans occurs in a juvenile or a young adult. It may develop between the ages of 10 and 50 years, but the peak incidence occurs between the ages of 10 and 20 years. Males are involved three times more frequently than females.[5,6]

Less than half the patients with osteochondritis dissecans give a history of trauma followed by an insidious or gradual onset of symptoms; acute onset is rare.[45,84] Radiologically, other than differences in location, there is often collapse of the osteonecrotic regions that are subjected to weightbearing force, whereas osteochondritis dissecans lesions rarely collapse. Because of its location it is mainly subjected to tangential force, which gives rise to the repetitive microtrauma theory of etiology. The development of osteoarthritis is a very frequent and often rapid consequence of osteonecrosis, whereas it is a rare complication in juvenile osteochondritis and a very slow and progressive one in the adult forms[45,46]; loose body formation frequently occurs in osteochondritis and is rare in osteonecrosis.

Bone marrow pressure studies in the condyles of patients with osteochondritis are infrequently altered and may indicate the localized nature of osteochondritis as compared with osteonecrosis,[10,11] which has been shown to be associated with increased intraosseous pressure. Histologically in osteochondritis dissecans, a fragment of bone that is separated does not show signs of necrosis unless it has been completely detached.[18] There is a clear-cut fibrocartilage layer retaining the fragment underlying the bone of the crater, with signs of attempt at repair by osteochondral ossification toward the ossific nucleus. The perifocal sclerotic reaction is narrow and does not deepen into the condyle.

Meniscal Tears

One must be careful when interpreting a degenerative meniscal tear as the cause of symptoms because degenerative tears of the medial meniscus are found with great frequency in the age groups under discussion.[68,69] Most tears must be noted. Because MRI is so sensitive, any intrasubstance degeneration will be manifested as a signal change within the meniscus, which frequently leads the orthopedist to consider arthroscopic débridement. This is a particular problem if MRI scans are obtained soon after the onset of symptoms and subchondral MRI changes have not had the chance to develop. The issue of whether degenerative changes or complex tears in the posterior corner of the meniscus are symptomatic and can be improved by removal or débridement is yet to be fully resolved.

Pes Anserinus Bursitis

Pes anserinus bursitis is believed to be a source of pain in the medial aspect of the knee[63]; however, with the development of MRI and the ability to visualize this area, bursitis or a fluid-filled bursa is only rarely noted. More commonly, the symptoms in the area of the pes anserinus bursa are related to underlying tibial osteonecrosis.

Insufficiency Fractures

Older osteopenic women may sustain a stress fracture on the medial side of the tibial metaphysis (Fig. 28–17). The typical location is just below the flare of the medial tibial plateau. By noting the location of the tenderness, a good examination should be able to suggest the diagnosis. However, the pain may initially be diffuse and radiographs will be negative for the first 7 to 10 days. Therefore, this diagnosis may be overlooked. Later, the typical fluffy new bone formation associated with a healing fracture will be apparent and help establish this diagnosis, but a follow-up radiograph and a good index of suspicion are required.

TREATMENT

Several treatment options are available.[50,80] Recognition of the entity is, of course, fundamental to instituting appro-

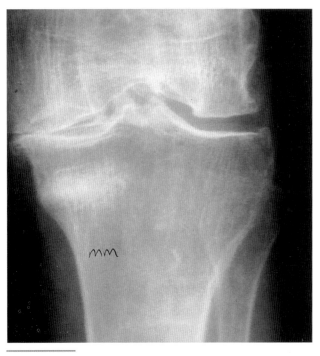

Figure 28–17. Healing insufficiency fracture on the medial side of the knee. Initially, the area was painful and tender; gradually, the symptoms resolved, and the radiograph shows new bone formation associated with healing of the stress fracture.

priate treatment. Even when MRI shows a degenerative meniscal tear and no marrow changes and even if the clinical indications are severe enough, defer surgery and re-evaluate in 6 weeks. A radionuclide bone scan may even be considered before proceeding with arthroscopic intervention. This is particularly important if the MRI scan was obtained within the first 6 weeks of the onset of symptoms because MRI changes may develop weeks after symptom onset.[67]

It should be noted that except for conservative treatment of small lesions and total knee replacement for large lesions, the efficacy of the intermediate procedures—numbers 2, 3, and 4 in the following list—has not been well documented, monitored, or stratified for the size of the lesion. Options include the following:
1. Conservative treatment
2. Core decompression of the distal end of the femur
3. Arthroscopic débridement
4. Proximal tibial osteotomy
5. Total knee replacement or unicompartmental arthroplasty

Conservative Treatment

Conservative treatment consists of protected weightbearing and analgesics or anti-inflammatory medications as needed, with performance of activities to tolerance. As the acute symptoms start to resolve, patients begin to return to a normal lifestyle. Excellent to good results can be obtained with these measures if the lesion is relatively small (i.e., less than 40% of the width of the condyle).[8,49,64,74] Over time, depending on the size of the lesion, degenerative changes begin to develop.[35] Patients whose condition resolves with these measures will continue to function very well with limited symptoms and slow progression of arthritis.[71] In the case of tibial osteonecrosis, conservative treatment should be tried first, especially for type A and type B lesions,[48] which almost universally improve, although it takes a long time (see Fig. 28–15). If the patients are very symptomatic and there appears to be a well-localized lesion, particularly on fat suppression views, extra-articular decompression may be considered for relief of pain. Unlike spontaneous osteonecrosis of the knee, secondary osteonecrosis tends to not respond well to nonoperative intervention. For instance, one study found only a 23% success rate in patients with steroid-induced osteonecrosis treated by nonoperative intervention at a mean 6-year follow-up as compared with a 74% success rate in patients treated by core decompression.[62]

Core Decompression

The concept of releasing intraosseous pressure to prevent further necrosis in the bone is an extension of the experience that some authors have had with decompression of the femoral head for the early stages of osteonecrosis in the hip (Fig. 28–18). The use of core decompression in

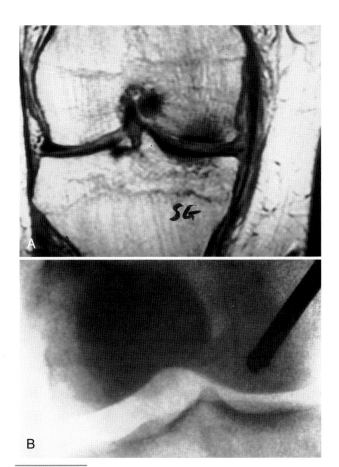

Figure 28–18. Small stage II osteonecrotic lesion of the femoral condyle treated by core decompression. **A,** T1-weighted image showing the relatively focal area of involvement in the medial femoral condyle. This is associated with intense pain. **B,** A trocar in place intraoperatively is decompressing the femoral condyle, with relief of acute symptoms.

the distal end of the femur was first reported by Jacobs et al.[37] They performed distal femoral core decompression and pathologically confirmed avascular necrosis in 28 knees. They treated seven stage I and II lesions, all with good results. Approximately half the stage III lesions had a good result after decompression. More recently, Forst et al[28,29] reported on 16 patients with an average age of 64 years who had spontaneous osteonecrosis of the femoral condyle verified by MRI. Fifteen lesions were stage I, with only one knee having radiological signs of stage II consisting of flattening of the femoral condyle. All patients were treated by surgical extra-articular drilling into the affected femoral condyle to achieve core decompression. The knee pain disappeared immediately after surgery in all patients. Successful healing was confirmed by normalization of the bone marrow signal on MRI at a 3-year follow-up. The authors recommended that core decompression by extra-articular drilling into the femoral condyle be considered as an effective treatment of osteonecrosis of the knee. If some flattening of the affected condyle was already apparent, progression of the disease could not always be avoided. Without a control group, it is not possible to know how these patients would have

done without core decompression because successful outcomes have been reported only for patients in stage I with MRI changes but without structural collapse.

In tibial osteonecrosis, type C and type D lesions in which there is definite evidence of osteonecrosis as shown by the low-signal serpiginous line extending into subchondral zone with or without collapse, treatment would depend on the time of recognition. If the lesion is still new with no collapse and the symptoms are intense, core decompression may be considered (Fig. 28–19). There are no hard data on the benefits of decompression of tibial lesions. If the lesion has already collapsed into the subchondral zone, the prognosis is generally much poorer. Most of these patients will eventually need either a unicompartmental or total knee arthroplasty. The choice between unicompartmental or total knee replacement depends on the status of the rest of the joint and the surgeon's preference.

Core decompression has also been considered for steroid-induced osteonecrosis. This is a different entity with a different anatomic location in the femoral condyle and does not necessarily involve the subchondral plate. It may have different mechanical ramifications. Mont et al[62] reviewed their experience with 79 knees that had steroid-induced osteonecrosis of the distal end of the femur, 47 of which underwent core decompression. They noted that a matched non–core decompression group had 23% survivorship of the knee without an arthroplasty whereas 74% of the knees in the core decompression group did well. At a mean follow-up of 11 years (range, 4 to 16 years), 17 of 47 knees (36%) treated by core decompression progressed radiographically, as opposed to 75% of knees treated nonoperatively.[62] They suggested that core decompression might slow the rate of symptomatic progression of steroid-induced avascular necrosis of the distal end of the femur.

At this time it appears that core decompression can relieve the initial acute pain that occurs with the onset of spontaneous osteonecrosis of the knee; however, it is still undetermined whether the disease process itself is altered or whether progression can be retarded or inhibited with early decompression.

Arthroscopic Débridement

In view of the intraosseous focus of the osteonecrotic lesion, it appears that arthroscopic débridement and chondroplasty will do little to alter the natural course and progression of this disease. Miller et al[58] reviewed a series of five patients with idiopathic osteonecrosis who underwent arthroscopic débridement and abrasion arthroplasty. A good postoperative result was reported in four of the five patients at an average follow-up of 31 months, but progression of the osteonecrosis was not halted.

Arthroscopy may be effective, however, in débriding unstable or delaminating chondral fragments, particularly in the setting of mechanical symptoms such as locking or catching. Retrograde drilling through overlying intact articular cartilage may theoretically stimulate revascularization of the osteonecrotic focus. It may be more advis-

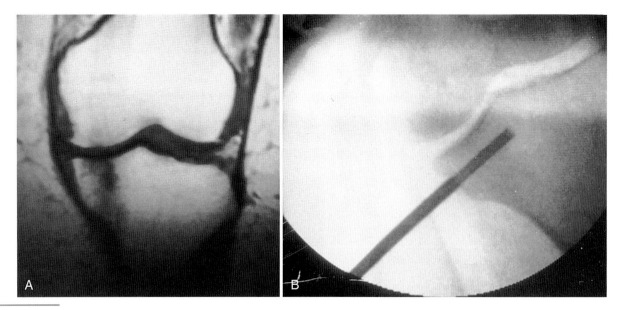

Figure 28–19. Tibial osteonecrosis with extreme pain treated by core decompression, with resolution of acute symptoms. Mild symptoms persist for many months. **A,** Midsized osteonecrotic defect involving the tibial metaphysis with a type B lesion. The low-signal area extends into tibial metaphysis below the epiphyseal line. **B,** Intraoperative image of core decompression with a trocar in the tibial metaphysis.

able to drill in an antegrade fashion because retrograde drilling risks traumatizing the articular cartilage. Arthroscopic débridement has been used to diagnose the osteonecrosis and to remove the fragments of articular cartilage. The results of these interventions are not well defined or controlled.[42]

In a few reports, osteonecrosis has been noted after arthroscopic treatment of meniscal or degenerative lesions.[16,76] Whether these lesions are new or were initially overlooked is still undetermined.

Osteochondral Allografts

There have been scattered reports and literature regarding the use of osteochondral allografts for osteonecrosis of the femoral condyle.[13,19,23,55,58,59] Fresh osteochondral allograft is conceived as an interim response to a localized loss of articular cartilage that has no other reasonable alternative after conservative procedures have failed.

Fresh osteochondral allografts have been successful in the treatment of post-traumatic defects of the knee. However, little has been written regarding the use of these grafts for the treatment of osteonecrosis. Bayne et al[13] reported on six knees requiring bipolar allografts (i.e., mating femoral condylar and tibial plateau grafts) for stage IV spontaneous osteonecrosis. The average age was 67 years. Five of the six patients had unsatisfactory results with early graft subsidence or fragmentation. The authors also reviewed three patients with steroid-induced osteonecrosis. Each had unsatisfactory results. Overall, the results were superior in patients who underwent treatment for post-traumatic injuries, with 76% successful outcomes in the steroid-induced osteonecrosis group and

46% satisfactory results in the spontaneous osteonecrosis group.

Meyers et al[59] reported on 59 fresh osteochondral allograft transplants, 5 of which were transplanted for osteonecrosis of the medial femoral condyle. Only three patients were available beyond 2 years' follow-up. Each of them was considered to have an excellent clinical result. The authors made no mention of the size of the lesions treated; four were steroid related. Patient age in this subset of patients was not identified.

Flynn et al[27] reviewed a series of 17 fresh frozen osteoarticular allografts used to treat distal femoral osteonecrosis. Seven patients had received corticosteroids; the remainder of cases were post-traumatic or developed spontaneously. The average patient age was 29.6 years, and follow-up averaged 51 months with a minimum 2-year follow-up. Results were considered good or excellent in 12 cases. Interestingly, 75% of the patients with steroid-induced osteonecrosis had good or excellent results versus only 67% of the patients with trauma-induced or spontaneous osteonecrosis. A fair result was achieved in a patient with spontaneous osteonecrosis, although the authors stated that this patient was limited by disease in the contralateral, unoperated side.

Osteochondral allografting may be an option for young patients with localized osteonecrosis, particularly osteochondritis dissecans; however, in elderly patients with collapse of subchondral bone, more predictable results may probably be achieved with arthroplasty. It is possible that the success of osteochondral allografts may be enhanced by simultaneous unloading procedures such as proximal tibial or distal femoral osteotomies, if associated malalignment of the mechanical axis exists. Since the results of total knee arthroplasty are so good for the older age groups, fresh osteochondral allografts do not seem to be indicated for this population because of the technical difficulties and possible immunogenic responses.

Proximal Tibial Osteotomy

Proximal tibial osteotomy may be considered for younger, active patients with osteonecrosis of the medial femoral condyle and a mechanical axis that has shifted medially because of collapse of the medial compartment (Fig. 28–20). The procedure can often be performed without arthroscopy or arthrotomy, unless an osteochondral loose body or chondral delamination is present. Soucacos et al[81] described their approach to stage III and IV osteonecrosis in which there is irreversible destruction of the subchondral bone and cartilage of the medial femoral condyle. Although the authors did not specifically detail the results of treatment, they reported better results in stage III osteonecrosis when less than 50% of the condyle was involved and in patients who were younger than 65 years. Larger lesions and older patients tended to do better with unicompartmental arthroplasty.

Koshino[41] reported on 37 knees treated by proximal tibial osteotomy. Concomitant retrograde drilling or bone grafting behind the lesion was performed in 23 patients. At a minimum 2-year follow-up (average, 61 months), the results were best when the proximal tibial osteotomy was combined with core decompression or bone grafting and with overcorrection of the femorotibial axis to at least 10 degrees of valgus. The necrotic lesion was noted to disappear radiographically in 13 patients and was improved in 17 knees. The results of proximal tibial osteotomy for osteonecrosis tend to be comparable to those observed after proximal tibial osteotomy for primary osteoarthritis. In the series by Koshino, only one patient subsequently required prosthetic replacement in the follow-up reported.

Periarticular osteotomy has not fared well and should generally not be considered in patients with diffuse secondary osteonecrosis. Similarly, hemiresurfacing with unicompartmental arthroplasty makes little sense in the presence of diffuse osteonecrosis, particularly in patients with compromised osseous support.

Prosthetic Replacement

Osteonecrosis with debilitating symptoms after failure of conservative treatment or other surgical efforts may be successfully treated by prosthetic resurfacing arthroplasty. It may also be a reasonable first-line treatment in elderly patients who are significantly disabled by their symptoms. This is particularly true when subchondral bone support has been compromised with subsequent collapse of the articular surface.

Proponents of unicompartmental arthroplasty can argue effectively that there is a role for unicompartmental replacement in patients with spontaneous osteonecrosis involving one condyle or one tibial plateau, but it is not a prudent endeavor in those with secondary osteonecrosis in view of the diffuse extent of osseous involvement (Fig. 28–21). Marmor[57] reported 89% good or excellent results in 34 knees treated by unicompartmental arthroplasty. Two of the four failures reported occurred because of the subsequent development of symptomatic osteonecrosis of the untreated compartment. The two other failures occurred because of subsidence into compromised bone stock. In the setting of osteonecrosis, it is critical to consider the possibility of synchronous or subsequent osteonecrosis of the opposite compartment. Preoperative MRI should be performed to carefully assess the contralateral compartment of the knee when considering unicompartmental arthroplasty. Additionally, involvement of the epiphyseal or metaphyseal bone should be considered because compromised osseous support may predispose to subsidence and compromise long-term survivorship. Therefore, in secondary osteonecrosis, stem extensions may be of value to reduce the risk for component subsidence (Figs 28–22).

Total knee arthroplasty has reportedly produced good and excellent results in well over 94% of patients into the second postoperative decade. Careful review of the literature detailing the results of total knee arthroplasty for spontaneous osteonecrosis suggests that although satisfactory results are attainable, a good deal of guarded optimism may be appropriate when treating this condition.[82] Ritter et al[73] reported on 32 knees with spontaneous osteonecrosis of the medial femoral condyle. With Kaplan-Meier survival analysis, the authors, using the posterior cruciate condylar prosthesis, reported results inferior to those seen in a comparable group of patients with osteoarthrosis. With pain relief used as an endpoint, the

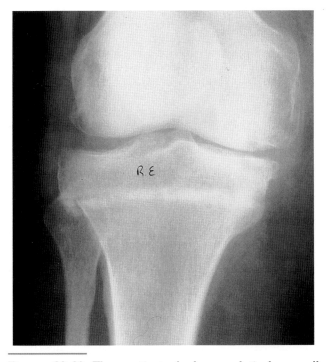

R E

Figure 28–20. The patient had a relatively small osteonecrotic defect in the medial femoral condyle that was treated by tibial osteotomy. This patient already has secondary degenerative arthritis and, in theory, will benefit from the osteotomy.

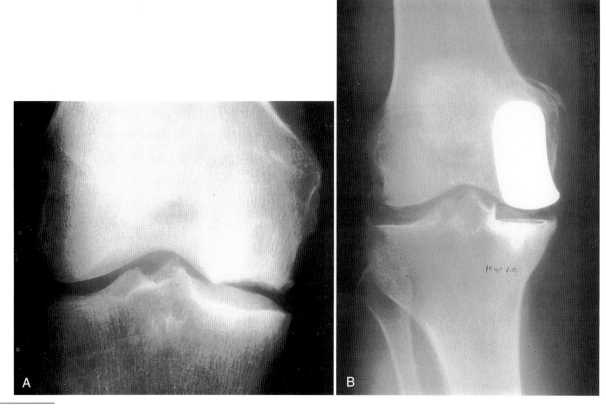

Figure 28–21. Treatment of a large osteonecrotic defect by unicompartmental arthroplasty. **A,** Large osteonecrotic defect in a 62-year-old man. Note that the lateral compartment is very well preserved. **B,** The patient continues to do well 10 years after the unicompartmental arthroplasty. There are some degenerative changes noted in the opposite compartment. The patient continued to do well at the latest follow-up of 18 years.

5-year postoperative success rate was 82% for osteonecrosis and 90% for osteoarthrosis. Although this difference was not statistically significant, the authors noted that small sample size prevented a significant difference between the two groups. At 7 years, 17% of the patients with osteonecrosis required revision as compared with 0% in the group with osteoarthrosis.

The results of total knee arthroplasty were equally concerning in a group of 36 patients with osteonecrosis of the femoral condyles reported by Bergman and Rand.[14] At a mean follow-up of 4 years, the authors reported good or excellent results in 87% of patients. Implant survivorship at 5 years was predicted to be 85% using an endpoint of revision arthroplasty but only 68% when moderate or severe pain was used as the criterion for failure. Although the authors did not find any clinical or radiographic evidence of loosening, it is possible that significant pain may result when subchondral or metaphyseal bone support is compromised by a focus of osteonecrosis.

In a series by Seldes and colleagues, 28 of 31 (90%) patients who underwent total knee arthroplasty had significant improvement in knee scores at a mean follow-up of 64 months when performed for secondary osteonecrosis of the knee; however, the results were inferior to those of comparable series of total knee arthroplasty performed for degenerative arthritis.[79] An additional series by Mont et al found that when total knee arthroplasty was performed in 31 knees for atraumatic osteonecrosis in patients younger than 50 years, only 55% had a good or excellent result.[61] In that series, 39% of knees were revised because of aseptic loosening at a mean follow-up of 8 years (range, 2 to 16 years), and 10% were revised because of deep infection. In their series, systemic lupus erythematosus was predictive of failure in 56% of cases. The authors surmised that there was generally poor-quality bone as a result of corticosteroid use and suggested enhanced fixation with cement and stem extensions.

SUMMARY

Osteonecrosis of the knee encompasses two distinct entities, and although the pathological appearance of involved bone is similar, spontaneous osteonecrosis differs enough from secondary osteonecrosis that they are typically easily distinguishable from each other. The characteristic ages at onset, associated risk factors, extent of bony involvement, and MRI appearance of the lesions differ between these two subsets of necrosis. The clinical course of these distinct entities and response to nonsurgical and surgical interventions also differ, thus making clinical distinction between the two that much more important. Although small lesions of focal osteonecrosis often resolve, its recognition may avoid unnecessary surgical intervention. There is a role for biological alternatives such as core decom-

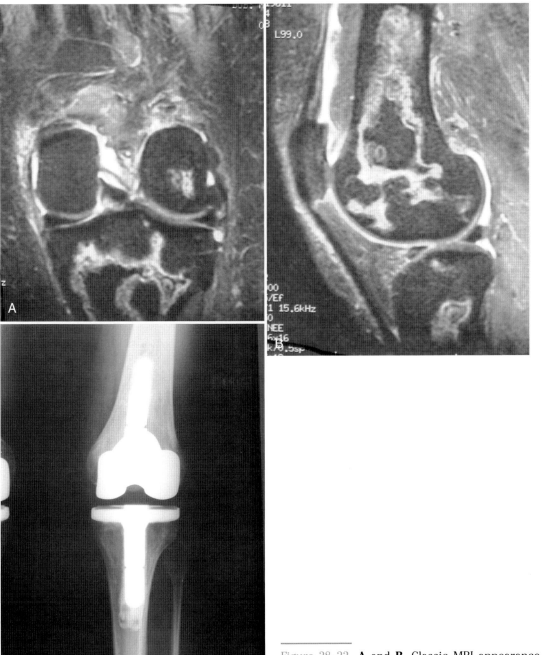

Figure 28–22. **A** and **B,** Classic MRI appearance of steroid-induced osteonecrosis. **C,** Total knee arthroplasty was performed with the use of short cemented stems to provide additional implant support.

pression; however, with progressive collapse and severe symptoms, prosthetic replacement may be necessary despite recognizing that the results of unicompartmental or total knee replacement for osteonecrosis tend to be inferior to those for degenerative arthritis.

References

1. Abeles M, Urman JD, Rothfield NF: Aseptic necrosis of bone in systemic lupus erythematosus. Relationship to corticosteroid therapy. Arch Intern Med 138:750, 1978.

2. Aglietti P, Insall J, Deschamps G, et al: The results of treatment of idiopathic osteonecrosis of the knee. J Bone Joint Surg Br 65:588, 1983.

3. Ahlback S, Bauer GCH, Bohne WH: Spontaneous osteonecrosis of the knee. Arthritis Rheum 11:705, 1968.

4. Ahuja SC, Bullough PG: Osteonecrosis of the knee. J Bone Joint Surg Am 60:191, 1978.

5. Aichroth P: Osteochondritis dissecans of the knee. A clinical survey. J Bone Joint Surg Br 53:440, 1971.

6. Aichroth P: Osteochondral fractures and the relationship to osteochondritis dissecans of the knee. J Bone Joint Surg Br 53:448, 1971.

7. Al-Rowaih A, Bjorkengren A, Egund N, et al: Size of osteonecrosis of the knee. Clin Orthop 287:68, 1993.

8. Al-Rowaih A, Lindstrand A, Bjorkengren A, et al: Osteonecrosis of the knee. Diagnosis and outcome in 40 patients. Acta Orthop Scand 62:19, 1991.

9. Al-Rowaih A, Wingstrand H, Lindstrand A, et al: Three phase scintimetry in osteonecrosis of the knee. Acta Orthop Scand 61:120, 1990.

10. Arlet P, Maziere B: Osteochondrite dissequante et osteonecros dela extremity inferior de femur. Sem Hap Pans 51:1907, 1975.

11. Arnoldi CC, Lemperg KR, Linderholm H: Intraosseous hypertension and pain in the knee. J Bone Joint Surg Br 57:360, 1975.

12. Bauer GCH: Osteonecrosis of the knee. Clin Orthop 130:210, 1978.

13. Bayne E, Lanner F, Pritzker KPH, et al: Osteochondral allografts in the treatment of ON of the knee. Orthop Clin North Am 16:727, 1985.

14. Bergman NR, Rand JA: Total knee arthroplasty in osteonecrosis. Clin Orthop 273:77, 1991.

15. Bjorkengren AG, Al-Rowaih A, Lindstrand A, et al: Spontaneous osteonecrosis of the knee: Value of MR imaging in determining prognosis. AJR Am J Roentgenol 154:331, 1990.

16. Brahme SK, Fox JM, Ferkel RD, et al: Osteonecrosis of the knee after arthroscopic surgery: Diagnosis with MR imaging. Radiology 178:851, 1991.

17. Braverman DL, Lachmann EA, Nagler W: Avascular necrosis of bilateral knees secondary to corticosteroid enemas. Arch Phys Med Rehabil 79:49, 1998.

18. Chiroff RT, Cooke CP: Osteochondritis dissecans: A histologic and microradiographic analysis of surgically excised lesions. J Trauma 15:689, 1975.

19. Convery FR, Meyers MH, Akeson WH: Fresh osteochondral allografting of the femoral condyle. Clin Orthop 273:139, 1991.

20. D'Anglejean G, Ryckewaert A, Glimet A: Osteonecrose du plateau tibial intern. Extr Rheum 8:253, 1976.

21. Daumont A, Deplante JP, Bouvier M, et al: L'ostenecrose des condyles femoraux chez l'adulte: A propos de 30 cas personnels. Rev Rhum Mal Osteoartic 43:27, 1976.

22. Defino C, Turrini P: Contributo allo studio della condrite dissecante dell'eta senile. Arch 1st Osp Santa Corona 31:516, 1966.

23. De la Caffiniere JY: La translocation osteocartilagineuse autogene dans les necroses condyliennes du genou chez le viellard. Rev Chir Orthop 64:653, 1980.

24. Dupare J, Alnot JY: Osteonecrose primitive du condyle femoral interne du sujet age. Rev Chir Orthop 55:615, 1969.

25. Ecker MI, Lotke PA: Spontaneous osteonecrosis of the knee. J Am Acad Orthop Surg 2:173, 1994.

26. Ecker MI, Lotke PA: Osteonecrosis of the medial part of the tibial plateau. J Bone Joint Surg Am 77:596, 1995.

27. Flynn JM, Springfield DS, Mankin HJ: Osteoarticular allografts to treat distal femoral osteonecrosis. Clin Orthop 303:38, 1994.

28. Forst J, Forst R, Heller KD, et al: Core decompression in Ahlback's disease: Follow-up and therapy control using MR tomography. Rofo Fortschr Geb Rontgenstr Neuen Bildgeb Verfahr 161:142, 1994.

29. Forst J, Forst R, Heller KD, et al: Spontaneous osteonecrosis of the femoral condyle: Causal treatment by early core decompression. Arch Orthop Trauma Surg 117:18, 1998.

30. Garino JP, Lotke PA, Sapega AA, et al: Osteonecrosis of the knee following laser-assisted arthroscopic surgery: A report of six cases. Arthroscopy 11:467, 1995.

31. Glueck CJ, Freilberg R, Tracy T, et al: Thrombophilia and hypofibrinolysis. Pathophysiologies of osteonecrosis. Clin Orthop 334:43, 1997.

32. Healy WL: Osteonecrosis of the knee detected only by magnetic resonance imaging. Orthopedics 14:703, 1991.

33. Houpt JB, Alpert B, Lotem M, et al: Spontaneous osteonecrosis of the medial tibial plateau. J Rheumatol 9:81, 1982.

34. Hungerford DS, Zizic TM: Alcoholism associated ischemic necrosis of the femoral head. Early diagnosis and treatment. Clin Orthop 130:144, 1978.

35. Insall JN, Aglietti P, Bullough PG, et al: Osteonecrosis. In Insall JN, Scott WN (eds): Surgery of the Knee, 2nd ed. New York, Churchill Livingstone, 1993, pp 609-633.

36. Isono SS, Woolson ST, Schurman DJ: Total joint arthroplasty for steroid-induced osteonecrosis in cardiac transplant patients. Clin Orthop 217:201, 1987.

37. Jacobs MA, Leob PE, Hungerford DS: Core decompression of the distal femur for avascular necrosis of the knee. J Bone Joint Surg Br 71:583, 1989.

38. Janzen DL, Kosarek FJ, Helms CA, et al: Osteonecrosis after contact neodymium:yttrium aluminum garnet arthroscopic laser meniscectomy. AJR Am J Roentgenol 169:855-858, 1997.

39. Jones JP: Risk factors potentially activating intravascular coagulation and causing nontraumatic osteonecrosis. In Urbaniak JR, Jones JP (eds): Osteonecrosis—Etiology, Diagnosis, and Treatment. Chicago, American Academy of Orthopaedic Surgeons, 1997, p 89.

40. Kelman GJ, William GW, Colwell CW Jr, et al: Steroid-related osteonecrosis of the knee. Two case reports and a literature review. Clin Orthop 257:171, 1990.

41. Koshino T: The treatment of spontaneous osteonecrosis of the knee by high tibial osteotomy with and without bone-grafting or drilling of the lesion. J Bone Joint Surg Am 64:47, 1982.

42. Koshino T, Okamoto R, Takamura K, et al: Arthroscopy in spontaneous osteonecrosis of the knee. Orthop Clin North Am 10:509, 1979.

43. La Prade RF, Nottsinger MA: Idiopathic osteonecrosis of the patella: An unusual cause of pain in the knee—a case report. J Bone Joint Surg Am 72:1414, 1990.

44. Lecouvet FE, van de Berg BC, Maldague BE, et al: Early irreversible osteonecrosis versus transient lesions of the femoral condyles: Prognostic values of subchondral bone and marrow changes on MR imaging. AJR Am J Roentgenol 170:71, 1998.

45. Linden B: The incidence of osteochondritis dissecans in the condyles of the femur. Acta Orthop Scand 47:664, 1976.

46. Linden B, Nilsson BE: Strontium-85 uptake in knee joints with osteochondritis dissecans. Acta Orthop Scand 59:769, 1977.

47. Lotke PA: Osteonecrosis of the knee: Current concepts review. J Bone Joint Surg Am 170:470, 1988.

48. Lotke PA: Tibial osteonecrosis. In Urbaniak JR, Jones JP (eds): Osteonecrosis—Etiology, Diagnosis, and Treatment. Chicago, American Academy of Orthopaedic Surgeons, 1997, p 425.

49. Lotke PA, Abend JA, Ecker ML: The treatment of osteonecrosis of the medial femoral condyle. Clin Orthop 171:109, 1982.

50. Lotke PA, Battish R, Nelson CL: Treatment of osteonecrosis of the knee. Instr Course Lect 50:483, 2001.

51. Lotke PA, Ecker ML: Osteonecrosis-like syndrome of the medial tibial plateau. Clin Orthop 176:148, 1983.

52. Lotke PA, Ecker ML: Osteonecrosis of the knee. Orthop Clin North Am 16:721, 1985.

53. Lotke PA, Ecker ML, Alavi A: Painful knees in older patients: Radionuclide diagnosis of possible osteonecrosis with spontaneous resolution. J Bone Joint Surg Am 59:617, 1977.

54. Lotke PA, Ecker ML, Barth P, et al: Subchondral magnetic resonance imaging changes in early osteoarthritis associated with tibial osteonecrosis. J Arthrosc Rel Surg 16:76, 2000.

55. Marco F, Lopez-Olivia F, Fernanadez-Arroyo JM, et al: Osteochondral allografts for osteochondritis dissecans and osteonecrosis of the femoral condyles. Int Orthop 17:104, 1993.

56. Marmor L: Fracture as a complication of osteonecrosis of the tibial plateau: A case report. J Bone Joint Surg Am 70:454, 1988.

57. Marmor L: Unicompartmental arthroplasty for osteonecrosis of the knee joint. Clin Orthop 294:247, 1993.

58. Miller GK, Maylan DJ, Drennan DM: The treatment of idiopathic ON of the medial femoral condyle with arthroscopic débridement. Arthroscopy 2:21, 1986.

59. Meyers MH, Ackeson W, Convery FR: Resurfacing of the knee with fresh osteochondral allograft. J Bone Joint Surg Am 71:704, 1989.

60. Mont MA, Baumgarten KM, Rifai A, et al: Atraumatic osteonecrosis of the knee. J Bone Joint Surg Am 82:1279, 2000.

61. Mont MA, Myers TH, Krackow KA, Hungerford DS: Total knee arthroplasty for corticosteroid associated avascular necrosis of the knee. Clin Orthop 338:124, 1997.

62. Mont MA, Tomek IM, Hungerford DS: Core decompression for avascular necrosis of the distal femur: Long term followup. Clin Orthop 334:124, 1997.

63. Moshowitz E: Bursitis of sartorius bursa: An undescribed malady stimulating chronic arthritis. JAMA 109:1362, 1937.

64. Motohashi M, Morii T, Koshino T: Clinical course and roentgenographic changes of osteonecrosis of the femoral condyle under conservative treatment. Clin Orthop 266:156, 1991.

65. Muheim G, Bohne WH: Prognosis in spontaneous osteonecrosis of the knee. J Bone Joint Surg Br 52:605, 1970.

66. Nakamura N, Horibe S, Nakamura S, Mitsuoka T: Subchondral microfractures of the knee without osteonecrosis after arthroscopic medial meniscectomy. Arthroscopy 18:538, 2002.

67. Nakamura T, Matsumoto T, Nishino M, et al: Early magnetic resonance imaging and histologic findings in a model of femoral head necrosis. Clin Orthop 334:68, 1977.

68. Negendank WC, Fernandez-Madrid FR, Heilbrun LK, et al: Magnetic resonance imaging of meniscal degeneration in asymptomatic knees. J Orthop Res 8:8, 1990.

69. Noble J, Hamblen DL: The pathology of the degenerate meniscus lesions. J Bone Joint Surg Br 57:180, 1975.

70. Papadopoulos E, Papagelopoulos PJ, Kaseta M, et al: Bone marrow edema syndrome of the knee. Knee 10:295, 2003.

71. Pape D, Seil R, Fritsch E, et al: Prevalence of spontaneous osteonecrosis of the medial femoral condyle in elderly patients. Knee Surg Sports Traumatol Arthrosc 10:233, 2002.

72. Pollack MS, Dalinka MK, Kressel HY, et al: Magnetic resonance imaging in the evaluation of suspected osteonecrosis of the knee. Skeletal Radiol 16:121, 1987.

73. Ritter MA, Eizember LE, Keating EM, Faris PM: The survival of total knee arthroplasty in patients with osteonecrosis of the medial condyle. Clin Orthop 267:108, 1991.

74. Rozing PM, Insall J, Bohne WH: Spontaneous osteonecrosis of the knee. J Bone Joint Surg Am 62:2, 1980.

75. Rubens-Dual A, Villiaumey J, Lubetzdi D, et al: L'osteochondrite du genou du sujet age: Interet de la biopsie synoviale. Rev Rhum Mal Osteoartic 33:709, 1964.

76. Santori N, Condello V, Adriani E, et al: Osteonecrosis after arthroscopic medial meniscectomy. Arthroscopy 11:220, 1995.

77. Satku K, Kumar RP, Chong SM, Thambyah A: The natural history of spontaneous osteonecrosis of the medial tibial plateau. J Bone Joint Surg Br 85:983, 2003.

78. Scaglietti O, Fineschi G: La condrite dissecante dell'eta senile. Arch Putti 20:1, 1965.

79. Seldes RM, Tan V, Duffy G, et al: Total knee arthroplasty for steroid induced osteonecrosis. J Arthroplasty 14:533, 1999.

80. Soucacos PN, Johnson EO, Soultauis K, et al: Diagnosis and management of the osteonecrotic triad of the knee. Orthop Clin North Am 35:371, 2004.

81. Soucacos PN, Xenakis TH, Beris AE: Idiopathic osteonecrosis of the medial femoral condyle. Classification and treatment. Clin Orthop 341:82, 1997.

82. Stern SH, Insall JN, Windsor RE: Total knee replacement in osteonecrotic knees. Orthop Trans 12:722, 1988.

83. Weissman BN, Hussain S: Magnetic resonance imaging of the knee. Rheum Dis Clin North Am 17:637, 1991.

84. Williams JS Jr, Bush-Joseph CA, Bach BR Jr: Osteochondritis dissecans of the knee. Am J Knee Surg 11:221, 1998.

CHAPTER 29

Osteonecrosis of the Knee

Michael A. Mont • Phillip S. Ragland

Osteonecrosis of the knee was first described by Ahlback and coworkers in 1968.[3] However, since that time, the term has come to refer to two separate disorders: spontaneous osteonecrosis of the knee (SPONK), which usually affects one condyle in patients older than 60 years,[2-6,18,19,37,42,54-56,83,90,96] and secondary osteonecrosis of the knee, which is seen in young patients, generally those younger than 45 years, with multiple condylar involvement.[34,44,46,58,66,70,76,85,91] Secondary osteonecrosis of the knee has been reported on less frequently than SPONK. Pathologically, these two entities are similar, with histology revealing necrotic or dead bone, and both have unknown pathophysiology. This chapter compares these two disorders in terms of their similarities and differences and then describes the evaluation, staging, and treatment of both these disorders individually.

COMPARISON OF SPONTANEOUS OSTEONECROSIS WITH SECONDARY OSTEONECROSIS OF THE KNEE

SPONK is a disorder that generally appears in patients older than 55 to 60 years and usually involves a single condyle or plateau. The medial femoral condyle is most often involved (Fig. 29–1), but lesions of the lateral femoral condyle or either tibial plateau have also been described.[19,38,55,56,57,92] SPONK patients have no associated risk factors (Fig. 29–2) for osteonecrosis, and they have unilateral involvement with no involvement of other joints (Table 29–1). In contrast, secondary osteonecrosis occurs in patients younger than 45 years and appears to be a completely different disease entity from SPONK. The disease typically affects multiple condyles simultaneously (medial and lateral femoral condyles or medial and lateral tibial plateaus, or both) and is bilateral more than 80% of the time. The femoral heads are commonly involved (approximately 90% of the time), and patients have associated risk factors for osteonecrosis, often including a history of alcohol or corticosteroid use. Other disorders that can be confused with these two entities include osteochondritis dissecans, bone bruises, and transient osteopenia of the knee, which will be discussed later in the section on differential diagnosis.[87] See Table 29–1 for a comparison of SPONK and secondary osteonecrosis.

DIFFERENTIAL DIAGNOSIS

Included in the differential diagnosis of osteonecrosis of the knee are osteochondritis dissecans, primary osteoarthritis, meniscal tears, transient osteonecrosis of the knee, bone bruises, and pes anserinus bursitis.

Osteochondritis dissecans of the knee occurs two to three times more commonly in men than women, either of whom is usually 15 to 20 years old. The lateral part of the medial femoral condyle toward the intercondylar notch is the area most often affected, and in some cases the lesion may extend into the weightbearing portion of this condyle. Its manifestation is usually insidious in nature with a gradual onset of symptoms. Approximately half the patients give a history of trauma, which is rare in osteonecrosis. If there is sudden detachment of an unstable fragment, the patient may complain of an acute onset of pain and locking of the knee. However, this scenario usually develops in an already symptomatic patient.

In osteoarthritis, the onset of symptoms and progression of the disease are slower than in osteonecrosis. Radiographic changes start at the joint line because the disease affects cartilage first. The bone is only secondarily affected. Osteoarthritis secondary to osteonecrosis, however, has a more rapid radiographic and clinical course.

Elderly patients with meniscal tears often have symptoms similar to those of osteonecrosis of the knee. A degenerative tear can be found at arthroscopy in patients with osteonecrosis, which may or may not be the cause of the patient's pain. Removal of a meniscus in an osteonecrotic patient may not result in pain relief and at times may worsen the patient's knee pain.[18]

Osteonecrosis after yttrium-aluminum-garnet (YAG) laser arthroscopic meniscectomy has been described.[25,82] A postulated cause is inappropriate depth and energy of the laser fields. The surgeon should be aware of this potential complication and the possibility of iatrogenic or traumatic osteonecrosis of the knee. In another recent report, osteonecrosis occurred after arthroscopic meniscectomy with a radiofrequency device.[20] There have, however, been reports of osteonecrosis occurring after meniscectomy without laser fields.[16,52] Middle-aged and elderly patients appear to be at risk, but the condition is still not clearly understood.

Patients with pes anserinus bursitis can also have pain over the medial aspect of the knee. The pain is localized over the proximal medial aspect of the tibia and is found well below the joint line. Swelling over the proximal

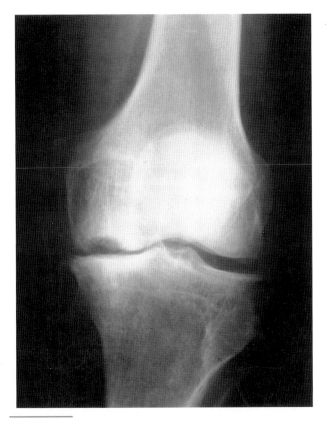

Figure 29–1. Anteroposterior radiograph of a patient with spontaneous osteonecrosis of the knee. Note the typical lesion of the medial femoral condyle.

medial part of the tibia, as well as a thickened bursa, can also be seen. Injection of lidocaine into the area may aid in differentiating between this entity and osteonecrosis, although in confusing cases a magnetic resonance imaging (MRI) examination is diagnostic.

Bone bruises and transient osteopenia of the knee[87] are self-limited disorders that can also be confused with osteonecrosis. These entities can be clearly differentiated with MRI, and the marrow findings resolve within 6 months.

PATHOLOGY OF BOTH DISORDERS

In the early stages of osteonecrosis, the gross appearance of the articular cartilage is relatively normal. There may be slight discoloration and flattening of the articular cartilage as the disease progresses. Eventually, a line of demarcation becomes evident, and an osteochondral flap will overlie an area of osteonecrosis (Figs. 29–3 and 29–4).[2,4,61] As secondary degenerative changes occur, the defect in the cartilage becomes filled with necrotic debris and fibrocartilage. The characteristic secondary changes seen in osteoarthritis will be evident in the surrounding joints and include osteophytes, synovial hypertrophy, and eburnated bone.

When specimens are examined with a microscope, a segment of dead bone is seen in the weightbearing part of the affected joint in association with subchondral fracture and collapse. Empty lacunae (Fig. 29–5) and fatty

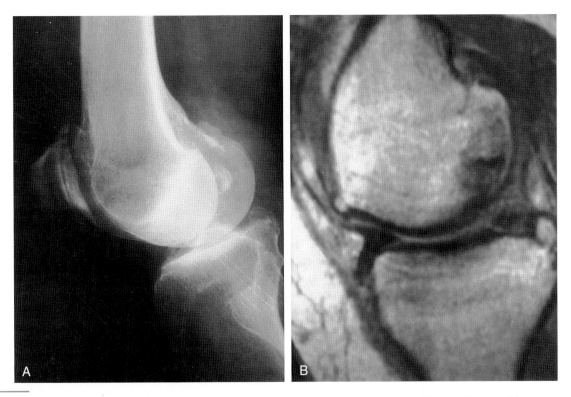

Figure 29–2. Lateral radiograph (**A**) with a corresponding magnetic resonance image (**B**) of a 70-year-old woman with left knee pain. The patient never used corticosteroids and has no medical problems. The diagnosis was spontaneous osteonecrosis of the knee.

Table 29–1. Comparison of Spontaneous Osteonecrosis with Secondary Osteonecrosis

CHARACTERISTIC	SPONTANEOUS OSTEONECROSIS OF THE KNEE	SECONDARY OSTEONECROSIS OF THE KNEE
Age	>55 to 60 years	<45 years
Pain onset	Acute	Gradual
Bilaterality	<5%	>80%
Lesion number	One	Multiple
Lesion size	Small	Large
Location	Usually medial femoral condyle	Multiple femoral and tibial condyles
Hip involvement	<1%	>90%
Associated factors	None	Corticosteroids, alcohol, tobacco
Associated diseases	None	Systemic lupus erythematosus and other disorders

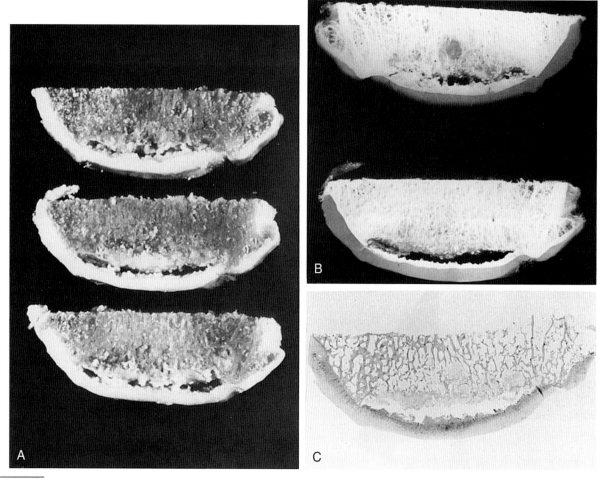

Figure 29–3. **A,** Gross inspection of the medial femoral condyle reveals smooth cartilage but with a focally depressed area demarcated by a well-defined circumferential groove. In frontal sections, a transarticular fracture can be seen. These changes give rise to the typical radiographic findings already illustrated. **B,** Radiograph of the same specimen showing the subchondral bone plate still attached to cartilage. The radiolucent crescent is similar to that seen in the hip in early osteonecrosis. **C,** Histological preparation of the same specimen.

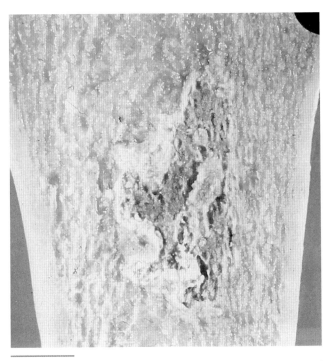

Figure 29–4. Gross pathological specimen showing area of osteonecrosis in the metaphyseal region of the distal end of the femur.

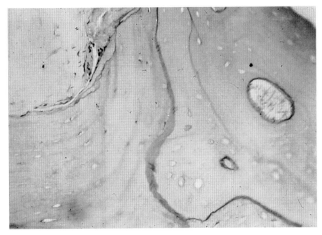

Figure 29–5. Photomicrograph of a pathological specimen of an osteonecrotic area showing empty lacunae. Original magnification ×1000, hematoxylin-eosin stain.

degeneration are noted within the center of the lesion. Osteoblastic activity, cartilage formation, and bands of fibrovascular granulation tissue are characteristic of the surrounding area where reparative bone formation takes place. The pathological characteristics and sequence of events for the knee are similar to those for the hip, for which the reader can seek further information.[39,47,61,77]

SPONTANEOUS OSTEONECROSIS OF THE KNEE

Etiology and Associated Factors

Most patients with spontaneous osteonecrosis are elderly women (three times more common in women than men), and a traumatic theory of origin has been applied to this disease. Many of these patients have osteoporotic bone, and therefore it is believed that minor trauma may lead to microfractures in the weak subchondral area. At this point, a bone scan would be positive but MRI might still be unremarkable. This phenomenon has been noted in several published reports and supports the traumatic theory of origin.[4,18,56] It has been hypothesized that fluid enters through the space caused by the microfractures, thereby leading to increasing edema and eventual osseous ischemia. However, in clinical practice it is noted that less than 10% of patients with SPONK give any history of trauma. Therefore, the exact etiology of SPONK is still unknown, and further studies are necessary to elucidate its pathophysiological mechanisms. Recently, multiple studies are supporting the "insufficiency stress fracture

in osteopenic bone" theory for the etiology of this disease.[75,80,98] In a recent MRI study of 39 patients with presumed SPONK lesions, the investigators found osteoarthritis and insufficiency fractures commonly associated.[75] These authors called into question the validity of the term "spontaneous osteonecrosis" and urged further investigation of possibly various causes for the MRI findings. Zanetti and coworkers determined bone mineral density by computed tomography in patients with MRI-diagnosed SPONK lesions.[98] They found osteopenia commonly, which the authors believed supports an insufficiency mechanism for this disease.

Clinical Features

The lesion in SPONK is three times more common in women than in men and typically occurs in patients older than 60 years. There is usually a history of acute onset of severe pain well localized to the area of the lesion. Because the medial femoral condyle is most commonly involved, pain occurs just proximal to the joint line. Often, the patient is able to recall the exact moment when the pain began. This pain is worse with weightbearing and is also usually worse at night and on using stairs. A small effusion may be present. Knee range of motion may be slightly limited secondary to pain, effusion, and muscle spasm. Examination of the knee for instability is normal. SPONK can also occur in either tibial plateau (medial more common).

Radiographic Evaluation

Anteroposterior and lateral plain radiographs (Fig. 29–6) should be obtained whenever a possible diagnosis of osteonecrosis is being considered (knee pain of sudden onset in older patients). Occasionally, skyline or Merchant views can be helpful to delineate a medial condylar lesion

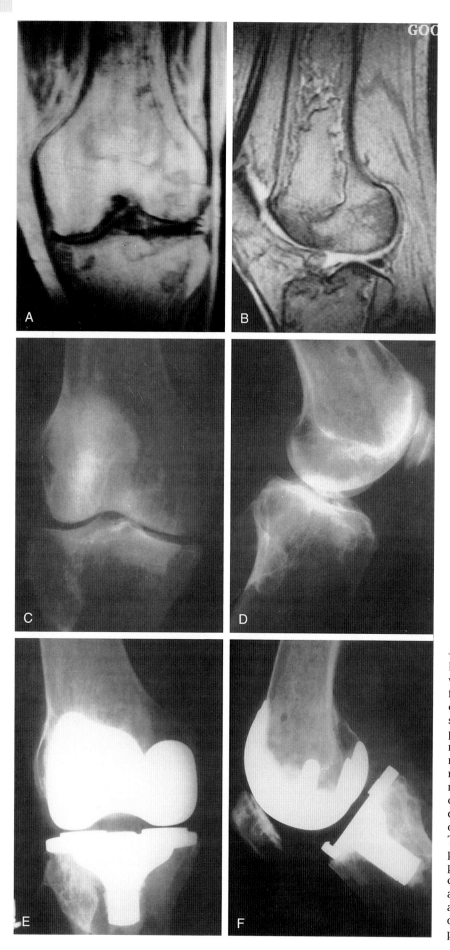

Figure 29–6. Knee of a 57-year-old woman with a history of pulmonary fibrosis who was taking high-dose corticosteroids. Extensive osteonecrosis of the distal end of the femur and proximal end of the tibia was diagnosed by clinical examination, plain radiographs, and (**A** and **B**) magnetic resonance imaging. Treatment was nonoperative for 6 months. Because of continued pain, she underwent core decompression and had lateral radiographs taken after surgery (**C** and **D**). Ten months later, arthroscopy was performed because of persistent pain. Findings included degenerative changes. Two months after arthroscopy, she required total knee arthroplasty (**E** and **F**) and is presently doing well (Knee Society score of 94 points).

or even a patellar lesion. Typically, roentgenograms may not show any abnormalities for many months after the onset of symptoms. Later in the disease process, abnormal findings on x-ray film may include subtle flattening of the weightbearing portion of the affected condyle and a radiolucent area of variable size located in the subchondral bone and bordered by a sclerotic halo (Fig. 29–7). As the disease progresses, the sclerotic halo thickens and the subchondral bone further collapses. Later, there is complete osseous destruction accompanied by secondary degenerative changes, including osteophyte formation, joint space narrowing, and sclerosis, with resultant degenerative changes on the opposite side of the joint (Fig. 29–8). Varus or valgus angulation may then be seen as a result of this degenerative process. In SPONK, these findings are encountered on the medial side of the knee joint (Fig. 29–9), whereas in secondary osteonecrosis, the medial or lateral side of the knee joint may be affected.

Many important parameters can be measured from plain radiographs and applied to patients with SPONK. Originally, the process was divided into five sequential stages. In stage I, radiographs are normal and lesions often resolve spontaneously. In stage II, there is subtle flattening of the condyle indicative of impending collapse. Stage III is the typical lesion with a subchondral lucent area bordered by

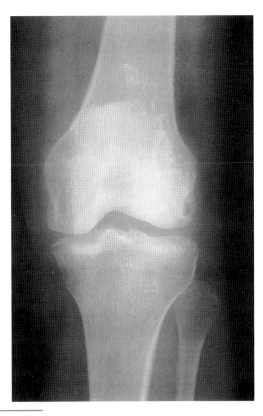

Figure 29–8. Plain radiograph of a knee with flattening of the femoral condyle and subchondral collapse. In this patient, the tibia also shows subchondral collapse.

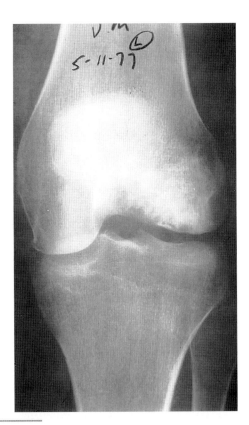

Figure 29–7. Plain radiograph of a knee depicting osteonecrosis of the lateral femoral condyle with typical flattening and subchondral collapse (Ficat and Arlet stage III).

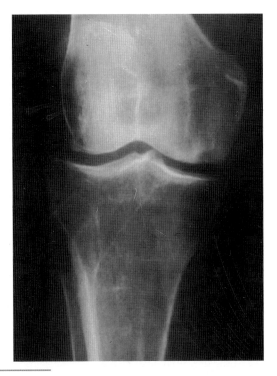

Figure 29–9. Plain radiograph of an 86-year-old woman with no associated risk factors but pain in the right medial side of her knee. Her diagnosis was spontaneous osteonecrosis of the medial femoral condyle.

a sclerotic halo. Stages IV and V denote progressive stages of collapse. In stage III the arc area of the lesion can have prognostic implications. It can be calculated by multiplying the greatest diameters on the anteroposterior and lateral radiographs and then determining the ratio of the width of the necrosis to the width of the entire condyle on the anteroposterior view. Lotke and coworkers[54,56] suggested that if this ratio is greater than 50%, the prognosis is poor. Their study reviewed 87 knees in 79 patients, including 64 women and 15 men with a mean age of 68 years (range, 46 to 83 years). Patients with systemic lupus erythematosus were excluded. The mean follow-up was 3.5 years (range, 1 to 17 years). Lotke and colleagues divided these patients into three groups based on the width of condylar involvement. There were 36 knees in group I (negative plain radiographs but positive bone scan). All these patients did well except one patient, who eventually required prosthetic replacement. Group II patients (23 knees) and group III patients (28 knees) all had radiographically evident lesions. In group II, a mean of 32% of the transverse width of the medial femoral condyle was affected, whereas in group III this mean was 57%. Sixteen knees in group II that were treated nonoperatively functioned well for as long as 7 years after diagnosis. Only five of the group II patients underwent total knee arthroplasty (22%), whereas all the patients in group III underwent prosthetic replacement. These studies were performed on patients with osteonecrosis of the femoral condyles. Though less common than femoral involvement, the same radiographic changes can occur in the medial tibial plateau.[86]

At the end stage of the disease it may be difficult to distinguish between osteonecrosis and osteoarthritis of the knee on plain radiographs (Fig. 29–10). Some authors have postulated that many cases of what was thought to be aggressive osteoarthritis are in fact missed or advanced examples of osteonecrosis.

MRI of the affected knee often reveals more extensive involvement than can be appreciated on plain radiographs (Fig 29–11).[10,14,35,48,78,80,85] On T1-weighted images, the high-intensity signal normally produced by fat in the marrow is replaced by a discrete subchondral area of low signal intensity that is at times surrounded by an area of intermediate signal intensity (Figs. 29–12 and 29–13). On T2-weighted images, there is an area of low signal intensity surrounded by a variable high-intensity signal. This high-intensity signal is thought to be the result of edema surrounding the lesion (Fig. 29–14). MRI studies, however, can be initially read as negative. Some have postulated that this negative finding may be a result of thickness of the imaging sections, a process other than osteonecrosis being involved, or the MRI study being normal early in the course of the disease.[10,14,35,61,78,93]

For SPONK, bone scans performed with technetium 99m have often been used for confirming the diagnosis.[31,33,72] A focally intense area of uptake is seen on static-phase images. Multiple authors have considered bone scans to be the definitive test over MRI. Bone scans can be positive even when MRI is negative because findings may not be apparent on MRI for a variable time after the onset of symptoms.

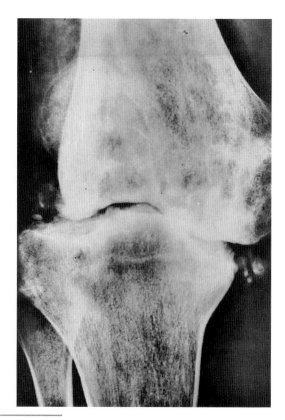

Figure 29–10. Plain radiograph of patient with severe osteonecrosis of the knee who presented a difficult problem for planning a total knee arthroplasty because of severe deformity and subluxation. At first glance, one might attribute this condition to osteoarthritis and not appreciate the cause of the disease.

Staging

Several staging systems have been used for SPONK. Koshino[49] first described a four-tiered system, including stage I (initial stage), in which no abnormalities are seen on roentgenograms but the patient has knee pain; stage II (avascular stage), in which a radiolucent oval shadow appears and osteosclerosis increases in the surrounding area; and stage III (developed stage), in which the radiolucent area is surrounded by a sclerotic halo. The subchondral bone plate is collapsed and is visible as a calcified plate. In stage IV (degenerative stage), osteophytes and osteosclerosis are seen in the ipsilateral tibia as well as in the femoral condyle. Aglietti and associates[2] modified the Koshino staging to include five categories (Fig. 29–15). In stage I, plain radiographs are normal. If no changes are seen after 6 months, the patient will remain in stage I. In stage II, an area of slight flattening can be appreciated on the convex portion of the condyle. In stage III, a radiolucency with distal sclerosis and a faint halo of bony reaction are seen. In stage IV, a calcified plate, sequestrum, or flap fragment with a radiolucency surrounded by a definite sclerotic halo is seen, and in stage V, narrowing of the joint space, subchondral (tibial and femoral) sclerosis, and osteophyte formation typical of osteoarthritis are apparent.

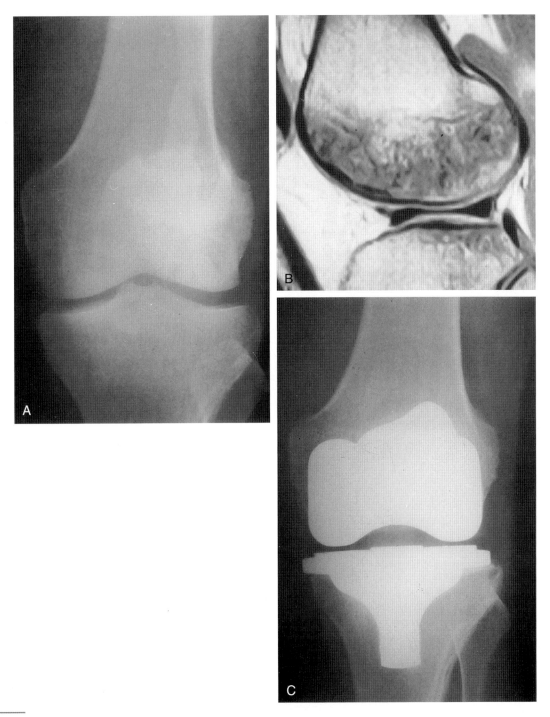

Figure 29–11. Plain radiograph of the left knee of a 45-year-old woman (history of corticosteroid use) with evidence of osteonecrosis (**A**). Magnetic resonance imaging reveals the osteonecrosis to be more involved than appreciated on plain films (**B**). The patient was treated nonoperatively for 2.5 years until she returned with pain and was treated by core decompression. This lasted 2 years, at which time she underwent total knee arthroplasty (**C**).

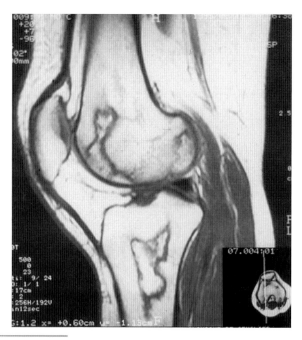

Figure 29–12. Magnetic resonance image of the knee of a 26-year-old woman with evidence of osteonecrosis of the distal end of the femur and proximal end of the tibia.

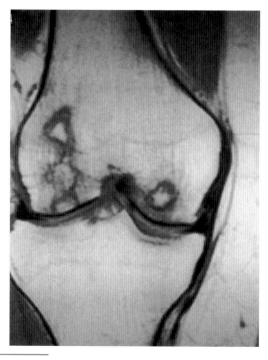

Figure 29–13. Magnetic resonance image of the knee of a 37-year-old woman with osteonecrosis of the knee.

TREATMENT

Nonoperative Treatment

Nonoperative management of SPONK consists of protected weightbearing with crutches, analgesics, and nonsteroidal anti-inflammatory medications, as well as physical therapy. Therapy may include straight-leg–raising exercises aimed at strengthening the quadriceps and hamstring muscles.

Excellent results have been reported with symptomatic treatment. Motohashi and coworkers[71] studied 15 knees in 14 patients—9 women and 5 men with an average age of 63 years (range, 23 to 79 years). SPONK was observed in 12 knees; the remaining 3 knees had steroid-associated secondary osteonecrosis. At a mean follow-up of 5 years (range, 1 to 12 years), five patients were able to walk continuously for 1 km without pain. Four patients had occasional pain, and one had mild pain while walking. The other four patients were restricted to walking less than 1 km because of pain. None required total knee arthroplasty. These results were found in SPONK patients with relatively small lesions. The knee score was not found to significantly increase; however, the necrotic lesion remained unchanged, improved, or got worse in equal proportions. The degenerative changes seen at the end stages are often not severe. The varus deformity increases with time. There was a slow progression of arthritis, and these patients functioned relatively well with limited symptoms. Lotke and coworkers[54] reported on 87 knees with SPONK, 36 of which (in group I) were treated nonoperatively. Only one patient progressed to prosthetic replacement, with the remaining 35 knees functioning well.

In a recent study involving SPONK of the medial plateau, Satku and coauthors reported on the natural history of 21 knees.[86] In contradistinction to the excellent prognosis of many femoral lesions, they found complete resolution in only four knees. Five of the knees progressed to needing a total knee replacement by 5.6 years, with symptoms and progression noted in most other knees. They concluded that osteonecrosis of the medial tibial plateau progresses in most cases to significant degenerative disease.

Operative Treatment

Various surgical procedures have been used, including arthroscopic débridement, osteochondral allografting and other bone grafting, high tibial osteotomy, core decompression, and unicompartmental and total knee arthroplasty.

ARTHROSCOPIC DÉBRIDEMENT

Arthroscopic débridement has had mixed results, at best, for the treatment of osteonecrosis of the knee.[50,62,97] In 1986, Miller and coworkers[62] showed that in five knees treated by arthroscopy, four were rated good at a mean follow-up of 31 months. They concluded that arthroscopy does not alter the natural course of the disease. Patients with SPONK may have degenerative tears of the menisci, but arthroscopic débridement of these tears has no effect on the osteonecrotic lesion of the bone. The partial meniscectomy performed at arthroscopy may actually cause

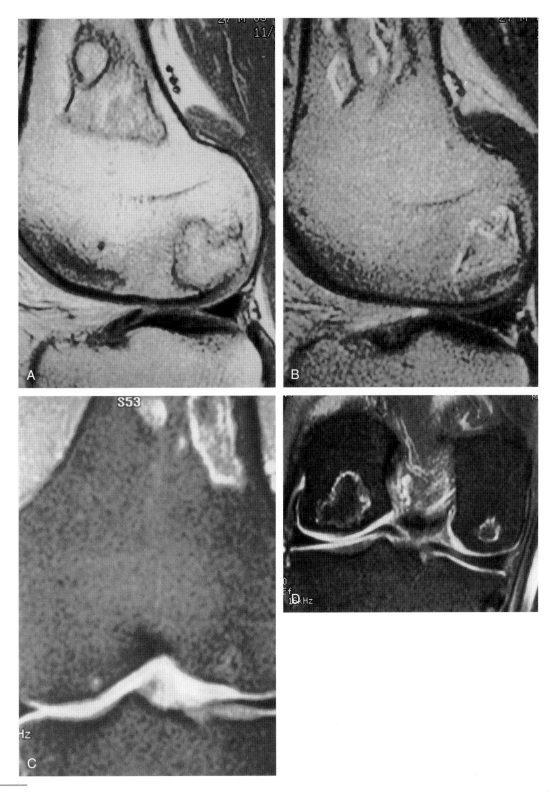

Figure 29–14. Magnetic resonance imaging studies of a 27-year-old man with a history of cerebrovascular accident and a possible coagulation disorder. **A**, T1-weighted image with typical findings of osteonecrosis. **B** to **D**, T2-weighted images.

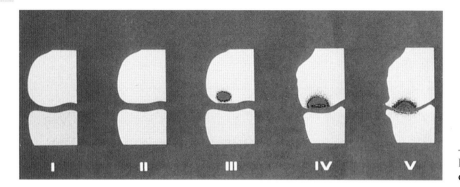

Figure 29–15. Five stages of osteonecrosis (see text).

further degeneration of the knee joint. Furthermore, the fluid used during arthroscopy may increase osseous pressure, which can lead to ischemia as a result of the fluid pumps that are commonly used and can potentially lead to further necrosis. Koshino and associates[50] reported on eight knees that had undergone arthroscopy, but these patients underwent the procedure as a diagnostic measure.

OSTEOCHONDRAL ALLOGRAFTS

Several studies using osteochondral allografts as a treatment option have been cited in the literature.[8,27,29,32,74] Bayne and colleagues[8] reported on a series of 21 knees in which fresh, nonfrozen allografts were used to treat condylar defects. Fifteen knees had post-traumatic osteonecrosis, with 10 (66%) having good or excellent results. Spontaneous osteonecrosis was the diagnosis in six knees, with only one good result. These authors believed that the SPONK patients did not do well with allografts because of the lack of compliance in these elderly patients, which resulted in subsidence and fragmentation of the graft. Three knees had a diagnosis of steroid-induced osteonecrosis; all failed. These authors attributed this high failure rate to the continued use of corticosteroids, which caused poor vascularization of the allograft and resulting subsidence. On the basis of this study and a study using this method in secondary osteonecrosis, the results with osteochondral allografts do not appear encouraging. A small number of patients have been treated with allografts, and there is only anecdotal mention of the use of other types of bone grafting (autogenous, vascularized fibula) for this disease. In addition, bone grafting has been used in an ancillary role with other procedures (accompanying high tibial osteotomy and core decompression). Further work will be necessary to determine the role of various bone grafts or the use of ancillary growth and differentiation factors for the treatment of these bony lesions.[67]

HIGH TIBIAL OSTEOTOMY

High tibial osteotomy has been performed on patients with SPONK and has produced satisfactory results.[49,56] However, many of these patients are older than 60 years,

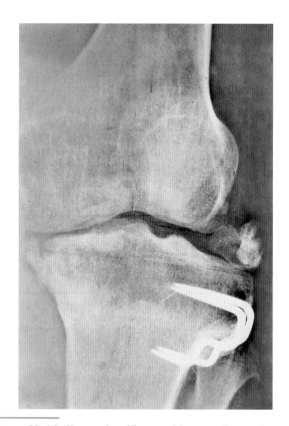

Figure 29–16. Knee of a 45-year-old man who underwent a high tibial osteotomy; after only 3 years, severe degenerative changes developed and required total knee arthroplasty.

and this population is treated more often with total knee arthroplasty, which reportedly yields more predictable results (Fig. 29–16). Koshino[49] reported on 37 knees treated by high tibial osteotomy for osteonecrosis. Thirty-five of these lesions were medial, and 2 were lateral. This author also used drilling or bone grafting concomitantly in 23 knees. At a follow-up of 2 to 8.5 years, 35 of 37 knees (95%) experienced relief of pain and improved walking ability. The necrotic lesion seemed to disappear in 13 knees and improved radiographically in 17 knees. After a mean follow-up of 5 years, only one patient underwent total knee arthroplasty. Aglietti and associates[2] described 31 patients who underwent high tibial osteotomy, with 21 knees having ancillary bone grafting.

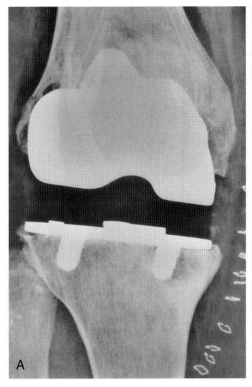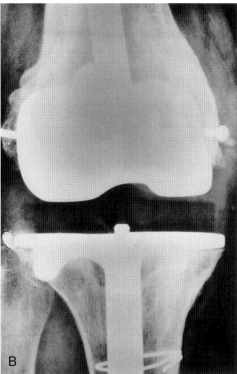

Figure 29–17. Total knee arthroplasty (**A**) is performed in a patient with severe osteonecrosis. Note that modern prostheses can use stems when the bone is severely necrotic (**B**).

These authors reported 27 excellent and good results (87%) at a mean follow-up of 6.2 years. Two knees underwent prosthetic replacement. In a recent long-term follow-up report (15- to 28-year follow-up), Koshino and colleagues described excellent results with high tibial valgus osteotomies.[51]

CORE DECOMPRESSION

See the section on core decompression in secondary osteonecrosis concerning the use of this procedure. This technique does not, however, seem to be successful with SPONK and should be reserved for recalcitrant cases.

UNICONDYLAR AND TOTAL KNEE REPLACEMENT

Some patients are initially seen in the later stages of disease and are not candidates for any procedures except prosthetic replacement. There has been debate on whether unicondylar or total knee replacement should be used. In SPONK, it may be possible to use unicondylar replacement because usually only one condyle is affected.

Marmor[60] reported on the use of unicondylar replacement in 34 knees with osteonecrosis of the medial femoral condyle. The mean follow-up was 5.5 years. Good or excellent results were found in 30 knees (88%). Of the four failures, two were attributed to the development of osteonecrosis in the lateral compartment. In a recent study by Radke et al, 23 patients treated with unicondylar knee

arthroplasty were compared with 16 treated with bicondylar implants. On a short-term basis, unicondylar implants had better results; however, on a long-term basis, bicondylar implants had better results. Revisions occurred only in the unicondylar group.[79] Reasons for the high failure rate of unicondylar implants were poor bone stock and arthritic changes.

Total knee arthroplasty has had variably reported outcomes (Fig. 29–17).[9,43,79,81] Bergman and Rand[9] reported 87% good or excellent results in 38 total knee arthroplasties with a short follow-up (4 ± 2 years. Twenty-nine of these knees had SPONK, and 9 had secondary osteonecrosis. The authors determined that implant survivorship can be predicted to be 85% with revision used as an endpoint or to be 68% with revision for moderate or severe pain used as an endpoint. These results were inferior to those of knee replacements for other diagnoses. Ritter and coworkers[81] compared 32 osteonecrotic knees with 63 osteoarthritic knees with follow-ups of 3.9 and 4.6 years, respectively. All the osteonecrosis patients had SPONK (medial femoral condyle). There was no statistical difference in results between the two groups, with a success rate of 82% for the osteonecrotic knees and 90% for the osteoarthritic knees when pain relief was used as an endpoint.

SECONDARY OSTEONECROSIS

Etiology and Associated Factors

The exact etiology of secondary osteonecrosis of the knee is also unknown. The leading candidate theories include

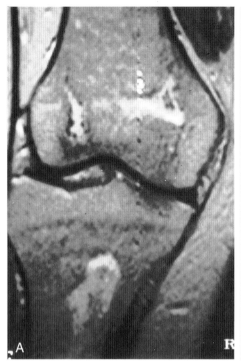 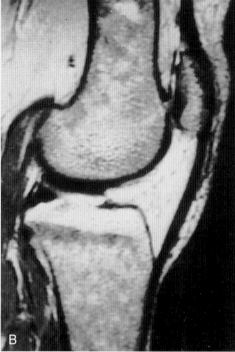

Figure 29–18. T1- and T2-weighted magnetic resonance imaging (MRI) scans of a 35-year-old woman with a history of corticosteroid use after renal transplantation. This patient has not required surgery 6 years after initial evaluation. Note the evidence on MRI of osteonecrosis of the distal end of the femur and proximal end of the tibia.

those of vascular or traumatic origin.* Interference with the microcirculation to subchondral bone is the main hypothesis in the vascular theory. Exactly what causes this vascular interruption is unknown, but experimental evidence from animal studies has implicated fat emboli,[26,94-96] microthrombi,[45] and coagulation disorders.[12,30] Edema in a nonexpandable compartment results in increased pressure within the bone marrow, which diminishes circulation and results in ischemia within the bone.[39] In secondary osteonecrosis it is noted that many of these patients are being treated with corticosteroids. These corticosteroids may cause an increase in the size of fat marrow cells, thereby resulting in decreased circulation, increased intraosseous pressure, and osseous ischemia. There have been multiple reports of heritable coagulation disorders leading to thrombophilia or hypofibrinolysis, or both, with the resultant emboli causing ischemia and subsequent bone necrosis.[30,66] More is known about these disorders from investigations of the hip.[30,66] A recent study[11] analyzed 38 consecutive patients for coagulation abnormalities and found that factor V Leiden and the prothrombin 20210A gene mutation might play a role in the pathogenesis of knee osteonecrosis.

Other factors that have been associated with secondary osteonecrosis of the knee include corticosteroid therapy;[1,15] systemic lupus erythematosus;[1,41,64] renal transplantation (Fig. 29–18);[43] alcoholism;[36,40] Caisson's decompression disease; Gaucher's disease;[45] hemoglobinopathies;[61] arthroscopic meniscectomy, especially with lasers;[13,25,73,82,84] and anterior cruciate reconstruction.

*References 7, 21, 22, 24, 39, 45, 47, 59, 89, 99.

Clinical Features

The lesion in secondary osteonecrosis is three to four times more common in women than in men and can occur at any age, although it is more common in patients younger than 55 years, with a mean occurrence in the mid-30s. The pain is insidious in onset and can be medial or lateral in location. Often, there is an association with an immunocompromising disorder such as systemic lupus erythematosus, renal transplantation, and sickle cell anemia, which may affect more of the clinical picture than just the knee. Examination of the knee for instability, as in SPONK, is also normal.

Radiographic Evaluation

As in SPONK, anteroposterior and lateral plain radiographs should be obtained whenever a possible diagnosis of osteonecrosis is being considered (patients with associated risk factors for osteonecrosis). In addition, skyline views can be helpful to delineate patellar lesions. Roentgenograms may not show any abnormalities for many months after the onset of symptoms.

To date, few prognostic radiographic features have been described for secondary osteonecrosis, but patients with extensive epiphyseal involvement have the worst prognosis.

On MRI, the sagittal sections can be divided into proximal, distal, anterior, and posterior sections (Fig. 29–19). In the frontal plane, the MRI sections can be divided into medial condyle, lateral condyle, epiphyseal, and metaphyseal regions. Making note of these areas on MRI scans may aid in the planning of treatment.

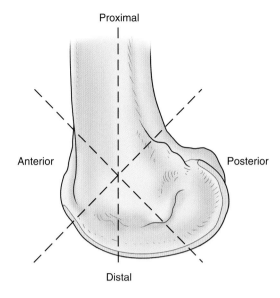

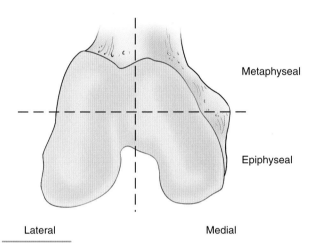

Figure 29–19. Magnetic resonance imaging schematic with the knee divided into various regions to aid in the planning of treatment (see text).

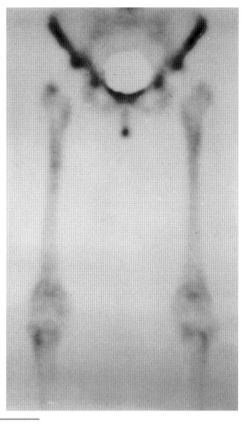

Figure 29–20. Bone scan of a 26-year-old woman with a history of osteonecrosis of the knee. This scan was read as negative by a radiologist. A magnetic resonance image that is positive for osteonecrosis is shown in Figure 29-12.

Bone scans do not have the same success in the diagnosis of secondary osteonecrosis as they do in SPONK. Bone scans are at times difficult to interpret because secondary osteonecrosis is manifested bilaterally and symmetric uptake may be read as degenerative changes or even as negative when uptake is not thought to be significant (Fig. 29–20). Mont and coworkers compared bone scans with MRI and histological diagnosis of osteonecrosis (Fig. 29–21). Twenty-four patients with 89 lesions were identified by MRI and histology. Only 48 of those lesions (54%) were identified by bone scan. These authors concluded that bone scans are unreliable and that initial radiographs are satisfactory and should be followed by MRI when necessary. MRI remains the diagnostic test of choice because it is 99% reliable in detecting early marrow changes.

Staging

The staging system used mainly for secondary osteonecrosis was described by Mont and colleagues[66,68] and is a modification of Ficat and Arlet's staging for osteonecrosis of the hip as applied to the knee.[23] In stage I, no changes are appreciated on plain radiographs, but MRI scans are positive. In stage II, sclerotic or cystic changes, or both, are present on plain radiographs. In stage III, subchondral collapse (crescent sign) is evident. In stage IV, there is evidence of degenerative changes on the opposite side of the joint, as well as joint space narrowing.

TREATMENT

Nonoperative Treatment

Nonoperative management, as in the treatment of SPONK, consists of protected weightbearing, analgesics, nonsteroidal anti-inflammatory medications, and physical therapy.

In contrast to SPONK, however, secondary osteonecrosis tends to fare poorly with nonoperative management. The lesions are larger and are in a younger, more active

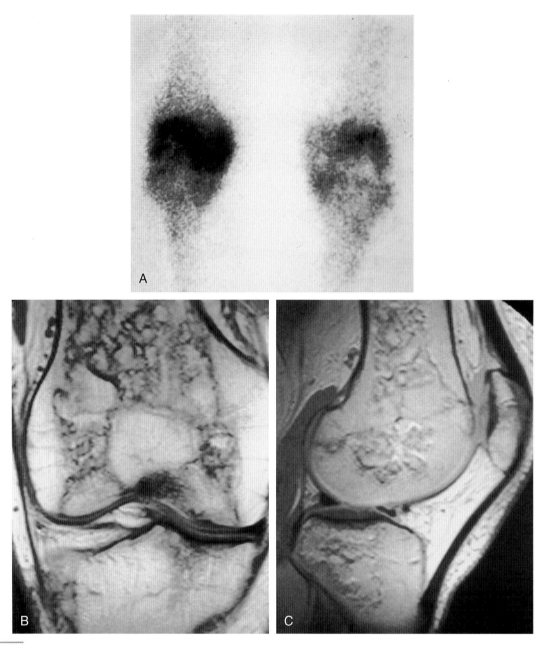

Figure 29–21. Bone scan (**A**) and magnetic resonance imaging studies (**B** and **C**) that are consistent with extensive osteonecrosis of the distal end of the femur and proximal end of the tibia. The patient is a 33-year-old man with a history of chronic corticosteroid use secondary to ulcerative colitis.

patient population often immunocompromised secondary to another disease process. In a series by Mont and coworkers,[70] of 32 knees treated nonoperatively, only 19 (59%) had good or excellent outcomes at 2 years' follow-up. At 6 years, only five knees (16%) survived nonoperative management. The lesions that did well with nonoperative management tended to be smaller. The stage had little effect on results, with a 25% success rate in Ficat and Arlet stage I lesions versus a 15% success rate with stage III lesions. Overall, 75% of the knees (24 of 32 knees) progressed one or two Ficat and Arlet radiographic

stages. Soucacos and coworkers reported spontaneous resolution of the lesions or no additional deterioration in only 20% of patients with secondary osteonecrosis.[90] Mont and coworkers reported on 51 patients treated nonoperatively out of a group of 136 patients with secondary osteonecrosis.[63] Overall, only 31% responded to nonoperative treatment. The subgroup of 10 patients who were asymptomatic at initial evaluation did better. Eight remained asymptomatic and two became symptomatic at 6 and 8 years, with femoral condylar collapse necessitating total knee arthroplasty.

Operative Treatment

ARTHROSCOPIC DÉBRIDEMENT

Arthroscopic débridement has rarely been reported for secondary osteonecrosis of the knee. Mont and coworkers reported 6 of 10 knees with clinically satisfactory results after a mean follow-up of 3 years (range, 2 to 5 years).[63] The four less than satisfactory results were treated by total knee arthroplasty. Arthroscopic débridement may be appropriate for relief of pain and mechanical symptoms and may delay arthroplasty in selected patients.

OSTEOCHONDRAL ALLOGRAFTS

Flynn and associates[27] evaluated 17 knees with secondary osteonecrosis in which fresh-frozen allografts were used. At a mean follow-up of 4.2 years (range, 2 to 9 years), 12 knees (71%) had good or excellent results. Fukui and associates reported the 6.5-year mean follow-up of 10 knees (eight patients) treated with autologous iliac bone grafts.[28] All patients had successful results. The present authors believe that bone grafting is more appropriate in patients with SPONK (single lesions) and would be more difficult in those with secondary osteonecrosis (multiple lesions).

HIGH TIBIAL OSTEOTOMY

The use of high tibial osteotomy in secondary osteonecrosis is not generally recommended because most of these patients have bicondylar femoral involvement and may have tibial involvement as well. Its use in this disease subset has been only anecdotally described in case reports.

CORE DECOMPRESSION

Core decompression (Fig. 29–22) has been used in the hip and other joints,[17,64,68] with success in the early stages of disease, and has been applied in the knee. The first report on such application was by Jacobs and coworkers[44] in 1989 on 28 knees. These patients had a mean age of 33 years and a mean follow-up of 54 months. They found that patients with Ficat and Arlet stage I and II disease (seven knees) all had successful outcomes. Knees with stage III disease (21 knees) had a success rate of 52%. Radiographically, Ficat and Arlet stage I or II knees progressed one stage or remained stable. Of the stage III knees, 11 of 21 had good radiographic results. These results were favorable considering the young age of these patients, who might otherwise require a total knee arthroplasty. Mont and coauthors[70] in 1997 reported on a series of 47 knees that were treated by core decompression for secondary osteonecrosis. The mean age in this group was 35 years, with osteonecrosis being bilateral in 88%. Their success rate was found to be 72% (34 of 47 knees) at a mean follow-up of 11 years (range, 4 to 16 years). Seventeen of 47 knees (36%) progressed to Ficat and Arlet stage III or IV disease as compared with 24 of 32 knees (75%) treated nonoperatively. In a later study the same authors reported clinical success with core decompression in 74 of 94 knees (79%) at a mean follow-up of 7 years (range, 2 to 24 years).[63]

Core decompression is a relatively minor procedure with little morbidity that has been shown to at least lengthen the time required before total knee arthroplasty. Many of the patients feel pain relief immediately in the recovery room; this relief has been found to be lasting in 74% of patients at a mean follow-up of 10.5 years.

Preoperative physical examination to determine the areas of pain (femoral or tibial, or both) should be performed. MRI scans are obtained before surgery (Fig. 29–23) to determine the areas that need to be cored and the extent of involvement. When femoral or tibial core decompression is performed, a tourniquet is applied but rarely inflated. For femoral cores, a small lateral or, alternatively, a medial incision (Fig. 29–24) can be made under fluoroscopic control just above the flare of the condyle. A 3- to 6-mm Michelle trephine (RMS International, Toulouse, France) (Fig. 29–25) is then introduced at the metaphyseal flare. It is guided into the medial and lateral condyles to within a few millimeters of the subchondral bone. For tibial cores, a small incision is made just medial to the tibial tubercle while avoiding the medial saphenous nerve. Under fluoroscopic control, the trephine is guided into the medial and lateral tibial plateaus, as for the femur. The trocar is turned within the bone as it is advanced to clear the teeth of the trocar and to obtain the best possible biopsy specimen. Postoperatively, patients ambulate with crutches or a cane at 50% weightbearing for 6 weeks, followed by full weightbearing.

UNICONDYLAR KNEE REPLACEMENT

Unicondylar knee replacement for secondary osteonecrosis has only infrequently been reported on in a few patients from a larger series of patients with SPONK. The authors do not recommend this approach for use in secondary osteonecrosis because these patients have bicondylar disease.

TOTAL KNEE ARTHROPLASTY

For secondary osteonecrosis, Mont and Hungerford[66] reported on 31 total knee replacements in patients younger than 50 years (mean of 36 years), all of whom had a history of corticosteroid use. Follow-up averaged 8.2 years (range, 2 to 16 years). The results in 55% were good or excellent. Thirty-seven percent had to be revised for aseptic loosening, and 10% were revised for deep infection. All the knees that did not have a diagnosis of systemic lupus erythematosus ($n = 6$) had excellent clinical results, whereas only 44% of lupus patients had a good clinical outcome. The authors proposed that the appropriate use of cement and stems might lead to improved results in the future. Seldes and colleagues reported

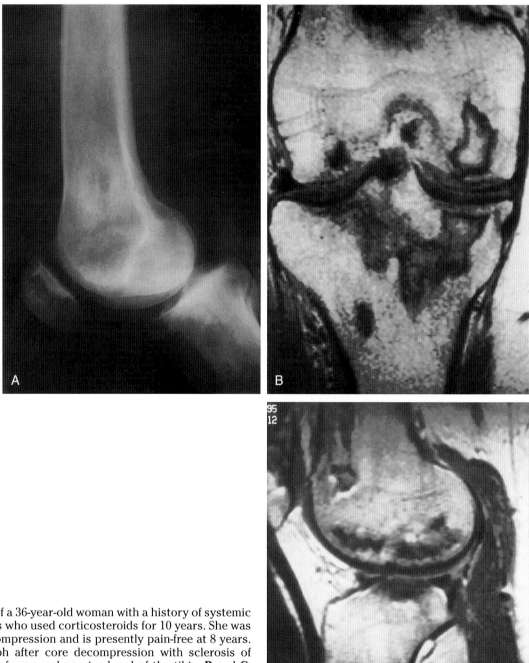

Figure 29–22. Knee of a 36-year-old woman with a history of systemic lupus erythematosus who used corticosteroids for 10 years. She was treated by core decompression and is presently pain-free at 8 years. **A,** Lateral radiograph after core decompression with sclerosis of the distal end of the femur and proximal end of the tibia. **B** and **C,** Magnetic resonance imaging scans with evidence of osteonecrosis.

slightly better outcomes for total knee arthroplasty in 31 knees (24 patients) with secondary osteonecrosis.[88] They still found that five knees (16%) required a revision procedure at a mean follow-up of 64 months. Survivorship was 84% at 5 years. In a recent report, Mont et al found that cemented implants with the use of auxiliary stems for bone stock loss led to excellent clinical and radiographic outcomes in 31 of 32 knee replacements (97%) at a mean follow-up of 9 years (range, 48 to 144 months).[69]

In summary, total knee arthroplasty with modern techniques and designs can be a successful procedure for patients with steroid-induced osteonecrosis.[63]

SUMMARY

Osteonecrosis of the knee denotes two distinct disorders: SPONK and secondary osteonecrosis, which can be clearly distinguished from each other by the age of the patient, condylar involvement, the incidence of bilateral involvement, and associated risk factors. Standard radiographs and MRI can clearly differentiate these diseases from other entities and can help plan treatment. Initial treatment is nonoperative, with various procedures (arthroscopic débridement, bone grafting, osteotomy, core

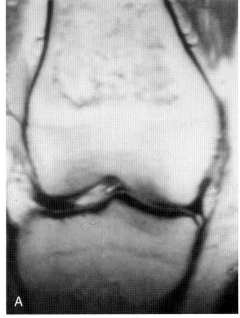
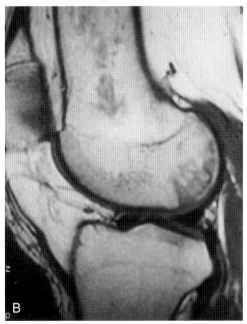

Figure 29–23. Knee of a 35-year-old woman with a history of ulcerative colitis, corticosteroid use, and right knee pain. **A**, Radiograph. **B**, Magnetic resonance imaging revealed osteonecrosis of the distal end of the femur and proximal end of the tibia.

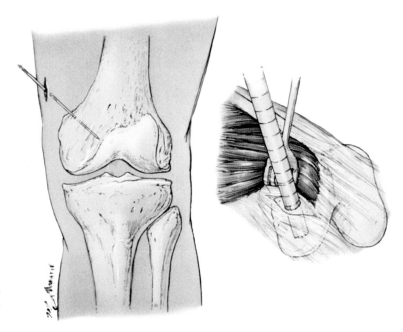

Figure 29–24. Schematic drawing depicting the technique of core decompression from the medial side of the knee.

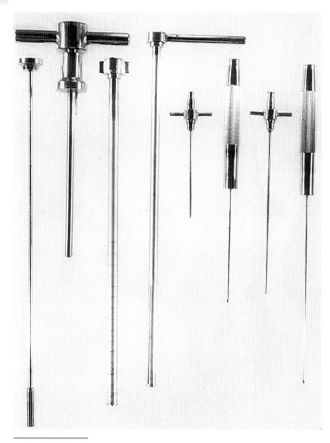

Figure 29–25. Michelle instrumentation used for core decompression. (Courtesy of RMS International, Toulouse, France.)

decompression) used in selected cases to forestall joint replacement. Unicondylar and tricompartmental knee arthroplasty have historically had results inferior to those in patients with other knee diagnoses. Present-day modern designs and techniques have led to improved results.

References

1. Abeles M, Urman JB, Rothfield N: Aseptic necrosis of bone in systemic lupus erythematosus: Relationship to corticosteroid therapy. Arch Intern Med 138:750, 1978.
2. Aglietti P, Insall JN, Buzzi R, et al: Idiopathic osteonecrosis of the knee. Etiology, prognosis and treatment. J Bone Joint Surg Br 65:588, 1983.
3. Ahlbäck S, Bauer GCH, Bohne WH: Spontaneous osteonecrosis of the knee. Arthritis Rheum 11:705, 1968.
4. Ahuja SC, Bullough PG: Osteonecrosis of the knee: A clinicopathological study in twenty-eight patients. J Bone Joint Surg Am 60:191, 1978.
5. Al-Rowaih A, Bjorkengren A, Egund N, et al: Size of osteonecrosis of the knee. Clin Orthop 287:68, 1993.
6. Al-Rowaih A, Lindstrand A, Bjorkengren A, et al: Osteonecrosis of the knee: Diagnosis and outcome in 40 patients. Acta Orthop Scand 62:19, 1991.
7. Arnoldi CC, Lemperg K, Linderholm H: Intraosseous hypertension and pain in the knee. J Bone Joint Surg Br 57:360, 1975.
8. Bayne O, Langer F, Pritzker KPH, et al: Osteochondral allografts in the treatment of osteonecrosis of the knee. Orthop Clin North Am 16:727, 1985.
9. Bergman NR, Rand JA: Total knee arthroplasty in osteonecrosis. Clin Orthop 273:77, 1991.
10. Bjorkengren AG, Al-Rowaih A, Linstrand A, et al: Spontaneous osteonecrosis of the knee: Value of MR imaging in determining prognosis. AJR Am J Roentgenol 154:331, 1990.
11. Bjorkman A, Burtscher IM, Svensson PJ, et al: Factor V Leiden and the prothrombin 20210A gene mutation: Osteonecrosis of the knee. Arch Orthop Trauma Surg 125:51, 2005.
12. Boettcher WG, Bonfiglio M, Hamilton HHG, et al: Non-traumatic necrosis of the femoral head, part I. Relation of altered hemostasis to etiology. J Bone Joint Surg Am 52:312, 1970.
13. Brahme SK, Fox JM, Ferkel RD: Osteonecrosis of the knee after arthroscopic surgery: Diagnosis with MR imaging. Radiology 178:851, 1991.
14. Burk DL Jr, Mitchell DG, Rifkin MD, et al: Recent advances in magnetic resonance imaging of the knee. Radiol Clin North Am 28:379, 1990.
15. Cruess RL: Steroid-induced osteonecrosis: A review. Can J Surg 24:567, 1981.
16. DeFalco RA, Ricci AR, Balduini FC: Osteonecrosis of the knee after arthroscopic meniscectomy and chondroplasty: A case report and literature review. Am J Sports Med 31:1013, 2003.
17. Delanois RE, Mont MA, Yoon TR, et al: Atraumatic osteonecrosis of the talus. J Bone Joint Surg Am 80:529, 1998.
18. Ecker ML, Lotke PA: Spontaneous osteonecrosis of the knee. J Am Acad Orthop Surg 2:173, 1994.
19. Ecker ML, Lotke PA: Osteonecrosis of the medial part of the tibial plateau. J Bone Joint Surg Am 77:596, 1995.
20. Encalada I, Richmond JC: Osteonecrosis after arthroscopic meniscectomy using radiofrequency. Arthroscopy 20:632, 2004.
21. Ficat RP: Aseptic necrosis of the femur head. Pathogenesis: The theory of circulation. Acta Orthop Belg 47:198, 1981.
22. Ficat RP: Idiopathic bone necrosis of the femoral head. Early diagnosis and treatment. J Bone Joint Surg Br 67:3, 1985.
23. Ficat RP, Arlet J: Functional investigation of bone under normal conditions. In Hungerford DS (ed): Ischemia and Necrosis of Bone. Baltimore, Williams & Wilkins, 1980, p 29.
24. Ficat RP, Arlet J: Necrosis of the femoral head. In Hungerford DS (ed): Ischemia and Necrosis of Bone. Baltimore, Williams & Wilkins, 1980, p 171.
25. Fink B, Schneider T, Braunstein S, et al: Holmium:YAG laser–induced aseptic bone necrosis of the femoral condyle. Arthroscopy 12:217, 1996.
26. Fisher DE: The role of fat embolism in the etiology of corticosteroid-induced avascular necrosis. Clin Orthop 130:68, 1978.
27. Flynn JM, Springfield DS, Mankin HJ: Osteoarticular allografts to treat distal femoral osteonecrosis. Clin Orthop 303:38, 1994.
28. Fukui N, Kurosawa H, Kawakami A, et al: Iliac bone graft for steroid-associated osteonecrosis of the femoral condyle. Clin Orthop 401:185-193, 2002.
29. Ganel A, Israeli A, Horoszowski H, et al: Osteochondral graft in the treatment of osteonecrosis of the femoral condyle. J Am Geriatr Soc 29:186, 1981.
30. Glueck CJ, Glueck HI, Welch M, et al: Familial idiopathic osteonecrosis mediated by familial hypofibrinolysis with high levels of plasminogen activator inhibitor. Thromb Haemost 71:195, 1994.
31. Greyson ND, Lotem MM, Gross AE, et al: Radionuclide evaluation of spontaneous femoral osteonecrosis. Radiology 142:729, 1982.
32. Gross AE, McKee NH, Pritzker KPH, et al: Reconstruction of skeletal deficits at the knee: A comprehensive osteochondral transplant program. Clin Orthop 179:96, 1983.
33. Gupta SM, Foster CR, Kayani N: Usefulness of SPECT in the early detection of avascular necrosis of the knee. Clin Nucl Med 12:99, 1987.
34. Havel PE, Ebraheim NA, Jackson WT: Steroid-induced bilateral avascular necrosis of the lateral femoral condyles. A case report. Clin Orthop 243:166, 1989.
35. Healy WL: Osteonecrosis of the knee detected only by magnetic resonance imaging. Orthopedics 14:703, 1991.
36. Hirota Y, Hirohata T, Fukuda K, et al: Association of alcohol intake, cigarette smoking and occupational report status with the risk of idiopathic osteonecrosis of the femoral head. Am J Epidemiol 137:530, 1993.
37. Houpt JB, Alpert B, Lotem M, et al: Spontaneous osteonecrosis of the medial tibial plateau. J Rheumatol 9:81, 1982.
38. Houpt JB, Pritzker KPH, Alpert B, et al: Natural history of spontaneous osteonecrosis of the knee (SPONK): A review. Semin Arthritis Rheum 13:212, 1983.

39. Hungerford DS: Pathogenetic considerations in ischemic necrosis of bone. Can J Surg 24:583, 1981.

40. Hungerford DS, Zizic TM: Alcoholism associated ischemic necrosis of the femoral head. Early diagnosis and treatment. Clin Orthop 130:144, 1978.

41. Hungerford DS, Zizic TM: The treatment of ischemic necrosis of bone in systemic lupus erythematosus. Medicine (Baltimore) 59:143, 1980.

42. Insall JN, Aglietti P, Bullough PG, et al: Osteonecrosis. In Insall JN, Windsor RE, Scott WN, et al (eds): Surgery of the Knee, 2nd ed. New York, Churchill-Livingstone, 1993, p 609.

43. Isono SS, Woolson ST, Schurman DJ: Total joint arthroplasty for steroid-induced osteonecrosis in cardiac transplant patients. Clin Orthop 217:201, 1987.

44. Jacobs MA, Loeb P, Hungerford DS: Core decompression of the distal femur in the treatment of avascular necrosis of the knee. J Bone Joint Surg Br 71:583, 1989.

45. Jones JP Jr: Etiology and pathogenesis of osteonecrosis. Semin Arthroplasty 2:160, 1991.

46. Kelman GJ, Williams GW, Colwell CW, et al: Steroid-related osteonecrosis of the knee. Two case reports and a literature review. Clin Orthop 257:171, 1990.

47. Kenzora JE, Glimcher MJ: Pathogenesis of idiopathic osteonecrosis: The ubiquitous crescent sign. Orthop Clin North Am 16:681, 1985.

48. Khanna AJ, Cosgarea AJ, Mont MA, et al: Magnetic resonance imaging of the knee. Current techniques and spectrum of disease. J Bone Joint Surg Am 83(Suppl 2):S128, 2001.

49. Koshino T: The treatment of spontaneous osteonecrosis of the knee by high tibial osteotomy with and without bone-grafting or drilling of the lesion. J Bone Joint Surg Am 64:47, 1982.

50. Koshino T, Okamoto R, Takamura K, et al: Arthroscopy in spontaneous osteonecrosis of the knee. Orthop Clin North Am 10:609, 1979.

51. Koshino T, Yushida T, Ara Y, et al: Fifteen to twenty-eight years' follow-up results of high tibial valgus osteotomy for osteoarthritic knees. Knee 11:439, 2004.

52. Kusayama T: Idiopathic osteonecrosis of the femoral condyle after meniscectomy. Tokai J Exp Clin Med 28:145, 2003.

53. La Prade RF, Noffsinger MA: Idiopathic osteonecrosis of the patella: An unusual cause of pain in the knee. A case report. J Bone Joint Surg Am 72:1414, 1990.

54. Lotke PA, Abend JA, Ecker ML: The treatment of osteonecrosis of the medial femoral condyle. Clin Orthop 171:109, 1982.

55. Lotke PA, Ecker ML: Osteonecrosis-like syndrome of the medial tibial plateau. Clin Orthop 176:148, 1983.

56. Lotke PA, Ecker ML: Current concepts review. Osteonecrosis of the knee. J Bone Joint Surg Am 70:470, 1988.

57. Lotke PA, Nelson CL, Lonner JH: Spontaneous osteonecrosis of the knee: Tibial plateaus. Orthop Clin North Am 35:365-370, 2004.

58. Mahood J, Bogoch E, Urowitz M, et al: Osteonecrosis of the knee in systemic lupus erythematosus. J Bone Joint Surg Br 72:541, 1990.

59. Mankin HJ: Non-traumatic necrosis of bone (osteonecrosis). N Engl J Med 326:1473, 1991.

60. Marmor L: Unicompartmental arthroplasty for osteonecrosis of the knee joint. Clin Orthop 294:247, 1993.

61. McCarthy EF, Frassica FJ: Pathology of Bone and Joint Disorders with Clinical and Radiographic Correlation. Philadelphia, WB Saunders, 1998, p 135.

62. Miller GK, Maylahn DS, Drennan DB: The treatment of idiopathic osteonecrosis of the medial femoral condyle with arthroscopic débridement. Arthroscopy 2:21, 1986.

63. Mont MA, Baumgarten KM, Rifai A, et al: Atraumatic osteonecrosis of the knee. J Bone Joint Surg Am 82:1279, 2000.

64. Mont M, Fairbank A, Petri M, et al: Core decompression for osteonecrosis of the femoral head in systemic lupus erythematosus. Clin Orthop 334:91, 1997.

65. Mont MA, Hungerford DS: Non-traumatic avascular necrosis of the femoral head. J Bone Joint Surg Am 77:459, 1995.

66. Mont MA, Hungerford DS: Osteonecrosis of the shoulder, knee, and ankle. In Urbaniak JR, Jones JP (eds): Osteonecrosis: Etiology, Diagnosis, and Treatment. Rosemont, IL, American Academy of Orthopaedic Surgeons, 1997, p 429.

67. Mont MA, Jones LC, Einhorn TA, et al: Osteonecrosis of the femoral head: Potential treatment with growth and differentiation factors. Clin Orthop 355:S314, 1998.

68. Mont MA, Maar DC, Urquhart M, et al: Results of core decompression for avascular necrosis of the humeral head. Average 7.4 year follow-up. J Bone Joint Surg Br 75:785, 1993.

69. Mont MA, Rifai A, Baumgarten KM, et al: Total knee arthroplasty for osteonecrosis. J Bone Joint Surg Am 84:599, 2002.

70. Mont MA, Tomek IM, Hungerford DS: Core decompression for avascular necrosis of the distal femur: Long-term followup. Clin Orthop 334:124, 1997.

71. Motohashi M, Morii T, Koshino T: Clinical course and roentgenographic changes of osteonecrosis in the femoral condyle under conservative treatment. Clin Orthop 266:156, 1991.

72. Muheim G, Bohne WH: Prognosis in spontaneous osteonecrosis of the knee: Investigation by radionuclide scintimetry and radiography. J Bone Joint Surg Br 52:605, 1970.

73. Muscolo DL, Costa-Paz M, Makino A, et al: Osteonecrosis of the knee following arthroscopic meniscectomy in patients over 50 years old. Arthroscopy 12:273, 1996.

74. Myers MH, Akeson W, Convery FR: Resurfacing the knee with fresh osteochondral allografts. J Bone Joint Surg Am 71:704, 1989.

75. Narvaez JA, Narvaez J, De Lama E, Sanchez A: Spontaneous osteonecrosis of the knee associated with tibial plateau and femoral condyle insufficiency stress fracture. Eur Radiol 13:1843, 2003.

76. Ochi M, Kimori K, Sumen Y, et al: A case of steroid-induced osteonecrosis of femoral condyle treated surgically. Clin Orthop 312:226, 1995.

77. Ono K, Sugioka Y: Epidemiology and risk factors in avascular necrosis of the femoral head. In Schoutens A (ed): Bone Circulation and Vascularization in Normal and Pathological Conditions. Reading, MA, Plenum, 1993, p 241.

78. Pollack MS, Dalinka MK, Kressel HY, et al: Magnetic resonance imaging in the evaluation of suspected osteonecrosis of the knee. Skeletal Radiol 16:121, 1987.

79. Radke S, Wollmerstedt N, Bischoff A, Eulert J: Knee arthroplasty for spontaneous osteonecrosis of the knee: Unicompartmental vs. bicompartmental knee arthroplasty. Knee Surg Sports Traumatol Arthrosc 13:158-162, 2005.

80. Ramnath RR, Kattapuram SV: MR appearance of SONK-like subchrondral abnormalities in the adult knee: SONK redefined. Skeletal Radiol 33:575-581, 2004.

81. Ritter MA, Eizember LE, Keating EM, et al: The survival of total knee arthroplasty in patients with osteonecrosis of the medial condyle. Clin Orthop 267:108, 1991.

82. Rozbruch SR, Wickiewicz TL, Di Carlo EF, et al: Osteonecrosis of the knee following arthroscopic laser meniscectomy. Arthroscopy 12:245, 1996.

83. Rozing PM, Insall J, Bohne WH: Spontaneous osteonecrosis of the knee. J Bone Joint Surg Am 62:2, 1980.

84. Santori N, Condello V, Adriani E, et al: Osteonecrosis after arthroscopic medial meniscectomy. Arthroscopy 11:220, 1995.

85. Sasaki T, Yagi T, Monji J, et al: Steroid-induced osteonecrosis of the femoral condyle: A clinical study of eighteen knees in ten patients. J Jpn Orthop Assoc 60:361, 1986.

86. Satku K, Kumar VP, Chong SM, Thambyah A: The natural history of spontaneous osteonecrosis of the medial tibial plateau. J Bone Joint Surg Br 85:983, 2003.

87. Schneider R, Goldman A, Pellicci P, et al: Transient regional osteoporosis of the knee. Presented at the 57th Annual Meeting of the American Academy of Orthopaedic Surgeons, 1990, New Orleans, p 96.

88. Seldes RM, Ran V, Duffy G, et al: Total knee arthroplasty for steroid-induced osteonecrosis. J Arthroplasty 14:533, 1999.

89. Solomon L: Idiopathic necrosis of the femoral head: Pathogenesis and treatment. Can J Surg 24:573, 1981.

90. Soucacos PN, Beris AE, Xenakis TH, et al: Knee osteonecrosis: Distinguishing features and differential diagnosis. In Urbaniak JR, Jones JP (eds): Osteonecrosis: Etiology, Diagnosis, and Treatment. Rosemont, IL, American Academy of Orthopaedic Surgeons, 1997, p 413.

91. Soucacos PN, Johnson EO, Soultanis K, et al: Diagnosis and management of the osteonecrotic triad of the knee. Orthop Clin North Am 35:371, 2004.

92. Soucacos PN, Xenakis TH, Beris AE, et al: Idiopathic osteonecrosis of the medial femoral condyle. Classification and treatment. Clin Orthop 341:82, 1997.

93. Stiehl JB, Erickson SJ: Magnetic resonance imagining in systemic corticosteroid-induced osteonecrosis of the knee. Am J Knee Surg 4:131, 1991.

94. Wang GJ, Lennox DW, Reger SI, et al: Cortisone-induced intrafemoral head pressure change and its response to a drilling decompression method. Clin Orthop 159:274, 1981.

95. Wang GJ, Mogra DB, Richemer WG, et al: Cortisone-induced bone changes and its response to lipid clearing agents. Clin Orthop 130:81, 1978.

96. Wang GJ, Sweet DE, Reger SI, et al: Fat-cell changes as a mechanism of avascular necrosis of the femoral head in cortisone-treated rabbits. J Bone Joint Surg Am 59:729, 1977.

97. Wiedel JD: Arthroscopy in steroid-induced osteonecrosis of the knee. Arthroscopy 1:68, 1985.

98. Zanetti M, Romero J, Danabacher MA, Hodler J: Osteonecrosis diagnosed on MR images of the knee. Relationship to reduced bone mineral density determined by high resolution peripheral quantitative CT. Acta Radiol 44:525, 2003.

99. Zizic TM, Hungerford DS: Avascular necrosis of bone. In Kelley WN, Harris ED, Ruddy S, et al (eds): Textbook of Rheumatology. Philadelphia, WB Saunders, 1985, p 1689.

CHAPTER 30

Healing of Knee Menisci

Matthew J. Crawford • Julie A. Dodds • Steven P. Arnoczky

Muscle, ligaments, and menisci complement the bony architecture of the knee and allow for normal kinematics throughout the range of motion. Functionally, the menisci serve to guide the femoral condyles in their articulation with the tibial plateau, distribute the weight more evenly, and act as shock absorbers. Structural damage to the menisci results in altered joint kinematics and joint forces, ultimately resulting in degenerative changes in the knee. Therefore, it is imperative to preserve the homeostatic balance within the knee through preservation of the meniscus.

It is the purpose of this chapter to review the basic science aspects of meniscal healing and meniscal repair techniques to provide a sound, fundamental basis for the care and treatment of meniscal injuries.

MENISCAL STRUCTURE AND FUNCTION

The menisci of the knee are C-shaped wedges of fibrocartilage interposed between the condyles of the femur and tibia. They are actually extensions of the tibia that serve to deepen the articular surfaces of the tibial plateau to better accommodate the condyles of the femur. The peripheral border of each meniscus is thick and convex and attached to the joint capsule, whereas the inner border tapers to a thin, free edge.[127] The proximal surfaces of the menisci are concave and in contact with the condyles of the femur; their distal surfaces are flat and rest on the tibial plateau (Fig. 30–1).

The medial meniscus is somewhat semicircular in form, approximately 3.5 cm in length and considerably wider posteriorly than anteriorly. The anterior horn of the medial meniscus is attached to the tibial plateau in the area of the anterior intercondylar fossa, anterior to the anterior cruciate ligament (ACL) (Fig. 30–2). The posterior fibers of the anterior horn merge with the transverse ligament, which connects the anterior horns of the medial and lateral menisci.[127] The posterior horn of the medial meniscus is firmly attached to the posterior intercondylar fossa of the tibia between the attachments of the lateral meniscus and the posterior cruciate ligament. The periphery of the medial meniscus is attached to the joint capsule throughout its length. The tibial portion of the capsular attachment is referred to as the coronary ligament. At its midpoint, the medial meniscus is more firmly attached to the femur and tibia through a condensation in the joint capsule known as the deep medial collateral ligament.[127]

The lateral meniscus is more circular in shape and covers a larger percentage of the articular surface of the tibial plateau than the medial meniscus does. The anterior and posterior horns are approximately the same width (Fig. 30–2). The anterior horn of the lateral meniscus is attached to the tibia anterior to the intercondylar eminence and posterior to the attachment of the ACL, with which it partially blends.[127] The posterior horn of the lateral meniscus is attached posterior to the intercondylar eminence of the tibia, anterior to the posterior horn of the medial meniscus. In addition to this posterior attachment to the tibia, two ligaments may run from the posterior horn of the lateral meniscus to the medial femoral condyle, passing either in front of or behind the origin of the posterior cruciate ligament.[127] These attachments are known as the anterior meniscofemoral ligament (ligament of Humphrey) and the posterior meniscofemoral ligament (ligament of Wrisberg). Although there is no attachment of the lateral meniscus to the lateral collateral ligament, it has a loose peripheral attachment to the joint capsule.[127]

Histologically, the meniscus is a fibrocartilaginous tissue composed primarily of an interlacing network of collagen fibers interposed with cells (Fig. 30–3).[7] The predominant type of collagen in the meniscus is type I, but types II, III, and V are present as well.[88] Although other components, such as proteoglycans, glycoproteins, and water, also contribute to the makeup of the extracellular matrix of the meniscus, it is the specific orientation of the collagen fibers that appears to be most directly related to the function of the meniscus.[88] Even though the principal orientation of the collagen fibers is circumferential, a few small, radially disposed fibers appear on both the femoral and tibial surfaces of the menisci, as well as within the substance of the tissue.[17] It is theorized that these radial fibers act as "ties" to provide structural rigidity and help resist longitudinal splitting of the menisci as a result of overcompression (Fig. 30–4).[17] Subsequent light and electron microscopic examination of the menisci has revealed three different collagen framework layers: a superficial layer composed of a network of fine fibrils woven into a mesh-like matrix; a surface layer just beneath the superficial layer composed, in part, of irregularly aligned collagen bundles; and a middle layer in which the collagen fibers are larger, coarser, and oriented in a parallel, circumferential direction (Fig. 30–5).[11,131] It is this middle layer that allows the meniscus to resist tensile forces and function as a transmitter of load across the knee joint.[11,17,131]

The function of the menisci may be clinically inferred by the degenerative changes that accompany their

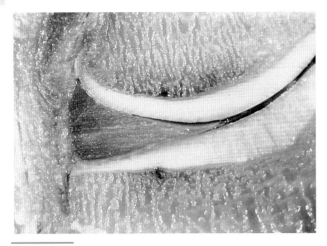

Figure 30–1. Frontal section of the medial compartment of a human knee illustrating the articulation of the menisci with the condyles of the femur and tibia. (From Warren R, Arnoczky SP, Wickiewicz TL: Anatomy of the knee. In Nicholas JA, Hershman EB [eds]: The Lower Extremity and Spine in Sports Medicine. St Louis, CV Mosby, 1986, p 657.)

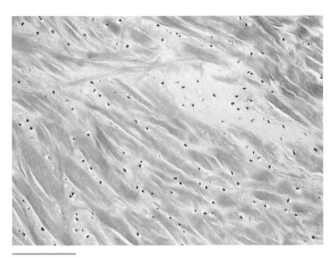

Figure 30–3. Photomicrograph of a longitudinal section of human meniscus showing the histological appearance of meniscal fibrocartilage (hematoxylin-eosin, ×100).

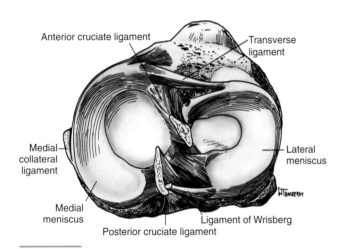

Figure 30–2. Human tibial plateau showing the relative size and attachments of the medial and lateral menisci. (From Warren R, Arnoczky SP, Wickiewicz TL: Anatomy of the knee. In Nicholas JA, Hershman EB [eds]: The Lower Extremity and Spine in Sports Medicine. St Louis, CV Mosby, 1986, p 657.)

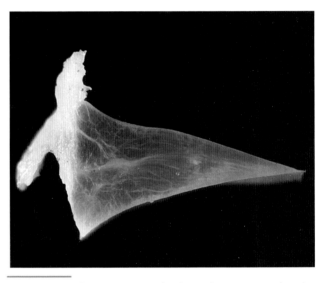

Figure 30–4. Cross-section of a lateral meniscus showing the radial orientation of fibrous ties within the substance of the meniscus. (From Arnoczky SP, Torzilli PA: The biology of cartilage. In Hunter LY, Funk FJ Jr [eds]: Rehabilitation of the Injured Knee. St Louis, CV Mosby, 1984, p 148.)

removal. Fairbank[40] described radiographic changes after meniscectomy that included narrowing of the joint space, flattening of the femoral condyle, and the formation of osteophytes. These changes were attributed to loss of the weightbearing function of the meniscus. Biomechanical studies have demonstrated that at least 50% of the compressive load of the knee joint is transmitted through the meniscus in extension and that approximately 85% of the load is transmitted in 90 degrees of flexion.[1] In a meniscectomized knee, the contact area is reduced approximately 50%.[1,45] This reduction significantly increases the load per unit area and results in articular damage and degeneration. Partial meniscectomy has also been shown to significantly increase contact pressure.[12] In an experi-

mental study, resection of as little as 15% to 34% of the meniscus increased contact pressure by more than 350%.[107] Thus, even partial meniscectomy does not appear to be a benign procedure.[3,24,26,27,41,68,79,104]

Another proposed function of the meniscus is that of shock absorption. By examining the compressive load-deformation response of normal and meniscectomized knees, it has been suggested that the viscoelastic menisci may function to attenuate the intermittent shock waves generated by impulse loading of the knee during gait.[126] Studies have shown that a normal knee has a shock-absorbing capacity about 20% higher than that of knees that have undergone meniscectomy.[126] Because the inability of a joint system to absorb shock has been implicated

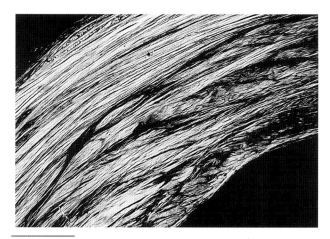

Figure 30–5. Photomicrograph of a longitudinal section of a meniscus under polarized light demonstrating the orientation of the coarse, deep, circumferentially oriented collagen fibers.

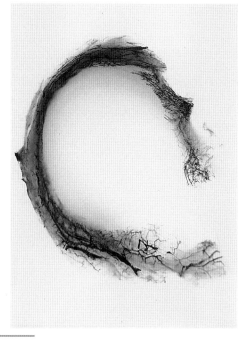

Figure 30–6. Superior aspect of a medial meniscus after vascular perfusion with India ink and tissue clearing with a modified Spalteholz technique. Note the vascularity at the periphery of the meniscus, as well as at the anterior and posterior horn attachments. (From Arnoczky SP, Warren RF: Microvasculature of the human meniscus. Am J Sports Med 10:90-95, 1982.)

in the development of osteoarthritis,[99] the shock absorption mechanism would appear to play a role in maintaining the health of the knee joint.

In addition to the role of the meniscus in load transmission and shock absorption, the menisci are thought to contribute to knee joint stability.[81,86] Although meniscectomy alone may not significantly increase joint instability, several studies have shown that meniscectomy in association with ACL insufficiency significantly increases anterior laxity of the knee.[2,81,96]

Because the menisci serve to increase congruity between the condyles of the femur and tibia, they contribute significantly to overall joint conformity. Posterior translation of the menisci (lateral greater than medial) during knee flexion has been demonstrated in magnetic resonance imaging studies.[69,120] Additionally, the anterior and posterior translation of the menisci during flexion and extension is hypothesized to protect the articular surfaces from injury.[70]

Finally, the menisci have been suggested as being proprioceptive structures that provide a feedback mechanism for joint position sense. This has been inferred from the observation of type I and type II nerve endings in the anterior and posterior horns of the meniscus.[47,71,130,135]

In summary, the proposed functions of the menisci include load bearing, shock absorption, joint stability, lubrication, and proprioception. Loss of the meniscus, partially or totally, significantly alters these functions and predisposes the joint to degenerative changes. Because acute, traumatic tears of the meniscus usually occur in young (13- to 40-year-old), active individuals, the need to preserve the meniscus, and thus minimize these degenerative changes, is of paramount importance.[7] The development of techniques to save the meniscus has all but replaced traditional total meniscectomy in the treatment of many meniscal lesions. Although partial meniscectomy may be the only option for some central avascular tears, research into new techniques of meniscal repair may eliminate even partial meniscectomy and the undesirable consequences of loss of this important structure.

BASIC SCIENCE OF MENISCAL REPAIR

Thomas Annandale was credited with the first surgical repair of a torn meniscus in 1883.[5] It was not until 1936, when King published his classic experiment on meniscus healing in dogs, that the actual biological limitations of meniscus healing were set forth. King demonstrated that for meniscus lesions to heal, they must communicate with the peripheral blood supply.[74] Enhancing vascularity at or near the site of meniscal injury has remained a major focus in the techniques of surgical repair. In addition, advances in cellular and molecular biology now allow researchers to investigate the role of specific growth factors and cytokines in the cellular response to injury. Further application of these findings will continue to provide for means of enhancing meniscal repair.

Vascular Anatomy of the Meniscus

The vascular supply to the medial and lateral menisci of the knee originates predominantly from the medial and lateral genicular arteries (inferior and superior branches).[8] Branches from these vessels give rise to a perimeniscal capillary plexus within the synovial and capsular tissues of the knee joint. The plexus is an arborizing network of vessels that supply the peripheral border of the meniscus about its attachment to the joint capsule (Figs. 30–6 and

30–7).[35] These perimeniscal vessels are oriented in a predominantly circumferential pattern, with radial branches being directed toward the center of the joint (Fig. 30–8). Anatomic studies have shown that the degree of peripheral vascular penetration is 10% to 30% of the width of the medial meniscus and 10% to 25% of the width of the lateral meniscus.[8] The middle genicular artery, along with a few terminal branches of the medial and lateral genicular vessels, also supplies vessels to the menisci through the vascular synovial covering of the anterior and posterior horn attachments.[8] These synovial vessels penetrate the horn attachments and give rise to smaller vessels that enter the meniscal horns for a short distance and end in terminal capillary loops.

A small reflection of the vascular synovial tissue is also present throughout the peripheral attachment of the medial and lateral menisci on the femoral and tibial articular surfaces.[8] This "synovial fringe" extends for a short distance over the peripheral surfaces of the meniscus and contains small, terminally looped vessels. Although the synovial fringe is adherent to the articular surfaces of the menisci, it does not contribute vessels to the meniscus per se.[8] The clinical significance of these fringe vessels lies in their potential contribution to the reparative response of the meniscus, as seen in "synovial abrasion" techniques.*

Vascular Response to Injury

The vascular supply of the meniscus is the essential element in determining its potential for repair. This blood supply must have the ability to support the inflammatory response characteristic of wound repair. Clinical and experimental observations have demonstrated that the peripheral meniscal blood supply is capable of producing a reparative response similar to that in other connective tissue.†

After injury within the peripheral vascular zone, a fibrin clot forms that is rich in inflammatory cells. Vessels from the perimeniscal capillary plexus proliferate through this fibrin "scaffold," accompanied by the proliferation of undifferentiated mesenchymal cells.[9] Eventually, the lesion is filled with a cellular, fibrovascular granulation tissue that "glues" the wound edges together and appears to be continuous with the adjacent normal meniscal fibrocartilage.[9,20] The initial strength of this repair tissue is minimal in comparison to a normal meniscus. Increased collagen synthesis within the granulation tissue slowly results in a fibrous scar (Fig. 30–9).

Experimental studies have shown that radial lesions of the meniscus that extend to the synovium are completely healed with fibrovascular scar tissue by 10 weeks (Fig. 30–10).[9,20] Modulation of this scar into normal-appearing fibrocartilage, however, requires several months.[20] Further study is required to delineate the biomechanical properties at each stage of the repair process.

The ability of meniscal lesions to heal has provided the rationale for the repair of peripheral meniscal injuries, and many reports have demonstrated excellent results after primary repair of peripheral meniscal injuries.[23,30-32,51,59,85,102,106,116] Follow-up examination of these peripheral repairs has revealed a process of repair similar to that noted in experimental models.

When examining injured menisci for potential repair, lesions are often classified by the location of the tear relative to the blood supply of the meniscus and the "vascular appearance" of the peripheral and central surfaces of the tear (Fig. 30–8).[6] The so-called *red-red* tear (periph-

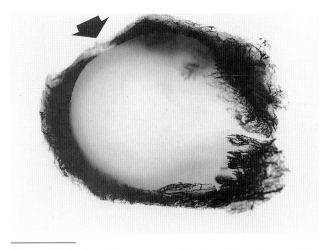

Figure 30–7. Superior aspect of a lateral meniscus after vascular perfusion with India ink and tissue clearing with a modified Spalteholz technique. Note the absence of vascularity at the posterior lateral aspect of the meniscus (*arrow*). This is adjacent to the popliteal hiatus. (From Arnoczky SP, Warren RF: Microvasculature of the human meniscus. Am J Sports Med 10:90-95, 1982.)

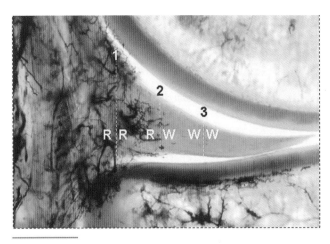

Figure 30–8. A 5-mm-thick frontal section of the medial compartment of a human knee (Spalteholz preparation). Branching radial vessels from the perimeniscal capillary plexus penetrate the peripheral border of the medial meniscus. RR, red-red zone; RW, red-white zone; WW, white-white zone. (From Arnoczky SP, Warren RF: Microvasculature of the human meniscus. Am J Sports Med 10:90-95, 1982.)

*References 13, 22, 34, 52, 55-59, 61, 62, 76, 84, 89, 90, 94, 95, 100, 105, 111, 112, 117, 119, 122.
†References 6, 9, 20, 23, 28-30, 51, 54, 59, 66, 75, 85, 102, 106, 116.

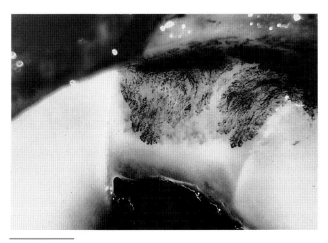

Figure 30–9. A meniscus 6 weeks after the creation of a radial lesion. Fibrovascular scar tissue has filled the defect, and vascular proliferation from the synovial fringe can be seen. (From Arnoczky SP, Warren RF: The microvasculature of the meniscus and its response to injury: An experimental study in the dog. Am J Sports Med 11:131-141, 1983.)

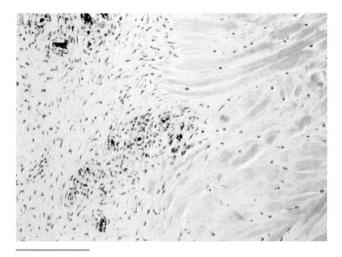

Figure 30–10. Photomicrograph of the junction of the meniscus and fibrovascular repair tissue at 10 weeks (hematoxylin-eosin, ×100). (From Arnoczky SP, Warren RF: The microvasculature of the meniscus and its response to injury: An experimental study in the dog. Am J Sports Med 11:131-141, 1983.)

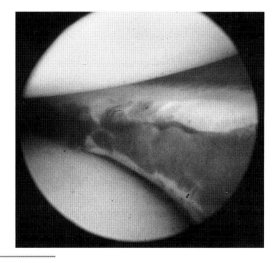

Figure 30–11. Arthroscopic view of a peripheral tear in a human meniscus. Note the vascular granulation tissue present at the margin of the lesion. This is classified as a red-white tear. Also note the proliferation of the synovial fringe over the femoral surface of the meniscus. (From Arnoczky SP, Torzilli PA: The biology of cartilage. In Hunter LY, Funk FJ Jr [eds]: Rehabilitation of the Injured Knee. St Louis, CV Mosby, 1984, p 148.)

Cellular Response to Injury

The ability of fibrochondrocytes within a meniscus to mount a reparative response is dependent in part on its cellular activity. Cytokines and growth factors present during the inflammatory response to injury may promote meniscal healing through enhancement of cell migration, cell division, and the production of extracellular matrix. Although no specific growth factor has been shown to enhance meniscus healing, researchers are beginning to identify how the meniscal fibrochondrocyte responds to various growth factors.[14,25,80,82,83,115,128] Meniscal repair augmentation methods such as fibrin clot and platelet-rich plasma (PRP) are based on the concept that growth factors have a positive impact on meniscal healing. Understanding which growth factors positively affect the healing potential of the meniscal fibrochondrocyte matrix will undoubtedly provide future strategies for treating meniscal injuries.

Indications for Meniscal Repair

As described earlier, the menisci perform several critical functions in the knee. For this reason, it is essential to try to preserve the meniscus via repair whenever feasible. Although it is most critical to perform meniscal repair on young patients in an attempt to decrease the eventual articular cartilage wear of a meniscectomized knee, meniscal repair can also be successful in older patients.[21] Well-vascularized longitudinal red-red tears and red-white tears are ideal for repair and also have the highest rate of healing.[21] Stable longitudinal tears (<1 cm in length) and partial-thickness tears often remain asymptomatic or heal

eral capsular detachment) has a functional blood supply to the capsular and meniscal side of the lesion and obviously has the best prognosis for healing. *Red-white* tears (meniscus tears through the peripheral vascular zone) have an active peripheral blood supply; however, the central (inner) surface of the lesion is devoid of functioning vessels (Fig. 30–11). These lesions have sufficient vascularity to heal by the aforementioned fibrovascular proliferation. *White-white* tears (meniscus lesions completely in the avascular zone) are without blood supply and theoretically cannot heal.[6] However, as will be discussed later, specific meniscal repair enhancement techniques have been developed to address tears in the white-white zone.

without suturing.[111] Even though degenerative tears and radial tears can also be repaired, the function of a repaired meniscus has yet to be proved.

The onset of degenerative change has been linked to the amount of meniscus removed.[3] Large bucket handle tears as seen in young, active patients would require a large portion of the meniscus to be removed if not repaired. In these younger patients, meniscal repair is often extended into the white-white (avascular) zone by using the vascular enhancement techniques that will be discussed later. A poorer prognosis in a meniscectomized knee has also been associated with varus alignment[18,41] and ACL deficiency,[18] so meniscal repair should likewise be considered in these situations, when possible. In addition, decreased healing rates are seen in ACL-deficient knees,[91,118] so any instability of the knee should also be addressed.

ENHANCEMENT OF MENISCAL REPAIR

The desire to preserve meniscal tissue has led to efforts to extend the region of viable meniscal repair to the central, avascular portion of the meniscus (white-white tears).[6] Experimental and clinical observations have shown that these lesions are incapable of healing under usual circumstances and have provided the rationale for partial meniscectomy.[8,75] In an effort to extend the level of repair into these avascular areas, techniques have been developed to provide vascularity to these white-white tears, as well as enhance the repair of red-white tears. Such techniques include débridement, creation of vascular access channels,[9,48] trephination, use of synovial pedicles, and synovial abrasion.[59] The use of fibrin clot and PRP products to improve meniscal healing will also be addressed.

Débridement

Débridement of devitalized or degenerative meniscal tissue at the repair site may expose a bleeding surface on at least one side of the tear. In theory, a white-white tear immediately adjacent to the peripheral vasculature can be débrided to yield a red-white tear, but extensive removal of tissue from either surface of the lesion could change the cross-sectional geometry of the meniscus and thus alter its mechanical function and create a critical gap too large to bridge with healing tissue.[15] Although no hard and fast rule exists regarding the amount of tissue that can be safely excised to expose a bleeding bed, débridement is usually limited to the most superficial tissue covering the wound surface.[95]

Vascular Access Channels and Trephination

Creation of vascular access channels (VACs) was one of the early techniques used to extend the vascular response into the avascular zone of the meniscus.[8,19,43,59] The premise of this technique is to create full-thickness channels connecting the avascular lesion to the peripheral vasculature of the meniscus. Experimental studies in animals demonstrated that lesions in the avascular portion of the meniscus, when connected to the peripheral vasculature by means of a full-thickness VAC, healed through the proliferation of fibrovascular scar tissue from the VAC into the tear (Figs. 30–12 and 30–13). VACs can allow for an extensive influx of vessels into a white-white tear, but they also cut across the predominately circumferential orientation of the collagen fibers of the meniscus. This disruption in collagen architecture may adversely affect the function of the meniscus, especially if the VAC is carried out through the peripheral rim of the meniscus. Consequently, the original VAC technique has not been used extensively in the clinical situation.

The technique of trephination was introduced as a means of creating a pathway for vascular migration without imparting significant damage to the collagen architecture of the meniscus.[7,42,101] In this procedure, a series of horizontally oriented trephinations are made with

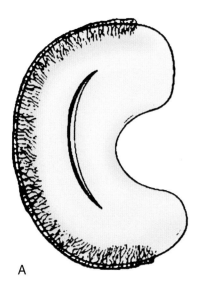
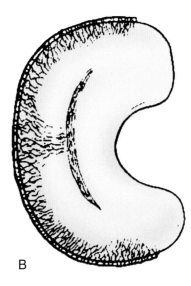

A   B

Figure 30–12. Schematic drawing showing the concept of connecting a lesion in the avascular portion of the meniscus with the peripheral blood supply through the use of a vascular access channel. **A**, Tear in an avascular zone. **B**, Vascular proliferation through an access channel. (From Arnoczky SP, Warren RF: The microvasculature of the meniscus and its response to injury: An experimental study in the dog. Am J Sports Med 11:131-141, 1983.)

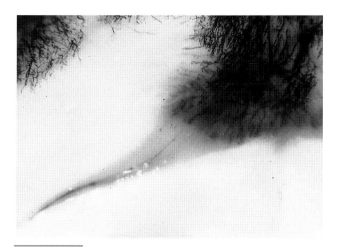

Figure 30–13. India ink–perfused medial meniscus 4 weeks after longitudinal incision and creation of a vascular access channel. Vessels progress within the fibrin clot in the anterior limb of the longitudinal lesion. (From Arnoczky SP, Warren RF: The microvasculature of the meniscus and its response to injury: An experimental study in the dog. Am J Sports Med 11:131-141, 1983.)

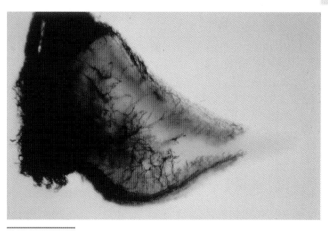

Figure 30–14. Cross-section through the fibrovascular scar pictured in Figure 30–9 showing the vascular pannus of the synovial fringe over the femoral and tibial surfaces. (From Arnoczky SP, Warren RF: The microvasculature of the meniscus and its response to injury: An experimental study in the dog. Am J Sports Med 11:131-141, 1983.)

a hypodermic needle (18-gauge or larger) through the peripheral aspect of the meniscal rim to produce a series of bleeding puncture sites, which provide an avenue for vascular ingrowth. This modification of the VAC technique minimizes the damage done to the collagen architecture of the meniscus but still allows the influx of a vascular response. Initially developed in an animal model,[133,134] clinical application of this technique has been described with and without the use of sutures. In the first clinical report of trephination, this technique was used to treat incomplete lesions in the peripheral and middle third of the meniscus.[43] Although a 90% success rate was reported in this series, there was no control group with which to compare the specific efficacy of the technique. More recently, controlled studies have found trephination alone to be successful in treating stable meniscal lesions,[15,111,112] as well as a means of augmenting traditional suture repair.[132]

Synovial Pedicles (Flaps)

An additional approach to extend the vascular supply to an avascular meniscal tear involves the use of a synovial pedicle or flap. In this technique, a pedicle of the highly vascular synovial tissue immediately adjacent to the peripheral attachment of the meniscus is rotated into the avascular lesion and sutured in place.[46,48,49,53,73,77,108,113,125] Laboratory animal models have demonstrated that both free synovial grafts[108,113] and vascularized synovial flaps[46,48,49,73,77,127] provide a sufficient stimulus for repair of meniscal tears in the avascular region. Although animal experiments using this technique suggest excellent potential for augmenting repairs in the white-white zone of the human meniscus, there is a paucity of clinical

research in this area, possibly because of the technical difficulties in adapting synovial pedicle use to an arthroscopic approach.

Synovial Abrasion

During the normal repair process of peripheral lesions, a vascular pannus develops from the synovial fringe and extends over the femoral and tibial surfaces of the meniscus (see Fig. 30–9). The combination of this vascular response with the peripheral meniscal blood supply provides support for the repair process (Fig. 30–14). Because the vascular pannus observed in the repair process is often extensive, it was theorized that stimulation of the synovial fringe could accentuate this response and help extend it into avascular or marginally vascularized areas.[7,59,60,66] To perform synovial abrasion, the synovial fringe of the femoral and tibial surfaces of the meniscus is abraded with a rasp to stimulate a proliferative response (Figs. 30–15 and 30–16). The ability of synovial abrasion to enhance the healing potential of tears in avascular areas of the meniscus has been demonstrated in several animal models.[94,100] Furthermore, cytokine induction has been shown after rasping of the parameniscal synovium in the rabbit, thereby providing the physiological mechanism to explain the enhanced vascular response.[93] Clinical application of synovial abrasion alone, as well as in conjunction with other enhancement techniques (including trephination and fibrin clot), has been shown to be effective in treating stable or partial-thickness meniscal tears.[57,59,112,117,119,122] Additionally, the efficacy of synovial abrasion and the simplicity of the surgical technique have led to recommendations for its use in augmenting suture repairs.[13,33,57,62,95,105]

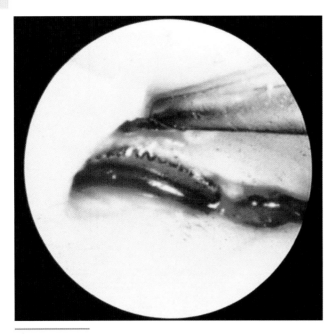

Figure 30–15. Arthroscopic photograph demonstrating abrasion of the synovial fringe on the surface of the meniscus with a rasp. (Courtesy of Dr. Charles Henning.)

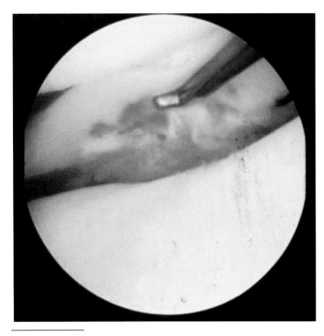

Figure 30–16. Arthroscopic photograph taken 8 weeks after synovial abrasion demonstrating a vascular pannus extending into a white-white tear. (Courtesy of Dr. Charles Henning.)

Marrow-Stimulating Techniques

Excellent rates of meniscal healing have been observed when meniscal repair is performed simultaneously with ACL reconstruction.[20,22,30,51,67,78,92,109-112] Cannon and Vittori found that meniscal healing rates improved from 53% to 93% when the repair was performed in conjunc-

tion with ACL reconstruction.[22] Shelbourne and Heinrich's long-term follow-up of lateral meniscal tears left in situ at time of ACL reconstruction demonstrated 96% normal or near-normal results.[111] These clinical findings suggest that blood and marrow elements may produce a milieu bathing the healing meniscus, thus providing essential mitogenic and chemotactic elements. Assuming that the cytokines and growth factors in the blood and marrow elements introduced into the knee after notchplasty in ACL reconstruction are responsible for the improved repair rates, there would be a theoretical advantage to reproducing the presence of blood and marrow elements during meniscal repair in an ACL-intact knee. Microfracture of the intercondylar notch has been proposed as a means of recreating the hemarthrosis present after ACL reconstruction in the hope of improving meniscal repair outcomes.[44] However, the clinical results of microfracture as a stimulus to enhance meniscal repair have not been documented.

Fibrin Clot

Several clinical studies have documented improved success rates for meniscal repair when they are associated with ACL reconstruction.[20,22,30,51,67,78,92] Although the precise reason for this improvement is unclear, one intriguing explanation is the possibility that the increased hemarthrosis associated with ACL reconstruction may provide a more favorable environment for meniscal repair because of the increased presence of various growth factors in the clot. An in vitro study has shown that when meniscal fibrochondrocytes are exposed to growth factors normally found in a blood clot the cells demonstrated a marked increase in proliferation and matrix synthesis.[128] An in vivo study in animals demonstrated that when a defect in the avascular portion of the meniscus was filled with a fibrin clot, the defect was able to heal with connective tissue that was similar to that seen in normal meniscal repair.[10] Thus, by providing the factors necessary for repair, as well as a substrate/scaffold on which the repair process could take place, the fibrin clot was able to induce and support a healing response in the avascular portion of the meniscus.[10] A fibrin clot is formed by gently stirring whole blood in a glass container. Approximately 50 to 60 mL of whole blood is obtained from the patient and placed in a sterile glass beaker. Then, with the sintered glass barrel from a 20-mL glass syringe, the blood is stirred gently until a fibrin clot is precipitated on the surface of the barrel (Fig. 30–17A). This process usually takes between 3 and 5 minutes. The consistency of the clot formed in this manner is similar to that of wet chewing gum and is capable of holding sutures placed through its substance (Fig. 30–17B). Although use of the fibrin clot technique in white-white tears has been limited, clinical studies have suggested improved healing rates in red-white meniscal tears in which a fibrin clot was used.[61,62,124]

Platelet-Rich Plasma

Another potential way to provide growth factors to the area of an avascular meniscal lesion, but in greater

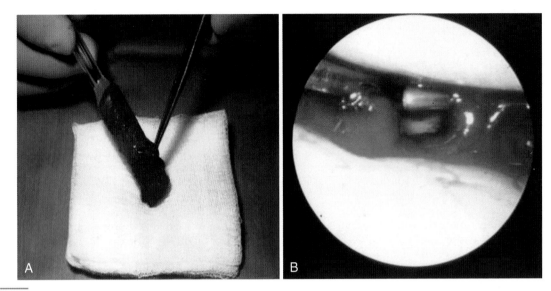

Figure 30–17. **A,** Fibrin clot precipitated on the surface of a glass syringe barrel. **B,** Arthroscopic photograph of a fibrin clot being sutured into a meniscal tear. (From McAndrews PT, Arnoczky SP: Meniscal repair enhancement techniques. Clin Sports Med 15:499-510, 1996.)

concentrations than possible in a normal fibrin clot, is through the use of platelet-rich plasma (PRP). PRP is defined as a platelet concentration of at least 1,000,000 platelets per microliter in 5 mL of plasma.[87] This represents a threefold to fivefold increase in concentration over normal circulating platelet numbers. Lesser concentrations cannot be relied on to enhance wound healing, and greater concentrations have not yet been shown to further enhance wound healing.[87] PRP is created through separation of the cellular components of citrated whole blood through centrifugation (plasmapheresis). The smaller, less dense platelets are separated from the other cellular components of blood and concentrated in the plasma fraction. Calcium chloride or exogenous thrombin can then be added to initiate the clotting cascade, and a platelet-rich fibrin construct can be formed.

PRP contains increased concentrations (above normal circulating plasma levels) of several growth factors, including platelet-derived growth factor (PDGF), transforming growth factor-β (TGF-β), epidermal growth factor (EGF), and insulin-like growth factor type I (IGF-I).[103,129] Although numerous clinical studies have shown improved healing in bone and soft tissue,[4,35,97,98,121] the use of PRP in meniscal repair has not been reported.

Fibrin Glue

A corollary to the use of a fibrin clot or PRP is the proposed use of a synthetic fibrin glue. The fibrin adhesive, which is formed by combining various factors in the normal clotting cascade (fibrinogen, thrombin, $CaCl_2$, and factor XIII) with an antifibrinolysate (aprotinin), has been used in other surgical applications to hold biological tissues in approximation. Although the adhesive property of fibrin glue is superior to that of a natural fibrin clot, the synthetic material lacks the biologically active growth

factors normally found in the clot. Thus, even though it may be able to hold wound edges in apposition more securely than a natural fibrin clot can, it has not been shown to play an active role in stimulating the repair process.[16] Several limited clinical studies have investigated the use of fibrin glue to repair longitudinal or bucket handle tears in the posterior segments of the medial and lateral menisci.[64,65] Through second-look arthroscopy of 25 repairs, 20 were rated good, 4 fair, and 1 poor.[65] A follow-up report included 40 patients (average follow-up, 8 years), with only 15% of the patients having residual meniscal symptoms requiring partial meniscectomy.[64] These studies concluded that fibrin glue may be an alternative to suture repair for relatively stable longitudinal lesions in the posterior horn of the medial and lateral menisci; however, its role in repair enhancement was not examined.

Thermal "Welding" of Meniscal Tissue

The use of thermal energy as a means of welding or soldering meniscal tears has been proposed.[36,42,63,123] In vitro transmission electron microscopy has demonstrated that treatment of meniscal tears at a temperature of 63° C will fuse the tissue without any necrotic nuclear changes.[63] Although the concept of thermal welding is an intriguing option for meniscal repair, in vitro studies have failed to demonstrate improved tensile strength over meniscal suture.[42] An in vivo rabbit model of avascular meniscal tears failed to demonstrate healing in tears treated with suture plus the neodymium:yttrium-aluminum-garnet (Nd:YAG) laser (or the laser alone).[123] To date, no controlled clinical studies have demonstrated the efficacy of thermal energy in the repair of meniscal tears, and its use cannot be supported.

MENISCAL REGENERATION

The concept that the meniscus will regenerate after removal has long provided the rationale for total meniscectomy.[38,39,74,114] However, the ability of a meniscus or a meniscus-like structure to regenerate after total meniscectomy has been the subject of much controversy. This controversy may have arisen from confusion about the extent of meniscectomy (partial versus total) or the fact that much of the data regarding meniscal regeneration has been derived from investigations in animals.[37,50,72] Studies in dogs[37,50] and rabbits[72] have demonstrated that after total meniscectomy, there is regrowth of a structure that is similar in shape and texture to the removed meniscus. Initially, this regenerated tissue has the histological appearance of fibrous connective tissue. However, with time, fibrocartilaginous metaplasia occurs within the tissue, and by 7 months it resembles fibrocartilage.[37]

For fibrocartilaginous tissue to regenerate after meniscectomy, an entire meniscus must be resected to expose the peripheral vascular connective tissue.[114] Experimental studies have shown the importance of this peripheral synovial tissue in meniscal regeneration.[72] In rabbits in which synovectomy accompanied total resection of the meniscus, there was no evidence of tissue regrowth at 12 weeks.[72] However, regrowth of a meniscus-like structure after total meniscectomy alone was observed in 83% of the animals.[72]

It appears, therefore, that the synovial and peripheral meniscal vasculature in the animal model is capable of generating a connective tissue replacement for a resected meniscus. However, in humans this regeneration is not thought to be complete and does not occur in all cases (Fig. 30–18). Furthermore, it is doubtful that any regenerate meniscus would functionally resemble the native meniscus. A better option for restoration of knee mechanics in patients requiring complete meniscectomy may be a meniscal allograft.

SUMMARY

Understanding the structure of the meniscus and its process of repair has been critical in advancing surgical techniques and increasing healing rates after meniscal repair. Knowledge of the circumferential orientation of the collagen fibers has led to the preferred position of sutures—vertical mattress sutures. Increasing knowledge of normal meniscal healing and meniscal vascularity has led to the application of vascular enhancement techniques and the ability to extend meniscal repair into the white-white zone.

When deciding which meniscal tears to repair, several factors should be taken into consideration. In active patients, all red-red and red-white tears (3 mm or less of rim width) should be repaired. When associated with ACL reconstruction, the indication for meniscal repair can be extended even farther because of the high healing rates associated with concomitant ACL reconstruction. In very young patients, an attempt at meniscal repair should be carried out whenever feasible, with possible consideration of vascular enhancement if healing potential appears low. Multiple techniques and devices are now available for meniscal repair, thus making it a skill that should be mastered by all arthroscopists.

Further understanding of basic science and meniscal healing has allowed us to expand the potential for meniscal repair. In the treatment of difficult fractures and nonunion, growth factors, such as bone morphogenic protein, have had a dramatic impact in increasing healing rates. Similarly, the future of meniscal repair will probably involve the use of growth factors as well as innovative vascular enhancement techniques to improve healing. Because no perfect substitute has been created to eliminate the problems seen after meniscal removal, we must continue to strive for meniscal preservation through meniscal repair.

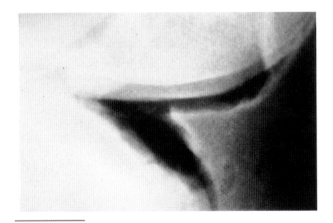

Figure 30–18. Arthrogram of a patient 8 years after total meniscectomy. Note the limited regeneration of the peripheral rim. (From Arnoczky SP: Meniscal healing, regeneration, and repair. Adv Orthop Surg 7:244, 1984.)

References

1. Ahmed AM, Burke DL: In-vitro measurement of static pressure distribution in synovial joints—Part I: Tibial surface of the knee. J Biomech Eng 105:216-225, 1983.
2. Allen CR, Wong EK, Livesay GA, et al: Importance of the medial meniscus in the anterior cruciate ligament–deficient knee. J Orthop Res 18:109-115, 2000.
3. Andersson-Molina H, Karlsson H, Rockborn P: Arthroscopic partial and total meniscectomy: A long-term follow-up study with matched controls. Arthroscopy 18:183-189, 2002.
4. Anitua E: Plasma rich in growth factors: Preliminary results of use in the preparation of future sites for implants. Int J Oral Maxillofac Implants 14:529-535, 1999.
5. Annandale T: An operation for displaced semilunar cartilage. Br J Med 1:1885, 1885.
6. Arnoczky SP: Meniscus healing. Contemp Orthop 10:31, 1985.
7. Arnoczky SP, Adams ME, DeHaven K: The meniscus. In Woo S-Y, Buckwalter J (eds): NIAMS/AAOS Workshop on the Injury and Repair of the Musculoskeletal Soft Tissues. Park Ridge, IL, American Academy of Orthopaedic Surgeons, 1988, p 487.
8. Arnoczky SP, Warren RF: Microvasculature of the human meniscus. Am J Sports Med 10:90-95, 1982.
9. Arnoczky SP, Warren RF: The microvasculature of the meniscus and its response to injury. An experimental study in the dog. Am J Sports Med 11:131-141, 1983.

10. Arnoczky SP, Warren RF, Spivak JM: Meniscal repair using an exogenous fibrin clot. An experimental study in dogs. J Bone Joint Surg Am 70:1209-1217, 1988.

11. Aspden RM, Yarker YE, Hukins DW: Collagen orientations in the meniscus of the knee joint. J Anat 140:371-380, 1985.

12. Baratz ME, Fu FH, Mengato R: Meniscal tears: The effect of meniscectomy and of repair on intraarticular contact areas and stress in the human knee. A preliminary report. Am J Sports Med 14:270-275, 1986.

13. Barrett GR, Treacy SH, Ruff CG: Preliminary results of the T-fix endoscopic meniscus repair technique in an anterior cruciate ligament reconstruction population. Arthroscopy 13:218-223, 1997.

14. Bhargava MM, Attia ET, Murrell GA, et al: The effect of cytokines on the proliferation and migration of bovine meniscal cells. Am J Sports Med 27:636-643, 1999.

15. Biedert RM: Treatment of intrasubstance meniscal lesions: A randomized prospective study of four different methods. Knee Surg Sports Traumatol Arthrosc 8:104-108, 2000.

16. Brunner FX: Histological findings in sutured and fibrin-glued microvascular anastomosis. Arch Otorhinolaryngol 240:311-318, 1984.

17. Bullough PG, Munuera L, Murphy J, et al: The strength of the menisci of the knee as it relates to their fine structure. J Bone Joint Surg Br 52:564-567, 1970.

18. Burks RT, Metcalf MH, Metcalf RW: Fifteen-year follow-up of arthroscopic partial meniscectomy. Arthroscopy 13:673-679, 1997.

19. Buseck MS, Noyes FR: Arthroscopic evaluation of meniscal repairs after anterior cruciate ligament reconstruction and immediate motion. Am J Sports Med 19:489-494, 1991.

20. Cabaud HE, Rodkey WG, Fitzwater JE: Medical meniscus repairs. An experimental and morphologic study. Am J Sports Med 9:129-134, 1981.

21. Cannon WD: Arthroscopic meniscal repair. In McGinty JB (ed): Operative Arthroscopy. New York, Lippincott Williams & Wilkins, 1996.

22. Cannon WD Jr, Vittori JM: The incidence of healing in arthroscopic meniscal repairs in anterior cruciate ligament–reconstructed knees versus stable knees. Am J Sports Med 20:176-181, 1992.

23. Cassidy RE, Shaffer AJ: Repair of peripheral meniscus tears. A preliminary report. Am J Sports Med 9:209-214, 1981.

24. Chatain F, Adeleine P, Chambat P, et al: A comparative study of medial versus lateral arthroscopic partial meniscectomy on stable knees: 10-year minimum follow-up. Arthroscopy 19:842-849, 2003.

25. Collier S, Ghosh P: Effects of transforming growth factor beta on proteoglycan synthesis by cell and explant cultures derived from the knee joint meniscus. Osteoarthritis Cartilage 3:127-138, 1995.

26. Cox JS, Cordell LD: The degenerative effects of medial meniscus tears in dogs' knees. Clin Orthop 125:236-242, 1977.

27. Cox JS, Nye CE, Schaefer WW, et al: The degenerative effects of partial and total resection of the medial meniscus in dogs' knees. Clin Orthop 109:178-183, 1975.

28. Curtis RJ, Delee JC, Drez DJ Jr: Reconstruction of the anterior cruciate ligament with freeze dried fascia lata allografts in dogs. A preliminary report. Am J Sports Med 13:408-414, 1985.

29. Danylchuk KD, Finlay JB, Krcek JP: Microstructural organization of human and bovine cruciate ligaments. Clin Orthop 131:294-298, 1978.

30. DeHaven KE: Peripheral meniscus repair: An alternative to meniscectomy. J Bone Joint Surg Br 63:463, 1981.

31. DeHaven KE: Meniscus repair in the athlete. Clin Orthop 198:31-35, 1985.

32. DeHaven KE: Meniscus repair—open vs. arthroscopic. Arthroscopy 1:173-174, 1985.

33. DeHaven KE: [Meniscus resection versus reattachment of the meniscus.] Orthopade 23:133-136, 1994.

34. DeHaven KE, Arnoczky SP: Meniscus repair: Basic science, indications for repair, and open repair. Instr Course Lect 43:65-76, 1994.

35. de Obarrio JJ, Arauz-Dutari JI, Chamberlain TM, Croston A: The use of autologous growth factors in periodontal surgical therapy: Platelet gel biotechnology—case reports. Int J Periodontics Restorative Dent 20:486-497, 2000.

36. Dew DK, Supik L, Darrow CR 2nd, et al: Tissue repair using lasers: A review. Orthopedics 16:581-587, 1993.

37. DeYoung DJ, Flo GL, Tvedten HW: Experimental medical meniscectomy in dogs undergoing cranial cruciate ligament repair. Am Anim Hosp Assoc 16:639, 1980.

38. Doyle JR, Eisenberg JH, Orth MW: Regeneration of knee menisci: A preliminary report. J Trauma 6:50-55, 1966.

39. Evans DK: Repeated regeneration of a meniscus in the knee. J Bone Joint Surg Br 45:748-749, 1963.

40. Fairbank TJ: Knee joint changes after meniscectomy. J Bone Joint Surg Br 30:644-670, 1948.

41. Fauno P, Nielsen AB: Arthroscopic partial meniscectomy: A long-term follow-up. Arthroscopy 8:345-349, 1992.

42. Forman SK, Oz MC, Lontz JF, et al: Laser-assisted fibrin clot soldering of human menisci. Clin Orthop 310:37-41, 1995.

43. Fox JM, Rintz KG, Ferkel RD: Trephination of incomplete meniscal tears. Arthroscopy 9:451-455, 1993.

44. Freedman KB, Nho SJ, Cole BJ: Marrow stimulating technique to augment meniscus repair. Arthroscopy 19:794-798, 2003.

45. Fukubayashi T, Kurosawa H: The contact area and pressure distribution pattern of the knee. A study of normal and osteoarthrotic knee joints. Acta Orthop Scand 51:871-879, 1980.

46. Fukushima K: [Meniscal transplantation with a synovial pedicle—an animal experiment.] Nippon Seikeigeka Gakkai Zasshi 67:1162-1169, 1993.

47. Gardner E: The innervation of the knee joint. Anat Rec 101:109-130, 1948.

48. Gershuni DH, Skyhar MJ, Danzig LA, et al: Experimental models to promote healing of tears in the avascular segment of canine knee menisci. J Bone Joint Surg Am 71:1363-1370, 1989.

49. Ghadially FN, Wedge JH, Lalonde JM: Experimental methods of repairing injured menisci. J Bone Joint Surg Br 68:106-110, 1986.

50. Ghosh P, Taylor TK, Pettit GD, et al: Effect of postoperative immobilisation on the regrowth of the knee joint semilunar cartilage: An experimental study. J Orthop Res 1:153-164, 1983.

51. Hamberg P, Gillquist J, Lysholm J: Suture of new and old peripheral meniscus tears. J Bone Joint Surg Am 65:193-197, 1983.

52. Hashimoto J, Kurosaka M, Yoshiya S, et al: Meniscal repair using fibrin sealant and endothelial cell growth factor. An experimental study in dogs. Am J Sports Med 20:537-541, 1992.

53. He L: [An experimental study on accelerating regeneration of meniscus with synovial flap implant in the rabbit knee.] Zhonghua Wai Ke Za Zhi 31:591-592, 1993.

54. Heatley FW: The meniscus—can it be repaired? An experimental investigation in rabbits. J Bone Joint Surg Br 62:397-402, 1980.

55. Henning CE: Arthroscopic repairs of meniscus tears. Orthopedics 6:1130-1132, 1983.

56. Henning CE: Current status of meniscus salvage. Clin Sports Med 9:567-576, 1990.

57. Henning CE, Clark JR, Lynch MA, et al: Arthroscopic meniscus repair with a posterior incision. Instr Course Lect 37:209-221, 1988.

58. Henning CE, Lynch MA: Current concepts of meniscal function and pathology. Clin Sports Med 4:259-265, 1985.

59. Henning CE, Lynch MA, Clark JR: Vascularity for healing of meniscus repairs. Arthroscopy 3:13-18, 1987.

60. Henning CE, Lynch MA, Yearout KM: Meniscal repair with rasp abrasion of both tear surfaces: A preliminary report. Presented at the Annual Meeting of the American Orthopaedic Society for Sports Medicine, Sun Valley, ID, 1990.

61. Henning CE, Lynch MA, Yearout KM, et al: Arthroscopic meniscal repair using an exogenous fibrin clot. Clin Orthop 252:64-72, 1990.

62. Henning CE, Yearout KM, Vequist SW, et al: Use of the fascia sheath coverage and exogenous fibrin clot in the treatment of complex meniscal tears. Am J Sports Med 19:626-631, 1991.

63. Imakiire N, Kotani A, Ishii Y: Experimental study on thermal welding for the knee meniscal white zone. J Orthop Sci 8:683-692, 2003.

64. Ishimura M, Ohgushi H, Habata T, et al: Arthroscopic meniscal repair using fibrin glue. Part II: Clinical applications. Arthroscopy 13:558-563, 1997.

65. Ishimura M, Tamai S, Fujisawa Y: Arthroscopic meniscal repair with fibrin glue. Arthroscopy 7:177-181, 1991.

66. Jakob RP, Staubli HU, Zuber K, et al: The arthroscopic meniscal repair. Techniques and clinical experience. Am J Sports Med 16:137-142, 1988.

67. Johnson L: Arthroscopic Surgery: Principles and Practice. St Louis, CV Mosby, 1986, pp 1034-1037.

68. Jorgensen U, Sonne-Holm S, Lauridsen F, et al: Long-term follow-up of meniscectomy in athletes. A prospective longitudinal study. J Bone Joint Surg Br 69:80-83, 1987.

69. Kawahara Y, Uetani M, Fuchi K, et al: MR assessment of movement and morphologic change in the menisci during knee flexion. Acta Radiol 40:610-614, 1999.

70. Kawahara Y, Uetani M, Fuchi K, et al: MR assessment of meniscal movement during knee flexion: Correlation with the severity of cartilage abnormality in the femorotibial joint. J Comput Assist Tomogr 25:683-690, 2001.

71. Kennedy JC, Alexander IJ, Hayes KC: Nerve supply of the human knee and its functional importance. Am J Sports Med 10:329-335, 1982.

72. Kim JM, Moon MS: Effect of synovectomy upon regeneration of meniscus in rabbits. Clin Orthop 141:287-294, 1979.

73. Kimura M, Shirakura K, Hasegawa A, et al: Second look arthroscopy after meniscal repair. Factors affecting the healing rate. Clin Orthop 314:185-191, 1995.

74. King D: Regeneration of the semilunar cartilage. Surg Gynecol Obstet 62:167, 1936.

75. King D: The healing of the semilunar cartilage. J Bone Joint Surg 64:883, 1936.

76. Klompmaker J, Jansen HW, Veth RP, et al: Porous polymer implant for repair of meniscal lesions: A preliminary study in dogs. Biomaterials 12:810-816, 1991.

77. Kobuna Y, Shirakura K, Niijima M: Meniscal repair using a flap of synovium. An experimental study in the dog. Am J Knee Surg 8:52-55, 1995.

78. Kocabey Y, Nyland J, Isbell WM, Caborn DN: Patient outcomes following T-Fix meniscal repair and a modifiable, progressive rehabilitation program, a retrospective study. Arch Orthop Trauma Surg 124:592-596, 2004.

79. Kruger-Franke M, Siebert CH, Kugler A, et al: Late results after arthroscopic partial medial meniscectomy. Knee Surg Sports Traumatol Arthrosc 7:81-84, 1999.

80. Kumagae Y: [Proteoglycan and collagen synthesis of cultured fibrochondrocytes from the human knee joint meniscus.] Nippon Seikeigeka Gakkai Zasshi 68:885-894, 1994.

81. Levy IM, Torzilli PA, Warren RF: The effect of medial meniscectomy on anterior-posterior motion of the knee. J Bone Joint Surg Am 64:883-888, 1982.

82. Lietman SA, Hobbs W, Inoue N, et al: Effects of selected growth factors on porcine meniscus in chemically defined medium. Orthopedics 26:799-803, 2003.

83. Lietman SA, Yanagishita M, Sampath TK, et al: Stimulation of proteoglycan synthesis in explants of porcine articular cartilage by recombinant osteogenic protein-1 (bone morphogenetic protein-7). J Bone Joint Surg Am 79:1132-1137, 1997.

84. Lipscomb AB, Anderson AF: Tears of the anterior cruciate ligament in adolescents. J Bone Joint Surg Am 68:19-28, 1986.

85. Lynch MA, Henning CE, Glick KR Jr: Knee joint surface changes. Long-term follow-up meniscus tear treatment in stable anterior cruciate ligament reconstructions. Clin Orthop 172:148-153, 1983.

86. Markolf KL, Kochan A, Amstutz HC: Measurement of knee stiffness and laxity in patients with documented absence of the anterior cruciate ligament. J Bone Joint Surg Am 66:242-252, 1984.

87. Marx RE: Platelet-rich plasma (PRP): What is PRP and what is not PRP? Implant Dent 10:225-228, 2001.

88. McDevitt CA, Webber RJ: The ultrastructure and biochemistry of meniscal cartilage. Clin Orthop 252:8-18, 1990.

89. Miller DB Jr: Arthroscopic meniscus repair. Am J Sports Med 16:315-320, 1988.

90. Mooney MF, Rosenberg TD: [Arthroscopic reattachment of the meniscus.] Orthopade 23:143-152, 1994.

91. Morgan CD, Wojtys EM, Casscells CD, et al: Arthroscopic meniscal repair evaluated by second-look arthroscopy. Am J Sports Med 19:632-637, discussion 637-638, 1991.

92. Noyes FR, Barber-Westin SD: Arthroscopic repair of meniscus tears extending into the avascular zone with or without anterior cruciate ligament reconstruction in patients 40 years of age and older. Arthroscopy 16:822-829, 2000.

93. Ochi M, Uchio Y, Okuda K, et al: Expression of cytokines after meniscal rasping to promote meniscal healing. Arthroscopy 17:724-731, 2001.

94. Okuda K, Ochi M, Shu N, et al: Meniscal rasping for repair of meniscal tear in the avascular zone. Arthroscopy 15:281-286, 1999.

95. O'Meara PM: Surgical techniques for arthroscopic meniscal repair. Orthop Rev 22:781-790, 1993.

96. Papageorgiou CD, Gil JE, Kanamori A, et al: The biomechanical interdependence between the anterior cruciate ligament replacement graft and the medial meniscus. Am J Sports Med 29:226-231, 2001.

97. Petrungaro PS: Using platelet-rich plasma to accelerate soft tissue maturation in esthetic periodontal surgery. Compend Contin Educ Dent 22:729-732, 734, 736 passim, quiz 746, 2001.

98. Petrungaro PS: Immediate restoration of multiple tooth implants for aesthetic implant restorations. Implant Dent 11:118-127, 2002.

99. Radin EL, Rose RM: Role of subchondral bone in the initiation and progression of cartilage damage. Clin Orthop 213:34-40, 1986.

100. Ritchie JR, Miller MD, Bents RT, et al: Meniscal repair in the goat model. The use of healing adjuncts on central tears and the role of magnetic resonance arthrography in repair evaluation. Am J Sports Med 26:278-284, 1998.

101. Rodeo SA, Warren RF: Meniscal repair using the outside-to-inside technique. Clin Sports Med 15:469-481, 1996.

102. Rosenberg TD, Scott SM, Coward DB, et al: Arthroscopic meniscal repair evaluated with repeat arthroscopy. Arthroscopy 2:14-20, 1986.

103. Sanchez AR, Sheridan PJ, Kupp LI: Is platelet-rich plasma the perfect enhancement factor? A current review. Int J Oral Maxillofac Implants 18:93-103, 2003.

104. Scheller G, Sobau C, Bulow JU: Arthroscopic partial lateral meniscectomy in an otherwise normal knee: Clinical, functional, and radiographic results of a long-term follow-up study. Arthroscopy 17:946-952, 2001.

105. Schmitz MA, Rouse LM Jr, DeHaven KE: The management of meniscal tears in the ACL-deficient knee. Clin Sports Med 15:573-593, 1996.

106. Scott GA, Jolly BL, Henning CE: Combined posterior incision and arthroscopic intra-articular repair of the meniscus. An examination of factors affecting healing. J Bone Joint Surg Am 68:847-861, 1986.

107. Seedholm BB, Hargreaves DJ: Transmission of the load in the knee joint with special reference to the role of the menisci. Eng Med 8:220, 1979.

108. Sekiya H: [Free synovium grafting for repair of the avascular portion of canine knee joint meniscus.] Nippon Seikeigeka Gakkai Zasshi 66:50-60, 1992.

109. Shelbourne KD, Carr DR: Meniscal repair compared with meniscectomy for bucket-handle medial meniscal tears in anterior cruciate ligament–reconstructed knees. Am J Sports Med 31:718-723, 2003.

110. Shelbourne KD, Dersam MD: Comparison of partial meniscectomy versus meniscus repair for bucket-handle lateral meniscus tears in anterior cruciate ligament reconstructed knees. Arthroscopy 20:581-585, 2004.

111. Shelbourne KD, Heinrich J: The long-term evaluation of lateral meniscus tears left in situ at the time of anterior cruciate ligament reconstruction. Arthroscopy 20:346-351, 2004.

112. Shelbourne KD, Rask BP: The sequelae of salvaged nondegenerative peripheral vertical medial meniscus tears with anterior cruciate ligament reconstruction. Arthroscopy 17:270-274, 2001.

113. Shirakura K, Niijima M, Kobuna Y, et al: Free synovium promotes meniscal healing. Synovium, muscle and synthetic mesh compared in dogs. Acta Orthop Scand 68:51-54, 1997.

114. Smilie IS: Observations on the regeneration of the semilunar cartilages in man. Br J Surg 31:398, 1944.

115. Spindler KP, Mayes CE, Miller RR, et al: Regional mitogenic response of the meniscus to platelet-derived growth factor (PDGF-AB). J Orthop Res 13:201-207, 1995.

116. Stone RG, VanWinkle GN: Arthroscopic review of meniscal repair: Assessment of healing parameters. Arthroscopy 2:77-81, 1986.

117. Talley MC, Grana WA: Treatment of partial meniscal tears identified during anterior cruciate ligament reconstruction with limited synovial abrasion. Arthroscopy 16:6-10, 2000.

118. Tenuta JJ, Arciero RA: Arthroscopic evaluation of meniscal repairs. Factors that affect healing. Am J Sports Med 22:797-802, 1994.

119. Tetik O, Kocabey Y, Johnson DL: Synovial abrasion for isolated, partial thickness, undersurface, medial meniscus tears. Orthopedics 25:675-678, 2002.

120. Thompson WO, Thaete FL, Fu FH, et al: Tibial meniscal dynamics using three-dimensional reconstruction of magnetic resonance images. Am J Sports Med 19:210-215, discussion 215-216, 1991.

121. Tischler M: Platelet rich plasma. The use of autologous growth factors to enhance bone and soft tissue grafts. N Y State Dent J 68:22-24, 2002.

122. Uchio Y, Ochi M, Adachi N, et al: Results of rasping of meniscal tears with and without anterior cruciate ligament injury as evaluated by second-look arthroscopy. Arthroscopy 19:463-469, 2003.

123. Vangsness CT Jr, Akl Y, Marshall GJ, et al: The effects of the neodymium laser on meniscal repair in the avascular zone of the meniscus. Arthroscopy 10:201-205, 1994.

124. van Trommel MF, Simonian PT, Potter HG, et al: Arthroscopic meniscal repair with fibrin clot of complete radial tears of the lateral meniscus in the avascular zone. Arthroscopy 14:360-365, 1998.

125. Veth RP, den Heeten GJ, Jansen HW, Nielsen HK: An experimental study of reconstructive procedures in lesions of the meniscus. Use of synovial flaps and carbon fiber implants for artificially made lesions in the meniscus of the rabbit. Clin Orthop 181:250-254, 1983.

126. Voloshin AS, Wosk J: Shock absorption of meniscectomized and painful knees: A comparative in vivo study. J Biomed Eng 5:157-161, 1983.

127. Warren R, Arnoczky SP, Wickiewicz TL: Anatomy of the knee. In Nicholas JA, Hershman EB (eds): The Lower Extremity and Spine in Sports Medicine. St Louis, CV Mosby, 1986, p 657.

128. Webber RJ, Harris MG, Hough AJ Jr: Cell culture of rabbit meniscal fibrochondrocytes: Proliferative and synthetic response to growth factors and ascorbate. J Orthop Res 3:36-42, 1985.

129. Weibrich G, Kleis WK, Hafner G: Growth factor levels in the platelet-rich plasma produced by 2 different methods: Curasan-type PRP kit versus PCCS PRP system. Int J Oral Maxillofac Implants 17:184-190, 2002.

130. Wilson AS, Legg PG, McNeur JC: Studies of the innervation of the medial meniscus in the human knee joint. Anat Rec 165:485-492, 1969.

131. Yasui K: The dimensional architecture of the human normal menisci. J Jpn Orthop Assoc 52:391, 1978.

132. Zhang Z, Arnold JA: Trephination and suturing of avascular meniscal tears: A clinical study of the trephination procedure. Arthroscopy 12:726-731, 1996.

133. Zhang Z, Arnold JA, Williams T, et al: Repairs by trephination and suturing of longitudinal injuries in the avascular area of the meniscus in goats. Am J Sports Med 23:35-41, 1995.

134. Zhang ZN, Tu KY, Xu YK, et al: Treatment of longitudinal injuries in avascular area of meniscus in dogs by trephination. Arthroscopy 4:151-159, 1988.

135. Zimny ML, Albright DJ, Dabezies E: Mechanoreceptors in the human medial meniscus. Acta Anat (Basel) 133:35-40, 1988.

Chapter 31

Arthroscopic Meniscus Regeneration with Collagen Scaffolding*

William G. Rodkey • J. Richard Steadman

Tissue engineering is a relatively new discipline that has received much recent attention.[12] It has provided a fundamental understanding and technology that have permitted the development of structures derived from biological tissues. Bioresorbable collagen matrices serve as one example of innovative new devices that have resulted from the discipline of tissue engineering.[2-4] These collagen matrix materials have many positive features that can be used to preserve and restore meniscus tissue, including a controlled rate of resorption based on the degree of cross-linking, processing of the collagen to minimize any immune response, and close approximation of the extremely complex biochemical composition of the normal meniscus during the production process.[2-4] If such a material could serve successfully as a scaffold for the regeneration of new tissue, many of the previously noted negative effects of losing meniscus cartilage might be prevented or at least minimized.[1]

When we commenced development of this collagen scaffold, which we refer to as the collagen meniscus implant (CMI), our goals were straightforward. The purpose was to generate or grow meniscus-like tissue in an effort to restore or preserve the critical functions of the meniscus.[6,8,10] We also wanted to prevent further degenerative joint disease and osteoarthritis, which would probably be progressive and lead to multiple surgeries, possibly including total joint replacement. Another goal of this new regenerated tissue was to enhance joint stability. Finally, we wanted the implant and the new tissue to have the effect of providing pain relief and preclude the necessity for constant medication. We also focused on several criteria for design of the CMI.[6,8,10] There was a requirement for a material that would be resorbable over time so that as the collagen of the scaffold was metabolized, new tissue would have the opportunity to replace it. We also wanted the CMI to maintain its structural integrity in the intraarticular environment for a period that would be adequate to support new matrix formation and maturation. It was essential that the implant be nonimmunogenic to minimize reactions that might cause rejection or destruction of the implant. Consequently, biochemical techniques were developed as part of the processing procedures to

minimize such reactions.[2-4] We designed the implant so that it would be technically straightforward to implant surgically with a minimum of sizing considerations. We believed that the implant would have to be nonabrasive, not produce any wear particles, and not incite an excessive inflammatory response. Finally, it was extremely critical that the implant be nontoxic to the cells that invaded the scaffold and eventually produced the new matrix.[6,8,10]

Hence, it was our hypothesis that if we could provide such an environment, the meniscus fibrochondrocytes, or perhaps other progenitor cells, would migrate into the scaffold, divide and populate the scaffold, produce extracellular matrix, and ultimately lead to the regeneration of new meniscus-like tissue. This new tissue would then preserve and help restore the damaged meniscus cartilage and would function like the meniscus in a chondroprotective role. We were able to affirm our hypothesis and confirm that our requirements had been met in various animal studies.[3,8,9]

COLLAGEN MENISCUS IMPLANT FABRICATION, INDICATIONS, AND SURGICAL TECHNIQUE

The CMI (Fig. 31–1) is fabricated from bovine Achilles tendons. The tendon tissue is trimmed and minced and then washed copiously with tap water to remove blood residue and water-soluble material. The type I collagen fibers are purified with various chemical treatments such as acid, base, and enzymatic processes to remove noncollagenous material and lipids. The isolated type I collagen fibers are then analyzed for purity. After further processing, terminal sterilization is carried out by gamma irradiation.[2-4]

At present, the CMI is designed only for use in the medial compartment of the knee. However, a lateral CMI is in the final stages of development. The CMI is indicated for use in acute or chronic irreparable meniscus injuries or after previous partial meniscectomy. There must be enough meniscus rim remaining to which the CMI can be sutured. The CMI is contraindicated after total meniscectomy, if there is uncorrected ligamentous instability, in patients with uncorrected axial malalignment, if there is full-thickness loss of articular cartilage with exposed bone, or in those with documented evidence of allergy to collagen. Other systemic conditions may also preclude use of the CMI.

*DISCLAIMER: The collagen meniscus implant (CMI) described in this presentation is not currently available (2005) for sale or distribution in the United States. Studies described in this presentation were performed under a U.S. Food and Drug Administration (FDA) Investigational Device Exemption (IDE). The FDA has classified the CMI as an investigational device, and it may be used in the United States only within the standards set forth in the IDE.

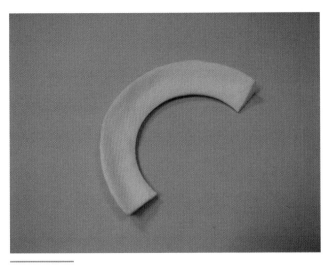

Figure 31–1. The collagen meniscus implant as it appears before implantation.

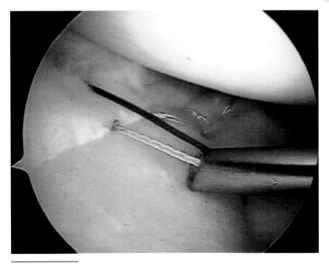

Figure 31–2. The collagen meniscus implant has been inserted into the lesion and is being sutured into place with an inside-out technique.

Routine arthroscopic surgical procedures are used to place the CMI.[5,7,11] The damaged meniscus tissue is débrided only until healthy tissue is reached. In cases in which the débridement does not reach the red zone of the meniscus, a microfracture awl is used to perforate the host meniscus rim until a bleeding bed is ensured.[5,7] A special Teflon measuring device developed for this procedure is then used to measure the exact size of the defect. The CMI is measured and trimmed to the correct size on the sterile field of the operating environment. A posterior medial incision is made approximately 3 cm in length parallel and just posterior to the medial collateral ligament and directly over the joint line so that the inside-out meniscus repair needles can be captured and the sutures tied over the capsule.[5,7] A specially designed introducer containing the CMI is inserted through the ipsilateral portal, and then a plunger pushes the implant out of the delivery device into the joint.

When positioning is satisfactory, the implant is sutured to the host meniscus rim with standard inside-out techniques and zone-specific meniscus repair cannulas (Fig. 31–2).[5,7] We prefer to use a suture "gun," called the Sharp-Shooter (ReGen Biologics, Franklin Lakes, NJ), to pass the sutures. Size 2-0 nonabsorbable braided polyester sutures are placed approximately 4 to 5 mm apart. Sutures are placed in a vertical mattress pattern around the rim of the meniscus remnant, and a horizontal pattern is used in the anterior and posterior horns.[5] Typically, 8 to 10 sutures are used to secure the implant in place. The sutures are then tied over the capsule in a standard manner. Alternatively, consideration might be given to the use of an all-inside fixation technique. However, care must be exercised to avoid damage to the CMI when using all-inside devices because they are usually larger and stiffer than needles and sutures.

CLINICAL STUDIES

In a phase II feasibility study, eight patients underwent arthroscopic placement of the CMI to reconstruct and restore the irreparably damaged medial meniscus of one knee during the first half of 1996.[5] Seven patients had undergone one or more previous medial meniscectomies, and one patient had an acute medial meniscus injury. Patients were observed with frequent clinical, serological, radiographic, and magnetic resonance imaging (MRI) examinations for at least 24 months (range, 24 to 32 months) initially. As part of the initial study, all patients underwent relook arthroscopy and biopsy of the CMI-regenerated tissue at either 6 or 12 months after implantation.[5] All patients improved clinically from their preoperative status to 1 and 2 years postoperatively with respect to pain, Lysholm scores, Tegner activity scale, and self-assessment. Relook arthroscopy revealed tissue regeneration in all patients with apparent preservation of the joint surfaces by visual observation. Based on measurements, the average amount of meniscus loss (defect) before placement of the CMI was 62%. That is, only 38% of the meniscus remained. At the initial relook surgery, the average filling of the meniscus defect was 77% with a range of 40% to 100%. Histological analysis of the CMI-regenerated tissue confirmed new fibrocartilage matrix formation. Radiographs confirmed no progression of degenerative joint disease in the medial compartment.[5]

As a part of a long-term (5 to 6 years) follow-up study, all eight patients previously described returned for clinical, radiographic, and MRI examinations.[7] Clinical outcome measurements were virtually unchanged from the 2-year follow-up examination. Radiographs confirmed that the medial compartment chondral surfaces continued to be protected from further degeneration. MRI revealed that the CMI-regenerated tissue continued to mature, and it was often indistinguishable from the native meniscus tissue. All eight patients underwent relook arthroscopy to assess the status of the CMI-regenerated tissue, as well as the condition of the chondral surfaces. The CMI-regenerated tissue appeared similar to that seen at the earlier relook arthroscopy, and its appearance was meniscus-like, both grossly and histologically (Fig. 31–3).[7]

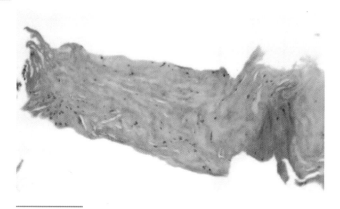

Figure 31–3. A biopsy sample obtained 6.3 years after placement of the collagen meniscus implant shows fibrocartilaginous tissue that is meniscus-like in appearance. The original magnification is 25×. The stain is hematoxylin-eosin.

At arthroscopy the amount of the original meniscus defect remaining filled by newly generated meniscus-like tissue was determined by physical measurements and comparison to video images of the index surgery and the first relook procedures. Physical measurements were made with the same arthroscopic measuring device that had been used during the index surgery. For example, if the original implant was 50 mm long and 7 mm wide, it covered an area of 350 mm². If the newly generated tissue was measured and determined to cover 300 mm², the original defect was calculated to remain 86% filled. The average amount of the original defect remaining filled at nearly 6 years after placement of the CMI was 69% with a range of 50% to 95%.[7] That is, only a small loss of tissue had occurred since the initial relook arthroscopy about 5 years earlier when 77% of the defect was filled on average.[5] By adding the amount of filled defect to the amount of meniscus remaining at the time of index surgery, this group of eight patients had 81% of their normal meniscus (range, 66% to 98%) at about 6 years after placement of the CMI.[7] The percentage of meniscus gain versus the index remnant (the quotient of the percentage of new tissue divided by the percentage of remaining meniscus at the index surgery) averaged 170% (range, 27% to 340%). No negative findings attributable to the implant were observed, such as damage to the chondral surfaces or exuberant tissue growth.[7]

The positive results of this phase II feasibility study after 2 years[5] led to Food and Drug Administration approval of a large multicenter randomized (CMI versus meniscectomy alone) clinical trial of about 300 patients in the United States. These patients were enrolled at 14 sites throughout the United States. Additionally, about 100 nonrandomized patients were enrolled at 10 sites in Europe and 2 sites in Japan. Patients who received the CMI had partial medial meniscus loss with an intact meniscus rim and no full-thickness chondral defects. Patients in the U.S. multicenter trial underwent frequent clinical examination and relook arthroscopy with biopsy 1 year after implantation.

For patients enrolled in this multicenter study at our institution (N = 41), no serious or unanticipated complications have been attributed to the CMI. Patients routinely returned to daily activities by 3 months, most were fully active by 6 months, and then they continued to improve through at least 2 years as evidenced by Tegner and Lysholm scores. Enzyme-linked immunosorbent assay failed to detect any increase in antibodies to the collagen material. No increased degenerative joint disease was observed, nor was there radiographic evidence of further joint space narrowing. Sequential MRI examinations revealed progressive signal intensity changes indicating ongoing tissue ingrowth, regeneration, and maturation of the new tissue. At relook arthroscopy, the gross appearance and shape of the regenerated tissue were generally similar to that of native meniscus cartilage, with a solid interface to the host meniscus rim in the majority of patients. The average amount of defect filled, calculated as described earlier, was greater than 70% with a range of 40% to 90%. Histologically, the collagen implant was progressively invaded and replaced by cells similar to meniscus fibrochondrocytes with production of new matrix. No inflammatory cells or histological evidence of immunological or allergic reactions was observed.

SUMMARY

Based on our personal experiences with the limited long-term feasibility study and the randomized multicenter clinical trial, we conclude that the CMI is implantable, biocompatible, and bioresorbable. It supports new tissue regeneration as it is resorbed, and the new tissue appears to function similar to normal meniscus tissue. Although the advantage of the CMI, as opposed to partial meniscectomy alone, in limiting the progression of degenerative joint disease over the long term has not been definitely proved yet, the results of the studies described earlier provide evidence that a CMI-based, tissue-engineered meniscus structure can survive within the joint. Based on the relook procedures, the chondral surfaces are protected by the CMI-regenerated tissue. No serious or unanticipated complications directly related to the CMI have thus far been observed, and most patients have functioned well based on clinical examination and assessment of outcomes. Relook arthroscopy results are positive and encouraging. These findings lend strong support to the concept that a CMI can be used to replace irreparable or removed meniscus tissue. Similar positive European observations resulted in obtaining the European Union CE mark for the CMI in 2000. Regulatory approval was obtained in Australia and Chile in 2002. Approval is pending in other non-U.S. countries at this time.

References

1. Arnoczky SP: Building a meniscus. Biologic considerations. Clin Orthop 367:S244-S253, 1999.
2. Li S-T: Biologic biomaterials: Tissue-derived biomaterials (collagen). In Bronzino J (ed): The Biomedical Engineering Handbook. Boca Raton, FL, CRC Press, 1995, pp 627-647.
3. Li S-T, Rodkey WG, Yuen D, et al: Type I collagen–based template for meniscus regeneration. In Lewandrowski K-U, Wise DL, Trantolo DJ, et al (eds): Tissue Engineering and Biodegradable Equiva-

lents. Scientific and Clinical Applications. New York, Marcel Dekker, 2002, pp 237-266.

4. Li S-T, Yuen D, Li PC, et al: Collagen as a biomaterial: An application in knee meniscal fibrocartilage regeneration. Mater Res Soc Symp Proc 331:25-32, 1994.

5. Rodkey WG, Steadman JR, Li S-T: A clinical study of collagen meniscus implants to restore the injured meniscus. Clin Orthop 367:S281-S292, 1999.

6. Rodkey WG, Stone KR, Steadman JR: Prosthetic meniscal replacement. In Finerman GAM, Noyes FR (eds): Biology and Biomechanics of the Traumatized Synovial Joint: The Knee as a Model. Rosemont, IL, American Academy of Orthopaedic Surgeons, 1992, pp 222-231.

7. Steadman JR, Rodkey WG: Tissue-engineered collagen meniscus implants: 5 to 6-year feasibility study results. Arthroscopy 21:515-525, 2005.

8. Stone KR, Rodkey WG, Webber RJ, et al: Future directions: Collagen-based prosthesis for meniscal regeneration. Clin Orthop 252:129-135, 1990.

9. Stone KR, Rodkey WG, Webber RJ, et al: Meniscal regeneration with copolymeric collagen scaffolds: In vitro and in vivo studies evaluated clinically, histologically, biochemically. Am J Sports Med 20:104-111, 1992.

10. Stone KR, Rodkey WG, Webber RJ, et al: Development of a prosthetic meniscal replacement. In Mow VC, Arnoczky SP, Jackson DJ (eds): Knee Meniscus: Basic and Clinical Foundation. New York, Raven Press, 1992, pp 165-173.

11. Stone KR, Steadman JR, Rodkey WG, Li S-T: Regeneration of meniscal cartilage with use of a collagen scaffold: Analysis of preliminary data. J Bone Joint Surg Am 79:1770-1777, 1997.

12. Vunjak-Novakovic G, Goldstein SA: Biomechanical principles of cartilage and bone tissue engineering. In Mow VC, Huiskes R (eds): Basic Orthopaedic Biomechanics and Mechano-Biology. Philadelphia, Lippincott William & Wilkins, 2005, pp 343-407.

CHAPTER 32

Meniscal Allograft Transplantation

J. Winslow Alford • Brian J. Cole

Meniscal allograft transplantation has moved into mainstream orthopedics. With proper patient selection and with careful analysis and treatment of comorbid conditions, meniscal allograft transplantation offers a solution that can decrease pain, increase function, and prevent or retard knee degeneration associated with a deficient meniscus, at least temporarily. In this chapter we review the basic science of meniscal mechanics, the pathomechanics of meniscal injury, meniscal allograft preparation, and the immunology of meniscal transplantation. We describe our indications for meniscal transplantation, as well as our method of patient evaluation and preoperative preparation. A description of various surgical techniques and their outcomes are presented as well.

REVIEW OF MENISCAL ANATOMY AND BIOMECHANICS

In a normal knee, the medial and lateral menisci contribute to the maintenance of articular cartilage health, provide mechanical protection to articular cartilage, and thereby help prevent degenerative joint disease. Meniscal removal or injury has been implicated in articular degeneration and the development of osteoarthritis.[74] Articular cartilage damage has been shown to occur as early as 12 weeks after meniscectomy in skeletally mature mongrel dogs, with a decreased tensile modulus for articular cartilage after meniscectomy, thus suggesting that changes in collagen composition, density, and structure may be early events in the pathogenesis of cartilage degeneration.[29] The many functions of menisci include shock absorption, load transmission, secondary mechanical stability, and joint lubrication and nutrition.

The anatomic configuration of the meniscus, which forms a semilunar, wedge-shaped structure, enhances tibial-femoral joint stability by filling the void created by the incongruous femoral condyle and tibial plateau.[40] Whereas the lateral meniscus forms a C-shaped, incomplete semicircle, the medial meniscus is more U shaped with slightly wider separation of its anterior and posterior horns than in the lateral meniscus. Through deepening of the tibial socket, menisci act as secondary stabilizers, particularly in the medial compartment, by enhancing positional control and alignment of the knee, as well as providing a mechanical block by the presence of the posterior horn of the medial meniscus.[101] The posterior horn of the medial meniscus contributes a substantial block to posterior-anterior translation of the tibia on the femur.[60,98] Previous medial meniscectomy or incompetence of the posterior horn of the medial meniscus in the setting of primary anterior cruciate ligament (ACL) reconstruction has been associated with graft elongation and joint laxity.[96] Loss of a significant portion of the posterior horn of the medial meniscus significantly increases rotatory instability of the knee and may ultimately accelerate the development of osteoarthritis in an ACL-deficient knee.[60,70]

During a normal gait pattern, the articular surface of the knee bears between 4.5 and 6.2 times body weight; 72.2% of that load is transmitted to the medial tibial plateau.[46,91] The menisci increase the contact area in the tibiofemoral joint and dissipate the compressive force at the articular cartilage. Given its slightly greater width and thickness and therefore greater surface area, the lateral meniscus carries the majority of the lateral compartment load, with up to 75% of the axial compressive load transmitted by the lateral meniscus versus just 40% by the medial meniscus. Meniscectomy increases peak articular contact stress at least twofold to threefold and has been shown to lead to the development of early degenerative changes.[2,11,81] An intact meniscus converts joint loading forces to radial-directed hoop stresses, which lead to tensile stress on circumferential collagen fibers. As a result, the menisci transmit 50% of the joint load when the knee is in extension and 90% when in flexion.[2,112] In vitro animal studies have demonstrated that loss of just 20% of a meniscus can lead to a 350% increase in contact force.[93] Meniscal transplantation has been demonstrated to improve contact force when compared with total meniscectomy, provided that the posterior and anterior horns are adequately anchored to bone.[4,21,81] Other studies imply that the soft viscoelastic meniscus has the ability to attenuate shock waves generated through the normal gait pattern and, through the intrinsic material properties of the meniscus, decrease the stress loading of articular cartilage.[28,103] The ultrastructure of the menisci contributes to the nutritional environment of the knee, as originally proposed by MacConaill,[66] and enhances lubrication of the joint by distributing synovial fluid within the knee.

MENISCAL ULTRASTRUCTURE

An understanding of the ultrastructure of a normal meniscus is necessary for a functional knowledge of the pathophysiology of meniscal dysfunction and of how to approach replacement of this function. For further information, Mow et al,[74] Thompson et al,[105] Skaggs et al,[100] and Spilker and Donzeley[101] are excellent sources of understandable meniscal biochemistry.

Meniscal tissue is composed of cells that are either elongated on the surface or ovoid in deeper layers and equipped with few mitochondria, thus suggesting anaerobic metabolism.[93] The extracellular matrix of menisci is 74% water by weight, but type I collagen constitutes about 65% of the dry weight, and glycosaminoglycans make up 2% of the dry weight. With this structure, the meniscus is able to resist tension, compression, and shear forces. Other collagens (II, III, V, and VI) make up about 5% of the dry weight. There are additional noncollagenous proteins, including elastin, fibronectin, and thromboplastin, that probably assist in organizing the matrix by binding molecules. The blood supply to the meniscus is derived from the inferior medial and lateral geniculate arteries, which form a plexus encompassing 10% to 30% of the width of the medial meniscus and 10% to 25% of the width of the lateral meniscus.[6] There is also a 1- to 3-mm cuff of vascular synovium that lies on both the femoral and tibial surfaces. This complex blood supply is key to successful meniscal repair or transplantation. In addition, a network of micropores permits synovial fluid to pump through the meniscal tissue with normal cyclic joint compression. This synovial fluid circulation is key to the function of articular cartilage.[73]

The structure of meniscal tissue allows it to behave as a fiber-reinforced, porous-permeable composite material containing both solids (matrix proteins) and fluid (water).[35,36] Collagen is responsible for the major structural scaffolding of the meniscus. Collagen fibers are arranged in multiple parallel circumferential bundles around the periphery of the entire meniscus. These circumferential collagen fibers provide the hoop stress resistance to strain. The parallel collagen fibers in the periphery of the meniscus provide increased stiffness in this region, in contrast to the central two-thirds, which has randomly oriented collagen fibers and a sheet-like arrangement of radial tie fibers, with correspondingly higher strain rates.

It is not surprising, then, that the periphery of the meniscus has a low proteoglycan-collagen ratio. The restraining collagen fibers, if undamaged, permit little swelling in this stiff region. In contrast, the less stiff central two-thirds of the meniscus has a high proteoglycan-collagen ratio, which promotes hydration and swelling. This hydration pressure within meniscal tissue affects compressive stiffness of the meniscus, which enables meniscal cartilage to effectively load-share with articular cartilage. It follows that abnormal meniscal hydration pressure indicates collagen or proteoglycan damage.

Collagen and proteoglycan damage can be caused by mechanical factors, enzymatic degradation, or the synthesis of new, poorly functioning molecules. Once collagen damage occurs, water of hydration increases, and an irreversible cascade of tissue alteration begins. When proteoglycans are damaged (but collagen remains intact), these tissue changes are reversible. For example, immobilization and lack of compressive loading lead to proteoglycan loss. Rehabilitation with increased range of motion and loading stimulates fibrochondrocytes to synthesize new proteoglycan molecules.

Central and peripheral tears occur with different mechanisms and have different consequences. With the higher strain rate and lack of stiffness of the central meniscus, collagen meshwork tears are relatively common (bucket handle tears), often resulting from low-energy mechanisms. Reparability is highly variable and depends on the location and orientation of the tear. The consequence of central tissue resection is far less than that of peripheral meniscal resection. Meniscal tears in the stiff peripheral region are more rare than central tears. In the periphery, the densely packed circumferential meniscal collagen fibers provide vital hoop strain resistance to joint compression. However, at higher-energy injury mechanisms that cause high shear loading and compression, tears can propagate radially through the peripheral rim. Once this outer rim loses continuity, that knee compartment is irreversibly meniscus deficient.

If the meniscal periphery is not intact, even over relatively short distances, meniscal allograft transplantation may be indicated.[58] In the setting of meniscal transplantation, the same ultrastructural principles that govern successful function of the original meniscus also apply to a transplanted meniscus.

When considering meniscal transplantation, the cause of the meniscal damage is most commonly mechanical rather than degenerative[113] or inflammatory. If the inciting feature of the meniscal demise was synovial disease (viral arthritis, enzymatic degradation, or neoplasm), the allograft will experience the same fate as the original meniscus. It has been demonstrated that circumferential bundles of collagen fibers of the transplanted meniscus must be intact from the anterior (bony) horn to the posterior (bony) horn. Adequate function of the meniscal transplant relies on secure bone fixation of the anterior and posterior horns.[5,21,81] Commonly, this is accomplished by using bone plugs or a slot-and-keyhole technique. Viable, functioning host fibrochondrocytes must survive within the lacunae of the implanted allograft to produce proteoglycans, which in turn are required to maintain hydration pressure and proper mechanical integrity. Physiological loads are required to stimulate the fibrochondrocytes. An accurately sized allograft must be anatomically oriented in the compartment to allow for congruent articulation and proper load sharing with articular cartilage. Conversely, the recipient compartment cannot lack congruency with the implant (e.g., mechanical malalignment or advanced Fairbank changes).[32]

MENISCECTOMY

Meniscal tears may create symptoms of pain and dysfunction in the knee and predispose the knee to osteoarthritis and cartilage degeneration. Depending on the size, location, and orientation of the tear, a torn meniscus may or may not retain its biomechanical function.[28] Currently, the gold standard of care for a meniscal disorder emphasizes that a meniscal tear be repaired when possible. However, partial and total meniscectomies are still necessary at times. In 1948, Fairbank[32] recognized the detrimental effects of altered biomechanics in a meniscectomized knee, and several studies have since examined the impact that partial and complete meniscectomies have in spurring the progression of degenerative changes.[47,53,64,65,78,104] Unique biomechanical and anatomic factors lead to a relatively higher risk for tibiofemoral degeneration in the lateral compartment than in the medial compartment after meniscectomy.[2,59,81,112] Under normal physiological conditions, the lateral meniscus carries most of the load in the lateral compartment, whereas in the medial compartment, the load is shared approximately equally between the meniscus and the exposed cartilage.[112] Furthermore, it has been shown that removal of the medial meniscus may cause a reduction in contact area by up to 70% and that absence of a meniscus increases the pressure gradient considerably near the margin of the articular contact area.[1] An important predictive factor in the development of degenerative arthritis is the time since meniscectomy.

HISTORICAL PERSPECTIVE

The limb-sparing reconstructions performed almost a century ago represent the first meniscal allograft transplantations, and they were combined with complete knee transplantation in 1908 by Lexer,[61] who reported a 50% success rate when allograft was incorporated into the host bone.[62] Meniscal allograft reconstruction has existed since 1972, when Zukor et al[116] reported on a series of 33 fresh meniscal allograft transplants. Since that time, fresh meniscus transplantation has been abandoned for several reasons, including the logistic challenges of size-matching a donor to a recipient within narrow time constraints. The concept of meniscus reconstruction might have been abandoned if not for the development of safe and effective allograft tissue preservation and storage techniques. The ability to store a meniscus allows tissue processors the opportunity to accumulate an inventory of menisci from which a surgeon can select an appropriately sized meniscus for a patient. Since that time, significant work has been done to establish animal models and develop reproducible surgical techniques for humans.

Animal Research

Animal studies have contributed greatly to our understanding of meniscal transplantation and the ability of a transplanted meniscus to function protectively and survive within the knee. In New Zealand white rabbits, Cummins et al[26] showed that both immediate and delayed meniscal allograft transplantation offered protection to the articular cartilaginous surfaces of the knee after meniscectomy and may even reverse some early degenerative changes.

In sheep, Milachowski et al[69-71] examined various methods of graft preparation and sterilization and showed that lyophilized, gamma–irradiated allografts demonstrated healing within 6 weeks and remodeling in a year, whereas frozen allografts took longer to heal and never demonstrated revascularization and remodeling. Irradiated allografts had a healed meniscal rim at 6 weeks and were fully remodeled at 48 weeks, whereas sheep receiving deep-frozen specimens were noted to have a healed meniscal rim at 48 weeks but little revascularization and disorganized remodeling over time.

Using canine models in which cryopreserved allografts were implanted, Arnoczky and colleagues[8,10] demonstrated an initial 2-week post-transplantation decrease in cellularity, with a return toward normal at 3 to 6 months. Evaluation of the cellular repopulation of deep-frozen meniscal autografts demonstrated that, although freezing killed all cells in the central portion of the graft, the peripheral region could still be repopulated with host cells. At 6 months there was persistent disruption of collagen orientation. In goats, Jackson et al[48] found no donor DNA but an abundance of host DNA in the revascularized cryopreserved allograft 4 weeks after implantation. Other goat revascularization studies have shown that in cryopreserved transplants there is a physiological distribution of vascular ingrowth in the peripheral third, whereas freeze-dried allografts demonstrate a more haphazard pattern associated with graft shrinkage.[9] Despite these differences, additional evidence has shown that both methods of preserving grafts result in some increase in uronic acid levels and increased water content, thus suggesting slight degeneration at 6 months.[49] Mikic et al[68] reported normal meniscal architecture 8 to 12 months after the implantation of fresh medial allografts. Despite the normal architecture, these menisci were noted to have less cellularity than those in controls.

Although a new signaling system for interleukin-17, a proinflammatory cytokine secreted by activated T cells, has recently been identified in meniscal tissue,[72] animal studies have not found a predictable immune response from implanted meniscal allografts. Fabbriciani et al[30] compared cryopreserved and deep-frozen meniscal allografts in goats. Follow-up at 2 weeks and 1, 3, 6, and 12 months showed a normal appearance of the grafts and adequate peripheral healing. An initial decrease in the cellularity of both graft types was followed by cellular proliferation and revascularization at 3 months. Additionally, they could find no evidence of immunological rejection; ultimately, no difference was found between deep-frozen and cryopreserved meniscal transplants.

In the previously described study by Jackson et al[48] in which DNA elimination from the meniscus was evaluated, there was no evidence of a humoral immune response, thus essentially eliminating an early immunological reaction as the cause of death of the cryopreserved fibrochondrocytes. Ochi et al[79] placed fresh meniscal allografts under the skin in mice. Using the stimulation index of mixed lymphocyte culture and a complement-dependent cytotoxicity test, no evidence existed over a 24-week period for either humoral or cell-mediated immune responses.

Human Immunogenicity

A brief description of human immunology in meniscal transplantation is warranted. The immunologic system responds to antigenic challenges either by humeral immunity, an antibody-mediated phenomenon, or by cell-mediated immunity, which is regulated by cytotoxic leukocytes.[56]

HUMORAL IMMUNITY

Proteins with antibody activity are synthesized by B lymphocytes and are called immunoglobulins. Electrophoresis of blood serum clearly bands gamma globulin apart from other serum immunoglobulins. A primary humoral-mediated response takes place over a period of several days and elicits the prodrome of a viral illness characterized by general malaise. Re-exposure to the same antigen permits a secondary response within hours that is often without constitutional symptoms and may remain subclinical. Humoral immunity, which mediates the immune response to pathogens, plays a less important and ill-defined role in responding to the antigen challenge from foreign tissue grafts. It is the cell-mediated immune system that is primarily responsible for graft rejection.[56]

CELL-MEDIATED IMMUNITY

Graft rejection is a cell-mediated immune response. On activation of cell-mediated, type IV delayed-type hypersensitivity, sensitized individuals respond to the challenge within 10 hours and reach a peak response in 48 to 72 hours. The cell-mediated immune response is mediated by T lymphocytes. Sensitized T lymphocytes release lymphokines on contact with a specific antigen, which in turn attract proportionally larger concentrations of nonspecific macrophages, lymphocytes, and other cytotoxic white blood cells to attack the foreign allograft material. Histologic examination of an allograft undergoing rejection by the host will show nonspecific leukocytes and macrophages within the tissue.

The major histocompatibility complex HLA is a closely linked set of loci on chromosome 6. These genetic alleles encode class I and class II histocompatibility antigens. Class I genes refer to the particular loci on each chromosome and are classified as A, B, or C (i.e., HLA-A, HLA-B, and HLA-C). These class I genes encode antigens, which are found on the surface of most cells in the body. Expression of class II genes is more limited than is the case for class I genes.[56] Class II antigens are found on only a few types of cells, such as dendritic cells, activated macrophages, and mature B cells. In response to foreign human leukocyte antigens, the host mounts a cell-mediated reaction.[16]

Even after deep-freezing, class I and II histocompatibility antigens are expressed on the cells of a meniscal allograft, thus indicating the potential for an immune response.[55] Attached bone plugs and synovial tissue also contain immunogenic cells, and it is well established that bone remains immunogenic even after freezing.[38] We are aware of only one report providing clinical and histological evidence of frank immunological rejection of a cryopreserved, non–tissue antigen–matched meniscal allograft.[45] Although frank immunological rejection is rarely seen, there is histological evidence of an immune response directed against the graft. For example, one study demonstrated sensitization to HLA class I and class II antigens in recipients of cryopreserved, non–tissue antigen–matched meniscal allografts; however, there was no clinical evidence of rejection in these patients[90,107] even though immunoreactive cells (B lymphocytes and cytotoxic T cells) were reported in 9 of 12 recipients of fresh frozen meniscal allografts. The effect of an immune response on graft incorporation is unknown, but such a reaction may modulate graft healing, incorporation, and revascularization.

Clinical Reports

With respect to articular allograft safety, Friedlaender et al compared immunological response and clinical outcome 10 years after the implantation of massive osteochondral allografts in 29 patients. Although these were articular cartilage osteochondral allografts, the low rate of meaningful immune reactions is relative to meniscal allograft transplants. In this series, eight patients (28%) had anti–class II HLA responses, but of those, five (63%) had good to excellent results. Of the 21 without an immune reaction, 18 (86%) had satisfactory outcomes. They concluded that the immune reactions found with even massive grafts were self-limited and did not preclude a satisfactory result.[39]

De Boer and Koudstall[27] implanted a non–tissue antigen–matched, cryopreserved meniscal allograft in the lateral compartment of a patient's knee. Evaluation of the nonmatched allograft showed that it remained metabolically active and did not differ from control specimens. Clinically, the postoperative result was classified as excellent.

Van Arkel et al[107] and Khoury et al[55] reported antibodies against the HLA complex in recipients without accompanying graft failure. These studies suggest a need for serological and biopsy monitoring to detect immunogenicity related to meniscal allograft transplantation. Van Arkel et al used non–tissue antigen–matched, cryopreserved meniscal allografts and demonstrated class I anti-HLA antibodies in 11 of 18 patients.[107] This finding was, however, without clinical or histological signs of rejection. (Class I HLA antigens are routinely found on the surface of fibrochondrocytes. No class II antigens exist on these cells.)

GRAFT PROCUREMENT AND PROCESSING

Because of the difficulty in locating, harvesting, and distributing fresh donor allografts to a size-matched recipient within a few days of harvest, fresh menisci suitable for allograft implantation have given way to bank-preserved meniscal allografts. The manner in which the menisci are preserved and stored and the subsequent clinical outcome constitute a major portion of what has been reported in the orthopedic literature.

Stringent donor selection plus screening, beginning with recording of a comprehensive medical and social history, is a critical first step in ensuring procurement of disease-free allograft tissue. The American Association of Tissue Banks has defined the recommended testing protocol.[67] Serological screening is performed for human immunodeficiency virus (HIV) p24 antigen, HIV-1/HIV-2 antibody, human T-cell lymphotropic virus-I (HTLV-I) and HTLV-II, hepatitis B surface antigen, hepatitis B core antibody, hepatitis C antibody, and syphilis. Most tissue banks perform polymerase chain reaction testing, which can detect 1 HIV-infected cell out of 10^6 cells. The current "window" of time for development of detectable antibodies to HIV is approximately 20 to 25 days (a donor may be infected but test negative for HIV). Blood cultures for aerobic and anaerobic bacteria are done, and lymph node sampling may be performed.

Graft processing, including débridement, ultrasonic/pulsatile washing, and the use of ethanol to denature proteins, further lowers the risk of disease transmission. Freezing lowers the risk even more, but HIV can survive washing, freezing, and freeze-drying.[75] It is evident that safety depends on donor screening and not graft processing. The current risk for transmission of HIV by frozen connective tissue allografts is estimated to be 1 in 8 million.[17]

The tissue is procured within 12 hours after death (fresh grafts) or within 24 hours after death if the body has been stored at 4°C. The tissue may be harvested with use of sterile surgical technique, or it may be procured in a clean, nonsterile environment. After harvest, tissue is preserved by one of four methods: it can be fresh, cryopreserved, fresh frozen, or lyophilized. Fresh and cryopreserved allografts contain viable cells, whereas fresh frozen and lyophilized tissues are acellular at the time of transplantation. Fresh tissue is harvested under sterile conditions within 12 hours after death. The tissue is stored in culture medium at 4°C or 37°F to maintain viable cells. Transplantation must be performed within several days of graft procurement, thus resulting in difficult logistics.[111] The proportion of cells that survive and the duration for which they survive after transplantation are unknown. The DNA probe study by Jackson et al[49] demonstrated that all the donor cells in a fresh meniscal transplant were rapidly replaced by host cells.

Cryopreservation includes the use of a cryoprotectant (such as dimethyl sulfoxide) in an attempt to maintain cell viability while allowing prolonged storage without affecting graft biomechanics.[7] Fresh frozen grafts are rapidly frozen to −80°C, which kills cells without an important effect on graft material properties. Lyophilization, or freeze-drying, kills cells and may adversely affect graft material properties and result in graft shrinkage.[71,114] Unlike the case with fresh osteochondral grafts, the morphological and biochemical characteristics of meniscal allografts do not seem to be improved by graft cell viability; thus, the most commonly implanted grafts are either fresh frozen or cryopreserved. Experimental studies in goats have suggested that there are no important differences between cryopreserved and deep-frozen grafts.[31,49]

Secondary sterilization with ethylene oxide, gamma irradiation, or chemical means may be used for fresh frozen or lyophilized grafts. The amount of gamma irradiation required to eliminate viral DNA (at least 3.0 Mrad [30,000 gray]) may adversely affect the material properties of the meniscus.[46] Lower doses of gamma irradiation (<2.0 Mrad [<20,000 gray]) may be used for bacterial sterilization. Ethylene oxide is used only for lyophilized grafts, but it is not recommended because the ethylene chlorohydrin byproduct has been found to induce synovitis.[50] Chemical sterilization may be done with use of proprietary bactericidal/virucidal solutions. In general, however, secondary sterilization is not preferred for meniscal allografts.

INDICATIONS FOR MENISCUS TRANSPLANTATION

The ideal patient for meniscal allograft transplantation is a young, but skeletally mature, nonobese individual with stable knee ligaments, normal anatomic alignment, and normal articular cartilage who seeks treatment for pain in a meniscus-deficient compartment. There must be no inflammatory arthritis, synovial disease, or history of infection in the involved knee.

The patient should be young enough that total knee arthroplasty is not an option. Although there is no upper chronological age limit, meniscus-deficient patients who are older than 50 to 55 years often already have a degree of arthritis that contraindicates the procedure. Skeletal maturity is necessary to avoid causing asymmetric physeal arrest and progressive angular deformity from metaphyseal tunnels and potential bony bar formation.

To maximize the potential for a good outcome, it is important to optimize the mechanical environment of the implanted meniscus. For this reason, obesity is a relative contraindication to meniscal transplantation. Untreated comorbid conditions of ligament instability, axial limb malalignment, and focal cartilage defects create a hostile mechanical environment for the meniscal allograft and are therefore relative contraindications. It is advisable to treat these comorbid conditions, often in combined procedures with ligament reconstruction, osteotomy, or cartilage restoration as indicated. Just a few degrees of deviation toward the involved compartment in comparison to the alignment in the contralateral limb may be an indication for osteotomy. The treatment of comorbid conditions as concomitant or staged procedures is discussed later in this chapter.

Fairbank[32] described the progression of arthritis in meniscectomized knees. Stage I is defined as the formation of an anteroposterior ridge projecting downward from the margin of the femoral condyle over the meniscal site. Stage II consists of a generalized flattening of the marginal half of the femoral articular surface of the involved compartment, and in stage III narrowing of the joint space on the involved side is often associated with varus-valgus deformity of the knee. Theoretically, restoration of the normal meniscal anatomy could decelerate or prevent such progressive degenerative change, but this has not been proven.

Serious articular disease (i.e., late grade III or IV)[80] and radiographic signs of flattening of the femoral condyle or marked osteophyte formation are associated with inferior results, however, and are considered the most common contraindications to meniscal transplantation. Several authors have suggested that advanced arthritis is an absolute contraindication to meniscal allograft transplantation, primarily because of questionable graft survival.[41,99,108]

It is of utmost importance to accurately identify the motivation of a patient seeking meniscal allograft transplantation. Although the procedure may be able to halt the rapid progression of osteoarthritis, it is primarily a pain-relieving effort. Reasonable patient expectations of partial, relatively short-term pain relief must be established. Therefore, the ideal patient seeks treatment of a painful condition referable to the meniscus-deficient compartment and understands that even the most successful meniscal transplantation does not obviate the potential for total knee arthroplasty in the future.

Any systemic physiological metabolic condition or local inflammatory condition in the affected knee is a contraindication to meniscal transplantation. Erosions from synovial disease or deposits from metabolic conditions will damage meniscal allografts and predict failure. Existing systemic immunodeficiency or a history of previous infection in the involved knee is a contraindication to meniscal transplantation because the risk for infection and the associated potential for devastating outcomes, especially in the setting of a deficient host immune system, outweigh the potential for benefit with this procedure.

Most patients, however, do not fall clearly into all of these categories. It may be that a patient with an absent lateral meniscus fits all these criteria but pain has not yet developed in the meniscus-deficient compartment. Earlier transplantation in certain asymptomatic patients could be appropriate. It is advisable for patients considering meniscal transplantation to seek a second opinion from a knee specialist. The benefit to the surgeon of receiving a fresh perspective and opinion from a knowledgeable colleague while evaluating a transplant candidate should not be underestimated.

PATIENT EVALUATION

Not uncommonly, patients who have had an open or arthroscopic meniscectomy report nearly immediate and complete resolution of symptoms, followed by a subtle increase, over time, in ipsilateral joint line pain, activity-related swelling, generalized aching affected by changes in ambient barometric pressure, and, occasionally, giving way and crepitus. A thorough history, including the mechanism of injury, associated injuries, and previous treatments such as ligament reconstruction or management of articular cartilage lesions, should be elicited.

Physical examination is essential to look for concomitant disorders (e.g., malalignment or ligament deficiency) that would modify treatment recommendations. The location of previous incisions is noted and may provide evidence of previous meniscectomy. An effusion may or may not be present. Typically, patients have tenderness along the ipsilateral joint line and may have palpable osseous change along the edge of the femoral or tibial condyle. If the patient is to receive a meniscal transplant, motion should be normal inasmuch as the degree of arthritis acceptable for meniscus transplantation is rarely associated with motion loss.

Diagnostic imaging is required and should begin with a standard weightbearing anteroposterior radiograph of both knees in full extension, a non-weightbearing 45-degree flexion lateral radiograph, and an axial radiograph of the patellofemoral joint. Additionally, a 45-degree flexion weightbearing posteroanterior radiograph is recommended to help identify the subtle joint narrowing that traditional extension views may fail to identify.[92]

It is often necessary to order special studies, such as a long-cassette mechanical axis radiograph if there is any degree of clinical malalignment or magnetic resonance imaging (MRI) if chondral injury is suspected. Generally, MRI is helpful when radiographs and/or previous operative reports are unavailable or are unable to reveal the status of the articular cartilage or the extent of a previous meniscectomy. Techniques include two-dimensional fast spin-echo and three-dimensional fat suppression with and without intra-articular gadolinium.[85] When questions remain about the source of symptoms, a three-phase technetium bone scan can be useful to assess for increased uptake in the involved compartment.

ALLOGRAFT SIZING

One should not use an MRI scan from the contralateral knee to measure the soft-tissue dimensions of a meniscal allograft. The work of Kohn and Moreno[57] demonstrated that the appropriate size of an absent meniscus cannot be determined by measuring the contralateral meniscus in the same compartment because meniscal allografts are side and compartment specific. In addition, they demonstrated that the size of a particular meniscus does not correlate predictably with a patient's height.

Several studies have assessed the accuracy and reliability of MRI, x-rays films, and computed tomography (CT) for sizing meniscus allografts.[19,54,108] Kennedy et al[54] compared x-ray films and MRI scans with cadaver dissections and concluded that the methods were comparable in accuracy and reliability, but that both overestimated meniscus size. In contrast, Carpenter et al[19] compared MRI, x-ray film, and CT in cadaver specimens. In this study, x-ray film and CT were more accurate than MRI, which tended to underestimate meniscus size. A similar study by Veltri et al[108] found that CT-arthrography underestimated 74% of menisci by a mean of 3.8 mm and overestimated 19% by 2.0 mm. MRI underestimated 54% of menisci by 2.8 mm and overestimated 34% by 4 mm.

Because of these potential inaccuracies, plain radiographs are most commonly used to size allografts.[84,95] Preoperatively, precise measurements are made on anteroposterior and lateral radiographs, with magnification markers placed on the skin at the level of the proximal end of the tibia. The surgeon should be familiar with the sizing techniques used by the tissue provider to minimize the chance of a size mismatch. Most commonly, the technique described by Pollard et al[84] is used for meniscal sizing. Meniscal width is determined on an anteroposterior radiograph, after correction for magnification, on the basis of a 1:1 relationship to the distance from the center of the respective tibial eminence to the periphery of the tibial plateau. Meniscal length is calculated on the lateral radiograph on the basis of the sagittal length of the tibial plateau. After correction for magnification, this length is multiplied by 0.8 for the medial meniscus and by 0.7 for the lateral meniscus. For example, if the tibial plateau measures 38 mm from the medial tibial eminence to the periphery of the tibia on an anteroposterior radiograph with 5% magnification, the width of the required meniscal graft is 36 mm (38 × 0.95). If the sagittal length of the tibial plateau from anterior to posterior is 50 mm on a lateral radiograph with 5% magnification, the length of the required medial meniscal graft is 38 mm ([50 × 0.95] × 0.8). With use of this technique, size mismatch occurs less than 5% of the time.

If the graft is judged perioperatively by the surgeon to be undersized or oversized or if the surgeon is presented with the incorrect meniscus altogether (e.g., a medial rather than a lateral meniscus or a left rather than a right meniscus), the meniscus should not be used. Small size mismatches can be handled with only minor modifications and are likely to have minimal effects on anatomic restoration, but accurate sizing remains important to maximize the chondroprotective effect of the graft.[110]

SURGICAL TECHNIQUES

The goal of meniscal allograft transplantation is to replace any absent or deficient meniscus in an anatomic position that restores the original meniscofemoral or meniscotibial articulation. The meniscus can be implanted using either an open or an arthroscopically assisted technique. Although the results of the two methods have been reported to be similar, arthroscopic techniques are routinely used because of the reduced surgical morbidity.[18,20,24,34,37,41,71,102,106]

The most common methods of anchoring the meniscal allograft use either bone plugs on the anterior and posterior horns, which are not attached to one another, or a bone bridge, which rigidly fixes the distance between the anterior and posterior horns. Regardless of the technique used, it is essential that the meniscus be placed in an anatomic position if it is to replicate an intact host meniscus. Even though it is technically easier to secure the graft with soft tissue alone, bone anchorage of the anterior and posterior horns is required to provide a biomechanically functional meniscus.[4,21,81]

Although a medial meniscus transplant may be anchored with either bone plugs in tunnels or a bone bridge in a slot, bone plugs are used only for medial meniscal transplants and are not recommended for use on the lateral side. Using bone plugs for a lateral meniscus transplant presents a risk of tunnel communication with compromised fixation because the distance between the lateral meniscus horns is only 1 cm or less.[52] Proponents of bone plugs on the medial side point out the variability in the anterior horn attachment site and the ability to make minor modifications in position.[13,57] Proponents of a bone bridge on the medial side point out the ease of

insertion and relative maintenance of the anatomic relationship between the anterior and posterior horns.[24,34] Thus, whereas a bone bridge is commonly used on the lateral side, the medial side can be reconstructed with either a bridge or plugs, depending on the surgeon's preference.

Patient Positioning and Initial Preparation

The patient is placed under general anesthesia and intravenous prophylactic antibiotics are administered. Before placing the patient in the desired leg holder, a thorough examination under anesthesia is performed to confirm the absence of ligamentous instability. The patient is positioned supine either with the leg unsupported and a lateral post placed just proximal to the knee or with the leg in a well-padded leg holder placed midthigh and a tourniquet on but not inflated. The position of the leg holder should be proximal enough to allow ample exposure to the posterolateral and posteromedial corners for an inside-out meniscal repair, but distal enough to allow considerable valgus or varus stress to be placed on the knee without undue concern of causing a femoral fracture as a result of an excessively long lever arm in the distal end of the femur. Standard arthroscopic portals are used, and standard diagnostic arthroscopy is performed to confirm the absence of grade III or greater chondral injuries in the recipient compartment. This step is particularly important if previous surgeries have been performed by another surgeon. We recommend that débridement of the residual meniscal tissue be performed without a tourniquet so that a vascularized recipient meniscocapsular interface can be verified during débridement.

Regardless of the fixation technique used, the initial steps for medial and lateral meniscal transplantation are similar and performed in the recipient compartment only. The host meniscus is débrided arthroscopically to a 1- to 2-mm peripheral rim until punctate bleeding occurs. A remnant of the anterior and posterior horns is left to clearly identify their location during tunnel creation or slot formation. A low modified notchplasty is recommended on either the medial or the lateral femoral condyle to assist with allograft passage and visualization. A standard inside-out meniscal repair exposure at the posterolateral or posteromedial corner is oriented one-third above and two-thirds below the joint line and placed in line with the respective femoral condyle.

Bone Plug Technique

Medial meniscal allograft transplantation is often performed with separate bone plug anchors of the anterior and posterior horns. For this procedure, the involved compartment is prepared in the same manner as though performing a bridge technique. Two separate 9-mm cylindrical bone plugs are cored from the meniscal allograft, with care taken to preserve all soft-tissue attachments of the meniscal horns to the bone plug. A 1.5-mm drill bit is used to create a suture hole in each bone plug, through which No. 2 braided nonabsorbable polyethylene sutures are passed. These sutures will be passed through the recipient tunnels and allow for secure anchorage of the bone plugs. Alternatively, the posterior horn bone plug is undersized by 1 mm to facilitate passage and seating within the tunnel. A monofilament suture is placed in the posterior medial corner of the allograft to act as a traction stitch at the time of implantation (Figs. 32–1 and 32–2).

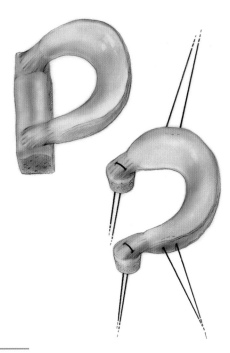

Figure 32–1. Sutures are preinserted into the posteromedial edge of the meniscus and through each bone plug.

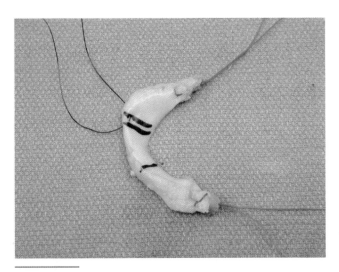

Figure 32–2. Nonabsorbable sutures are centered within each bone block. Guide sutures (which help spread out the meniscus within the medial compartment) are preinserted into the posteromedial and anterior portions of the allograft.

To assist in visualization of the posterior horn and facilitate passage of the posterior bone plug, it is advisable to perform a modified low notchplasty between the fibers of the posterior cruciate ligament and the medial femoral condyle. To drill the recipient tunnels, an ACL guide is used to pass a pin from medial to the tibial tuberosity to the exact center of the posterior horn and the tunnel then reamed to 9 mm. The same technique can be used to position and create the anterior horn tunnel. The location of the anterior horn attachment is anterior to the footprint of the ACL at the anterior margin of the tibial plateau (Fig. 32–3). The anterior tunnel is generally made after the meniscus is seated posteriorly and repaired peripherally with inside-out sutures.

Viewing from the lateral portal, the medial portal is expanded to receive the allograft. Next, the posteromedial traction stitch is passed into the knee joint and out the posteromedial corner of the knee. The posterior bone plug stitch is then passed into the knee and out through the posterior horn tunnel with a suture-passing device. With tension maintained on the traction stitches at the posteromedial corner and the posterior bone plug, valgus stress is placed on the knee to open the medial compartment while the allograft is guided through the expanded medial portal and into the medial side of the joint (Fig 32–4). The bone plug is manipulated into the posterior horn tunnel, a task that takes patience and persistence, but is facilitated by removal of the top of the medial tibial eminence by medial low notchplasty (Fig. 32–5) and firm traction on the traction stitch with the knee positioned in about 30 degrees of flexion. After the meniscus is reduced in the medial compartment, the knee is cycled several times to properly position the meniscus.

The anterior horn bone plug is press-fit into a blind tunnel, which ideally has been reamed in the center of the footprint of the host anterior horn after the meniscus is secured posteriorly. Minor adjustments in position are made as required. Sutures are passed through the anterior cortex of the proximal end of the tibia with a free cutting needle and tied over bone (Fig. 32–6). This technique

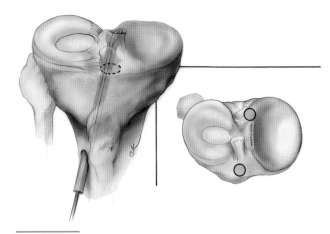

Figure 32–3. The anterior horn attachment is at the anterior margin of the tibial plateau. The posterior horn attachment is on the posterior slope of the medial intercondylar eminence. The "top" of the medial tibial eminence is removed.

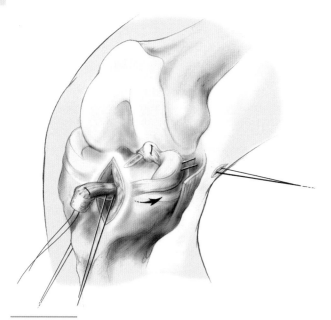

Figure 32–4. The allograft is gently urged through the expanded medial portal. The posteromedial suture and the anterior suture are tensioned to spread out the meniscus within the compartment.

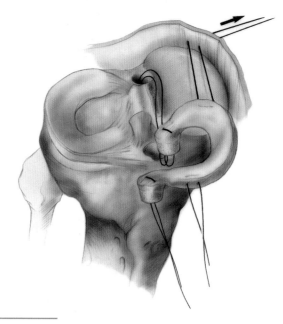

Figure 32–6. The posteromedial preinserted suture is passed into the joint through the medial portal and out the joint through a hole in the posteromedial capsule.

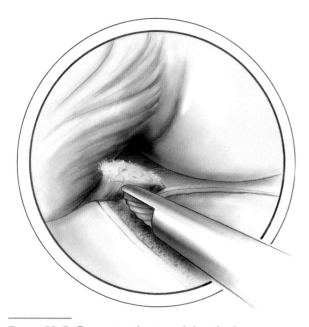

Figure 32–5. Removing the top of the tibial eminence.

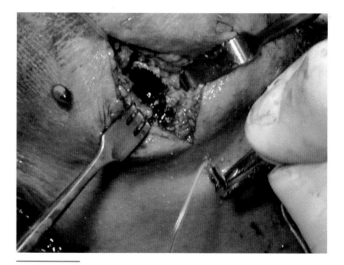

Figure 32–7. The anterior horn plug is pulled into a blind tunnel with sutures passed through the anterior cortex.

avoids an additional stress riser in the tibial metaphysis and allows for a tibial ACL tunnel if a simultaneous ACL reconstruction is performed.

Eight to ten vertically placed 2-0 nonabsorbable mattress sutures are placed in a posterior-to-anterior direction with use of a standard inside-out meniscal repair technique (Fig. 32–7). On the medial side, all-inside bioabsorbable devices are a reasonable choice to secure the most posterior aspect of the meniscus to minimize the risk of neurovascular injury, but their pull-out strength is less

than that of vertical sutures and they provide only single-point fixation.[3,14]

Bridge-in-Slot Technique

An exact description of this technique is available elsewhere.[24,34] Exposure for creation of the slot is made directly in line with the anterior and posterior meniscal horns of the recipient compartment. A miniarthrotomy is made either directly adjacent to the patellar tendon or by splitting the tendon in line with its fibers and preserving a paratenon layer for closure.

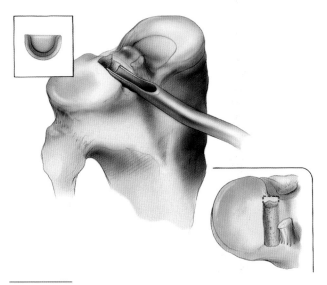

Figure 32–8. Drawing of a quarter-round gouge removing a posterior trough.

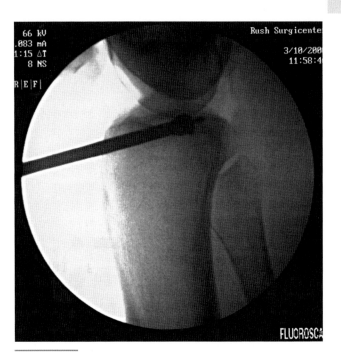

Figure 32–9. Fluoroscopic lateral visualization of the location of a reamer with respect to the posterior tibial cortex.

To create a slot in the proper anatomic location, the centers of the anterior and posterior horns are identified, and electrocautery is used to mark a line between the centers of the horns. Next, a 4-mm bur is used to create a superficial reference slot along this line. This reference slot should be the depth of the bur and should match the sagittal slope of the tibia. A depth gauge is placed into the slot and hooked onto the posterior of the tibia to confirm that it is of uniform height and depth and to accurately measure the anteroposterior dimension of the slot. A drill guide chucked at the measured depth is used to insert a guide pin parallel to the tibial slope, with care taken to not penetrate the posterior cortex of the tibial plateau (Fig. 32–8). It is recommended that guide wire placement and reaming be performed under fluoroscopic control (Fig. 32–9). The guide pin is advanced, but not through the posterior cortex of the tibial plateau. An 8-mm cannulated reamer is advanced over the guide wire. Next, a box cutter 8 mm wide (equal to the diameter of the reamer) and 10 mm deep is used to create a slot 8 mm wide and 10 mm deep. A rasp is used to smoothe the surface and edges of the slot to ensure uniformity in width and depth and prevent impingement of the prepared allograft bone bridge.

ALLOGRAFT PREPARATION

The allograft arrives from the tissue bank as a hemiplateau with the meniscus attached. All nonmeniscal soft tissue is débrided from the hemiplateau, and the exact locations of the anterior and posterior horn anchors are clearly identified (Fig. 32–10). The anchors are typically 5 or 6 mm in diameter. Using a commercially available cutting jig, the bone bridge is then cut to a width of 7 mm and a depth of 10 mm. We recommend undersizing the full length of the bridge by 1 mm to facilitate passage through the slot,

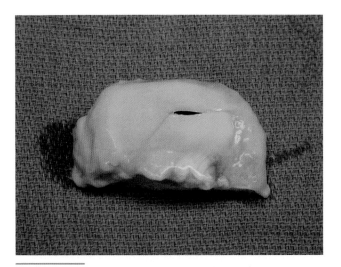

Figure 32–10. The thawed lateral meniscal allograft is prepared on the back table simultaneously with trough preparation in the lateral tibial plateau of the recipient. Each preplaced suture has a dual function: (1) to guide the meniscus around the lateral femoral condyle and (2) to critically support the graft in zones where sewing is difficult. Each suture placed in the bone blocks will be pulled into transosseous holes in the depths of the trough.

unless the host medial anterior horn anchor is particularly wide, in which case the anterior slot is slightly widened and only the posterior portion of the bridge is undersized. The prepared bridge is tested for ease of passage through calibrated troughs on the back table (Fig. 32–11). The posterior wall of the bridge should be flush or slanted slightly anterior to the fibers of the posterior horn attach-

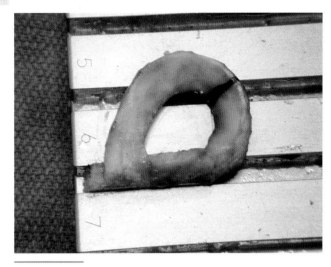

Figure 32–11. Lateral meniscus bridge measured carefully to confirm width.

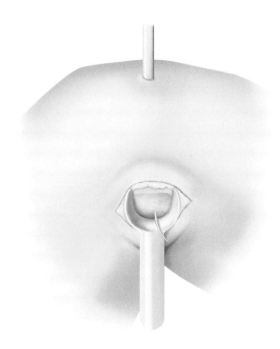

Figure 32–13. The posterolateral sutures on a long flexible needle are passed through the posterolateral capsule, glancing off a curved retractor that protects the posterior neurovascular structures.

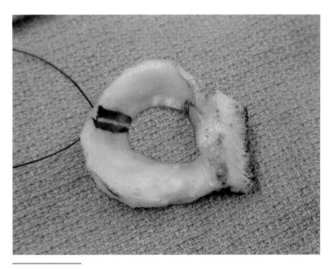

Figure 32–12. Prepared bone bridge demonstrating lack of bone posterior to the posterior horn insertion.

ment to allow for insertion at the most posterior edge of the prepared slot. Bone anterior to the anterior horn should be left in place to allow for safer graft manipulation during insertion (Fig. 32–12). A No. 0 polydioxanone vertical mattress traction suture is placed at the junction of the posterior and middle thirds.

GRAFT INSERTION

With a protective retractor placed in the posteromedial or posterolateral exposure, zone-specific cannulas are inserted in the contralateral portal, and a long nitinol needle is placed through the posteromedial capsule and retrieved through the posterior incision. The trailing end of the nitinol pin is then pulled out through the arthrotomy, and the traction sutures are inserted into the nitinol loop and withdrawn through the posterior incision

(Fig. 32–13). The meniscus is inserted through the arthrotomy and pulled under the condyle as the bone bridge is carefully guided into the slot. Care is taken to align the allograft with the recipient slot and to fully reduce the meniscus under the femoral condyle by pulling on the traction suture while cycling the knee to allow the femoral condyle to engage and position the allograft meniscus. Applying varus or valgus stress will open the recipient compartment. The slightly undersized meniscal bone bridge allows the meniscus to achieve its proper position by sliding freely within the tibial slot. Once the proper bone bridge position is achieved, a guide wire is inserted between the bone bridge and the more midline wall of the slot. A tap is used over the guide wire to create a path for an interference screw, and the bone bridge held firmly in place with an elevator placed through the arthrotomy. A bioabsorbable interference screw 7 or 8 mm by 20 mm is inserted while maintaining meticulous rotational control of the bone bridge. Of particular importance is fixation of the allograft bone bridge within the host tibial slot to maintain proper anatomic position of the meniscal horns. We have had recent success with allograft interference screws created from cortical allograft bone (Fig. 32–14).[34] However, bioabsorbable screws offer an acceptable alternative.

The final arthroscopic examination of the implanted allograft should confirm not only that the graft is anatomically reduced under the condyle but also that the proper size was selected. The lack of undulation on the surface indicates that the tissue is not distorted in situ (Fig. 32–15).

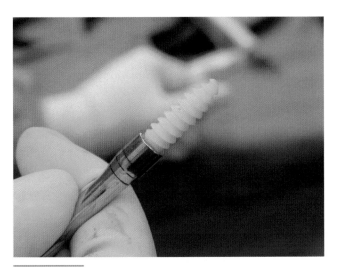

Figure 32–14. An interference screw machined from allograft bone is used for fixation of the bone bridge in the slot.

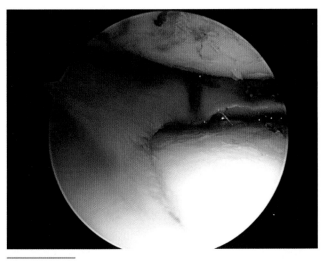

Figure 32–15. Arthroscopic image of a transplanted meniscus demonstrating proper reduction under the femoral condyle and proper size selection as evidenced by the smooth contour in situ.

ADVANCED COMBINED PROCEDURES

It is often advisable to perform simultaneous or staged procedures to treat any comorbid conditions that may coexist in the setting of meniscal transplantation. Limb axis malalignment, ligament instability, or cartilage defects may require an osteotomy, ligament reconstruction, or a cartilage-resurfacing procedure. When combining a meniscus transplant with other procedures, it is important to plan the exact sequence of events in a detailed preoperative plan.

Corrective Osteotomy

It is commonly believed that in the setting of an allograft transplantation, realignment osteotomy should be per-

formed as an adjunct procedure if the compartment receiving the allograft is under more than physiological compression.[43] In the setting of medial meniscal deficiency and varus alignment, a combined meniscus transplantation and high tibial osteotomy may be performed. In contrast to a standard high tibial osteotomy for isolated medial compartment osteoarthritis, in which the aim is to correct the mechanical axis laterally to 66% of the width of the tibial plateau in the lateral compartment,[63] high tibial osteotomies combined with medial meniscus transplantation should correct the mechanical axis to just beyond neutral. We recommend the use of an opening medial osteotomy to create a valgus correction rather than the more traditional closing lateral osteotomy. Commercially available instrumentation (Arthrex, Naples, FL) allows for a technically precise, simple, rapidly performed osteotomy with rigid fixation.

For meniscal allograft transplantation, a bridge-and-slot technique will prevent communication of the metaphyseal tunnels with the osteotomy. If bone plugs are used, the tunnels should exit as far proximal as possible to avoid traversing the osteotomy. Arthroscopic evaluation, soft-tissue preparation, notchplasty, and slot or tunnel creation for the meniscal transplant technique are performed first and then followed by the osteotomy. Osteotomies should be performed as far distally as possible. Rigid fixation is necessary to withstand manipulation of the leg during introduction of the meniscal graft and application of the valgus moment required for graft insertion and arthroscopic meniscal repair after the osteotomy. Proximal screw placement under fluoroscopic guidance is helpful to direct screws away from the previously prepared meniscal tunnels or trough.

For valgus angulation of a knee joint with lateral compartment disease, a distal femoral osteotomy is required to restore a normal mechanical axis. As with a high tibial osteotomy to treat varus disease, the goal with a distal femoral osteotomy is to correct the mechanical axis to neutral. Care must be taken to not overcorrect and create a varus alignment. Generally, we recommend an opening lateral distal femoral osteotomy with rigid plate fixation, although other techniques and fixation methods have been described, including a percutaneous dome osteotomy combined with temporary external fixation and intramedullary nail fixation.[44]

Meniscal Allograft Transplantation and ACL Reconstruction

Uncorrected ligamentous instability is a contraindication to meniscal transplantation. Preoperative evaluation of a meniscus-deficient knee includes careful analysis of the ligamentous instability, including a history of the injury, familiarity with previous surgical procedures, MRI and radiographic information, and ideally, KT arthrometry evaluation (see Chapter 36). Examination of the ACL under anesthesia is more reliable than while the patient is awake. Ideally, if a patient had previous surgeries, documentation of that examination would be available from those surgeries.

The biomechanical interdependence between an ACL reconstruction and the presence or condition of functional menisci is well documented[82] and has been shown to play an important role in obtaining a successful outcome after primary ACL reconstruction. Successful results are expected after primary ACL reconstruction, but they are still not universally predictable and may be related to the condition of the meniscus at the time of revision. A review of 482 patients with up to 15 years' follow-up (mean, 7.6 years) after primary ACL reconstruction demonstrated that the condition of the menisci at the time of ACL reconstruction was a key factor in predicting long-term outcome.[51,96] Thus, a successful ACL reconstruction relies on an intact medial meniscus to minimize anterior-posterior stress,[59,96] and an intact ACL, in turn, protects the menisci and articular cartilage.[12,15] Simultaneous meniscus transplantation plus ACL reconstruction has been shown to be mutually beneficial in properly selected patients.[22,115] This important interdependence is specifically highlighted in patients who have failure of their ACL reconstruction and a history of previous meniscectomy with complaints of instability and/or pain.

If a meniscus transplant is combined with either primary reconstruction or revision of the ACL, several issues related to the three-dimensional relationship of tunnels in the tibial metaphysis should be considered. Previous tunnel expansion and position, intended locations of new tunnels, ACL graft selection, and the meniscus anchor method offer variability to address the needs of each particular patient. With the medial double–bone plug technique, all soft-tissue and osseous portions of the meniscal transplant technique are performed first. The tibial tunnel for the ACL reconstruction is then drilled slightly more medially than usual to avoid confluence between it and the tunnel for the posterior horn of the meniscus. The remaining portions of the ACL reconstruction are performed as usual. With a bone bridge technique, the tibial tunnel for the ACL reconstruction is reamed after placement of the meniscal allograft. Placing the tunnel entrance slightly distally and medially on the tibia without compromising the anatomic position of the ACL footprint can avoid or minimize confluence between the tunnel and the lateral slot. The meniscal bone bridge may, however, be partially compromised without untoward effects during creation of the tibial tunnel.[22] Use of a hamstring graft for reconstruction of the ACL may facilitate graft passage and allow for a smaller-diameter tibial ACL tunnel.

Occasionally, patients have combined varus alignment, ACL deficiency, and an absent medial meniscus with relatively intact articular cartilage. These patients are typically managed with reconstruction of the ACL at the time of a high tibial osteotomy. The meniscal transplantation is performed simultaneously with these procedures only in rare situations, such as in very young patients. More commonly, meniscal allograft reconstruction is done in a delayed fashion in patients with persistent symptoms after recovery from the initial procedures.

Meniscal Allograft Transplantation and Cartilage Restoration Procedures

When combining cartilage restoration with meniscal transplantation in the same compartment, it is important to plan the exact sequence of events in a detailed preoperative plan. It is typically easier and safer for chondral procedures to be performed after all steps of the meniscal transplant have been completed to avoid inadvertent damage to the periosteal patch or osteochondral graft during meniscal instrumentation or suture repair.[23] On the other hand, the anterior horn of the transplanted meniscus could be damaged by a subsequent cartilage procedure on the ipsilateral femoral condyle. For example, implanting an osteochondral allograft and performing a meniscal transplant to treat a deep articular cartilage defect on the medial femoral condyle in a knee after previous medial meniscectomy will require that the posterior horn anchor be established before preparing the articular cartilage defect and implanting the osteochondral allograft plug. The bone plug and anterior horn of the meniscal allograft are gently retracted out of harm's way during implantation of the osteochondral graft and inserted in a blind tunnel at the anatomic site of the anterior horn after the osteochondral graft implantation is completed.

OUTCOMES

After meniscal allograft transplantation, good to excellent results are achieved in nearly 85% of cases, and patients have a measurable decrease in pain and an increase in activity level. Table 32–1 summarizes the outcomes of several series. From these series there appears to be a greater risk for graft failure in irradiated grafts, in patients with grade III to IV osteoarthritic changes, and in patients without bone anchorage in the anterior and posterior horns.[76] There is a trend toward better results in more recent series, which reflects collective improvement in patient selection, graft processing, and surgical technique over the last 15 years.

In 1989, Milachowski et al[71] reported a series of 22 patients with 6 fresh frozen and 16 freeze-dried meniscus allografts. At a mean of 14 months postoperatively, 18 grafts were evaluated by second-look arthroscopy, and 15 demonstrated peripheral healing. In the whole series of 22 there were only 3 failures that required removal (1 fresh frozen graft and 2 freeze-dried grafts). Generally, the fresh frozen grafts were found to have a more normal gross appearance than the freeze-dried grafts.

In 1993, Garrett[41] reported a minimum 2-year follow-up of 43 patients after complex meniscal allograft transplantation. Of the 16 fresh and 27 cryopreserved transplants, only 6 were isolated procedures. In this series there were 24 concomitant ACL reconstructions, 13 osteotomies, and 11 osteochondral allografts; 28 patients underwent second-look arthroscopy at 2 years. Twenty of these patients were asymptomatic and were considered to have a successful result, with healing of the meniscus to the host and no meniscal shrinkage or degeneration. Eight

Table 32–1. Selected Clinical Results of Meniscal Allograft Transplantation Series

AUTHOR	FOLLOW-UP DURATION	RESULTS
Milachowski et al,[71] 1989	14 months mean	19 of 22 (86%) successful
Garrett,[41] 1993	2-7 years	35 of 43 (81%) successful
Noyes and Barber-Weston,[76] 1995	30 months mean (22-58 months)	56 of 96 (58%) failed
Van Arkel and de Boer,[106] 1995	2-5 years	20 of 23 (87%) successful
Wilcox et al,[113] 1996	2 years minimum	17 of 18 (94%) successful
Cameron and Saha,[18] 1997	31 months mean (12-66 months)	58 of 63 (92%) successful
Carter,[20] 1999	48 months mean	45 of 51 (88%) successful
Rodeo et al,[90] 2000	2 years minimum	22 of 33 (67%) successful 14 of 16 (88%) bone fixation 8 of 17 (47%) no bone fixation
Rath et al,[87] 2001	5.4 years mean (2-8 years)	14 of 22 (64%) successful
Noyes et al,[77] 2004	40 months mean	34 of 38 (89%) successful

transplant failures were associated with grade IV chondromalacia revealed at second-look arthroscopy. The 15 patients who did not have repeat arthroscopy were asymptomatic and considered to have a clinically successful outcome. One of the six patients with isolated transplants experienced graft failure. No differences were found between the results associated with fresh and cryopreserved grafts. Other than failure in 8 of 43 grafts, no other complications were noted.

Zukor et al[116] implanted 33 fresh meniscal and osteochondral allografts for knee injuries that resulted in focal chondral defects and a deficient meniscus. At 1 year, 26 implantations (79%) were considered clinically successful, with no meniscal failures. In all 10 patients who underwent second-look arthroscopy, their meniscal allograft had healed to the meniscocapsular junction, although there were small foci of degenerative changes on the graft.

Veltri et al[108] reviewed their results of 16 deep-frozen or cryopreserved meniscal transplantations in which 11 of the reported cases underwent either ACL or posterior cruciate ligament reconstruction at surgery. At follow-up, only 2 of 14 patients complained of persistent joint line tenderness in the affected articular compartment. Seven of 11 patients at 6 months or greater follow-up underwent arthroscopic evaluation; five menisci were revealed to have complete healing at the periphery. It was, however, noted that one of the well-healed grafts had undergone a significant amount of degeneration in the midportion of the meniscus. The remaining two patients showed evidence of impaired healing at the posterior horn attachment. Four patients were not arthroscopically examined while remaining clinically asymptomatic.[108]

In 1994, Shelton and Dukes[97] reported on a 4-year experience with 20 patients in whom cryopreserved meniscal allografts with bone plugs were used. Four of the 20 patients had allografts implanted in advanced degenerative (grade IV) compartments. Two of the four patients who received meniscal allografts in grade IV compartments reported no reduction in pain, whereas the other two experienced a mild reduction in symptoms. Of the 16 patients with less than grade II arthritic changes, 15 reported a significant decrease in pain and no recurrent effusion. Seven patients underwent second-look

arthroscopy, which revealed complete peripheral healing and bone plug incorporation. All seven cases were described as having a 10% to 15% decrease in meniscal size, but cellular viability was confirmed by biopsy.

A larger series was reported by Noyes and Barber-Weston in 1995[76]; they evaluated 96 fresh frozen irradiated grafts implanted in 82 patients. Many grafts were secured with bone at the posterior horn, but none had bone anchorage in the anterior and posterior horns. The mean age of the patients was 29 years (range, 13 to 45 years). Twenty-nine menisci had to be removed less than 2 years after the operation, which left 67 menisci (57 medial and 10 lateral) in 63 patients followed for a mean of 30 months (range, 22 to 58 months). Arthroscopy and/or MRI was performed on all patients to evaluate healing. Overall, 9% of the 96 grafts healed, 31% were partially healed, and 58% failed clinically. Rates of failure were much higher in knees with arthrosis ($p < .001$). Knees with grade IV arthrosis had a 50% failure rate. Of the knees that were considered to be normal on postoperative MRI, 70% healed and 30% were partially healed. The relatively high failure rates in this series reflect the importance of using nonirradiated menisci, selecting patients with no worse than grade III arthrosis, and maintaining the osseous attachment of the meniscal horns.

In the same year, van Arkel and de Boer[106] reported their prospective outcomes of 23 patients 2 to 5 years after receiving cryopreserved meniscal transplants. A successful result was reported in 20 of 23 patients (87%), and peripheral healing was demonstrated in all but 3 of the patients examined by second-look arthroscopy. Histological analysis demonstrated revascularization with viable meniscal chondrocytes. Three patients with uncorrected malalignment failed before 2 years.

In 1996, Goble et al[113] reported on a series of 18 patients 2 years after cryopreserved meniscal allograft transplantation. Seventeen of 18 (94%) patients reported a significant decrease in knee pain and improvement in function. A yearly survey of their pain, knee motion, limitations in activities of daily life, changes in lifestyle, and general social or emotional effect was conducted. The results showed that 70% to 89% of patients improved at least one grade in each of the five categories just listed; 100% of patients beyond 2 years responded that they would "do it again," and 20% of this group were determined to be class III or class IV.[80] Complications include one case of infection and removal, three cases of removal because of pain, and partial meniscectomy in three patients. Improper sizing was blamed for two failures. Second-look arthroscopy was performed on 13 patients (13 grafts), 10 (77%) of whom had a well-healed and functional meniscus. Four of the grafts demonstrated a noticeable pattern of degenerative wear or peripheral detachment at the posterior horn. It was believed that the failure of healing at the posterior horn was secondary to inadequate anchorage in the early cases. Biopsy performed on 8 of 14 grafts revealed an average of 80% viable meniscal tissue.

In 1997, Cameron and Saha[18] reported the results of 67 deep-frozen, gamma ray–irradiated meniscal transplants without bone anchors, many in patients with advanced unicompartmental arthritis. Despite such disadvantages, 87% of the patients had a good or excellent result at an average of 31 months (range, 1 to 5.5 years) according to a 100-point functional knee score. The most frequent complication was a traumatic tear of the posterior horn, which occurred in six knees at a mean of 21 months. Twenty-one of the patients received isolated meniscal allografts, and 19 achieved good to excellent results (90.5%).

In 1999, Carter[20] reported the results of 46 cryopreserved transplants at a minimum of 2 years. Second-look arthroscopy in 38 cases demonstrated 4 with failure, 4 with visible shrinkage of the graft, and 2 with progression of arthritis. There was significant pain relief and functional improvement in 32 of these 38, and only 1 patient indicated an unwillingness to undergo the procedure again under similar circumstances.

Stollsteimer et al[102] reported on 22 patients treated with a total of 23 cryopreserved allografts and monitored for 1 to 5 years. All patients reported substantial pain relief. When compared with the normal menisci, the allografts demonstrated an average shrinkage of 37% (range, 0% to 69%) as seen on MRI. This finding, however, was not associated with an adverse outcome.

In 2001, Rodeo[89] reported a 2-year minimum follow-up with overall 22 of 33 (67%) successful results. Further analysis of the outcomes reveals that successful results were obtained in 14 of the 16 (88%) transplants that were anchored to bone at the anterior and posterior horns, whereas only 8 of the 17 (47%) non–bone anchorage transplants were successful.

Rath et al[87] in 2001 reported on their series 2 to 8 years after cryopreserved meniscal allograft transplantation for compartmental pain after total meniscectomy. Eight of 22 allograft menisci (36%) tore during the study period and necessitated 6 partial and 2 total meniscectomies. Two patients subsequently underwent reimplantation. Histological examination of the removed tissue revealed reduced cellularity in comparison to normal or torn native menisci. A successful result was reported in 14 of 22 patients.

Most recently, Noyes et al[77] prospectively evaluated the results of cryopreserved meniscal transplantation in a consecutive series of younger patients treated for pain in meniscus-deficient knees. Forty cryopreserved menisci were implanted into 38 patients. Sixteen knees also had an osteochondral autograft transfer, and 9 underwent knee ligament reconstruction. At a mean of 40 months, meniscal allograft characteristics were determined with the use of a rating system that combined subjective, clinical, and MRI factors. Thirty-four (89%) of the 38 patients rated their knee condition as improved. Although 30 patients (79%) had pain with daily activities before surgery, only 4 (11%) had similar symptoms postoperatively. In fact, 27 knees (68%) had no pain and 13 (33%) had only mild compartment pain at the time of latest follow-up. Twenty-nine patients (76%) returned to light low-impact sports without problems. By treating comorbid conditions, concomitant osteochondral autograft transfer and knee ligament reconstruction procedures improved knee function without increasing the rate of complications. Meniscal allograft characteristics, including MRI data, were normal in 17 knees (43%), were altered in 12 (30%), and resulted in failure in 11 (28%). The authors concluded that the short-term results of meniscal transplantation are encouraging in terms of reducing knee pain and increasing function and that these results do not always strictly correlate with the radiographic appearance of the meniscus. Also evident is the benefit of effectively treating comorbid conditions.

Series reporting ACL reconstruction and meniscus transplantation demonstrate the synergistic effect of combined procedures, particularly with successful transplantation of a medial meniscus to reconstitute a key secondary restraint to anterior tibial translation. Sekiya et al[94] and Yoldas et al[115] in 2003 reported their series of patients who had received meniscal transplants in conjunction with ACL reconstruction. In the report of Sekiya and colleagues, 28 patients who underwent ACL reconstruction along with meniscal transplantation were evaluated postoperatively at an average of 2.8 years (range, 1.8 to 5.6). Twenty-four of 28 (86%) had normal or nearly normal International Knee Documentation Committee scores, and nearly 90% had normal or nearly normal Lachman and pivot-shift test scores. The maximum manual KT arthrometer testing demonstrated a mean side-to-side difference of 1.5 mm. Joint space narrowing of the transplanted compartments was not significantly different from that of the contralateral knee. From these results the authors concluded that restoration of meniscal function may provide protection for the articular cartilage and improve joint stability and that correcting ligament instability eliminates a contraindication to meniscal transplantation.

The report by Yoldas et al[115] described the results of 31 patients after meniscal allograft transplantation with and without combined ACL reconstruction. In this group, 11 underwent isolated meniscal transplantation and 20, meniscal transplantation combined with ACL reconstruction. Bony fixation was performed with bone plugs for medial transplants and the use of a bone bridge for lateral transplants. At a mean of 2.9 years, flexion weightbearing radiographs were compared with preoperative radiographs. In addition, several validated knee-specific scoring systems were used. In this study there were no significant differences in these scores based on which meniscus (medial or lateral) was transplanted, concurrent ACL reconstruction, or the degree of chondrosis at arthroscopy. Assessment with the KT-1000 arthrometer revealed a side-to-side difference of 2 mm (range, −2 mm to 7 mm). No statistically significant joint space narrowing was observed by radiography over time. From this series the authors concluded that allograft transplantation with and without combined ACL reconstruction in patients with complaints of compartmental joint line pain and/or instability appears able to provide relief of symptoms and restore relatively high levels of function, particularly during activities of daily living.

Between 1997 and 2003, the senior author (BJC) has performed 96 meniscus transplants, 17 of which were performed in conjunction with an ACL reconstruction. Seven of the transplants were performed with a primary ACL reconstruction (6 medial and 1 lateral), and 10 of the transplants (all medial) were performed in combination with ACL revision. Nine of the ACL revisions were performed with a bone-tendon-bone allograft. Eight of the meniscus transplants were performed with the bone plug technique and two with the bone bridge in slot technique. Three patients failed within the first year because of recurrent instability (two patients whose ACL grafts were being revised for the third time) or persistent pain despite arthroscopic evidence of complete healing of the meniscus and intact articular cartilage (in a workers' compensation patient). Only the workers' compensation patient was revised to a partial knee replacement, with complete resolution of his pain. The remaining two patients (one at 3 years' and one at 6 years' follow-up) have not undergone additional surgery but continue to complain of some instability.

Of the remaining seven patients, there were three females and four males with an average age of 27 years (range, 19 to 46 years) and an average follow-up of 12 months (range, 3 to 27 months). All seven patients had statistically significant improvements in the International Knee Documentation Committee, Lysholm, Tegner, and SF-12 physical component scores. All patients stated that they were satisfied with their results and would undergo the surgery again given similar circumstances. Of the seven patients, all denied complaints of instability, and as a group, there was a mean 50% reduction of pain in comparison to their preoperative pain scores as measured on a 10-point visual analog scale.

DISCUSSION

Meniscus deficiency is considered by some authors to be the number one problem in orthopedics today.[76] To patients, meniscal deficiency is a problem leading to pain, swelling, arthritic changes, and limitation of activity. To physicians, meniscal deficiency is a problem because of the relative lack of suitable solutions for their patients. To society, the sequelae of a meniscus-deficient knee translate into loss of productivity and an increase in monetary expenditures for health care benefits. It is evident that many patient- and surgeon-specific variables differ among studies, such as the degree of arthrosis, method of graft

processing, surgical technique, types of concomitant procedures, and method of evaluation. Thus, it is difficult to make comparisons or draw conclusions on the basis of the existing literature.

The average age of the patient affected by knee ligament instability is 21 years. The average age of the patient undergoing total knee arthroplasty is 70 years. The average age for meniscal allograft transplantation is 33 years (range, 27 to 44 years).[25] Knee instability primarily disables young athletes. Knees requiring salvage procedures, such as total knee arthroplasty, primarily affect retirement-age individuals, whereas patients with meniscus-deficient knees represent a greater percentage of individuals within the day-to-day workforce who have parental responsibilities. It should therefore be medically understandable that even a documented short-term improvement in an otherwise disabled population could be defined as a success.

It is clear that obtaining secure bone anchorage of both the anterior and posterior horns, though technically more demanding, is necessary to maximize the potential for a successful outcome. Rodeo's series, in which overall there were only 22 (66%) of 33 successful outcomes, demonstrated a much higher rate of successful outcomes, 14 (88%) of 16, in patients in whom bone anchorage had been obtained as compared with only 8 (47%) of the 17 patients without bone anchorage.[89] These clinical results coincide with our biomechanical understanding of the potential for benefit from a meniscal allograft.[5,21,81]

The degree of arthrosis at the time of allograft transplantation is possibly the most important factor predicting outcome, with advanced arthrosis being associated with the highest failure rates.[42,76,106] Using MRI, Rodeo[89] demonstrated that knees with advanced arthrosis had a greater propensity for graft extrusion, a finding believed to be associated with an increased risk for failure.

Correcting limb malalignment is another factor believed to be critical for success.[18] Van Arkel and de Boer[106] attributed their three graft failures to uncorrected limb alignment. Cameron and Saha[18] performed osteotomy in 34 of 63 patients. By realigning the knees to "unload" the involved compartment, they achieved a success rate comparable to that in the group as a whole, with a good or excellent result in 85% and 87%, respectively.

Pain relief was the most consistent benefit experienced in most series. Stollsteimer et al[102] reported pain relief in all patients in their series. Garrett and Stevenson[42] noted the difficulty in objectively evaluating meniscal transplants clinically. Although relief of pain was a common finding in their series, they relied on second-look arthroscopy in 28 of 43 cases to establish meniscal healing and success.

Meniscal shrinkage is difficult to assess, even at second-look arthroscopy, because of inconsistencies when visually estimating size. At second-look arthroscopy in 22 cases, Carter[20] believed that only 3 showed a significant size reduction. Milachowski et al[71] noted shrinkage from 33% to 66% in 14 of 23 menisci examined by second-look arthroscopy at an average of 8 months postoperatively. The finding of loss of meniscal volume as shown by MRI is troubling. It is not known why grafts shrink. Shrinkage could be due to a subclinical immune response with graft remodeling during cellular repopulation, a poor-quality graft, excessive graft loading during healing, the surgical technique, the extent of knee arthrosis, or some variable not currently recognized. Some MRI scans have demonstrated that the grafts can look similar to a normal meniscus, whereas others have shown signals consistent with degenerative changes.[20,76,90,102]

The use of MRI as a postoperative tool to determine graft healing is still questionable, but improving. Second-look arthroscopy is often necessary to define the exact quality of graft healing.[33,83,86,109]

Whether meniscal grafts prevent arthritis is not known. Unfortunately, many investigators have not reported the findings on weightbearing radiographs, whereas others have obtained radiographs at only early postoperative time points. Rath et al[87] reported that the compartment space of the involved knees of 11 patients averaged 5.2 mm before surgery and 4.5 mm at 2 to 8 years after surgery. Carter[20] stated that only 2 of 46 knees demonstrated radiographic progression at a mean of 34.5 months (range, 24 to 73 months) postoperatively, but their results were not quantified. To our knowledge, a longer-term prospective, randomized study comparing the progression of arthritis with and without an allograft has not been completed in humans. In rabbits, Rijik et al[88] demonstrated that meniscectomized animals and those undergoing meniscal transplantation had equal rates of degenerative changes on radiographs at 1 year. This study is clearly limited by the fact that the mechanics and anatomy of the rabbit knee are different from those of human knees, and drawing conclusions from a feature directly responsible for proper biomechanical function of the meniscal allograft should be done with caution.

We have recently reported (Alford, Cole, case report, *Arthroscopy*) two cases of rapid onset of lateral compartment arthritis after subtotal meniscectomy that was halted by meniscus transplantation and osteochondral autologous transfer in a 16-year-old and by an osteochondral allograft plug and meniscus transplantation in a 33-year-old athletic professional. Both patients have not only demonstrated halt of a preoperative rapid radiographic progression of arthritis but have also returned to athletic participation without reports of pain.

With respect to combined procedures, it is clear that uncorrected comorbid conditions are a contraindication to meniscal transplantation. An awareness of the mutually beneficial effect of combined procedures is emerging, and the synergy of concomitant reconstructions is evident. When a cartilage restoration or ligament reconstruction protects a meniscal transplant, the healthy functioning meniscus transplant will protect the ligament reconstruction or cartilage-resurfacing procedure.

SUMMARY

Despite encouraging intermediate-term benefits, the true long-term function of a transplanted meniscus remains unknown. The transplant appears to remodel and experience changes in its collagen fiber architecture that affect its load-sharing capabilities and long-term survival. It is important that the meniscal transplant surgeon advise patients that this procedure is indicated for those who have few other options and that it is probably not curative in the long term. However, establishing a pain-free and mechanically stable environment for even an intermediate period (i.e., 5 or 10 years), as supported by the literature, seems entirely justified given the lack of alternatives and the added benefit of placing a patient chronologically at an age more appropriate for arthroplasty in the unlikely event that the meniscus allograft fails.

References

1. Ahmed AM: The load bearing of the knee meniscus. In Mow VC, Arnoczky SP, Jackson DW (eds): DDS: Knee Meniscus—Basic and Clinical Foundations. New York, Raven Press, 1992, p 59.
2. Ahmed AM, Burke DL: In-vitro measurement of static pressure distribution in synovial joints—Part I: Tibial surface of the knee. J Biomech Eng 105:216-225, 1983.
3. Albrecht-Olsen P, Lind T, Kristensen G, Falkenberg B: Failure strength of a new meniscus arrow repair technique: Biomechanical comparison with horizontal suture. Arthroscopy 13:183-187, 1997.
4. Alhalki MM, Howell SM, Hull ML: How three methods for fixing a medial meniscal autograft affect tibial contact mechanics. Am J Sports Med 27:320-328, 1999.
5. Alhalki MM, Hull ML, Howell SM: Contact mechanics of the medial tibial plateau after implantation of a medial meniscal allograft. A human cadaveric study. Am J Sports Med 28:370-376, 2000.
6. Arnoczky SP, McDevitt CA: The meniscus: Structure, function, repair and replacement. In Buckwalter JA, Einhorn TA, Simon SR (eds): Orthopedic Basic Science: Biology and Biomechanics of the Musculoskeletal System. Rosemont, IL, American Academy of Orthopaedic Surgeons, 2000, pp 531-545.
7. Arnoczky SP, McDevitt CA, Schmidt MB, et al: The effect of cryopreservation on canine menisci: A biochemical, morphologic, and biomechanical evaluation. J Orthop Res 6:1-12, 1988.
8. Arnoczky SP, Milachowski KA: Meniscal allografts: Where do we stand? In Ewing JW (ed): Articular Cartilage and the Knee Joint Function: Basic Science and Arthroscopy. New York, Raven Press, 1990, p 129.
9. Arnoczky SP, O'Brian S, DeCarlo E, et al: Cell survival after transplantation of fresh meniscal allograft: DNA probe analysis in goat model. Am J Sports Med 21:540, 1988.
10. Arnoczky SP, Warren RF, McDevitt CA: Meniscal replacement using cryopreserved allograft: An experimental study in the dog. Clin Orthop 252:121-128, 1990.
11. Baratz ME, Fu FH, Mengato R: Meniscal tears: The effect of meniscectomy and of repair on intraarticular contact areas and stress in the human knee. A preliminary report. Am J Sports Med 14:270-275, 1986.
12. Barrack RL, Bruckner JD, Kneisl J, et al: The outcome of nonoperatively treated complete tears of the anterior cruciate ligament in active young adults. Clin Orthop 259:192-199, 1990.
13. Berlet GC, Fowler PJ: The anterior horn of the medial meniscus. An anatomic study of its insertion. Am J Sports Med 26:540-543, 1998.
14. Boenisch UW, Faber KJ, Ciarelli M, et al: Pull-out strength and stiffness of meniscal repair using absorbable arrows or Ti-Cron vertical and horizontal loop sutures. Am J Sports Med 27:626-631, 1999.
15. Bonamo JJ, Fay C, Firestone T: The conservative treatment of the anterior cruciate deficient knee. Am J Sports Med 18:618-623, 1990.
16. Brown KL, Cruess RL: Bone and cartilage transplantation in orthopedic surgery review. J Bone Joint Surg Am 64:270-279, 1982.
17. Buck BE, Resnick L, Shah SM, Malinin TI: Human immunodeficiency virus cultured from bone. Implications for transplantation. Clin Orthop 251:249-253, 1990.

18. Cameron JC, Saha S: Meniscal allograft transplantation for unicompartmental arthritis of the knee. Clin Orthop 337:164-171, 1997.

19. Carpenter JE, Wojtys EM, Huston LJ: Pre-operative sizing of meniscal replacements. Presented at the 12th Annual Meeting of the Arthroscopy Association of North America, Palm Desert, CA, April 1, 1993.

20. Carter TR: Meniscal allograft transplantation. Sports Med Arthrosc Rev 7:51-62, 1999.

21. Chen MI, Branch TP, Hutton WC: Is it important to secure the horns during lateral meniscal transplantation? A cadaveric study. Arthroscopy 12:174-181, 1996.

22. Cole BJ, Carter TR, Rodeo SA: Allograft meniscal transplantation: Background, techniques, and results. Instr Course Lect 52:383-396, 2003.

23. Cole BJ, Cohen B: Chondral injuries of the knee: A contemporary view of cartilage restoration. Orthop Spec Ed 6:71-76, 2000.

24. Cole BJ, Fox JA, Lee SJ, Farr J: Bone bridge in slot technique for meniscal transplantation. Op Tech Sports Med 11:2, 144-155, 2003.

25. Cole BJ, Rodeo S, Carter T: Allograft meniscus transplantation: Indications, techniques, results. J Bone Joint Surg Am 84:1236-1250, 2002.

26. Cummins JF, Mansour JN, Howe Z, Allan DG: Meniscal transplantation and degenerative articular change: An experimental study in the rabbit. Arthroscopy 13:485-491, 1997.

27. De Boer HH, Koudstaal J: The fate of meniscus cartilage after transplantation of cryopreserved nontissue-antigen– matched allograft. A case report. Clin Orthop 266:145-151, 1991.

28. DeHaven KE: Meniscectomy vs. repair: Clinical report of arthroscopic findings. In Surgery and Arthroscopy of the Knee. Proceedings of the Second Congress of the European Society. Berlin, Springer, 1992, p 131.

29. Elliott DM, Guilak F, Vail TP, et al: Tensile properties of articular cartilage are altered by meniscectomy in a canine model of osteoarthritis. J Orthop Res 17:503-508, 1999.

30. Fabbriciani C, Lucania L, Milano G, et al: Meniscal allografts: Cryopreservation vs. deep-frozen technique. An experimental study in goats. Knee Surg Sports Traumatol Arthroscopy 5:124-134, 1997.

31. Fabbriciani C, Lucania L, Milano G, et al: Meniscal allografts: Cryopreservation vs deep-frozen technique. An experimental study in goats. Knee Surg Sports Traumatol Arthrosc 5:124-134, 1997.

32. Fairbank TJ: Knee joint changes after meniscectomy. J Bone Joint Surg Br 30:664-670, 1948.

33. Farley TE, Howell SM, Love KF, et al: Meniscal tear: MR and arthrographic findings after arthroscopic repair. Radiology 180:517-522, 1991.

34. Farr J, Meneghini RM, Cole BJ: Allograft interference screw fixation in meniscus transplantation. Arthroscopy 20:322-327, 2004.

35. Favenesi JA, Shaffer JC, Mow VC: Biphasic mechanical properties of knee meniscus. Trans Orthop Res Soc 8:57, 1983.

36. Fithian DC, Kelly MA, Mow VC: Material properties and structure-function relationships in the menisci. Clin Orthop 252:19-31, 1990.

37. Fox JA, Lee SJ, Cole BJ: Bone plug technique for meniscal transplantation. Op Tech Sports Med 11:2, 161-169, 2003.

38. Friedlaender GE, Strong DM, Sell KW: Studies on the antigenicity of bone. I. Freeze-dried and deep-frozen bone allografts in rabbits. J Bone Joint Surg Am 58:854-858, 1976.

39. Friedlaender GE, Strong DM, Sell KW: Studies on the antigenicity of bone. II. Donor-specific anti-HLA antibodies in human recipients of freeze-dried allografts. J Bone Joint Surg Am 66:107-112, 1984.

40. Fu FH, Thompson WO: Motion of meniscus during knee flexion. In Mow VC, Arnoczky SP, Jackson DW (eds): Knee Meniscus—Basic and Clinical Foundations. New York, Raven Press, 1992, p 75.

41. Garrett JC: Meniscal transplantation: Review of forty-three cases with two-to-seven year follow up. Sports Med Am Arthrosc Rev 1:164-167, 1993.

42. Garrett JC, Stevenson RN: Meniscal transplantation in the human knee: A preliminary report. Arthroscopy 7:57-62, 1991.

43. Gross AE: Fresh osteochondral allografts for post-traumatic knee defects: Surgical technique. Op Tech Orthop 7:334-339, 1997.

44. Gugenheim JJ Jr, Brinker MR: Bone realignment with use of temporary external fixation for distal femoral valgus and varus deformities. J Bone Joint Surg Am 85:1229-1237, 2003.

45. Hamlet W, Liu SH, Yang R: Destruction of a cyropreserved meniscal allograft: A case for acute rejection. Arthroscopy 13:517-521, 1997.

46. Hsu RWW, Himeno S, Coventry MB (eds): Transactions of the 34th Annual Meeting of the Orthopedic Research Society, vol 13. Park Ridge, IL, Orthopaedic Research Society, 1988, p 282.

47. Huckle JR: Is meniscectomy a benign procedure? A long-term follow-up study. Can J Surg 8:254, 1965.

48. Jackson DW, McDevitt CA, Simon TM, et al: Meniscal transplantation using fresh and cryopreserved allograft: An experimental study in goats. Am J Sports Med 20:644-656, 1992.

49. Jackson DW, Whelan J, Simon TM: Cell survival after transplantation of fresh meniscal allografts: DNA probe analysis in a goat model. Am J Sports Med 21:540-550, 1993.

50. Jackson DW, Windler GE, Simon TM: Intraarticular reaction associated with the use of freeze-dried, ethylene oxide–sterilized bone–patella tendon–bone allografts in the reconstruction of the anterior cruciate ligament. Am J Sports Med 18:1-10, 1990.

51. Jager A, Welsch F, Braune C, et al: [Ten year follow-up after single incision anterior cruciate ligament reconstruction using patellar tendon autograft.] Z Orthop Ihre Grenzgeb 141:42-47, 2003.

52. Johnson DL, Swenson TM, Livesay GA, et al: Insertion-site anatomy of the human menisci: Gross, arthroscopic, and topographical anatomy as a basis for meniscal transplantation. Arthroscopy 11:386-394, 1995.

53. Johnson RJ, Kettlekamp DB, Clark W, Leaverton P: Factors affecting late results after meniscectomy. J Bone Joint Surg Am 56:719-729, 1974.

54. Kennedy S, Shaffer B, Yao L: Preoperative planning in meniscal allograft reconstruction. Presented at the 24th Annual Meeting of the American Orthopaedic Society for Sports Medicine, Vancouver, British Columbia, July 12, 1998.

55. Khoury MA, Goldberg VM, Stevenson S: Demonstration of HLA and ABH antigens in fresh and frozen human menisci by immunohistochemistry. J Orthop Res 12:751-757, 1994.

56. Kimball JW: Introduction to Immunology, 2nd ed. New York, Collier Macmillan, 1978.

57. Kohn D, Moreno B: Meniscus insertion anatomy as a basis for meniscus replacement: A morphological cadaveric study. Arthroscopy 11:96-103, 1995.

58. Lee SJ, Aadalen KJ, Lorenz EP, et al: Tibiofemoral contact mechanics following serial medial meniscectomies in the human cadaveric knee. Presented at the Annual Meeting of the American Orthopaedic Society for Sports Medicine, Quebec City, Canada, June 24-27, 2004.

59. Levy IM, Torzilli PA, Gould JD, et al: The effect of lateral meniscectomy on motion of the knee. J Bone Joint Surg Am 71:401-406, 1989.

60. Levy IM, Torzilli PA, Warren RF: The effect of medial meniscectomy on anterior-posterior motion of the knee. J Bone Joint Surg Am 64:883-888, 1982.

61. Lexer E: Substitution of whole or half joints from freshly amputated extremities by free plastic operation. Surg Gynecol Obstet 6:601-607, 1908.

62. Lexer E: Joint transplantations and arthroplasty. Surg Gynecol Obstet 40:782-809, 1925.

63. Lobenhoffer P, Agneskirchner JD: Improvements in surgical technique of valgus high tibial osteotomy. Knee Surg Sports Traumatol Arthrosc 11:132-138, 2003.

64. Lynch MA, Henning CE: Osteoarthritis in the ACL deficient knee. In Feagin JA Jr (ed): The Cruciate Ligaments. New York, Churchill Livingstone, 1988, p 385.

65. Lynch MA, Henning CE, Glick KR Jr: Knee joint surface changes: Long-term follow-up of meniscus tear treatment and stable anterior cruciate ligament reconstruction. Clin Orthop 172:148-153, 1983.

66. MacConaill MA: The movements of bones and joints; the mechanical structure of articulating cartilage. J Bone Joint Surg Br 33:251-257, 1951.

67. Standards for Tissue Banking. American Association of Tissue Banks, McLean, VA, 2002.

68. Mikic ZD, Brankoy MZ, Tubic MV, Lazetic AB: Allograft meniscal transplantation in a dog. Acta Orthop Scand 64:329-332, 1993.

69. Milachowski KA, Kohn D, Wirth CJ: [Transplantation of allogeneic menisci.] Orthopade 23:160-163, 1984.

70. Milachowski KA, Weismeier K, Worth CJ, et al: Meniscus transplantation: Experimental study, clinical report and arthroscopic findings. In Surgery and Arthroscopy of the Knee. Proceedings of the Second Congress of the European Society. Berlin, Springer, 1988, p 131.

71. Milachowski KA, Weismeier K, Worth CJ, et al: Homologous meniscus transplantation: Experimental and clinical results. Int Orthop 13:1-11, 1989.

72. Moseley TA, Haudenschild DR, Rose L, Reddi AH: Interleukin-17 family and IL-17 receptors. Cytokine Growth Factor Rev 14:155-174, 2003.

73. Mow VC, Holmes MH, Lai WM: Fluid transport and mechanical properties of articular cartilage: A review. J Biomech 17:377-394, 1984.

74. Mow VC, Ratcliff A, Chern KY, et al: Structure and function relationships of the menisci of the knee. In Mow VC, Arnoczky SP, Jackson DW (eds): Knee Meniscus—Basic and Clinical Foundations. New York, Raven Press, 1992, p 37.

75. Nemzek JA, Arnoczky SP, Swenson CL: Retroviral transmission by the transplantation of connective-tissue allografts. An experimental study. J Bone Joint Surg Am 76:1036-1041, 1994.

76. Noyes FR, Barber-Weston SC: Irradiated meniscal allografts in the human knee: A two- to five-year follow-up study. Orthop Trans 19:417, 1995.

77. Noyes FR, Barber-Westin SD, Rankin M: Meniscal transplantation in symptomatic patients less than fifty years old. J Bone Joint Surg Am 86:1392-1404, 2004.

78. O'Brien WR: Degenerative arthritis of the knee following anterior cruciate ligament injury: Role of the meniscus. Sports Med Arthrosc Rev 1:114, 1993.

79. Ochi M, Ishida O, Daisaku H, et al: Immune response to fresh meniscal allografts in mice. J Surg Res 58:478-484, 1995.

80. Outerbridge RE: The etiology of chondromalacia patellae. J Bone Joint Surg Br 43:752-757, 1961.

81. Paletta GA Jr, Manning T, Snell E, et al: The effect of allograft meniscal replacement on intraarticular contact area and pressures in the human knee. A biomechanical study. Am J Sports Med 25:692-698, 1997.

82. Papageorgiou CD, Gil JE, Kanamori A, et al: The biomechanical interdependence between the anterior cruciate ligament replacement graft and the medial meniscus. Am J Sports Med 29:226-231, 2001.

83. Patten RM, Rolfe BA: MRI of meniscal allografts. J Comput Assist Tomogr 19:243-246, 1995.

84. Pollard ME, Kang Q, Berg EE: Radiographic sizing for meniscal transplantation. Arthroscopy 11:684-687, 1995.

85. Potter HG, Linklater JM, Allen AA, et al: Magnetic resonance imaging of articular cartilage in the knee. An evaluation with use of fast-spin-echo imaging. J Bone Joint Surg Am 80:1276-1284, 1998.

86. Potter HG, Rodeo SA, Wickiewicz TL, Warren RF: MR imaging of meniscal allografts: Correlation with clinical and arthroscopic outcomes. Radiology 198:509-514, 1996.

87. Rath E, Richmond JC, Yassir W, et al: Meniscal allograft transplantation. Two- to eight-year results. Am J Sports Med 29:410-414, 2001.

88. Rijk PC, de Rooy TP, Coerkamp EG, et al: Radiographic evaluation of the knee joint after meniscal allograft transplantation. An experimental study in rabbits. Knee Surg Sports Traumatol Arthrosc 10:241-246, 2002.

89. Rodeo SA: Meniscal allografts—where do we stand? Am J Sports Med 29:246-261, 2001.

90. Rodeo SA, Seneviratne A, Suzuki K, et al: Histological analysis of human meniscal allografts. A preliminary report. J Bone Joint Surg Am 82:1071-1082, 2000.

91. Rohrie H, Scholten R: Joint forces in the human pelvis-leg skeleton during walking. J Biomech 17:409-424, 1984.

92. Rosenberg TD, Paulos LE, Parker RD, et al: The forty-five-degree posteroanterior flexion weight-bearing radiograph of the knee. J Bone Joint Surg Am 70:1479-1483, 1988.

93. Seedhom BB, Hargreaves DJ: Transmission of load in the knee joint with special reference to the role of the menisci: Part II. Experi-

mental results, discussions, and conclusions. Eng Med Biol 8:220-228, 1979.

94. Sekiya JK, Giffin JR, Irrgang JJ, et al: Clinical outcomes after combined meniscal allograft transplantation and anterior cruciate ligament reconstruction. Am J Sports Med 31:896-906, 2003.

95. Shaffer B, Kennedy S, Klimkiewicz J, Yao L: Preoperative sizing of meniscal allografts in meniscus transplantation. Am J Sports Med 28:524-533, 2000.

96. Shelbourne KD, Gray T: Results of anterior cruciate ligament reconstruction based on meniscus and articular cartilage status at the time of surgery. Five- to fifteen-year evaluations. Am J Sports Med 28:446-452, 2000.

97. Shelton WR, Dukes AD: Meniscus replacement with bone anchors: A surgical technique. Arthroscopy 10:324-327, 1994.

98. Shoemaker SC, Markolf KL: The role of the meniscus in the anterior-posterior stability of the loaded anterior cruciate– deficient knee. Effects of partial versus total excision. J Bone Joint Surg Am 68:71-79, 1986.

99. Siegel MG, Roberts CS: Meniscal allografts. Clin Sports Med 12:59-80, 1993.

100. Skaggs DL, Warden WH, Mow VC: Radial tie fibers influence the tensile properties of the bovine medial meniscus. J Orthop Res 12:176-185, 1994.

101. Spilker RL, Donzeley PS: A biphasic finite element model of the meniscus for stress-strain analysis. In Mow VC, Arnoczky SP, Jackson DW (eds): Knee Meniscus—Basic and Clinical Foundations. New York, Raven Press, 1992, p 91.

102. Stollsteimer GT, Shelton WR, et al: Meniscal allograft transplantation: A 1- to 5-year follow-up of 22 patients. Arthroscopy 16:343-347, 2000.

103. Szomor ZL, Martin TE, Bonar F, et al: The protective effects of meniscal transplantation on cartilage. An experimental study in sheep. J Bone Joint Surg Am 82:80-88, 2000.

104. Tapper EM, Hoover NW: Late results after meniscectomy. J Bone Joint Surg Am 51:517-526, 1969.

105. Thompson WO, Thaette FL, Fu FH, Dye SF: Tibial meniscal dynamics using three-dimensional reconstruction of magnetic resonance images. Am J Sports Med 19:210-215, discussion 215-216, 1991.

106. van Arkel ER, de Boer HH: Human meniscal transplantation. Preliminary results at 2 to 5-year follow-up. J Bone Joint Surg Br 77:589-595, 1995.

107. van Arkel ER, van den Berg-Loonen EM, van Wersch JW, de Boer HH: Human leukocyte antigen sensitization after cryopreserved human meniscal transplantations. Transplantation 64:531-533, 1997.

108. Veltri DM, Warren RF, Wickiewicz TL, O'Brien SJ: Current status of allograft meniscal transplantation. Clin Orthop 303:44-55, 1994.

109. Verdonk R: Alternative treatments for meniscal injuries. J Bone Joint Surg Br 79:866-873, 1997.

110. Verdonk R, Kohn D: Harvest and conservation of meniscal allografts. Scand J Med Sci Sports 9:158-159, 1999.

111. Verdonk R, Van Daele P, Claus B, et al: [Viable meniscus transplantation.] Orthopade 23:153-159, 1994.

112. Walker BF, Erkman MJ: The role of the menisci in forced transmission across the knee. Clin Orthop 109:184-192, 1975.

113. Wilcox TR, Goble EM, Doucette SA: Goble technique of meniscus transplantation. Am J Knee Surg 9:37-42, 1996.

114. Yahia LH, Drouin G, Zukor D: The irradiation effect on the initial mechanical properties of meniscal grafts. Biomed Mater Eng 3:211-221, 1993.

115. Yoldas EA, Sekiya JK, Irrgang JJ, et al: Arthroscopically assisted meniscal allograft transplantation with and without combined anterior cruciate ligament reconstruction. Knee Surg Sports Traumatol Arthrosc 11:173-182, 2003.

116. Zukor DJ, Cameron JC, Brooks PJ, et al: The fate of human meniscal allografts. In Ewing JW (ed): Articular Cartilage and Knee Joint Function: Basic Science and Arthroscopy. New York, Raven Press, 1990, p 147.

CHAPTER 33

Osteotomy in the Sports Knee

James M. Leone • Mark W. Pagnano

Lower extremity realignment procedures around the knee are most commonly used to treat isolated unicompartmental osteoarthritis. The use of proximal tibial osteotomies for the treatment of knee osteoarthritis was first introduced by Jackson and Gariepy and later popularized in North America by Coventry.[20,21,24,56,57] Through the 1970s and early 1980s osteotomies were the mainstay for treatment of isolated advanced unicompartmental osteoarthritis. With the reported success rates of total joint replacement approaching 94% at 10-year follow-up,[26] coupled with the resurgence of unicompartmental replacements with equally impressive outcomes,[5,9,108] the popularity of osteotomies has been on the decline (Fig. 33–1). Importantly, this declining trend reflects the treatment of an older population of patients, and osteotomy continues to have a role for the younger, more active subset of patients.

For these younger individuals, the use of osteochondral allografting techniques, autologous chondrocyte transplantation, and meniscal allograft transplantation has shown promising early outcomes[97]; however, in the presence of significant limb malalignment, these procedures may be best accompanied by a realignment osteotomy. Moreover, in the younger population of patients with symptomatic leg malalignment associated with chronic ligament deficiencies, realignment osteotomy remains the preferred treatment either in isolation or combined with ligament reconstruction. Younger patients with high functional demands and localized arthritis in a malaligned limb treated by realignment osteotomy often experience both pain relief and improved function.[26,53,78,81,113,119]

The key to success with realignment procedures involves proper patient selection, careful preoperative planning, and precise surgical technique.[67,118] This chapter focuses on the younger population of patients and discusses the process of patient selection, preoperative planning, operative techniques, complications, and results of realignment osteotomy of the knee.

PATIENT SELECTION

The initial steps in defining the ideal candidate for a realignment procedure involve a very detailed history and an accurate and thorough physical examination. The nature of the symptoms must be well understood to better anticipate what procedure or combination of procedures will yield the most favorable results. The exact correction angle and order of surgical interventions are often influenced by whether the patient complains of localized joint line pain versus instability or a combination of both. The presence of diffuse, nonspecific knee pain probably decreases the chance of a successful outcome after realignment osteotomy. Patient selection as a process might be better understood by outlining specific indications and limitations for this intervention.

Indications

Osteotomy for the treatment of unicompartmental knee arthrosis associated with limb malalignment in young active individuals who are thin, have localized activity-related knee pain and a stable knee with good range of motion, and do not have significant patellofemoral symptoms is well established.* Less commonly described is the role of realignment procedures in a malaligned limb with a chondral or osteochondral injury or a limb with confounding ligamentous disruption in the absence of frank gonarthrosis.[50,64,82,87,97,107] These latter conditions are among the more difficult treatment entities that exist, and the optimal treatment of them remains less clear.[75,85]

The biomechanical advantage of osteotomy and limb realignment has previously been described in detail.[15,48] In brief, malalignment of the limb has been attributed to increased stress on previously damaged articular cartilage leading to further loss of articular surface area and increased angular deformity. This process creates a perpetual cycle of progressive deformity and loss of cartilage over time. With realignment osteotomy, stress on the damaged cartilage is reduced by redistributing the load to the contralateral compartment of the knee, and such load redistribution has been shown to reliably reduce pain and increase function in appropriately selected patients for up to 7 to 10 years.[26,53,78,81,113,119]

The role of osteotomy about the knee continues to evolve and has led to the development of considerable interest in applying these advantageous mechanical principles to a broader set of indications. Preexisting full-thickness chondral injuries or osteochondritis dissecans in adolescents and adults, if left alone, have long been presumed to progress to frank gonarthrosis. Though not clearly defined, the rate of disease progression is probably affected by chondral defect size, depth, and location or

---

* References 1, 13, 15, 19, 20, 23, 26, 32, 34, 44, 53, 62, 70, 71, 73, 78, 79, 81, 103, 113, 119.

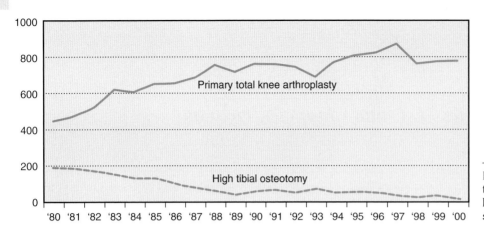

Figure 33–1. Number of upper tibial osteotomies versus total knee arthroplasties performed since 1980 at the Mayo Clinic.

specific factors such as patient age, weight, and limb alignment. An isolated study following 31 knees with Outerbridge grade III or IV lesions larger than 1 cm^2 did show a significant rate of joint space narrowing at long term follow-up.[74]

Late osteotomy has been shown to be a reliable procedure in the treatment of de generative arthrosis secondary to osteochondritis dissicans.[26,53,78,81] Because limb malalignment has been implicated as a cause of osteochondritis dissecans, it makes some intuitive sense to address this problem early.[2,39] In a small study evaluating the use of high tibial osteotomy (HTO) for adult osteochondritis dissecans by Slawski, seven knees treated with appropriate correction before the onset of marked degenerative arthrosis showed early clinical promise at a mean follow-up of 2.5 years.[107]

Present treatment modalities to address osteochondral defects in young active patients include subchondral microfracture, periosteal grafting, osteochondral autografting, osteochondral allografting, and autologous cultured chondrocyte transplantation. The prerequisite for the success of any of these techniques is that the limb remain well aligned. In fact, Odenbring et al studied the effects of realignment osteotomy in patients with isolated compartment gonarthrosis via arthroscopic, roentgenographic, and histological analysis.[94] They showed that cartilage in the previously overloaded compartment did eventually repair itself to some degree after osteotomy alone.[94] Though weighted toward an older population of patients, our institution has not found any benefit to adding arthroscopic abrasion arthroplasty to upper tibial osteotomy procedures in patients with isolated unicompartmental gonarthrosis.[79]

The benefits of offloading full-thickness articular cartilage defects with realignment procedures based on purely mechanical implications are clear. Therefore, it follows that malaligned limbs that are treated with a cartilage augmentation procedure will also benefit from realignment osteotomy either before or concomitantly with that augmentation. What remains unanswered at this time is whether osteotomy alone or in conjunction with a cartilage augmentation technique will yield more satisfying results.

Previously, HTO was considered contraindicated in the presence of significant instability.[26,83] The indications for realignment osteotomy have gradually expanded to include the treatment of this very difficult clinical problem.[50,64,82,87] Noyes and Simon have previously devised the terms primary-, double-, and triple-varus knee syndromes to classify various degrees of limb malalignment in young patients with confounding ligament and soft-tissue deficiencies.[92] These terms take into account leg alignment, knee motion, joint position, and specific ligament deficits (Fig. 33–2).

Primary varus refers to the tibiofemoral osseous alignment and geometry of the knee joint, including the added varus alignment that occurs with loss of the medial meniscus and confounding damage to the articular cartilage.[31] Double varus is a progression to increased lateral joint opening secondary to lateral soft-tissue laxity. Therefore, both tibiofemoral alignment and separation of the lateral tibiofemoral space are occurring simultaneously. With further trauma or stress, the limb may progress to a varus recurvatum position.[49] The three components that come into play as part of the triple-varus analogy are tibiofemoral osseous alignment, marked separation of the lateral tibiofemoral compartment, and increased external tibial rotation and hyperextension associated with an abnormal varus recurvatum position.[92] Previously, some surgeons have reported poor results with soft-tissue procedures alone for the treatment of knee instability associated with varus malalignment.[82] Various treatment algorithms have been proposed to deal with each of these entities individually and will be outlined later in the chapter. These algorithms involve correcting the varus alignment with or without the addition of ligament reconstructive procedures.

Contraindications

Although contraindications to corrective osteotomy are less commonly encountered in a young active patient, it remains paramount that these entities be understood because they will ultimately result in an outcome that is unsatisfactory to both the patient and the surgeon. Specific contraindications have been well delineated in the literature.[79] These contraindications vary from knee symptoms to patient expectations (Table 33–1). Symp-

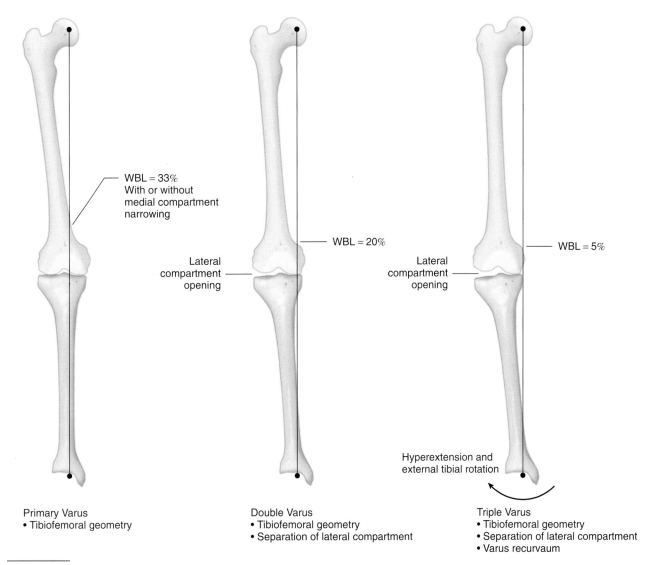

WBL = 33%
With or without
medial compartment
narrowing

WBL = 20%

WBL = 5%

Lateral
compartment
opening

Lateral
compartment
opening

Hyperextension and
external tibial rotation

Primary Varus
• Tibiofemoral geometry

Double Varus
• Tibiofemoral geometry
• Separation of lateral compartment

Triple Varus
• Tibiofemoral geometry
• Separation of lateral compartment
• Varus recurvaum

Figure 33–2. Schematic illustration of primary-, double-, and triple-varus knee angulation. WBL, weightbearing line. (From Noyes FR, Simon R: The role of high tibial osteotomy in the anterior cruciate ligament–deficient knee with varus alignment. In DeLee JC, Drez D [eds]: Orthopaedic Sports Medicine, Principles and Practice. Philadelphia, WB Saunders, 1993.)

Table 33–1. Contraindications to Corrective Osteotomy

Diffuse nonspecific knee pain
Meniscectomy in the compartment intended for weightbearing
Arthrosis in the compartment intended for weightbearing
Underlying diagnosis of inflammatory joint disease
Patellofemoral pain as a primary complaint
Weight more than 1.5 times ideal body weight
Physiological age older than 60 (relative)
Range-of-motion arc less than 90 degrees
Extension deficit greater than 10 degrees
Significant lateral tibial subluxation
Unrealistic patient expectations

toms of osteoarthritis as an underlying cause of cartilage degeneration are more likely to improve after an osteotomy than are symptoms attributed to inflammatory arthritis.[21,43,61] Degenerative arthritis of the patellofemoral joint may be a cause of failure after corrective osteotomy.[32,51] Conversely, patellofemoral pain can also improve after upper tibial osteotomy because the realignment may favorably alter patellofemoral mechanics.[25,30,44,66] Therefore, patients with mild patellofemoral pain may still be considered for realignment provided that their primary source of pain rests in the tibiofemoral joint.

Age assessment must be individualized for each patient and should be thought of in terms of physiological status and lifestyle requirements. In patients older than 60 years, arthroplasty provides more complete pain relief and shorter rehabilitation.[53] Body weight may also contribute to a compromised result. Weight that exceeds 1.5 times ideal body weight has been associated with higher early failure rates.[26] Other considerations less frequently discussed are gender and gait. Females who undergo realignment, especially when overcorrection is the goal, may be unhappy with the cosmetic appearance of their limb postoperatively. With regard to gait, the adductor moment (lateral thrust) must be accounted for in the preoperative planning because it will alter the degree of correction required. This will be discussed further in the section to follow.

PREOPERATIVE PLANNING

Recommendations for corrective osteotomy are based on a number of considerations acquired through a clear understanding of subjective symptoms, findings on physical examination, radiographic findings accounting for alignment and arthrosis, and gait analysis or biomechanical motion studies if available.

Counseling

Defining patient expectations and future desired activity level remains the cornerstone to the anticipated success that will follow any type of realignment intervention. Patients need to be aware of all associated risks, benefits, alternatives, and limitations that follow this intervention. They must be informed that the goal of surgery is to improve their symptoms; however, it will not leave them with a normal joint, and subsequent pain relief is oftentimes incomplete or time limited. A number of confounding factors have been associated with a less satisfactory outcome, including sex, obesity, chronicity of symptoms, and severity of disease.[26,46,72,78,81,95]

Examination

As pointed out previously by Noyes et al, a comprehensive physical examination must be performed on each patient and a number of key factors addressed.[88] During the examination the following parameters should be checked: (1) patellofemoral tracking and the presence of crepitus; (2) extensor mechanism alignment; (3) presence of crepitus at the tibiofemoral joint with varus and valgus loading; (4) detection of gait hyperextension abnormalities (often amenable to preoperative retraining); (5) examination for significant joint subluxation; (6) examination for range of motion; (7) a general soft-tissue examination to evaluate for ligament deficits, edema, masses, or the presence of confounding neuromas; (8) gait assessment to detect abnormalities such as a varus thrust or hyperextension position during the stance phase[91]; and (9) detection of any neurovascular abnormalities in the limb.

Several special tests have been used to identify specific ligamentous injuries. Anterior-posterior translation maneuvers are commonly performed to look for cruciate ligament deficiencies. Collateral ligament assessment is performed by applying varus and valgus stress to the knee in positions of 0 and 30 degrees of flexion. Though somewhat subjective, the examiner must quantify the amount of joint opening from an initial closed contact position to maximal opening. Integrity of the lateral and posterolateral ligamentous structures is best evaluated by performing tibiofemoral rotation tests at 30 and 90 degrees of knee flexion.[90] Arthroscopy with the use of a calibrated nerve hook as a direct measuring device is occasionally a useful adjunct to accurately record the amount of joint space opening. A functional classification has previously been described to rate the integrity of the lateral and posterolateral structures.[86] Less than a 3-mm increase in lateral joint opening or less than a 5-degree increase in external tibial rotation was considered functional, between a 3- and 5-mm increase in lateral joint opening or a 6- and 10-degrees increase in external tibial rotation was considered partially functional, and more than a 5-mm increase in lateral joint opening or more than a 10-degree increase in external tibial rotation was considered nonfunctional or failed.[86] These findings can help formulate a treatment plan, which must be individualized for each patient. This algorithm will be discussed later in the chapter.

Radiographic Evaluation

Weightbearing, anteroposterior, lateral, intercondylar notch, and skyline patellar views should be used to determine the presence, location, and severity of arthritis in the knee. It is important to systematically approach all films to look for contralateral tibiofemoral joint involvement, tibiofemoral subluxation, osteophytes, chondrocalcinosis, and excessive bone loss secondary to erosion. These factors have previously been correlated with less satisfactory outcomes after realignment procedures.[21,32,42,54,60]

Varus and valgus stress films are helpful in assessing the collateral ligamentous restraints and the condition of individual compartments. Marked narrowing of a compartment intended for weightbearing based on these stress films has previously been cited as a relative contraindication to the procedure.[58]

Hip-knee-ankle standing radiographs are the workhorse films for planning an osteotomy. Most centers are using bipedal standing films, which give a correct estimation of axial alignment and can easily be obtained.[112] These films are used to determine the existing anatomic and mechanical axes. They also help detect preexisting deformities of the tibia or femur and the effect of these deformities on overall leg alignment. Care must be taken to avoid errors in rotational positioning of the limb because such errors will alter the reliability of the standing radiographs.[6,41,59,93,101,111,114]

On the bipedal standing radiograph several landmarks are identified and used for subsequent measurement, including the center of the hip, the center of the ankle, the mechanical axis of the femur (joining the center of the hip to the center of the intracondylar notch),[37] the mechanical axis of the tibia (joining the center of the tibial epiphysis to the center of the ankle),[37] and the mechanical axis of the lower extremity (joining the center of the hip to the center of the ankle).[100] These landmarks allow for the assessment of several angles, including (1) the hip-knee-ankle angle (between the mechanical axis of the femur and the mechanical axis of the tibia); this angle approaches 0 degrees in a normally aligned limb;[17,77,101] (2) the transcondylar angle (between a line tangent to the condyles and the mechanical axis of the femur);[18,99,120] (3) the tibial plateau–tibial shaft angle (between a line tangent to the tibial plateau and the mechanical axis of the tibia);[17,99,120] and (4) the tibiofemoral separation angle (between a line tangent to the distal aspect of the femoral condyles and a line tangent to the tibial plateau).[17,31] These angles help identify the present physiological status and alignment of the limb from which further planning can be made.

Treatment Algorithm

After the preceding workup has been completed, the surgeon must now assimilate the information and decide what individual or combination of procedures will provide the most benefit to the patient in the long term.

MALALIGNMENT WITH ISOLATED GONARTHROSIS

In planning an osteotomy for isolated malalignment with unicompartmental degeneration, one must account for the location, direction, and degree of malalignment. Perhaps the single most common reason for failed treatment after realignment osteotomy is either undercorrection or overcorrection.[33,44,72,103,116] Although a number of different techniques can be used for the realignment itself, the concepts that must be considered are ubiquitous. Because varus malalignment is most commonly encountered, we will concentrate our discussion on the treatment of medial-sided gonarthrosis.

The present treatment of varus deformity associated with symptomatic medial-sided arthrosis is HTO. A well-accepted goal of this procedure is to obtain a slight overcorrection of the mechanical axis (or weightbearing line).[26,53] Typically, this goal means overcorrecting the mechanical axis 3 to 5 degrees, which oftentimes leaves the limb in 8 to 10 degrees of anatomic valgus (Fig. 33–3). The normal femoral-tibial angle approaches 6 degrees of anatomic valgus, whereas the mechanical axis normally measures 1.2 degrees of varus. From the standing full-length roentgenogram, one must determine overall limb alignment, with particular attention paid to joint line obliquity and ligamentous laxity. Ligamentous laxity corresponds to the amount of tibiofemoral joint separation noted on the bipodal standing films. For a proximal tibia width of 56 mm, each millimeter of extra tibiofemoral separation results in approximately 1 degree of additional angular deformity. Therefore, one must subtract approximately 1 degree per millimeter (or proportionally less for tibias wider than 56 mm) from the preoperative calculations for angular correction to avoid overcorrection.[31]

We frequently use the weightbearing line method to plan uncomplicated realignment osteotomies. First, the centers of the femoral head and tibiotalar joint are marked

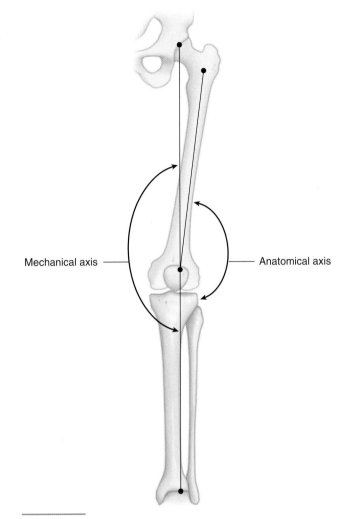

Figure 33–3. The mechanical axis represents a line drawn between the center of the femoral head and the center of the tibiotalar joint and averages 1.2 degrees varus. The anatomic axis represents the difference between the longitudinal axes of the femur and tibia and normally averages 6 degrees valgus. (Modified from Trousdale RT: Osteotomy: Patient selection, preoperative planning, and results. In Callaghan JJ, Rosenberg AG, Rubash HE, et al. (eds): The Adult Knee, Vol. 1, Lippincott, Williams & Wilkins, 2003, pp 985-990. Artwork originally prepared by Mayo Foundation.)

Mechanical axis — Anatomical axis

on the full-length radiograph. Then the selected weight-bearing line coordinate of the tibial plateau is marked. To facilitate this step, the tibial plateau is divided from 0% to 100% in a medial-to-lateral direction. To allow for slight overcorrection (usually 2 to 4 degrees of mechanical or 8 to 10 degrees of anatomic valgus), the 62% coordinate is marked out. One line is drawn from the center of the femoral head to the proximal tibial coordinate, and a second line is drawn from the center of the tibiotalar joint to the proximal tibial coordinate. The angle resulting from the intersection of these two lines corresponds to the intended angular correction (Fig. 33–4). This angle must then be revised to account for the magnitude of tibiofemoral joint separation as previously described; otherwise, unintended overcorrection will result. A wedge is then calculated by tracing directly on the radiograph. The height of the wedge must be normalized to account

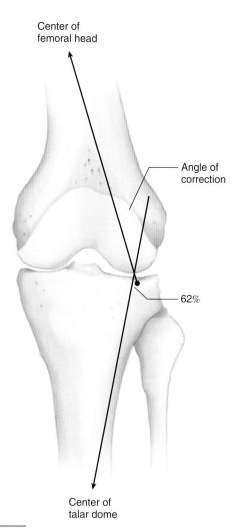

Figure 33–4. The weightbearing line method of preoperative planning is useful for straightforward osteotomy cases. The 62% coordinate is identified just lateral to the lateral tibial spine. The angle that is subtended by lines from the femoral head center and the tibiotalar center to the 62% coordinate is the proposed angle of correction. (Modified from Trousdale RT: Osteotomy: Patient selection, preoperative planning, and results. In Callaghan JJ, Rosenberg AG, Rubash HE, et al. (eds): The Adult Knee, Vol. 1, Lippincott, Williams & Wilkins, 2003, pp 985-990. Artwork originally prepared by Mayo Foundation.)

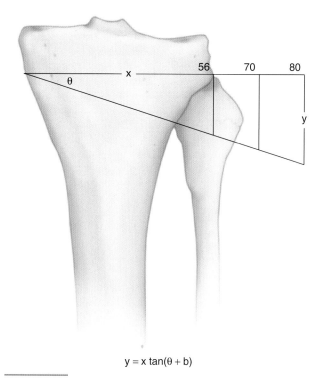

$$y = x \tan(\theta + b)$$

Figure 33–5. The amount of correction can be determined by using trigonometric methods. The size of the wedge in millimeters equals degrees of correction only when the width of the tibia equals 56 mm. (Modified from Trousdale RT: Osteotomy: Patient selection, preoperative planning, and results. In Callaghan JJ, Rosenberg AG, Rubash HE, et al. (eds): The Adult Knee, Vol. 1, Lippincott, Williams & Wilkins, 2003, pp 985-990. Artwork originally prepared by Mayo Foundation.)

for radiographic magnification. If the size of the wedge is to be derived from the angle by trigonometric methods, it is important to account for the exact width of the tibia (Fig. 33–5). The traditional rule of 1 degree equates to 1 mm will lead to undercorrection in virtually every tibia.[3] Finally, if available, it may be beneficial to incorporate specific information acquired through gait analysis to the correction angle planned. It has previously been suggested that patients with a high preoperative adduction moment will probably benefit in the long term from either a larger overcorrection or possibly gait training to reduce high adduction moments.[98]

Periarticular osteotomies are also used in symptomatic patients with excessive valgus malalignment and associated lateral compartment arthrosis. In contrast to varus malalignment, valgus knees often have superolateral obliq-

uity of the joint line. Wedge resections at the proximal end of the tibia will result in an increase in joint obliquity and should be avoided in deformities that exceed 12 degrees of valgus.[8,21,25,43,73,105] As a general rule, it may be best to approach valgus malalignment by identifying where the maximal deformity exists. Most commonly, this deformity is noted at the distal end of the femur.[17,99,120] Therefore, many surgeons prefer to use a distal femoral realignment procedure for any magnitude of valgus malalignment because this technique will correct the joint line obliquity. The most commonly performed procedure is a medial closing wedge osteotomy of the distal end of the femur with either lateral or medial rigid fixation to align the transcondylar line perpendicular to the mechanical axis and minimize medial collateral ligament laxity.[13,32,43]

In valgus malaligned knees, most surgeons aim to correct the alignment to an anatomic axis of 0 degrees. Such alignment will create a varus mechanical axis with 80% of body weight being transmitted through the medial compartment and 20% through the lateral compartment. As with varus knees, full-length standing, hip-to-ankle films are used for preoperative planning. The resultant postoperative mechanical axis should transect the knee joint just medial to the medial tibial spine.

In cases with confounding factors such as excessive extra-articular deformities, deformities in various planes, or excessive joint line obliquity, it may be helpful to use a computer software program in the preoperative planning. The Osteotomy Analysis Simulation Software (OASIS) (Zona Japan, Inc.) conducts a two-dimensional static analysis of the full-length standing radiograph. Anatomic landmarks are manually digitized to enable the program to formulate a two-dimensional rigid-body spring model. From this model a simulation is carried out to determine the exact location, magnitude, and type of knee osteotomy that most accurately reproduces the desired final limb alignment.

ASSOCIATED CARTILAGE REPAIR

Although little has been published that addresses the role of osteotomy in conjunction with articular cartilage repair techniques in a malaligned limb, it seems reasonable to apply the treatment algorithm just presented to this clinical entity. As previously discussed in the chapter, the natural history of full-thickness chondral or osteochondral lesions in the knee based on defect size, depth, and location or specific factors such as patient age, weight, and limb alignment has not been clearly defined. Nor is it clear whether performing an osteotomy alone or in conjunction with articular cartilage repair can prevent or delay the development of gonarthrosis. Nonetheless, a symptomatic patient with a large chondral injury superimposed on a maligned limb will probably benefit from the favorable biomechanical changes associated with a periarticular osteotomy about the knee.

ASSOCIATED LIGAMENT DEFICIENCIES

Symptomatic malaligned limbs with associated ligament deficiencies in the presence or absence of unicompartmental arthrosis present some of the most difficult diagnostic and treatment dilemmas that a surgeon must manage. The emerging literature on this topic would suggest that treatment of these cases must be individualized for any given patient. Because this topic contains a myriad of different clinical scenarios, we will concentrate on those encountered most commonly.

HTO with or without ligament reconstruction for varus-angulated anterior cruciate ligament (ACL)-deficient knees will be the focus of discussion. As previously outlined, it is imperative that the treating physician clearly discern the true character of the patient's complaints. The first question that must be clarified is whether the patient is complaining of arthritic-type symptoms versus instability. Symptomatic unicompartmental arthritis without instability can be treated with osteotomy alone by following the algorithm that we have previously discussed. Such patients are best served by a realignment osteotomy that is carried out with the goal of overcorrection to unload the symptomatic compartment without creating functional instability.

Subjective complaints of activity-related instability in a malaligned limb introduce a new set of clinical dilemmas. As pointed out by Noyes et al, there are a number of reasons for instability, and each presents a different set of problems.[88] Among the reasons cited are (1) subluxation of the anterior of the tibia, (2) separation of the lateral tibiofemoral joint with ambulation (varus thrust), (3) posterior subluxation, and (4) excessive hyperextension or varus recurvatum. In a malaligned limb, a combination of the first three reasons for subluxation will probably benefit from realignment osteotomy with or without subsequent cruciate ligament reconstruction, whereas a triple-varus knee will probably require a more complex approach consisting of HTO, ACL reconstruction, and posterolateral ligamentous reconstruction. Addressing the coronal and sagittal plane with an osteotomy as the initial procedure in a complex reconstruction might be considered in light of a recent study reporting satisfactory outcomes in patients with symptomatic hyperextension-thrust who were treated with an isolated opening wedge osteotomy.[82] In these cases, the posterior tibial slope was increased enough to correct for the hyperextension.[82]

In the setting of malalignment and instability, the timing (combined or staged) and types (opening versus closing wedge osteotomy, autograft versus allograft ligament reconstruction) of reconstructive options remain a source of both debate (for experienced surgeons) and confusion (for less experienced surgeons). First, it is commonly agreed that HTO should precede or be included with ligament reconstruction to safeguard the graft from undue tension.[82,86] Moreover, in the presence of minimal or no medial arthrosis, it is not necessary to produce a valgus overcorrection, and the goal of realignment should be a normal 50% weightbearing line.[82] Planning of the osteotomy beyond these recommendations has not been clearly defined.

Previous work by Dejour and Bonnin coupled with a biomechanical study carried out by Bonnin has helped clarify the relationship between tibial slope and tibial translation of the knee with weightbearing.[28] These authors suggested that decreasing the posterior tibial slope in the sagittal plane will result in less joint contact force in that plane and reduce anterior subluxation of the tibia relative to the femur, thus improving symptoms of anterior instability. Likewise, increasing the tibial slope will increase the anteroposterior component of the joint contact force and reduce posterior subluxation of the tibia with the potential for improving symptoms of posterior instability. The advantage of treating separate problems of malalignment and instability with a single procedure must be weighed against the potential long-term implications of changing the degree and location of joint contact pressure and increasing the tension or altering the kinematics of the opposing cruciate ligament.

Follow-up studies have noted that lateral closing wedge osteotomies about the tibia tend to decrease the posterior tibial slope.[4,65] Conversely, medial opening wedge osteotomies have been associated with an increase in tibial slope.[4,65] These concepts are in support of recommendations that closing wedge HTOs are effective in the treatment of chronic ACL-deficient knees.[29,35,65,85,87] Therefore, with anterior instability, decreasing the tibial slope several degrees may be beneficial if the surgeon is not planning on reconstructing the ACL. Likewise, with posterior instability, increasing the slope may compensate for the ligamentous deficiency. Increasing the slope for posterior instability beyond 10 degrees has been cautioned against because such an increase will cause chronic insufficiency of the ACL.[106] If planning to reconstruct the ACL as a supplement to the realignment procedure, the normal tibial slope should not be altered. Numerous studies have reported satisfactory results of treating younger patients with varus malalignment and ACL deficiency by both HTO and ACL reconstruction.[29,64,65,84,85,87]

The timing of combined surgical interventions remains a topic of controversy. To facilitate this discussion, treatment options will be discussed in the context of whether the treatment is addressing a primary-varus, double-varus, or triple-varus knee. Primary-varus knees can be treated by either HTO alone or HTO in combination with an ACL reconstruction performed simultaneously. The advantages and disadvantages of using a specific graft source (allograft, autograft, bone–patellar tendon–bone, quadriceps tendon–patellar bone, or hamstrings graft) depend on whether the procedures are performed simultaneously or in staged fashion and are beyond the scope of this overview.

For double-varus knees, it has been recommended that an ACL reconstruction not be performed simultaneously in knees with concomitant excessive abnormal lateral joint opening (best measured with a gap test during arthroscopy), which would expose the graft to excessive stress.[87] It has been suggested that staging the procedures may allow an opportunity for the posterolateral tissues to undergo adaptive shortening.[87]

In a triple-varus knee, recommendations to stage the operative procedure are based on concerns regarding the length of time needed for combined operative procedures, the increased propensity for postoperative complications, prolonged rehabilitation, and less satisfactory knee range of motion.[12,64,110] Therefore, it is recommended that the HTO be performed first with adequate time allowed for healing, followed by an arthroscopically assisted ACL reconstruction and open posterolateral ligament reconstruction.[87] The objective of the osteotomy is to eliminate the hyperextension-varus thrust during gait.[82] Discussion of the various techniques and indications for repair or reconstruction of the posterolateral structures (proximal advancement, allograft augmentation, double-graft substitution) is beyond the scope of this overview, and interested readers can find this information elsewhere in this text.

Whether to carry out a valgus closing wedge versus an opening wedge osteotomy for the treatment of persistent instability in a varus malaligned limb is also a topic of controversy. Satisfactory clinical outcomes with both techniques have been reported for the treatment of primary-, double-, and triple-varus knees either as a single procedure or in conjunction with other interventions.* The advantages and disadvantages specific to each technique will be discussed in the section to follow.

SURGICAL TECHNIQUES

Although a variety of osteotomy techniques about the knee have been described for the treatment of deformity, a number of key principles remain universal. The importance of proper incision placement, careful handling

*References 7, 29, 35, 40, 50, 64, 65, 82, 85, 86, 115.

of tissues, protection of neurovascular structures, accurate placement and manipulation of the osteotomy, and definitive fixation cannot be overemphasized. These techniques require meticulous surgical attention and are best performed by a surgeon who has a good understanding of knee anatomy and biomechanics. The use of alignment and cutting jigs to assist with placement and orientation of the osteotomy should be considered, especially if the surgeon is not performing a high volume of these procedures. Intraoperative radiographs or fluoroscopy is also strongly recommended to ensure that the final alignment of the limb reflects the intended preoperative templating.

Varus Deformity

The most common procedure for correcting varus deformity at the knee remains a closing wedge osteotomy, although opening wedge osteotomies are increasing in popularity.[44,68] Surgeons are best advised to use a technique that they are most comfortable with and have achieved satisfactory results with in the past.

Perhaps the greatest advantage of a closing wedge osteotomy is that it remains a time-honored procedure with a well-defined long-term track record.[11,22,26,38,45,80] Other advantages include a high rate of healing because of the large cancellous surfaces and the ability to be more aggressive with postoperative weightbearing. Potential disadvantages include removal of a large piece of native bone, the requirement for a concomitant fibular procedure, increased risk of causing damage to the common peroneal nerve, risk for avascular necrosis of the proximal fragment, and potential for lateral collateral laxity, shortening of the limb, and change in patellar height relative to the proximal end of the tibia.

Medial-sided opening wedge osteotomies have been reported with equally successful results.[27,36,44,69] Advantages associated with this type of osteotomy include a small incision with limited dissection, preservation of proximal tibial bone stock, no requirement for a concomitant procedure to address the proximal end of the fibula, decreased risk to the peroneal nerve, and the ability to simultaneously tighten the often lax medial collateral ligaments. Disadvantages include the need for bone grafting (autograft versus allograft or combined allograft and bone graft substitute) and a postulated increased risk for nonunion, patella baja, and lengthening of the extremity.

Though less commonly performed, dome osteotomies allow for correction of deformity in various planes, avoid limb length alterations, and can be used for larger corrections while still safeguarding against resultant joint line obliquity. This procedure is technically demanding and has been associated with a high rate of complications.[47] Likewise, dual osteotomies are less common but often required for complex deformities that cannot be corrected with a single procedure without creating an unacceptable amount of joint line obliquity. Dual osteotomies have been associated with fewer successful outcomes, a higher incidence of complications, and less satisfactory knee range of motion postoperatively.[55]

CLOSING WEDGE OSTEOTOMY

We continue to use a modification of a technique that has previously been described by Coventry.[19,20] The procedure is performed through a slightly oblique skin incision placed from the fibular head toward the tibial tubercle (Fig. 32–6). Subperiosteal dissection of the anterior compartment is done to expose the proximal end of the tibia and the tibiofibular joint. The inner third of the fibular head along with its cartilage is then removed for a standard uncomplicated realignment osteotomy. In cases of double- or triple-varus knees, disruption of the proximal tibiofibular joint is avoided to prevent proximal migration

and laxity of the posterolateral structures as recommended by Noyes et al.[87] These cases require that the osteotomy of the fibula be performed at the fibular neck, with bone removed to allow for compression after removal of bone from the proximal end of the tibia.

Malleable retractors are then carefully positioned behind the patellar tendon and the posterior of the tibia. Two guide pins are inserted, one parallel and 2 cm distal to the joint surface and the other at a precalculated distance distal to the first pin and angled to intersect at the medial tibial cortex. Pin placement is done with fluoroscopic guidance. The first saw cut is made under the first pin with the saw slightly tilted to match the patient's

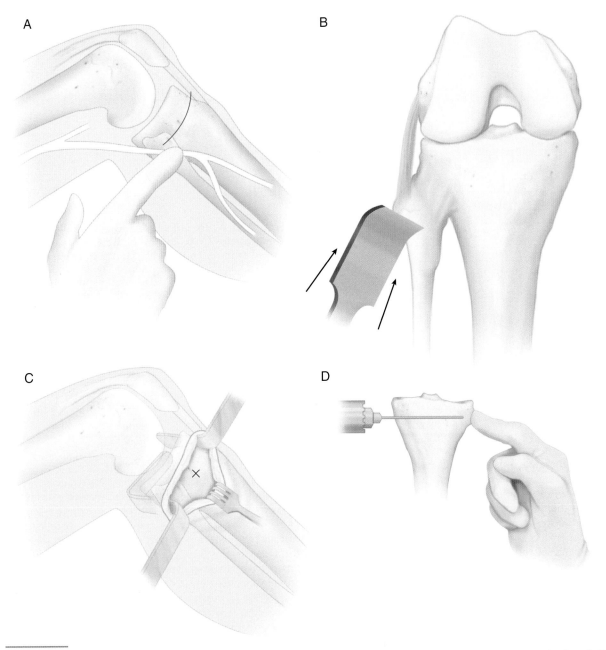

Figure 33–6. High tibial osteotomy technique. **A**, Skin incision. **B**, Resection of the inner third of the fibular head. **C**, Retractors placed anteriorly and posteriorly. **D**, Pin No. 1 placed parallel to the joint, 2.0 cm distal to the joint line.

(Figure continues)

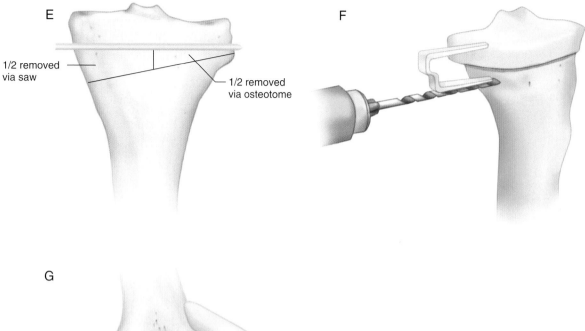

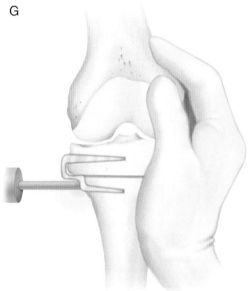

Figure 33–6, cont'd. **E,** Wedge cut with a saw proximally, then distally, but traversing only 50% to 75% of the tibial width. The inner wedge is removed with osteotomes. **F,** Step staples are applied, and a hole is drilled just distal to the inferior tine to promote compression of the osteotomy site. **G,** Firm counterpressure applied to avoid medial hinge disruption during final staple insertion. (Modified from Pagnano MW, Hanssen AD: Periarticular osteotomy of the knee for chondral and osteochondral lesions. Seminars in Arthroplasty 19(1):37-43, 1999. Artwork originally prepared by Mayo Foundation.)

posterior tibial slope (unless otherwise planned). The second saw cut is made above the second pin and traverses only 50% to 75% of the tibial width. After removal of the outer wedge of bone, osteotomes and curets are used to remove the remaining inner wedge. Care is taken to ensure that the medial periosteal sleeve and cortex are left intact. This medial column is then perforated with a drill or osteotome as required.

The knee is then brought out into extension and a controlled valgus stress is applied to close the osteotomy. Using the cautery cord and fluoroscopy, a plumb line is dropped intraoperatively to landmark the new mechanical axis and ensure that the amount of bone removed is correct. Fixation then follows with two stepped staples (or a single specialized plate), the first placed adjacent to the fibular head and the second more anterior. Any drilling or impacting requires that counterpressure be applied along the contralateral cortex to avoid medial cortex disruption. Wounds are closed in layers over a temporary drain.

Postoperatively, the patient is placed in a hinged knee brace that allows for knee range of motion and quadriceps

exercises. Partial weightbearing is allowed for the first 6 to 8 weeks, followed by progression to full weightbearing.

OPENING WEDGE OSTEOTOMY

An opening wedge osteotomy is performed through a small vertical incision over the pes anserinus insertion halfway between the medial border of the patellar ligament and the posterior margin of the tibia to expose the sartorial fascia (Fig. 33–7). This fascia is incised to expose the hamstring tendons. The osteotomy is planned above the tibial tubercle. Retractors are carefully placed anterior and posterior to protect the patellar tendon and posterior neurovascular structures along with the hamstring tendons and medial collateral ligament. The superficial medial collateral ligament inserts 5 to 7 cm distal to the joint and is usually elevated subperiosteally.

Under fluoroscopic imaging, a guide wire is drilled across the proximal end of the tibia in a medial-to-lateral

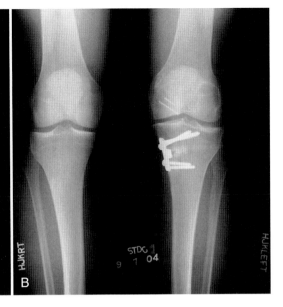

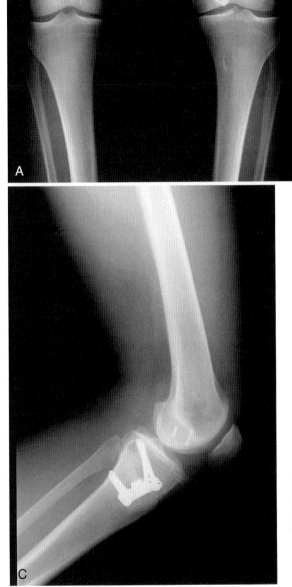

Figure 33-7. Preoperative and postoperative knee alignment in a young active patient with a previous history of medial-sided left knee pain. **A**, Anteroposterior radiograph of the knees revealing degenerative arthritis in the left knee with medial compartment narrowing and varus deformity. Screw fixation of an old osteochondral defect in the left medial femoral condyle is also apparent. One-year postoperative anteroposterior (**B**) and lateral (**C**) films are seen after an opening wedge high tibial osteotomy with plate and screw fixation.

direction. The guide is positioned at the level of the superior aspect of the tibial tubercle and oriented obliquely to end approximately 1 cm below the joint line at the lateral tibial cortex. The tip of the fibular head can be used as a reference point. The saw cut is then made on the underside of the pin and advanced to within 1 cm of the lateral edge of the tibia. Oftentimes, the cortical cut is made with a small sagittal saw, and flexible osteotomes are used to deepen the osteotomy under fluoroscopic guidance. Once the osteotomy is completed, the medial opening is created with an osteotomy wedge to the predetermined size. The anteroposterior slope can be matched or changed in accor-

dance with the amount of deformity present and the preoperative goals. If replicating the native slope, it is important to understand that the distraction anteriorly at the tubercle should be less than that at the posteromedial corner; otherwise, the slope will be increased.[3,106] In cases in which the anterior opening is greater than 1 cm, a tibial tubercle osteotomy can be performed to advance the tubercle the same height as the osteotomy.[82]

Fluoroscopic imaging is used in conjunction with the cautery cord to trace out the mechanical axis and ensure that it is appropriate. When the desired opening is achieved, the osteotomy is secured with a plate and a bone graft. The type of osteotomy plate and bone graft selected is dependent on the individual preferences of the surgeon. A drain is then inserted and the wound closed in layers.

Alternatively, an external fixator can be used to achieve a gradual correction. This technique has a number of advantages, including the potential for correcting larger deformities that may be technically impossible with standard closing or opening wedge procedures (because of excessive loss of bone or overtensioning of soft tissues), the ability to address angular and translational correction in multiple planes, and the ability to continue to manipulate the osteotomy site postoperatively and throughout the healing process to achieve optimal correction.[3] These advantages must be weighed against the cumbersome nature of this treatment and the potential risk for development of a deep pin site infection, which if not adequately treated can compromise the results of later arthroplasty should it be necessary.

After an opening wedge osteotomy with acute plate fixation and bone grafting, the patient is protected in a hinged knee brace and kept feather weightbearing with crutches for 6 to 8 weeks postoperatively. The patient is then gradually advanced to full weightbearing by 12 weeks if there is radiographic confirmation of bony union.

Valgus Deformity

The most common treatment of symptomatic valgus deformity with associated lateral compartment gonarthrosis is a medial closing wedge osteotomy of the distal end of the femur and either lateral or medial rigid fixation. The reasons for the continued popularity of this technique have been outlined earlier in the chapter. At our center, we frequently use a modification of the original technique described by the AO group.[1,73,76,79]

DISTAL FEMORAL CLOSING WEDGE OSTEOTOMY

A 12- to 15-cm skin incision is placed medially or in the midline. The vastus medialis is elevated anteriorly to expose the metaphyseal region of the distal end of the femur. An initial guide pin is placed across the knee joint parallel to the joint surface (Fig. 33–8). A second pin is placed 2.5 cm proximal to the joint line, parallel to its surface, and inserted in an anteromedial-to-posterolateral direction to accommodate for distal femoral geometry. The second more proximal pin provides a guide for the direction of the blade plate chisel to follow. The medial cortex is perforated in advance of inserting the chisel to prevent comminution. The chisel is advanced parallel to the guide pin. Before completing the osteotomy, it is helpful to mark the medial cortex to keep track of the native femoral rotation.

The osteotomy is carried out proximal to the adductor tubercle with a saw. The lateral cortex is safeguarded but later perforated multiple times with a 7-mm osteotome while leaving an intact periosteal hinge. A 5-mm wedge of

bone is removed to allow a 90-degree angle between the chisel and the medial femoral cortex. Varus stress is then applied to the limb in a controlled fashion, and the proximal cortical fragment is impacted into the distal cancellous bone. This maneuver is done under fluoroscopic imaging to confirm adequate correction of the malalignment. A 90-degree blade plate is used for definitive fixation. The autogenous bone removed earlier is used as local graft at the site of the osteotomy. Also described is placement of the blade plate along the lateral femoral cortex. Proponents of this technique argue that laterally based fixation is biomechanically superior and allows for fixation along the tensile side of the bone.[76] The need for this additional support is questioned in a young active patient population with good bone quality. The wound is then closed in layers over a drain.

Postoperative management restricts the patient to toe-touch weightbearing for 4 to 6 weeks, followed by progressive weightbearing in a hinged knee brace locked in extension for 12 weeks. If the osteotomy is well healed at 12 weeks, weightbearing is allowed as tolerated. Provided that the fixation achieved intraoperatively is adequate, early active range of motion is allowed.

COMPLICATIONS

Because the majority of the chapter focuses on proximal tibial osteotomies (HTOs), the discussion of complications will likewise. Most of the present literature focuses on experiences with HTO in treating the more common unicompartmental arthritic patient with associated malalignment. Reports of complications in patients who have undergone HTO for the specific indications of instability, as an adjunct to a cartilage repair technique, or in conjunction with combined procedures to address a myriad of instability scenarios are less common inasmuch as these indications are only presently becoming more popular. Moreover, comparing the reported complications between these groups is difficult because reported rates of complications with combined procedures are highly variable. Part of the difficulty with combined procedures is the inability to sort out which individual procedure is responsible for the noted complication.

A number of cited complications are inherent to the HTO procedure on its own (Table 33–2). Perhaps the most common is overcorrection or undercorrection, which often reflects failure in planning or execution of the osteotomy.[33,44,72,103,116] The literature supports less pain relief and decreased durability of the osteotomy after undercorrection.[19,22,26] Overcorrection beyond an anatomic angle of 10 degrees is also detrimental because it will have an impact on gait[104] and can be cosmetically displeasing. Scarring of the patellar ligament has been linked to patella baja. This complication has not been clearly shown to result in less satisfactory clinical outcomes; however, it will make exposure more difficult in patients who subsequently require total knee replacement. Intra-articular fractures at the time of surgery can be considered technical flaws. Either the surgeon has left the

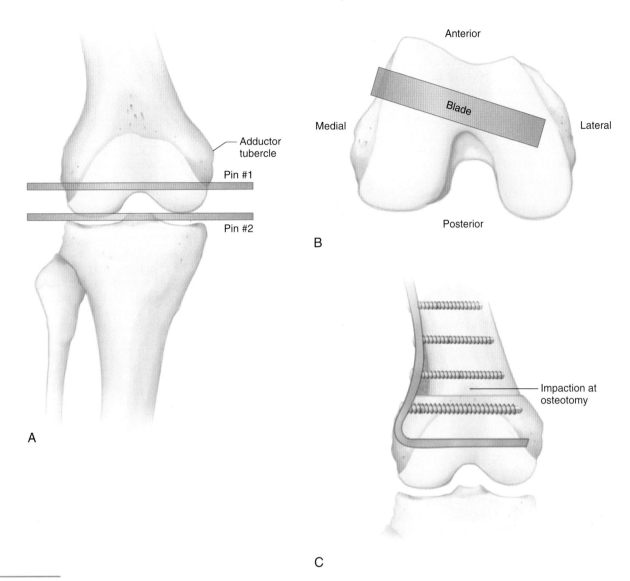

Figure 33–8. Distal femoral osteotomy. **A**, Pin No. 1 placed across the joint and pin No. 2 placed 2.5 cm from the joint line parallel to the joint surface. **B**, Pin No. 2 and a chisel directed in an anteromedial-to-posterolateral direction to accommodate the geometry of the distal end of the femur. **C**, Small wedge of bone removed medially to accommodate the 90-degree blade plate and the proximal fragment impacted into distal cancellous bone.

Table 33–2. Complications Associated with High Tibial Osteotomy

MAJOR	MINOR
Overcorrection or undercorrection	Superficial wound problem
Loss of correction	Postoperative hematoma
Neurovascular injury	Painful hardware
Deep infection	Arthrofibrosis
Compartment syndrome	Patellar shift
Intra-articular fracture	Delayed union
Hardware failure	Osteonecrosis of the tibial plateau
Thromboembolic event	Joint line obliquity
Nonunion or malunion	Painful neuroma

proximal tibial fragment too thin,[52] or the osteotomy before manipulation was not adequate. Nonunion and malunion are also potentially the result of technical shortcomings. Leaving the proximal tibial fragment too thin has been associated with avascular necrosis with a subsequent increased risk for nonunion.[19,63] Inadequate fixation can result in nonunion or a delayed shift of the opposing surfaces. Any rotational shift can substantially change patellofemoral kinematics. If not identified, rotational shifts can also result in malpositioning of total knee components. Finally, infection, though rare, is very debilitating for the patient and might best be treated with the same principles that are applied to infected fractures. Treatment goals should include eradication of the infection, establishment of union, and relief of pain.

Complications specific to cases in which an osteotomy has been used to treat instability rather than arthritis are not well understood. With a variety of treatment combinations for the management of often similar problems, the reporting of perioperative and long-term complications remains highly variable. For instance, reported complication rates for combined HTO/ACL reconstruction in several different studies range from no complications[96] to major complication rates of 5%, 7%, and 37%.[29,64,85] In general, performing a number of procedures in a single setting for the treatment of patients with complex knee instability has been associated with prolonged operating time, an increase in postoperative complications, prolonged rehabilitation, and less satisfactory range of motion.[12,64,110] The nature and rate of complications after realignment procedures performed for indications other than arthritis will be better defined as this practice continues to evolve.

RESULTS AND CONCLUSIONS

Periarticular osteotomy of the knee has a proven record in the treatment of symptomatic, malaligned limbs. Both proximal tibial valgus osteotomy and distal femoral varus osteotomy produce reliable and reproducible improvements in pain and function for appropriately selected patients with gonarthrosis.[26,32,34,53,73,78,81,113,119] The importance of patient selection and meticulous surgical technique is paramount for success of the procedure. In the absence of precise indications, osteotomy has been less successful.[10] Similarly, a study reporting 57% compromised results, despite rigid patient selection criteria, has clearly demonstrated a direct correlation between suboptimal surgical technique and poor clinical outcome.[16] A number of the cases with poor outcomes were linked to undercorrection or overcorrection. The natural history of this procedure based on pooled data suggests that there is a marked drop-off in success between 5- and 10-year follow-up.[14,44,102] At the Mayo Clinic, the 5-year success rate is approximately 87% for HTOs, but the rate drops to 69% by 10 years.[14] Success was based on pain symptoms and limitations in activity.[14] Preoperative alignment and postoperative alignment are two of the most common variables attributed to long-term success.[22,25] The optimal postoperative alignment remains somewhat controversial. Recommendations range from 3 to 6 degrees of valgus using hip-knee-ankle alignment by Hernigou et al, to 10 to 12 degrees of anatomic valgus by Cass and Bryan, to 6 to 14 degrees of femorotibial valgus by Rudan and Simurda.[14,44,103] Work by Coventry et al revealed a 94% survival rate when postoperative anatomic femorotibial alignment was 8 degrees or greater versus 63% if the anatomic valgus alignment was 5 degrees or less.[26] In the literature, the most common reason cited for long-term failure is progressive degenerative arthritis in the medial or lateral compartments.[109] The severity of preexisting arthritis has clearly been implicated in the progression of arthritis with the passage of time.[66]

In the case of symptomatic articular cartilage injury with confounding limb malalignment, it seems reasonable to offer a patient earlier intervention with a corrective osteotomy in advance of progressing arthritis. This recommendation is based on the principle that realignment will provide favorable biomechanical changes to a previously overloaded compartment coupled with the understanding that intervening before the progression of arthritis will have favorable long-term implications.[66] The protective role of osteotomy alone or osteotomy coupled with cartilage repair in preventing the development of gonarthrosis is not clear at this time.

In contrast to our present knowledge of the favorable outcomes with realignment procedures in the presence of symptomatic malaligned limbs with marked unicompartmental arthritis, there is little information on the functional outcome of patients undergoing osteotomy primarily for instability.[7,35,40,82,115] As previously discussed, the realignment goals will differ, depending on whether the procedure is being done primarily to address arthritic symptoms or instability. Slight overcorrection (anatomic axis of 8 to 10 degrees) is desired for the treatment of unicompartmental arthrosis versus neutral alignment for instability (anatomic axis of approximately 6 degrees). Soft-tissue procedures alone to address instability in a malaligned limb will result in repetitive stress and failure of the surgically reconstructed structures.[82,86] Therefore, realignment should precede ligament reconstruction in an attempt to re-create a more physiological environment with respect to knee kinematics and biomechanical properties. Various protocols have been proposed for the treatment of symptomatic malaligned knees and chronic ligament deficiencies with predominant symptoms of instability. The reported short-term outcomes in these studies have been comparable[7,35,40,50,64,82,87,115,117]; however, we need longer-term evaluation before definitive recommendations can be made.

The ability of a well-planned osteotomy as a single procedure to compensate for ligamentous deficits is also being explored. Good functional outcomes have been reported with the use of a lateral closing wedge osteotomy alone for ACL instability and malalignment[35] and a medial opening wedge osteotomy alone to treat patients with confounding posterolateral instability and a hyperextension-varus thrust.[82] Conversely, reports of combined techniques that include both bony and soft-tissue procedures for the treatment of various degrees of instability have also been encouraging.[12,50,64,85,87,89] In cases in which combined procedures are indicated, it may be wise to stage them because simultaneous combined treatment protocols have been associated with significant complication rates.[64] Current recommendations to address coronal and sagittal plane alignment first in these cases and deal with residual ligamentous laxity on a required basis seem to be reasonable.[82]

In summary, the treatment of young active patients with limb malalignment who complain of pain and instability secondary to ligament deficiencies in the presence or absence of unicompartmental gonarthrosis continues to evolve. Treating these patients requires that the physician conduct a thorough assessment of various parameters, including but not limited to pain, instability, alignment, and patient expectations. The ultimate goal for these patients will be the ability to return to a level of recreational activities.

References

1. Aglietti P, Stringa G, Buzzi R, et al: Correction of the valgus deformity with a supracondylar V osteotomy. Clin Orthop 217:214-220, 1987.
2. Aichroth P: Osteochondritis dissecans of the knee: A clinical survey. J Bone Joint Surg Br 53:440-447, 1971.
3. Amendola A: Unicompartmental osteoarthritis in the active patient: The role of high tibial osteotomy. Arthroscopy 19(Suppl 1):109-116, 2003.
4. Amendola A, Rorabeck CH, Bourne RB, et al: Total knee arthroplasty following high tibial osteotomy for osteoarthritis. J Arthroplasty 4:S11-S17, 1989.
5. Argenson JN, Chevrol-Benkeddache Y, Aubaniac JM: Modern unicompartmental knee arthroplasty with cement: A three to ten-year follow-up study. J Bone Joint Surg Am 84:2235-2239, 2002.
6. Augereau B: Radiological assessment before femoral and tibial osteotomies. Ann Radiol Paris 36:252-255, 1993.
7. Badne NP, Forster IW: High tibial osteotomy in knee instability: The rationale of treatment and early results. Knee Surg Sports Traumatol Arthrosc 10:38-43, 2002.
8. Bauer BC, Insall J, Koshino T: Tibial osteotomy in gonarthrosis (osteo-arthritis of the knee). J Bone Joint Surg Am 51:1545-1563, 1969.
9. Berger RA, Nedeff DD, Barden RM, et al: Unicompartmental knee arthroplasty. Clinical experience at 6- to 10-year follow-up. Clin Orthop 367:50-60, 1999.
10. Berman AT, Bosacco SJ, Kirshner S, et al: Factors influencing long-term results in high tibial osteotomy. Clin Orthop 272:192-198, 1991.
11. Billings A, Scott D, Camargo M, et al: High tibial osteotomy with a calibrated osteotomy guide, rigid internal fixation, and early motion. Long-term follow-up. J Bone Joint Surg Am 81:70-79, 2000.
12. Boss A, Stutz G, Oursin C, et al: Anterior cruciate ligament reconstruction combined with valgus tibial osteotomy (combined procedure). Knee Surg Sports Traumatol Arthrosc 3:187-191, 1995.
13. Cameron HU, Botsford DJ, Park YS: Prognostic factors in the outcome of supracondylar femoral osteotomy for lateral compartment osteoarthritis of the knee. Can J Surg 40:114-118, 1997.
14. Cass JR, Bryan RS: High tibial osteotomy. Clin Orthop 230:196-199, 1988.
15. Chao EYS: Biomechanics of high tibial osteotomy. In American Academy of Orthopaedic Surgeons Symposium on Reconstructive Surgery of the Knee. St Louis, CV Mosby, 1978, pp 143-153.
16. Chillag KJ, Nicholls PJ: High tibial osteotomy. A retrospective analysis of 30 cases. Orthopedics 7:1821-1826, 1984.
17. Cooke TD, Bryant JT, Scudamore RA: Biomechanical factors in alignment and arthritic disorders of the knee. In Fu FH, Harner CD, Vince KG (eds): Knee Surgery. Baltimore, Williams & Wilkins, 1994, p 1061.
18. Cooke TD, Li J, Scudamore RA: Radiographic assessment of bony contributions to knee deformity. Orthop Clin North Am 25:387-393, 1994.
19. Coventry MB: Osteotomy of the upper portion of the tibia for degenerative arthritis of the knee: A preliminary report. J Bone Joint Surg Am 47:984-990, 1965.
20. Coventry MB: Stepped staple for upper tibial osteotomy. J Bone Joint Surg Am 51:1011, 1969.
21. Coventry MB: Osteotomy about the knee for degenerative and rheumatoid arthritis. J Bone Joint Surg Am 55:23-48, 1973.
22. Coventry MB: Upper tibial osteotomy for osteoarthritis. J Bone Joint Surg Am 67:1136-1140, 1985.
23. Coventry MB: Proximal tibial varus osteotomy for osteoarthritis of the lateral compartment of the knee. J Bone Joint Surg Am 69:32-38, 1987.
24. Coventry MB: Osteotomy of the upper portion of the tibia for degenerative arthritis of the knee. A preliminary report. Clinical Orthop 248:4-8, 1989.
25. Coventry MB, Bowman PW: Long-term results of upper tibial osteotomy for degenerative arthritis of the knee. Acta Orthop Belg 48:139-156, 1982.
26. Coventry MB, Ilstrup DM, Wallrichs SL: Proximal tibial osteotomy: A critical long-term study of 87 cases. J Bone Joint Surg Am 75:196-201, 1993.
27. Debeyre J, Patte D: Traitment chirurgical des gonarthroses déviations laterals. Rev Rhum Mal Osteoartic 33:327-336, 1966.
28. Dejour H, Bonnin M: Tibial translation after anterior cruciate ligament rupture: Two radiological tests compared. J Bone Joint Surg Br 76:745-749, 1994.
29. Dejour H, Neyret P, Boileau P, et al: Anterior cruciate reconstruction combined with valgus tibial osteotomy. Clin Orthop 299:220-228, 1994.
30. Dohin B, Migaud H, Gougeon F, et al: Effect of a valgization osteotomy with external wedge removal on patellar height and femoro-patellar arthritis. Acta Orthop Belg 59:69-75, 1993.
31. Dugdale TW, Noyes FR, Styer D: Preoperative planning for high tibial osteotomy: The effect of lateral tibiofemoral separation and tibiofemoral length. Clin Orthop 274:248-264, 1992.
32. Edgerton BC, Mariani EM, Morrey BF: Distal femoral varus osteotomy for painful genu valgum: A 5-11 year follow-up. Clin Orthop 288:263-269, 1993.
33. Engel GM, Lippert FG III: Valgus tibial osteotomy: Avoiding the pitfalls. Clin Orthop 160:137-143, 1981.
34. Finkelstein J, Gross A, Davis A: Varus osteotomy of the distal part of the femur. J Bone Joint Surg Am 78:1348-1352, 1996.
35. Fowler PJ, Kirkley A, Roe J: Osteotomy of the proximal tibia in the treatment of chronic anterior cruciate ligament insufficiency. J Bone Joint Surg Br 76(Supp):26, 1994.
36. Fowler P, Tan J, Brown G: Medial opening wedge high tibial osteotomy. Op Tech Sports Med 8:32-38, 2000.
37. Frain PH: Retentissement sur le genou des atteintes de la hanche: Bases théoriques. Rev Chir Orthop 53:713-717, 1967.
38. Fujisawa Y, Masuhara K, Shiomi S: The effect of high tibial osteotomy for arthritis of the knee. Orthop Clin North Am 10:585-608, 1979.
39. Garrett JC: Osteochondritis dissecans. Clin Sports Med 10:569-593, 1991.
40. Goradia VK, Van Allen J: Chronic lateral knee instability treated with a high tibial osteotomy. Arthroscopy 18:807-811, 2002.
41. Green SA, Green HD: The influence of radiographic projection on the appearance of deformities. Orthop Clin North Am 25:467-475, 1994.
42. Hanssen AD: Osteotomy about the knee: American perspective. In Insall JN, Scott WN (eds): Surgery of the Knee, vol 2, 3rd ed. Philadelphia, Churchill Livingstone, 2001, pp 1447-1464.
43. Healy WL, Anglen JO, Wasilewski SA, et al: Distal femoral varus osteotomy. J Bone Joint Surg Am 70:102-109, 1988.
44. Hernigou PL, Medevielle D, Debeyre J, et al: Proximal tibial osteotomy for osteoarthritis with varus deformity: A ten to thirteen year follow-up study. J Bone Joint Surg Am 69:332-353, 1987.
45. Hofmann A, Wyatt R, Beck S: High tibial osteotomy. Use of osteotomy jig, rigid fixation, and early motion versus conventional surgical technique and cast immobilization. Clin Orthop 271:212-217, 1991.
46. Holden DL, James SL, Larson RL, et al: Proximal tibial osteotomy in patients who are 50 years old or less. A long-term follow-up study. J Bone Joint Surg Am 70:977-982, 1988.
47. Hsu R: The study of Maquet dome high tibial osteotomy. Arthroscopic-assisted analysis. Clin Orthop 243:280-285, 1989.
48. Hsu RWW, Himeno S, Coventry MB, Chao EY: Normal axial alignment of the lower extremity and load bearing distribution at the knee. Clin Orthop 255:215-227, 1990.
49. Hughston JC, Jacobson KE: Chronic posterolateral rotatory instability of the knee. J Bone Joint Surg Am 67:351-359, 1985.
50. Imhoff AB, Linke RD, Agneskirchner J: [Corrective osteotomy in primary varus, double varus and triple varus knee instability with cruciate ligament replacement.] Orthopade 33:201-207, 2004.
51. Insall JN: High tibial osteotomy in the treatment of osteoarthritis of the knee. South Surg Ann 7:347-359, 1975.
52. Insall JN: Osteotomy. In Insall JN, Windsor RE, Scott WN, et al (eds): Surgery of the Knee. New York, Churchill Livingstone, 1993, p 635.
53. Insall JN, Joseph D, Msika C: High tibial osteotomy for varus gonarthrosis: A long-term follow-up study. J Bone Joint Surg Am 66:1040-1048, 1984.
54. Insall JN, Shoji H, Mayer V: High tibial osteotomy. J Bone Joint Surg Am 56:1397-1405, 1974.

55. Iveson JM, Longton EB, Wright V: Comparative study of tibial (single) and tibiofemoral (double) osteotomy for osteoarthrosis and rheumatoid arthritis. Ann Rheum Dis 36:319-326, 1977.

56. Jackson JP: Osteotomy for osteoarthritis of the knee. J Bone Joint Surg Br 40:826, 1958.

57. Jackson JP, Waugh W: The technique and complications of upper tibial osteotomy: A review of 226 operations. J Bone Joint Surg Br 56:236-245, 1974.

58. Jacob R: Prognostic Features and Proximal Tibial Osteotomy. Atlanta, AAOS Instructional Course, 1990.

59. Jiang CC, Insall JN: Effect of rotation on the axial alignment of the femur: Pitfalls in the use of femoral intramedullary guides in total knee arthroplasty. Clin Orthop 248:50-56, 1989.

60. Job-Deslandre C, Languepin A, Benvenuto M, Menkes CJ: [Tibial valgization osteotomy in gonarthrosis with or without chondrocalcinosis: Results after 5 years.] Rev Rhum Mal Osteoarth 58:491-496, 1991.

61. Johnson EW Jr, Bodell LS: Corrective supracondylar osteotomy for painful genu valgus. Mayo Clin Proc 56:87-92, 1981.

62. Keene JS, Monson DK, Roberts JM, et al: Evaluation of patients for high tibial osteotomy. Clin Orthop 243:157-165, 1989.

63. Kettelkamp DB, Leach RE, Nasca R: Pitfalls of proximal tibial osteotomy. Clin Orthop 106:232-241, 1975.

64. Lattermann C, Jakob RP: High tibial osteotomy alone or combined with ligament reconstruction in anterior cruciate ligament–deficient knees. Knee Surg Sports Traumatol Arthrosc 4:32-38, 1996.

65. Lerat JL, Moyen B, Garin C, et al: Anterior laxity and medial compartment osteoarthritis of the knee: Results of reconstruction of the anterior cruciate ligament with upper tibial osteotomy. J Orthop Surg 7:333-342, 1993.

66. Lootvoet L, Massinon A, Rossillon R, et al: Upper tibial osteotomy for gonarthrosis in genu varum. Apropos of a series of 193 cases. Rev Chir Orthop Reparatrice Appar Mot 79:375-384, 1993.

67. Mabrey JD, McCollum DE: High tibial osteotomy: A retrospective review of 72 cases. South Med J 80:975, 1987.

68. Magyar G, Ahl TL, Vibe P: Open-wedge osteotomy by hemicallostasis or the closed-wedge technique for osteoarthritis of the knee: A randomized study of 50 operations. J Bone Joint Surg Br 81:444-448, 1999.

69. Magyar G, Toksvig LS, Lindstrand A: Hemicallotasis open wedge osteotomy for osteoarthritis of the knee. J Bone Joint Surg Br 81:449-451, 1999.

70. Maquet P: Valgus osteotomy for osteoarthritis of the knee. Clin Orthop 120:143-148, 1976.

71. Maquet P: The treatment of choice in osteoarthritis of the knee. Clin Orthop 192:108-112, 1985.

72. Matthew LS, Goldstein SA, Malvitz TA, et al: Proximal tibial osteotomy: Factors that influence the duration of satisfactory function. Clin Orthop 229:193-200, 1988.

73. McDermott AG, Finkelstein JA, Farine I, et al: Distal femoral varus osteotomy for valgus deformity of the knee. J Bone Joint Surg Am 70:110-116, 1988.

74. Messner K, Maletius W: The long-term prognosis for severe damage to weight-bearing cartilage in the knee. Acta Orthop Scand 67:165-168, 1996.

75. Miller MD, Fu FH: The role of osteotomy in anterior cruciate ligament–deficient knee. Clin Sports Med 12:697-708, 1993.

76. Miniacci A, Grossman SP, Jakob RP: Supracondylar femoral varus osteotomy in the treatment of valgus knee deformity. Am J Knee Surg 2:65-73, 1990.

77. Moreland JR, Basset LW, Hanker GJ: Radiographic analysis of the axial alignment of the lower extremity. J Bone Joint Surg Am 69:745-749, 1987.

78. Morrey BF: Upper tibial osteotomy for secondary osteoarthritis of the knee. J Bone Joint Surg Br 71:554-558, 1989.

79. Morrey BF: Medial compartment disease: Tibial osteotomy. In Morrey BF (ed): Reconstructive Surgery of the Joints, vol 2, 2nd ed. New York, Churchill Livingstone, 1996, pp 1449-1468.

80. Mynerts R: Optimal correction in high tibial osteotomy for varus deformity. Acta Orthop Scand 51:689-694, 1980.

81. Nagel A, Insall JN, Scuderi GR: Proximal tibial osteotomy: A subjective outcome study. J Bone Joint Surg Am 78:1353-1358, 1996.

82. Naudie DD, Amendola A, Fowler PJ: Opening wedge high tibial osteotomy for symptomatic hyperextension-varus thrust. Am J Sports Med 32:60-70, 2004.

83. Naudie D, Bourne RB, Rorabeck CH, et al: Survivorship of the high tibial valgus osteotomy: A 10 to 22 year follow-up study. Clin Orthop 367:18-27, 1999.

84. Neuschwander DC, Drez D Jr, Paine RM: Simultaneous high tibial osteotomy and ACL reconstruction for combined genu varum and symptomatic ACL tear. Orthopedics 16:679-684, 1993.

85. Noyes FR, Barber SD, Simon R: High tibial osteotomy and ligament reconstruction in varus angulated, anterior cruciate ligament–deficient knees: A two- to seven-year follow-up study. Am J Sports Med 21:2-12, 1993.

86. Noyes FR, Barber-Westin SD: Surgical restoration to treat chronic deficiency of the posterolateral complex and cruciate ligaments of the knee joint. Am J Sports Med 24:415-426, 1996.

87. Noyes FR, Barber-Westin SD, Hewett TE: High tibial osteotomy and ligament reconstruction for varus angulated anterior cruciate ligament–deficient knees. Am J Sports Med 28:282-296, 2000.

88. Noyes FR, Barber-Westin SD, Roberts CS: High tibial osteotomy in knees with associated chronic ligament deficiencies. In Jackson DW (ed): Master Techniques in Orthopaedic Surgery: Reconstructive Knee Surgery, 2nd ed. Philadelphia, Lippincott Williams & Wilkins, 2002, pp 229-260.

89. Noyes FR, Berrios-Torres S, Barber-Westin SD, et al: Prevention of permanent arthrofibrosis after anterior cruciate ligament reconstruction alone or combined with associated procedures: A prospective study of 443 knees. Knee Surg Sports Traumatol Arthrosc 8:196-206, 2000.

90. Noyes FR, Cummings JR, Grood ES, et al: The diagnosis of knee motion limits, subluxations, and ligament injury. Am J Sports Med 19:163-171, 1991.

91. Noyes FR, Dunworth LA, Andriacchi TP, et al: Knee hyperextension gait abnormalities in unstable knees. Recognition and preoperative gait retraining. Am J Sports Med 24:35-45, 1996.

92. Noyes FR, Simon R: The role of high tibial osteotomy in the anterior cruciate ligament–deficient knee with varus alignment. In DeLee JC, Drez D (eds): Orthopaedic Sports Medicine. Principles and Practice. Philadelphia, WB Saunders, 1994, pp 1401-1443.

93. Odenbring S, Berggren AM, Peil L: Roentgenographic assessment of the hip-knee-ankle axis in medial gonarthrosis: A study of reproducibility. Clin Orthop 289:195-196, 1993.

94. Odenbring S, Egund N, Lindstrand A, et al: Cartilage regeneration after proximal tibial osteotomy for medial gonarthrosis: An arthroscopic, roentgenographic, and histologic study. Clin Orthop 277:210-216, 1992.

95. Odenbring S, Tjornstrand B, Egund N, et al: Function after tibial osteotomy for medial gonarthrosis below aged 50 years. Acta Orthop Scand 60:527-531, 1989.

96. O'Neill D, James S: Valgus osteotomy with anterior cruciate ligament laxity. Clin Orthop 278:153-159, 1992.

97. Pagnano MW, Hanssen AD: Periarticular osteotomy of the knee for chondral and osteochondral lesions. Semin Arthroplasty 10:37-47, 1999.

98. Poilvache P: Osteotomy for the arthritic knee: A European perspective. In Insall JN, Scott WN (eds): Surgery of the Knee, vol 2, 3rd ed. Philadelphia, Churchill Livingstone, 2001, pp 1465-1505.

99. Poilvache PL, Insall J, Scuderi GR, et al: Rotational landmarks and sizing of the distal femur in total knee arthroplasty. Clin Orthop 331:35-46, 1996.

100. Ramadier JO: Etude radiologique des déviations dans la gonarthrose. Rev Chir Orthop 53:139-147, 1967.

101. Ramadier JO, Buard JE, Lortat-Jacob A, et al: Mesure radiologique des déformations frontales du genou: Procédé du profil vrai radiologique. Rev Chir Orthop 68:75-78, 1982.

102. Ritter MA, Fechtman RA: Proximal tibial osteotomy. A survivorship analysis. J Arthroplasty 3:309-311, 1988.

103. Rudan JF, Simurda MA: High tibial osteotomy: A prospective clinical and roentgenographic review. Clin Orthop 255:251-256, 1990.

104. Segal P, Burdin PH, Cartier PH, et al: Les échecs des ostéotomies tibiales de valgisation pour gonarthrose et leurs reprises: Symposium. Rev Chir Orthop 78(Suppl):85, 1992.

105. Shoji H, Insall J: High tibial osteotomy for osteoarthritis of the knee with valgus deformity. J Bone Joint Surg Am 55:963-973, 1973.

106. Silverton CD, Kentsch ARW, Muller W: Osteotomies about the knee. In Callaghan JJ, Rosenberg AG, Rubash HE, et al (eds): The Adult Knee, vol 1. Philadelphia, Lippincott Williams & Wilkins, 2003, pp 991-1015.

107. Slawski DP: High tibial osteotomy in the treatment of adult osteo-chondritis dissecans. Clin Orthop 341:155-161, 1997.
108. Squire MW, Callaghan JJ, Goetz DD, et al: Unicompartmental knee replacement. A minimum 15 year follow-up study. Clin Orthop 367:61-72, 1999.
109. Stuart MJ, Grace JN, Ilstrup DM, et al: Late recurrence of varus deformity after proximal tibial osteotomy. Clin Orthop 260:61-65, 1990.
110. Stutz G, Boss A, Gachter A: Comparison of augmented and non-augmented anterior cruciate ligament reconstruction combined with high tibial osteotomy. Knee Surg Sports Traumatol Arthrosc 4:143-148, 1996.
111. Thomine JM, Boudjemaa A, Gibon Y, et al: Les écarts varisants dans la gonarthrose: Fondement théorique et essai d'évaluation pratique. Rev Chir Orthop 67:319-327, 1981.
112. Trousdale RT: Osteotomy: Patient selection, preoperative planning, and results. In Callaghan JJ, Rosenberg AG, Rubash HE, et al (eds): The Adult Knee, vol 1. Philadelphia, Lippincott Williams & Wilkins, 2003, pp 985-990.
113. Vainionpaa S, Laide E, Kirbes P, et al: Tibial osteotomy for osteoarthritis of the knee: A five to ten-year follow-up study. J Bone Joint Surg Am 63:938-941, 1981.
114. Van De Berg AJ, Collard PH, Quiriny M: Gonarthrose et déviation angulaire du genou dans le plan frontal. Acta Orthop Belg 48:8, 1982.
115. Veltri DM, Warren RF: Operative treatment of posterolateral instability of the knee. Clin Sports Med 13:615-627, 1994.
116. Wada M, Imura S, Nagatani K, et al: Relationship between gait and clinical results after high tibial osteotomy. Clin Orthop 354:180-188, 1998.
117. William RJ III, Rohrbough JT: Management of the arthritic, anterior cruciate–insufficient knee. In Callaghan JJ, Rosenberg AG, Rubash HE, et al (eds): The Adult Knee, vol 1. Philadelphia, Lippincott Williams & Wilkins, 2003, pp 1033-1046.
118. Windsor RE, Insall JN, Vince KG: Technical considerations of total knee arthroplasty after proximal tibial osteotomy. J Bone Joint Surg Am 70:547-555, 1988.
119. Yasuda K, Majima T, Tsuchida T, et al: A ten to fifteen year follow-up observation of high tibial osteotomy in medial compartment osteoarthritis. Clin Orthop 282:186-195, 1992.
120. Yoshioka Y, Siu D, Cooke TD: The anatomy and functional axes of the femur. J Bone Joint Surg Am 69:873-880, 1987.

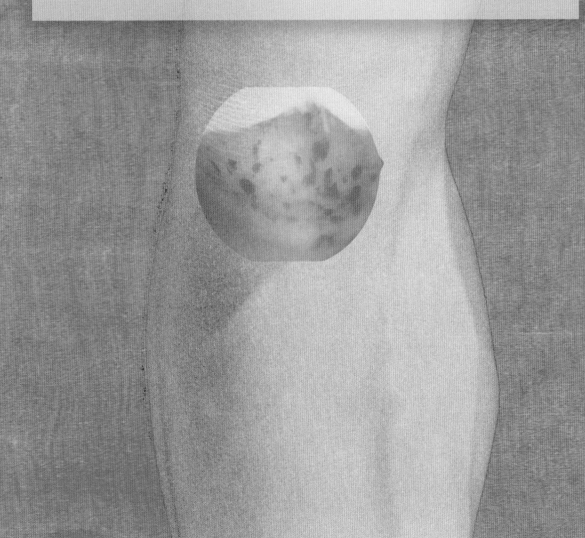

SECTION V

Ligament Injuries

CHAPTER 34

Classification of Knee Ligament Injuries

Craig S. Radnay • Giles R. Scuderi • W. Norman Scott

Given the extensive investigation of ligamentous injuries of the knee, the descriptive terminology has been challenged and modified. However, the specific definitions and classifications have not altered much since the last edition of this textbook was published. The current literature is reviewed and discussed as necessary. Clinical examination findings, operative findings, and anatomic studies have been correlated in an attempt to clarify the classification of these injuries. For accurate assessment and comparison, it is essential that a standardized, valid, reproducible, and universally accepted classification system be adopted. Effective systems of classification necessitate agreement on both the meaning and appropriate use of terms to describe abnormal knee kinematics such that there is no ambiguity. This chapter discusses the relationship of knee anatomy and kinematics, defines terms, and attempts to classify knee ligament injuries in an understandable fashion.

RELATIONSHIP OF CAPSULAR AND LIGAMENTOUS STRUCTURES

Critical to defining stability of the knee is understanding the relationship of the surrounding capsular and ligamentous structures.

Medial Structures

Hughston and colleagues[32] and Warren and Marshall[81] clearly described the supporting structures on the medial side of the knee (Fig. 34–1). The medial collateral ligament (MCL) and the posteromedial capsular ligament, termed the posterior oblique ligament, are augmented by the dynamic stabilizing effect of the capsular arm of the semimembranosus tendon and its aponeurosis, the oblique popliteal ligament. The medial head of the gastrocnemius provides dynamic support to the medial compartment. Brantigan and Voshell[10] described the MCL as having vertical and oblique portions that behave differently as the knee flexes. The parallel anterior fibers of the superficial medial ligament are arranged around the axis of flexion so that tension remains constant throughout the arc of motion. Posteriorly, the oblique fibers of the superficial ligament blend with the deeper layer within the posteromedial corner to form the posterior oblique ligament, which relaxes in flexion (Fig. 34–2).

Hughston and colleagues[31,32,37] believe that the posterior oblique ligament is the primary medial support against valgus stress to the knee. Though somewhat lax as the knee goes into flexion, the posterior oblique ligament is dynamized by the muscular attachment to the semimembranosus tendon, and it has a significant influence on stability throughout the first 60 degrees of flexion (Fig. 34–3). Muller[55] also believes that the posterior oblique ligament is paramount in abolishing any valgus laxity in the extended knee. He claims that even though the posterior oblique ligament and tibial collateral ligament are functionally independent, they are both dynamized, the former by the semimembranosus tendon and the latter by the vastus medialis. Muller also claims that the MCL has some function in preventing external rotation of the tibia on the femur with the knee flexed. However, the main deterrent to external rotation is the posterior oblique ligament.

In contrast to Hughston and Muller, Warren and coworkers[82] believe that most fibers of the MCL are the prime static stabilizers on the medial side of the knee. The anterior 5 mm of the MCL remains tight in flexion and thus resists valgus stress in external rotation in this position (Fig. 34–4). The posterior two-thirds of the superficial MCL is, according to the authors, slightly lax with the knee in flexion and therefore serves as a backup restraint against valgus and external rotatory forces. The oblique or posterior aspect of the superficial MCL was labeled by Hughston as the posterior oblique ligament. This is a thickening of the posteromedial capsule of the knee, and it is firmly attached to and contiguous with the medial meniscus in this location.

Still another viewpoint, presented by Kennedy and Fowler,[43] identifies the deep medial capsular ligament as a primary restraint against external rotatory instability. They concluded that external rotatory instability is caused by a tear in the medial capsular ligament, with or without a partial or a complete tear of the MCL. Grood et al,[29] in a biomechanical study of cadaveric knees, concluded that the long parallel-oriented fibers of the tibial collateral ligament are the prime medial static stabilizers of the knee that resist medial opening to valgus stress. Although this ligament contributes to medial support with the knee close to full extension, as the knee flexes, the importance of this ligament increases from providing 57% of the restraining force to providing 78% of the restraining force. This increase is due to the relaxation or laxity that develops with flexion in the other contributing structures, mainly the posteromedial capsule. The deep medial capsular ligament, though important in that it provides a firm attachment site for the medial meniscus, does not serve as a primary restraint against straight medial opening.[29,38]

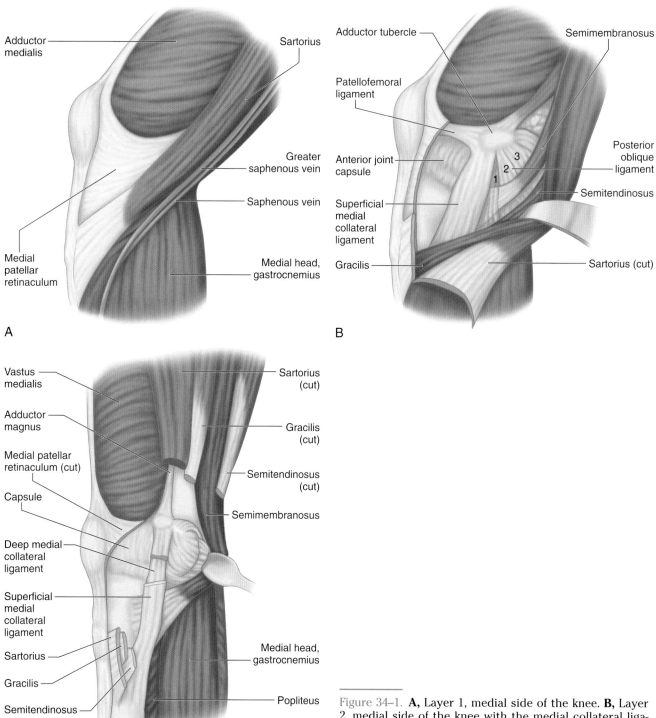

Figure 34–1. **A,** Layer 1, medial side of the knee. **B,** Layer 2, medial side of the knee with the medial collateral ligament and posterior oblique ligament. **C,** Layer 3, medial side of the knee.

Lateral Structures

The lateral supporting structures have been described by Hughston et al[33] and by Seebacher et al[67] (Fig. 34–5). The lateral collateral ligament (LCL) is the major static support to varus stress, whereas the iliotibial tract provides both dynamic and static support. Terry and associates[75] investigated the role of the iliotibial tract, iliopatellar band, and iliotibial band as both dynamic and static stabilizers of the lateral side of the knee. The posterolateral capsule is composed of the LCL, the arcuate ligament, and the aponeurosis of the popliteus muscle. These structures form the arcuate complex, whose function is augmented by the dynamic effects of the biceps femoris, popliteus, and lateral head of the gastrocnemius.[5] Tria and colleagues,[78] however, found that the popliteus tendon has no role in retraction and protection of the lateral meniscus.

Anterior Cruciate Ligament

The anterior cruciate ligament (ACL) (Fig. 34–6) is the primary structure that controls anterior displacement in the unloaded knee. The anatomic and functional aspects of the ACL have undergone extensive investigation.[51-53,74] It has been described as a single ligament with different portions taut throughout the range of motion (ROM).[6] In investigating the functional anatomy of the ACL, Odensten and Gillquist[61] found no anatomic separation of the ligament into different bundles. However, they did find that the ligament is twisted through 90 degrees and that both the length[45,76,79] and the tension[23] of different fibers in the ligament change as knee flexion occurs. Therefore, they believe that there are different functional portions of the ACL.[61,83] Based on this concept of different functional portions of the ACL, Girgis and colleagues[25] divided the ACL into anteromedial and posterolateral bands. Norwood and Cross[56] further divided the ACL into three functional bundles and described their different actions in

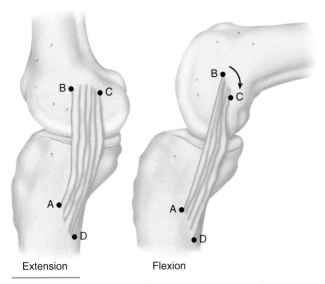

Extension   Flexion

Figure 34–2. Medial collateral ligament in flexion and extension. (From Scott WN [ed]: The Knee. St Louis, CV Mosby, 1994.)

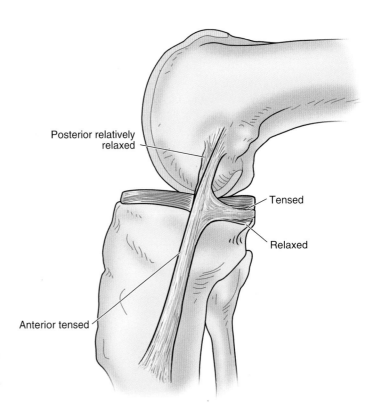

Figure 34–3. The posterior oblique fibers become more tense in flexion. (From Palmer I: On the injuries to ligaments of the knee joint. A clinical study. Acta Chir Scand 81[Suppl 53]:3, 1938.)

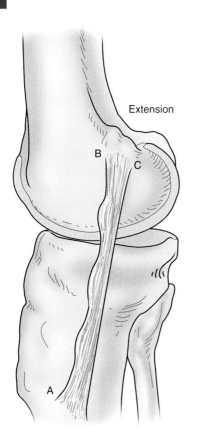
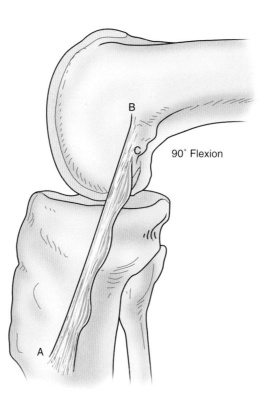

Figure 34–4. Diagram of the superficial medial ligament with flexion and extension of the knee. Because point B moves superiorly, the anterior border is tightened in flexion. Conversely, in extension, point C moves proximally, and the posterior margin of the ligament is tightened. (From Warren RF, Marshall JL, Girgis F: The prime static stabilizer of the medial side of the knee. J Bone Joint Surg Am 56:665, 1974.)

resisting rotatory instability. Amis and Dawkins[3,4] support this multifascicular structure of the ACL: though not necessarily separate entities, the bundles interact as three functional bundles. Amis and Dawkins found that the fiber bundles were not isometric; the anteromedial bundle lengthens, and the posterolateral bundle shortens during flexion (Fig. 34–7). These changes in fiber length correlate with their changing participation in total ACL action as the knee is flexed.

Tibial rotation is better resisted by a combination of capsular structures, collateral ligaments, the joint surface, and meniscal geometry, whereas the cruciates play only a secondary role.[3,4,59] The MCL is anatomically better suited than the ACL and has the mechanical advantage to control torsion or laxity because its attachments are further removed from the axis of tibial rotation.[69] The MCL will provide significant resistance to the anterior drawer test only after the ACL is gone and when both ligaments are lost. In this scenario, the knee will exhibit large tibial excursions and response to anterior force if it is unchecked by muscle action.[69] Injuries to the medial structures further compromise anterior stability when they accompany ACL injuries.[72]

Posterior Cruciate Ligament

The posterior cruciate ligament (PCL) (Fig. 34–8) is believed to be the most important of the knee ligaments because of its cross-sectional area, tensile strength, and location in the central axis of the knee joint.[11,12,14,15,35,36] Its position provides 95% of the total resistance to posterior displacement of the tibia. Both James and colleagues[40] and Kennedy and colleagues[44] have shown that the tensile strength of the PCL is almost twice that of the ACL. Hughston and coworkers[32] describe the PCL as the fundamental stabilizer of the knee because it is located in the center of the knee joint and functions as the axis about which the knee moves in flexion and extension, as well as in rotation.

The PCL prevents posterior translation at all angles of flexion.[11,22,30] Patients who have an isolated injury of the PCL may maintain fairly good function of the knee in positions that are closer to extension. Gollehon et al[26] found that isolated sectioning of the PCL produces increased posterior translation of the tibia at all degrees of flexion of the knee, with the greatest increase occurring from 75 to 90 degrees. Absence of the PCL has no effect on primary varus or external rotation of the tibia as long as the LCL and capsular structures are intact.

Like the ACL, the PCL is a continuum of fascicles with different portions being taut throughout ROM. The anterior portion, which forms the bulk of the ligament, tightens in flexion, whereas the smaller posterior portion tightens in extension (Fig. 34–9).[6] The PCL originates from the posterior part of the lateral aspect of the medial femoral condyle and inserts on the posterior surface of the tibia. The insertion reaches approximately 1 cm below the articular surface in a nonarticular area that Jacobsen[39] termed the "area intercondylaris posterior." Lying anterior to the PCL and connecting the posterior horn of the lateral

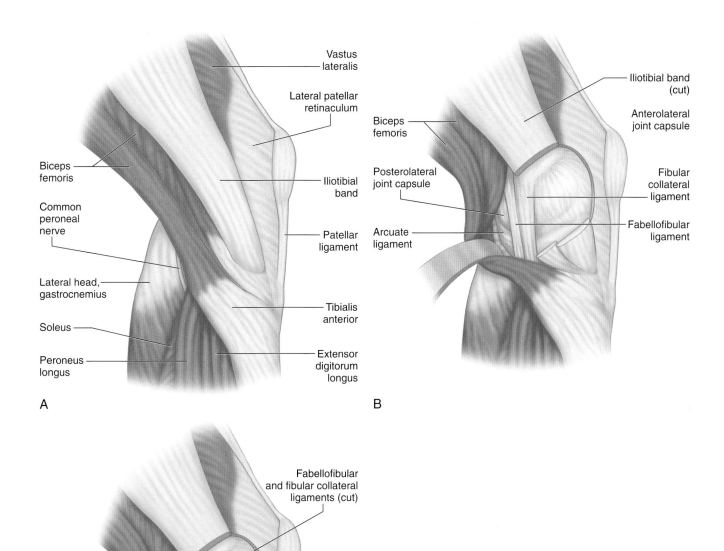

Figure 34–5. **A,** Layer 1, lateral side of the knee. **B,** Layer 2, lateral side of the knee with the lateral collateral ligament. **C,** Layer 3, lateral side of the knee with the arcuate complex. (From Scott WN: Ligament and Extensor Mechanism Injuries of the Knee: Diagnosis and Treatment. St Louis, Mosby–Year Book, 1991.)

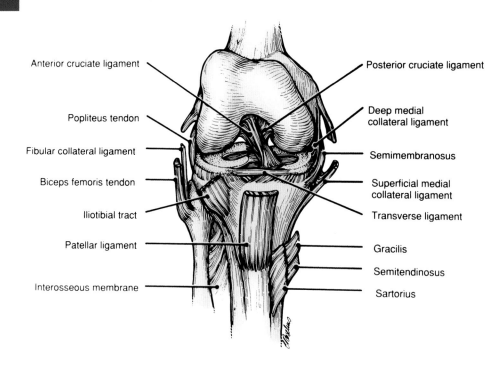

Anterior cruciate ligament

Popliteus tendon

Fibular collateral ligament

Biceps femoris tendon

Iliotibial tract

Patellar ligament

Interosseous membrane

Posterior cruciate ligament

Deep medial collateral ligament

Semimembranosus

Superficial medial collateral ligament

Transverse ligament

Gracilis

Semitendinosus

Sartorius

Figure 34–6. The anterior cruciate ligament has been described as a single ligament with different portions taut throughout the range of motion. (From Scott WN: Ligament and Extensor Mechanism Injuries of the Knee: Diagnosis and Treatment. St Louis, Mosby–Year Book, 1991.)

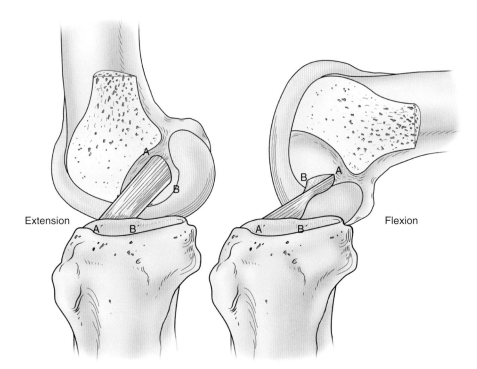

Extension

Flexion

Figure 34–7. Diagram of the anterior cruciate ligament in extension and flexion. Note that in extension the posterolateral bulk is taut, whereas in flexion the anteromedial band is tight and the posterolateral bulk is relatively relaxed. (From Girgis FG, Marshall JL, Al Monajem ARS: The cruciate ligaments of the knee joint: Anatomical, functional and experimental analysis. Clin Orthop 106:216, 1975.)

meniscus to the medial femoral condyle is the ligament of Humphrey (Fig. 34–10). The ligament of Wrisberg passes posterior to the PCL to attach on the PCL. The ligaments of Humphrey and Wrisberg (Fig. 34–11) are so intimately related that early authors described them as separate por- tions of a single ligament.[49] Clancy et al[12] believed that the meniscofemoral ligament may serve as a secondary stabi- lizer in a posterior cruciate–deficient knee. The presence of these structures may account for the absence of poste- rior drawer in isolated PCL tears.

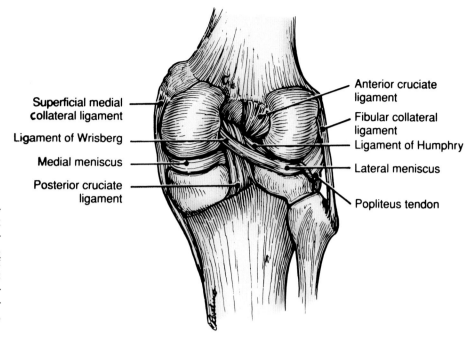

Figure 34–8. The posterior cruciate ligament is an important ligament because of its cross-sectional area, tensile strength, and location in the central axis of the knee joint. (From Scott WN: Ligament and Extensor Mechanism Injuries of the Knee: Diagnosis and Treatment. St Louis, Mosby–Year Book, 1991.)

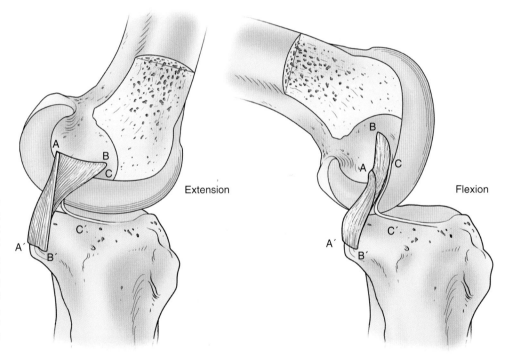

Figure 34–9. Posterior cruciate ligament. In flexion the bulk of the ligament becomes tight, whereas in extension it is relaxed. (From Girgis FG, Marshall JL, Al Monajem ARS: The cruciate ligaments of the knee joint: Anatomical, functional and experimental analysis. Clin Orthop 106:216, 1975.)

KINEMATICS

In classifying knee ligamentous instabilities, it is important that the terms be clearly understood and used in a lucid and universally accepted manner. The terms in the literature should be specific to define positions of the knee, motions of the knee, and ligamentous injury. Noyes and coworkers[60] have taken the time to review the literature and define terms that are in common orthopedic usage.

Position

Position refers to the orientation of the tibia with respect to the femur and determines the tension in each of the ligaments and supporting structures. *Dislocation* is a term indicating a complete noncontact position of both the tibia and the femur or the patellofemoral joint. Dislocations of the knee are classified by the final tibial position—anterior, posterior, medial, lateral, or rotary.[46] *Subluxation* is defined as an incomplete partial dislocation and does not have limits. It can be described in an anteroposterior, medial lateral, or rotary position.

Motion

Motion is the process of changing position and describes the displacement between the starting and ending points. *Displacement* is the change in position and is described according to 6 degrees of freedom, a combination of three translations, and three rotations. *Translation* is the parallel displacement of a rigid body or, in the case of the knee joint, the tibia with respect to the femur. Translation of the tibia is composed of three independent components or translational degrees of freedom: medial lateral translation, anteroposterior translation, and proximal distal

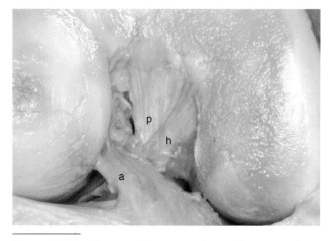

Figure 34–10. Close-up of an anatomic specimen seen from the anterior aspect demonstrating the relationship of the ACL (a), ligament of Humphry (h), and PCL (p) from anterior to posterior in the intercondylar notch.

translation. *Rotation* describes motion or displacement about an axis and in the knee has 3 degrees of freedom: flexion-extension, internal-external rotation, and abduction-adduction. *Range of motion* is defined as the displacement that occurs between the two limits of movement for each degree of freedom. There is a ROM for each of the translational and rotational degrees of freedom. For motions other than flexion-extension, ROM generally depends on the angle of knee flexion. The limits of motion are defined as the extreme positions of movement that are possible in each of the 6 degrees of freedom. Injury to the ligamentous and osseous structures about the knee alters the limits of motion. By convention, the limits of flexion and extension are termed relative to the neutral position or extension of 0 degrees, with flexion described in positive terms and hyperextension in negative terms. *Coupled displacement* concerns motion in 1 or more degrees of freedom that is caused by a load applied in another degree of freedom. The amount of coupled rotation depends on where the force is applied to the tibia or on whether the center of rotation is constrained or allowed to move freely. An example is the internal rotation that results when an anterior load is applied to the tibia.[22] When assessing ligamentous stability, motion of the knee joint may occur freely or be constrained, based on the integrity of the ligamentous structures. The ligaments determine the constraint of the knee joint. Elongation or stretching of the ligament limits joint motion and is also supported by compressive joint contact forces that act in an opposite direction. Two ligaments are required to limit translation and rotation, one for each direction. A single ligament alone is unable to resist rotation. If the motion is unconstrained, the tibia displaces into its maximum position. Most clinical tests performed on the knee, however, are constrained.

The force that displaces the knee has three properties: an orientation or line of action, a sense (forward or backward) along its line of action, and a magnitude. The effect

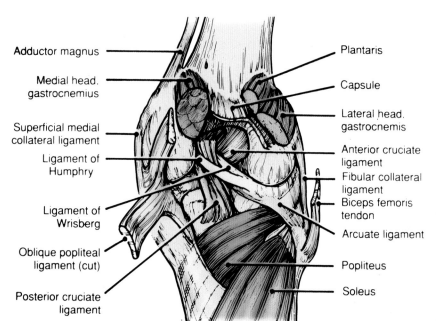

Figure 34–11. The ligaments of Humphry and Wrisberg are so intimately related that early authors described them as separate portions of a single ligament. (From Scott WN: Ligament and Extensor Mechanism Injuries of the Knee: Diagnosis and Treatment. St Louis, Mosby–Year Book, 1991.)

of a force depends on all three of its properties and its point of application. The moment causes an angular or rotational acceleration and has three properties: an orientation or line of action, a sense (clockwise or counterclockwise) about its line of action, and a magnitude. When indicating the moment of the knee joint, it is essential that the axis of rotation be defined.

Laxity

Laxity is a term used to describe the looseness of the joint, which can be normal or abnormal. To avoid confusion, it is better to measure the amount of displacement in millimeters of translation and rotation. The differences between the involved and uninvolved knee should also be reported clearly. Instability is characterized by increased or excessive displacement of the tibia caused by a traumatic injury.

LIGAMENT INJURY TESTS

The joint motion assessed on clinical examination determines the classification of knee ligament instability. It is important that the objective findings on the clinical examination correlate with the pathological knee motion and allow standardized classification of knee ligament instability. Clinical findings have been substantiated by biomechanical studies.

Valgus Stress Test

This test should be performed first on the normal extremity for later comparison. The involved knee is flexed to 30 degrees, and a gentle valgus stress is applied to the knee,

with one hand placed on the lateral aspect of the thigh and the other hand grasping the foot and ankle (Fig. 34–12). Placing the hip in relative extension helps relax the hamstring musculature. The valgus stress test must also be performed with the knee in full extension or in the amount of recurvatum present in the opposite uninvolved limb. The degree of opening of the medial side of the knee should be quantified, graded, and recorded.

Varus Stress Test

This test is similar to the valgus stress test. The varus stress test is carried out with the knee in full extension and in 30 degrees of flexion. The degree of lateral opening should be quantified, graded, and recorded (Fig. 34–13).

Anterior Drawer Test

This test has been the standard examination for evaluating the integrity of the ACL. The hip is flexed to 45 degrees with the knee flexed to 80 to 90 degrees (Fig. 34–14). The examiner sits on the table and, using the buttocks, stabilizes the foot. The examiner places hands about the upper part of the tibia and palpates the hamstrings to make sure that they are relaxed. Then the examiner gently pulls and pushes the proximal portion of the tibia in a to-and-fro manner. The test is performed in a neutral, internal, and external rotated posture of the foot. The degree and type of anterior drawer should be reported.

Lachman Test

This clinical test is used to assess anterior knee laxity and stiffness with the knee in about 20 degrees of flexion

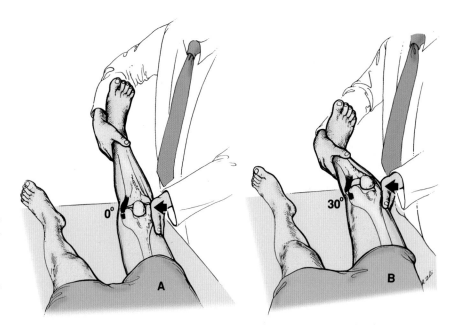

Figure 34–12. Valgus stress in extension tests the medial collateral ligament and the posteromedial capsule. Stress in 30 degrees of flexion tests only the medial collateral ligament. (From Tria AJ Jr, Klein KS: An Illustrated Guide to the Knee. New York, Churchill Livingstone, 1992.)

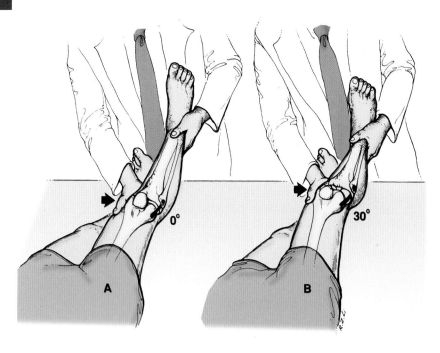

Figure 34–13. Varus stress in extension tests the lateral collateral ligament and the posterolateral capsule. Stress in 30 degrees of flexion tests only the lateral collateral ligament. (From Tria AJ Jr, Klein KS: An Illustrated Guide to the Knee. New York, Churchill Livingstone, 1992.)

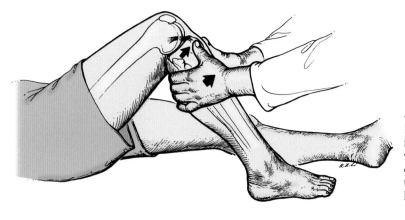

Figure 34–14. The anterior drawer test is performed with the knee flexed to 90 degrees and with anterior force applied to the proximal end of the tibia. (From Tria AJ Jr, Klein KS: An Illustrated Guide to the Knee. New York, Churchill Livingstone, 1992.)

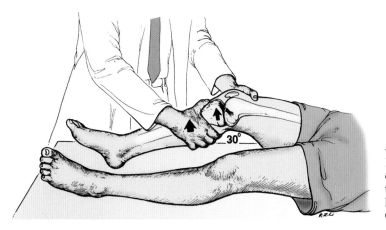

Figure 34–15. The Lachman test is performed in 30 degrees of flexion with anterior force exerted on the proximal end of the tibia. (From Tria AJ Jr, Klein KS: An Illustrated Guide to the Knee. New York, Churchill Livingstone, 1992.)

(Fig. 34–15). In this position, an anterior drawer is applied to the proximal part of the calf, at which time the examiner perceives displacement of the tibia and assesses the endpoint stiffness.[41] The slightest increase in anterior displacement of the tibia would be considered a positive test when compared with the contralateral knee. Endpoint stiffness should be clearly documented.

Pivot-Shift Test

The pivot-shift test[24] (Fig. 34–16) and the Losee test[47] (Fig. 34–17) demonstrate anterior subluxation and reduction of the tibia with knee in flexion-extension from 10 to 40 degrees as a result of ACL disruption. Patients with an

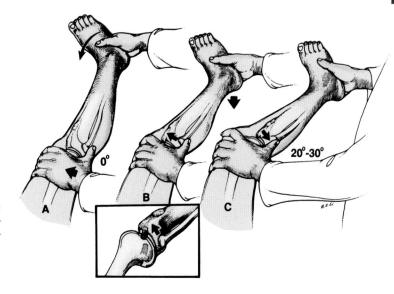

Figure 34–16. The pivot-shift test begins with the knee in full extension and applies internal rotation and valgus stress to demonstrate anterolateral subluxation. (From Tria AJ Jr, Klein KS: An Illustrated Guide to the Knee. New York, Churchill Livingstone, 1992.)

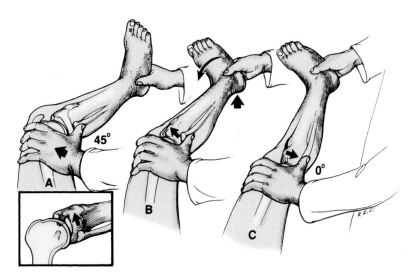

Figure 34–17. The Losee test begins with the knee in flexion but externally rotates the foot. Valgus stress is applied, and the tibia is internally rotated as the knee is extended. (From Tria AJ Jr, Klein KS: An Illustrated Guide to the Knee. New York, Churchill Livingstone, 1992.)

MCL disruption or previous iliotibial tract surgery may have less dramatic findings on physical examination.[17]

Posterior Drawer Test

The standard test to assess the PCL has been the posterior drawer test. The knee is flexed to 90 degrees, and posterior force is exerted on the tibia in an attempt to sublux it posteriorly in relation to the femur (Fig. 34–18). A posterior Lachman test has been described for acute PCL injuries (Fig. 34–19). The knee is held in 30 degrees of flexion, and the tibia is forced posteriorly. Any motion in this direction correlates with a tear of the PCL.[77] A knee with chronic PCL deficiency may demonstrate posterior sag when the knee and hip are flexed to 90 degrees. To perform the 90-degree quadriceps active test, the clinician sits beside the examining table with the patient's knee flexed to 90 degrees at eye level (Fig. 34–20). The foot is stabilized by the clinician, and the patient is asked to slide the foot gently down the table. The clinician's hand pre-

vents the foot from moving forward, thereby allowing anterior translation of the tibia, which occurs when the tibia is posteriorly subluxated secondary to PCL disruption.

Reverse Pivot-Shift Test

This test is used to diagnose injuries to the posterolateral ligament complex. The clinician supports the limb with a hand under the heel with the knee in full extension and neutral rotation (Fig. 34–21). A valgus stress is applied, and the knee is flexed. In a positive test, at about 20 to 30 degrees of flexion the tibia will rotate externally, and the lateral tibial plateau will subluxate posteriorly and remain in this position during further flexion. When the knee is then extended, the tibia reduces. In the standard pivot-shift test, the tibia is subluxated anteriorly in early flexion and reduces between 20 and 40 degrees of flexion. In the reverse pivot-shift test, the tibia is initially reduced, and then the lateral tibial plateau posteriorly subluxates at 20

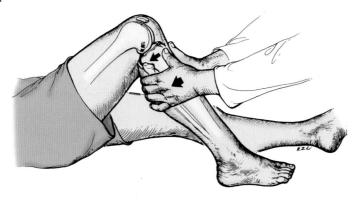

Figure 34–18. The posterior drawer test is performed in 90 degrees of flexion with posterior force applied to the proximal end of the tibia. (From Tria AJ Jr, Klein KS: An Illustrated Guide to the Knee. New York, Churchill Livingstone, 1992.)

Figure 34–19. The "posterior" Lachman test applies posterior force to the proximal end of the tibia with the knee flexed 30 degrees. (From Tria AJ Jr, Klein KS: An Illustrated Guide to the Knee. New York, Churchill Livingstone, 1992.)

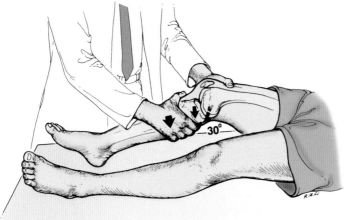

A

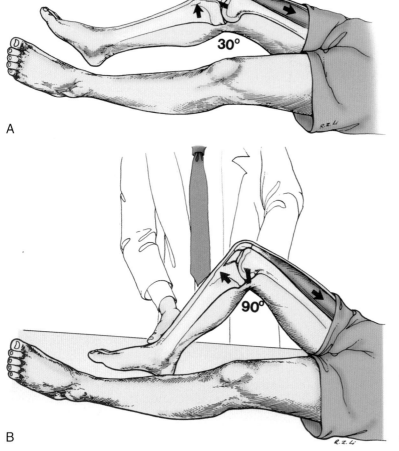

B

Figure 34–20. Quadriceps active test for the anterior cruciate ligament in 30 degrees of flexion (**A**) and for the posterior cruciate ligament in 90 degrees of flexion (**B**). (From Scott WN [ed]: The Knee, St Louis, CV Mosby, 1994.)

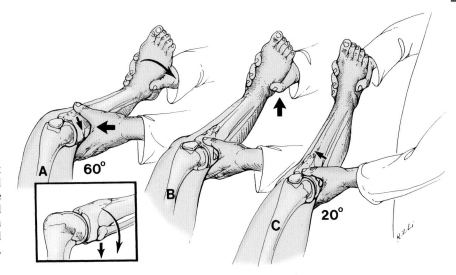

Figure 34–21. The reverse pivot-shift test begins with the knee flexed and the tibia externally rotated. The knee is then extended and posterolateral capsular laxity demonstrated. (From Tria AJ Jr, Klein KS: An Illustrated Guide to the Knee. New York, Churchill Livingstone, 1992.)

to 30 degrees of flexion. In a patient with a combined ACL and posterolateral ligament complex injury, one may observe the tibia go from anterior subluxation to a reduced position and then to a posterior subluxated position.[17] A knee with a posterolateral injury should be tested at 0 to 30 degrees of flexion for maximum primary posterior translation and at 75 to 90 degrees of external rotation for minimum translation. A knee in which an isolated PCL injury is suspected should be tested at 75 to 90 degrees of flexion for maximum primary posterior translation and at 0 to 30 degrees for minimum translation. In an isolated PCL injury, no change should be expected in primary external rotation. If both the posterolateral structures and the PCL are ruptured, there will be a substantial increase in primary posterior translation, external rotation, and varus rotation at all angles of flexion of the knee as compared with an intact knee or one in which either structure has been injured in isolation.[26]

CLASSIFICATION OF LIGAMENT INJURIES

Several terms have been used to describe an injury to a ligament.

Sprain

A sprain is an injury to a joint ligament that stretches or tears ligamentous fibers but does not completely disrupt the ligament. In the handbook *Standard Nomenclature of Athletic Injuries*,[1] the Committee on Medical Aspects of Sports of the American Medical Association characterized sprains on the basis of indirect evidence of ligament injury, including the history, symptoms, and physical examination (Fig. 34–22). A first-degree sprain is a tear involving a minimal number of fibers of a ligament, with localized tenderness and no instability. A second-degree sprain tears more ligamentous fibers, with slight to moderate abnormal motion. In a third-degree sprain, there is

a complete tear of the ligament, with disruption of fibers and demonstrable instability. Third-degree sprains are further subdivided as follows: grade I, less than a 0.5-cm opening of the joint surfaces; grade II, 0.5- to 1-cm opening of the joint surfaces; and grade III, rupture greater than a 1-cm opening. Rupture of a ligament implies complete tearing of the ligament with concomitant loss of function. Because a ligament may undergo a complete tear but still retain continuity between displaced fibers, it is the loss of function (resistance to displacement) that defines a tear, not the property of continuity.[60] Deficiency of a ligament implies that the ligament is absent or that there is loss of function, such as when the ligament still exists but is stretched and nonfunctional.[54]

Instability

The most elaborate classification system of knee ligament instability was developed by Hughston and colleagues[32,33] and the American Orthopaedic Society of Sports Medicine Research and Education Committee in 1976.[2] This classification system attempts to describe the instability by the direction of tibial displacement and, when possible, by structural deficits. The classification of knee ligament instability is based on rotation of the knee about the central axis of the PCL. All rotatory instabilities indicate subluxation about the intact PCL. Once the PCL is damaged, the instability is designated as straight instability, which indicates subluxation or translation without rotation around a central axis. The subluxation hinges on the intact MCL or LCL.

ROTATORY INSTABILITY

Rotatory instability includes anteromedial, anterolateral, posterolateral, posteromedial, and combined (Fig. 34–23).[65] Combined instability is not as clearly defined as rotatory or straight instability.

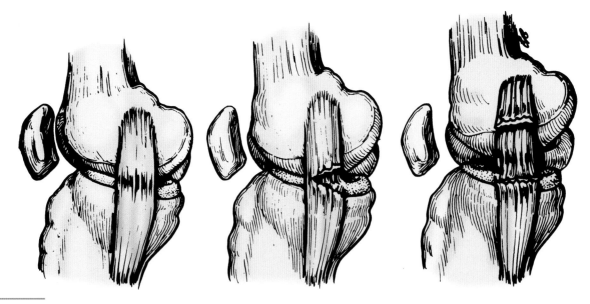

Figure 34–22. Sprains have been characterized on the basis of ligament injury: first degree (**A**), second degree (**B**), and third degree (**C**). (From Scott WN: Ligament and Extensor Mechanism Injuries of the Knee: Diagnosis and Treatment. St Louis, Mosby–Year Book, 1991.)

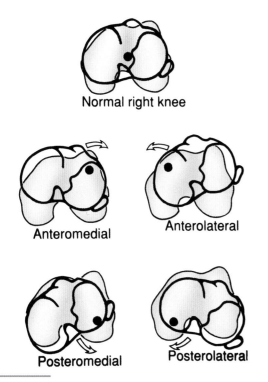

Figure 34–23. Rotatory instability includes anteromedial, anterolateral, posteromedial, and posterolateral instability, which are described in terms of abnormal tibial rotation. (From Scott WN: Ligament and Extensor Mechanism Injuries of the Knee: Diagnosis and Treatment. St Louis, Mosby–Year Book, 1991.)

Anteromedial Rotatory Instability

External tibial rotation plus anterior translation is manifested as anteromedial rotatory instability, which causes the medial tibial plateau to sublux anteromedially on the medial femoral condyle.[34] This motion implies disruption of the medial capsular ligament, MCL, posterior oblique ligament, and ACL.[37,42,43,71] The medial meniscus is considered an important stabilizing structure and may also be injured.[34,64] On clinical examination, the abduction stress test result is positive, with abnormal excess opening of the medial joint space 30 degrees, along with positive anterior drawer and Lachman test results.

Anterolateral Rotatory Instability

This instability results in excessive internal tibial rotation and anterior subluxation, which implies disruption of the lateral capsular ligament, the arcuate complex, and the ACL. The iliotibial band may be damaged to a varying degree, with most of the injury occurring to the deep fibers, which are attached to the posterior cortex of the lateral femoral condyle. Clinical examination reveals positive results for an adduction test at 30 degrees of flexion and for the anterior drawer, Lachman, and pivot-shift tests. The anterior drawer result with the tibia rotated externally will be negative because the tibia will not be able to rotate internally. The radiographic presence of a Segond fracture implies an avulsion fracture of the attachment of the anterior oblique band of the lateral capsule from the tibia. This finding, associated with a tear of the ACL, is pathognomonic for anterolateral rotatory instability.[66]

Posterolateral Rotatory Instability

This instability is apparent when the lateral tibial plateau rotates posterior to the lateral femoral condyle.[9,13,33] The pathological condition involves tears of the arcuate ligament, popliteus tendon, and LCL, with possible injury to the biceps tendon.[9] The PCL is not torn and is the axis on which the knee rotates. The anterior drawer, Lachman, and pivot-shift results will be negative. The patient may be observed walking with a lateral thrust.

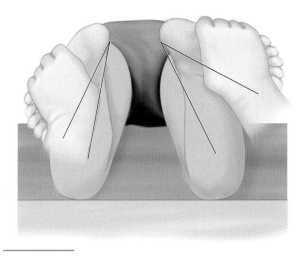

Figure 34–24. The prone external rotation test, which is performed at both 30 and 90 degrees of knee flexion. Forceful external rotation is exerted by the examiner, and the amount of external rotation is measured by comparison of the axis of the medial border of the foot with the femur. (From Veltri DM, Warren RF: Isolated and combined posterior cruciate ligament injuries. J Am Acad Orthop Surg 1:70, 1993.)

On examination, numerous specific tests to help diagnose injuries of the posterolateral corner of the knee have been described; most should be performed without any posterior subluxation of the knee reduced.[14] The posterior drawer test should be performed at 30 and 90 degrees of flexion. If posterior translation, varus rotation, and external rotation are increased at 90 degrees but are normal at 30 degrees, a tear of the PCL should be suspected. With posterior translation increased at 30 degrees but normal at 90 degrees, posterolateral injury should be assumed. Combined injury should be suspected if posterior translation, varus rotation, and external rotation are increased at all degrees of flexion. The Dial test (tibial external rotation test) is best done with the patient prone at both 30 and 90 degrees of flexion (Fig. 34–24).[79] Increased external rotation at 30 but not 90 degrees is characteristic of injury to the posterolateral corner; increased external rotation at both angles suggests injury to both the PCL and the posterolateral corner. The posterolateral external rotation test is performed with the knee flexed 30 and 90 degrees, with components of posterior and external force applied to the proximal end of the tibia while palpating for posterolateral tibial subluxation. Again, subluxation at 90 degrees implies injury only to the PCL; subluxation at both 30 and 90 degrees suggests injury to both the PCL and posterolateral corner. Veltri and Warren have reported that the most useful tests for the diagnosis of posterolateral knee injury are the Dial test at 30 and 90 degrees of flexion and the varus stress test at 0 and 30 degrees of flexion.[14,79]

Posteromedial Rotatory Instability

This instability is manifested by posterior rotation of the medial tibial plateau on the medial femoral condyle. It implies disruption of the MCL, the medial capsular ligament, the posterior oblique ligament, the ACL, and the posteromedial capsule. There may be stretching or major injury to the semimembranosus tendon. The PCL is intact. Hughston et al do not believe that posteromedial rotatory instability occurs if the PCL is intact because the tightening of the PCL that accompanies internal rotation would prevent this type of instability.[32] If the PCL is disrupted, there would be no fixed axis of rotation, and the instability would be straight posterior.

Combined Anteromedial and Anterolateral Rotatory Instability

This instability results in simultaneous anterior subluxation of both the medial and lateral tibial plateaus. It implies injury to the medial and lateral supporting structures, along with a tear of the ACL. Medially, the injury involves the middle third of the medial capsular ligament, the posterior oblique ligament, and the MCL. Laterally, there is a tear of the middle third of the lateral capsular ligament, the iliotibial band, and the short head of the biceps. Clinically, the knee demonstrates positive results for the anterior drawer, Lachman, pivot-shift, and abduction stress tests at 30 degrees of flexion; the adduction stress test at 30 degrees is equivocal.

Combined Anterolateral and Posterolateral Rotatory Instability

This instability is the result of disruption of all of the lateral capsular ligaments, with or without a tear of the iliotibial band. Although the ACL is torn, the PCL remains intact. There is a high incidence of lateral meniscal tears. On clinical examination, results of the adduction stress test are markedly positive, along with positive results for the Lachman and the anterior drawer tests.

Combined Anteromedial and Posteromedial Rotatory Instability

This instability occurs when all the medial and posteromedial structures, including the semimembranosus complex, are torn along with an injury to the ACL. The PCL is intact.

STRAIGHT INSTABILITY

The four types of straight instability are medial, lateral, posterior, and anterior.

Straight Medial Instability

This instability is caused by disruption of the medial supporting structures, including the MCL, middle third of the medial capsular ligament, and the posterior oblique ligament. Although the ACL is usually torn, Hughston believes that the PCL must be torn for straight medial instability to exist. This opinion is not held by all clinicians; some investigators believe that the PCL may not be disrupted.[70] Because the axis of rotation is the LCL, the clinical examination will demonstrate medial joint space opening with an abduction stress test at both 30 and 0 degrees. If the ACL is torn, the anterior drawer result will be positive in all three rotational positions. With a torn PCL, the posterior drawer result is positive.

Straight Lateral Instability

This instability is the result of a tear of the lateral supporting structures and the PCL with an axis hinging on the MCL. It is manifested by lateral opening with an adduction stress test in the fully extended position. The injury involves disruption of the lateral capsular ligament, the LCL, the arcuate complex, and the PCL. Clinically, the adduction stress test result is positive at 30 and at 0 degrees, but the degree of opening depends on the level of injury to the iliotibial band. The posterior drawer result is positive in the neutral position and will show increased translation with the knee rotated externally. If there is an ACL tear, the anterior drawer and the Lachman test results will be positive. The pivot-shift result may not be positive if there is an injury to the iliotibial band.

Straight Posterior Instability

This instability occurs in patients with isolated injury to the PCL. Although there might be injury to the arcuate ligament and the posterior oblique ligament, the MCL, LCL, and ACL are intact. On examination, the knee demonstrates a posterior drop-back of the tibia without evidence of rotation. Whereas the posterior drawer test result is markedly positive, medial, lateral, and anterior test results are negative.

Straight Anterior Instability

This instability is the result of disruption of the ACL and is demonstrated by a positive result of the anterior drawer test in neutral rotation with an equal amount of medial and lateral subluxation. There is no evidence of rotational displacement. In contrast, Hughston and colleagues defined straight instability as an injury to the PCL and related supporting structures, with loss of the central axis of rotation. Therefore, they did not regard straight anterior instability as an injury to the ACL, but rather as an injury to the PCL. With this in mind, Hughston et al claimed not to have encountered any anterior displacement great enough to rupture the PCL without also rupturing the MCL and LCL.[32,33]

NOYES AND GROOD ROTATORY INSTABILITY MODEL

Noyes and Grood[28,58,59] maintain that the terms for rotatory instability as discussed earlier are imprecise and do not represent a specific definable motion or set of motions. An almost infinite number of combinations of joint motion actually exist and can occur, depending on the abnormalities in any of 1, 2, or 3 of the degrees of freedom. Accurate diagnosis requires knowledge of the precise abnormalities and biomechanical data as to which ligaments limit the use of motion. As a result of such information, Noyes and Grood developed the "bumper model" of the knee. They found this model to be useful in understanding how the ligaments and capsular structures limit anterior and posterior translation and internal and external rotation.

They developed a knee ligament evaluation form (Fig. 34–25). The clinician examines and tests the knee for integrity of the primary and secondary ligament restraints. It is important to select a laxity test to diagnose a specific ligament injury. The extent of damage to each structure is reported: I, partial damage, still functional; II, partial damage, compromised function; and X, complete damage, nonfunctional. The assessment of functional capacity of the injured ligaments and capsule is only an approximation. Ultimately, it is necessary to quantitate the damaged structures. In the bumper model, the bumpers do not represent exact ligament structures; instead, they represent the final restraints to tibial motion, with summation of the effect of the ligament, menisci, and capsular structures.

Type I motion is described as normal, and there are three clinically identifiable types of anterior knee subluxation that can occur after a rupture of the ACL. Noyes and Grood recommend performing the anterior drawer and Lachman tests in a neutral position without rotation to initially evaluate the ACL. The anterior drawer test is then repeated with internal and external rotation to determine the maximum excursion of the lateral and medial tibiofemoral compartments in order to provide information on the laxity of the extra-articular ligamentous restraints.[58] The results of the laxity tests are indicated on the evaluation form by recording, first, the amount of central subluxation and, second, the amount of translation of the medial and lateral compartments when tibial rotation is added. The clinical significance of identifying these three types of anterior subluxation rests in their different natural histories and treatment programs. Type II subluxation is characterized by tight extra-articular structures; the amount of anterior and lateral tibial translation is only slightly increased. Type III subluxation consists of anterior subluxation with increased translation of the medial and lateral tibial compartments. The translation of the lateral tibial compartment will be greater because of associated increases in the internal rotation units. Type IV anterior subluxation indicates gross subluxation with increased translation of the medial and lateral compartments. As the degree of subluxation increases, the axis of rotation is shifted medially outside the joint.

The final diagnosis of a ligament defect must be made in precise anatomic terms; in cases of partial disruption or after healing occurs, the clinician must analyze the remaining functional capacity of the ligaments. It has been suggested that identifying these types of anterior subluxation has clinical significance because each carries a different prognosis. Type II subluxation, characterized by tight extra-articular structures, has a better prognosis than that of types III and IV subluxation; ACL reconstruction is recommended.[58] With type IV subluxation, it is impor-

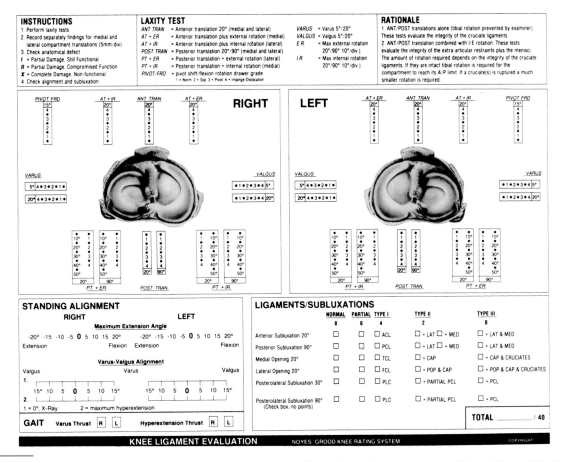

Figure 34–25. The knee ligament evaluation form used in the Noyes-Grood rating system. (From Noyes FR, Grood ES: Classification of ligament injuries: Why an anterolateral laxity or anteromedial laxity is not a diagnostic entity. Instr Course Lect 36:185, 1987.)

tant to restore the associated damaged ligamentous structures, especially the lateral extra-articular structures.

Recent Ligament Testing Devices Used in Classification

It is important that the classification of ligament injuries be precise and that the clinician understand the remaining functional capacity of the ligaments. Difficulties still remain in the evaluation of these injuries, and it is anticipated that newer diagnostic devices will provide detailed information to enable the clinician to determine the different types of instability under defined loading conditions.

In the 1980s, several ligament testing devices were developed in an attempt to objectively quantitate anteroposterior displacement of the knee joint.[16,20,21,50,62,63,68] The variability in subjective clinical grades given to many testing maneuvers makes it difficult to compare injuries and clinical results. Objective quantitative ligament testing devices provide the opportunity to more accurately compare populations of patients. The pathological anteroposterior motion of cruciate ligament injuries can be diagnosed with the KT-1000 arthrometer (MEDmetric Corporation, San Diego, CA). Daniel and coworkers[20] reported that 97% of 120 normal subjects tested with the

KT-1000 arthrometer demonstrated less than 3-mm right-left difference whereas the right-left difference in 33 patients with an acute ACL injury was 3 mm or greater in 90% with the manual maximum test. Miyasaka et al[53] found that use of the KT-1000 arthrometer and quadriceps active tests helped them diagnose a PCL injury with high accuracy. In another study, 40 of 41 patients with documented PCL rupture were found to have pathological laxity by this method.[18] Objective quantification of knee laxity in ACL and PCL injury with instrumented testing is useful. Daniel and coworkers showed that 96% of patients with an arthroscopically confirmed tear of the ACL had a maximum manual KT-1000 test with a greater than 3-mm side-to-side difference.[19] It has been suggested that further quantitative reporting should include 89 N, maximum manual, compliance index, and side-to-side difference because variation in testing parameters has been noted.[7] There are pitfalls and limitations with the use of current instrumented testing devices. Bach and colleagues[8] found that the KT-1000 is useful only for anteroposterior translation because it does not allow assessment of rotational or varus-valgus instability. The clinical applicability of the Genucom system appears to be limited by variability in measurements of knee laxity.[27] The problem is that this device assumes that the change in stiffness of the soft tissues can be accurately predicted from one angle of flexion of the knee to another. However, major variations in the effect of the position of the knee are expected between subjects and even between repeated examinations of the same individual.

Objective quantitation of knee laxity in ligamentous injuries is an important diagnostic adjunct. Testing devices that objectively measure laxity permit the clinician to evaluate the injured or postsurgical knee and predict the functional outcome. In a prospective study, Daniel et al showed that the early KT grade was a predictor of the late KT grade.[19]

KNEE LIGAMENT RATING SYSTEMS

In the course of developing knee ligament rating systems, investigators have attempted to correlate function and clinical findings. Although universal acceptance has not been achieved, several rating systems have been popularized. The Lysholm scale[48] (Table 34–1) is based solely on the patient's subjective evaluation of function, with no weight given to objective findings. In an effort to rate a patient's level of function, Tegner and Lysholm[73] developed a knee activity assessment that questions patients about their participation in sports and work (Table 34–2).

Table 34–1. Lysholm Scale

Limp		
	None	5
	Slight or periodic	3
	Severe and constant	0
Support		
	None	5
	Stick or crutch needed	2
	Weightbearing impossible	0
Locking		
	None	15
	None, but catching sensation present	10
	Occasional	6
	Frequent	2
	At examination	0
Stairs		
	No problem	10
	Sight problem	6
	One step at a time	3
	Impossible	0
Instability		
	Never	25
	Rarely during athletic activities	20
	Frequently during athletic activities	15
	Occasionally during daily activities	10
	Often during daily activities	5
	Every step	0
Pain		
	None	25
	Inconstant and slight during strenuous activities	20
	Marked during or after walking more than 2 km	10
	Marked during or after walking less than 2 km	5
	Constant	0
Swelling		
	None	10
	After strenuous activities	6
	After ordinary activities	3
	Constant	0
Squatting		
	No problem	5
	Slight problem	4
	Not beyond 90 degrees of knee flexion	2
	Impossible	0

From Lyholm J, Gillquist J: Evaluation of knee ligament surgery results with special emphasis on using a scoring scale. J Sports Med 10:150, 1982.

Table 34–2. The Tegner and Lysholm Activity Scale

10 Competitive sports
    Soccer—national or international level

9 Competitive sports
    Soccer—lower divisions
    Ice hockey
    Wrestling
    Gymnastics

8 Competitive sports
    Bandy
    Squash or badminton
    Athletics (e.g., jumping)
    Downhill skiing

7 Competitive sports
    Tennis
    Athletics (e.g., running)
    Motocross or speedway
    Handball or basketball
  Recreational sports
    Soccer
    Bandy or ice hockey
    Squash
    Athletics (e.g., jumping)
    Cross-country track finding (orienteering), both
      recreational and competitive

6 Recreational sports
    Tennis or badminton
    Handball or basketball
    Downhill skiing
    Jogging at least five times weekly

5 Work
    Heavy labor (e.g. construction, forestry)
  Competitive sports
    Cycling
    Cross-country skiing
  Recreational sports
    Jogging on uneven ground at least twice weekly

4 Work
    Moderately heavy work (e.g., truck driving, scrubbing
      floors)
  Recreational sports
    Cycling
    Cross-country skiing
    Jogging on uneven ground at least weekly

3 Work
    Light work (e.g., nursing)
  Competitive and recreational sports
    Walking on rough forest terrain

2 Work
    Light work
    Walking on uneven ground

1 Work
    Sedentary work
    Walking on uneven ground

0 Sick leave or disability pension because of knee problems

From Tegner Y, Lysholm J: Rating systems in evaluation of knee ligament injuries. Clin Orthop 198:43, 1985.

Because it is important to include objective clinical findings with the level of activity, Noyes designed a knee rating system that uses both subjective and objective criteria (Table 34–3).[57] The subjective criteria include a system rating scale, assessment of function, and sports rating scale. Objective testing includes ROM, the presence of crepitus, KT-1000 testing, and a radiographic review. The scale includes a scheme for a final rating of excellent, good, fair, or poor. Although these rating systems have gained regional or institutional acceptance, the American Orthopaedic Society of Sports Medicine and its European equivalent, under the auspices of the International Knee Documentation Committee, have published a knee ligament injury evaluation form (Fig. 34–26).

Table 34–3. Cincinnati Knee Rating System

A. Assessment of Function

ACTIVITIES OF DAILY LIVING

Activity	Function	Points
Walking		
	Normal, unlimited	40
	Some limitations	30
	No more than 3–4 blocks possible	20
	Less than 1 block with cane or crutch	0
Stair Climbing		
	Normal, unlimited	40
	Some limitations	30
	No more than 11–30 steps possible	20
	No more than 1–10 steps possible	0
Squatting/Kneeling		
	Normal, unlimited	40
	Some limitations	30
	No more than 6–10 possible	20
	No more than 0–5 possible	0

SPORTS ACTIVITIES

Activity	Function	Points
Straight Running		
	Fully competitive	100
	Some limitations, guarding	80
	Run half-speed, definite limitations	60
	Not able to do so	40
Jumping/Landing on Affected Leg		
	Fully competitive	100
	Some limitations, guarding	80
	Definite limitations, half-speed	60
	Not able to do so	40
Hard Twisting/ Cutting/Pivoting		
	Fully competitive	100
	Some limitations, guarding	80
	Definite limitations, half-speed	60
	Not able to do so	40

B. Symptom Rating Scale

SYMPTOMS	ACTIVITES	POINTS
None	Able to do strenuous work/sports with jumping and hard pivoting	10
With strenuous work/sports	Able to do moderate work/sports with running, turning, and twisting	8
With moderate work/sports	Able to do light work/sports with no running, twisting, or jumping	6
With light work/sports	Able to perform activities of daily living alone	4
Frequent and limiting	Activities of daily living produce moderate symptoms	2
Constant and not relieved	Activities of daily living produce severe symptoms	0

C. Sports Activities Rating Scale

LEVEL	PARTICIPATION	MOTION	SPORT	POINTS
I	4–7 days per week	Jumping, hard pivoting, cutting	Basketball, volleyball, football, gymnastics, soccer	100
		Running, twisting, turning	Tennis, racquetball, handball, baseball, ice hockey, field hockey, skiing, wrestling	95
		No running, twisting, jumping	Cycling, swimming	90
II	1–3 days per week	Jumping, hard pivoting, cutting	Basketball, volleyball, football, gymnastics, soccer	85
		Running, twisting, turning	Tennis, racquetball, handball, baseball, ice hockey, field hockey, skiing, wrestling	80
		No running, twisting, jumping	Cycling, swimming	75

Table 34-3. Cincinnati Knee Rating System—cont'd

III	1–3 times per month	Jumping, hard pivoting, cutting	Basketball, volleyball, football, gymnastics, soccer	65
		Running, twisting, turning	Tennis, racquetball, handball, baseball, ice hockey, field hockey, skiing, wrestling	60
		No running, twisting, jumping	Cycling, swimming	55
IV	None	No problems with activities of daily living		40
		Moderate problems with activities of daily living		20
		Severe problems with activities of daily living (uses crutches, full disability)		0

D. Scheme for Final Rating

SIGNS	EXCELLENT	GOOD	FAIR	POOR
Pain	10	8	6-4	2-0
Swelling	10	8	6-4	2-0
Partial giving way	10	8	6-4	2-0
Full giving way	10	8	6-4	2-0
Walking	40	30	20	0
Stairs or squatting (choose lower score)	40	30	20	0
Running	100	80	60	40
Jumping	100	80	60	40
Hard twists, cuts, pivots	100	80	60	40
Effusion (mL)	Normal	<25	26–60	>60
Lack of flexion (degrees)	0–5	6–15	16–30	>30
Lack of extension (degrees)	0–3	4–5	6–10	>10
Tibiofemoral crepitus*	Normal	—	Moderate	Severe
Patellofemoral crepitus*	Normal	—	Moderate	Severe
Anterior displacement (KT-1000)	<3 mm	3–5 mm	6 mm	>6 mm
Pivot-shift test Joint space narrowing	Negative	Slip	Definite	Severe
Medial tibiofemoral (radiographs)[†]	Normal	Mild	Moderate	Severe
Lateral tibiofemoral (radiographs)[†]	Normal	Mild	Moderate	Severe
Patellofemoral (radiographs)[†]	Normal	Mild	Moderate	Severe
Functional testing (limb symmetry, percent)[‡]	100–85	75–84	65–74	<65

*Moderate indicates definite fibrillation and cartilage abnormality of 25 to 50 degrees, and severe, cartilage abnormality of more than 50 degrees.
[†]Moderate indicates narrowing of less than half the joint space, and severe, more than half the joint space.
[‡]Use an average of at least three one-legged hop-type tests.
Adapted from Noyes FR, Barber SD, Mangine RE: Bone–patellar ligament–bone and fascia lata allografts for reconstruction of the anterior cruciate ligament. J Bone Joint Surg Am 72:1125, 1990.

THE SEVEN GROUPS | THE FOUR GRADES | GROUP GRADE (see footnotes)

	A: normal	B: nearly normal	C: abnormal	D: sev. abnorm.	A	B	C	D
1 Patient subjective assessment								
On a scale of 0 to 3 how did you rate your pre-injury activity level?	☐ 0	☐ 1	☐ 2	☐ 3				
On a scale of 0 to 3 how did you rate your current activity level?	☐ 0	☐ 1	☐ 2	☐ 3				
If your normal knee performs 100%, what percentage does your operated knee perform?	_____ %				☐	☐	☐	☐

2 Symptoms (Grade at highest activity level known by patient)

	I Strenuous activities	II Moderate activities	III ADL/Light activities	IV ADL problems	A	B	C	D
Pain	☐	☐	☐	☐				
Swelling	☐	☐	☐	☐				
Partial giving way	☐	☐	☐	☐				
Full giving way	☐	☐	☐	☐	☐	☐	☐	☐

3 Range of motion Flex/Ext: Index side: __ / __ / __ Opposite side: __ / __ / __

					A	B	C	D
Lack of extension (from zero degrees)	☐ <3°	☐ 3–5°	☐ 6–10°	☐ >10°				
Δ Lack of flexion	☐ 0–5°	☐ 6–15°	☐ 16–25°	☐ >25°	☐	☐	☐	☐

4 Ligament examination

					A	B	C	D
Δ Lachman (25° flex) (manual, instrumented, x-ray)	☐ 1 to 2 mm	☐ 3 to 5 mm	☐ 6 to 10 mm	☐ >10 mm				
Endpoint: ☐ firm ☐ soft	☐ firm		☐ soft					
Δ Total a.p. transl. (70° flex)	☐ 0 to 2 mm	☐ 3 to 5 mm	☐ 6 to 10 mm	☐ >10 mm				
Δ Post. sag in 70° flex	☐ 0 to 2 mm	☐ 3 to 5 mm	☐ 6 to 10 mm	☐ >10 mm				
Δ Med. joint opening (valgus rotation)	☐ 0 to 2 mm	☐ 3 to 5 mm	☐ 6 to 10 mm	☐ >10 mm				
Δ Lat. joint opening (varus rotation)	☐ 0 to 2 mm	☐ 3 to 5 mm	☐ 6 to 10 mm	☐ >10 mm				
Pivot shift	☐ neg.	☐ + (glide)	☐ ++ (clunk)	☐ +++ (gross)				
Reversed pivot shift	☐ equal	☐ glide	☐ marked	☐ gross	☐	☐	☐	☐

5 Compartmental findings

					A	B	C	D
Crepitus patellofemoral	☐ none		☐ moderate	☐ severe				
Crepitus medial compartment	☐ none		☐ moderate	☐ severe				
Crepitus lateral compartment	☐ none		☐ moderate	☐ severe (palpable & audible)	☐	☐	☐	☐

6 X-ray findings

					A	B	C	D
Med. joint space narrowing	☐ none		☐ <50%	☐ >50%				
Lat. joint space narrowing	☐ none		☐ <50%	☐ >50%				
Patellofemoral joint space narrowing	☐ none		☐ <50%	☐ >50%	☐	☐	☐	☐

7 Functional test

					A	B	C	D
Δ One leg hop (% of opposite side)	☐ 100–90%	☐ 90–76%	☐ 75–50%	☐ <50%	☐	☐	☐	☐
Final evaluation					☐	☐	☐	☐

Footnotes:
- Group grade: The lowest grade within a group determines the group grade.
- Final evaluation: The worst group determines the final evaluation.
- In a final evaluation all 7 groups are to be evaluated; for a quick knee profile the evaluation of groups 1–4 are sufficient.

Figure 34–26. International Knee Documentation Committee knee rating system. (From The International Knee Documentation Committee: Knee ligament injury and reconstruction evaluation. In Knee Surgery Current Practice. New York, Martin Dunitz/Raven Press, 1992, p 760.)

558 SECTION V Ligament Injuries

References

1. American Medical Association, Committee of the Medical Aspects of Sports: Standard Nomenclature of Athletic Injuries. American Medical Association, Chicago, 1966.
2. American Orthopaedic Society of Sports Medicine Research and Education Committee: 1976.
3. Amis AA: Anterior cruciate ligament replacement: Knee stability of the effect of implants. J Bone Joint Surg Br 71:819, 1989.
4. Amis AA, Dawkins GPC: Functional anatomy of the anterior cruciate ligament. J Bone Joint Surg Br 73:260, 1991.
5. Andrews JR, Baker CL, Curl WW, et al: Surgical repair of acute and chronic lesions of the lateral capsular ligamentous complex of the knee. In Feagin JA Jr (ed): The Crucial Ligaments. New York, Churchill Livingstone, 1987, p 425.
6. Arnoczky SP, Warren RF: Anatomy of the cruciate ligaments. In Feagin JA Jr (ed): The Crucial Ligaments. New York, Churchill Livingstone, 1987, p 179.
7. Bach BR, Johnson JC: Ligament testing devices. In Scott WN (ed): Ligament and Extensor Mechanism Injuries of the Knee: Diagnosis and Treatment. St Louis, Mosby–Year Book, 1991, p 135.
8. Bach BR, Warren RF, Flynn WM, et al: Arthrometric evaluation of knees that have a torn anterior cruciate ligament. J Bone Joint Surg Am 72:1299, 1990.
9. Baker CL, Norwood LA, Hughston JC: Acute posterolateral rotatory instability of the knee. J Bone Joint Surg Am 65:614, 1983.
10. Brantigan OC, Voshell AF: The mechanics of the ligaments and menisci of the knee joint. J Bone Joint Surg 23:44, 1941.
11. Butler DL, Noyes FR, Grood ES: Ligamentous restraints to anterior posterior drawer in the human knee: A biomechanical study. J Bone Joint Surg Am 62:259, 1980.
12. Clancy WG, Shelbourne KD, Zoellner GB, et al: Treatment of knee joint instability secondary to rupture of the posterior cruciate ligament. J Bone Joint Surg Am 65:310, 1983.
13. Copper DE: Tests for posterolateral instability of the knee in the normal subjects: Results of examination under anesthesia. J Bone Joint Surg Am 73:30, 1991.
14. Covey DC: Injuries of the posterolateral corner of the knee. J Bone Joint Surg Am 83:106, 2001.
15. Dandy DJ, Pusey RS: The long-term results of unrepaired tears of the posterior cruciate ligament. J Bone Joint Surg Br 64:92, 1982.
16. Daniel DM, Malcom LL, Losse G, et al: Instrumented measurement of anterior laxity of the knee. J Bone Joint Surg Am 67:720, 1985.
17. Daniel DM, Stone ML: Diagnosis of knee ligament injury: Tests and measurements of joint laxity. In Feagin JA Jr (ed): The Crucial Ligaments. New York, Churchill Livingstone, 1987, p 287.
18. Daniel DM, Stone ML, Barnett P, et al: Use of the quadriceps active tests to diagnose posterior cruciate ligament disruption and measure posterior laxity of the knee. J Bone Joint Surg Am 70:386, 1988.
19. Daniel DM, Stone ML, Dobson BE, et al: Fate of the ACL-injured patient: A prospective outcome study. Am J Sports Med 22:632, 1994.
20. Daniel DM, Stone ML, Sachs R, et al: The measurement of anterior knee laxity in patients with acute anterior cruciate ligament disruption. Am J Sports Med 13:401, 1985.
21. Fowler PJ, Messieh SS: Isolated posterior cruciate ligament injuries. Am J Sports Med 15:553, 1987.
22. Fukubayashi T, Torzilli PA, Sherman MF, et al: An in vitro biomechanical evaluation of anterior posterior motion of the knee: Tibial displacement, rotation and torque. J Bone Joint Surg Am 64:258, 1982.
23. Furman W, Marshall JL, Girgis FG: The anterior cruciate ligament: A functional analysis based on postmortem studies. J Bone Joint Surg Am 58:179, 1976.
24. Galaway RD, Beaupre A, MacIntosh DL: Pivot shift: A clinical sign of symptomatic anterior cruciate insufficiency. J Bone Joint Surg Br 54:763, 1972.
25. Girgis FG, Marshall JL, Al Monajem ARS: The cruciate ligaments of the knee joint: Anatomical, functional and experimental analysis. Clin Orthop 106:216, 1975.
26. Gollehon DL, Torzilli PA, Waren RF: The role of the posterolateral and cruciate ligaments in the stability of the human knee: A biomechanical study. J Bone Joint Surg Am 69:233, 1987.

27. Granberry WM, Noble PC, Woods GW: Evaluation of electrogoniometric instrument for measurement of laxity of the knee. J Bone Joint Surg Am 72:1316, 1990.
28. Grood ES, Noyes FR: Diagnosis and classifications of knee ligament injuries: Biomechanical precepts. In Feagin JA Jr (ed): The Crucial Ligaments. New York, Churchill Livingstone, 1987, p 245.
29. Grood ES, Noyes FR, Butler DL, et al: Ligamentous and capsular restraints preventing straight medial and lateral laxity in intact human cadaver knees. J Bone Joint Surg Am 63:1257, 1981.
30. Hseieh HH, Walker PS: Stabilizing mechanisms of the loaded and unloaded knee joint. J Bone Joint Surg Am 58:87, 1976.
31. Hughston JC: Acute knee injuries in athletes. Clin Orthop 23:114, 1962.
32. Hughston JC, Andrews JR, Cross MJ, et al: Classification of knee ligament instabilities: The medial compartment and cruciate ligaments. J Bone Joint Surg Am 58:159, 1976.
33. Hughston JC, Andrews JR, Cross MJ, et al: Classification of knee ligament instabilities: The lateral compartment. J Bone Joint Surg Am 58:173, 1976.
34. Hughston JC, Barrett GR: Acute anteromedial rotatory instability: Long-term results of surgical repair. J Bone Joint Surg Am 65:145, 1983.
35. Hughston JC, Bowden JA, Andrews JR, et al: Acute tears of the posterior cruciate ligament: Results of operative treatment. J Bone Joint Surg Am 62:438, 1980.
36. Hughston JC, Degenhardt TC: Reconstruction of the posterior cruciate ligament. Clin Orthop 164:59, 1982.
37. Hughston JC, Eilers AF: The role of the posterior oblique ligament in repair of acute medial collateral ligament tears of the knee. J Bone Joint Surg Am 55:923, 1973.
38. Indelicato PA: Injury to the medial capsuloligamentous complex. In Feagin JA Jr (ed): The Crucial Ligaments. New York, Churchill Livingstone, 1987, p 197.
39. Jacobsen K: Area intercondylaris tibial: Osseous surface structure and its relation to soft tissue structures and applications to radiography. J Anat 177:605, 1974.
40. James SL, Wood GW, Homsy CA, et al: Cruciate ligament stents in reconstruction of the unstable knee. Clin Orthop 143:90, 1979.
41. Jonsson T, Althoff B, Peterson L, et al: Clinical diagnosis of ruptures of the anterior cruciate ligament: A comparative study of the Lachman test and the anterior drawer sign. Am J Sports Med 10:100, 1982.
42. Kaplan E: Some aspects of the functional anatomy of the human knee joint. Clin Orthop 23:18, 1962.
43. Kennedy JC, Fowler PJ: Medial and anterior instability of the knee: An anatomical and clinical study using stress machine. J Bone Joint Surg Am 53:257, 1971.
44. Kennedy JC, Hawkins RJ, Willis RB, et al: Tension studies of human knee ligaments: Yield point, ultimate failure and disruption of the cruciate and tibial collateral ligaments. J Bone Joint Surg Am 58:350, 1976.
45. Kurosawa H, Yamakoshi K, Yasuda K, et al: Simultaneous measurement of changes in length of the cruciate ligaments during knee motion. Clin Orthop 265:233, 1991.
46. Larson RL, Jones DC: Dislocation and ligamentous injuries of the knee. In Rockwood CA Jr, Green DP (eds): Fractures in Adults, vol 2, 2nd ed. Philadelphia, JB Lippincott, 1984, pp 1, 480, 591.
47. Losee RE, Jonson TR, Southwick WO: Anterior subluxation of the lateral tibial plateau. J Bone Joint Surg Am 60:1015, 1978.
48. Lysholm J, Gillquist J: Evaluation of knee ligament surgery results with special emphasis on using a scoring scale. J Sports Med 10:150, 1982.
49. Main WK, Scott WN: Posterior cruciate ligament insufficiency. In Scott WN (ed): Ligament and Extensor Mechanism Injuries of the Knee: Diagnosis and Treatment. St Louis, Mosby–Year Book, 1991, p 361.
50. Malcom LL, Daniel DM, Stone ML, et al: The measurement of anterior knee laxity after anterior cruciate ligament reconstructive surgery. Clin Orthop 169:35, 1985.
51. Markolf KL, Kochaan A, Amstutz HC: Measurement of knee stiffness and laxity in patients with documented absence of the anterior cruciate ligament. J Bone Joint Surg Am 66:242, 1984.
52. Markolf KL, Mensch JS, Amstutz HC: Stiffness and laxity of the knee: Contributions of the supporting structures—a quantitative in vitro study. J Bone Joint Surg Am 58:583, 1976.

53. Miyasaka KC, Daniel DM, Stone ML, et al: The incidence of knee ligament injuries in the general population. Am J Knee Surg 4:3, 1991.

54. Mont NA, Scott WN: Classification of ligament injuries. In Scott WN (ed): Ligament and Extensor Mechanism Injuries of the Knee: Diagnosis and Treatment. St Louis, Mosby–Year Book, 1991, p 83.

55. Muller W: The Knee: Form, Function and Ligament Reconstruction. New York, Spring-Verlag, 1983.

56. Norwood LA, Cross MJ: Anterior cruciate ligament: Functional anatomy of its bundles in rotatory instabilities. Am J Sports Med 7:23, 1979.

57. Noyes FR, Barber SD, Mangine RE: Bone–patellar ligament–bone and fascia lata allografts for reconstruction of the anterior cruciate ligament. J Bone Joint Surg Am 72:1125, 1990.

58. Noyes FR, Grood ES: Classification of ligament injuries: Why an anterolateral laxity or anteromedial laxity is not a diagnostic entity. Instr Course Lect 36:185, 1987.

59. Noyes FR, Grood ES: Diagnosis of knee ligament injuries: Clinical concepts. In Feagin JA Jr (ed): The Crucial Ligaments. New York, Churchill Livingstone, 1987, p 261.

60. Noyes FR, Grood ES, Torzilli PA: Current concepts review: The definition of terms for motion and position of the knee and injuries of the ligaments. J Bone Joint Surg Am 71:465, 1989.

61. Odensten M, Gillquist J: Functional anatomy of the anterior cruciate ligament and a rationale for reconstruction. J Bone Joint Surg Am 67:257, 1985.

62. Oliver JH, Coughlin LP: Objective knee evaluation using the Genucom knee analysis system: Clinical implications. Am J Sports Med 15:571, 1987.

63. Parolie JM, Bergfeld TA: Long-term results of nonoperative treatment of isolated posterior cruciate ligament injuries in the knee. Am J Sports Med 14:35, 1986.

64. Price CT, Allen WC: Ligament repair in the knee with preservation of the meniscus. J Bone Joint Surg Am 60:61, 1978.

65. Scott WN: Ligament and Extensor Mechanism Injuries to the Knee: Diagnosis and Treatment. St Louis, Mosby–Year Book, 1991.

66. Scuderi GR: The second fracture. Am J Knee Surg 4:32, 1991.

67. Seebacher JR, Linglis AE, Marshall JL, et al: The structure of the posterolateral aspect of the knee. J Bone Joint Surg Am 64:536, 1982.

68. Sherman OH, Markolf KL, Ferkel RD: Measurements of anterior knee laxity in normal and anterior cruciate absent knees with two instrumented test devices. Clin Orthop 215:156, 1987.

69. Shoemaker SC, Markolf KL: Effects of joint load on the stiffness and laxity of ligament deficient knees: An in vitro study of the anterior cruciate and medial collateral ligament. J Bone Joint Surg Am 67:136, 1985.

70. Sisk TD: Knee injuries. In Crenshaw AH (ed): Campbell's Operative Orthopedics, 7th ed. St Louis, CV Mosby, 1987, p 2283.

71. Slocum DB, Larson RL: Rotatory instability of the knee. J Bone Joint Surg Am 50:211, 1968.

72. Sullivan D, Levy IM, Sheskier S, et al: Medial restraints to anterior-posterior motion of the knee. J Bone Joint Surg Am 66:930, 1984.

73. Tegner Y, Lysholm J: Rating systems in evaluation of knee ligament injuries. Clin Orthop 198:43, 1985.

74. Terry GC, Hughston JC: Associated joint pathology in the anterior cruciate ligament–deficient knee with emphasis on a classification system and injuries to the meniscocapsular ligament: Musculo-tendinous unit complex. Orthop Clin North Am 16:29, 1985.

75. Terry GC, Hughston JC, Norwood LA: The anatomy of the iliopatellar band and iliotibial tract. Am J Sports Med 14:39, 1986.

76. Trent PS, Walker PS, Wolf B: Ligament length patterns: Strength and rotational axes of the knee joint. Clin Orthop 117:263, 1976.

77. Tria AJ, Hosea TM: Diagnosis of knee ligament injuries. In Scott WN (ed): Ligament and Extensor Mechanism Injuries of the Knee. St Louis, Mosby–Year Book, 1991, p 87.

78. Tria AJ, Jonson CD, Zawadsky JP: The popliteus tendon. J Bone Joint Surg Am 71:714, 1989.

79. Veltri DM, Warren RF: Anatomy, biomechanics, and physical findings in posterolateral knee instability. Clin Sports Med 13:599, 1994.

80. Wang CJ, Walker PS: The effects of flexion and rotation on the length patterns of the ligaments of the knee. J Biomech 6:587, 1973.

81. Warren RF, Marshall JL: The supporting structures and layers on the medial side of the knee: An anatomical analysis. J Bone Joint Surg Am 61:56, 1979.

82. Warren RF, Marshall JL, Girgis F: The prime static stabilizer of the medial side of the knee. J Bone Joint Surg Am 56:665, 1974.

83. Welsh RP: Knee joint structure and function. Clin Orthop 147:7, 1980.

CHAPTER 35

Knee Outcome Scales

Lynanne J. Foster • Sanjiv Bansal • Vipool K. Goradia
Leslie S. Matthews

Surgical management of a ligament-deficient knee has drastically changed over the past 25 years, and surgical reconstruction has proved effective in restoring stability to such knees. However, assessing the results of ligament reconstruction has been difficult because of the multitude of rating systems, each of which emphasizes different criteria, and the inconsistencies inherent in subjective and objective evaluations among various observers. It is extremely difficult to completely eliminate such variables from any rating system, but the best knee rating system will have the fewest biases and the most objective reproducible data. To date, no single sports knee rating system has been accepted universally. Thus, it is imperative that a consistent and uniform evaluation be developed to determine the ideal treatment for individual knee injuries.

HISTORICAL PERSPECTIVE

O'Donoghue[38] was among the first to formulate a rating scale in the search for a standardized means of evaluating postoperative results of ligament surgery. This evaluation consisted of a questionnaire that required yes or no answers to four main questions: (1) does your operated knee bother you, (2) is it as good as your other knee, (3) are you completely happy with the result of your operation, and (4) has your knee kept you from participating in athletics? If the patient answered no to question 2, there were 10 subquestions (10 points each) for a total of 100 points: (1) does it hurt, (2) is it loose or wobbly, (3) is knee motion restricted, (4) does it swell, (5) does it seem weak, (6) does it catch or snap, (7) does it bother you to squat, (8) do you have trouble with stairs, (9) does it limit your activities (if so, how), and (10) does it handicap you in your work?

The initial O'Donoghue study[38] laid the foundation for contemporary sports knee rating systems. O'Donoghue[39] realized the limitations of his initial study and expanded the parameters to include a greater number of concrete observations, such as stability, swelling, range of motion, functional return, and patient disability, which were graded from + to ++++. Investigators such as Slocum and Larson[43] subsequently realized the importance of critical evaluation in knee injury and surgery and incorporated a preoperative examination for the purpose of postoperative comparison. Slocum and Larson[43] were the first to introduce rotatory instability into the evaluation form; Larson[24] incorporated functional tests such as running, squatting, and jumping; and Hughston and Eilers,[15] Ellsasser et al,[6]

and Godshall and Hansen[10] quantified tibiofemoral excursion in terms of millimeters as a means of grading ligament injury. Ellsasser et al,[6] in performing a valgus stress to determine medial collateral ligament injury, further classified ligament integrity as a soft or hard endpoint.

Hospital for Special Surgery Knee Score

In 1977, Marshall and colleagues[26] published the first comprehensive knee rating system, the Hospital for Special Surgery Knee Score (HSSKS) evaluation form (Fig. 35–1). They, like other investigators in the early 1970s, recognized the need for a universal, standardized method of ligament injury examinations and follow-up. This standardized form had several goals: (1) determine a natural history of recovery after a specific injury and, thus, an appropriate course of treatment; (2) define long-term functional goals of a specific type of injury; (3) provide the means of studying a specific type of injury under various treatment modalities; (4) facilitate objective assessment of therapeutic modalities; and (5) allow a rapid and new means of communication between physicians and patients.

The HSSKS evaluation form is used only for patients with a definitive diagnosis of ligament injury. This form is not used for patients with meniscal tears or patellofemoral pathology unassociated with ligament injury. The form consists of two separate sheets: the Knee Discharge Summary and the Follow-up Sheet.

The Knee Discharge Summary (see Fig. 35–1) is designed to parallel a general medical examination. It divides patients into two categories: those with an acute first-time injury and those with multiple knee injuries. The date of injury refers to the most clinically significant injury and not to the most recent injury. Physical examination includes observing the patient's ability to perform a functional test, followed by inspection and palpation of the joint. In testing ligaments, no specific unit of displacement is used; rather, measurement includes quality with quantity of instability. Quality of endpoint, deemed important, is quantified as being soft or hard. These findings, along with diagnostic studies and surgical findings, are recorded on the form. The surgical findings provide an internal check with which to evaluate preoperative diagnostic techniques.

The Follow-up Sheet (see Fig. 35–1) consists of three parts: subjective, objective, and functional tests to evaluate the integrity of the anterior cruciate ligament (ACL),

560

THE HOSPITAL FOR SPECIAL SURGERY
SPORTS MEDICINE SERVICE
KNEE INJURIES DISCHARGE SUMMARY
FOLLOW-UP SCORE SHEET

NAME _____ TEL: HOME ( ) ___ WORK ( ) ___

CHART NO.: HSS# ___ PVT# ___ AGE: ___ SEX: ___

DATE OF INJURY: ___ DATE OF SURGERY: ___

DIAGNOSIS: ___

TREATMENT: ___ NON-OP: ___

SURGICAL FINDINGS: ___

SURGICAL PROCEDURES: ___

INSTRUCTIONS: NORMAL PERSON HAS HIGHEST SCORE. AWARD POINTS WHEN NO PATHOLOGY.

DATE OF EXAMINATION:

TIME: POST INJURY/POST SURGERY:

A. PATIENT'S OWN EVALUATION.
N = normal   I = improved
S = severe   W = worse

B. PAIN 0 = yes, 1 = no
SWELLING: 0,1 — 0,1
STAIRS DIFFICULTY: — 0,1
CLICKING-NUMBNESS: — 0,1
Giving way: — 0–4
 4 = normal, none
 2 = with stress only
 1 = with stress upon daily activity
 0 = regularly upon daily activity
RETURN TO SPORTS OR WORK: 0–3
 3 = full return
 2 = return to orig. with limitations
 1 = return to different
 0 = no return

C. 1) FUNCTIONAL TESTS
DUCK WALK:* — 0, 1, 2
RUN IN PLACE: — 0, 1, 2
JUMP ON ONE LEG:* — 0, 1, 2
HALF SQUAT: — 0, 1, 2
FULL SQUAT: — 0, 1, 2
* = for C1–0 = cannot perform
 1 = can perform but with discomfort
 2 = can perform

2) SPECIFIC KNEE EXAM
TENDERNESS: — 0,1
JOINT EFFUSION — 0,1
SWELLING (soft tissue) — 0,1
CREPITATIONS — 0,1
MUSCLE POWER — 0–3
 3 = normal
 2 = diminished flex. or ext.
 1 = diminished flex. and ext.
 0 = very week
THIGH SIZES — 0–2
 2 = equal
 1 = 1–2 cm difference
 0 = < 2 cm different
RANGE OF MOTION — 0–3
 3 = normal
 2 = limited flex. or ext.
 1 = limited flex. and ext.
 0 = > 90
STABILITY — 0–5 (a/b)
LCL: 5 = normal
 4 = mild inst. in flex.
 3 = moderate inst. in flex.
 2 = inst. in flex. and ext.
 0 = gross instability
 *a = hard end point
 *b = soft or no end point
MCL: 5 = normal — 0–5 (a/b)
 4 = mild inst. in flex.
 3 = moderate inst. in flex.
 2 = inst. in flex. and ext.
 0 = gross instability
 *a = hard end point
 *b = soft or no end point
ACL: 5 = normal (= opp. leg)
 4 = slight jog
 3 = moderate jog
 2 = severe in neutral
 0 = severe in neu. and rot. (Pivot Shift, Slocum, Jerk Test)
 *a = hard end point
 *b = soft or no end point
PCL: 5 = normal (= opp. leg)
 4 = slight jog
 3 = moderate jog
 2 = severe in neutral
 0 = severe in neu. and rot.
 *a = hard end point
 *b = soft or no end point
D. TOTAL SCORE max. 50 pts.
E. PHYSICIAN'S INITIALS
* = For all stability scores the answer must include both number and letter, e.g., 4a.

Figure 35–1. Hospital for Special Surgery Knee Score (HSSKS) form. (Redrawn from Marshall JL, Fetto JF, Botero PM: Knee ligament injuries: A standardized evaluation method. Clin Orthop 123:115, 1977.)

posterior cruciate ligament (PCL), medial collateral ligament, and lateral collateral ligament. The subjective section consists of questions to be answered with yes or no and a patient evaluation of the knee as normal, improved, worse, or severe. The objective section includes functional tests (duck walk, running in place, jumping on one leg, half squat, and full squat) and specific knee examination (knee tenderness, joint effusion, swelling, crepitations, muscle power, range of motion, and thigh circumference). The third section, ligament testing, is the most important.

A normal knee receives a total of 50 points; 20 (40%) of those 50 points are related to stability because the system's primary goal is to measure ligament stability and stability is the most critical determinant of successful and functional return. A patient receives a normal score when there is no evidence of any hesitation to participate in all activities. For example, athletes would receive a normal knee rating if the knee did not prevent them from participating in any activity with full confidence, irrespective of not returning to the original sport in which the injury occurred. A follow-up examination is performed at 3 months and then at 1 year.

There are two major problems with the HSSKS: first, it gives patients a higher score because they do not have to return to their original sport; and second, a large percentage of the score (40%) is dedicated to ligament stability, thus assuming that ligaments are the most important aspect of the knee for all activities.

Noyes Knee Profile

In 1983, Noyes et al[37] developed another knee scale (Fig. 35–2) in an attempt to determine the outcome of an ACL-deficient knee that was treated by rehabilitation and activity modification rather than by surgery. The scale consisted of three parts: subjective rating, knee examination, and laxity examination. Each of the three parts were

Cincinnati Sports Medicine and Orthopaedic Center
Knee Examination   R   L

NAME _____ M ___ F ___ AGE _____ TELEPHONE _____ DATE _____
DIAGNOSIS _____
DATE OF INJURY _____ DATE OF SURGERY _____ WEEKS POSTOP. _____
PROCEDURE _____

SUBJECTIVE KEY (50 points)

10 = Normal knee, no symptoms

8 = Vigorous athletics possible, some guarding and limitations, still rare symptoms

6 = Light recreational athletics possible with rare symptoms: higher activity level causes frequent symptoms

4 = Activities of daily living possible with rare symptoms: any athletics causes frequent symptoms

2 = ADL causes moderate symptoms, frequent limitation

0 = ADL causes severe problem, persistent symptoms

	NL	VIG	REC	ADL	ADL-FREQ	ADL-SEV
Pain*	10	8	6	4	2	0
Activity Limits*	20	16	12	8	4	0
Giving-Way*	10	8	6	4	2	0
Swelling*	10	8	6	4	2	0

TOTAL R _____ L _____

* No or rare symptoms at highest level

KNEE EXAMINATION

VARIABLES	RIGHT (1)	(2)	(3)	(4)	LEFT (1)	(2)	(3)	(4)
1. Effusion	NL	MIN	MOD	SEV	NL	MIN	MOD	SEV
2. Total ROM	NL	110	90	<90	NL	110	90	<90
3. Flexion Contracture	NL	5–10	11–15	>15	NL	5–10	11–15	>15
4. Pat. Fem. Crepitus	NL	MIN	MOD	SEV	NL	MIN	MOD	SEV
5. Pat. Fem. Pain	NO	YES			NO	YES		
6. Tibial Fem. Crepitus	NL	MIN	MOD	SEV	NL	MIN	MOD	SEV
7. Meniscal Click	NO	MED	LAT	BOTH	NO	MED	LAT	BOTH
8. Plica	NO	YES			NO	YES		
9. Fat Pad	NL	SWOLLEN	TENDER	BOTH	NL	SWOLLEN	TENDER	BOTH
10. Quad. Weakness	NL	MIN	MOD	SEV	NL	MIN	MOD	SEV
11. Local Tenderness	NO	YES	SITE _____		NO	YES	SITE _____	

R TOTAL [   ]   L TOTAL [   ]

CONSTANTS:

	RIGHT				LEFT			
P.F. Lat. Sublux. (% width)	0–25%	26–50	51–75	>75	0–25%	26–50	51–75	>75
P.F. Med. Sublux. (30)	15 mm	11–15	6–10	0–5	15 mm	11–15	6–10	0–5
Patellar Tilt	>45	+ 15	0	–15	>45	+ 15	0	–15
Q Angle 0	0–10	11–15	16–20	>20	0–10	11–15	16–20	>20
Q Angle Max 30	15	20	25	>25	15	20	25	>25
Alignment	VARUS	VALGUS			VARUS	VALGUS		
Degrees of Varus/Valgus	0–10	11–15	16–20	>20	0–10	11–15	16–20	>20

R TOTAL [   ]   L TOTAL [   ]

LAXITY EXAM (50 points)

POINTS	GRADE	STRAIGHT	ROTATORY
10 9 8	I	5 mm	Mild/Physiologic
7 6 5	II	6–10 mm	Moderate
4 3 2	III	11–15 mm	Severe
0	IV	15 mm	Gross

Other _____
_____
_____
_____
_____
_____

Signature _____ M.D.

RIGHT

ACL   I II III IV ___ mm
      9 6   3   0

ALRI I II III IV

MED   I II III IV
      9 6   3   0

AMRI [I | II | III | IV]

LAT   I II III IV
      9 6   3   0

PCL   I II III IV
      9 6   3   0

PLRI I II III IV
      9 6   3   0

[P] [C]
TOTAL [   ]

LEFT

ACL   I II III IV ___ mm
      9 6   3   0

ALRI I II III IV

MED   I II III IV
      9 6   3   0

AMRI [I | II | III | IV]

LAT   I II III IV
      9 6   3   0

PCL   I II III IV
      9 6   3   0

PLRI I II III IV
      9 6   3   0

[P] [C]
TOTAL [   ]

Figure 35–2. Noyes Knee Profile form. (Redrawn from Noyes FR, Matthews DS, Mooar PA, et al: The symptomatic anterior cruciate–deficient knee. Part II: The results of rehabilitation, activity modification, and counseling on functional disability. J Bone Joint Surg Am 65:163, 1983.)

analyzed separately; the total of the parts has less meaning than the individual parts.

The subjective section specifically analyzed symptoms as reported by patients at varying levels of activity. Noyes et al[37] were the first to recognize that if a symptomatic ACL-deficient athlete continues to participate at a high level of sports, the athlete will not receive any points in this category because such participation would result in long-term damage to the knee. This scale also unmasks athletes who have reduced their athletic activities to the point at which they have no symptoms. In addition, it differentiates between symptoms occurring during sports and those occurring during activities of daily living. Symptoms such as pain, activity limitation, giving way, and swelling are evaluated at different levels of activity rather than in a binary manner. A total of 50 points (range, 0 to 50 points) is given in this category of the knee scale.

The knee examination section, designed to determine factors not associated with ligaments, is divided into variables and constants. It evaluates the patellofemoral joint, medial and lateral compartments, meniscus, and extensor mechanism. Eight categories from the variables and constants section specifically evaluate the patellofemoral joint and extensor mechanism for crepitus, pain, patellar subluxation, patellar tilt, and quadriceps (Q) angle.

In the laxity examination, each knee is examined, and the difference between the two is noted for two reasons: normal or inherent laxity is defined in the unaffected knee, and laxity is expressed in terms of absolute laxity and increased laxity as compared with the unaffected knee. This is true only if the contralateral knee is uninjured.

American Orthopaedic Society for Sports Medicine Study Group Knee Score

In 1983, Feagin and Blake[7] in conjunction with American Orthopaedic Society for Sports Medicine (AOSSM) study group published their A.C.L. Follow-up Form (Fig. 35–3). This system evaluates results after soft-tissue knee reconstruction through strength and endurance testing, radiography, and Lachman testing. It emphasizes joint function, subjective pain, stability, and range of motion.

According to the AOSSM study group, this form provides a convenient means of preoperative and postoperative documentation in the office for comparison of results. Like Noyes et al,[37] the AOSSM study group recommended that each category be evaluated separately, and a total score lacked discrimination. This score consists of subjective symptoms, subjective function, and an objective section.

In addition to ligament testing, the AOSSM study group recommended that radiographs of the knee be obtained to evaluate for degenerative joint changes and stability of the knee be assessed by instrumented examination; the latter would provide reproducible results among physicians. We agree with the AOSSM study group that instrumented testing provides a more reliable and accurate measurement of ligament stability than manual testing does. Instrumented machines such as the KT-1000 arthrometer (MEDmetric Corp., San Diego, CA) have been shown to be extremely reliable in the objective evaluation of ligamentous laxity.[21]

Lysholm Knee Scoring Scale

The Lysholm Knee Scoring Scale (Fig. 35–4A) was introduced by Lysholm and Gillquist[25] in 1982. According to Weitzel and Richmond,[47] this scale is the most widely used patient-reported outcome measure. The scale redistributes the points in the original Larson scale[24] (Fig. 35–4B) and includes the concept of "giving way" or "instability."[25] This subjective rating scale primarily focuses on symptoms during daily and athletic activities. Of the eight items for which points are assigned, the only objective category is thigh atrophy. This 100-point scale was administered to 130 patients 1 to 8 years after an acute knee injury.[25] All patients were also asked to rate their overall knee function as excellent, good, fair, or poor. The investigators found that the final score correlated with the patients' overall perception of their knee function. In 1985, Tegner and Lysholm[44] modified the scale (Fig. 35–4C) by decreasing "instability" and "pain" by 5 points each, eliminating "thigh atrophy," and adding "locking." This modified score was compared with the first HSSKS form (see Fig. 35–1) in 76 patients with ACL injuries. The binary questions (yes/no) in the HSSKS were found to provide less detail than the graded Lysholm Knee Scoring Scale. The conclusion was that stability testing (e.g., Lachman test), functional scores (e.g., Lysholm Knee Scoring Scale), performance tests (e.g., single-leg hop), and activity levels should not be included in the same scoring scale. Tegner and Lysholm[44] believed that each evaluation was important at different times in the treatment of knee ligament injuries and thus should be reported separately. We agree that each should be reported separately but also believe that all should be reported at various intervals for better comparison during a patient's postoperative or treatment course.

The Lysholm Knee Scoring Scale has been proved to be valid, reliable, and responsive, and its use is facilitated by its ease of administration, with approximately 4 minutes required.[28,29,48] It is often used in conjunction with another instrument such as the Tegner Activity Score,[44] but even alone it gives a more differentiated view of patients' disabilities than a binary system does. The Lysholm score has been shown to yield statistically higher scores than other scales do[48] and is more related to activities of daily living than to sports.[29,47] Additional criticism points out that 50% of the total score is based on pain and instability, with no objective data used to support this system,[19] and that fewer items are associated with less internal consistency.[27]

Tegner Activity Score

This 10-point score (Fig. 35–5) was introduced in 1985 by Tegner and Lysholm.[44] They recommended its use as a complement to the modified Lysholm Knee Scoring Scale because it allows discrimination between sedentary

Text continued on p. 591

SIDE 1
To be filled out
by patient

A.C.L. FOLLOW-UP FORM
A.O.S.S.M. STUDY GROUP

Date _____

IDENTIFICATION

PLEASE PRINT

Name _____   SS # _____   OFF # _____
        (LAST)   (FIRST)   (INITIAL)

Age _____   Sex ☐ M ☐ F   Knee involved ☐ Right   ☐ Left

Phone # _____   Phone # and name ⎫ Name _____
          (AREA CODE)   of someone   ⎬
Sport Causing Injury _____   who can reach you ⎭ Phone # _____
                                       if you have moved   (AREA CODE)

Date of Surgery _____   Number of months since surgery: 6   12   18   24   36
                (MO.) (DATE) (YEAR)   (CIRCLE ONE)

POST-OP COURSE

Cast? # weeks in rigid cast _____   # weeks in flexible/hinged cast _____

                              Current
Brace? ☐ Yes ☐ No   **Brace Use?** ☐ All the Time   ☐ Sports Only   ☐ No Longer Use

Physical Therapy? # months in supervised program (Cybex Orthotron etc.) _____

                Are you still doing a **regular** home program? ☐ Yes   ☐ No

SYMPTOMS

Knee Pain?   ☐4 None   ☐3 Mild   ☐2 Moderate (with activity)   Score
                 ☐1 Severe (at rest & preventing activity)   _____

Giving Way? ☐8 None   ☐6 Only with Cutting (stop & turn) Sports
                 ☐4 Occasional (only with awkward step)   ☐2 With Normal Daily Activities   _____

Swelling?   ☐4 None   ☐3 With Strenuous Activity   ☐2 With Moderate Activity
                 ☐1 With Any Activity   _____

Stiffness?   ☐4 None   ☐2 Occasional   ☐1 Frequent   _____

("X" in appropriate box)   Symptom Summary = Total/4 [   ]

FUNCTION

Activity level?   ☐1 No sports   ☐3 Active, but   [   ]
                                                    different sports
                       ☐2 Sports activities   ☐4 Same sports, but lower   Function Summary
                          significantly limited   performance level   (Activity Level)

Problems with Specific Activities?   ☐5 Equal performance at same
("X" in appropriate box)   sports as before injury

              NONE   MILD   MODERATE   CAN'T DO
Walking   ☐   ☐   ☐   ☐

Running   ☐   ☐   ☐   ☐   If your prior injury activity level rates at 10,
                                                     what does your current activity level rate? ____
Turn/Cut   ☐   ☐   ☐   ☐
                                                     If your normal knee performs at 100%, at what
Jumping   ☐   ☐   ☐   ☐   % does your operated knee perform? _____

Stairs   ☐   ☐   ☐   ☐

A

Figure 35–3. American Orthopaedic Society for Sports Medicine A.C.L. Follow-up Form. (Redrawn from Feagin JA, Jr, Blake WP: Postoperative evaluation and result recording in the anterior cruciate ligament–reconstructed knee. Clin Orthop 172:143, 1983.)

SIDE 2
To be filled out by physician
(make sure Side 1 is complete)

SURGICAL H$_X$

Type of ACL Injury: ☐ Acute (<1 wk)   ☐ Sub Acute (1–6 wks)   ☐ Chronic (>6 wks)   ☐ Acute or Chronic

Associated Injury (acute or chronic):   ☐ MCL   ☐ PCL   ☐ LCL   ☐ Med Men   ☐ Lat Men

ACL Surgery:
☐ No Repair   ☐ Primary Repair Aug with _____
☐ Primary Repair without Augmentation   ☐ Reconstruction with _____

Subsequent Injury: ☐ None   ☐ Medical Meniscus   ☐ Lateral Meniscus
☐ ACL   ☐ MCL   ☐ LCL   ☐ PCL

Subsequent Surgery: ☐ None   ☐ Hardware removal   ☐ MUA   ☐ Meniscectomy   ☐ Ligament repair

STABILITY

R   **Ant Draw/Lachmans**   L
_____ 15 _____
_____ 90 _____

Sublux (Pivot, Shift, Jerk, etc.)
_____ _____
record as 0 tr 1$^+$ 2$^+$ 3$^+$

Varus   **Valgus**   **Varus**
_____ 0 _____
_____ 30 _____

ROM
R −10 / 0
140 / 45 / 90

−10 / 0
L
45 / 140 / 90

ADDITIONAL STUDIES

Xray: NONE   MILD   MOD   SEVERE   **Cybex/Orthotron** (if available)
Med joint DJD   ☐ ☐ ☐ ☐
Lat joint DJD   ☐ ☐ ☐ ☐
P/F joint DJD   ☐ ☐ ☐ ☐
ICN osteophytes ☐ ☐ ☐ ☐

Other (your favorite test):

Strength _____ (rate)   Power _____ (rate)
R   L   R   L
Q   Q
H   H

Thigh Circ   R _____   L _____
(10cm ? patella)

CAPSULE SUMMARY *

Symptoms _____   Function _____   Stability _____

1) The **Symptom** score is the total score/4 of the entire symptom section.
2) The **Function** score is the score of the activity level question only.
3) The **Stability** score comes from only the Ant Draw/Lach/Sublux portion of the P.E. as follows: 5 = none of the 3 tests>trace; 4 = none of the 3 tests >1$^+$; 3 = two tests 1$^+$ on test 2$^+$; 2 = two tests 2$^+$ one test 1$^+$; 1 = all tests 2$^+$.

* The Capsule Summary is intended to give a brief picture of the patient NOT summarize all of the above data.

B

Figure 35–3, cont'd.

The modified Larson scoring scale (left column) and our scoring scale (right column)

Function (55 points)

Gait (10 points)

Limp:
None	5
Slight	3
Marked	0

Support:
Full support	5
Stick or crutch	3
Weight bearing impossible	0

Activities (45 points)

Stairs:
No difficulty	10
Slight difficulty	6
One step at a time	2
Unable	0

Squatting:
No difficulty	5
Slight difficulty	4
Not past 90	2
Unable	0

Walking:
Unlimited	20
More than 2 km	15
1–2 km	5
Unable	0

Running:
No difficulty	5
Slight difficulty	4
Straight ahead only	2
Unable	0

Jumping:
No difficulty	5
Slight difficulty	3
Unable	0

Pain (30 points)
None	30
Not incapacitating	25
Incapacitating	10
Severe	0

Anatomy (5 points)

Swelling (3 points)
None	3
Slight and occasional	1
Frequent	0

Atrophy of thigh (2 points)
None	2
1–2 cm	1
More than 2 cm	0

Range of motion (10 points)
0–45, deduct for each 10 loss	1
45–90, deduct for each 15 loss	1
90–100 deduct for each 20 loss below 130	1

Limp (5 points)
None	
Slight or periodical	5
Severe and constant	3

Support (5 points) — 0
Full support	
Stick or crutch	5
Weight bearing impossible	3

Stairclimbing (10 points) — 0
No problems	
Slightly impaired	
One step at a time	10
Unable	6

Squatting (5 points) — 2
No problems	0
Slightly impaired	
Not past 90	5
Unable	4
	2

Walking, running and jumping (70 points) — 0

A. Instability
Never giving way	
Rarely during athletic or other severe exertion	30
Frequently during athletic or other severe exertion (or unable to participate)	25
Occasionaly in daily activities	
Often in daily activities	20
Every step	10
	5

B. Pain — 0
None	
Inconsistent and slight during severe exertion	
Marked on giving way	30
Marked during severe exertion	
Marked on or after walking more than 2 km	25
	20
Marked on or after walking less than 2 km	15
Constant and severe	10

C. Swelling — 5
None	0
With giving way	
On severe exertion	
On ordinary exertion	10
Constant	7
	5

Atrophy of thigh (5 points) — 2
None	0
1–2 cm	
More than 2 cm	

5
3
0

A

Figure 35–4. **A,** Original Lysholm Knee Scoring Scale form. (**A,** From Lysholm J, Gillquist J: Evaluation of knee ligament surgery results with special emphasis on use of a scoring scale. Am J Sports Med 10:150, 1982.)

Rating sheet for knee function. (Dr. Robert L. Larson, Eugene, Oregon, 1972.)

Name _____

Hospital or chart no. _____   Date _____

Age _____   Sex: M.   F.   Knee: R.   L.

Occupation _____

Examiner _____ M.D.

Diagnosis _____

Primary aim of procedure (circle):   Relieve pain   Regain stability   Eradicate sepsis, tumor
                                        Restore motion   1. Everyday activities   Correct deformity
                                                           2. Vigorous activities   Other _____

Secondary aim of procedure _____

Operative procedure _____   Date _____

Results evaluation date _____

RATING (Circle one in each group)

Function (50 points)

GAIT (10 points)	*Limp*	
	None	5
	Mild	3
	Moderate	1
	Marked	0
	Support	
	None	5
	Cane	3
	Crutches	1
	Unable to bear wt.	0

ACTIVITIES (40 points)	*Walking*	
	Unlimited	20
	Mildly limited (over 1 mile)	15
	Moderately limited (over 1/2 mile)	10
	Severely limited (over 1/4 mile)	5
	Unable to walk	0
	Up-down stairs or inclines	
	No difficulty	8
	Slight difficulty	6
	One step at a time (instability)	4
	Unable	0
	Squatting	
	No difficulty	5
	Slight difficulty	4
	Moderate limitation (not past 90)	3
	Unable	0
	Running	
	No difficulty	5
	Slight difficulty	4
	Straight only (unable to cut)	3
	Unable	0
	Jumping	
	No difficulty	2
	Unable	0

Range of Motion

0 to 45
    Deduct 1 for each 10 of loss. Max. 5 points.
45 to 90
    Deduct 1 for each 15 of loss. Max 3 points.
90 to 130
    Deduct 1 for each 20 of loss. Max 2 points.
                                Total _____

Anatomy (10 points)

ABSENCE OF DEFORMITY

(5 points)	*Genu valgus or varum*	
	0 to 15	2
	15 to 30	1
	Over 30	0
	Recurvatum	
	None	0
	Over 5	0
	Flexion contracture	
	None	1
	Over 15	0
	Patellar abnormality	
	None	1
	Lateral positions	0
	High riding	0
	Increased mobility	0

ATROPHY—THIGH (2 points)	None	2
	Less than 1 cm	1 1/2
	1 to 3 cm	1
	3 cm or more	0

SWELLING (3 points)	None	3
	Slight or occasional	1
	Moderate or frequent	1/2
	Marked or persistent	0

Pain

(30 points)	None	30
	Slight (no compromise in activity)	25
	Mild	20
	Moderate	15
	Severe	5
	Disabled	0

TOTAL MOTION POINTS
(Nearest whole number)   _____

SUBTOTAL   1. FUNCTION   _____
               2. ANATOMY   _____
               3. PAIN   _____
               4. RANGE OF MOTIONS   _____

               TOTAL RATING _____

B
_____

Figure 35–4, cont'd. **B**, Original Larson Knee Scale. (**B**, From Larson R: Rating sheet for the knee function. In Smillie IS [ed]: *Diseases of the Knee Joint*, 2nd ed. New York, Churchill Livingstone, 1979.)

ADDITIONAL CRITERIA
Graded but not included in number rating. Check appropriate analysis

A. FUNCTIONAL TESTS

1. *Ligamentous laxity*

Medial at 0
- _ _ _ _ _ _ _ _ _ _ none
- _ _ _ _ _ _ _ _ _ _ slight
- _ _ _ _ _ _ _ _ _ _ moderate
- _ _ _ _ _ _ _ _ _ _ severe

Medial at 30
- _ _ _ _ _ _ _ _ _ _ none
- _ _ _ _ _ _ _ _ _ _ slight
- _ _ _ _ _ _ _ _ _ _ moderate
- _ _ _ _ _ _ _ _ _ _ severe

Lateral
- _ _ _ _ _ _ _ _ _ _ none
- _ _ _ _ _ _ _ _ _ _ slight
- _ _ _ _ _ _ _ _ _ _ moderate
- _ _ _ _ _ _ _ _ _ _ severe

Posterior cruciate
- _ _ _ _ _ _ _ _ _ _ none
- _ _ _ _ _ _ _ _ _ _ slight
- _ _ _ _ _ _ _ _ _ _ moderate
- _ _ _ _ _ _ _ _ _ _ severe

Anterior cruciate
- _ _ _ _ _ _ _ _ _ _ none
- _ _ _ _ _ _ _ _ _ _ slight
- _ _ _ _ _ _ _ _ _ _ moderate
- _ _ _ _ _ _ _ _ _ _ severe

Rotary—30 internal
- _ _ _ _ _ _ _ _ _ _ none
- _ _ _ _ _ _ _ _ _ _ slight
- _ _ _ _ _ _ _ _ _ _ moderate
- _ _ _ _ _ _ _ _ _ _ severe

Rotary—15 external
- _ _ _ _ _ _ _ _ _ _ none
- _ _ _ _ _ _ _ _ _ _ slight
- _ _ _ _ _ _ _ _ _ _ moderate
- _ _ _ _ _ _ _ _ _ _ severe

2. *Muscle weakness*

Extensor mechanism
- _ _ _ _ _ _ _ _ _ _ strong
- _ _ _ _ _ _ _ _ _ _ weak to resistance
- _ _ _ _ _ _ _ _ _ _ able to extend against gravity
- _ _ _ _ _ _ _ _ _ _ extends with gravity
- _ _ _ _ _ _ _ _ _ _ eliminated
- _ _ _ _ _ _ _ _ _ _ flail

Flexor mechanism
- _ _ _ _ _ _ _ _ _ _ strong
- _ _ _ _ _ _ _ _ _ _ weak to resistance
- _ _ _ _ _ _ _ _ _ _ able to extend against gravity
- _ _ _ _ _ _ _ _ _ _ extends with gravity
- _ _ _ _ _ _ _ _ _ _ eliminated
- _ _ _ _ _ _ _ _ _ _ flail

B. X-RAY

1. Congruity of joint
- _ _ _ _ _ _ _ _ _ _ good
- _ _ _ _ _ _ _ _ _ _ fair
- _ _ _ _ _ _ _ _ _ _ poor

2. Osteophyte formation
- _ _ _ _ _ _ _ _ _ _ none
- _ _ _ _ _ _ _ _ _ _ slight
- _ _ _ _ _ _ _ _ _ _ moderate
- _ _ _ _ _ _ _ _ _ _ marked

3. Joint separation on stress

Valgus stress
- _ _ _ _ _ _ _ _ _ _ none
- _ _ _ _ _ _ _ _ _ _ slight
- _ _ _ _ _ _ _ _ _ _ moderate
- _ _ _ _ _ _ _ _ _ _ marked

Varus stress
- _ _ _ _ _ _ _ _ _ _ none
- _ _ _ _ _ _ _ _ _ _ slight
- _ _ _ _ _ _ _ _ _ _ moderate
- _ _ _ _ _ _ _ _ _ _ marked

4. Patellar-femoral congruity
- _ _ _ _ _ _ _ _ _ _ nomal
- _ _ _ _ _ _ _ _ _ _ fair
- _ _ _ _ _ _ _ _ _ _ poor

5. Osteopenia
- _ _ _ _ _ _ _ _ _ _ none
- _ _ _ _ _ _ _ _ _ _ mild
- _ _ _ _ _ _ _ _ _ _ moderate
- _ _ _ _ _ _ _ _ _ _ severe

6. Fracture or arthrodesis
- _ _ _ _ _ _ _ _ _ _ union
- _ _ _ _ _ _ _ _ _ _ non-union

C. PATIENT'S EVALUATION
- _ _ _ _ _ _ _ _ _ _ Enthusiastic
- _ _ _ _ _ _ _ _ _ _ Satisfied
- _ _ _ _ _ _ _ _ _ _ Non-committal
- _ _ _ _ _ _ _ _ _ _ Dissatisfied

D. PSYCHOSOCIAL
- _ _ _ _ _ _ _ _ _ _ Better ability in desired activities
- _ _ _ _ _ _ _ _ _ _ Same ability in activities
- _ _ _ _ _ _ _ _ _ _ Lessened ability in activities

E. MOTIVATION
- _ _ _ _ _ _ _ _ _ _ Excellent
- _ _ _ _ _ _ _ _ _ _ Good
- _ _ _ _ _ _ _ _ _ _ Average
- _ _ _ _ _ _ _ _ _ _ Poor

F. COMPENSATION–LITIGATION
- _ _ _ _ _ _ _ _ _ _ Present
- _ _ _ _ _ _ _ _ _ _ Not present

G. COMPLICATIONS
- _ _ _ _ _ _ _ _ _ _ Post-op. infection
- _ _ _ _ _ _ _ _ _ _ Post-op. hematoma
- _ _ _ _ _ _ _ _ _ _ Nerve damage
- _ _ _ _ _ _ _ _ _ _ Vascular damage
- _ _ _ _ _ _ _ _ _ _ Thrombophlebitis
- _ _ _ _ _ _ _ _ _ _ Growth disturbance
- _ _ _ _ _ _ _ _ _ _ Mal-union of fracture

B2

Figure 35–4, cont'd.

Lysholm Knee Scoring Scale

Limp (5 points)	
None	5
Slight or periodical	3
Severe and constant	0
Support (5 points)	
None	5
Stick or crutch	2
Weight-bearing impossible	0
Locking (15 points)	
No locking and no catching sensations	15
Catching sensation but no locking	10
Locking	
Occasionally	6
Frequently	2
Locked joint on examination	0
Instability (25 points)	
Never giving way	25
Rarely during athletics or other severe exertion	20
Frequently during athletics or other severe exertion (or incapable of participation)	15
Occasionaly in daily activities	10
Often in daily activities	5
Every step	0

Pain (25 points)	
None	25
Inconstant and slight during severe exertion	20
Marked during severe exertion	15
Marked on or after walking more than 2 km	10
Marked on or after walking less than 2 km	5
Constant	0
Swelling (10 points)	
None	10
On severe exertion	6
On ordinary exertion	2
Constant	0
Stair-climbing (10 points)	
No problems	10
Slightly impaired	6
One step at a time	2
Impossible	0
Squatting (5 points)	
No problems	5
Slightly impaired	4
Not beyond 90	2
Impossible	0

C

Figure 35–4, cont'd. **C,** Modified Lysholm Knee Scoring Scale. (**C,** From Tegner Y, Lysholm J: Rating systems in the evaluation of knee ligament injuries. Clin Orthop 198:43, 1985.)

patients with few symptoms and symptomatic, highly active individuals. It categorizes the relative activity level of various recreational and competitive sports and types of labor (light, moderate, or heavy). Tegner and Lysholm[44] discovered that approximately 20% of patients with low activity had a high modified Lysholm Knee Scoring Scale score. Inclusion of the Tegner Activity Score with the modified Lysholm Knee Scoring Scale prevents a sedentary patient from receiving a higher score. The score does not discriminate between participation in activities on a daily basis and the occasional athlete. It assumes that competitive athletes are active on a regular schedule. However, a recreational athlete, for example, may play basketball 5 days per week or once a month (this rating system would give both the same score). Nevertheless, the system does thoroughly delineate between various sports activities. In addition, unlike many other activity scores, this one includes different levels of labor for patients who do not participate in sports. This scale has been determined to have high intrarater reliability ($rp = .97$) and to be a valuable addition to the Lysholm score because patients could rate highly subjectively without participating in their former activities.[34] Effects of age or health status are not included.

The Revised HSSKS

Hanley and Warren[11] updated the HSSKS in 1987. In 1988, Windsor and coworkers[49] revised the HSSKS (Fig. 35–6) to update and improve the original form and to facilitate the orthopedic surgeon's assessment of ligament injuries. This 100-point system is composed of subjective symptoms, subjective function, and objective functional sections.

The first section of the knee ligament rating form is assessment of the patient's symptoms. This section is given a total of 5 points: 2 for the absence of swelling and 3 for the absence of locking symptoms. The second section (total of 20 points) assesses the symptom of giving way. This section is weighted heavily because the scale primarily measures instability, as did the original HSSKS. Giving way is divided into severity and frequency. Severity of giving way is measured by the length of time required for the patient to recover from each episode. Frequency of giving way is also assigned points. The more frequently the giving way occurs, the fewer points are given. The third and final part of the subjective section is the functional assessment, which is divided into activities of daily living and work, sports, and ability to perform specific maneuvers with the knee, each of which is assigned a point value (see Fig. 35–6).

The objective examination consists of determination of range of motion, effusion, thigh circumference, and ligament stability. Points are given on the basis of 5-mm excursions: 1+ (0 to 5 mm), 2+ (5 to 10 mm), and 3+ (>10 mm); the endpoint is noted. Pivot shift and reverse pivot shift are documented. Pivot shift is classified as negative or equal to that in the unaffected knee. Grind, crepitus, or a "grinding" sensation is detected rather than any movement: 1+, slight movement of the tibia; 2+, definite movement without locking; and 3+, definite movement with a locking sensation.

The next section of this score is the functional examination (total, 10 points). A single-leg standing broad jump is used as the functional test. Windsor et al[49] believe that this test reliably discriminates functional ability related to

Activity Score	

10. Competitive sports
    Soccer—national and international elite
9. Competitive sports
    Soccer, lower divisions
    Ice hockey
    Wrestling
    Gymnastics
8. Competitive sports
    Bandy
    Squash or badminton
    Athletics (jumping, etc.)
    Downhill skiing
7. Competitive sports
    Tennis
    Athletics (running)
    Motorcross, speedway
    Handball
    Basketball
  Recreational sports
    Soccer
    Bandy and ice hockey
    Squash
    Athletics (jumping)
    Cross-country track findings both
      recreational and competitive
6. Recreational sports
    Tennis and badminton
    Handball
    Basketball
    Downhill skiing
    Jogging, at least five times per week
	5. Work
	    Heavy labor (e.g., building, forestry)
	  Competitive sports
	    Cycling
	    Cross-country skiing
	  Recreational sports
	    Jogging on uneven ground at least twice
	      weekly
	4. Work
	    Moderately heavy labor
	      (e.g., truck driving, heavy domestic
	      work)
	  Recreational sports
	    Cycling
	    Cross-country skiing
	    Jogging on even ground at least twice
	      weekly
	3. Work
	    Light labor (e.g., nursing)
	  Competitive and recreational sports
	    Swimming
	    Walking in forest possible
	2. Work
	    Light labor
	  Walking on even ground possible but
	      impossible to walk in forest
	1. Work
	    Sedentary work
	    Walking on uneven ground possible
	0. Sick leave or disability pension because of
	      knee problems

Figure 35–5. Tegner Activity Scale form. (From Tegner Y, Lysholm J: Rating systems in the evaluation of knee ligament injuries. Clin Orthop 198:43, 1985.)

cruciate function. The score is expressed as a percentage. The patient jumps as far as possible on the unaffected leg (numerator). The best of three jumps is measured in centimeters, and this is compared with the best of three attempts completed on the injured or the involved knee (denominator). This test requires the patient to perform maximum acceleration and deceleration movements on each knee. This tests the stability of the ligament as the patient lands on one leg, thereby causing knee torsion. The patient must land firmly on the affected leg and not be allowed to quickly transfer weight to the uninvolved leg.

The last section of the score is the deduction section; it is divided between derotation brace and pain. Points are deducted if a brace is required for stability and/or if a patient has pain. A weighting factor of 3 is used if the pain is secondary to a PCL deficiency because the only symptom that a PCL-deficient patient manifests is pain. Thus, if a patient has continuous pain secondary to PCL deficiency, a total of 30 points is deducted from the total score.

The last section of this knee rating system is not assigned a point value. Patients are placed in a sports category depending on their level of involvement. The level of involvement is divided into very stressful, moderately stressful, and mildly stressful categories (see Fig. 35–6). Placing a patient in a particular category allows the physician to recognize at what activity levels the symptoms are occurring. The final score is rated as excellent (90 to 100 points), good (80 to 89 points), fair (70 to 79 points), or poor (<70 points). This system takes about 14 minutes to administer and is probably less frequently used. Notably,

it is more sensitive to PCL injury, but has not been justified statistically.[23]

Swiss Orthopaedic Society Knee Study Group Evaluation

In the same year as the revised HSSKS, the Swiss Orthopaedic Society Knee (Orthopaedische Arbeitsgruppe Knie [OAK]) study group, led by Muller et al,[33] developed a knee evaluation form based on "shells" of instability. This short form (Fig. 35–7) can be conveniently completed in the clinic, and it identifies technical problems of the knee rather than giving a knee score. Before the form is completed, the patient is classified according to preinjury activity level and assigned to one of the three groups: little stress (no sports), moderate stress (sports with controlled movements), and substantial stress (construction worker, contact sports).

A normal knee scores 100 points. The form has four columns that represent four categories of problems: category A, parameters connected with pain and swelling; category B, parameters concerning strength and range of motion; category C, stability parameters; and category D, function.

Four different factors have to be taken into account to rate the results as excellent, good, fair, or poor. The first factor is the total score: 91 to 100 points (excellent), 81 to 90 points (good), 71 to 80 points (fair), and less than 70 points (poor). The second factor is that each category is also evaluated separately. The maximum possible scores

THE HOSPITAL FOR SPECIAL SURGERY KNEE LIGAMENT RATING FORM

NAME _____ HSS# _____ AGE _____ SEX: M F

DIAGNOSIS: ACL PCL MM LM MCL LCL ACUTE CHRONIC PREVIOUS SURGERY _____

INJURY DATE _____   OPERATIVE DATE _____   TYPE _____

		LEFT						RIGHT				
SYMPTOMS (5)	Score	pre	6mo	1yr	2yr	3yr	4yr	pre	6mo	1yr	2yr	3yr	4yr

SYMPTOMS (5)

SWELLING:
No _____ 2
Yes _____ 0
LOCKING:
No _____ 3
Yes _____ 0

GIVING WAY (20)
SEVERITY:
None _____ 10
Transient _____ 8
Recovery < 1 day _____ 6
Recovery < 1 week _____ 2
Recovery > 1 week _____ 0
FREQUENCY:
None _____ 10
1 per year _____ 8
2–6 per year _____ 6
1 per month _____ 4
1 per week _____ 2
Daily _____ 0

FUNCTION (20)
ADL AND WORK:
Full return _____ 4
Limited, or job change _____ 2
Unable due to knee _____ 0
SPORTS:
Full return _____ 4
Same but modified _____ 3
Different sport _____ 2
No return _____ 0
ABILITY TO:
Decelerate _____ 4
Cut side-to-side _____ 4
Jump _____ 4

EXAMINATION (45)
ROM:
Normal _____ 3
Limited flexion or extension ___ 1
Both _____ 0
EFFUSION:
No _____ 4
Yes _____ 0
THIGH CIRCUMFERENCE:
Equal to 1cm difference _____ 2
> 1cm difference _____ 0
LACHMAN: (note end point)
Negative _____ 4
1+ (0–5 mm) _____ 3
2+ (5–10 mm) _____ 2
3+ (10–15 mm) _____ 0

Figure 35–6. Revised Hospital for Special Surgery Knee Score (HSSKS) form. (From Windsor RE, Insall JN, Warren RF, et al: The Hospital for Special Surgery knee ligament rating form. Am J Knee Surg 1:140, 1988.)

		LEFT						RIGHT					
EXAMINATION (45)	Score	pre	6mo	1yr	2yr	3yr	4yr	pre	6mo	1yr	2yr	3yr	4yr
ANTERIOR DRAWER:													
Negative	2												
1+ (0–5mm)	2												
2+ (5–10mm)	0												
3+ (10–15mm)	0												
POSTERIOR DRAWER:													
Negative	5												
1+ (0–5mm)	3												
2+ (5–10mm)	2												
3+ (10–15mm)	0												
PIVOT SHIFT:													
Negative (or equal to Unaffected side)	10												
Grind, no movement	8												
1+, slight movement	4												
2+, definite movement	2												
3+, movement and locks	0												
MCL:													
Normal	5												
1+	3												
2+	2												
3+	0												
LCL:													
Normal	5												
1+	3												
2+	2												
3+	0												
REVERSE PIVOT SHIFT:													
Negative	5												
Positive	0												
FUNCTIONAL EXAM (10)													
STANDING FORWARD JUMP %													
DIFFERENCE BETWEEN LEGS:													
90–100%	10												
75–90%	7												
50–75%	5												
50%	0												

SCORE: _____

DEDUCTIONS		
DEROTATION BRACE:		
Security of mind	2	
Due to instability	4	
PAIN: (if PCL, X3)		
None	0	
Occasional aching	2	
After stressful sports	5	
After daily activities	8	
Continuous	10	

TOTAL SCORE: _____

SPORTS CATEGORIES (A = Very Stressful, B = Moderately Stressful, C = Mildly Stressful)

A	B	C
Basketball	Professional Dance	X-Country Skiing
Volleyball	Football	Jogging
Gymnastics	Rugby	Tennis (doubles)
Soccer	Racquetball	Swimming
	Squash	Bicycling
	Handball	Fencing
	Tennis (singles)	Boxing
	Downhill Skiing	Golf

Figure 35–6, cont'd.

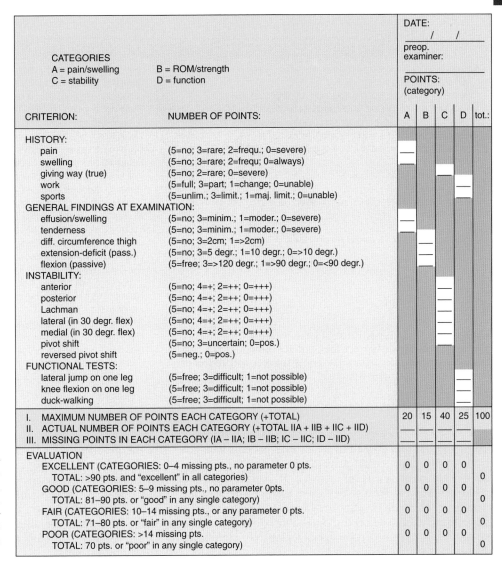

CATEGORIES							
A = pain/swelling B = ROM/strength							
C = stability D = function							

DATE: ___/___/___
preop.
examiner: _____

POINTS: (category)

CRITERION:	NUMBER OF POINTS:	A	B	C	D	tot.:
HISTORY:						
pain	(5=no; 3=rare; 2=frequ.; 0=severe)					
swelling	(5=no; 3=rare; 2=frequ; 0=always)					
giving way (true)	(5=no; 2=rare; 0=severe)					
work	(5=full; 3=part; 1=change; 0=unable)					
sports	(5=unlim.; 3=limit.; 1=maj. limit.; 0=unable)					
GENERAL FINDINGS AT EXAMINATION:						
effusion/swelling	(5=no; 3=minim.; 1=moder.; 0=severe)					
tenderness	(5=no; 3=minim.; 1=moder.; 0=severe)					
diff. circumference thigh	(5=no; 3=2cm; 1=>2cm)					
extension-deficit (pass.)	(5=no; 3=5 degr.; 1=10 degr.; 0=>10 degr.)					
flexion (passive)	(5=free; 3=>120 degr.; 1=>90 degr.; 0=<90 degr.)					
INSTABILITY:						
anterior	(5=no; 4=+; 2=++; 0=+++)					
posterior	(5=no; 4=+; 2=++; 0=+++)					
Lachman	(5=no; 4=+; 2=++; 0=+++)					
lateral (in 30 degr. flex)	(5=no; 4=+; 2=++; 0=+++)					
medial (in 30 degr. flex)	(5=no; 4=+; 2=++; 0=+++)					
pivot shift	(5=no; 3=uncertain; 0=pos.)					
reversed pivot shift	(5=neg.; 0=pos.)					
FUNCTIONAL TESTS:						
lateral jump on one leg	(5=free; 3=difficult; 1=not possible)					
knee flexion on one leg	(5=free; 3=difficult; 1=not possible)					
duck-walking	(5=free; 3=difficult; 1=not possible)					
I. MAXIMUM NUMBER OF POINTS EACH CATEGORY (+TOTAL)		20	15	40	25	100
II. ACTUAL NUMBER OF POINTS EACH CATEGORY (+TOTAL IIA + IIB + IIC + IID)						
III. MISSING POINTS IN EACH CATEGORY (IA – IIA; IB – IIB; IC – IIC; ID – IID)						

EVALUATION	A	B	C	D	
EXCELLENT (CATEGORIES: 0–4 missing pts., no parameter 0 pts.	0	0	0	0	
TOTAL: >90 pts. and "excellent" in all categories)					0
GOOD (CATEGORIES: 5–9 missing pts., no parameter 0pts.	0	0	0	0	
TOTAL: 81–90 pts. or "good" in any single category)					0
FAIR (CATEGORIES: 10–14 missing pts., or any parameter 0 pts.	0	0	0	0	
TOTAL: 71–80 pts. or "fair" in any single category)					0
POOR (CATEGORIES: >14 missing pts.	0	0	0	0	
TOTAL: 70 pts. or "poor" in any single category)					0

Figure 35–7. Swiss Orthopaedic Society Knee (OAK) evaluation form. (Redrawn from Muller W, Biedert R, Hefti F, et al: OAK knee evaluation: A new way to assess knee ligament injuries. Clin Orthop 232:37, 1988.)

are 20 points in category A, 15 points in category B, 40 points in category C, and 25 points in category D. The third factor depends on the missing points in each category: 0 to 4 missing points (excellent), 5 to 9 missing points (good), 10 to 14 missing points (fair), and more than 14 missing points (poor). The overall result can never be better than that in the worst category. The fourth factor is that if there is even a single parameter with zero, the overall result cannot be better than fair.

Muller et al[33] compared the OAK evaluation form with the revised HSSKS and found that the HSSKS gave the patient a higher rating (82.7% versus 75%). They concluded that the OAK evaluation provides a more accurate assessment of knee function. The OAK form is not widely used in the United States.[48]

Cincinnati Knee Ligament Rating Scale

In 1990, Noyes and colleagues[35] stated that major sources of error in existing scoring scales include the combination of different variables into an overall score and the random allocation of point ranges into categories such as excellent, good, fair, and poor. They introduced a sports activity rating scale, assessment of function, and symptom rating. The activity scale (Fig. 35–8) addresses the frequency of participation and specific knee functions required. It includes four basic levels based on the frequency of participation (level I, 4 to 7 days per week; level II, 1 to 3 days per week; level III, 1 to 3 times per month; and level IV, no sports). Within levels I to III, the scale is further classified according to the type of activity. Jumping and pivoting receive the highest number of points, followed by running and twisting and finally activities that require no pivoting, jumping, or twisting (e.g., swimming and cycling). Patients who do not participate in sports are penalized in the activity rating scale, but they can be evaluated in the symptom and functional rating scales; therefore, it is important to report each separately. The assessment of function (see Fig. 35–8) includes both activities of daily living (walking, stairs, and squatting) and sports activity (running, jumping, and twisting). Even if patients do not run, jump, or twist on a regular basis, they are asked whether they could. Again, this permits separate evaluation of patients who cannot participate in sports.

SYMPTOM-RATING SCALE*	
Description	Points
Normal knee; able to do strenuous work/sports with jumping, hard pivoting	10
Able to do moderate work/sports with running, turning, twisting; symptoms with strenuous work/sports	8
Able to do light work/sports with no running, twisting, jumping; symptoms with moderate work/sports	6
Able to do activities of daily living alone; symptoms with light work/sports	4
Moderate symptoms (frequent, limiting) with activities of daily living	2
Severe symptoms (constant, not relieved) with activities of daily living	0

* The symptoms that are rated are pain, swelling, partial giving-way and full giving-way.

A

Figure 35–8. Cincinnati Knee Ligament Rating Scale form. (From Noyes FR, Barber SD, Mangine RE: Bone-patellar, ligament-bone, and fascia lata allografts for reconstruction of the anterior cruciate ligament. J Bone Joint Surg Am 72:1125, 1990.)

SPORTS ACTIVITIES RATING SCALE	
	Points
Level I (participates 4–7 days per wk.)	
Jumping, hard pivoting, cutting (basketball, volleyball, football, gymnastics, soccer)	100
Running, twisting, turning (tennis, racquetball, handball, baseball, ice hockey, field hockey, skiing, wrestling)	95
No running, twisting, jumping (cycling, swimming)	90
Level II (participates 1–3 days per wk.)	
Jumping, hard pivoting, cutting (basketball, volleyball, football, gymnastics, soccer)	85
Running, twisting, turning (tennis, racquetball, handball, baseball, ice hockey, field hockey, skiing, wrestling)	80
No running, twisting, jumping (cycling, swimming)	75
Level III (participates 1–3 days per mo.)	
Jumping, hard pivoting, cutting (basketball, volleyball, football, gymnastics, soccer)	65
Running, twisting, turning (tennis, racquetball, handball, baseball, ice hockey, field hockey, skiing, wrestling)	60
No running, twisting, jumping (cycling, swimming)	55
Level IV (no sports)	
Performs activities of daily living without problems.	40
Has moderate problems with activities of daily living.	20
Has severe problems with activities of daily living—on crutches, full disability.	0

B

The symptoms scale (see Fig. 35–8) asks patients whether pain, swelling, or partial or complete giving way occurs during different levels of activity. If patients do not perform certain activities, they are to predict whether they would be able to do so without symptoms if required. The scale is intended to detect the "knee abuser" who performs strenuous activities despite having clinically significant symptoms such as giving way.

This rating scale, along with the final rating scheme (see Fig. 35–8), was applied to a group of 47 consecutive patients who underwent ACL reconstruction.[36] An important aspect of this study was that the final rating did not arbitrarily assign point ranges to categories of excellent, good, and so on. Instead, the overall rating was determined by the lowest scores in any single area. For example, if the patient has an excellent rating for everything but has some limitations with jumping, the final rating would be good instead of excellent. We agree with Noyes and associates[35,36] that this scheme provides for the most valid assessment of treatment results.

Barber-Westin et al[3] and Marx et al[29] have confirmed the validity, reliability, and responsiveness of the Cincinnati Knee Ligament Rating Scale. Sgaglione et al[41] found it to be more precise and specific than the Lysholm, Tegner, and HSSKS for athletic patients. However, the 17 minutes required to administer the test deters some from using it.

Visual Analog Scale

Flandry and colleagues[8] emphasized the use of a continuous method of magnitude expression to eliminate many of the problems associated with knee rating systems that use a point rating (Fig. 35–9). These problems include investigator bias, patient compliance, interpretation bias, and sensitivity. Because subjective complaints are difficult to measure and analyze, unlike objective testing such as range of motion or thigh circumference, they recommended using a visual analog scale (VAS) to analyze subjective knee data.

The VAS is a graphic, continuous method of expression by which the patient describes the magnitude of a subjective symptom. It consists of a line of specified length, in this case 100 mm, with polar descriptors of the two extremes of a given experience at each end of the line (see Fig. 35–9). Patients read the question and place a mark on the line at the point that they feel best represents their symptom relative to the two extremes. This mark can be converted to a numerical value by simple measurement techniques.

Flandry et al[8] cited several advantages to use of the VAS, such as validity, increased patient compliance, greater sensitivity of measurement, reduced bias, graphic representation, and numerical analysis.

International Knee Documentation Committee Knee Ligament Standard Evaluation Form

Because of the lack of standard nomenclature and scoring systems for evaluation of ligament pathology, the International Knee Documentation Committee (IKDC) was

ASSESSMENT OF FUNCTION			
Activities of Daily Living	Points	Sports	Points
Walking		Straight running	
Normal, unlimited	40	Fully competitive	100
Some limitations	30	Some limitations, guarding	80
Only 3–4 blocks possible	20	Run half-speed, definite limitations	60
Less than 1 block, cane, crutch	0	Not able to do	40
Stair-climbing		Jumping/landing on affected leg	
Normal, unlimited	40	Fully competitive	100
Some limitations	30	Some limitations, guarding	80
Only 11–30 steps possible	20	Definite limitations, half-speed	60
Only 1–10 steps possible	0	Not able to do	40
Squatting kneeling		Hard twisting/cutting/pivoting	
Normal, unlimited	40	Fully competitive	100
Some limitations	30	Some limitations, guarding	80
Only 6–10 possible	20	Definite limitations, half-speed	60
Only 0–5 possible	0	Not able to do	40

C

SCHEME FOR FINAL RATING*				
	Excellent	Good	Fair	Poor
Pain	10	8	6–4	2–0
Swelling	10	8	6–4	2–0
Partial giving-way	10	8	6–4	2–0
Full giving-way	10	8	6–4	2–0
Walking	40	30	20	0
Stairs / Squatting } (score lowest)	40	30	20	0
Running	100	80	60	40
Jumping	100	80	60	40
Hard twists, cuts, pivots	100	80	60	40
Effusion (ml)	Normal	< 25	26–60	> 60
Lack of flexion (degrees)	0–5	6–15	16–30	> 30
Lack of extension (degrees)	0–3	4–5	6–10	> 10
Tibiofemoral crepitus†	Normal		Mod.	Severe
Patellofemoral crepitus†	Normal		Mod.	Severe
Anterior displacement (KT-1000)	< 3 mm	3–5 mm	6 mm	> 6 mm
Pivot-shift test	Neg.	Slip	Definite	Severe
Joint-space narrowing				
Medial tibiofemoral (radiographs)‡	Normal	Mild	Mod.	Severe
Lateral tibiofemoral (radiographs)‡	Normal	Mild	Mod.	Severe
Patellofemoral (radiographs)‡	Normal	Mild	Mod.	Severe
Functional testing (limb symmetry)§ (per cent)	100–85	84–75	74–65	< 65

* Rating for pain, swelling, partial giving-way, and full giving-way—see Table I. Rating for walking, stairs, squatting, running, jumping, hard twists, cuts, and pivots—see Table III.
† Moderate indicates definite fibrillation and cartilage abnormality of 25 to 50 degrees, and severe, cartilage abnormality of more than 50 degrees.
‡ Moderate indicates narrowing of less than one-half of the joint space, and severe, of more than one-half of the joint space.
§ Use of average of at least three one-legged hop-type tests.

D

Figure 35–8, cont'd.

formed in 1987. This committee consisted of 11 North American members (from the AOSSM) and 11 European members (from the European Society for Knee Surgery and Arthroscopy). They met over the course of several years to analyze existing scoring scales and attempted to define valid and reliable criteria for measurement. In an effort to improve communication among physicians, the committee also developed and defined standard terminology used in the literature and in scoring scales.[36]

The IKDC Knee Ligament Standard Evaluation Form, along with instructions for use (Fig. 35–10), was introduced in 1993. Hefti et al[12] published the first version, and

KNEE DISORDERS SUBJECTIVE HISTORY

NAME _____

CHART _____ DATE _____ SIDE: L R

For each question, shade in a box between the two descriptions which you think describes your knee relative to the two extremes. Please complete both sides of this form.

1. How often does your knee hurt?
never [ ] daily, even at rest

2. How bad is the pain at its worst?
none [ ] severe, requiring pain pills every few hours

3. Do you have swelling in your knee?
never [ ] daily, even at rest

4. Does your knee give way or buckle?
never [ ] I must guard my knee to prevent giving way even with normal everyday activity

5. Does your knee lock up so you are unable to straighten it?
never [ ] I must guard my knee to prevent locking even with normal everyday activity

6. Does your knee catch or hang up when moving?
never [ ] I must guard my knee to prevent catching even with normal everyday activity

7. Is your knee stiff?
none [ ] I can barely move my knee because of stiffness

8. Are you able to walk on level ground?
no problem [ ] unable

9. Are you able to walk on rough ground, inclines, or negotiate curves?
no problem [ ] unable

10. Do you ever need crutches, cane or walker to walk?
never [ ] always

11. Do you feel grinding when your knee moves?
none [ ] severe

12. Do you have problems twisting or pivoting on your injured knee?
none [ ] unable

13. Do you have problems carrying heavy objects because of your knee?
none [ ] unable   ☐ not attempted

14. Do you have problems climbing stairs?
none [ ] unable   ☐ not attempted

15. Do you have problems going down stairs?
none [ ] unable   ☐ not attempted

16. Do you have problems running?
none [ ] unable   ☐ not attempted

17. Do you have problems decelerating (slowing down) after running or jogging?
none [ ] unable   ☐ not attempted

18. Do you have problems cutting (changing directions while running by pivoting on affected knee)?
none [ ] unable   ☐ not attempted

19. Do you have problems jumping?
none [ ] unable   ☐ not attempted

20. Do you have problems taking part in competitive sports?
none [ ] unable   ☐ not attempted

21. Do you have night pain?
none [ ] severe

22. Do you have problems kneeling?
no problem [ ] unable   ☐ not attempted

23. Do you have problems squatting?
no problem [ ] unable   ☐ not attempted

24. Do you have problems getting in and out of a car?
no problem [ ] unable

25. Does your knee ache while you are sitting?
never [ ] always

26. Do you have problems getting in or out of a chair?
no problem [ ] unable

27. Do you have stiffness or discomfort when you first start to walk?
none [ ] always

28. Do you have problems turning over in bed?
none [ ] unable

HUGHSTON SPORTS MEDICINE FOUNDATION, INC.   HUGHSTON SPORTS MEDICINE FOUNDATION, INC.

Figure 35–9. Visual analog scale (VAS) form. (Redrawn from Flandry F, Hunt JP, Terry GC, et al: Analysis of subjective knee complaints using visual analog scales. Am J Sports Med 19:112, 1991.)

it has been updated several times.[1,17,47] The Standard Knee Evaluation Form is a patient-reported system based on a 100-point scale that includes 18 questions covering symptoms, sports activities, and function. Its content validity, test-retest reliability, and responsiveness were demonstrated by Irrgang et al in 2001,[17] with a score change of 11.5 representing a true change over time. The overall rating was similar to that used by Noyes and colleagues[36] in the Cincinnati Knee Ligament Rating Scale in that the lowest grade in any single category determines the final score. In the IKDC form, the activity level and eight sections are recorded; each is to be reported separately for publication.[18] However, only the first four sections are required to determine the final rating. Activity is recorded on four levels (level I, strenuous; level II, moderate; level III, light; and level IV, sedentary) at three time periods (preinjury, pretreatment, and post-treatment), which is important for assessing improvement in chronically deficient patients. A grade of normal (A), nearly normal (B), abnormal (C), or severely abnormal (D) is given in each category. In addition to subjective functions and symptoms, range of motion, ligament examination, compartmental findings, harvest site pathology, radiographic degeneration, and functional testing (single-leg

hop) are recorded. Manual labor is included, but the frequency of activity participation is not. Recording both preinjury and pretreatment activity levels is particularly important for patients with chronic ligamentous deficiencies. For example, a patient who had an ACL deficiency for 5 years and participated in level I activities before injury had to decrease to level III activities before treatment because of the injury. After treatment, the patient is able to perform level II activities. When compared with preinjury status, the patient has had a decline in activity level; however, because of the operation, the patient has improved from the preoperative level. Recording only the preinjury and post-treatment activity levels would not have shown this improvement.

Quality of Life Outcome Measure

The Quality of Life Outcome Measure was introduced in 1998 by Mohtadi[32] as a patient-reported subjective survey designed to evaluate the quality of life in patients with ACL-deficient knees. Using a 100-point base, it consists of 35 items divided into five categories: (1) symptoms, (2)

THE IKDC KNEE LIGAMENT STANDARD EVALUATION FORM *[1]

Name: _____   First name: _____   DOB: _/_/_ Med. rec. #: _____

Examiner: _____   Date of examination: _/_/_   Date of injury/ies: _/_/_ ; _/_/_   Date of surgeries: _/_/_ ; _/_/_

Cause of injury   : □ADL *[2] □traff. □non-pivoting non-contact sports □pivoting non-contact sp. □contact sp. □ work

Time inj. to surg. : _____ (months)   □ acute (0–2 weeks) □ subacute (2–8 weeks)   □ chronic (>8 weeks)

Knee involved   : □r. □l.   opposite knee: □norm. □injured   exam. under anesthes.: □ yes □no

Postop. diagnosis: _____

Surgical proced. : _____

Status menisci   : norm□med.□lat. 1/3 removed:□med.□lat. 2/3 removed:□med□lat. compl. rem.□med.□lat.

Morphotype   :   □lax.   □ normal   □ tight   □varus   □ valgus

Activ. level *[3]   :   preinjury: □I   □II   □III   □ IV   pretreatment: □ I □II   □III   □ IV
                       present: □I   □II   □III   □ IV   Eventual change knee-related: □yes □ no

GROUPS (PROBLEM AREA)	QUALIFICATION WITHIN GROUPS *[4] A: normal B: nearly norm. C: abnormal D: sev. abnorm.				GROUP QUALIFIC. A B C D*[4]
1. PATIENT SUBJECTIVE ASSESSMENT					
How does your knee function?	□ normally	□near norm.	□ abnormally	□ sev. abnorm.	
On a scale of 0 to 3 how does your knee affect your activity level?	□ 0	□ 1	□ 2	□ 3	□ □ □ □
2. SYMPTOMS (absence of significant symptoms, at highest activity level known by patient) *[5]					
No pain at activity level *[3]	□I	□II	□III	□ IV or worse	
No swelling at activity level *[3]	□I	□II	□III	□ IV or worse	
No partial giving way at activity level *[3]	□I	□II	□III	□ IV or worse	
No complete giving way at activity level *[3]	□I	□II	□III	□ IV or worse	□ □ □ □
3. RANGE OF MOTION: Flex./ext.: documented side _/_/_ opposite side: _/_/_ *[6]					
Lack of extension (from zero anatomic)	□ <3°	□3–5°	□ 6–10°	□ >10°	
Δ *[7] lack of flexion	□ 0–5°	□6–15°	□ 16–25°	□ >25°	□ □ □ □
4. LIGAMENT EXAMINATION *[8]		3 to 5mm or	6 to 10mm		
Δ *[7] Lachman (in 25 flex.) *[9]	□ –1 to 2mm	□ –1 to –3mm[10]	□ or <–3mm	□ >10mm	
idem (alternative measurement, optional)	□ –1 to 2mm	□ 3–5/–1 to –3mm	□ 6–10/<–3mm	□ >10mm	
Endpoint: □ firm □ soft					
Δ *[7] total a.p. transl. in 70 flex. *[9]	□ 0 to 2mm	□ 3 to 5mm	□ 6 to 10mm	□ >10mm	
idem (alternative measurement, optional)	□ 0 to 2mm	□ 3 to 5mm	□ 6 to 10mm	□ >10mm	
Δ *[7] post. sag in 70 flex.	□ 0 to 2mm	□ 3 to 5mm	□ 6 to 10mm	□ >10mm	
Δ *[7] med. joint opening (valgus rotation)	□ 0 to 2mm	□ 3 to 5mm	□ 6 to 10mm	□ >10mm	
Δ *[7] lat. joint opening (varus rotation)	□ 0 to 2mm	□ 3 to 5mm	□ 6 to 10mm	□ >10mm	
Pivot shift *[11]	□ neg.	□ + (glide)	□ + + (clunk)	□ + + + (gross)	
Δ *[7] reversed pivot shift	□ equal (neg.) □ equal (pos.)	□ slight	□ marked	□ gross	□ □ □ □
5. COMPARTMENTAL FINDINGS *[12]					
Δ *[7] Crepitus patellofemoral	□ none/equal	□ moderate	□ painful	□ severe	
Δ *[7] Crepitus medial compartment	□ none	□ moderate	□ painful	□ severe	
Δ *[7] Crepitus lateral compartment	□ none	□ moderate	□ painful	□ severe	
6. HARVEST SITE PATHOLOGY *[13]					
Tenderness, irritation, numbness	□ none	□ slight	□ moderate	□ severe	
7. X-RAY FINDINGS (DEGENERATIVE JOINT DISEASE) *[14]					
Patellofemoral cartilage space	□ normal	□ >4mm	□ 2–4mm	□ <2mm	
Medial compartment cartilage space	□ normal	□ >4mm	□ 2–4mm	□ <2mm	
Lateral compartment cartilate space	□ normal	□ >4mm	□ 2–4mm	□ <2mm	
8. FUNCTIONAL TEXT *[15]					
Δ One leg hop (percent of opposite side)	□ 90–100%	□ 76–90%	□ 50–75%	□ <50%	
FINAL EVALUATION					□ □ □ □

Figure 35–10. International Knee Documentation Committee (IKDC) form. (Redrawn from Irrgang JJ, Ho H, Harner CD, et al: Use of the International Knee Documentation Committee guidelines to assess outcome following anterior cruciate ligament reconstruction. Knee Surg Sports Traumatol Arthrosc 6:107, 1998.)

work-related problems, (3) sports and recreational activities, (4) lifestyle, and (5) social and emotional factors. Scores are determined with a visual analog scale, and input from patients, athletic trainers, and physical therapists was used to confirm its face validity. Content validity was confirmed by orthopaedic surgeons. Acceptable test-retest reliability error (<6%) and responsiveness (84%) were shown. An average score of 31 in a chronically ACL-deficient patient determined a potential benefit from reconstructive surgery, whereas patients who could continue to be treated conservatively had an average score of 79.

Knee Injury and Osteoarthritis Outcome Score

Roos et al[40] developed the Knee Injury and Osteoarthritis Outcome Score in 1998 as a self-administered questionnaire. Five subsections consist of a 42-question scale rating pain, symptoms, activities of daily living, sports and recreational function, and knee-related quality of life. This outcome score was designed to assess young patients with ACL and meniscal injuries and traumatic osteoarthritis. Observer bias is eliminated by the administrative method, which takes about 10 minutes. Content validity was confirmed by a pilot study literature review and expert panel. Reliability intraclass correlation coefficients were .75 to .93 for the five sections, and responsiveness was high.

The Knee Outcome Survey

In 1998, Irrgang and colleagues[19] developed a patient-reported measure-of-function survey (Fig. 35–11) and suggested that in the clinical setting, it avoids the increased normative data misinterpretation. Two branches, the Activities of Daily Living Scale and the Sports Activity Scale, are included in the Knee Outcome Survey.

The patient-reported measure of function includes both general and specific measures of health status. General measures of health status include the Short Form-36 and the Sickness Impact Profile.[30,31,44] Specific measures of health status focus on the primary condition of interest, with the intent of creating a more responsive measure. Specific patient-reported measures of function of the knee include the Lysholm Knee Scoring Scale, the Cincinnati Knee Ligament Rating Scale, and the Western Ontario and McMaster Universities Osteoarthritis Index. The IKDC form was used in measuring physical impairment in combination with patient-reported measure of function. Knee Society[16] guidelines were used for assessment of outcome after total knee arthroplasty. This scale, developed for specific pathological conditions (such as osteoarthrosis and ligament injuries), attempts to be useful in patients with concomitant ligamentous and patellofemoral symptoms or osteoarthrosis. The alternative is to use multiple scales, as proposed by Tegner and Lysholm,[44] but comparisons across different disease states are difficult.

The Knee Outcome Survey is a patient-reported instrument for the measurement of functional limitations commonly experienced by individuals who have various pathological disorders of the knee. This survey consists of two separate scales, the Activities of Daily Living Scale and the Sports Activity Scale, which include items related to symptoms and functional limitations experienced during activities of daily living and sports activities, respectively. The Activities of Daily Living Scale was developed as a combination of various existing scales such as the Cincinnati Knee Ligament Rating Scale, the Lysholm Knee Scoring Scale, the Western Ontario and McMaster Universities Osteoarthritis Index, and the IKDC form. The underlying construct that this scale is intended to measure is the level of function that the pathological conditions or impairment of the knee imposes during activities of daily living. The symptoms included in this scale are pain, crepitus, stiffness, swelling, instability, and weakness. Responses range from absence of the symptom to complete loss of function as a result of the symptom. The functional limitations included in this scale are difficulty with regard to walking on level surfaces and stairs, standing, kneeling, squatting, sitting, and rising from a sitting position. An ordinal scoring system is used to assign a value to the responses, with a lower level of function resulting in a lower score.

The score on the Activities of Daily Living Scale is calculated by summing the point values for the responses to all 17 items on the scale. This sum is then divided by 80, which is the total possible number of points for all the items on the scale. Finally, this value is multiplied by 100, with the final total store expressed as a percentage.

The Sports Activity Scale is composed of 10 items on a 50-point scale and involves the use of sport-specific measures of pain, grinding, stiffness, swelling, giving way, buckling, running, jumping, cutting, and stopping. The scale is valid, reliable, and correlates well with sports-related function. Borsa et al[5] also determined it to be a viable alternative to the Cincinnati Knee Ligament Rating Scale or the Lysholm Knee Scoring Scale. The Knee Outcome Survey is well designed and clearly validated,[29] but it not widely used outside Pittsburgh at this time.[47]

PATELLOFEMORAL INSTRUMENTS

Beyond the scope of this chapter, but worthy of mention, are a few patellofemoral instruments. Although numbers are small, the IKDC and Cincinnati Knee Ligament Rating Scale have been used for patients with patellofemoral disorders despite having been designed for ligamentous instability.

Turba et al[45] devised a subjective and clinical scale for patients after extension mechanism reconstruction in 1979 that involved the use of a fairly complex formula. Then in 1984, Kelly et al[20] used functional symptoms, clinical evaluation, and Cybex testing to report on patients with jumper's knee. Fulkerson et al[9] modified the Lysholm scale in 1990, with 45% of this subjective study related to pain. In 1993 Kujala et al[22] developed a new patient-reported scale consisting of 13 questions similar in content, but weighted differently from Fulkerson's scale. Finally, Shelbourne and Trumper[42] in 1997 described an instrument with five equally weighted items: (1) retropatellar symptoms during strenuous sports or work, (2) symptoms during stair climbing, (3) symptoms after sitting, (4) symptoms during activities of daily living, and (5) symptoms during kneeling. To our knowledge, no statistical testing has been published on these scales.

COMPARISON OF KNEE SCORES

The various scales have been compared in several studies. The modified Lysholm Knee Scoring Scale has been shown

Knee Outcome Survey
Activities of Daily Living Scale

Instructions: The following questionnaire is designed to determine the symptoms and limitations that you experience because of your knee while you perform your usual *daily activities.* Please answer each question by *checking the statement that best describes you over the last 1 to 2 days.* For a given question, more than one of the statements may describe you, but please mark ONLY the statement that best describes you during your usual daily activities.

Symptoms

1. To what degree does pain in your knee affect your daily activity level?
   _5_ I never have pain in my knee.
   _4_ I have pain in my knee, but it does not affect my daily activity.
   _3_ Pain affects my activity slightly.
   _2_ Pain affects my activity moderately.
   _1_ Pain affects my activity severely.
   _0_ Pain in my knee prevents me from performing all daily activities.

2. To what degree does grinding or grating in your knee affect your daily activity level?
   _5_ I never have grinding or grating in my knee.
   _4_ I have grinding or grating in my knee, but it does not affect my daily activity.
   _3_ Grinding or grating affects my activity slightly.
   _2_ Grinding or grating affects my activity moderately.
   _1_ Grinding or grating affects my activity severely.
   _0_ Grinding or grating in my knee prevents me from performing all daily activities.

3. To what degree does stiffness in your knee affect your daily activity level?
   _5_ I never have stiffness in my knee.
   _4_ I have stiffness in my knee, but it does not affect my daily activity.
   _3_ Stiffness affects my activity slightly.
   _2_ Stiffness affects my activity moderately.
   _1_ Stiffness affects my activity severely.
   _0_ Stiffness in my knee prevents me from performing all daily activities.

4. To what degree does swelling in your knee affect your daily activity level?
   _5_ I never have swelling in my knee.
   _4_ I have swelling in my knee, but it does not affect my daily activity.
   _3_ Swelling affects my activity slightly.
   _2_ Swelling affects my activity moderately.
   _1_ Swelling affects my activity severely.
   _0_ Swelling in my knee prevents me from performing all daily activities.

5. To what degree does slipping of your knee affect your daily activity level?
   _5_ I never have slipping of my knee.
   _4_ I have slipping of my knee, but it does not affect my daily activity.
   _3_ Slipping affects my activity slightly.
   _2_ Slipping affects my activity moderately.
   _1_ Slipping affects my activity severely.
   _0_ Slipping of my knee prevents me from performing all daily activities.

6. To what degree does buckling of your knee affect your daily activity level?
   _5_ I never have buckling of my knee.
   _4_ I have buckling of my knee, but it does not affect my daily activity.
   _3_ Buckling affects my activity slightly.
   _2_ Buckling affects my activity moderately.
   _1_ Buckling affects my activity severely.
   _0_ Buckling of my knee prevents me from performing all daily activities.

7. To what degree does weakness or lack of strength of your leg affect your daily activity level?
   _5_ My leg never feels weak.
   _4_ My leg feels weak, but it does not affect my daily activity.
   _3_ Weakness affects my activity slightly.
   _2_ Weakness affects my activity moderately.
   _1_ Weakness affects my activity severely.
   _0_ Weakness of my leg prevents me from performing all daily activities.

Functional Disability with Activities of Daily Living

8. How does your knee affect your ability to walk?
   _5_ My knee does not affect my ability to walk.
   _4_ I have pain in my knee when walking, but it does not affect my ability to walk.
   _3_ My knee prevents me from walking more than 1 mile.
   _2_ My knee prevents me from walking more than 1/2 mile.
   _1_ My knee prevents me from walking more than 1 block.
   _0_ My knee prevents me from walking.

9. Because of your knee, do you walk with crutches or a cane?
   _3_ I can walk without crutches or a cane.
   _2_ My knee causes me to walk with 1 crutch or a cane.
   _1_ My knee causes me to walk with 2 crutches.
   _0_ Because of my knee, I cannot walk even with crutches.

10. Does your knee cause you to limp when you walk?
    _2_ I can walk without a limp.
    _1_ Sometimes my knee causes me to walk with a limp.
    _0_ Because of my knee, I cannot walk without a limp.

11. How does your knee affect your ability to go up stairs?
    _5_ My knee does not affect my ability to go up stairs.
    _4_ I have pain in my knee when going up stairs, but it does not limit my ability to go up stairs.
    _3_ I am able to go up stairs normally, but I need to rely on use of a railing.
    _2_ I am able to go up stairs one step at a time with use of a railing.
    _1_ I have to use crutches or a cane to go up stairs.
    _0_ I cannot go up stairs.

12. How does your knee affect your ability to go down stairs?
    _5_ My knee does not affect my ability to go down stairs.
    _4_ I have pain in my knee when going down stairs, but it does not limit my ability to go down stairs.
    _3_ I am able to go down stairs normally, but I need to rely on use of a railing.
    _2_ I am able to go down stairs one step at a time with use of a railing.
    _1_ I have to use crutches or a cane to go down stairs.
    _0_ I cannot go down stairs.

Figure 35–11. Knee Outcome Survey form.

13. How does your knee affect your ability to stand?

_5_ My knee does not affect my ability to stand. I can stand for unlimited amounts of time.

_4_ I have pain in my knee when standing, but it does not limit my ability to stand.

_3_ Because of my knee I cannot stand for more than 1 hour.

_2_ Because of my knee I cannot stand for more than 1/2 hour.

_1_ Because of my knee I cannot stand for more than 10 minutes.

_0_ I cannot stand because of my knee.

14. How does your knee affect your ability to kneel on the front of your knee?

_5_ My knee does not affect my ability to kneel on the front of my knee. I can kneel for unlimited amounts of time.

_4_ I have pain when kneeling on the front of my knee, but it does not limit my ability to kneel.

_3_ I cannot kneel on the front of my knee for more than 1 hour.

_2_ I cannot kneel on the front of my knee for more than 1/2 hour.

_1_ I cannot kneel on the front of my knee for more than 10 minutes.

_0_ I cannot kneel on the front of my knee.

15. How does your knee affect your ability to squat?

_5_ My knee does not affect my ability to squat. I can squat all the way down.

_4_ I have pain when squatting, but I can still squat all the way down.

_3_ I cannot squat more than 3/4 of the way down.

_2_ I cannot squat more than 1/2 of the way down.

_1_ I cannot squat more than 1/4 of the way down.

_0_ I cannot squat at all.

16. How does your knee affect your ability to sit with your knee bent?

_5_ My knee does not affect my ability to sit with my knee bent. I can sit for unlimited amounts of time.

_4_ I have pain when sitting with my knee bent, but it does not limit my ability to sit.

_3_ I cannot sit with my knee bent for more than 1 hour.

_2_ I cannot sit with my knee bent for more than 1/2 hour.

_1_ I cannot sit with my knee bent for more than 10 minutes.

_0_ I cannot sit with my knee bent.

17. How does your knee affect your ability to rise from a chair?

_5_ My knee does not affect my ability to rise from a chair.

_4_ I have pain when rising from the seated position, but it does not affect my ability to rise from the seated position.

_2_ Because of my knee, I can only rise from a chair if I use my hands and arms to assist.

_0_ Because of my knee I cannot rise from a chair.

Figure 35–11, cont'd.

to consistently produce higher scores than those produced by the Cincinnati Knee Ligament Rating Scale. In 41 patients with documented ACL deficiencies, Bollen and Seedhom[4] showed a linear relationship between the two (modified Lysholm Knee Scoring Scale = 30 + 0.72 Cincinnati Knee Ligament Rating Scale). Using multiple scales, Anderson and coworkers[2] evaluated 70 patients at a minimum of 5 years after ACL reconstruction. The results according to the modified Lysholm Knee Scoring Scale were 43 excellent, 16 good, 8 fair, and 3 poor; according to the Cincinnati Knee Ligament Rating Scale, the results were 18 excellent, 49 good, and 3 fair. The correlation coefficient between these scales was .595; that between the modified Lysholm and revised HSSKS was .762, and that between the Cincinnati Knee Ligament Rating Scale and the revised HSSKS was .684. When the overall scores for each scale were normalized to a maximum of 100, the revised HSSKS resulted in the lowest scores. Anderson and associates[2] found that it was very difficult to compare the different scales. Each scale evaluates subjective and objective factors in different ways and assigns different relative weights to the individual criteria. This discrepancy introduces error in the final score. They appropriately concluded that separate scores for each category should be reported and that the IKDC form should be universally adopted to facilitate comparisons between studies.

Sgaglione and coworkers[41] retrospectively compared the revised HSSKS, modified Lysholm, and Cincinnati Knee Ligament Rating Scale systems in 65 patients who underwent ACL reconstruction (minimum of 2 years' follow-up). The modified Lysholm Knee Scoring Scale produced the highest score, the revised HSSKS score was intermediate, and the Cincinnati Knee Ligament Rating Scale score was the lowest. They concluded that the low activity levels of some patients might not have been identified in the modified Lysholm Knee Scoring Scale and revised HSSKS scores. Again, the recommendation was to report individual category scores rather than the overall score. They favored the Noyes rating scheme in which individual scores are reported and the final rating is based on the lowest score in any single category.

We compared the components of the modified Lysholm Knee Scoring Scale, revised HSSKS, Cincinnati Knee Ligament Rating Scale, and IKDC form in Table 35–1. Each category in the Cincinnati Knee Ligament Rating Scale (see Fig. 35–8) was given a maximum score of 4 points. Although the profile shows 10 points for pain, 40 for walking, and 100 for running, each of these actually receives equal weight in the final rating. Each category is rated as excellent, good, fair, or poor (four levels); thus, we assigned a maximum of 4 points to each, except for tibiofemoral and patellofemoral crepitation, which are graded as excellent, fair, or poor (maximum of 3 points each). Similarly, the IKDC form (see Fig. 35–10A) receives a maximum of 4 points for each category (normal, nearly normal, abnormal, and severely abnormal).

It is readily apparent from Table 35–1 that the modified Lysholm Knee Scoring Scale is purely subjective, with a high relative weight assigned to pain (25%), giving way (25%), and locking (15%). These three combined to account for 65% of the score. The subjective part of the revised HSSKS is 45% of the total possible 100-point score. The subjective portion of the Cincinnati Knee Ligament Rating Scale is 40 points (49% of the total), and that of the IKDC form is 24 points (40% of the total). The revised HSSKS is heavily weighted to giving way (20 of the 45 points). "Return to sports," "return to work," and the "ability to decelerate" are not included in any of the other three rating systems. Both the Cincinnati Knee Ligament Rating Scale and the IKDC form include pain, swelling, and partial and complete giving way. Because there are

Table 35–1. Relative Weights of Various Knee Rating Scale Components

COMPONENTS	MODIFIED LYSHOLM	REVISED HSSKS	CINCINNATI KNEE LIGAMENT RATING SCALE	IKDC
Subjective				
Pain	25		4	4
Swelling	10	2	4	4
Clicking				
Giving way	25	20	4*	4*
Locking	15	3		
Limp	5			
Support needed	5			
Function				
Difficulty with stairs	10		4	
Difficulty walking			4	
Difficulty running			4	
Return to work		4		
Return to sports		4		4†
Ability to decelerate		4		
Cutting		4	4‡	
Jumping		4	4‡	
Pivoting			4‡	
Squatting	5		4‡	
Composite knee function				4
Knee effect on activity level				4
Total Subjective Score	100	45	40*	24
Objective Examination Findings				
Effusion		4	4	
Crepitation			3§	4†
Atrophy		2		
Motion		3	4¶	4¶
Patellofemoral radiograph			4*	4†
Medial tibial radiograph			4*	4†
Lateral tibial radiograph			4*	4†
Function				
Forward jump		10	4*	4†
Stability				
Lachman		4	4	4
Anterior drawer		2		4†
Posterior drawer		5		4†
Pivot shift		10	4	4†
Reverse pivot shift		5		4†
Valgus laxity		5		4†
Varus laxity		5		4†
Total Objective Score	0	55	42*	36

*Includes 4 points for partial and 4 points for complete giving way.
†Items recorded but not included in the final overall rating.
‡Pivoting and cutting are both combined into a single category.
§Separate categories for patellofemoral and tibiofemoral crepitus with 3 points each.
¶Four points each for flexion and extension.
HSSKS, Hospital for Special Surgery Knee Score; IKDC, International Knee Documentation Committee.

fewer categories in the subjective part of the IKDC, these four symptoms account for 16 of the 24 points as compared with 16 of 40 points for the Noyes scale. The Cincinnati Knee Ligament Rating Scale includes functional activities (such as walking, climbing stairs, running, cutting, jumping, and squatting) that are not included in the IKDC form. Instead, the IKDC asks two global questions: how does your knee function, and how does your knee affect your activity level?

The objective section of the scales contributes 55 of 100 points (55%) for the revised HSSKS, 42 of 82 points (51%) for the Cincinnati Knee Ligament Rating Scale, and 36 of 60 points (60%) for the IKDC form. The ligamentous aspect of the objective section is heavily weighted by the ligamentous examination in the revised HSSKS (65%) and IKDC (78%) systems, whereas only 19% of the Cincinnati Knee Ligament Rating Scale is allocated to this topic. Crepitation and radiographic findings are recorded in both the Cincinnati Knee Ligament Rating Scale and IKDC systems, but they contribute to the final rating only in the Cincinnati scale. Overall, the categories assessed in the objective section are most similar for the revised HSSKS and IKDC form. However, the method of determining the final rating is identical for the Cincinnati Knee Ligament Rating Scale and IKDC form (i.e., the lowest score of any individual criterion determines the final rating). Although groups 1 to 4 are sufficient to determine the final rating in the IKDC system, an investigator should also document the other groups for future comparisons. If compartmental findings, radiographic findings, and the functional test were included, the IKDC form would be similar to the Cincinnati Knee Ligament Rating Scale.

Concurring that the Cincinnati scale is more sports specific and the Lysholm scale better represents activities of daily living, Borsa et al[5] also compared the Knee Outcome Survey in 1998. They determined that the Knee Outcome Survey was superior in distinguishing symptomatic and functional limitations between activities of daily living and sports involvement. After comparing the Lysholm, HSSKS, OAK, Cincinnati, and IKDC systems in 2000, Hrubesch et al[14] decided that the IKDC correlated best with instrumented knee laxity measurements. Other findings included higher scores for Lysholm and Cincinnati scales, lower for the IKDC. In 2001, Marx and colleagues[29] determined that the Activities of Daily Living Scale of the Knee Outcome Survey had better construct validity and responsiveness than did the Lysholm, Cincinnati, and AOSSM instruments. He granted that the other instruments were all acceptable for clinical use based on satisfactory criteria for validity, reliability, and responsiveness, but that the Activities of Daily Living Scale of the Knee Outcome Survey was easy to understand and administer.

In December 2003, Marx[28] compared the same instruments with the Single Assessment Numeric Evaluation, the Knee Injury and Osteoarthritic Outcome Score (which includes the Western Ontario and McMaster Universities Osteoarthritis Index used for degenerative knee patients), and the Quality of Life Outcome Measure. He confirmed the validity of these instruments and emphasized the importance of measuring activity level to compare groups meaningfully because two people with the same injury may have different levels of disability.

Comparative studies are sometimes published by the authors of one particular system and must be carefully evaluated. Furthermore, different centers value different aspects of outcome, which is easily demonstrated by the diverse amount of weight placed on any single measured component. In addition, older papers have fewer tests to compare.

FUTURE DIRECTION

There is clearly a need for a more uniform evaluation system that must be imposed universally. We agree with Labs and Paul[23] that a new form that combines the IKDC and the VAS would be the best sports knee rating system, both subjectively and objectively. Although the inclusion or exclusion of specific criteria in the final evaluation can be argued, we believe that the IKDC form has several advantages. First, a committee of experienced investigators from North America and Europe met over a period of several years, determined definitions of individual criteria, evaluated existing rating scales, and developed a consensus form. Second, after careful study of the instructions, the form can be easily administered. Third, patients with persisting knee problems cannot be hidden behind high numerical scores added for other unrelated parameters. Finally, the eight groups assessed in the form are inclusive, but also allow some flexibility.

The first two categories in the IKDC form (patient subjective assessment and symptoms) can be changed to the VAS format. Advantages of including the VAS in the IKDC,

as previously stated, are that it is user-friendly and offers increased validity, increased patient compliance, greater sensitivity of measurement, reduced bias, and graphic representation. Self-administered, standardized data collection of the subjective items may improve the accuracy of the IKDC score.[13]

It is hoped that this new form will facilitate comparison of treatment methods. To critically evaluate the most appropriate knee injury management, one universal sports knee rating system should be used.

References

1. Anderson AF: Rating scales. In Fu FH, Harner CD, Vince KL, (eds): Knee Surgery. Baltimore, Williams & Wilkins, 1994, p 275.
2. Anderson AF, Federspiel CF, Snyder RB: Evaluation of knee ligament rating systems. Am J Knee Surg 6:67, 1993.
3. Barber-Westin SD, Noyes FR, McCloskey JW: Rigorous statistical reliability, validity, and responsiveness testing of the Cincinnati knee rating system in 350 subjects with uninjured, injured or anterior cruciate ligament–reconstructed knees. Am J Sports Med 27:402, 1999.
4. Bollen S, Seedhom BB: A comparison of the Lysholm and Cincinnati knee scoring questionnaires. Am J Sports Med 19:189, 1991.
5. Borsa PA, Lephart SM, Irrgang JJ: Sports-specificity of knee scoring systems to assess disability in anterior cruciate ligament–deficient athletes. J Sports Rehabil 7:44, 1998.
6. Ellsasser JC, Reynolds FC, Omohundro JR: The non-operative treatment of collateral ligament injuries of the knee in professional football players. An analysis of seventy-four injuries treated non-operatively and twenty-four injuries treated surgically. J Bone Joint Surg Am 56:1185, 1974.
7. Feagin JA Jr, Blake WP: Postoperative evaluation and result recording in the anterior cruciate ligament–reconstructed knee. Clin Orthop 172:143, 1983.
8. Flandry F, Hunt JP, Terry GC, et al: Analysis of subjective knee complaints using visual analog scales. Am J Sports Med 19:112, 1991.
9. Fulkerson JP, Becker GJ, Jeaney JA, et al: Anteromedial tibial tubercle transfer without bone graft. Am J Sports Med 18:490, 1990.
10. Godshall RW, Hansen CA: The classification, treatment, and follow-up evaluation of medial collateral ligament injuries of the knee [abstract]. J Bone Joint Surg Am 56:1316, 1974.
11. Hanley ST, Warren RF: Arthroscopic meniscectomy in the anterior cruciate ligament–deficient knee. Arthroscopy 3:59, 1987.
12. Hefti F, Muller W, Jakob RP, et al: Evaluation of knee ligament injuries with the IKDC form. Knee Surg Sports Traumatol Arthrosc 1:226, 1993.
13. Hoher J, Bach T, Munster A, et al: Does the mode of data collection change result in a subjective knee score? Self-administration versus interview. Am J Sports Med 25:642, 1997.
14. Hrubesch R, Rangger C, Reichkendler M, et al: Critical analysis of knee ligament rating systems. Am J Sports Med 28:850, 2000.
15. Hughston JC, Eilers AF: The role of the posterior oblique ligament in repairs of acute medial (collateral) ligament tears of the knee. J Bone Joint Surg Am 55:923, 1973.
16. Insall JN, Dorr LD, Scott RD, et al: Rationale of the Knee Society clinical rating system. Clin Orthop 248:13, 1989.
17. Irrgang JJ, Anderson AF, Boland AL, et al: Development and validation of the International Knee Documentation Committee Subjective Knee Form. Am J Sports Med 29:600, 2001.
18. Irrgang JJ, Ho H, Harner CD, et al: Use of the International Knee Documentation Committee guidelines to assess outcome following anterior cruciate ligament reconstruction. Knee Surg Sports Traumatol Arthrosc 6:107, 1998.
19. Irrgang JJ, Snyder-Mackler L, Wainner RS, et al: Development of a patient-reported measure of function of the knee. J Bone Joint Surg Am 80:1132, 1998.
20. Kelly DW, Carter VS, Jobe FW, et al: Patellar and quadriceps tendon ruptures—jumper's knee. Am J Sports Med 12:375, 1984.
21. Kowalk DL, Wojtys EM, Disher J, et al: Quantitative analysis of the measuring capabilities of the KT-1000 knee ligament arthrometer. Am J Sports Med 21:744, 1993.

22. Kujala UM, Jaakkola LH, Koskinen, et al: Scoring of patellofemoral disorders. Arthroscopy 9:159, 1993.
23. Labs K, Paul B: To compare and contrast the various evaluation scoring systems after anterior cruciate ligament reconstruction. Arch Orthop Trauma Surg 116:92, 1997.
24. Larson R: Rating sheet for the knee function. In Smillie IS (ed): Diseases of the Knee Joint, 2nd ed. New York, Churchill Livingstone, 1979.
25. Lysholm J, Gillquist J: Evaluation of knee ligament surgery results with special emphasis on use of a scoring scale. Am J Sports Med 10:150, 1982.
26. Marshall JL, Fetto JF, Botero PM: Knee ligament injuries: A standardized evaluation method. Clin Orthop 123:115, 1977.
27. Marx RG: Patient-reported measure of knee function. J Bone Joint Surg Am 82:1199, 2000.
28. Marx RG: Knee rating scales. Arthroscopy 19:1103-1108, 2003.
29. Marx RG, Jones EC, Allen AA, et al: Reliability, validity, and responsiveness of four knee outcome scales for athletic patients. J Bone Joint Surg Am 83:1459, 2001.
30. McHorney CA, Ware JE Jr, Lu JFR, et al: The MOS 36-Item Short-Form Health Survey (SF-36): III. Tests of data quality, scaling assumptions, and reliability across diverse patient groups. Med Care 32:40, 1994.
31. McHorney CA, Ware JE Jr, Raczek AE: The MOS 36-Item Short-Form Health Survey (SF-36): II. Psychometric and clinical tests of validity in measuring physical and mental health constructs. Med Care 31:247, 1993.
32. Mohtadi N: Development and validation of the quality of life outcome measure (questionnaire) for chronic anterior cruciate ligament deficiency. Am J Sports Med 26:350, 1998.
33. Muller W, Biedert R, Hefti F, et al: OAK knee evaluation: A new way to assess knee ligament injuries. Clin Orthop 232:37, 1988.
34. Neeb TB, Aufdemkampe G, Wagener JHD, Mastenbroek L: Assessing anterior cruciate ligament injuries: The association and differential value of questionnaires, clinical tests, and functional tests. J Orthop Sports Phys Ther 26:324, 1997.
35. Noyes FR, Barber SD, Mangine RE: Bone-patellar, ligament-bone, and fascia lata allografts for reconstruction of the anterior cruciate ligament. J Bone Joint Surg Am 72:1125, 1990.
36. Noyes FR, Grood ES, Torzilli PA: Current concepts review. The definitions of terms for motion and position of the knee and injuries of the ligaments. J Bone Joint Surg Am 71:465, 1989.
37. Noyes FR, Matthews DS, Mooar PA, et al: The symptomatic anterior cruciate–deficient knee. Part II: The results of rehabilitation, activity modification, and counseling on functional disability. J Bone Joint Surg Am 65:163, 1983.
38. O'Donoghue DH: An analysis of end results of surgical treatment of major injuries to the ligaments of the knee. J Bone Joint Surg Am 37:1, 1955.
39. O'Donoghue DH: A method for replacement of the anterior cruciate ligament of the knee: Report of twenty cases. J Bone Joint Surg Am 45:905, 1963.
40. Roos EM, Roos HP, Lohmander LS, et al: Knee Injury and Osteoarthritis Outcome Score (KOOS): Development of a self-administered outcome measure. J Orthop Sports Phys Ther 78:88, 1998.
41. Sgaglione NA, Del Pizzo W, Fox JM, et al: Critical analysis of knee ligament rating systems. Am J Sports Med 23:660, 1995.
42. Shelbourne KD, Trumper RV: Preventing anterior knee pain after anterior cruciate ligament reconstruction. Am J Sports Med 25:41, 1997.
43. Slocum DB, Larson RL: Pes anserinus transplantation. A surgical procedure for control of rotatory instability of the knee. J Bone Joint Surg Am 50:226, 1968.
44. Tegner Y, Lysholm J: Rating systems in the evaluation of knee ligament injuries. Clin Orthop 198:43, 1985.
45. Turba JE, Walsh WM, McLoed W: Long-term results of extensor mechanism reconstruction, a standard for evaluation. Am J Sports Med 7:91, 1979.
46. Ware JE Jr, Sherbourne CD: The MOS 36-Item Short-Form Health Survey (SF-36): I. Conceptual framework and item selection. Med Care 30:473, 1992.
47. Weitzel PP, Richmond JC: Critical evaluation of different scoring systems of the knee. Sports Med Arthrosc Rev 10:183, 2002.
48. Williams GN, Taylor DC, Gangel TJ, et al: Comparison of the single assessment numeric evaluation method and the Lysholm score. Clin Orthop 373:184, 2000.
49. Windsor RE, Insall JN, Warren RF, et al: The Hospital for Special Surgery knee ligament rating form. Am J Knee Surg 1:140, 1988.

CHAPTER 36

Instrumented Ligamentous Laxity Testing

J. Winslow Alford • Bernard R. Bach Jr.

During the last 4 decades, advances in the understanding and treatment of knee instability have progressed at a rapid rate. Refinements in physical examination techniques, improved radiographic modalities, advances in the principles of ligament healing and rehabilitation, improved surgical techniques, and the constant integration of new technology as it becomes available have contributed to an improved ability to care for patients with an anterior cruciate ligament (ACL)-deficient knee or a knee with a more complex instability pattern. During the 1980s, several ligament testing devices were developed in an attempt to quantize anteroposterior (AP) displacement of the knee joint. The Lachman, pivot-shift, and anterior drawer tests often vary from examiner to examiner, thus making comparison difficult. Objective, quantitative ligament testing devices provide the opportunity to compare populations of patients more accurately. Clinical studies that evaluate the results of knee stability procedures should use quantifiable instrumented ligament testing in addition to the clinical grading reported by various authors, especially when evaluating new technology or novel graft sources. To accurately interpret the results of instrumented ligament testing it is important to have baseline comparison data for various physiological and anatomic conditions for various surgical scenarios. Two ligament testing devices have commonly been used: the KT-2000 arthrometer (MEDmetric, San Diego, CA) and the Stryker knee laxity tester (Stryker Co., Kalamazoo, MI).[11,38,60,78] The KT-2000 arthrometer and its predecessor the KT-1000 have most often been reported in the literature and provide the basis for most of this chapter.

OBJECTIVES

This chapter discusses the KT-2000 and its application to the assessment of knee stability. It includes a description of the testing device and testing protocol, a review of the literature, a comparison between acute and chronic ACL injuries, and a comparison of data obtained from patients examined while awake and while under anesthesia. Since the publication of the last edition of this chapter, several new developments in knee reconstruction have been evaluated by KT testing. Data evaluating various allograft and autograft sources for ACL reconstruction are now available and will be presented. Recent developments in knee reconstruction technology and various clinical scenarios, including posterior cruciate ligament (PCL) reconstruc-

tion, fracture repair, arthroplasty, cartilage restoration, and meniscus transplantation, have been evaluated by instrumented ligamentous laxity testing, and an update on the available data will be presented. In addition, several alternative methods of knee stability assessment have been developed and will be compared with KT-2000 arthrometry.

DEFINITIONS AND TERMINOLOGY

KT-2000 arthrometer: This instrumented testing machine for quantitating AP knee displacement differs from its predecessor, the KT-1000, only in its data-recording capability (Figs. 36–1 and 36–2).

Passive Lachman test: Sequential amounts of force are applied through the KT-2000 force handle with the knee flexed to above 30 ± 5 degrees. The direction of force applied may be either anterior or posterior. The amount of force applied includes 15 lb (67 N), 20 lb (89 N), and 30 lb (133 N).

Maximum manual test: With the KT-2000 properly positioned, maximum anterior force is applied by the examiner's hand on the calf, thereby passively displacing the tibia relative to the femur. This test clinically approximates the Lachman test. Estimated force generated by the maximum manual test ranges from 135 to 180 N (Fig. 36–3), depending on examiner's strength.

Compliance index determination: Difference in millimeters between the 89-N and the 67-N testing results.

Involved-uninvolved differences: Also referred to as side-to-side difference, this parameter quantifies the difference between the involved (injured) and the uninvolved knee. It may be reported at any of the force values, including maximum manual, or compliance I-N (involved minus noninvolved).

Quadriceps active test: This test is performed by asking the patient to gently lift the heels off the bed while the knee is resting at approximately 30 degrees of flexion, thus causing contraction of the quadriceps muscles. The resulting displacement of the KT-2000 dial needle is recorded.

Quadriceps neutral angle[23]: Knee flexion angle at which quadriceps contraction results in neither anterior nor posterior tibial translation (Figs. 36–4 to 36–6). At this position (approximately 70 degrees of knee flexion) the patellar tendon is perpendicular to the joint surface of the tibia.

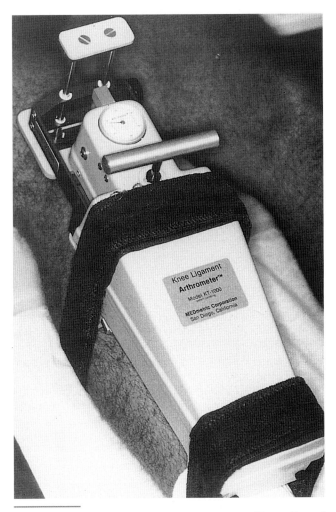

Figure 36–1. Arthrometer model KT-1000. (From Daniel DM, Stone ML: Diagnosis of knee ligament injury: Tests and measurements of joint laxity. In Feagin JA Jr [ed]: The Crucial Ligaments: Diagnosis and Treatment of Ligamentous Injuries about the Knee. New York, Churchill Livingstone, 1988, pp 287-300.)

DESCRIPTION OF THE KT-2000 ARTHROMETER

The KT-2000 is an instrumented device that was developed to measure anterior and posterior translation of the tibia relative to the femur in a clinical setting (see Figs. 36–1 and 36–2). A complete description of the testing protocol was originally provided for its predecessor, the KT-1000, by Daniel and Malcom and colleagues,[22,23,25,62] as well as in the manufacturer's manual. The protocol for use of the KT-1000 and KT-2000 differs only in the ability of the KT-2000 to graphically record output data on an X-Y plotter. Patient positioning, device application, and force generation for the KT-1000 and KT-2000 are identical. Users of these devices should review their protocols before use.

The patient is placed in the supine position on the examination table with the thighs resting on the bolster provided to maintain the knees at approximately 30 degrees of flexion. The heels are positioned symmetrically on the positioning cup to maintain the tibia in symmetric external rotation of approximately 15 degrees. The examiner must make certain that the patient's thighs remain relaxed throughout the examination. The device's two force-sensing pads are positioned on the patella and the tibial tubercle, and the body of the device is secured to the lower part of the leg with straps. When an anterior force is applied to the tibia, relative motion between the two properly positioned pads is displayed as AP displacement by the gauge on the KT-2000, which is calibrated to the nearest 0.5 mm. Next, the examiner must determine and set the point at which the knee rests naturally, the zero point. To determine the zero point, the examiner grasps the device's handle, located 10 cm below the joint line, and performs several anterior and posterior translations. After several repetitions, the zero point is determined, and the device is calibrated to reflect this determination. An audible characteristic tone is heard at 15 lb (67 N) and

Figure 36–2. Components of the arthrometer: A, force handle; B, patellar sensor pad; C, tibial tubercle sensor pad; D, Velcro strap; E, arthrometer case; F, displacement dial indicator; G, thigh support; H, foot support. (1) A constant pressure of 4 to 6 lb applied to the patellar sensor pad keeps it in contact with the patella; (2) posterior force applied; (3) anterior force applied. (From Daniel DM, Stone ML: Diagnosis of knee ligament injury: Tests and measurements of joint laxity. In Feagin JA Jr [ed]: The Crucial Ligaments: Diagnosis and Treatment of Ligamentous Injuries about the Knee. New York, Churchill Livingstone, 1988, pp 287-300.)

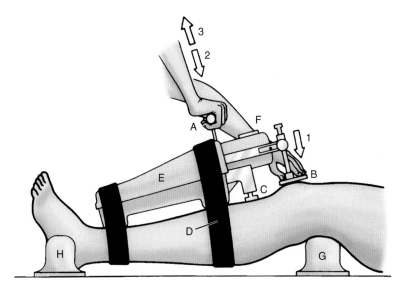

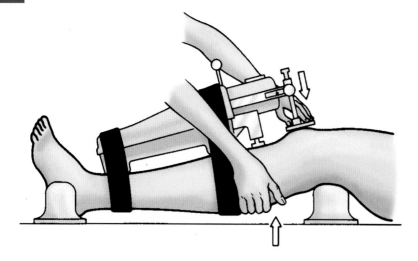

Figure 36–3. Manual maximum anterior displacement test. High anterior displacement force is applied directly to the proximal part of the calf, and displacement is measured with the arthrometer. (From Daniel DM, Stone ML: Diagnosis of knee ligament injury: Tests and measurements of joint laxity. In Feagin JA Jr [ed]: The Crucial Ligaments: Diagnosis and Treatment of Ligamentous Injuries about the Knee. New York, Churchill Livingstone, 1988, pp 287-300.)

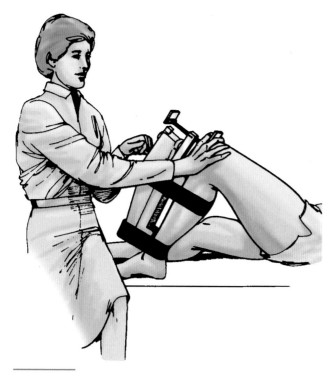

Figure 36–4. Arthrometer position for testing at the quadriceps neutral angle (mean, 70 degrees). (From Daniel DM, Stone ML: Diagnosis of knee ligament injury: Tests and measurements of joint laxity. In Feagin JA Jr [ed]: The Crucial Ligaments: Diagnosis and Treatment of Ligamentous Injuries about the Knee. New York, Churchill Livingstone, 1988, pp 287-300.)

20 lb (89 N) of anterior force in the KT-1000, and an additional tone has been added to the KT-2000 at 30 lb for larger patients requiring additional force. Newer KT-1000 and all KT-2000 models feature posterior force tones as well.

The compliance index is the difference between displacements at 20 and 15 lb. This test should be performed at least twice and the results averaged. After each test, the arthrometer must be recalibrated to the zero position. By reversing the direction of application of force, posterior knee stability may be evaluated as well. The quadriceps active test as described by Daniel et al[24] and the quadriceps neutral position may also be evaluated and quantified with the KT-2000. Accurate and reproducible results of KT-2000 testing require an experienced examiner using identical patient and device positioning and force application.

TECHNICAL POINTS AND PITFALLS

Proper technique is necessary to obtain accurate measurements and ensure reproducibility. The MEDmetric user manual is an important reference guide for KT-2000 and KT-1000 users. An entire section of the manual is devoted to potential pitfalls and technical errors. Ensuring that variables such as the knee flexion angle and force vector angles are reproduced and controlled will enhance the accuracy of measurements.

Patient relaxation must be maintained throughout the entire test to obtain meaningful data. The physician must periodically check the patient's thighs to make certain that they are relaxed and there is no guarding. If the dial needle is noted to "float" or shift erratically, the examiner must re-evaluate for patient guarding because this will confound the results. Maintaining the patient in a comfortable symmetric supine position helps keep the quadriceps and abdominal muscles relaxed.

Errors in *arthrometer placement* and the *angle of force vector* can also occur and cause significant variations in measurements. Kowalk et al[59] demonstrated that positioning the device 1 cm proximal to the joint line produces larger anterior translations when measured in vivo than does positioning the device at the joint line (5.8 versus 5.4 mm), whereas positioning it 1 cm distal to the joint line produces smaller measurements (4.4 mm). Both these measurements, one taken 1 cm above the joint line and the other taken 1 cm below the joint line, were

RESTING POSITION–Normal knee

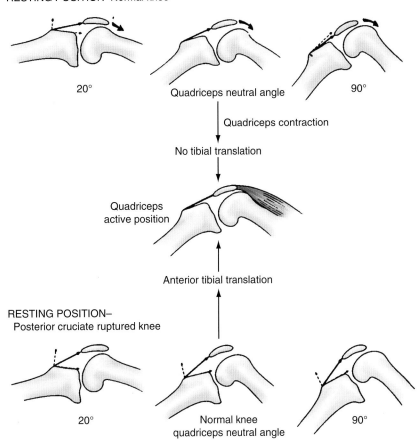

Figure 36–5. Resting position of a normal knee and a knee with rupture of a posterior cruciate ligament (PCL). In 20 degrees of flexion, the patellar ligament passes anteriorly from the tibial tubercle to the patella, relative to a line drawn perpendicular to the surface of the tibial plateau. In a normal knee in 90 degrees of flexion, the patellar ligament is directed more posteriorly. In a knee with rupture of the PCL, the patellar ligament is still directed anteriorly. In a normal knee there is an angle of flexion (quadriceps neutral angle: mean, 70 degrees) at which the patellar ligament is perpendicular to the joint surface. The position of the knee with the quadriceps contracted (quadriceps active position) at the quadriceps neutral angle is independent of the integrity of the cruciate ligaments and may be used as a neutral position to distinguish anterior from posterior laxity. (From Daniel DM, Stone ML, Barnett P, et al: Use of the quadriceps active test to diagnose posterior cruciate ligament disruption and measure posterior laxity of the knee. J Bone Joint Surg Am 70:386, 1988.)

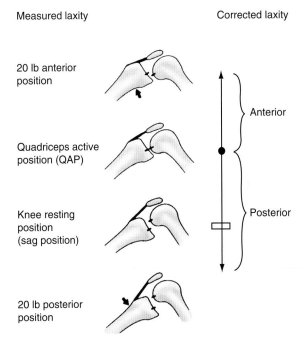

Figure 36–6. In an injured knee, the measured anterior tibial displacement is the distance from the resting position (*rectangle*) to the *superior arrowhead* (10 mm), and the measured posterior displacement is the distance from the resting position to the *inferior arrowhead* (3 mm). With contraction of the quadriceps, the tibia moves forward from the resting position to the quadriceps active position (*black circle*). Determinations of laxity calculated from the quadriceps active position (corrected laxity) are presented. (From Daniel DM, Stone ML, Barnett P, et al: Use of the quadriceps active test to diagnose posterior cruciate ligament disruption and measure posterior laxity of the knee. J Bone Joint Surg Am 70:386, 1988.)

shown to be statistically significant ($p = .05$). In addition, that study demonstrated that changing the angle of force vector by only 10 degrees off the direct perpendicular causes a larger range of measurements, thus indicating that the vector of pull should be oriented along the axis of the device's handle to provide the most reproducible results.

Soft-tissue considerations and the resulting *position of the patella* must also be taken into account during testing, especially in patients with patella alta. In patients with abnormal extensor mechanism tracking or patellar height, slight adjustments in the knee flexion angle may allow the patella to sit more concentrically within the trochlea. The examiner must also stabilize the patellar reference pad manually and maintain consistent pressure while testing.

Tibial rotation errors may also result in testing discrepancies. Anterior force results in anterior displacement and internal rotation of the tibia; posterior force results in posterior displacement and external rotation of the tibia. These AP displacements and rotations of the tibia are coupled motions in the knee joint that may change dramatically as a result of injury. During KT testing, internal rotation of the tibia will cause decreased translation. Therefore, it is critical to ensure that both tibiae are in proper and symmetric rotation when testing. Under general anesthesia, muscle relaxation will result in excess external rotation of the thigh and thus effectively place the tibia in excessive internal rotation. In this scenario, it is recommended that an assistant hold the thigh internally rotated or that a derotation strap be used. Other technical pitfalls include rotational orientation of the arthrometer, variations in patellar pad pressure, testing reference position (must be reset after each test), and temperature effects on the device itself. These technical points must be remembered to ensure accuracy and reproducibility.

The *rate of force application* has been demonstrated by Gross et al[42] to affect compliance and stiffness measurements, but not to have a significant effect on absolute displacement measurements. Slower rates of anterior force application resulted in lower compliance and higher stiffness measurements.

TESTING REPRODUCIBILITY AND DEVICE COMPARISON

The utility of instrumented ligament laxity testing is based on the ability to translate and compare reproducible data from study to study and to evaluate patients within a reliable reference data set. To evaluate the reproducibility of KT measurements, Hanten and Pace[44] determined interexaminer, intraexaminer, and intraclass reliability coefficients for KT measurements on 43 uninjured college athletes. The authors noted high reliability coefficients ($r = .85$) and intraclass coefficients ($r = .92$) and concluded that the KT-1000 had good interexaminer and intraexaminer reliability. These values were slightly lower than the results obtained by Malcom et al[62] ($r = .93$). Bach

reviewed 16 normal knees tested by one examiner twice on one day, with repeat examinations performed twice 1 week later. No statistically significant differences in compliance index or displacement at 67-N, 89-N, or maximum manual testing were noted, thus illustrating excellent reliability within time and examiner variables. Edixhoven et al[29] noted that reproducibility was directly affected by changes in subject positioning when using a more rudimentary laboratory testing apparatus not commercially available, which made it difficult to standardize patient positioning.

Several studies have evaluated other commercially available arthrometers. Neuschwander et al[68] compared side-to-side results at 20 lb and maximum manual results with the KT-1000 and the Acufex Knee Signature System in 21 ACL-deficient patients. In that study, no statistically significant differences between these two devices were noted for side-to-side testing or maximum manual testing. Anderson et al[3] prospectively randomized 50 normal and 50 ACL-deficient patients to be measured with five different testing devices: the KT-1000, Stryker knee laxity tester, Acufex Knee Signature System, Dyonics Dynamic Cruciate Tester, and Genucom Knee Analysis System. In normal subjects, the authors did not find any significant differences in side-to-side testing among the five devices, but reported significant differences in anterior translations between devices. Translations with the Dyonics and Acufex were 50% less than those with the other devices, whereas the Genucom tended to overestimate translations in normal knees. For ACL-deficient knees, measurements were almost twice those in normal knees, except for the Genucom device, which had overestimated translations in normal knees. There was significant variation among devices in their measurements of side-to-side differences in patients with ACL-deficient knees. Diagnostic accuracy was improved with the maximum manual test for all devices in both ACL-deficient and normal knees. Overall, the KT-1000 and Stryker devices had the highest diagnostic accuracy. They concluded that measurements cannot be generalized from one device to another.

Steiner et al[80] compared the test reproducibility of four knee laxity testing devices (KT-1000, Stryker, Acufex, and Genucom) in 13 normal and 15 ACL-deficient patients at 20- and 30-lb force. They observed significant ($p < .01$) differences in device measurement reproducibility. Measurements with the Acufex, KT-1000, and Stryker devices were more reproducible than with the Genucom and were capable of correctly identifying normal and abnormal knees approximately 90% of the time. The diagnostic accuracy of the Genucom was 60%. Testing sensitivity (65%) and specificity (45%) were lowest for the Genucom, whereas the KT-1000 and Stryker ranged between 75% and 85% and the Acufex between 85% and 95%.

Wroble et al[90] addressed the testing reproducibility of the Genucom system in 10 normal subjects and 3 with ACL-deficient knees. This study compared the results of multiple testing of normal subjects on 3 consecutive days and interexaminer and intraexaminer testing of three ACL-deficient patients on six occasions by two examiners.

Analysis of variance testing demonstrated no significant differences when normal subjects were multiply examined on a given day. There were, however, significant day-to-day differences within these normal subjects. For patients with ACL-deficient knees, there were significant interexaminer differences within a given day. They also observed a significant interaction between the day and the subject, indicative of day-to-day variation within individual subjects. The authors concluded that when using the Genucom, care must be taken in interpreting the data of a single measurement or even repeated measurements within a single seating because of day-to-day measurement variance.

Another analysis of the Genucom system was performed by Granberry and coworkers,[41] who used the system in eight cadaver lower extremities and compared their results with radiographic measurements. They noted that the Genucom overestimated internal and external rotation by approximately 10 degrees and that AP translations were overestimated in the Lachman test position (30 degrees of knee flexion). They attributed these errors to inaccuracies in adjustment for soft-tissue compression and concluded that the Genucom system was clinically of limited value.

Torzilli et al[84] prospectively compared the testing reproducibility of the KT-1000 versus the Genucom in 20 normal subjects. They studied between-subject variance and within-subject variance by performing repeat tests on the same day and repeating the examination 1 week later. The authors observed no statistically significant differences ($p < .05$) between the two testing dates and agreed with the conclusions of Edixhoven et al[29] that patient positioning could greatly affect measurement. However, they observed large variations for a given subject at different measurement points, which they quantified as a coefficient of variance. The authors noted a coefficient of variance that was two to three times greater with the Genucom device than with the KT-1000, with increased variance observed as larger force was applied across the knee. The authors concluded that the testing reproducibility of the KT-1000 was superior to that of the Genucom device. Repeated tests and large force resulted in better testing reproducibility, and the maximum manual test produced lower measurement variability.

Wroble et al[91] addressed the issue of testing repeatability with the KT-1000 in six normal subjects evaluated three times daily for 6 consecutive days with 20- and 30-lb force. Although there were no significant differences within a given day, significant ($p < .01$) differences were observed from one day to the next, with the greatest variation occurring on the first day of testing. Side-to-side comparisons were more repeatable than absolute translations.

In summary, these studies illustrate technical pitfalls and specific scenarios that could lead to inaccurate data or misinterpretation of data. Because the KT-1000 and its successor the KT-2000 have the most consistent reliability, it has become the most widely used instrumented arthrometer and is the recommended gold standard for outcome reporting and comparison of knee ligament laxity.

COMPARISON OF ARTHROMETRY WITH MAGNETIC RESONANCE IMAGING, CLINICAL EXAMINATION, OTHER METHODS

To better understand the relative accuracy of KT arthrometers, clinicians and researchers should be familiar with studies comparing this instrument's ability to accurately measure and diagnose knee laxity with the measurement and diagnostic ability of magnetic resonance imaging (MRI), clinical examination, stress radiography, and roentgen stereophotogrammetric analysis (RSA).

In 1995, Liu et al[61] reviewed 38 patients with arthroscopically proven ACL tears (complete). The results of physical examination, KT-1000 testing, and MRI were analyzed. MRI had an overall sensitivity of 97% for detecting ACL injuries; however, 6 of the 38 tears were classified as partial and 1 as intact. In fact, MRI had an overall sensitivity for differentiating between complete and partial tears of only 82%. KT-1000 testing based on a 2-mm side-to-side difference rather than a 3-mm difference classified two additional patients as having an ACL tear. The threshold for diagnosis was lowered to 2 mm and the sensitivity of the manual maximum test was 100%, whereas at a 3-mm threshold the sensitivity was 97%. Sensitivity increased with progressively larger amounts of force used for testing. Lachman test results yielded a sensitivity of 95%, with only two being recorded as negative. There were no statistically significant differences between the Lachman and the KT-1000 maximum manual and active displacement testing. This study illustrates the potential of arthrometry and careful physical examination to accurately diagnose an ACL tear. It is noted that though more expensive, MRI reveals a wealth of information regarding anatomic structures not evaluated by arthrometry.

A recently performed comparison of KT arthrometry, RSA, and stress radiography was reported by Fleming et al.[32] RSA is a technique that has been demonstrated to have a high level of accuracy in measuring joint kinematics and was used as the gold standard for comparison in this study. Fifteen patients were prospectively monitored after ACL reconstruction with a patellar autograft; stress radiography, KT arthrometry, and RSA analysis were performed at each postoperative evaluation. Mean AP laxity measurements for all time points were 11.4 ± 3.0, 10.2 ± 3.3, and 6.9 ± 3.0 mm (mean $\pm$ standard deviation) for the KT-1000, planar stress radiography, and RSA, respectively. These results were significantly different ($p < .001$), with the KT-1000 slightly overestimating the absolute AP excursion distance. The KT-1000 ($p = .04$) and the RSA techniques ($p = .04$) detected significant increases in AP laxity values over time, but the planar stress radiography technique did not ($p = .89$). The authors concluded that the KT-1000 and RSA documented temporal changes in AP laxity after ACL reconstruction that were not documented by planar stress radiography.

Margheritini et al[63] and others[47,73] have compared planar stress radiography with KT-2000 arthrometry for evaluation of PCL injuries. In these studies, planar stress radiography was shown to be superior to KT measurements in accurately determining the amount of posterior displacement. Margheritini and coworkers evaluated 60 patients with arthroscopically or MRI-confirmed complete PCL injuries with four different commercially available stress radiograph devices and techniques and compared these evaluations with KT-2000 assessment of PCL injuries. In these patients, stress radiographs were shown to be superior to arthrometric evaluation in quantifying posterior tibial translation. Stress radiographs performed with the knee in 90 degrees of flexion allowed for greater posterior tibial displacement than did tests performed in other positions. Consequently, quantification of ligament insufficiency was easier in this position. Stress radiographs performed through hamstring contraction gave the same results as those performed with Telos at 90 degrees of knee flexion.

IN VITRO KT-1000 TESTING

Several in vitro cadaver studies have examined the uninjured ACL with respect to arthrometry in an effort to understand the specific parameters in a normal ACL without a tear. Markolf and coworkers[64] used an instrumented testing device in a selective cutting study. In 35 normal cadaver knees tested at 20 degrees of flexion, they noted a mean translation of 6.6 mm ($\pm$2.5 mm) with a force of 100 N before ACL failure. Anterior displacement was studied in nine autopsy specimens by Fukubayashi et al,[36] who used a materials testing system machine in which the mean anterior displacement in intact specimens with a 100-N load was 7 mm (range, 5 to 7 mm). A large increase in displacement occurred after transection of the ACL (range, 12 to 17 mm). The authors noted that maximal anterior displacement occurred in all specimens at 30 degrees of knee flexion. In a subsequent study, Bach et al[10] noted that anterior displacement at 30 $\pm$ 5 degrees was statistically greater than that at 90 degrees because of relaxation of secondary stabilizers. This observation reinforces the importance of proper patient positioning to obtain accurate arthrometry data.

Daniel et al[22] quantified the restraining effect of the ACL in 31 fresh frozen cadaver knees by performing KT analysis before and after ACL sectioning. Mean anterior displacement before transection was 5.8 $\pm$ 2.3 mm (range, 2.8 to 11 mm). After complete ACL transection, mean anterior displacement was 12.1 mm. The mean difference between the two testing conditions was 6.3 $\pm$ 2.0 mm (range, 2 to 10 mm).

In a study of 10 fresh frozen cadaver knees to determine graft tension before fixation in ACL reconstruction, Burks and Leland[17] used the KT-1000 to assess displacement before and after ACL sectioning. At 89 N, the intact specimen had a mean displacement of 6.8 mm (range, 4.5 to 13 mm); on sectioning the ACL, the mean displacement was 13.1 mm (range, 8.5 to 20 mm). The mean difference was 6.3 mm (range, 3.5 to 9.5 mm), identical to Daniel's reported mean difference. The authors noted that these data were similar to their data in a previous study[16] in which the KT-1000 was used to measure displacement after ACL reconstruction in cadaver knees and the effects

of continuous passive motion. These cadaver-derived data of Burks et al, Fukubayashi et al, and Daniel et al closely parallel the in vivo data noted by Malcom, Daniel, and Bach.[12,16,22,23,25,36] These studies support the classic article of Butler et al[18] in which it was confirmed that the ACL is the primary restraint to anterior translation at 25 to 30 degrees of flexion.

NORMAL AND ACL-DEFICIENT KNEES

In 1985 and 1988 Daniel and colleagues[22-25,62] published several classic articles that introduced the KT-1000 arthrometer to the orthopedic community. These articles are valuable because they determined the parameters of *normal and abnormal* knees, thus establishing instrumented laxity testers as an important objective component in clinical knee laxity evaluation. In one study, normal ($n = 328$) and chronic ACL-deficient ($n = 89$) patients were compared.[22] A second study characterized the KT-1000 measurements in acute ACL-deficient patients ($n = 138$).[25] Another study compared KT-1000 measurements before and after ACL reconstruction.[62] They reported a mean anterior displacement at 89 N of 5.8 mm and 5.5 mm for left and right control knees, respectively. Of interest, displacement in the normal knee of chronic ACL-deficient patients was increased, with a mean anterior displacement of 7.4 mm. The injured knees had a mean translation of 13 mm. At 89 N, the side-to-side difference was noted to be 0.3 mm for control subjects versus a mean of 5.6 mm for chronic ACL-deficient patients. The mean compliance in normal subjects was 0.9 mm. In the normal knees of ACL-deficient patients, the mean compliance index was 1.2 mm, whereas the mean compliance was 2.9 mm in the injured knee. In the group of normal controls, neither gender nor age had an effect on mean displacement. They reported that 92% of subjects with normal knees had a side-to-side difference of less than 2 mm whereas 96% of patients with a unilateral ACL tear had a side-to-side difference of greater than 2 mm. Ninety-three percent of the normal subjects had a side-to-side difference in compliance of less than 0.5 mm, and 85% of the patients with unilateral ACL tears had a side-to-side difference in compliance of greater than 0.5 mm. Figure 36–7 demonstrates the distributions and side-to-side differences in normal ($n = 240$) and unilateral chronic ACL-deficient knees ($n = 74$).[23]

Daniel et al[25] studied 138 *acute* unilateral ACL-deficient patients and used 69-N, 89-N, compliance index, maximum manual, and injured-uninjured data in their evaluations. Their normal control knees ($n = 120$) had translations of 7.2 mm (range, 3 to 13.5 mm) at 89 N. The mean anterior displacement increased slightly when compared with the normal controls of their initial study, and the authors attributed this increase to improved testing technique and modification in the limb support system. The contralateral normal knee of the acute ACL-deficient patients had a mean translation of 7.3 mm (range, 3 to 13 mm) at 89 N, and this value was similar to that in the normal knees of chronic ACL-deficient patients reported earlier.[22] The mean maximum manual displacement was

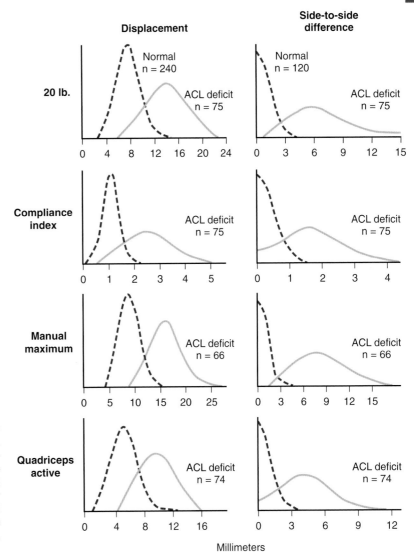

Figure 36–7. Frequency distribution curves of anterior laxity in a normal knee at 30 degrees of flexion and in knees with unilateral chronic anterior cruciate ligament (ACL) disruption. (From Daniel DM, Stone ML: Diagnosis of knee ligament injury: Tests and measurements of joint laxity. In Feagin JA Jr [ed]: The Crucial Ligaments: Diagnosis and Treatment of Ligamentous Injuries about the Knee. New York, Churchill Livingstone, 1988, pp 287-300.)

8.5 mm (range, 5 to 15 mm) in the control knees, and the mean compliance index was 0.9 mm (range, 0 to 2.5 mm). A key finding with the displacement measurements was that normal subjects have a wide range of normal laxity, but small side-to-side differences. For example, the 89-N anterior displacement range was 3 to 13.5 mm with a right knee–left knee mean difference of only 0.8 mm. Table 36–1 summarizes the data of the normal group.

In their acute ACL-deficient patients, Daniel et al[25] reported that the mean anterior displacement on the injured side was 11.4 mm (range, 6 to 19 mm) at 89 N (Fig. 36–8). The mean injured-uninjured difference at 89 N was 5 mm (range, 2 to 12 mm). The authors established a range of equivocal diagnostic and diagnostic laxity ranges for 89 N, maximum manual, compliance index, and side-to-side differences (Table 36–2). They reported that side-to-side differences were more important than absolute translations and concluded that a side-to-side difference of 3 mm or greater was diagnostic at 89 N or at maximum manual testing (Fig. 36–9). The authors noted that the side-to-side difference in normal knees at 89 N was less than 2 mm in 88% of patients. The maximum

Table 36–1. Normal Anterior Laxity (mm)

	MEAN	SD	RANGE
Joint displacement (n = 240)			
20 lb	7.2	1.9	3.0-13.5
Manual maximum	8.5	2.2	5.0-15.0
Compliance index	0.9	0.4	0-2.5
Joint displacement (n = 120), right-left difference			
20 lb	0.8	0.7	0-3.5
Manual maximum	0.8	1.0	0-3.5
Compliance index	0.2	0.3	0-1.0

From Daniel DM, Stone ML, Sachs R, et al: Instrumented measurement of anterior knee laxity in patients with acute anterior cruciate ligament disruption. Am J Sports Med 13:401, 1985.

manual difference was suggestive or diagnostic in 91% of patients. The mean injured-uninjured difference in the acute subjects at 89 N was 3.8 mm (range, 0 to 8 mm). On maximum manual testing, the mean difference was 5.2 mm (range, 1 to 10 mm). The mean compliance difference was 1.3 mm (range, 0 to 3 mm). Daniel et al also

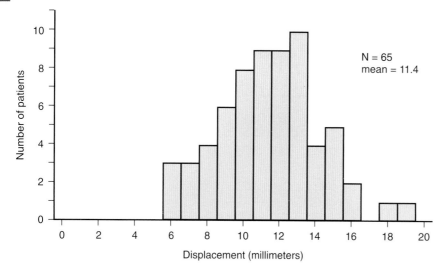

Figure 36–8. Twenty-pound anterior drawer displacement differences (without anesthesia) in 65 patients with findings of anterior cruciate ligament injury on arthroscopic examination. (From Daniel DM, Stone ML, Sachs R, et al: Instrumented measurement of anterior knee laxity in patients with acute anterior cruciate ligament disruption. Am J Sports Med 13:401, 1985.)

Table 36–2. Anterior Laxity (mm) Indicative of ACL Disruption in an Acutely Injured Knee

TEST	EQUIVOCAL LAXITY	DIAGNOSTIC LAXITY
20-lb anterior drawer	10.0-13.5	≥14.0
Manual maximum	12.0-15.0	≥15.5
Compliance index	2.0-2.5	≥3.0
Right-left difference (I-N)		
20-lb anterior drawer	2.0-2.5	≥3.0
Manual maximum	2.0-2.5	≥3.0
Compliance index	1	≥1.5

From Daniel DM, Stone ML, Sachs R, et al: Instrumented measurement of anterior knee laxity in patients with acute anterior cruciate ligament disruption. Am J Sports Med 13:401, 1985.

included 26 patients who were examined under anesthesia, and an increase in the mean 89-N difference and maximum manual difference was noted (Fig. 36–9) in this population.

Malcom et al[62] prospectively reviewed KT-1000 measurements in preoperative and postoperative ACL reconstruction patients. Four different surgical procedures were studied in 43 patients, including the Mott semitendinosus reconstruction, the Insall iliotibial band-over-the-top reconstruction, the Lambert bone–patellar tendon–bone (BPTB) reconstruction, and the Marshall-MacIntosh patellar tendon over-the-top reconstruction. The reader is referred to Malcom et al[62] for specific data regarding these procedures. The authors noted a mean translation of 8.5 mm at 89 N in the contralateral normal knees of chronic patients ($n = 19$). The mean side-to-side difference was 6.8 mm at 89 N before reconstruction. In the 24 acute patients, the mean displacement of the normal knees was 7.3 mm, and the mean injured-uninjured difference was 4 mm. In the operating room, patients were examined under anesthesia before reconstruction. The chronic patients ($n = 19$) had a mean injured-uninjured difference of 6.4 mm at 89 N (range, 1.5 to 16 mm). The acute

patients ($n = 24$) had a mean injured-uninjured difference of 5.6 mm at 89 N (range, 1.5 to 14.5 mm). After reconstruction, the immediate mean 89-N side-to-side difference was −1.4 mm for the chronic patients and 0.8 mm for the acute patients, thus indicating that the reconstructed knees were initially tighter than the contralateral normal knees. Figures 36–10 and 36–11 summarize these data.

Bach et al[4,10] used the KT-1000 to differentiate normal and abnormal ACL populations, to define the differences in translation between acute and chronic ACL-deficient knees, and to assess whether the uninjured knees of patients with unilateral ACL tears differed from those of a control population with normal knees. In this study, 141 controls, 107 patients with acute isolated ACL tears, and 153 chronic isolated ACL-deficient patients were evaluated. The authors reported their data regarding 30-degree anterior Lachman testing, 69-N and 89-N testing, maximum manual testing, compliance index determination, and side-to-side differences. ACL deficiency was confirmed by an abnormal asymmetric Lachman test, a positive pivot-shift phenomenon, or surgical verification.

Table 36–3 summarizes the authors' reported mean translations and ranges for normal, acute, and chronic ACL-deficient knees. Although mean translations were greater for acute and chronic knees at 69 N, 89 N, and maximum manual testing than for normal knees, there were wide ranges noted for both normal and abnormal knees, which concurs with Daniel's reported data of normal knees discussed earlier.

In Bach's series, only 6% of normal subjects exceeded 11-mm displacement at 89 N, thus leading the authors to conclude that 10 mm or less of anterior translation at this level of force was a predictor of a normal ACL. It should be emphasized, however, that an ACL-deficient knee may have 10 mm or less of translation. Table 36–3 demonstrates the distribution of translation in normal, acute, and chronic ACL-deficient patients. At 89 N, 99% of normal subjects had 10 mm or less of translation, whereas 62% of the acute and 56% of the chronic patients had 10 mm or less of anterior translation. On maximum manual testing, 94% of control subjects had 10 mm or less of translation,

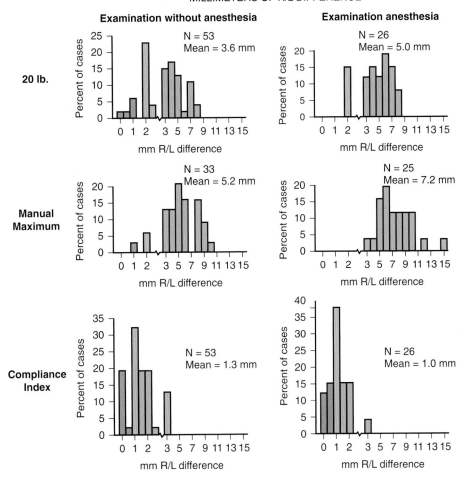

Figure 36–9. Instrumented measurements of anterior laxity in patients with acute anterior cruciate ligament disruption. (From Daniel DM, Stone ML, Sachs R, et al: Instrumented measurement of anterior knee laxity in patients with acute anterior cruciate ligament disruption. Am J Sports Med 13:401, 1985.)

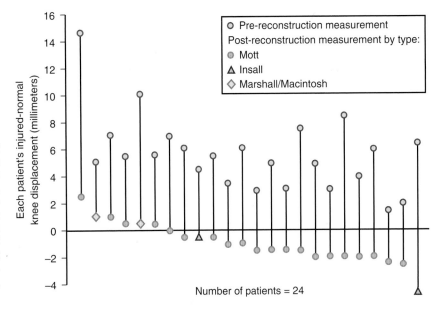

Figure 36–10. Results of three types of reconstruction in 24 patients with anterior cruciate ligament disruption operated on within 4 weeks of injury. Preoperative and postoperative reconstruction displacement differs between the injured knee and the normal knee in each patient. (From Malcom LL, Daniel DM, Stone ML, et al: The measurement of anterior knee laxity after ACL reconstructive surgery. Clin Orthop 196:35, 1985.)

CHRONIC PRE- AND POST-RECONSTRUCTION KNEE
ANTERIOR LAXITY UNDER ANESTHESIA

Arthrometer measurements: 30˚ flexion/20 lb. anterior force

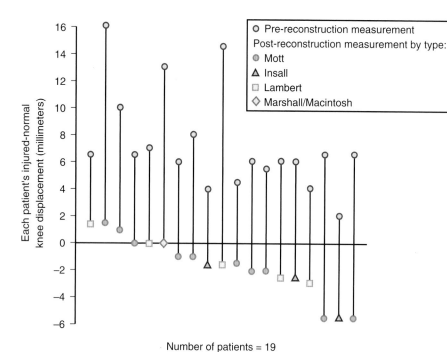

Number of patients = 19

Figure 36–11. Results of four types of reconstruction in 19 patients with chronic anterior cruciate ligament disruption. Preoperative and postoperative reconstruction displacement differs between the injured knee and the normal knee in each patient. (From Malcom LL, Daniel DM, Stone ML, et al: The measurement of anterior knee laxity after ACL reconstructive surgery. Clin Orthop 196:35, 1985.)

Table 36–3. Profiles of Normal, Acute, and Chronic ACL-Deficient Knees (mm)

	MEAN	RANGE	SD
89 N at 30 degrees of flexion			
Normal ($n = 141$)	6.3	2-12	1.84
Acute ($n = 107$)	9.6	4.5-19	3.1
Chronic ($n = 153$)	11.4	3-21	3.7
Maximum manual at 30 degrees of flexion			
Normal	7.0	4-11	ND
Acute	13.0	5-22	ND
Chronic	13.5	7-22	ND
Compliance at 30 degrees of flexion			
Normal	1.1	0.5-2.0	0.4
Acute	2.2	0.5-4.0	0.96
Chronic	2.1	0.5-6.0	1.05

ND, not determined; SD, standard deviation.
From Bach BR Jr, Warren RF, Flynn WM, et al: Arthrometric evaluation of knees that have a torn anterior cruciate ligament. J Bone Joint Surg Am 72:1299, 1990.

Table 36–4. Comparison of Involved-Uninvolved Differences (mm) in Acute and Chronic ACL-Insufficient Knees

	ACUTE (%)	CHRONIC (%)
30 Degrees (67 N)		
≤2.0	28	15
≥2.0	72	85
≥3.0	50	69
30 Degrees (89 N)		
≤2.0	16	12
≥2.0	84	88
≥3.0	69	79
30 Degrees maximum manual		
≤2.0	10	23
≥2.0	90	77
≥3.0	87	72

normal knees of chronic ACL-deficient patients were compared with those of control subjects at 67 N ($p < .003$), 89 N ($p < .002$), maximum manual ($p < .006$), and compliance index determination ($p < .001$). The authors did not have a specific explanation for these observations.

Differences between injured and uninjured knees, so-called side-to-side differences, were studied as well (Table 36–4). Side-to-side differences of 2 mm or less were noted in only 16% of acute and 12% of chronic ACL-deficient subjects. Maximum manual testing revealed that 91% of control subjects had 2 mm or less and 99% had 3 mm or less of involved-uninvolved differences. Of acute patients, 90% had 2-mm or greater side-to-side differences, and 87%

in contrast to 23% of acute and 22% of chronic ACL-deficient patients. Ninety-nine percent of normal subjects had a compliance index of 2 mm or less, whereas 43% of acute and 39% of chronic patients had a compliance index of 2 mm or greater.

Bach et al[4,10] also compared control knees with the uninjured knees of acute and chronic ACL-deficient subjects. No significant differences were found between the normal knees of acute subjects versus control subjects. However, statistically significant differences were noted when the of these patients had differences of 3 mm or greater. The authors also noted that the compliance side-to-side difference was 1 mm or less in 99% of the control subjects.[4,10] The mean, range, and standard deviations of side-to-side differences in control, acute, and chronic subjects are presented in Table 36–5. The differences between control subjects and ACL-deficient patients are statistically significant ($p < .001$), but there were no significant differences between acute and chronic ACL-deficient patients.

In that same study,[10] Lachman and pivot-shift grades were compared with the maximum manual test measurements of the KT-1000 in an attempt to correlate objective measurements with clinical grades. It was interesting to note that a statistically significant difference ($p < .003$) was noted when Lachman grades 1, 2, and 3 were compared with the maximum manual test results (Table 36–6). Mean translations were 12, 13, and 16 mm, respectively, for Lachman grades 1, 2, and 3. For pivot-shift grades 1, 2, and 3, statistically significant differences were also noted ($p < .027$). The pivot-shift grades (1 to 3) correlated with 13, 14, and 17 mm of anterior translation.

These findings for maximum manual differences were correlated with the Lachman and pivot-shift grades (Table 36–6). Though not statistically significant, an increasing trend was associated with increasing Lachman grade. Lachman grades 1, 2, and 3 correlated with 3, 4, and 8 mm of anterior side-to-side difference on maximum manual testing. The same trend was noted when compared with pivot-shift grades. The mean maximum manual side-to-side differences were 4, 5, and 8 mm, respectively, for pivot-shift grades 1, 2, and 3.

These data allowed a determination of the sensitivity, specificity, positive predictive accuracy, and negative predictive accuracy for side-to-side differences, the results of which are shown in Table 36–7. In general, the authors found that the most sensitive test was the maximum manual test in acute ACL-deficient patients (90%) when a side-to-side difference of 2 mm or greater was used. In both acute and chronic patients, a diagnostic cutoff of greater than 2 mm had higher sensitivity and higher negative predictive accuracy but less specificity than when a diagnostic cutoff of 3 mm or greater was used. In acute ACL-deficient patients, the authors noted that the maximum manual test was the best screening test (89%). A diagnostic cutoff of 3 mm or greater in side-to-side difference was found to be highly specific (90% to 94%) but less sensitive in the acute and chronic ACL-deficient subjects. At that diagnostic cutoff, the maximum manual test was a better screening test in the acute ACL-deficient subjects (84%). When an absolute displacement of 10 mm or less was selected as a diagnostic cutoff, the maximum manual test was determined to be highly specific and sensitive for both acute (93%) and chronic (91%) subjects. It also had high positive predictive accuracy (92% and 94%). On compliance index determination, the authors noted that a diagnostic cutoff of 1.6 mm or less was more sensitive than a cutoff of 2 mm or less. However, the positive

Table 36–5. Maximum Manual Involved-Uninvolved Difference in Normal and in Acute and Chronic ACL-Insufficient Knees (mm)

	MEAN	SD	RANGE
Normal ($n = 141$)	0.2	±1.6	(–4 to +4)
Acute ($n = 107$)	4.8	±3.7	(–7 to +12)
Chronic ($n = 153$)	5.5	±4.5	(–6 to +16)

Table 36–6. Comparison of Maximum Manual and Maximum Manual Involved-Uninvolved Differences (mm) with Clinical Lachman and Pivot-Shift Grades

	MAXIMUM MANUAL	MAXIMUM MANUAL DIFFERENCE
Lachman		
1	12	3
2	13	4
3	16	8
Pivot shift		
1	13	4
2	14	5
3	17	8

Table 36–7. Sensitivity (%) and Specificity (%) of Involved-Uninvolved Differences in Acute and Chronic ACL Deficiency

	ACUTE ACL DEFICIENCY			CHRONIC ACL DEFICIENCY		
	15 lb	20 lb	Maximum Manual	15 lb	20 lb	Maximum Manual
>2 mm						
Sensitivity	72	84	90	85	88	77
Specificity	75	73	64	75	73	64
PPA	69	71	65	72	78	68
NPA	74	86	89	84	84	73
>3 mm						
Sensitivity	50	49	77	69	79	72
Specificity	94	93	90	94	94	90
PPA	88	66	86	93	94	98
NPA	64	84	84	74	81	76

NPA, negative predictive accuracy; PPA, positive predictive accuracy.
Adapted from Bach BR Jr, Warren RF, Flynn WM, et al: Arthrometric evaluation of knees that have a torn anterior cruciate ligament. J Bone Joint Surg Am 72:1299, 1990.

predictive accuracy was higher in both acute and chronic patients when the 2-mm cutoff was used.

In consideration of these findings, Bach et al used a maximum manual difference of 3 mm and absolute displacement of 10 mm as criteria for diagnosing an ACL tear and ran these criteria against normal and injured populations. For these parameters, the sensitivity was 99% (chi-square test, 65.2). With regard to whether a 3-mm side-to-side difference or an absolute displacement of 10 mm is a better criterion for diagnosing an ACL tear, there was no statistically significant difference in the diagnostic ability of these two criteria when applied to normal and abnormal populations. The maximum manual test was the best parameter for differentiating normal from abnormal knees ($p < .001$) as determined by a stepwise discriminate analysis using 16 factors, whereas compliance index determination was the most important testing parameter for differentiating between acute and chronic ACL-deficient knees.

In 1994, Rijke et al[74] reported on the use of instrumented arthrometry for diagnosing partial versus complete ACL tears. They used a KT-1000 equipped with a strain gauge and processor that monitored the force required to increase anterior displacement by 1-mm increments, which was then read on a light-emitting diode. They examined 19 patients with the clinical diagnosis of ACL injury via the modified KT-1000 before arthroscopy. The authors reported that the results of KT testing of partially torn and completely torn ligaments were similar to those obtained by graded stress radiography. Partial tears could be differentiated from complete tears with a sensitivity and specificity of 80% and 100%, respectively, whereas for complete tears, the figures were 100% and 80%. The authors note that because of large patient-to-patient variables, only side-to-side comparisons can provide diagnostic distinction and then only in the presence of a normal opposite knee.

KT-1000 COMPARISON EXAMINATION: PATIENTS AWAKE AND UNDER ANESTHESIA

Several published works have examined the effect of anesthesia on physical examination and arthrometry of the knee, specifically with respect to the evaluation of ligamentous laxity. Combined, these studies demonstrate the value of examination under anesthesia and identify the maximum manual anterior KT arthrometry displacement test as the single best test to measure anterior displacement in both acute and chronic ACL injuries, as well as knees without ligament injuries.

Highgenboten et al[49] used the KT-1000 to measure anterior laxity in the knees of 68 unilateral ACL-deficient patients while they were awake and again while under anesthesia. They reported a significant increase ($p < .01$) in the measured displacement in normal and uninjured knees while under anesthesia. In addition, when compared with awake measurements, there was an increase ($p < .01$) in the side-to-side difference in patients while they were under anesthesia.

Bach et al analyzed KT measurements in ACL patients undergoing reconstruction while awake and while under anesthesia, but unlike Highgenboten et al[49] and others,[28,55,56,93] this study included an analysis of the diagnostic accuracy of the anterior drawer, Lachman, and pivot-shift tests as well.[87,92] A hundred patients with surgically confirmed ACL deficiency were evaluated. In acute patients, all demonstrated an abnormal Lachman test preoperatively and under anesthesia. The sensitivity of the anterior drawer test improved from 36% to 76% when examined under anesthesia in the acute subgroup. The pivot-shift phenomenon improved from 24% while awake to 92% while under anesthesia in the acute subjects. In the chronic subjects, all patients had an abnormal Lachman test while awake preoperatively and under anesthesia, the anterior drawer test improved from 61% to 83%, and the pivot-shift test improved from 71% to 100%.

The mean translations in the acute, chronic, and total populations in this study are shown in Tables 36–8 and 36–9. The mean displacement at 89 N increased from 8.4 mm while awake to 9.8 mm under anesthesia. The mean maximum manual difference increased from 12 to 15.8 mm. The mean compliance index determination did not appear to change significantly from the awake state (2.2 mm) to examination under anesthesia (2.3 mm). Mean side-to-side differences increased at 89 N and maximum manual testing, but compliance index differences did not (Table 36–10). At 89 N, the mean side-to-side difference was 4.4 mm while awake and 5 mm under anesthesia. For the combined acute and chronic ACL-deficient populations, the mean maximum manual side-to-side difference between the injured and uninjured knees was 7 mm while awake and 9 mm under anesthesia.

Table 36–8. KT-1000 Data in 50 Contralateral Normal Knees

| | 15 lb | | | | 20 lb | | | | MAXIMUM MANUAL | | | |
| | Preoperative | | Under Anesthesia | | Preoperative | | Under Anesthesia | | Preoperative | | Under Anesthesia | |
ACL DEFICIENCY	Mean	Range	Mean	Range	Mean	Range	Mean	Range	Mean	Range	Mean	Range
Acute ($n = 10$)	3.0	1-7	4.4	3.0-6.5	3.8	1.5-8.0	5.2	3.5-7.5	4.6	2.0-10.0	6.9	4.0-9.0
Chronic ($n = 40$)	3.2	1-8	4.1	1.5-8.0	4.0	1.0-9.5	5.0	2.0-9.0	5.1	2.0-10.5	6.8	3.0-12.0
Total ($n = 50$)	3.2	3.0	4.2	1.0-9.5	4.0	2.0-9.0	5.0	2.0-9.0	5.0	3.0-10.5	6.8	3.0-12.0

Values are in millimeters.
From Wang CW, Bach BR Jr: Clinical diagnosis of ACL-deficient knees. J Orthop Surg 7:139, 1990.

Table 36–9. KT-1000 Data in 50 ACL-Deficient Knees

| | 15 lb | | | | 20 lb | | | | MAXIMUM MANUAL | | | |
| | Preoperative | | Under Anesthesia | | Preoperative | | Under Anesthesia | | Preoperative | | Under Anesthesia | |
ACL DEFICIENCY	Mean	Range	Mean	Range	Mean	Range	Mean	Range	Mean	Range	Mean	Range
Acute ($n = 10$)	6.0	3.5-8.5	7.2	4.0-9.0	8.0	4.5-10.5	9.2	7.0-12.5	10.8	7.5-14.0	15.2	12.0-19.5
Chronic ($n = 40$)	6.4	2.5-14.5	7.7	2.5-13.0	8.5	4.0-16.5	9.9	3.5-16.0	12.3	6.0-21.0	16.0	9.5-24.0
Total ($n = 50$)	6.3	2.5-14.5	7.6	2.5-13.0	8.4	4.0-16.5	9.8	3.5-16.0	12.0	6.0-21.0	15.8	9.5-24.0

Values are in millimeters.
From Wang CW, Bach BR Jr: Clinical diagnosis of ACL-deficient knees. J Orthop Surg 7:139, 1990.

Table 36–10. Compliance Index Determination in Normal and ACL-Deficient Knees

| | PREOPERATIVE | | UNDER ANESTHESIA | |
	Mean (mm)	Range (mm)	Mean (mm)	Range (mm)
Normal knees ($n = 50$)	0.85	0.5-2.0	0.89	0.5-2.0
ACL-deficient knees ($n = 50$)	2.17	0.5-4.0	2.27	0.5-4.0

From Wang CW, Bach BR Jr: Clinical diagnosis of ACL-deficient knees. J Orthop Surg 7:139, 1990.

Wang and Bach[87] and Wu et al[92] applied the diagnostic criteria established by Daniel et al.[25] Daniel et al established a *diagnostic* cutoff of 14 mm or greater for 89 N, 15.5 mm or greater for maximum manual testing, and 3 mm or greater for compliance index determination (see Table 36–2). *Equivocal* diagnostic cutoffs were 10 to 13.5 mm (89 N), 11 to 15 mm (maximum manual), and 2 to 3 mm (compliance index). Table 36–11 summarizes the results of these criteria. Of particular note is that the maximum manual test under anesthesia was the only test that was diagnostic in more than 50% of our patients, although the sum of the equivocal and diagnostic patients was 95%. We applied the modified criteria of Bach et al[10] to this study (Table 36–12) and used the diagnostic criteria of an absolute translation of 10 mm or greater for either the 89-N or maximum manual test and 2 mm or greater for the compliance index. This previously described modification significantly improved the diagnostic accuracy; the maximum manual test correctly diagnosed 75% of the patients examined while awake and 98% of those examined under anesthesia (Table 36–12).

In this study, Bach et al evaluated the criteria of Daniel et al and their own modified criteria by applying these criteria to the 89-N, maximum manual, and compliance tests to determine whether no, one, two, or all three diagnostic criteria were met (Table 36–13).[10] The results showed that 53% of the patients met only one diagnostic criterion (chronic; examination under anesthesia) and 45% to 95% failed to meet any of these criteria. In contrast, when the modified criteria were applied, fewer patients failed to meet any diagnostic criteria (0% to 25%). Seventy-five percent to 100% met at least one diagnostic criterion, and 64% to 74% met at least two diagnostic criteria. It should be recalled that the modified criteria were based on the observation that nearly all normal patients have a maximum manual translation of 10 mm or less. Based on the findings of this study, we support the observation of Bach et al that 10 mm or greater translation on 89-N or maximum manual testing implies ACL injury until proved otherwise, and we concur that the KT arthrometer instrumented ligamentous laxity maximum manual test is the single best physical examination test for evaluation of ACL injury.

Anderson and Lipscomb[2] conducted a prospective study of 50 subjects awake and under anesthesia with the KT-1000, Stryker knee ligament laxity tester, and the Genucom. The objective of this study was to compare laxity differences in subjects while awake and while under anesthesia and to compare the three different testing devices. The authors tested 30 acute, 9 subacute (2 weeks to 3 months), and 11 chronic injuries. The Lachman test was abnormal in 91% of acute and 100% of chronic patients while awake, whereas the anterior drawer test was positive in only 20% of acute and 60% of chronic patients. The authors reported 130-N readings and compliance index determination results; they did not report maximum manual results because they could not be compared with the Stryker and Genucom readings. They used a side-to-side difference of 3 mm or greater as a diagnostic criterion (Table 36–14). The mean side-to-side difference was 0.4 mm in normal knees and 4.3 mm in isolated ACL injuries with the KT-1000. No statistically significant differences were noted in acute and chronic ACL-deficient patients. The diagnosis after clinical examination under anesthesia was correct in 98% of patients. Using side-to-side difference criteria, the KT-1000 was correct in 75% (Table 36–15). Daniel et al[25] noted an increase in their diagnostic accuracy from 62% to 91% when the maximum manual test was used for awake patients, but if the authors had used the maximum manual test under anesthesia, it is likely that the diagnostic accuracy would have improved for that series. Anderson and Lipscomb reported that their diagnostic accuracy was better than that of Daniel et al, but it is important to note that Daniel et al reported their data in an acute ACL-deficient population whereas the series reported by Anderson and Lipscomb included chronic ACL-deficient patients.

Table 36-11. Analysis of ACL-Deficient Knees with Negative or Equivocal Diagnostic Testing Criteria*

	ACUTE (N = 40)						CHRONIC (N = 40)						TOTAL (N = 50)					
	Neg		Eq		Diag		Neg		Eq		Diag		Neg		Eq		Diag	
	n	%	n	%	n	%	n	%	n	%	n	%	n	%	n	%	n	%
20 lb																		
Awake	9	90	1	10	0		30	75	8	20	2	5	39	78	9	18	2	4
Under anesthesia	6	60	4	40	0		20	50	15	38	5	12	26	52	19	38	5	10
Maximum manual																		
Awake	4	40	6	60	0		15	38	18	45	7	17	19	38	24	48	7	14
Under anesthesia	0		7	70	3	30	2	5	18	45	20	50	2	4	25	50	23	46
Compliance index																		
Awake	3	30	6	60	1	10	15	38	16	40	9	22	18	36	22	44	10	20
Under anesthesia	3	30	5	50	2	20	14	35	16	40	10	25	17	34	21	42	12	24

*Equivocal diagnostic criteria (Eq): 20 lb, 10.0 to 13.5 mm; maximum manual, 11 to 15 mm; compliance index, 2.0 to 3.0 mm. Negative (Neg) indicates values less than the range; diagnostic (Diag) indicates values greater than the range.
From Wang CW, Bach BR Jr: Clinical diagnosis of ACL-deficient knees. J Orthop Surg 7:139, 1990.

Table 36-12. KT-1000 Diagnostic Criteria: Acute and Chronic ACL Deficiency

	CRITERIA OF DANIEL ET AL[24]*		MODIFIED CRITERIA[†]	
	n	%	n	%
Acute (n = 10)				
20 lb				
Awake	0	0	1	10
Under anesthesia	0	0	4	40
Maximum manual				
Awake	0	0	8	80
Under anesthesia	3	30	10	100
Compliance index				
Awake	1	10	7	70
Under anesthesia	2	20	7	70
Chronic (n = 40)				
20 lb				
Awake	2	5	12	30
Under anesthesia	5	12.5	20	50
Maximum manual				
Awake	7	17.5	30	75
Under anesthesia	20	50	39	98
Compliance index				
Awake	9	22.5	25	63
Under anesthesia	10	25	26	65

*Criteria of Daniel et al[24]: 20 lb, ≥14 mm; maximum manual, ≥15.5 mm; compliance index, ≥3.0 mm.
[†]Modified criteria: 20 lb, ≥10 mm; maximum manual, ≥10 mm; compliance index, ≥2.0 mm.
From Wang CW, Bach BR Jr: Clinical diagnosis of ACL-deficient knees. J Orthop Surg 7:139, 1990.

Table 36-13. Diagnostic Categories: Assessment of Patients Meeting Zero to Three Diagnostic Criteria

	CRITERIA OF DANIEL ET AL[24]*		MODIFIED CRITERIA[†]	
	n	%	n	%
Acute (n = 10)				
Awake				
0	9	90	2	20
≥1	1	10	8	80
≥2	0	7	70	
≥3	0	1	10	
Under anesthesia				
0	7	70	0	
≥1	3	30	10	100
≥2	2	20	7	70
≥3	0	4	40	
Chronic (n = 40)				
Awake				
0	27	67.5	10	25
≥1	13	32.5	30	75
≥2	5	12.5	25	63
≥3	0	12	30	
Under anesthesia				
0	18	45	0	
≥1	22	53	40	100
≥2	9	22.5	28	70
≥3	4	10	17	43
Total (N = 50)				
Awake				
0	9	90	12	24
≥1	14	28	38	76
≥2	5	10	32	64
≥3	0	13	26	
Under anesthesia				
0	36	72	0	
≥1	25	50	50	100
≥2	11	22	35	70
≥3	4	8	21	42

*Criteria of Daniel et al[24]: 20 lb, ≥14 mm; maximum manual, ≥15.5 mm; compliance index, ≥3.0 mm.
[†]Modified criteria: 20 lb, ≥10 mm; maximum manual, ≥10 mm; compliance index, ≥2.0 mm.
From Wang CW, Bach BR Jr: Clinical diagnosis of ACL-deficient knees. J Orthop Surg 7:139, 1990.

From this study, Anderson and Lipscomb concluded that the KT-1000 and Stryker knee ligament laxity testers were similar in their diagnostic abilities but that the KT-1000 most clearly paralleled the clinical examination and was more versatile. The authors believed that the versatility of the KT-1000 included the ability to determine the quadriceps neutral position and the diagnosis of PCL deficiency. Anderson and Lipscomb pointed out that the Genucom was more versatile for collateral and rotatory

Table 36–14. Side-to-Side Differences in Patients with ACL Tears

DEVICE	20- TO 30-DEGREE ANTERIOR DRAWER (89 N)			COMPLIANCE INDEX		
	Acute	Chronic	All	Acute	Chronic	All
KT-1000	4.35	4.4	4.4	2.1	1.4	1.7
Stryker	4.4	5.2	4.6	1.4	1.1	1.2
Genucom	1.7	1.5	2.0			

From Anderson AF, Lipscomb AB: Preoperative instrumented testing of anterior and posterior knee laxity. Am J Sports Med 17:387, 1989.

Table 36–15. Accuracy of Instrumented Examination in All ACL Tears

	KT-1000	STRYKER	GENUCOM	CLINICAL EXAMINATION
Correct	75	75	70	95
Equivocal*	12	12	5	0
Incorrect	13	13	25	5
False positive	0	10	10	0

*Equivocal: passive anterior drawer of 2 to 3 mm or compliance of 1.0 to 1.55 mm.
From Anderson AF, Lipscomb AB: Preoperative instrumented testing of anterior and posterior knee laxity. Am J Sports Med 17:387, 1989.

Table 36–16. Mean Arthrometric Values (mm) in Injured Knees and Contralateral Uninjured Knees Examined with the Patient Awake and under Anesthesia

	AWAKE	UNDER ANESTHESIA	p
Acute injury ($n = 23$)			
AD I	9.6	11.7	<.001
AD IUD	3.1	4.8	<.001
Comp I	2.3	2.6	NS
Comp IUD	1.1	1.4	NS
MM I	12.8	15.9	<.001
MM IUD	4.8	7.4	<.001
Chronic injury ($n = 18$)			
AD I	12.1	13.8	<.001
AD IUD	5.6	7.1	<.001
Comp	2.6	2.8	NS
Comp IUD	1.2	1.3	NS
MM I	15.1	17.4	<.001
MM IUD	7.7	9.2	<.002
Contralateral uninjured knee ($n = 41$)			
AD U	6.5	6.8	<.05
Comp U	1.3	1.3	NS
MM U	7.7	8.4	<.001

AD, anterior displacement at 89 N; AD IUD, anterior displacement difference, injured-uninjured knee at 89 N; Comp, compliance; Comp IUD, compliance difference, injured-uninjured knees; I, injured; MM, maximum manual displacement; MM IUD, maximum manual displacement difference, injured-uninjured knees; NS, not significant; U, uninjured.
From Dahlstedt LJ, Dalen N: Knee laxity in cruciate ligament injury: Value of examination under anesthesia. Acta Orthop Scand 60:181, 1989.

Table 36–17. Mean Differences (mm) between Injured and Uninjured Knees When Examined with an Arthrometer under Anesthesia

	MEAN DIFFERENCE
Acute ACL injury ($n = 23$)	
Anterior displacement (89 N)	4.8
Compliance	1.4
Maximum manual displacement	7.4
Chronic ACL injury ($n = 41$)	
Anterior displacement (89 N)	7.1
Compliance	1.3
Maximum manual displacement	9.1

From Dahlstedt LJ, Dalen N: Knee laxity in cruciate ligament injury: Value of examination under anesthesia. Acta Orthop Scand 60:181, 1989.

insufficiency and nearly as accurate as the KT-1000 and Stryker but that the recorded displacements were less (mean involved-uninvolved differences, 2.2 mm). Clinical examination yielded the most accurate approach to the ACL diagnosis, but the authors concluded that instrumented testing was beneficial.[2]

Dahlstedt and Dalen[21] demonstrated the value of examination under anesthesia by performing KT-1000 evaluations under anesthesia in 41 patients. They noted statistically significant increases ($p < .001$) for uninvolved knees in both acute and chronic ACL patients when side-to-side differences were performed at 89-N and maximum manual testing (Table 36–16). No statistically significant differences were noted for the compliance index in patients examined while awake or under anesthesia for normal or injured knees. At 89 N, the mean anterior displacement in acute and chronic ACL-deficient knees was 9.6 and 12.1 mm, respectively, while awake. This value increased to 11.7 and 13.8 mm, respectively, when examined under anesthesia. For the maximum manual test, displacement in acute knees increased from 12.8 mm while awake to 15.9 mm while under anesthesia, whereas in chronic ACL-deficient knees, displacement increased from 15.1 mm while awake to 17.4 mm under anesthesia. The mean side-to-side difference at 89 N while awake was 4.8 mm in acute patients and 7.4 mm in chronic patients. The side-to-side differences in chronic patients increased while under anesthesia. A mean involved-uninvolved difference of 7.1 mm was noted at 89 N, and an involved-uninvolved difference of 9.1 mm was noted on maximum manual testing (Table 36–17). The authors' results led them to conclude that the maximum manual test was the best diagnostic test for ACL deficiency. Their conclusion agrees with those of Bach et al,[5] Daniel et al,[22] and Wang and Bach.[87]

APPLICATION OF KNEE LAXITY TESTERS TO SURGICAL RESULTS

Several studies have examined the arthrometric results of surgical treatment of ACL injuries. Correlations to knee function and outcomes after ACL reconstruction by various techniques, including fracture repair[58] and graft sources, are now available and will be reviewed here. Familiarity with these studies and their results is important to clinicians and researchers for proper interpretation of arthrometry results.

Giannotti et al[37] reported a study in which they correlated arthrometric measurements with functional knee scores. Immediate and 1-, 2-, and 3-year postoperative reconstruction KT-1000 maximum manual test results, as well as Tegner, Lysholm, and Hospital for Special Surgery knee scores, were compared in 28 patients who underwent ACL reconstruction. The average immediate postoperative reconstruction maximum manual side-to-side difference was −2.1 mm, with the reconstructed side tighter than the uninvolved knee. The 1-year postoperative side-to-side difference was 2.3 mm, with the reconstructed knee demonstrating more laxity than the uninvolved knee. Evaluation of the various functional knee scores showed uniformly excellent results despite a wide range of laxity at 2 and 3 years. The authors concluded that an increase in laxity does not preclude excellent functional results and proposed that the follow-up side-to-side differences are more important than the time-dependent increase in laxity.

Although direct primary ACL repair was popular in the mid-1980s, ACL repair has fallen out of favor in the last 2 decades, in large part because of the use of carefully measured KT arthrometry data that allow for meticulous analysis of outcomes and the formation of carefully supported conclusions based on objective evaluations of persistent anterior laxity after attempted repair. In 1987, Higgins and Steadman[48] retrospectively reviewed 24 elite-level skiers who underwent acute ACL repair (nonaugmented) and were evaluated at a mean of 57 months postoperatively. Nineteen patients underwent extra-articular iliotibial band tenodesis. Five of the patients had sustained knee dislocations. The authors evaluated the knees with the KT-1000 arthrometer and reported KT-1000 data at 69 N, 89 N, and maximum manual testing, as well as compliance index determination and quadriceps active displacement. Their KT data demonstrated a persistent mean maximum manual side-to-side difference of 1.8 mm, with a mean translation of 9.0 mm (range, 4.5 to 13.5 mm ± 2.3). Although the mean is below the cutoff

established by Bach et al[4] for ACL deficiency, with a standard deviation of 2.3, a large portion of these arthrometry maximum manual side-to-side differences were above the threshold for ACL deficiency, thus indicating a failed repair. In addition, of the 24 patients in the repair group, 4 had positive pivot-shift or Lachman examinations suggestive of a failed ACL, and 5 patients required re-repair.

Autograft Reconstruction

In 1988, Harter et al[46] retrospectively reviewed 51 patients at an average of 48 months after a variety of repairs and reconstructions, both intra- and extra-articular. The authors used KT-1000 measurements at 67 N and 89 N and compliance index data, but not maximum manual. They found a statistically significant difference ($p < 0.001$) between surgical and control knees at 89 N. The mean anterior displacement of the surgical knees at 89 N was 8 mm, as compared with 6.2 mm for the control knees. The KT data gathered in this study were part of a comprehensive evaluation that consisted of questionnaires, physical examination, including objective measurement of strength and proprioception, patient activity rating scales, and other experimental variables. The authors concluded that the results of static and dynamic clinical tests to assess knee stability and function were independent of the patient's perception of the knee.

Harter and coworkers[45] used the KT-1000 arthrometer to measure anterior laxity in the knees of 50 patients at a minimum of 2 years after ACL reconstruction by either patellar tendon or semitendinosus autograft reconstruction. The authors reported 67-N, 89-N, and compliance index tests, but not the maximum manual test. Statistically significant differences ($p < .001$) were noted between normal knees and reconstructed knees, but not between the types of grafts used. For patellar tendon reconstructions, the mean translation was 8.1 mm at 67 N and 8.5 mm at 89 N. The mean compliance was 0.5 mm. For the semitendinosus graft (combined with an extra-articular tenodesis in 20 patients), the mean translations were 6.6, 7.3, and 0.8 mm, respectively (Table 36–18). In their

Table 36–18. Anterior Laxity and Anterior Compliance Indices according to Type of Reconstruction and Duration of Follow-up*

	TYPE OF RECONSTRUCTION[†]		DURATION OF POSTOPERATIVE FOLLOW-UP	
	Central Third of Patellar Tendon (n = 30)	*Semitendinosus Tendon* (n = 20)	*Intermediate*[‡] (n = 24)	*Long Term*[§] (n = 26)
Laxity (mm)				
68-N Lachman test	8.1 ± 3.5	6.6 ± 2.5	7.6 ± 3.1	7.4 ± 3.4
90-N Lachman test	8.5 ± 3.8	7.3 ± 3.0	8.1 ± 3.4	8.0 ± 3.7
Anterior compliance index (mm)	0.5 ± 0.4	0.8 ± 0.6	0.5 ± 0.5	0.7 ± 0.5

*Values represent mean and standard deviation. Differences between groups (classified according to type of reconstruction and duration of follow-up) were not significant (p > .01), as shown by analyses of variance.
[†]All patients also had one of four types of extra-articular iliotibial band tenodesis at the time of ACL reconstruction (see text).
[‡]Twenty-four to 40 months after reconstruction; mean, 31.6 months.
[§]More than 40 months after reconstruction; mean, 63 months.
From Harter RA, Osternig LR, Singer KM: Instrumented Lachman tests for the evaluation of anterior laxity after reconstruction of the anterior cruciate ligament. J Bone Joint Surg Am 71:975, 1989.

intermediate follow-up group, monitored 24 to 40 months postoperatively, there was no statistically significant differences from the 26 patients monitored for a mean of 63 months. In their series, 44% had flexion contractures ranging from 1 to 10 degrees, so they compared the effect of flexion contractures on laxity measurements. No statistically significant difference was noted in anterior displacement (89 N) or compliance index determination (Table 36–19) as a result of flexion contracture. Although the mean difference between normal and reconstructed knees was found to be significant ($p < .001$), it should be noted that the normal reconstructed difference was 2 mm. Daniel et al[22] noted that 92% of *normal* subjects have a right-left difference of 2 mm or less. Harter et al,[45] in fact, noted that 66% of their patients had normal reconstructive differences of less than 3 mm.

This debate of the relative benefits of a patellar tendon graft versus a hamstring autograft continues today. Freedman et al[35] performed a meta-analysis of 34 studies evaluating KT arthrometer data in 1976 patients at a minimum of 2 years after ACL reconstruction with either a patellar tendon or hamstring autograft. In the cumulative analysis of KT data, 79% of the patellar tendon autograft patients had a maximum manual side-to-side difference of less than 3 mm, whereas only 73% of the hamstring autograft patients had a side-to-side difference of less than 3 mm. This difference was statistically significant and led the authors to conclude that the patellar tendon graft choice resulted in greater static stability at 2 years than did the hamstring graft. In this meta-analysis, the improved arthrometer scores correlated with improved patient satisfaction with the patellar tendon graft at 2 years despite a higher incidence of anterior knee pain.

Another recent KT arthrometer evaluation of the hamstring autograft was performed by Feller and Webster.[30] Sixty-five patients were evaluated at a minimum 36 months after being randomized to receive either a patellar tendon autograft or a quadruple hamstring autograft for primary ACL reconstruction. This analysis revealed a greater side-to-side difference in anterior laxity at maximum manual testing for the hamstring autograft

group than for the patellar tendon autograft group. This increased laxity in the hamstring autograft group was associated with increased femoral tunnel widening, but there were no statistically significant differences in Cincinnati outcome scores, International Knee Documentation Committee (IKDC) ratings, and return-to-play rates between the patellar tendon and hamstring groups.

Tibone and Antich[83] reviewed 11 patients at a minimum of 2 years after intra-articular patellar tendon reconstruction and extra-articular augmentation. The patients were studied objectively by gait analysis, Cybex, and KT-1000 arthrometer assessment. No patients demonstrated a pivot shift, but instrumented arthrometry testing revealed the operated knee to be significantly looser only during maximum manual testing (7.2 mm versus 5.3 mm, $p < .01$). For all other KT measurements, there was no significant difference between the normal and surgical knees. The mean side-to-side differences were 1 mm (67 N), 1.1 mm (89 N), 0 mm (compliance index), and 1.9 mm (maximum manual).

Andriacchi's group[14] reported on the functional results via gait analysis after ACL reconstruction. Ten patients were studied in a gait analysis laboratory at a 22-month mean postoperative follow-up. KT-1000 data were used preoperatively and postoperatively in clinical follow-up. All patients had a preoperative clinical evaluation consistent with ACL deficiency. The mean translations of involved and uninvolved knees preoperatively and postoperatively are shown in Table 36–20. The mean maximum manual side-to-side difference (0.4 mm), the mean displacements at 89-N and maximum manual testing, and the compliance indices were significantly reduced ($p < .001$) in comparison to preoperative KT-1000 measurements. These data paralleled their clinical evaluation in which 90% of the patients had a negative pivot-shift phenomenon.

Grana and Hines[40] used the Stryker system to evaluate their results of 54 ACL reconstructions at an average of 3.4 years after arthroscopically assisted semitendinosus reconstruction without extra-articular augmentation. At a 13.5-kg force, side-to-side differences of 5 mm or greater were noted in five patients (9%).

Table 36–19. Anterior Laxity and Anterior Compliance Indices according to Postoperative Extension of Knee*

LAXITY	68-N LACHMAN TEST (mm)	90-N LACHMAN TEST (mm)	ANTERIOR COMPLIANCE INDEX (mm)
Full extension ($n = 28$)			
Involved knees	8.2 ± 3.5	8.6 ± 3.9	0.4 ± 0.5
Contralateral knees	5.8 ± 1.9	6.4 ± 2.1	0.6 ± 0.5
Right knee–left knee differences	2.4 ± 2.6	2.2 ± 2.6	-0.2 ± 0.4
Lack of full extension[†] ($n = 22$)			
Involved knees	6.7 ± 2.7	7.1 ± 4.0	0.4 ± 0.5
Contralateral knees	5.3 ± 1.9	5.8 ± 2.3	0.5 ± 0.6
Right knee–left knee differences	1.4 ± 2.1	1.3 ± 2.3	-0.1 ± 0.6

*Values represent mean and standard deviation. Differences in anterior tibial displacement and anterior compliance index between patients who did and did not have full extension at follow-up (mean, 48 months after reconstruction) were not significant ($p > .05$).
[†]Fifteen knees lacked 1 to 5 degrees, and 7 lacked 6 to 10 degrees.
From Harter RA, Osternig LR, Singer KM: Instrumented Lachman tests for the evaluation of anterior laxity after reconstruction of the anterior cruciate ligament. J Bone Joint Surg Am 71:975, 1989.

Table 36–20. KT-1000 Preoperative and Postoperative Data (mm) in 10 Patients

	INVOLVED SIDE			UNINVOLVED SIDE			INVOLVED-UNINVOLVED DIFFERENCE
	89 N	Maximum Manual	Compliance	89 N	Maximum Manual	Compliance	
Preoperative							
Mean	9.2	14.0	2.3	4.4	5.7	0.8	8.3
SD	±0.8	±1.9	±0.4	±1.5	±1.7	±0.2	±1.3
Postoperative							
Mean	4.0	5.3	0.9	3.6	4.9	0.6	0.4
SD	±1.5	±1.7	±1.3	±1.7	±2.3	±0.3	±1.3

From Birac D, Bach BR Jr, Andriacchi TP: Functional results following ACL reconstruction. Presented at the Annual Meeting of American Orthopaedic Society for Sports Medicine, Traverse City, MI, June 1989.

O'Brien et al[70] reported their clinical results in 80 patients at a minimum of 2 years after open ACL reconstruction using a patellar tendon autograft, with extra-articular augmentation in 32 (40%) patients. The authors reported that 61 (76%) patients had side-to-side differences of 3 mm or less on maximum manual testing, 16 (20%) had 3- to 5-mm differences, and 3 (4%) had greater than 5 mm. No statistically significant differences were noted between their subgroups of augmented and unaugmented patients.

In 1995 Bach et al[6] reported on 62 of 75 patients who underwent ACL reconstruction with an autologous patellar tendon via a two-incision arthroscopic technique without extra-articular augmentation. The patients were evaluated at a minimum of 2 years and an average of 3.1 years postoperatively. Preoperatively, 94% of the patients had a maximum manual side-to-side difference of 3 mm or greater. Postoperatively, 56 patients (90%) had a maximum manual side-to-side difference of 3 mm or less; 3 (5%) had 3 to 5 mm, and 3 (5%) had greater than 5 mm. Of the three patients with a side-to-side difference of greater than 5 mm, two had a demonstrable pivot shift. Arthrometric parameters were statistically reduced ($p < .0001$) from preoperative status and were consistent with the diagnostic criteria established for normal knees. Table 36–21 summarizes the preoperative and postoperative KT-1000 data in the involved and uninvolved knees for 20-lb, maximum manual, 20-D, and MM-D testing. Figures 36–12 through 36–15 summarize the distributions and reductions of postoperative KT-1000 parameters from their preoperative status. Figures 36–16 and 36–17 graphically depict the preoperative examination under anesthesia, 6-month follow-up, and final follow-up translations at a minimum of 2 years postoperatively for 20-lb and maximum manual testing. Of note is the significant reduction in translations from the preoperative examination under anesthesia testing, with a plateau in translations between 6 months and at final follow-up.

In 1998, Bach et al[8,9] published two articles on the surgical results of ACL reconstruction with patellar tendon autografts. The first was a retrospective 2-year minimum follow-up assessment of a single-incision technique that included arthrometric evaluation.[8] In this study, 103 patients were evaluated at a mean follow-up of 36 months (range, 24 to 55 months). KT-1000 results were recorded on 86 patients preoperatively and on all patients postoperatively. These results showed statistically significant

Table 36–21. Comparison of Preoperative and Postoperative KT-1000 Arthrometer Results (mm)

TEST	N	MEAN	SD	RANGE
Preop 20 Inv	52	8.6	±2.4	4-14
Preop 20 Uninv	52	4.2	±2.0	1-9.5
Postop 20 Inv	62	4.0	±2.4	1-15
Postop 20 Uninv	62	3.4	±1.5	0.5-7.5
Preop MM Inv	52	12.7	±3.1	7-21
Preop MM Uninv	62	5.6	±2.3	2-10.5
Postop MM Inv	62	5.5	±3	1.5-20
Postop MM Uninv	62	4.8	±1.7	1.5-9.5
Preop 20-D	52	4.4	±2	−1-8
Postop 20-D	62	0.5	±2.6	−5-11.5
Preop MM-D	52	7.1	±2.9	2-14
Postop MM-D	62	0.7	±3.2	−6-16

20, 20-lb anterior translation; 20-D, 20-lb injured minus uninjured difference; Inv, involved; MM, maximum manual anterior translation; MM-D, maximum manual injured minus uninjured difference; Uninv, uninvolved.

reductions in maximum manual anterior translation and side-to-side differences ($p < .0001$). The mean maximum manual translation preoperatively was 11.9 mm (range, 5.0 to 23 mm), and the mean side-to-side difference preoperatively was 6.5 mm (range, −5 to 15 mm). At postoperative follow-up, the mean maximum manual translation was reduced to 6.3 mm (range, 2 to 16 mm), and the mean side-to-side difference was reduced to 1.1 mm (range, −6 to 7 mm). Eighty-six patients (83%) had side-to-side differences of 3 mm or less, 14 patients (14%) had differences between 3 and 5 mm, and 3 patients (3%) had differences of 5 mm or more.

Bach et al[9] retrospectively reviewed their results of ACL reconstruction with a patellar tendon autograft via an arthroscopically assisted two-incision technique at an interval intermediate follow-up of 5 to 9 years postoperatively. Preoperative KT-1000 data were recorded on 76 patients. The mean preoperative maximum manual translation was 13.1 mm (range, 4 to 22 mm), and the maximum manual side-to-side difference was 7.6 mm (range, 0.5 to 13.5 mm). The mean postoperative maximum manual translation was 6.3 mm (range, 1 to 12 mm). The mean side-to-side difference was 1 mm (range, −11.5 to 7 mm). At the final follow-up in 94 knees,

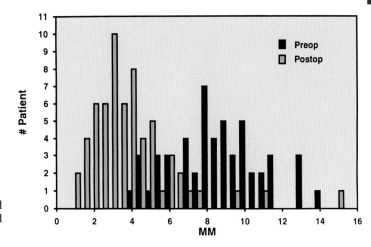

Figure 36–12. The 20-lb anterior preoperative and postoperative translation distributions are depicted in this bar graph. MM, millimeters.

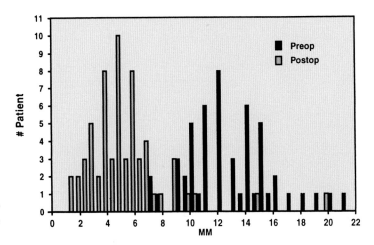

Figure 36–13. Maximum manual anterior preoperative and postoperative translation distributions. MM, millimeters.

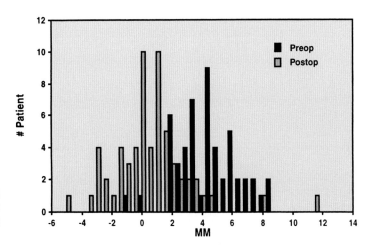

Figure 36–14. The 20-D anterior preoperative and postoperative translation distributions for the study group. 20-D, 20-lb injured minus uninjured difference; MM, millimeters.

the maximum manual side-to-side difference was less than 3 mm in 66 patients (70%), 3 to 5 mm in 24 patients (26%), and more than 5 mm in 4 patients (4%). The anterior maximum manual translation was significantly reduced postoperatively ($p < .001$). The average postoperative decrease in side-to-side difference from preoperative values was 6.6 mm (range, 3 to −16 mm). The reductions in absolute translation and side-to-side differences were statistically significant ($p < .001$).

Allograft Reconstruction

Noyes and Mangine[69] prospectively reported on the effects of early motion after open and arthroscopically assisted ACL reconstructions in 18 patients. In this series, direct repair and fascia allograft or patellar tendon allograft were used in all but one patient. The authors incorporated KT-1000 data into their objective evaluation of patients and reported side-to-side differences at 89 N. In this small

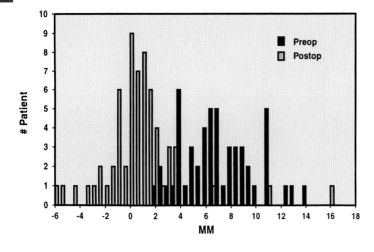

Figure 36–15. The MM-D anterior preoperative and postoperative translation distributions. MM, millimeters; MM-D, maximum manual injured minus uninjured difference.

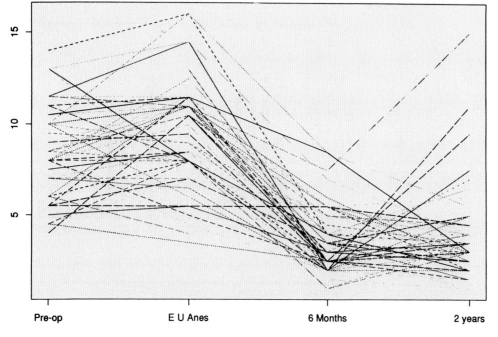

Figure 36–16. The individual KT-1000 arthrometer 20-lb translations over time are depicted. Each *line* represents one patient. Preoperative, examination under anesthesia (E U Anes), 6-month, and minimum 2-year follow-up translations clearly reveal a marked reduction from preoperative and examination under anesthesia results. As a population, there are few changes from the 6-month data to the final follow-up.

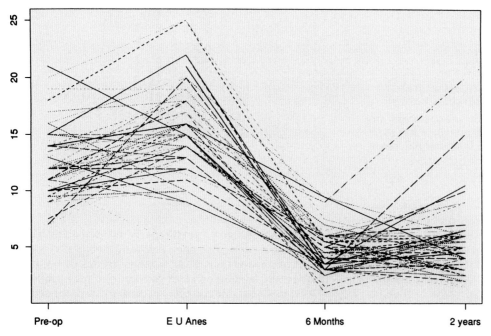

Figure 36–17. The individual KT-1000 arthrometer maximum manual translations over time are depicted. Each *line* represents one patient. Preoperative, examination under anesthesia (E U Anes), 6-month, and minimum 2-year follow-up translations clearly reveal a marked reduction from preoperative and examination under anesthesia results.

series of 10 acute and 8 chronic ACL-deficient knees, the mean involved knee had 5.4-mm greater anterior displacement than the uninjured knee did preoperatively. At 1 month postoperatively, the surgical knee had a −1.9-mm less anterior displacement, and at 3 months the knees were nearly symmetric at a −0.6-mm difference. At 6 months, 15 patients had an injured-uninjured difference of 3 mm or less at 89 N. At 1-year follow-up, three patients had injured-uninjured differences of 5.0 mm.

Wainer et al[86] reported the short-term results in 23 patients after ACL reconstruction with several sources of fresh frozen allograft tendons, including the flexor hallucis longus, posterior tibialis, and toe extensors. The authors reported KT-1000 anterior translation results of 4.4 mm on the postoperative knee and 3.5 mm on the contralateral knee, but they did not specify the forces used to obtain these readings.

More recently, Bach et al[5] reported the results of the use of patellar tendon allografts for primary ACL reconstruction. In this study, 59 patients were evaluated at a mean follow-up of 51 months (range, 26 to 170) after primary ACL reconstruction with a patellar tendon allograft. The indications for using patellar tendon allografts for primary ACL reconstruction were (1) age older than 40 years, (2) radiographic evidence of mild degenerative joint disease, (3) moderate patellofemoral crepitation or pain symptoms, (4) petite stature with donor graft tissue of questionable quality, or (5) patient request for allograft reconstruction. The fresh frozen, nonirradiated allografts were all obtained from the same tissue bank (Allosource Tissue Bank, Denver). A 10-mm, middle third patellar tendon allograft was fashioned with 25-mm bone plugs.

In this study, patients were evaluated by comprehensive physical examination, functional testing, radiographic studies, and patient questionnaire, in addition to KT-2000 arthrometry. Anterior maximum manual and maximum manual side-to-side differences were calculated. Arthrometric failure was defined as a side-to-side difference of 5 mm. Results were stratified into 3 mm or less, 3.1 to 4.9 mm, and 5 mm or greater. Knee-rating questionnaires included the 2000 IKDC Subjective Knee Evaluation Form, Knee Injury and Osteoarthritis Outcome Score (KOOS), Noyes Sports Activity Scale, Tegner, Lysholm, and SF-12. The questionnaire also included a visual analog scale for pain ratings. The average age of the 59 patients at the time of reconstruction was 41 years (range, 18 to 61; SD 10), there were 21 men and 38 women, and 27 right knees and 33 left knees were evaluated. One patient underwent single-stage bilateral reconstruction.

KT-1000 arthrometric testing was recorded on 39 patients preoperatively. The mean maximum manual translation of the affected knees was 14 mm (range, 6 to 21 mm; SD 3) before surgery and 7.5 mm (range, 4 to 13 mm; SD 2) for the unaffected knee. These differences were significant ($p < .001$). Stratification of side-to-side differences preoperatively revealed that 15% had less than 3-mm, 26% had 3.1- to 4.9-mm, and 59% had greater than 5-mm differences. KT-1000 arthrometric testing was performed on all patients except one postoperatively. The mean maximum manual translation was 7.6 mm (range, 4 to 16 mm; SD 2) for the affected knee and 6.9 mm (range, 2 to 15 mm; SD 2) for the unaffected knee, a significant

improvement when compared with preoperative translation of the affected knee ($p < .001$). No significant differences were found between the reconstructed knee and the nonaffected knee postoperatively. Stratification of side-to-side differences postoperatively revealed that 95% had 3-mm or less side-to-side differences and 5% had greater than 3-mm but less than 5-mm side-to-side differences. The side-to-side reductions were statistically significant ($p = .001$). This KT-2000 arthrometric testing showed a significant reduction in maximum manual anterior translation and side-to-side differences at follow-up. There were no statistically significant differences between the affected and unaffected knees postoperatively with regard to arthrometric testing. High patient satisfaction rates correlated with excellent KT-2000 measurements. Ninety-five percent of the patients were completely or mostly satisfied with the results of their surgical procedure. Sixty-five percent were completely satisfied, 30% were mostly satisfied, 5% were somewhat satisfied, and no patients were dissatisfied. Ninety-six percent of the patients stated that they would have the surgery again if the injury occurred to the opposite knee.

In this study, graft failure was defined as the presence of a pivot shift of any grade or KT-1000 maximum manual test of 5-mm or greater side-to-side difference. Five patients had a grade 1 pivot shift, and one had a grade 3 pivot shift (10%). The overall failure rate was 10%. There were no infections, no evidence of any acute or chronic rejection of the grafts, and no evidence of disease transmission. No patients had chronic effusions or synovitis. No patients had significant tunnel expansion (>20 mm) on radiographic evaluation.

Although the evidence in the literature is conflicting with regard to outcomes after allograft reconstruction, the allograft results compare favorably with those of the previously studied autograft cohort from Rush Medical Center.[7-9] In this study, 92% of patients in the autograft group were mostly or completely satisfied versus 94% in the allograft group. A positive pivot-shift test (grade 1 and higher) was present in 9% of our autograft group and 10% of the allograft group. In the autograft group, 74% had a negative Lachman test versus 72% in the allograft group (Table 36–22).

These results of primary patellar tendon allograft use are significantly better than the previous experience with nonirradiated allograft for revision ACL surgery after a failed primary patellar tendon autograft.[5,34] The authors concluded that the use of allograft tissue for ACL reconstruction is a viable alternative to autograft in certain patient populations. Patients in this ACL-deficient population often include older athletes or those with preexisting chondral disease. These patients must be counseled about realistic expectations of pain and functional outcome despite successful ACL reconstruction confirmed by KT arthrometry.

The use of both patellar tendon and other allograft tissues sources for primary ACL reconstruction has increased dramatically in the last decade. As various allograft sources have moved into mainstream orthopedics, the use of instrumented arthrometry has allowed objective evaluation of these ACL graft sources through standardized measurements of anterior ligamentous laxity after

Table 36–22. Primary Allograft Patellar Tendon ACL Reconstruction Outcomes Compared with Primary Autograft ACL Reconstructions: The Rush Medical Center Experience

	AADALEN ET AL	BACH ET AL*	BACH ET AL[†]	BACH ET AL[‡]
Age	41 (18-61)	27 (16-45)	25 (10-52)	26 (12-53)
MMD-STS postop				
<3 mm	95%	92%	83%	70%
3-5 mm	5%	4%	14%	26%
>5 mm	0%	4%	3%	4%
Negative pivot shift	90%	92%	91%	84%
Pain with stair climbing				
Mild/moderate	46%	NA	14%	13%
Severe	2%	NA	0%	0%
Tegner	6.3 (2-10)	6.3 (1-9)	6.5 (2-9)	6.3 (2-9)
Lysholm	82 (43-100)	88 (52-100)	89 (43-100)	87 (34-100)
Noyes Sports Activity Scale	71 (20-100)	90 (50-100)	90 (33-100)	89 (27-100)
Would repeat surgery	96%	95%	95%	94%
Mostly or completely satisfied	94%	90%	92%	97%

*Two- to 4-year retrospective follow-up.
[†]Minimum 2-year retrospective follow-up.
[‡]Five- to 9-year retrospective follow-up.
MMD-STS, maximum manual difference side to side.

ACL reconstruction. The majority of these evaluations have been performed with the KT-1000 and KT-2000 arthrometer. Indelli et al[54] evaluated the outcome of 50 patients 3 to 5 years after primary ACL reconstruction with Achilles tendon allografts. Patients were evaluated by physical examination, IKDC outcome questionnaire, radiographs, and KT-1000 arthrometry. KT-1000 testing revealed a mean side-to-side difference of 2.3 mm in AP translation. The side-to-side difference was less than 2 mm in 33 patients (66%), between 3 and 5 mm in 16 patients (32%), and greater than 6 mm in 1 patient. These results with Achilles allografts for primary ACL reconstruction were comparable, but less favorable than those of several series from Rush Medical Center in which patellar tendon allografts and autografts were used for primary ACL reconstruction (see Table 36–22).

To compare patellar tendon and Achilles allografts, Siebold et al[79] evaluated the outcomes of 251 patients at a minimum of 2 years after primary ACL reconstruction with either patellar tendon or Achilles tendon allografts. In this study, stability measured with the KT-1000 showed an average side-to-side difference of 2.1 mm in the patellar tendon group and 2.0 mm in the Achilles tendon group. Despite these equivalent laxity measurements, there was a higher failure rate ($p < .001$) in the patellar tendon group, with a 10% ACL retear rate in the patellar tendon group versus a 5% rate in the Achilles tendon group. The authors concluded that because of the higher failure rate in both allograft tissues, autograft tissue should be used routinely for primary ACL reconstruction and the use of allograft tissue be reserved for revision reconstructions or scenarios with multiple ligament injuries. The results in this series do not agree with those of Bach et al with respect to patellar tendon allografts, nor with the results of Indelli with respect to Achilles tendon allografts. It should be considered, however, that the KT data in these studies serve well to offer objective comparison specifically concerning anterior laxity after ACL

reconstruction. The good KT arthrometry results obtained by Siebold et al eliminate concerns of allograft tissue laxity and suggest that there may be other reasons for the failure.

Revision ACL Reconstruction

KT arthrometry has permitted increased precision in the quantitative assessment of outcomes of revision ACL reconstruction. In a revision scenario, a variety of graft sources must often be considered. Taggart et al[82] retrospectively reviewed 20 patients after ACL revision reconstruction with varied graft sources. In this study, patients underwent a thorough clinical evaluation as well as arthrometry measurements. There was a significant maximum manual side-to-side difference after the revision ACL reconstruction, but these results did not correlate with high patient subjective ratings. The results of this study indicate that despite residual AP laxity on clinical assessment and KT-1000 instrumentation after revision ACL reconstruction, the majority of patients subjectively rated the results as good or excellent. The poor correlation between objective KT measurements and patient subjective rating of the surgery follows the trend reported in primary ACL reconstruction by Harter et al,[46] who found in 1988 that postoperative laxity measurements did not correlate with patients' perception of knee function.

In another study from Rush Medical Center, Fox et al[34] retrospectively reviewed a cohort of 39 patients 2 to 11 years after revision ACL reconstruction with nonirradiated fresh frozen patellar tendon allograft. In this review, Tegner, Lysholm, Noyes, KOOS, IKDC, and SF-12 rating scales were used in addition to KT-2000 arthrometry. The KT-2000 tester revealed that 84% had a maximum manual side-to-side difference of less than 3 mm and 6% had greater than a 5-mm side-to-side difference. With the use of KT-2000 data to objectively evaluate the status of anterior knee laxity after ACL reconstruction, this study demonstrates that the results of revision ACL reconstruction with a nonirradiated patellar tendon allograft are less favorable than those of primary ACL reconstruction, and the authors concluded that it should be considered a salvage situation.

Several studies[39,53,76] have used the precise quantitative reproducibility of instrumented arthrometry to carefully evaluate the results of ACL reconstruction with synthetic prostheses. Generally, these studies demonstrated poor outcomes, and since the last edition of this text, the routine use of Gore-Tex prosthetic grafts has fallen out of favor. In several studies there was no improvement in objective measurements of side-to-side differences in preoperative versus postoperative testing despite subjective and functional improvement. These studies serve as historic examples of the benefit of objective instrumented arthrometry in evaluating new technology. Future studies evaluating outcomes should use objective measurements to support the findings made by more subjective means such as questionnaires and functional scoring systems.

THE ROLE OF KT ARTHROMETRY IN POSTERIOR CRUCIATE LIGAMENT INSUFFICIENCY

In 1986 and 1987, Parolie and Bergfeld[72] and Fowler and Messieh[33] independently reviewed their long-term follow-up of isolated PCL injuries in athletes. Clinical examinations, subjective questionnaires, Cybex evaluations, and KT-1000 assessments were performed by both studies at an average follow-up of more than 2 years. Parolie and Bergfeld used the KT-1000 at 90 degrees of flexion and applied passive and active posterior translations to 25 patients with isolated PCL injuries that were treated nonoperatively. The authors reported a mean side-to-side difference of 7.1 mm (range, 2.5 to 14.5 mm) in posterior displacement of the tibia relative to the femur. In this group, the mean side-to-side difference for the *active* pos-

terior drawer test was 1.3 mm. In this series, despite the posterior laxity measured by KT arthrometry, 80% of the patients were satisfied with their knees and 84% had returned to their previous sport (68% at the same level of performance, 16% at a decreased level of performance). This finding led the authors to conclude that athletes with isolated PCL injuries who maintain strength in musculature can return to sports without functional disability. In the series reported by Fowler and Messieh, 13 patients had arthroscopically confirmed PCL injuries that were not reconstructed. KT arthrometry revealed no significant side-to-side difference in three patients, nine patients had up to a 5-mm side-to-side difference, and one patient had a side-to-side difference of greater than 5 mm. In this series, all patients were able to return to their previous activity and experienced no limitations with their injured knees. The authors concluded that with respect to isolated PCL injuries, acceptable functional stability in these patients does not necessarily require absolute static stability. These studies illustrate the value of correlating objective arthrometer measurements with clinical and functional outcomes to draw conclusions regarding the ability of patients to function with nonoperative treatment of isolated PCL injuries.

To understand the magnitude of posterior laxity in PCL-injured knees, it is valuable to have an understanding of the posterior displacement in knees without PCL injuries. Daniel et al[25] reported a mean posterior side-to-side difference of 1.5 mm in patients with acute PCL insufficiency and 0.6 mm in those with chronic PCL insufficiency when tested at 30 degrees of knee flexion (Table 36–23). To provide a reference point for this quantifiable posterior laxity, Daniel examined several series of noninjured knees as well. In a separate control group (n = 338), Daniel et al noted a mean posterior translation of 2.7 ± 0.9 mm at 25 degrees of flexion with 89-N testing. In another group of ACL-deficient patients, the contralateral normal knee had a mean posterior displacement at 25 degrees of flexion (89 N) of 2.5 ± 0.8 mm. Bach et al[10] noted a mean posterior displacement of 2.5 ± 0.8 mm in 141 control subjects at 25 degrees (89 N), 2.6 ± 1 mm in the contralateral

Table 36–23. Passive Laxity Measurements with 89-N Push or Pull

	NORMAL	CHRONIC ANTERIOR CRUCIATE LIGAMENT RUPTURE	ACUTE POSTERIOR CRUCIATE LIGAMENT RUPTURE	CHRONIC POSTERIOR CRUCIATE LIGAMENT RUPTURE
30 Degrees				
Anterior	0.0	4.9*	2.6*	4.1*
Posterior	0.3	0.0	1.5	0.6
Quadriceps neutral angle (mean, 71 degrees)				
Measured from resting position				
Anterior	−0.1	1.0	4.4†	5.9†
Posterior	0.6	0.0	3.4	2.1
Referenced to neutral position (quadriceps active position)				
Anterior	−0.1	1.0	0.7	0.7
Posterior	0.6	0.0	7.1*†	7.3*†

Values are in millimeters of displacement of the injured knee minus that of the contralateral knee (right minus left knee in normal subjects).
*p < .001 versus normal subjects.
†p < .001 versus subjects with ACL injury.
From Daniel DM, Stone ML, Barnett P, et al: Use of the quadriceps active test to diagnose posterior cruciate ligament disruption. J Bone Joint Surg Am 70:386, 1988.

Table 36–24. Posterior Translation in Normal Knees (Displacement at 89 N)

	MEAN POSTERIOR TRANSLATION (mm)
Daniel et al[24]	
Control (n = 338)	2.8 ± 0.9
Contralateral normal (chronic ACL; n = 89)	2.5 ± 0.8
Bach et al[6]	
Control (n = 141)	2.5 ± 0.8
Contralateral normal (acute ACL; n = 107)	2.6 ± 1.0
Contralateral normal (chronic ACL; n = 132)	2.6 ± 1.1

Table 36–25. Posterior Knee Translation (mm) in Normal Knees

	MEAN	RANGE	SD
Normal controls (n = 141)			
(30) 89 N, posterior	2.5	1-5.5	±0.8
(90) 89 N, posterior*	1.9	1-4.0	±0.7
(90) Compliance	0.6	0.5-1.5	±0.2
Normal knees in patients with acute ACL (n = 107)			
(30) 89 N, posterior	2.0	0.5-6.0	±0.9
(90) 89 N, posterior	2.2	0.1-9.0	±1.4
(90) Compliance	0.9	0.3-3.0	±0.4
Normal knees in patients with chronic ACL (n = 153)			
(30) 89 N, posterior	2.6	0.3-7.0	±1.1
(90) 89 N, posterior	1.9	0.1-7.0	±0.9
(90) Compliance	0.7	0.3-2.0	±0.3

Degrees of flexion are in parenthesis.
*Tests performed passively.
From Bach BR Jr, Warren RF, Flynn WM, et al: Arthrometric evaluation of knees that have a torn ACL. J Bone Joint Surg Am 72:1299, 1990.

normal knees of 104 acute ACL-deficient subjects, and 2.6 ± 1.1 mm in the contralateral normal knees of 132 chronic ACL-deficient patients (Tables 36–24 and 36–25). At 90 degrees of knee flexion, Bach et al[10] noted a mean passive posterior displacement of 1.9 ± 0.7 mm in 128 control knees. In the normal knees of the acute ACL subpopulation, the mean posterior translation was 1.9 ± 0.9 mm, and in the chronic ACL subgroup, the mean posterior displacement at 89 N was 1.9 ± 0.9 mm. Table 35–25 summarizes the data of Bach et al at 30 and 90 degrees of knee flexion with passive posteriorly applied force in three patient populations. It is clear from these data and the study by Daniel et al that mean passive posterior displacement is less than mean anterior displacement in normal knees at 25 or 90 degrees.

Huber et al[50] were the first to assess posterior translation with the KT-1000 by incorporating use of the quadriceps neutral angle. They measured tibial translation in the knees of 22 subjects with PCL tears or reconstructions with the KT-1000. Two testers were used to assess the reliability of the device, one being a novice and the other having substantial clinical experience. They determined the quadriceps neutral angle on the uninvolved knee and then repeated the measurement on the involved knee. Anterior and posterior translation and total AP excursion were then measured. The intraclass correlation coefficient values for novice, experienced, and intertester reliability were 0.67, 0.79, and 0.62, respectively, for corrected posterior translation; 0.59, 0.68, and 0.64, respectively, for corrected anterior translation; 0.70, 0.74, and 0.29, respectively, for the quadriceps neutral angle; and 0.84, 0.83, and 0.62, respectively, for total AP excursion. This intraclass variability demonstrates the benefit of having consistent personnel collecting KT data and places additional emphasis on side-to-side differences rather than absolute translations when making comparisons between series. Ninety-five percent confidence intervals for novice, experienced, and intertester reliability were ±2.95, ±2.53, and ±3.27 mm, respectively, for corrected posterior translation; ±3.99, ±3.89, and ±3.74 mm, respectively, for corrected anterior translation; and ±10.7 degrees, ±11.73 degrees, and ±16.25 degrees, respectively, for the quadriceps neutral angle.

Hewett et al[47] compared KT-1000 testing with stress radiography and posterior drawer testing for the diagno-

sis of complete and partial PCL injuries. They studied 21 patients with acute and chronic isolated PCL injuries (10 with complete tears and 11 with partial tears), with the testing performed at an average of 4 years after injury. A posteriorly directed 89-N load was applied to the proximal end of the tibia with the knee in 70 degrees of flexion, and lateral radiographs were taken. The relative amount of sagittal translation was determined at both the medial and lateral tibial plateaus from the radiographs. Arthrometric (KT-1000) and posterior drawer tests were also performed. The mean relative posterior translation by stress radiographs averaged 12.2 ± 3.7 mm for knees with complete tears; for partially torn PCLs, the mean relative translation measured on stress radiographs was 5.6 ± 1.5 mm, which was a statistically significant difference from knees with complete tears. Arthrometer testing of the same knees showed 7.6 ± 2.5 mm of translation, and posterior drawer testing demonstrated 9.2 ± 3.3 mm of posterior translation. The arthrometer and posterior drawer test results were not statistically different in distinguishing between knees with complete or partial tears of the PCL. These data suggest that stress radiographs are more sensitive in differentiating between complete and partial PCL injuries. The authors concluded that 8 mm or more of increased posterior translation on stress radiographs is indicative of complete rupture.

Complete PCL injuries requiring reconstruction are unusual, but Deehan et al[26] were able to evaluate 31 patients at a minimum of 2 years after reconstruction of isolated PCL injuries via endoscopic techniques in which four-strand hamstring tendon autografts were used without removal of the torn PCL stump. These patients were prospectively evaluated by physical examination, knee scoring questionnaires, and KT-1000 instrumented arthrometry. At 2 years, the side-to-side difference in total anterior and posterior translation was 2 mm or less in 17 patients (74%) and between 3 and 4 mm in the remaining 6 patients (26%). At 2 years, no patient rated their knee as normal, and although 94% of patients participated in moderate or strenuous activity, only 63% had returned to that level at review despite small posterior translations by KT arthrometry. The study demonstrates the value of correlating KT data with clinical outcomes and contrasts ACL reconstruction data from several studies[46,58,82] in which high patient function and subjective rating are demonstrated despite persistent anterior laxity.

Colosimo et al[19] evaluated 11 patients at an average of 28 months after simultaneous ACL and PCL reconstruction for either acute ($n = 7$) or chronic ($n = 4$) knee dislocations. Seven patients received a BPTB autograft for ACL and an Achilles allograft for PCL reconstruction, three patients received bilateral BPTB autografts, and one patient received BPTB and Achilles allografts. In addition to physical examination and knee scoring scales, KT arthrometer data were collected for both anterior and posterior laxity. The average anterior active difference on the KT-1000 was 2.6 (range, 0 to 6), although the authors conceded that it was technically difficult to determine where the starting point was because of the combined PCL injury. No patient required postoperative manipulation to regain range of motion, and 10 of the 11 returned to their previous activity level postoperatively. The authors concluded that simultaneous reconstruction of the ACL and PCL, though technically difficult, is feasible and yields good to excellent functional results.

SPECIAL CIRCUMSTANCES

The KT arthrometer has become an important adjunct for evaluating various techniques of knee reconstruction. Recently, the arthrometer has been used to evaluate special circumstances that go beyond the realm of strict ligament reconstruction. Its use in these areas is critical to making careful objective measurements and rational comparisons of the outcomes of various techniques, thereby allowing for techniques to be improved after scrutiny of data that can be translated from one study to another.

A tibial spine fracture is considered the pediatric equivalent of an ACL injury.[51] After fixation of type III tibial spine fractures in children, Kocher et al[58] evaluated six patients at a minimum of 2 years after arthroscopic reduction and 3.5-mm screw fixation of Meyers and McKeever[65] type III tibial spine avulsion fractures. Patients were evaluated by comprehensive physical examination, knee outcome questionnaires, and KT arthrometry. Instrumented knee laxity (KT-1000) showed greater than 3-mm manual maximum side-to-side difference in four of six patients. Functional assessment, however, revealed excellent function, with a mean Lysholm score of 99.5 (range, 98 to 100), mean Marshall score of 49.0 (range, 47 to 50), and mean Tegner score of 8.7 (range, 7 to 9). The authors concluded that arthroscopic reduction plus internal fixation of type III tibial spine fractures in skeletally immature patients results in persistent laxity but excellent functional outcomes.

Meniscus transplantation has moved into mainstream orthopedics over the last decade. In the setting of both meniscus and ACL deficiency, combined meniscus transplantation and ACL reconstruction are indicated. Sekiya et al[77] evaluated 28 patients retrospectively at a mean of 2.8 years after combined simultaneous ACL reconstruction and meniscus transplantation. Patients were evaluated by physical examination, IKDC scores, SF-36, and KT-1000 arthrometry. Eighty-six percent of patients had normal or near-normal IKDC scores, with 90% rated as normal or nearly normal on Lachman and pivot examination. At both 30-lb and maximum manual testing, there was an average side-to-side difference of 1.5-mm anterior laxity. The authors concluded that concomitant meniscal transplantation and ACL reconstruction could restore meniscal function, protect articular cartilage, and by restoring a key secondary stabilizer, protect the ACL reconstruction. Using KT arthrometry measurements, future studies may be able to compare the results of revision ACL reconstruction with or without meniscal transplantation.

Osteochondral allograft (OCA) implantation for the treatment of focal chondral defects has become more commonplace in the last decade.[1] In the setting of combined ACL deficiency, treatment of a symptomatic focal chondral defect by OCA implantation must be combined with ACL reconstruction. Klinger et al[57] prospectively reviewed 21 patients for longer than 32 months after OCA implantation of cartilage defects with a mean area of 3.5 cm². KT arthrometry revealed a decrease in the side-to-side difference from 5.9 mm before reconstruction to 1.9 mm after combined OCA implantation and ACL reconstruction. All but two patients had returned to full activities without restriction and were asymptomatic. The authors concluded that symptomatic full-thickness articular cartilage defects associated with ACL instability can be effectively treated by performing ACL reconstruction and osteochondral autologous grafting in one procedure.

Arthrometry has been instrumental in evaluating both anterior and posterior ligamentous laxity after both complex and simple ligament reconstruction in primary and revision scenarios. Recently, the arthrometer has been applied to knee arthroplasty to obtain an objective measurement of true stability in the AP plane. Nabeyama et al[67] prospectively evaluated the changes in AP stability after PCL-retaining and PCL-substituting total knee arthroplasty (TKA) in 29 knees of 24 patients for an average of 3 years after surgery. They found no significant difference in AP translation after PCL-retaining TKA, and translation was similar to that in a cohort of normal knees measured as controls. For PCL-substituting TKA, however, there was increased stability in the AP plane, and this increased stability was significantly greater than that of normal subjects an average of 3 years after surgery.

NONANATOMIC VARIABLES AFFECTING MEASUREMENTS

The KT arthrometer's ability to make accurate comparisons is rooted in its ability to standardize objective data and eliminate subjective evaluation by clinicians, patients, and researchers. Despite considerable effort to standardize positioning, technique, and anatomic considerations, it remains challenging to control for the multitude of nonanatomic variables that can affect ligament laxity testing. An understanding of the magnitude and direction of variation caused by certain biological and social conditions will allow for more accurate interpretation of the data obtained from the test.

Workers' Compensation

A general perception exists that outcomes of orthopedic procedures in patients with worker's compensation claims fair worse than those of patients without such claims. Bach et al[88] evaluated KT-2000 arthrometry results in 22 patients with workers' compensation claims who underwent ACL reconstruction between 1987 and 1995. They showed a mean maximum manual difference of 1. 9 mm, with 15 patients (68%) having a maximum manual difference of 3 mm or less and 7 patients (32%) having a difference of 3 to 5 mm. These data compare comparably with historical data at Rush and other institutions.[7-9] This study did not find that the presence of a workers' compensation claim negatively affects the outcome of ACL surgery, nor does it significantly alter KT measurements.

Gender Differences

The higher incidence of ACL tears in women has been proposed to be due to multiple factors, among them gender differences in ligamentous laxity. Neuromuscular gender differences include less total muscle mass, delayed muscle activation, and slower force generation than in men,[13] as well as decreased ability to generate muscle force in female athletes in comparison to male athletes, even when corrected for differences in size.[43] In addition, the muscle recruitment patterns of female athletes are different from those of men, with a tendency to recruit quadriceps muscles rather than hamstrings or gastrocnemius muscles,[52] a pattern that places the female ACL at additional risk. Estrogen and progesterone receptors have been demonstrated within the ACL,[60] and female athletes are at greater risk for ACL injury during the ovulatory phase of their menstrual cycle.[89] It is reasonable to predict that female knee laxity would fluctuate with hormone cycles and affect the ACL.

Van Lunen et al[85] examined ACL laxity by arthrometry during female subjects' menstrual cycle. In this study, 12 college-age women not currently receiving hormone therapy with regular cycles for 12 months before initiating the study underwent KT-2000 measurement of normal knees at the onset of menses, near ovulation, and on day 23 of the midluteal phase of the menstrual cycle. At each measurement, blood was drawn to monitor hormone levels. There were no differences noted in KT measurements relative to hormone changes during their cycles. This study found no association between hormone concentrations during any phase of the menstrual cycle and ACL laxity as measured on the KT-2000 arthrometer.

More recently, however, Romani et al[75] examined normal knees in 20 college-age women with normal cycles who were not taking oral contraception. Each woman underwent regular blood donations to assay for estradiol, estrone, and progesterone levels, and their normal knee underwent KT-2000 arthrometer measurements. This study identified a significant correlation between estradiol and estrone levels and ACL laxity during the ovulation phase of the cycle. Deie et al[27] examined the normal knees of 16 college-age women experiencing normal cycles. In addition to hormone levels, basal body temperatures were recorded to assist in identifying the follicular, ovulatory, and luteal phases of the menstrual cycle. In addition, the normal knees of eight college-age men were measured for comparison. For the women there were significant changes in anterior displacement at the 89-N and 134-N force levels during the follicular and luteal phases, but no change in laxity during the testing period for the male subjects. It is possible that the hormone changes that occur in conjunction with fluctuations in ACL laxity take place in a narrow window of time around the ovulation event and that Van Lunen and colleagues' investigation did not draw blood during the correct window of hormone level changes. Each of these studies is limited by the small number of subjects and the complex physiological variables present during the normal menstrual cycle. Notwithstanding these limitations, the KT-2000 data presented in these studies provide compelling evidence that cyclic hormone-driven fluctuation in ACL laxity is one of many factors that explain gender differences in rates of ACL injury.

To investigate gender differences after ACL reconstruction, Bach et al presented KT data for matched populations of men and women undergoing ACL reconstruction with patellar tendon grafts. In that study, 200 patients consisting of 137 men and 63 women were evaluated by physical examination, questionnaire, functional testing, radiographic evaluation, and KT-1000 arthrometry at a mean of 5 years after ACL reconstruction with BPTB autografts. Male patients had a significantly greater mean KT-1000 maximum manual side-to-side difference (0.76 versus 1.73 mm, $p = .014$) than women did. However, no differences were noted in the percentage of patients with greater than 5-mm side-to-side difference, with five men (4%) and two women (3%) classified as arthrometric failures.[30] This study illustrates that despite significant physiological differences between the ACL in male and female knees, good long-term outcomes after ACL reconstruction can be achieved in both men and women.

In an effort to understand the factors leading to differences in ACL injury rates between men and women athletes, Medrano and Smith[66] used KT measurements of male and female college-age soccer players and compared these measurements with those of male and female nonathletes. In this study, the Lachman test and both active and passive anterior translation of the tibia were performed. Although females demonstrated greater laxity than their male counterparts did for the Lachman test, the nonathletic group had overall higher displacement than the athletes did in all tests performed. They concluded that although gender has an independent effect on knee laxity, the effect of conditioning is a greater cause of knee laxity than gender differences are.

Table 36–26. Effect of Exercise on Anteroposterior Knee Laxity

	ANTERIOR LAXITY			POSTERIOR LAXITY			TOTAL AP LAXITY		
	Pre	Post	CHANGE (%)	Pre	Post	CHANGE (%)	Pre	Post	CHANGE (%)
Sedentary controls	2.8 ± 1.7	2.8 ± 1.6	1	3.5 ± 1.5	3.7 ± 1.5	4	6.3 ± 2.4	6.5 ± 2.6	3
Squat powerlifters	3.8 ± 1.6	3.9 ± 1.9	5	2.5 ± 1.6	2.4 ± 1.5	−3	6.2 ± 2.1	6.3 ± 2.7	2
Basketball players	2.9 ± 1.5	3.4 ± 1.4	19	4.0 ± 2.1	4.7 ± 1.9	18*	6.8 ± 2.5	8.1 ± 1.8	19
Distance runners	1.6 ± 1.3	2.0 ± 1.5	20	3.4 ± 1.6	4.0 ± 1.8	19*	5.0 ± 2.2	6.0 ± 2.1	19
General anesthesia	3.3 ± 1.7	3.5 ± 1.8	6	4.8 ± 2.4	4.7 ± 2.2	−3*	8.1 ± 3.1	8.1 ± 2.6	1

Values represent mean and standard deviation. Percent change is calculated with absolute values.
*$p \le .05$.
From Steiner ME, Brown C, Zarins B, et al: The effect of exercise on AP knee laxity. Am J Sports Med 14:24, 1986.

Exercise

Steiner et al[81] studied the immediate effect of exercise on AP laxity of the knee in college-age athletes. A displacement force of 30 lb (133 N) was applied with a Stryker knee laxity testing device. Four groups were evaluated (sedentary, squat powerlifters, basketball players, and distance runners). Table 36–26 summarizes the authors' data. For the distance runners and basketball players ($p < .01$) but not the powerlifters, up to 20% increased laxity was demonstrated after exercise. This study incorporated the use of a knee laxity tester and demonstrated that exercises that cause repetitive physiological stress at a high strain rate can result in a transient immediate increase in laxity whereas exercises involving a relatively low number of large stresses at a low strain rate do not significantly change laxity.

Generalized Ligamentous Laxity

The extent to which a patient's inherent generalized ligamentous laxity will affect a KT measurement is important to understand. In the patient population reported by Bach et al,[4,10] generalized ligamentous laxity was assessed in normal controls and ACL-deficient populations to determine whether this factor affected KT-2000 displacements. Thumb-to-forearm laxity (TFL), metacarpophalangeal extension (MPE), elbow recurvatum, and knee recurvatum were measured and graded. The grades of these various parameters of ligamentous laxity were summarized in a total laxity score (TLS), and an attempt was made to correlate increased KT arthrometer displacement with generalized ligamentous laxity in the test population.

Chi-square analysis revealed that the condition of the ACL (normal controls versus ACL deficiency) was dependent on MPE ($p < .001$), TFL ($p < .001$), recurvatum of the involved knee ($p < .001$), and recurvatum of the uninvolved knee ($p < .05$), but not on elbow recurvatum. In patients with TFL, statistically significant differences were noted at 67 N and 89 N ($p < .001$). For example, at 89 N, patients without TFL had a mean anterior displacement of 11.3 mm, whereas those with positive TFL had a mean anterior displacement of 14.6 mm.

The combined TLS was not statistically significant in the normal or acute populations but was statistically significant in the chronic patients. For example, at 89 N of force, KT measurement increases correlated with higher grades of generalized ligamentous laxity as reflected by a higher TLS. Patients with a TLS of 0 had a mean translation of 10.7 mm on the injured side; TLS of 1, 11 mm; TLS of 2, 13.1 mm; TLS of 3, 14.3 mm; and TLS of 4, 15 mm. This was statistically significant ($p < 0.01$) for involved and uninvolved knees. For uninvolved knees, there was a trend toward greater displacement as the TLS increased at both 89-N and maximum manual test levels. For example, at 89 N of force, patients with a TLS of 0 had a mean displacement of 5 mm; TLS of 1, 6.2 mm; and TLS of 3, 7.5 mm. For maximum manual testing, a similar increased trend of displacements was noted: TLS of 0, 12.6 mm; TLS of 1, 13.8 mm; and TLS of 2, 16.3 mm. However, only two patients had a TLS of 3 with a mean displacement of 12.2 mm, and for this reason the trend did not reach statistical significance. The trend witnessed in displacement and the correlation with higher TLS were also seen with respect to the compliance calculations.

With compliance index determination, trends for increased compliance correlated with a higher TLS, but they were not statistically significant. For example, in patients with a TLS of 0, the mean compliance was 2.0 mm; TLS of 1, 1.9 mm; TLS of 2, 2.4 mm; TLS of 3, 2.6 mm; and TLS of 4, 3.6 mm. Compliance was the only statistically significant testing parameter ($p < .001$) in chronic patients with knee recurvatum on the involved or uninvolved side. Similarly, compliance was the only statistically significant testing parameter in chronic patients with elbow recurvatum ($p < .001$).

Based on these observations, it appears that MPE and TFL were the most important parameters of the four tested. It has been observed by many surgeons that a patient with generalized ligamentous laxity is analogous to a "double-edged sword" in that this patient often fails conservative treatment yet is at high risk for failing surgical stabilization, possibly because of the biological composition of autograft tissue, as well as the composition of the secondary restraints. Future ACL outcome studies should consider quantifying ligamentous laxity and incorporating this nonanatomic biological feature of laxity into the analysis.

INSTRUMENTED TESTING OF KNEE BRACES

Several authors have studied the effects of bracing on ACL-deficient knees and have studied instrumented laxity testers for quantitating translations.[12,15,20] Beck et al[12] used both the KT-1000 and Stryker testers. Branch et al[15] used the KT-1000, whereas Colville et al[20] used a custom-designed testing apparatus and indirectly compared its accuracy with that of the KT-1000.

Beck et al[12] studied the effects of seven different braces on surgically confirmed chronic ACL-deficient subjects. The authors compared the maximum manual difference in braced versus normal knees and noted no statistically significant difference. The maximum manual difference ranged from 2.0 to 7.6 mm. The data allowed the authors to rank the braces according to their effectiveness in reducing the maximum manual difference. It should be noted that prebracing at 89 N and maximum manual translations was not reported in this study. The authors analyzed the percent reduction of the involved (braced) knee versus the normal knee and noted no statistically significant difference at 89 N, but on maximum manual testing a significant relationship ($p < 0.05$) was noted. Similar results were observed between the KT-1000 and Stryker test results.

SUMMARY

Instrumented laxity testers, particularly the KT-1000, have been used to evaluate normal and ACL-deficient knees in both in vitro and in vivo studies. Objective quantification of knee laxity in ACL-deficient or PCL-deficient patients is an important treatment adjunct. Although it has not been established whether KT-1000 displacements increase temporarily after ACL reconstruction as a result of strain on secondary restraints, it is clear that KT measurements after meniscal transplantation and ACL reconstruction seem to normalize this trend of gradually increasing displacements after reconstruction. Increasing numbers of clinicians are using knee laxity testers to objectively report anterior displacements. Subsequent reports should include 89-N, maximum manual, compliance index, and side-to-side differences because variations in testing parameters have been highlighted in the previously reviewed papers. KT arthrometry (KT-1000 or KT-2000) allows the orthopedic community worldwide to accurately compare and evaluate reported results in a more objective fashion because these measurements eliminate the subjectivity of graded clinical tests. It should be noted that in several studies,[45,58,82] patient satisfaction and subjective evaluations by the examiner and patient tended to overestimate the presumed ligamentous stability, and in these cases, the KT arthrometer provides important objective information regarding the integrity of ligament stability. Knee laxity testing data should be incorporated into the objective postoperative evaluation of the patient, and we believe that the surgeon should strive to match the contralateral normal knee. These testing devices are important clinical and research tools for the treatment of a ligament-injured knee.

References

1. Alford JW, Cole BJ: Cartilage restoration, part 1: Basic science, historical perspective, patient evaluation, treatment options. Am J Sports Med 33:295, 2005.
2. Anderson AF, Lipscomb AB: Preoperative instrumented testing of anterior and posterior knee laxity. Am J Sports Med 17:387, 1989.
3. Anderson AF, Snyder RB, Federspiel CF, et al: Instrumented evaluation of knee laxity: A comparison of five arthrometers. Am J Sports Med 20:135, 1992.
4. Bach BR Jr: KT-1000 arthrometer evaluation of normal, acute and chronic anterior cruciate ligament patients. Orthop Trans 12:194, 1988.
5. Bach BR Jr, Aadalen KJ, Dennis M, et al: Primary anterior cruciate ligament reconstruction using fresh frozen, non-irradiated patellar tendon allograft. Minimum two year follow-up. Am J Sports Med 32:1, 2004.
6. Bach BR Jr, Jones GT, Hager CA, et al: Arthrometric results of arthroscopically assisted anterior cruciate ligament reconstruction using autograft patellar tendon substitution. Am J Sports Med 23:179, 1995.
7. Bach BR Jr, Jones GT, Sweet FA, et al: Arthroscopy-assisted anterior cruciate ligament reconstruction using patella tendon substitution. Two-to-four year follow-up results. Am J Sports Med 22:758, 1994.
8. Bach BR Jr, Levy ME, Bojchuk J, et al: Single-incision endoscopic anterior cruciate ligament reconstruction using patellar tendon autograft: Minimum two-year follow-up evaluation. Am J Sports Med 26:30, 1998.
9. Bach BR Jr, Tradonsky S, Bojchuk J, et al: Arthroscopically assisted anterior cruciate ligament reconstruction using patellar tendon autograft: Five- to nine-year follow-up evaluation. Am J Sports Med 26:20, 1998.
10. Bach BR Jr, Warren RF, Flynn WM, et al: Arthrometric evaluation of knees that have a torn anterior cruciate ligament. J Bone Joint Surg Am 72:1299, 1990.
11. Baxter MD: Assessment of normal pediatric knee ligament laxity using the Genucom. J Pediatr Orthop 8:546, 1988.
12. Beck C, Drez D Jr, Young J, et al: Instrumented testing of functional knee braces. Am J Sports Med 14:253, 1986.
13. Bell DG, Jacobs I: Electro-mechanical response times and rate of force development in males and females. Med Sci Sports Exerc 18:31, 1986.
14. Birac D, Bach BR Jr, Andriacchi TP: Functional results following ACL reconstruction. Presented at the Annual Meeting of the American Orthopaedic Society for Sports Medicine, June 1989, Traverse City, MI.
15. Branch T, Hunter R, Reynolds P: Controlling anterior tibial displacement under static load: A comparison of two braces. Orthopedics 11:1249, 1988.
16. Burks R, Daniel D, Losse G: The effect of continuous passive motion on anterior cruciate ligament reconstruction stability. Am J Sports Med 12:323, 1984.
17. Burks RT, Leland R: Determination of graft tension before fixation in anterior cruciate ligament reconstruction. Arthroscopy 4:260, 1988.
18. Butler DL, Noyes FR, Grood ES: Ligamentous restraints to anterior-posterior drawer in the human knee. J Bone Joint Surg Am 62:259, 1980.
19. Colosimo AJ, Carroll PF, Heidt RS Jr, Carlonas RL: Simultaneous ACL and PCL reconstruction. J Knee Surg 16:191, 2003.
20. Colville MR, Lee CS, Ciullo JV: The Lenox Hill brace: An evaluation of effectiveness in treating knee instability. Am J Sports Med 14:257, 1986.
21. Dahlstedt LJ, Dalen N: Knee laxity in cruciate ligament injury: Value of examination under anesthesia. Acta Orthop Scand 60:181, 1989.
22. Daniel DM, Malcom LL, Losse G, et al: Instrumented measurement of anterior laxity of the knee. J Bone Joint Surg Am 67:720, 1985.

23. Daniel DM, Stone ML: Diagnosis of knee ligament injury: Tests and measurements of joint laxity. In Feagin JA Jr (ed): The Crucial Ligament: Diagnosis and Treatment of Ligamentous Injuries about the Knee. New York, Churchill Livingstone, 1988, pp 287-300.

24. Daniel DM, Stone ML, Barnett P, et al: Use of the quadriceps active test to diagnose posterior cruciate ligament disruption and measure posterior laxity of the knee. J Bone Joint Surg Am 70:386, 1988.

25. Daniel DM, Stone ML, Sachs R, et al: Instrumented measurement of anterior knee laxity in patients with acute anterior cruciate ligament disruption. Am J Sports Med 13:401, 1985.

26. Deehan DJ, Salmon LJ, Russell VJ, Pinczewski LA: Endoscopic single-bundle posterior cruciate ligament reconstruction: Results at minimum 2-year follow-up. Arthroscopy 19:955, 2003.

27. Deie M, Sakamaki Y, Sumen Y, et al: Anterior knee laxity in young women varies with their menstrual cycle. Int Orthop 26:154, 2002.

28. Donaldson WF, Warren RF, Wickiewicz T: A comparison of acute anterior cruciate ligament examinations: Initial vs. examination under anesthesia. Am J Sports Med 13:5, 1985.

29. Edixhoven P, Huiskes R, de Graaf R, et al: Accuracy and reproducibility of instrumented knee drawer tests. J Orthop Res 5:378, 1987.

30. Feller JA, Webster KE: A randomized comparison of patellar and hamstring tendon anterior cruciate ligament reconstruction. Am J Sports Med 31:564, 2003.

31. Ferrari JD, Bach BR Jr, Bush-Joseph CA, et al: Anterior cruciate ligament reconstruction in men and women: An outcome analysis comparing gender. Arthroscopy 17:588, 2001.

32. Fleming BC, Brattbakk B, Peura GD, et al: Measurement of anterior-posterior knee laxity: A comparison of three techniques. J Orthop Res 20:421, 2002.

33. Fowler PJ, Messieh SS: Isolated posterior cruciate ligament injuries. Am J Sports Med 15:553, 1987.

34. Fox JA, Pierce M, Bojchuk J, et al: Revision anterior cruciate ligament reconstruction with nonirradiated fresh frozen patellar tendon allograft. Arthroscopy 20:787, 2004.

35. Freedman KB, D'Amato MJ, Nedeff DD, et al: Arthroscopic anterior cruciate ligament reconstruction: A metaanalysis comparing patellar tendon and hamstring tendon autografts. Am J Sports Med 32:2, 2003.

36. Fukubayashi T, Torzilli PA, Sherman MF, et al: An in vitro biomechanical evaluation of anterior-posterior motion of the knee: Tibial displacement, rotation, and torque. J Bone Joint Surg Am 64:258, 1982.

37. Giannotti BF, Fanelli GC, Barrett TA, et al: The predictive value of intraoperative KT-1000 arthrometer measurements in single incision anterior cruciate ligament reconstruction. Arthroscopy 12:660, 1996.

38. Gillquist J, Odensten M: Arthroscopic reconstruction of the anterior cruciate ligament. Arthroscopy 4:5, 1988.

39. Glousman R, Shields C Jr, Kerlan R, et al: Gore-Tex prosthetic ligament in anterior cruciate deficient knees. Am J Sports Med 16:321, 1988.

40. Grana WA, Hines R: Arthroscopic assisted semitendinosus reconstruction of the anterior cruciate ligament. Am J Knee Surg 5:16, 1992.

41. Granberry WM, Noble PC, Woods W: Evaluation of an electrogoniometric instrument for measurement of laxity after reconstruction of the knee. J Bone Joint Surg Am 72:1316, 1990.

42. Gross SM, Carcia CR, Gansneder BM, Shultz SJ: Rate of force application during knee arthrometer testing affects stiffness but not displacement measurements. J Orthop Sports Phys Ther 34:132, 2004.

43. Hakkinen K: Force production characteristics of leg extensor, trunk flexor and extensor muscles in male and female basketball players. J Sports Med Phys Fitness 31:325, 1991.

44. Hanten WP, Pace MB: Reliability of measuring anterior laxity of the knee joint using a knee ligament arthrometer. Phys Ther 67:357, 1987.

45. Harter RA, Osternig LR, Singer KM: Instrumented Lachman tests for the evaluation of anterior laxity after reconstruction of the anterior cruciate ligament. J Bone Joint Surg Am 71:975, 1989.

46. Harter RA, Osternig LR, Singer KM, et al: Long-term evaluation of knee stability and function following surgical reconstruction for anterior cruciate ligament insufficiency. Am J Sports Med 16:434, 1988.

47. Hewett TE, Noyes FR, Lee MD: Diagnosis of complete and partial posterior cruciate ligament rupture: Stress radiography compared with KT-1000 arthrometer and posterior drawer testing. Am J Sports Med 25:648, 1997.

48. Higgins RW, Steadman JR: Anterior cruciate ligament repairs in world class skiers. Am J Sports Med 15:439, 1987.

49. Highgenboten CL, Jackson AW, Jansson KA, et al: KT-1000 arthrometer: Conscious and unconscious test results using 15, 20, and 30 pounds of force. Am J Sports Med 20:450, 1992.

50. Huber FE, Irrgang JJ, Harner C, et al: Intratester and intertester reliability of the KT-1000 arthrometer in the assessment of posterior laxity of the knee. Am J Sports Med 25:479, 1997.

51. Hunter RE, Willis JA: Arthroscopic fixation of avulsion fractures of the tibial eminence: Technique and outcome. Arthroscopy 20:113, 2004.

52. Huston LJ, Wojtys EM: Neuromuscular performance characteristics in elite female athletes. Am J Sports Med 24:427, 1996.

53. Indelicato PA, Pascale MS, Huegel MO: Early experience with the Gore-Tex polytetrafluoroethylene anterior cruciate ligament prosthesis. Am J Sports Med 17:55, 1989.

54. Indelli PF, Dillingham MF, Fanton GS, Schurman DJ: Anterior cruciate ligament reconstruction using cryopreserved allografts. Clin Orthop 420:268, 2004.

55. Jonsson T, Althoff B, Peterson L, et al: Clinical diagnosis of ruptures of the anterior cruciate ligament: A comparative study of the Lachman test and the anterior drawer sign. Am J Sports Med 10:100, 1982.

56. Katz JW, Fingeroth RJ: The diagnostic accuracy of ruptures of the anterior cruciate ligament comparing the Lachman test, the anterior drawer sign, and the pivot shift test in acute and chronic knee injuries. Am J Sports Med 14:88, 1986.

57. Klinger HM, Baums MH, Otte S, Steckel H: Anterior cruciate reconstruction combined with autologous osteochondral transplantation. Knee Surg Sports Traumatol Arthrosc 11:366, 2003.

58. Kocher MS, Foreman ES, Micheli LJ: Laxity and functional outcome after arthroscopic reduction and internal fixation of displaced tibial spine fractures in children. Arthroscopy 19:1085, 2003.

59. Kowalk DL, Wojtys EM, Disher J, et al: Quantitative analysis of the measuring capabilities of the KT-1000 knee ligament arthrometer. Am J Sports Med 21:744, 1993.

60. Liu SH, al-Shaikh R, Panossian V, et al: Primary immunolocalization of estrogen and progesterone target cells in the human anterior cruciate ligament. J Orthop Res 14:526, 1996.

61. Liu SH, Osti L, Henry M, et al: The diagnosis of acute complete tears of the anterior cruciate ligament: Comparison of MRI, arthrometry and clinical examination. J Bone Joint Surg Br 77:586, 1995.

62. Malcom LL, Daniel DM, Stone ML, et al: The measurement of anterior knee laxity after ACL reconstructive surgery. Clin Orthop 169:35, 1985.

63. Margheritini F, Mancini L, Mauro CS, Mariani PP: Stress radiography for quantifying posterior cruciate ligament deficiency. Arthroscopy 19:706, 2003.

64. Markolf KL, Mensch JS, Amstutz HC: Stiffness and laxity of the knee: The contributions of the supporting structures—a quantitative in vitro study. J Bone Joint Surg Am 58:583, 1976.

65. Meyers MH, McKeever FM: Fracture of the intercondylar eminence of the tibia. J Bone Joint Surg Am 41:209, 1959.

66. Medrano D Jr, Smith D: A comparison of knee joint laxity among male and female collegiate soccer players and non-athletes. Sports Biomech 2:203, 2003.

67. Nabeyama R, Matsuda S, Miura H, et al: Changes in anteroposterior stability following total knee arthroplasty. J Orthop Sci 8:526, 2003.

68. Neuschwander DC, Drez D Jr, Paine RM, et al: Comparison of anterior laxity measurements in anterior cruciate deficient knees with two instrumented testing devices. Orthopedics 13:299, 1990.

69. Noyes FR, Mangine RE: Early knee motion after open and arthroscopic anterior cruciate ligament reconstruction. Am J Sports Med 15:149, 1987.

70. O'Brien SJ, Warren RF, Pavlov H, et al: Reconstruction of the chronically insufficient anterior cruciate ligament with the central third of the patellar ligament. J Bone Joint Surg Am 73:278, 1991.

71. Oliver JH, Coughlin LP: Objective knee evaluation using the Genucom knee analysis system: Clinical implications. Am J Sports Med 15:571, 1987.

72. Parolie JM, Bergfeld TA: Long-term results of nonoperative treatment of isolated posterior cruciate ligament injuries of the knee. Am J Sports Med 14:35, 1986.

73. Puddu G, Gianni E, Chambat P, De Paulis F: The axial view in evaluating tibial translation in cases of insufficiency of the posterior cruciate ligament. Arthroscopy 16:217, 2000.

74. Rijke AM, Perrin DH, Goitz HT, et al: Instrumented arthrometry for diagnosing partial versus complete anterior cruciate ligament tears. Am J Sports Med 22:294, 1994.

75. Romani W, Patrie J, Curl LA, Flaws JA: The correlations between estradiol, estrone, estriol, progesterone, and sex hormone–binding globulin and anterior cruciate ligament stiffness in healthy, active females. J Womens Health (Larchmt) 12:287, 2003.

76. Roth JH, Kennedy JC, Lockstadt H, et al: Polypropylene braid augmented and nonaugmented intraarticular anterior cruciate ligament reconstruction. Am J Sports Med 13:321, 1985.

77. Sekiya JK, Giffin JR, Irrgang JJ, et al: Clinical outcomes after combined meniscal allograft transplantation and anterior cruciate ligament reconstruction. Am J Sports Med 31:896, 2003.

78. Sherman OH, Markolf KL, Ferkel RD: Measurements of anterior laxity in normal and anterior cruciate–absent knees with two instrumented test devices. Clin Orthop 215:156, 1987.

79. Siebold R, Buelow JU, Bos L, Ellermann A: Primary ACL reconstruction with fresh-frozen patellar versus Achilles tendon allografts. Arch Orthop Trauma Surg 123:180, 2003.

80. Steiner ME, Brown C, Zarins B, et al: Measurement of anterior-posterior displacement of the knee: A comparison of the results with instrumented devices and with clinical examination. J Bone Joint Surg Am 72:1307, 1990.

81. Steiner ME, Grana WA, Chillag K, et al: The effect of exercise on anterior-posterior knee laxity. Am J Sports Med 14:24, 1986.

82. Taggart TF, Kumar A, Bickerstaff D: Revision anterior cruciate ligament reconstruction: A midterm patient assessment. Knee 11:29, 2004.

83. Tibone JE, Antich JJ: A biomechanical analysis of anterior cruciate ligament reconstruction with the patellar tendon: A two-year follow-up. Am J Sports Med 16:332, 1988.

84. Torzilli PA, Panariello RA, Forbes A, et al: Measurement reproducibility of two commercial knee test devices. J Orthop Res 9:730, 1991.

85. Van Lunen BL, Roberts J, Branch JD, Dowling EA: Association of menstrual-cycle hormone changes with anterior cruciate ligament laxity measurements. J Athl Train 38:298, 2003.

86. Wainer RA, Clarke TJ, Poehling GG: Reconstruction of the anterior cruciate ligament using allograft tendon. Arthroscopy 4:199, 1988.

87. Wang CW, Bach BR Jr: Clinical diagnosis of ACL deficient knees. J Orthop Surg 7:139, 1990.

88. Wexler G, Bach BR Jr, Bush-Joseph CA, et al: Outcomes of anterior cruciate ligament reconstruction in patients with workers' compensation claims. Arthroscopy 16:49, 2000.

89. Wojtys EM, Huston LJ, Lindenfeld et al: Association between the menstrual cycle and anterior cruciate ligament injuries in female athletes. Am J Sports Med 26:614, 1998.

90. Wroble RR, Grood ES, Noyes FR, et al: Reproducibility of Genucom knee analysis system testing. Am J Sports Med 18:387, 1990.

91. Wroble RR, Van Ginkel LA, Grood ES, et al: Repeatability of the KT-1000 arthrometer in a normal population. Am J Sports Med 18:396, 1990.

92. Wu CD, Bach BR Jr, Johnson JC: Arthrometric comparisons of ACL deficiency: Examined while awake and while under anesthesia. Am J Knee Surg 5:9, 1992.

93. Zelko RR: The Lachman sign vs. the anterior drawer sign in the diagnosis of acute tears of the anterior cruciate ligament. Orthop Trans 6:196, 1982.

CHAPTER 37

Medial Ligament Injuries of the Knee

Craig S. Radnay • Stephen G. Silver

Management of injuries to the medial aspect of the knee has evolved during the past 25 years. This evolution is mainly due to much better understanding of the functional anatomy, biomechanics, and physiological healing of the important extracapsular structures.

Whereas the focus of management of cruciate ligament injuries has been directed toward surgical reconstruction, the approach to collateral ligament injuries has been conservative, nonoperative management. The purpose of this chapter is to describe the functional anatomy, mechanism of injury, diagnosis, and nonoperative and operative treatment of injuries to the medial ligaments of the knee.

FUNCTIONAL ANATOMY

Over the past 15 years, the nomenclature has remained relatively consistent regarding the medial stabilizing structures of the knee joint. Dynamic medial stabilizers include the pes anserinus muscles (sartorius, gracilis, and semimembranosus muscles), which flex and internally rotate the knee, and the medial head of the gastrocnemius. The medial collateral ligament (MCL) is the major static stabilizer of the medial side of the knee joint,[24] in addition to the capsuloligamentous complex. Three different layers have been described by Warren and Marshall.[23] The superficial MCL is located in layer 2 (Fig. 37–1). The proximal attachment site of this important structure is somewhat circular and located on the medial femoral epicondyle. The ligament is between 10 and 12 cm in length, and the distal attachment site is much larger and is located 4 to 5 cm below the joint line on the medial metaphyseal area of the tibia (Fig 37–2A).[17] Posterior and deep to the MCL is the posterior oblique ligament, which is, in fact, a thickening of the deep posterior capsule of the knee (layer 3) (Fig. 37–3).

Biomechanical studies have shown that the MCL is the primary medial stabilizer of the knee that resists valgus loading.[6,24] At 25 degrees of flexion, the MCL provides up to 78% of the restraint to valgus stress; although it has a decreasing role in extension, it still provides up to 57% of the restraint at 5 degrees of extension[17] because of the relaxation or laxity that develops with flexion in the other contributing structures, mainly the posteromedial capsule. As a result of the parallel arrangement of the collagen that composes the MCL, only a relatively small increase in laxity (approximately 5 to 8 mm) is indicative of complete failure of the ligament.[5] One needs to keep this important

point in mind when examining the knee for possible medial ligament damage. Another key point to remember is that the deep capsular ligament (layer 3) serves as an important anchoring location for the medial meniscus; damage to this deep layer could extend into the substance of the meniscus and thereby add to the disorder encountered as a result of a valgus force applied to the knee.

The location of the proximal attachment site of the MCL places it near the instant center of rotation of the knee. Consequently, some aspect of its fan-shaped structure is always under tension during knee flexion (Fig. 37–4). As the knee goes into flexion, the anterior fibers of the MCL tighten whereas the posterior fibers slacken (Fig. 37–5). The posterior oblique ligament blends in with the posterior edge of the MCL. This ligament, which is tense in extension and loose in flexion, helps prevent medial opening with valgus loading when the knee is in full extension. In a flexed position, the anterior aspect of the posterior oblique ligament actually lies underneath the MCL. A bursa separates these two structures and allows for the 1- to 2-cm anteroposterior excursion that must occur to the MCL during flexion/extension of the knee. When surgically repairing damage to this area, one must keep this relationship in mind. Suturing the anterior aspect of the posterior oblique ligament to the posterior fibers of the MCL with the knee in more than 30 degrees of flexion could limit the necessary anteroposterior excursion of the MCL, thus inviting development of a significant flexion contracture postoperatively.

The posteromedial capsule is also specifically reinforced by insertions of the semimembranosus[13] (Fig. 37–6). The semimembranosus musculotendinous unit stabilizes the posteromedial corner and provides capsular reinforcement as a result of its various attachment sites, thereby helping to stabilize the knee during active flexion (Fig. 37–7). In addition to providing resistance to valgus stress, the MCL and posterior oblique ligament provide resistance to abnormal external tibial rotation.[5,13,24] Damage to this area of the knee leads to an increase in external tibial rotation, but not to the same extent that occurs when there is combined damage to the MCL, posterior oblique ligament, and anterior cruciate ligament (ACL). The origin and insertion of the MCL are also reinforced by attachments of the vastus medialis obliquus muscle to the adductor tubercle and tibia.[13] A fibrous connection between this muscle and the proximal end of the MCL helps keep the ligament taut during active knee extension; this tautness decreases the residual abnormal valgus laxity that may exist as a result of previous damage to the MCL (see Fig. 37–2B).

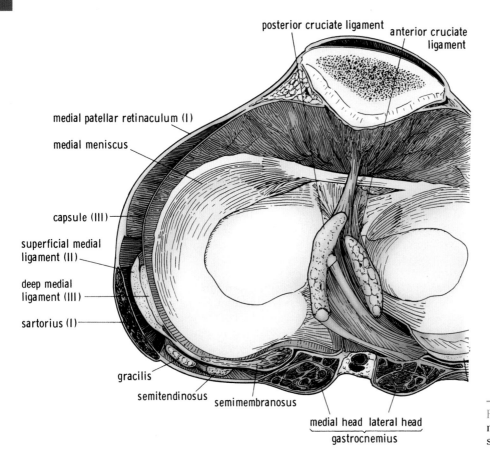

Figure 37–1. Cross-section of the medial side of the knee demonstrating the three-layer concept.

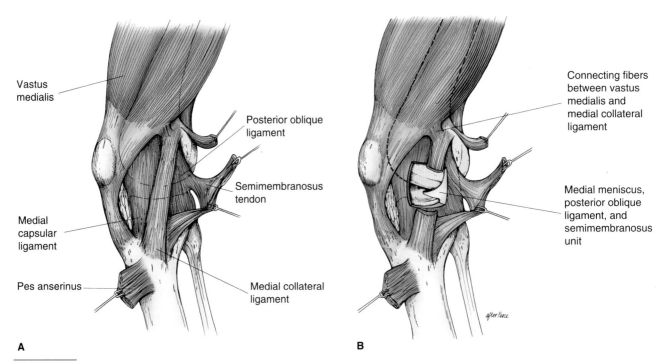

Figure 37–2. **A,** Medial capsuloligamentous complex. **B,** According to Muller,[13] the MCL is dynamized by the connecting fibers of the vastus medialis, and the posterior oblique ligament is dynamized by the semimembranosus. (From Indelicato PA: Isolated medial collateral ligament injuries in the knee. J Am Acad Orthop Surg 3:9, 1995.)

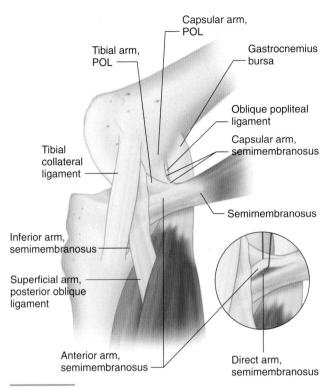

Figure 37–3. Posterior oblique ligament (POL). Note the more posterior origin, expansile insertions, and relationship with the posteromedial capsule and semimembranosus expansions. (From Sims WF, Jacobson KE: The posteromedial corner of the knee: Medial-sided injury patterns revisited. Am J Sports Med 32:337, 2004.)

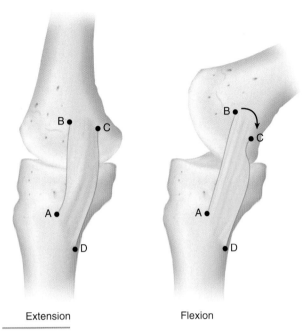

Figure 37–4. Medial collateral ligament in flexion and extension.

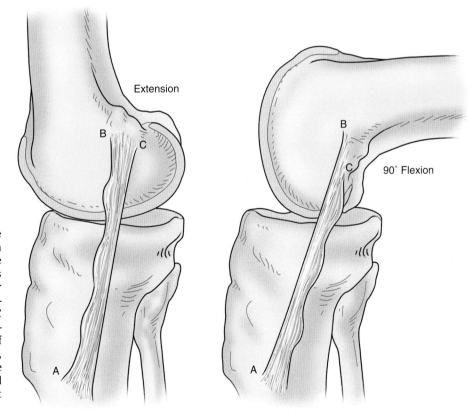

Figure 37–5. Diagram of the superficial medial ligament with flexion and extension of the knee. Because point B moves superiorly, the anterior border is tightened in flexion. Conversely, in extension, point C moves proximally, thereby tightening the posterior margin of the ligament. (From Warren LF, Marshall JL, Girgis F: The prime static stabilizer of the medial side of the knee. J Bone Joint Surg Am 56:665, 1974.)

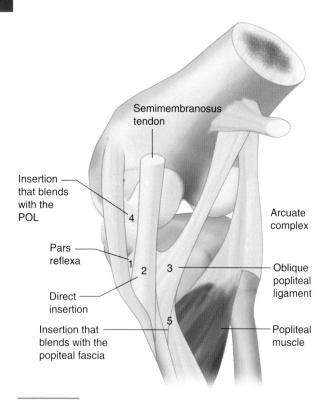

Figure 37–6. Semimembranosus expansions. The five insertions are (1) the pars reflexa, (2) direct posteromedial tibial insertion, (3) oblique popliteal ligament insertion, (4) expansion to the posterior oblique ligament (POL), and (5) popliteus aponeurosis expansion. Note the investment into the POL. (From Sims WF, Jacobson KE: The posteromedial corner of the knee: Medial-sided injury patterns revisited. Am J Sports Med 32:337, 2004.)

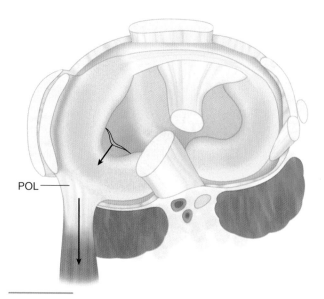

Figure 37–7. Bird's-eye view of the proposed dynamizing action of the semimembranosus. The *large arrow* represents tension created in the posterior meniscocapsular complex by the semimembranosus. Note the ability of the semimembranosus to tension the posterior oblique ligament (POL) and aid in posterior meniscal retraction, represented by the *small arrow*. (From Sims WF, Jacobson KE: The posteromedial corner of the knee: Medial-sided injury patterns revisited. Am J Sports Med 32:337, 2004.)

MECHANISM OF INJURY

An important aspect of the history is to try to establish the mechanism of injury to the knee joint. The majority of injuries to the medial supporting structures of the knee are caused by a blow to the lateral aspect of the lower part of the thigh or the upper part of the leg, which may occur in a traumatic setting or during sports. Among alpine skiers, for example, the MCL has been reported to be the most commonly injured ligament, with such injuries accounting for 60% of all knee injuries.[2,17,22] Rotational noncontact force usually results in damage to the posterior oblique ligament and posterior fibers of the MCL. If sufficiently strong, this rotational force could cause significant structural damage to the ACL as well. Because most injuries are a combination of valgus/external rotation, it is not unusual to discover damage to the MCL, posterior oblique ligament, and ACL in the same knee.

DIAGNOSIS

When examining the knee it is critical to keep in mind some important principles. First, the patient must be relaxed to accurately assess the amount of structural damage to the medial and posteromedial aspect of the knee joint, including the MCL, cruciate ligaments, and surrounding muscles and tendons. Second, always use the uninjured contralateral knee as a control to determine the presence of asymmetric medial joint opening when valgus stress is applied. Third, the examination should be performed as gently as possible. Valgus stress testing with the knee in 30 degrees of flexion is still the key physical test for determining the extent of damage to the medial supporting structures of the knee. In larger patients, this degree of knee flexion can easily be achieved by resting the thigh on the examining table and dropping the foot over the edge of the table a few inches (Fig. 37–8). This position allows the patient the opportunity to relax more easily and maintain a flaccid thigh instead of the examiner attempting to hold the extremity suspended with the hip flexed while applying valgus stress to the medial knee joint. To test the MCL, secure the ankle with one hand and place the other hand around the knee with the thenar eminence abutting the fibular head. The amount of medial opening detected with the application of valgus stress and the knee in 30 degrees of flexion in comparison to the uninjured knee is a direct reflection of damage to the MCL.

Fourth, the examiner should also record the quality of the endpoint to valgus stress. It can be graded from I to III or by the number of millimeters that the joint opens as determined by the examiner.[6] Neither approach is very objective; therefore, we prefer to use the grading system. With a grade I tear, the stress examination produces minimal to no opening with stress, but the manipulation causes pain along the line of the collateral ligament, most especially at the site of the tear. A grade II tear corresponds to a physical examination that shows some opening of the joint but with a distinct endpoint to the test. In a grade III tear, the stress examination shows no distinct endpoint to the evaluation, with the knee opening almost an unlimited degree. It is worth re-emphasizing that a difference of more than 5 to 8 mm is indicative of significant structural

damage to the MCL.[7] When a complete, isolated disruption of the MCL is present, the endpoint identified is, in fact, that of the intact ACL. In other words, the endpoint encountered is beyond the point where it should be felt when compared with the opposite knee. This is a subtle, but significant finding. Fifth, one needs to distinguish between soft-tissue swelling, which normally accompanies damage to the medial supporting structures of the knee, and hemarthrosis, which is frequently seen with ACL rupture. When there is combined damage to the MCL and ACL, the size of the hemarthrosis may be paradoxically small because of extravasation of blood into the soft tissues through the coexisting tear in the medial capsular ligament (layer 3).

The medial knee examination is not complete without examining the joint for structural damage in full extension. In extension, additional structures in the knee contribute to valgus restraint, including the capsule, ACL, posterior oblique ligament, medial meniscus, and semimembranosus (Fig. 37–9). Once again, the examination must be performed gently. Asymmetric medial joint space opening with valgus stress that occurs in full extension is indicative of combined MCL and posterior oblique ligament damage and should caution the examiner to suspect associated ACL and/or posterior cruciate ligament involvement. One can safely assume that if the knee is stable to valgus stress in full extension, there is probably no significant damage to the posterior oblique ligament.

Finally, the posteromedial capsule is evaluated with the Slocum test (anterior drawer at 90 degrees of flexion with external rotation of the lower part of the leg).[2,24] When the tibia is rotated externally, the posteromedial capsule should tighten and allow less anterior excursion than the drawer test in neutral rotation. When the posteromedial capsule is torn, the Slocum test demonstrates an increase in anterior motion of the tibia versus the drawer test in neutral, and the tibia tends to "roll out" (Fig. 37–10). External tibial rotation and anterior translation are mani-

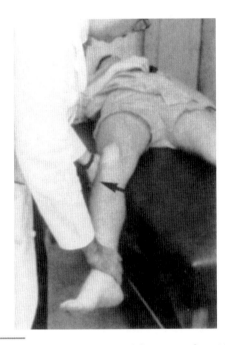

Figure 37–8. Placing the injured leg over the side of the table will help the patient relax while allowing the knee to flex the necessary 30 degrees. (From Indelicato PA: Isolated medial collateral ligament injuries in the knee. J Am Acad Orthop Surg 3:9, 1995.)

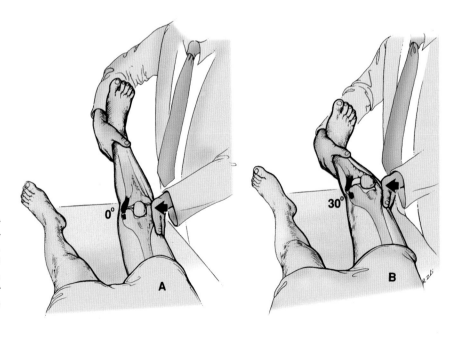

Figure 37–9. Valgus stress in extension tests the medial collateral ligament and the posteromedial capsule. Stress in 30 degrees of flexion tests only the medial collateral ligament. (From Tria AJ Jr, Klein KS: An Illustrated Guide to the Knee. New York, Churchill Livingstone, 1992.)

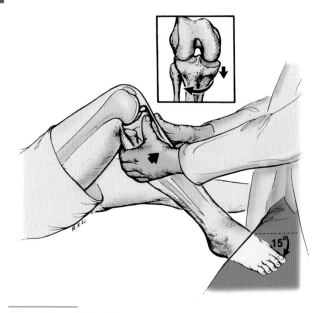

Figure 37–10. The Slocum test is performed in 90 degrees of flexion with the foot externally rotated and anterior proximal tibial force applied to test the posteromedial capsule. (From Tria AJ Jr, Klein KS: An Illustrated Guide to the Knee. New York, Churchill Livingstone, 1992.)

fested as anteromedial rotatory instability, which causes the medial tibial plateau to sublux anteromedially on the medial femoral condyle. On clinical examination, the abduction stress test result is positive with abnormal excess opening of the medial joint space at 30 degrees, along with positive anterior drawer and Lachman test results.

Sometimes, even to the most experienced knee examiner, pain, swelling, and muscle spasm preclude an adequate examination. When this situation exists, one should splint the extremity and reexamine the individual a few days later when the pain and swelling have subsided. Magnetic resonance imaging (MRI) can provide an advantage in four circumstances: (1) when the status of the ACL remains uncertain despite repeated physical examinations, (2) when the status of the meniscus is in question, (3) when surgical repair of the MCL is indicated and the location of the tear may limit the need for a large exposure, and (4) when an unexplainable effusion develops during the rehabilitation program. The need to perform MRI should be infrequent when the status of the ACL and meniscus can be ascertained by physical examination. However, Nakamura et al recently postulated that the location of the injury and the superficial MCL appearance on MRI can potentially predict the outcome of nonoperative treatment of MCL injury in terms of residual valgus laxity.[14] Diagnostic arthroscopy is rarely helpful in deciding the amount of damage to the medial supporting structures of the knee joint. Furthermore, postarthroscopic complications may develop as a result of fluid extravasation if the arthroscopy is performed in a knee with an acute complete medial disruption by a relatively inexperienced arthroscopist using a pressurized pump.

TREATMENT

Treatment of collateral ligament injuries of the knee can be divided into nonoperative and operative approaches. As stated previously, the trend over the past 30 years has been toward a conservative, nonsurgical method, particularly when there is no coexisting damage to the ACL.

Isolated partial tears of the collateral ligaments universally do well with nonoperative management. The healing process, as described by Frank et al, consists of an inflammatory phase (72 hours), a repair and regeneration phase (6 weeks), and a remodeling phase (1 year).[5] In general, incomplete tears are managed by temporary immobilization and protective weightbearing, with crutches used for pain control. Progressive resistive exercises, including isometric, isotonic, and when available, isokinetic strengthening programs, are begun as soon as the pain begins to subside. Early weightbearing is encouraged, with the joint held in full extension in the knee immobilizer. Once comfortable motion is achieved, the immobilizer is removed and progressive weightbearing is allowed, but crutch-free ambulation is not permitted until the patient can walk without a noticeable limp. Infrequently, patients experience pain near the attachment site of the MCL that prevents them from achieving early, full, pain-free extension. If this occurs, the knee should be immobilized longer until this discomfort spontaneously subsides.

It is very unusual for an effusion to develop during the course of the rehabilitation program. If one is noted, the possibility of coexisting meniscus and/or articular damage should be suspected. Once a patient recovers all motion, no longer experiences an effusion, and regains 80% of strength, return to competitive sports can be safely initiated. Patients with grade I sprains are usually able to return to unrestricted sports within 2 weeks and those with grade II injuries within 3 weeks. The author has not found it necessary to recommend the routine use of a brace, even when the patient returns to contact sports. The prognosis after conservative management is generally good.[1,12] If joint line tenderness persists beyond 3 weeks, the index of suspicion for an associated meniscal tear should increase, and MRI may be indicated in these circumstances.

The older literature supports surgical repair of complete tears of the MCL. O'Donoghue[16] strongly advocated suture repair of such lesions as soon as possible after injury. Hughston and Barrett[8] supported primary repair of all MCL and posterior oblique tears. They believed that anterior advancement of the posterior oblique ligament was the key to restoring medial stability and advocated correct tension and placement of each suture, best accomplished under direct visualization. Some recent animal studies have also shown the repair tissue in the nonoperative setting to be composed of primarily type III collagen, which has inferior mechanical properties, increased laxity, and only 70% of maximum tensile strength.[17] However, the bulk of the current literature concurs that surgical treatment is not commonly advised for isolated acute MCL injuries. Current reports that recommend operative repair of the MCL do so only for cases of severe instability greater than 10 mm.[9]

The nonoperative approach to management of complete tears of the MCL was first advocated by Ellsasser et al.[3] Fetto and Marshall[4] also reported excellent results after complete isolated MCL tears, irrespective of whether they were treated in open or closed fashion. In 1983 a series of isolated, complete MCL tears of the knee treated nonoperatively showed no advantage to direct suture repair when compared with a nonoperative approach that involved a structured rehabilitation program.[10] In a subsequent article it was shown that the conservative approach was successful, even in highly competitive athletes who returned to contact sports.[11] More recently, Reider et al[18] furthered the idea of early functional rehabilitation of isolated tears of the MCL in athletes. They reported excellent results in 35 athletes monitored for more than 5 years. Nineteen patients were able to return to full, unlimited sports in less than 8 weeks after their injury. Sixteen of the 19 football players were able to return to the sport within 4 weeks after injury.

Our method for treating isolated, complete rupture (grade III) of the MCL has evolved over the past 15 years. The old method was to immobilize the knee in a cast brace in 30 degrees of flexion for 2 weeks, limit range of motion from 30 to 90 degrees of flexion in the cast brace after 2 weeks, limit weightbearing for 6 weeks, and keep the cast brace on for 6 to 8 weeks. Now, we prefer to place the leg in a commercially available splint in full extension for 2 weeks. The patient is then able to start motion throughout a comfortable range with no limitations and is allowed to bear weight as tolerated. Independent walking without crutches is limited until the patient can walk without a noticeable limp. The knee splint should be discontinued within the first 3 to 4 weeks. Once isokinetic studies show that the extremity has recovered at least 80% of its strength, power, and endurance, an on-the-field agility program is begun. If the patient desires to go back and play contact sports such as football, soccer, or rugby, it is recommended that a double-upright knee orthosis be worn for the remainder of the season. The brace becomes optional the following season.

The likelihood of detecting a significant intrasubstance tear of the medial meniscus is also small when complete isolated disruption of the MCL occurs. Meniscocapsular separation occurs frequently in complete MCL tears, but this damage occurs within the vascular perimeter of the meniscus and thus can heal spontaneously without direct suture repair. One explanation may be that the fulcrum required to load the medial compartment and subsequently tear the meniscus is lost when the MCL tears completely.

Although the treatment of combined MCL and ACL injuries has evolved during the past 20 years, the issues of surgically repairing a concurrent MCL tear and the timing of that repair remain controversial. The ACL is the primary restraint to anterior tibial displacement; however, it also serves as a secondary restraint, along with the PCL, to valgus instability. Therefore, injury to both the ACL and MCL will result in anterior and valgus instability. When there is incomplete damage to the MCL, surgical reconstruction of the ACL alone appears to be necessary to provide a good functional result.[7] Additionally, early ACL reconstruction has not led to functional improvement in outcomes but instead has been associated with an increased rate of complications (Petersen). Because complete tears of the MCL have been shown to heal well without surgery, certain authors have claimed that with combined MCL/ACL injuries, one needs only to surgically address the ACL and treat the MCL nonoperatively.[20] Excellent subjective and objective results have been reported with ACL reconstruction and nonoperative management of the MCL, even in a high-demand athlete, with no advantages identified from the additional surgery.[15,21] Furthermore, combined reconstruction of both ligaments does not alter the prevalence of late valgus laxity when compared with ACL reconstruction alone,[7,21] although MCL repair has been associated with increased knee stiffness. Pressman and Johnson recently evaluated alpine skiers with combined injuries (which they noted was a rare combination) and also concluded that most MCL injuries do not require surgical repair if the ACL is reconstructed after a combined injury. Operative repair was considered only with a grade III MCL injury that was grossly unstable both in 30 degrees of flexion and in extension.[17] Others reports favor operative repair of the medial structures and meniscus in high-demand athletes with extensive medial joint space opening secondary to gross medial ligament damage and associated ACL disruption.

Our approach in managing combined MCL/ACL injuries has also evolved. When faced with this combined injury, the knee is immobilized in extension for a period of 3 to 4 weeks to allow early primary healing of the MCL. Patients are then started on a rehabilitation program to recover most of their motion. This approach may take up to 4 to 6 weeks or longer, particularly if the MCL damage is proximal. Once a patient has recovered most of the motion, an ACL reconstruction is performed. Intraoperatively, after ACL reconstruction, the knee is reexamined for medial laxity, both in full extension and in 30 degrees of flexion. If the knee remains grossly unstable, particularly in full extension, a small posteromedial incision is made, with avoidance of injury to the saphenous vein and nerve, and the posterior oblique ligament is tightened. Care is taken to avoid any significant anterior advancement or reefing of this ligament because of the risk for flexion contracture postoperatively. Suture tension is tested under direct observation, and the knee is placed in full extension. Immediate range-of-motion exercises are begun, and the patient continues with an ACL rehabilitation protocol. Some reports advocate the use of a hinged orthosis for 8 to 10 weeks after surgery to protect the MCL repair.

Again, if it is necessary to repair the medial ligaments of the knee surgically, the potential complication of loss of motion postoperatively is quite high, particularly if the lesion in the MCL is near the femoral condyle and/or proximal to the joint line. Robins and colleagues[19] demonstrated that when damage occurs to the proximal half of the MCL in combined ACL/MCL tears, recovery of full motion may be a problem and an aggressive program should be designed that focuses on regaining full extension. Once again, it needs to be stressed that the majority of cases do not require direct suture repair of the medial supporting structures.

SUMMARY

The method of managing injury to the medial structures of the knee has evolved over the past several years. The MCL is the primary restraint to valgus loading. When injured, a nonoperative approach appears to provide predictably good results in most cases. Imaging studies may be necessary when the presence of coexisting ACL, meniscus, and/or articular damage is suspected. In the setting of combined injury to the ACL and MCL, good clinical results and knee stability are achieved with nonsurgical management of the MCL and late ACL reconstruction. In the few instances when repair of the MCL is performed, effort should be undertaken to prevent postoperative stiffness, especially with proximal injuries to the MCL.

References

1. Dersheid GL, Garrick JG: Medial collateral ligament injuries in football: Nonoperative management of grade I and grade II sprains. Am J Sports Med 9:365, 1981.
2. Duncan J, Hunter R, Purnell M, et al: Meniscal injuries associated acute anterior cruciate ligament tears in alpine skiers. Am J Sports Med 23:170, 1995.
3. Ellsasser JC, Reynolds FC, Omohundro JR: The non-operative treatment of collateral ligament injuries of the knee in professional football players: An analysis of seventy-four injuries treated non-operatively and twenty-four injuries treated surgically. J Bone Joint Surg Am 56:1185, 1974.
4. Fetto JF, Marshall JL: Medial collateral ligament injuries of the knee: A rationale for treatment. Clin Orthop 132:206, 1978.
5. Frank C, Woo SL-Y, Amiel D, et al: Medial collateral ligament healing: A multi-disciplinary assessment in rabbits. Am J Sports Med 11:379, 1983.
6. Grood ES, Noyes FR, Butler DL, et al: Ligamentous and capsular restraints preventing straight medial and lateral laxity in intact human cadaver knees. J Bone Joint Surg Am 63:1257, 1981.
7. Hillard-Sembell D, Daniel DM, Stone ML, et al: Combined injuries to the anterior cruciate and medial collateral ligaments of the knee. J Bone Joint Surg Am 78:169, 1996.
8. Hughston JC, Barrett GR: Acute anteromedial rotatory instability: Long-term results of surgical repair. J Bone Joint Surg Am 65:145, 1983.
9. Hughston JC, Eilers AF: The role of the posterior oblique ligament in repairs of the acute medial ligament tears of the knee. J Bone Joint Surg Am 55:923, 1973.
10. Indelicato PA: Non-operative treatment of complete tears of the medial collateral ligament of the knee. J Bone Joint Surg Am 65:323, 1983.
11. Indelicato PA, Hermansdorfer J, Huegel M: Nonoperative management of complete tears of the medial collateral ligament of the knee in intercollegiate football players. Clin Orthop 256:191, 1990.
12. Lundberg M, Messner K: Long-term prognosis of isolated partial medial collateral ligament ruptures. Am J Sports Med 24:160, 1996.
13. Muller W: The Knee: Form, Function, and Ligament Reconstruction. New York, Springer-Verlag, 1983.
14. Nakamura N, Horibe S, Toritsuka Y, et al: Acute grade III medial collateral ligament injury of the knee associated with anterior cruciate ligament tear. Am J Sports Med 31:261, 2003.
15. Noyes FR, Barber-Weston SD: The treatment of acute combined ruptures of the anterior cruciate and medial ligaments of the knee. Am J Sports Med 23:380, 1995.
16. O'Donoghue DH: Surgical treatment of fresh injuries to the major ligaments of the knee. J Bone Joint Surg Am 32:721, 1950.
17. Pressman A, Johnson DH: A review of ski injuries resulting in combined injury to the anterior cruciate ligament and medial collateral ligaments. Arthroscopy 19:194, 2003.
18. Reider B, Sathy MR, Talkington J, et al: Treatment of isolated medial collateral ligament injuries in athletes with early functional rehabilitation: A five-year follow-up study. Am J Sports Med 22:470, 1993.
19. Robins AJ, Newman AP, Burks RT: Postoperative return of motion in anterior cruciate ligament and medial collateral ligament injuries: The effect of medial collateral ligament rupture location. Am J Sports Med 21:20, 1993.
20. Shelbourne KD, Porter DA: Anterior cruciate ligament/medial collateral ligament injury: Nonoperative management of medial collateral ligament tears with anterior cruciate ligament reconstruction: A preliminary report. Am J Sports Med 20:283, 1992.
21. Sims WF, Jacobson KE: The posteromedial corner of the knee: Medial-sided injury patterns revisited. Am J Sports Med 32:337, 2004.
22. Warme W, Feagin J, King P, et al: Ski injury statistics, 1982-1993, Jackson Hole Ski Resort. Am J Sports Med 23:597, 1995.
23. Warren F, Marshall J: The supporting structures and layers on the medial side of the knee. J Bone Joint Surg Am 61:56, 1979.
24. Warren LF, Marshall JL, Girgis F: The prime static stabilizer of the medial side of the knee. J Bone Joint Surg Am 56:665, 1974.

CHAPTER 38

Lateral Collateral Ligament Injuries

Michael J. Stuart

The fibular collateral ligament (FCL), popliteus tendon, and popliteofibular ligament (PFL) are the main static stabilizers of the lateral and posterolateral aspect of the knee. Recent experimental and clinical studies have further elucidated the anatomy, biomechanics, and surgical treatment of these important structures. FCL sprain may occur as an isolated injury, but it is often associated with disruption of the posterolateral corner and cruciate ligaments.[2,4] Accurate diagnosis and prompt treatment are critical because persistent posterolateral pathological laxity can result in persistent symptoms and failure of cruciate ligament reconstruction.

ANATOMY

The lateral and posterolateral knee anatomy is quite complex, but anatomic dissections combined with recent descriptions of the ligament and tendon attachments have established a consistent pattern.[18,38,39,43,44] Individual structures include the layers of the iliotibial tract, the long and short heads of the biceps femoris muscle and combined tendon, the FCL, the midthird lateral capsular ligament, the fabellofibular ligament, the posterior arcuate ligament, the lateral coronary ligament, the posterolateral capsule, and the popliteus muscle complex, including the PFL and popliteus tendon (Fig. 38–1). Seebacher et al defined three distinct lateral knee anatomic layers.[35] Layer I includes the superficial fascia, iliotibial band, biceps femoris tendon, and peroneal nerve. Layer II is the FCL. Layer III consists of the popliteus, PFL, arcuate ligament, fabellofibular ligament, coronary ligament, and posterolateral capsule. Cadaveric dissections and quantitative measurements with a digitizing motion analysis system by LaPrade et al precisely located the attachment sites in relation to bony landmarks[18] (Fig. 38–2). The FCL is a round, cord-like structure with an average total length of 69.6 mm (range, 62.6 to 73.5 mm). It attaches in a small bony depression located slightly proximal and posterior to the lateral femoral epicondyle. This origin has a cross-sectional area of 0.48 cm² and is positioned 18.5 mm (range, 16.8 to 22.9 mm) from the popliteus insertion. The FCL attaches to the lateral aspect of the fibular head with a cross-sectional area of 0.43 cm². The popliteus muscle originates from the posteromedial part of the tibia, with the PFL arising from the musculotendinous junction and the popliteus tendon continuing on to attach to the lateral femoral condyle. This tendon is an intra-articular, extrasynovial structure coursing through the popliteus hiatus, then deep to the FCL before inserting in the ante-

rior portion of the popliteal sulcus. The average tendon length from the musculotendinous junction to the femoral insertion measures approximately 55 mm. The femoral attachment site has an average cross-sectional area of 0.59 cm² and is always anterior to the FCL origin. The popliteus tendon is located anterior to the popliteus sulcus with the knee in extension and then enters the sulcus between 105 and 130 degrees of knee flexion. The PFL courses from the popliteus musculoskeletal junction to the fibular styloid process. This ligament consists of an anterior division and a larger posterior division. The anterior division inserts on the medial styloid with some fibers extending to the lateral part of the tibia. The posterior division inserts at the tip and posteromedial aspect of the styloid process. The cross-sectional area of the PFL (6.9 mm²) is nearly equal to that of the FCL (7.2 mm²).[29] The lateral gastrocnemius tendon is adherent to the lateral capsule and inserts at or very near the femoral supracondylar process, approximately 14 mm posterior to the FCL origin and 28 mm posterior to the popliteus tendon insertion. The fabellofibular ligament is the distal edge of the capsular arm of the short head of the biceps femoris.

BIOMECHANICS

Numerous researchers have performed selective sectioning studies of the lateral and posterolateral structures in the human cadaver knee.[6,32,33,36,46,47,51] Improved understanding of knee biomechanics has helped establish physical examination and surgical treatment principles. Selective cutting techniques have revealed that sectioning of all the posterolateral structures results in larger increases in primary posterior translation, varus rotation, external rotation, and coupled external rotation. The FCL is the primary static restraint to varus rotation, and the PFL and popliteus tendon limit external tibial rotation. Ulrich et al showed that the PFL becomes lax when the tibia is internally rotated and tense when externally rotated. Therefore, the popliteus muscle-tendon unit stabilizes the lateral meniscus and balances neutral tibial rotation.[45] Selective sectioning of the PFL and FCL has revealed that the PFL has a significant role in preventing posterior translation and varus angulation and restricting excessive primary and coupled external rotation.[13] The FCL was a primary restraint against varus angulation and secondary restraint against external rotation and posterior displacement. Pasque et al, on the other hand, proposed that the popliteus muscle-tendon unit, FCL, and posterolateral capsular structures function as a unit. Their

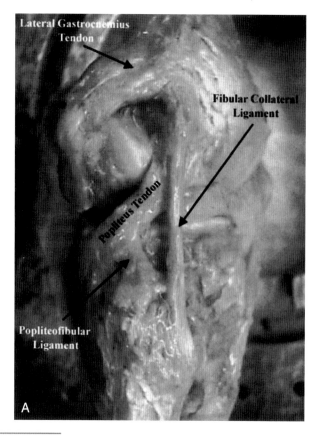

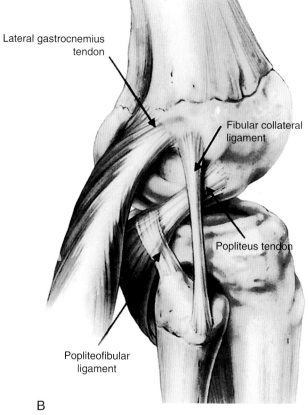

Figure 38–1. Cadaveric knee dissection (**A**) and diagram (**B**) delineating the fibular collateral ligament, popliteus tendon, popliteofibular ligament, and lateral gastrocnemius tendon. (From LaPrade RF, Ly TV, Wentorf FA, Engebretsen L: The posterolateral attachments of the knee: A qualitative and quantitative morphologic analysis of the fibular collateral ligament, popliteus tendon, popliteofibular ligament, and lateral gastrocnemius tendon. Am J Sports Med 31:854-860, 2003.)

conclusions were based on the fact that sectioning the PFL produced no significant changes in external rotation, varus rotation, or posterior translation and that sectioning of the PFL and popliteus tendon produced an increase of only 5 to 6 degrees in external rotation from flexion of 30 to 120 degrees.[33] Wang and colleagues measured coupled posterolateral displacement at 299% of the intact knee after cutting the popliteus tendon and FCL with the knee at 90 degrees of flexion and the posterior cruciate ligament (PCL) intact. Subsequent cutting of the PCL increased posterolateral displacement to 367%.[50] Veltri et al combined sectioning of the posterolateral ligaments and the anterior cruciate ligament (ACL), which resulted in maximal increases in primary anterior and posterior translation at 30 degrees of flexion.[47] Primary varus, primary internal rotation, and coupled external rotation also increased and were maximal at 30 degrees of knee flexion. Combined sectioning of the posterolateral structures with the PCL resulted in primary posterior translation, primary varus and external rotation, and coupled external rotation at all angles of flexion. The authors concluded that physical examination of the knee at 30 and 90 degrees can differentiate between an isolated posterolateral injury and combined PCL and posterolateral involvement. Posterolateral tibial subluxation by the voluntarily evoked

posterolateral drawer test was demonstrated by electromyography in 10 patients and revealed that the biceps femoris muscle acts as a major subluxator and the popliteus as a reducer.[37]

MECHANISM OF INJURY

An FCL sprain results from a varus stress, and posterolateral injuries typically occur as a result of a direct blow to the proximal medial aspect of the tibia with the knee in extension. Simulated varus stress testing in a human cadaver model revealed that the FCL consistently failed first, followed by the PFL and then the popliteus muscle.[29] Lateral and posterolateral capsule and ligament injuries often occur in combination with ACL and/or PCL injuries. Combined injuries to the ACL, PCL, FCL, and posterolateral structures may represent a reduced knee dislocation. Prompt recognition plus treatment of associated neurovascular involvement in a multiple ligament–injured knee is essential.[40] In addition, identification of posterolateral knee injuries is imperative to avoid chronic instability problems and failure of ACL and/or PCL reconstruction.[19,20]

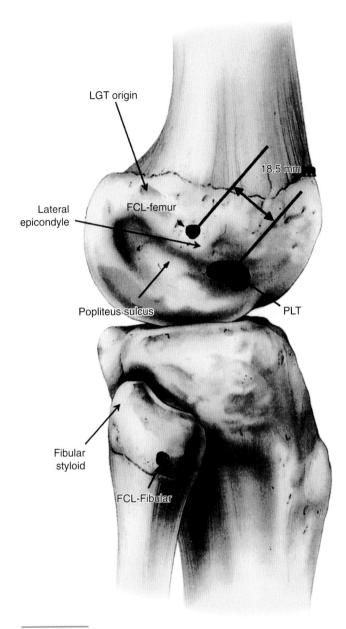

Figure 38–2. Diagram of the fibular collateral ligament (FCL) and popliteus tendon attachments and their relationship to bony landmarks. PLT, popliteus tendon. (From LaPrade RF, Ly TV, Wentorf FA, Engebretsen L: The posterolateral attachments of the knee: A qualitative and quantitative morphologic analysis of the fibular collateral ligament, popliteus tendon, popliteofibular ligament, and lateral gastrocnemius tendon. Am J Sports Med 31:854-860, 2003.)

DIAGNOSIS

Patients with injuries to the lateral and posterolateral knee structures may seek medical assistance after an acute traumatic event or because of complaints of recurrent pain and giving way. Symptoms may reflect the associated ligament injuries, including involvement of the cruciate ligaments.

Numbness, paresthesia, or weakness in the lower part of the leg and foot signifies damage to the peroneal nerve.[48]

Physical Examination

Severe pathological laxity in an acutely injured knee requires careful assessment and documentation of the limb's neurovascular status.[40] Check for capillary refill, skin color, and temperature; palpate and compare the pedal pulses (dorsalis pedis, posterior tibial); and test skin sensation to light touch on the dorsum of the foot, as well as the first web space. Perform manual muscle strength testing of the anterior tibial, peroneal, and extensor hallucis longus to document peroneal nerve function. The ligament examination should systematically identify injury to each specific anatomic structure, especially the FCL, popliteus tendon, PFL, ACL, and PCL.[21,22] Increased lateral joint space opening to varus stress at 30 degrees of flexion signifies an FCL injury. Increased lateral joint space to varus stress with the knee in full extension is consistent with combined cruciate ligament and FCL injuries. Integrity of the ACL is determined by the Lachman test and integrity of the PCL by the posterior sag and drawer tests. Increased external rotation of the tibia (>15 degrees) in comparison to the contralateral limb at 30 degrees of flexion is consistent with injury to the posterolateral structures, namely, the PFL and popliteus tendon. Increased external rotation at 90 degrees of flexion signifies combined PCL and posterolateral injuries. The posterolateral drawer test describes posterior subluxation of the lateral tibial plateau with the knee flexed at 80 degrees. This subluxation is maximal at 15 degrees of external tibial rotation, and the test is negative on maximum internal tibial rotation if the PCL is intact.[9] The external rotation recurvatum test is performed by suspending the limb against gravity to cause varus, hyperextension, and external rotation, which also indicates the combined injury pattern.[9] Examination under anesthesia may further define the pattern and extent of the damage. Comparison of physical examination findings in 71 consecutive patients who had posterolateral knee injuries with injury patterns detected at the time of surgery determined that the FCL was injured in only 23% of the knees.[15] The reverse pivot-shift test was associated with involvement of the FCL, popliteus, and midthird lateral collateral ligament, and the posterolateral drawer test at 30 degrees of knee flexion was associated with injury to the FCL and lateral gastrocnemius tendon.

Imaging

Anteroposterior, lateral, oblique, and patellar radiographs are important to confirm satisfactory joint position, but they may also identify periarticular and osteochondral fractures. In addition, radiographs can help in the diagnosis of specific ligament injuries when avulsion fractures occur. An osseous fibular head fragment represents an FCL, PFL, or biceps femoris avulsion. Comparison views while applying varus/valgus or anterior/posterior translation stress may detect a physeal injury in a skeletally immature patient or help determine the extent of ligamentous damage in an adult.

Improvement in magnetic resonance imaging (MRI) software and imaging sequences has resulted in better delineation of the lateral and posterolateral anatomic structures.[16,26,30,34] MRI provides insight on meniscal tears, intraosseous contusions, occult fractures, capsular disruptions, and muscle strains. LaPrade reported sensitivity, specificity, and accuracy data for thin-slice coronal oblique T1-weighted MRI scans, including the FCL (94%, 100%, 95%), popliteus tendon (93%, 80%, 90%), and PFL (69%, 67%, 68%). A study of the injury patterns in the fibular head according to specific ligament and tendon injuries by Lee et al diagnosed injury to the arcuate ligament or PFL in eight patients with a small avulsion fracture of the styloid process of the fibula, bone marrow edema in the medial aspect of the fibular head, or both.[26] Injury to the conjoined tendon or FCL was associated with a larger avulsion fragment and more diffuse proximal fibular edema. MRI can also assist in surgical planning, including the location of incisions, the extent of exposure, the specific procedures required (reattachment or reconstruction), and the number and types of grafts needed. Ross et al correlated MRI findings, examination under anesthesia, and open lateral reconstruction in six consecutive patients. MRI outlined the extent of injury in each case and identified a characteristic bone contusion on the anteromedial femoral condyle.[34]

Arthroscopy

Diagnostic arthroscopy provides direct visualization and palpation of the popliteus tendon, popliteomeniscal fascicles, and lateral meniscus. The "drive-through sign" refers to arthroscopic appreciation of excessive lateral joint space opening with varus stress (Fig. 38–3). LaPrade and Terry compared the arthroscopic and open surgical findings in 33 consecutive knees with grade 3 posterolateral complex injuries.[21] Identification of injured structures by open surgical exploration was incomplete. Arthroscopy added to diagnostic accuracy by visualization of the popliteomeniscal fascicles (83%), coronary ligament (83%), meniscotibial portion of the midthird lateral capsular ligament (73%), posterior capsule (37%), and Wrisberg ligament (33%). Aronowitz et al identified the PFL arthroscopically in the cadaver knee as vertically oriented fibers descending from the inferior surface of the intraarticular portion of the popliteus tendon at the popliteal hiatus.[1]

TREATMENT

Acute Injuries

Clinical observations and biomechanical analysis in the animal model support the belief that complete posterolat-

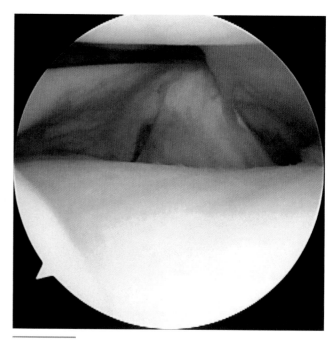

Figure 38–3. Arthroscopic photograph of the intact lateral compartment of the knee with a probe lifting the lateral meniscus to help identify the popliteus tendon. The excessive lateral joint space widening with the application of varus stress is referred to as the "drive-through sign."

eral corner injuries have limited healing potential and generally result in poor outcomes if untreated.[12,23] Nonoperative management is indicated only for isolated grade 1 and grade 2 FCL sprains.[4,12] Partial ligament tears will heal after a 6-week period of early motion and protected weightbearing. A rehabilitation brace is typically used to protect a grade 2 sprain. Kannus reported on 23 patients treated without surgery for an FCL injury.[12] Nine of the 11 patients with a grade 2 sprain returned to their preinjury activity level; however, only 1 of 12 patients with a grade 3 sprain was asymptomatic. All 12 of these knees were unstable on physical examination; therefore, nonoperative treatment was not recommended for grade 3 FCL injuries. Isolated injury to the popliteus complex is uncommon. Nakhostine and coauthors reported on four patients who sustained an external rotation injury with the knee in slight flexion that resulted in isolated avulsion of the popliteus tendon.[31] Radiographs showed a small fragment in the area of the lateral femoral condyle. Anatomic reduction and fixation of the femoral attachment of the popliteus tendon resulted in an excellent knee score for all patients.

Surgical exploration plus treatment of all involved structures provides the most reliable result, and early surgery is always advised when the cruciate ligaments are torn in conjunction with the FCL. The posterolateral structures are important secondary restraints to anterior and posterior translation; therefore, cruciate ligament injuries must be addressed.[6,11] Posterolateral repair or reconstruction is at risk for attenuation if the ACL and/or PCL is not reconstructed. In addition, cadaver studies have shown that posterolateral deficiency results in increased ACL and PCL graft force.[19,20] These biomechanical principles have resulted in the recommendation that posterolateral repair or reconstruction be performed at the time of ACL or PCL reconstruction to decrease the chance of ACL or PCL graft failure.[7] The timing of surgery is important because anatomic repair of the lateral and posterolateral structures is more difficult if surgery is delayed because of tissue retraction and scarring. Arthroscopically assisted cruciate ligament reconstruction together with lateral side anatomic repair within 2 weeks of the traumatic event is advised. The FCL, PFL, posterolateral corner, and associated tendinous injuries to the biceps, popliteus, and iliotibial band are repaired and augmented if necessary.

Veltri and Warren recommend acute surgical treatment of a posterolateral knee injury when possible because the results are better than treatment in the chronic setting.[49] Associated cruciate ligament injuries are reconstructed first, and then the posterolateral corner is exposed through an open lateral incision. The FCL, popliteus tendon, and PFL are anatomically repaired, advanced and recessed, augmented, or reconstructed as indicated. A retrospective review of 25 patients treated for acute lateral knee ligament injuries by Krukhaug et al included 7 with isolated FCL/capsular injuries and 19 with concomitant ligament injuries.[14] Twelve of the 18 surgically treated patients had a stable knee or only mild varus laxity at a medial follow-up of 7.5 years. These authors concluded that early surgery provided the best results and that nonoperative management should be considered only in patients with mild varus laxity and no associated cruciate ligament injury.

RECOMMENDED SURGICAL TECHNIQUE

The arthroscope is valuable for meniscal treatment, tunnel drilling for cruciate ligament reconstruction, graft passage, and femoral fixation before definitive repair of the lateral and posterolateral structures.[41] The ACL and PCL grafts are both fixed on the femoral side, but tensioning and tibial fixation are delayed until after the lateral and posterolateral repairs. This sequence is important because ACL graft tension may cause increased tibial external rotation if the posterolateral structures are incompetent.[52] The open portion of the surgical technique includes a straight, anterolateral paramedian skin incision or a posterolateral incision combined with small anteromedial incisions for the cruciate ligament reconstructions. Full-thickness skin flaps are developed and the peroneal nerve is protected throughout the procedure. Exposure windows are established by splitting the iliotibial band in line with its fibers in addition to developing the interval between the posterior iliotibial band and the biceps femoris. A more extensile exposure detaches the iliotibial band insertion with a block of bone from Gerdy's tubercle to allow proximal retraction. Each injured ligament and tendon is systematically identified with a locking whipstitch (No. 2 nonabsorbable suture) in each structure for later repair or augmentation. Proximal avulsions of the FCL and the popliteus tendon are repaired back to their anatomic attachment sites into a 4- to 6-mm bone trough in an attempt to restore isometry and proper tension. The ligament and tendon are secured with a locking whipstitch, and nonabsorbable suture is passed through femoral drill holes and tied over a medial bone bridge or with a screw and ligament washer combined with sutures tied around the screw. Distal avulsions of the FCL, PFL, and the biceps tendon are reattached to the fibular head through drill holes or with suture anchors. The coronary ligament, arcuate ligament, midthird lateral capsular ligament, menisci, popliteomeniscal fascicles, and osteochondral fractures are repaired anatomically whenever possible. When the FCL and/or PFL cannot be repaired, a free semitendinosus autograft reconstruction is performed.[3,24] The graft is passed through a 6-mm fibular head tunnel and fixed at both ends into a 25-mm socket at the lateral epicondyle with an interference screw or by tying the lead sutures over a button on the medial part of the femur. Figure 37–4 shows a postoperative anteroposterior radiograph after allograft reconstruction of the ACL and PCL along with repair and semitendinosus tendon augmentation of the FCL.

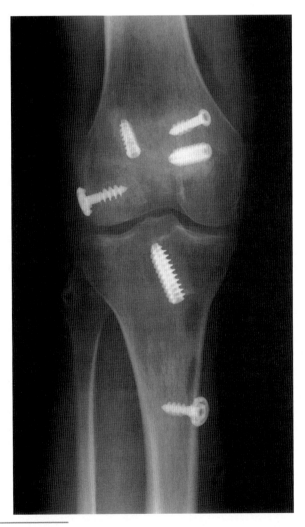

Figure 38–4. Postoperative anteroposterior radiograph after fibular collateral ligament repair and semitendinosus augmentation combined with anterior and posterior cruciate ligament reconstructions.

Chronic Injuries

Before any ligament reconstruction surgery, lower extremity alignment must be analyzed and corrected as necessary. Failure to rectify malalignment and gait abnormalities may compromise any reconstructive soft-tissue procedures.

Gait analysis identifies the dynamic component of the deformity, such as a varus (lateral) thrust or hyperextension that may not be apparent on standing radiographs. Bracing, heel lifts, muscle strengthening, and gait retraining can correct hyperextension before surgery. Malalignment in the coronal plane is treated with a valgus-producing (antivarus), proximal medial tibial opening wedge osteotomy. Static analysis of a full-length standing roentgenogram (51 × 14 inches) includes measurement of the anatomic axis, mechanical axis, and weightbearing line. The mechanical axis of the limb is the angle formed between a line drawn from the hip center to the knee center (femoral mechanical axis) and a line drawn from the knee center to the ankle center (tibial mechanical axis). The normal mechanical axis is approximately 1.2 degrees of varus.[8] The weightbearing line method is a simple and reproducible technique for determining the desired correction angle.[5] Divide the lateral tibial plateau from 0% to 100% from the medial to the lateral margins. Draw lines from the center of the femoral head and the center of the tibiotalar joint to the 62% coordinate on the tibial plateau. The resultant angle formed by these two lines equals the calculated angle of correction. The use of standing radiographs can overestimate the magnitude of correction as a result of ligament attenuation. Each millimeter of lateral tibiofemoral joint separation causes approximately 1 degree of varus angular deformity. Compare the amount of lateral joint space opening (in millimeters) with that in the contralateral knee and subtract the difference from the calculated angle (1 degree per millimeter) to obtain the final angle of correction. This adjustment is important to avoid overcorrection. Figure 38–5 is an intraoperative, anteroposterior fluoroscopic view during an opening wedge osteotomy that shows slight overcorrection of the weightbearing line into the lateral compartment. In addition to valgus correction in the coronal plane, the proximal tibial osteotomy should maintain a neutral tibial slope in the sagittal plane. Sagittal plane alignment is important because increased posterior tibial slope places excessive strain on an ACL graft and increased anterior tibial slope places excessive strain on a PCL graft.

After 4 to 6 months, when the osteotomy has healed, FCL, PFL, and popliteus tendon reconstructions are performed as necessary. Occasionally, the FCL and popliteus tendon can be tensioned by advancement if these structures are intact but retracted from their femoral attachments. The isometric point is nearly maintained by recessing the ligament and tendon into a 4- to 6-mm bone trough that is slightly proximal and anterior to the lateral epicondyle. Fixation is achieved by tying nonabsorbable locking whipstitch sutures around a screw combined with a ligament washer.

The important contribution of the PFL to knee stability has been well documented. Cadaver testing has shown that the PFL is dominant when the knee is flexed because

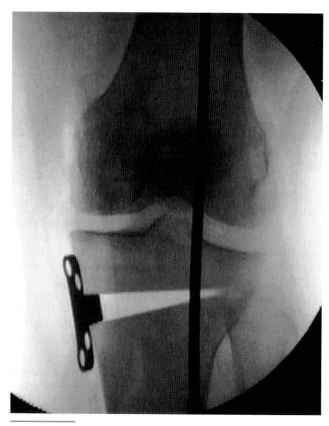

Figure 38–5. Intraoperative, anteroposterior fluoroscopic view during an opening wedge osteotomy showing slight overcorrection of the weightbearing line into the medial compartment.

of slackening of the FCL.[42] Reconstruction of the PFL is important to withstand tibial external rotation forces at higher knee flexion angles. Anatomic reconstruction of the FCL, PFL, and popliteus tendon is the preferred technique, and biceps tenodesis has fallen out of favor. Biceps tenodesis in the cadaver model overconstrained external tibial rotation at all flexion positions and varus angulation at 60 and 90 degrees of flexion.[51]

A robotic/universal force moment sensor testing system compared biceps tenodesis and PFL reconstruction in the cadaver. PFL reconstruction restored intact knee external tibial rotation values at any angle tested, but those after biceps tenodesis remained as much as 5.7 times greater.[10]

Reconstruction graft sources include an Achilles tendon allograft and semitendinosus or patellar tendon autograft/allograft. Lee and coworkers used a split Achilles tendon allograft to reconstruct the posterolateral corner by restoring isometry of the FCL and repositioning the reconstructed popliteus into its original position.[27] Lill et al described an arthroscopically assisted technique of simultaneous reconstruction of the PCL with a four-stranded hamstring tendon graft and the FCL with a looped semitendinosus graft from the contralateral knee.[28] Latimer et al retrospectively reviewed 10 patients treated by reconstruction of the FCL with a bone–patellar tendon–bone allograft secured with interference screws, as well as cruciate ligament reconstruction with autograft or allograft tendons.[25] At 28 months' average follow-up, excessive external rotation and varus laxity at 30 degrees knee flexion were corrected in nine and six patients, respectively. LaPrade and colleagues used 10 cadaver specimens to study static varus and external rotatory stability in a knee with intact structures; with the FCL, PFL, and popliteus tendon cut; and also with the FCL, PFL, and popliteus tendon reconstructed.[17] The surgical procedure used a split Achilles tendon to create two allografts. One graft was used to reconstruct the popliteus tendon and the other to reconstruct both the PFL and the FCL. No significant differences were found between the intact and reconstructed knees for varus translation at 0, 60, and 90 degrees or for external rotation at any flexion angle.

RECOMMENDED SURGICAL TECHNIQUE

The Achilles tendon provides excellent strength and bone block fixation at the femoral attachment for reconstruction of the FCL, PFL, and popliteus tendon as necessary.[17] This tendon is split into two grafts with 9-mm bone plugs. Two 9 × 20-mm bone tunnels are drilled into the lateral femoral condyle at the attachments sites of the FCL and popliteus tendon. A 7-mm tunnel is drilled at the FCL attachment site on the lateral fibular head and exits posteromedially at the attachment site of the PFL. A 9-mm tibial tunnel is drilled in an anteroposterior direction from a point just distal and medial to Gerdy's tubercle to the

posterior popliteal sulcus at the level of the popliteus musculotendinous junction (Fig. 38-6). The bone blocks are each fixed in the femoral tunnels with 7 × 20-mm interference screws. The first graft, which reconstructs the popliteus tendon, is pulled through the tibial tunnel in a posterior-to-anterior direction (Fig. 38-7). The second graft, which reconstructs both the FCL and PLF, is passed deep to the iliotibial band, through the fibular head, in a lateral-to-posteromedial direction and then pulled through the tibial tunnel in a posterior-to-anterior direction. The graft is fixed in its fibular tunnel with a 7-mm bioabsorbable interference screw with the knee flexed 30 degrees and slight valgus stress and neutral rotation. Both grafts emerging from the tibia are then tensioned simultaneously and fixed with a 9-mm bioabsorbable interference screw. Additional fixation is achieved with a staple or screw and ligament washer on the tibia.

A soft compressive dressing with plaster splints is applied after surgery to maintain the knee in slight flexion. A custom polypropylene knee-ankle-foot orthosis or a rehabilitation brace with an extension lock and a 90-degree flexion stop then protects against varus and external rotation stress. The brace is locked in extension at all times except when performing range-of-motion exercises. During the first 4 weeks, general rehabilitation guidelines include prone passive flexion from 0 to 90 degrees, touchdown weightbearing with the brace locked in extension, patellar mobilization, isometrics and straight-leg lifts, and

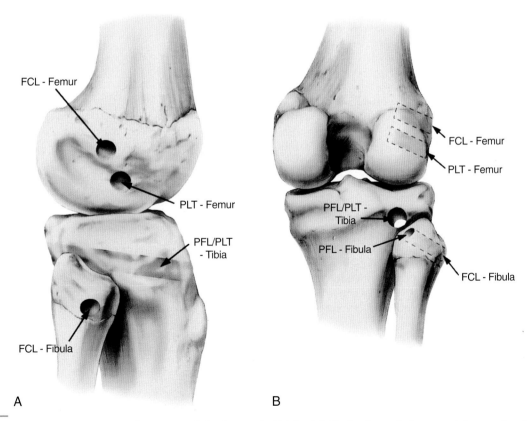

A   B

Figure 38–6. Lateral and posterior diagrams of the femoral, tibial, and fibular tunnel placement for posterolateral knee reconstruction. FCL, fibular collateral ligament; PFL, popliteofibular ligament; PLT, popliteus tendon. (From LaPrade RF, Johansen S, Wentorf FA, et al: An analysis of an anatomical posterolateral knee reconstruction. An in vitro biomechanical study and development of a surgical technique. Am J Sports Med 32:1405-1414, 2004.)

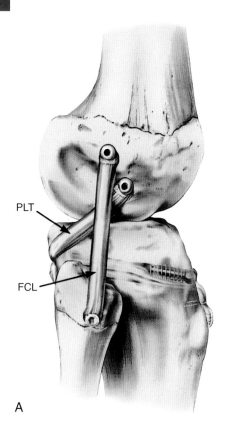

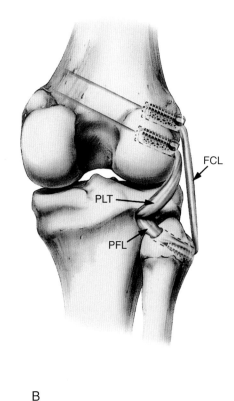

Figure 38–7. Lateral and posterior diagrams of fibular collateral ligament (FCL), popliteofibular ligament (PFL), and popliteus tendon (PLT) allograft reconstructions. (From LaPrade RF, Johansen S, Wentorf FA, et al: An analysis of an anatomical posterolateral knee reconstruction. An in vitro biomechanical study and development of a surgical technique. Am J Sports Med 32:1405-1414, 2004.)

electrical muscle stimulation as necessary. After 4 weeks, progress to passive and active assisted gradual full flexion, partial weightbearing with the brace locked in extension, and low-resistance closed-chain strengthening exercises, including mini squats and leg presses. After 8 weeks, begin full active range of motion, full weightbearing with the brace locked in extension, progressive-resistance closed-chain strengthening exercises, low-resistance bicycling, and swimming. After 3 months, allow full weightbearing with the brace unlocked, low-resistance bicycling, swimming, and hamstring strengthening. At 4 to 5 months after surgery, patients wear an unloader with a slight valgus moment and continue their strengthening and proprioceptive training exercises.

Isolated injury to the FCL is uncommon, and only partial sprains are treated nonoperatively. Complete disruption requires early repair of the involved lateral and posterolateral structures along with reconstruction of the cruciate ligaments as necessary. Augmentation or reconstruction of the FCL, PFL, and popliteus tendon is necessary if the tissues are inadequate. Late reconstruction is more challenging and may require a proximal tibial osteotomy to correct limb alignment before any ligament surgery. Improved surgical techniques with anatomic placement of high-strength allografts will probably provide the most reliable results.

References

1. Aronowitz ER, Parker RD, Gatt CJ: Arthroscopic identification of the popliteofibular ligament. Arthroscopy 17:932-939, 2001.

2. Baker CL Jr, Norwood LA, Hughston JC: Acute combined posterior cruciate and posterolateral instability of the knee. Am J Sports Med 12:204-208, 1984.

3. Buzzi R, Aglietti P, Vena LM, Giron F: Lateral collateral ligament reconstruction using a semitendinosus graft. Knee Surg Sports Traumatol Arthrosc 12:36-42, 2004.

4. Covey DC: Injuries of the posterolateral corner of the knee. J Bone Joint Surg Am 83:106-118, 2001.

5. Dugdale TW, Noyes FR, Styer D: Preoperative planning for high tibial osteotomy. The effect of lateral tibiofemoral separation and tibiofemoral length. Clin Orthop 274:248-264, 1992.

6. Gollehon DL, Torzilli PA, Warren RF: The role of the posterolateral and cruciate ligaments in the stability of the human knee: A biomechanical study. J Bone Joint Surg Am 69:233-242, 1987.

7. Harner CD, Vogrin TM, Hoher J, et al: Biomechanical analysis of a posterior cruciate ligament reconstruction. Deficiency of the posterolateral structures as a cause of graft failure. Am J Sports Med 28:32-39, 2000.

8. Hsu RWW, Himeno S, Coventry MB, et al: Normal axial alignment of the lower extremity and load-bearing distribution at the knee. Clin Orthop 255:215-227, 1990.

9. Hughston JC, Norwood LA Jr: The posterolateral drawer test and external rotational recurvatum test for posterolateral rotatory instability of the knee. Clin Orthop 147:82-87, 1980.

10. Kanamori A, Lee JM, Haemmerle MJ, et al: A biomechanical analysis of two reconstructive approaches to the posterolateral corner of the knee. Knee Surg Sports Traumatol Arthrosc 11:312-317, 2003.

11. Kanamori A, Sakane M, Zeminski J, et al: In-situ force in the medial and lateral structures of intact and ACL-deficient knees. J Orthop Sci 5:567-571, 2000.

12. Kannus P: Nonoperative treatment of grade II and III sprains of the lateral ligament compartment of the knee. Am J Sports Med 17:83-88, 1989.

13. Krudwig WK, Witzel U, Ullrich K: Posterolateral aspect and stability of the knee joint. II. Posterolateral instability and effect of isolated and combined posterolateral reconstruction on knee stability: A biomechanical study. Knee Surg Sports Traumatol Arthrosc 10:91-95, 2002.

14. Krukhaug Y, Molster A, Rodt A, Strand T: Lateral ligament injuries of the knee. Knee Surg Sports Traumatol Arthrosc 6:21-25, 1998.

15. LaPrade RF: Arthroscopic evaluation of the lateral compartment of knees with grade 3 posterolateral knee complex injuries. Am J Sports Med 25:596-602, 1997.

16. LaPrade RF, Gilbert TJ, Bollom TS, et al: The magnetic resonance imaging appearance of individual structures of the posterolateral knee. A prospective study of normal knees and knees with surgically verified grade III injuries. Am J Sports Med 28:191-199, 2000.

17. LaPrade RF, Johansen S, Wentorf FA, et al: An analysis of an anatomical posterolateral knee reconstruction. An in vitro biomechanical study and development of a surgical technique. Am J Sports Med 32:1405-1414, 2004.

18. LaPrade RF, Ly TV, Wentorf FA, Engebretsen L: The posterolateral attachments of the knee: A qualitative and quantitative morphologic analysis of the fibular collateral ligament, popliteus tendon, popliteofibular ligament, and lateral gastrocnemius tendon. Am J Sports Med 31:854-860, 2003.

19. LaPrade RF, Resig S, Wentorf F, Lewis JL: The effects of grade III posterolateral knee complex injuries on anterior cruciate ligament graft force. A biomechanical analysis. Am J Sports Med 27:469-475, 1999.

20. LaPrade RF, Resig S, Wentorf FA, Lewis JL: The effect of injury to the posterolateral structures of the knee on force in a posterior cruciate ligament graft: A biomechanical analysis. Am J Sports Med 30:233-238, 2002.

21. LaPrade RF, Terry GC: Injuries to the posterolateral aspect of the knee. Association of anatomic injury patterns with clinical instability. Am J Sports Med 25:433-438, 1997.

22. LaPrade RF, Wentorf F: Diagnosis and treatment of posterolateral knee injuries. Clin Orthop 402:110-121, 2002.

23. LaPrade RF, Wentorf FA, Crum JA: Assessment of healing of grade III posterolateral corner injuries: An in vivo model. J Orthop Res 22:970-975, 2004.

24. Larson RV: Isometry of the lateral collateral and popliteofibular ligaments and techniques for reconstruction using a free semitendinosus graft. Op Tech Sports Med 9:84-90, 2001.

25. Latimer HA, Tibone JE, El Attrache NS, McMahon PJ: Reconstruction of the lateral collateral ligament of the knee with patellar tendon allograft. Report of a new technique in combined ligament injuries. Am J Sports Med 26:656-662, 1998.

26. Lee J, Papakonstantinou O, Brookenthal KR, et al: Arcuate sign of posterolateral knee injuries: Anatomic, radiographic, and MR imaging data related to patterns of injury. Skeletal Radiol 32:619-627, 2003.

27. Lee MC, Park YK, Lee SH, et al: Posterolateral reconstruction using split Achilles tendon allograft. Arthroscopy 19:1043-1049, 2003.

28. Lill H, Glasmacher S, Korner J, et al: Arthroscopic-assisted simultaneous reconstruction of the posterior cruciate ligament and the lateral collateral ligament using hamstrings and absorbable screws. Arthroscopy 17:892-897, 2001.

29. Maynard MJ, Deng X, Wickiewicz TL, Warren RF: The popliteofibular ligament. Rediscovery of a key element in posterolateral stability. Am J Sports Med 24:311-316, 1996.

30. Munshi M, Pretterklieber ML, Kwak S, et al: MR imaging, MR arthrography, and specimen correlation of the posterolateral corner of the knee: An anatomic study. AJR Am J Roentgenol 180:1095-1101, 2003.

31. Nakhostine M, Perko M, Cross M: Isolated avulsion of the popliteus tendon. J Bone Joint Surg Br 77:242-244, 1995.

32. Nielsen S, Helmig P: The static stabilizing function of the popliteal tendon in the knee. An experimental study. Arch Orthop Trauma Surg 104:357-362, 1986.

33. Pasque C, Noyes FR, Gibbons M, et al: The role of the popliteofibular ligament and the tendon of popliteus in providing stability in the human knee. J Bone Joint Surg Br 85:292-298, 2003.

34. Ross G, Chapman AW, Newberg AR, Scheller AD Jr: Magnetic resonance imaging for the evaluation of acute posterolateral complex injuries of the knee. Am J Sports Med 25:444-448, 1997.

35. Seebacher JR, Inglis AE, Marshall JL, Warren RF: The structure of the posterolateral aspect of the knee. J Bone Joint Surg Am 64:536-541, 1982.

36. Shahane SA, Ibbotson C, Strachan R, Bickerstaff DR: The popliteofibular ligament. An anatomical study of the posterolateral corner of the knee. J Bone Joint Surg Br 81:636-642, 1999.

37. Shino K, Horibe S, Ono K: The voluntarily evoked posterolateral drawer sign in the knee with posterolateral instability. Clin Orthop 215:179-186, 1987.

38. Staubli HU, Birrer S: The popliteus tendon and its fascicles at the popliteal hiatus: Gross anatomy and functional arthroscopic evaluation with and without anterior cruciate ligament deficiency. Arthroscopy 6:209-220, 1990.

39. Staubli HU, Rauschning W: Popliteus tendon and lateral meniscus: Gross and multiplanar cryosectional anatomy of the knee. Am J Knee Surg 4:110-121, 1991.

40. Stuart MJ: Evaluation and treatment principles of knee dislocations. Op Tech Sports Med 9:91-95, 2001.

41. Stuart MJ: Surgical treatment of ACL/PCL/lateral side knee injuries. Op Tech Sports Med 11:257-262, 2003.

42. Sugita T, Amis AA: Anatomic and biomechanical study of the lateral collateral and popliteofibular ligaments. Am J Sports Med 29:466-472, 2001.

43. Terry GC, LaPrade RF: The posterolateral aspect of the knee. Anatomy and surgical approach. Am J Sports Med 24:732-739, 1996.

44. Terry GC, LaPrade RF: The biceps femoris muscle complex at the knee. Its anatomy and injury patterns associated with acute anterolateral-anteromedial rotatory instability. Am J Sports Med 24:732-739, 1996.

45. Ullrich K, Krudwig WK, Witzel U: Posterolateral aspect and stability of the knee joint. I. Anatomy and function of the popliteus muscle-tendon unit: An anatomical and biomechanical study. Knee Surg Sports Traumatol Arthrosc 10:86-90, 2002.

46. Veltri DM, Deng XH, Torzilli PA, et al: The role of the cruciate and posterolateral ligaments in stability of the knee. A biomechanical study. Am J Sports Med 23:436-443, 1995.

47. Veltri DM, Deng XH, Torzilli PA, et al: The role of the popliteofibular ligament in stability of the human knee. A biomechanical study. Am J Sports Med 24:19-27, 1996.

48. Veltri DM, Warren RF: Anatomy, biomechanics, and physical findings in posterolateral knee instability. Clin Sports Med 13:599-614, 1994.

49. Veltri DM, Warren RF: Operative treatment of posterolateral instability of the knee. Clin Sports Med 13:615-627, 1994.

50. Wang CJ, Chen CY, Chen LM, Yeh WL: Posterior cruciate ligament and coupled posterolateral instability of the knee. Arch Orthop Trauma Surg 120:525-528, 2000.

51. Wascher DC, Grauer JD, Markoff KL: Biceps tendon tenodesis for posterolateral instability of the knee. An in vitro study. Am J Sports Med 21:400-406, 1993.

52. Wentorf FA, LaPrade RF, Lewis JL, Resig S: The Influence of the integrity of posterolateral structures on tibiofemoral orientation when an anterior cruciate ligament graft is tensioned. Am J Sports Med 30:796-769, 2002.

Anterior Cruciate Ligament Reconstruction with Bone–Patellar Tendon–Bone Autograft: Indications, Technique, Complications, and Management

Stephen G. Manifold • Fred D. Cushner • W. Norman Scott

Injury to the anterior cruciate ligament (ACL) is the most common ligament injury in the knee and results in approximately 50,000 reconstructions per year in the United States.[39] Greater participation in sporting and recreational activities by the general population continues to expose more individuals to the risk of ACL rupture. As the experience of orthopedic surgeons with ACL injuries has expanded, so have the science and technique of ACL reconstruction. Numerous methods for reconstructing the ligament exist, including the use of patellar tendon autograft, hamstring tendons, and allograft material. The most extensive research has been performed on the use of patellar tendon autograft, and this technique remains the gold standard for ACL reconstruction.

HISTORY OF ANTERIOR CRUCIATE LIGAMENT RECONSTRUCTION

Use of the central third of the patellar tendon for reconstructing a torn ACL was first described by Jones[53] in an effort to provide a more physiological procedure than those previously described. His technique involved transferring the patellar tendon with a patella bone block to the intercondylar region of the femur while maintaining the distal attachment of the tendon to the tibial tubercle. Other authors subsequently modified Jones' technique by using the medial third of the patellar tendon.[4,36] Marshall et al[60] described using the central third of the patellar tendon along with the prepatellar fascia and the central portion of the quadriceps tendon. These modifications of Jones' technique also involved creating a more anatomic placement of the reconstructed ligament by passing it through a tibial tunnel from the anterior aspect of the tibia to the normal tibial ACL insertion site and leaving the distal attachment of the patellar tendon in place on the tubercle. The femoral side of the graft was passed either through bone tunnels in the femur or "over the top" of the lateral femoral condyle and secured with sutures or staples. Clancy et al,[28] in an effort to obtain bony union at the femoral fixation site, first described harvesting a

block of patellar bone along with the proximal portion of the patellar tendon. They also described detaching the tibial origin of the graft along with a block of bone when the graft was found to be too short. The bone–patellar tendon–bone graft is now the gold standard in ACL reconstruction. Advantages of this type of autograft include its increased stiffness and energy to failure,[76] as well as its ability to revascularize.[9] It has been shown that a 14- to 15-mm-wide bone–patellar tendon–bone graft has a mean strength that is approximately 168% that of a normal ACL.[76] In addition, the bone–patellar tendon–bone autograft has a superior ability to achieve stable initial fixation because of the bone plugs. Noyes et al[74] recommended avoiding the use of bone–patellar tendon–bone autografts in patients with preexisting chondrosis of the patellofemoral joint, malalignment of the extensor mechanism, or a narrow-width patellar tendon.

CLINICAL RESULTS

Early results of open reconstruction of the ACL were encouraging in terms of restoration of knee stability.[28,36,57,60,79,91] Marshall et al[60] reported on 40 patients with an average follow-up of 22 months. Four patients were considered failures because of recurrent giving way in two, inability to return to sports in one, and persistent synovitis in one. Clancy et al[28] reported good or excellent results in 94% of 50 patients at an average 33-month follow-up. None of the patients had any postoperative episodes of instability, and all but six were able to return to full sports activity. O'Brien et al[79] reviewed 79 patients undergoing intra-articular ACL reconstruction with use of a free, non-vascularized autologous graft from the central third of the patellar tendon. Augmentation with an extra-articular lateral sling of iliotibial band was performed in 60% of the reconstructions. Episodes of giving way were eliminated in 95% of the patients; however, nine were unable to return to previous activity levels, and 40% of those who did maintain previous levels of activity continued to wear a brace. Addition of a lateral sling had no effect on the outcome.

Despite these early results, persistent problems associated with ACL reconstruction became evident and included flexion contracture, patellofemoral pain, limited range of motion, and quadriceps muscle atrophy, in addition to a prolonged rehabilitation period. Technological advances in orthopedic surgery resulted in the emergence of arthroscopically assisted ACL reconstruction. This reduced the surgical morbidity associated with open reconstruction and facilitated rehabilitation and return to activity. Several studies showed that when compared with open reconstruction, the arthroscopically assisted technique resulted in a decreased incidence of patella symptoms, knee stiffness, and need for manipulation, with no difference in knee stability.[2,12,23] Current techniques of ACL reconstruction have evolved further and now involve the use of a single-incision endoscopic approach that further reduces the surgical morbidity and has been shown to yield consistently good results.[11,81,99] Despite concern with this newer technique regarding potential divergence of interference screw fixation, graft breakage, and posterior cortical violation, comparison studies between the arthroscopically assisted technique and the endoscopic technique showed similar results in terms of outcome and complications.[7,46,86,93]

Harner et al[46] prospectively compared patients undergoing the two-incision "rear entry" technique for ACL reconstruction with another group undergoing the single-incision endoscopic reconstruction technique. At an average follow-up of 35 months, no significant functional or radiographic differences were noted between the two groups. The authors concluded that the single-incision technique yielded reliable results, provided that tunnel placement and graft fixation were accurately performed, and that this technique was less invasive and more cosmetic. They also suggested that less postoperative pain and therefore a faster rehabilitation period were other potential benefits of this technique. Reat and Lintner[86] prospectively studied 30 patients with chronic ACL injuries. The patients were randomly assigned to undergo reconstruction with either the one-incision or the two-incision technique. At a mean follow-up of 17 months, no statistically significant differences were found between the two groups, including early postoperative pain and range of motion. They concluded that the two techniques are interchangeable and that both should be familiar to surgeons because the two-incision technique allows for salvage of intraoperative loss of endoscopic fixation of the femoral bone plug.

Sgaglione and Schwartz[93] retrospectively reviewed 90 patients who underwent ACL reconstruction with either the endoscopic single-incision or the arthroscopically assisted two-incision technique. Similar outcomes were noted in subjective, functional, and objective data for the two groups. Four cases of posterior cortical violation occurred in the endoscopic group; however, all of them occurred early in the series. The authors also noted a 33% rate of screw divergence in the endoscopic group versus 14% in the two-incision group but found no clinical differences in these patients and those with parallel screw placement.

Several studies reported on the longer-term follow-up of ACL reconstruction with autologous patellar tendon graft.[12,81,95] Bach et al[12] retrospectively reviewed the results of 97 patients 5 to 9 years after arthroscopically assisted ACL reconstruction with patellar tendon autograft. A manual maximum side-to-side difference of 3 mm or less was noted in 70% of the patients, and 82% had excellent or good results according to the modified Hospital for Special Surgery scoring system. In addition, all patients had a pivot-shift result of 1+ or less, and no patient demonstrated clinical findings of chronic patella tendinitis. The authors concluded that this technique of ACL reconstruction yields reliable stability and a high level of patient satisfaction. Shelbourne and Gray[95] reported on the 2- to 9-year follow-up of ACL reconstructions performed through a medial miniarthrotomy, followed by accelerated rehabilitation. A total of 1057 patients were prospectively monitored, and objective data were available for 806 of these patients. The mean manual maximum KT-1000 knee arthrometer score was 2.0 mm, and quadriceps muscle strength testing revealed 94% strength after acute reconstruction and 91% strength after chronic reconstruction. Patients were able to return to sports-specific activities at a mean of 6.2 weeks postoperatively. Otto et al[81] retrospectively reviewed the 5-year results of 68 patients who underwent single-incision ACL reconstruction with patellar tendon autograft. Three patients experienced rerupture of their ACL grafts before the 5-year evaluation; of the remaining patients, 98% exhibited 5 mm or less of laxity on the Lachman test, and 77% were participating in level I or level II activities according to the International Knee Documentation Committee scale. Extension loss of more than 3 degrees was seen in 5% of the patients; however, the postoperative therapy regimen consisted of the use of a brace, which did not allow full extension for the first 4 weeks after reconstruction. The authors concluded that this technique results in excellent stability of the knee and allows return to a high level of function and that even better results are anticipated with newer postoperative therapy regimens.

When comparing surgical results, one must also consider the postoperative rehabilitation protocol. Previous ACL reconstruction rehabilitation was characterized by periods of immobilization and non-weightbearing in casts. More recent protocols now emphasize early range of motion and full weightbearing as tolerated with or without brace support. These aggressive programs have been shown to restore range of motion, reduce patellofemoral complications, and hasten return to activities without compromising knee stability.[95,96] As a result, overall outcomes of ACL reconstruction have improved (see Chapter 40).

Other factors in ACL reconstruction that have received significant attention in the literature include the timing of surgery, optimum position for the femoral and tibial tunnels, importance of graft isometry, and the ideal method of graft fixation. Further advances in these areas will facilitate attaining the ultimate goal of ACL reconstruction surgery, which is to provide a stable knee under physiological loads that allows the patient a full and rapid return to function and activity level while avoiding the postoperative complications that can interfere with these goals.

PREDISPOSING FACTORS

Several studies have attempted to identify factors predisposing to ACL injury and found an association between such injury and intercondylar notch stenosis.[47,58,94,103,104] Souryal and Freeman[103] prospectively examined 902 high-school athletes and noted that athletes who sustained ACL tears had statistically significant stenosis of the intercondylar notch when compared with those who did not have such injuries. Harner et al[47] compared 31 patients with noncontact, bilateral ACL injuries with 23 controls who had no history of knee injury. Computed tomographic analysis of the lower extremities revealed that the width of the lateral femoral condyle was significantly larger in the injured knee group and was the predominant contributor to intercondylar notch stenosis. A study comparing notch width measurements in men and women with and without ACL tears revealed a narrower intercondylar notch width in women than in men, as well as a narrower width in patients with ACL tears than in controls.[94] These results may enable identification of individuals at increased risk for unilateral and, in particular, bilateral ACL tears, which have an overall incidence of approximately 4%. In addition, this may be one factor responsible in part for the increased incidence of ACL tears in female athletes.

Much attention has been focused on the cause of ACL tears in women. Studies investigating injury rates noted that women sustain four to eight times the number of ACL injuries as men in the same sports.[8,17] Possible reasons for this discrepancy include both extrinsic factors, such as muscle strength, and intrinsic factors, such as joint laxity and notch dimensions.[8] Little objective evidence is currently available, however, to support a single hypothesis. Wojtys et al[109] examined the association between female athletes' menstrual cycle and ACL injuries. More injuries than expected were noted during the ovulatory phase of the cycle, when a surge in estrogen production occurs. This finding suggests that noncontact ACL tears in female athletes may be related in part to hormonal fluctuations. The hormones responsible for this observed association and the effect of the mechanism of action on the mechanical properties of the ACL have yet to be determined.

INDICATIONS FOR RECONSTRUCTION

Identification of patients with an ACL injury can usually be made on the basis of the history and physical examination. Patients commonly describe a history of a deceleration injury, with or without contact, during such maneuvers as cutting and pivoting. Patients with this injury mechanism associated with an audible "pop," severe pain, and significant swelling of the knee can be assumed to have a torn ACL. Physical examination confirms the diagnosis by demonstrating a positive Lachman test[106] or the anterior drawer sign in the injured knee as opposed to the opposite normal knee (Fig. 39–1).

After the acute phase of knee pain and swelling subsides, symptomatic patients complain of persistent instability and giving way of the knee, which can be associated with intermittent episodes of swelling. Once a torn ACL is diagnosed, one must decide whether to recommend nonoperative or operative treatment. Satisfactory results from conservative treatment of ACL tears have been reported.[22,40,41,65] McDaniel and Dameron[65] noted that 70% of patients with complete ACL tears treated conservatively returned to strenuous sports. Similarly, Giove et al[41] reported a 59% rate of return to sports activities after a program emphasizing hamstring strengthening. However, sports requiring sudden stopping and pivoting had the lowest rate of return to participation. Buss et al[22] evaluated the results of conservative treatment of acute, complete ACL injuries in older, lower-demand patients. They noted that 70% of patients were able to continue with moderate-demand sports at an average follow-up of 46 months. They concluded that conservative treatment in this group of patients can be successful despite a modest amount of residual instability.

Numerous other studies, however, have reported less successful outcomes of nonoperative treatment.[6,14,32,38,48,54,77,78,101] Noyes et al[78] studied 103

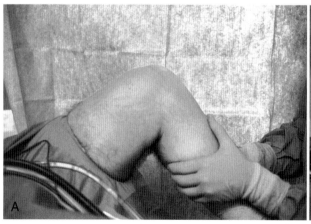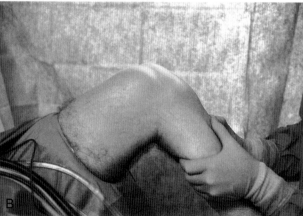

Figure 39–1. Demonstration of the anterior drawer sign. **A,** Knee in neutral position. **B,** Increased anterior translation of the knee secondary to anterior cruciate ligament rupture.

athletically active patients an average of 5.5 years after ACL injury. Despite an initial return to sports activity by 82% of the participants, 51% sustained a significant reinjury within 1 year of the original injury and only 35% were participating in strenuous sports at the most recent follow-up. Hawkins et al[48] reported on 40 patients treated nonoperatively with an average follow-up of 4 years and noted 87.5% fair or poor results; only 14% of patients were fully able to return to unlimited athletic activity. Similarly, Barrack et al[14] reported 69% fair or poor results after nonoperative treatment in an active naval midshipmen population. Daniel et al[32] determined that the best predictor for later meniscal or ligament reconstruction surgery was total hours per year of level I and level II sports participation before injury. This observation highlights the fact that individuals who engage in demanding recreational or vocational activities do not respond well to nonoperative treatment of ACL injuries.

The decision to reconstruct an ACL tear should be based not only on the presence of symptomatic instability but also on the lifestyle and activity level of the patient. We do not use guidelines based on age in our practice because the more important factor is the overall level of activity. It is generally agreed that younger individuals have higher levels of activity and, therefore, place greater demands on their knees. However, many older individuals are participating in higher levels of recreational sports and are doing so for longer periods. Consequently, age itself should not be a contraindication to ACL reconstruction. Plancher et al[85] reported 97% good or excellent results after ACL reconstruction in patients older than 40 years at a mean follow-up of 55 months. All the patients were satisfied with the procedure, and the majority were able to return fully to their sports activities, including tennis and skiing.

Symptomatic patients with a more sedentary lifestyle and those who are willing to modify their level of activity can be considered for nonoperative treatment consisting of a supervised rehabilitation program. It is reasonable to initially treat all patients with an ACL rupture nonoperatively and perform reconstruction on those in whom this form of treatment fails. This approach can involve several months of rehabilitation followed by several more months if reconstruction is ultimately performed. In our experience, we have found that most patients are unwilling to accept this amount of time away from their recreational activities; therefore, we recommend early reconstruction for symptomatic patients with greater lifestyle demands. The goal of early reconstruction in this patient population is to provide stability, which allows a return to previous activity levels without further damage to the knee, such as meniscal tears and arthrosis. The significant reinjury rate in the study of Noyes et al[78] emphasizes the potential sequelae of continued high levels of activity in patients with ACL injury. There is still a lack of definitive evidence, however, that reconstruction of the ligament prevents long-term degenerative changes.

TIMING OF SURGERY

The timing of ACL reconstruction has also been debated; however, no consensus has yet been reached regarding the ideal timing. Initial concern existed over reconstruction of the ACL during the early postinjury period because of the increased risk for arthrofibrosis and difficulty gaining full motion of the knee postoperatively. Shelbourne et al[100] demonstrated a higher rate of arthrofibrosis in patients undergoing ACL reconstruction within the first week after injury than in those who underwent reconstruction 21 days or longer after injury. The same authors noted, however, that when an accelerated rehabilitation protocol was followed postoperatively, the rates of arthrofibrosis in the two groups were comparable. Noyes and Barber-Westin[75] reported that 69% of knees with chronic rupture scored in the normal or very good range after reconstruction as compared with 100% of knees with an acute rupture. Other studies also found earlier return to sporting activities as well as better clinical and laxity testing results in knees undergoing early reconstruction.[59] Hunter et al[51] showed that the use of modern arthroscopic surgical techniques and an aggressive rehabilitation protocol can yield results that are independent of the timing of surgery. We agree that the specific number of days after injury when the reconstruction should be performed is not as important as the preoperative condition of the knee. Criteria for successful results of ACL reconstruction are minimal or no swelling, good leg control, and full range of motion, including full hyperextension.[97]

SURGICAL TECHNIQUE

Endoscopic reconstruction of a torn ACL with a bone–patellar tendon–bone autograft is our procedure of choice and is the technique described here. Steps of the reconstructive procedure include diagnostic arthroscopy, harvesting the graft, preparing the graft, performing the notchplasty, drilling of the tibial and femoral tunnels, passing the graft, and femoral and tibial fixation of the graft. Before beginning the reconstructive procedure, however, the knee is examined under anesthesia. A positive Lachman test and a pivot-shift sign are sought on the injured knee as clinical evidence of a torn ACL. These maneuvers are repeated on the uninjured contralateral knee for comparison and to determine the degree of "normal" laxity in the knee for the individual patient. The injured extremity is then prepared and draped in the usual sterile fashion after the application of a thigh tourniquet well above the operative site.

Diagnostic Arthroscopy

After inflation of the thigh tourniquet, the arthroscope is inserted into the knee through a standard lateral portal, and the ACL is visualized to confirm the injury. The ACL is most commonly torn from its proximal attachment on the femur, which results in a stump of tissue that is usually easily visualized through the arthroscope. At times, however, the appearance of the ACL can be deceiving. A torn ACL can become scarred to the surface of the posterior cruciate ligament (PCL) and give the erroneous impression of an intact ligament. Visualization of the ACL with the leg in the figure-four position enables adequate assessment of its proximal attachment site in these cases. This view clearly demonstrates absence of the ACL attachment to the femur in ACL-deficient knees.

Meniscal resection or repair can also be performed at the diagnostic examination or can be addressed during preparation of the graft. A second medial working portal is established if the menisci are addressed at this stage. Otherwise, the arthroscope is removed and attention turned to the graft.

Graft Harvesting

The patella and tibial tubercle landmarks are drawn on the skin, and a vertical incision is made from the inferior pole of the patella to 1 cm medial to the tibial tubercle. Skin flaps are developed to identify the full width of the tendon, and the paratenon is incised in line with the skin incision and reflected. A 9- or 10-mm catamaran blade is used to make the incision in the tendon from the patella to the tibial tubercle, with care taken to remain parallel to the tendon fibers. In general, no more than a third of the patellar tendon is used. The incision is carried proximally over the patella for a distance of 25 mm from the tendon insertion, as well as distally over the tibial tubercle, also 25 mm from the attachment site of the tendon. A small oscillating saw is used to cut bone plugs to a depth of approximately 8 mm, and these plugs are then carefully removed with an osteotome.

We have examined the effect of graft diameter on postoperative knee stability by testing ACL-reconstructed knees with the KT arthrometer after the use of either a 9- or 10-mm-diameter graft.[42] The average time from surgery to KT arthrometer testing was 6.6 months, and at the time of testing the average side-to-side difference for the 9-mm group was 1.02 mm. The average side-to-side difference for the group receiving 10-mm grafts was 1.14 mm. No significant differences between the two groups could be identified with regard to knee stability.

Graft Preparation

Excess soft tissue is first removed from the graft, and the diameter of the bone plugs is trimmed with a rongeur to the appropriate width (9 or 10 mm). The plug from the tibial tubercle is prepared for placement in the femoral tunnel, where its anatomy provides maximum bone fill. The edges of the plugs are rounded to permit smooth passage of the graft, and the diameters are checked by passing the graft through a tunnel template of the correct size. Three drill holes are then made in the patellar bone plug and one in the tibial tubercle bone plug, followed by passage of No. 5 nonabsorbable suture through these holes (Fig. 39–2). The suture facilitates passage and tensioning of the graft. Finally, the total length of the graft is measured. In general, if the total length is less than 95 mm, fixation with interference screws can be achieved. Fixation with a screw and washer on the tibial side is usually required for grafts measuring more than 95 mm in length.

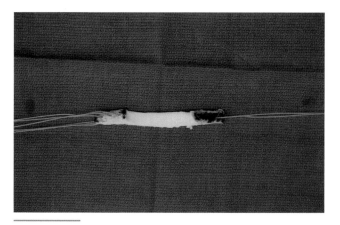

Figure 39–2. Completed preparation of a bone–patellar tendon–bone graft. Methylene blue ink is placed on the cancellous surfaces of the plugs to facilitate their orientation during graft passage.

Notchplasty

A second arthroscopic portal is made medial to the patellar tendon, if not done previously, as well as a superomedial inflow portal to improve visualization. The remnants of the ACL are then removed with an intra-articular punch and motorized shaver. The lateral wall of the intercondylar notch is cleared of soft-tissue attachments while taking care to not injure the adjacent PCL. The motorized bur is then inserted into the medial portal, and the notchplasty is begun. The amount of bone to be removed remains controversial and ultimately depends on intraoperative assessment by the surgeon.

Several studies have attempted to establish guidelines for assessing the adequacy of the notchplasty.[15,43,80,105] Odensten and Gillquist[80] noted an average maximum distance of 21 mm between the inner surfaces of the medial and lateral femoral condyles in 20 normal cadaver knees. As a result, they suggested that the notchplasty should restore the notch width to this diameter. Berg[15] defined an adequate notchplasty on the basis of the notch-width index[104] and stated that this index, which is the ratio of the intercondylar width to the total femoral condylar width at the level of the popliteal groove, should be at least 0.250 to prevent impingement of the graft. Howell et al[50] described the relationship between the placement of the tibial tunnel and the required size of the notchplasty. A more anteriorly placed tibial tunnel required up to 6 mm of bone removal from the intercondylar roof as compared with only minimal removal of bone for tunnels placed 2 to 3 mm posterior to the ACL tibial insertion site. Berns and Howell[16] further defined the requirements for notchplasty by determining the flexion angle at which the graft contacted the roof through the use of a force transducer in cadaver knees. The angle at which contact occurred averaged 12.8 degrees for knees with an eccentrically placed tibial tunnel and required 4.6 mm of bone removal to achieve zero impingement. This angle of contact decreased to 4.1 degrees when the tibial tunnel was placed 4 to 5 mm posterior to the slope of the intercondylar roof and required only 1.3 mm of bone removal to prevent impingement. We prefer a generous notchplasty in which up to 6 mm of bone is removed from the anterior edge of the lateral wall of the notch to prevent any possible impingement on the graft (Fig. 39–3).

The effect of the extent of the notchplasty on the patellofemoral articulation has been investigated. Morgan et al[68] measured patellofemoral contact area and pressure after increasing degrees of notchplasty (3, 6, and 9 mm) and found no statistical differences between the groups. The authors concluded that routine notchplasty, including up to 9 mm, does not affect the patellofemoral articulation. Patellofemoral complications related to the size of the notchplasty have likewise not been a problem in our experience.

The notchplasty is continued posteriorly to the posterior edge of the lateral wall. It is important to identify and remove the "resident's ridge" to prevent inadvertent anterior placement of the femoral tunnel. This ridge is located at the level of the anterior border of the PCLI. Therefore, care must be taken to extend the notchplasty posterior to this border. A hooked probe is useful in ensuring that the over-the-top position and the posterior edge of the lateral wall have been reached. The surface of the lateral wall should be smooth with no rough edges, which could impinge on and abrade the graft.

Tunnel Placement

The choice of location for the tibial and femoral tunnels can have a significant effect on the outcome of ACL reconstructive surgery. Several studies have examined the effect of tunnel site on graft impingement,[49,110] range of motion,[87] and overall clinical results.[55] It is recognized that anterior placement of the femoral tunnel is to be avoided to prevent excessive tightness of the graft and thus limit full knee flexion. Similarly, excessive anterior placement of the tibial tunnel may result in graft impingement and early failure. In an attempt to identify definitive landmarks for reproducible tibial tunnel placement, Morgan et al[68] determined that the ACL central insertion point on the intercondylar floor averages 7 mm anterior to the anterior border of the PCL with the knee flexed to 90 degrees; therefore, this is the ideal location for the tibial tunnel.

We set the tibial drill guide at 55 degrees because a more posterior tunnel is preferred to prevent impingement. The guide tip is placed through the medial portal and positioned with the use of several landmarks, including the anterior border of the PCL, the posterior border of the anterior horn of the lateral meniscus, and the interspinous area of the tibial plateau. The tunnel is positioned to enable the graft to drape the PCL (Fig. 39–4). The starting point for the guide pin on the proximal end of the tibia is approximately one fingerbreadth medial to the tibial tubercle and two fingerbreadths distal to the medial joint line. After insertion of the guide pin, the tunnel is drilled with a reamer, and the intra-articular edges of the tunnel are smoothed with a rasp to prevent abrasion of the graft (Fig. 39–5). Attempts have been made to produce the correct tibial tunnel length consistently to prevent graft

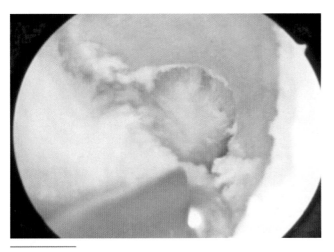

Figure 39–3. Arthroscopic view of a completed femoral notchplasty. The posterior edge of the notch roof must be visualized for correct femoral tunnel position.

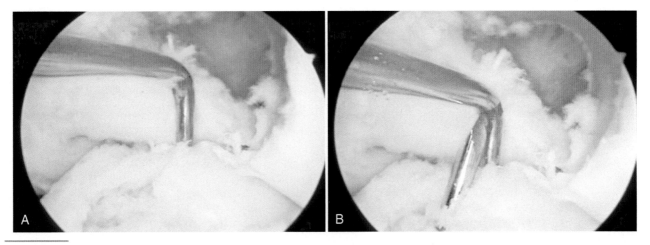

Figure 39–4. Optimal position of the tibial guide. **A,** Proper positioning of the tibial pin guide adjacent to the posterior cruciate ligament. **B,** The tip of the guide pin should be at the level of the posterior edge of the anterior horn of the lateral meniscus such that the graft will drape over the posterior cruciate ligament.

extrusion with tunnels that are too short, as well as prevent difficult distal fixation and femoral tunnel placement with tunnels that are too long.[67] We have found, however, that this is not always accurate and may be altered by small variations in operative technique.[82]

Attention is then turned to the femoral tunnel. The guide pin, which represents the center of the tunnel, is placed in the 1-o'clock position for the left knee or the 11-o'clock position for the right knee and 6 or 7 mm anterior to the over-the-top position, depending on whether a 9- or 10-mm graft, respectively, is used (Fig. 39–6). It is inserted to a depth of 35 mm, or 1{1/2} inches, to ensure room for the tunnel without violating the posterior cortex (Fig. 39–7). An indentation in the bone is then made with the reamer over the guide pin to confirm the correct position in relation to the posterior cortex. This also ensures that the posterior cortex is intact (Fig. 39–8). The tunnel is then reamed to fit the length of the bone plug. The integrity of the posterior cortex is once again verified by directly visualizing the tunnel with the arthroscope before passage of the graft (Fig. 39–9).

Testing for isometry can be performed at this point or just before committing to the femoral tunnel. Isometer readings are obtained to determine the position of the graft that will result in equal length and tension throughout a full range of motion. However, it has been shown that these readings may vary widely from the final graft isometry because of eccentric placement of the graft within the bone tunnels.[29] Additionally, because the normal ACL is nonisometric, intra-articular testing for isometry is not required if anatomic zones are maintained.[108]

GRAFT PASSAGE

A Beath needle is drilled through the femoral tunnel while maintaining the knee in a flexed position. The tip of the needle is pushed through the soft tissues and exits the skin on the anterolateral aspect of the distal part of the thigh. The Beath needle is used to pull the suture in the femoral bone plug through the femoral tunnel. The graft is then passed through the tunnels by grasping the sutures on either end of the bone plugs and pulling the graft into the joint. The graft is inserted so that the cancellous bone of the femoral plug is facing superolaterally in the femoral tunnel (Fig. 39–10). Insertion of a fixation screw on the cortical surface of the plug may lead to disruption of the ligamentous attachment. Tension is applied to the graft through manual pull on the bone plug sutures, and the orientation of the graft is assessed (Fig. 39–11). The arthroscope is used to visualize the intra-articular side of the tibial tunnel to verify that the tibial bone plug does not enter into the joint. Assessment of graft clearance from the notch roof is performed both at 30 degrees of flexion and in full knee extension (Fig. 39–12).

The position of the tunnels can be checked with intraoperative or, more commonly, postoperative radiographs. Yoshiya et al[111] reported on the optimal orientation of the bone tunnels to minimize the bending and strain imposed on the graft throughout the range of motion. Their ideal

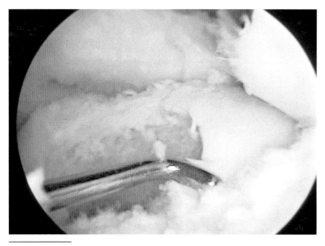

Figure 39–5. Arthroscopic view of the intra-articular rim of the tibial tunnel showing the relationship to the posterior edge of the anterior horn of the lateral meniscus (located at the tip of the probe).

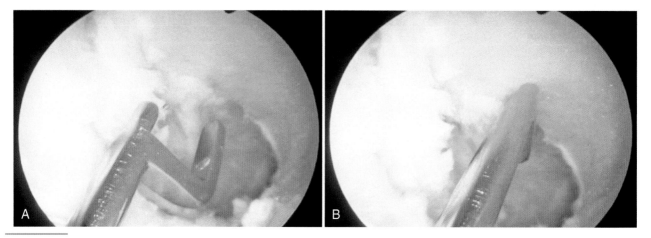

Figure 39–6. **A,** Femoral guide with a 6-mm offset. **B,** Positioning of the femoral guide in the 11-o'clock position for a right knee. The guide is placed in the 1-o'clock position for a left knee. Note that the posterior tip of the guide is in the over-the-top position on the femur.

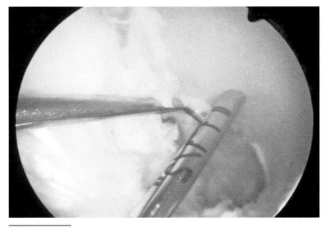

Figure 39–7. Femoral pin inserted to a depth of $1^1/_2$ inches.

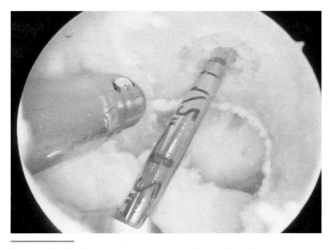

Figure 39–8. Initial reaming over the guide pin to create a femoral "footprint." This allows visual inspection of the posterior rim to verify adequate wall thickness before completion of the reaming.

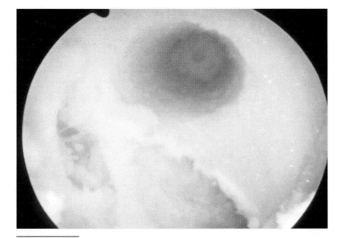

Figure 39–9. Arthroscopic view of a reamed femoral tunnel to confirm the integrity of the posterior wall. The distance between the posterior rim of the tunnel and the posterior edge of the notch roof should be approximately 2 mm.

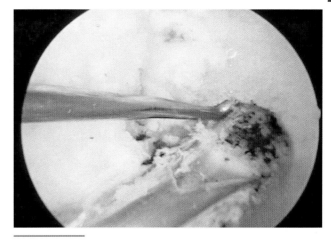

Figure 39–10. Passage of the femoral bone plug into the femoral tunnel with the cancellous surface oriented superolaterally in the tunnel.

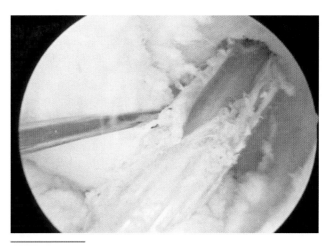

Figure 39–11. Appearance of the graft under manual tension before fixation.

tibial tunnel position was angled 30 degrees medial to the isometric point in the coronal plane and 20 degrees anterior to the isometric point in the sagittal plane. The femoral tunnel should ideally be angled 25 degrees anterior to the isometric point in the sagittal plane and 15 degrees lateral to this point in the coronal plane.

Graft Fixation

Kurosaka et al[56] introduced the self-tapping interference screw, which demonstrated improved mechanical properties when compared with buttons or staples. In their study, comparison between 6.5-mm AO cancellous interference screw fixation and sutures tied over a button demonstrated no difference in ultimate failure load. However, interference fixation with the 6.5-mm AO screw resulted in greater graft stiffness. The same study demonstrated that both maximum graft strength and stiffness are greater with 9-mm interference screw fixation than with the 6.5-mm AO interference screw. Paschal et al[83] compared

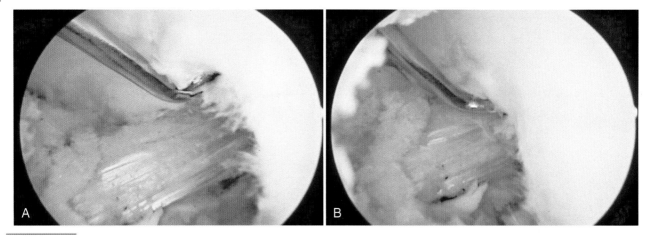

Figure 39–12. An arthroscopic probe is used to assess graft clearance from the roof of the notch with the knee in 30 degrees of flexion (**A**) and in the fully extended position (**B**). No impingement should occur in either position.

fixation strengths between 9-mm interference screws and sutures tied over a cancellous screw and washer (post fixation) in porcine knees. Higher ultimate failure loads and less displacement of the bone graft were noted with interference screw fixation. Matthews et al[63] found no difference in the force to failure of patellar tendon–bone grafts in cadaveric knees when comparing interference screw fixation with post fixation. The authors did note, however, that post fixation strength is dependent on the type of suture used; No. 5 nonabsorbable suture material provided optimal strength. No studies to date have demonstrated any differences in clinical outcome when comparing interference screw fixation with post fixation.

Absorbable interference screws have been introduced, and several studies have examined the biomechanical properties and clinical results of these screws versus standard metal interference screws.[25,26,52,84] Pena et al[84] investigated the insertional torque and failure load for metallic and absorbable interference screws in young and middle-aged cadaveric knees. They noted a higher mean insertional torque for the metal screws as well as a greater mean failure load. Other laboratory studies, however, did not demonstrate any differences between the two types of screws.[25,26,52] Caborn et al[26] compared the maximum load to failure of titanium alloy interference screws with that of absorbable screws in a human cadaveric model with the approximate physiological strain rate of in vivo bone–patellar tendon–bone graft loading. No statistical differences were noted between the two groups in the failure mode or the maximum load to failure. Similarly, clinical studies did not demonstrate significant differences in use of the screw types.[13,61] Barber et al[13] performed a randomized, prospective, multicenter comparison of bioabsorbable and metallic interference screws in 110 patients undergoing arthroscopic ACL reconstruction with patellar tendon autografts. At a minimum 12-month follow-up, postoperative Tegner and Lysholm scores and KT arthrometer maximum side-to-side differences were not statistically different between the two groups. The authors concluded that the absorbable screw is a reasonable alternative to the metal interference screw for bone plug fixation.

Potential problems with the use of interference screws include length mismatch in the tunnel, graft, and screw; divergence of the screw; graft fracture; and suture laceration.[10] Screw divergence has been implicated in failure of graft fixation[63]; however, others have observed that screw divergence less than 30 degrees does not appear to lead to early failure provided that intraoperative stability is noted.[35] Similarly, we examined the effect of divergence between the femoral interference screw and the femoral bone plug.[92] Radiographs and KT-2000 values from 100 consecutive endoscopic autologous bone–patellar tendon–bone ACL reconstructions were reviewed at a minimum follow-up of 1 year. The mean anteroposterior divergence angle was 6.6 degrees (range, 0 to 32 degrees), and no association was found between the divergence angle and KT-2000 measurements.

The guide pin for the femoral interference screw should be inserted between the edge of the femoral tunnel and the cancellous surface of the bone plug in a direction parallel to the orientation of the graft. The interference screw is passed over the guide pin and advanced into the femoral tunnel. The screw should engage at least 75%, if not 100% of the bone block (Fig. 39–13). A 7-mm interference screw is recommended if the bone plug–tunnel gap is 2 mm or less. A gap greater than 2 mm requires the use of a 9-mm screw.

Several studies have examined the effect of twisting the graft 90 to 180 degrees before fixation of the tibial plug in an attempt to reproduce the normal helicoid orientation of the ACL fibers. In vitro studies noted enhanced isometry of the graft fibers,[34] improved graft strength,[30] and restoration of normal tibial rotation in relation to the femur[90] as a result of graft twisting. The clinical significance of these findings, however, remains unclear. Diduch et al[33] performed a prospective, randomized study examining the clinical and arthrometric results of patients undergoing ACL reconstruction with and without pretwisting of the graft. The authors reported no clinical failures in either group and no statistically significant differences clinically or by arthrometry between the two groups. The study concluded that pretwisting of the graft has no short-term effect on knee laxity.

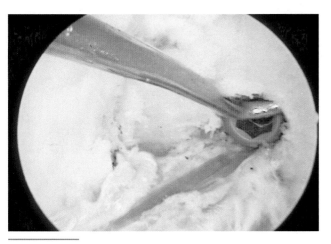

Figure 39–13. Fixation of the femoral bone plug with an interference screw. The screw should be fully seated with no protrusion from the rim of the tunnel into the joint.

The precise amount of initial tension applied to the graft before fixation has not been determined. This will have a direct effect on the stability of the knee because inadequate tension will lead to persistent instability whereas excessive tensioning may lead to elongation of the graft or early fixation failure. Previous studies investigating graft tension concluded that excessive tightness may result in abrasion on the edges of the bone tunnels or the intercondylar roof; in addition, revascularization of these overly tight grafts may be impaired.[19,112]

Burks and Leland[20] noted that the tension applied to an ACL graft to obtain normal anteroposterior translation was dependent on the graft tissue; less stiff grafts required more tension. They determined that 3.6 lb of tension applied to the knee at 20 to 25 degrees of flexion was required for patellar tendon grafts.

In addition to the amount of tension, the position of the knee during application of the tension has also been investigated. Bylski-Austrow et al[24] reconstructed cadaveric knees with a flexible cable and examined the effect of varying degrees of tension and knee position during tensioning. They noted that knees tensioned in 30 degrees of flexion were overconstrained and that this was independent of the initial tension used. Similarly, Melby et al[66] also reported overconstraint of reconstructed cadaveric knees when tensioned at 30 degrees of flexion. In addition, greater quadriceps force was necessary to achieve full extension as the graft tension increased, particularly when tensioned in 30 degrees of flexion. Nabors et al[70] evaluated 57 patients after ACL reconstruction with a patellar tendon autograft in which the graft was tensioned by a maximal sustained one-handed pull on the tibial end with the knee in full passive extension. At a minimum 2-year follow-up, the Lysholm score improved from 65 preoperatively to 90 postoperatively, the mean side-to-side difference on instrumented laxity testing was reduced from 7.6 mm to 0.8 mm, and only one patient had a postoperative contracture. The authors concluded that tensioning of the graft in full extension ensures that the knee will come to full extension without compromising the stability of the knee. We use a similar technique of graft tensioning in which a manual pull is exerted on the sutures

in the tibial end of the graft such that there is no laxity in the suture strands. Fixation of the graft is then performed with the knee in full extension.

Fixation of the tibial plug is dependent on the length of the plug with respect to the extra-articular edge of the tibial tunnel. Interference screw fixation is used when the end of the plug is within 5 mm of the extra-articular edge of the tibial tunnel. The bone plug can be visualized in the tibial tunnel with the arthroscope to ensure that the interference screw is placed on the cancellous side of the bone plug. If the tibial plug is positioned more than 5 mm from the extra-articular tunnel edge (long or short), fixation is achieved by tying the sutures over a tibial post.

The functional adequacy of the graft is then tested by performing a manual Lachman test and by directly visualizing the graft with the arthroscope and probing the graft to verify proper tension throughout a range of motion. Bone graft is placed in the patella defect, followed by closure of the paratenon and skin in successive layers. Radiographs can be obtained in the recovery room to assess placement of the bone tunnels, if not done intraoperatively (Fig. 39–14).

All patients undergo a standardized, postoperative rehabilitation protocol that focuses on immediate weightbearing and obtaining full range of motion, including early full extension. Rehabilitation of the knee is considered complete when equal quadriceps strength is achieved, which is defined as being within 10% of the strength of the contralateral, uninjured leg by isokinetic testing. When this goal has been attained, the patient may return to full activities, including return to sports.

COMPLICATIONS

Complications associated with ACL reconstruction can be classified as intraoperative and postoperative. Intraoperative complications include patella fracture, incorrect tunnel placement, violation of the posterior cortex of the femur, graft fracture, and suture laceration. Postoperative complications can include patella or quadriceps tendon avulsion, loss of motion, graft stretching and failure, patellofemoral symptoms, and quadriceps weakness.

Patella fracture after ACL reconstruction is infrequent, and the literature on this complication consists mostly of case reports.[27,64,102] Both direct force and indirect force have been implicated in the cause of this fracture. Simonian et al[102] suggested that an indirect force can result in different patella fracture patterns, depending on the time elapsed from harvesting. They determined that stellate fractures can occur without direct injury in the early postoperative period (within 5 weeks). After this period, the fracture pattern is more likely to be transverse. Fracture of the patella during graft harvesting can be avoided by not deepening the cuts more than 8 mm and by maintaining a 45-degree orientation of the sagittal saw blade to the perpendicular surface of the patella. The cuts should also not extend beyond the limits of the fragment to avoid a possible stress riser. In the event of an intraoperative patella fracture, the patella fragments should be rigidly fixed to facilitate early range of motion postoperatively.

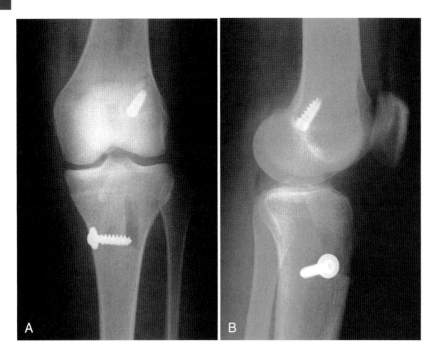

Figure 39–14. Postoperative anteroposterior (**A**) and lateral (**B**) radiographs after anterior cruciate ligament reconstruction showing correct placement of the bone tunnels. In this case, fixation of the femoral plug was achieved with an interference screw and the tibial plug was secured by tying sutures over a screw and washer.

Correct placement of the tunnels is crucial to the outcome of ACL reconstruction. Careful evaluation of the position of the guide pins before reaming can prevent erroneous tunnel placement. It is much easier to reposition the guide pin than to correct the position of a tunnel that has already been reamed. If, however, a reamed tunnel is noted to be slightly malpositioned, the orientation of the graft plug and the interference screw may compensate. For example, if the tibial tunnel is noted to be slightly anterior, placing the graft posteriorly and the screw anteriorly in the tunnel will effectively move the insertion site of the graft posterior to the center of the hole.[10] When there is gross malpositioning of the reamed tunnel, re-reaming of the tunnel in the correct position should be performed, followed by the use of a larger-diameter interference screw and bone graft, if necessary, to achieve adequate fixation.

Violation of the posterior cortex of the femur can occur from inadvertently reaming too far into the femoral tunnel and not maintaining the femur in a flexed position during the reaming. When this complication occurs, fixation with an interference screw is no longer possible because the graft will be pushed out of the posterior aspect of the femur by the screw. Fixation with a screw and post on the lateral aspect of the distal end of the femur through a separate incision is necessary, or alternatively, the traditional two-incision technique with a more anteriorly placed tunnel can be used.[21] This problem can be avoided by maintaining clear visualization during advancement of the reamer into the femoral tunnel and not exceeding 30 mm in the depth of insertion.

Both graft fracture and suture laceration can be caused by inadequate space for the plug and screw in the tunnel. In this situation, as the screw is inserted, the graft becomes overly compressed and can fracture. A tight fit can also predispose to the screw engaging the sutures and causing laceration and loss of tension on the graft. Over-reaming of the tunnels by 1 mm can prevent an overly tight fit of

the interference screw. In addition, we routinely place a single suture in the end of the femoral bone plug and use an interference screw that is shorter than the length of the plug. This prevents the screw from reaching the suture and possibly causing laceration. On the tibial side, the screw should be inserted under direct visualization to avoid entangling the sutures. If laceration occurs at this end, the tibial plug can be passed into the joint and pulled through the patellar tendon defect, and new holes can be drilled. The plug is then passed back into the joint and pulled through the tibial tunnel from inside out. In the event of bone plug fracture, sutures can be placed in the end of the tendon with a Krackow-type stitch and tied over a screw and post.

Despite initially good results after ACL reconstructive surgery, postoperative complications may occur that are detrimental to the long-term outcome. Fortunately, patella and quadriceps avulsions are rare, but they are devastating when they do occur. Several case reports have documented this complication, with some occurring up to 6 years after the reconstructive surgery.[18,62] Nixon et al[73] noted that the patellar tendon donor site, left open at the time of surgery, was histologically identical to normal tendon at 2 years. Others have shown that the ultrasound signal of the tendon returns to normal by 1 year.[1] This time frame may explain why the majority of these avulsions occur within the first 10 months after surgery.

Much attention has been focused on postoperative loss of motion after ACL reconstruction. This complication may result from preoperative, intraoperative, or postoperative factors. The presence of an effusion, limited range of motion, and concomitant ligamentous injuries of the knee preoperatively are factors that predispose to poor postoperative motion.[45,97] Intraoperative factors include erroneous tunnel placement and inadequate notchplasty. Anterior placement of the femoral tunnel results in overtightening of the graft and loss of full flexion (Fig. 39–15).

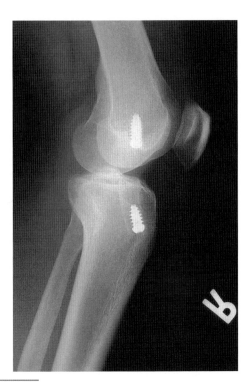

Figure 39–15. Lateral radiograph after anterior cruciate ligament reconstruction showing anterior femoral placement of the graft and interference screw.

Placement of the tibial tunnel too far anteriorly can result in impingement of the graft and lead to loss of full extension. Similarly, an inadequate notchplasty can also lead to extension loss secondary to impingement. Finally, postoperative immobilization and the rehabilitation protocol can have a significant effect on ultimate range of motion. Previous methods of cast immobilization after reconstruction and therapy emphasizing limited knee extension resulted in significant rates of postoperative arthrofibrosis. The trend toward limited or no immobilization and more aggressive rehabilitation has decreased these rates.[31,44,96] The concern over possible stretching and failure of the graft as a result of aggressive rehabilitation has not been realized. Histological analysis of the patellar tendon autografts used for ACL reconstruction reveals that the grafts undergo "ligamentization" over a period of months to years,[5,37] but that a necrotic stage may not occur and the grafts may be viable as early as 3 weeks postoperatively.[88]

The incidence of arthrofibrosis after ACL reconstructive surgery has decreased as postoperative rehabilitative protocols emphasizing early motion have been instituted. The cause of the arthrofibrosis may be due to poor patient motivation or compliance with the therapy regimen or other factors such as incorrect bone tunnel placement or the development of reflex sympathetic dystrophy. Treatment of postoperative arthrofibrosis begins with recognition of the problem. Initial treatment with physical therapy should focus on stretching exercises and may also involve the use of static or dynamic braces to regain motion, particularly extension. Manipulation under anesthesia may be necessary if no significant improvement is noted with physical therapy alone. Manipulation is most effective if performed within the first 6 weeks after reconstructive surgery, and aggressive physical therapy must follow the manipulation to prevent recurrence. Adequate anesthesia with an indwelling epidural catheter can facilitate this early rehabilitation. If the manipulation is unsuccessful or it is more than 6 weeks after surgery, arthroscopic or possibly open release of the adhesions will be required. Revision of the notchplasty may be needed at this time if scar tissue has developed in this area. Once again, aggressive physical therapy must follow any release to prevent recurrence. If the limited range of motion is due to improper tunnel placement, revision of the tunnels will need to be performed to prevent recurrence.

Stretching of the graft results in recurrence of instability symptoms and a positive Lachman test on examination. This may occur acutely or gradually over time and may be the result of improper tunnel placement, inadequate tension at the time of the reconstruction, or loss of fixation. Treatment of this complication must start with determining the reason for the failure. Graft incompetence immediately postoperatively is most likely due to inadequate tensioning at surgery. Tunnel-graft mismatch may result in incarceration of the plug in the tunnel and lead to fixation of the plug with laxity in the graft. Proper tunnel sizing and evaluation of graft tension after fixation is achieved should prevent this unnecessary complication. Early (within 6 weeks) acute failure indicates a loss of fixation of one of the plugs because this is the weak link in the construct until bony union occurs. Removal of the interference screw and insertion of a larger-diameter screw or fixation with the screw and post technique are required. Improper tunnel placement can result in either loss of motion, as noted previously, or stretching and failure of the graft. In the latter case, treatment consists of graft revision with correct tunnel placement.

The most common and persistent complication of ACL reconstruction may be postoperative patellofemoral pain. The exact cause of this problem has not been determined, but several studies have suggested that a relationship exists among persistent flexion contracture, patellofemoral pain, and quadriceps weakness.[3,89] Sachs et al[89] reported on 126 patients undergoing ACL reconstruction and noted a 19% rate of patellofemoral pain, which correlated positively with the presence of a flexion contracture. Similarly, Aglietti et al[3] noted a 5% incidence of patellofemoral pain and a 20% incidence of patellofemoral crepitus without pain in 226 patients after ACL reconstruction. A positive correlation was found between patellofemoral symptoms and flexion and extension losses. Although some studies have suggested that the morbidity of the donor site in autologous patellar tendon reconstructions may contribute to patellofemoral pain,[107] Shelbourne and Trumper[98] showed that the incidence of anterior knee pain is related more to failure to obtain full knee hyperextension. In their study, 602 patients who underwent ACL reconstruction followed by a rehabilitation protocol emphasizing full knee hyperextension were compared with 122 control patients with no history of knee injury. No differences in patellofemoral symptoms were found between the two groups. The authors concluded that anterior knee pain can be prevented through a program of early motion and full knee hyperextension.

No detrimental effects on stability of the knee from the hyperextension protocol have been noted, provided that precise location of the graft is achieved.

NEW DIRECTIONS

Although numerous options exist for treatment of cartilage injuries of the knee, each has its own limitations and benefits.

Cartilage transplantation requires an arthrotomy, as well as significant costs associated with cell culturing. Osteochondral allografts have shown some promise, but cell viability as well as graft availability remains a concern. Thus, no optimal procedure exists, and certainly new products are being evaluated to aid in the treatment of these osteochondral lesions.

At our institution we have begun using cartilage scaffolding (Tru-Fit Plugs, OsteoBiologics, San Antonio, TX) for numerous osteochondral lesions about the knee.[71,72] Placement of these biological scaffolds can be done arthroscopically, and they have been used to supplement osteochondral autograft transfers for large lesions and single lesions, as well as primary repair of large defects at both the trochlea and condyle.

These plugs were initially developed to back-fill bony defects resulting from osteochondral harvest in the hope of decreasing excessive bleeding and donor site morbidity.

Second-look arthroscopies, as well as animal studies, have demonstrated healing at the level of the cartilage surface. Several animal studies have examined the healing of these defects, and gross observations at various time points up to 1 year have demonstrated no significant cratering or osteophytosis, findings indicative of a stable articulating joint. Histological analysis of these studies has shown the gross observation that the predominant repair tissue was mostly hyaline cartilage and not fibrocartilage repair.

These biomechanical scaffolds are designed to support normal biological healing and are hydrophilic to absorb blood, cells, marrow, and proteins. These implants are cylindrical with a length of 18 mm and come in a variety of diameters. Tru-Fit Plugs are composed of PLG copolymer as well as calcium sulfate at the level of the cartilage surface. The estimated time of resorption is 6 to 9 months. These scaffolds are structurally sound to effectively fill defects and, because of their porous nature, may provide conduits for tissue ingrowth.

Thus far, we have been quite happy with the results, and certainly the results are preliminary and further studies are needed to document the degree of cartilage healing, as well as the long-term durability of this repair. In the future, enhancements of the scaffolds may be devised to further expedite osteochondral healing.

CONCLUSION

The goal of ACL reconstruction is to provide stability of the knee without loss of motion and thereby allow return of patients to their preinjury level of function. The patellar tendon autograft has proved to be a reliable substitute for the native ligament and has yielded good long-term results. Refinements in surgical technique and postoperative therapy regimens have reduced complication rates and decreased recovery times after the procedure. The challenge for the future is to determine the optimal time for return to full activities without jeopardizing incorporation of the graft and the overall stability of the knee.

ACKNOWLEDGMENT

We thank Henrik Bo Pedersen, M.D., for his valuable assistance in preparation of the illustrations in this chapter.

References

1. Adriani E, Mariani PP, Maresca G, et al: Healing of the patellar tendon after harvesting of its mid-third for anterior cruciate ligament reconstruction and evolution of the unclosed donor site defect. Knee Surg Traumatol Arthrosc 3:138, 1995.
2. Aglietti P, Buzzi R, D'Andria S, et al: Arthroscopic anterior cruciate ligament reconstruction with patellar tendon. Arthroscopy 8:510, 1992.
3. Aglietti P, Buzzi R, D'Andria S, et al: Patellofemoral problems after intraarticular anterior cruciate ligament reconstruction. Clin Orthop 288:195, 1993.
4. Alm A, Gillquist J: Reconstruction of the anterior cruciate ligament by using the medial third of the patellar ligament. Acta Chir Scand 140:289, 1974.
5. Amiel D, Kleiner JB, Akeson WH: The natural history of the anterior cruciate ligament autograft of patellar tendon origin. Am J Sports Med 14:449, 1986.
6. Andersson C, Odensten M, Gillquist J: Knee function after surgical or nonsurgical treatment of acute rupture of the anterior cruciate ligament: A randomized study with a long-term follow-up period. Clin Orthop 264:255, 1991.
7. Arciero RA, Scoville CR, Snyder RJ, et al: Single versus two-incision arthroscopic anterior cruciate ligament reconstruction. Arthroscopy 12:462, 1996.
8. Arendt E, Dick R: Knee injury patterns among men and women in collegiate basketball and soccer. NCAA data and review of literature. Am J Sports Med 23:694, 1995.
9. Arnoczky SP, Tarvin GB, Marshall JL: Anterior cruciate ligament replacement using patellar tendon. An evaluation of graft revascularization in the dog. J Bone Joint Surg Am 64:2172, 1982.
10. Bach BR Jr: Potential pitfalls of Kurosaka screw interference fixation for ACL surgery. Am J Knee Surg 2:76, 1989.
11. Bach BR Jr, Levy ME, Bojchuk J, et al: Single-incision endoscopic anterior cruciate ligament reconstruction using patellar tendon autograft. Am J Sports Med 26:30, 1998.
12. Bach BR Jr, Tradonsky S, Bojchuk J, et al: Arthroscopically assisted anterior cruciate ligament reconstruction using patellar tendon autograft. Am J Sports Med 26:202, 1998.
13. Barber FA, Elrod BF, McGuire DA, Paulos LE: Preliminary results of an absorbable interference screw. Arthroscopy 11:537-548, 1995.
14. Barrack RL, Bruckner JD, Kneisl J, et al: The outcome of nonoperatively treated complete tears of the anterior cruciate ligament in active young adults. Clin Orthop 259:192, 1990.
15. Berg EE: Assessing arthroscopic notchplasty. Arthroscopy 7:275, 1991.
16. Berns GS, Howell SM: Roofplasty requirements in vitro for different tibial hole placements in anterior cruciate ligament reconstruction. Am J Sports Med 21:292, 1993.
17. Bjordal JM, Arnly F, Hannestad B, et al: Epidemiology of anterior cruciate ligament injuries in soccer. Am J Sports Med 25:341, 1997.
18. Bonamo JJ, Krinick RM, Sporn AA: Rupture of the patellar ligament after use of its central third for anterior cruciate reconstruction. J Bone Joint Surg Am 66:1294, 1984.

19. Burks RT, Daniel D, Losse G: The effect of continuous passive motion on anterior cruciate ligament reconstruction stability. Am J Sports Med 12:323, 1984.

20. Burks RT, Leland R: Determination of graft tension before fixation in anterior cruciate ligament reconstruction. Arthroscopy 4:260, 1988.

21. Bush-Joseph CA, Bach BR Jr, Bryan J: Posterior cortical violation of the femoral tunnel during endoscopic anterior cruciate ligament reconstruction. Am J Knee Surg 8:130, 1995.

22. Buss DD, Min R, Skyhar M, et al: Nonoperative treatment of acute anterior cruciate ligament injuries in a selected group of patients. Am J Sports Med 23:160, 1995.

23. Buss DD, Warren RF, Wickiewicz TL, et al: Arthroscopically assisted reconstruction of the anterior cruciate ligament with use of autogenous patellar-ligament grafts. Results after twenty-four to forty-two months. J Bone Joint Surg Am 75:1346, 1993.

24. Bylski-Austrow DI, Grood ES, Hefzy MS, et al: Anterior cruciate ligament replacements: A mechanical study of femoral attachment location, flexion angle at tensioning, and initial tension. J Orthop Res 8:522, 1990.

25. Caborn DN, Coen M, Neef R, et al: Quadrupled semitendinosus-gracilis autograft fixation in the femoral tunnel: A comparison between a metal and a bioabsorbable interference screw. Arthroscopy 14:241, 1998.

26. Caborn DN, Urban WP Jr, Johnson DL, et al: Biomechanical comparison between Bioscrew and titanium alloy interference screws for bone–patellar tendon–bone graft fixation in anterior cruciate ligament reconstruction. Arthroscopy 13:229, 1997.

27. Christen B, Jakob RP: Fractures associated with patellar ligament grafts in cruciate ligament surgery. J Bone Joint Surg Br 74:617, 1992.

28. Clancy WG Jr, Nelson DA, Reider B, et al: Anterior cruciate ligament reconstruction using one-third of the patellar ligament, augmented by extra-articular tendon transfers. J Bone Joint Surg Am 64:352, 1982.

29. Colville MR, Bowman RR: The significance of isometer measurements and graft position during anterior cruciate ligament reconstruction. Am J Sports Med 21:832, 1993.

30. Cooper DE: Biomechanical properties of the central third patellar tendon graft: Effect of rotation. Knee Surg Sports Traumatol Arthrosc 6:16, 1998.

31. Cosgarea AJ, Sebastianelli WJ, DeHaven KE: Prevention of arthrofibrosis after anterior cruciate ligament reconstruction using the central third patellar tendon autograft. Am J Sports Med 23:87, 1995.

32. Daniel DM, Stone ML, Dobson BE, et al: Fate of the ACL-injured patient: A prospective outcome study. Am J Sports Med 22:632, 1994.

33. Diduch DR, Mann J, Geary SP, et al: The effect of pretwisting the ACL autograft on knee laxity. Am J Knee Surg 11:15, 1998.

34. Draganich LF, Hsieh YF, Reider B: Strategies for attachment site locations and twist of the intraarticular anterior cruciate ligament graft. Am J Sports Med 24:342, 1996.

35. Dworsky BD, Jewell BF, Bach BR Jr: Interference screw divergence in endoscopic anterior cruciate ligament reconstruction. Arthroscopy 12:45, 1996.

36. Eriksson E: Reconstruction of the anterior cruciate ligament. Orthop Clin North Am 7:167, 1976.

37. Falconiero RP, DiStefano VJ, Cook TM: Revascularization and ligamentization of autogenous anterior cruciate ligament grafts in humans. Arthroscopy 14:197, 1998.

38. Fetto JF, Marshall JL: The natural history and diagnosis of anterior cruciate ligament insufficiency. Clin Orthop 147:29, 1980.

39. Frank CB, Jackson DW: The science of reconstruction of the anterior cruciate ligament. J Bone Joint Surg Am 79:1556, 1997.

40. Friden T, Zatterstrom R, Lindstrand A, et al: Anterior-cruciate–insufficient knees treated with physiotherapy. Clin Orthop 263:190, 1991.

41. Giove TP, Miller SJ III, Kent BE, et al: Non-operative treatment of the torn anterior cruciate ligament. J Bone Joint Surg Am 65:184, 1983.

42. Gotlin R, Cushner FD, Scott WN: Influence of graft diameter on knee stability: KT arthrometry study. Unpublished data.

43. Good L, Odensten M, Gillquist J: Precision in reconstruction of the anterior cruciate ligament. A new positioning device compared with hand drilling. Acta Orthop Scand 58:658, 1987.

44. Graf B, Uhr F: Complications of intra-articular anterior cruciate reconstruction. Clin Sports Med 7:835, 1988.

45. Harner CD, Irrgang JJ, Paul J, et al: Loss of motion after anterior cruciate ligament reconstruction. Am J Sports Med 20:499, 1992.

46. Harner CD, Marks PH, Fu FH, et al: Anterior cruciate ligament reconstruction: Endoscopic versus two-incision technique. Arthroscopy 10:502, 1994.

47. Harner CD, Paulos LE, Greenwald AE, et al: Detailed analysis of patients with bilateral anterior cruciate ligament injuries. Am J Sports Med 22:37, 1994.

48. Hawkins RJ, Misamore GW, Merritt TR: Followup of the acute non-operated isolated anterior cruciate ligament tear. Am J Sports Med 14:205, 1986.

49. Howell SM, Clark JA: Tibial tunnel placement in anterior cruciate ligament reconstruction and graft impingement. Clin Orthop 283:187, 1992.

50. Howell SM, Clark JA, Farley TE: A rationale for predicting anterior cruciate graft impingement by the intercondylar roof. A magnetic resonance imaging study. Am J Sports Med 19:276, 1991.

51. Hunter RE, Mastrangelo J, Freeman JR, et al: The impact of surgical timing on postoperative motion and stability following anterior cruciate ligament reconstruction. Arthroscopy 12:667, 1996.

52. Johnson LL, Van Dyk GE: Metal and biodegradable interference screws: Comparison of failure strength. Arthroscopy 12:452, 1996.

53. Jones KJ: Reconstruction of the anterior cruciate ligament. J Bone Joint Surg Am 45:925, 1963.

54. Kannus P, Jarvinen M: Conservatively treated tears of the anterior cruciate ligament. J Bone Joint Surg Am 69:1007, 1987.

55. Khalfayan EE, Sharkey PF, Alexander AH, et al: The relationship between tunnel placement and clinical results after anterior cruciate ligament reconstruction. Am J Sports Med 24:335, 1996.

56. Kurosaka M, Yoshiya S, Andrish JT: A biomechanical comparison of different surgical techniques of graft fixation in anterior cruciate ligament reconstruction. Am J Sports Med 15:225, 1987.

57. Lambert KL: Vascularized patellar tendon graft with rigid internal fixation for anterior cruciate ligament insufficiency. Clin Orthop 172:85, 1983.

58. LaPrade RF, Burnett QM II: Femoral intercondylar notch stenosis and correlation to anterior cruciate ligament injuries. A prospective study. Am J Sports Med 22:198, 1994.

59. Marcacci M, Zaffagnini S, Iacono F, et al: Early versus late reconstruction for anterior cruciate ligament rupture: Results after five years of followup. Am J Sports Med 23:690, 1995.

60. Marshall JL, Warren RF, Wickiewicz TL, et al: The anterior cruciate ligament: A technique of repair and reconstruction. Clin Orthop 143:97, 1979.

61. Marti C, Imhoff AB, Bahrs C, et al: Metallic versus bioabsorbable interference screw for fixation of bone–patellar tendon–bone autograft in arthroscopic anterior cruciate ligament reconstruction. A preliminary report. Knee Surg Sports Traumatol Arthrosc 5:217, 1997.

62. Marumoto JM, Mitsunaga MM, Richardson AB, et al: Late patellar tendon ruptures after removal of the central third for anterior cruciate ligament reconstruction. Am J Sports Med 24:698, 1996.

63. Matthews LS, Lawrence SJ, Yahiro MA, et al: Fixation strengths of patellar tendon–bone grafts. Arthroscopy 9:76, 1993.

64. McCaroll JR: Fracture of the patella during a golf swing following reconstruction of the anterior cruciate ligament. A case report. Am J Sports Med 11:26, 1983.

65. McDaniel WJ Jr, Dameron TB Jr: Untreated ruptures of the anterior cruciate ligament: A followup study. J Bone Joint Surg Am 62:696, 1980.

66. Melby A III, Noble JS, Askew MJ, et al: The effects of graft tensioning on the laxity and kinematics of the anterior cruciate ligament reconstructed knee. Arthroscopy 7:257, 1991.

67. Miller MD, Hinkin DT: The "N+7 rule" for tibial tunnel placement in endoscopic anterior cruciate ligament reconstruction. Arthroscopy 12:124, 1996.

68. Morgan CD, Kalman VR, Grawl DM: Definitive landmarks for reproducible tibial tunnel placement in anterior cruciate ligament reconstruction. Arthroscopy 11:275, 1995.

69. Morgan EA, McElroy JJ, DesJardins JD, et al: The effect of intercondylar notchplasty on the patellofemoral articulation. Am J Sports Med 24:843, 1996.

70. Nabors ED, Richmond JC, Vannah WM, et al: Anterior cruciate ligament graft tensioning in full extension. Am J Sports Med 23:488, 1995.

71. Niederauer GG, Leatherbury NC, Simon TM, Aberman HM: Treatment of osteochondral autograph donor sites using porous biodegradable scaffolds. Presented at a meeting of the International Cartilage Repair Society, 2004, p 666.

72. Niederauer GG, Slivka MA, Leatherbury NC, et al: Evaluation of multiphase implants for repair of focal osteochondral defects. Biomaterials 22:2561, 2000.

73. Nixon RG, SeGall GK, Sax SL, et al: Reconstitution of the patellar tendon donor site after graft harvest. Clin Orthop 317:162, 1995.

74. Noyes FR, Barber SD, Mangine RE: Bone–patellar ligament–bone and fascia lata allografts for reconstruction of the anterior cruciate ligament. J Bone Joint Surg Am 72:1125, 1990.

75. Noyes FR, Barber-Westin SD: A comparison of results in acute and chronic anterior cruciate ligament ruptures of arthroscopically assisted autogenous patellar tendon reconstruction. Am J Sports Med 25:460, 1997.

76. Noyes FR, Butler DL, Grood ES, et al: Biomechanical analysis of human ligament grafts used in knee-ligament repairs and reconstructions. J Bone Joint Surg Am 66:344, 1984.

77. Noyes FR, Matthews DS, Mooar PA, et al: The symptomatic anterior cruciate–deficient knee. Part II: The results of rehabilitation, activity modification, and counseling on functional disability. J Bone Joint Surg Am 65:163, 1983.

78. Noyes FR, Mooar PA, Matthews DS, et al: The symptomatic anterior cruciate–deficient knee: Part I. The long-term functional disability in athletically active individuals. J Bone Joint Surg Am 65:154, 1983.

79. O'Brien SJ, Warren RF, Pavlov H, et al: Reconstruction of the chronically insufficient anterior cruciate ligament with the central third of the patellar ligament. J Bone Joint Surg Am 73:278, 1991.

80. Odensten M, Gillquist J: Functional anatomy of the anterior cruciate ligament and a rationale for reconstruction. J Bone Joint Surg Am 67:257, 1985.

81. Otto D, Pinczewski LA, Clingeleffer A, et al: Five-year results of single-incision arthroscopic anterior cruciate ligament reconstruction with patellar tendon autograft. Am J Sports Med 26:181, 1998.

82. Pagnano MW, Kim CW, Huie G, et al: Difficulties with the "N+7 rule" in endoscopic anterior cruciate ligament reconstruction. Arthroscopy 13:597, 1997.

83. Paschal SO, Seemann MD, Aschman RB, et al: Interference fixation versus post fixation of bone–patellar tendon–bone grafts for anterior cruciate ligament reconstruction. Clin Orthop 300:281, 1994.

84. Pena F, Grontvedt T, Brown GA, et al: Comparison of failure strength between metallic and absorbable interference screws. Influence of insertion torque, tunnel–bone block gap, bone mineral density, and interference. Am J Sports Med 24:329, 1996.

85. Plancher KD, Steadman JR, Briggs KK, et al: Reconstruction of the anterior cruciate ligament in patients who are at least forty years old. A long-term follow-up and outcome study. J Bone Joint Surg Am 80:184, 1998.

86. Reat J-FP, Lintner DM: One- versus two-incision ACL reconstruction. Am J Knee Surg 10:198, 1997.

87. Romano VM, Graf BK, Keene JS, et al: Anterior cruciate ligament reconstruction. The effect of tibial tunnel placement on range of motion. Am J Sports Med 21:415, 1993.

88. Rougraff B, Shelbourne KD, Gerth PK, et al: Arthroscopic and histologic analysis of human patellar tendon autografts used for anterior cruciate ligament reconstruction. Am J Sports Med 21:277, 1993.

89. Sachs RA, Daniel DM, Stone ML, et al: Patellofemoral problems after anterior cruciate ligament reconstruction. Am J Sports Med 17:760, 1989.

90. Samuelson TS, Drez D Jr, Maletis GB: Anterior cruciate ligament graft rotation. Reproduction of normal graft rotation. Am J Sports Med 24:67, 1996.

91. Sandberg R, Balkfors B: The durability of anterior cruciate ligament reconstruction with the patellar tendon. Am J Sports Med 16:341, 1988.

92. Scuderi GR, Alicea JA, Scott WN: Effect of divergence between the femoral interference screw and the femoral bone block in endoscopic anterior cruciate ligament reconstructions. Presented at the Annual Meeting of the American Academy of Orthopaedic Surgeons, 1995, Orlando, FL.

93. Sgaglione NA, Schwartz RE: Arthroscopically assisted reconstruction of the anterior cruciate ligament: Initial clinical experience and minimal 2-year follow-up comparing endoscopic transtibial and two-incision techniques. Arthroscopy 13:156, 1997.

94. Shelbourne KD, Facibene WA, Hunt JJ: Radiographic and intraoperative intercondylar notch width measurements in men and women with unilateral and bilateral anterior cruciate ligament tears. Knee Surg Sports Traumatol Arthrosc 5:229, 1997.

95. Shelbourne KD, Gray T: Anterior cruciate ligament reconstruction with autogenous patellar tendon graft followed by accelerated rehabilitation: A two- to nine-year followup. Am J Sports Med 25:786, 1997.

96. Shelbourne KD, Nitz P: Accelerated rehabilitation after anterior cruciate ligament reconstruction. Am J Sports Med 18:292, 1990.

97. Shelbourne KD, Patel DV: Timing of surgery in anterior cruciate ligament–injured knees. Knee Surg Traumatol Arthrosc 3:148, 1995.

98. Shelbourne KD, Trumper RV: Preventing anterior knee pain after anterior cruciate ligament reconstruction. Am J Sports Med 25:41, 1997.

99. Shelbourne KD, Whitaker HJ, McCarroll JR, et al: Anterior cruciate ligament injury: Evaluation of intraarticular reconstruction of acute tears without repair—two to seven year followup of 155 athletes. Am J Sports Med 18:484, 1990.

100. Shelbourne KD, Wilckens JH, Mollabashy A, et al: Arthrofibrosis in acute anterior cruciate ligament reconstruction. The effect of timing of reconstruction and rehabilitation. Am J Sports Med 19:332, 1991.

101. Sherman MF, Warren RF, Marshall JL, et al: A clinical and radiographical analysis of 127 anterior cruciate insufficient knees. Clin Orthop 227:229, 1988.

102. Simonian PT, Mann FA, Mandt PR: Indirect forces and patella fracture after anterior cruciate ligament reconstruction with the patellar ligament. Case report. Am J Knee Surg 8:60, 1995.

103. Souryal TO, Freeman TR: Intercondylar notch size and anterior cruciate ligament injuries in athletes. A prospective study. Am J Sports Med 21:535, 1993.

104. Souryal TO, Moore HA, Evans JP: Bilaterality in anterior cruciate ligament injuries: Associated intercondylar notch stenosis. Am J Sports Med 16:449, 1988.

105. Tanzer M, Lenczner E: The relationship of intercondylar notch size and content to notchplasty requirement in anterior cruciate ligament surgery. Arthroscopy 6:89, 1990.

106. Torg JS, Conrad W, Kalen V: Clinical diagnosis of anterior cruciate ligament instability in the athlete. Am J Sports Med 4:84, 1976.

107. Weiss RA, Re LP, Rintz KG, et al: Incidence of anterior knee pain after treatment for anterior cruciate ligament rupture. Arthroscopy 9:366, 1993.

108. Wiztzs EM: The ACL Deficient Knee. Rosemont, IL, American Academy of Orthopaedic Surgeons, 1994, p 1-10.

109. Wojtys EM, Huston LJ, Lindenfeld TN, et al: Association between the menstrual cycle and anterior cruciate ligament injuries in female athletes. Am J Sports Med 26:614, 1998.

110. Yaru NC, Daniel DM, Penner D: The effect of tibial attachment site on graft impingement in an anterior cruciate ligament reconstruction. Am J Sports Med 20:217, 1992.

111. Yoshiya M, Kurosaka M, Yamada M, et al: Optimal orientation of bone tunnels in the anterior cruciate ligament reconstruction. Trans Orthop Res Soc 16:602, 1991.

112. Yoshiya S, Andrish JY, Manley MT, et al: Graft tension in anterior cruciate ligament reconstruction. Am J Sports Med 15:464, 1987.

CHAPTER 40

Arthroscopic Anterior Cruciate Reconstruction with Hamstring Tendons: Indications, Surgical Technique, and Complications and Their Treatment

Timothy S. Mologne • Marc J. Friedman

Anterior cruciate ligament (ACL) reconstruction in which a free tendon graft is substituted for the torn ligament is a common surgical procedure for the orthopedic surgeon. Although some patients can function exceptionally well with an ACL-deficient knee,[14,105] most experience pain and recurrent episodes of instability. Because the menisci, articular surfaces, and other restraining structures around the knee are susceptible to injury during episodes of instability, it is generally accepted that ACL reconstruction should be offered to patients who have or are at risk for having recurrent knee instability.

The goal of ACL reconstruction is to restore normal anterior knee stability, and when deciding on surgical intervention, the orthopedist has to determine which graft substitute best accomplishes this goal. The ideal graft is one that retains strength at least equivalent to that of the normal ACL, allows for secure fixation, enables unrestricted rehabilitation, and is associated with minimal graft harvest morbidity.

The majority of orthopedists prefer an autogenous graft, and historically, the patellar tendon has been the most popular graft source.* However, given the associated morbidity,[3,39,94,122,125,134,135,137] many surgeons have turned to autogenous semitendinosus/gracilis (ST/G) tendons.

ACL reconstruction with autogenous hamstring tendons has been well described.† The four-stranded ST/G graft has many advantages over other grafts, including its strength. Biomechanical testing has shown the strength of a four-stranded ST/G graft to vary from 3880 to 4213 N,[24,63,65,69,102,103,145] which makes it approximately 240% stronger than the normal ACL[24,102,103,123,155] and at least 138% stronger than a 10-mm-wide patellar tendon graft.[24,37,102,103]

Another advantage of the four-stranded ST/G graft is its stiffness, which has been measured to be between 805 and 954 N/mm.[63,65,69,145] This property makes it nearly three times stiffer than the normal ACL[37,104,123,155] and twice as stiff as a central-third patellar tendon.[37]

The four-stranded ST/G graft has a large cross-sectional area that closely resembles that of the normal ACL, which has been measured to be 44.4 to 56.5 mm^2.[102,104,123] An 8-mm-diameter hamstring graft has a cross-sectional area of 50 mm^2, which is 1.5 times that of a 10-mm-wide patellar tendon. This larger area is advantageous for maximizing vascular ingrowth and ligamentization.

The biggest advantage of the hamstring graft over autogenous patellar or quadriceps tendon grafts is preservation of the extensor mechanism. As a result, postoperative problems such as patellar fracture,[137] patellar tendon rupture,[94] patellofemoral pain,[2,3,23,26,39,75,109,113,125] patellar tendonitis, quadriceps weakness,[122,125] and flexion contracture[114,125] are minimized. Patellofemoral pain has been a problem when autogenous patellar tendon grafts are used, with a 17% to 56% postoperative incidence of pain.[2,23,109,113] Pain on kneeling has been reported to occur in 42%[26] of those who undergo ACL reconstruction with autogenous bone–patellar tendon–bone grafts. Quadriceps weakness, believed to be a result of graft harvest and to be associated with flexion contracture and patellar irritability, has been reported to occur in as many as 65% of patients.[122,125] Deterioration of the patellofemoral articular surfaces, documented by second-look arthroscopy, has been reported in as many as 57% of patients after the use of an autogenous patellar tendon graft.[135]

The literature is replete with clinical studies of ACL reconstruction using a hamstring tendon graft.* Although various techniques have been described, these studies have reported a negative pivot shift in 69% to 100% of patients.[4,5,13,35,38,56,62,69,70,91,93,111,112,121,136,154] In studies that have provided KT-1000 (MEDmetric, San Diego, CA) data, most have reported a manual maximum side-to-side difference of 3 mm or less in 70% to 100% of patients.†

A review of ACL reconstruction with an autogenous patellar tendon reveals mostly excellent and good results, with several studies reporting greater than 90% excellent and good results.[23,109,113,131-133] On casual comparison with the hamstring graft studies, it appears that the results are improved with a patellar tendon graft. However, keep in mind that some of the poor results previously reported

*References 2, 8, 15, 23, 31, 39, 75-77, 109, 113, 131-134.
†References 4, 10, 13, 15, 20-22, 28, 30, 32, 35, 38, 56, 57, 62, 68-70, 85, 88, 89, 96, 97, 100, 119, 121, 128, 136, 146, 154, 159.

*References 4, 5, 10, 13, 15, 18, 20-22, 26, 28, 30, 32, 35, 38, 56, 57, 62, 67-70, 85, 88-91, 93, 95-97, 100, 111, 112, 119, 121, 128, 136, 139, 146, 154, 159.
†References 22, 28, 35, 38, 62, 69, 70, 91, 93, 111, 112, 121, 128, 136, 154.

with the use of a hamstring graft resulted from the use of an inadequate graft (single-, double-, or triple-stranded graft) and the lack of strong, stiff fixation on both ends of the graft. Studies that have used a four-stranded graft with adequate fixation on both the tibia and femur have reported 90% with an absent pivot shift and 90% with less than 3 mm of side-to-side difference on KT-1000 manual maximum testing.[35,69,70,121,128]

Several clinical studies have compared the results of autogenous hamstring versus patellar tendon ACL reconstructions. Although many of the earlier studies showed improved results with the patellar tendon graft, these studies were not prospective and lacked any form of randomization.[67,112,139] Meta-analyses[49,157] have reported greater stability, higher activity levels, and a lower incidence of graft failure in patients reconstructed with a patellar tendon graft. Some of the nonrandomized comparison studies have shown similar objective results with respect to postoperative laxity, but greater compromise in functional performance and evidence of arthritis in patients reconstructed with patellar tendon grafts.[40,118,124] In the prospective comparison studies,* most have not shown any functional difference between the two grafts. A few of the studies, however, do show a trend toward increased objective laxity in female patients despite equal subjective outcomes.[15,38,55,100] In some of the prospective randomized studies, a higher incidence of patellofemoral pain and quadriceps weakness has been reported in patients who received patellar tendon grafts.[5,26,38,44,47,82,95,129] In some, this morbidity has prevented or delayed return to full activities.[39,95]

Historically, one of the biggest disadvantages of using the hamstring tendons was fixation. To allow for unrestricted rehabilitation, graft fixation should be stronger than the force experienced by the normal ACL during activities of daily living, which has been estimated to be nearly 500 N.[29,39,66,69,81,95] The metal interference screw, with a fixation strength of 416 to 640 N,[80,115,123] has proved to be reliable fixation for the bone–patellar tendon–bone graft and the accepted standard by which other fixations are measured. In the past, because of the lack of bone in the hamstring graft, the fixation had to be outside the bone tunnels. Outside fixation has the potential disadvantage of increasing graft construct length and thereby increasing the chance for graft elongation with cyclic loading.[71] In addition, many outside fixation devices were minimally strong or stiff enough to allow for unrestricted rehabilitation. A recent study comparing femoral fixation on the cortex with aperture fixation, however, found no difference in outcomes.[88] Newer fixation methods have been and continue to be developed to allow the hamstring tendons to be adequately fixated in the femoral and tibial tunnels.

Biomechanical data have shown slippage and lack of stiffness to be problematic for many soft-tissue fixation devices.[42,54,92] In an attempt to increase fixation strength and stiffness, femoral cross-pin fixation has been developed. Many companies market these devices, including Arthrotek (Warsaw, IN), Arthrex (Naples, FL), Stryker

Endoscopy (San Jose, CA) and Mitek (Mansfield, MA). Femoral cross-pin fixation is the strongest and stiffest fixation in ACL reconstruction surgery, irrespective of the graft source. Fixation strength varies from 1002 to 1600 N,[32,145] and stiffness has been measured at 176 to 224 N/mm.[46,145] Newer tibial fixation methods, including the Intrafix and Bio-Intrafix (Mitek) and the WasherLoc (Arthrotek), have been developed, and these newer methods of fixation have also helped increase the ultimate strength and stiffness of the graft fixation construct (see Table 40–1).

Another potential disadvantage of hamstring ACL reconstruction is the lack of bone-to-bone healing. Animal studies have demonstrated that the tendons are incorporated into the bone tunnel by 12 weeks.[59,61,120] In addition, animal studies have shown that a semitendinosus autograft is histologically transformed into a structure that is similar to the native ACL.[60] Biopsy specimens from human knees have confirmed this incorporation and the formation of Sharpey-like fibers in the bone tunnels,[117] whereas in another study, the biopsied tissue from the tendon-bone interface resembled granulation tissue without fibers between the tendon and bone.[99] A lack of biological fixation can lead to postoperative instability.[147] In theory, therefore, graft fixation, in most cases, needs to be secure for a minimum of 12 weeks, until such time that the tendons have healed in the bone tunnel.

A four-stranded ST/G graft looped over a femoral cross-pin and secured on the tibia with a central sheath and screw (Intrafix) or washer plate (WasherLoc) is a strong and stiff graft construct that easily allows for unrestricted and aggressive rehabilitation without the risk of graft elongation or failure. We currently recommend this graft fixation construct for ACL reconstruction.

The four-stranded ST/G graft is our graft of choice for patients less than 200 lb, women, patients with open physes, low-demand patients, patients with small patellar tendons, patients with vocations/avocations that require "bent-knee" activities (such as carpet layers, carpenters, plumbers), and those with preoperative patellofemoral pain. Some authors have reported less successful results with use of the hamstring graft in female patients.[15,38,100] We have not had the same experience. We advocate use of the bone–patellar tendon–bone graft in some high-performance athletes who require an early return to training and those who may require strong knee flexors for their sport or occupation.

SURGICAL TECHNIQUE

Graft Harvest

The semitendinosus and gracilis tendons are harvested through a 1.5-inch incision centered approximately 2 cm medial to the tibial tubercle (Fig. 40–1). Dissection is carried down to the sartorius fascia, which is incised parallel and distal to the palpable semitendinosus tendon. The semitendinosus and gracilis tendons are then released from their tibial attachment and reflected proximally to visualize the undersurface and their natural separation

---

*References 5, 7, 12, 15-18, 26, 38, 41, 44, 45, 47, 74, 82, 93, 95, 111, 129.

Table 40–1. Fixation Options

	ULTIMATE STRENGTH (N)	STIFFNESS (N/mm)	SLIPPAGE UNDER CYCLIC LOAD	EXTENSION AT FAILURE (mm)
Metal interference screw with bone–patellar tendon graft	416-640 N[80,115,123]	51-58 N/mm[80,123]		12.6 mm[123]
Knotted loop of Mersilene tape	493 N[140]			
Knotted loop of No. 5 Ethibond	302 N[140]			
Femoral Devices for Hamstring Grafts				
Arthrex Bio-TransFix	746-1392 N[6,46]	176 N/mm[46]	1.4 mm after 100 s of 250 N cyclic loading[6] 3.1 mm after 100 cycles of 150 N[46]	
Arthrex TransFix	1002-1235 N[42,46]	181 N/mm[46]	1.7-3.4 mm after 1000 cycles of 150 N[42,46]	
Continuous-loop EndoButton (CL)	Single: 864-1086 N[6,42,78] Double: 1324 N	106 N/mm[46]	Single: 3.9 mm after 1500 cycles of 200 N[78] 1.8 mm at 1000 cycles of 150 N[42] 1.75 mm after 100 s of 250-N cyclic loading[6] Double: 1.6 mm at 1000 cycles of 150 N[42]	
Bone Mulch Screw (Arthrotek)	1112-1126 N[78,145]	115-225 N/mm[78,145]	2.2 mm after 1500 cycles of 200 N[78]	
Mitek-Depuy Cross Pin	35-mm pin: 1003 N[32] 70-mm pin: 1604 N[32]			
Mitek RIGIDfix (bioabsorbable cross-pins)	638-868 N[6,78,158]	77-226 N/mm[78,158]	3.7 mm after 1500 cycles of 200 N[78] 5.07 mm after 1000 cycles of 250 N[158] 8.6 mm after 1000 cycles of 450 N[158] 6.02 mm after 100 s of 250-N cyclic loading[6]	
EndoButton	352-703 N[20,58,123,145]	8-98 N/mm[20,58,123,145]	Failure occurred in 5 of 5 trials between 1041 and 29,260 cycles of 155 N. None withstood the testing condition of 250,000 cycles.[43] (Note: Graft tunnel motion increases as the length of the loop of tape increases[50])	23.6 mm[123]
RCI screw	336-546 N[46,56,78,116]	51-68 N/mm[46,78]	6.8 mm after 1100 cycles of 150 N[56,116] 3.9 mm after 1500 cycles of 200 N[78]	
Arthrex metal soft screw	226 N[56,116]			
Bioabsorbable screw (Arthrex)	327-539 N[6,11]		5.4 mm with cyclic loading for 100 s of 250 N[6]	
Bioscrew (Linvatec)	310-589 N[42,78,153]	26-66 N/mm[78,153]	4.0 mm after 1500 cycles of 200 N[78] 4 of 5 failed before 1000 cycles of 150 N[42]	
Bioscrew with EndoPearl	659 N[153]	42 N/mm[153]		
FastLok (Neoligaments)	11 mm with ST/G: 600 N[34] 11 mm with Leeds-Keio Lig.: 1258 N[34] 8 mm with Leeds-Keio Lig.: 1027 N[34] 6 mm with No. 2 Ethibond: 483-510 N[34] 6 mm with No. 5 Ethibond: 735 N[34]	55-66 N/mm[34] 149 N/mm[34]	1.1 mm after 1.5 million cycles of 200-500 N[34] 1.4 mm after 1.5 million cycles of 200-500 N[34]	7.4-9.4 mm[34] 4.9 mm[34]

Table continues on next page

Table 40–1. Fixation Options—Cont'd.

	ULTIMATE STRENGTH (N)	STIFFNESS (N/mm)	SLIPPAGE UNDER CYCLIC LOAD	EXTENSION AT FAILURE (mm)
Clawed washer with 6-mm screw	502 N[54]		6.7 mm after 300 cycles of 150 N[54]	
Two 6-mm soft-tissue washers	821 N[142]	29 N/mm[142]		26 mm[142]
Sutures tied over a 6.5-mm screw post	573 N[142]	18 N/mm[142]		22 mm[142]
20-mm spiked washer with 6.5-mm screw	248 N[72]			
Tibial Fixation for Hamstring Grafts				
Intrafix (Mitek)	796-1332 N[25,79] Force required to produce 2 mm of laxity = 216 N[141]	49-223 N/mm[25,79]	1.5 mm after 1500 cycles[79]	17.3 mm[25]
Bio-Intrafix (Mitek)	1275 N[138]			
WasherLoc plate/screw (Arthrotek)	903-975 N[79,92]	87-273 N/mm[79,92]	0.8-2 mm at 500 N[92] 3.2 mm after 1500 cycles[79]	
Tandem AO washers/screws	1159 N[92]	259 N/mm[92]	0.5 mm at 500 N[92]	
Evolgate device	1237 N[48]	168 N/mm[48]		
AO washer/screw and sutures around screw post	768 N[92]	181 N/mm[92]	0.9 mm at 500 N[92]	
Tandem bicortical screws with spiked washers (Linvatec)	769 N[79]	69 N/mm[79]	4.2 mm after 1500 cycles[79]	
RCI screw	350-419 N[92,151] Force required to produce 2 mm of laxity = 167 N[141]	40-248 N/mm[92,151]	3.7 mm at 500 N (4 of 7 failed at 500 N)[92]	
Arthrex bioabsorbable screw (35-mm length)	647 N[25]	64.5 N/mm[25]		10.9 mm[25]
Various bioabsorbable screws	439-830 N[79,149,150,152] Increasing screw length improves fixation strength[149]	41-115 N/mm[79,150,152]	3.8-4.7 mm after 1500 cycles[79] Corticocancellous fixation stronger than cancellous-only fixation[64]	
Sutures over a screw post	374-442 N[92,101]	24-60 N/mm[92,101]	4.9 mm at 500 N	
Double soft-tissue staple	785 N[92]	118 N/mm[92]	3.3 mm at 500 N[92]	
20-mm spiked washer/screw	724 N[92]	126 N/mm[92]	3.5 mm at 500 N[92]	
Stirrup (Corifix)	898 N[54]		2.1 mm after 1100 cycles of 150 N[54]	

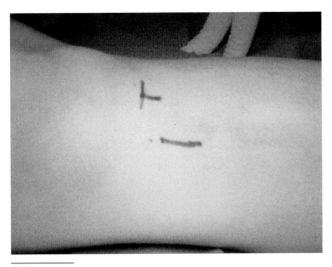

Figure 40–1. Picture of a skin incision for hamstring tendon harvest. The 1.5-inch incision is made approximately 2 cm medial to the tibial tubercle.

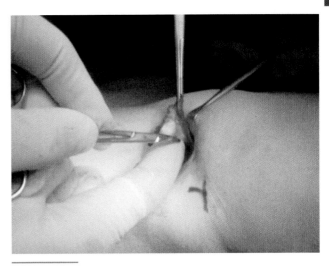

Figure 40–3. Extratendinous bands from the semitendinosus tendon.

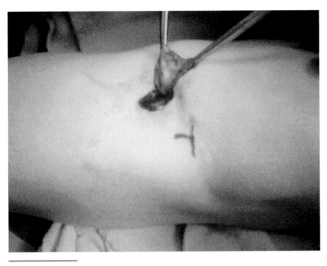

Figure 40–2. Visualization of the undersurface of the semitendinosus and gracilis tendons. Note the natural separation.

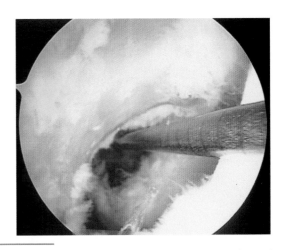

Figure 40–4. Arthroscopic view of the posterolateral wall of the notch after débridement of scar and the ACL remnant.

Arthroscopy and ACL Reconstruction

All arthroscopies are videotaped so that the surgeon can review the case. Standard anterolateral and anteromedial arthroscopic portals in the knee are fashioned, and diagnostic arthroscopy is performed. A pressurized fluid delivery system is routinely used for all ACL reconstructions. Articular and meniscal cartilage lesions are treated as indicated. After exsanguination and application of a thigh tourniquet, the notch is débrided of scar and the old ACL remnant to clearly visualize the ACL footprint on the tibia, as well as the posterolateral wall of the notch (Fig. 40–4). A bony notchplasty or roofplasty is not routinely performed unless there is evidence of notch stenosis or notch/roof impingement on the graft.

A tibial guide is used to aim and drill a guide pin through the ACL footprint, approximately 5 to 7 mm anterior to the posterior cruciate ligament (Fig. 40–5). Before the surgeon drills the tibial tunnel, the knee is placed in

(Fig. 40–2). The tendons are separated, and each tendon is whipstitched with nonabsorbable suture. Using blunt dissection, the tendons are freed from surrounding adventitia. In addition, Intrafix extratendinous bands are incised to completely free up the tendons to their respective sheaths (Fig. 40–3). It is important to incise these fascial bands to prevent premature amputation of the tendon short of its muscle belly. The tendons are then harvested with a blunt-ended tendon stripper and taken to the back table, where they are prepared by removing attached muscle. The tendons are cut to give an overall length of 24 cm, and the free ends are whipstitched with No. 2 braided polyester suture. The tendons are looped to give a four-stranded graft, and the graft is sized in preparation for tunnel drilling.

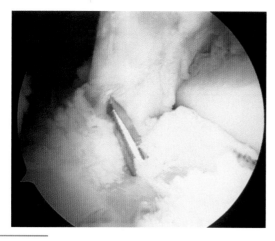

Figure 40–5. Arthroscopic view of a drill pin through the ACL footprint, approximately 5 to 7 mm anterior to the PCL.

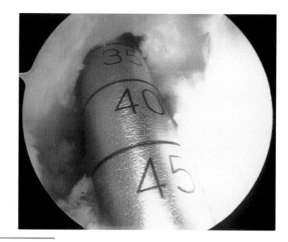

Figure 40–7. Femoral tunnel cannulated reamer, drilled to 35 to 40 mm.

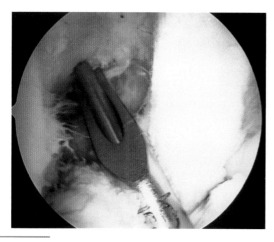

Figure 40–6. Five-millimeter offset femoral tunnel guide inserted through the tibial tunnel and locked in the over-the-top position by flexing the knee to 90 degrees.

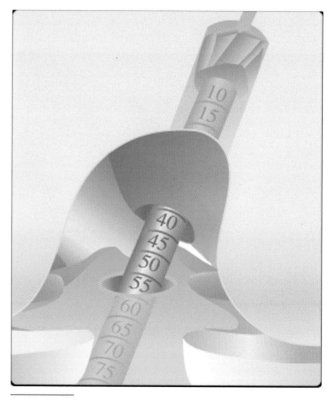

Figure 40–8. Femoral tunnel cannulated reamer, drilled to 35 to 40 mm. (Courtesy of Arthrex.)

full extension and checked for any roof impingement by the guide pin. The tibial tunnel is initially drilled with a cannulated drill corresponding to the diameter of the four-stranded graft. Previously, we sequentially enlarged the tibial tunnel with tunnel impactors to the desired tunnel diameter to, theoretically, increase the strength of tibial tunnel interference screw fixation as a result of increased bone density in the tunnel. Recent cadaveric studies,[106,107] however, have shown that tunnel impaction does not increase fixation strength, and thus we have abandoned this technique. After tibial tunnel drilling, the intra-articular entrance of the tunnel is smoothed with a hand rasp or powered chamfering tool.

Attention is then directed to making the femoral tunnel. A transtibial offset guide is used to direct a guide pin in the desired location of the femoral tunnel. The guide is inserted through the tibial tunnel and locked in the over-the-top position by flexing the knee to 90 degrees (Fig. 40–6). The guide pin is directed at the 10-o'clock (right

knee) or the 2-o'clock (left knee) position and drilled to the anterior femoral cortex. In the past, we attempted to create the insertion point at the 11- and 1-o'clock positions, respectively. However, recent data suggest that a more obliquely oriented femoral tunnel is better at resisting complex rotatory loads.[87,126] The femoral tunnel is drilled to 35 to 40 mm with the appropriately sized cannulated reamer (Figs. 40–7 and 40–8). The guide pin and cannulated reamer are then removed from the knee.

The Arthrex TransFix II femoral guide, with a tunnel hook that corresponds to the diameter of the femoral tunnel, is placed through the tibial tunnel and into the femoral tunnel. A small stab incision is made over the lateral femoral condyle, and dissection is carried down through the iliotibial band to the cortex. The guide pin sleeve is then seated onto the lateral femoral condyle. (Note: The femoral drill pin will enter the femoral tunnel eccentrically if the guide sleeve is positioned too firmly against the lateral femoral condyle.) A 3-mm drill pin is then drilled through the guide sleeve and tunnel hook and made to exit out on the medial side of the knee (Fig. 40–9). A cortex broach is used to open the lateral cortex to 5 mm (Fig. 40–10). A nitinol graft-passing wire is connected to the 3-mm guide pin slot. The guide pin is pulled medially to pull the nitinol wire through the tunnel hook and across the knee (Fig. 40–11). The TransFix II femoral guide is retracted out of the knee, thereby pulling a loop of the nitinol wire out of the tibial tunnel (Fig. 40–12). The semitendinosus and gracilis tendons are looped over the wire, and the wire is then tensioned medially and laterally, which pulls the graft into the femoral tunnel (Fig. 40–13). The Bio-TransFix Dilator may be inserted over the nitinol wire to ensure proper graft positioning (Fig. 40–14). A 40- or 50-mm Bio-TransFix implant is then inserted over the nitinol wire and made to seat flush on the lateral femoral cortex (Fig. 40–15). To aid in passing of the TransFix device, the wire should be tensioned by pulling on the wire both medially and laterally. The wire is then removed. If a metallic cross-pin device is used, adequate seating of the cross-pin on the lateral femoral condyle can be ensured by fluoroscopy (Fig. 40–16).

The knee is taken through several cycles of motion before tibial fixation. Cycling of the graft theoretically helps precondition the graft and eliminate creep and is also a means for the surgeon to assess the tension behav-

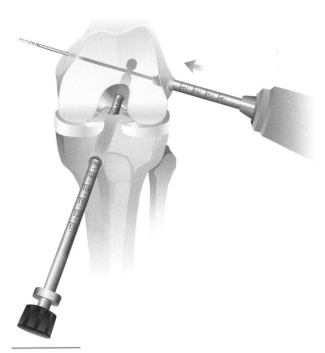

Figure 40–10. The lateral cortex is opened to 5 mm with a cannulated cortex broach. (Courtesy of Arthrex.)

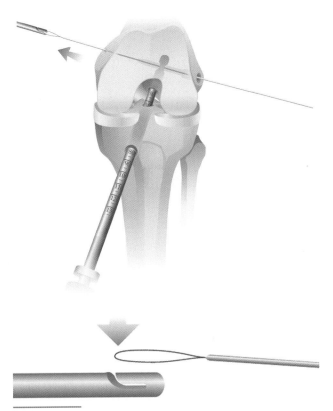

Figure 40–11. A nitinol wire is connected in the slot on the 3-mm drill pin and pulled across the femoral tunnel. (Courtesy of Arthrex.)

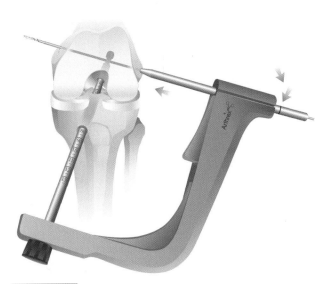

Figure 40–9. TransFix II femoral guide with a pin guide sleeve against the lateral femoral cortex and a 3-mm drill pin drilled across the femoral tunnel. (Courtesy of Arthrex.)

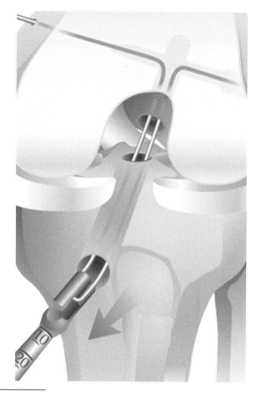

Figure 40–12. The TransFix II guide is retracted out of the knee, with a loop of the nitinol wire pulled out of the tibial tunnel. (Courtesy of Arthrex.)

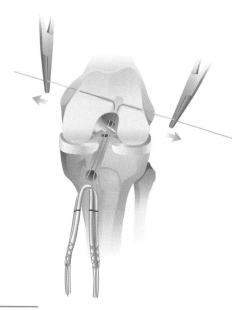

Figure 40–13. The semitendinosus and gracilis tendons are looped over the nitinol wire and pulled into place in the femoral tunnel by tensioning the nitinol wire both medially and laterally. (Courtesy of Arthrex.)

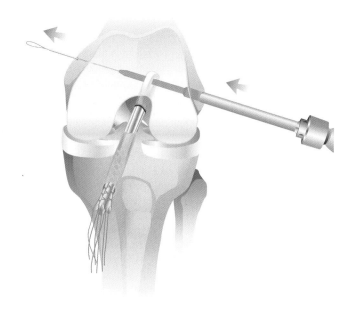

Figure 40–14. A TransFix dilator can be inserted over the nitinol wire to ensure proper graft positioning. (Courtesy of Arthrex.)

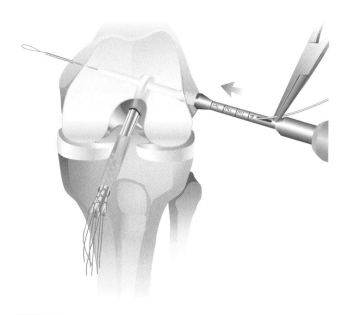

Figure 40–15. The Bio-TransFix implant is inserted over the nitinol wire and made to seat flush with the lateral femoral cortex. (Courtesy of Arthrex.)

ior of the graft with flexion and extension. Initial graft tension has been demonstrated to decrease with cyclic loading.[19,108] A recent study showed a 60% decrease in graft tension within 60 minutes after fixation and thus has called into question the ability of preconditioning of

the graft to eliminate its intrinsic viscoelasticity.[108] Nevertheless, we continue to precondition and cycle the graft before tibial fixation. The knee is positioned between full extension and approximately 20 degrees of flexion. Tibial fixation is achieved by using the Mitek Intrafix device. The four-limb graft tie tensioner is connected to the limbs of the graft, and 25 lb of longitudinal tension is applied (Fig. 40–17). The tunnel is dilated with the Intrafix Sheath Trial

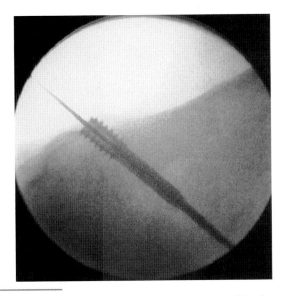

Figure 40–16. Fluoroscopic view of a metallic femoral cross-pin to ensure that the pin is adequately seated on the lateral femoral condyle.

Dilator (Fig. 40–18), and the 30-mm Intrafix tibial sheath is then inserted so that each limb of the graft is in one of the four quadrants (Fig. 40–19). A tapered polyethylene screw, an 8/10-mm tapered screw in most cases, is then inserted into the center of the sheath to compress the graft limbs against the sides of the tibial tunnel (Figs. 40–20 and 40–21).

The wounds are irrigated well and closed in layers, and a sterile dressing is applied. A range-of-motion brace and cold flow therapy are routinely used in all patients.

POSTOPERATIVE MANAGEMENT

ACL reconstructions are performed on an outpatient basis. Patients are encouraged to use the ice therapy unit as much as tolerable and to bear weight as tolerated with the use of crutches. Patients are instructed to change their dressing after 48 hours.

The excellent graft strength and fixation, as well as the lack of extensor mechanism disruption, allow patients to rehabilitate the knee aggressively. An accelerated rehabilitation program, originally described for use after ACL reconstructions with a patellar tendon autograft,[131-133] has been shown to be equally successful after ACL reconstructions with a hamstring graft.[68-70,89] In cases in which fixations are not as strong or stiff as the femoral TransFix or tibial Intrafix, aggressive and early return to sports may lead to postoperative laxity.[51] Unlimited range of motion, with an emphasis on full extension, and weightbearing are encouraged immediately postoperatively. Physical therapy is started at the 1-week postoperative visit. The goal of therapy is to allow a return to unlimited sporting activities by 4 to 6 months postoperatively. Our current postoperative rehabilitation protocol is shown in Table 40–2.

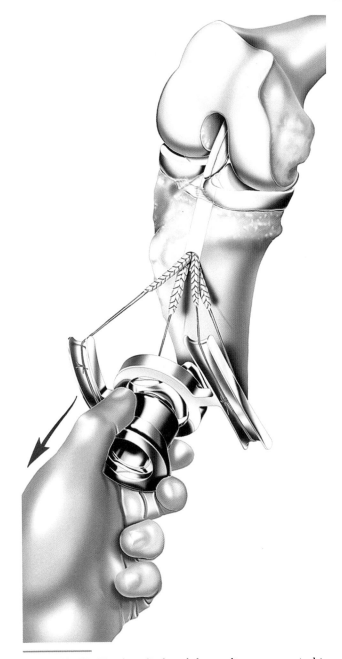

Figure 40–17. The four limbs of the graft are connected to the tie tensioner, and 25 lb of traction is applied. (Courtesy of Arthrex.)

COMPLICATIONS AND THEIR TREATMENT

Complications in ACL surgery can be classified as intraoperative complications (errors in technique) and postoperative complications. Intraoperative complications, such as improper tunnel placement, and postoperative complications, such as arthrofibrosis, motion problems, infection, hemarthrosis, injury to the infrapatellar branch of the saphenous nerve, and deep venous thrombosis, are not unique to ACL reconstructions with hamstring tendons and are not discussed in this chapter.

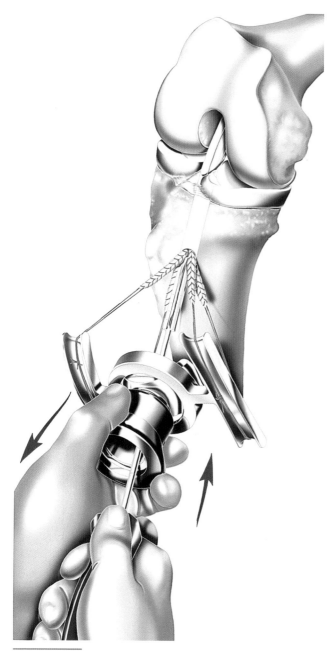

Figure 40–18. The tibial tunnel is dilated to 8 mm with the Intrafix Sheath Trial Dilator. (Courtesy of Mitek.)

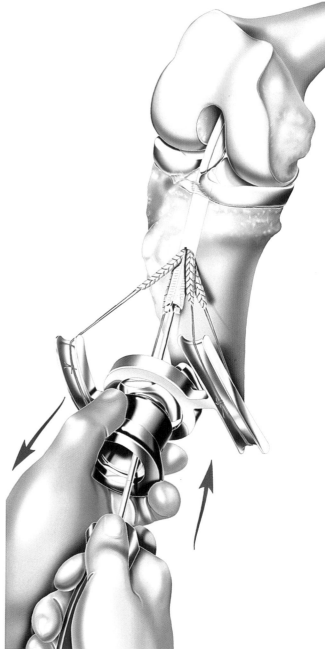

Figure 40–19. A 30-mm Intrafix tibial sheath is inserted into the tibial tunnel with one limb of the graft in each of the four quadrants. (Courtesy of Mitek.)

One of the most common complications seen in hamstring ACL reconstructions is that of premature amputation of the pes tendons because of the surgeon's failure to incise all extratendinous fascial bands (see Fig. 40–3). If these bands are not appreciated or recognized, the tendon stripper can take an aberrant path, and the tendons will be cut short of their muscle belly. If this occurs, the tendon can still be used in the reconstruction, provided that at least 12 cm of tendon is harvested, which is the minimum length that will allow the tendon to be doubled and still have at least 15 mm of graft in the femoral and tibial tunnels. Short grafts can be accommodated by using fixation devices with polyester tape (EndoButton, Acufex,

Smith and Nephew, Mansfield, MA, or FastLok, Neoligaments, Ltd., Leeds, UK) or by using a fixation device that secures the graft in the femoral tunnel, such as a femoral cross-pin. A short graft can be accommodated on the tibial side by extending the graft with polyester tape woven through the tendons and secured onto the tibial cortex with FastLok or a similar device. Sutures and polyester tape are relatively elastic.[140] By incorporating these materials into the graft, the entire construct (fixation–polyester tape–graft–polyester tape–fixation) dramatically loses

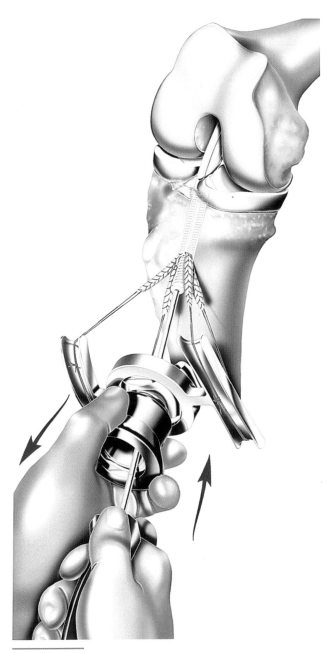

Figure 40–20. A tapered polyethylene screw in inserted into the center of the Intrafix sheath to compress the graft against the sides of the tunnel. (Courtesy of Mitek.)

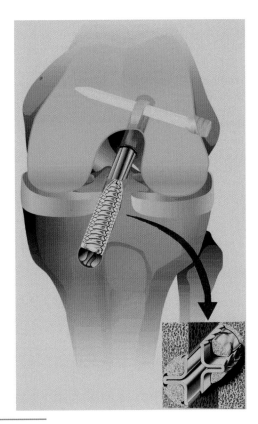

Figure 40–21. Final graft fixation in the femur and tibia. (Courtesy of Arthrex and Mitek.)

stiffness to the point that it may not withstand the force seen with full range of active motion and full weightbearing. Consideration should be given to modifying the postoperative rehabilitation protocol should this situation arise.

Failure of fixation, which includes loss and slippage, has been a concern of many of the surgeons who perform ACL reconstructions with hamstring tendons and probably the biggest reason that some surgeons are reluctant to change from the patellar tendon graft. Loss of fixation[42,43,58] and slippage of fixation[56,92,142] have been a problem only with fixations that relied on a polyester suture or tape interface with the tendon graft. The Bio-

TransFix femoral fixation technique and the tibial fixation technique of Intrafix avoid the suture/tape interface and, as such, are strong enough to withstand the force seen during activities of daily living. In addition, these fixation methods are less susceptible to graft slippage during these applied loads.[6,42,46,79] All ACL surgeons, however, must be familiar with various fixation options, including the suture post, screw/washer devices, FastLok, and others, should the primary fixation method prove to be unsatisfactory during the procedure. Failure of fixation can occur in the femoral tunnel if the surgeon plans to use a soft-tissue interference screw and the posterior wall of the femoral tunnel is disrupted (back wall blowout). If such disruption occurs, the surgeon must be familiar with the cross-pin technique, the EndoButton technique, and the two-incision technique to allow for fixation on the femoral cortex.

Another theoretical concern of ACL reconstructions with hamstring tendons is that of postoperative hamstring weakness. Some authors[86,91,156] have demonstrated that postoperative hamstring weakness is of little functional significance, whereas others[27,36,143] have shown persistent knee flexor weakness postoperatively. Regrowth of the semitendinosus has been reported to occur,[53,83,143] and the regenerate tendon may have an effect on minimizing postoperative weakness. Several recent articles[1,98,110,143,144] have suggested that the peak flexion torque and total work performed are not different from that in the nonoperative limb postoperatively. However, the flexion angle at peak torque is shifted to a shallower angle. From a practical standpoint, patients may complain of knee flexor weak-

Table 40–2. Hamstring ACL Reconstruction Rehabilitation Protocol

GOALS	EXERCISES
Phase I (Initial 2 Weeks Postoperatively)	
Alleviate pain/inflammation	ROM, PROM positioning for knee extension
Full, symmetric extension by 1 week	Hamstring stretch
90 degrees of flexion by 1 week	Heel slides/wall slides without brace
Weightbearing as tolerated with crutches	1/2 revolutions on nonresistant bicycle
Discard crutches at 2 weeks	Patellar/soft-tissue and scar mobilization
	Multiple-angle closed-chain isometrics
	Prone knee flexion
	Theraband to ankle
	4-quadrant hip exercises (weight above knee)
	Standing weight shifts and minisquats (0-30)
	Electrical stimulation as needed
Phase II (2-6 Weeks Postoperatively)	
Decrease swelling/prevent quadriceps atrophy	Continue PROM at 0-125 degrees, emphasis on full extension
Full symmetric extension	Continue phase I exercises
Flexion to 125 degrees	Stairmaster/Nordic Track at 2-3 weeks
Increase quadriceps/hamstring strength	Leg press
Increase hip strength	Trampoline and BAPS board for balance
	Electrical stimulation as needed
	Continue closed kinetic chain exercises
	Calf raises
	Pool therapy at 3 weeks
	Hinged brace for prolonged ambulation
Phase III (6 Weeks to 4 Months Postoperatively)	
Full, symmetric ROM	Continue phase II exercises
Independent ambulation without brace	Increased closed kinetic chain rehabilitation (step-ups, minisquats)
	Increase proprioception training (sport cord, body blade, Plyoballs)
	Light jogging at 3 months
Phase IV (4 Months to Full Activity)	
Development of strength, power, and endurance	Continue strengthening exercises
Prepare for return to full activity	Initiate hard running and agility drills
Begin sport-specific training	Sport-specific training and drills
	Return to full sports at 5-6 months

BAPS, biomechanical ankle platform system; PROM, passive range of motion; ROM, range of motion.

ness in activities that require high flexion angles, such as removing a cowboy boot. Persistent weakness in internal rotation has also been reported.[9,127,148] The clinical implications of internal rotation weakness have not been determined.

Tunnel expansion and widening appear to occur universally after ACL reconstruction with autogenous hamstring tendons[33,52,73,84,88,154] and to a greater degree than seen with the use of autogenous patellar tendon grafts.[33] Expansion of the femoral tunnel diameter by up to 77% and the tibial tunnel diameter by up to 42% has been reported.[33,88] Tunnel expansion, however, has not been shown to correlate with outcome[33,52,73,84,88,154] and occurs despite the presence or absence of aperture fixation.[88] Magnetic resonance imaging studies have shown that this tunnel expansion is due, in part, to an accumulation of periligamentous tissue around the graft.[73] Although tunnel expansion does correlate with outcome, it can be a treatment challenge in patients who require a revision ACL reconstruction.

The final complication that can occur after ACL reconstruction with the semitendinosus and gracilis tendons is that of graft failure. Graft failure is usually due to improper

tunnel placement, tension, or fixation. However, the surgeon can expect an approximately 2% retearing rate per year after reconstruction, even when the procedures are performed satisfactorily.[130] Freedman and colleagues' meta-analysis of hamstring and patellar tendon grafts showed graft failure to be less common in patellar tendon patients.[49] A recent article by Williams[154] reported a 11% failure rate at a mean of 28 months' follow-up, 7% of which were thought to be due to traumatic reinjury/tearing of the graft and 4% not due to any further trauma. Toritsuka et al[146] reported on the findings of second-look arthroscopy 5 to 51 months after ACL reconstruction with a hamstring graft. They found that although all patients were considered a clinical success, 11% of the grafts showed evidence of laxity and 34% had partial tearing.[146]

Graft failure because of technical error can occur for a variety of reasons, including graft impingement on the roof or lateral sidewall of the notch and improper tunnel placement leading to overtension in the graft. It is important for the surgeon to check pin placement before drilling the tibial and femoral tunnels. It is also important to check that there is ample clearance for the tibial guide pin from the roof and lateral sidewall when the knee is fully extended. A roofplasty and lateral notchplasty should be performed if there is any concern of graft impingement. However, graft impingement should not be a common problem, provided that the tibial and femoral tunnels are properly placed. As mentioned, the tibial tunnel should be in the center of the ACL footprint, approximately 5 to 8 mm anterior to the posterior cruciate ligament and 70 to 80 degrees in the coronal plane. The femoral tunnel should be at the 10-o'clock (right knee) or 2-o'clock (left knee) position and should have a posterior wall 1 to 2 mm thick.

SUMMARY

ACL reconstruction is a common procedure in the orthopedic community and is successful in restoring anterior stability to the knee in 75% to 90% of patients. ACL reconstruction with hamstring tendons is an excellent surgical option for most patients. The hamstring graft has many advantages, including strength, stiffness, and relative lack of donor site morbidity. Hamstring graft fixation with a femoral cross-pin (Bio-TransFix) and an interference screw/sheath device (Intrafix) on the tibial side is a strong and stiff ACL construct that easily allows patients to begin an aggressive rehabilitation program immediately postoperatively.

References

1. Adachi N, Ochi M, Uchio Y: Harvesting hamstring tendons for ACL reconstruction influences postoperative hamstring muscle performance. Arch Orthop Trauma Surg 123:460, 2003.
2. Aglietti P, Buzzi R, D'Andria S: Arthroscopic anterior cruciate ligament reconstruction with patellar tendon. Arthroscopy 8:510, 1992.
3. Aglietti P, Buzzi R, D'Andria S: Patellofemoral problems after intraarticular anterior cruciate ligament reconstruction. Clin Orthop 288:195, 1993.
4. Aglietti P, Buzzi R, Menchetti P: Arthroscopically assisted semitendinosus and gracilis tendon graft in reconstruction for acute anterior cruciate ligament injuries in athletes. Am J Sports Med 24:726, 1996.
5. Aglietti P, Buzzi R, Zaccherotti G: Patellar tendon versus semitendinosus and gracilis tendons for anterior cruciate ligament reconstruction. Am J Sports Med 22:211, 1994.
6. Ahmad C, Gardner T, Groh M: Mechanical properties of soft tissue femoral fixation devices for anterior cruciate ligament reconstruction. Am J Sports Med 32:635, 2004.
7. Anderson A, Snyder R, Lipscomb A: Anterior cruciate ligament reconstruction. A prospective randomized study of three surgical methods. Am J Sports Med 29:272, 2001.
8. Arendt EA, Hunter RE, Schneider WT: Vascularized patellar tendon anterior cruciate ligament reconstruction. Clin Orthop 244:222, 1989.
9. Armour T, Forwell L, Litchfield R, et al: Isokinetic evaluation of internal/external tibial rotation strength after the use of hamstring tendons for anterior cruciate ligament reconstruction. Am J Sports Med 32:1639, 2004.
10. Arneja S, Froese W, MacDonald P: Augmentation of femoral fixation in hamstring anterior cruciate ligament reconstruction with a bioabsorbable bead. Am J Sports Med 32:159, 2004.
11. Athanasiou K: Arthrex Bio-Interference Screw. Arthrex, Inc., Naples, FL.
12. Aune A, Holm I, Risberg M: Four-strand hamstring tendon autograft compared with patellar tendon–bone autograft for anterior cruciate ligament reconstruction. A randomized study with two-year follow-up. Am J Sports Med 29:722, 2001.
13. Barber F, Small N, Click J: Anterior cruciate ligament reconstruction by semitendinosus and gracilis tendon autograft. Am J Knee Surg 4:84, 1991.
14. Barrack R, Bruckner J, Kneisl J: The outcome on nonoperatively treated complete tears of the anterior cruciate ligament in active young adults. Clin Orthop 259:192, 1990.
15. Barrett G, Noojin F, Hartzog C: Reconstruction of the anterior cruciate ligament in females: A comparison of hamstring versus patellar tendon autograft. Arthroscopy 18:46, 2002.
16. Beard D, Anderson A, Davies S: Hamstrings vs. patella tendon for anterior cruciate ligament reconstruction: A randomised controlled trial. Knee 8:45-50, 2001.
17. Beynnon B, Johnson R, Fleming B: Anterior cruciate ligament replacement: Comparison of bone–patellar tendon–bone grafts with two-strand hamstring grafts. J Bone Joint Surg Am 84:1503, 2002.
18. Beynnon B, Johnson R, Kannus P: A prospective, randomized clinical investigation of anterior cruciate ligament reconstruction: A comparison of the bone–patellar tendon–bone and semitendinosus-gracilis autograft. Arthroscopy 14:20, 1998.
19. Boylan D, Greis P, West J: Effects of initial graft tension on knee stability after anterior cruciate ligament reconstruction using hamstring tendons: A cadaver study. Arthroscopy 19:700, 2003.
20. Brown C, Sklar J: Endoscopic anterior cruciate ligament reconstruction using quadrupled hamstring tendons and endobutton femoral fixation. Tech Orthop 13:281, 1998.
21. Brown C, Steiner M, Carson E: The use of hamstring tendons for anterior cruciate ligament reconstruction: Technique and results. Clin Sports Med 12:723, 1993.
22. Buelow J, Siebold R, Ellermann A: A new bicortical tibial fixation technique in anterior cruciate ligament reconstruction with quadruple hamstring graft. Knee Surg Sports Traumatol Arthrosc 8:218, 2000.
23. Buss D, Warren R, Wickiewicz T: Arthroscopically assisted reconstruction of the anterior cruciate ligament with use of autogenous patellar-ligament grafts. J Bone Joint Surg Am 75:1346, 1993.
24. Butler D, Grood E, Noyes F: On the interpretation of our anterior cruciate ligament data. Clin Orthop 196:26, 1985.
25. Caborn D, Brand J, Nyland J: A biomechanical comparison of initial soft tissue tibial fixation devices. The Intrafix versus a tapered 35 mm bioabsorbable interference screw. Am J Sports Med 32:956, 2004.
26. Calloway G, Nicholas S, Cavanaugh J: Hamstring augmentation versus patella tendon reconstruction of acute anterior cruciate ligament disruption: A randomized prospective study. Orthop Trans 18:1017, 1994.
27. Carter T, Edinger S: Isokinetic evaluation of anterior cruciate ligament reconstruction: Hamstring versus patellar tendon. Arthroscopy 15:169, 1999.
28. Charlton W, Randolph D, Lemos S: Clinical outcome of anterior cruciate ligament reconstruction with quadrupled hamstring tendon graft and bioabsorbable interference screw fixation. Am J Sports Med 31:518, 2003.
29. Chen E, Black J: Materials design analysis of the prosthetic anterior cruciate ligament. J Biomed Mater Res 14:567, 1980.
30. Cho K: Reconstruction of the anterior cruciate ligament by semitendinosus tenodesis. J Bone Joint Surg Am 57:608, 1975.
31. Clancy W, Nelson D, Reider B: Anterior cruciate ligament reconstruction using one-third of the patellar ligament, augmented by extra-articular tendon transfers. J Bone Joint Surg Am 64:352, 1982.
32. Clark R, Olsen R, Larson B: Cross-pin femoral fixation: A new technique for hamstring anterior cruciate ligament reconstruction on the knee. Arthroscopy 14:258, 1998.
33. Clatworthy M, Annear P, Bulow J, Bartlett R: Tunnel widening in anterior cruciate ligament reconstruction: A prospective evaluation of hamstring and patella tendon grafts. Knee Surg Sports Traumatol Arthrosc 7:138, 1999.
34. Collins S, Tresnan J: FastLoc Fixation System. Neoligaments, Ltd., Leeds, UK.

35. Cooley V, Deffner K, Rosenberg T: Quadrupled semitendinosus anterior cruciate ligament reconstruction: 5-year results in patients without meniscus loss. Arthroscopy 17:795, 2001.

36. Coombs R, Cochrane T: Knee flexor strength following anterior cruciate ligament reconstruction with the semitendinosus and gracilis tendons. Int J Sports Med 22:618, 2001.

37. Cooper D, Deng X, Burnstein A: The strength of the central third patellar tendon graft. Am J Sports Med 21:818, 1993.

38. Corry I, Webb J, Clingeleffer A: Arthroscopic reconstruction of the anterior cruciate ligament. A comparison of patellar tendon autograft and four-stranded hamstring tendon autograft. Am J Sports Med 27:444, 1999.

39. Cullison T, O'Brien T, Getka K: Anterior cruciate ligament reconstruction in the military patient. Mil Med 163:17, 1998.

40. Doral M, Leblebicioglu G, Atay O: Arthroscopy-assisted anterior cruciate ligament reconstruction with patellar tendon or hamstring autografts. Bull Hosp Jt Dis 59:81, 2000.

41. Ejerhed L, Kartus J, Sernert N: Patellar tendon or semitendinosus tendon autografts for anterior cruciate ligament reconstruction? A prospective randomized study with a two-year follow-up. Am J Sports Med 31:19, 2003.

42. Ellis B, Weiss J: Cyclic stability of the Smith and Nephew continuous loop endobutton when used for hamstring-grafted ACL reconstruction. Smith and Nephew Endoscopy. Mansfield, MA.

43. Ellis B, Weiss J: In vitro evaluation of initial pullout strength of the Innovasive Devices Inc LinX HT hamstring tendon fastener in cancellous bone. Innovasive Devices. Marlborough, MA.

44. Eriksson K, Anderberg P, Hamberg P: There are differences in early morbidity after ACL reconstruction when comparing patellar tendon and semitendinosus tendon graft. A prospective randomized study of 107 patients. Scand J Med Sci Sports 11:170, 2001.

45. Eriksson K, Anderberg P, Hamberg P: A comparison of quadruple semitendinosus and patellar tendon grafts in reconstruction of the anterior cruciate ligament. J Bone Joint Surg Br 83:348, 2001.

46. Fabbriciani C, Milano G, Fadda S: Comparison of different femoral fixation devices for ACL reconstruction with hamstring tendon grafts. A biomechanical study on porcine knees. University of Sassari, Sassari, Italy. On file, Arthrex, Inc., Naples, FL, 2001.

47. Feller J, Webster K: A randomized comparison of patellar tendon and hamstring tendon anterior cruciate ligament reconstruction. Am J Sports Med 31:564, 2003.

48. Ferretti, A, Conteduca, F, Morelli F, et al: The Evolgate: A method to improve the pullout strength of interference screws in tibial fixation of anterior cruciate ligament reconstruction with doubled gracilis and semitendinosus tendons. Arthroscopy, 19:936, 2003.

49. Freedman K, D'Amato M, Nedeff D: Arthroscopic anterior cruciate ligament reconstruction: A metaanalysis comparing patellar tendon and hamstring tendon autografts. Am J Sports Med 31:2, 2003.

50. Fu F, Hoher J, Withrow J: Early stress causes graft-tunnel motion in hamstring grafts. In ACL Study Group. Beaver Creek, CO, 1998.

51. Fujimoto E, Sumen Y, Urabe Y: An early return to vigorous activity may destabilize anterior cruciate ligaments reconstructed with hamstring grafts. Arch Phys Med Rehabil 85:298, 2004.

52. Fules P, Madhav R, Goddard R: Evaluation of tibial bone tunnel enlargement using MRI scan cross-sectional area measurement after autologous hamstring tendon ACL replacement. Knee 10:87, 2003.

53. Gill S, Turner M, Battaglia T: Semitendinosus regrowth: Biochemical, ultrastructural, and physiological characterization of the regenerate tendon. Am J Sports Med 32:1173, 2004.

54. Giurea M, Zorilla P, Amis A: Comparative pull-out and cyclic-loading strength tests of anchorage of hamstring tendon grafts in anterior cruciate ligament reconstruction. Am J Sports Med 27:621, 1999.

55. Gobbi A, Domzalski M, Pascual J: Comparison of anterior cruciate ligament reconstruction in male and female athletes using the patellar tendon and hamstring autografts. Knee Surg Sports Traumatol Arthrosc 12:534, 2004.

56. Gomes J, Marczyk L: Anterior cruciate ligament reconstruction with a loop or double thickness of semitendinosus tendon. Am J Sports Med 12:199, 1984.

57. Goradia V, Grana W: A comparison of outcomes at 2 to 6 years after acute and chronic anterior cruciate ligament reconstruction using hamstring tendon grafts. Arthroscopy 17:383, 2001.

58. Goradia V, Rochat M, Grana W: Strength of ACL reconstructions using semitendinosus tendon grafts. J Okla State Med Assoc 91:275, 1998.

59. Goradia V, Rochat M, Grana W: Tendon-to-bone healing of a semitendinosus tendon autograft used for ACL reconstruction in a sheep model. Am J Knee Surg 13:143, 2000.

60. Goradia V, Rochat M, Kida M, Grana W: Natural history of a hamstring tendon autograft used for anterior cruciate ligament reconstruction in a sheep model. Am J Sports Med 28:40, 2000.

61. Grana W, Egle D, Mahnken R: An analysis of autograft fixation after anterior cruciate ligament reconstruction in a rabbit model. Am J Sports Med 22:344, 1994.

62. Grana W, Hines R: Arthroscopically-assisted semitendinosus reconstruction of the anterior cruciate ligament. Am J Knee Surg 5:16, 1992.

63. Hamner D, Brown C, Steiner M: Hamstring tendon grafts for reconstruction of the anterior cruciate ligament: Biomechanical evaluation of the use of multiple strands and tensioning techniques. J Bone Joint Surg Am 81:549, 1999.

64. Harvey A, Thomas N, Amis A: The effect of screw length and position on fixation of four-stranded hamstring grafts for anterior cruciate ligament reconstruction. Knee 10:97, 2003.

65. Hecker A, Brown C, Deffner K: Tensile properties of young multi-stranded hamstring grafts. Presented at a meeting of the American Orthopaedic Society for Sports Medicine, 1997, San Francisco.

66. Holden J, Grood E, Korvick D: In vivo forces in the anterior cruciate ligament: Direct measurements during walking and trotting in a quadruped. J Biomech 27:517, 1994.

67. Holmes P, James S, Larson R: Retrospective direct comparison of three intraarticular anterior cruciate ligament reconstructions. Am J Sports Med 19:596, 1991.

68. Howell S, Deutsch M: Comparison of endoscopic and two-incision technique for reconstructing a torn anterior cruciate ligament using hamstring tendons. Arthroscopy 15:594, 1999.

69. Howell S, Hull M: Aggressive rehabilitation using hamstring tendons. Am J Knee Surg 11:120, 1998.

70. Howell S, Taylor M: Brace-free rehabilitation, with early return to activities, for knees reconstructed with a double-looped, semitendinosus and gracilis graft. J Bone Joint Surg Am 78:814, 1996.

71. Ishibashi Y, Rudy T, Livesay G: The effect of anterior cruciate ligament graft fixation site at the tibia on knee stability: Evaluation using a robotic testing system. Arthroscopy 13:177, 1997.

72. Ivey M, Li F: Tensile strength of soft tissue fixations about the knee. Am J Knee Surg 4:18, 1991.

73. Jansson K, Harilainen A, Sandelin J: Bone tunnel enlargement after anterior cruciate ligament reconstruction with the hamstring autograft and endobutton fixation technique. A clinical, radiographic, and magnetic resonance imaging study with 2 years follow-up. Knee Surg Sports Traumatol Arthrosc 7:290, 1999.

74. Jansson K, Linko E, Sandelin J: A prospective randomized study of patellar versus hamstring tendon autografts for anterior cruciate ligament reconstruction. Am J Sports Med 31:12, 2003.

75. Johnson R, Eriksson E: Five-to ten-year follow-up evaluation after reconstruction of the anterior cruciate ligament. Clin Orthop 183:122, 1984.

76. Jones K: Reconstruction of the anterior cruciate ligament. J Bone Joint Surg Am 45:925, 1963.

77. Jones K: Reconstruction of the anterior cruciate ligament using the central one-third of the patellar ligament. J Bone Joint Surg Am 52:1302, 1970.

78. Kousa P, Jarvinen T, Vihavainen M: The fixation strength of six hamstring tendon graft fixation devices in anterior cruciate ligament reconstruction. Part I: Femoral site. Am J Sports Med 31:174, 2003.

79. Kousa P, Jarvinen T, Vihavainen M: The fixation strength of six hamstring tendon graft fixation devices in anterior cruciate ligament reconstruction. Part II: Tibial site. Am J Sports Med 31:182, 2003.

80. Kurosaka M, Yoshiya S, Andrish J: A biomechanical comparison of different surgical techniques of graft fixation in anterior cruciate ligament reconstruction. Am J Sports Med 15:225, 1987.

81. Kuster M, Wood G, Sakurai S: Downhill walking: A stressful task for the anterior cruciate ligament reconstructive surgery. Knee Surg Sports Traumatol Arthrosc 4:84, 1996.

82. Laxdal G, Kartus J, Hansson L: Patellar tendon or multiple-strand hamstring tendon autografts for anterior cruciate ligament reconstruction? A prospective randomised study using three different graft types with a two-year follow-up. Presented at the 11th ESSKA

Congress and 4th World Congress on Sports Trauma, 2004, Athens, Greece.

83. Leis H, Sanders T, Larsen K: Hamstring regrowth following harvesting for ACL reconstruction: The lizard tail phenomenon. J Knee Surg 16:159, 2003.

84. L'Insalata J, Klatt B, Fu F: Tunnel expansion following anterior cruciate ligament reconstruction: A comparison of hamstring and patellar tendon autografts. Knee Surg Sports Traumatol Arthrosc 5:234, 1997.

85. Lipscomb A, Johnston R, Snyder R: Secondary reconstruction of anterior cruciate ligament in athletes using the semitendinosus tendon. Am J Sports Med 7:81, 1979.

86. Lipscomb A, Johnston R, Snyder R: Evaluation of hamstring strength following use of semitendinosus and gracilis tendons to reconstruct the anterior cruciate ligament. Am J Sports Med 10:340, 1982.

87. Loh J, Fukuda Y, Tsuda E: Knee stability and graft function following anterior cruciate ligament reconstruction: Comparison between 11 o'clock and 10 o'clock femoral tunnel placement. Arthroscopy 19:297, 2003.

88. Ma C, Francis K, Towers J: Hamstring anterior cruciate ligament reconstruction: A comparison of bioabsorbable interference screw and endobutton-post fixation. Arthroscopy 20:122, 2004.

89. MacDonald P, Hedden D, Huebert D: Effects of an accelerated rehabilitation program after anterior cruciate ligament reconstruction with combined semitendinosus-gracilis and a ligament augmentation device. Am J Sports Med 23:588, 1995.

90. Macey H: A new operative procedure for repair of ruptured cruciate ligaments of the knee joint. Surg Gynecol Obstet 69:108, 1939.

91. Maeda A, Shino K, Horibe S: Anterior cruciate ligament reconstruction with multistranded autogenous semitendinosus tendon. Am J Sports Med 24:504, 1996.

92. Magen H, Howell S, Hull M: Structural properties of six tibial fixation methods for anterior cruciate ligament soft tissue grafts. Am J Sports Med 27:35, 1999.

93. Marder R, Raskind J, Carroll M: Prospective evaluation of arthroscopically assisted anterior cruciate ligament reconstruction: Patellar tendon versus semitendinosus and gracilis tendons. Am J Sports Med 19:478, 1991.

94. Marumoto J, Mitsunaga M, Richardson A: Late patellar tendon rupture after removal of the central third for anterior cruciate ligament reconstruction. Am J Sports Med 24:698, 1996.

95. Mologne T, Crabb I, Grover, I: Hamstring versus patellar tendon ACL reconstruction in the active duty patient: Preliminary results of a prospective, randomized study. Orthop Trans 20:912, 1996.

96. Mott H: Semitendinosus anatomic reconstruction for cruciate ligament insufficiency. Clin Orthop 172:90, 1983.

97. Moyer R, Betz R, Iaquinto J: Arthroscopic anterior cruciate reconstruction using the semitendinosus and gracilis tendons: Preliminary report. Contemp Orthop 12:17, 1986.

98. Nakamura N, Horibe S, Sasaki S: Evaluation of active knee flexion and hamstring strength after anterior cruciate ligament reconstruction using hamstring tendons. Arthroscopy 18:598, 2002.

99. Nebelung W, Becker R, Urback D: Histological findings of tendon-bone healing following anterior cruciate ligament reconstruction with hamstring grafts. Arch Orthop Trauma Surg 123:158, 2003.

100. Noojin F, Barrett G, Hartzog C: Clinical comparison of intraarticular anterior cruciate ligament reconstruction using autogenous semitendinosus and gracilis tendons in men versus women. Am J Sports Med 28:783, 2000.

101. Novak P, Wexler G, Williams J: Comparison of screw post fixation and free bone block interference fixation for anterior cruciate ligament soft tissue grafts: Biomechanical considerations. Arthroscopy 12:470, 1996.

102. Noyes F, Butler D, Grood E: Biomechanical analysis of human ligament grafts used in knee-ligament repairs and reconstructions. J Bone Joint Surg Am 66:344, 1984.

103. Noyes F, Butler D, Paulos L: Intra-articular cruciate reconstruction I: Perspectives of graft strength, vascularization, and immediate motion after replacement. Clin Orthop 172:71, 1983.

104. Noyes F, Grood E: The strength of the anterior cruciate ligament in humans and rhesus monkeys. J Bone Joint Surg Am 58:1074, 1976.

105. Noyes F, Matthews D, Mooar P: The symptomatic anterior cruciate deficient knee II: The success of rehabilitation, activity modification and counseling on functional disability. J Bone Joint Surg Am 65:163, 1983.

106. Nurmi J, Kannus P, Sievanen H: Compaction drilling does not increase the initial fixation strength of the hamstring tendon graft in anterior cruciate ligament reconstruction in a cadaver model. Am J Sports Med 31:353, 2003.

107. Nurmi J, Kannus P, Sievanen H: Interference screw fixation of soft tissue grafts in anterior cruciate ligament reconstruction: Part I. Effect of tunnel compaction by serial dilators versus extraction drilling on the initial fixation strength. Am J Sports Med 32:411, 2004.

108. Nurmi J, Kannus P, Sievanen H: Interference screw fixation of soft tissue grafts in anterior cruciate ligament reconstruction: Part II. Effect of preconditioning on graft tension during and after screw insertion. Am J Sports Med 32:418, 2004.

109. O'Brien S, Warren R, Pavlov H: Reconstruction of the chronically insufficient anterior cruciate ligament with the central third of the patellar tendon. J Bone Joint Surg Am 73:278, 1991.

110. Ohkoshi Y, Inoue C, Yamane S: Changes in muscle strength properties caused by harvesting of autogenous semitendinosus tendon for reconstruction of contralateral anterior cruciate ligament. Arthroscopy 14:580, 1998.

111. O'Neill D: Arthroscopically assisted reconstruction of the anterior cruciate ligament: A prospective randomized analysis of three techniques. J Bone Joint Surg Am 78:803, 1996.

112. Otero A, Hutcheson L: A comparison of the doubled semitendinosus/gracilis and central third of the patellar tendon autografts in arthroscopic anterior cruciate ligament reconstruction. Arthroscopy 9:143, 1993.

113. Otto D, Pinczewski L, Clingeleffer A: Five-year results of single-incision arthroscopic anterior cruciate ligament reconstruction with patellar tendon autograft. Am J Sports Med 26:181, 1998.

114. Paulos L, Rosenberg T: Infrapatellar contracture syndrome: An unrecognized cause of knee stiffness with patellar entrapment and patella infra. Am J Sports Med 15:331, 1987.

115. Pena F, Grontvedt T, Brown G: Comparison of failure strength between metallic and absorbable interference screws. Am J Sports Med 24:329, 1996.

116. Pflaster D: Pull out test: Pinczewski endoscopic hamstring technique utilizing the DonJoy RCI ACL fixation screw. Smith and Nephew DonJoy, Mansfield, MA.

117. Pinczewski, L, Clingeleffer A, Otto D: Integration of hamstring tendon graft with bone in reconstruction of the anterior cruciate ligament. Arthroscopy 13:641, 1997.

118. Pinczewski L, Deehan D, Salmon L: A five-year comparison of patellar tendon versus four-strand hamstring tendon autograft for arthroscopic reconstruction of the anterior cruciate ligament. Am J Sports Med 30:523, 2002.

119. Puddu G: Method for reconstruction of the anterior cruciate ligament using the semitendinosus tendon. Am J Sports Med 8:402, 1980.

120. Rodeo S, Arnoczky S, Torzilli P: Tendon healing in a bone tunnel. J Bone Joint Surg Am 75:1795, 1993.

121. Rosenberg T, Deffner K: Quadrupled semitendinosus ACL reconstruction: 5-year results in patients without meniscus loss. Arthroscopy 13:386, 1997.

122. Rosenberg T, Franklin J, Baldwin G: Extensor mechanism function after patellar tendon graft harvest for anterior cruciate ligament reconstruction. Am J Sports Med 20:519, 1992.

123. Rowden N, Sher D, Rodgers G: Anterior cruciate ligament graft fixation: Initial comparison of patellar tendon and semitendinosus autografts in young fresh cadavers. Am J Sports Med 25:472, 1997.

124. Rudroff T: Functional capability is enhanced with semitendinosus than patellar tendon ACL repair. Med Sci Sports Exerc 35:1486, 2003.

125. Sachs R, Daniel D, Stone M: Patellofemoral problems after anterior cruciate ligament reconstruction. Am J Sports Med 17:760, 1989.

126. Scopp J, Jasper L, Belkoff S: The effects of oblique femoral tunnel placement on rotational constraint of the knee reconstructed using patellar tendon autografts. Arthroscopy 20:294, 2004.

127. Segawa H, Omori G, Koga Y: Rotational muscle strength of the limb after anterior cruciate ligament reconstruction using semitendinosus and gracilis tendons. Arthroscopy 18:177, 2002.

128. Sgaglione N, Del Pizzo W, Fox J: Arthroscopically assisted anterior cruciate ligament reconstruction with pes anserine tendons. Am J Sports Med 21:249, 1993.

129. Shaieb M, Kan D, Chang S: A prospective randomized comparison of patellar tendon versus semitendinosus and gracilis tendon auto-

grafts for anterior cruciate ligament reconstruction. Am J Sports Med 30:214, 2002.

130. Shapiro M, Farzadmehr A, Davis B: Survivorship analysis of ACL reconstruction. Presented at a meeting of the American Orthopaedic Society for Sports Medicine, 1998, Vancouver, British Columbia, Canada.

131. Shelbourne K, Gray T: Anterior cruciate ligament reconstruction with autogenous patellar tendon graft followed by accelerated rehabilitation: A two- to nine-year followup. Am J Sports Med 25:786, 1997.

132. Shelbourne K, Klootwyk T, Wilckens J: Ligament stability two to six years after anterior cruciate ligament reconstruction with autogenous patellar tendon graft and participation in accelerated rehabilitation program. Am J Sports Med 23:575, 1995.

133. Shelbourne K, Nitz P: Accelerated rehabilitation after anterior cruciate ligament reconstruction. Am J Sports Med 18:292, 1990.

134. Shelbourne K, Trumper R: Preventing anterior knee pain after anterior cruciate ligament reconstruction. Am J Sports Med 25:41, 1997.

135. Shino K: Deterioration of patellofemoral articular surfaces after anterior cruciate ligament reconstruction. Am J Sports Med 21:206, 1993.

136. Siegel M, Barber-Westin S: Arthroscopically-assisted outpatient anterior cruciate ligament reconstruction using the semitendinosus and gracilis tendons. Arthroscopy 14:268, 1998.

137. Simonian P, Mann F, Mandt P: Indirect forces and patellar fracture after anterior cruciate ligament reconstruction with the patellar ligament: Case report. Am J Knee Surg 8:60, 1995.

138. Sklar J: Bio-Intrafix Cadaver Testing. Mitek, Inc. Springfield, MA, 2004.

139. Specchiulli F, Laforgia R, Mocci A: Anterior cruciate ligament reconstruction: A comparison of 2 techniques. Clin Orthop 311:142, 1995.

140. Spencer E, Chissell H, Spang J: Behavior of sutures used in anterior cruciate ligament reconstructive surgery. Knee Surg Sports Traumatol Arthrosc 4:84, 1996.

141. Starch D, Alexander J, Noble P: Multistranded hamstring tendon graft fixation with a central four-quadrant or a standard tibial interference screw for anterior cruciate ligament reconstruction. Am J Sports Med 31:338, 2003.

142. Steiner M, Hecker A, Brown C: Anterior cruciate ligament graft fixation: Comparison of hamstring and patellar tendon grafts. Am J Sports Med 22:240, 1994.

143. Tadokoro K, Matsui N, Yagi M, et al: Evaluation of hamstring strength and tendon regrowth after harvesting for anterior cruciate ligament reconstruction. Am J Sports Med 32:1644, 2004.

144. Tashiro T, Kurosawa H, Kawakami A: Influence of medial hamstring tendon harvest on knee flexor strength after anterior cruci-

ate ligament reconstruction. A detailed evaluation with comparison of single- and double-tendon harvest. Am J Sports Med 31:522, 2003.

145. To J, Howell S, Hull M: Contributions of femoral fixation methods to the stiffness of anterior cruciate ligament replacements at implantation. Arthroscopy 15:379, 1999.

146. Toritsuka Y, Shino K, Horibe S: Second-look arthroscopy of anterior cruciate ligament grafts with multi-stranded hamstring tendons. Arthroscopy 20:287, 2004.

147. Uchio Y, Ochi M, Adachi N: Determination of time of biologic fixation after anterior cruciate ligament reconstruction with hamstring tendons. Am J Sports Med 31:345, 2003.

148. Viola R, Sterett W, Newfield D: Internal and external tibial rotation strength after anterior cruciate ligament reconstruction using ipsilateral semitendinosus and gracilis tendon autografts. Am J Sports Med 28:552, 2000.

149. Weiler A, Hoffman R, Siepe C: The influence of screw geometry on hamstring tendon interference fit fixation. Am J Sports Med 28:356, 2000.

150. Weiler A, Hoffman R, Stahelin A: Hamstring tendon fixation using interference screws: A biomechanical study in calf tibial bone. Arthrex, Inc., Naples, FL.

151. Weiler A, Hoffman R, Stahelin A: Hamstring tendon fixation using interference screws: A biomechanical study in calf tibial bone. Arthroscopy 14:29, 1998.

152. Weiler A, Hoffman R, Winhagen H: Biomechanical evaluation of different biodegradable screws. Arthroscopy 13:403, 1997.

153. Weiler A, Richter M, Schmidmaier G: The endopearl device increases fixation strength and eliminates construct slippage of hamstring tendon grafts with interference screw fixation. Arthroscopy 17:353, 2001.

154. Williams R: Anterior cruciate ligament reconstruction with a four-strand hamstring tendon autograft. J Bone Joint Surg Am 86:225, 2004.

155. Woo S, Hollis M, Adams D: Tensile properties of the human femur–anterior cruciate ligament–tibia complex. Am J Sports Med 19:217, 1991.

156. Yasuda K, Tsujino J, Ohkoshi Y: Graft site morbidity with autogenous semitendinosus and gracilis tendons. Am J Sports Med 23:706, 1995.

157. Yunes M, Richmond J, Engels EA, Pinczewski LA: Patellar versus hamstring tendons in anterior cruciate ligament reconstruction: A meta-analysis. Arthroscopy 17:248, 2001.

158. Zantop T, Weimann A, Rummler M: Initial fixation strength of two bioabsorbable pins for the fixation of hamstring grafts compared to interference screw fixation. Am J Sports Med 32:641, 2004.

159. Zaricznyj B: Reconstruction of the anterior cruciate ligament of the knee using a doubled tendon graft. Clin Orthop 220:162, 1987.

CHAPTER 41

Allograft Anterior Cruciate Ligament Reconstruction

Chang Haw Chong • David N. M. Caborn

Allograft tissues have been used for anterior cruciate ligament (ACL) reconstruction for more than 20 years. Shino,[82] Noyes,[66,67] and their colleagues independently reported good clinical results with allografts in the 1980s. Since then, there have been numerous reports reinforcing the success of ACL reconstruction using allograft tissue both with and without bone blocks: freeze-dried (lyophilized) or cryopreserved patellar tendon, Achilles tendon, and fascia lata, in addition to tibialis tendon.[41,52,53,70,88] Good clinical experience has been reported with the use of allograft tissue in reconstruction of the ACL in skeletally immature patients,[5] as well as those older than 40 years.[50]

GRAFT CHOICES IN ACL RECONSTRUCTION

Jones first described the use of autogenous patellar tendon graft for ACL reconstruction in 1970.[47] Advantages of patellar tendon grafts are high initial strength, early bone-to-bone healing by 6 weeks, and predictable success in restoring stability to the knee.[2,8,19,22,59,69] This graft rapidly became the gold standard graft. Disadvantages of autogenous bone–patellar tendon–bone (BPTB) grafts are all the problems associated with graft harvest,[11,26,60,62,73,85] including quadriceps femoris inhibition, patellar tendon shortening, infrapatellar fat pad fibrosis, and patellar fracture. Other problems include functional deficits such as decreased quadriceps strength, reduced knee range of motion, increased patellofemoral pain, chondromalacia patellae, and altered patellar alignment.[37,48,65] With improvements in soft-tissue bone tunnel fixation, autogenous medial hamstring tendons have become a popular choice for grafts because of less harvest site morbidity with the extensor mechanism.[56] However, ACL reconstruction with semitendinosus and gracilis tendons results in a significant limitation in knee flexion and hip extension strength that is detrimental to the performance of any sprinting athlete or any athlete who requires knee flexion strength above 90 degrees, such as wrestlers, sprinters, gymnasts, and judo participants.[93] The ACL-hamstring reflex arc is a protective ligamentous-muscular pathway found in normal human knees, and sacrificing the medial hamstring tendons will disrupt this ACL–hamstring muscle reflex arc.[10] In a study comparing knee flexor and extensor strength in patients after either autograft BPTB or hamstring ACL reconstruction with that of an age- and activity level–matched control group,[37] the combined ACL group had a global 25.5% deficit in extensor strength, with eccentric regional (angle and velocity matched) deficits of up to 50% of control values. In addition, the BPTB group demonstrated a concentric, low-velocity knee extensor strength deficit at 60 to 95 degrees that was not observed in the hamstring group. Significant graft site–dependent regional knee flexor deficits of up to 50% of controls were observed for the hamstring group.

There are several advantages to the use of allograft ligaments for reconstruction of the ACL as opposed to autografts. By doing away with the need for graft harvesting, smaller incisions are used, surgical times are shortened, postoperative pain is reduced, and there is no morbidity associated with loss of donor graft function. Our group looked at the lower extremity muscle activation latencies of patients after rehabilitated unilateral ACL reconstruction (allograft or autograft BPTB tissue) and normal control subjects.[71] Patients who received allografts demonstrated muscle latency, activation, and recruitment patterns that more closely approximated those of normal controls than did patients who received BPTB autografts. The availability of a range of graft sizes allows the surgeon to choose the most appropriate graft. Allografts also serve as a source of ligaments when more than one ligament is required for multiligament knee reconstruction.[51,54,79,98]

The biomechanical properties in terms of ultimate failure load and stiffness of doubled tibialis anterior, doubled tibialis posterior, doubled peroneus longus, native ACL, 14-mm BPTB, 10-mm BPTB, and quadrupled semitendinosus/gracilis grafts are represented in Figures 41–1 and 41–2, respectively. The doubled tibialis anterior, doubled tibialis posterior, and doubled peroneus longus tendons showed ultimate tensile strength and stiffness that were equal to or exceeded those of nearly all currently described ACL graft sources.[72] The patellar tendon component of BPTB grafts may be less than two-thirds the diameter of the attached bone plugs. The average tendon mass available for ACL reconstruction is approximately 65% more when using a doubled tibialis tendon in comparison to BPTB with standard clinical constructs and sizes.[24]

However, the risk of disease transmission with the use of allografts cannot be ignored.[42,78,97] The failure rate is potentially higher.[44,58] There is also the potential for a subclinical immunological reaction. Lack of tissue availability and high cost have fueled recent interest in xenograft tissue. The technology involves enzymatic removal of the specific carbohydrates that cause rejection. Xenograft

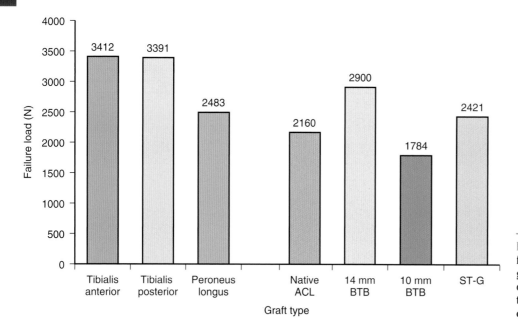

Figure   41–1. Ultimate failure loads of different grafts compared with doubled tibialis anterior, tibialis posterior, and peroneus longus tendons.

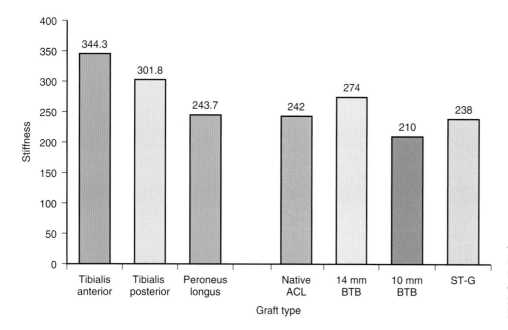

Figure 41–2. Stiffness of different grafts compared with doubled tibialis anterior, tibialis posterior, and peroneus longus tendons.

BPTB grafts have been used to reconstruct a torn ACL in humans.

BIOLOGY OF ALLOGRAFT ACL RECONSTRUCTION

Immune Response

An immune response to the allograft usually occurs in recipients but is subclinical and does not appear to affect the success of the reconstruction.[77]

Arnoczky et al used an animal model to study the immune response to the implantation of fresh and fresh frozen allografts versus autogenous tendon grafts.[6] Fresh grafts prompted a vigorous immune response with rejection of the tissue, whereas fresh frozen grafts showed histological changes identical to those of autografts with no evidence of immune response or rejection. Similarly, no immunological reactions were detected on histological examination as reported by Shino and colleagues with the use of fresh frozen allografts in dogs,[84] as well as independently by Drez et al[25] and Jackson et al[43] in goats. Freezing tendons to −70° C kills fibroblasts, which are the loci for the major histocompatibility antigens, and such processing reduces the immunogenicity of the graft.[16,28,33,61] Deep-freezing does not appear to alter the biomechanical properties of ligament tissues. In a study comparing the biomaterial properties of fresh and deep-frozen cruciate ligaments from monkeys,[9] the results suggested that changes in the material properties of deep-frozen ligaments were not statistically different from those in the fresh controls. Caution is advised when extrapolating the findings of this study to clinical practice, however, because the deep-frozen allografts are usually frozen, thawed, and refrozen as part of the processing. The formation of ice crystals in tissue from repeated deep-freezing may be detrimental to tissue properties without cryoprecipitant protection. Cryopreserved allografts have been shown in animal studies to excite less immune response,[29] especially when used with dimethyl sulfoxide.[100]

Pinkowski and coworkers[74] demonstrated an assayable immune response with ethylene oxide–processed, freeze-dried BPTB allografts in human ACL reconstruction. Lymphocytes drawn from six patients (75%) showed an immunological reaction to goat xenograft tendon homogenate, whereas four patients (50%) had a reaction to at least one of a panel of human allograft tendon homogenates. All four autograft controls had a nonimmunogenic response to testing. However, the poor clinical outcome of two of eight patients with allografts could also be due to the use of ethylene oxide. Jackson et al[46] showed that 6.4% of 109 patients who received the same type of allograft for ACL reconstruction had a persistent intra-articular reaction characterized by synovial effusion with collagenous particulates and a cellular inflammatory response. Synovial biopsy samples in all cases showed a similar chronic inflammatory process characterized by fibrin, collagen, and phagocytic cells. The intra-articular white cells were predominantly lymphocytes. Removal of the allograft resulted in resolution of the reaction in all the patients. Three of the seven patients demonstrated HLA conversion. Gas chromatography showed detectable levels of ethylene chlorhydrin, a toxic reaction product of ethylene oxide, within the allograft and synovium 14 months after the implantation of one graft.

Both humoral and cellular immune responses have been documented in patients who received ACL allografts. Thompson and coworkers investigated the cellular and humoral immune response to fresh frozen ACL allograft with bone plugs in 41 recreational athletes with chronic ACL deficiency who underwent reconstruction.[94] Patients were self-selected into two groups: allograft and control autograft. Immune parameters were determined at regular intervals over a 1-year postoperative period. The cellular response was characterized by increased interleukin-6 levels in both groups and increased serum activation of CD4- and CD8-positive cells in the allograft group only. A humoral immune response (lymphocytotoxic antidonor IgG production) was present in 38% of the allograft recipients and not evident in those who received autografts. Schulte et al[77] prospectively investigated whether the presence of a detectable immune response affects the clinical outcome of patients undergoing ACL reconstruction. In that study they detected the presence of a humoral immune response in 43% of the patients who received fresh frozen, nonirradiated allografts, but there was no difference in clinical outcome when compared with those who did not show a response and those in the autograft control group.

Fate of Implanted Allografts

Implanted allografts remodel over time with histological changes that closely parallel the healing of autografts, including phases of central hypocellularity, revascularization, fibroblast invasion, and collagen synthesis. Drez and associates[25] showed that the histology and graft strength of freeze-dried patellar tendon allografts were similar to those of autografts for up to 52 weeks in a goat model. However, Jackson et al,[43] using a similar model, found a more gradual rate of incorporation of allografts at 6 months, which raised concern that allografts may be weaker than autografts at the same time interval after implantation. In an analysis of nine allografts used for ACL reconstruction that were retrieved between 20 days and 10 years after implantation, Malinin and colleagues found that 2 years after transplantation, the central portions of the grafts remained acellular and that complete attachment was not present but was found in a 3.5-year post-transplantation specimen.[58] Studies by Shino et al showed that the surface blood flow of human ACL allografts was higher in the 6-month grafts, gradually declined toward a plateau by 12 months, reached maturity by 18 months, and maintained a level similar to that of normal ACLs thereafter.[83] The allograft ACL consisted predominantly of a unimodal profile of small-diameter collagen fibrils (30 to 80 nm) 12 months after implantation,[87] which is similar to that found in autograft ACL.[1] In cryopreserved allografts, the living donor cells were replaced by recipient cells by 4 weeks after implantation.[32,45]

The mechanical strength of implanted allografts has been investigated only in animal models. Using a canine model, Shino et al estimated that the mean maximum tensile strength of fresh frozen allografts 30 months after implantation was only 30% of the strength of the ACL in the control limb.[84] Interestingly, there were no significant differences in mechanical properties between allograft and autograft at the same time intervals. Similarly, Curtis and coworkers demonstrated that freeze-dried fascia lata allografts achieved a mean maximum load to failure at 24 weeks of 536 N as opposed to 801 N in the contralateral knee, which had an intact ACL.[23] Similar findings of inferior mechanical strength after implantation in comparison to normal ACL but similar properties when compared with autografts are seen in other studies.[99,104] It has been shown in large animal studies that even in autograft ACL reconstruction, the implanted ACLs do not attain mechanical properties comparable to those of the control ACL up to 3 years after surgery.[64,90] Remodeling of reconstructed ACLs is a lengthy process and is demonstrated in both allografts and autografts.

ALLOGRAFTS AND INFECTION

Although tissue allografts can substantially improve the quality of life in many patients, infections associated with bacterial contamination of allografts can result in serious morbidity and death.[42,78,97] Another major concern with the use of an allograft for ACL reconstruction is the transmission of viral infections such as human immunodeficiency virus (HIV) and hepatitis B or C by the donor tissue, from which fatal outcomes might occur in the recipient. The risk of transmission of infectious disease by musculoskeletal grafts is estimated to be 1 in 1.5 million.[4,7,13,17]

Viral Infection

The risk of implanting allograft tissue from an undetected HIV carrier can be reduced to less than 1 in 1 million by aseptic processing and strict adherence to donor screening and testing. With the use of polymerase chain reaction (PCR), the risk of HIV transmission from screened and tested donors can be reduced to 1 in 1.6 million.[13] Tissue banks that routinely use PCR to test for HIV can reduce the window period from 6 months to 19 days.[80] There have been two documented cases of HIV transmission as a result of musculoskeletal allograft tissue transplantation.[95] One involved a fresh frozen BPTB allograft in 1985[89] that had cleared donor screening as well as an enzyme-linked immunosorbent assay for HIV. The graft was fresh frozen and did not undergo processes to remove bone marrow or blood. Fascia lata, Achilles tendon, and patellar tendon from the same donor were processed, freeze-dried, and implanted into three other recipients but did not result in HIV infection.

Transmission of hepatitis C virus (HCV) via fresh frozen allograft patellar tendon grafts has been reported in two separate cases by Conrad and coauthors in 1995.[20] In both instances, the grafts were not processed by removal of blood or marrow elements, and there was also no secondary sterilization. In contrast, 12 other musculoskeletal allografts from the same donor that were processed and irradiated did not transmit the virus. A third case of HCV transmission occurred in 2002 in a patient who had received a patellar tendon with bone allograft from a donor approximately 6 weeks before the onset of illness.[36] The donor serum tested anti-HCV negative at the time of death. However, subsequently tested stored serum was HCV RNA positive. The donor was the probable source of HCV infection for at least eight recipients of organs or tissues. All cases occurred in recipients of organs or soft tissues; no infections were found in those who received skin or irradiated bone.

Bacterial Infection

After the reported death of a recipient of an allograft contaminated with Clostridium (an anaerobic spore- and toxin-forming organism) in 2001, the Centers for Disease Control and Prevention (CDC) investigated this case and solicited additional reports of allograft-associated infection.[97] A case of allograft-associated bacterial infection was defined by the CDC as any surgical site infection at the site of allograft implantation that occurs within 12 months of implantation in an otherwise healthy patient with no known risk factors for such infection (e.g., diabetes). Cases could be culture negative if diagnosed by an infectious disease specialist or surgeon and diagnostic (e.g.,

knee aspirate) if operative findings supported the diagnosis of surgical site infection. If only Staphylococcus aureus or Staphylococcus species were isolated, patients were excluded unless additional epidemiological or microbiological evidence suggested allograft contamination.

Twenty-six cases were identified. Thirteen (50%) of the 26 patients were infected with Clostridium species (C. septicum [12], C. sordellii [1]). Allografts implicated in the Clostridium infections were tendons used for ACL reconstruction (eight), femoral condyles (two), bone (two), and meniscus (one). Eleven (85%) of the allografts were frozen and two (15%) were fresh (femoral condyles). All allografts were processed aseptically but did not undergo terminal sterilization. In 11 of these 13 cases, additional evidence (e.g., common donors or cultures of nonimplanted tissue) implicated the allograft as the source of the infection. Eleven patients were infected with gramnegative bacilli; five had polymicrobial infections. Cultures from two patients were negative. The transplanted tissues included ACL (10), femoral condyle (1), meniscus (1), and bone (1). One tissue was fresh (femoral condyle), one was freeze-dried (bone), and the rest were frozen. For 8 (62%) of these 13 cases, additional evidence implicated the allograft (e.g., common donors or positive preimplantation or processing cultures with matching microorganisms). Eight patients received allografts that had undergone aseptic processing but not terminal sterilization. Three patients received allografts that were reported to have undergone gamma irradiation.

As a result of this audit, the CDC recommended that when possible, a method that can kill bacterial spores should be used to process tissue. Existing sterilization technologies used for tissue allografts, such as gamma irradiation, or new technologies effective against bacterial spores should be considered. Unless a sporicidal method is used, aseptically processed tissue should not be considered sterile, and health care providers should be informed of the possible risk of bacterial infection.

If no sporicidal method is available (e.g., for certain tissues such as fresh femoral condyles), effort should be made to minimize the potential for clostridial and other bacterial contamination. First, tissue should be cultured before suspension in antimicrobial solutions,[101] and if Clostridium or other bowel flora are isolated, all tissue from that donor that cannot be sterilized should be discarded. Second, culture methods should be validated to ensure that residual antimicrobials do not result in falsenegative culture results.[96] Performance of both destructive and swab cultures should be considered. Third, the recommended time limits for tissue retrieval should be followed.[101]

After receiving a report of potential allograft-associated infection, the remaining tissue from that donor should not be released until it is determined that the allograft is not the source of infection.[101] Tissue processors should contact health care providers of recipients of tissue from the same donor implicated in an allograft-associated infection. In these cases, a sample of nonimplanted tissue that underwent the same processing method should be cultured by an independent laboratory with a validated method.

Malinin and colleagues investigated the incidence of clostridial contamination in donor musculoskeletal tissue.[57] They found that 64 of 795 (8.1%) consecutive donors had clostridia, commonly *C. sordellii*. They also found that the incidence of clostridial infection increased with increasing time between death and tissue excision. Multiple microbiological cultures, including blood, were needed to identify clostridial contamination in their series.

A case of invasive group A streptococcal (*Streptococcus pyogenes*) infection was reported in 2003 from a contaminated hemipatellar tendon allograft used for ACL reconstruction.[42] Preprocessing cultures obtained by the tissue bank yielded group A streptococci, but all postprocessing cultures were reported as negative. The bank processed the allografts with an aseptic technique and an antimicrobial solution, but no sterilization procedure (e.g., gamma irradiation) was performed.

The presence of group A streptococci in donor tissue should prompt rejection of the tissue unless a sterilizing procedure can be used. The American Association of Tissue Banks (AATB), a voluntary accreditation organization, has proposed sterilizing or discarding certain tissues if specified organisms, including group A streptococci, are detected given the apparent ability of the organism to endure tissue processing with antimicrobial treatment. Because the prevalence of group A streptococci in donor cultures is low, this recommendation should not substantially limit the supply of tissue available for transplantation.

The occurrence of these allograft-associated infections must be seen in light of the amount of allograft tissues used by surgeons. It is reported that about 1 million allograft tissues were distributed for transplantation in orthopedic cases in 2002 alone.[42]

Minimizing the Risk of Infection through Controlling Bodies

The American Association of Tissue Banks (AATB) is a nonprofit organization founded in 1976. It was formed to establish and promulgate voluntary standards to encourage the provision of transplantable cells and tissue of uniform high quality. The AATB strives to prevent disease transmission and to ensure optimum clinical performance of transplanted tissues. The AATB first published its *Standards for Tissue Banking* in 1984 to help ensure that the conduct of tissue banks met their safety and ethical standards.[39] These standards are reviewed periodically and have been revised and updated several times by the AATB standards committee to incorporate current member practice. In 1986, the AATB began offering inspection and accreditation of tissue banks to its members. The Food and Drug Administration (FDA) has the power to shut down a tissue bank and fine or imprison its owner/operators and can force a recall and destruction of all its tissues. The Center for Biologics Evaluation and Research (CBER) was formed in 1987 by the U.S. government. In 1993, the CBER published an "interim rule" mandating that all tissue intended for transplantation be tested for HIV and hepatitis B and C virus "for the prevention of spread of communicable diseases."[40] Since 1993, there has been only one reported case of viral transmission with the use of musculoskeletal allograft tissue.[36]

Minimizing Risk of Infection by Tissue Processing

Because of the potential for exposure to pathogens, the safety of allograft tissue remains a primary focus for tissue banks, clinicians, the FDA, and patients. Tissue processing should eliminate all pathogens and yet preserve the biomechanical properties of the graft. Current methods of terminal sterilization of these tissues are limited to gamma irradiation and ethylene oxide. Gamma irradiation from a cobalt 60 source effectively penetrates tissue and can sterilize pathogens, but the dose required to reliably kill cell-associated viruses can be so high that the tendon graft is weakened by separation of collagen bundles and denaturing of protein, thereby rendering the tendon graft unsuitable for ligament reconstruction.[14,31,75] Conway et al estimated that 3.6 mrad is required to inactivate free HIV-1 virus by gamma irradiation and that higher doses are needed to eliminate cell-associated viruses.[21] Fideler and colleagues found a dose-dependent effect of irradiation on the biomechanical properties of human BPTB allografts.[27] A 10% to 24% and 19% to 46% reduction in all biomechanical properties was found after 3 and 4 mrad of irradiation, respectively. The ultimate load of human tendon allograft was less than that of reported values for the human ACL after 4 mrad. More importantly, irradiation of allografts with doses at or below 2 mrad will not significantly affect the mechanical properties of the tissue, and it is an effective bacterial sterilizer.[40,75] In practice, the AATB recommends a radiation dosage of between 1.5 and 2.5 mrad.

Tissue sterilization by exposure to ethylene oxide has been used, but ethylene chlorhydrin residues in the allograft can provoke an inflammatory reaction after implantation.[46,76] Reports of studies that do not favor ethylene oxide as a method of sterilization have led to a trend for tissue banks to limit the use of ethylene oxide for sterilization. A survey of tissue banks in 1987 and 1988 by the AATB reported that ethylene oxide was used for sterilization in two-thirds of the banks and irradiation in one-third[63]; in 1992, in contrast, ionizing irradiation was used twice as often as ethylene oxide.[91] Therefore, although ethylene oxide continues to be used by hospitals and industry, many tissue banks now rely on other methods of sterilization, such as gamma irradiation.

Current Directions and Future Trends in Tissue Processing

The current direction in research and development is to devise sterilization methods that do not degrade the mechanical properties of allografts.

The Allowash technology from LifeNet (Virginia Beach, VA) is designed to facilitate the removal of cellular elements from musculoskeletal tissue while maintaining structural integrity. Bioburden is reduced by both mechanical and chemical methods. It provides up to a 3-log reduction in residuals of bone marrow and blood elements in bone grafts (cleaning) and an additional 5- to 20-log reduction in potential microbial and viral bioburden through disinfection. This technique has been in use by the LifeNet Tissue Bank since 1995 with no reported incident of disease transmission.

Tutoplast processing of bone-tendon-bone and soft-tissue allografts is another method of reducing bioburden. It consists of a proprietary tissue-processing system designed to significantly reduce the amount of cells, bone marrow, and lipid components from processed allograft bone and connective tissue while preserving the extracellular matrix (collagen and mineral components). It involves the sequential processes of delipidization, osmotic contrast treatment, oxidation in hydrogen peroxide, and limited-dose gamma irradiation. This method inactivates and removes bacteria and viruses and thereby produces cleaner and safer allograft tissue. A biomechanical analysis of solvent-dehydrated (Tutoplast) and freeze-dried human fascia lata allograft showed significantly higher stiffness and higher maximum load in the Tutoplast group.[38]

New low-temperature chemical sterilization methods (BioCleanse Tissue Sterilization Process, Regeneration Technologies, Inc., Gainesville, Florida) with good tissue penetration have been developed. These methods appear to be sporicidal and do not seem to adversely affect the biomechanical properties of tissue.[92] After cleansing by disinfectant treatment, the tissues are then sterilized with gamma radiation and stored by freezing or freeze-drying. Over 400,000 allografts have been sterilized and distributed for implantation through the BioCleanse process over the last 4 years without a single reported case of recipient infection.

The Clearant process (Clearant, Inc., Los Angeles) uses antioxidants in conjunction with gamma irradiation[3,34] to inactivate pathogens with retention of allograft integrity. This process delivers 50 kGy of gamma radiation to the allografts with the use of a patented medium (containing radioprotectants) and set conditions such as temperature and pressure to achieve a sterility assurance level of 10^{-6}. Using such high radiation levels, it is effective against all forms of pathogens, including both enveloped and nonenveloped viruses, bacteria, molds, spores, and prions. King and coworkers showed that despite the high radiation levels used, there was no significant difference in the tensile strength of nonirradiated tendons and those irradiated to 50 kGy under controlled conditions with radioprotectants.[49] Similarly, there was no change in Young's modulus between groups. Biochemical analysis indicated no collagen degradation after 50-kGy irradiation in the presence of radioprotectants. This process is designed for allograft tissue in the final container, thus making the product ready for use in the operating room. The concept of end user sterilization in a final container is attractive because it removes variables that may contribute to infection, such as lack of standardized procurement, inadequate culture methods, and emerging infections. Clinical evaluation of allografts for ACL reconstruction that were treated by this process is still ongoing.

Other sterilization methods are under development, including terminal sterilization with supercritical carbon dioxide. This patented process uses the physicochemical properties of supercritical carbon dioxide in a novel reactor design together with innovative processing and proprietary additives. The new technique of "supercritical carbon dioxide bone sterilization" reported by NovaSterilis (Ithaca, NY) at the 27th Annual Meeting of the AATB in August 2003 in San Diego, California, is the first effective method of bacterial decontamination of bone without radiation, but with preservation of structural integrity.

Others are attempting to develop acellularized human tendon grafts for ACL reconstruction. By doing so, all the cells that may cause an immune response are removed, whereas the main structural proteins responsible for mechanical integrity of the ligament remain intact and unaltered. Fibroblasts from a patient's own damaged ACL can be "seeded" into the acellularized ACL graft to re-create a living replacement that will be accepted after implantation and be capable of growth and self-maintenance. The living ACL graft can then be implanted into the patient by the standard arthroscopic surgical techniques currently used for ACL replacement. There is the advantage of having an intact, naturally derived extracellular matrix to repopulate with cells. The intact matrix has the required mechanical and biological properties, as opposed to synthetic tissue engineering scaffolds, which do not contain the proper the "biological signals" required by living cells and/or do not posses the structural and mechanical properties required for proper tissue function.

Peracetic acid has been shown to provide reliable sterilization of bone allografts and has recently been evaluated for processing of soft-tissue allografts. Research conducted at Humboldt Universität Berlin by Weiler's group has shown no significant mechanical differences between fresh frozen nonsterilized human BPTB grafts versus those treated with peracetic acid and ethanol (personal communication).

It remains to be seen whether these novel techniques of allograft tissue processing will translate into lower risk of disease transmission.

CLINICAL RESULTS

The earliest published series on allograft ACL reconstruction were from Dr. Shino (Osaka, Japan) and Dr. Noyes (Cincinnati, OH), who independently started using allografts for ACL reconstruction in 1981. Shino et al published their results of 84 patients who underwent ACL reconstruction with fresh frozen allogeneic tendon in 1990.[82] They were reviewed and evaluated by subjective and functional rating scales, physical examination, instrumented anterior drawer tests, isokinetic testing, and arthroscopy. The average follow-up was 57 months (range, 36 to 90 months), and the average age at surgery was 22 years (range, 16 to 37 years). The subjective and functional results were rated as excellent in 48 patients (57%), good in 31 (37%), and fair in 2 (2%). Three patients (4%) experienced a retear of the ACL. Physical examination and instrumented anterior drawer tests showed that satisfactory anterior stability was restored in 88% of the patients. Isokinetic evaluation demonstrated that the extension torque of the involved knee recovered to a slightly lower level than that of controls, although flexion torque recovered to a level equivalent to that of controls. Arthroscopic evaluation revealed that the allografts were elaborately remodeled, viable, and taut. There was no sign of immunological rejection at any time postoperatively. In a different study, Shino and colleagues compared their results of allograft ACL versus autograft ACL reconstruction.[86] The subjects were divided into two groups according to the type of graft: fresh frozen allogenic tendon (n = 47) or central third of the ipsilateral patellar tendon (n = 45). Instrumented drawer tests in the Lachman position were performed to measure anterior tibial displacement at 200 N (anterior laxity). Thigh muscle power was isokinetically measured with a Cybex II dynamometer. Significantly increased anterior laxity was found in the reconstructed knees when compared with the contralateral normal knees regardless of graft material (paired t-test, $p < 0.01$), except for the male allograft patients. Although the mean anterior laxity difference between sides for the allograft patients was less than that for the autograft patients, analysis of variance failed to demonstrate a statistically significant difference between the two groups if comparison was made strictly within the same sex. Thigh muscle tests revealed that extension torque in the reconstructed knees was significantly less than that in the contralateral knees, and analysis of variance showed that knee extension torque at 60 deg/sec in the allograft patients was significantly better than that in the autograft patients ($p < 0.05$). They concluded that the allograft procedure is more advantageous than the patellar tendon autograft procedure in terms of better restoration of anterior stability. Shino's 10-year follow-up results for 41 patients[81] who underwent arthroscopic ACL reconstruction with nonirradiated fresh tendon allograft showed 29% normal and 71% nearly normal based on the International Knee Documentation Committee (IKDC) Knee Ligament Standard Evaluation Form. The mean side-to-side difference in anterior laxity measured with the KT-2000 arthrometer was 1.7 mm, and 83% had less than 3-mm translation.

In a prospective study, Noyes' group reported good to excellent results in 89% of 47 patients who underwent ACL reconstruction with either freeze-dried, ethylene oxide–treated fascia lata or fresh frozen, nonirradiated BPTB allografts assessed at a mean and minimum follow-up of 3 years and 2 years, respectively.[68] In just one patient, the only one in whom the fascia lata graft failed, did giving way develop. They published the 7-year follow-up of their patients and compared the 7-year results with those at 2 years.[65] A noteworthy finding was the apparent ability of the allograft to provide stability for at least 5 to 9 years postoperatively. At the 2-year evaluation, the result was rated excellent in 13 (21%) of 63 patients, good in 25 (40%), fair in 21 (33%), and poor in 4 (6%). The results in four patients were not rated because of incomplete data. At the 7-year evaluation, the result was rated excellent in 15 (22%) of the 68 patients, good in 30 (44%), fair in 18 (26%), and poor in 5 (7%). Only three patients (4%) had an increase in displacement between the early and the later evaluation that resulted in failure of the graft. Five additional patients had a slight increase in displacement but still had a partially functioning graft according to

KT-1000 arthrometric and pivot-shift test criteria. Both studies[65,68] showed that a small number (4% to 5%) of allografts may stretch slightly over time. However, this stretching amounted to only 2 to 3 mm in most of the knees and did not inevitably lead to failure or a poor result. The overall rate of failure for these 73 patients was 10% (7 patients) for the early period and 14% (10 patients) for the later period. Noyes' group also highlighted the use of allografts for arthroscopically assisted ACL reconstruction in patients with symptomatic and advanced arthrosis[66] and showed improvement in the Cincinnati Knee Rating System from a preoperative score of 55 to a postoperative score of 77. There was no clinical evidence of rejection of the allografts or transmission of disease in any of the knees. Overall, 55% of their study patients returned to light athletic activities and were asymptomatic with regard to pain and knee giving way.

Harner's group looked at their midterm, 3- to 5-year results of nonirradiated allografts versus autografts for ACL reconstruction and found no statistically significant difference in results between the two groups.[35] Interestingly the allograft group had better results than the autograft group did with the use of two different knee scores, but this difference was not statistically significant. In this study, the autograft group had a higher incidence of terminal extension loss. In a separate study, Chang and coworkers compared the minimum 2-year outcome of ACL reconstruction with fresh frozen BPTB allografts and BPTB autografts[18] and found no significant difference in results.

Investigators have also looked at the clinical performance of different allografts in terms of tissue type and processing and storage methods. Levitt and associates reported the results of 214 patients who underwent arthroscopically assisted ACL reconstruction with either freeze-dried or fresh frozen BPTB or Achilles tendon allografts.[52] Of these 214 patients, 181 were available for follow-up testing and examination. The minimum follow-up time was 4 years, and they reported that 79% of the patients had satisfactory results. No difference was noted between Achilles and patellar tendon allografts. Siebold et al compared the results of primary ACL reconstruction with fresh frozen patellar versus Achilles tendon allografts in a large series of 251 patients with a mean follow-up of 38 months and found a significantly lower failure rate in the group that received Achilles tendon allografts (4.8%) than in the group that received fresh frozen BPTB allografts (10.4%) based on rerupture rates.[88] They did comment that the total failure rate appears to be higher than reported failure rates with autogenous ACL reconstruction. Indelicato's group compared freeze-dried and fresh frozen patellar tendon allografts and showed marked improvement in their patients after allograft ACL reconstruction, with fresh frozen allografts doing slightly better than freeze-dried ones.[41] Our group prefers to use cryopreserved tibialis anterior allograft in a single-looped bundle technique for ACL reconstruction.[15,70] Nyland et al reviewed our 2-year results of ACL reconstruction with tibialis anterior cryopreserved allografts and found 13 of 18 with an IKDC grade of normal, 4 of 18 with an IKDC grade of nearly normal, and 1 of 18 with an IKDC grade of abnormal.[70] Ninety-four percent of the subjects (17/18) had normal or nearly normal results on manual knee ligament tests.

Poor results have been reported in the literature with regard to allograft ACL reconstruction. Roberts and coworkers from New Orleans published their early experience of ACL reconstruction with freeze-dried, ethylene oxide–treated BPTB allografts in 36 patients in 1991.[76] Only 17 of 36 patients (47%) did well and returned to their desired level of activity. Nine patients had episodes of recurrent synovitis. Eight (22%) had complete loss of stability with graft resorption on repeat arthroscopy. The authors agreed with Jackson et al[46] that the probable cause of failure is ethylene oxide and its byproducts ethylene glycol and ethylene chlorhydrin.

Enlargement of the osseous tunnels has been highlighted in allograft ACL reconstruction.[46,53,87] Ethylene oxide–treated grafts were used in two of the series,[46,76] and the authors believed that the terminal sterilization agent may have been responsible for the tunnel enlargement. In Linn and colleagues' series,[53] the allografts were fresh frozen Achilles tendons and were not treated with ethylene oxide. Even though worrisome radiographic tunnel enlargement of various degree was seen in that series, the clinical outcome was not adversely affected, with 85% of the patients having a good outcome. In contrast, Shino's group obtained follow-up radiographs for 84 patients and reported that the tunnels became less obvious with time and eventually were not visible.[82] The etiology of tunnel enlargement in allograft ACL reconstruction is still not understood and might be a problem involving biomechanical and biological issues rather than allograft tissues per se.

For skeletally immature ACL-deficient patients with open physes, soft-tissue allografts (fascia lata or Achilles tendon) have been used by Noyes' group with clinical success and no growth plate disturbance.[5] Kuechle and coworkers reviewed ACL allograft reconstructions in patients older than 40 years and found the results to be comparable to those in younger patients.[50] In their study 94% of patients had negative Lachman tests, negative pivot-shift tests, and less than 2-mm side-to-side difference in translation on maximum-effect KT-1000 testing.

In general, allograft ACL reconstruction is stable in the majority of patients, with satisfactory results demonstrated at 7- to 10-year follow-up. Although no randomized controlled trials have been conducted, multiple case series comparing allograft with autograft ACL reconstruction show comparable outcomes.

ACL RECONSTRUCTION WITH TIBIALIS ANTERIOR TENDON ALLOGRAFT

The tibialis anterior tendon is a thick, strong tendon that can be prepared with one doubling of the graft, has a large cross-sectional area, and has been shown to be stronger than semitendinosus, gracilis, and patellar tendons and native ACL. We have routinely been using this graft for ACL reconstructions since 1998. Our detailed surgical technique for single–anteromedial bundle ACL reconstruction has been published.[15]

Indications

The indication for allograft ACL reconstruction is the same as that for autograft ACL reconstruction in our practice. In high-performance athletes, preservation of medial hamstring function is important. We believe that the advantages of using soft-tissue tendon allograft outweigh the small risk of disease transmission. To date, there has been no published report of infectious disease transmission in ACL reconstruction with a soft-tissue allograft without bone plugs. All the reports of disease transmission related to allograft ACL reconstruction have involved soft-tissue allografts together with bone plugs. Surgeons should educate themselves on the differences in tissue processing to make a good selection for their patients.

Surgical Technique for Single–Anteromedial Bundle ACL Reconstruction

GRAFT PREPARATION

The tibialis anterior allograft is thawed 30 minutes before beginning surgery. The graft had been harvested aseptically and deep-frozen in glycerol to −70° C and stored at −135° C. Grafts harvested in this manner can be stored to give time for serological testing and provide for an on-demand source of grafts. The patient is prepared and draped in the usual sterile fashion for knee arthroscopy with a tourniquet and leg holder. The assistant can begin preparing the graft simultaneously at the beginning of arthroscopy. The average length of an unprepared tibialis tendon allograft should be 220 mm. This allows for a total finished graft length of 100 mm. The length should include 30 mm of sutured tendon on the femoral end, 40 mm on the tibial end, and 30 mm of intra-articular tissue. It is important to presize the tendon by folding it over a No. 2 Fiberwire (Arthrex, Naples, FL) suture and passing it through a sizer without excessive force. This allows for preoperative tunnel planning. Sizing to the nearest 0.5 mm is recommended for more accurate matching of the graft and tunnel. After suture placement, the allograft is resized because the dimensions may be the same or reduced by 0.5 to 1 mm. It is recommended that the tunnel size be correlated with the final graft size to allow for the best graft-tunnel match. The folded graft is mounted on a workstation and both ends secured. From the folded end we measure 100 mm for the total graft length and place a mark to represent the end of the prepared graft. A mark is made 30 mm from the free ends and 40 mm from the folded end to indicate the areas to be sutured. The graft is tensioned to 10 lb during preparation. Baseball-type sutures with No. 2 Fiberwire are placed at both ends of the graft. The folded end of the graft is usually larger than the fanned end, but suturing the flaps together over the single shaft can augment the fanned end. The sutures are pulled tight during suturing to compress the graft and allow for a smaller tunnel size. The sutures are interdigitated so that the interference screw edges will have a path to follow without splitting the tendon fibers. On the folded end, the pull-through sutures are retained and tied over an EndoPearl (Linvatec, Fort Myers, FL). The excess tissue from the fanned end after the 100-mm mark is trimmed off. The finished graft is sized by passing it through an appropriate sizer without excessive force. It may be the same size or 0.5 to 1 mm less than the preliminary sizing. The smaller end is placed in the femoral tunnel; otherwise, the tibial tunnel will demonstrate a size mismatch with the graft. The graft is wrapped in moist gauze and pretensioned on the graft preparation board on the back table.

PROCEDURE

Standard anteromedial and anterolateral portals are created and all other procedures such as meniscal procedures are performed as needed. The ACL stump is minimally débrided with a motorized shaver to ensure adequate visualization of the femur and the ACL footprint. To prevent any possible impingement of the graft and provide better visualization for tunnel placement, a limited notchplasty of the lateral condyle and roof is performed while making certain that the posterior extent of the notch is visualized. The tibial tunnel is reamed through the anteromedial aspect of the tibia by first using an arthroscopic guide to place the guide pin just through the posteromedial ACL footprint. The guide is set at 50 degrees and placed midway front to back from the tibial tubercle at an angle of 60 to 65 degrees to the coronal plane to allow for a tunnel length of 45 to 60 mm. The tunnel is reamed with the appropriately sized reamer for the graft. A guide pin is then placed through this tunnel and through the femur at the 10- or 2-o'clock position, depending on the side, to allow retention of a 1-mm shelf of bone posteriorly after the femoral tunnel is reamed. The graft is pulled into position by placing the smaller end through the femur to allow for a wedging effect in the tibia. A notch is created for the 8 × 28-mm bioabsorbable interference screw, which is placed anterior to the graft and its overlapping sutures through the anteromedial portal. The distal end of the graft is then pulled to tension by hand, and the knee is flexed and extended with tension 25 times before fixation. This maneuver helps work the crimp out of the graft and ensures that the femoral fixation is adequate. The tibial bioabsorbable interference screw is inserted with the knee in full extension; it is placed posterior to the graft and advanced until the back end of the screw is in contact with cortical bone. The measured insertion torque should be greater than 15 in-lb, which correlates to a pullout strength of more than 400 N.[12] The arthroscope is reintroduced into the joint to rule out impingement, and adequacy of the tension of the graft is determined with a probe and anterior drawer maneuver. Wounds are closed with absorbable suture.

REHABILITATION

Rehabilitation begins the first night after surgery and consists of continuous passive motion from 0 to 45 degrees and advanced to 90 degrees as tolerated. Patients are allowed to ambulate with their knee brace locked in extension and are weaned from crutches in a few days to a week as the quadriceps becomes stronger and the effusion decreases. Strict rehabilitation and return-to-function protocols are followed during the first month and focus on early weightbearing, intensive range of motion, early extension, and gradual strengthening. The last phase is variable and dependent on the individual progress of each different athlete. Functional evaluation is performed at 3 months, and patients are usually released to full competition between 4 and 6 months, depending on functional ability. We also place our patients on the Gary Gray chain reaction matrix program, which conditions their body to offload force to the knee during sports activities.

Surgical Technique for Single–Femoral Socket, Two-Bundle ACL Reconstruction with a Tibialis Anterior Tendon Allograft

The human ACL is functionally divided into two bundles, the anteromedial bundle and the posterolateral bundle, which stabilize the knee in flexion and near extension respectively. Current single-bundle techniques cannot restore these two portions, and therefore complete restoration of knee stability is not possible. The biomechanical function of ACL reconstructions with quadruple-loop semitendinosus and gracilis tendon grafts and BPTB grafts was evaluated in a cadaveric study using a robotic/universal force-moment sensor testing system.[102] The resulting data revealed that these ACL reconstruction procedures were successful in limiting anterior tibial translation in response to an anterior tibial load but were insufficient to control a combined rotatory load of internal and valgus torque. Using the same robotic/universal force-moment sensor testing system, Yagi and coworkers showed that anatomic ACL reconstruction could more closely restore knee kinematics, especially during rotatory loads.[103] In addition, the in situ force in the ACL grafts was closer to that in the intact ACL when compared with single-bundle reconstruction. Our present indication for using a double-bundle technique is ACL insufficiency together with medial collateral ligament injury.

GRAFT PREPARATION

Graft preparation is similar to that for the single–anteromedial bundle reconstruction except that the graft is not folded over during suturing. Each tail end of the fold is sutured separately as two separate bundles. Initially, the graft is folded and mounted on the graft preparation board with both ends secured. From the folded end, ink marks are made at 100 mm for the total graft length, 40 mm from the free ends for the tibial tunnel, and 30 mm from the folded end for the femoral tunnel to indicate the areas to be sutured. This leaves 30 mm of intra-articular graft. The graft is unfolded and mounted on a workstation with both ends secured with 10 lb of tension during preparation. Baseball-type sutures with No. 2 Fiberwire are applied at one end of the graft until 40 mm of graft is sutured. This is repeated with a new No. 2 Fiberwire at the opposite end. The sutures are pulled taut during suturing to compress the graft and thereby allow for a smaller tunnel size. The sutures are overlapped so that they are interdigitated. This provides a path for the interference screw edges to follow without splitting the tendon fibers. At the central 60 mm of the graft, similar stitches are applied with another No. 2 Fiberwire. At the fanned end, excess tissue is trimmed off beyond the 100-mm mark. The graft is then folded over a free No. 2 Fiberwire, and an EndoPearl is tied to the looped end. A picture of the prepared graft is shown in Figure 41–3.

PROCEDURE

The arthroscopic portals, notchplasty, ACL stump débridement, and tibial tunnel preparations are the same as for the single-bundle technique. Any meniscal pathology is appropriately managed before graft passage. The critical difference is in preparation of the femoral tunnels. A guide pin is placed through the tibial tunnel and through the femur at the 10:30 and 1:30 clock face positions for the right and left knee, respectively, to allow for a 1-mm shelf of bone posteriorly after the femoral tunnel is reamed. After the initial femoral tunnel has been reamed to approximately 40 to 45 mm, the opening of the femoral tunnel is notched eccentrically with a combination of motorized shaver and curet to create the trough for each of the bundles. The nomenclature of anteromedial bundle femoral socket opening and posterolateral bundle femoral socket opening is taken in reference to the operated knee in 90 degrees of flexion (Fig. 41–4). The bulkier limb of the prepared graft will be designated the anteromedial bundle, whereas the smaller limb will be the posterolateral bundle. The graft is passed up the tibial tunnel into the femoral tunnel with a Beath pin. An assistant applies tension to each limb of the graft at the tibial opening to ensure that the anteromedial limb stays anterior to the posterolateral bundle in the tibial tunnel as well as at the

tibial footprint (Fig. 41–5). This technique re-creates the position of the bundles at the level of the tibial footprint. A blunt trocar introduced from the anteromedial arthroscopic portal is used to orientate the two bundles of the ACL during entry into the femoral tunnel to achieve proper positioning of the anteromedial and posterolateral bundle (Fig. 41–6). The cannulated screw driver for the femoral tunnel interference screw is passed up the tibial tunnel between the two limbs of the graft bundles, into the joint, and positioned at the femoral socket opening anterior to the axilla of the two graft bundles. A cannulated nitinol guide wire is passed up the screwdriver and

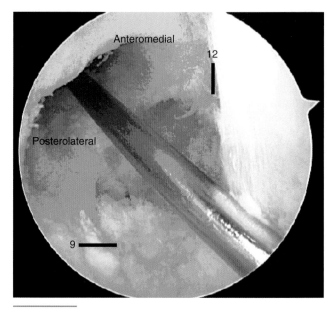

Figure 41–4. The aperture of the single femoral tunnel is notched to allow seating of the anteromedial and posterolateral bundles of the graft for a right knee.

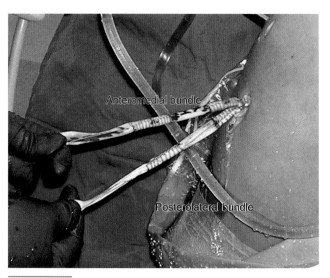

Figure 41–5. The interference screws for femur and tibia fixation are passed up the tibial tunnel. For the tibia side, the screw is positioned between the two bundles to spread the footprint out.

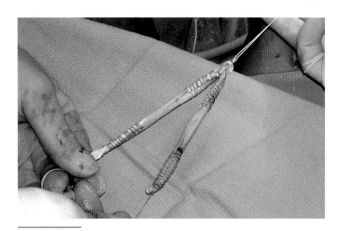

Figure 41–3. Graft preparation for the double-tunnel technique with a tibialis anterior allograft.

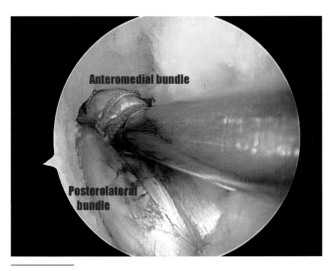

Figure 41-6. The two bundles of the anterior cruciate ligament seated at the troughs.

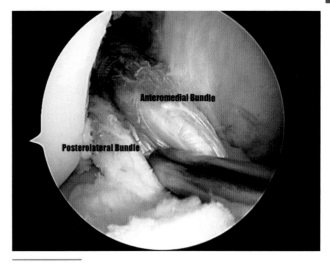

Figure 41-8. The two reconstructed bundles of the anterior cruciate ligament.

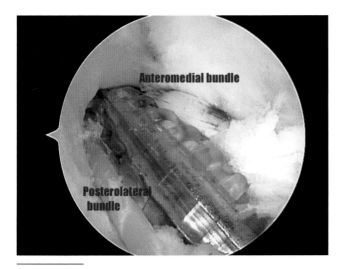

Figure 41-7. An 8 × 23-mm bioabsorbable interference screw is inserted.

seated into the femoral socket. The screwdriver is carefully withdrawn while leaving the nitinol guide wire in place. An 8 × 23-mm bioabsorbable interference screw is introduced into the femoral tunnel via the tibial tunnel once the two bundles of the graft have been correctly seated (Fig. 41-7). The screw is positioned anterior to the loop of the graft to compress the two separate bundles into their desired position. The screw will compress the graft posteriorly and sit between the two bundles to create a larger footprint on the femoral side. Fine-tuning of the final position of the two bundles at the opening of the single femoral socket can be done with a clockwise turn of the interference screw for the right knee and a counterclockwise turn of a reverse-threaded interference screw for the left knee. The distal end of the graft is then tensioned by hand, and the knee is flexed and extended 25 times before fixation to help work the crimp out of the graft and ensure that the femoral fixation is adequate. The tibial bioabsorbable interference screw is inserted with the knee in 15 degrees of flexion; it is placed between

the two limbs of the graft and advanced until the back end of the screw is in contact with cortical bone. The final appearance of the two newly reconstructed bundles of the ACL is shown in Figure 41-8. We tension the final fixation at 15 degrees of knee flexion in accordance with elegant studies by Mae et al[55] and Gabriel et al.[30] Mae and colleagues have shown that under a 100-N anterior load, the anteromedial and posterolateral bundles reach equal tension at approximately 15 degrees of knee flexion. Gabriel and coworkers showed that under a combined rotatory load, the in situ force of the posterolateral bundle is higher at 15 degrees and lower at 30 degrees of flexion whereas the in situ force in the anteromedial bundle is similar at 15 degrees and 30 degrees of knee flexion. Fixation of the grafts at full knee extension may lead to difficulty achieving full knee flexion during rehabilitation, and there is a possibility of the anteromedial bundle being overconstrained, which may predispose it to stretching out over time as the knee achieves full flexion. The arthroscope is reintroduced, impingement is ruled out, and reciprocal tensioning of each bundle of the graft is determined with a probe while the knee is brought from full extension to 90 degrees of flexion. At full extension, the posterolateral bundle should tighten while the anteromedial bundle is lax, and at 90 degrees of flexion, the anteromedial bundle should tighten while the posterolateral bundle relaxes.

REHABILITATION

The rehabilitation protocol after double-bundle ACL reconstruction is the same as that after single-bundle ACL reconstruction.

CONCLUSION

Allograft ACL single-bundle reconstruction is a reliable and reproducible technique to achieve anteroposterior stability of an ACL-deficient knee. To establish sagittal, frontal, and transverse plane stability in an ACL-deficient knee, double-bundle reconstruction may be a better option. The advantages of using an allograft have clearly been shown. The implanted allograft remodels over time with histological changes that closely parallel the healing of autografts, although it is accepted that the rate of remodeling is slower than with autografts. Clinical series comparing allografts with autografts do not show significant differences in clinical outcome even when reviewed over a period of 10 years.

More than 1 million musculoskeletal allografts were distributed in the United States in 2003. The risk of disease transmission, though very small, does exist, with documented cases of disease transmission with a fatal outcome. However, it is notable that none of these infections occurred when the allograft used consists solely of soft tissue without any bony component. It is hoped that the development of sterilization techniques that preserve the vital mechanical properties of musculoskeletal grafts will provide a safer and a wider range of options for surgeons and patients. Orthopedic surgeons who intend to use allografts in their patients need to know the tissue bank. Surgeon knowledge of tissue bank practices regarding donation and screening, serological testing, and processing is important when making the decision to use these allograft tissues.

Ultimately, clinical success in allograft ACL reconstruction depends on meticulous graft preparation, tunnel sizing, accurate positioning of the tibial and femoral tunnels, avoidance of impingement, appropriate graft tension, and secure fixation addressing both load to failure and graft slippage to reproduce the physiometry of the original ACL.

References

1. Abe S, Kurosaka M, Iguchi T, et al: Light and electron microscopic study of remodeling and maturation process in autogenous graft for anterior cruciate ligament reconstruction. Arthroscopy 9:394, 1993.
2. Aglietti P, Buzzi R, Zaccherotti G, et al: Patella tendon versus doubled semitendinosus and gracilis tendons for anterior cruciate ligament reconstruction. Am J Sports Med 22:211, 1994.
3. Amareld RW Jr, Wersocki M, Drohan M, et al: Controlled gamma-irradiation mediated pathogen inactivation of human urokinase preparations with significant recovery of enzymatic activity. Biologicals 31:261, 2003.
4. American Association of Tissue Banks: HIV transmission incident described by LifeNet's Bottenfield. Am Assoc Tissue Banks NL 14:1, 1991.
5. Andrews M, Noyes FR, Barber SD: Anterior cruciate ligament allograft reconstruction in the skeletally immature athlete. Am J Sports Med 22:48, 1994.
6. Arnoczky SP, Warren RF, Ashlock MA: Replacement of the anterior cruciate ligament using a patella tendon allograft. An experimental study. J Bone Joint Surg Am 68:376, 1986.
7. Asselmeier MA, Caspari RB, Bottenfield S: A review of allograft processing and sterilization techniques and their role in transmission of the human immunodeficiency virus. Am J Sports Med 21:170, 1993.
8. Ballock RT, Woo SLY, Lyon RM, et al: Use of patellar tendon autograft for anterior cruciate ligament reconstruction in the rabbit: A long-term histologic and biomechanical study. J Orthop Res 7:474, 1989.
9. Barad S, Cabaud HE, Rodrigo JJ: The effect of storage at −80 degrees C as compared to 4 degrees C on the strength of rhesus monkey anterior cruciate ligament. Trans Orthop Res Soc 7:378, 1982.
10. Biedert RM, Zwick EB: Ligament-muscle reflex arc after anterior cruciate ligament reconstruction: Electromyographic evaluation. Arch Orthop Trauma Surg 118:81, 1998.
11. Bonatus TJ, Alexander AH: Patellar fracture and avulsion of the patellar ligament complicating arthroscopic anterior cruciate ligament reconstruction. Orthop Rev 20:770, 1991.
12. Brand JC Jr, Pienkowski D, Steenlage E, et al: Interference screw fixation: Strength of a quadrupled hamstring tendon graft is directly related to bone mineral density and insertion torque. Am J Sports Med 28:705, 2000.
13. Buck BE, Malinin TI, Brown MD: Bone transplantation and human immunodeficiency virus: An estimate of risk of acquired immunodeficiency syndrome (AIDS). Clin Orthop 240:129, 1989.
14. Butler DL, Noyes FR, Walz KA: Biomechanics of human knee ligament allograft treatment. Trans Orthop Res Soc 12:128, 1987.
15. Caborn DN, Selby JB: Allograft anterior tibialis tendon with bioabsorbable interference screw fixation in anterior cruciate ligament reconstruction. Arthroscopy 18:102, 2002.
16. Cameron RR, Conrad RN, Sell KW, et al: Freeze-dried composite tendon allografts: An experimental study. Plast Reconstr Surg 47:39, 1971.
17. Caspari RB, Bottenfield S, Hurwitz RL, et al: HIV transmission via allograft organs and tissues. Sports Med Arthrosc Rev 1:42, 1993.
18. Chang KY, Egami DK, Shaieb MD et al: Anterior cruciate ligament reconstruction: Allograft versus autograft. Arthroscopy 19:453, 2003.
19. Clancy WG, Narechania RG, Rosenberg TD, et al: Anterior and posterior cruciate ligament reconstruction in rhesus monkeys. A histological, microangiographic, and biomechanical analysis. J Bone Joint Surg Am 63:1270, 1981.
20. Conrad EU, Gretch DR, Obermeyer KR, et al: Transmission of the hepatitis-C virus by tissue transplantation. J Bone Joint Surg Am 77:214, 1995.
21. Conway B, Tomford W, Mankin HJ, et al: Radiosensitivity of HIV-1: Potential application to sterilization of bone allografts. AIDS 5:608, 1991.
22. Cooper DE, Deng XH, Burstein AL, et al: The strength of the central third patellar tendon graft. A biomechanical study. Am J Sports Med 21:818, 1993.
23. Curtis RJ, Delee JC, Drez DJ Jr: Reconstruction of the anterior cruciate ligament with freeze dried fascia lata allografts in dogs. A preliminary report. Am J Sports Med 13:408, 1985.
24. DeConciliis GP, Choi K, Balint C, et al: Quantitative comparison of bone–patellar tendon–bone and tibialis tendon allografts [poster P308]. Presented at the Annual Meeting of the Academy of Orthopaedic Surgery, 2004, San Francisco.
25. Drez DJ, DeLee J, Holden JP, et al: Anterior cruciate ligament reconstruction using bone–patellar tendon–bone allografts. A biological and mechanical evaluation in goats. Am J Sports Med 19:256, 1991.
26. DuMontier TA, Metcalf MH, Simonian PT, et al: Patellar fracture after anterior cruciate ligament reconstruction with the patellar tendon: A comparison between different shaped bone block excisions. Am J Knee Surg 14:9, 2001.
27. Fideler BM, Vangsness CT Jr, Lu B, et al: Gamma irradiation: Effects on biomechanical properties of human bone–patellar tendon–bone allografts. Am J Sports Med 23:643, 1995.
28. Friedlaender GE, Strong DM, Sell KW: Studies on the antigenicity of bone. I. Freeze-dried and deep-frozen bone allografts in rabbits. J Bone Joint Surg Am 58:854, 1976.
29. Fromm B, Schafer B, Parsch D, et al: Reconstruction of the anterior cruciate ligament with a cyropreserved ACL allograft. A microangiographic and immunohistochemical study in rabbits. Int Orthop 20:378, 1996.
30. Gabriel MT, Wong EK, Woo SL-Y, et al: Distribution of in situ forces in the anterior cruciate ligament in response to rotatory loads. J Orthop Res 22:85, 2004.
31. Gibbons MJ, Butler DL, Grood ES, et al: Effects of gamma irradiation on the initial mechanical and material properties of goat bone–patellar tendon–bone allografts. J Orthop Res 9:209, 1991.
32. Goertzen MJ, Buitkamp J, Clahsen H, et al: Cell survival following bone–anterior cruciate ligament–bone allograft transplantation:

DNA fingerprints, segregation, and collagen morphological analysis of multiple markers in the canine model. Arch Orthop Trauma Surg 117:208, 1998.

33. Graham WC, Smith DA, McGuire MP: The use of frozen stored tendons for grafting: An experimental study. In Proceedings of the Orthopaedic Research Society. J Bone Joint Surg Am 37:624, 1955.

34. Grieb T, Forng RY, Brown R, et al: Effective use of gamma irradiation for pathogen inactivation of monoclonal antibody preparations. Biologicals 30:207, 2002.

35. Harner CD, Olson E, Irrgang JJ, et al: Allograft versus autograft anterior cruciate ligament reconstruction: 3- to 5-year outcome. Clin Orthop 324:134, 1996.

36. Hepatitis C virus transmission from an antibody-negative organ and tissue donor—United States, 2000-2002. MMWR Morb Mortal Wkly Rep 52(13):273, 2003.

37. Hiemstra LA, Webber S, MacDonald PB, et al: Knee strength deficits after hamstring tendon and patellar tendon anterior cruciate ligament reconstruction. Med Sci Sports Exerc 32:1472, 2000.

38. Hinton R, Jinnah RH, Johnson C, et al: A mechanical analysis of solvent-dehydrated and freeze-dried human fascia lata allografts. A preliminary report. Am J Sports Med 20:607, 1992.

39. Hornicek FJ, Woll JE, Kasprisin D (eds): Standards for Tissue Banking, 10th ed. McLean, VA, American Association of Tissue Banks, 2002.

40. Human tissue intended for transplantation: Interim rule. Fed Reg 58:65514, 1993.

41. Indelicato PA, Bittar ES, Prevot TJ, et al: Clinical comparison of freeze-dried and fresh frozen patellar tendon allografts for anterior cruciate ligament reconstruction of the knee. Am J Sports Med 18:335, 1990.

42. Invasive Streptococcus pyogenes after allograft implantation—Colorado, 2003. MMWR Morb Mortal Wkly Rep 52(48):1174, 2003.

43. Jackson DW, Grood ES, Arnoczky SP, et al: Freeze dried anterior cruciate ligament allografts. Preliminary studies in a goat model. Am J Sports Med 15:295, 1987.

44. Jackson DW, Grood ES, Goldstein JD, et al: A comparison of patellar tendon autograft and allograft used for anterior cruciate ligament reconstruction in the goat model. Am J Sports Med 21:176 1993.

45. Jackson DW, Simon TM, Rosen MA, el al: Survival of cells after intraarticular transplantation of fresh allografts of the patellar and anterior cruciate ligaments. J Bone Joint Surg Am 74:112, 1992.

46. Jackson DW, Windler GE, Simon TM: Intraarticular reaction associated with the use of freeze-dried, ethylene oxide–sterilized bone–patella tendon–bone allografts in the reconstruction of the anterior cruciate ligament. Am J Sports Med 18:1, 1990.

47. Jones KG: Reconstruction of the anterior cruciate ligament using the central one-third of the patellar ligament. J Bone Joint Surg Am 52:838, 1970.

48. Kartus J, Movin T, Karlsson J: Donor-site morbidity and anterior cruciate ligament reconstruction using autografts. Arthroscopy 17:971, 2001.

49. King WD, Grieb TA, Forng RY, et al: Pathogen inactivation of soft tissue allografts using high dose gamma irradiation with early clinical results [poster P106]. Presented at the Annual Meeting of the Academy of Orthopaedic Surgery, 2004, San Francisco.

50. Kuechle DK, Pearson SE, Beach WR, et al: Allograft anterior cruciate ligament reconstruction in patients over 40 years of age. Arthroscopy 18:845, 2002.

51. Latimer HA, Tibone JE, El Attrache NS, et al: Reconstruction of the lateral collateral ligament of the knee with patellar tendon allograft. Report of a new technique in combined ligament injuries. Am J Sports Med 27:269, 1998.

52. Levitt RL, Malinin T, Posada A, et al: Reconstruction of anterior cruciate ligaments with bone–patellar tendon–bone and Achilles tendon allografts. Clin Orthop 303:67, 1994.

53. Linn RM, Fischer DA, Smith JP, et al: Achilles tendon allograft reconstruction of the anterior cruciate ligament–deficient knee. Am J Sports Med 21:825, 1993.

54. Liow RY, McNicholas MJ, Keating JF, et al: Ligament repair and reconstruction in traumatic dislocation of the knee. J Bone Joint Surg Br 85:845, 2003.

55. Mae T, Shino K, Miyama T, et al: Single– versus two–femoral socket anterior cruciate ligament reconstruction technique: Biomechanical analysis using a robotic simulator. Arthroscopy 17:708, 2001.

56. Mahfouz MR, Traina SM, Komistek RD, et al: In vivo determination of knee kinematics in patients with a hamstring or patellar tendon ACL graft. J Knee Surg 16:197, 2003.

57. Malinin TI, Buck BE, Temple HT, et al: Incidence of clostridial contamination in donors' musculoskeletal tissue. J Bone Joint Surg Br 85:1051, 2003.

58. Malinin TI, Levitt RL, Bashore C, et al: A study of retrieved allografts used to replace anterior cruciate ligament. Arthroscopy 18:163, 2002.

59. Marder RA, Raskind JR, Carroll M: Prospective evaluation of arthroscopically assisted anterior cruciate ligament reconstruction. Patellar tendon versus semitendinosus and gracilis tendons. Am J Sports Med 19:478, 1991.

60. Miller MD, Nichols T, Butler CA: Patella fracture and proximal tendon rupture following arthroscopic anterior cruciate ligament reconstruction. Arthroscopy 15:640, 1999.

61. Minami A, Ishii S, Ogino T, et al: Effect of the immunological antigenicity of the allogeneic tendons on tendon grafting. Hand 14:111, 1982.

62. Moebius UG, Georgoulis AD, Papageorgiou CD, et al: Alterations of the extensor apparatus after anterior cruciate ligament reconstruction using the medial third of the patellar tendon. Arthroscopy 17:953, 2001.

63. Mowe J: Survey of Tissue Banks—1988. McLean, VA, American Association of Tissue Banks, 1989.

64. Ng GY, Oakes BW, Deacon OW, et al: Biomechanics of patellar tendon autograft for reconstruction of the anterior cruciate ligament in the goat: Three-year study. J Orthop Res 13:602, 1995.

65. Noyes FR, Barber SD: Reconstruction of anterior cruciate ligament with human allograft. Comparison of early and later results. J Bone Joint Surg Am 78:524, 1996.

66. Noyes FR, Barber SD: Arthroscopic-assisted allograft anterior cruciate ligament reconstruction in patients with symptomatic arthrosis. Arthroscopy 13:24, 1997.

67. Noyes FR, Barber SD, Craig SR: Use of allografts after failed treatment of rupture of the anterior cruciate ligament. J Bone Joint Surg Am 7:1019, 1994.

68. Noyes FR, Barber SD, Mangine RE. Bone–patellar ligament–bone and fascia lata allografts for reconstruction of the anterior cruciate ligament. J Bone Joint Surg Am 72:1125, 1990.

69. Noyes FR, Butler DL, Grood ES, et al: Biomechanical analysis of human ligament grafts used in knee-ligament repairs and reconstructions. J Bone Joint Surg Am 66:344, 1984.

70. Nyland J, Caborn DNM, Rothbauer, et al: Two-year outcomes following ACL reconstruction with allograft tibialis anterior tendons: A retrospective study. Knee Surg Sports Traumatol Arthrosc 11:212, 2003.

71. Oeffinger DJ, Shapiro R, Nyland J, et al: Delayed gastrocnemius muscle response to sudden perturbation in rehabilitated patients with anterior cruciate ligament reconstruction. Knee Surg Sports Traumatol Arthrosc 9:19, 2001.

72. Pearsall AW, Hollis JM, Russell GV, et al. A biomechanical comparison of three lower extremity tendons for ligamentous reconstruction about the knee. Arthroscopy 19:1091, 2003.

73. Petsche TS, Hutchinson MR: Loss of extension after reconstruction of the anterior cruciate ligament. J Am Acad Orthop Surg 7:119, 1999.

74. Pinkowski JL, Reiman PR, Chen S: Human lymphocyte reaction to freeze-dried allograft and xenograft ligamentous tissue. Am J Sports Med 17:595, 1989.

75. Rasmussen TJ, Feder SM, Butler DL, et al: The effects of 4 mrad of Tau irradiation on the initial mechanical properties of bone–patellar tendon–bone grafts. Arthroscopy 10:188, 1994.

76. Roberts TS, Drez D Jr, McCarthy W, et al: Anterior cruciate ligament reconstruction using freeze-dried, ethylene oxide– sterilized, bone–patellar tendon–bone allografts. Two year results in thirty-six patients. Am J Sports Med 19:35, 1991.

77. Schulte K, Thompson W, Jamison J, et al: The immune response to allograft anterior cruciate ligament reconstruction: Clinical correlation. Presented at the Academy of Orthopaedic Surgery Specialty Day, 1996, Atlanta.

78. Septic arthritis following anterior cruciate ligament reconstruction using tendon allografts—Florida and Louisiana, 2000. MMWR Morb Mortal Wkly Rep 50(48):1081, 2001.

79. Shapiro MS, Freedman EL: Allograft reconstruction of the anterior and posterior cruciate ligaments after traumatic knee dislocation. Am J Sports Med 23:580, 1995.

80. Shelton WR, Treacy SH, Dukes AD, et al: Use of allografts in knee reconstruction: II Surgical considerations. J Am Acad Orthop Surg 6:169, 1998.

81. Shino K: Allograft anterior cruciate ligament reconstruction. In Insall JN, Scott WN (eds): Surgery of the Knee, 3rd ed. Philadelphia, Churchill Livingstone, 2001, p 712.

82. Shino K, Inoue M, Horibe S, et al: Reconstruction of the anterior cruciate ligament using allogeneic tendon. Long-term followup. Am J Sports Med 18:457, 1990.

83. Shino K, Inoue M, Horibe S, et al: Surface blood flow and histology of human anterior cruciate ligament allografts. Arthroscopy 7:171, 1991.

84. Shino K, Kawasaki T, Hirose H, et al: Replacement of the anterior cruciate ligament by an allogeneic tendon graft. An experimental study in the dog. J Bone Joint Surg Br 66:672, 1984.

85. Shino K, Nakagawa S, Inoue M, et al: Deterioration of patellofemoral articular surfaces after anterior cruciate ligament reconstruction. Am J Sports Med 21:206, 1993.

86. Shino K, Nakata K, Horibe S, et al: Quantitative evaluation after arthroscopic anterior cruciate ligament reconstruction. Allograft versus autograft. Am J Sports Med 21:609, 1993.

87. Shino K, Oakes BW, Horibe S, et al: Collagen fibril populations in human anterior cruciate ligament allografts. Electron microscopic analysis. Am J Sports Med 23:203, 1995.

88. Siebold R, Buelow JU, Bos L, et al: Primary ACL reconstruction with fresh-frozen patellar versus Achilles tendon allografts. Arch Orthop Trauma Surg 123:180, 2003.

89. Simmons RJ, Holmberg SD, Huriwtz RL, et al: Transmission of human immunodeficiency virus type 1 from a seronegative organ and tissue donor. N Engl J Med 326:726, 1992.

90. Smith JJ, Lewis JL, Mente PL, et al: Intraoperative force-setting did not improve the mechanical properties of an augmented bone-tendon-bone anterior cruciate ligament graft in a goat model. J Orthop Res 14:209, 1996.

91. Strong DM, Eastlund T, Mowe J: Tissue bank activity in the United States: 1992 survey of accredited tissue banks. Tissue Cell Rep 3:15, 1996.

92. Summitt M, Bianchi J, Keesling J, et al: Biomechanical testing of bone treated through a new tissue cleaning process. In 25th Annual Meeting of the American Association of Tissue Banks. Washington, DC, American Association of Tissue Banks, 2001, pp 55, s-15.

93. Tashiro T, Kurosawa H, Kawakami A, et al: Influence of medial hamstring tendon harvest on knee flexor strength after anterior cruciate ligament reconstruction. A detailed evaluation with comparison of single- and double-tendon harvest. Am J Sports Med 31:522, 2003.

94. Thompson W, Schulte K, Jamison J, et al: Immunologic response to allograft anterior cruciate ligament reconstruction: Part I: Humoral and cellular parameters. Presented at the Academy of Orthopaedic Surgery Specialty Day, Atlanta, 1996.

95. Tomford WW: Transmission of disease through musculoskeletal transplantation. In Portland Bone Symposium. Portland, OR, Oregon Health Sciences University, 1997, p 410.

96. United States Pharmacopeia: Sterility tests. In United States Pharmacopeia XXV. Rockville, Md, United States Pharmacopeial Convention, 2001, p 1878.

97. Update: Allograft-associated bacterial infections—United States, 2000. MMWR Morb Mortal Wkly Rep 51(10):207, 2002.

98. Wascher DC, Becker JR, Dexter JG, et al: Reconstruction of the anterior and posterior cruciate ligaments after knee dislocation. Results using fresh-frozen nonirradiated allografts. Am J Sports Med 27:189, 1999.

99. Webster DA, Werner FW: Freeze-dried flexor tendons in anterior cruciate ligament reconstruction. Clin Orthop 181:238, 1983.

100. Wingenfeld C, Egli RJ, Hempfing A, et al: Cryopreservation of osteochondral allografts: Dimethyl sulfoxide promotes angiogenesis and immune tolerance in mice. J Bone Joint Surg Am 84:1420, 2002.

101. Woll JE, Kasprisin D: Standards for Tissue Banking. McLean, VA, American Association of Tissue Banks, 2001.

102. Woo SL-Y, Kanamori A, Zeminski J, et al: The effectiveness of reconstruction of the anterior cruciate ligament with hamstrings and patellar tendon: A cadaveric study comparing anterior tibial and rotational loads. J Bone Joint Surg Am 84:907, 2002.

103. Yagi M, Wong EK, Kanamori A, et al: Biomechanical analysis of an anatomic anterior cruciate ligament reconstruction. Am J Sports Med 30:660, 2002.

104. Zimmerman MC, Contiliano JH, Parsons JR, et al: The biomechanics and histopathology of chemically processed patellar tendon allografts for anterior cruciate ligament replacement. Am J Sports Med 22:378, 1994.

CHAPTER 42

Double-Bundle Anterior Cruciate Ligament Reconstruction

Paolo Aglietti • Pierluigi Cuomo • Francesco Giron

Anterior cruciate ligament (ACL) reconstruction with standard single-bundle techniques provides satisfactory subjective results and restores anteroposterior stability in the vast majority of patients in the short term. Long-term sequelae of the operation have not yet been defined, and some believe that such ligament reconstruction does not protect the knee joint from osteoarthritis.[22] Moreover, many authors have clinically detected residual minimal rotatory instability (pivot shift) in almost a fifth of cases independent of the graft, surgical technique, and choice of fixation device.

Freedman et al[14] in a meta-analysis of 34 ACL reconstruction studies with a 2-year minimum follow-up performed between 1990 and 2000 found that a pivot-shift glide was present in 14.5% of the patellar tendon grafts and 13.7% of the hamstring grafts. It is worthy of note that only 24 of the 34 studies clinically addressed rotational stability of the knee.

Our experience[2] with single-bundle reconstruction has yielded similar results: in a prospective randomized study comparing patellar tendon and quadrupled hamstring grafts after a minimum of 2 years, a pivot-shift glide was present in 17% of patients with patellar tendon grafts and 18% with hamstrings grafts.

In addition, several authors have studied the in vivo kinematics of ACL-reconstructed knees. Logan et al[26] used dynamic multiple resonance imaging to compare the ACL-reconstructed and the uninjured contralateral knee during weightbearing flexion and a Lachman test. Although anteroposterior stability did not differ significantly, the reconstructed knee showed increased tibial internal rotation throughout the range of motion. Tashman et al[42] used a stereoradiographic system to evaluate six subjects during downhill jogging and compared the ACL-reconstructed knee with the uninjured contralateral one. In the reconstructed knee, rotation was not restored. With a similar stereoradiographic system, Brandsson et al[8] studied knee kinematics during a step in nine patients and found that preoperative and postoperative measurements of femorotibial reciprocal rotation and translation did not differ after single-bundle transtibial ACL reconstruction. Other investigators[9,38] have used a gait analysis system to compare pivoting and cutting activities in ACL-reconstructed patients and a matched control group and similarly found that surgery did not restore perfect knee rotational stability.

Based on these observations, it is evident that single-bundle ACL reconstruction does not perfectly restore normal knee kinematics. Several solutions have been proposed to increase rotational control of a reconstructed graft, including a more horizontal graft orientation through a lower femoral tunnel entry point (such as the 10:00-o'clock position)[27,41] and additional anterolateral extra-articular backup procedures.[11]

This chapter discusses the anatomic and biomechanical background of double-bundle ACL reconstruction, as well as the surgical technique.

ANATOMY AND BIOMECHANICS OF THE NATIVE ANTERIOR CRUCIATE LIGAMENT

Girgis et al[17] in 1975 were the first to describe ACL functional anatomy with respect to its main bundles. In 19 cadaver knees they found that, while in extension, the whole ligament was taut and, while in deep flexion, only a small anterior part was in tension and the bulk of the ligament was loose. The term anteromedial bundle (AMB) was introduced to describe the most isometric part of the ligament.

In 1979 Norwood and Cross[34] studied ACL anatomy and function in 18 freshly amputated knees. They isolated and distinguished the bundles on a purely anatomic basis, and in some knees they found that synovium divided the bundles. Three main bundles were identified and differentiated according to their tibial insertion: the AMB, intermediate bundle, and posterolateral bundle (PLB). The tibial insertion was described as a triangle with a posterior apex (PLB insertion) and two anterior corners (AMB and intermediate bundle). On the femur, the AMB insertion was described as being posterior and superior in the notch, whereas the PLB was anterior and inferior; the intermediate bundle had an intermediate position between the other two. Selective cutting of the bundles was performed to investigate the influence of the bundles on knee stability. The AMB and intermediate bundle were described as primary restraints to anteroposterior translation, whereas when the PLB was selectively cut, tibial external rotation and recurvatum increased.

Other investigators[3,4,10,12,15,21,31,35] have subsequently studied ACL anatomy, and a different number of bundles ranging from one to six have been described from an anatomic point of view. Synovial separation between bundles cannot always be identified. Age-dependent changes have been described, with actual interbundle cleavage being more easily observed in older specimens.[3]

Despite the aforementioned variability and difficulties, great consensus now exists that ACL complexity should be considered from a functional rather than an anatomic point of view as a continuum of fascicles that are differentially recruited throughout the range of motion even if two main components (AMB and PLB) can be distinguished on the basis of their differential behavior.

Amis and Dawkins[3] in 1991 used a transducer to measure the changes in length of the AMB and PLB in flexion-extension and with tibial rotation. Neither was found to be isometric: the PLB was taut in extension, whereas the AMB was taut in flexion. Tibial internal or external rotation had no significant effect on bundle length. Similarly, Kurosawa et al[24] used four elongation transducers to measure the change in length of the anterior and posterior portions of the ACL. Two transducers were positioned in the anterolateral and anteromedial portions of the ligament and two in the posterolateral and posteromedial portions. The anteromedial and anterolateral fibers, as well as the posteromedial and posterolateral fibers, showed the same elongation behavior. Close to extension, the anterior fibers were shorter and the posterior fibers lengthened, whereas at higher degrees of flexion, the posterior became shorter and the anterior lengthened.

Bach et al[6] implanted a strain gauge in the AMB and PLB and measured changes in strain during range of motion. The AMB exhibited quasi-isometric behavior from 10 to 90 degrees with changes of less than 1%. At full extension and full flexion the AMB stretched. The PLB, in contrast, was relaxed from 40 degrees onward, whereas in extension it elongated more than 12% of its initial length.

In vivo, the differential lengthening behavior of the two bundles has been addressed only by Li et al,[25] who used a computed reconstruction of a fluoroscopic movie obtained during lunge activity in five young volunteers. The AMB showed quasi-isometric behavior with no statistical differences in length at different flexion angles. The PLB, in contrast, was significantly longer in extension.

Sakane et al[40] used robotics to measure the in situ force of the bundles in response to applied anterior tibial loads ranging from 22 to 110 N. Whereas the AMB was found to have a relatively constant in situ force that did not change with the flexion angle, the PLB showed larger in situ force between 0 and 45 degrees of knee flexion with a peak at 15 degrees.

With a similar robotic device, Gabriel et al[16] analyzed the in situ force of the bundles in two loading conditions: a 134-N anterior tibial load at different knee flexion angles and a combined rotatory load of 10 N·m valgus and 5 N·m internal tibial torque at 15 and 30 degrees of flexion. Under an isolated anterior tibial load the PLB showed greater in situ force during extension, whereas the in situ force of the AMB increased with flexion and reached a peak at 60 degrees. Under the combined rotatory load the PLB had a larger in situ force at 15 than at 30 degrees. The AMB, instead, showed a similar magnitude of in situ force at both angles that was superior to the PLB. None of the bundles alone could, in any case, reproduce the in situ force of the entire intact ACL.

Based on the aforementioned studies, evidence exists that ACL native bundles show load-sharing behavior. Neither of the two bundles alone can reproduce the mechanical properties of the intact ACL. The AMB by itself is not sufficient to control both translation and rotation in extension. In flexion, however, the function of the AMB alone is similar to that of the intact ACL. The effect of the PLB on both translation and rotation is more evident during extension. Therefore, to address residual laxity in extension after ACL reconstruction, it seems reasonable to reconstruct both bundles.

BIOMECHANICS OF TWO-BUNDLE ANTERIOR CRUCIATE LIGAMENT RECONSTRUCTION

Radford and Amis[37] in 1990 were the first to assess double-bundle reconstruction in the laboratory and compare it with single-bundle reconstruction and the intact ACL. The AMB and PLB were replicated by using two synthetic polyester grafts that were passed through two distinct tibial tunnels; on the femur, the AMB graft was passed over the top, whereas the PLB graft was passed in a transcondylar tunnel. Anteroposterior stability at 20 and 90 degrees of flexion was assessed with an Instron machine. Double-bundle reconstruction was found to better restore anteroposterior stability of the native ACL, whereas single-bundle reconstruction showed increased laxity.

Using a differential variable reluctance transducer, Edwards et al[13] measured changes in length in the native AMB and PLB and after reconstruction with the single- and double-bundle techniques in cadaver knees. Three double-bundle techniques that differed according to the number of tunnels produced were compared: single tibial and dual femoral, dual tibial and single femoral, and dual tibial and dual femoral. Single-bundle reconstruction did not reproduce the functional behavior of the native ACL. Only dual-tibial and dual-femoral tunnel reconstruction more closely restored native bundle strain. Other double-bundle techniques (single tibial/dual femoral and single femoral/dual tibial) not only failed to restore normal kinematics but also tended to overconstrain the knee.

Mae et al[28] used a robotic simulator to compare single- and double-bundle reconstruction in seven cadaver knees and studied anterior translation and in situ force. Double-bundle reconstruction was found to be more effective than single-bundle reconstruction in reducing anteroposterior laxity. The in situ force in the reconstructed bundles showed a load-sharing behavior that is similar to that of the native AMB and PLB: the PLB was more effective in extension and the AMB in flexion. The authors did not, however, measure the in situ force in the native bundles before cutting them.

Using a similar robotic apparatus, Yagi et al[43] compared single- and double-bundle reconstruction with intact and ACL-deficient knees. Single-bundle reconstruction was performed by positioning the femoral tunnel in the 11:00-o'clock position. Anteroposterior laxity throughout the range of motion and rotational stability after a combined valgus and rotatory load at 15 and 30 degrees were measured. Double-bundle reconstruction reduced antero-posterior laxity better than single-bundle reconstruction did. In extension, residual laxity significantly differed from that in the intact knee. Under the combined valgus and rotatory load, in situ force was higher in the double-bundle reconstruction than in the single and, close to extension, did not differ from that in the intact knee.

The same group of researchers[44] again used a robot to compare double-bundle with single-bundle reconstruction. In this study, single-bundle reconstruction was performed with a lower femoral tunnel (10:00 o'clock), which in practice was positioned at the insertion of the native PLB. In extension, single- and double-bundle reconstruction did not differ in terms of rotatory and anteroposterior stability. From 60 degrees onward, the single-bundle procedure was less effective than the double-bundle procedure in reducing anteroposterior laxity.

In conclusion, it appears from several laboratory studies that double-bundle reconstruction is biomechanically more advantageous than single-bundle reconstruction performed with either an 11:00- or even a 10:00-o'clock femoral position. When performing double-bundle reconstructions, the two–tibial tunnel techniques seem to be advisable.

SURGICAL TECHNIQUE

Double-bundle ACL reconstruction should reproduce the native AMB and PLB insertions. A quantitative analysis of bundle insertions has been performed by Harner et al,[21] who showed that the AMB and PLB insertion area is approximately the same, 47 mm^2 on the femur and 55 mm^2 on the tibia. ACL insertion landmarks (i.e., the posterior cruciate ligament and the anterior horn of the lateral meniscus on the tibia and the over-the-top on the femur) have been described for the whole ligament,[18,23,32] but no investigator up to now has described individual bundle insertion landmarks. Consequently, it is not an easy task to replicate the native insertions because ACL remnants can rarely be seen at surgery, especially with chronic lesions.

Tibial Tunnels

Although it is agreed that two femoral tunnels are mandatory, it is still debated whether one or two tibial tunnels are needed. "One-tunnel" supporters maintain that two tunnels are not necessary because the tension behavior of the bundles is mainly driven by their femoral insertion. Most of the published laboratory studies[28,43,44] on double-bundle ACL reconstruction used one tibial tunnel, and this solution controlled translation and rotation more effectively than single-bundle reconstructions did. Only one study[13] has compared one– and two–tibial tunnel reconstructions in vitro, and it demonstrated superiority of the latter, which more closely restores the native bundles' behavior. Yasuda,[45] using a transtibial technique in vivo, compared one– and two–tibial tunnel double-bundle reconstructions with single-bundle reconstruction:

only when two tibial tunnels were used and a more precise femoral position for the PLB was found was anterior tibial translation reduced significantly better than with single-bundle reconstruction. No differences were noted between the various techniques in terms of residual pivot shift.

In addition to the findings in the studies just presented, we are in favor of two–tibial tunnel reconstruction for several other reasons. First, it more closely replicates the anatomy of the AMB and PLB, which have separate tibial insertions.[21] Second, two tibial tunnels allow one to achieve differential bundle tensioning and fixation to more closely restore the different functional behaviors of the AMB and PLB. Finally, two tibial tunnels with different directions are useful to surgeons who prefer to drill the two femoral tunnels through a transtibial approach.

The intra-articular exit of the tibial tunnels should reproduce the footprint of the native bundles. The native ACL footprint is about 20 mm long in the anteroposterior direction and is therefore large enough to allow the placement of two 6-mm tunnels. The reconstructed graft cannot reproduce the "dovetail" aspect of the most anterior fibers of the native ACL, and the most anterior part of the anteromedial tibial insertion is not useful for tunnel placement because the graft would impinge against the roof of the intercondylar notch. The AMB tunnel should be placed in the posterior part of the anteromedial insertion. Similarly, the PLB tunnel should be drilled in the posterior part of the posterolateral native insertion in order to leave a bony bridge between the two tunnels, which should limit tunnel confluence and ensure graft independence.

At surgery we use the 65-degree Howell guide (Arthrotek, Warsaw, IN) to drill the anteromedial guide wire. This guide has a nose that is inserted into the joint through the anteromedial arthroscopic portal with the knee flexed. When the knee is extended, the nose is locked within the intercondylar notch (Fig. 42–1) and the guide

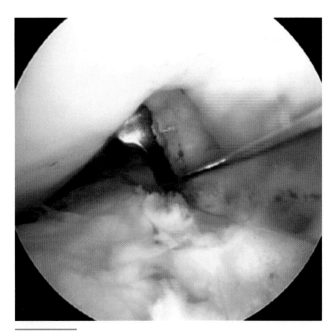

Figure 42–1. The nose of the 65-degree Howell guide, which takes as a reference off the roof of the intercondylar notch.

wire is drilled from the anteromedial aspect of the tibia, thereby automatically avoiding roof impingement.

For double-bundle reconstruction we rotate the guide barrel to position the guide wire 2 mm more anterior than the standard single-bundle position; this adjustment would not subject the AMB graft to roof impingement because its diameter is usually small (6 mm). We have checked this method in 21 cadaver knees (unpublished data) and have found it to be reproducible and effective in positioning the guide wire in the posterior aspect of the AMB insertion.

The posterolateral tibial wire should be placed about 8 mm posterior to the AMB and slightly more lateral. This position usually leaves only a small bony bridge between the two tunnels, which is important because the intra-articular exit of the tunnels is slightly oval rather than circular. More posterior posterolateral tunnel placement should be avoided because it is less anatomic and less functional. We have developed a system to drill the posterolateral tunnel in view of these considerations. It consists of a guide attached to a rod that is inserted into the anteromedial tunnel. The posterolateral guide wire is preset to exit at a fixed distance of 8 mm from the center of the anteromedial tunnel (Fig. 42–2).

The orientation of the posterolateral tunnel is important, especially for surgeons who prefer to drill the femoral tunnels through the tibial ones. In such cases the posterolateral tunnel should be angulated around 45 degrees in the coronal plane (Fig. 42–3).

Care must be taken to not damage the medial collateral ligament when drilling this tunnel (Fig. 42–4).

Femoral Tunnels

Femoral tunnel positioning is critical because it will be the main determinant of bundle tension behavior. Therefore, one should aim to replicate the femoral insertions. As for the tibia, the main difficulty is that up to now no definitive landmarks have been described for anatomic placement of the tunnels. Furthermore, native bundle insertions show some variability in their position. If a true anatomic position cannot always be achieved in view of native bundle variability, at least the positioning should be as safe as possible and avoid dangerous areas. It is important to look at the notch through different angles to have a two-dimensional perception of it and to become confident with the region where the native ACL insertion is located. It is useful at this point to recall the notch nomenclature that we are using in this chapter, as described in Figure 42–5.

Most surgeons usually rely on a single portal view, the anterolateral one, which is useful for varying the tunnel

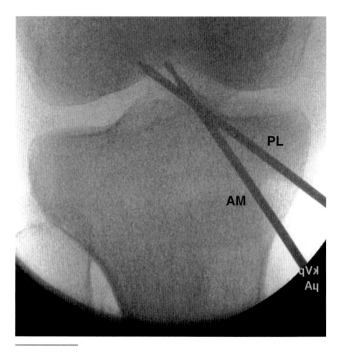

Figure 42–3. The frontal orientation of the tibial tunnels is important when drilling the femoral tunnels through the tibia. AM, anteromedial; PL, posterolateral.

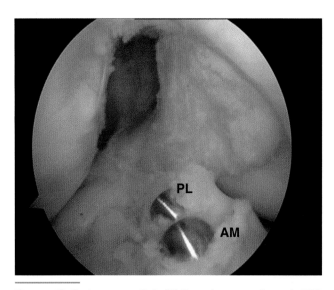

Figure 42–2. Anteromedial (AM) and posterolateral (PL) tibial tunnels.

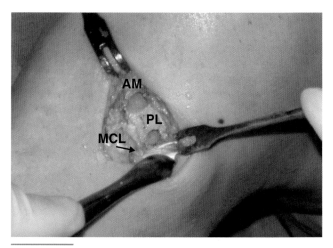

Figure 42–4. Care must be taken to not damage the medial collateral ligament (MCL) when drilling the tibial tunnels. AM, anteromedial; PL, posterolateral.

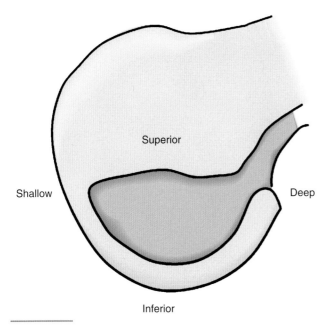

Figure 42–5. Notch nomenclature: superior (anterior), inferior (posterior), deep (proximal), shallow (distal).

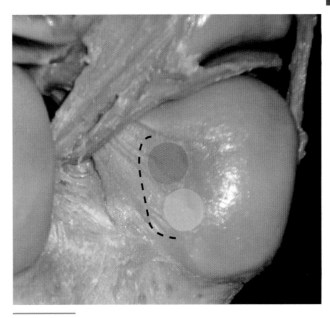

Figure 42–7. The femoral insertion is wide, and replication is difficult with only one tunnel.

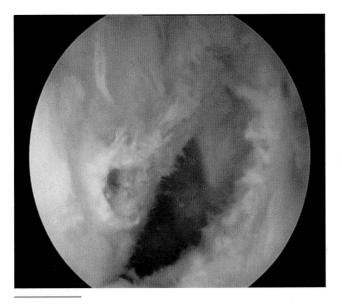

Figure 42–6. Chronic anterior cruciate ligament lesion. Femoral insertion remnants are present.

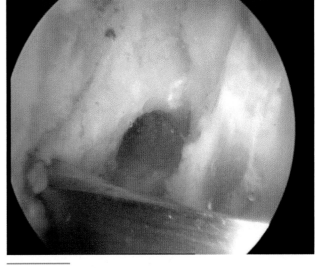

Figure 42–8. The posterolateral tunnel is drilled in flexion through the transportal approach. In flexion, visualization is poor.

position superoinferiorly and adjusting the o'clock position of the tunnels. The view from the anteromedial portal, in contrast, is particularly useful for adjustment of the deep-shallow position of the tunnel (Fig. 42–6).

In this light we advise placement of the tunnels as deep as possible within the notch and along the articular cartilage contour to mimic the fan-shaped appearance and position of the native fibers (Fig. 42–7).

Three different surgical approaches can be used to drill the femoral tunnels: the transportal, the transtibial, and the two-incision outside-in technique. The transportal technique is performed by drilling the femoral tunnel through the anteromedial portal with the knee in hyperflexion. It is a very easy and simple method, but accuracy

is totally dependent on the experience of the surgeon, and furthermore, visualization in deep flexion is not optimal. In addition, the posterolateral tunnel is rather short (Fig. 42–8).

The transtibial technique is very popular in single-bundle reconstruction because of its simplicity, reproducibility, and efficacy in placing the femoral tunnel in a relatively safe position, even if the positioning has not been demonstrated to be very anatomic.[5,18] The femoral tunnel is usually placed in a slightly more shallow and superior position with respect to the native insertion; nonetheless, this position has been demonstrated to be safe for the graft throughout the range of motion, and the graft has nearly isometric behavior.[48] An attempt at more

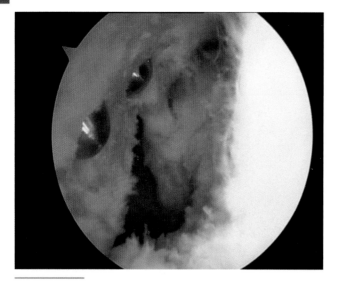

Figure 42–9. Anteromedial and posterolateral tunnels drilled through the tibial tunnel. The posterolateral tunnel is rather superior and shallow.

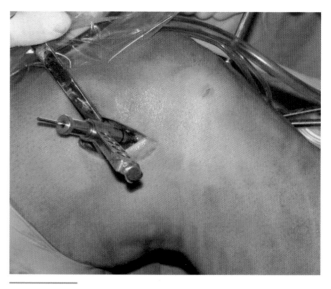

Figure 42–10. The rear entry guide is inserted into the joint through a second incision.

anatomic placement can be made by rotating the femoral aimer externally so that it is deeper and inferior in the notch. In the laboratory we have verified the efficacy of this adjustment, but it was still not precise in replicating the femoral anteromedial insertion, although it was very reproducible (unpublished data). Drilling the femoral posterolateral tunnel through the tibial tunnel is appealing as well; however, proper angulation of the tibial tunnel is mandatory. No specific aimers are available. It is not easy to find the proper angulation of the tibial tunnel to reach the anatomic point on the femur, and a tendency to be superior and more shallow than the native posterolateral insertion has been observed by the authors (Fig. 42–9).

Proper external loading conditions are important as well. We found (unpublished data) that tibial external rotation and posterior tibial drawer allow the femoral wire to be more anatomic. Malposition of the posterolateral tunnel in this direction would lead to increased graft tension with flexion and possible risk of failure.

The last option for drilling the femoral tunnels is the dual-incision outside-in technique. A second incision is needed on the lateral aspect of the distal part of the thigh. Several jigs for drilling the tunnel from the outside are available on the market, and the technique can be performed simply either by using jigs that are introduced into the joint in an anterior direction or by using jigs that pass posterior to the condyle. We prefer the latter technique with the rear entry guide (Acufex Microsurgical) (Fig. 42–10), which we are currently using in double-bundle reconstruction.

The rear entry guide is very precise in placing the guide wire along the posterior border and has been shown to position the guide wire in the superior and central aspect of the native ACL insertion, where the anteromedial fibers are.[18] Furthermore, while handling the guide it is very easy to look at the notch through the anteromedial portal and have wider visualization of the wall (Fig. 42–11).

Positioning is safe because the curvature of the guide arm follows the shape of the condyle and thus shallow

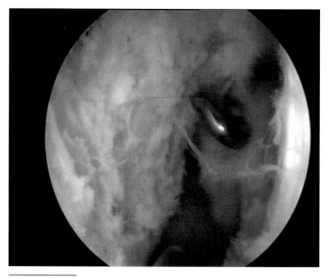

Figure 42–11. The tip of the rear entry guide to position the anteromedial guide wire.

positions are avoided (Fig. 42–12). The posterolateral insertion is not easily reached with the same conventional rear entry guide. Systems that use the anteromedial wire as a point of reference can be developed.

An advantage of the outside-in technique versus the transtibial technique is that the entrance of the tunnel in the notch is more round and less oval because of the direction of drilling.

Tensioning and Fixation

The aim of double-bundle ACL reconstruction is to replicate the anatomic and functional complexity of the native ACL. Provided that the anatomy is restored, effort must

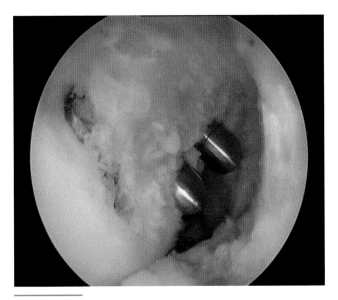

Figure 42–12. The anteromedial and posterolateral femoral tunnels drilled through the outside-in approach. Both tunnels are within the remnants of the native anterior cruciate ligament.

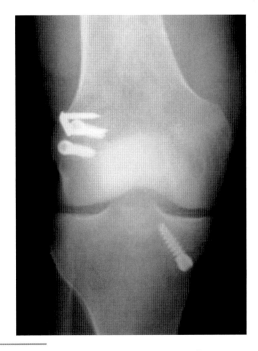

Figure 42–13. Postoperative radiograph after anterior cruciate ligament double-bundle reconstruction with the outside-in approach on the femur. The grafts are fixed with three interference screws, which are secured with a staple on the femur.

be undertaken to restore the reciprocal behavior of the native AMB and PLB. The AMB works mainly in flexion or is nearly isometric, whereas the PLB works mainly in extension. For this reason we believe that the two bundles should be tensioned and fixed separately. To do so we tension and fix the PLB close to extension (15 degrees) and the AMB at about 45 degrees of flexion. Further studies are needed to demonstrate which graft should be fixed first and in which loading condition to ensure reciprocal function and avoid the risk of overconstraining the joint.

At present we first pass single semitendinosus and gracilis tendons in the posterolateral tunnels and fix them on the femur with a 6-mm soft-tissue interference screw. Tibial side PLB graft fixation is achieved at 15 degrees of flexion and posterior tibial drawer with another interference screw after 3 minutes of pretensioning. The graft is then passed into the anteromedial tunnels. Tibial fixation of the AMB graft is achieved through the bony bridge on the anterior aspect of the tibia. AMB femoral fixation is obtained with a third interference screw at 45degrees of flexion. Both bundles are finally secured to the femur with a staple (Fig. 42–13).

Most fixation devices are presently borrowed from single-bundle reconstruction, but smaller sizes are required. We believe that once the technique has been standardized and validated, both anatomically and biomechanically, dedicated double-bundle fixation devices will be designed.

RESULTS

Several authors in the last decades have described double-bundle techniques for ACL reconstruction. Mott[33] was the first to perform the so-called STAR technique (semitendinosus anatomic reconstruction). It was an open procedure that included osteotomy of the lateral femoral condyle. Two tibial and two femoral tunnels were drilled.

In 1987 Zaricznyj[47] proposed a double-bundle technique in which two tibial tunnels and one femoral tunnel were created. His idea did not gain much support because the differential bundle behavior is driven by the femoral insertion rather than the tibial one. Pederzini et al[36] in 2000 reproposed this tunnel combination with use of the quadriceps tendon. Other authors[20,29] have tried to reproduce the multistrand shape of the ACL by combining an "over-the-top" graft to reproduce the AMB and a transcondylar tunnel to reproduce the PLB. Only one tibial tunnel is used.

In the 1990s Rosenberg and Graf[39] popularized their double-bundle reconstruction technique, which consisted of one tibial tunnel and two femoral tunnels drilled through the anteromedial portal. Recently, Bellier et al[7] modified the technique by using a second tibial tunnel for the PLB.

All the aforementioned authors have not yet published their long-term results. Only a few outcome studies on double-bundle reconstructions are available in the literature.

Hamada et al[19] showed no clinical difference when prospectively comparing single- versus double-bundle reconstruction in 106 patients. A single tibial tunnel was used. On the femur, AMB wire position was determined with a tensioning device in an attempt to achieve graft tensioning in extension like that of the intact ACL.[30] The PLB wire was drilled at the 9-o'clock position without checking tension. In contrast, we believe that the AMB and PLB have tension behavior that is different from that of the intact ACL. As a result, the authors have not shown any clinical difference at 2 years' follow-up between single- and double-bundle reconstruction. We believe that this could probably be explained on the basis of nonanatomic placement.

Adachi et al[1] compared single- and double-bundle reconstruction in a prospective randomized study. Antero- medial and posterolateral tunnels were drilled at the 11:00 and 9:30 positions. Both bundles were tensioned and fixed together at 90 degrees of flexion. At a mean follow-up of 32 months no clinical differences were detected between the groups.

Recently, Yasuda et al[46] reported their results with a transtibial technique. The authors validated their tech- nique in cadaver knees with respect to the native inser- tions and found it to be anatomic. In the femur, according to their anatomic findings, the Navitip guide was used to position the PLB guide wire with the knee at 90 degrees of flexion and the femur horizontal, 5 to 8 mm superior to the cartilage border at the point where the femoral condyle contacts the tibial plateau. The anteromedial guide wire was positioned by using a conventional 5- or 6-mm offset femoral aimer. A hybrid graft (semitendin- osus and gracilis plus polyester tape augmentation) was used. Both bundles were fixed at 20 degrees of flexion. Fifty-seven consecutive patients were monitored for at least 24 months. No control group has been included. The average 20-lb KT side-to-side difference from the con- tralateral unaffected knee was 1.0 mm. Only one patient showed a positive pivot-shift test (glide).

AUTHORS' EXPERIENCE

At our institution, double-bundle ACL reconstruction has been performed since the beginning of 2003. A laboratory and clinical study is being performed.

The procedure has been tested in cadaver knees in coop- eration with the Imperial College of London group headed by Professor Andrew A. Amis. With electromagnetic sensors (Nest of Birds), the range of kinematics in six knees was tested. Six loading conditions were investi- gated: posterior drawer with either neutral, internal, or external rotation (5-N·m torque) and 60-N anterior drawer with either neutral, internal, or external rotation (5-N·m torque). Lachman and pivot-shift tests were per- formed as well. All the tests were performed in the same knee in intact conditions, with a deficient ACL, and after single- and double-bundle two-incision rear entry ACL reconstruction. Anterior translation and rotation were cal- culated. Double-bundle ACL reconstruction significantly better controlled anterior translation during extension. No differences were detected in flexion. A trend toward better rotational control in extension was observed in double- bundle reconstruction. In conclusion, the operation seems to benefit from a second PLB, which works mainly in extension.

Fifty patients have undergone the procedure up to now. In 25 patients the procedure was performed through a transtibial approach (group 1), and in 25 the femoral

tunnels were drilled through a second-incision outside-in approach (group 2). A contemporary single-bundle group of 25 patients is prospectively being monitored (group 3). Fifteen patients in each double-bundle group underwent volumetric magnetic resonance imaging to study femoral tunnel position. The outside-in technique resulted in more anatomic positioning, whereas in the transtibial group, both the anteromedial and the posterolateral tunnel showed a tendency to be more superior and shallow than the native insertion. At a minimum follow-up of 1 year, the KT side-to-side differences in groups 1, 2, and 3 were 1.7, 1.5, and 1.9 mm, respectively. The incidences of pivot- shift glide in groups 1, 2, and 3 were 15%, 12%, and 20%, respectively. One failure per group was recorded in groups 1 and 3.

CONCLUSIONS

Double-bundle ACL reconstruction is a fascinating proce- dure that was devised to replicate ACL function and anatomy and restore normal knee kinematics and patient activity level. The surgical technique is more demanding, and the possibility of malposition is doubled; nonetheless, the desire for an easy technique suitable to every surgeon should not circumvent the need for anatomic accuracy. Before popularizing the technique, further in vivo and in vitro studies are needed to definitely demonstrate the superiority of the technique over standard single-bundle reconstruction, which produces satisfactory results in the vast majority of the cases. The classic single-bundle techniques should not be abandoned in favor of the more modern two-bundle reconstruction until we have clear evidence of its superiority. Further investigations are nec- essary to evaluate in vivo kinematics.

References

1. Adachi N, Ochi M, Uchio Y, et al: Reconstruction of the anterior cru- ciate ligament. Single- versus double-bundle multistranded ham- string tendons. J Bone Joint Surg Br 86:515-520, 2004.
2. Aglietti P, Giron F, Buzzi R, et al: Anterior cruciate ligament recon- struction: Bone–patellar tendon–bone compared with double semi- tendinosus and gracilis tendon grafts. A prospective, randomized clinical trial. J Bone Joint Surg Am 86:2143-2155, 2004.
3. Amis AA, Dawkins GP: Functional anatomy of the anterior cruciate ligament. Fibre bundle actions related to ligament replacements and injuries. J Bone Joint Surg Br 73:260-267, 1991.
4. Arnoczky SP: Anatomy of the anterior cruciate ligament. Clin Orthop 172:19-25, 1983.
5. Arnold MP, Kooloos J, van Kampen A: Single-incision technique misses the anatomical femoral anterior cruciate ligament insertion: A cadaver study. Knee Surg Sports Traumatol Arthrosc 9:194-199, 2001.
6. Bach JM, Hull ML, Patterson HA: Direct measurement of strain in the posterolateral bundle of the anterior cruciate ligament. J Biomech 30:281-283, 1997.
7. Bellier G, Christel P, Colombet P, et al: Double-stranded hamstring graft for anterior cruciate ligament reconstruction. Arthroscopy 20:890-894, 2004.
8. Brandsson S, Karlsson J, Sward L, et al: Kinematics and laxity of the knee joint after anterior cruciate ligament reconstruction: Pre- and postoperative radiostereometric studies. Am J Sports Med 30:361- 367, 2002.

9. Bush-Joseph CA, Hurwitz DE, Patel RR, et al: Dynamic function after anterior cruciate ligament reconstruction with autologous patellar tendon. Am J Sports Med 29:36-41, 2001.

10. Butler DL, Guan Y, Kay MD, et al: Location-dependent variations in the material properties of the anterior cruciate ligament. J Biomech 25:511-518, 1992.

11. Chol C, Ait Si Selmi T, Chambat P, et al: Seventeen year outcome after anterior cruciate ligament reconstruction with an intact or repaired medial meniscus. Rev Chir Orthop Reparatrice Appar Mot 88:157-162, 2002.

12. Dodds JA, Arnoczky SP: Anatomy of the anterior cruciate ligament: A blueprint for repair and reconstruction. Arthroscopy 10:132-139, 1994.

13. Edwards TB, Guanche CA, Petrie SG, Thomas KA: In vitro comparison of elongation of the anterior cruciate ligament and single- and dual-tunnel anterior cruciate ligament reconstructions. Orthopedics 22:577-584, 1999.

14. Freedman KB, D'Amato MJ, Nedeff DD, et al: Arthroscopic anterior cruciate ligament reconstruction: A metaanalysis comparing patellar tendon and hamstring tendon autografts. Am J Sports Med 31:2-11, 2003.

15. Fuss FK: Optimal replacement of the cruciate ligaments from the functional-anatomical point of view. Acta Anat (Basel) 140:260-268, 1991.

16. Gabriel MT, Wong EK, Woo SL, et al: Distribution of in situ forces in the anterior cruciate ligament in response to rotatory loads. J Orthop Res 22:85-89, 2004.

17. Girgis FG, Marshall JL, Monajem A: The cruciate ligaments of the knee joint. Anatomical, functional and experimental analysis. Clin Orthop 106:216-231, 1975.

18. Giron F, Buzzi R, Aglietti P: Femoral tunnel position in anterior cruciate ligament reconstruction using three techniques. A cadaver study. Arthroscopy 15:750-756, 1999.

19. Hamada M, Shino K, Horibe S, et al: Single- versus bi-socket anterior cruciate ligament reconstruction using autogenous multiple-stranded hamstring tendons with EndoButton femoral fixation: A prospective study. Arthroscopy 17:801-807, 2001.

20. Hara K, Kubo T, Suginoshita T, et al: Reconstruction of the anterior cruciate ligament using a double bundle. Arthroscopy 16:860-864, 2000.

21. Harner CD, Baek GH, Vogrin TM, et al: Quantitative analysis of human cruciate ligament insertions. Arthroscopy 15:741-749, 1999.

22. Hogervorst T, Pels Rijcken TH, Rucker D, et al: Changes in bone scans after anterior cruciate ligament reconstruction: A prospective study. Am J Sports Med 30:823-833, 2002.

23. Hutchinson MR, Bae TS: Reproducibility of anatomic tibial landmarks for anterior cruciate ligament reconstructions. Am J Sports Med 29:777-780, 2001.

24. Kurosawa H, Yamakoshi K, Yasuda K, Sasaki T: Simultaneous measurement of changes in length of the cruciate ligaments during knee motion. Clin Orthop 265:233-240, 1991.

25. Li G, DeFrate LE, Sun H, Gill TJ: In vivo elongation of the anterior cruciate ligament and posterior cruciate ligament during knee flexion. Am J Sports Med 32:1415-1420, 2004.

26. Logan MC, Williams A, Lavelle J, et al: Tibiofemoral kinematics following successful anterior cruciate ligament reconstruction using dynamic multiple resonance imaging. Am J Sports Med 32:984-992, 2004.

27. Loh JC, Fukuda Y, Tsuda E, et al: Knee stability and graft function following anterior cruciate ligament reconstruction: Comparison between 11 o'clock and 10 o'clock femoral tunnel placement. Arthroscopy 19:297-304, 2003.

28. Mae T, Shino K, Miyama T, et al: Single– versus two–femoral socket anterior cruciate ligament reconstruction technique: Biomechanical analysis using a robotic simulator. Arthroscopy 17:708-716, 2001.

29. Marcacci M, Molgora AP, Zaffagnini S, et al: Anatomic double-bundle anterior cruciate ligament reconstruction with hamstrings. Arthroscopy 19:540-546, 2003.

30. Markolf KL, Burchfield DM, Shapiro MM, et al: Biomechanical consequences of replacement of the anterior cruciate ligament with a patellar ligament allograft. Part I: Insertion of the graft and anterior-posterior testing. J Bone Joint Surg Am 78:1720-1727, 1996.

31. Mommersteeg TJ, Kooloos JG, Blankevoort L, et al: The fibre bundle anatomy of human cruciate ligaments. J Anat 187:461-471, 1995.

32. Morgan CD, Kalman VR, Grawl DM: Definitive landmarks for reproducible tibial tunnel placement in anterior cruciate ligament reconstruction. Arthroscopy 11:275-288, 1995.

33. Mott HW: Semitendinosus anatomic reconstruction for cruciate ligament insufficiency. Clin Orthop 172:90-102, 1983.

34. Norwood LA, Cross MJ: Anterior cruciate ligament: Functional anatomy of its bundles in rotatory instabilities. Am J Sports Med 7:23-26, 1979.

35. Odensten M, Gillquist J: Functional anatomy of the anterior cruciate ligament and a rationale for reconstruction. J Bone Joint Surg Am 67:257-262, 1985.

36. Pederzini L, Adriani E, Botticella C, Tosi M: Technical note: Double tibial tunnel using quadriceps tendon in anterior cruciate ligament reconstruction. Arthroscopy 16(5):E9, 2000.

37. Radford WJ, Amis AA: Biomechanics of a double prosthetic ligament in the anterior cruciate deficient knee. J Bone Joint Surg Br 72:1038-1043, 1990.

38. Ristanis S, Giakas G, Papageorgiou CD, et al: The effects of anterior cruciate ligament reconstruction on tibial rotation during pivoting after descending stairs. Knee Surg Sports Traumatol Arthrosc 11:360-365, 2003.

39. Rosenberg T, Graf B: Techniques for ACL Reconstruction with Multi-Trac Drill Guide. Mansfield, MA, Acufex Microsurgical, 1994.

40. Sakane M, Fox RJ, Woo SL, et al: In situ forces in the anterior cruciate ligament and its bundles in response to anterior tibial loads. J Orthop Res 15:285-293, 1997.

41. Simmons R, Howell SM, Hull ML: Effect of the angle of the femoral and tibial tunnels in the coronal plane and incremental excision of the posterior cruciate ligament on tension of an anterior cruciate ligament graft: An in vitro study. J Bone Joint Surg Am 85:1018-1029, 2003.

42. Tashman S, Collon D, Anderson K, et al: Abnormal rotational knee motion during running after anterior cruciate ligament reconstruction. Am J Sports Med 32:975-983, 2004.

43. Yagi M, Wong EK, Kanamori A, et al: Biomechanical analysis of an anatomic anterior cruciate ligament reconstruction. Am J Sports Med 30:660-666, 2002.

44. Yamamoto Y, Hsu WH, Woo SLY, et al: Knee stability and graft function after anterior cruciate ligament reconstruction: A comparison of a lateral and an anatomical femoral tunnel placement. Am J Sports Med 32:1825-1832, 2004.

45. Yasuda K: Double bundle ACL reconstruction. Presented at the 11th Congress of the European Society of Sports Traumatology, Knee Surgery and Arthroscopy, May 4-8, 2004, Athens, Greece.

46. Yasuda K, Kondo E, Ichiyama H, et al: anatomic reconstruction of the anteromedial and posterolateral bundles of the anterior cruciate ligament using hamstring tendon grafts. Arthroscopy 20:1015-1025, 2004.

47. Zaricznyj B: Reconstruction of the anterior cruciate ligament of the knee using a doubled tendon graft. Clin Orthop 220:162-175, 1987.

48. Zavras TD, Race A, Bull AM, Amis AA: A comparative study of "isometric" points for anterior cruciate ligament graft attachment. Knee Surg Sports Traumatol Arthrosc 9:28-33, 2001.

CHAPTER 43

The Safe and Effective Use of Allograft Tissue

Scott A. Barbour • Warren King

The use of allograft tissue in orthopedic surgery has been a tremendous advance in the management of a variety of orthopedic problems. Today, allograft tissues are commonly used for a number of procedures, including limb salvage procedures, ligament reconstruction, cartilage resurfacing, and as osteoconductive and inductive substrates. The role of allograft tissue is constantly expanding and its use becoming more common. In 1999 alone, U.S. tissue banks distributed over 750,000 allografts.[24]

The use of allograft tissue has many advantages over autografts, including unlimited size, lack of donor site morbidity, and availability for revision surgery. However, allograft tissue is not without some disadvantages. It has decreased osteoinductive and osteoconductive characteristics, as well as increased incorporation times when compared with autograft tissue.[24,54] The most significant disadvantage is the risk of disease transmission.

Currently, the risk of viral transmission through allograft tissue transplantation is extremely low. Proper donor screening and tissue processing help prevent the transmission of viral disease. However, window periods of infection where detection is missed through serological tests and human error make transmission still possible.[45,55]

As of 1995, two documented human immunodeficiency virus (HIV)-, one hepatitis B virus–, and four hepatitis C virus–infected donors had been used for the transplantation of musculoskeletal allografts and resulted in several cases of disease transmission.[1,45,55] It is important to note that if adherence to the screening methods available today had been in effect, most, if not all of these infections would have been avoided.[1,45]

The risk for bacterial infection from allograft tissue is unknown because of several factors[12]: lack of a standardized procurement protocol for tissue harvesting, failure of surgeons to recognize or confirm the allograft as the source of infection, and lack of reporting when this complication does occur.

As of March 2003, the Centers for Disease Control and Prevention (CDC) had received 62 reports of allograft-associated infection. Ninety-three percent of these allografts were musculoskeletal tissues. Cases of infection were reported from 20 states and 12 different tissue processors; 45% of the infections were the result of graft material from one tissue processor.[55]

HISTORY OF ALLOGRAFTS

MacEwen reported the first use of musculoskeletal allograft in 1880.[6] Lexer reported on 23 articular cartilage transplantations performed between 1908 and 1925. These reports included phalangeal, elbow, and knee joints, and he claimed a 50% success rate.[41] Noyes et al reported allograft ligament reconstructions in 1981,[47] and Milachowski reported on transplanted menisci in 1984.[46] Today, the use of allograft tissues is extremely common, and thus the demand for tissue is increasing. Consequently, surgeons must keep informed of the risks and benefits of this ever-expanding technology.

TISSUE PROCESSING

Musculoskeletal allografts are processed with a variety of methods, depending on the tissue being transplanted and the requirements of the surgeon. Fresh allograft refers to tissue that is harvested under sterile conditions and transplanted directly from the host to the recipient. This is most effective type of tissue required for successful osteochondral transplantation. The tissue is normally maintained in lactated Ringer's solution at 2° C to 4° C for a period of up to 7 days. Many studies show that viable cartilage cells diminish substantially in culture media after 24 hours and are virtually nonexistent after 7 days.[53] However, numerous animal studies have shown that cell viability can be maintained for up to 28 days.[49] Pearsall et al demonstrated that refrigerated osteochondral allograft can be maintained up to 44 days with 67% cell viability.[49]

Although these tissues are thoroughly washed before transplantation, they still contain some marrow elements and viable cells from the donor; thus, an immune response does occur.[31,39] This immune reaction is usually clinically insignificant. However, anecdotally speaking, the authors have had experience with allograft Achilles tendon failure over a several-month period after anterior cruciate ligament (ACL) reconstruction. On follow-up arthroscopy of these patients, only connective tissue debris remained. An immunological reaction was believed to be the source of the failure by the authors. Currently, no standard of processing these tissues with regard to washing, antibiotic treatment, or sterilization treatment (gamma radiation, ethylene oxide, etc.) exists.[17]

Cryopreservation is a process of controlled-rate freezing in which dimethyl sulfoxide and glycerol are used to remove water during the freezing process in an attempt to preserve viable cells. The process works by altering water crystallization during the freezing process, which preserves up to 80% of cells.[53] Grafts are cooled to 0° C and processed within 48 hours. They are then incubated in an antibiotic solution for 24 hours at 37° C, frozen to −135° C, and packed in a cryoprotectant solution for up to 10 years.[53] This technique works well for meniscal cartilage; however, the process damages articular cartilage. Meniscal allografts may be obtained as fresh, cryopreserved, fresh frozen, or lyophilized. Cryopreserved and fresh meniscal allograft contains live cells at the time of transplantation, but studies have demonstrated that graft cells are rapidly replaced with host cells soon after transplantation.[37] It is not known what percentage of cells survive the transplant procedure or for how long they survive. In addition, fresh grafts require transplantation soon after harvest, which results in difficult logistics. The increased cost prohibits the use of fresh grafts for other types of tissue, but other less expensive techniques appear to have similar success rates.[53]

Fresh frozen tissue is the most common technique for processing ligament allografts and is becoming the most common technique for meniscal allografts. Studies of fresh frozen meniscal allografts include patients with follow-up of 15 years. Review of the literature demonstrates that over time, knees that have undergone transplantation more closely resemble intact knees than do knees that have undergone meniscectomy.[66] After tissue harvest under sterile conditions, the tissue is usually cultured and frozen while serological tests are carried out, a process that takes 2 to 4 weeks. It is then soaked in an antibiotic solution at room temperature for 1 hour, packaged, and frozen without solution for up to 5 years.[53] No viable cells reliably survive this process,[53] which has several important clinical ramifications. Loss of cells decreases the likelihood of immune reaction and disease transmission; however, the effectiveness of this treatment is controversial.

Finally, freeze-dried (lyophilized) allograft tissues are also commonly used in ligament reconstruction. Attempts have been made to use them for meniscal allografts, but the tissue undergoes shrinkage after transplantation and such use is not currently recommended.[3,66] After harvest under sterile conditions, the tissue is frozen pending serological and bacterial culture results. They are then subjected to a 1-hour soak in antibacterial solution at room temperature. A process of refreezing and lyophilization to a residual moisture of less than 5%, followed by packaging and storage for up to 5 years, is then carried out. Even though the color and strength of the tissues are altered, studies have shown no deleterious effects on clinical outcomes of ligament reconstruction.[53] A period of rehydration is required before implantation.[3]

ALLOGRAFT PHYSIOLOGY

Allogeneic tissues function as a scaffold that is eventually incorporated into the host. Incorporation generally occurs through three stages. First, death of cells from the donor tissue occurs. This stage is usually considered to be a characteristic of fresh or cryopreserved tissues because other processing methods (fresh frozen or freeze-dried) are considered to have already caused cell death in donor tissues. The second stage includes revascularization of the donor tissue with repopulation of the donor tissue by host cells.[53] These first two stages occur relatively rapidly when compared with the final stage, remodeling, which occurs more slowly. Jackson et al demonstrated complete replacement of donor cells by host cells in goat ACLs in 4 weeks.[36] It has been shown that complete remodeling of allograft tissue may take one and a half times as long as autograft tissue to regain comparable strength.[15] Prolongation of the remodeling phase may be a consequence of tissue antigen mismatch resulting in a subclinical immune response.[53] Several studies in dogs and goats have noted similar gross and histological patterns of tissue in native and allograft ligaments at 6 months to 1 year after transplantation.[23,43,67]

STERILIZATION

In addition to proper donor screening, adherence to sterile technique during procurement and processing, and appropriate serological and bacteriological testing, postharvest sterilization can improve the safety of allograft tissue. Currently, the two most common methods of sterilization are ethylene oxide treatment and gamma irradiation. Unfortunately, both these treatments can have deleterious side effects and are therefore not universally used. Ethylene oxide leaves behind a chemical residue that may cause chronic synovitis and graft failure,[38] and gamma irradiation greater than 3.0 Mrad weakens collagen tissue.[50] Tissues are weakened by irradiation as a result of the destruction of collagen chains, probably mediated by oxygen free radicals.[30]

Recent literature suggests that gamma radiation can be efficaciously used to sterilize allograft material without a deleterious clinical effect. In 1951, Meeker and Gross reported that 1.5 Mrad destroyed 95% of bacterial organisms, but 3.0 Mrad caused significant tissue damage.[45] Fideler et al showed that 30 kGy was necessary to eradicate HIV in bone–patella tendon–bone allograft at −70° C.[21] In 1956 Turner et al reported that bone grafts sterilized at 2.0 Mrad underwent abnormal absorption and fragmentation, but reported only 2 infections in 100 patients receiving 189 allografts, thus demonstrating the effective sterilizing properties of gamma radiation.[61] In 1959, Bassett and Packard reported less than a 1% infection rate in 1037 patients receiving bone grafts sterilized with 2.0 Mrad of gamma radiation.[26] Fideler showed in 1995 that the initial biomechanical strength of fresh frozen bone–patellar tendon–bone allograft was reduced by 15% after sterilization with 2.0 Mrad of gamma radiation, but that stiffness, elongation, and strain were not reduced with statistical significance.[20] Goertzen reported that canine bone–patellar tendon–bone allograft treated with 2.0 Mrad of gamma radiation protected with argon gas compared favorably with nonirradiated controls with regard to maximum load to failure at 12 months.[27] The irradiated group failed at 718.3 N (63.8% of normal ACLs), and the control group failed at 780.1 N (69.1% of normal). In addition, histological studies showed no difference between the groups with regard to collagen structure. Silver staining showed the presence of Golgi tendon organs and free nerve endings in both groups, and only slight hypervascularity was noted in the controls versus the irradiated group.[27]

Currently, research is in progress to develop new techniques to effectively sterilize allografts without affecting the clinical biomechanical integrity of the tissue. One such process is known as the Clearant process, which involves irradiation of tissue at low temperatures and reduced hydration in the presence of free radical scavengers. Early clinical results are promising and have demonstrated the effectiveness of this treatment.[10,28,29] The literature on sterilization has shown that no technique is 100% effective in rendering allogeneic tissues sterile, but that improved sterility with certain treatment protocols can be used to improve the quality of these tissues without adversely affecting clinical outcomes.[1]

Toritsuka et al studied the effect of 25 kGy of gamma irradiation and freeze-drying on patella tendon graft remodeling after transplantation in the rat model.[60] They studied four groups, including fresh frozen, freeze-dried, fresh frozen gamma irradiated, and freeze-dried gamma irradiated. They discovered that freeze drying and gamma irradiation temporarily accelerated graft remodeling in the early phase (first 12 weeks), accompanied by an increase in newly synthesized collagen and a decrease in donor collagen.[60] Histologically, no difference in the progression of cellular repopulation was observed between the four groups. It was thus assumed that the chemotactic properties of the graft materials were unaffected and that accelerated graft remodeling was potentiated. Although it can be assumed that the rapid decrease in donor collagen would initially weaken grafts treated in this manner, further studies would be required to determine whether this phenomenon has any clinical significance that requires modification of rehabilitation protocols. One can conclude that grafts treated in this manner would be safer and less likely to promote immunological reactions and thus accelerate incorporation of the grafts.

TISSUE BANKING

Our current knowledge of the safe procurement of allogeneic tissues was originally adapted from procedures developed by the U.S. Navy Tissue Bank[7] and has been modified through clinical experience over many years. Inclan reported on the first dedicated bone bank in 1942, and in the 1950s bone banks began to appear across the United States.[18,32,33]

As our understanding of the risks and means by which disease is transmitted is further delineated, efforts have been made to modify techniques to ensure the highest possible safety of allograft tissue. Current understanding of safe tissue-banking procedures has led to the development of a comprehensive screening process for potential donors, including a detailed medical and social history; serological tests for HIV I/II antibodies and HIV antigen; polymerase chain reaction for detection of HIV, hepatitis B surface antigen, hepatitis B surface antibodies, hepatitis B core antibodies, and hepatitis C virus antibodies; and the rapid plasmin reagin test for syphilis. In addition, an autopsy of potential donors, with a separate study of the lymph nodes, completes the screening process. Currently, only the medical history, social history, and serological testing are required by the Food and Drug Administration (FDA).[1,62] It is also pointed out by Malinin et al that procurement of tissue is a surgical skill requiring strict adherence to sterile technique.[9,42] Procurement is also a clinical service that carries with it the responsibilities incumbent on any physician providing medical care. As such, it would seem logical that personnel who procure tissue be held to the same standard as other medical professionals.

Buck and Malinin reported on their experience at the University of Miami Tissue Bank.[8] They discussed the reasons for exclusion of 187 of 1000 consecutive donors over a 6½-year period. Eighty-five were excluded on the basis of bacteriological criteria alone. Seventeen had bacteriological exclusionary criteria, as well as serological and/or morphological exclusionary criteria. Sixty-eight cases were excluded for hepatitis detected by serological markers or morphological changes, and 1 case was excluded because of histological changes alone.[8] Documented or suspected HIV accounted for 10 exclusions. In one case a donor was excluded because of classic non-specific changes of HIV noted in the lymph nodes.[48,51] Another donor was excluded as a result of birefringent material consistent with drug abuse noted in granulomas located in the liver and lungs.[56] Seven donors were rejected for granulomatous disease, four for unsuspected malignancies, and two for myocarditis.[56] The experience of Buck and Malinin clearly demonstrates the need for screening beyond serological tests to ensure the safety of allograft tissue.[9]

In January 2001, The Office of the Inspector General, Department of Health and Human Services, convened an oversight committee to profile the current state of tissue banking in this country. It was noted that oversight of tissue-banking practices occurs at three levels, the FDA, the American Association of Tissue Banks (AATB), and the state level. The FDA requires donor screening and testing to prevent the transmission of communicable diseases. It had conducted 188 inspections of 118 tissue banks known to the government at that time (since 1993). The AATB conducts a voluntary accreditation program that evaluates the procurement practices of each tissue bank. As of January 2001, 58 tissue banks had been accredited and another 90 identified banks were not. According to the oversight committee's report, only New York and Florida require licensing and inspection of tissue banks, although authorities in California report that AATB certification is required in that state. Furthermore, the oversight committee pointed out that many tissue banks do not seek AATB accreditation because there is no incentive to do so.[1,17]

The committee reported that no cases of disease transmission had been identified since the FDA's regulation regarding donor screening and testing in 1993. However, in 2001, a 23-year-old man in Minnesota underwent reconstructive knee surgery with a femoral condyle allograft. Three days later, severe pain developed at the surgical site that rapidly progressed to shock and resulted in death the following day. Culture of blood obtained before death grew *Clostridium sordelli*.[13] Six days after the Minnesota case, a 17-year-old male in Illinois received a fresh femoral condyle and a fresh frozen meniscus for reconstructive knee surgery. The following day a fever developed, and 8 days later the patient was readmitted for septic arthritis of the postsurgical knee. No cultures were obtained for the Illinois patient. Follow-up investigation by the CDC determined that both patients received graft material from the same donor. It was learned that the body of the donor was refrigerated 19 hours after death and that one tissue procurement organization harvested the tissue 23.5 hours after death.[13]

Shortly after the Minnesota case was investigated by the CDC, Barbour and King reported a similar case in which *Clostridium septicum* infection developed in two different patients after ACL reconstruction with bone–patella tendon–bone allografts from the same donor. A 50-year-old man sustained a torn right ACL while playing baseball and received a hemipatellar tendon allograft reconstruction in March 1998. The fresh frozen graft was removed from the package on the back table, and a sample of the bone and tendon was sent for aerobic and anaerobic culture before implantation. The patient was seen in follow-up 4 days later and was doing well; physical therapy was prescribed.

On the 10th postoperative day the patient was evaluated in the clinic and found to have an erythematous, warm right knee. The patient complained of a significant increase in pain and reported feeling febrile. Culture results of purulent fluid aspirated from his right knee identified the gram-positive rod as *C. septicum*. The patient was immediately taken to the operating room for arthroscopic débridement and for removal of the graft and bioabsorbable fixation screws in the femur and tibia. The patient was admitted to the hospital and administered intravenous antibiotics, and his right knee was subsequently débrided multiple times in the operating room. Several intraoperative cultures confirmed *C. septicum* infection.

The patient completed a 4-week course of intravenous antibiotics followed by a 2-week course of oral antibiotics, as well as physical therapy. His case was further complicated by arthrofibrosis with a range of motion of 15 to 90 degrees. Three months after the initial operation he was again taken to the operating room for arthroscopic lysis of adhesions and manipulation under anesthesia, which improved his range of motion to 5 to 100 degrees.

The primary surgeon routinely sends allograft tissue for culture before implantation to determine whether any subsequent postoperative infections originated from contaminated tissue. In this case, the preoperative tissue culture results correlated with the rare organism cultured from the patient's knee aspirate, thus suggesting that the tissue was contaminated before delivery to the hospital and subsequent implantation. The tissue bank was contacted and informed of the incident; they responded that

their testing revealed no evidence of contamination of the allograft tissue and held the position that the infection was the result of contamination at the time of surgery. The tissue bank was not forthcoming with information regarding the methods used to harvest the tissue or the circumstances of the donor's death and medical history.

The patient subsequently filed a lawsuit against the tissue bank, which allowed the senior surgeon to access the donor's autopsy report and the harvesting methods of the tissue bank. These documents let us track other tissues from the same donor to other recipients around the country. It was learned that a patient in another part of the country received the other half of the hemipatellar tendon allograft from this donor and contracted a postoperative infection with the same rare organism, *C. septicum*.

Despite the medical evidence, the tissue bank still maintained the position that the infections were separate complications resulting from perioperative tissue contamination. The tissue bank ultimately reached an out-of-court settlement with the patient that included a confidentiality clause prohibiting disclosure of the facts of this case.[1]

It is believed that bacterial infections have occurred as a result of contaminated allograft tissue as demonstrated by the two cases just presented. Lack of reporting and failure to recognize allograft tissue as a source of infection are believed to be the reason for missing allograft-associated bacterial infections in the past. At the time of the case report, Barbour and King were treating two other patients who underwent ACL allograft transplantation by other surgeons that was complicated by postoperative clostridial infections. In addition, they were aware of a fourth patient who received the other half of the hemipatellar tendon graft that caused one of their patient's infections and that patient contracted the same rare *C. septicum* infection. In these particular cases, no preoperative graft tissue was taken for culture to confirm that the graft was the source of infection, but three patients received a legal settlement from the tissue bank with a nondisclosure clause. Despite the lack of preoperative culture results from three of these cases, *Clostridium* is an extremely rare organism in postoperative wound infections, and it seems likely that the graft material was the source of infection. We believe that the rarity of contamination, failure of surgeons to recognize the allograft as a source of infection, and the tissue bank's failure to properly investigate these complications resulted in subsequent infections that may have been otherwise avoided.[1]

In 2001, the oversight committee found 36 tissue banks that have never been inspected out of 154 identified tissue banks and noted that the actual number and location of all tissue banks are unknown. Although the FDA does regulate donor screening and testing, no regulations exist for quality and handling of tissue.[17] Of the 118 tissue banks inspected by the FDA since 1993 as reported by the 2001 committee, 26 official notices requiring the banks to take corrective action were issued.[17] In 72 others, notices were issued that suggested changes to improve quality.[17] The FDA reported a list of examples of safety and qualities problems found in the tissue banks inspected, including "lack of adequate controls to assure product sterility, lack of standard operating procedures to prevent cross contamination of human tissue during manufacture, and distribution and implantation of soft tissue grafts from a single donor with possible bacterial contamination," just to name a few.

In 2002, approximately 1 million allografts were distributed for implantation.[14] In March 2002, the *Morbidity and Mortality Weekly Report* of the CDC reported an update of allograft-associated bacterial infections.[13] They had received 26 reports of bacterial infection associated with musculoskeletal allograft transplantation.[13] Thirteen (50%) of the 26 cases were infected with *Clostridium* species. Allografts implicated in *Clostridium* infection consisted of eight tendons used for ACL reconstruction, two femoral condyles, two bones, and one meniscus.[13] Eleven of the grafts were fresh frozen, and 2 were fresh. All the allografts were processed aseptically; however, none had received terminal sterilization. Eighty-five percent of the tissue had been procured by one tissue processor.[13]

In June 2002, a physician reported to the Oregon Department of Health Services a case of acute hepatitis C infection in a patient who had received a patellar tendon from a donor approximately 6 weeks before the onset of illness. No detectable antibody to hepatitis C had been found in the donor's serum before his death in October 2000. An investigation conducted by the CDC determined that although the donor was seronegative at the time of tissue harvest, he was infected with hepatitis C and was the "probable" source of the infection.[55] Based on these findings, the CDC has instituted additional steps with regard to tissue procurement to help ensure tissue sterility.[13]

BACTERIAL CONTAMINATION OF ALLOGRAFTS

To understand the potential risks of bacterial infection with the use of allograft tissue, one must first identify the manner in which these tissues become contaminated. A review of the literature reports a 5% to 44% rate of bacterial contamination of allograft tissue.[2,4,5,19,35,42,57-59,65] Because of variability of the culture techniques used, it is not possible to compare the contamination rates.[64] Deijkers et al analyzed the incidence and predisposing factors for bacterial contamination of allograft tissue.[16] They evaluated 1999 bone and soft-tissue grafts from 200 cadaver donors under sterile operating conditions. After removal of the grafts from the cadaver donors, they were rinsed with an antibiotic solution in the first 150 donors and with saline only in the last 50 donors. Swabs were then taken from the entire graft surface and placed in a transport medium. The swabs were subsequently inoculated onto blood agar and chocolate agar plates and cultured under aerobic and anaerobic conditions. The entire swab sticks were then placed in a brain-heart infusion broth and cultured for another 72 hours under both aerobic and anaerobic conditions. Blood samples from the cadaver donors were cultured aerobically and anaerobically for 7 days. Microbial load was considered low if

microorganisms grew only in the broth and high if growth occurred directly on the plates. They found that 50% of the grafts cultured positive for organisms of low pathogenicity and 69% had a low microbial load. Three percent of the grafts grew organisms of high pathogenicity.

The authors determined that organisms of low pathogenicity (e.g., coagulase-negative staphylococci, *Corynebacterium*, *Propionibacterium acnes*) were likely to have contaminated the grafts exogenously during procurement. Organisms of high pathogenicity originated endogenously from the donor, were usually contaminants from the gastrointestinal or the upper respiratory tract, and were more likely to cause a clinically significant infection in the recipient. They found that contamination with organisms of high pathogenicity was 3.4 times higher in donors with a traumatic cause of death and 5.2 times higher in those with positive blood cultures. It was also noted that although washing the grafts with antibiotic solution reduced the organisms of low pathogenicity by a factor of 2, organisms of high pathogenicity were not reduced with antibiotic soaks. The authors concluded that exogenous contamination was most affected by the procurement team and that endogenous contamination was best controlled through careful donor selection.[16,57,65]

Martinez et al reported on microbiological cultures of blood and bone from 239 cadaver donors and 58 "beating heart donors" who had been aseptic before tissue harvest. The incidence of positive blood cultures was significantly lower in the "beating-heart donors" (8.6%) than in the cadaver donors (38%).[44] Agonal bacteremia is a well-described process whereby endogenous bacteria such as normal intestinal flora are disseminated throughout the body after death in cadaver donors.[22,25,34] This process is thought to be facilitated by loss of the barrier function of gut capillaries and may also result from trauma or manipulation procedures during resuscitation attempts around the time of death.[16,22,25,63] The difference in blood culture results between the two groups in this study was attributed to the persistence of anatomic barriers to microbial invasion and competent microbial clearing mechanisms in the "beating heart donor" group.

Microorganisms were isolated from the tissues of 55.4% of the cadaver donors and 67.9% of the "beating-heart donors" who had negative blood cultures. *Clostridium* species were the second most commonly isolated group behind coagulase-negative staphylococci. It was also noted that 60% of donors with positive blood cultures for *Clostridium* species also cultured positive in tissue samples.[40,44] They found the predictive value of positive blood cultures to be 83.5%; however, the predictive value of negative blood cultures was only 44.5% in the two groups. These results demonstrate that blood cultures are ineffective in confirming the sterility of allograft tissue and that *Clostridium* species seem to be disseminated at the time of death in cadaver donors and often seed tissues before harvest.[4,65]

The tremendous increase in allograft tissue applications and thus demand has resulted in failure to adequately supervise the safety of this industry. Generally, allograft tissues are extremely safe, and complications resulting from disease transmission are extremely low. However, when they do occur, the consequences are often catastrophic, but potentially avoidable with strict adherence to known protocols designed to ensure safety.

SUMMARY

The use of allogeneic tissue in orthopedic surgery is generally safe and efficacious. The indications for these tissues continue to expand and represent a marked advance in the implementation of medical care. Recently, recognition of the risk for bacterial infection from contaminated grafts and for devastating consequences has prompted the CDC and other government agencies to scrutinize the tissue-banking industry.[52]

Several changes in the practice of tissue banking and the use of allograft tissue will be required to improve the quality of allogeneic tissue. First, it is imperative that tissue banks be closely regulated to ensure that proper practices for safe tissue banking are being followed. Furthermore, research needs to be conducted to develop safer methods for tissue procurement. A review of the literature demonstrates that blood and swab cultures and antibiotic washes are ineffective in confirming the sterility of donor tissue. In addition, the current literature on known methods of sterilization, such as gamma irradiation, demonstrate efficacy when used, thus necessitating that standard protocols be implemented for all tissue banks. We also suggest that only trained professionals, held to the same standards as other medical professionals, be allowed to harvest tissue. Moreover, it is necessary that donor medical records be made available to surgeons using their graft material to aid in clinical decision making. Finally, reporting of bacterial infections to a central agency for monitoring future outbreaks should be mandatory. When complications do occur, these cases need to be investigated rather than buried by legal sanctions to improve tissue-banking techniques. Based on these case reports, we would recommend that the implanting surgeon obtain cultures of allograft tissue so that appropriate action may be taken should high-pathogenic bacteria such as *Clostridium* be encountered.

These changes are likely to increase the cost of tissue banking and may create difficulty in obtaining graft material. However, even though the complication rate associated with the use of allograft tissue is extremely low, the devastating impact on morbidity and mortality under the current system is unacceptable.[52]

Additionally, it is incumbent on the orthopedic surgeon to keep informed on the various tissue types and indicated uses. Understanding these factors will allow orthopedic surgeons to better inform their patients about the potential risks and to use the various graft types available in the most efficacious manner.

References

1. Barbour SA, King W: The safe and effective use of allograft tissue—an update. Am J Sports Med 31:791-797, 2003.
2. Barrios RH, Leyes M, Amillo S, Oteiza C: Bacterial contamination of allografts. Acta Orthop Belg 60:152-154, 1994.
3. Bechtold JE, Eastlund TD, Butts MK, et al: The effects of freeze-drying and ethylene oxide sterilization on the mechanical properties of human patellar tendon. Am J Sports Med 22:562-566, 1994.
4. Bennett L: Gas gangrene and other *Clostridium*-associated diseases. In Mandell G, Bennett J, Raphael D (eds): Mandell, Douglas, and Bennett's Principles and Practice of Infectious Disease, 5th ed. Philadelphia, Churchill Livingstone, 2000, pp 2549-2561.
5. Betten D, Dethloff M, Steinbeck J, Polster J: Organization of a bone and tissue bank. Z Orthop Grengeb 132:453-458, 1994.
6. Bolano L, Kopta JA: The immunology of bone and cartilage transplantation. Orthopedics 14:987-996, 1991.
7. Bright RW, Friedlaender GE, Sell KW: Current concepts: Tissue banking: The United States Navy Tissue Bank. Milit Med 142:503-510, 1977.
8. Buck BE, Malinin TI: Human bone and tissue allografts, preparation and safety. Clin Orthop 303:8-17, 1994.
9. Buck BE, Malinin TI, Brown MD: Bone transplantation and human immunodeficiency virus: An estimate of risk of acquired immunodeficiency syndrome (AIDS). Clin Orthop 240:129-136, 1989.
10. Burgess WH, Lin J: Optimized high-dosed gamma irradiation of cadaveric tissue: Structural integrity comparable to conventional irradiation. Presented at the Pittsburgh Bone Symposium, 2003.
11. Centers for Disease Control and Prevention: Unexplained deaths following knee surgery—Minnesota, November 2001. MMWR Morb Mortal Wkly Rep 50:1035-1036, 2001.
12. Centers for Disease Control and Prevention: Septic arthritis following anterior cruciate ligament reconstruction using tendon allografts—Florida and Louisiana, 2000. MMWR Morb Mortal Wkly Rep 50(48):1081-1083, 2001.
13. Centers for Disease Control and Prevention: Allograft-associated bacterial infections—United States, 2002. MMWR Morb Mortal Wkly Rep 51(10):207-210, 2002.
14. Centers for Disease Control and Prevention: Invasive *Streptococcus pyogenes* after allograft implantation—Colorado, 2003. MMWR Morb Mortal Wkly Rep 52(48):1173-1176, 2003.
15. Cordrey LI, McCorkle H, Hilton E: A comparative study of fresh autogenous and preserved homogenous tendon grafts in rabbits. J Bone Joint Surg Am 45:182-195, 1963.
16. Deijkers RL, Bloem RM, Petit PL, et al: Contamination of bone allografts, analysis of incidence and predisposing factors. J Bone Joint Surg Br 79:161-166, 1997.
17. Department of Health and Human Services, Office of Inspector General, Oversight of Tissue Banking, January 2001.
18. Doppelt SH, Tomford WW, Lucas AD, Mankin HJ: Operational and financial aspects of a hospital bone bank. J Bone Joint Surg Am 63:1472-1481, 1981.
19. Farrington M, Matthews I, Foreman J, et al: Microbial monitoring of bone grafts: Two years experience at a tissue bank. J Hosp Infect 38:261-271, 1998.
20. Fideler BM, Vangsness CT Jr, Lu B, et al: Gamma irradiation: Effects on biomechanical properties of human bone–patellar tendon–bone allografts. Am J Sports Med 23:643-646, 1995.
21. Fideler BM, Vangsness CT Jr, Moore T, et al: Effects of gamma irradiation on the human immunodeficiency virus: A study in frozen human bone–patellar tendon–bone grafts obtained from infected cadavera. J Bone Joint Surg Am 76:1032-1035, 1994.
22. Finegold SM, Attebery HR, Sutter VL: Effect of diet on human fecal flora: Comparison of Japanese and American diets. Am J Clin Nutr 27:1456-1469, 1974.
23. Garrett JC: Osteochondral allografts for reconstruction of articular defects. In McGinty JB, Caspari RB, Jackson RW, Poehling GG (eds): Operative Arthroscopy, 2nd ed. Philadelphia, Lippincott-Raven, 1996, pp 395-403.
24. Gazdag AR, Lane JM, Glaser D, Forster RA: Alternatives to autogenous bone graft: Efficacy and indications. J Am Acad Orthop Surg 3:1-8, 1995.
25. George WL, Finegold SM: *Clostridia* in the human gastrointestinal flora. In Boriello SP (ed): Clostridia in Gastrointestinal Disease. Boca Raton, FL, CRC Press, 1985, pp 1-37.
26. Godette GA, Kopta, JA, Egle DM: Biomechanical effects of gamma irradiation on fresh frozen allografts in vivo. Orthopedics 19:649-653, 1996.
27. Goertzen MJ, Clahsen H, Burrig KF, Schulitz KP: Sterilization of canine anterior cruciate allografts by gamma irradiation in argon.

Mechanical and neurohistological properties retained one year after transplantation. J Bone Joint Surg Br 77:205-212, 1995.

28. Grieb TA, Forng RY, Stafford RE, et al: Effective use of optimized, high-dose (50 kGy) gamma irradiation for pathogen inactivation of human bone allografts. Biomaterials 26:2033-2042, 2005.

29. Grieb TA, Lin J, et al: A novel processing for sterilizing allografts using 50 kgy of gamma irradiation. NASS 2003.

30. Hamer AJ, Stockley I, Elson RA: Changes in allograft bone irradiated at different temperatures. J Bone Joint Surg Br 81:342-344, 1999.

31. Hirn MY, Salmela MP, Vuento RE: High-pressure saline washing of allografts reduces bacterial contamination. Acta Orthop Scand 72:83-85, 2001.

32. Hyatt G, Turner T, Bassett CA, et al: New methods for preserving bone, skin and blood vessels. Postgrad Med 12:239-254, 1952.

33. Inclan A: The use of preserved bone grafts in orthopaedic surgery. J Bone Joint Surg 24:81-96, 1942.

34. Isenberg HD, D'Amato RF: Indigenous and pathogenic microorganisms in humans. In Murray PR, Baron EJ, Pfaller MA, et al (eds): Manual of Clinical Microbiology, 6th ed. Washington, DC, ASM Press, 1995, pp 5-18.

35. Ivory JP, Thomas IH: Audit of a bone bank. J Bone Joint Surg Br 75:355-357, 1993.

36. Jackson DW, Simon TM, Kurzweil PR, Rosen MA: Survival of cells after intraarticular transplantation of fresh allograft of the patellar and anterior cruciate ligaments: DNA-probe analysis in a goat model. J Bone Joint Surg Am 45:182-195, 1963.

37. Jackson DW, Whelan J, Simon TM: Cell survival after transplantation of fresh meniscal allografts. DNA probe analysis in a goat model. Am J Sports Med 21:540-550, 1993.

38. Jackson DW, Windler GE, Simon TM: Intraarticular reaction associated with the use of freeze-dried, ethylene oxide–sterilized bone–patella tendon–bone allografts in the reconstruction of the anterior cruciate ligament. Am J Sports Med 18:1-10, 1990.

39. Langer, F, Czitrom A, Pritzker KP, Gross AE: The immunogenicity of fresh and frozen allogeneic bone. J Bone Joint Surg Am 57:216-220, 1975.

40. Larson CM, Brubrick MP, Jacobs DM, West MA: Malignancy, mortality, and medicosurgical management of *Clostridium septicum* infection. Surgery 118:592-597, discussion 597-598, 1995.

41. Lexer E: Joint transplantations and arthroplasty. Surg Gynecol Obstet 40:782-809, 1925.

42. Malinin TI, Martinez OV, Brown MD: Banking of massive osteoarticular and intercalary bone allografts: 12 years' experience. Clin Orthop 197:44-57, 1985.

43. Mankin HJ, Doppelt SH, Tomford WW: Clinical experience with allograft implantation: The first ten years. Clin Orthop 174:69-86, 1983.

44. Martinez OV, Malinin TI, Valla PH, Floros A: Postmortem bacteriology of cadaver tissue donors: An evaluation of blood cultures as an index of tissue sterility. Diagn Microbiol Infect Dis 3:193-200, 1985.

45. Meeker IA Jr, Gross RE: Low-temperature sterilization of organic tissue by high-voltage cathode ray irradiation. Science 114:283-285, 1951.

46. Milachowski KA, Weismeier K, Wirth CJ: Homologous meniscus transplantation: Experimental and clinical results. Int Orthop 13:1-11, 1989.

47. Noyes FR, Barber SD, Mangine RE: Bone–patellar ligament–bone and fascia lata allografts for reconstruction of the anterior cruciate ligament. J Bone Joint Surg Am 72:1125-1136, 1990.

48. O'Murchadha MT, Wolf BC, Neiman RS: The histologic features of hyperplastic lymphadenopathy in AIDS-related complex are nonspecific. Am J Surg Pathol 11:94-99, 1987.

49. Pearsall AW 4th, Tucker JA, Hester RB, Heitman RJ: Chondrocyte viability in refrigerated osteochondral allografts used for transplantation within the knee. Am J Sports Med 32:125-131, 2004.

50. Pelker RR, Friedlaender GE: Biomechanical aspects of bone autografts and allografts. Orthop Clin North Am 18:235-239, 1987.

51. Racz P, Tenner-Racz K, Kahl C, et al: Spectrum of morphologic changes of lymph nodes from patients with AIDS or AIDS-related complexes. Prog Allergy 37:81-181, 1986.

52. Rodeo SA: Meniscal allografts—where do we stand? Am J Sports Med 29:246-261, 2001.

53. Shelton WR, Treacy SH, Dukes AD, Bomboy AL: Use of allografts in knee reconstruction: I. Basic science aspects and current status. J Am Acad Orthop Surg 6:165-168, 1998.

54. Shelton WR, Treacy SH, Dukes AD, Bomboy AL: Use of allografts in knee reconstruction: II. Surgical considerations. J Am Acad Orthop Surg 6:169-175, 1998.

55. Solomon SL: Director, Division of Healthcare Quality Promotion, CDC's National Center for Infectious Disease. Committee on Governmental Affairs, US Senate, May 14, 2003.

56. Tomashefski JF Jr, Hirsch CS: The pulmonary vascular lesions of intravenous drug abuse. Hum Pathol 11:133-145, 1989.

57. Tomford W: Current concepts review: Transmission of disease through transplantation of musculoskeletal allografts. J Bone Joint Surg Am 77:1742-1757, 1995.

58. Tomford WW, Dopplet SH, Mankin HJ, Friedlaender GE: 1983 bone bank procedures. Clin Orthop 174:15-21, 1983.

59. Tomford WW, Thongphasuk J, Mankin HJ, Ferraro MJ: Frozen musculoskeletal allografts: A study of the clinical incidence and causes of infection associated with their use. J Bone Joint Surg Am 72:1137-1143, 1990.

60. Toritsuka Y, Shino K, Horibe S, et al: Effect of freeze-drying or gamma-irradiation on remodeling of tendon allograft in a rat model. J Orthop Res 15:294-300, 1997.

61. Turner TC, Bassett CAL, Pate JW, et al: Sterilization of allografts by high-voltage cathode irradiation. J Bone Joint Surg Am 38:862-884, 1956.

62. Vangsness CT Jr, Garcia IA, Mills CR, et al: Allograft transplantation in the knee: Tissue regulation, procurement, processing, and sterilization. Am J Sports Med 31:474-481, 2003.

63. Veen MR: Bone Allografts: A Study into Bacterial Contamination, Sensitivity of Cultures, Decontamination, and Contribution to Postoperative Infection [thesis]. University of Leiden, The Netherlands, 1994.

64. Veen MR, Bloem RM, Petit PL: Sensitivity and negative predictive value of swab cultures in musculoskeletal allograft procurement. Clin Orthop 300:259-263, 1994.

65. Vehmeyer SBW, Bloem RM, Petit PL: Microbiological screening of post-mortem bone donors—two case reports. J Hosp Infect 47:193-197, 2001.

66. Wirth CJ, Peters G, Milachowski KA, et al: Long-term results of meniscal allograft transplantation. Am J Sports Med 30:174-181, 2002.

67. Zukor DJ, Paitich B, Oakeshott RD, et al: Reconstruction of post-traumatic articular surface defects using fresh small-fragment osteochondral allografts. In Aebi M, Regazzoni P (eds): Bone Transplantation. Berlin, Springer-Verlag, 1989, pp 293-305.

CHAPTER 44

"Criteria"-Based Rehabilitation of Surgically Reconstructed and Nonsurgically Treated Anterior Cruciate Ligament Injuries

Lonnie E. Paulos • Anastassios Karistinos • James A. Walker

In the past two decades our understanding of the basic science of the anterior cruciate ligament (ACL)-deficient knee and ACL reconstruction has increased dramatically. Such knowledge has allowed surgeons to develop techniques and materials that allow more reliable reconstruction of the missing ligament. Perhaps the biggest gain from these developments has been realized in the rehabilitation strategy for injured and surgically reconstructed knees. We came to understand that prolonged periods of protection of the knee are not necessary and in fact may be detrimental to the graft.[2,4] Conservative rehabilitation approaches prolonged the physiological imbalance of the knee and not infrequently led to stiffness and arthrofibrosis, thereby adversely affecting the outcome of ACL reconstruction.[58] The beneficial effect of early motion and rehabilitation after ACL reconstruction had been suggested as early as 1981.[55,58] Protocols that advocated bracing or casting for 6 to 8 weeks and crutch use for up to 12 weeks were gradually replaced by more aggressive regimens[16]; this change in treatment led to the development of accelerated rehabilitation programs that improved the results and minimized complications after ACL reconstruction.[66,67]

Even though ACL reconstruction has become the most widely performed treatment after ACL injury, nonoperative management is still indicated for patients who are willing to modify their activities.

In this chapter we discuss factors that influence the design of a rehabilitation program and present criteria-based knee rehabilitation protocols that we have successfully used in the treatment of ACL-deficient or reconstructed knees.

CONSIDERATIONS IN DEVELOPING A REHABILITATION PROGRAM

Choice of Graft, Graft Strength, and Fixation

The bone–patellar tendon–bone (BPB), quadrupled hamstring tendon, and quadriceps tendon–bone are the most frequently used grafts in ACL reconstruction. The first two have emerged as the gold standards, with equal results reported in several studies.[29,61,65] All three demonstrate higher ultimate strength to failure and higher stiffness than the native ACL does. Woo et al[80] reported an ultimate strength of 2160 N and stiffness of 242 N/mm for the native ACL. Cooper et al[23] reported values of 2977 N and 455 N/mm, respectively, for the central 10 mm of the BPB graft. The corresponding values for the quadrupled hamstring tendon graft (semitendinosus and gracilis) are 4140 N and 807 N/mm.[39] The quadriceps tendon–bone graft has values between the two: an ultimate strength to failure of 2353 N and stiffness of 326 N/mm.[70] Although the force applied to an ACL graft during rehabilitation programs that emphasize early range-of-motion (ROM) and weightbearing exercises is unknown, Noyes et al[54] estimated that during daily activities the native ACL is subjected to loads of 454 N. Morrison's calculations[52,53] were similar and ranged between 27 and 445 N. It appears that all three grafts have sufficient strength to counteract the force anticipated during the early rehabilitation phase.

The weak link in the reconstructed ligament, regardless of graft choice, is the interface between the graft, bone tunnel, and fixation device. There is agreement among most investigators that the BPB graft provides more reliable and faster healing in the bone tunnel and therefore rehabilitation protocols can be more aggressive when this graft is used. In a study of BPB grafts in rhesus monkeys, Clancy et al[21] noted evidence of histological healing by 8 weeks. In a histological and biomechanical analysis of doubled semitendinosus tendon graft in sheep hind limbs, Goradia et al[37] found evidence of histological healing at 12 weeks. During failure testing the authors found that up to 12 weeks, all the failures occurred by pullout from the bone tunnel. After 24 weeks all specimens ruptured through the intra-articular portion of the graft. However, tendon healing in the tunnel may occur earlier. Grana et al,[38] in a rabbit model using semitendinosus autograft reconstruction, found that by 3 weeks, failures of the bone-graft-bone construct occurred through the intra-articular portion of the graft and not as a result of pullout from the bone tunnel. The type of healing of tendon grafts in the bone tunnels is thought to be indirect with the formation of Sharpey fibers.[38] However, it appears that the type of healing is related to the type of fixation. Anatomic or aperture fixation allows direct healing to occur in the articular opening of the tunnel and, interestingly, prevents the tunnel expansion seen with soft-tissue graft ACL reconstruction.[77]

Present graft fixation constructs are less stiff than the native ACL or the grafts used to reconstruct the ligament. The majority of the devices used to achieve fixation of tendon or tendons in bone tunnels are less stiff than the interference screw–bone plug construct that is considered the standard for BPB fixation.[18] The more commonly used femoral fixation techniques for hamstring grafts include fixation buttons (EndoButton), interference screws (metallic or biodegradable), and transfixation techniques. For tibial fixation, biodegradable interference screws, often augmented with other forms of fixation (sutures over a post, tibial fixation buttons, washers, etc.), are used more commonly. In addition, there is significant variability in failure strength and stiffness among tendon fixation devices. Kousa et al[47] studied six different devices used for femoral fixation of quadrupled human hamstring grafts: Bone Mulch Screw (Arthrotec, Warsaw, IN), EndoButton CL (Acufex Microsurgical, Mansfield, MA), RIGIDfix (Mitek Products, Norwood, MA), SmartScrew ACL (Bionx Implants, Blue Bell, PA), BioScrew (Linvatec, Largo, FL), and RCI screw (Acufex). The suspensory fixation methods (Bone Mulch Screw, Endobutton CL, and RIGIDfix) generally provided better strength of fixation than did the apertural fixation methods (interference screws). The same authors[48] reported on the fixation strength of six tibial tendon fixation devices: Intrafix (Innovasive Devices, Marlborough, MA), WasherLoc (Arthrotec), tandem spiked washer (Linvatec), SmartScrew ACL (Bionx Implants), BioScrew (Linvatec), and SoftSilk (Acufex). Intrafix provided clearly superior strength in the fixation of hamstring tendon grafts to the tibial drill hole. In a different study, Coleridge and Amis[22] tested five tibial tendon fixation devices: WasherLoc, Intrafix fastener, and the RCI, Delta Tapered, and Bicortical interference screws. All devices performed well under cyclic loading, but WasherLoc gave the highest ultimate strength. When the two fixation points of tendon grafts are compared, the tibial side is more vulnerable to graft slippage, especially when an interference screw is used, and thus backup or hybrid fixation is recommended.[64] Although the majority of the fixation techniques have performed well clinically, the surgeon should be familiar with the biomechanical properties of the system being used and adjust the rehabilitation program accordingly.

The changes in the graft that take place after implantation represent another consideration in the rehabilitation of an ACL-reconstructed knee. The graft is stronger at the time of implantation. Animal studies on patellar tendon grafts have shown that the initially avascular graft is repopulated by cellular elements of extrinsic origin as early as 2 to 3 weeks[1] and is revascularized at approximately 6 to 8 weeks.[3,21,75] The graft undergoes restructuring of its collagen fibers and proteoglycan content until it resembles the normal ACL. This "ligamentization" process is evident by 30 weeks and is accompanied by a decline in the structural properties of the graft. Butler et al[19] demonstrated a decrease in stiffness of the graft to 24% of ACL control values at 7 weeks and to 57% at 1 year. To

what extent this change can be extrapolated to human grafts is a matter of debate. Rougraff et al[63] conducted a study on human patellar tendon grafts and concluded that human autografts are viable as early as 3 weeks and may not go through a necrotic stage. They mature through a prolonged process of ligamentization that may take as long as 3 years to complete. Although a reduction in the structural properties must be assumed, it may not be as pronounced as the one observed in animal studies. A case report of a patient who committed suicide 8 months after ACL reconstruction with a BPB autograft revealed that the ultimate failure strength of the graft remained at 87% of the normal contralateral ligament.[15]

Mobility and Ligamentous Healing

In an effort to protect the healing graft, immobilization and avoidance of weightbearing used to be common practice after ACL injury or reconstruction. The detrimental effects of this approach now have long been recognized. All the anatomic structures of the immobilized joint are affected by the ensuing disuse, even if it occurs for a short period.

Among the first changes occurring with immobilization is muscle atrophy. The weight of the entire muscle is decreased, and this decline is exponential, with more weight loss observed in the initial period of immobilization. The loss of muscle mass results in loss of strength and an increase in fatigability of the muscle.[17] Eriksson and Haggmark[30] showed 40% quadriceps atrophy after 5 weeks of immobilization and noted a decrease in oxidative fast-twitch and slow-twitch endurance fibers. Immobilization in a shortened position accentuates the described changes.

Hyaline cartilage and menisci are also sensitive to disuse and immobility. Reduced joint loading and immobilization lead to atrophy or degeneration of articular cartilage. Changes observed in the immobilized and noncontact areas of articular cartilage include fibrillation, decreased proteoglycan content and synthesis, and altered proteoglycan conformation, such as a decrease in the size and amount of aggregates. These effects are due to decreased stress, which disrupts normal nutritive transport to articular cartilage from the synovial fluid by means of diffusion and convection.[49]

Alteration of the bone-ligament-bone complex after immobilization has been studied primarily in extraarticular ligaments. With disuse, significant reabsorption occurs at ligament insertion sites. Lack of stress leads to random deposition of collagen with a resultant decrease in the structural properties of the ligament. After 8 weeks of immobilization, Noyes found a 40% decrease in strength and a 30% decrease in stiffness at the ligament insertion sites. These changes were reversible, but recovery of the strength and stiffness of the ligament took more than a year. Immobility also facilitates the formation of interfibrillar connections between new collagen fibrils that restrict the normal parallel sliding of ligament fibers, thereby leading to joint contractures. Studies on tendon repairs have demonstrated that controlled loading can enhance the rate and strength of healing.[35] There is sufficient experimental evidence to use motion and mechanical stimuli as means to improve the structural properties of repaired ligaments or tendons.[72] Whether these observations can be applied to intra-articular ligaments such as the ACL is unclear. In a histological animal study, Yamakado et al[82] found that tensile stress enhances the healing process of the tendon-bone junction. Numerous clinical studies have demonstrated no deleterious effect from early motion and weightbearing after ACL reconstruction.[44,56,74]

In an effort to counterbalance the adverse effects of immobility, many authors advocate continuous passive motion (CPM) as a way to achieve early motion. However, there are no studies that show a better long-term outcome with CPM. Noyes et al[56] found that patients treated with CPM regained motion earlier than a group not treated with CPM for the first postoperative week but that by the 14th postoperative day, both groups had the same motion. Therefore, we do not routinely use CPM. In addition, CPM can be dangerous to the ACL reconstruction if the equipment is inappropriately placed on the patient or if the limits for ROM are inappropriately set. Design characteristics of the specific CPM equipment and in particular the level of calf support can influence the amount of anterior tibial translation and place undesired strain on the healing graft.[28] It is our preference to encourage active and passive ROM exercises as soon as possible. We have found that this is more beneficial to the patient because rather than relying on equipment that for a variety of reasons may not be appropriately used or even be available, the patient gets actively involved in the early rehabilitation and becomes part of the healing process.

Biomechanical Considerations

From the moment of insertion the graft, as well as the fixation method, is subjected to loads that must be withstood for a successful outcome. The process starts with intraoperative tensioning of the graft, which aims to reduce laxity as a result of stress relaxation. Although the optimal amount of initial tensioning is not known, most authors agree that hamstring grafts require higher initial tensioning than BPB grafts do. In a prospective, randomized study performed at our laboratory (Orthopaedic Biomechanics Institute), we evaluated laxity and postoperative flexion results at different degrees of initial graft tension. We found higher tensioning loads to be associated with higher side-to-side laxity and slower return of flexion postoperatively.[40] In addition, the position of the joint during tensioning influences the force applied to the graft. Preloading the graft in full or nearly full extension limits the risk of capturing the knee and subsequent difficulty in regaining full extension during the rehabilitation process.

Traumatic overload can injure a graft and is most likely to occur during the initial healing period when the graft is weakest. The maximum load that a graft can withstand during its incorporation is unknown, as well as the magnitude of load that is imposed on the graft during various rehabilitation exercises. Submaximal overloading can also

render the graft nonfunctional through elongation. Cyclic loading can cause loosening of the fixation device or migration of the graft past the fixation device. Simonian et al,[69] in a study of the response of hamstring and patellar tendon grafts during cyclic tensile loading, did not notice statistically significant differences in tissue strain between graft types. For both types of grafts, overall length significantly increased after 3600 cycles but tissue creep was not significant. Knowledge of the behavior of the fixation device under cyclic loading in addition to careful planning of the number of repetitions of various exercises is important in designing the rehabilitation protocol. Caution should be exercised during rehabilitation programs that introduce high loads or an excess of repetitive exercises within the first few weeks or months after surgery. Barber-Westin et al[7] performed sequential arthrometer testing and noted that 38% of the knees that demonstrated abnormal displacement did so in the early phases of rehabilitation before the institution of strenuous exercises.

Patient Factors

The healing process is known to vary among patients. Patients with generalized ligamentous laxity (i.e., hyperextension of the elbows, knees, and hand metacarpophalangeal joints) tend to be "slow healers" and may need to be protected longer. These patients typically have little pain and swelling after their injury or surgical reconstruction and regain motion fast. In contrast, patients who tend to be "scar formers" are at greater risk for arthrofibrosis and need a faster and more aggressive effort to restore ROM.[59]

Associated knee pathology or preexisting disease may dictate modifications of the rehabilitation program in terms of both speed of progression and intensity. A characteristic example is the presence of patellofemoral disease, where exercises at low flexion angles decrease patellofemoral joint reaction force and may be better tolerated by the patient.

The patient's professional and/or recreational aspirations also dictate the rehabilitative approach. Professional athletes are more likely to participate in an accelerated program where more time will be spent in the strengthening phase and emphasis will be placed on sport-specific exercises.

Compliance and motivation of the patient are important considerations. A noncompliant or poorly motivated patient can compromise the outcome of an otherwise perfectly executed reconstruction.

REHABILITATION OF THE OPERATIVE ANTERIOR CRUCIATE LIGAMENT

Preoperative Phase

The rehabilitation program begins in the preoperative phase, immediately after the injury. The goal is to resolve the acute inflammation present in the knee, restore ROM, and normalize gait. ACL reconstruction in an acutely injured, reactive knee that has not regained full motion can result in postoperative arthrofibrosis.[24]

To control the edema and post-traumatic pain, a classic regimen of rest, ice, compression, and elevation is instituted. Both after the acute injury and postoperatively we like to use a continuous-flow cold therapy device. It circulates cold water into a pad on the patient's knee, which cools the joint and at the same time keeps the dressings dry. In addition, it allows adjustment of the temperature to a comfortable level and thus reduces the risk of skin frostbite. In a study comparing continuous-flow cold therapy and crushed ice after ACL reconstruction, Barber[5] found that continuous-flow cold therapy was more effective in reducing postoperative pain and decreasing the use of analgesics. Patients in the continuous-flow cold therapy group used the modality more than patients used crushed ice, had higher flexion in the first postoperative week, and rated performance of the device higher than crushed ice.

A preoperative physical therapy session in which the rehabilitation program will be reviewed is particularly useful. The patient will learn specific exercises and their proper execution, become familiar with equipment that will be used, and establish a working relationship with the therapist. Educational materials in the form of pamphlets or video demonstration of the surgical procedure enhances the patient's understanding, lessens anxiety, and increase compliance with the treatment.

Postoperative Phase

Immediately after the operation the patient is assigned to a rehabilitation protocol. The decision is based primarily on the type of graft that was used. We currently use two specific protocols. Both protocols are criteria based and advance the patient through the different phases only when specific goals have been achieved. It is important to realize that trying to advance the patient to the next phase based on strict adherence to timetables, while the knee is not physiologically ready, can have an effect opposite that desired and lead to difficulty and frustration. The "bone-to-bone, rapid-healing protocol," or protocol A (Fig. 44–1), is initiated in cases in which a BPB autograft is used. Patients who received a hamstring autograft or any type of allograft are allocated to the "soft-tissue–healing protocol," or protocol B (Fig. 44–2). Patients who undergo ACL reconstruction follow the same protocol. The main difference between the two is that the patients in protocol A are advanced to phase II in 3 to 4 weeks and patients in protocol B are advanced in approximately 6 weeks to accommodate for the slower healing of tendon grafts in the bone tunnels. A copy of the particular protocol is attached to the physical therapy prescription and provides a framework for the physical therapist.

Individual modifications are made in both protocols, depending on additional pathology that was encountered and/or addressed during the surgery and the connective tissue profile of the patient (i.e., "slow healer" versus "scar former."). Group-specific instructions (weightbearing status, use of crutches, brace settings, etc.) are outlined on the first page of the protocol. In an attempt to enhance communication between the surgeon and therapist, website addresses where the therapist can find demonstrations of exercises and forward any questions are provided.

BRACING, CONTROL OF EDEMA, AND RANGE OF MOTION

All patients are placed postoperatively in a hinged knee brace. The brace is locked at 0 degrees if the patient does not have hyperextension in the opposite knee and at −10 degrees if the opposite knee can be hyperextended. In patients who fit in the "slow healer" profile, the brace is kept locked at 0 degrees. We believe that keeping the knee in extension or hyperextension reduces the tibia under the femur, pushes the fat pad and the anterior soft tissue away from the graft and thus prevents scarring, and facilitates quadriceps contraction and patellar mobilization exercises. The brace can be adjusted to the desired ROM and allows access for patellar mobilization exercises. It is removed during exercising sessions but it is kept locked for ambulation during the first postoperative week. During the second postoperative week, flexion is gradually increased as tolerated and the patient is allowed to shower and sleep without the brace. In most cases of isolated ACL reconstruction the brace is discontinued by the fourth postoperative week.

The primary focus in the first phase is reversal of the physiological imbalance in the knee after surgery. Aggressive control of postoperative inflammation, effusion, and pain is paramount. This can be accomplished through cryotherapy, elastic compressive dressings, oral analgesics, periarticular muscle activation, and passive ROM exercises. To combat the inhibitory effect of the acute inflammation and swelling on the quadriceps muscle and the vastus medialis obliquus in particular, modalities such as neuromuscular electrical stimulation and electromyographic biofeedback can be used as necessary.

Since one of the most common problems after ACL reconstruction is loss of motion, nonmanual, slow passive and active or active assisted ROM exercises are begun immediately after surgery. Particular emphasis is placed on regaining full extension or hyperextension if this is present in the opposite knee as soon as possible. Specific exercises to achieve full extension include hamstring stretching; supine extension with a bolster under the ankle, with or without a small weight over the knee; prone hangs; and opposite leg active assisted leg extension. Flexion is achieved through wall slides, heel slides, sitting knee flexion, and opposite leg active assisted knee flexion exercises. Patellar mobilization exercises, glides and tilts, are started in the first week to prevent patellar entrapment syndrome. The exercises should be performed gently to avoid causing pain and reaction of the knee because this can actually increase the risk for patellar entrapment.

An important determination during the first phase is the connective tissue profile of the patient. If ROM criteria are

Text continued on p. 727

CRITERIA-BASED
KNEE REHABILITATION PROTOCOL

Group A–Rapid Healing Protocol

INTRODUCTION

The criteria-based knee rehabilitation protocol for a Group A patient is based on rapid healing without need for time constraints to allow significant tissue or bone healing. We expect the physical therapist to use his best judgment, training, and skills to advance the patient as tolerated, based on normal physiologic criteria. Criteria for advancement as well as modifiers for each phase are provided as suggestions but not "rules." Should any phase or instructions be confusing or not clear, please contact us by telephone and/or email. Using our email address you can send each patient's progress per advancement from Phase 1 through the completion of the rehab protocol. In this way we can keep it as part of the patient record.

For questions or clarification toapearson@aosmgroup.com. For progress notes please email to tokkreb@aosmgroup.com.

Group Specific instructions:

Begin protocol post-op week _____

Weight-bearing restrictions:_____

ROM restrictions_____

Category: Slow RPM for_____wks. Begin unlimited RPM in time on_____post-op wk

Squatting > 90°: after_____post-op wks

Crutch guidelines: Toe Touch for_____wks

        Start 25% WB in_____post-op wk
        Start 50% WB in_____post-op wk
        1 crutch on_____ post-op wk
        Off crutches_____ post-op wk
Bracing: Extension_____ post-op wk
          Flexion_____ post-op wk
D/C brace on_____post-op wk

PHASE I GOALS:

1. Reverse physiologic imbalances in the knee
2. Determine if patient is fast healer (+stiffness) or slow healer (–stiffness) ***See Below**
3. Prepare for unaided ambulation

PHASE I Exercises:

1. Patella glides and tilts
2. Decrease swelling
3. Quad sets
4. Straight leg raises
5. Short arc quads 90°–40°
6. Move to aquatic therapy after wound is ***completely*** healed or a protective waterproof dressing is available
7. Modalities as necessary (EGS, e-stim, biofeedback, etc.)
8. Passive Range of Motion (non-manual, slow, full extension) **ASAP**
9. Opposite Leg Active Assist Leg Extension (OLAALE)
10. Hamstring PRE
11. Proprioception exercises
12. Prone terminal knee extensions

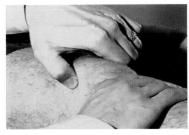 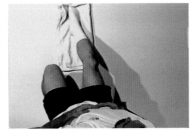 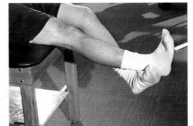

A   Patellar glides/tilts   B   Wall slides   C   OLAALE

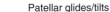

Figure 44–1. Criteria-based knee rehabilitation protocol: group A—rapid-healing protocol. **A,** Patella glides/tilts. **B,** Wall slides. **C,** Opposite leg active assisted leg extension.

CRITERIA FOR ADVANCEMENT TO PHASE II

1. Knee flexion = at least 110°
2. Straight leg raise with **no quad lag**
3. Full passive knee extension
4. Minimal swelling and pain
5. Good or improving patellar mobility

MODIFIERS FOR PHASE I

*1. If ROM criteria is **not** met within 4 weeks, refer to physician for evaluation and possible change in protocol and refrain from maximum manual pushing for range of motion
*2. If patient who has had a HTO, proximal-distal realignments, meniscal transplants, or ACL achieves ROM quickly, with little or no swelling and stiffness,–DO NOT advance to Phase II, refer to MD.

PHASE II

1. Off crutches (unless otherwise noted)
2. Bicycle with resistance
3. Leg press progressive resistive exercises
4. 0°–30° leg extension exercises
5. Increase flexion as fast as possible
6. Discontinue brace (unless otherwise noted)
7. Continue hamstring PREs
8. Move to independent program and check patient every two wks for progress

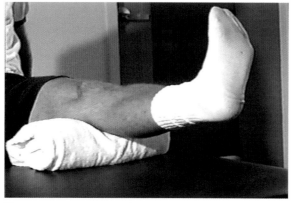

D   0–30° Short arc quad

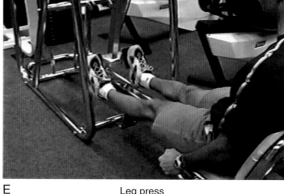

E   Leg press

CRITERIA FOR ADVANCEMENT TO PHASE III

1. Near normal ROM is established
2. No persistant swelling
3. No pain with extension
4. Positive patellar glides and tilts

MODIFIERS FOR PHASE II

1. If ROM criteria is **not** met within 4 weeks, refer to physician.
2. Recurrence of swelling, pain, etc. Return to phase I—add anti-inflammatories. Two failures to advance—refer to physician.

PHASE III

1. Full PRE's
2. Hamstrings and quads
3. Open and closed chain
4. Stair stepper
5. Patient may golf and hike
6. KT 1000 evaluation (If ACL surgery)
7. Isokinetic testing
8. Plyometrics (ground based)

Figure 44–1, cont'd. **D,** Short-arc quads. **E,** Leg press.

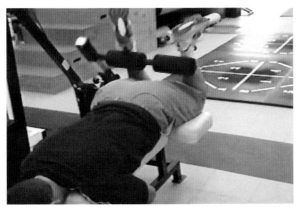

F   Open Chain Hamstrings Strengthening

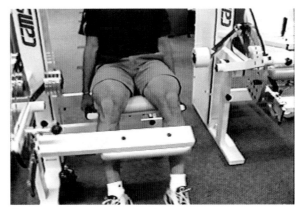

G   Open Chain Quadriceps Strengthening

CRITERIA FOR ADVANCEMENT TO PHASE IV

1. Quad strength at 75%
2. Wait 16 weeks (post-op) for HTO, proximal-distal patellar realignments, meniscal transplants, and ACL

MODIFIERS FOR PHASE III

1. Recurrence of swelling, pain, stiffness, etc. Return to Phase II—add anti-inflammatories. Two failures to advance—refer to physician.

PHASE IV—Transition to Sport and Work

1. No contact or competition
2. Full weight lifting program–See front sheet for restrictions
3. Advanced balance exercises
4. Begin progressive running program

CRITERIA FOR ADVANCEMENT TO PHASE V—Sport/Work

1. Quads at 90% strength (isokinetic or manual strength test)
2. Hamstrings at 90% strength (isokinetic or manual strength test)
3. No swelling with activities
4. Pass functional tests

MODIFIERS FOR PHASE IV

1. Recurrence of swelling, pain, stiffness, etc. Returns to Phase III—refer to physician.
2. Advance PRN

PHASE V—Return to Play

1. Run up and down (stairs and hills)
2. Progress to cutting, jumping, and sport-specific drills
3. Transition to sport
4. Isokinetic testing
5. Quad strength must be 90% of opposite side (90% to body weight)
6. Hamstring strength must be 90% of opposite side
7. No swelling with or after activities
8. Pass a battery of functional tests
9. Sports brace is optional for HTO, proximal-distal alignments, meniscal transplants, or ACL unless:
   • KT 1000 is greater than 3mm
   • Quad/Ham strength is less than 90%
   • Participating in contact sports, aerial sports, soccer, or basketball

Figure 44–1, cont'd. **F,** Open-chain hamstring strengthening. **G,** Open-chain quadriceps strengthening.

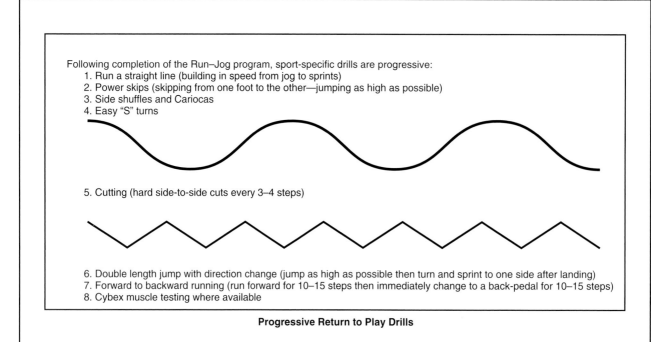

Following completion of the Run–Jog program, sport-specific drills are progressive:
1. Run a straight line (building in speed from jog to sprints)
2. Power skips (skipping from one foot to the other—jumping as high as possible)
3. Side shuffles and Cariocas
4. Easy "S" turns

5. Cutting (hard side-to-side cuts every 3–4 steps)

6. Double length jump with direction change (jump as high as possible then turn and sprint to one side after landing)
7. Forward to backward running (run forward for 10–15 steps then immediately change to a back-pedal for 10–15 steps)
8. Cybex muscle testing where available

Progressive Return to Play Drills

MODIFIERS FOR PHASE V

1. Recurrence of swelling, pain, stiffness, etc. Return to Phase IV. Two failures to advance—refer to physician.

Figure 44–1, cont'd.

CRITERIA-BASED
KNEE REHABILITATION PROTOCOL

Group B–Soft Tissue Healing Protocol

INTRODUCTION

Group B is a more prolonged protocol designed to allow soft tissue healing and generally has a time constraint of approximately 6 weeks prior to entering into the CRITERIA-BASED PROTOCOL. We expect the physical therapist to use his best judgment, training, and skills to advance the patient as tolerated, based on normal physiologic criteria. Criteria for advancement as well as modifiers for each phase are provided as suggestions but not "rules." Should any phase or instructions be confusing or not clear, please contact us by telephone and/or email. Using our email address you can send each patient's progress per advancement from Phase 1 through the completion of the rehab protocol. In this way we can keep it as part of the patient record.

For questions or clarification toapearson@aosmgroup.com. For progress notes please email to tokkreb@aosmgroup.com.

Group Specific instructions:

Begin protocol post-op week _____

Weight-bearing restrictions: _____

ROM restrictions _____

Category: Slow RPM for_____wks. Begin unlimited RPM in time on_____post-op wk

Squatting > 90°: after_____post-op wks

Crutch guidelines: Toe Touch for_____wks

     Start 25% WB in_____post-op wk
     Start 50% WB in_____post-op wk
     1 crutch on_____ post-op wk
     Off crutches_____ post-op wk
Bracing: Extension_____ post-op wk
         Flexion_____ post-op wk
D/C brace on_____post-op wk

PHASE I GOALS:

1. Reverse physiologic imbalances in the knee
2. Determine if patient is fast healer (+stiffness) or slow healer (–stiffness) ***See Below**
3. Prepare for unaided ambulation

PHASE I Exercises:

1. Patella glides and tilts
2. Decrease swelling
3. Quad sets
4. Straight leg raises
5. Short arc quads 90°–40°
6. Move to aquatic therapy after wound is ***completely*** healed or a protective waterproof dressing is available
7. Modalities as necessary (EGS, e-stim, biofeedback, etc.)
8. Passive Range of Motion (non-manual, slow, full extension) **ASAP**
9. Opposite Leg Active Assist Leg Extension (OLAALE)
10. Hamstring PRE
11. Proprioception exercises
12. Prone terminal knee extensions

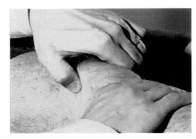

A   Patellar glides/tilts

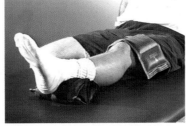

B   Terminal knee extension

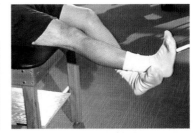

C   OLAALE

Figure 44–2. Criteria-based knee rehabilitation protocol: Group B—soft-tissue–healing protocol. **A,** Patella glides/tilts. **B,** Terminal knee extension. **C,** Opposite leg active assisted leg extension.

CRITERIA FOR ADVANCEMENT TO PHASE II

1. Knee flexion = at least 110°
2. Straight leg raise with **no quad lag**
3. Full passive knee extension
4. Minimal swelling and pain
5. Good or improving patellar mobility

MODIFIERS FOR PHASE I

*1. If ROM criteria is **not** met within 4 weeks, refer to physician for evaluation and possible change in protocol and refrain from maximum manual pushing for range of motion.
*2. If range of motion criteria are achieved early this means faster healing therefore advancement to Phase II must be delayed until **post-op week 8. STOP** manual pushing for ROM

PHASE II

1. Off crutches (unless otherwise noted)
2. Bicycle with resistance
3. Leg press, progressive resistive exercises
4. 0°–30° leg extension exercises
5. Increase flexion as fast as possible
6. Discontinue brace (unless otherwise noted)
7. Continue hamstring PREs
8. Move to independent program and check patient every two wks for progress

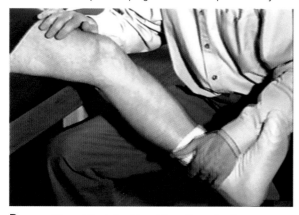

D   Manual Resistive Hamstrings Strengthening

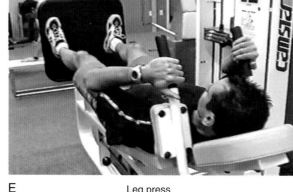

E   Leg press

CRITERIA FOR ADVANCEMENT TO PHASE III

1. Near normal ROM is established
2. No persistant swelling
3. No pain with extension
4. Positive patellar glides and tilts

MODIFIERS FOR PHASE II

1. Recurrence of swelling, pain, etc. Return to Phase I—add anti-inflammatories. Two failures to advance—refer to physician.

PHASE III

1. Full PREs
2. Hamstrings and quads
3. Open and closed chain
4. Stair stepper
5. Patient may golf and hike
6. KT 1000 evaluation (If ACL surgery)
7. Isokinetic testing
8. Plyometrics (ground based)

Figure 44–2, cont'd. **D,** Manual resistive hamstring strengthening. **E,** Leg press.

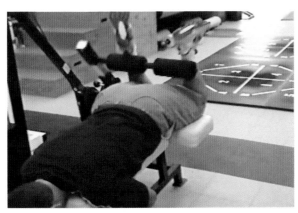

F   Open Chain Hamstrings Strengthening

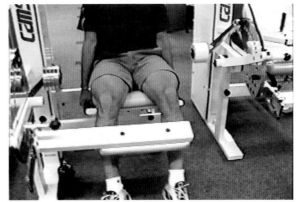

G   Open Chain Quadriceps Strengthening

CRITERIA FOR ADVANCEMENT TO PHASE IV

1. Quad strength at 75%
2. Wait 16 weeks (post-op) for HTO, proximal-distal patellar realignments, meniscal transplants, and ACL

MODIFIERS FOR PHASE III

1. Recurrence of swelling, pain, stiffness, etc. Return to Phase II—add anti-inflammatories. Two failures to advance—refer to physician.

PHASE IV—Transition to Sport and Work

1. No contact or competition
2. Full weight lifting program—See front sheet for restrictions
3. Advanced balance exercises
4. Begin progressive running program

CRITERIA FOR ADVANCEMENT TO PHASE V—Sport/Work

1. Quads at 90% strength (isokinetic or manual strength test)
2. Hamstrings at 90% strength (isokinetic or manual strength test)
3. No swelling with activities
4. Pass functional tests

MODIFIERS FOR PHASE IV

1. Recurrence of swelling, pain, stiffness, etc. Returns to Phase III—refer to physician.

PHASE V—Return to Play

1. Run up and down (stairs and hills)
2. Progress to cutting, jumping, and sport-specific drills
3. Transition to sport
4. Isokinetic testing
5. Quad strength must be 90% of opposite side (90% to body weight)
6. Hamstring strength must be 90% of opposite side
7. No swelling with or after activities
8. Pass a battery of functional tests
9. Sports brace is optional unless:
    • KT 1000 is greater than 3mm
    • Quad/Ham strength is less than 90%
    • Participating in contact sports, aerial sports, soccer, or basketball

Figure 44–2, cont'd. **F,** Open-chain hamstring strengthening. **G,** Open-chain quadriceps strengthening.

Following completion of the Run–Jog program, sport-specific drills are progressive:
   1. Run a straight line (building in speed from jog to sprints)
   2. Power skips (skipping from one foot to the other—jumping as high as possible)
   3. Side shuffles and Cariocas
   4. Easy "S" turns

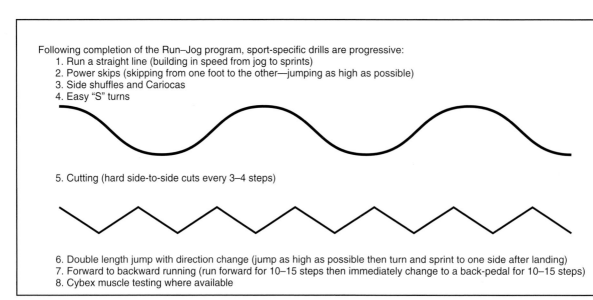

   5. Cutting (hard side-to-side cuts every 3–4 steps)

   6. Double length jump with direction change (jump as high as possible then turn and sprint to one side after landing)
   7. Forward to backward running (run forward for 10–15 steps then immediately change to a back-pedal for 10–15 steps)
   8. Cybex muscle testing where available

Progressive Return to Play Drills

MODIFIERS FOR PHASE V

1. Recurrence of swelling, pain, stiffness, etc. Return to Phase IV. Two failures to advance—refer to physician.

Figure 44–2, cont'd.

achieved early with little or no swelling and stiffness, the patient is a slow healer and therefore advancement to Phase II must be delayed until postoperative week 8. At the same time the therapist should stop manual pushing for ROM.

WEIGHTBEARING

Weightbearing is started immediately in most cases. The patient is allowed 50% weightbearing in the first postoperative week, with increases as tolerated thereafter. Patients are usually free of crutches by the end of the third postoperative week. Repair of a stable meniscal tear does not alter our weightbearing protocol. Although studies have found no difference in the outcome of the repair after early weightbearing,[6,36] we prefer to protect the repair of unstable tears. Concomitant chondral restoration procedures (microfracture, mosaicplasty, etc.) are treated with non-weightbearing for 4 to 6 weeks to avoid damaging the treated area by axial compression and shear forces. Revision ACL reconstructions in which bone quality is deemed poor are also protected with non-weightbearing for 6 weeks.

STRENGTH

Isometric Exercises. Isometric exercises are those in which muscle contraction occurs without a change in the length of the muscle or joint position. These are the first strengthening exercises allowed after ACL reconstruction. Quadriceps sets and straight-leg raises are the mainstay of this program. These exercises can be performed with or without the brace. They are performed by both legs for cross-education. This concept refers to the carryover of strength gains in the uninvolved limb to the contralateral injured or untrained limb. The effects are attributed to simultaneous neural adaptations in the trained and untrained muscles. There is evidence that eccentric strength training of the uninvolved quadriceps can provide greater gains for the injured or recently operated limb.[41] For patients who have difficulty in this initial strengthening phase, electromyographic biofeedback and neuromuscular electrical stimulation can be used. We prefer the first because it gives a visual guide as to when the quadriceps has successfully contracted and therefore gets the patient more involved with the rehabilitation effort.

Isotonic Exercises (Progressive Resistance Exercises). In progressive resistance exercises (PREs), muscle contraction produces constant tension over a given ROM. They can be done with manual resistance, free weights, or machines. PREs must be carefully instituted, with strict attention paid to the arc of motion. The first PREs are those that isolate the agonist muscles, predominantly the hamstrings. They should be performed in seated and prone positions to target the hamstring-to-quadriceps torque ratios at functional activity-specific hip and knee angles[27,43,76] and should be performed on the surgical and nonsurgical limbs. Open kinetic chain exercises are of

value because they isolate the quadriceps and hamstrings. However, open kinetic chain quadriceps isotonic exercises can place excessive stress on the graft if performed at low angles. Therefore, we initially use short-arc quads from 90 to 40 degrees without resistance in the early rehabilitative period and incorporate long-arc quads and 0- to 30-degree leg extension exercises without resistance in the second phase of the rehabilitation program, generally between the third and fourth postoperative week. Zero- to 30-degree leg extension isotonic exercises have the advantage of minimizing patellofemoral compressive force and creating less discomfort in patients with patellofemoral joint disease. Close kinetic chain PREs train agonist and antagonist muscles in a cocontraction, such as in a leg press, and are followed by antagonist muscle work. All PREs are prescribed according to the universally accepted principles of periodization, or cycling of the training load. The progression is modified to place greater emphasis and amount of time spent on the initial joint preparation–anatomic adaptation stage of strength training. This period is characterized by a high volume of low- to moderate-intensity repetitions of each exercise that are quantified in terms of minutes rather than repetitions per set. The purpose of this phase is to facilitate articular surface integrity and enhance the vascularity and strength of musculotendinous junctions in preparation for the hypertrophy, strength, and power stages to follow. The length of this phase will vary, depending on the specific diagnosis and length of the non-weightbearing or limited weightbearing phase. Closed kinetic chain PREs are emphasized during this stage of rehabilitation because they place less tension on the ACL graft than open kinetic chain exercises do because of the posterior force applied by the hamstrings during the cocontraction.[12,31,62,81] These exercises appear to better imitate functional tasks and enhance functional performance to a greater extent than open kinetic chain exercises do.[57] They appear to be less demanding on the patellofemoral joint, an important consideration in patients with patellofemoral pathology.[71] Another benefit of closed chain activities is that while strengthening agonist and antagonist muscles, they also enhance coordination and proprioception through the cocontraction mentioned previously. A variety of closed chain exercises can be incorporated into the rehabilitation program.

Patients can begin using four-way hip machines and performing isolated trunk exercises as soon as possible. When the weightbearing status reaches 50%, minisquats and bilateral neuromuscular control exercises can be added. Once the wound has healed, aquatic exercises are an excellent way to stimulate muscle activity and reeducate the neural system, especially in a patient in whom full weightbearing will be delayed for any of the reasons mentioned earlier. Gait training, minisquats, hamstring curls, and aqua-jogging exercises are all early activities that patients can begin in the water. Flutter kicking with fins is avoided because of the marked strain placed on the ACL graft by a whip kick. Cycling is started when the patient has reached at least 105 degrees of flexion.

As the patient progresses to full weightbearing, the preparation phase is fully implemented by increasing the number of exercises, sets, and repetitions completed.

The hypertrophy phase is initiated when the patient has spent sufficient time preparing the joint surfaces, musculotendinous junctions, graft harvest sites, and muscular firing patterns to function efficiently under increased load. The hypertrophy phase serves the purpose of enhancing muscle girth and is distinguished by multiple sets of each exercise that result in exhaustion after 10 to 15 repetitions. By inducing fatigue, additional muscle fibers are recruited to complete the work, thereby resulting in more thorough training of the involved musculature. Most patients will remain in the hypertrophy phase for the duration of their rehabilitation. Increasing the load through strength and power training is not necessary if this capacity is not needed by the patient.

The strength and power phases of the PREs, with their increased resistance and velocity of movement, are initiated when it has been decided that the patient is going to return to sport-specific activities. The goals of the strength phase are to increase motor unit activation and fast-twitch fiber recruitment, increase neural output, provide a base for increased muscular endurance, and improve coordination and synchronization of muscle groups. Loads of 85% to 100% of one repetition maximum are performed during the strength phase (one to four repetitions). The power phase is designed to transform strength gains into sport-specific strength. Power refers to the ability of the neuromuscular system to produce the greatest possible force in the shortest time. As such, movements performed during the power phase are reserved until the patient has been cleared to perform explosive, high-velocity training. Movements common to power training include very fast PREs and ballistic exercises, such as plyometric activities, which take advantage of the stretch reflex and series elastic component properties of the musculotendinous unit and result in increased contractile force with each repetition.

Isokinetics. Isokinetics are exercises in which the speed of motion is fixed and resistance to motion adapts to the amount of force applied to the machine. They require access to isokinetic machines. Isokinetics are the last strengthening exercises introduced after ACL reconstruction, usually between the fifth or sixth postoperative month, because they produce high joint reactive force, especially at slow speeds. Our preferred exercising program is pyramid-like and starts at 180 degrees/sec, increases at a 30-degree/sec interval until reaching 300 degrees/sec, and then works back to 180 degrees/sec. Exercises in the 60- to 180-degree/sec range are avoided until very late in the rehabilitation schedule because of their increased joint reactive force. These open kinetic chain exercises may be particularly uncomfortable to patients with patellofemoral chondrosis.

Although decisions regarding return to play are aided by the results of isokinetic testing when available, it has been demonstrated that maximum isokinetic quadriceps strength may not be as important a predictor of function as initially thought. Keays et al[45] have demonstrated a decrease in isokinetic quadriceps strength 6 months after ACL reconstruction when compared with preoperative values despite improvement in functional tests. For these reasons and because of limited availability of the appropriate equipment in different rehabilitation facilities, we tend to use isokinetic strengthening less often.

REHABILITATION AFTER ANTERIOR CRUCIATE LIGAMENT RECONSTRUCTION COMBINED WITH OTHER PROCEDURES

Meniscal Repairs. The incidence of concomitant meniscal injury after an acute ACL tear is high. Combining the incidence reported in different series, Fithian et al[33] found that meniscal injury was present in 58% of acute ACL tears and 84% of chronic ACL tears. A high percentage of these tears are expected to be repairable, and ACL reconstruction creates an environment that promotes healing. After repair of a stable meniscal tear we generally allow early weightbearing and do not pose any restrictions in ROM. Repair of unstable tears is treated more conservatively. The patient is kept non-weightbearing for 6 weeks, and the brace is adjusted to block flexion beyond 90 degrees for 4 to 6 weeks. Squatting beyond 90 degrees is not allowed for 4 to 6 months.

Posterior Cruciate Ligament Reconstruction. If ACL reconstruction is combined with posterior cruciate ligament (PCL) reconstruction, the patient follows the PCL criteria–based protocol, or protocol C (Fig. 44–3). Hamstring PREs are not allowed for 24 weeks. The patient is fitted with a Jack PCL Brace (Albrecht Gmbh, Germany), which is used for 3 months. The brace prevents posterior sagging of the tibia by applying an anteriorly directed translation force through an adjustable spring tension mechanism incorporated at the level of the hinges.

Collateral Ligament Repair or Reconstruction. In cases in which collateral ligament repair or reconstruction is undertaken at the same time as ACL reconstruction, our preference is to protect the knee with a brace and non-weightbearing status for a period of 4 to 6 weeks, depending on the extent of injury. An unloading brace (medial for lateral repairs and lateral for medial repairs) can be particularly useful since it may allow resumption of weightbearing earlier. Multiligament reconstructions, especially those that involve the medial collateral ligament, have greater potential for postoperative stiffness, so restoration of ROM is pursued more aggressively than for isolated ACL reconstruction. Exercises that may stress the collateral ligament repair or reconstruction are avoided for 6 to 8 weeks.

REHABILITATION LOGISTICS

In an era of medical cost containment it is important for the rehabilitation program to be structured so that the benefit of the available resources is maximized for the time that they are available. Various studies have documented the efficacy of home-based rehabilitation after ACL reconstruction.[8,26,32] Frosch et al[34] compared two groups of patients who attended a regular physiotherapy program or an extended and supervised rehabilitation program. Despite higher initial cost associated with the intensive rehabilitation program, they documented better functional outcome and earlier return to work. Treacy et al[73] found that poor compliance and infrequent physiotherapy attendance are associated with suboptimal outcome. We believe that supervised physical therapy is important during the

CRITERIA-BASED
KNEE REHABILITATION PROTOCOL

Group C—PCL Protocol

INTRODUCTION

Group C is a combination of rapid and constrained PCL healing. We expect the physical therapist to use his best judgment, training, and skills to advance the patient as tolerated, based on normal physiologic criteria. Criteria for advancement as well as modifiers for each phase are provided as suggestions but not "rules." Should any phase or instructions be confusing or not clear, please contact us by telephone and/or email. Using our email address you can send each patients progress per advancement from Phase 1 through the completion of the rehab protocol. In this way we can keep it as part of the patient record.

For questions or clarification toapearson@aosmgroup.com. For progress notes please email to tokkreb@aosmgroup.com.

Group Specific instructions:

Begin protocol post-op week _____

Weight-bearing restrictions:_____

ROM restrictions_____

Category: Slow RPM for_____wks. Begin unlimited RPM in time on_____post-op wk

Squatting > 90°: after_____post-op wks

Crutch guidelines: Toe Touch for_____wks. Non-weightbearing for_____weeks

    Start 25% WB in_____post-op wk
    Start 50% WB in_____post-op wk
    1 crutch on_____ post-op wk
    Off crutches_____ post-op wk
Bracing: Extension_____ post-op wk
        Flexion_____ post-op wk
D/C brace on_____post-op wk

PHASE I GOALS:

1. Reverse physiologic imbalances in the knee
2. Determine if patient is fast healer (+stiffness) or slow healer (−stiffness) ∗**See Below**
3. Prepare for unaided ambulation

PHASE I Exercises:

1. Patella glides and tilts
2. Decrease swelling
3. Quad sets
4. Straight leg raises
5. Short arc quads 90°–40°
6. Move to aquatic therapy after wound is ***completely*** healed or a protective waterproof dressing is available
7. Modalities as necessary (EGS, e-stim, biofeedback, etc.)
8. Passive Range of Motion (non-manual, slow, full extension) **ASAP**
9. Opposite Leg Active Assist Leg Extension (OLAALE)
10. No hamstring PREs
11. Proprioception exercises
12. Prone terminal knee extension

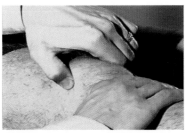

A   Patellar glides/tilts

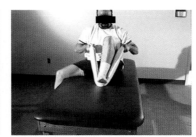

B   Heel slides

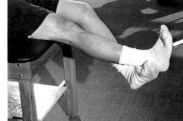

C   OLAALE

Figure 44–3. Criteria-based knee rehabilitation protocol: Group C—posterior cruciate ligament protocol. **A,** Patella glides/tilts. **B,** Heel slides. **C,** Opposite leg active assisted leg extension.

CRITERIA FOR ADVANCEMENT TO PHASE II

1. Knee flexion = at least 110°
2. Straight leg raise with **no quad lag**
3. Full passive knee extension
4. Minimal swelling and pain
5. Good or improving patellar mobility

MODIFIERS FOR PHASE I

*1. If ROM criteria is **not** met within 4 weeks, refer to physician for evaluation and possible change in protocol and refrain from maximum manual pushing for range of motion.
*2. If range of motion criteria are achieved early this means fast healer; therefore advancement to Phase II must be delayed until **post-op week 8. STOP** manual pushing for ROM.

PHASE II

1. Off crutches (unless otherwise noted)
2. Bicycle with resistance
3. Leg press progressive resistive exercises
4. 0°–30° leg extension exercises
5. Increase flexion as fast as possible
6. Discontinue brace (unless otherwise noted)
7. Move to independent program and check patient every 2 wks for progress

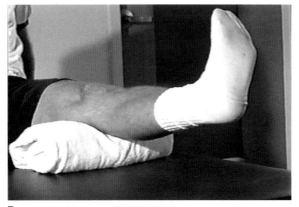

D   Short arc quads

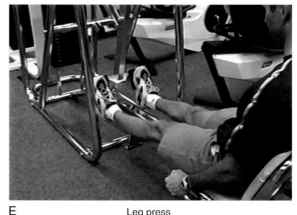

E   Leg press

CRITERIA FOR ADVANCEMENT TO PHASE III

1. Near normal ROM is established
2. No persistent swelling
3. No pain with extension
4. Positive patellar glides and tilts

MODIFIERS FOR PHASE II

1. If ROM criteria is **not** met within 12 weeks of starting protocol, refer to physician. Go to Phase III 16 weeks after starting protocol, except for PCL-Posterolateral corner, PCL-MCL (female), unstable meniscus repair, meniscal transplant, opening wedge HTO, patellar arthritis, or chondral restoration which should progress to Phase III at 24 weeks after start of protocol.
2. Recurrence of swelling, pain, etc. Return to Phase I—add anti-inflammatories. Two failures to advance—refer to physician.
3. NO hamstrings PREs until 24 week post-op.

PHASE III

1. Full PRE's
2. Hamstrings and quads
3. Open and closed chain
4. Stair stepper
5. Patient may golf and hike
6. KT 1000 evaluation
7. Isokinetic testing
8. Plyometrics ground based

Figure 44–3, cont'd. **D,** Short-arc quads. **E,** Leg press.

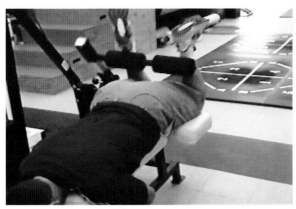

F   Open Chain Hamstrings

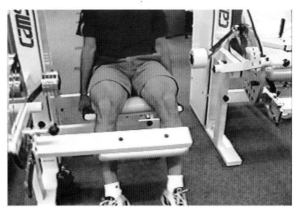

G   Open Chain Quadriceps Strengthening

CRITERIA FOR ADVANCEMENT TO PHASE IV

1. Quad strength at 75%
2. 24 weeks post-op for PCL auto, PCL-MCL, ACL-PCL

MODIFIERS FOR PHASE III

1. Recurrence of swelling, pain, stiffness, etc. Return to Phase II—add anti-inflammatories. Two failures to advance—refer to physician.

PHASE IV—Transition to Sport and Work

1. No contact or competition
2. Hamstring PRE's are ok for PCL auto, PCL-MCL, ACL-PCL, repair or reconstruction
3. Full unrestricted weight program
4. Start run/jog program

CRITERIA FOR ADVANCEMENT TO PHASE V–Sport/Work

1. Quads at 90% strength (isokinetic or manual strength test)
2. Hamstrings at 90% strength (isokinetic or manual strength test)
3. No swelling with activities
4. Pass functional tests

MODIFIERS FOR PHASE IV

1. Recurrence of swelling, pain, stiffness, etc. Returns to Phase III—refer to physician

PHASE V—Return to Play

1. Run up and down (stairs and hills)
2. Progress to cutting, jumping, and sport-specific drills
3. Transition to sport
4. Isokinetic testing
5. Quad strength must be 90% of opposite side (90% to body weight)
6. Hamstring strength must be 90% of opposite side
7. No swelling with or after activities
8. Pass a battery of functional tests
9. Sports brace is optional unless:
    • KT 1000 is greater than 3mm
    • Quad/Ham strength is less than 90%
    • Participating in contact sports, aerial sports, soccer, or basketball

Figure 44–3, cont'd. **F,** Open-chain hamstring strengthening. **G,** Open-chain quadriceps strengthening.

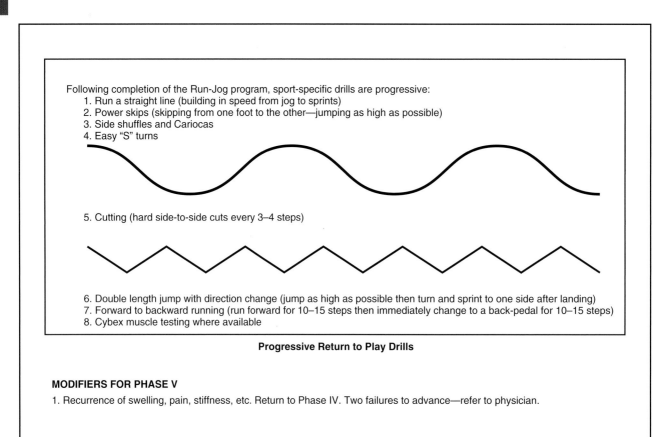

Following completion of the Run-Jog program, sport-specific drills are progressive:
1. Run a straight line (building in speed from jog to sprints)
2. Power skips (skipping from one foot to the other—jumping as high as possible)
3. Side shuffles and Cariocas
4. Easy "S" turns

5. Cutting (hard side-to-side cuts every 3–4 steps)

6. Double length jump with direction change (jump as high as possible then turn and sprint to one side after landing)
7. Forward to backward running (run forward for 10–15 steps then immediately change to a back-pedal for 10–15 steps)
8. Cybex muscle testing where available

Progressive Return to Play Drills

MODIFIERS FOR PHASE V

1. Recurrence of swelling, pain, stiffness, etc. Return to Phase IV. Two failures to advance—refer to physician.

Figure 44–3, cont'd.

period that the physiological imbalance in the knee is reversed. It is our experience that during this phase most patients need the assistance and expertise of a skilled therapist. In the criteria-based rehabilitation protocol that we propose, patients are moved to an independent program as soon as the physiological imbalance of the knee has been reversed and the exercises of the early strengthening phase have been mastered. This can be accomplished in the majority of cases in about 12 visits. After these initial phases, quite often the patient is allowed to return to the rehabilitation facility and use equipment or other resources for the exercise routine without having formal supervision from a therapist. Further supervised visits are required when the patient transitions through phases or reaches pivotal points, such as functional testing before return to play. Programs designed to bridge the gap between discharge from therapy and return to sports, though beneficial for the majority of patients, impose extra financial burden and are therefore generally reserved for competitive athletes. The components of such a program will be discussed in the section "Return to Sports."

REHABILITATION OF A NONOPERATIVELY TREATED ANTERIOR CRUCIATE LIGAMENT

Although the main focus on treatment of ACL injuries has been on operative management, there is still place for nonoperative treatment. In fact, studies on the natural history of ACL injury with follow-up between 5 and 15 years indicate that most patients with ACL injury do well with activities of daily living and the majority will be able to participate in light sports with no more than mild or occasional pain, giving way, and swelling. Participation in vigorous sports that involve hard cutting, jumping, and pivoting place the patient at increased risk for reinjury, especially meniscal tear. Although the presence of degenerative changes is a frequent finding on follow-up of a chronic ACL-deficient knee, arthrosis is more strongly associated with meniscal loss than with absence of the ACL. Patients unwilling to modify their activity level are unlikely to be satisfied with nonoperative management. An increased level of preinjury participation in high-demand sports correlates negatively with successful outcome after nonoperative treatment.[25] In view of current knowledge on the natural history of an ACL-deficient knee, it appears that before embarking on nonoperative management, appropriate counseling of the patient is critical for success.

Our criteria-based approach is used in rehabilitation of a nonoperative ACL as well. We use the "rapid-healing protocol," or Protocol A, that we use for ACL reconstruction with a BPB graft. The protocol is modified so that the patient does not have to wait 3 to 4 weeks before entering Phase II of resistance strengthening since graft healing is not a consideration in this case.

To reverse the physiological imbalance present in the joint as a result of the injury, the joint is kept at rest, and crutches and a knee immobilizer are used for comfort as needed. Oral anti-inflammatory medications and a continuous-flow cold therapy device are used to control pain and swelling. As the patient becomes more comfortable, ROM and patellar mobilization exercises are begun. Isometric quadriceps and hamstring exercises are instituted as soon as possible to prevent disuse atrophy. Once the patient has achieved full or nearly full ROM, has minimal swelling and pain, and is able to ambulate unaided, advancement to the strengthening and proprioception enhancement phases is initiated.

The strengthening phase emphasizes a high hamstring-to-quadriceps strength ratio. The strengthening program should include the gastrocnemius and soleus. The importance of these muscles is probably under-recognized, but nevertheless, they contribute to dynamic stabilization of the knee.[68] Open and closed kinetic chain exercises are instituted with progression from high volume/low load to low volume/high load. Since there are no concerns regarding straining of a healing graft, more liberal use of open kinetic chain strengthening exercises, which can produce greater strength gains,[51] is allowed.

Equally and perhaps more important in rehabilitation of an ACL-deficient knee is proprioception enhancement. Functional instability has been attributed at least in part to loss of proprioception, and studies have documented a significant correlation between the latency of reflex hamstring contraction and the frequency of "giving way."[10] In a prospective, double-blind, randomized clinical trial, Beard et al[9] investigated the efficacy of two regimens of rehabilitation for knees with ACL deficiency. Patients were randomly assigned to a program of muscle strengthening or to a program designed to enhance proprioception and improve hamstring contraction reflexes. The authors found greater functional gains in the second group of patients. In addition, in both groups functional gains were positively correlated with improvement in reflex hamstring contraction latency, which the authors used as a measure of proprioceptive function.

To enhance proprioceptive function we use weight-bearing closed kinetic chain exercises. The proprioceptive response can be further challenged with a progressive reduction in the stability of the supporting surface through the use of various training boards. Since muscle fatigue affects the dynamic stability of the knee,[70] the training program should include enough exercising sequences to elicit fatigue and train these responses.[20]

Bracing in the nonoperative treatment of an ACL-deficient knee remains a controversial issue. Although many studies have shown that functional bracing decreases the amount of anterior tibial translation in patients with an ACL tear, it does not eliminate it.[11,13,78] It has been suggested that the use of a functional brace, neoprene sleeve, or even an elastic bandage can improve the position sense and the ability to detect passive knee motion.[50,60] However, the proprioceptive benefits of these interventions are of questionable clinical and functional significance.[14] Kocher et al,[46] in a study on subsequent knee injury in ACL-deficient professional skiers, found that a significantly higher proportion of injuries occurred in nonbraced skiers than in braced skiers. Despite the lack of sufficient scientific evidence that functional braces can prevent injury in an ACL-deficient knee, they continue to be popular, and it has been our experience that patients report improved function when wearing a brace. This is especially true in patients who do not cope well with their injury.

It must be noted that conservative management of an ACL injury does not necessarily mean nonoperative treatment. Failure of the patient to advance through the various phases of the rehabilitation program may be due to meniscal or chondral pathology that has to be addressed surgically. The incidence of such pathology after acute ACL injury has been found to be as high as 68% and 23%, respectively.[42]

RETURN TO SPORTS

It is important to have a well-organized and supervised program to facilitate the athlete's program after discharge from physical therapy and before return to functional, recreational, and athletic independence. The program must be personalized to an individual's abilities and should provide a consistent progression of stages that become increasingly more challenging. There are several components of a comprehensive return-to-sport program.

Strength training is a major component of a return-to-sport program. It should specifically target the core musculature (hip girdle, abdominals) and legs and focus on appropriate hamstring-to-quadriceps ratios, as well as good postural and proprioceptive control. It should incorporate resistive equipment in addition to functional activities such as the use of balance boards, medicine balls, physioballs, and other devices.

Forward incline running on a quality treadmill will improve overall conditioning, improve speed and flexibility, and aid the athlete in relearning proper running mechanics without the impact force associated with running over ground. The treadmill incline provides additional advantages over level running, such as increased muscular loading of the hip flexors and extensors and reinforcement of the appropriate foot-strike position. Treadmill velocity should be adjusted to accommodate the individual's ability and to maintain appropriate running mechanics at all times. Special attention should be paid to ensuring that the stride of the involved leg is not shorter than the stride of the contralateral leg because of inadequate knee flexion. It is also important to watch for internal rotation at the hip compensating for decreased motor control and strength and resulting in increased valgus stress at the knee.

Backward or retrograde treadmill walking and running are another excellent means of enhancing motor control, coordination pattern, and strength improvement in a functional and safe manner at sport-specific velocities. The administrator must emphasize and enforce proper biomechanics by making sure that the athlete maintains an "athletic stance" with the shoulders balanced over the knees. The foot should be in alignment with the knee and hip, and bilateral symmetry is emphasized at all times. If the athlete is unable to perform more than half of a particular repetition without being spotted or assisted, the treadmill must be slowed to accommodate performance with appropriate biomechanics. An unequal stride length may indicate inadequate strength, decreased motor control, a lack of flexion at the knee, decreased hamstring flexibility, or any combination of these factors. The program administrator must assess and treat accordingly to attain symmetry of gait.

The benefits and popularity of plyometric exercises are well documented and accepted in the training of athletes and need not be described in this text. Suffice it to say that a well-designed progression of appropriate plyometrics given the individual's functional status and sport requirements will challenge the body to improve the neuromuscular efficiency and kinesthetic awareness needed for sport and recreational activities. All weightbearing sports include plyometric movements that load and unload the limbs during movement patterns. Therefore, a progressive program of these activities is essential in a return-to-sport program. Plyometrics should not be significantly painful to perform, and the administrator must be conscientious in observing and correcting any improper biomechanics by being aware of the role of fatigue and deconditioning in the decay of proper execution as a session progresses. Valgus moments about the knee in excess of 10 degrees, especially with single-leg activities, should be specifically avoided. If valgus stress persists, additional stabilization exercises for the core, hip, and knee should be integrated into the overall program. Accuracy and proper biomechanics are more important than speed during these exercises, and if the athlete is unable to properly perform the drills, the protocol should be adjusted to ensure success.

Agility and multidirectional movements are key components of sport performance and must be included in the program. These drills should be designed to improve kinesthetic awareness, reinforce proper movement mechanics, and enhance the neuromuscular pathways for improving sport- or work-specific performance. Progression of these activities should not occur too quickly. It is important to maintain control of the progression according to the individual's ability to ensure success and confidence in performing the appropriate drills as determined by the needs of the athlete's particular sport. This will reduce the potential for pain-related inhibition and the establishment of substitution patterns.

Training sessions on consecutive days should be avoided to accommodate the body's recovery requirements and adaptations by the involved knee's healing tissues and structures. Strength training should be performed three times per week. Finally, nonimpact cardiovascular exercise should be performed a minimum of 15 to 20 minutes, two times per week, in addition to the sport-specific training program. Periodic strength and performance testing correlating to the types of training being performed should be included at logical stages throughout the program to assess progress and allow modification of the program according to the individual's status at these time points.

SUMMARY

Increased understanding of the basic science surrounding ACL injury and reconstruction together with advances in fixation devices has allowed surgeons to successfully pursue more aggressive rehabilitation schemes. The weak link in the reconstruction continues to be the fixation interface, and the surgeon should be familiar with the biomechanical behavior of the fixation device chosen. The "criteria-based rehabilitation protocols" we propose represent a rational approach that instead of strict adherence to timetables, advance the patient through the various phases when the knee is physiologically ready. The protocols allow wise utilization of available resources and account for variations that have to be made for any additional pathology that is addressed at the time of ACL reconstruction. Counseling, activity modification, rehabilitation, and bracing continue to be the mainstays of conservative management of ACL injuries. The rehabilitation process continues to be an important link in the chain of events that aim to return the patient safely and expediently to full activity.

References

1. Amiel D, Kleiner JB, Roux RD, et al: The phenomenon of "ligamentization": Anterior cruciate ligament reconstruction with autogenous patellar tendon. J Orthop Res 4:162-172, 1986.
2. Arem AJ, Madden JWA: Effects of stress on healing wounds: I: Intermittent noncyclical tension. J Surg Res 20:93-102, 1976.
3. Arnoczky SP, Tarvin GB, Marshall JL: Anterior cruciate ligament replacement using patellar tendon. An evaluation of graft revascularization in the dog. J Bone Joint Surg Am 64:217-224, 1982.
4. Bair GR: The effect of early mobilization versus casting on anterior cruciate ligament reconstruction. Trans Orthop Res Soc 5:108, 1980.
5. Barber FA: A comparison of crushed ice and continuous flow cold therapy. Am J Knee Surg 13:97-101, 2000.
6. Barber FA, Click SD: Meniscus repair rehabilitation with concurrent anterior cruciate reconstruction. Arthroscopy 13:433-437, 1997.
7. Barber-Westin SD, Noyes FR, Heckmann TP, et al: The effect of exercise and rehabilitation on anterior-posterior knee displacements after anterior cruciate ligament autograft reconstruction. Am J Sports Med 27:84-93, 1999.
8. Beard DJ, Dodd CA: Home or supervised rehabilitation following anterior cruciate ligament reconstruction: A randomized controlled trial. J Orthop Sports Phys Ther 27:134-143, 1998.
9. Beard DJ, Dodd CA, Trundle HR, et al: Proprioception enhancement for anterior cruciate ligament deficiency. A prospective randomized trial of two physiotherapy regimes. J Bone Joint Surg Br 76:654-659, 1994.
10. Beard DJ, Kyberd PJ, Fergusson CM, et al: Proprioception after rupture of the anterior cruciate ligament. An objective indication of the need for surgery? J Bone Joint Surg Br 75:311-315, 1993.
11. Beck C, Drej D Jr, Young J, et al: Instrumented testing of functional knee braces. Am J Sports Med 14:253-256, 1986.
12. Beynnon BD, Fleming BC: Anterior cruciate ligament strain in-vivo: A review of previous work. J Biomech 31:519-525, 1998.
13. Beynnon BD, Fleming BC, Churchill DL, et al: The effect of anterior cruciate ligament deficiency and functional bracing on translation of the tibia relative to the femur during nonweightbearing and weightbearing. Am J Sports Med 31:99-105, 2003.
14. Beynnon BD, Good L, Risberg MA: The effect of bracing on proprioception of knees with anterior cruciate ligament injury. J Orthop Sports Phys Ther 32:11-15, 2002.
15. Beynnon BD, Risberg MA, Tjomsland O, et al: Evaluation of knee joint laxity and the structural properties of the anterior cruciate ligament graft in the human. A case report. Am J Sports Med 25:203-206, 1997.
16. Blackburne TA: Rehabilitation of anterior cruciate ligament injuries. Orthop Clin North Am 16:240-269, 1985.
17. Booth FW: Physiologic and biochemical effects of immobilization on muscle. Clin Orthop 219:15-20, 1987.
18. Brand J Jr, Weiler A, Caborn DN, et al: Graft fixation in cruciate ligament reconstruction. Am J Sports Med 28:761-774, 2000.
19. Butler DL, Grood ES, Noyes FR, et al: Mechanical properties of primate vascularized vs. nonvascularized patellar tendon grafts; changes over time. J Orthop Res 7:68-79, 1989.
20. Cerulli G, Benoit DL, Caraffa A, et al: Proprioceptive training and prevention of anterior cruciate ligament injuries in soccer. J Orthop Sports Phys Ther 31:655-660, 2001.
21. Clancy WG Jr, Narechania RG, Rosenberg TD, et al: Anterior and posterior cruciate ligament reconstruction in rhesus monkeys. A histological microangiographic and biomechanical analysis. J Bone Joint Surg Am 63:1270-1284, 1981.
22. Coleridge SD, Amis AA: A comparison of five tibial-fixation systems in hamstring-graft anterior cruciate ligament reconstruction. Knee Surg Sports Traumatol Arthrosc 12:391-397, 2004.
23. Cooper DE, Deng XH, Burstein AL, et al: The strength of the central third patellar tendon graft: A biomechanical study. Am J Sports Med 21:818-823, 1993.
24. Cosgarea AJ, Sebastianelli WJ, DeHaven KE: Prevention of arthrofibrosis after anterior cruciate ligament reconstruction using the central third patellar tendon autograft. Am J Sports Med 23:87-92, 1995.
25. Daniel DM, Stone ML, Dobson BE, et al: Fate of the ACL-injured patient. A prospective outcome study. Am J Sports Med 22:632-644, 1994.
26. De Carlo MS, Sell KE: The effects of the number and frequency of physical therapy treatments on selected outcomes of treatment in patients with anterior cruciate ligament reconstruction. J Orthop Sports Phys Ther 26:332-339, 1997.
27. Deffner KT, Johnson SC, Walker JA, et al: Joint angle specific knee flexor-extensor torque ratios of active woman. Med Sci Sports Exerc 30:S252, 1998.
28. Drez D Jr, Paine RM, Neuschwander DC, et al: In vivo measurement of anterior tibial translation using continuous passive motion devices. Am J Sports Med 19:381-383, 1991.
29. Eriksson K, Anderberg P, Hamberg P, et al: A comparison of quadruple semitendinosus and patellar tendon grafts in reconstruction of the anterior cruciate ligament. J Bone Joint Surg Br 83:348-354, 2001.
30. Eriksson E, Haggmark T: Comparison of isometric muscle training and electrical stimulation supplementing isometric muscle training in the recovery after major knee ligament surgery. A preliminary report. Am J Sports Med 7:169-171, 1979.
31. Escamilla RF, Fleisig GS, Zheng N, et al: Biomechanics of the knee during closed kinetic chain and open kinetic chain exercises. Med Sci Sports Exerc 30:556-569, 1998.
32. Fischer DA, Tewes DP, Boyd JL, et al: Home based rehabilitation for anterior cruciate ligament reconstruction. Clin Orthop 347:194-199, 1998.
33. Fithian DC, Paxton LW, Goltz DH: Fate of the anterior cruciate ligament-injured knee. Orthop Clin North Am 33:621-636, 2002.
34. Frosch KH, Habermann F, Fuchs M, et al: Is prolonged ambulatory physical therapy after anterior cruciate ligament-plasty indicated? Comparison of costs and benefits. Unfallchirurg 104:513-518, 2001.
35. Gelberman RH, Woo SL-Y, Lothringer K, et al: Effects of early intermittent passive mobilization on healing canine flexor tendons. J Hand Surg [Am] 7:170-175, 1982.
36. Gill SS, Diduch DR: Outcomes after meniscal repair using the Meniscus Arrow in knees undergoing concurrent anterior cruciate ligament reconstruction. Arthroscopy 18:569-577, 2002.
37. Goradia VK, Rochat MC, Grana WA et al: Tendon-to-bone healing of a semitendinosus tendon autograft used for ACL reconstruction in a sheep model. Am J Knee Surg 12:143-151, 2000.
38. Grana WA, Egle DM, Mahnken R, et al: An analysis of autograft fixation after anterior cruciate ligament reconstruction in a rabbit model. Am J Sports Med 22:344-351, 1994.
39. Hamner DL, Brown CH Jr, Steiner ME, et al: Hamstring tendon grafts for reconstruction of the anterior cruciate ligament: Biomechanical evaluation of the use of multiple strands and tensioning techniques. J Bone Joint Surg Am 81:549-557, 1999.
40. Heis FT, Paulos LE: Tensioning of the anterior cruciate ligament graft. Orthop Clin North Am 33:697-700, 2002.
41. Hortobagyi T, Lambert NJ, Hill JP: Greater cross education following training with muscle lengthening than shortening. Med Sci Sports Exerc 29:107-112, 1997.

42. Indelicato PA, Bittar ES: A perspective of lesions associated with ACL insufficiency of the knee. A review of 100 cases. Clin Orthop 198:77-80, 1985.

43. Johnson SC, Walker JA, Deffner KT, et al: Effect of hip angle on knee angle specific hamstrings to quadriceps torque ratios. Med Sci Sports Exerc 30:S47, 1998.

44. Jorgensen U, Jensen CM, Scavenius M, Bak K: Rehabilitation with or without initial weightbearing: A prospective randomized study. Presented at a conference on Sports Medicine, 1995, Stockholm, p 76.

45. Keays SL, Bullock-Saxton J, Keays AC: Strength and function before and after anterior cruciate ligament reconstruction. Clin Orthop 373:174-183, 2000.

46. Kocher MS, Sterett WI, Briggs KK, et al : Effect of functional bracing on subsequent knee injury in ACL-deficient professional skiers. J Knee Surg 16:87-92, 2003.

47. Kousa P, Jarvinen TL, Vihavainen M, et al: The fixation strength of six hamstring tendon graft fixation devices in anterior cruciate ligament reconstruction. Part I: The femoral site. Am J Sports Med 31:174-181, 2003.

48. Kousa P, Jarvinen TL, Vihavainen M, et al: The fixation strength of six hamstring tendon graft fixation devices in anterior cruciate ligament reconstruction. Part II: The tibial site. Am J Sports Med 31:182-188, 2003.

49. Mankin HJ, Mow VC, Buckwalter JA, et al: Articular cartilage structure, composition, and function. In Buckwalter JA, Einhorn TA, Simon SR (eds): Orthopaedic Basic Science Biology and Biomechanics of the Musculoskeletal System, 2nd ed. American Academy of Orthopaedic Surgeons, 2000.

50. McNair PJ, Stanley SN, Strauss GR: Knee bracing: Effects of proprioception. Arch Phys Med Rehabil 77:287-289, 1996.

51. Mikkelsen C, Werner S, Eriksson E: Closed kinetic chain alone compared to combined open and closed kinetic chain exercises for quadriceps strengthening after anterior cruciate ligament reconstruction with respect to return to sports: A prospective matched follow-up study. Knee Surg Sports Traumatol Arthrosc 8:337-342, 2000.

52. Morrison JB: Function of the knee joint in various activities. Biomed Eng 4:573-580, 1969.

53. Morrison JB: The mechanics of the knee joint in relation to normal walking. J Biomech 3:51-61, 1970.

54. Noyes FR, Butler DL, Grood ES, et al: Biomechanical analysis of human ligament grafts used in knee-ligament repairs and reconstructions. J Bone Joint Surg Am 66:344-352, 1984.

55. Noyes FR, Butler DL, Paulos LE, et al: Intra-articular cruciate ligament reconstruction. I: Perspectives on graft strength, vascularization, and immediate motion after replacement. Clin Orthop 172:71-77, 1983.

56. Noyes FR, Mangine RE, Barber SD: Early knee motion after open and arthroscopic anterior cruciate ligament reconstruction. Am J Sports Med 15:149-160, 1987.

57. Palmitier RA, An KN, Scott SG, et al: Kinetic chain exercise in knee rehabilitation. Sports Med 11:402-413, 1991.

58. Paulos LE, Noyes FR, Grood ES: Knee rehabilitation after anterior ligament reconstruction and repair. Am J Sports Med 9:140-149, 1981.

59. Paulos LE, Payne FC, Rosenberg TD: Rehabilitation following anterior cruciate ligament surgery. In Jackson DW, Drez D (eds): The Anterior Cruciate Ligament Deficient Knee. St Louis, CV Mosby, 1987.

60. Perlau R, Frank C, Fick G: The effect of elastic bandages on human knee proprioception in the uninjured population. Am J Sports Med 23:251-255, 1995.

61. Pinczewski LA, Deehan DJ, Salmon LJ: A five -year comparison of patellar tendon versus four-strand hamstring tendon autograft for arthroscopic reconstruction of anterior cruciate ligament. Am J Sports Med 30:523-536, 2002.

62. Renström P, Arms SW, Stanwyck TS, et al: Strain within the anterior cruciate ligament during hamstring and quadriceps activity. Am J Sports Med 14:83-87, 1986.

63. Rougraff B, Shelbourne KD, Gerth PK, et al: Arthroscopic and histologic analysis of human patellar tendon autografts used for anterior cruciate ligament reconstruction. Am J Sports Med 21:277-284, 1993.

64. Scheffler SU, Sudkamp NP, Gockenjan A et al: Biomechanical comparison of hamstring and patellar tendon graft anterior cruciate ligament reconstruction techniques: The impact of fixation level and fixation method under cyclic loading. Arthroscopy 18:304-315, 2002.

65. Shaieb MD, Kan DM, Chang SK et al: A prospective randomized comparison of patellar tendon versus semitendinosus and gracilis tendon autografts for anterior cruciate ligament reconstruction. Am J Sports Med 30:214-220, 2002.

66. Shelbourne KD, Klootwyk TE, Wilckens JH, et al: Ligament stability two to six years after anterior cruciate ligament reconstruction with autogenous patellar tendon graft and participation in accelerated rehabilitation program. Am J Sports Med 23:575-579, 1995.

67. Shelbourne KD, Nitz P: Accelerated rehabilitation after anterior cruciate ligament reconstruction. Am J Sports Med 18:292-299, 1990.

68. Sherbondy PS, Queale WS, McFarland EG, et al: Soleus and gastrocnemius muscle loading decreases anterior tibial translation in anterior cruciate ligament intact and deficient knees. J Knee Surg 16:152-158, 2003.

69. Simonian PT, Levine RE, Wright TM, et al: Response of hamstring and patellar tendon grafts for anterior cruciate ligament reconstruction during cyclic tensile loading. Am J Knee Surg 13:8-12, 2000.

70. Stäubli HU, Schatzmann L, Brunner P, et al: Quadriceps tendon and patellar ligament: Cryosectional anatomy and structural properties in young adults. Knee Surg Sports Traumatol Athrosc 4:100-110, 1996.

71. Steinkamp LA, Dillingham MF, Markel MD, et al: Biomechanical considerations in patellofemoral joint rehabilitation. Am J Sports Med 21:438-444, 1993.

72. Tipton CM, Vailas AC, Matthes RD: Experimental studies on the influences of physical activity on ligaments, tendons and joints: A brief review. Acta Med Scand Suppl 711:157-168, 1986.

73. Treacy SH, Barron OA, Brunet ME, et al: Assessing the need for extensive supervised rehabilitation following arthroscopic ACL reconstruction. Am J Orthop 26:25-29, 1997.

74. Tyler TF, McHugh MP, Gleim GW, et al: The effect of immediate weightbearing after anterior cruciate ligament reconstruction. Clin Orthop 357:141-148, 1998.

75. Unterhouser FN, Bail HJ, Hoher J, et al: Endoligamentous revascularization of an anterior cruciate ligament graft. Clin Orthop 414:276-288, 2003.

76. Walker JA, Johnson SC, Motl RW, et al: Effect of knee and hip angles on concentric and eccentric hamstrings-to-quadriceps torque ratios in semiprofessional football players. J Athletic Training 33:S13, 1998.

77. Weiler A, Hoffmann RF, Bail HJ, et al: Tendon healing in a bone tunnel. Part II: Histologic analysis after biodegradable interference fit fixation in a model of anterior cruciate ligament reconstruction in sheep. Arthroscopy 18:124-135, 2002.

78. Wojtys EM, Kothari SU, Husto LJ: Anterior cruciate ligament functional brace use in sports. Am J Sports Med 24:539-546, 1996.

79. Wojtys EM, Wylie BB, Huston LJ: The effects of muscle fatigue on neuromuscular function and anterior tibial translation in healthy knees. Am J Sports Med 24:615-621, 1996.

80. Woo SL, Hollis JM, Adams DJ, et al: Tensile properties of the human femur–anterior cruciate ligament–tibia complex: The effects of specimen age and orientation. Am J Sports Med 19:217-225, 1991.

81. Yack HJ, Collins CE, Whieldon TJ: Comparison of closed and open kinetic chain exercise in the anterior cruciate ligament–deficient knee. Am J Sports Med 21:49-54, 1993.

82. Yamakado K, Kitaoka K, Yamada H, et al: The influence of mechanical stress on graft healing in a bone tunnel. Arthroscopy 18:82-90, 2002.

CHAPTER 45

Knee Bracing for Athletic Injuries

R. Alexander Creighton • Bernard R. Bach, Jr.

Knee injuries in athletics are a major problem facing the sports medicine community. As sports participation continues to increase, so does the likelihood of sustaining a knee injury. Successful prevention of knee injuries has not paralleled the substantial advances in diagnosis and treatment of these knee problems.

The use of braces in sports medicine has long been surrounded by controversy. A brace is a device that functions to clasp or connect objects so that they can resist deforming forces and provide support for ligament reconstruction. Part of the controversy is that there are a multitude of braces for a multitude of uses. This chapter focuses on prophylactic, rehabilitative, functional, patellofemoral, and unloader braces. After reading this chapter, the reader should be familiar with the types of braces available, historical data and studies concerning braces, and how to evaluate and prescribe braces appropriately.

PROPHYLACTIC KNEE BRACES

There are two basic types of prophylactic knee braces designed to prevent or reduce the severity of knee injuries (Fig. 45–1). One type includes lateral bars with a single axis, dual axis, or polycentric hinges. The second type uses a plastic shell that encircles the thigh and calf and has polycentric hinges.

Epidemiologic studies regarding the efficacy of prophylactic knee braces must take into consideration many variables. The ideal study should be randomized and prospective. Controls ideally should be simultaneous rather than historical. The time a study was conducted is crucial because prevailing orthopedic attitudes may affect diagnoses or frequency of surgery. Also, many studies in the literature use cadavers and mechanical surrogate knee models, not fully assimilating real-life conditions.

Nowalski[48] studied 20 patients who had anteroposterior radiographs of the knee before and with 40 lb of valgus stress applied below the knee. A second radiograph was obtained with the patient wearing a variety of lateral-sided braces, hinged in the middle, and offset from the knee. Less medial gaping of the braced knee was noted. This was the first published study evaluating prophylactic knee braces to protect the knee from valgus forces.

The Anderson Knee Stabler was developed in 1978 by Anderson, head trainer of the Oakland Raiders, to protect medial collateral ligaments (MCLs) from reinjury.[3] Anderson's colleagues in the professional and college ranks were impressed with the reports of its effectiveness and began using it on their athletes who had sustained MCL injuries. Subsequently the medical staffs of several teams decided that, more importantly, the brace could be used prophylactically. As the word about the potential to protect the MCL spread, some physicians were not careful to discern between MCL and total knee protection. Considerable controversy remains on how effective these braces are in preventing such injuries (Tables 45–1 and 45–2).

Hewson,[28] Rovere,[58] Teitz,[67] Paulos[51,52] and their colleagues reported epidemiologic studies that have been nonsupportive in substantiating decreased incidence of MCL and anterior cruciate ligament (ACL) injuries. A medical record review was presented by Hewson and colleagues[28] concerning the University of Arizona intercollegiate football teams over an 8-year period (1977-1985). "Exposure to injury" was defined as one player at each practice session or game. The nonbraced period was reviewed from 1977 to 1981. Following this, the Anderson Knee Stabler was mandatory for all practices and games for players at greatest risk, including linemen, linebackers, and tight ends, from 1981 to 1985. In the mandatory brace group, 28,191 exposures occurred, and in the nonbraced group, 29,293 exposures occurred. Information was analyzed by type of injury, severity of injury, player's position, days lost from practice or games, and rate of knee injury per season per 100 players at risk. Results showed that the number of knee injuries was similar for the braced and nonbraced groups, and the type and severity of injury were similar in all categories. Knee bracing did not reduce significantly the number or type of knee injuries or reduce the practice time missed for an entire team or players at risk. Although practice time missed because of third-degree MCL and medial meniscus injuries was significantly lower, this was a result of improved techniques in treating these conditions. The type and severity of injury were similar for braced and nonbraced players at risk; each player faced a 23% chance of knee injury each season and a 64% chance during a 4-year football career.

Rovere and associates[58] performed a 2-year study including all players on the Wake Forest football team using the Anderson Knee Stabler prophylactically during practice and games. A 2-year nonbrace group control period (2 years prior) also was evaluated. Braces were applied with elastic foam under wrap over the distal thigh and proximal leg, then secured with two neoprene straps, Velcro fasteners, or adhesive tape. The time and mechanism of injury, diagnosis, and treatment were noted. Results showed 24 knee injuries during the control period compared with 29 knee injuries with brace wearing. Grade I MCL sprains accounted for 67% of injuries in the nonbrace period and 62% of injuries in the brace period.

Table 45–1. Summary of Principal Scientific Investigators of the Anderson Knee Stabler

SUPPORTIVE	NONSUPPORTIVE
Hansen et al[25]: 4-year University of Southern California injury review showed reduction in injuries and surgery for braced players	*Hewson et al[28]:* Reduction in injury frequency and severity at University of Arizona owing to better care, not braces
Schriner and Schriner[59]: Review of 25 Michigan high schools found 5% injury rate for unbraced players and no injuries for braced players	*Rovere et al[58]:* Increase in MCL strains and ACL tears during bracing of Wake Forest University football players
Taft et al[66]: University of North Carolina study, 3 years before bracing (no bracing) and 3 years after bracing (100%), showed some injury reduction and significant severity reduction (grade III MCL injuries decreased 70%)	*Paulos et al[50]:* Biomechanical testing suggested potential preloading of MCL; now stated as clinically insignificant
Paulos et al[51,52]: Braces that increased impact duration protect ACL more than MCL. Most braces provide some degree of protection to the ACL with direct lateral impact	*Baker et al[6]:* Biomechanical testing showed reduction in abduction angle using functional brace, but little or no protection with prophylactic braces
Sitler et al[62]: Most highly controlled study; in a prospective 2-year study of 1396 West Point cadets, braced defensive players had a significant decrease in number, but not severity, of knee injuries; no difference in foot and ankle injuries	*Garrick and Requa[20]:* Evaluated 6 studies, finding significant methodologic problems and conflicting results: "Impossible to state with assurance the role of prophylactic knee bracing at this time"
	Grace et al[21]: 2-year high school study showed 4 times more knee injuries in the braced group; dramatic increase in foot and ankle injuries in braced group (3 times)

ACL, anterior cruciate ligament; MCL, medial collateral ligament.

Table 45–2. Studies of Prophylactic Knee Braces

STUDY	YEAR	POSITION	MECHANISM OF INJURY	SEVERITY OF INJURY	LEVEL OF SKILL	NONBRACED	BRACED	CONCLUSION
Hansen et al[25]	1980-1984	Not specified	Not specified	Not specified	College	329	148	Less surgery and injuries for braced players
Taft et al[66]	1980-1985	Not specified	Not specified	Operative versus nonoperative	College	Not specified	Not specified	Some injury and severity reduction
Schriner and Schriner[59]	1984	Not specified	Not specified	Not specified	High school	1049	197	Nonbraced 5%; braced 0% injury
Hewson et al[28]	1977-1985	Linemen, linebackers	Not specified	MCL, ACL, meniscus	College	226	224	No difference
Rovere et al[58]	1981-1984	All	76% body contact	MCL, ACL, meniscus	College	368	374	Increase in ACL and MCL braced players
Teitz et al[67]	1984-1985	All	Not specified	MCL, ACL, mensicus	College	3001	2387	More injuries in braced players
Grace et al[21]	1985-1986	Not specified	Not specified	Time lost (1-21 days)	High school	250	330	Knee injuries more severe in braced group
Sitler et al[62]	1986-1987	Offense versus defense	47% direct lateral knee contact	MCL, ACL	College	705	691	Defensive braced players had fewer knee injuries

ACL, anterior cruciate ligament; MCL, medial collateral ligament.

During the brace period, nine knees had surgery compared with five during the control period. There were three ACL repairs during the brace period and one in the nonbrace period. During both periods, offensive team members (especially linemen) had the most knee injuries, and defensive backs had the fewest. Brace use did not alter significantly the relative frequency of injuries by player or position. This study concluded that the Anderson Knee Stabler was ineffective for prophylaxis. Knee injuries were more common when braces were worn. Brace wearing also was associated with cramping and added financial expenditures. The authors concluded that they could not recommend the use of a prophylactic knee brace without further study.

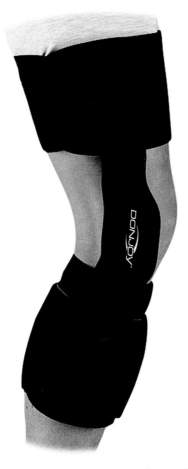

Figure 45–1. Lateral hinge prophylactic brace. (Courtesy of djorthopedics, Inc., Vista, CA.)

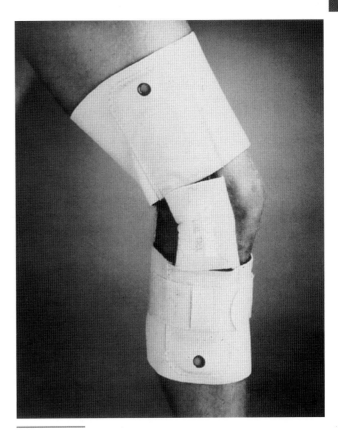

Figure 45–2. McDavid lateral hinge prophylactic knee brace. (Courtesy of McDavid Knee Guard, Inc., Chicago, IL.)

Teitz and coworkers[67] used the members of Division I of the National Collegiate Athletic Association as its study population. The authors reviewed statistics from 71 colleges in 1984 and 61 colleges in 1985; 6307 players in 1984 and 5445 players in 1985 were analyzed. Player's position; incidence of injury; type, mechanism, and severity of injury; playing surface; level of skill; and prior knee injury were considered contributing factors. The results showed that in 1984 and 1985 players who wore braces had a significantly higher injury rate than players who did not wear braces. Four different types of prophylactic knee braces were worn, and no attempt was made to differentiate between them with data analysis. The severity of injuries did not differ between the two groups. Player position, playing surface, mechanism of injury, or type of brace did not affect the rates of injury. Injuries were more common during contact and at every skill level among players who used braces. Incidence of ACL injury was similar in both groups, but braced players had more meniscal injuries. The severity of injury was assessed by measuring playing time lost and the need for surgery. Surgical rates were similar for both groups. Although the average playing time lost was less for players who used braces, the increased incidence of injury produced an overall time lost greater in players using braces. Teitz and coworkers[67] concluded that prophylactic bracing would not prevent injuries and may be harmful. They did not advise preventive bracing among collegiate football players.

Paulos and colleagues,[51,52] in a biomechanical study using fresh frozen cadaveric knees, measured ligament tension and joint displacement at static, nondestructive valgus forces and at low rated destructive forces. After nonbraced controls were examined, knees were braced with two different laterally applied preventive braces: the McDavid Knee Guard (Fig. 45–2) and the Anderson Knee Stabler. The effects of lateral bracing were analyzed according to valgus force, joint line opening, and ligament tension. Valgus applied forces, with or without braces, consistently produced MCL disruption at ligament tension surprisingly higher than the ACL and higher than or equal to the posterior cruciate ligament (PCL). In the first part of their study, no significant protection could be documented with the two preventive braces used. Also, four potentially adverse effects were noted: MCL preloading, center axis shift, premature joint line contact, and brace slippage.[51] In the second part of their study, brace-induced MCL preload in vivo was negated by joint compressive forces. Paulos and colleagues[51,52] concluded that most prophylactic knee braces presently available are biomechanically inadequate. They believed that before prophylactic knee braces can be categorically recommended, more biomechanical and clinical studies should be initiated. They believed that prophylactic lateral knee bracing could be effective if the proper type of brace were used.

Paulos and colleagues[52] recommended that prophylactic lateral knee bracing not be abandoned, but improved and evaluated further in well-controlled prospective studies.

Scientific investigators supporting the use of prophylactic bracing include Hansen,[25] Taft,[66] Schriner[59] and their colleagues. These reviews showed reduction in injuries and surgery for braced players. The study by Hansen and colleagues[25] involved players on the University of Southern California football team from 1980 to 1984. There were 329 players nonbraced and 148 braced. Neither the criteria for brace usage nor the exposure of players braced or unbraced was defined. No definition of knee injury was given. Only injuries requiring surgical intervention were included. Diagnoses apparently were made by the operating surgeons. The authors concluded that prophylactic bracing was better than no bracing in reducing injuries and surgery.

The University of North Carolina experience was reported by Taft and associates.[66] This study documented the football team's experience from 1980 through 1982, when no braces were used, and from 1983 to 1985, when all team members were required to wear braces. Injuries were defined as those that "modified or prevented practice for at least 1 week." MCL injuries were graded by an orthopedic surgeon as operative or nonoperative. The authors concluded that bracing was helpful in decreasing severity and frequency of injuries.

Schriner and coworkers[59] reported a survey of 1246 players from 25 high schools in Michigan during the 1984 season. From 12 of the schools, 197 players volunteered for bracing. Diagnoses were made by physicians as reported by coaches, and only injuries from lateral forces and from hyperextension were analyzed. Schriner and coworkers[59] found a 5% injury rate for unbraced players and no injuries for braced players.

Garrick and Requa[20] evaluated six studies (Hansen, Hewson, Rovere, Schriner, Taft, and Teitz) designed to determine the effectiveness of prophylactic knee bracing in preventing MCL injury in football. Criteria useful for evaluating studies included the probability of confounding factors, bias in selecting cases and controls, and variations in defining injury and exposure. Cost and ethical issues associated with mandated use were discussed. Four of the studies found a reduction in MCL injuries associated with using a brace; two studies reported increases. No consensus arose from these studies, and conflicting results and methodologic problems were apparent, which makes it impossible to state with assurance the role of prophylactic knee bracing in football at that time.

More recently, two prospective, randomized studies evaluated prophylactic knee braces, resulting in contradictory conclusions. Grace and coworkers[21] evaluated 580 high school football players over a 2-year period; 250 nonbraced athletes were matched according to size, weight, and position with 247 athletes wearing single-hinged braces and 83 athletes wearing double-hinged braces. The athletes wearing prophylactic single-hinged braces had a significantly higher knee injury rate ($p < 0.001$), and the athletes wearing double-hinged braces had a greater number of injuries (no statistical significance). Foot and ankle injuries occurred three times more frequently in the braced group ($p < 0.01$). Different playing surfaces were used, and no documentation of prophylactic ankle taping was noted. The study results questioned the efficacy of prophylactic knee braces and called attention to the potential adverse effects on adjacent joints.

A study by Sitler and associates[62] from West Point noted a decrease in frequency, but not severity, of knee injuries. This prospective 2-year study evaluated 1396 intramural tackle football players with an average age of 19.3 years. Strict definitions of athlete exposure (every athlete participating in a practice or game), identical athletic shoes, and uniform playing surface (natural grass) were involved. The study comprised 705 controls and 691 braced (double-hinged single lateral upright) athletes. All athletes underwent a preparticipation physical examination. A significant decrease in frequency and total number of MCL knee injuries was noted in defensive, but not offensive, players. Retrospectively the authors assessed all players for foot and ankle injuries and noted no significant difference between the two groups.

In 1991, Paulos and colleagues[50] evaluated the effects of six different prophylactic knee braces on ACL ligament strain under valgus loads using a mechanical surrogate limb. The results indicated that these braces have a beneficial effect in protecting the knee against direct lateral blows, greater for the ACL than for the MCL. Brace hinge contact with the lateral joint line of the knee reduced the effectiveness. These results should be confirmed clinically, and there is a definite need for improved designs.

Prevention of injuries is important to athletes, but they still are most concerned with performance. Greene and associates[23] evaluated 30 college football players in full gear and had them run a 40-yard dash and perform a four-cone agility drill wearing braces on both knees or no braces. The athletes performed the tasks in six different types of braces. Select knee braces did perform better, not significantly reducing speed or agility. Braces showed a variable tendency to migrate, possibly affecting their protective function and the athlete's performance.

Prophylactic knee bracing remains controversial. A review of the literature shows that current prophylactic knee braces can provide 20% to 30% greater resistance to a lateral blow.[1] These braces have not been shown consistently to prevent or reduce the severity of injuries to the ACL or menisci. Several studies have shown a trend toward a reduced incidence of serious MCL injuries, but other studies have shown no change in the incidence of these injuries. With the exception of the West Point study, most have overgeneralized and cannot document that prophylactic knee braces are the cause of increased or decreased injuries. Biomechanical data proved braces clinically applicable, but some prophylactic braces may result in an increased incidence of ACL injuries.

The American Academy of Orthopaedic Surgeons[2] in 1985 stated, "Efforts need to be made to eliminate the unsubstantiated claims of currently available prophylactic braces and to curtail the inevitable misuse, unnecessary costs, and medical legal problems." The American Orthopaedic Society of Sports Medicine and the *Journal of Bone and Joint Surgery* (in an editorial, January 1987) have taken the same position.[17a] The American Academy of Pediatrics went further with its position statement, recommending that prophylactic lateral knee bracing not be considered standard equipment for football players because of lack of efficacy and the potential of causing harm.[40]

Factors such as rule changes, including no downfield or below-the-waist blocking, crack-back, or high-low double-team blocking and clipping, have helped to make players aware of the serious knee injuries that result from these techniques.[53] Additional rule changes may help to decrease the frequency and severity of knee injuries in football. Certain players, particularly offensive linemen, are at marked increased risk of sustaining knee injuries. Further study and improvements in brace design are warranted.

REHABILITATIVE KNEE BRACES

Rehabilitative knee braces are designed to allow protected motion of surgically repaired or injured knees. These are for the most part off-the-shelf types of braces, with thigh and calf enclosures, hinges, hinge-brace arms, and straps that encircle the brace components on the thigh and calf (Fig. 45–3). Footplates are an option that can be used to control tibial rotation and prevent brace migration. The hinges allow the ability to limit motion of the knee to varying degrees.

Cawley and associates[14] performed a biomechanical comparison of eight commonly used rehabilitative knee braces using a mechanical surrogate limb. Most of the braces significantly reduced translations and rotations compared with the unbraced limb under static test conditions. Factors believed to be important in brace design included overall brace stiffness; the use of nonelastic straps, which adapt to leg contour better; and hinge design, including the presence or absence of joint line contact.

After a repair or reconstruction of certain knee ligaments, it may be necessary to prevent certain knee motions. Stevenson and colleagues[63] presented data that showed the knee joint extended approximately 20 degrees more than the setting on the rehabilitative knee brace hinges. Hoffman and coworkers[30] reported one rehabilitation knee brace to be better than the others in providing stability to static anterior forces. This study did not control for tightness of brace application, however.

In a survey from the American Orthopaedic Society of Sports Medicine, most surgeons after ACL reconstruction prefer early postoperative weightbearing with an average of 3.8 weeks of postoperative bracing.[19] Harilainen and colleagues[26] prospectively evaluated 60 patients undergoing bone–patellar tendon–bone reconstructions and found that there was no difference in laxity, isokinetic muscle torque, or functional outcome scores at 2 years' follow-up between bracing and not bracing in the first 12 weeks after surgery. Kartus and associates[32] also looked at patellar tendon autografts treated with 4 weeks of postoperative bracing and compared them with without bracing. Bracing or not bracing made no difference in KT-1000 laxity, one-hop testing, functional activity scores, and International Knee Documentation Committee scores. Muellner and colleagues[46] found no differences in regard to KT-1000 laxity or flexion/extension strength at 1 year when evaluating braced patients in the first 6 weeks postoperatively versus unbraced patients. Melegati and coworkers[42] showed that locking the knee in full extension for the first week compared with locking the brace from 0 to 90 degrees showed improved extension at 4 months, but no difference in KT-1000 laxity measures. Mikkelsen and coworkers,[43] in a prospective study of ACL-reconstructed knees, compared the differences between a hyperextension brace (−5 degrees) and an extension brace (0 degrees) postoperatively. No significant differences were found between the groups in terms of knee flexion, sagittal knee laxity, or postoperative pain. Only 2 of 22 patients in the hyperextension brace group had an extension loss of greater than 2 degrees, however, compared with 12 of 22 in the extension brace group. Risberg and colleagues,[57] in a prospective, randomized study, compared an unbraced population with a braced population that included the use of a postoperative rehabilitative knee brace for 2 weeks, then a functional brace for an additional 10 weeks. There were no differences between the groups except at the 3-month point. Despite greater thigh atrophy, the braced group showed an improved Cincinnati knee score. Otherwise, KT-1000 laxity, Cincinnati knee score, goniometry-measured range-of-motion testing, computed tomography, thigh atrophy measurement, Cybex testing, functional knee tests, and visual analog pain scale all were equal at 6 weeks, 3 and 6 months, and 1 and 2 years. Although the literature shows no difference in final outcomes of ACL-reconstructed knees in which braces were worn, many orthopedic surgeons still apply them in the early postoperative period. It is still questionable whether brace use under special circumstances (collagen disorders, suboptimal fixation, revision surgery) is truly beneficial.

Rehabilitative knee braces are used routinely in the early rehabilitative period. They are easily applied and adjusted, are lightweight, and provide easy access to incisions, and patients seem to feel more comfortable in them until their quadriceps strength improves. Caution should be exercised when allowing motion in rehabilitative knee

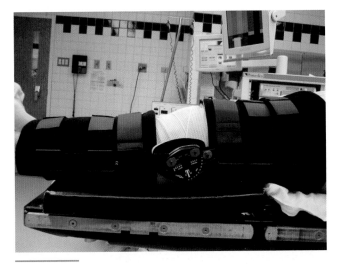

Figure 45–3. Postoperative brace by DonJoy. (Courtesy of DonJoy, Inc., Carlsbad, CA.)

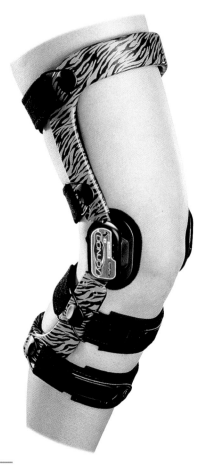

Figure 45–4. Custom DonJoy functional orthosis. (Courtesy of djorthopedics, Inc., Vista, CA.)

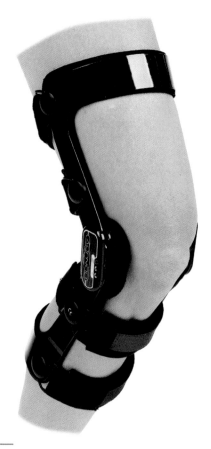

Figure 45–5. Off-the-shelf functional orthosis. (Courtesy of djorthopedics, Inc., Vista, CA.)

braces because more knee joint motion than expected can occur, and little static anteroposterior control is obtained. With modern reconstructed ACL grafts with initial strong graft fixation, postoperative bracing may have little effect, however, on the clinical outcomes and the healing of the graft. The American Academy of Orthopaedic Surgeons believes that rehabilitative braces neither improve nor degrade clinical outcomes, and their use should be individualized to each particular patient.

FUNCTIONAL KNEE BRACES

Functional knee braces are designed to aid in the control of unstable knees (Figs. 45–4 through 45–6). Although many companies manufacture custom-made and off-the-shelf ACL orthoses, only a few companies have developed orthoses for PCL insufficiency (Fig. 45–7). The two basic construction types have similar design features. Both types use unilateral or bilateral hinges and posts; the difference is whether they use thigh and calf shell enclosures or straps for suspension.

ACL injuries are common in athletes and physically active persons. Normal gait patterns at a low cadence rate generally do not pose any difficulty to such patients, but

instability and risk of further injury are possible if above-normal cadence or sudden deceleration movements are encountered. Instability is primarily due to knee subluxation and tibial rotation during the terminal aspect of knee extension.[69] The contributing factor for such instability seems to be the increased angular velocity of the knee during fast cadence rates when anatomic deficiencies allow increased impact energy at extension, resulting in anterior displacement and rotation of the tibia relative to the femur.[4]

Braces to improve the stability of the ACL-deficient knee are designed to prevent full extension by mechanical limits to avoid the instability episode. Some braces also incorporate a derotation benefit or attempt to control varus based on a closed-chain concept. The designers of this brace believe that the femur displaces anteriorly on the tibia and uses a different axis of rotation to control the instability event.[7]

To determine the effectiveness of functional knee braces, numerous studies have been performed. Beck and coworkers[8] tested seven functional knee braces on three ACL-deficient knees with KT-1000 and Stryker knee laxity testers. They found that the hinge, post, and shell types of braces performed consistently better in controlling anterior tibial displacement at low loads. As these forces increased, the effectiveness of the functional knee braces in controlling anterior tibial displacement decreased. Liu

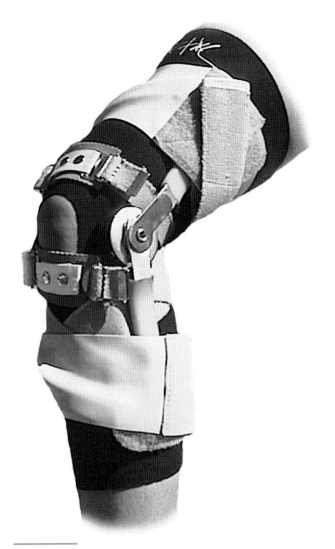

Figure 45–6. Custom Lenox Hill anterior cruciate ligament orthosis by 3M. (Courtesy of 3M Health Care, St. Paul, MN.)

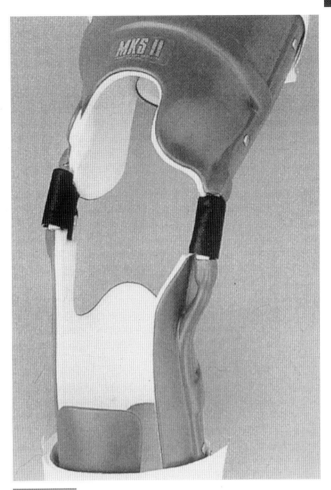

Figure 45–7. Posterior cruciate ligament orthosis, custom MKS II brace.

and colleagues[37] evaluated 10 functional knee braces on a surrogate knee model and found the post/bilateral hinge/shell models provided the greatest resistance to anterior displacement, whereas the post/unilateral hinge/shell models provided the least resistance. None of these braces were capable of controlling displacement at high loads comparable to strenuous activities (i.e., >150 to 400 N). Baker and associates[6] evaluated commercially available athletic braces for their effect on abduction forces applied to a cadaveric knee with no instability and with experimentally created medial instability. Under computer control, abduction forces were applied, while simultaneous data were obtained from an electrogoniometer and transducers applied to the ACL and superficial MCL at 0, 15, and 30 degrees of flexion. Results showed a reduction in abduction angle using functional braces, whereas prophylactic braces showed little or no protective effect.

Concern that functional knee braces prestrain the ACL and place the patient at additional risk for wearing the brace was evaluated by Beynnon and coworkers.[11] Five patients with normal ACLs underwent diagnostic arthroscopy and had placement of the Hall Effect Strain Transducer within the anteromedial bundle of their ACL. Measurements were performed braced and unbraced. The authors concluded that for active range of motion, application of a functional knee brace does not increase the normal ACL strain pattern.

Studies of the Lenox Hill brace by Colville and associates[16] showed that the absolute laxity of the deficient knee was unchanged by the brace, but that the relative resistance to displacement was increased. Hunter and colleagues[31] compared the restraining effect of the Lenox Hill and the CTi brace (Innovation Sports, Foothill Ranch, CA) to static loading using the KT-1000. Both braces controlled anterior translation at 15 lb, whereas only the CTi controlled it at 20 lb. Neither the Lenox Hill nor the CTi brace was effective in controlling anterior tibial translation when higher loading forces were used in the active anterior drawer test.

Branch and colleagues[13] evaluated the contribution of functional bracing to muscle-firing amplitude, duration, and timing, which may result in improved dynamic stability. Ten ACL-deficient subjects and five normal controls were evaluated using footswitches and dynamic electromyography. Bracing did not alter the relative electromyography activity and it did not change firing patterns compared with the unbraced situation. All muscles showed a similar reduction in activity, suggesting that functional braces do not have a proprioceptive influence.

Birmingham and coworkers[12] evaluated the effect of a functional knee brace on knee flexion and extension strength after ACL reconstruction in 27 patients. These patients were fitted with a custom ACL functional knee brace. Knee flexion strength during concentric exercises, as measured by peak torque, decreased significantly (−7.3%). The authors concluded that a functional knee brace may inhibit knee flexion strength of stronger patients, but results in no change or slight improvements in weaker patients.

Cook and associates[17] performed a dynamic analysis of functional knee braces for ACL-deficient athletes. Footswitch, high-speed photography, and force plate data were recorded with and without the custom-fitted CTi braces. Cutting angle, approach time to cut, and time on the force plate showed no significant differences during brace wear. Athletes who did not achieve 80% of the isokinetic quadriceps torque of the sound limb generated significantly more forces during cutting maneuvers while wearing their braces. Athletes also reported better subjective results while snow skiing and waterskiing compared with playing basketball and racquet sports. They noted subjectively fewer subluxation episodes and better performances with the brace. Improvements were even more significant in the quadriceps-deficient patients, suggesting athletes who rehabilitate incompletely may obtain increased benefit from functional knee bracing.

Scott and coworkers[60] compared the CTi, OTI (DJ Orthopedics, Vista, CA), and TS7 (Omni Scientific, Springfield, UT) knee braces in 14 patients with arthroscopically shown ACL-deficient knees. The subjects evaluated the braces and underwent testing with physical examination, KT-1000 arthrometry, and timed running events. All braces reduced subjective symptoms of knee instability, and a reduction in anterior tibial displacement was seen with all braces at low loads. This reduction decreased, however, as forces increased. A timed figure-eight running event did not show any functional advantage, and five subluxation events occurred in four subjects while braced.

Mishra and associates[45] evaluated four functional knee braces and their effect on anterior knee laxity. All braces reduced giving-way episodes and the grade of pivot shift testing. Brace use decreased anterior displacement on KT-1000 measurements at 89-N, high-load passive anterior displacement and with quadriceps contraction active displacement. There was no significant effect on functional test results. Patients with the most functional limitations improved the most, whereas patients minimally affected had diminished performance.

Loubert and colleagues[38] examined the ability of 14 different functional knee braces to control tibial rotation and translation under rigid mechanical loading conditions on fresh human cadaveric legs. They found that braces were more effective at decreasing anteroposterior translation than at decreasing rotation. Braces also were more effective at decreasing displacement at 60 degrees of knee flexion as opposed to 30 degrees. Loubert and colleagues[38] pointed out that their model was not a real-life situation and lacked the muscular contribution during testing.

In another study, Wojtys and colleagues[71] evaluated relative restraints of 14 functional knee braces, using six

cadaveric limbs. Three trends were noted: (1) Braces were more effective in decreasing internal and external rotation than anteroposterior translation, (2) they were more effective at decreasing displacement at 60 degrees than at 30 degrees, and (3) they more effectively decreased translation in combined MCL/ACL rather than isolated ACL injuries. The study showed that functional knee braces provide a variable restraining influence that may be beneficial in the control of abnormal knee displacements.

In a more recent study, Beynnon and associates[10] critically evaluated nine ACL-deficient subjects looking at the transition between non-weightbearing and weightbearing conditions and the effect of three different functional knee braces. They used the Vermont Knee Laxity Device (DJ Orthopedics, Vista, CA) and recorded tibial translation relative to the femur in the simulated conditions. Bracing resulted in significant reduction of anterior translation values, to a level within normal limits in the non-weightbearing and weightbearing states. As the knees transitioned from non-weightbearing to weightbearing, however, the translation increased 3.5 times greater in the braced knee than in the normal knee, and bracing did not reduce this translation to within normal limits. Beynnon and associates[10] concluded that this is why patients gain partial control of their pathologic laxity, but may continue to experience subluxation episodes during activity.

Several studies have evaluated metabolic costs of knee brace wear. Highgenboten and coworkers[29] studied four braces in 14 normal subjects undergoing horizontal treadmill running. The braces caused increases in oxygen consumption, heart rate, and ventilation of 3% to 8% compared with running without the brace. Subjective exertion also was increased 9% to 13%. They concluded that these braces cause a consistent increase in metabolic cost, which was related to their weight. These results are consistent with past research on braced ACL-deficient or reconstructed patients.[72]

An increase in intramuscular pressures in the anterior leg compartment also has been associated with functional knee brace wear. Styf and coworkers[65] evaluated three braces in eight healthy subjects and noted significant increases in anterior tibial muscle pressures regardless of posture. Additionally, during exercise, muscle relaxation pressures were increased. The pressure levels reached could decrease muscle blood significantly (40 mm Hg in 9 of 18 subjects) and possibly induce premature muscle fatigue secondary to decreased perfusion.

Patient noncompliance prompted Zvijac and colleagues[73] to perform a study of the postoperative use of derotation knee braces. Patients underwent arthroscopy-assisted ACL reconstruction and at 6 weeks postoperatively were placed in braced or nonbraced groups. Results of follow-up lasting 6 to 30 months, including Lachman, pivot shift, anterior drawer test, and KT-1000 measurements, were identical. Range of motion was slightly greater in the nonbraced group, but not statistically significant. The authors concluded that postoperative functional knee bracing is not required, although it may benefit some patients from a psychological standpoint.

In a survey of orthopedic surgeons in the American Orthopaedic Society of Sports Medicine, certain bracing prescription patterns were revealed. Descriptive analysis found 13% of physicians never brace ACL-reconstructed patients, whereas only 3% never brace ACL-deficient patients. Physicians prescribe off-the-shelf braces more frequently for ACL-deficient patients as opposed to ACL-reconstructed patients. Half of the responding physicians reported bracing less frequently than 5 years ago. The varying range of responses reflects the lack of scientific knowledge for bracing decisions.[18]

Factors to consider when looking at a brace or a study evaluating a brace are the use of extension stops, thigh size, body fat percentage of the subjects, and effect and type of exercise used for the study.[22] An additional factor is compliance, which may be related to the appearance, comfort, and effect on performance of the brace.[64] In athletic competition with conditions of high loading, the ability of the brace to control pathologic instability is minimal at best.[70] The functional brace may play a role in the overall treatment plan for the ACL-deficient knee, although it does not restore normal stability.

PATELLOFEMORAL BRACES

Anterior knee pain is one of the most common musculoskeletal disorders affecting adults and is frustrating to patients and the treating physician. The patella's function is to improve the quadriceps force during knee extension by increasing the moment arm from the knee center of rotation. Despite this primary function, the many variations of anatomy make treatment of this problem difficult and often not straightforward. Few prospective randomized clinical studies have evaluated the treatment and outcomes of patients with anterior knee pain. Conservative treatment, including rest, quadriceps strengthening, activity modification, nonsteroidal anti-inflammatory drugs, injections of steroids or glycosaminoglycan polysulfate, and bracing, should be exhausted before considering surgery. Bracing for patellofemoral pain syndrome and patellar instability has shown some promise in the literature; however, studies are not always conclusive.

A patellofemoral brace (Figs. 45–8 through 45–10) can function by maintaining the patella within the trochlear groove, improving tracking and alignment. It can displace a patella medially in a laterally subluxating patella, can stretch the lateral retinacular soft tissue in a tight lateral retinaculum, dissipate forces, and possibly provide neuroproprioception.[15] Patellar braces range from simple neoprene sleeves to more involved components with straps, rings, pads, and lateral hinged arms.

Levine[35] looked at a simple patellar strap in patients with anterior knee pain. This bracing strategy was less effective in younger, more active patients, but did help 77% of the patients evaluated, who reported relief of pain and return to normal function. Villar[68] also looked at the infrapatellar strap in military recruits. The brace was effective in only 24% of recruits in the short-term and 22% at 1 year. Despite these less than ideal results, the strap seems to help some individuals and is inexpensive.

Palumbo[49] evaluated a brace used for lateral patellar subluxation. This brace provided a medially directed force to improve the tracking of the patella. The brace

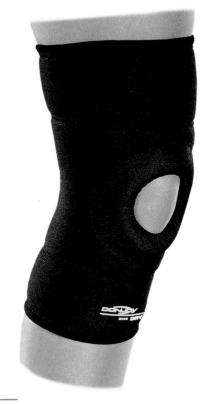

Figure 45–8. Universal orthosis by DonJoy. (Courtesy of djorthopedics, Inc., Vista, CA.)

reduced symptoms in 93% of 62 patients with active knee motion.

Lysholm and colleagues[39] assessed knee extension strength in 24 patients with patellofemoral pain. Strength was measured by Cybex testing. Of the patients wearing a patellofemoral brace, 88% improved their extension strength an average of 14% compared with the unbraced condition. Also, more than half of the patients obtained 95% of leg extension strength compared with the unaffected knee.

Greenwald and coworkers[24] evaluated the effect of a patellofemoral knee brace on healthy volunteers and symptomatic patients. Subjectively the brace was believed to improve knee stability and decrease the level of pain with activities of daily living. The objective results showed no change, however, on knee flexion angle during stair ascent, stair descent, or level walking.

BenGal and associates[9] prospectively looked at the value of a patellar sleeve with a ring support to prevent knee pain in 60 military recruits; 27 recruits were assigned to the brace group and 33 to the nonbrace control group. The brace significantly reduced the development of anterior knee pain. In addition, the brace did not hamper the ability of the recruits to perform their training regimen. Miller and coworkers[44] found the opposite in their study of military recruits. Two different patellar braces had no effect in improving knee pain in this recruit population.

MRI of a patellofemoral realignment brace effect on the kinematics of the patella has been performed. Shellock and associates[61] studied 21 patellofemoral joints with the

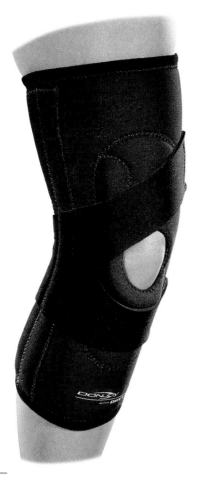

Figure 45–9. Patellofemoral brace with lateral buttress by DonJoy. (Courtesy of djorthopedics, Inc., Vista, CA.)

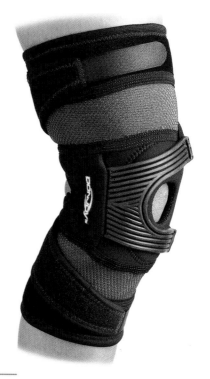

Figure 45–10. Tru-pull advanced system patellofemoral brace by DonJoy. (Courtesy of djorthopedics, Inc., Vista, CA.)

with a strengthening program to improve patellar kinematics. It is hoped that improved studies evaluating this difficult patient population will continue to appear in the literature.

UNLOADER BRACES

Unloader braces (Fig. 45–11) are designed to provide pain relief in arthritic knees. These braces decompress the medial compartment in varus knees and the lateral compartment in valgus knees. The valgus-producing braces for medial gonarthrosis have been much more extensively studied.

Lindenfeld and colleagues[36] used automated gait analysis to study the adductor moment of a valgus-producing brace. Eleven patients with confined medial arthritis were custom fitted with a valgus-producing brace and compared with 11 healthy controls. The mean adduction moment with the use of the brace decreased 10%, approaching the normal controls. The visual analog pain scale decreased 48%, and the Cincinnati Knee Rating System increased 79%. This study shows that pain, function, and biomechanics of the knee are improved with the use of an appropriately fitted unloader brace.

Hewett and associates[27] prospectively evaluated 18 patients with symptomatic medial compartment arthritis and fitted them with a valgus-producing brace. All subjects were evaluated after 9 weeks of brace use, and 13 subjects were evaluated at 1 year. At the 9-week evaluation, pain with activities of daily living decreased from 78% to 39%, and walking tolerance improved from 51

brace in place. There was restraint to lateral displacement of the patella in 16 knees. They concluded that the other four knees did not have a change because these subjects had patella alta. Muhle and coworkers[47] also used MRI data to evaluate the usefulness of a brace in altering patella kinematics. They looked at 24 knees and found no significant improvement in patellar tilt angle, bisect offset, or lateral patellar displacement before or after wearing the patellar brace. Using a dynamic MRI evaluation of the knee, Powers and colleagues[55] found no improvement in patellar tracking, only a change in the sulcus angle of the knee while wearing the brace. MRI for evaluation of these types of braces may be helpful in settling this debate, but controversy still exists.

Powers and colleagues[56] more recently studied 15 patients with patellofemoral pain. They critically evaluated these patients with MRI and gait analysis. The subjects reported a 56% reduction in pain with the use of the brace. The brace reduced peak stress during free and fast walking, 17% and 27%, respectively. Bracing seemed to increase the patellofemoral contact area, resulting in a decrease in stress.

Despite the contradictions of data, patients routinely find subjective improvement in anterior knee pain with the use of a knee brace.[5] The use of a brace also is coupled

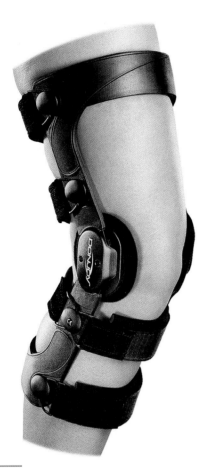

Figure 45–11. Custom off-loading brace by DonJoy. (Courtesy of djorthopedics, Inc., Vista, CA.)

minutes to 138 minutes. At the 1-year evaluation, pain with activities decreased to 31%, and walking tolerance was 107 minutes. A gait analysis also was performed for this study, but no differences were found in dynamic gait parameters.

Matsuno and coworkers[41] studied an unloader brace in 20 subjects with varus arthritis wearing the brace full-time for 12 months. Of 20 patients, 19 had decreased pain when ascending and descending stairs. Also, 17 of 20 showed improved strength in their quadriceps.

Komistek and associates[34] used fluoroscopic surveillance to study 15 patients diagnosed with symptomatic unicompartmental arthritis. Twelve of 15 patients (80%) reported relief of pain and showed condylar separation of the degenerative compartment. The average changes in condylar separation and condylar separation angle were 1.2 mm and 2.2 degrees, respectively. The three patients who did not obtain relief or separation were obese, making fitting of the brace difficult.

In a well-designed prospective study, Kirkley and associates[33] randomized 119 patients with varus gonarthrosis to a control group of medical treatment alone, a combined group of medical treatment and a neoprene sleeve, and a combined group of medical treatment and an unloader brace. At 6-month evaluation, there was a significant improvement in the quality of life and function of the neo-

prene-sleeve group and the unloader brace group. The unloader brace group had significant improvement over the neoprene-sleeve group with regard to pain after a 6-minute walking test and a 30-second stair-climbing test. The combination of an unloader brace and medical treatment was the best treatment regimen for varus gonarthrosis.

Pollo and coworkers[54] studied 11 patients with medial compartment arthritis. The subjects were custom fitted with a valgus brace. Pain and activity level improved in all patients. Using gait analysis, the varus moment about the knee was decreased an average of 13% (7.1 N-m), and the medial compartment load decreased 11% (114 N) in the 4-degree calibrated brace setting.

Unloader bracing for the arthritic knee seems to be helpful in decompressing the diseased compartment. This decompression is appreciated in these subjects by decreasing pain and improving function. These braces seem to be useful in patients with unicompartmental arthritis who do not wish to undergo, or cannot undergo for medical reasons, an osteotomy or total knee arthroplasty.

SUMMARY

Five types of knee braces are used for the athlete's knee (Table 45–3). Prophylactic braces remain controversial and for the most part have been shown to be ineffective in preventing knee injuries in collegiate and high school players. Biomechanical studies have shown some preloading of the ligaments in vivo, but this has not been shown in vitro. Most studies have design flaws and bias, and no definitive conclusions can be drawn at this time. Prophylactic knee bracing cannot be recommended until further prospective and biomechanical studies can show benefit. Rehabilitative braces provide little or no static anteroposterior control of motion, and the hinge setting may not affect true joint motion by a factor of 15 to 20 degrees. They are useful, however, for the operative and nonoperative treatment of ligamentous knee injuries as long as this limitation is kept in mind. Functional knee braces alone are inadequate to control the pathological laxity resulting from ACL injury with higher, more active loads. Combined with an adequate rehabilitation program and activity modification or surgery, these braces limit excessive anterior tibial translation under low loads. Patellofemoral braces are similar to functional braces in that, when coupled with a rehabilitative program, many athletes find a subjective improvement of symptoms. Unloader braces have some good scientific studies providing supportive evidence and are promising modalities for patients with unicompartmental arthritis. They are limited at times by patient factors, such as degree of mechanical axis, body habitus, and compliance.

Knee bracing remains a complex topic in orthopedics. It is difficult to assess the data pertaining to clinical, epidemiologic, or biomechanical studies of knee braces. The treating physician always must use these braces in conjunction with rehabilitative protocols, patient individualization, and patient education, understanding their limitations, uses, and appropriate application.

Table 45–3. Summary of Knee Braces

BRACE CATEGORY	DEFINITION	INDICATION	COMMENT
Prophylactic	Designed to prevent or reduce severity of knee injury	Use in contact sports to protect MCL and ACL	Limited scientific evidence proving protection
Rehabilitative	Designed to allow protected motion of injured or surgically reconstructed knees	Used most commonly after ACL or multiple ligament reconstructed knee	May play a role in early postoperative phase and acute injury phase for comfort and improved knee extension
Functional	Provide stability for ligament-deficient knee or protection for surgically reconstructed knee	ACL or PCL deficient knee	Offer limited functional control of instability; have not been shown to limit meniscal or cartilage injury; negatively affect some aspects of athletic performance
Patellofemoral	Provide pain relief or improve stability of patellofemoral joint	Patellofemoral pain syndrome and patellar instability	Offer subjective relief of many symptoms
Unloader	Provide pain relief and improved function of patients with arthritic knees	Osteoarthritic/malaligned knees	Properly fitted unloader braces provide significant pain relief in selected patients

ACL, anterior cruciate ligament; MCL, medial collateral ligament; PCL, posterior cruciate ligament.

References

1. Albright JP, Powell J, Smith S, et al: Medial collateral ligament knee sprains in college football: Effectiveness of preventative braces. Am J Sports Med 22:12-18, 1999.
2. American Academy of Orthopedic Surgeons: Knee Braces. Seminar Report. St Louis, CV Mosby, 1985.
3. Anderson G, Zeman SC, Rosenfeld RT: The Anderson knee stabler. Phy Sports Med 7:125-127, 1979.
4. Arcierno SP, D'Ambrosia C, Solomonow M, et al: Electromyography and biomechanics of a dynamic knee brace for anterior cruciate deficiency. Orthopaedics 18:1101-1107, 1995.
5. Arroll B, Ellis-Peagler E, Edwards A, et al: Patellofemoral pain syndrome: A critical review of the clinical trials on nonoperative therapy. Am J Sports Med 25:207-212, 1997.
6. Baker BE, VanHanswyk E, Bogosian S, et al: The effect of knee braces on lateral impact loading of the knee. Am J Sports Med 17:182-186, 1989.
7. Bassett GS, Fleming BW: The Lenox Hill Brace and anterolateral rotatory instability. Am J Sports Med 11:345-348, 1983.
8. Beck C, Drez D Jr, Young J, et al: Instrumented testing of functional knee braces. Am J Sports Med 14:253-256, 1986.
9. BenGal S, Lowe J, Mann G, et al: The role of the knee brace in the prevention of anterior knee pain syndrome. Am J Sports Med 25:118-122, 1997.
10. Beynnon BD, Fleming BC, Churchill DL, et al: The effect of anterior cruciate ligament deficiency and functional bracing on translation of the tibia relative to the femur during nonweightbearing and weightbearing. Am J Sports Med 31:99-105, 2003.
11. Beynnon B, Wertheimer C, Fleming A, et al: The effect of functional knee bracing on the anterior cruciate ligament in the weightbearing and non-weightbearing knee. Am J Sports Med 25:353-359, 1997.
12. Birmingham TB, Kramer JF, Kirkley A: Effect of a functional knee brace on knee flexion and extension strength after anterior cruciate ligament reconstruction. Arch Phys Med Rehabil 83:1472-1475, 2002.
13. Branch TP, Hunter R, Donath M: Dynamic EMG analysis of anterior cruciate deficient legs with and without bracing during cutting. Am J Sports Med 17:35-41, 1989.
14. Cawley PW, France EP, Paulos LE: Comparison of rehabilitative knee braces: A biomechanical investigation. Am J Sports Med 17:141-146, 1989.
15. Cherf J, Paulos LE: Bracing for patellar instability. Clin Sports Med 9:813-821, 1990.
16. Colville MR, Lee CL, Ciullo JV: The Lenox Hill Brace: An evaluation of effectiveness in treating knee instability. Am J Sports Med 14:257-261, 1986.

17. Cook F, Tibone JE, Redfern NF: A dynamic analysis of a functional brace for anterior cruciate ligament insufficiency. Am J Sports Med 17:519-524, 1989.
17a. Cowell HR: College football: To brace or not to brace. J Bone Joint Surg [Am] 69:1, 1987.
18. Decoster LC, Vailas JC: Functional anterior cruciate ligament bracing: A survey of current brace prescription patterns. Orthopaedics 26:701-706, 2003.
19. Delay BS, Smolinski RJ, Wind WM, et al: Current practices and opinions in ACL reconstruction and rehabilitation: Results of a survey of the American Orthopaedic Society of Sports Medicine. Am J Knee Surg 14:85-91, 2001.
20. Garrick JG, Requa RK: Prophylactic knee bracing. Am J Sports Med 15:471-476, 1987.
21. Grace TG, Skipper BJ, Newberry JC, et al: Prophylactic knee braces and injury to the lower extremity. J Bone Joint Surg Am 70:422-427, 1988.
22. Grana WA, Steiner ME, Chillage E: The effect of exercise on A-P knee laxity. Am J Sports Med 14:24-29, 1986.
23. Greene DL, Hamson KR, Bay RC, et al: Effects of protective knee bracing on speed and agility. Am J Sports Med 28:453-459, 2000.
24. Greenwald AE, Bagley AM, France EP, et al: A biomechanical and clinical evaluation of a patellofemoral knee brace. Clin Orthop 324:453-459, 2000.
25. Hansen BL, Ward JC, Diehl RC: The preventive use of the Anderson Knee Stabler. Phys Sports Med 13:75-81, 1985.
26. Harilainen A, Sandelin J, Vanhanen I, et al: Knee brace after bone-tendon-bone anterior cruciate ligament reconstruction: Randomized, prospective study with 2-year follow-up. Knee Surg Sports Traumatol Arthrosc 5:10-13, 1997.
27. Hewett TE, Noyes FR, Barber-Westin SD, Heckmann TP: Decrease in knee joint pain and increase in function in patients with medial compartment arthrosis: A prospective analysis of valgus bracing. Orthopaedics 21:131-138, 1998.
28. Hewson GF, Mendini RA, Wang JB: Prophylactic knee bracing in college football. Am J Sports Med 14:262-266, 1986.
29. Highenboten CL, Jackson A, Meske N, et al: The effects of knee brace wear on perceptual and metabolic variables during horizontal treadmill running. Am J Sports Med 19:639-643, 1991.
30. Hoffman AA, Wyatt RWB, Bourne MH: Knee stability in orthotic knee braces. Am J Sports Med 12:371-374, 1984.
31. Hunter R, Branch T, Reynolds P: Controlling anterior tibial displacement under static load: A comparison of two braces. Orthopedics 11:1249-1252, 1988.
32. Kartus J, Stener S, Kohler K, et al: Is bracing after anterior cruciate ligament reconstruction necessary? A 2-year follow-up of 78 consecutive patients rehabilitated with or without a brace. Knee Surg Sports Traumatol Arthrosc 5:157-161, 1997.

33. Kirkley A, Webster-Bogaert S, Litchfield R, et al: The effect of bracing on varus gonarthrosis. J Bone Joint Surg Am 81:539-548, 1999.

34. Komistek RD, Dennis DA, Northcut EJ, et al: An in-vivo analysis of the effectiveness of the osteoarthritic knee brace during heel-strike of gait. J Arthroplasty 14:738-742, 1999.

35. Levine J: A new brace for chondromalacia patella and kindred conditions. Am J Sports Med 3:137-140, 1978.

36. Lindenfeld TN, Hewett TE, Andriacchi TP: Joint loading with valgus bracing in patients with varus gonarthrosis. Clin Orthop 344:290-297, 1997.

37. Liu SH, Lunsford TR, Vangsness T: Comparison of functional knee braces for control of anterior tibial displacement. Clin Orthop 303:203-210, 1994.

38. Loubert PV, Wojtys EM, Viviano DM, et al: A quantitative assessment of the efficacy of fourteen functional knee braces. Presented at Orthopedic Research Society, Las Vegas, NV, February 1989.

39. Lysholm J, Nordin M, Ekstrand J, Gillquist J: The effect of a patella brace on performance in a knee extension strength test in patients with patellar pain. Am J Sports Med 12:110-112, 1984.

40. Martin TJ: Technical report: Knee brace use in the young athlete. Pediatrics 108:503-506, 2001.

41. Matsuno H, Kadowaki KM, Tsuji H: Generation II knee bracing for severe medial compartment osteoarthritis of the knee. Arch Phys Med Rehabil 78:745-749, 1997.

42. Melegati G, Tornese D, Bandi M, et al: The role of the rehabilitation brace in restoring knee extension after anterior cruciate ligament reconstruction: A prospective controlled study. Knee Surg Sports Traumatol Arthrosc 11:322-326, 2003.

43. Mikkelsen C, Cerulli G, Lorenzin M, et al: Can a post-operative brace in slight hyperextension prevent extension deficit after anterior cruciate ligament reconstruction? A prospective randomized study. Knee Surg Sports Traumatol Arthrosc 11:318-321, 2003.

44. Miller MD, Hinkin DT, Wisnowski JW: The efficacy of orthotics for anterior knee pain in military trainees: A preliminary report. Am J Knee Surg 10:10-13, 1997.

45. Mishra DK, Daniel DM, Stone ML: The use of functional knee braces in the control of pathologic anterior knee laxity. Clin Orthop 241:213-220, 1989.

46. Muellner T, Alacamlioglu Y, Nikolic A, et al: No benefit of bracing on the early outcome after anterior cruciate ligament reconstruction. Knee Surg Sports Traumatol Arthrosc 6:88-92, 1998.

47. Muhle C, Brinkmann G, Skaf A, et al: Effect of a patellar realignment brace on patients with patellar subluxation and dislocation: Evaluation with kinematic magnetic resonance imaging. Am J Sports Med 27:350-353, 1999.

48. Nowalski ED: Alternative methods of knee stabilization in sports: A comparative analysis. J Can Athletic Therapists Assn 5:13-17, 1978.

49. Palumbo P: Dynamic patellar brace: A new orthosis in the management of patellofemoral disorders. Am J Sports Med 1:45-49, 1976.

50. Paulos LE, Cawley PW, France EP: Impact biomechanics of lateral knee bracing. Am J Sports Med 19:337-342, 1991.

51. Paulos LE, France EP, Rosenberg TD, et al: The biomechanics of lateral knee bracing: Part I. Response of valgus restraints to loading. Am J Sports Med 15:419-428, 1987.

52. Paulos LE, France EP, Rosenberg TD, et al: The biomechanics of lateral knee bracing: Part II. Impact response of the braced knee. Am J Sports Med 15:430-438, 1987.

53. Peterson TR: The cross body block: Major cause of knee injuries. JAMA 211:449-452, 1970.

54. Pollo FE, Otis JC, Backus SI, et al: Reduction of medial compartment loads with valgus bracing of the osteoarthritic knee. Am J Sports Med 30:414-421, 2002.

55. Powers CM, Shellock FG, Beering TV, et al: Effect of bracing on patellar kinematics in patients with patellofemoral joint pain. Med Sci Sports Exerc 31:1714-1720, 1999.

56. Powers CM, Ward SR, Chen Y, et al: The effect of bracing on patellofemoral joint stress during free and fast walking. Am J Sports Med 32:224-231, 2004.

57. Risberg MA, Holm I, Eriksson J, et al: The effect of knee bracing after anterior cruciate ligament reconstruction: A prospective randomized study with two years' follow-up. Am J Sports Med 27:76-83, 1999.

58. Rovere GD, Haupt HA, Yates CS: Prophylactic knee bracing in college football. Am J Sports Med 15:111-116, 1987.

59. Schriner JL, Schriner DK: The effectiveness of knee bracing in high school athletes. Presented at American Academy of Orthopedic Surgeons Meeting, San Francisco, January 22, 1987.

60. Rink PC, Scott RA, Lupo RI, Guert SJ: A comparative study of functional bracing in the anterior cruciate deficient knee. Orthop Rev 18:719-727, 1989.

61. Shellock FG, Mink JH, Deutsch AL, et al: Effect of a newly designed patellar realignment brace on patellofemoral relationships. Med Sci Sports Exerc 27:469-472, 1995.

62. Sitler M, Ryan J, Hopkinson W, et al: The efficacy of a prophylactic knee brace to reduce knee injuries in football. Am J Sports Med 18:310-315, 1990.

63. Stevenson DV, Shields CL, Perry J, et al: Rehabilitative knee braces control of terminal knee extension in the ambulatory patient. Trans Orthop Res Soc 34:517, 1988.

64. Styf JR: The effects of functional knee bracing on muscle function and performance. Sports Med 28:77-81, 1999.

65. Styf JR, Nakhostine M, Gershuni DH: Functional knee braces increase intramuscular pressures in the anterior compartment of the leg. Am J Sports Med 20:46-49, 1992.

66. Taft TN, Hunter SL, Funderburk CH: Preventative lateral knee bracing in football. Presented at the Eleventh Annual Meeting of the American Orthopedic Society for Sports Medicine, Nashville, TN, July 1985.

67. Teitz CC, Hermanson BK, Kronmal RA, et al: Evaluation of prophylactic braces to prevent injury to the knee in collegiate football players. J Bone Joint Surg Am 69:2-9, 1987.

68. Villar R: Patellofemoral pain and the infrapatellar brace. Am J Sports Med 13:313-315, 1985.

69. Wojtys EM, Goldstein SA, Matthews LS: A biomechanical evaluation of the Lenox Hill knee brace. Clin Orthop 220:179-184, 1987.

70. Wojtys EM, Kothari SU, Huston LJ: Anterior cruciate ligament functional brace use in sports. Am J Sports Med 24:539-546, 1996.

71. Wojtys EM, Loubert PV, Samson SY, et al: Use of a knee brace for control of tibial translation and rotation. J Bone Joint Surg Am 72:1323-1329, 1990.

72. Zetterlung AE, Serfass RC, Hunter RE: The effect of wearing the complete Lenox Hill derotation brace on energy expenditure during horizontal treadmill running at 161 meters per minute. Am J Sports Med 14:73-76, 1986.

73. Zvijac JE, Janecki CJ, Uribe JW, et al: Functional bracing after ACL reconstruction. Presented at the Fifty-seventh Annual Meeting of the American Academy of Orthopaedic Surgeons, New Orleans, 1990.

CHAPTER 46

Revision Anterior Cruciate Ligament Surgery: How We Do It

Nikhil Verma • Michael Battaglia • Thomas L. Wickiewicz

Anterior cruciate ligament (ACL) reconstruction continues to be one of the most common procedures performed in orthopedics.[27] Although primary reconstruction results in a satisfactory outcome more than 75% to 90% of the time, a significant number of patients may still require revision procedures.[1,11,14,15,31] The approach to revision surgery should follow the same principles as those applied to primary reconstruction. The cause of the failure initially should be identified to allow the surgeon to plan the revision procedure so that deficiencies that led to failure of the primary reconstruction can be addressed. Results of revision surgery to date have been inferior to those of primary reconstruction. However, as experience with revision cases expands and arthroscopic techniques improve, we believe that good results can be achieved.

ETIOLOGY OF FAILURE

The factor or factors leading to failure of the index ACL reconstruction must be pursued aggressively before considering revision surgery.[11-14,21,31] This is necessary not only to avoid repetition of the same error but also, in a broader sense, to advance knowledge of factors leading to failure. Clinical failures have been defined and classified by several authors.[11,12,21] The majority of preventable poor results are due to errors in surgical technique or lack of recognition of associated disorders (Table 46–1). Poor outcomes can be categorized into one of three areas: motion loss, persistent pain, and recurrent instability.

Loss of Motion

Loss of motion is among the more common causes of a poor outcome after ACL reconstruction.[14,31] The timing of surgery, graft malposition, excessive graft tension, capsulitis, scarring of the extensor mechanism, and prolonged immobilization have been implicated as causative factors.[11,14,31] Loss of extension is more commonly reported than loss of flexion, possibly because loss of flexion is better tolerated in most activities.

The cause of loss of motion must be determined and corrected before revision surgery. At the authors' institution, emphasis is placed on avoiding primary or revision reconstruction when the knee is inflamed or stiff. In the early phase, only gentle motion exercises and nonsteroidal anti-inflammatory drugs may be necessary to regain motion. As the knee becomes fibrosed, after approximately 3 months, arthroscopic or even open débridement becomes warranted and a staged revision procedure may be indicated.

Persistent Pain

Persistent pain after reconstruction may result from a variety of sources, including a prolonged inflammatory response, osteochondral defects, nonhealed meniscal tears, arthritic changes, graft site morbidity, and neuromas and painful scars.[11,28] The natural history of bone contusions commonly seen with ACL tears is not well understood,[37] but contusions may have a role in postoperative pain. Symptoms arising from persistent instability may be difficult to differentiate from painful arthritic conditions. However, selection of an optimal treatment plan depends on the surgeon making this distinction.

Recurrent Instability

The remainder of this chapter focuses on addressing and correcting recurrent instability. In our experience, return of instability after ACL reconstruction can be classified into three broad categories. Classification of patients into one of these three categories based primarily on the history and physical examination can be helpful when planning the revision surgery. The first category is traumatic graft rerupture. This group of patients has a complaint of recurrent instability after a single trauma event in a previously stable knee. The mechanism of failure is the same as that occurring in a native ACL rupture, and the primary reconstruction can be assumed to have been optimally performed. Important considerations in these cases include identification of the graft used for the primary reconstruction and appropriate graft selection for the revision procedure. The surgeon may choose to avoid grafts that have been associated with slightly higher failure rates, such as four-stranded hamstring tendon grafts,[39] in favor of autograft patellar tendon or allograft tissue.[1,15] Given that the primary reconstruction resulted in a stable knee, it is assumed that the primary procedure was technically well done and the same tunnels used for the primary surgery can be used for the revision.

Table 46–1. Common Technical Errors and Results

Femoral tunnel malposition
  Anterior
  Vertical (coronal plane)
	Graft impingement/loss of extension
	Excessive graft length changes (graft tension in flexion)
	Rotational instability

Tibial tunnel malposition
  Anterior
  Posterior
	Graft impingement/loss of extension
	Excessive graft length changes (graft tension in flexion)
	Excessive graft length changes (graft tension in extension)

Inadequate notchplasty	Graft impingement/loss of extension
Inadequate graft tensioning	Translational/rotational instability
Unrecognized ligament injury	Translational/rotational instability
Unrecognized chondral/meniscal injury	Persistent pain/mechanical symptoms
Poor fixation	Translational/rotational instability

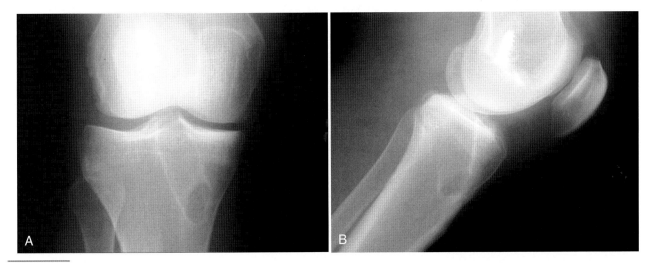

Figure 46–1. Anteroposterior (**A**) and lateral (**B**) radiographs demonstrating significant tibial tunnel widening after primary anterior cruciate ligament reconstruction.

The second category of recurrent instability is atraumatic graft failure. These patients have had a technically well done reconstruction, but with progressive return of instability in the absence of trauma. Potential sources of failure in these cases include failure of graft biological integration, improper graft tension, failure of bone healing, or missed associated instabilities such as persistent medial laxity or posterolateral corner deficiency.[2,8,23,24,29] In such cases, the surgeon must again be cognizant of the graft used for primary reconstruction when choosing an appropriate graft for the revision procedure. Furthermore, a careful physical examination should be performed to assess for other instability patterns that can predispose an ACL reconstruction to early failure. These secondary instability patterns must also be corrected at the time of revision surgery to achieve a successful outcome.

If no coexisting pathology is identified, tunnels are assessed with preoperative radiographs and magnetic resonance imaging (MRI) or computed tomography. In most cases, the tunnel position is optimal and the same tunnels may be used for the revision procedure. If tunnel widening is present, a decision should be made whether the widening can be addressed at the time of revision with techniques such as larger bone plugs, stacked interference

screws, or single-stage bone grafting or whether a two-stage procedure is required (Fig. 46–1). If tunnel widening exceeds 15 mm, serious consideration should be given to a staged procedure (Fig. 46–2). If a single-stage procedure is undertaken, careful attention should be paid to thorough graft removal, proper graft tensioning, and secure graft fixation.

The third category of recurrent instability is graft failure caused by a malpositioned graft or failure of fixation. Loss of fixation can occur secondary to poor bone quality, screw breakage, screw divergence, or graft damage during screw insertion.[7,25] If recognized early (within the first week), it may be amenable to revision fixation. However, in most cases, revision reconstruction is necessary. If bone quality is poor, options include compaction drilling or bone grafting. Supplementary fixation such as EndoButton (Acufex, Mansfield, OH) fixation on the femoral side or soft-tissue button fixation on the tibial side can also be used. Whenever possible, aperture fixation should be achieved. If graft injury has occurred during femoral screw placement, the graft can be reversed such that the tibial bone block is placed on the femoral side and soft-tissue fixation techniques are used on the tibial side.

Graft malposition can occur in either the femoral or the tibial tunnel. Most commonly, this technical error occurs

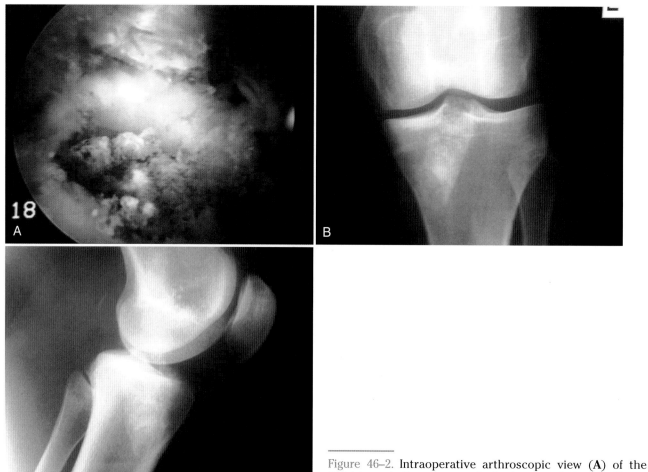

A

B

C

Figure 46–2. Intraoperative arthroscopic view (**A**) of the tibial tunnel after placement of a bone graft for significant tunnel widening. Anteroposterior (**B**) and lateral (**C**) radiographs after successful tibial tunnel grafting.

on the femoral side with incorrect femoral tunnel placement. Anterior femoral tunnel placement results in flexion deficits and early graft failure as a result of impingement in extension.[4] In this case, a proper posterior tunnel may be placed posterior to the original anterior tunnel (Fig. 46–3). If preexisting hardware is not impeding proper tunnel placement, it should be left in place to avoid creating a larger defect. If sufficient room is not available to place a correct posterior tunnel, a two-stage procedure may be necessary in which initial bone grafting is followed by revision reconstruction in 12 weeks. A posterior femoral tunnel position with femoral cortical compromise can be revised by using a two-incision technique to create divergent tunnels. If this technique is not possible, a two-stage revision should be considered. A central femoral tunnel position results in a vertical graft that provides anteroposterior stability without rotation control (Fig. 46–4). This problem can be manifested on physical examination with a negative Lachman examination and a persistent pivot shift. If adequate bone stock remains, a proper femoral tunnel should be created with either an endoscopic or a two-incision technique. Otherwise, a two-stage revision should be considered.

Tibial tunnel malposition can also lead to failure of primary ACL reconstruction.[17-19,40] An anteriorly placed tibial tunnel will result in graft impingement in extension and early graft failure. A posterior position will result in a vertical graft and loss of rotational control. It is important to note that when using an endoscopic technique, the coronal plane obliquity of the tibial tunnel will affect femoral tunnel position. In cases of tibial tunnel malposition, an attempt can be made to drill a properly oriented tibial tunnel if bone stock is present, but most cases require a two-stage revision with initial bone grafting.

PATIENT EVALUATION

A detailed history must be obtained, including a thorough description of the index procedure. The mechanism of the initial injury may suggest the presence of an undiagnosed injury. Noting the timing of the procedure in relation to the injury can be useful, particularly in the case of motion loss.[36] The rehabilitation program and the patient's progress should be ascertained. The patient should be questioned regarding traumatic episodes after the reconstruction, along with symptoms before and after this event. When available, operative notes should be obtained. They may indicate important information of

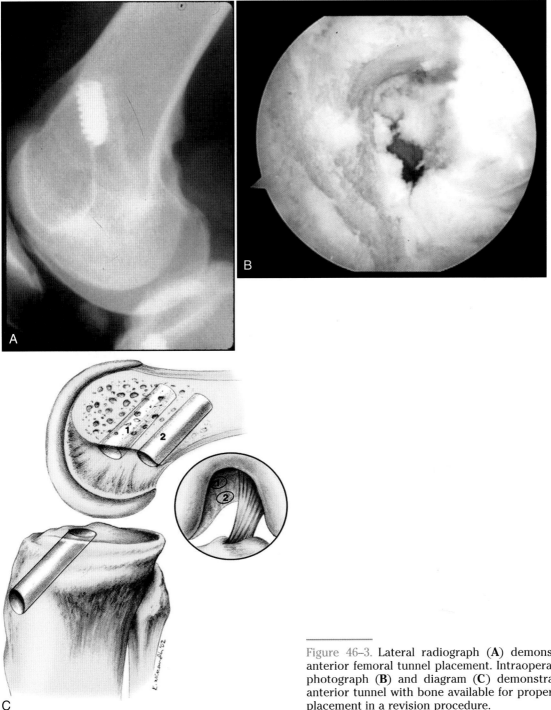

Figure 46–3. Lateral radiograph (**A**) demonstrating improper anterior femoral tunnel placement. Intraoperative arthroscopic photograph (**B**) and diagram (**C**) demonstrating the original anterior tunnel with bone available for proper posterior tunnel placement in a revision procedure.

which the patient is not aware, such as the condition of the articular surfaces and menisci, the type of graft and fixation used, and whether a notchplasty was performed.

A thorough physical examination should be performed on all patients with a failed a primary reconstruction. The patient should be examined standing and during gait to assess alignment and evaluate for varus or valgus thrust. Range of motion should be accurately evaluated, particularly to ensure that full extension is present. Instability examination, including Lachman and pivot-shift testing, should be performed. Finally, a thorough evaluation of the

integrity of the medial structures and posterolateral corner should be performed because failure to address injuries to these structures has been reported as a cause of early failure after ACL reconstruction.[9,24,29]

Plain radiographs should be obtained in all cases of failed ACL reconstruction. Specific views required include standing anteroposterior and lateral views, a Merchant view, a notch view, and a weightbearing anteroposterior 45-degree flexion view.[24] The tibial and femoral tunnels can be evaluated on both the anteroposterior and lateral views to assess for tunnel widening and position, as well

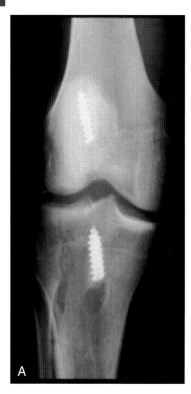
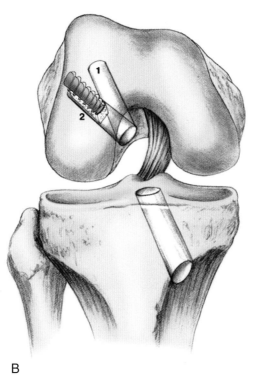

Figure 46–4. **A**, Anteroposterior radiograph demonstrating vertical graph placement. **B**, Schematic diagram demonstrating revision of a vertical graft with a divergent tunnel technique.

as the presence of retained hardware. The flexion weight-bearing view can be used to evaluate for early degenerative disease, which can affect the prognosis.[33] Additional views to assess for objective evidence of instability in the valgus plane can be obtained to quantify side-to-side differences.[16,38] Finally, if any malalignment is appreciated on physical examination, a full-length standing mechanical axis view should be obtained to determine whether an alignment-correcting osteotomy is necessary in addition to or in place of ligament reconstruction.

In most cases, MRI should also be obtained as a routine preoperative study. MRI allows for direct evaluation of the integrity of the ligament graft (Fig. 46–5).[34] Tunnel position as well as tunnel widening can also be assessed in both the sagittal and coronal plane. The integrity of the menisci can be evaluated to allow for planning of any alternative procedures that may be required at the time of revision surgery. The competency of the medial and lateral structures can be assessed and correlated with the physical examination findings. The integrity of the menisci has a direct effect on the long-term outcome of ACL reconstruction, and MRI provides a valuable clinical tool in predicting outcome.[35,38] Finally, with the development of newer cartilage-sensitive MRI techniques, the integrity of the articular cartilage can be evaluated to help identify any degenerative changes that may affect prognosis.[10,26,32]

SURGICAL TECHNIQUE

Preoperative Planning

Once the cause of the failure has been identified and the need for revision surgery confirmed, proper preoperative

---

Box 46-1. Considerations in Planning Revision ACL Reconstruction

Motion loss: rehabilitation, arthroscopic or open débridement
Malalignment: previous or concurrent high tibial osteotomy
Tunnel osteolysis: débridement, possible autogenous bone grafting
Graft removal (en block for synthetic grafts)
Hardware removal (if necessary for tunnel placement)
Revision tunnel placement
Remaining graft sources/selection
Graft fixation
Associated injuries: menisci, chondral defects, other ligaments

---

planning is essential to obtain a successful outcome. Important factors that should be considered when planning for revision procedures are listed in Box 46–1. The first step is to identify the graft material to be used for the revision procedure. Current options for revision graft selection are listed in Box 46–2. At our institution, we prefer allograft tissue as our graft of choice for revision procedures. The main advantages of allograft tissue are the absence of morbidity associated with graft harvest and decreased operative time. Second, the large bone blocks provide with allograft tissue provide the surgeon with the flexibility to create bone blocks of a size and shape necessary to fill preexisting bone tunnels. Finally, although allograft tissue has been demonstrated to require increased time for graft neovascularization and remodeling in

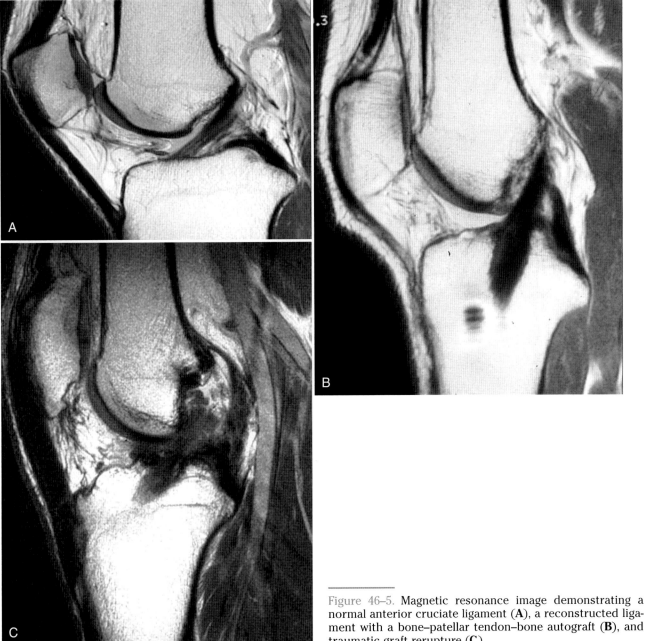

Figure 46–5. Magnetic resonance image demonstrating a normal anterior cruciate ligament (**A**), a reconstructed ligament with a bone–patellar tendon–bone autograft (**B**), and traumatic graft rerupture (**C**).

Box 46-2. Graft Sources

Autogenous
  Patellar tendon–bone
    Ipsilateral
    Contralateral
  Hamstring tendons—semitendinosus, gracilis
  Quadriceps tendon–bone
Allograft
  Patellar tendon–bone
  Achilles tendon–bone
Synthetic
  Gore-Tex
  Dacron
  Ligament augmentation devices

animal models, clinical outcomes after reconstruction with an allograft have been reported to be equivalent to those after reconstruction with an autograft.[3,6,20,30]

The second step is to identify potential problems secondary to existing tunnel and hardware placement. If possible, operative reports from the primary surgery should be reviewed to identify the size and manufacturer of the implants used during the primary surgery. Tibial-sided hardware can often be removed directly through the old anterior tibial incision. Removal of femoral hardware can be more difficult, but in many cases, femoral screws do not need to be removed. If a two-incision technique is planned, the divergent nature of the new femoral tunnel often avoids the existing femoral screw. In cases in which the femoral tunnel is placed too anterior, there is often room to drill the new femoral tunnel in the proper posterior position without obstruction from the existing hardware. In many cases, removal of the femoral hardware can actually be detrimental because it may create a larger femoral defect that can be difficult to fill. However, in all cases, a wide variety of screw drivers and instruments to remove stripped screws should be available if hardware removal becomes necessary.

Anesthesia and Setup

The patient is placed on the operating table in a supine position. Anesthesia can be general or regional. At our institution, we prefer to use a combined spinal/epidural anesthetic with a femoral nerve block for postoperative pain management. One the patient is anesthetized, the positioning is the same as for a primary ACL reconstruction. The leg is placed in a cradle leg holder, or a lateral post is used. Care should be taken to position the patient such that the knees fall below the distal break in the table. This position enables the bottom of the table to be dropped during surgery, thus allowing knee flexion. Routine use of antibiotic prophylaxis is recommended.

Before surgical preparation, a thorough examination under anesthesia is performed. Range of motion is determined and any flexion or extension deficits noted. Varus and valgus instability is determined both in full extension and in 30 degrees of flexion. Posterolateral corner integrity is assessed with the posterolateral drawer test and external rotation spin at 30 degrees of knee flexion. It is important to recognize and address persistent varus, valgus, or posterolateral instability because it may be a cause of early ACL graft failure. The integrity of the posterior cruciate ligament is determined with the posterior drawer test.

The integrity of the ACL graft is determined with both the pivot-shift and the Lachman tests. The Lachman test is used to check graft function in the anterior-posterior plane. A graft that is intact but placed in a vertical position may have a negative Lachman examination. The pivot-shift test is used to assess rotational forms of instability. A positive pivot-shift examination defines a failed primary reconstruction. In all revision cases the pivot shift should be abnormal, indicative of either graft failure or malposition with persistent rotational instability.

Technique

Once the examination under anesthesia is completed, the leg is prepared and draped and diagnostic arthroscopy is performed. Special attention is paid to assessment of the integrity of the menisci, as well as the integrity of the graft. The graft is best assessed with the leg in the figure-four position, which places the graft under maximal tension. If necessary, an arthroscopic Lachman examination can be performed. Finally, the position of the graft on both the tibial side and the femoral side should be critically evaluated. However, the decision to proceed with revision reconstruction is based primarily on the examination

under anesthesia, with a positive pivot-shift test indicating graft failure or malfunction.

Once the decision to proceed with revision has been made, the existing graft is removed with a combination of arthroscopic scissors or biters, a motorized shaver, and a radiofrequency device. On the femoral side, the over-the-top position and the back wall of the femur should be clearly identified. If necessary, a revision notchplasty is performed to provide proper clearance for the new graft with knee extension. The existing femoral tunnel and hardware can now usually be visualized and a decision made whether the existing hardware needs to be removed. In many cases of graft malposition or cases in which a two-incision technique is planned, the old hardware can often be left in place and the new tunnel drilled in a different location. However, if the hardware conflicts with proper femoral tunnel positioning, it should be removed. Removal can be accomplished through the standard inferomedial portal and accessory inferomedial portal or a miniarthrotomy. The surgeon should be cognizant that removal of femoral hardware may create a larger femoral tunnel defect.

On the tibial side, the remaining stump of the existing graft is removed with a motorized shaver and radiofrequency device. The appropriate landmarks for tibial tunnel positioning, including the anterior edge of the posterior cruciate ligament, the tibial spines, and the posterior border of the anterior horn of the lateral meniscus, should be identified. Again, the position of the existing tibial tunnel should be evaluated to determine whether it can be used or a new tunnel should be drilled.

Next, the tibial tunnel entrance site is exposed. Usually, the old tibial incision is opened and dissection carried sharply down to bone. Subperiosteal dissection is performed to expose the existing tibial tunnel and hardware. The tibial screw is removed. Again, a wide variety of screwdrivers and screw removal tools should be available to assist with hardware removal. Often, a guide wire can be placed either manually or on power and its position evaluated arthroscopically in the joint. In this manner, a decision can be made whether the existing tibial tunnel can be used or a new tunnel should be created.

At this point, based on the intraoperative findings and the preoperative radiographs, a decision can be made whether to proceed with primary reconstruction or a staged reconstruction. This decision is primarily based on significant tunnel widening, which requires primary bone grafting. If a staged procedure is indicated, the tunnels are cleared of any remaining soft tissue, which can be done with a motorized shaver and radiofrequency device. Next, the tunnels are reamed over a guide wire with the use of compaction reamers to preserve as much bone stock as possible. Care must be taken to follow the path of the existing tunnel and not create new tunnels. Any other intra-articular pathology should be addressed before proceeding with bone grafting.

Bone grafting is initially performed in the femoral tunnel. Graft choices include either allograft or autograft. At our institution we used a calcium sulfate–based allograft substitute (Vitoss, Orthovita, Malvern, PA), which is mixed with 5 mL of bone marrow aspirate before implantation. To access the femoral tunnel, a Yankower suction tip is cut to the appropriate length and placed through either the tibial tunnel or an accessory inferomedial portal and into the femoral tunnel. Graft is then packed into the femoral tunnel through the suction catheter. Graft should be firmly impacted with a bone tamp or similar device. In our experience, no covering of the tunnel entrance site is necessary.

The tibial tunnel is grafted next. A large periosteal elevator is placed over the tunnel exit site on the tibial plateau. The graft is then impacted through the tibial tunnel entrance site and packed against the periosteal elevator, followed by closure of the periosteum over the tibial tunnel entrance site. Incisions are closed in standard manner. The patient is allowed to bear weight as tolerated with the knee locked in extension. Unrestricted active and passive range of motion is allowed. Second-stage revision graft reimplantation can be carried out in 8 to 12 weeks.

In the case of primary revision reconstruction, the tibial tunnel is created first. The position of the existing tunnel is addressed. If necessary, the angled ACL guide is used to place a new guide wire. The tibial tunnel is then created with standard reaming techniques. Compaction reamers should be used when possible to maintain bone stock. All excess bone shavings should be removed from the joint and the tunnel exit site débrided with a motorized shaver.

The femoral tunnel is addressed next. Based on the position of the existing tunnel, a decision is made whether to use the existing tunnel, drill a new tunnel via an endoscopic technique, or drill a new tunnel with a two-incision technique. Similarly, the existing femoral hardware can be either retained or removed, based on the position of the new tunnel. Again, compaction reamers should be used to maintain bone stock.

Once the tunnels have been placed, the graft is passed via standard techniques. Fixation on the femoral side is carried out most commonly with an interference screw. Options for filling a femoral tunnel defect include use of a larger bone plug on the graft, use of a larger interference screw, or stacking of interference screws. If necessary, secondary forms of fixation such as EndoButton fixation can be used.

When femoral fixation has been achieved, the graft is tensioned and the knee is cycled to remove creep. The graft is visualized arthroscopically with the knee in full extension to confirm that no impingement on the femoral notch exists. Fixation on the tibial side is most commonly achieved with an interference screw. At our institution, the soft-tissue side of the Achilles tendon allograft is placed in the tibial tunnel, and fixation is carried out with a soft-tissue interference screw and a soft-tissue button or staple as secondary fixation. Options for dealing with a large tibial tunnel include using a large bone block with a bone–patellar tendon–bone allograft, using stacked interference screws, or using a bone block autograft or allograft.

Once the graft has been secured in place, the Lachman and pivot-shift examinations are rechecked to ensure that instability has been eliminated. Wounds are closed in standard fashion with nylon suture in the portal sites and a layered closure for the skin incisions. Local anesthetic can be used in the joint to improve patient comfort postoperatively. Sterile dressings are applied and the leg is wrapped

in a compressive dressing from the heel to the thigh. The leg is then placed in a hinged knee brace that can be locked in extension.

TECHNICAL ALTERNATIVES AND PITFALLS

The key to success with revision ACL reconstruction is to be familiar with multiple different techniques for tunnel placement and fixation. With regard to the femoral tunnel, the most important factor is proper tunnel placement. The tunnel must be correctly placed as close to the back wall as possible, but also in a lateralized position. If this cannot be accomplished with a standard endoscopic technique, the easiest alternative is to switch to a two-incision technique. This technique involves making an accessory incision over the lateral femoral condyle and placing a guide from behind the posterior lateral femoral condyle, through the femoral notch, and then along the lateral femoral wall. The guide pin and tunnel are drilled from outside-in, and fixation is achieved at the lateral femoral cortex. This technique allows proper positioning of the femoral tunnel in cases of tibial tunnel malposition, helps bypass an improperly positioned femoral tunnel or femoral hardware, and can be used to achieve fixation when the back wall is compromised.

Interference screw fixation is the standard method used on the femoral side. However, alternative forms of fixation may be required in patients with significant tunnel widening or compromise of the back wall. In cases of tunnel expansion, fixation alternatives include the use of a longer screw, the use of a larger allograft bone plug, or placement of multiple screws in a "stacked" configuration to fill the defect. In cases in which the back wall is compromised, alternative forms of fixation include the use of an EndoButton, the use of suspension fixation techniques, or drilling of an alternate tunnel with a two-incision technique.

On the tibial side, alternative forms of fixation may be required in the case of significant tunnel expansion. In this situation, alternatives include the use of a larger interference screw or a "stacked" screw configuration. A second alternative is to fill the defect with an allograft plug, followed by interference screw fixation. Finally, alternative or supplemental forms of fixation outside the tunnel, such as a screw and washer, a soft-tissue button, or staple fixation, can be considered. However, we do not recommend that these devices be used as the primary method of tibial fixation.

REHABILITATION

Although the ideal goal of rehabilitation after revision ACL reconstruction is return to athletics, the primary goal is to return to activities of daily living. The protocol is similar to that used for primary reconstruction, but it should be amended depending on the quality of fixation achieved at revision surgery. Furthermore, secondary procedures such as meniscal surgery or osteotomy must also be considered when developing a rehabilitation program.

In general, for isolated revision ACL reconstruction with an allograft, our immediate postoperative protocol consists of partial weightbearing with the knee locked in extension. Early range of motion with an emphasis on extension is started immediately. At 6 weeks postoperatively, the brace is discontinued and the patient is allowed to bear weight as tolerated. Stationary bike riding is also allowed at this point once adequate flexion is achieved. Straight-ahead jogging is allowed at 4 months, followed by sport-specific rehabilitation. Return to athletics is allowed at 6 months if the knee is stable on examination and quadriceps strength is 80% of the opposite side.

SUMMARY

Revision reconstruction of the ACL can be a very complex undertaking. The cause of the failure must be addressed. Associated disorders must also be diagnosed and treated, occasionally as a separate stage. With multiple reasonable options available, one can expect a high likelihood of success from revision, provided that a systematic approach is maintained.[5,22]

References

1. Bach BR Jr, Levy ME, Bojchuk J, et al: Single-incision endoscopic anterior cruciate ligament reconstruction using patellar tendon autograft. Am J Sports Med 26:30-40, 1998.
2. Berg EE: Tibial bone plug nonunion: A cause of anterior cruciate ligament reconstructive failure. Arthroscopy 8:380-384, 1992.
3. Buck BE, Resnick L, Shah SM, et al: Human bone and tissue allografts; preparation and safety. Clin Orthop 303:8-17, 1994.
4. Bylski-Austrow DI, Grood ES, Hefzy MS, et al: Anterior cruciate ligament replacements: A mechanical study of femoral attachment location, flexion angle at tensioning, and initial tension. J Orthop Res 8:522-531, 1990.
5. Carson EW, Simonian PT, Wickiewicz TL, et al: Revision anterior cruciate ligament reconstruction. Instr Course Lect 43:137-140, 1994.
6. Daniel DM: Use of allografts after failed treatment of rupture of the anterior cruciate ligament. J Bone Joint Surg Am 77:1290, 1995.
7. Doerr AL Jr, Cohn BT, Ruoff MJ, et al: A complication of interference screw fixation in anterior cruciate ligament reconstruction. Orthop Rev 19:997-1000, 1990.
8. Fahey M, Indelicato PA: Bone tunnel enlargement after anterior cruciate ligament replacement. Am J Sports Med 22:410-414, 1994.
9. Gersoff WK, Clancy WG Jr: Diagnosis of acute and chronic anterior cruciate ligament tears. Clin Sports Med 7:727-738, 1988.
10. Gold GE, McCauley TR, Gray ML, et al: What's new in cartilage? Radiographics 23:1227-1242, 2003.
11. Graf B, Uhr F: Complications of intra-articular anterior cruciate ligament reconstruction. Clin Sports Med 15:331-341, 1987.
12. Greis PE, Johnson DL, Fu FH: Revision anterior cruciate ligament surgery: Causes of graft failure and technical considerations of revision surgery. Clin Sports Med 12:839-852, 1993.
13. Harner CD, Griffin JR, Dunteman RC, et al: Evaluation and treatment of recurrent instability after anterior cruciate ligament reconstruction. J Bone Joint Surg Am 82:1652-1664, 2000.
14. Harner CD, Irrgang JJ, Paul J, et al: Loss of motion after anterior cruciate ligament reconstruction. Am J Sports Med 20:499-506, 1992.
15. Harter RA, Osternig LR, Singer KM, et al: Long-term evaluation of knee stability and function following surgical reconstruction for

16. Hillard-Sembell D, Daniel DM, Stone ML, et al: Combined injuries of the anterior cruciate and medial collateral ligaments of the knee. J Bone Joint Surg Am 78:169-175, 1996.
17. Howell SM, Barad SJ: Knee extension and its relationship to the slope of the intercondylar roof: Implications for positioning the tibial tunnel in anterior cruciate ligament reconstructions. Am J Sports Med 23:288-294, 1995.
18. Howell SM, Clark JA: Tibial tunnel placement in anterior cruciate ligament reconstructions and graft impingement. Clin Orthop 283:187-195, 1992.
19. Jackson DW, Gasser SI: Tibial tunnel placement in ACL reconstruction. Arthroscopy 10:124-131, 1994.
20. Jackson DW, Grood ES, Goldstein JD, et al: A comparison of patellar tendon autograft and allograft used for anterior cruciate ligament reconstruction in the goat model. Am J Sports Med 21:176-185, 1993.
21. Johnson DL, Fu FH: Anterior cruciate ligament reconstruction: Why do failures occur? Instr Course Lect 44:391-406, 1995.
22. Johnson DL, Swenson TM, Irrgang JJ, et al: Revision anterior cruciate ligament surgery: Experience from Pittsburgh. Clin Orthop 325:100-109, 1996.
23. Linn RM, Fischer DA, Smith JP, et al: Achilles tendon allograft reconstruction of the anterior cruciate ligament–deficient knee. Am J Sports Med 21:825-831, 1993.
24. Marks PH, Harner CD: The anterior cruciate ligament in the multiple ligament–injured knee. Clin Sports Med 12:825-838, 1993.
25. Matthews LS, Soffer SR: Pitfalls in the use of interference screws for anterior cruciate ligament reconstruction: Brief report. Arthroscopy 5:225-226, 1989.
26. McGibbon CA, Trahan CA: Measurement accuracy of focal cartilage defects from MRI and correlation of graded lesions with histology: A preliminary study. Osteoarthritis Cartilage 11:483-493, 2003.
27. Miyaska KC, Daniel DM, Stone ML, et al: The incidence of knee ligament injuries in the general population. Am J Knee Surg 4:3-8, 1991.
28. Noyes FR, Barber-Westin SD: Anterior cruciate ligament reconstruction with autogenous patellar tendon grafts in patients with articular cartilage damage. Am J Sports Med 25:626-634, 1997.
29. O'Brien SJ, Warren RF, Pavlov H, et al: Reconstruction of the chronically insufficient anterior cruciate ligament with the central third of the patellar ligament. J Bone Joint Surg Am 73:278-286, 1991.
30. Olson EJ, Harner CD, Fu FH, et al: Clinical use of fresh frozen soft tissue allografts. Orthopedics 15:1225-1232, 1992.
31. Paulos LE, Rosenberg D, Drawbert J, et al: Infrapatellar contracture syndrome: An unrecognized cause of knee stiffness with patella entrapment and patella infra. Am J Sports Med 15:331-341, 1987.
32. Potter HG, Linklater JM, Allen AA, et al: Magnetic resonance imaging of articular cartilage in the knee. An evaluation with the use of fast-spin-echo imaging. J Bone Joint Surg Am 80:1276-1284, 1998.
33. Rosenberg TD, Paulos LE, Parker RD, et al: The forty-five-degree posteroanterior flexion weight-bearing radiograph of the knee. J Bone Joint Surg Am 70:1479-1483, 1988.
34. Schatz JA, Potter HG, Rodeo SA, et al: MR imaging of anterior cruciate ligament reconstruction. AJR Am J Roentgenol 80:1276-1284, 1998.
35. Shelbourne KD, Gray T: Results of anterior cruciate ligament reconstruction based on meniscus and articular cartilage status at the time of surgery. Am J Sports Med 28:446-452, 2000.
36. Shelbourne KD, Wilckens JH, Mollabash A, et al: Arthrofibrosis in acute anterior cruciate ligament reconstruction: The effect of timing of reconstruction and rehabilitation. Am J Sports Med 19:332-336, 1991.
37. Spindler KP, Schils JP, Bergfeld JA, et al: Prospective study of osseous, articular, and meniscal lesions in recent anterior cruciate ligament tears by magnetic resonance imaging and arthroscopy. Am J Sports Med 21:551-557, 1993.
38. Warren RF, Marshall JL, Girgis F: The prime static stabilizer of the medial side of the knee. J Bone Joint Surg Am 56:665-674, 1974.
39. Williams RJ 3rd, Hyman J, Petrigliano F, et al: Anterior cruciate ligament reconstruction with a four-strand hamstring tendon autograft. J Bone Joint Surg Am 86:225-232, 2004.
40. Yaru NC, Daniel DM, Penner D: The effect of tibial attachment site on graft impingement in an anterior cruciate ligament reconstruction. Clin Orthop 185:197-202, 1984.

anterior cruciate ligament insufficiency. Am J Sports Med 16:434-443, 1988.

CHAPTER 47

Current Concepts in Posterior Cruciate Ligament Reconstruction

Joshua Baumfeld • Diane L. Dahm

Despite many recent advances in our understanding of the anatomy and biomechanics of the posterior cruciate ligament (PCL), treatment of PCL injuries remains controversial. The goals of PCL reconstruction include the restoration of knee stability, function, and biomechanical properties beyond what could be achieved with nonoperative management. As such, PCL reconstruction continues to be a challenging operation with varying published opinions regarding surgical indications, techniques, and postoperative rehabilitation. In this chapter we provide a summary of the anatomy and biomechanics of the PCL, operative indications, and surgical techniques, including specific technical options and rationale for the use of each. We focus primarily on treatment of isolated PCL deficiency because the technique for surgical reconstruction of combined ligament insufficiency is discussed elsewhere in this book.

ANATOMIC AND BIOMECHANICAL CONSIDERATIONS

The PCL is an intracapsular structure that is contained within its own synovium. It averages between 32 and 38 mm in length between insertions.[22] The femoral footprint is elliptical in shape. It is approximately 32 mm in length and terminates 3 mm proximal to the articular cartilage margin of the femoral condyle.[27] The tibial insertion lies approximately 1 to 1.5 cm inferior to the posterior rim of the tibia in a depression between the medial and lateral tibial plateaus called the PCL facet or fovea.[21] The PCL has three main components: the anterolateral bundle, posteromedial bundle, and meniscofemoral ligaments. The larger anterolateral bundle demonstrates increasing tension with knee flexion and is most important for preventing abnormal posterior tibial displacement at 90 degrees of flexion. The posteromedial bundle becomes taut in extension.[32] The third component of the PCL complex, the meniscofemoral ligaments, is variably present and may contribute up to 30% to 40% of the PCL complex's total volume.[43] With an intact PCL, the meniscofemoral ligaments contribute 28% of the total force resisted during a posterior drawer test at 90 degrees. After sectioning of the PCL this contribution increases to 70%.[26] This information suggests that the meniscofemoral ligaments play an important functional role in knee stability;

however, their role with respect to PCL reconstruction has not been well defined. Some authors have suggested preserving the meniscofemoral ligaments during PCL reconstruction to improve posterior stability.[1]

The PCL is the primary restraint to posterior translation at 90 degrees of flexion and a secondary restraint to external rotation.[62] The degree of pathologic posterior and rotatory displacement noted on examination is indicative of isolated versus combined injury. Normal physiologic posterior laxity is approximately 3 mm.[33,53] Greater than 12 mm of posterior translation may be indicative of an associated injury to the posterolateral corner structures (popliteus, lateral collateral ligament, popliteofibular ligament, posterolateral joint capsule, iliotibial band, and biceps femoris).[28,33] Studies have shown that associated insufficiency of the posterolateral corner structures will increase force in the PCL, as well as in a PCL replacement graft, by up to 30%.[31,63] Combined PCL and posterolateral corner injuries are more common than initially recognized and are present in up to 60% of patients with significant PCL injuries.[15] Failure to treat this associated injury may lead to failure of the PCL reconstruction.[60]

Unlike the anterior cruciate ligament, the PCL has only a very small zone of isometric fibers located in the center of the femoral attachment.[24] In the laboratory, so-called isometric reconstruction has demonstrated poor resistance to posterior translation and has largely been abandoned in favor of anatomic reconstruction.[52] Because of its favorable biomechanical properties, surgeons have traditionally chosen to reconstruct the anterolateral bundle of the PCL.[14,28] More recently, surgical techniques involving double-bundle reconstruction have been described, and there is laboratory evidence that these reconstructions may more closely replicate the function of the native PCL.[23,30,44,52]

With respect to articular contact pressure, PCL deficiency has been reported to result in increased patellofemoral and medial femoral condyle contact pressure with increasing flexion angles.[20,42,58] In a biomechanical study, Gill et al[20] found that PCL reconstruction using a single-bundle technique did not significantly reduce the increased contact pressure observed in a PCL-deficient knee. The clinical effectiveness of current PCL reconstruction techniques in restoring normal knee kinematics and consequently preventing increased contact pressure and subsequent articular cartilage degeneration is not yet known.

MECHANISM OF INJURY

The most common mechanism of injury to the PCL is an anterior blow to the proximal end of the tibia. This is most commonly seen in motor vehicle accidents (dashboard injuries) but may also occur as a result of a fall on a flexed knee with the foot in plantar flexion, as often occurs in athletics.[17] High-energy injuries, such as those seen with motor vehicle accidents, often lead to multiple-ligament involvement, whereas athletic injuries are more likely to result in an isolated lesion of the PCL.[17] Additionally, hyperextension has also been described as a mechanism and may result in a combined injury to the PCL and posterolateral corner.[38] Fanelli and Edson reported a 38% incidence of PCL injury in knees with an acute hemarthrosis seen in a trauma setting, with a high percentage of patients demonstrating a combined pattern of injury.[15]

EVALUATION

The most accurate clinical test for detecting a PCL injury is the posterior drawer test.[12] A posteriorly directed force is applied to the proximal end of the tibia, and the extent of translation is evaluated by noting the change in step-off between the medial tibial plateau and the medial femoral condyle (Fig. 47–1). Grade I injuries have a palpable, but diminished step-off (0 to 5 mm). Grade II injuries allow 5 to 10 mm of posterior translation; however, the medial tibial plateau cannot be pushed beyond the medial femoral condyle. Grade III (complete) PCL injuries allow the medial tibial plateau to be displaced posterior to the medial femoral condyle (greater than 10-mm posterior translation) and demonstrate an osseous posterior sag of the tibia.[28] It is essential to rule out injury to the posterolateral corner structures, particularly when posterior tibial translation is greater than 10 mm. It is important to reduce the tibia to neutral and then test the posterolateral corner at both 90 and 30 degrees of flexion.[28] It is especially crucial to recognize combined PCL and posterolateral corner injuries because reconstruction of the PCL alone in the presence of an unrecognized posterolateral corner injury will lead to increased force on the PCL graft and the potential for subsequent graft failure.[31]

After a thorough physical examination is completed, plain radiographs should be obtained, including anteroposterior, lateral, and oblique views. In the chronic setting, posteroanterior flexion weightbearing views and patellar views may be helpful in evaluating degenerative changes. Radiographs should be examined for avulsion fracture fragments, tibial plateau fractures, and posterior subluxation. Lateral stress radiographs may be helpful to evaluate for tibia-femur step-off, particularly when compared with the normal knee (Fig. 47–2).[14,33,57] Magnetic resonance imaging (MRI) provides useful information regarding the PCL, as well as other potentially injured structures. MRI is highly sensitive and specific in the diagnosis and description of acute PCL tears (Fig. 47–3).[25] PCL tears may heal with time in an elongated fashion and

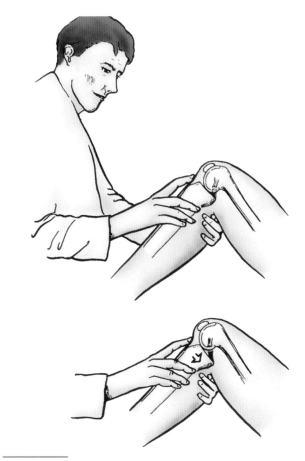

Figure 47–1. Assessing tibial step-off by performing the posterior drawer examination. (Adapted from Miller MD, Harner CD, Koshiwaguchi S: Acute posterior cruciate ligament injuries. In Fu FH, Harner CD, Vince KG [eds]: Knee Surgery, vol 1. Baltimore, Williams & Wilkins, 1994.)

result in a nearly normal appearance on MRI.[55] For this reason, clinical examination is superior to MRI in chronic cases.

NATURAL HISTORY

The natural history of isolated PCL injuries remains a source of continued debate. It is clear that nonoperative treatment of isolated PCL disruption generally results in satisfactory function in the short term.[17,51] The ultimate fate of a PCL-deficient knee is less clear. It has been demonstrated that the increase in posterior displacement occurring with PCL injuries leads to abnormal tibiofemoral and patellofemoral forces.[20,42,59] Geissler and Whipple performed arthroscopy in symptomatic patients with isolated PCL injuries.[19] In the acute setting, 12% of patients had chondral injuries and 27% had meniscal pathology. In the chronic population, the numbers increased to 49% and 36%, respectively. Lateral meniscal tears were more common in the acute setting, whereas medial meniscal tears were more common in the chronic setting. Medial femoral chondral defects were common in

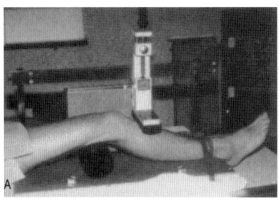
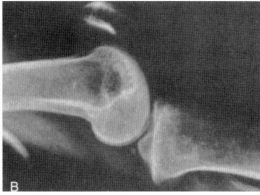

Figure 47–2. **A** and **B,** Stress test radiography performed with the patient under anesthesia. (From Jakob RP, Staubli HU [eds]: The Knee and Cruciate Ligaments. Berlin, Springer-Verlag, 1992.)

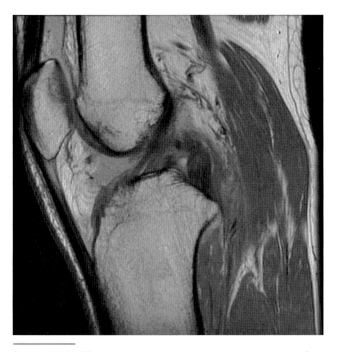

Figure 47–3. Magnetic resonance imaging appearance of an acute complete posterior cruciate ligament tear.

both settings. This trend suggests that instability secondary to a PCL tear may lead to compromised kinematics and intra-articular injury with the potential for early arthrosis. Dejour et al reported the longest follow-up of nonoperatively treated PCL tears, with a mean of 15 years. Despite remarkable functional tolerance seen in patients with isolated rupture, significant degenerative changes were observed in 17%, whereas lesser changes were noted in 69% at an average of 25 years' follow-up.[13] Boynton and Tietjens reported that as time from injury increased, progressive articular degeneration was seen on radiographs. They were unable, however, to identify any specific factors that predicted outcome.[6]

Parolie and Bergfeld monitored 25 patients with isolated tears of the PCL for an average of 6 years and concluded that 80% were subjectively satisfied with their outcome and 84% returned to their previous sport.[51] However, only 68% returned to sports at their preinjury level. They noted

a correlation between quadriceps atrophy and low subjective outcome rating. Additionally, they found no correlation between residual laxity and patient satisfaction or return to sports. Keller and colleagues reviewed 40 patients treated nonoperatively with an average follow-up of 6 years and found that increased posterior instability led to greater subjective complaints.[39] There was, however, no correlation found between isokinetic testing and knee score. Ninety percent of the patients complained of some pain with activity. In a more recent prospective study, Shelbourne et al found no correlation between objective and subjective knee scores and the PCL laxity grade at a mean interval of 5.4 years. Regardless of the laxity grade, 50% of the patients were able to resume sports at the same level or higher.[54]

Torg and associates demonstrated improved results in patients with unidirectional posterior instability versus combined multidirectional instability, with 86% of knees with unidirectional instability demonstrating good or excellent results versus 48% of knees with multidirectional instability.[61] Factors that influenced the prognosis included the degree of instability, a history of meniscectomy, quadriceps muscle insufficiency, and patellofemoral problems. The authors concluded that although patients with unidirectional instability as a result of PCL deficiency can be treated nonoperatively, those with multidirectional instability should be considered for reconstruction because of both a higher incidence of unacceptable function and roentgenographic degenerative changes.

In summary, it appears that patients with isolated grade I or II PCL injuries do well functionally in the short term. Some patients will experience increasing pain, instability, and deterioration in function, as well as progressive degenerative changes, most marked in the medial and patellofemoral compartments. It is still unknown whether operative management will prevent such long-term sequelae in these patients.

OPERATIVE INDICATIONS

In general, the decision to proceed operatively in the setting of PCL injury depends on patient age and activity level, severity of the knee injury (isolated versus combined), timing of the injury (acute versus chronic), and symptomatology. Most authors advise early operative management of displaced bony avulsions of the PCL insertion. Good results have been reported with screw fixation through a posterior or posteromedial approach (Fig. 47–4).[40,47] Additionally, combined ligament injuries involving the PCL and, in particular, those involving the PCL and posterolateral corner structures require surgical reconstruction. Early surgical management (within the first 2 weeks) is typically recommended in the case of combined injuries to avoid significant capsular scarring and allow for anatomic repair of the collateral structures.[15,29]

Operative indications for isolated PCL injuries are less clear. In general, isolated grade I and grade II PCL injuries can be treated nonoperatively.[12,17,28,39] Nonoperative treatment involves a period of protected weightbearing with immobilization in extension, typically using a posterior

tibial pad to prevent posterior subluxation. This is followed by progressive quadriceps-strengthening exercises.[14,28] Treatment of isolated grade III PCL injuries is somewhat controversial. In general, surgical management is recommended for chronic grade III PCL injuries that become symptomatic because of pain or instability despite an appropriate rehabilitation program. In these patients, it is important to rule out occult posterolateral corner injury because reconstruction of the PCL alone in such cases probably carries a higher risk for failure.[31] Additionally, patients with symptomatic grade III PCL insufficiency should be evaluated for varus malalignment and, in particular, varus thrust during gait. In this case a proximal tibial osteotomy to correct the varus deformity and perhaps reduce posterior tibial translation by increasing the posterior tibial slope should be considered.[48,50]

SURGICAL TECHNIQUE

Multiple different methods of PCL reconstruction have been described. Variables exist with respect to graft choice, graft placement, and graft fixation. Because of the large size and anatomic and biomechanical complexity of the PCL, reproducing the position and function of the native PCL remains challenging. The most commonly performed reconstruction techniques include the transtibial and tibial inlay techniques. Both can be performed with a single-bundle or double-bundle construct. Graft choices include autograft sources, including patellar tendon, hamstring tendon, and quadriceps tendon grafts. The structural properties of the three common autografts are summarized in Table 47–1. Allograft alternatives include Achilles tendon, patellar tendon, and more recently, tibialis anterior grafts. Potential advantages of allograft tissue include reduced donor site morbidity and surgical time, as well as availability for use of multiple grafts, which may be particularly important when treating combined injuries or in the case of a double-bundle reconstructive technique. Potential weakening of the quadriceps mechanism, which is synergistic with the PCL, has been cited as a particular concern with the use of patellar tendon and quadriceps autografts.[34] Proponents of autograft tissue cite increased cost, increased risk of disease transmission, and delayed remodeling and maturation of allograft tissue as

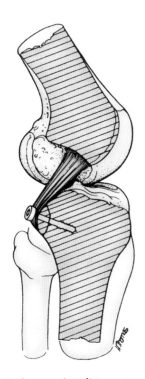

Figure 47–4. Posterior cruciate ligament avulsion from the tibia fixed with a screw.

Table 47–1. Comparison of Structural Properties of the Intact PCL and BPTB, Quadriceps Tendons, and Hamstring Tendons,

GRAFT	MAXIMUM STRENGTH (N)	STIFFNESS (N/mm)	CROSS-SECTIONAL AREA (mm²)	LENGTH (mm)
PCL-ACL bundle	1494 ± 390	306 ± 130		38-42
PCL-PM bundle	242 ± 66	75 ± 31		
BPTB (10 mm)	2977 ± 516	455 ± 56	36.8 ± 5.7	52.2 ± 4.8
Quadriceps tendon (10 mm)	2352 ± 495	325 ± 70	64.6 ± 8.4	86.4 ± 9.0
Quadruple semitendinosus/gracilis	4090 ± 295	776 ± 204	52 ± 5	100-120 mm

ACL, anterior cruciate ligament; BPTB, bone–patellar tendon–bone; PCL, posterior cruciate ligament; PM, posteromedial.
Modified from Hoher J, Scheffler S, Weiler A: Graft choice and graft fixation in PCL reconstruction. Knee Surg Sports Traumatol Arthrosc 11:297-306, 2003.

reasons for consideration of the use of an autograft in PCL reconstruction.[34,36,56]

Transtibial Tunnel Technique

As is common to all surgical techniques, examination under anesthesia is performed first to confirm the diagnosis. The patient is placed supine. Diagnostic arthroscopy is performed to document the PCL injury and address any associated intra-articular pathology. A common finding is pseudolaxity of the anterior cruciate ligament, which is seen at arthroscopy and is due to posterior translation of the tibia (Fig. 47–5). In the acute setting, the use of gravity inflow rather than a fluid pump is generally recommended to avoid fluid extravasation and reduce the risk for compartment syndrome. After diagnostic arthroscopy, the tibial stump of the torn PCL is identified and débrided. A 70-degree arthroscope is helpful in visualization of the PCL insertion site. A posteromedial portal is used to assist with débridement and visualization of the PCL insertion site, as well as for insertion of a curet to protect the posterior structures from an advancing drill or guide wire. Use of a posterior transseptal portal has been described and may provide improved visualization of the PCL tibial attachment.[1] The entrance to the tibial tunnel is placed approximately 2 cm distal to the traditional ACL tibial tunnel and midway between the tibial tubercle and the posterior border of the tibia.[28] Use of an anterolateral tibial entry point has also been described as a means of theoretically reducing graft angulation at the margin of the proximal end of the tibia.[35] The tibial guide wire is placed under arthroscopic and preferably fluoroscopic guidance such that the guide wire exits the posterior tibial cortex approximately 10 mm inferior to the posterior tibial plateau. Care is taken to avoid overpenetration of the guide wire into the posterior soft tissues. The guide pin is placed with the knee flexed to at least 90 degrees, at an angle of approximately 50 degrees

to the tibial plateau surface. A tibial tunnel of 10 or 11 mm is drilled. A large curet is placed through the posteromedial portal to prevent advancement of the guide pin and/or drilling into the posterior soft tissues (Fig. 47–6). Traditionally, a single-bundle reconstruction is performed, with reproduction of the anterolateral bundle of the PCL. For femoral tunnel placement via an outside-in technique, an incision approximately 3 cm in length is made 1 cm medial to the medial patellar border, over the medial femoral condyle.[28] The fibers of the vastus medialis obliquus are split to allow placement of a standard femoral drill guide. The guide pin is placed such that the femoral tunnel is centered 6 mm off the articular margin, at the 1 : 30 position in the right knee or the 10 : 30 position in the left knee. This technique should result in femoral tunnel placement through the anterior aspect of the femoral footprint just under the subchondral bone of the medial femoral condyle (Fig. 47–7). A 10- or 11-mm femoral tunnel is drilled. An inside-out technique can be used in which the guide pin is inserted in a lateral-to-medial direction through an accessory anterolateral portal.

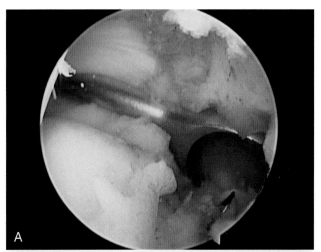

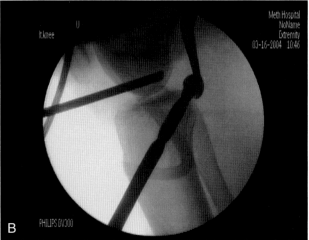

Figure 47–6. **A,** Arthroscopic visualization of the tibial guide pin during tibial tunnel preparation. A large curet has been placed through the posteromedial portal to prevent advancement of the guide pin. **B,** Fluoroscopic view during tibial tunnel preparation.

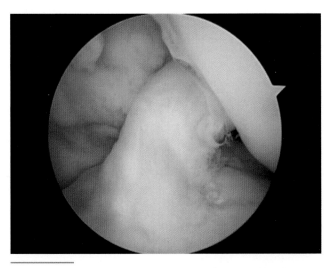

Figure 47–5. Anterior cruciate ligament pseudolaxity seen at the time of knee arthroscopy for chronic posterior cruciate ligament insufficiency.

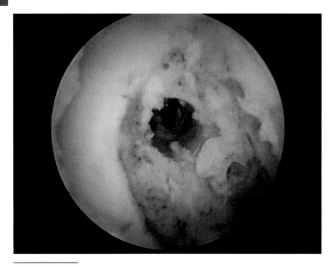

Figure 47–7. Arthroscopic view of the femoral tunnel for single-bundle posterior cruciate ligament reconstruction.

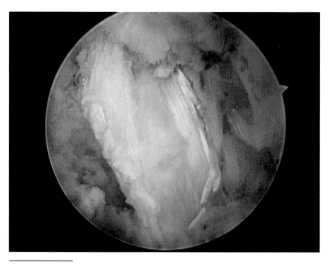

Figure 47–8. Arthroscopic view of single-bundle posterior cruciate ligament reconstruction with an Achilles allograft.

With the inside-out technique there is some concern regarding an acute angle between the intra-articular portion of the graft and the bony femoral tunnel.[10] It has been shown by Kim et al that the results of inside-out (one incision) and outside-in (two incision) PCL reconstruction are similar after 2 years.[41] The edges of the tunnels are chamfered, and the graft may be passed from the tibia to the femur or vice versa. A blunt instrument such as a switching stick is placed through the posteromedial portal anterior to the graft and used to assist graft passage around the posterior corner of the tibia. When passing the graft from the tibia to the femur, it is helpful to drill the tibial tunnel slightly larger than the femoral tunnel to facilitate graft passage. Of course, the diameters of the tunnels ultimately depend on graft size. At our institution, we use Achilles tendon allograft for single-bundle PCL reconstruction (Fig. 47–8). Graft fixation is typically performed with an interference screw on the femoral side first. The graft is cycled multiple times before final fixation on the tibial side to minimize graft elongation. The graft is fixed on the tibial side while holding the knee in 70 to 90 degrees of flexion and applying an anterior drawer force to recreate the normal step-off between the medial femoral condyle and the medial tibial plateau. At our institution, tibial fixation is performed with a biodegradable soft-tissue interference screw, as well as a bicortical screw and soft-tissue washer. This so-called backup fixation is used to achieve additional pullout strength on the tibial side.[49] If a patellar tendon graft is used, interference screw fixation can be performed on both the tibial and femoral sides. It should be noted that titanium fixation devices in the back of the tibia may cause a problem in revision PCL surgery.[34]

Tibial Inlay Technique

The tibial inlay technique involves the use of a posterior or posteromedial approach to the knee to allow for direct placement of the tibial portion of the graft in a trough placed in the tibial PCL footprint. The technique was devised, in theory, to avoid acute graft passage around the articular margin of the tibia, such as occurs with the transtibial technique, and it was originally described by Berg.[3] This technique has been shown to biomechanically result in less graft laxity with cyclic loading.[4,45] Disadvantages of this technique include difficulty with patient positioning, along with the potential morbidity of a posterior incision. The procedure is performed either by converting from the prone to the supine position intraoperatively or by carrying out the entire procedure in the lateral decubitus position (Fig. 47–9). Arthroscopic preparation of the tibial and femoral insertion sites is performed, and the femoral tunnel is drilled in routine fashion. The patient is then repositioned as needed for the posterior approach, which can be performed either through a direct posterior approach or, more commonly, through a posteromedial approach as described by Burks and Schaffer.[7] Lateral retraction of the medial gastrocnemius muscle protects the neurovascular structures and allows access to the posterior capsule. The inlay technique is most commonly performed with a patellar tendon autograft or allograft; however, quadriceps tendon autograft or allograft or Achilles tendon allograft may be used. The posterior capsule is incised vertically to allow visualization of the PCL insertion. A unicortical window is prepared according to the dimensions of the bone block. The bone block is typically predrilled to accept one or more screws. The graft is placed flush with the prepared surface and fixed with or without washers. The graft is then passed intra-articularly and into the femoral tunnel with the aid of a wire loop or commercial graft passer. After cycling the graft multiple times, it is tensioned and fixed in 70 to 90 degrees of knee flexion on the femoral side. Fixation is generally achieved with an interference screw in the femoral tunnel. Alternatively, if an Achilles or quadriceps graft is used, the soft-tissue end of the graft is fixed on the femoral side with a screw and spiked washer or staple, with or without a biodegradable soft-tissue interference

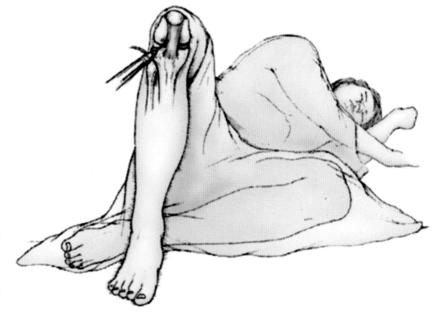

Figure 47–9. Tibial inlay technique. The patient is placed in the lateral decubitus position for initial arthroscopy and femoral tunnel preparation. The knee is extended and abducted for exposure of the tibial insertion site. (From Berg EE: Posterior cruciate ligament tibial inlay reconstruction. Arthroscopy 11:69-76, 1995.)

screw. We choose to avoid the use of interference screws alone for soft-tissue graft fixation because of decreased pullout strength with cyclic loading.[49]

Double-Femoral Bundle Technique

The double-bundle PCL reconstruction involves the use of two femoral tunnels to theoretically replace both the anterolateral and posteromedial bundles of the native PCL. Several authors have hypothesized that this technique is superior to single-bundle techniques because of restoration of more normal knee mechanics throughout flexion and extension.[23,31,44,52] Short-term results of the double-bundle technique are encouraging.[8,9] Long-term follow-up studies are needed to compare the outcome of a more "physiological" double-bundle PCL reconstruction with both single-bundle techniques and historical controls.[8] The double-bundle procedure can be performed with either a transtibial or tibial inlay technique. The anterolateral bundle is re-created by drilling a femoral tunnel as described earlier. A smaller, posteromedial tunnel is placed within the PCL footprint inferior and slightly posterior to the anterolateral tunnel. The femoral tunnels may be drilled from either inside out or outside in. The tunnels should diverge, and an adequate bone bridge should be preserved between the two tunnels to prevent collapse of the tunnels during fixation (Fig. 47–10). Graft choices include a split Achilles tendon allograft, tibialis anterior allograft, quadriceps tendon graft, or quadruple hamstring tendon grafts (Fig. 47–11).[5,9,59] Alternatively, a double-looped semitendinosus autograft may be used to reconstruct the posteromedial bundle, in addition to the surgeon's preferred graft of choice for reconstruction of the anterolateral bundle.[30] The method of graft fixation for the double-bundle technique includes the use of biodegradable soft-tissue interference screws or EndoButtons when using an inside-out technique. The use

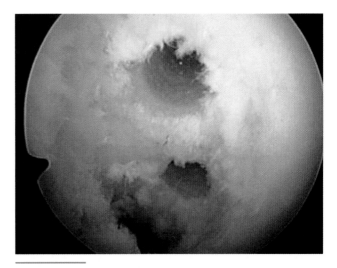

Figure 47–10. Arthroscopic view of femoral tunnel placement for two-bundle posterior cruciate ligament reconstruction.

of an EndoButton requires modification when drilling the femoral tunnels.[34] Alternatively, when using an outside-in technique, fixation can be achieved with an interference screw and/or a screw and spiked washer.

POSTOPERATIVE MANAGEMENT

Most postoperative PCL reconstruction protocols recommend immobilizing the knee in full extension for a period of 2 to 4 weeks. Both the force of gravity and the force of hamstring contraction are potentially dangerous during the early phases of rehabilitation. The tibia should be supported to prevent posterior translation and excessive graft stress. In the early postoperative period, prone passive

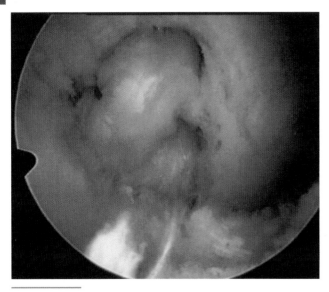

Figure 47–11. Arthroscopic view after double-bundle posterior cruciate ligament reconstruction with a quadriceps tendon autograft.

flexion exercises are performed to minimize hamstring activation. Partial weightbearing as tolerated and quadriceps exercises are begun immediately. Closed kinetic chain exercises typically begin at 6 weeks, and hamstring strengthening is delayed for at least 4 months to avoid excessive posterior stress on the graft. Patients generally return to full activities 9 to 12 months postoperatively.

COMPLICATIONS

Potential complications include infection, arthrofibrosis, neurological injuries, vascular complications, osteonecrosis of the medial femoral condyle, and the development of residual posterior laxity. With respect to arthrofibrosis, approximately 20% of cases require manipulation under anesthesia approximately 2 months after reconstruction to increase terminal flexion.[37] The use of rehabilitation programs that incorporate immediate full knee extension and early range of motion may help decrease this complication. Neurological injuries may occur in the form of a neuropraxia, which is most common after prolonged tourniquet time. Avoidance of tourniquet use altogether should prevent this complication. Direct injury to the tibial nerve can result from penetration by either the tibial guide pin or drill and can be prevented by the use of a posterior curet or retractor along with direct visualization of the tip of the guide pin and drill at all times during preparation of the tibial tunnel in the transtibial technique. Similarly, vascular complications such as laceration or intimal injury to the popliteal artery may occur during tibial tunnel preparation and are also prevented by direct visualization of the tibial pin and drill. Flexing the knee to at least 90 degrees decreases, but does not eliminate neurovascular risk when creating the tibial tunnel.[46] Fluid extravasation into the soft tissues with subsequent risk of compartment syndrome is a potential problem with

arthroscopically assisted reconstruction of the PCL, particularly in the setting of multiple-ligament injury. The use of gravity inflow combined with diligent preoperative, intraoperative, and postoperative examination should help prevent this complication. Osteonecrosis of the medial femoral condyle after PCL reconstruction has been described.[2] It is unknown whether the incidence of osteonecrosis of the medial femoral condyle is greater with the double–femoral tunnel technique; however, it is a theoretical concern. The most common complication after PCL reconstruction is residual laxity.[11] A significant percentage of patients undergoing PCL reconstruction experience some degree of delayed posterior laxity that may or may not be manifested clinically. It appears to be more common with combined injuries.[16,18] It is hoped that with accurate and anatomic tunnel placement, optimal fixation, and repair or reconstruction of associated ligamentous injuries, the incidence of clinically significant posterior laxity after PCL reconstruction will be minimized.

References

1. Ahn JH, Chung YS, Oh I: Arthroscopic posterior cruciate ligament reconstruction using the posterior transeptal portal. J Arthroscopy 19:101-107, 2003.
2. Athanasian EA, Wickiewicz TL, Warren RF: Osteonecrosis of the femoral condyle after arthroscopic reconstruction of a cruciate ligament. Report of two cases. J Bone Joint Surg Am 77:1418-1422, 1995.
3. Berg EE: Posterior cruciate ligament tibial inlay reconstruction. Arthroscopy 11:69-76, 1995.
4. Bergfeld JA, McAllister DR, Parker RD, et al: A biomechanical comparison of posterior cruciate ligament reconstruction techniques. Am J Sports Med 29:129-136, 2001.
5. Borden PS, Nyland JA, Caborn DN: Posterior cruciate ligament reconstruction (double bundle) using anterior tibialis tendon allograft. Arthroscopy 17(4):E14, 2001.
6. Boynton MD, Tietjens BR: Long-term follow-up of the untreated isolated posterior cruciate ligament–deficient knee. Am J Sports Med 24:306-310, 1996 .
7. Burks RT, Schaffer JJ: A simplified approach to the tibial attachment of the posterior cruciate ligament. Clin Orthop 254:216-219, 1990.
8. Cain EL Jr, Clancy WG Jr: Posterior cruciate ligament reconstruction: Two-bundle technique. J Knee Surg 15:108-113, 2002.
9. Chen CH, Chen WJ, Shih CH: Arthroscopic double-bundled posterior cruciate ligament reconstruction with quadriceps tendon–patellar bone autograft. Arthroscopy 16:780-782, 2000.
10. Christel P: Basic principles for surgical reconstruction of the PCL in chronic posterior knee instability. Knee Surg Sports Traumatol Arthrosc 11:289-296, 2003.
11. Clancy WG, Dison LJ: Double tunnel technique for reconstruction of the posterior cruciate ligament. Op Tech Sports Med 7:110-117, 1999.
12. Covey CD, Sapega AA: Injuries of the posterior cruciate ligament. J Bone Joint Surg Am 75:1376-1386, 1993.
13. Dejour H, Walch G, Peyrot J, Eberhard P: The natural history of rupture of the posterior cruciate ligament. Rev Chir Orthop 74:35-43, 1988.
14. Dowd GS: Reconstruction of the posterior cruciate ligament. Indications and results. J Bone Joint Surg Br 86:480-491, 2004.
15. Fanelli GC, Edson CJ: Posterior cruciate ligament injuries in trauma patients: Part II. Arthroscopy 11:526-529, 1995.
16. Fanelli GC, Giannotti BF, Edson CJ: Arthroscopically assisted combined posterior cruciate ligament/posterior lateral complex reconstruction. Arthroscopy 12:521-530, 1996.
17. Fowler PJ, Messieh SS: Isolated posterior cruciate ligament injuries in athletes. Am J Sports Med 15:553-557, 1987.
18. Freeman RT, Duri ZA, Dowd GS: Combined chronic posterior cruciate and posterolateral corner ligamentous injuries: A comparison

of posterior cruciate ligament reconstruction with and without reconstruction of the posterolateral corner. Knee 9:309-312, 2002.

19. Geissler WB, Whipple TL: Intraarticular abnormalities in association with posterior cruciate ligament injuries. Am J Sports Med 21:846-849, 1993.

20. Gill TJ, DeFrate LE, Wang C, et al: The effect of posterior cruciate ligament reconstruction on patellofemoral contact pressures in the knee joint under simulated muscle loads. Am J Sports Med 32:109-115, 2004.

21. Girgis FG, Marshall JL, Monajem A: The cruciate ligaments of the knee joint. Anatomical, functional and experimental analysis. Clin Orthop 106:216-231, 1975.

22. Gollehon DL, Torzilli PA, Warren RF: The role of the posterolateral and cruciate ligaments in the stability of the human knee. A biomechanical study. J Bone Joint Surg Am 69:233-242, 1987.

23. Giffin JR, Haemmerle MJ, Vogrin TM, Harner CD: Single- versus double-bundle PCL reconstruction: A biomechanical analysis. J Knee Surg 15:114-120, 2002.

24. Grood ES, Hefzy MS, Lindenfield TN: Factors affecting the region of most isometric femoral attachments. Part I: The posterior cruciate ligament. Am J Sports Med 17:197-207, 1989.

25. Gross ML, Grover JS, Bassett LW, et al: Magnetic resonance imaging of the posterior cruciate ligament. Clinical use to improve diagnostic accuracy. Am J Sports Med 20:732-737, 1992.

26. Gupte C, Bull A, Thomas R, Amos A: The meniscofemoral ligaments: Secondary restraints to the posterior drawer. Analysis of anteroposterior and rotatory laxity in the intact and posterior-cruciate–deficient knee. J Bone Joint Surg Br 85:765-773, 2003.

27. Harner CD, Baek GH, Vogrin TM, et al: Quantitative analysis of human cruciate ligament insertions. Arthroscopy 15:741-749, 1999.

28. Harner CD, Hoher J: Evaluation and treatment of posterior cruciate ligament injuries. Am J Sports Med 26:471-482, 1998.

29. Harner CD, Hoher J, Vogrin TM, et al: The effect of sectioning the posterolateral structures on in situ forces in the human posterior cruciate ligament. Trans Orthop Res Soc 23:47, 1998.

30. Harner CD, Janaushek MA, Kanamori A, et al: Biomechanical analysis of a double-bundle posterior cruciate ligament reconstruction. Am J Sports Med 28:144-151, 2000.

31. Harner CD, Vogrin TM, Hoher J, et al: Biomechanical analysis of a posterior cruciate ligament reconstruction. Deficiency of the posterolateral structures as a cause of graft failure. Am J Sports Med 28:32-39, 2000.

32. Harner CD, Xerogeanes JW, Livesay GA, et al: The human posterior cruciate ligament complex: An interdisciplinary study. Ligament morphology and biomechanical evaluation. Am J Sports Med 23:736-745, 1995.

33. Hewett TE, Noyes FR, Lee MD: Diagnosis of complete and partial posterior cruciate ligament ruptures. Stress radiography compared with KT-1000 arthrometer and posterior drawer testing. Am J Sports Med 25:648-655, 1997.

34. Hoher J, Scheffler S, Weiler A: Graft choice and graft fixation in PCL reconstruction. Knee Surg Sports Traumatol Arthrosc 11:297-306, 2003.

35. Huang T, Wang C, Weng L, Chan Y: Reducing the "killer turn" in posterior cruciate ligament reconstruction. Arthroscopy 19:712-716, 2003.

36. Jackson DW, Corsetti J, Simon TM: Biologic incorporation of allograft anterior cruciate ligament replacements. Clin Orthop 324:126-133, 1996.

37. Janousek AT, Jones DG, Clatworthy M, et al: Posterior cruciate ligament injuries of the knee joint. Sports Med 28:429-441, 1999.

38. Kannus P, Bergfeld J, Jarvinen M, et al: Injuries to the posterior cruciate ligament of the knee. Sports Med 12:110-131, 1991.

39. Keller PM, Shelbourne KD, McCarroll JR, Rettig AC: Nonoperatively treated isolated posterior cruciate ligament injuries. Am J Sports Med 21:132-136, 1993.

40. Kim SJ, Shin SJ, Choi NH, et al: Arthroscopically assisted treatment of avulsion fractures of the posterior cruciate ligament from the tibia. J Bone Joint Surg Am 83:698-708, 2001.

41. Kim SJ, Shin SJ, Kim HK, et al: Comparison of 1- and 2-incision posterior cruciate ligament reconstructions. Arthroscopy 16:268-278, 2000.

42. MacDonald P, Miniaci A, Fowler P, et al: A biomechanical analysis of joint contact forces in the posterior cruciate deficient knee. Knee Surg Sports Traumatol Arthrosc 3:252-255, 1996.

43. Makris CA, Georgoulis AD, Papageorgiou CD, et al: Posterior cruciate ligament architecture: Evaluation under microsurgical dissection. Arthroscopy 16:627-632, 2000.

44. Mannor DA, Shearn JT, Grood ES, et al: Two-bundle posterior cruciate ligament reconstruction. An in vitro analysis of graft placement and tension. Am J Sports Med 28:833-845, 2000.

45. Markolf KL, Zemanovic JR, McAllister DR: Cyclic loading of posterior cruciate ligament replacements fixed with tibial tunnel and tibial inlay methods. J Bone Joint Surg Am 84:518-524, 2002.

46. Matava MJ, Sethi NS, Totty WG: Proximity of the posterior cruciate ligament insertion to the popliteal artery as a function of the knee flexion angle: Implications for posterior cruciate ligament reconstruction. Arthroscopy 16:796-804, 2000.

47. Meyers MH: Isolated avulsion of the tibial attachment of the posterior cruciate ligament of the knee. J Bone Joint Surg Am 57:669-672, 1975.

48. Miller MD, Bergfeld JA, Fowler PJ, et al: The posterior cruciate ligament injured knee: Principles of evaluation and treatment. Instr Course Lect 48:199-207, 1999.

49. Nargarkatti DG, McKeon DT, Donahue BS, Fulkerson JP: Mechanical evaluation of a soft tissue interference screw in three tendon anterior cruciate ligament graft fixations. Am J Sports Med 29:67-71, 2001.

50. Noyes FR, Barber-Westin SD: Treatment of complex injuries involving the posterior cruciate and posterolateral ligaments of the knee. Am J Knee Surg 9:200-214, 1996.

51. Parolie JM, Bergfeld JA: Long-term results of nonoperative treatment of isolated posterior cruciate ligament injuries in the athlete. Am J Sports Med 14:35-38, 1986.

52. Race A, Amis AA: PCL reconstruction. In vitro biomechanical comparison of 'isometric' versus single and double-bundled 'anatomic' grafts. J Bone Joint Surg Br 80:173-179, 1998.

53. Ritchie JR, Bergfeld JA, Kambic H, Manning T: Isolated sectioning of the medial and posteromedial capsular ligaments in the posterior cruciate ligament–deficient knee. Influence on posterior tibial translation. Am J Sports Med 26:389-394, 1998.

54. Shelbourne KD, Davis TJ, Patel DV: The natural history of acute, isolated, nonoperatively treated posterior cruciate ligament injuries. A prospective study. Am J Sports Med 27:276-283, 1999.

55. Shelbourne KD, Jennings RW, Vahey TN: Magnetic resonance imaging of posterior cruciate ligament injuries: Assessment of healing. Am J Knee Surg 12:209-213, 1999.

56. Shino K, Inoue M, Horibe S, et al: Maturation of allograft tendons transplanted into the knee. An arthroscopic and histological study. J Bone Joint Surg Br 70:556-560, 1988.

57. Shino K, Mitsuoka T, Horibe S, et al: The gravity sag view: A simple radiographic technique to show posterior laxity of the knee. Arthroscopy 16:670-672, 2000.

58. Skyhar MJ, Warren RF, Ortiz GJ, et al: The effects of sectioning of the posterior cruciate ligament and the posterolateral complex on the articular contact pressures within the knee. J Bone Joint Surg Am 75:694-699, 1993.

59. Stahelin AC, Sudkamp NP, Weiler A: Anatomic double-bundle posterior cruciate ligament reconstruction using hamstring tendons. Arthroscopy 17:88-97, 2001.

60. Sugita T, Amis AA: Anatomic and biomechanical study of the lateral collateral and popliteal fibular ligament. Am J Sports Med 29:466-472, 2001.

61. Torg JS, Barton TM, Pavlov H, Stine R: Natural history of the posterior cruciate ligament–deficient knee. Clin Orthop 246: 208-216, 1989.

62. Veltri DM, Deng XH, Torzilli PA, et al: The role of the cruciate and posterolateral ligaments in stability of the knee. A biomechanical study. Am J Sports Med 23:436-443, 1995.

63. Vogrin TM, Hoher J, Aroen A, et al: Effects of sectioning the posterolateral structures on knee kinematics and in situ forces in the posterior cruciate ligament. Knee Surg Sports Traumatol Arthrosc 8:93-98, 2000.

CHAPTER 48

Posterior Cruciate Ligament Reconstruction

Gregory C. Fanelli

Posterior cruciate ligament (PCL) injuries are reported to account for 1% to 40% of acute knee injuries. This range is dependent on the patient population and is approximately 3% in the general population and 38% in reports from regional trauma centers.[3,4,10] Our practice at a regional trauma center has a 38.3% incidence of PCL tears in acute knee injuries, and 56.5% of these PCL injuries occur in multiple-trauma patients. A total of 45.9% of these PCL injuries are combined anterior cruciate ligament (ACL)/PCL tears, whereas 41.2% are PCL/posterolateral corner tears. Only 3% of acute PCL injuries seen in the trauma center are isolated.

This chapter illustrates my surgical technique of arthroscopic single-bundle, single–femoral tunnel, transtibial PCL reconstruction and presents the Fanelli Sports Injury Clinic 2- to 10-year results of PCL reconstruction with this technique. The information presented in this chapter has also been published elsewhere, and the reader is referred to these sources for additional information on this topic.[1,5-9,11-19,21,22]

SURGICAL INDICATIONS

The single-bundle/single–femoral tunnel, transtibial tunnel PCL reconstruction is an anatomic reconstruction of the anterolateral bundle of the PCL. The anterolateral bundle tightens in flexion, and this reconstruction reproduces that biomechanical function. Although the single-bundle/single–femoral tunnel, transtibial tunnel PCL reconstruction does not reproduce the broad anatomic insertion site of the normal PCL, certain factors lead to success with this surgical technique:
1. Identification and treatment of all pathology (especially posterolateral instability)
2. Accurate tunnel placement
3. Anatomic graft insertion sites
4. Strong graft material
5. Minimization of graft bending
6. Final tensioning at 70 to 90 degrees of knee flexion
7. Graft tensioning (e.g., with the Arthrotek mechanical tensioning device)
8. Primary and backup fixation
9. Appropriate rehabilitation program

Our indications for surgical treatment of acute PCL injuries include insertion site avulsions, tibial step-off decreased 10 mm or greater, and PCL tears combined with other structural injuries. Our indications for surgical treatment of chronic PCL injuries are isolated PCL tears that become symptomatic and the development of progressive functional instability.

SURGICAL TECHNIQUE

Patient Positioning and Initial Setup

The patient is positioned on the operating table in the supine position, and the surgical and nonsurgical knees are examined under general anesthesia. A tourniquet is applied to the operative extremity, and the surgical leg is prepared and draped in sterile fashion. Allograft tissue is prepared before beginning the surgical procedure, whereas autograft tissue is harvested before beginning the arthroscopic portion of the procedure. The arthroscopic instruments are inserted with the inflow through the superior lateral patellar portal, the arthroscope in the inferior lateral patellar portal, and the instruments in the inferior medial patellar portal. The portals are interchanged as necessary. The joint is thoroughly evaluated arthroscopically and the PCL evaluated via the three-zone arthroscopic technique.[14] The PCL tear is identified, and the residual stump of the PCL is débrided with hand tools and a synovial shaver.

Initial Incision

An extracapsular posteromedial safety incision approximately 1.5 to 2.0 cm long is created (Fig. 48–1). The crural fascia is incised longitudinally, with precautions taken to protect the neurovascular structures. The interval is developed between the medial head of the gastrocnemius muscle (posterior) and the posterior capsule of the knee joint (anterior). The surgeon's gloved finger is positioned so that the neurovascular structures are posterior to the finger and the posterior aspect of the joint capsule is anterior to the finger. This technique enables the surgeon to monitor surgical instruments such as the over-the-top PCL instruments and the PCL-ACL drill guide as they are positioned in the posterior aspect of the knee. The surgeon's finger in the posteromedial safety incision also confirms accurate placement of the guide wire before tibial

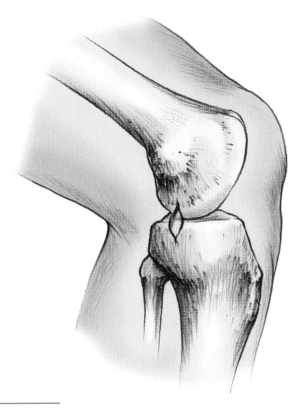

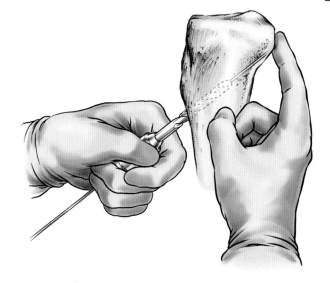

Figure 48–2. The surgeon is able to palpate the posterior aspect of the tibia through the extracapsular, extra-articular posteromedial safety incision. Palpation enables the surgeon to accurately position guide wires, create the tibial tunnel, and protect the neurovascular structures. (Courtesy of Arthrotek, Inc., Warsaw, IN.)

Figure 48–1. Posteromedial extra-articular extracapsular safety incision. (Courtesy of Arthrotek, Inc., Warsaw, IN.)

tunnel drilling in the medial-lateral and proximal-distal directions (Fig. 48–2).

Posterior Capsule Elevation

The curved, over-the-top PCL instruments are used to carefully lyse adhesions in the posterior aspect of the knee and to elevate the posterior knee joint capsule away from the tibial ridge on the posterior aspect of the tibia. This capsular elevation enhances correct drill guide and tibial tunnel placement (Fig. 48–3).

Drill Guide Positioning

The arm of the Arthrotek Fanelli PCL-ACL drill guide is inserted into the knee through the inferomedial patellar portal and positioned in the PCL fossa on the posterior aspect of the tibia (Fig. 48–4). The bullet portion of the drill guide contacts the anteromedial aspect of the proximal end of the tibia approximately 1 cm below the tibial tubercle, at a point midway between the tibial crest anteriorly and the posterior medial border of the tibia. This drill guide positioning creates a tibial tunnel that is relatively vertically oriented and has its posterior exit point in the inferior and lateral aspect of the PCL tibial anatomic insertion site. This positioning creates an angle of graft orientation such that the graft will turn two very smooth 45-degree angles on the posterior aspect of the tibia,

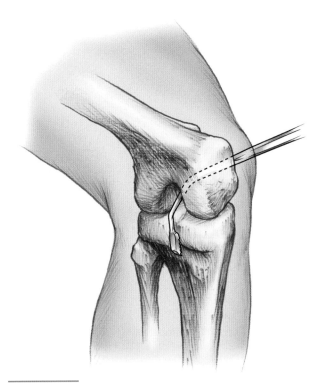

Figure 48–3. Posterior capsular elevation using the Arthrotek PCL instruments. (Courtesy of Arthrotek, Inc., Warsaw, IN.)

thereby eliminating the "killer turn" of 90-degree graft angle bending (Fig. 48–5).

The tip of the guide in the posterior aspect of the tibia is confirmed with the surgeon's finger through the extracapsular posteromedial safety incision. Intraopera-

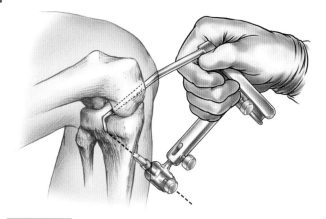

Figure 48–4. Arthrotek Fanelli PCL-ACL drill guide positioned to place a guide wire in preparation for creation of the transtibial PCL tibial tunnel. (Courtesy of Arthrotek, Inc., Warsaw, IN.)

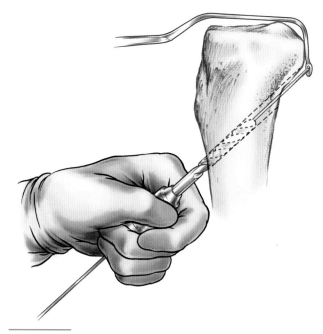

Figure 48–6. The Arthrotek PCL closed curet is used to cap the guide wire during tibial tunnel drilling. (Courtesy of Arthrotek, Inc., Warsaw, IN.)

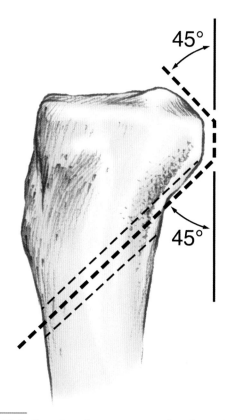

Figure 48–5. Drawing demonstrating the desired turning angles that the PCL graft will make after creation of the tibial tunnel. (Courtesy of Arthrotek, Inc., Warsaw, IN.)

tive anteroposterior and lateral radiographs may also be used, as well as arthroscopic visualization, to confirm drill guide and guide pin placement. A blunt, spade-tipped guide wire is drilled in an anterior-to-posterior direction and can be visualized with the arthroscope, in addition to being palpated with the finger in the posteromedial safety incision. We consider the finger in the posteromedial safety incision the most important step for accuracy and safety.

Tibial Tunnel Drilling

The appropriately sized, standard cannulated reamer is used to create the tibial tunnel. A closed, curved PCL curet may be positioned to cap the tip of the guide wire (Fig. 48–6). The arthroscope, when positioned in the posteromedial portal, visualizes the guide wire being captured by the curet and protecting the neurovascular structures, in addition to the surgeon's finger in the posteromedial safety incision. The surgeon's finger in the posteromedial safety incision is monitoring the position of the guide wire. The standard cannulated drill is advanced to the posterior cortex of the tibia. The drill chuck is then disengaged from the drill, and completion of the tibial tunnel reaming is performed by hand. This sequence gives an additional margin of safety for completion of the tibial tunnel. The tunnel edges are chamfered and rasped with the PCL-ACL system rasp (Fig. 48–7).

Femoral Tunnel Drilling

The Arthrotek Fanelli PCL-ACL drill guide is positioned to create the femoral tunnel (Fig. 48–8). The arm of the guide is introduced into the knee through the inferomedial patellar portal and positioned such that the guide wire will exit through the center of the stump of the anterolateral bundle of the PCL. The blunt, spade-tipped guide wire is drilled through the guide, and just as it begins to emerge through the center of the stump of the anterolateral bundle of the PCL, the drill guide is disengaged. The accuracy of guide wire position is confirmed arthroscopically by probing and direct visualization. Care must be taken to

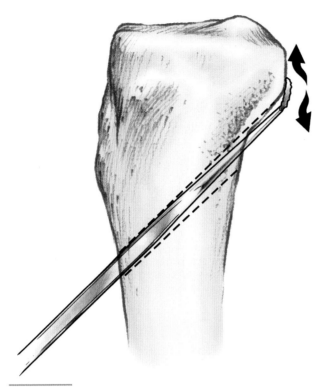

Figure 48–7. The tunnel edges are chamfered after drilling to smooth any rough edges. (Courtesy of Arthrotek, Inc., Warsaw, IN.)

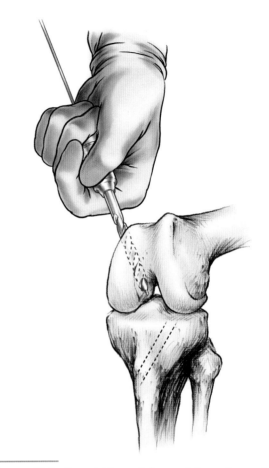

Figure 48–9. Completion of femoral tunnel reaming by hand for an additional margin of safety. (Courtesy of Arthrotek, Inc., Warsaw, IN.)

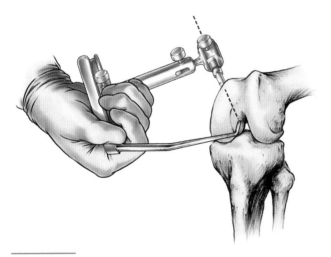

Figure 48–8. The Arthrotek Fanelli PCL-ACL drill guide is positioned to drill the guide wire from outside in. The guide wire begins at a point halfway between the medial femoral epicondyle and the medial femoral condyle trochlea articular margin, approximately 2 to 3 cm proximal to the medial femoral condyle distal articular margin, and exits through the center of the stump of the anterolateral bundle of the PCL. (Courtesy of Arthrotek, Inc., Warsaw, IN.)

the tip of the guide so that inadvertent advancement of the guide wire does not cause damage to the articular surface, the ACL, or other intra-articular structures. As the reamer is about to penetrate the wall of the intercondylar notch, it is disengaged from the drill, and the final femoral tunnel reaming is completed by hand for an additional margin of safety (Fig. 48–9). The reaming debris is evacuated with a synovial shaver to minimize any fat pad inflammatory response and a subsequent risk of arthrofibrosis. The tunnel edges are chamfered and rasped.

Tunnel Preparation and Graft Passage

The Arthrotek Magellan suture-passing device is introduced through the tibial tunnel and into the knee joint and retrieved through the femoral tunnel with an arthroscopic grasping tool (Fig. 48–10). A 7.9-mm Gore-Tex Smoother (W.L. Gore, Inc., Flagstaff, AZ) flexible rasp may be used and, when used, is attached to the Magellan suture-passing device; the Gore-Tex Smoother is then pulled into the femoral tunnel, into the joint, and into and out the tibial tunnel opening (Fig. 48–11). The tunnel edges are chamfered and rasped at 0, 30, 60, and 90 degrees of knee flexion. Care must be taken to

ensure that the patellofemoral joint has not been violated by arthroscopically examining the patellofemoral joint before drilling the femoral tunnel.

The appropriately sized standard cannulated reamer is used to create the femoral tunnel. A curet is used to cap

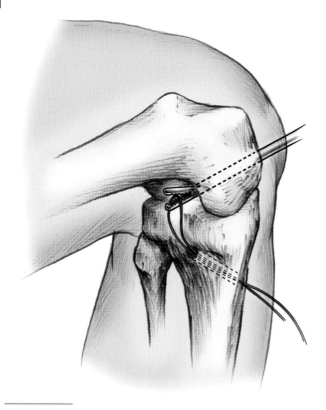

Figure 48–10. Retrieval of suture-passing wire. (Courtesy of Arthrotek, Inc., Warsaw, IN.)

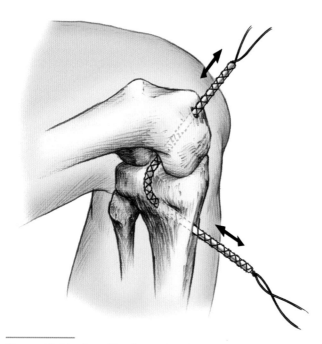

Figure 48–11. Gore-Tex Smoother flexible rasp in position. Note the tibial tunnel position, which allows a smooth transition of the graft around the posterior aspect of the proximal end of the tibia. Proper tibial tunnel positioning completely eliminates the effects of graft attrition around sharp tunnel edges. (Courtesy of Arthrotek, Inc., Warsaw, IN.)

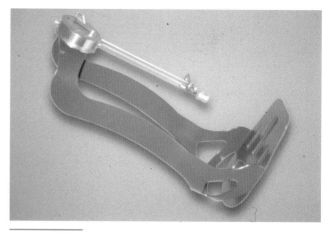

Figure 48–12. Arthrotek knee ligament graft tensioning boot. This mechanical tensioning device uses a ratcheted torque wrench device to assist the surgeon during graft tensioning. (Courtesy of Arthrotek, Inc., Warsaw, IN.)

avoid excessive pressure with the Gore-Tex Smoother, or the tunnel configuration could be altered or the bone destroyed. The traction sutures of the graft material are attached to the loop of the flexible rasp, and the PCL graft material is pulled into position.

Graft Tensioning and Fixation

Fixation of the PCL substitute is accomplished with primary and backup fixation on both the femoral and tibial sides. Our preferred graft source for PCL reconstruction is an Achilles tendon allograft. Femoral fixation is accomplished with press-fit fixation of a wedge-shaped calcaneal bone plug and aperture opening fixation with the Arthrotek Gentle Thread bioabsorbable interference screw, or primary aperture opening fixation is accomplished with the Arthrotek Gentle Thread bioabsorbable interference screw and backup fixation with a ligament fixation button, screw and spiked ligament washer, or screw and post assembly when there is no bone plug on the Achilles tendon allograft. The Arthrotek tensioning boot is applied to the traction sutures of the graft material on its distal end, set for 20 lb, and the knee cycled through 25 full flexion-extension cycles for graft pretensioning and settling (Fig. 48–12). The knee is placed in approximately 70 degrees of flexion, and tibial fixation of the Achilles tendon allograft is achieved via primary aperture opening fixation with the Arthrotek Gentle Thread bioabsorbable interference screw and backup fixation with a ligament fixation button or a screw and post or screw and spiked ligament washer assembly (Fig. 48–13).

Additional Surgery

When multiple ligament surgeries are performed at the same operative session, PCL reconstruction is

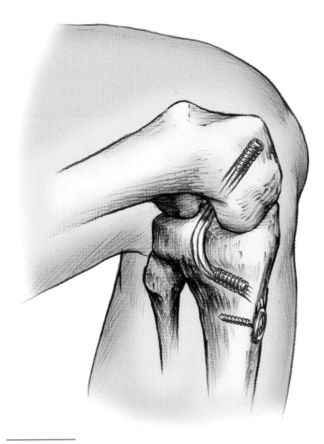

Figure 48–13. Final graft fixation with primary and backup fixation. (Courtesy of Arthrotek, Inc., Warsaw, IN.)

performed first, followed by ACL reconstruction and then collateral ligament surgery. One surgical technique for posterolateral reconstruction is split biceps tendon transfer to the lateral femoral epicondyle. Requirements for this procedure include an intact proximal tibiofibular joint, intact posterolateral capsular attachments to the common biceps tendon, and intact biceps femoris tendon insertion into the fibular head. This technique creates a new popliteofibular ligament and lateral collateral ligament, tightens the posterolateral capsule, and provides a post of strong autogenous tissue to reinforce the posterolateral corner.

A lateral hockey stick incision is made. The peroneal nerve is dissected free and protected throughout the procedure. The long head and common biceps femoris tendon is isolated, and the anterior two-thirds is separated from the short head muscle. The tendon is detached proximally and left attached distally to its anatomic insertion site on the fibular head. The strip of biceps tendon should be 12 to 14 cm long. The iliotibial band is incised in line with its fibers, and the fibular collateral ligament and popliteus tendons are exposed. A hole is drilled 1 cm anterior to the femoral insertion of the fibular collateral ligament. A longitudinal incision is made in the lateral capsule just posterior to the fibular collateral ligament. The split biceps tendon is passed medial to the iliotibial band and secured to the lateral femoral epicondylar region with a screw and spiked ligament washer at the aforementioned point. The residual tail of the transferred split biceps tendon is passed

medial to the iliotibial band and secured to the fibular head. The posterolateral capsule that had previously been incised is then shifted and sewn into the strut of transferred biceps tendon to eliminate posterolateral capsular redundancy. In cases in which the proximal tibiofibular joint has been disrupted, a two-tailed allograft reconstruction is used to control the tibia and fibula independently.

Posterolateral reconstruction with the free graft figure-of-eight technique uses semitendinosus autograft or allograft, Achilles tendon allograft, or other soft-tissue allograft material. A curvilinear incision is made in the lateral aspect of the knee and extends from the lateral femoral epicondyle to the interval between Gerdy's tubercle and the fibular head. The fibular head is exposed and a tunnel created in an anterior-to-posterior direction at the area of maximal fibular diameter. The tunnel is created by passing a guide pin followed by a cannulated drill, usually 7 mm in diameter. The peroneal nerve is protected during tunnel creation and throughout the procedure. The free tendon graft is then passed through the fibular head drill hole. An incision is next made in the iliotibial band in line with the fibers directly overlying the lateral femoral epicondyle. The graft material is passed medial to the iliotibial band, and the limbs of the graft are crossed to form a figure of eight. A hole is drilled 1 cm anterior to the femoral insertion of the fibular collateral ligament. A longitudinal incision is made in the lateral capsule just posterior to the fibular collateral ligament. The graft material is passed medial to the iliotibial band and secured to the lateral femoral epicondylar region with a screw and spiked ligament washer at the aforementioned point. The posterolateral capsule that had previously been incised is then shifted and sewn into the strut of the figure-of-eight graft tissue to eliminate posterolateral capsular redundancy. The anterior and posterior limbs of the figure-of-eight graft material are sewn to each other to reinforce and tighten the construct. The iliotibial band incision is closed. The procedures described are intended to eliminate posterolateral and varus rotational instability (Fig. 48–14).

Posteromedial and medial reconstructions are performed through a medial hockey stick incision. Care is taken to maintain adequate skin bridges between incisions. The superficial medial collateral ligament (MCL) is exposed and a longitudinal incision made just posterior to the posterior border of the MCL. Care is taken to not damage the medial meniscus during the capsular incision. The interval between the posteromedial capsule and medial meniscus is developed. The posteromedial capsule is shifted anterosuperiorly. The medial meniscus is repaired to the new capsular position, and the shifted capsule is sewn into the MCL. When superficial MCL reconstruction is indicated, it is performed with allograft tissue or semitendinosus autograft. This graft material is attached at the anatomic insertion sites of the superficial MCL on the femur and tibia. The posteromedial capsular advancement is performed and sewn into the newly reconstructed MCL (Fig. 48–15). At the completion of the procedure, the tourniquet is deflated and the wounds copiously irrigated. The incisions are closed in standard fashion.

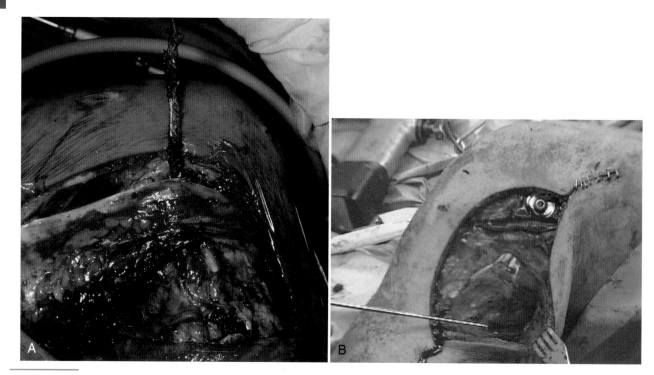

Figure 48–14. The surgical technique for posterolateral and lateral reconstruction involves the use of split biceps tendon transfer (**A**) or allograft or autograft figure-of-eight reconstruction (**B**) combined with posterolateral capsular shift and primary repair of the injured structures as indicated. These complex surgical procedures reproduce the function of the popliteofibular ligament and the lateral collateral ligament and eliminate posterolateral capsular redundancy. The split biceps tendon transfer uses anatomic insertion sites and preserves the dynamic function of the long head and common biceps femoris tendon. (Courtesy of Gregory C. Fanelli, M.D.)

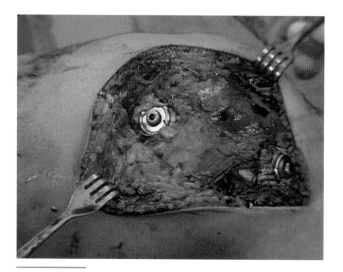

Figure 48–15. Severe medial side injuries are successfully treated by primary repair with a suture anchor technique, combined with medial collateral ligament (MCL) reconstruction with allograft tissue and a posteromedial capsular shift procedure. The Achilles tendon allograft's broad anatomy can anatomically reconstruct the superficial MCL. The Achilles tendon allograft is secured to the anatomic insertion sites of the superficial MCL with screws and spiked ligament washers. The posteromedial capsule can then be secured to the allograft tissue to eliminate posteromedial capsular laxity. This technique will address all components of the medial side instability (Courtesy of Gregory C. Fanelli, M.D.).

POSTOPERATIVE REHABILITATION

The knee is kept locked in a long-leg brace in full extension for 6 weeks with non-weightbearing and the use of crutches. Progressive range of motion occurs during weeks 4 through 6. The brace is unlocked at the end of 6 weeks, and progressive weightbearing is initiated at 25% body weight per week during postoperative weeks 7 through 10. The crutches are discontinued at the end of postoperative week 10. Progressive closed kinetic chain strength training and continued-motion exercises are performed. Return to sports and heavy labor occurs after the sixth to ninth postoperative month, when sufficient strength, range of motion, and proprioceptive skills have returned.

FANELLI SPORTS INJURY CLINIC RESULTS

We have previously published the results of our arthroscopically assisted combined ACL/PCL and PCL/posterolateral complex reconstructions using the reconstructive technique described in this chapter.[12,13,15,16] Our most recently published 2- to 10-year results of combined ACL/PCL reconstructions are presented here.[12]

This study presented the 2- to 10-year results of 35 arthroscopically assisted combined ACL/PCL reconstructions evaluated preoperatively and postoperatively with the Lysholm, Tegner, and Hospital for Special Surgery (HSS) knee ligament rating scales; KT-1000 arthrometer testing; stress radiography; and physical examination.

This study population included 26 males and 9 females with 19 acute and 16 chronic knee injuries. Ligament injuries included 19 ACL/PCL/posterolateral instabilities, 9 ACL/PCL/MCL instabilities, 6 ACL/PCL/posterolateral/MCL instabilities, and 1 ACL/PCL instability. All knees had grade 3 preoperative ACL/PCL laxity and were assessed preoperatively and postoperatively by arthrometry testing, three different knee ligament rating scales, stress radiography, and physical examination. Arthroscopically assisted combined ACL/PCL reconstructions were performed by using the single-incision endoscopic ACL technique and the single–femoral tunnel/single-bundle transtibial tunnel PCL technique. PCLs were reconstructed with Achilles tendon allografts (26), bone–patellar tendon–bone (BTB) autografts (7), and semitendinosus/gracilis autografts (2). ACLs were reconstructed with BTB autografts (16), BTB allografts (12), Achilles tendon allografts (6), and a semitendinosus/gracilis autograft (1). MCL injuries were treated with bracing or open reconstruction. Posterolateral instability was treated by biceps femoris tendon transfer, with or without primary repair, and posterolateral capsular shift procedures as indicated.

Postoperative physical examination revealed normal posterior drawer/tibial step-off in 16 of 35 (46%) knees. Lachman and pivot-shift tests were normal in 33 of 35 (94%) knees. Posterolateral stability was restored to normal in 6 of 25 (24%) knees and tighter than the normal knee in 19 of 25 (76%) knees evaluated with the external rotation thigh foot angle test. Thirty-degree varus stress testing was normal in 22 of 25 (88%) knees, with grade 1 laxity present in 3 of 25 (12%) knees. Thirty-degree valgus stress testing was normal in 7 of 7 (100%) surgically treated MCL tears and normal in 7 of 8 (87.5%) brace-treated knees. The postoperative mean side-to-side difference by KT-1000 arthrometer testing was 2.7 mm (PCL screen), 2.6 mm (corrected posterior), and 1.0 mm (corrected anterior), a statistically significant improvement from the preoperative status ($p = .001$). The postoperative stress radiographic side-to-side difference at 90 degrees of knee flexion and 32 lb of posteriorly directed proximal force was 0 to 3 mm in 11 of 21 (52.3%), 4 to 5 mm in 5 of 21 (23.8%), and 6 to 10 mm in 4 of 21 (19%) knees. Postoperative Lysholm, Tegner, and HSS knee ligament rating scale mean values were 91.2, 5.3, and 86.8, respectively, a statistically significant improvement from preoperative status ($p = .001$).

The conclusions drawn from the study were that combined ACL/PCL instabilities could be successfully treated with arthroscopic reconstruction and the appropriate collateral ligament surgery. Statistically significant improvement from the preoperative condition was noted at 2- to 10-year follow-up with the use of objective parameters of knee ligament rating scales, arthrometer testing, stress radiography, and physical examination. Postoperatively, these knees are not normal, but they are functionally stable. Continuing technical improvements will most likely improve future results.

Another group of multiple-ligament reconstructions that warrant attention are our 2- to 10-year results of combined PCL-posterolateral reconstruction.[18] This study presented the 2- to 10-year results of 41 chronic, arthroscopically assisted combined PCL/posterolateral reconstructions evaluated preoperatively and postoperatively with the Lysholm, Tegner, and HSS knee ligament rating scales; KT-1000 arthrometer testing; stress radiography; and physical examination.

This study population included 31 males and 10 females with 24 left and 17 right chronic PCL/posterolateral knee injuries with functional instability. The knees were assessed preoperatively and postoperatively by arthrometer testing, three different knee ligament rating scales, stress radiography, and physical examination. PCL reconstructions were performed with the arthroscopically assisted, single–femoral tunnel/single-bundle, transtibial tunnel PCL reconstruction technique using fresh frozen Achilles tendon allografts in all 41 cases. Reconstruction for posterolateral instability was performed with combined biceps femoris tendon tenodesis and posterolateral capsular shift procedures in all cases. The paired t-test and power analysis were the statistical tests used. Ninety-five percent confidence intervals were used throughout the analysis.

Postoperative physical examination revealed normal posterior drawer/tibial step-off in 29 of 41 (70.7%) knees in the overall group and normal posterior drawer and tibial step-off in 11 of 12 (91.7%) knees tensioned with the Arthrotek tensioning boot. Posterolateral stability was restored to normal in 11 of 41 (26.8%) knees and tighter than the normal knee in 29 of 41 (70.7%) knees evaluated with the external rotation thigh foot angle test. Thirty-degree varus stress testing was normal in 40 of 41 (97.6%) knees, with grade 1 laxity present in 1 of 41 (2.4%) knees. Postoperative mean side-to-side differences by KT-1000 arthrometer testing were 1.80 mm (PCL screen), 2.11 mm (corrected posterior), and 0.63 mm (corrected anterior). These measurements represent a statistically significant improvement from preoperative status for the PCL screen and the corrected posterior measurements ($p = .001$). The postoperative stress radiographic mean side-to-side difference at 90 degrees of knee flexion and 32 lb of posterior-directed force applied to the proximal end of the tibia with the Telos device was 2.26 mm, a statistically significant improvement from preoperative measurements ($p = .001$). Postoperative Lysholm, Tegner, and HSS knee ligament rating scale mean values were 91.7, 4.92, and 88.7, respectively, a statistically significant improvement from preoperative status ($p = .001$).

Conclusions drawn from this study were that chronic combined PCL/posterolateral instabilities could be successfully treated by arthroscopic PCL reconstruction with fresh frozen Achilles tendon allograft combined with posterolateral corner reconstruction via biceps tendon transfer and a posterolateral capsular shift procedure. Statistically significant improvement from the preoperative condition ($p = .001$) was noted at 2- to 10-year follow-up with the use of objective parameters of knee ligament rating scales, arthrometer testing, stress radiography, and physical examination.

ALTERNATIVE POSTERIOR CRUCIATE LIGAMENT RECONSTRUCTION SURGICAL TECHNIQUES

Two alternative surgical techniques for PCL reconstruction are the tibial inlay technique and the double-bundle, double–femoral tunnel technique. Theoretic advantages of the tibial inlay technique include elimination of acute graft angle turns at the tibial tunnel opening, easier graft passage, protection of neurovascular structures, a shorter graft creating a stiffer construct, and ease of revision PCL surgery. Potential disadvantages of the tibial inlay technique include lateral or prone positioning, posterior incisions, difficult future hardware removal, and graft tunnel mismatch. Promising clinical results with this technique have been published.[2]

The double-bundle, double–femoral tunnel PCL reconstruction technique attempts to more closely reproduce the broad femoral anatomic insertion site of the native PCL. This technique endeavors to reconstruct both the anterolateral and posteromedial bundles of the PCL. Personal communication with experienced PCL surgeons indicates promising clinical results; however, there are currently no long-term clinical studies published.

COMPLICATIONS

PCL reconstruction is technically demanding surgery. Complications encountered with this surgical procedure include failure to recognize associated ligament injuries, neurovascular problems, persistent posterior sag, osteonecrosis, knee motion loss, anterior knee pain, and fractures.[8,17-20] A comprehensive preoperative evaluation, including an accurate diagnosis, a well-planned and carefully executed surgical procedure, and a supervised postoperative rehabilitation program, will help reduce the incidence of these complications.

Our PCL-related reconstructions have included ACL/PCL reconstructions, PCL/posterolateral corner reconstructions, ACL/PCL/posterolateral reconstructions, ACL/PCL/MCL reconstructions, and PCL/MCL reconstructions. Our complications include loss of flexion requiring arthroscopic lysis of adhesions and manipulation (5 cases), removal of painful prominent hardware used for graft fixation (21 cases), and superficial suture abscess (1 case). We have had no incidence of nerve injuries, vascular injuries, deep infections, fractures, osteonecrosis, or skin slough complications. Our clinical results evaluated with the Lysholm, Tegner, and HSS knee ligament rating scales and KT 1000 arthrometer have previously been published.[12,13,15,16]

Analysis of our patients with loss of flexion requiring arthroscopic lysis of adhesions and manipulation is as follows. The first patient had ACL, PCL, MCL, and posterolateral complex tears and an acutely dislocated patella. Repair/reconstruction of all four ligaments plus extensor mechanism repair was performed as an open procedure. Adhesions developed and required arthroscopic adhesiolysis and manipulation. The second case was a patient with right knee ACL/PCL/MCL tears and an ipsilateral tibial shaft fracture. The tibial shaft fracture was treated by open reduction and internal fixation with a plate and screws. The MCL was treated in a brace for 6 weeks and healed with normal valgus stability. Arthroscopic combined ACL/PCL reconstruction was then performed with a double-loop semitendinosus/gracilis hamstring autograft and a BTB autograft. Suprapatellar pouch adhesions developed postoperatively and required arthroscopic adhesiolysis and manipulation.

Case 3 was a 20-year-old patient with a right PCL/posterolateral complex tear combined with a hip fracture and multiple fractures of the foot. The fractures were addressed by open reduction and internal fixation, followed by arthroscopic PCL/posterolateral complex reconstruction with BTB autograft and biceps tendon transfer. Postoperative suprapatellar pouch adhesions developed but responded well to arthroscopic lysis of the adhesions and manipulation.

Cases 4 and 5 were females aged 15 and 22 with PCL/posterolateral complex tears (one acute, one chronic); they underwent arthroscopic PCL/posterolateral reconstruction with an Achilles tendon allograft and Clancy biceps tendon tenodesis in one case and a BTB autograft and split biceps tendon transfer in the second case. Suprapatellar pouch adhesions developed in both patients postoperatively and required arthroscopic lysis of the adhesions and manipulation. Both patients returned to full unrestricted activity with stable knees.

We were not able to identify any trends to predict the patients in whom motion loss might develop postoperatively, with the exception of arthrotomy versus arthroscopy. Arthrotomy seems more likely to be associated with postoperative range-of-motion problems. However, motion loss developed and required surgical intervention and manipulation in only 5 of 92 (5.4%) patients, thus indicating a low rate for this complication.

CONCLUSIONS

The arthroscopically assisted, single-bundle transtibial PCL reconstruction technique is a reproducible surgical procedure. It has documented results demonstrating statistically significant improvements from preoperative to postoperative status as evaluated by physical examination, knee ligament rating scales, arthrometer measurements, and stress radiography. Factors contributing to the success of this surgical technique include identification and treatment of all pathology (especially posterolateral instability), accurate tunnel placement, placement of strong graft material at anatomic graft insertion sites, minimization of graft bending, final graft tensioning at 70 to 90 degrees of knee flexion with the Arthrotek graft tensioning boot, use of primary and backup fixation, and implementation of the appropriate postoperative rehabilitation program. Alternative techniques for PCL reconstruction such as the tibial inlay technique and the double-bundle, double–femoral tunnel technique provide additional methods for treating PCL injuries. As PCL surgeons we should be prepared to perform any and all of the PCL reconstructive operations, especially in the context of revision PCL surgery.

References

1. Arthrotek PCL Reconstruction Surgical Technique Guide. Fanelli PCL-ACL Drill Guide System. Warsaw, IN, Arthrotek, Inc., 1998.
2. Cooper DE, Stewart D: Posterior cruciate ligament reconstruction using single bundle patella tendon graft with tibial inlay fixation. 2 to 10 year follow-up. Am J Sports Med 32:346-360, 2004.
3. Daniel DM, Akeson W, O'Conner J (eds): Knee Ligaments—Structure, Function, Injury, and Repair. New York, Raven Press, 1990.
4. Fanelli GC: PCL injuries in trauma patients. Arthroscopy 9:291-294, 1993.
5. Fanelli GC: Point counter point. Arthroscopic posterior cruciate ligament reconstruction: Single bundle/single femoral tunnel. Arthroscopy 16:725-731, 2000.
6. Fanelli GC: Arthroscopic evaluation of the PCL. In Fanelli GC (ed): Posterior Cruciate Ligament Injuries. A Guide to Practical Management. New York, Springer-Verlag, 2001, pp 95-108.
7. Fanelli GC: Arthroscopic PCL reconstruction: Transtibial technique. In Fanelli GC (ed): Posterior Cruciate Ligament Injuries. A Guide to Practical Management. New York, Springer-Verlag, 2001, pp 141-156.
8. Fanelli GC: Complications in PCL surgery. In Fanelli GC (ed): Posterior Cruciate Ligament Injuries. A Guide to Practical Management. New York, Springer-Verlag, 2001, pp 291-302.
9. Fanelli GC: Combined ACL-PCL-medial-lateral side injuries of the knee. In Fanelli GC (ed): The Multiple Ligament Injured Knee. A Guide to Practical Management. New York, Springer-Verlag, 2004, pp 111-132.
10. Fanelli GC, Edson CJ: PCL injuries in trauma patients. Part II. Arthroscopy 11:526-529, 1995.
11. Fanelli GC, Edson CJ: Management of posterior cruciate ligament and posterolateral instability of the knee. In Chow J (ed): Advanced Arthroplasty. New York, Springer-Verlag, 2001.
12. Fanelli GC, Edson CJ: Arthroscopically assisted combined ACL/PCL reconstruction. 2-10 year follow-up. Arthroscopy 18:703-714, 2002.
13. Fanelli GC, Edson CJ: Combined posterior cruciate ligament–posterolateral reconstruction with Achilles tendon allograft and biceps femoris tendon tenodesis: 2-10 year follow-up. Arthroscopy 20:339-345, 2004.
14. Fanelli GC, Giannotti B, Edson C: Current concepts review. The posterior cruciate ligament: Arthroscopic evaluation and treatment. Arthroscopy 10:673-688, 1994.
15. Fanelli GC, Giannotti BF, Edson CJ: Arthroscopically assisted combined anterior and posterior cruciate ligament reconstruction. Arthroscopy 12:5-14, 1996.
16. Fanelli GC, Giannotti B, Edson C: Arthroscopically assisted posterior cruciate ligament/posterior lateral complex reconstruction. Arthroscopy 12:521-530, 1996.
17. Fanelli GC, Monahan TJ: Complications of posterior cruciate ligament reconstruction. Sports Med Arthrosc Rev 7:296-302, 1999.
18. Fanelli GC, Monahan TJ: Complications and pitfalls in posterior cruciate ligament reconstruction. In Malek MM, Fanelli GC, Johnson D, Johnson D (eds): Knee Surgery: Complications, Pitfalls, and Salvage. New York, Springer-Verlag, 2001.
19. Fanelli GC, Monahan TJ: Complications in posterior cruciate ligament and posterolateral complex surgery. Op Tech Sports Med 9:96-99, 2001.
20. Fanelli GC, Orcutt DR: Complications in posterior cruciate ligament reconstruction. Sports Med Arthrosc Rev 12:196, 2004.
21. Malek MM, Fanelli GC: Technique of arthroscopic PCL reconstruction. Orthopedics 16:961-966, 1993.
22. Miller MD, Cooper DE, Fanelli GC, et al: Posterior cruciate ligament: Current concepts. Instr Course Lect 51:347-351, 2002.

CHAPTER 49

The Dislocated Knee

Anikar Chhabra • John J. Klimkiewicz • Russell S. Petrie
Christopher D. Harner

Traumatic knee dislocations are serious injuries with devastating complications secondary to damage to multiple soft-tissue and stabilizing structures. Associated injuries may include the cruciate ligaments, collateral ligaments, medial and lateral capsular structures, menisci and articular cartilage, neurovascular injuries, and compartment syndrome. Because of the potential devastating complications from a missed knee dislocation, these injuries require timely and accurate diagnosis, stabilization, and treatment. Historically, these injuries occur predominantly from motorcycle and car accidents versus pedestrian accidents and football injuries.[22,52] Low-velocity knee dislocations also are prevalent, however.

In the acute setting, treatment goals include prompt reduction of the knee joint and, if necessary, revascularization. The severity of these injuries is emphasized by the fact that, despite modern vascular reconstructive techniques, 13% of knee dislocations result in amputation secondary to vascular compromise.[12] Although the need for treatment of arterial injury is well documented and accepted, the method of classifying and treating the ligamentous component of these injuries remains controversial. Limitations of studies addressing this area include small sample sizes, retrospective evaluations, and multiple treatment and rehabilitation protocols. Comparison of studies is complicated by the fact that classification according to the actual structures injured is not uniform among reports. Kennedy[23] described his classification according to the direction of the tibia in relation to the femur. More recently, an anatomically based classification has been proposed that more accurately reflects the degree of injury.[49,67] Lastly, the outcome analyses, with a few exceptions, often do not address return to high-level athletics, the ultimate test of knee function.[52,56]

Nonoperative management is the traditional treatment of choice because good results have been reported with cast immobilization.[60] This belief has changed, however, as history has shown that nonoperative treatment results in poor outcomes. More recently, with advances in ligament reconstruction and primary collateral ligament repair or reconstruction, better results have been shown.[46,52,56]

It is difficult to conceive that a knee with chronic bicruciate deficiency over the long-term would have a better result than a knee having undergone cruciate reconstruction, although this possibility exists. The trend in orthopedic surgery has been to address ligamentous instability after knee dislocations by early reconstruction or repair, typically with autograft or allograft tissue, and aggressive rehabilitation. This early reconstruction or repair is done to achieve the greatest stability of the knee and to minimize loss of motion. Surgical treatment remains controversial with respect to timing of surgery, specific surgical techniques, which structures to repair versus reconstruct, and choice of grafts.

Because of the severity of these injuries, the patient must undergo an extensive preoperative workup to discern the details of the injury and to ensure the patient is medically stable for surgery. Inherent in this evaluation is detailed attention to factors that may predicate emergent surgical intervention. Evaluation in the trauma bay revealing an open dislocation, irreducible dislocation, or arterial injury requires an emergent trip to the operating room. In the case of arterial injury, an orthopedic surgeon is helpful in the execution of the vascular repair because external fixation may be needed to stabilize the vascular graft. In addition, the location of future incision sites for ligamentous reconstruction should be discussed with the vascular surgeon. Recovery of associated soft tissue injury dictates the ability to perform later reconstruction or repair of the ligaments.

INCIDENCE

The rate of knee dislocations has been reported to be 0.001% to 0.013% per year at various institutions.[17,33,48,54] True incidence data are difficult to obtain, however, because it is now appreciated that approximately 50% of knee dislocations reduce spontaneously and are not diagnosed at time of injury.[37,38] A dislocation should be suspected in a knee with gross instability of two or more ligaments after trauma, despite a reduced joint on radiographs.[52] Subsequent evaluation and treatment should be performed on the assumption that a dislocation has occurred.[22]

MECHANISM

Knee dislocations occur as a result of severe direct or indirect violence to the knee. Most of these injuries occur as a result of vehicular accidents.[22] Knee dislocations also occur as a result of sports-related trauma. Shelbourne and colleagues[52] reported that the most commonly involved sports are football (35%), wrestling (15%), and running (10%).

Distinguishing between high-velocity trauma, such as automobile accidents, and low-velocity, sports-related injuries may have prognostic value because low-velocity injuries may be less severe. Shelbourne and colleagues,[52] in their series of low-velocity injuries, noted a lower incidence of vascular injuries (4.6%) than was reported by Green and Allen[12] (32%) in their series, in which high-velocity trauma was the inciting traumatic event.

VASCULAR INJURIES

The incidence of vascular injuries associated with knee dislocations varies in the literature from 4.6% to 80%.[17,21,52] If arterial injury is suspected in a multiligament-injured knee, its presence and subsequent treatment should take precedence over musculoskeletal management. Timing is critical for such an injury, and the existence of ischemic compromise to an extremity after reduction mandates emergent exploration by a vascular surgeon to restore arterial flow.[11,22,37,63] Green and Allen[12] showed the necessity of restoring the arterial blood supply in a timely fashion, as 86% of patients treated after 8 hours from the time of injury required amputation. This compares with an amputation rate of 13% when arterial repair is performed within 8 hours.

The popliteal artery is the main blood supply to the lower leg and is the vascular structure requiring attention. The popliteal artery traverses the popliteal space and is tethered to the femur proximally at the adductor hiatus and distally by the fibrous arch covering the soleus (Fig. 49–1).[37] Within the popliteal space, the medial superior, lateral superior, medial inferior, lateral inferior, and middle geniculate arteries branch from the popliteal artery. These vessels do not provide adequate collateral flow to the lower extremity in the case of a severe popliteal artery injury.[12]

For a limb to be considered vascularly competent, the pedal pulses must be normal to palpation after reduction. Normal pulses do not rule out a vascular injury, however. A foot that is warm with good capillary refill with abnormal pulses is considered to have a major vascular injury and requires immediate attention. Capillary refill is a poor indicator of vascular viability because significantly less blood flow is required to sustain the skin than the muscle.[63] Failure of the pulses to return to normal by palpation after reduction should not be attributed to vascular spasm in this setting.[12] Given the known incidence of vascular injuries associated with knee dislocations and the severe consequences of delayed treatment, all potential vascular injuries in this setting should be evaluated fully and treated aggressively.

Vascular injuries are typically either a traction injury with intimal tearing or a complete disruption. Kennedy[23] pointed out that anterior dislocations are more likely associated with intimal injuries because the vessel is stretched over the distal femur. He showed that popliteal artery injury occurs at 50 degrees of hyperextension (Fig. 49–2A). Vascular insufficiency in this setting may present acutely or in a delayed fashion because clot can form slowly on the injured intimal wall, resulting in occlusion hours or days after injury. Posterior dislocations are more likely, however, to be associated with complete artery disruption (Fig. 49–2B). Vascular injury can occur with all types of dislocations and can present in a delayed fashion. Repeated vascular examinations are necessary for at least the first 24 hours after injury.[63]

Multiple studies have focused on evaluation of vascular injury in knee dislocations. We, along with many other surgeons, advocate arteriography in all suspected knee dislocations, to avoid the potential devastating complications of a missed vascular injury.[46] Other authors have published studies questioning the need for arteriography in the face of a normal neurovascular examination. Mills and associates[35] published a study looking at the value of

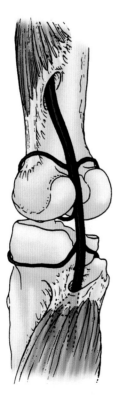

Figure 49–1. Anatomy of the popliteal artery posterior to the knee joint. (From Bloom MH: Traumatic knee dislocation. In Chapman MW: Operative Orthopaedics. Philadelphia, JB Lippincott, 1988, p. 1636.)

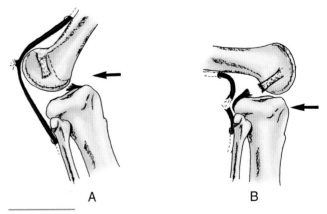

A   B

Figure 49–2. Mechanism for popliteal artery injury for anterior **(A)** and posterior **(B)** dislocations.

the ankle-brachial index (ABI) in diagnosing arterial injury in the dislocated knee. In a prospective study comprising 38 patients with acute knee dislocations, 11 were found to have ABIs of less than 0.90, and 27 had ABIs of greater than 0.90. The authors found that all 11 patients with ABIs less than 0.90 had vascular injuries requiring surgical treatment, whereas none of the 27 patients with ABIs greater than 0.90 were found to have vascular injury on either clinical examination or duplex ultrasound. Mills and associates[35] reported sensitivity, specificity, and positive predictive value of 100% for an ABI of less than 0.90 and a negative predictive value of 100% for an ABI greater than 0.90.

Other more recent studies have looked at the clinical neurovascular examination as a predictor of vascular injury. Klineberg and colleagues[25] reported a retrospective series of 57 knee dislocations, in which 32 had a normal vascular examination compared with the contralateral side (including ABIs), and 25 had abnormal examinations. None of the 32 knees with initially normal vascular examinations were found later to have vascular damage requiring surgical intervention. As such, the authors determined that all knee dislocations might not require arteriography if the initial neurovascular examination is normal. These data were corroborated by a study by Stannard and coworkers[58] that looked at the role of physical examination in determining the need for arteriography. They used an algorithm in which all affected limbs were examined carefully for dorsalis pedis and posterior tibial pulses and were examined grossly for color and temperature. Any patients who had an examination that was asymmetric with respect to the contralateral side underwent subsequent arteriography. None of the patients with an initially normal vascular examination went on to have vascular complications requiring intervention. Stannard and coworkers[58] recommended the selective use of arteriography in an acutely dislocated knee.

No clear consensus has been met regarding the need for angiography in the evaluation of the dislocated knee. Regardless of whether it is a standard policy to pursue angiography in all patients with knee dislocations versus selectively ordering studies based on serial examination findings, all patients with a suspected dislocation require close attention to vascular status to avoid potentially devastating consequences.

NEUROLOGICAL INJURY

Neurological injury also has been reported in 16% to 50% of knee dislocations.[33,54,67] Although most common in posterolateral dislocations, injury to the peroneal or posterior tibial nerve has been reported in all types of dislocations. The peroneal nerve is at greater risk because it is held tightly against the fibular head, whereas the tibial nerve is free within the popliteal space (Fig. 49–3). Most often a traction-type mechanism affecting the common peroneal nerve causes varying degrees of neurological injury, ranging from neurapraxia to axonotmesis. Treatment options for nerve dysfunction vary depending on the nature and degree of the injury.

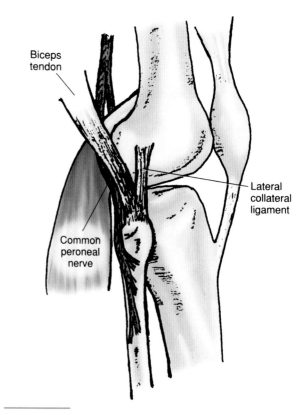

Figure 49–3. Anatomy of peroneal nerve near the knee joint.

CLASSIFICATION

Two accepted classification systems describe knee dislocations: descriptive and anatomic. These classifications can help in predicting associated injuries and planning surgical intervention.

Descriptive

Historically, knee dislocations have been classified according to the direction of the tibia in relation to the femur.[23] Commonly, five types are described: anterior, posterior, medial, lateral, and rotatory (Fig. 49–4). Common associated injuries include popliteal artery intimal tears with anterior dislocations, popliteal artery disruptions with posterior dislocations, and peroneal nerve injury with posterolateral dislocations (i.e., rotatory injuries). These associations are by no means absolute. Neurological and vascular injuries have been described with every type of dislocation.

This classification system is limited by the fact that spontaneous reductions are known to occur, and unless the patient or a witness can describe the mechanism of injury accurately, the type of dislocation remains unknown. Additionally, this classification does not help with planning the reconstructive procedure because the degree of injury to the individual ligaments can vary dramatically.

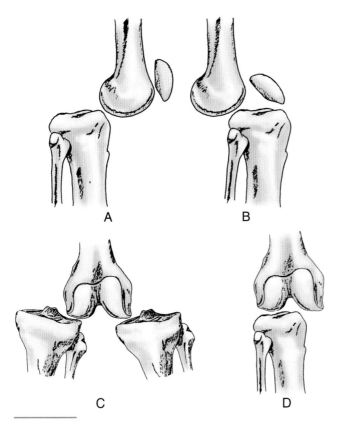

Figure 49–4. Descriptive classification system of knee joint dislocations. **A,** Posterior. **B,** Anterior. **C,** Medial or lateral. **D,** Rotatory.

ANTERIOR DISLOCATION

In their series, Green and Allen[12] found that anterior dislocations account for about 40% of knee dislocations. It is thought that the mechanism is hyperextension. Because the anterior cruciate ligament (ACL) is the primary structure preventing anterior displacement of the tibia, it is always disrupted. Biomechanical studies have shown that, with hyperextension, the posterior capsule ruptures first, followed by the ACL and the posterior cruciate ligament (PCL).[40] At approximately 50 degrees of hyperextension, the popliteal artery sustains injury.[23] Arterial injury in this setting is typically a traction injury causing an intimal tear, which can lead to acute or delayed thrombosis.

The force required to produce an anterior dislocation may be high or low energy. Anterior dislocations have been described after multiple mechanisms, ranging from vehicular trauma to simply missing a step.

POSTERIOR DISLOCATION

Posterior dislocation accounts for slightly fewer dislocations (33%) than its anterior counterpart (40%).[23] In contrast to anterior dislocation, posterior dislocation requires a significant force, which may be the reason it is less frequent. In his biomechanical study, Kennedy[23] had difficulty producing a posterior dislocation. These dislocations most commonly are associated with automobile accidents as "dashboard" injuries. In this setting, a seated passenger's proximal tibia is driven into the dashboard, creating a posteriorly directed force on the flexed knee.

The PCL is the primary stabilizer to posterior tibial translation; by definition, it is disrupted in these injuries. The ACL is frequently torn, although there are reports of posterior dislocation without ACL disruption.[54] Injury to the medial collateral ligament (MCL) and lateral collateral ligament (LCL) varies. Appreciating the degree of injury to the collateral ligaments helps with preoperative planning.

Injury to the popliteal artery in this setting traditionally has been described as a transection injury, as the posteriorly translated tibia tears the popliteal artery owing to the fact that it is constrained proximally and distally. Intimal tears also can occur with posterior dislocations, however.

MEDIAL AND LATERAL DISLOCATIONS

Medial and lateral dislocations are considerably less common, accounting for 18% and 4% of all dislocations.[12] It is difficult to produce pure ligamentous medial and lateral dislocation injuries experimentally. Most case reports describe high-energy varus or valgus trauma. Pure ligamentous injuries are perhaps the exception and not the rule, as many people have fractures associated with these injuries.

In contrast to anterior and posterior dislocations, in medial and lateral dislocations, both collateral ligaments are injured and at least one of the cruciate ligaments. Lateral dislocations can be additionally problematic because they can be irreducible as a result of infolding of the MCL.

ROTATORY DISLOCATION

Rotatory dislocations account for about 5% of knee dislocations and are produced by a rotational force.[12] Rotation occurs around one of the collateral ligaments, with rupture of both cruciate ligaments and the other collateral ligament. The most common rotatory dislocation is the posterolateral dislocation.[16] This type of dislocation can be irreducible as a result of "buttonholing" of the medial femoral condyle through the capsule and invagination of the MCL. Physical examination is remarkable for subcutaneous palpation of the medial femoral condyle and a furrow or skin dimple along the medial joint line (Fig. 49–5). Attempted reduction may accentuate these physical findings. Expeditious open reduction is indicated in this setting because prolonged vascular compromise to the overlying skin may result in significant skin loss.

Some dislocations cannot be classified according to the descriptive schema. Other times, classification is impossible because spontaneous reduction may occur.

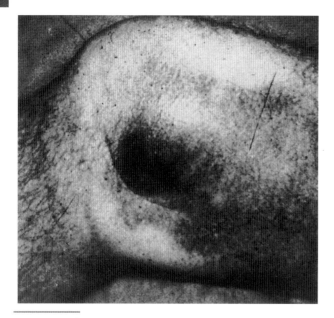

Figure 49–5. Irreducible posterolateral knee dislocation with characteristic dimple of skin. (From Reckling FW, Peltier LF: Acute knee dislocations and their complications. J Trauma 9:181, 1969.)

Anatomic

More recently, classification of knee dislocations has focused on which structures are injured and the degree to which these structures are injured (e.g., total versus partial tear).[49] This system facilitates preoperative planning with respect to specifying the structures requiring attention. There are significant differences in the healing potential between the MCL and LCL.[52] The MCL heals much more readily than the LCL, and instability is much less of a problem with the MCL.[52] MCL avulsions off the tibia heal less readily, however, than MCL avulsions off the femur. Stiffness in flexion can be a problem with operative repair of the MCL. Knowing and understanding these differences and appreciating the full extent of the injury can help with surgical approach and timing when addressing these injuries.

This classification system is limited by the difficulty in obtaining an accurate examination in the face of a severely traumatized knee. Often, despite the physical examination and MRI, the true extent of the injury may not be appreciated until an examination under anesthesia is performed. Nevertheless, some recognized patterns of injury have been established. Typically, the ACL and PCL are disrupted, although this is not universally true (case reports of knee dislocations without either an ACL or a PCL tear have been published[4,7]). Common recognized patterns include injury to the following: ACL/PCL/MCL, ACL/PCL/LCL, ACL/PCL/posterolateral corner (PLC), ACL/PCL/LCL/PLC, and ACL/PCL/LCL/PLC/MCL.[18]

EVALUATION

Acute knee dislocations require an expeditious but thorough evaluation consisting of a targeted history and physical examination, with particular attention to the mechanism of injury and potential associated injuries. Evaluation of patients with multiple ligamentous injuries to the knee requires a high index of suspicion to exclude the possibility of knee dislocation with spontaneous reduction. Figure 49–6 shows our algorithm for the evaluation and management of these injuries. After clearance by the trauma team of any life-threatening or associated injuries, a directed physical examination of the knee should be performed, looking for any signs of gross dislocation. It is imperative to perform and document a detailed neurovascular examination at the time of initial evaluation, before reduction, and after reduction because a significant number of knee dislocations lead to injury of the popliteal artery or the peroneal nerve. The extremity distal to the involved knee should be examined thoroughly for color, temperature, and capillary refill. Posterior tibial and dorsalis pedis pulses should be palpated and compared with the contralateral side. The ABI and arteriography play important roles in assessing potential vascular injury. In any case in which popliteal artery injury is suspected, an early and urgent consultation with the vascular surgery team is needed. Also, the presence of pulses does not definitively rule out a vascular injury. With regards to the peroneal nerve, sensation in the distribution of the superficial and deep peroneal nerves should be assessed, and peroneal nerve motor function should be graded and documented. After performing a detailed history and physical examination, initial radiographs should be obtained to determine the direction of dislocation and to look for concomitant osseous injury.

The rapid increase in amputation rate in cases of ischemia beyond 8 hours must be kept in mind when deciding whether and where to obtain an arteriogram (e.g., in the angioplasty suite versus the operating room). Depending on the center, significant delays can occur with obtaining arteriograms not performed in the operating room. It is advisable to obtain an arteriogram in the operating room, should one be deemed necessary in these cases. Valuable ischemia time is preserved without adding the additional delay of performing this study in the radiology suite. Vascular injury takes precedence over musculoskeletal injury in the acute setting, and the role of the orthopedic surgeon may be limited to reducing the joint and applying external fixation.

Because greater than 50% of acute knee dislocations may reduce spontaneously in the field, it is imperative to have a high index of suspicion. In any knee injury resulting in laxity of two or more of the major knee ligaments, a dislocation must be suspected. Any knee that is found to be grossly dislocated requires an urgent neurovascular examination, followed by reduction via traction/countertraction under conscious sedation. Postreduction neurovascular status must be assessed, documented, and followed closely. After reduction, the limb should be stabilized in a long-leg splint.

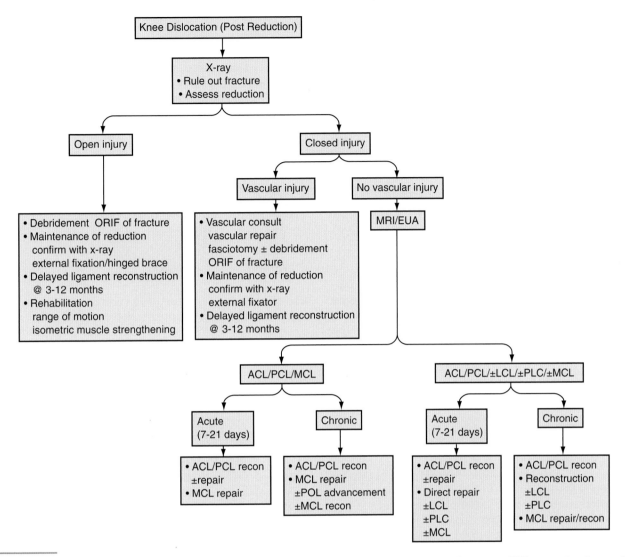

Figure 49–6. Evaluation and management of the dislocated knee. ACL, anterior cruciate ligament; EUA, examination under anesthesia; LCL, lateral collateral ligament; MCL, medial collateral ligament; ORIF, open reduction with internal fixation; PCL, posterior cruciate ligament; PLC, posterolateral corner; POL, posterior oblique ligament; recon, reconstruction.

When the patient is medically stable and a complete neurovascular evaluation is performed, more attention can be focused on the ligamentous damage to the knee. In the acute setting, it often is difficult to perform a thorough clinical examination because of the significant pain and edema. The usual tests for ligamentous laxity should be performed. The gold standard for testing of the ACL is the Lachman test, performed with the knee in 30 degrees of flexion.[8] The PCL integrity is tested with the posterior drawer and sag tests.[30,34] The collateral ligaments are tested with varus/valgus stress to the knee joint in full extension and 30 degrees of flexion.[8] PLC injuries should be evaluated by the external rotation dial test at 30 and 90 degrees.[30]

Radiographs should be obtained to confirm a reduction and to look for any associated bony injuries. MRI to evaluate these injuries is performed when the patient has been acutely stabilized. MRI enables one to visualize and characterize better the pattern of soft-tissue and occult osseous injury.[44,57,70] The actual site of cruciate and collateral liga-ment injury (i.e., avulsion versus midsubstance rupture) can be defined and be of tremendous help in planning operative reconstruction or primary repair. Also, MRI enables visualization of a potential meniscal disorder and the status of the popliteus tendon in suspected injuries to the PLC.[70] This study always is obtained at our institution before operative reconstruction, and we have found it extremely useful in planning our operative approach.

TREATMENT

The treatment of dislocations of the knee has been slow to evolve, secondary to the low incidence and hetero-geneity of these injuries. As Meyers and Harvey[32] stated in 1971, "It is, therefore, unlikely that any single physician personally cares for more than a few of these injuries in a lifetime of practice." Consequently, many different treat-ment recommendations, nonoperative and operative, have been proposed with differing rehabilitation protocols. Although there is no consensus on the exact method of treatment for these injuries, more recent studies have emphasized early operative stabilization. The following sections analyze the early results of nonoperative management along with the more contemporary results of different surgical techniques for stabilizing acute knee dislocations. Additionally, we address the indications for acute operative management and the approach to neurovascular injuries that frequently accompany these injuries. Finally, we describe in detail our approach to evaluating and treating knee dislocations.

Urgent Surgical Intervention

Several instances require immediate surgical intervention. As mentioned earlier, any evidence for vascular injury requires the immediate attention by a vascular surgeon. Patients with prolonged vascular compromise also should undergo fasciotomies at the time of revascularization. Open dislocations demand immediate surgical attention, with serial irrigation and débridements, intravenous antibiotics, and soft-tissue coverage procedures as needed.[46] Ligament repair or reconstruction should be delayed until the soft-tissue envelope has healed, especially in the face of complex soft-tissue reconstructions.

Irreducible dislocations provide a unique case in which urgent surgical intervention is required. The most commonly described irreducible dislocation is posterolateral with buttonholing of the medial femoral condyle through the medial joint capsule with subsequent invagination of the capsule into the joint.[64] Multiple other causes of irreducible knee dislocation have been described; several case reports include interposition of the vastus medialis,[26] muscular buttonholing,[24] and interposed menisci.[3]

Nonoperative Management

Immediate reduction and casting at one time was the preferred treatment. Much of the support for this approach was based on the experience of Taylor and colleagues,[60] who described 26 cases without neurovascular injury in 1972. After immediate reduction, these patients were immobilized in slight flexion for approximately 6 weeks, then given aggressive physical therapy. Eighteen of 26 patients were judged as having good results with this approach, as defined by motion of 90 degrees or more of flexion, in combination with a stable, painless knee. Only two patients had a poor result by their criteria, mainly as a result of stiffness. Based on this study, at that time, nonoperative treatment was thought to be the method of choice for uncomplicated knee dislocations. Subsequently, many studies have criticized the clinical outcome measurements chosen to evaluate these patients, questioning the proper method of treatment.

An infrequently reported complication of nonoperative treatment is chronic dislocation. To date, this complication has received little attention in the literature, likely because of its rare occurrence. Henshaw and associates[15] reported on one case treated by operative reduction and crossed Steinmann pin stabilization with a resultant 5 to 40 degrees range of motion. More recently, Simonian and colleagues[55] reported two cases of chronic posterior dislocation treated with operative reduction, ligament (ACL and PCL) reconstruction, and application of a hinged external fixator, with a resultant better final range of motion of 0 to 90 degrees. Petrie and coworkers[43] reported two additional cases of chronic posterior dislocation with arthrosis and severe bone loss treated with a semiconstrained total knee arthroplasty. Final range of motion in both patients was 10 to 90 degrees; neither patient had significant pain or instability at follow-up.

Operative Management

Historically, various types of operative stabilization have been proposed for treatment of knee dislocations with generally good results.[2,10,32,33,56] It has been difficult, however, to establish a consensus regarding these injuries: These reports generally contain few patients with different degrees of knee injury approached in different ways. Early reports emphasized primary ligamentous repair of collateral and cruciate ligament injuries. This recommendation later was modified for cruciate injuries as described by Marshall and colleagues,[31] in which ligament repair was performed with multiple looped sutures brought out through drill holes in the tibia and femur.[37,56] Meyers and associates[33] recognized the shortcomings of these previous studies and, in 1975, published a follow-up article to their original report on 33 patients treated with immobilization (13 patients) or early ligamentous primary repair (20 patients). Outcomes were based on the patients' pain, stability, and ability to perform their previous occupation. The types of injuries in each group were thought to be equivalent and without complications. The patients who underwent early operative primary repair of all the ligamentous injuries had the best results as measured by the authors' criteria. Subsequently, other studies have supported this approach. Sisto and Warren[56] reported on 20 knee dislocations. Similarly, patients treated with early primary repair had results superior to those from immobilization. These authors stressed generally modest clinical results in both groups, however, and clinical instability was generally not a problem. Almekinders and Logan[2] also showed modest results for these injuries regardless of the treatment method employed. Although the operatively treated group seemed to have superior motion and increased objective stability in the anteroposterior plane compared with nonoperatively treated patients, resultant pain, swelling, and degenerative changes by radiographic criteria were similar for both groups.

As techniques in single-ligament surgery have advanced for isolated anterior and posterior cruciate intrasubstance ruptures, reconstruction (as opposed to primary ligamentous repair) has produced the best functional results.[5,6,42,51] A similar approach to multiligament surgery for knee dislocations using allograft and autograft tissue for intrasubstance cruciate rupture has been documented. Shapiro and

Freedman[50] reported on seven patients treated with early allograft stabilization of both cruciates in combination with primary repair of other injured structures. Results at 4 years were graded as good or excellent in six patients, with arthrofibrosis being the most common postoperative complication encountered in four patients. Similarly, Noyes and Barber-Westin[39] reported on 11 patients with combined allograft and autograft reconstruction for bicruciate knee dislocations. At 5 years' follow-up, 8 of 11 patients (73%) were asymptomatic with daily activities, and 6 of 11 returned to sporting activities. Reconstructive approaches to cruciate injury in knee dislocations involving only one of the two cruciate ligaments in combination with medial or lateral injuries have been reported with good results.[4,7]

More recent studies show improved outcomes for multiligament-injured knees with operative intervention. A retrospective study by Richter and associates[45] looked at 89 traumatic knee dislocations, 63 of which were treated surgically and 26 of which were treated conservatively. At an average follow-up of more than 8 years, the Lysholm and Tenger scores were found to be better in the surgical group. Functional rehabilitation after ligament repair/reconstruction was the most important prognostic factor. Another study by Rios and coworkers[47] looked at the results after 26 traumatic dislocations. Eight of the patients (31%) were determined to have a poor result based on the Lysholm scoring system. Five of the eight patients with poor results underwent conservative management because of associated visceral or skeletal injuries that made immediate surgery inadvisable. The other three poor results occurred in patients who underwent primary repair of avulsed LCL and posterolateral structures, without addressing the cruciate ligaments. Rios and coworkers[47] advocated acute reconstruction of all injured structures to allow for the best postoperative result. Wong and colleagues[69] also published a study showing superior results in knee dislocations treated operatively compared with conservative management. In addition, the operative group did not show any decreased range of motion compared with the conservative management group. The authors recommended surgical treatment with repair of all ligamentous structures to achieve the most stable knee and the greatest degree of patient satisfaction.[69] These studies confirm the current trend that acute ligament repair or reconstruction is indicated in all but the most severely debilitated patients to achieve the most stable, functional result.[1,9,50,69]

There are other reports in the literature with a slightly different operative approach to these injuries. Several authors recommend reconstructing only the PCL, with autograft or allograft tissue, in combination with primary medial or lateral ligament repair. These reports are based on Hughston's experience[19] of addressing the PCL first when both cruciate ligaments are ruptured. In doing so, one reestablishes the center of rotation on which to base all subsequent repairs.[19] This approach delays reconstruction of the ACL for a later time if persistent instability remains a problem. In approaching bicruciate knee dislocations in this manner, the risk of postoperative arthrofibrosis may be less. Advocates of this theory believe stability is much less a problem than knee stiffness and

pain.[56,62] Shelbourne and colleagues[52] reported on 16 low-velocity knee dislocations treated with reconstruction either of both cruciate ligaments or of only the PCL, in combination with anatomic medial or lateral repairs and aggressive postoperative therapy. The patients in this series who underwent isolated PCL reconstruction in combination with collateral repair had less postoperative stiffness compared with the simultaneous bicruciate reconstructions. Walker and associates[66] reported on nine patients treated in a similar manner in combination with aggressive postoperative physiotherapy. The average range of motion for these patients averaged 0 to 130 degrees at 3 years, with three patients (all with injury to the lateral structures in combination with ACL/PCL rupture) requiring manipulation at 4 weeks for flexion less than 90 degrees.

Vascular Injuries

Typically, treatment of an injury to the popliteal artery requires repair. The most popular method involves resection of the damaged portion of the vessel, with reverse saphenous vein interposition grafting. Four-compartment fasciotomy also should be performed at this time. The edema caused as a result of the vascular reconstruction and acute restoration of flow in combination with the magnitude of injury often associated with these injuries makes a fasciotomy crucial in these settings.[10] Injury to the popliteal vein, if present, also should be addressed, if possible. Repair of the ligamentous structures is unnecessary at this time because prolonged operative time and manipulation potentially could jeopardize the arterial repair. Reduction of the knee joint is mandatory, however. Often an external fixator can be placed before or after revascularization to ensure skeletal stability to protect the vascular repair. Definitive ligamentous repair often can be performed within the next 10 to 14 days without significant risk to the vascular structures, but this is controversial.[37]

Neurological Injuries

Treatment of neurological injuries remains controversial with comparably poor results regardless of treatment. Immediate and delayed treatment of nerve injuries varies, depending on the physician and setting. In general, recovery is unpredictable, with more than 50% of these injuries having residual (partial to complete) nerve damage.[27,56,59] In the acute setting, repair is not possible secondary to the diffuse nature of the injury without the presence of a specific lesion benefiting from repair. Most authors approach these injuries nonoperatively for the first 3 months after injury.[68] A patient with a footdrop should be treated with an ankle-foot orthosis to prevent an equinus contracture during the recovery phase. If spontaneous resolution does not occur, reconstructive procedures, including nerve grafting, tendon transfers, and permanent bracing, are considered at that time. Results of operative decompression of the peroneal nerve have been reported after an initial period of observation, showing improvement in 97% of the patients studied.[36] Although this study suggests better results with early exploration and decompression, this may be misleading. Only a small subset of the patients included in this study had traumatically induced peroneal nerve injuries, and direct comparisons should not be made with previous reports.

Our approach to these injuries in the acute setting involves exploration and decompression of the peroneal nerve at the time of the initial operative procedure. Postoperatively the foot is braced, and recovery is monitored during the next 3 months. If residual deficits are present at this time, tendon transfers are discussed with the patient. In our experience, nerve grafting has been less successful and has not been performed for these injuries.

Current Surgical Controversies

Although most authors currently agree that ligamentous instability necessitates surgical treatment, there is no consensus regarding the timing of surgery, the need for staging of the repair, which ligaments to repair or reconstruct, and which grafts to use. Some authors in the past advocated a staged ligamentous repair/reconstruction after knee dislocation as mentioned previously, with early PCL reconstruction followed by reconstruction of the ACL and lateral injuries several months later.[41] These authors cited a theoretically decreased risk of postoperative stiffness with a staged repair and reported good results at follow-up with full range of motion and no varus/valgus instability. We and many other authors believe that concomitant reconstruction of the ACL and PCL, with repair or reconstruction of the collaterals or PLC, can be done in the acute setting (<3 weeks) without increasing the risk of late arthrofibrosis.[14,28,69] Tissue quality, severity of the injury, and stability dictate the ability to repair the MCL, LCL, or PLC injury. If the repair is inadequate, it is augmented or reconstructed. This single-stage procedure eliminates the morbidity of a second surgical procedure. Several studies have shown good results with acute ligament repair or reconstruction. Liow and coworkers[28] looked at a series of 22 knee dislocations, 8 of which were treated with acute ligament repair/reconstruction (<2 weeks), whereas the remainder were reconstructed at greater than 6 months postinjury. They showed that at an average follow-up of 32 months, the mean Lysholm score was 87 in the acute group versus 75 in the delayed group. Likewise, the Tenger activity rating was 5 in the acute group versus 4.4 in the delayed group. In addition to the improved results in the acute group, Liow and coworkers[28] did not see an increased risk of arthrofibrosis in the acute group compared with the delayed group.

These results were corroborated by a study by Harner and associates.[14] Following knee dislocation, 31 patients were followed for a minimum of 24 months after operative management. Of these patients, 19 underwent acute repair/reconstruction (within 3 weeks), whereas the remaining 12 patients underwent delayed reconstruction. The mean Lysholm scores, Knee Outcome Survey Activities of Daily Living scores, and Knee Outcome Survey Sports Activity scores all were significantly higher in the acute group versus the delayed group. Overall, by the Meyers ratings, 23 patients had an overall excellent or good score, whereas 8 had a fair or poor score. Sixteen of 19 patients with acutely treated knees and 7 of 12 with delayed reconstructions achieved an excellent or good Meyers score. All poor results were found in the delayed reconstruction group. Additionally, there was no difference in the postoperative range of motion between the acute and delayed reconstruction groups. Laxity tests showed improved stability in all patients, with more predictable results seen in the acute surgical group. Overall, patients treated acutely within 3 weeks of injury showed better subjective ratings and objective knee stability than patients who underwent delayed reconstruction.

AUTHORS' APPROACH

The goals in treating knee dislocations include restoration of knee motion and stability. It is important to counsel the patient preoperatively regarding the severity of the injury and the expected outcomes. Associated injuries, patient age, and preoperative level of function often influence the ultimate result. From a technical perspective, variables including timing, operative technique, graft selection, and postoperative rehabilitation all are crucial components of the overall treatment plan. A generalized treatment algorithm is presented in Figure 49–7.

Timing

Optimal timing for repair of multiligamentous injuries to the knee that include the collateral ligaments is within 10 to 14 days from the time of injury. At this time, the soft tissues surrounding the knee have had an appropriate time to heal, and the knee's range of motion has been partially restored. Anatomic definition and repair of the collateral ligament structures is often possible at this time after initial injury. After reduction and confirmation of vascular integrity, the patient is placed into a long-leg hinged knee brace and is instructed to begin range-of-motion exercises in the brace in conjunction with quadriceps-strengthening exercises until definitive surgical treatment is performed. Because postoperative stiffness is a potential concern with early surgical intervention, patients are informed preoperatively that a later manipulation may be necessary. Although manipulation under anesthesia may be necessary in 50% of these injuries, rarely has further reoperation for stiffness been necessary.[27]

In the presence of collateral ligament injuries requiring surgical intervention, operative treatment can be delayed 3 weeks in the face of vascular or other associated injuries, without compromising the surgeon's ability to perform a primary repair. After this time, the surgical approach becomes more difficult secondary to the abundant scar formation that occurs, making anatomic reattachment of the collateral ligaments difficult and imprecise in nature.[59]

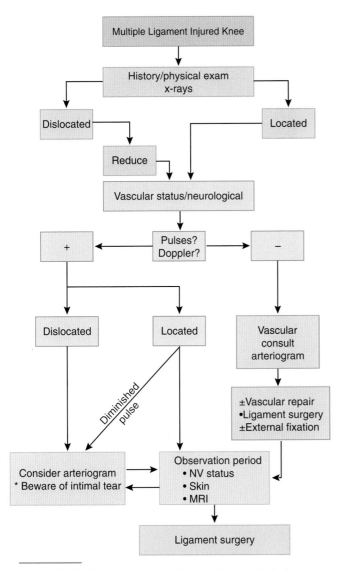

Figure 49–7. Treatment algorithm for the multiple-ligament injured knee. NV, neurovascular.

Reconstruction of the cruciate ligaments is less affected by such a delay. In situations where the sequence of events prohibits operative treatment before this time, it is best to take a more conservative approach to the knee, allowing full restoration of motion in a long-leg hinged brace before making further decisions regarding surgical treatment.

In the presence of any vascular injury, orthopedic management is secondary until vascular perfusion has been restored. The definitive repair of the ligamentous structures is a major undertaking requiring manipulation and dissection of the extremity that potentially could threaten the vascular repair if done simultaneously. Provided that normal perfusion has been reestablished, it is usually acceptable and safe to perform the definitive ligamentous repair at 10 to 14 days after the vascular repair.[21,37] The use of a tourniquet is intuitively unappealing in this setting because of the concern over iatrogenic thrombosis. For this reason, and owing to the length of these cases, we no longer use a tourniquet for any of these reconstructions.

Open injuries can occur in 20% to 30% of these injuries and require immediate surgical irrigation and débridement.[59] Ligament reconstruction in the presence of these injuries also should be delayed until the soft tissues allow a safe surgical approach. In severe soft-tissue injuries in which reconstruction is not possible within the first 3 weeks, it is better to treat these injuries nonoperatively until the patient regains full motion. Often in these cases it is necessary to obtain a plastic surgery consultation to assist in reconstructive efforts.

Anesthesia, Positioning, Surface Anatomy, and Examination Under Anesthesia

The choice of anesthesia is made in conjunction with the surgeon, the anesthesiologist, and the patient. It often depends on the age of the patient, the patient's comorbid medical problems, and the previous anesthesia history of the patient. Most commonly, we use general anesthesia or an epidural anesthetic with concomitant intravenous sedation. At our institution, preoperative femoral or sciatic nerve blocks or both are routinely performed as an adjunct for additional postoperative pain relief.[29,61] Additionally, we recommend that a vascular surgeon be "on call" during the procedure because unexpected injuries to the vessels may occur.

The patient is seen in the preoperative holding area, and the surgeon, patient, and nurse identify and mark the correct extremity. In the preoperative holding area, the status of the popliteal, dorsalis pedis, and posterior tibial pulses and the function of the tibial and peroneal nerves are documented.

The patient is placed in the supine position on the operating room table. Our goal is to have a full free range of motion of the knee during the procedure with the ability to have the knee statically flexed at 80 to 90 degrees without any manual assistance. We accomplish this by placing a small gel pad bump under the ipsilateral hip with a post placed on the side of the bed just distal to the greater trochanter; a sterile bump of towels or drapes is wedged between the post and the thigh. The heel rests on a 10-lb sandbag that is taped to the bed during the initial positioning with the knee at 90 degrees (Fig. 49–8).

A marker is used to identify the surface anatomy and the incisions that will be used during the procedure. The important osseous landmarks include the patella, the tibial tubercle, Gerdy's tubercle, and the fibular head. The peroneal nerve is palpated, and its course is marked superficial to the fibular neck. The medial and lateral joint lines are identified. The anterolateral arthroscopy portal is placed adjacent to the lateral border of the patella above the joint line. The anteromedial arthroscopy portal is placed approximately 1 cm medial to the patellar tendon at the same level. A superolateral outflow portal is placed proximal to the superior border of the patella and posterior to the quadriceps tendon. The posteromedial portal, if needed, is made under direct visualization from an inside-out technique and is not marked initially. A longitudinal 3-cm incision approximately 2 cm distal to the joint line and 2 cm medial to the tibial tubercle is drawn

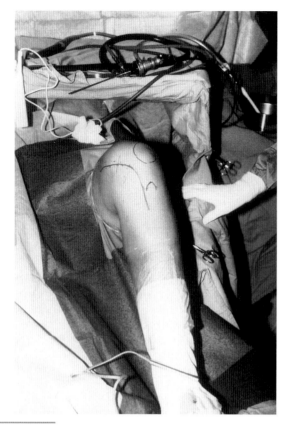

Figure 49–8. Supine operative positioning that includes a tourniquet, arthroscopic assistance, mini C-arm fluoroscopy, and intraoperative Doppler ultrasound capability, when indicated.

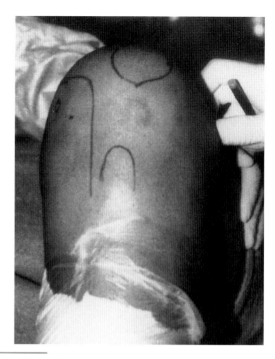

Figure 49–9. Skin incision for combined surgical exposure of a medial-sided injury, anterior cruciate ligament, and posterior cruciate ligament.

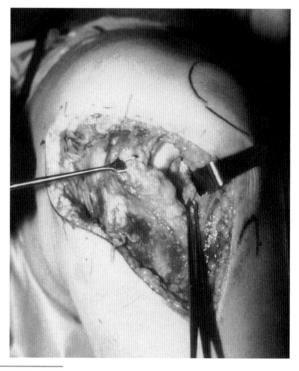

Figure 49–10. Skin incision for combined surgical exposure of a lateral-sided injury, anterior cruciate ligament, and posterior cruciate ligament.

on the anteromedial proximal tibia for the ACL and PCL tibial tunnels. Also, a 2-cm incision is placed medial to the medial trochlear articular surface along the subvastus interval for the PCL femoral tunnel. If there is a medial ligament injury, the distal incision for the tibial tunnels is traced proximally to the medial epicondyle and extended to the level of the vastus medialis in a curvilinear fashion (Fig. 49–9). The incision for the lateral and posterolateral injuries is a curvilinear 12-cm incision that is drawn midway between Gerdy's tubercle and the fibular head and traced proximally just inferior to the lateral epicondyle while the knee is flexed 90 degrees. The proximal extent of this incision parallels the plane between the biceps femoris tendon and the iliotibial band (Fig. 49–10). When both collateral ligaments are disrupted, we prefer the above medial and lateral incisions opposed to a midline incision owing to potential complications of skin breakdown over the patella and limited access to the collateral ligaments.

After successful induction of anesthesia in the operating room, a thorough examination under anesthesia is performed and correlated with the preoperative impression. It is crucial to examine the opposite extremity and use it as a reference. The knee range of motion is documented. The anterior drawer, Lachman's test, and pivot shift test reveal any deficits to the ACL. The PCL is examined by appreciating any posterior sag with associated step-off and by testing a posterior drawer at 90 degrees of flexion. The MCL is examined with a valgus stress at 0 and 30 degrees. The LCL is palpated in the figure-four position and tested with a varus stress at 0 and 30 degrees. The PLC, which consists of the LCL and the popliteus complex, is tested at 30 degrees and by holding the proximal tibia and externally rotating the leg. In addition, applying an external rotation force on the proximal tibia tests the PLC and fibula while the knee is flexed 90 degrees to feel for lateral dropout. Additionally, the mini C-arm fluoroscopy machine is in the operating suite and draped, and a sterile Doppler is used on the surgical field before the initial incision and throughout the case to confirm the presence of the dorsal pedis and posterior tibial pulses.

Surgical Approach

The two most common combined injury patterns with knee dislocations include the cruciate ligaments and MCL or the cruciate ligaments, LCL, and the PLC. Less commonly, the PCL is intact or only partially torn and does not require reconstruction. At our institution, we attempt to preserve specific bundles of the PCL that are not injured. Most commonly, we observe the anterolateral bundle ruptured, but the meniscofemoral ligament and the posteromedial bundle remain intact. If this injury pattern is present, we preserve the intact portion of the PCL and meniscofemoral ligament and simply reconstruct the ruptured portion via a single bundle technique.

Our approach is to reconstruct or repair all injured structures. The decision to repair or reconstruct the injured structures depends on numerous factors. Concerning cruciate injuries, most are intrasubstance tears that are not amenable to surgical repair and are treated best with ligament reconstruction. We recommend primary repair of ACL and PCL tibial avulsions, however, if a there is a large bony fragment. The primary repair can be accomplished by passing large nonabsorbable sutures into the bony fragment and through bone tunnels in the tibia. Also, a primary repair of the PCL insertion may be advocated in the case of a "peel off" or a soft-tissue avulsion of the PCL at its femoral insertion by a similar technique.

Concerning the MCL, LCL, and PLC, it is our experience that a primary repair is possible if performed within 3 weeks of injury. Chronic injuries are limited by scar formation and soft-tissue contractures and often require a ligament reconstruction. The MCL can be repaired directly with intrasubstance sutures or with suture anchors if avulsed off the bone. Repair of the PLC structures and the LCL can be accomplished with direct suture repair or by repair to bone via drill holes versus suture anchors. If direct repair is not possible because of the quality of the tissue, the involved structures should be augmented with hamstring tendons, biceps femoris, iliotibial band, or allograft; otherwise the involved structures should be reconstructed. In addition, concomitant injuries to the articular cartilage and menisci are operatively addressed at the time of surgery.

Graft Selection

There are many options for graft selection for the multiple-ligament knee injury. Graft choice is based on the extent of the injury, timing of the surgery, and experience of the surgeon. Autograft tissue may be harvested from the ipsilateral or contralateral extremity and has the advantage of better graft incorporation and remodeling. At our institution, we recommend the use of allograft over autograft in multiple-ligament reconstruction surgery. The advantages of using allograft tissue include decreased operative time, decreased skin incisions in a knee that has been severely traumatized, and no donor site morbidity.[53] We also believe that the use of allograft decreases pain and stiffness postoperatively. One must be willing to assume the risks of using allograft tissue, however, which include an increase in cost, a delay in the incorporation of the graft, and a risk of disease transmission.[13] When the grafts are fashioned, they are wrapped in a sponge and bathed in warm saline.

We prefer to use an allograft bone–patellar tendon–bone for ACL reconstructions. The bone–patellar tendon–bone allograft provides adequate biomechanical strength with rigid bony fixation at the femoral and the tibial attachment sites.

We recommend the use of Achilles tendon allograft for PCL reconstruction. If a double-bundle technique is indicated, an ipsilateral hamstring tendon (semitendinosus) autograft also is harvested. The allograft Achilles tendon is an attractive choice for reconstruction of the PCL because it is a long graft, it has a significant cross-sectional area, and it has a calcaneal bone plug that provides rigid fixation in the femoral tunnel.

The LCL is reconstructed with an Achilles tendon allograft with a calcaneal bone plug. The bone plug can be fixed into the LCL insertion at the fibula through a bone tunnel. We do not tubularize the tendon because it is often reinforced to the native LCL tissue. Alternatively the remaining bone–patellar tendon allograft may be used for the LCL reconstruction.

For the PLC, our graft choice for reconstructing the popliteofibular ligament (PFL) is a tibialis anterior soft-tissue allograft or an ipsilateral hamstring (semitendinosus) autograft. These are fashioned with a whipstitch on both ends.

Intra-articular Preparation

The arthroscope is introduced into the anterolateral portal, and gravity inflow is used with a superolateral outflow. Care must be taken to avoid a compartment syndrome, and the posterior leg and calf region must be palpated intermittently during the procedure. Factors that influence a potential compartment syndrome include an acute reconstruction (<2 weeks from the time of injury) in which the capsular healing was insufficient to maintain joint distention or if the capsule has been breeched iatrogenically during the procedure. If extravasation is noted, and a potential compartment syndrome is suspected, the arthroscopic technique is abandoned, and the remainder of the procedure is performed by an open technique.

All compartments within the knee are assessed. A posteromedial portal is needed to visualize the tibial insertion of the PCL completely. This portal is established under direct visualization by placing the 70-degree arthroscope into the anterolateral portal and through the intercondylar notch adjacent to the posterior aspect of the medial femoral condyle. The spinal needle and trocar is delivered just anterior to the saphenous nerve and vein.

When the intra-articular pathology is confirmed, any concomitant articular cartilage or meniscal injury is addressed. Every effort is made to preserve the meniscal tissue. Peripheral meniscal tears are repaired via the inside-out technique, whereas central or irreparable meniscal tears are débrided to a stable rim. Should the meniscus require a repair, the sutures are tied down directly onto the capsule at 30 degrees of flexion at the end of the procedure after the grafts are passed and secured.

The notch and the stumps of the torn cruciates are débrided, preserving any remaining intact PCL tissue as previously described. The tibial insertion of the PCL is removed by introducing a shaver or a curette or both into the posteromedial portal and gently developing the plane between the PCL and the posterior capsule, while looking through the anterolateral portal with a 70-degree arthroscope. Alternatively, the 30 degree arthroscope may be introduced through the posteromedial portal and a PCL curet and rasp may be introduced through the anterolateral or anteromedial portals. Every attempt is made to débride the distal-most aspect of the tibial insertion of the PCL because this helps with the eventual placement of the guide wire for the tibial tunnel.

Cruciate Tunnel Preparation, Graft Passage, and Proximal Fixation

We prefer to address the PCL tibial tunnel initially because it is the most dangerous portion of the procedure. We introduce an offset PCL guide via the anteromedial portal and place the tip of the guide at the distal and lateral third of the insertion site of the PCL on the tibia. A medial proximal tibia skin incision is made, and the periosteum is sharply dissected from the bone. The starting point of the Kirschner wire is approximately 3 to 4 cm distal to the joint line. The trajectory of the tibial PCL tunnel roughly parallels the angle of the proximal tibiofibular joint. We then pass a Kirschner wire into the desired position and perforate the far cortex of the tibia at the PCL insertion; this is done under direct arthroscopic visualization. Caution must be taken when passing the guide wire through the cortex of the tibial insertion of the PCL because of the close proximity of the neurovascular structures. Often the PCL tibial insertion site has a "cancellous feel" when the far cortex is breached, and no hard cortex can be felt while the Kirschner wire is advanced. The location of this pin placement is confirmed with the mini C-arm fluoroscopy machine on the true lateral projection of the knee (medial and lateral condyles of the femur are overlapping). Occasionally the wire is too proximal on the PCL tibial insertion site, and a 3-mm or a 5-mm parallel pin guide is used to obtain the ideal placement of the PCL tibial tunnel. The Kirschner wire for the PCL tibial tunnel is left in place, and attention is turned to the ACL tibial tunnel.

The ACL tibial guide is introduced into the anteromedial portal, and a guide wire is placed in the center of the ACL tibial footprint. The guide wire should rest posterior to Blumensaat's line on the full extension lateral mini C-arm projection to ensure proper placement of the ACL tibial tunnel. The ACL tibial tunnel is proximal and anterior to the PCL tibial tunnel.

After acceptable placement of the ACL and PCL tibial tunnel guide wires is confirmed (Fig. 49–11), the PCL tunnel is drilled to the desired graft size. A curet is placed directly on top of the guide wire over the area of the drill site. The PCL tibial tunnel is expanded using dilators in 0.5-mm increments to the size of the graft. Next the ACL tibial tunnel is drilled in a similar manner. We prefer at least a 1- to 2-cm bone bridge between the ACL and PCL tibial tunnels anteriorly on the tibia (Fig. 49–12).

Attention is then turned to the ACL and PCL femoral tunnels. For a single-bundle PCL reconstruction, the insertion of the PCL on the intercondylar notch is identified, and the Kirschner wire is placed from the anterolateral portal to a point approximately 7 to 10 mm from the articular margin within the anterior portion of the PCL femoral footprint. The Kirschner wire is overdrilled, and the tunnel is dilated to the size of the graft by 0.5-mm increments. If a double-bundle PCL reconstruction is chosen (in the delayed setting), the anterolateral tunnel is drilled at the 1 o'clock position approximately 5 to 6 mm

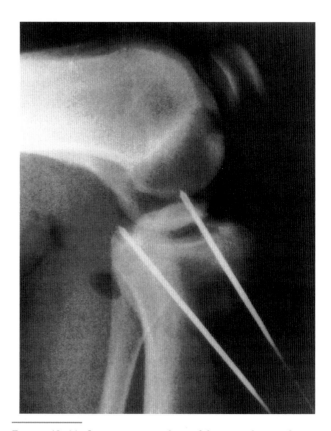

Figure 49–11. Intraoperative lateral knee radiograph confirms proper placement of anterior cruciate ligament and posterior cruciate ligament tunnels.

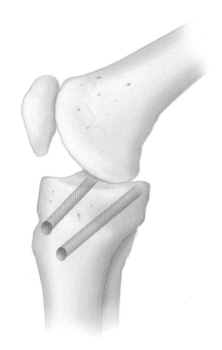

Figure 49–12. Lateral knee schematic shows anterior cruciate ligament and posterior cruciate ligament tibial tunnels.

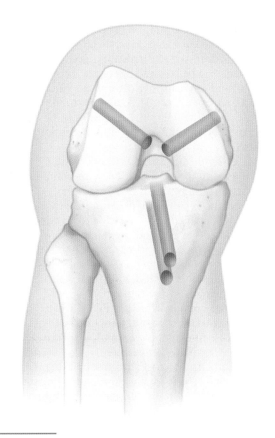

Figure 49–13. Anteroposterior knee schematic shows anterior cruciate ligament and posterior cruciate ligament femoral and tibial tunnels.

off the articular cartilage, and the posteromedial bundle is placed at the 3 to 4 o'clock position approximately 4 mm off the articular cartilage. These tunnels are drilled to a depth of 25 to 30 mm.

The ACL femoral tunnel is established while the knee is flexed to 120 degrees. The anteromedial portal is used to introduce the Kirschner wire into the desired position on the posterolateral portion of the intercondylar notch. The Kirschner wire is placed in the center of the anatomic insertion of the ACL, which is approximately 6 mm anterior to the back wall or over the top position of the femur and at the 2 and 10 o'clock positions for left and right knees. We prefer the medial portal technique to the traditional transtibial technique because the location of the femoral tunnel is not limited by the position or angulation of the tibial tunnel (Fig. 49–13). If there is any question about femoral tunnel placement, the mini C-arm fluoroscopic machine is used for visualization.

The Achilles allograft PCL graft is passed first. A long looped 18-gauge wire is passed retrograde into the PCL tibial tunnel and retrieved out the anterolateral arthroscopy portal with a pituitary rongeur. The no. 5 suture that has secured the tendon portion of the graft is shuttled into the joint with the looped 18-gauge wire via the anterolateral portal and antegrade down the PCL tibial tunnel to exit on the anteromedial tibia. The calcaneus portion of the graft is passed out the anteromedial femur via a Beath pin through the PCL femoral tunnel and out the anteromedial thigh. With arthroscopic assistance, a probe is used to direct the graft in the joint to facilitate passage of the graft.

The ACL graft is passed using the medial portal technique. The Beath pin with a no. 5 suture attached to the eyelet is passed through the femoral tunnel via the medial portal. A pituitary rongeur is passed retrograde through the tibial tunnel, and the no. 5 suture is retrieved. The graft is passed from the tibial tunnel into the femoral tunnel with arthroscopic assistance.

The femoral fixation of the PCL and ACL grafts is done at this time, but the cruciate grafts are not tensioned or fixed to the tibial side until the end of the case. The PCL femoral grafts are fixed with a 4.5-mm AO screw and washer, or the grafts are tied and secured over a button. The anteromedial incision is extended proximally and distally adjacent to the exiting Beath pins. The vastus medialis obliquus is split in line with the fibers, or a small subvastus approach is used to gain access to the graft sutures and the bone. Alternatively an interference screw may be used for the femoral fixation to the calcaneal bone plug for single-bundle PCL reconstructions. For the ACL femoral fixation, a metal interference screw secures the femoral bone plug via the medial portal technique. Other types of fixation are feasible and depend on the type of graft and the comfort level of the surgeon.

Cruciate and Medial Sided Injury

If the cruciate ligaments are injured in combination with a medial-sided injury, a standard medial curvilinear incision is made. The PCL femoral tunnel, the ACL and PCL tibial tunnels, medial meniscal repairs, or medial capsular tears can be addressed through this incision. Peripheral meniscal tears can be repaired by standard meniscal repair techniques, and any capsular disruptions can be repaired with suture anchors. During the approach, the infrapatellar branch of the saphenous nerve should be identified approximately 1 cm above the joint line and protected throughout the procedure.

The MCL should be repaired or reconstructed only for grade 3 injuries to the MCL that open up in full extension to valgus stress testing. In the acute setting (<3 weeks), the MCL can be repaired at the time of cruciate reconstruction. MCL avulsions off the tibial or femoral surface are reattached to bone via suture anchors, and intrasubstance tears are repaired primarily with no. 2 braided nonabsorbable sutures using a modified Kessler stitch configuration. In the chronic setting, a reconstruction may be required to augment the repair.

The posterior oblique ligament (POL), which is confluent with the posterior edge of the superficial MCL, is reinforced by the semimembranosus and is critical to medial knee stability. The plane between the posterior edge of the MCL and the POL is incised longitudinally, and the two flaps are elevated. The medial meniscus attachments to the POL must be released to the posteromedial corner of the knee. The peripheral border of the medial meniscus is rasped to prepare the bed for the eventual repair to the POL. The medial meniscus is repaired to the anteriorly advanced POL with full thickness outside-in no. 0 cottony Dacron sutures through the meniscus. The POL is advanced anteriorly and imbricated to the MCL in a pants-over-vest fashion using no. 2 cottony Dacron sutures (Fig. 49–14). If needed, the reconstruction can be augmented with a soft-tissue graft at the anatomic origin and insertion of the MCL. The graft is inserted directly to bone on the femoral and the tibial surfaces with suture anchors and reinforced to the native MCL in a side-to-side fashion.

Cruciate and Lateral Sided Injury

After femoral fixation of the cruciates, a standard lateral "hockey-stick" incision is made. The plane between the posterior edge of the iliotibial band and the biceps femoris is incised longitudinally, and the insertion of the iliotibial band at Gerdy's tubercle is partially released to increase visibility of the LCL and the popliteus insertions. The peroneal nerve is identified proximally as it travels posterior to the biceps femoris and distally as it travels along the fibular neck and into the anterior tibialis muscle belly. A formal neurolysis generally is not performed unless there is evidence of compromise of the nerve at the time of surgery.

If reparable lateral meniscal tears or lateral capsular avulsions are visualized during diagnostic arthroscopy, a longitudinal capsular incision is made just posterior to the ⊺ CL. The meniscus is repaired using standard meniscal repair techniques depending on the type and location of the tear, whereas capsular avulsions are repaired with suture anchors. Next the LCL and the PFL are identified.

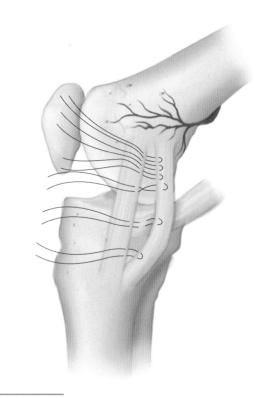

Figure 49–14. Schematic shows the posterior oblique ligament imbrication procedure.

If tissue quality allows, avulsions of the biceps, iliotibial band insertion, LCL, or popliteus are repaired directly with no. 2 braided nonabsorbable sutures acutely (Fig. 49–15). If interstitial injury occurs to these structures or the injury is chronic, reconstruction is usually necessary.

Our preferred method for LCL reconstruction involves an Achilles tendon allograft with an imbrication of the native LCL. The tendinous portion of the Achilles allograft is secured to the LCL insertion by means of drill holes or suture anchors. The native LCL is imbricated to the tendinous portion of the allograft using a whipstitch. The injured LCL is dissected free from its distal insertion on the fibular head, and a tunnel is drilled along the longitudinal axis of the fibula. The allograft calcaneal bone plug is tensioned and secured in the tunnel using a metal interference screw (Fig. 49–16). Alternatively the calcaneal bone plug can be fixed initially into the fibular tunnel, and the tendinous portion can be recessed into the lateral femoral epicondyle via a small bone tunnel and tied over a post or a button on the medial femur.

The goal of reconstruction of the popliteus complex is to re-create its static component, the PFL.[65] We prefer a tibialis anterior allograft, although hamstring autograft can be used. The lateral epicondyle of the femur is exposed, and the popliteus tendon is dissected off of its anatomic insertion. A whipstitch is placed in the popliteus tendon with a no. 2 braided nonabsorbable suture. Verification of the correct placement of the whipstitch is confirmed if the whole popliteus complex becomes taut when tension is placed on the suture. A 6-mm femoral drill tunnel is placed at the lateral epicondyle to the depth of

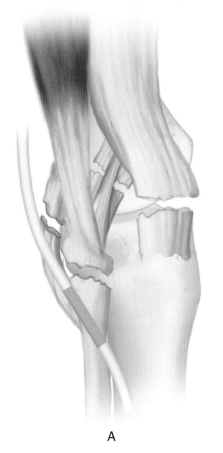
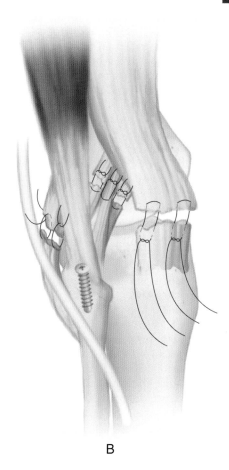

Figure 49–15. **A** and **B,** Schematic shows direct repair of the lateral structures.

A

B

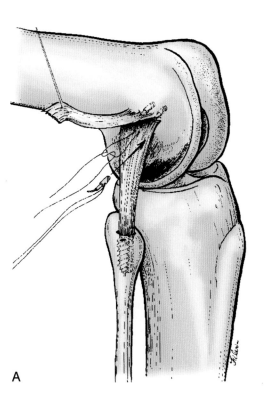
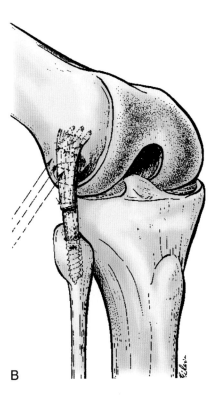

Figure 49–16. Schematic shows lateral collateral ligament (LCL) reconstruction with Achilles tendon allograft. **A,** The torn or stretched LCL is detached and elevated from its fibular insertion, and the allograft bone block is fixed in a tunnel in the proximal fibula using an interference screw. The tensioned graft is fixed at the lateral femoral epicondyle using multiple suture anchors. **B,** The native LCL is tensioned and sutured to the allograft.

A

B

25 to 30 mm, and the tunnel is expanded to 7 mm in diameter with the serial dilators. The posterior border of the fibula at the insertion of the PFL is exposed by incising horizontally just below the biceps insertion proximal to the peroneal nerve. The anterior border of the fibula also is exposed, and a guide wire is passed by hand with it loaded on a chuck from anterior to posterior across the fibular head in an attempt to match the oblique angle of the fibular head. The PFL tunnel rests more medial and closer to the proximal tibiofibular joint than the previously drilled LCL tunnel. The fibular head tunnel for the PFL graft is obliquely drilled over the guide wire with a 6-mm drill by hand and dilated to a diameter of 7 mm. The graft is passed from posterior to anterior through the tunnel with a Heuson suture passer, but it is not fixed to the fibula until the graft is tensioned properly. The graft is passed underneath and medial to the LCL and into the previously drilled tunnel out the popliteus tendon insertion via a Beath pin. The graft and the native popliteus tendon that was subperiosteally dissected are pulled into the tunnel. Approximately 25 mm of the allograft and approximately 10 mm of the popliteus tendon end up in the femoral tunnel. The graft and the popliteus tendon are tied over an AO screw and a washer or a button on the anteromedial distal femur. The reconstructed tendon is fixed to the fibula with either a bioabsorbable interference screw or over a button at the end of the case (Fig. 49–17). In certain cases, the LCL and PFL complexes need to be reconstructed, and the techniques described here are used.

Cruciate, Medial, and Lateral Sided Injuries

The combination of cruciate, medial, and lateral sided injuries is potentially the most unstable of injuries and is approached through bilateral hockey-stick incisions as described earlier. Cruciate reconstruction is performed first as described earlier, followed by medial and lateral repairs or reconstructions. Proximal fixation is the same as described earlier, followed by tensioning and distal fixation in a similar sequence.

Tensioning and Distal Fixation

After all grafts are successfully passed and fixed to the femur, the final tensioning and distal fixation of the grafts can be accomplished. In a stepwise fashion, we prefer to tension and fix the PCL, ACL, lateral structures, and medial structures. For the PCL, the knee is brought to 90 degrees of flexion, and a bolster is placed under the tibia to support its weight against gravity. The medial step-off is reduced with an anterior drawer so that the anterior edge of the medial tibial plateau rests approximately 10 mm anterior to the medial femoral condyle. The graft is fixed to the tibia with a bioabsorbable interference screw or an AO screw or both with a soft-tissue washer. The ACL graft is tensioned and fixed in full extension. We prefer a

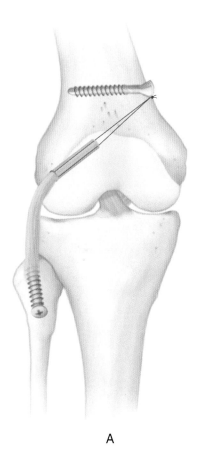

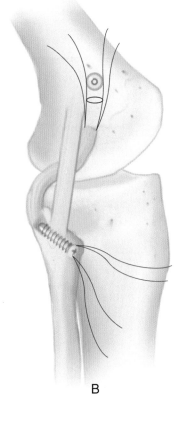

Figure 49–17. Schematic shows popliteofibular ligament reconstruction. The graft is fixed into a tunnel in the lateral femoral condyle over a post at the medial femoral condyle. It is passed deep to the lateral collateral ligament and through a tunnel in the fibula from posterior to anterior, where it is fixed with an interference screw. **A,** Anterior. **B,** Lateral.

A   B

metal interference screw for the bone–patellar tendon–bone allograft fixation in the tibia. The PLC of the knee is reduced with an internal rotation force to the tibia relative to the fixed femur, and the LCL and the PFL are tensioned at 30 degrees of flexion. The LCL is fixed with a metal interference screw into the fibular head. The PFL is fixed with a bioabsorbable interference screw in the fibula, and the remaining graft is reapproximated to itself or over the insertion of the biceps in the figure-eight pattern with a no. 2 braided absorbable suture. Alternatively the PFL graft is fixed to the fibula with sutures tied over a button. The MCL is fixed at 30 degrees of knee flexion, and the POL is fixed near full extension. This method prevents overconstraining of the knee during the repair/reconstruction.

After adequate tensioning and fixation, the knee is taken through a range of motion, and examination under anesthesia is performed to ensure proper fixation. An intraoperative x-ray is obtained to confirm that all of the hardware is intact and that the knee is adequately reduced.

Postoperative Regimen

In the early postoperative period, the main goals are to protect the healing structures, maximize quadriceps firing, and restore full passive extension. We place the limb locked in full extension for the first 4 weeks (Fig. 49–18). Exercises immediately after surgery include passive knee extension to neutral and isometric quadriceps sets with the knee in full extension. At 2 weeks postoperatively, the physical therapist begins passive flexion limited to 90 degrees and should prevent posterior tibial subluxation by applying an anterior force to the proximal tibia. For the first 6 weeks, active flexion is avoided to prevent posterior tibial translation, which results from hamstring contraction. At 6 weeks, passive and active-assisted range of motion and stretching exercises are begun to increase knee flexion. The brace is discontinued after 6 weeks. Depending on the combination of injury and the degree of insta-

bility as determined by the examination under anesthesia, a reasonable goal for range of motion in these patients is 0 to 120 degrees of flexion. Reports in the literature indicate that 37% to 54% of patients require manipulation after reconstruction of all damaged structures, despite aggressive postoperative rehabilitation.[39,50,56]

Quadriceps exercises are progressed to limited-arc, open-chain, knee-extension exercises only from 60 to 75 degrees of knee flexion as tolerated after 4 weeks. These exercises are performed to prevent excessive stress on the reconstructed grafts. Open-chain hamstring exercises are avoided for 12 weeks to prevent posterior tibial translation and excessive stress on the PCL graft. Crutch weightbearing is progressed from partial to weightbearing as tolerated over the first 4 weeks, unless a lateral repair/reconstruction was performed. In this case, we maintain partial weightbearing until the patient has regained good quadriceps control, at which time the brace may be unlocked for controlled gait training. Running is permitted at 6 months if 80% of quadriceps strength has been achieved. Patients may return to sedentary work in 2 to 3 weeks, heavy labor in 6 to 9 months, and sports in 9 to 12 months.

CONCLUSION

Knee dislocations are uncommon but serious injuries that require prompt evaluation and treatment to prevent major complications or poor results. Although the practicing orthopedist may encounter only few of these injuries throughout a career, it is imperative that a high initial index of suspicion exists for a patient who presents with a multiple-ligament knee injury. As the approach toward isolated ligamentous injuries of the knee continues to evolve, so has the treatment of knee dislocations. Treatment now involves early reconstruction of the cruciate ligaments combined with reconstruction or repair of the collateral structures with aggressive rehabilitation. This approach has improved knee function with regards to stability and range of motion.

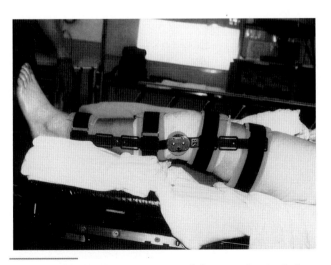

Figure 49–18. Postoperative immobilization that includes a fixed hinged knee brace.

References

1. Almekinders LC, Dedmond BT: Outcomes of the operatively treated knee dislocation. Clin Sports Med 19:503-518, 2000.
2. Almekinders LC, Logan TC: Results following treatment of traumatic dislocations of the knee joint. Clin Orthop 284:203, 1992.
3. Baxamusa TH, Galloway MT: Irreducible knee dislocations secondary to interposed menisci. Am J Orthop 30:141-143, 2001.
4. Bellabarba C, Bush-Joseph CA, Bach BR: Knee dislocation without anterior cruciate ligament disruption: A report of three cases. Am J Knee Surg 9:167, 1996.
5. Clancy WG: Repair and reconstruction of the posterior cruciate ligament. In: Chapman MW (ed): Operative Orthopaedics. Philadelphia, JB Lippincott, 1988, pp 1651-1655.
6. Clancy WG Jr, Ray JM, Zoltan DJ: Acute tears of the anterior cruciate ligament: Surgical versus conservative treatment. J Bone Joint Surg Am 70:1483, 1988.
7. Cooper DE, Speer KP, Wickiewicz TL, et al: Complete knee dislocation without posterior cruciate ligament disruption: A report of four cases and review of the literature. Clin Orthop 284:228, 1992.

8. Donaldson WF, Warren RF, Wickiewicz T: A comparison of acute anterior cruciate ligament examinations. Am J Sports Med 10:100-102, 1992.

9. Fanelli GC, Edson CJ: Arthroscopically assisted combined anterior and posterior cruciate ligament reconstruction in the multiple ligament injured knee: 2- to 10-year follow-up. Arthroscopy 18:703-714, 2002.

10. Frassica FJ, Staeheli JW, Pairolero PC: Dislocation of the knee. Clin Orthop 263:200, 1991.

11. Good L, Johnson, RJ: The dislocated knee. J Am Acad Orthop Surg 3:284, 1995.

12. Green NE, Allen BL: Vascular injuries associated with dislocation of the knee. J Bone Joint Surg Am 59:236, 1977.

13. Harner CD, Olson E, Irrgang JJ, et al: Allograft versus autograft anterior cruciate ligament reconstruction: 3- to 5-year outcome.Clin Orthop 324:134, 1996.

14. Harner CD, Waltrip RL, Bennett CH: Surgical management of knee dislocations. J Bone Joint Surg Am 86:262-273, 2004.

15. Henshaw RM, Shapiro MS, Oppenheim WL: Delayed reduction of traumatic knee dislocation: A case report and literature review. Clin Orthop 330:152, 1996.

16. Hill JA, Rana NA: Complications of posterolateral knee dislocations: Case report and review of the literature. Clin Orthop 154:212, 1981.

17. Hoover NW: Injuries of the popliteal artery associated with fractures and dislocations. Surg Clin North Am 41:1099, 1961.

18. Hughston JC, Andrews JR: Classification of knee ligamentous instabilities: Part II. The lateral compartment. J Bone Joint Surg Am 58:173, 1976.

19. Hughston JC, Bowben JA, Andrews JR: Acute tears of the posterior cruciate ligament: Results of operative treatment. J Bone Joint Surg Am 62:438, 1980.

20. Hughston JC, Jacobsen KE: Chronic posterolateral rotatory instability of the knee. J Bone Joint Surg Am 67:351, 1985.

21. Jones RE, Smith EC, Bone GE: Vascular and orthopedic complications of knee dislocation. Surg Gynecol Obstet 149:554, 1979.

22. Kendall RW, Taylor DC, Salvian AJ, et al: The role of arteriography in assessing vascular injuries associated with dislocations of the knee. J Trauma 35:875, 1993.

23. Kennedy JC: Complete dislocation of the knee. J Bone Joint Surg Am 45:889, 1963.

24. Kilicoglu O, Akman S, Demirham M, Berkman M: Muscular buttonholing: An unusual cause of irreducible knee dislocation. Arthroscopy 17:E22, 2001.

25. Klineberg EO, Crites BM, Flinn WR, et al: The role of arteriography in assessing popliteal artery injury in knee dislocations. J Trauma 56:786-790, 2004.

26. Kontakis GM, Christoforakis JJ, Katonis PG, Hadjipavlou AG: Irreducible knee dislocation due to interposition of the vastus medialis associated with neurovascular injury. Orthopaedics 26:645-646, 2003.

27. L'Insalata JC, Harner CD: The dislocated knee: Approach to treatment. Pittsburgh Orthop J 7:32, 1996.

28. Liow RY, McNicholas MJ, Keating JF, Nutton RW: Ligament repair and reconstruction in traumatic dislocation of the knee. J Bone Joint Surg Br 85:845-851, 2003.

29. Lynch J, Trojan S, Arhelger S, et al: Intermittent femoral nerve blockade for anterior cruciate ligament repair: Use of a catheter technique in 208 patients. Acta Anaesth Belg 42:207, 1991.

30. Mariani PP, Becker R, Rihn J, Margheritini F: Surgical treatment of posterior cruciate ligament and posterolateral corner injuries: An anatomical, biomechanical and clinical review. Knee 10:311-324, 2003.

31. Marshall JL, Warren RF, Wickiewicz TL, et al: The anterior cruciate ligament: A technique of repair and reconstruction. Clin Orthop 143:97, 1979.

32. Meyers MH, Harvey JP: Traumatic dislocation of the knee joint. J Bone Joint Surg Am 53:16, 1971.

33. Meyers MH, Moore TM, Harvey JP: Follow-up notes on articles previously published in the journal: Traumatic dislocation of the knee joint. J Bone Joint Surg Am 57:430, 1975.

34. Miller MD, Cooper DE, Fanelli GC, et al: Posterior cruciate ligament: Current concepts. Instr Course Lect 51:347-351, 2002.

35. Mills WJ, Barei DP, McNair P: The value of the ankle-brachial index for diagnosing arterial injury after knee dislocation: A prospective study. J Trauma 24:403-407, 2004.

36. Mont MA, Dellon AL, Chen F, et al: The operative treatment of peroneal nerve palsy. J Bone Joint Surg Am 78:863, 1996.

37. Montgomery JB: Dislocation of the knee. Orthop Clin North Am 18:149, 1987.

38. Muscat W, Rogers W, Cruz A, et al: Arterial injuries in orthopedics: True posteromedial approach for vascular control about the knee. J Orthop Trauma 10:476, 1996.

39. Noyes FR, Barber-Westin S: Reconstruction of the anterior and posterior cruciate ligaments after knee dislocation. Am J Sports Med 25:769, 1997.

40. Noyes FR, Grood ES: The strength of the anterior cruciate ligament in humans and rhesus monkeys: Age-related and species-related changes. J Bone Joint Surg Am 58:1074, 1974.

41. Ohkoshi Y, Nagasaki S, Shibata N, et al: Two-stage reconstruction with autografts for knee dislocations. Clin Orthop 398:169-175, 2002.

42. O'Neill DB: Arthroscopically assisted reconstruction of the anterior cruciate ligament. J Bone Joint Surg Am 78:803, 1996.

43. Petrie RS, Trousdale RT, Cabanela ME: Total knee arthroplasty for chronic posterior knee dislocation: Report of two cases with technical considerations. J Arthroplasty 15(3):380-386, 2000.

44. Reddy PK, Posteraro RH, Schenck RC: The role of MRI in evaluation of the cruciate ligaments in knee dislocations. Orthopedics 19:166, 1996.

45. Richter M, Bosch U, Wippermann B, et al: Comparison of surgical repair or reconstruction of the cruciate ligaments versus nonsurgical treatment in patients with traumatic knee dislocations. Am J Sports Med 30:718-727, 2002.

46. Rihn JA, Cha PS, Groff YJ, Harner CD: The acutely dislocated knee: Evaluation and management. J Am Acad Orthop Surg 12:334-346, 2004.

47. Rios A, Villa A, Fahandezh H, et al: Results after treatment of traumatic knee dislocations: A report of 26 cases. Trauma 55:489-494, 2003.

48. Schenck RC: The dislocated knee. Instr Course Lect 43:127, 1994.

49. Schenck RC: Classification and treatment of knee dislocations. Orthop Spec Educ 4:35, 1998.

50. Shapiro MS, Freedman EL: Allograft reconstruction of the anterior and posterior cruciate ligaments after traumatic knee dislocations. Am J Sports Med 23:580, 1995.

51. Shelbourne KD, Nitz P: Accelerated rehabilitation after anterior cruciate reconstruction. Am J Sports Med 18:292, 1990.

52. Shelbourne KD, Porter DA, Clingman JA: Low velocity knee dislocation. Orthop Rev 20:995, 1991.

53. Shelton WR, Papendick L, Dukes AD: Autograft versus allograft anterior cruciate ligament reconstruction. Arthroscopy 13:446, 1997.

54. Shields L, Mital M, Cave EF: Complete dislocations of the knee: Experience at the Massachusetts General Hospital. J Trauma 9:192, 1969.

55. Simonian PT, Wickiewicz TL, Hotchkiss RN, et al: Chronic knee dislocation-reduction, reconstruction and application of a skeletally fixed knee-hinge: A report of two cases. Am J Sports Med 26:591, 1998.

56. Sisto DJ, Warren RF: Complete knee dislocation: A follow-up study of operative treatment. Clin Orthop 198:94, 1985.

57. Speer KP, Spitzer CE, Bassett FH, et al: Osseous injury associated with acute tears of the anterior cruciate ligament. Am J Sports Med 20:382, 1992.

58. Stannard JP, Sheils TM, Lopez-Ben RR, et al: Vascular injuries in knee dislocation: The role of physical examination in determining the need for arteriography. J Bone Joint Surg Am 86:910-915, 2004.

59. Taft TN, Almekinders LC: The dislocated knee. In Fu HC, Fu FH, Vince KG (eds): Knee Surgery. Baltimore, Williams & Wilkins, 1994, pp 837-858.

60. Taylor AR, Arden GP, Rainey HA: Traumatic dislocation of the knee: A report of forty-three cases with special reference to conservative treatment. J Bone Joint Surg Br 54:96, 1972.

61. Tetzlaff JE, Andrish J, O'Hara J, et al: Effectiveness of bupivacaine administered via femoral nerve catheter for pain control after anterior cruciate ligament repair. J Clin Anesth 9:542, 1997.

62. Thomsen PB, Rudd B, Jensen UH: Stability and motion after traumatic dislocation of the knee. Acta Orthop Scand 55:278, 1984.

63. Treiman GS, Yellin AE, Weaver FA, et al: Examination of the patient with a knee dislocation: The case for selective angiography. Arch Surg 127:1056, 1992.

64. Urguden M, Bilbasar H, Ozenci AM, et al: Irreducible posterolateral knee dislocation resulting from a low-energy trauma. Arthroscopy 20:S50-S53, 2004.
65. Veltri DM, Deng XH, Torzilli PA, et al: The role of the popliteofibular ligament in stability of the human knee. Am J Sports Med 24:19, 1996.
66. Walker DN, Hardison RR, Schenck RC: A baker's dozen of knee dislocations. Am J Knee Surg 7:117, 1994.
67. Wascher DC, Dvirnak PC, DeCoster DC: Knee dislocation: Initial assessment and implications for treatment. J Orthop Trauma 11:525, 1997.
68. White KS: The results of traction injury to the common peroneal nerve. J Bone Joint Surg Br 50:346, 1968.
69. Wong CH, Tan JL, Chang HC: Knee dislocations—a retrospective study comparing operative versus closed immobilization treatment outcomes. Knee Surg Sports Traumatol Arthrosc 12:540-544, 2004.
70. Yu JS, Goodwin D, Salonen D, et al: Complete dislocation of the knee: Spectrum of associated soft-tissue injuries depicted by MR imaging. AJR Am J Roentgenol 164:135, 1995.

CHAPTER 50

Posterolateral Corner Injuries

David A. McGuire

Injuries to the posterolateral corner (PLC) of the knee, though infrequent, often present the most complex problems and can result in severe disability because of the relationship between rotatory instability, other ligamentous injury, and cartilage degeneration.[29,38,85] The PLC is stabilized by a single functional unit known as the arcuate ligament complex.[29,38] It is rare that injuries to the PLC occur in isolation, and indeed, they are often found in conjunction with posterior or anterior cruciate ligament (PCL, ACL) disruption.

Evolutionary anatomic development of the PLC has contributed significantly to its complex anatomy. Over time, developmental changes between the fibular head, biceps femoris muscle, and popliteus tendon have resulted in significantly intricate relationships. Particularly evident is the eventual descent over time of the fibular head from its initial articulation with the femur, which has contributed to speculation that its meniscus probably evolved into the popliteus attachment of the fibular styloid or the popliteus tendon. Anatomic comparisons with nonhuman mammalian species have identified similarities as well as variations in ligament attachments.

Fabricianni et al[17] observed in their anatomic studies that the popliteus muscle continues into a complex aponeurosis consisting of popliteofibular, popliteocapsular (*popliteal aponeurosis*), and popliteomeniscal fibers (*popliteomeniscal fascicles*). Thereafter, it forms a strong tendon attached to the lateral femoral condyle with superior and inferior popliteomeniscal fibers. In these authors' comparative anatomy study of lower-order vertebrates, they presented evidence of tibial and fibular articulation with the femur, with each having its respective menisci. They also identified popliteus muscle fiber attachment on the head of the fibula posteriorly. The fibular head recedes in higher species and the corresponding meniscus disappears. In later stages of evolution, the popliteus muscle attaches to the femorofibular meniscus, even later it becomes the popliteus tendon, and the popliteus muscle develops a tendinous attachment to the fibular head (popliteofibular ligament [PFL]). The popliteus tendon, during these developments, maintained its association with the lateral meniscus (popliteal aponeurosis).

ANATOMY

Anatomic descriptions of the PLC have been inconsistent. Accordingly, there is confusion surrounding the anatomic structures and their function.[83,87] The PFL has been defined by no less than five terms: popliteofibular fibers,[17]

the popliteus muscle with fibular head origin,[87] the short external lateral ligament,[46] the popliteofibular fascicles,[74] and the fibular origin of the popliteus.[76] This structure, notably absent in mid-20th century anatomy texts and orthopedic journals, has been rediscovered in the recent literature.[51]

The static stabilizers of the PLC include the lateral collateral ligament (LCL), PFL, arcuate ligament complex, fabellofibular ligament (FFL), and the posterolateral capsule. Dynamic stabilizing contributions[68] to the PLC include the biceps tendon, iliotibial tract (IT), and popliteus muscle-tendon complex. Injury to this complex can cause laxity that can result in posterolateral or anterolateral rotatory instability. The PLC controls anterolateral and posterolateral tibial rotation relative to the femur.[22,50,73,79,91]

Seebacher et al[68] in 1982 described the knee lateral structures as being composed of three distinct layers (Fig. 50–1). The most superficial layer (layer I) consists of two parts, the superficial portion of the biceps and its expansion posteriorly and the IT, including its anterior expansion. The middle layer (layer II—an incomplete layer) contains the patellomeniscal ligament and, anteriorly, is composed of the quadriceps retinaculum but is incomplete posteriorly, where it consists of the two PFLs. The deepest (layer III) of the three layers forms the lateral part of the joint capsule. This layer is divided into superficial and deep laminae. The superficial (*lateral aponeuroses of the long and short heads, capsular arm of the short head of the biceps femoris*) lamina includes the LCL and terminates at the FFL. The deep lamina passes along the edge of the lateral meniscus, where a hiatus forms for the popliteus tendon and the coronary ligament, and terminates at the arcuate ligament complex.

The anatomy of the PLC is significantly variable. Seebacher et al[68] noted three anatomic variations in their study of 35 cadaver knees. The FFL independently reinforced the PLC portion of the capsule in 20%, the arcuate ligament complex reinforced it unaided in 13% of the knees, and both structures reinforced it in 67%. Sudasna and Harnsiriwattanagit[76] found variation in PLC structures in their dissection of 50 knees. They identified the fibular origin of the popliteus tendon (presently known as the PFL) in 98%, an FFL in 68%, and a thin, membranous arcuate ligament in 24%. In a study of 115 cadaver knees, Watanabe et al[87] used a classification scheme that identified the presence or absence of the "popliteus muscle" with origin from the fibular head (the PFL); seven anatomic variants were recognized, with variations of the arcuate ligament complex and FFL previously noted by Seebacher et al also being included. They found an LCL and a popliteus tendon in all knees and a PFL in 93%.

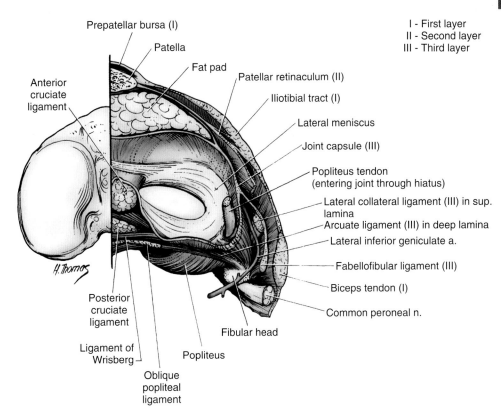

Figure 50–1. Coronal sectioned anatomy of the posterolateral corner of the knee. (From Seebacher JR, Inglis AE, Marshall JL, Warren RF: The structure of the posterolateral aspect of the knee. J Bone Joint Surg Am 64:536-541, 1982.)

BLOOD SUPPLY AND INNERVATION

The blood supply of the PLC is provided by the popliteal artery and its branches. Of the lateral superior genicular artery's three branches, the articular branch anastomoses with the ascending branch of the lateral inferior genicular artery, which runs anteriorly, deep to the LCL,[78,84] and supplies the LCL and the lateral region of the knee. The middle genicular artery supplies the posterior capsular region,[67] with additional supply derived from the posterior tibial recurrent artery, which segregates into small branches supplying the tibial condyle, popliteus muscle, and the area superior to the fibular head.[84] Small branches off the popliteal artery also supply the posterior capsular region.[84]

Injury to the PLC affects afferent signals to the central nervous system and knee kinematics. The PLC and the external portion of the lateral meniscus are supplied by the popliteal plexus, with aid from the terminal portions of the obturator nerve and the posterior articular nerve (a significant branch of the posterior tibial nerve).[34,39] Proprioception in this knee region is facilitated by mechanoreceptors performing complex reflex arc roles. Golgi tendon organ–like endings and pacinian corpuscles serve a regulatory function for PLC structures in resisting external rotation and excessive varus force. Golgi endings, as slowly adapting high-threshold mechanoreceptors, are activated during extremes in knee range of motion (ROM) and when high stress is generated in ligaments. Pacinian corpuscles adapt and signal rapidly to changes in joint deceleration and acceleration.[37,93]

By their location in and connection to ligaments, the capsule, and menisci, Ruffini endings provide static and dynamic mechanoreceptor input that signals the direction and amplitude of knee movement velocity, as well as changes in intra-articular pressure.[37,93] The high-threshold free nerve endings that are ubiquitously present in most articular tissue are pain receptors that respond directly to inflammatory mediators and mechanical deformation.[37,93]

BIOMECHANICAL STUDIES

Knowledge of the function and contribution to stability of individual PLC knee components has been derived largely from biomechanical studies. These studies provide a scientific basis for clinical assessment of a knee with PLC injury. Most research seeks to determine primary and combined function by measurement of knee motion in response to known forces with increasing anatomic defects in the knee.[62]

In cadaver knee studies involving selective ligament sectioning, Nielsen et al[55-58] illustrated the role of the PLC structures in opposing posterolateral rotational and varus forces. Collectively, the PLC and the LCL resist posterolateral rotation and varus displacement. The PLC plays the greater role in restricting posterolateral rotation, whereas the LCL plays a greater role in resisting varus displacement of the tibia.[57] Sectioning both the posterolateral part of the capsule and the LCL resulted in more posterolateral rotatory instability than did isolated resection of either structure.[58] The popliteus tendon resisted external tibial rotation between 20 and 130 degrees ROM, and it resisted varus displacement of the tibia from 0 to 90 degrees.[56] The PLC structures contributed secondary constraint to posterior translation. Isolated sectioning of the PCL did not affect external rotation or varus stability.[55,57]

A study by Gollehon et al[23] expanded on the work of Nielson and colleagues by selective transection of the ACL, PCL, LCL, and the "popliteus-arcuate (deep) ligament complex" (DLC), which included the arcuate ligament complex and the FFL, the popliteus tendon, and the posterolateral part of the joint capsule.[23,83] From 0 to 90 degrees ROM, the PCL was the principal structure resisting posterior translation, whereas the DLC and the LCL were the principal structures constraining posterolateral rotation and varus displacement. If either the DLC or the LCL were sectioned individually, there was no increase in posterior translation; however, their combined resection resulted in small increases in posterior translation throughout all ROM. A small varus displacement occurred at all knee angles in response to isolated LCL cutting, and when combined with resection of the DLC, varus displacement increased further in all ROM and was greatest at 30 degrees. With the addition of PCL sectioning, larger increases in varus displacement (from 15 to 19 degrees) occurred. When the DLC was sectioned, posterolateral rotation increased at 90 degrees, and when combined with LCL sectioning, posterolateral rotation increased at all angles, maximally at 30 degrees. When the PCL was also sectioned, additional increases in posterior translation and varus displacement occurred at all flexion angles, and posterolateral rotation increased at greater than 30 degrees of flexion. Isolated sectioning of the PCL did not affect posterolateral or varus displacement at any knee angle. When the ACL was sectioned along with the LCL and the DLC, tibial anterolateral rotation and anterior translation increased at 30 and 60 degrees of flexion. Isolated sectioning of the ACL or combined sectioning of the LCL and the DLC did not increase anterolateral rotation of the tibia.

In a study by Markolf et al,[50] sectioning of the PLC structures and subsequent posterolateral rotation or tibial varus produced increased force on the PCL at flexion between 45 and 90 degrees. Posterior tibial force and posterolateral rotation produced significantly increased stress on the PCL at all angles except full extension. With applied anterolateral rotation, there was no effect on the PCL. However, stress increased on the ACL from 0 to 20 degrees of flexion.

Noyes et al[63] quantified increases in abnormal posterior subluxation of the tibial plateau subsequent to ligament sectioning and specified loading conditions. Transection of both the PCL and PLC structures increased posterior subluxation of both the lateral and medial tibial plateau at 30 and 90 degrees of flexion. Subsequent to cutting the PLC structures, posterior translation of the lateral tibial plateau increased at 30 but not at 90 degrees of flexion.

LaPrade et al[44] measured the stress in ACL grafts in cadaver knees in which the PLC structures had been selectively cut. Graft force increased with varus loading, and it increased further with coupled varus and posterolateral rotation at 0 and 30 degrees of flexion.

In their study of articular contact pressure with the use of pressure-sensitive film, Skyhar et al[72] reported that combined sectioning of the PCL and PLC produced significantly more patellofemoral joint contact pressure than did isolated sectioning of the PCL ($p < .05$). Their cadaver knee model simulated non-weightbearing, resistive extension of the knee.

CLINICAL RELEVANCE

Isolated Ligament Injuries

Although PLC injury may be isolated or occur as part of a multiligament injury, isolated PLC injury is rare. In their report of 735 knees treated for ligament injuries, DeLee et al[16] identified only 12 (1.6%) that had acute isolated posterolateral rotatory instability. The most common mechanisms of injury to the PLC of the knee include athletic trauma, falls, and motor vehicle accidents.[3,16,21,24,41,60,81] If posterolateral force is directed to the proximal part of the tibia with the knee at or near full extension, an isolated PLC injury can result.[16,29] Knee hyperextension and a varus force combined can disrupt the PLC structures.[3,4,21] When isolated PLC injury occurs, the following conditions are typically found:

1. Posterior tibial translation = minimum (same as the reference knee)
2. External rotation at 30 degrees of knee flexion = maximum
3. Stable examination at 90 degrees

An isolated complete injury of the PLC results in maximally increased varus and external rotation at 30 degrees of flexion if the PCL is intact. At low knee flexion angles, only 10% to 15% of the PCL's fibers are taut, and it is accordingly unable to significantly resist such force.[14,15] In contrast, the fibers of an intact PCL are tight at 90 degrees and are able to exert an effective secondary restraint against posterolateral rotatory torque, or a varus force, and to exert a primary restraint against posterior translation.[25,50,66]

Signs of isolated PLC injury differ significantly from those associated with isolated LCL injury. Isolated LCL injury is manifested as mildly increased varus displacement at 0 degrees but as maximal displacement at 30 degrees of knee flexion. It is best assessed with adduction stress testing at 30 degrees.

Isolated tears of the PCL produce increases in posterior translation of the tibia that correlate positively with knee flexion. However, there is no correlation with posterolateral or anterolateral rotatory instability or varus displacement. The posterior drawer test at 90 degrees is the most accurate means of diagnosing such an injury.[14] Accordingly, an isolated PCL injury will have the following findings:

1. Abnormal posterior laxity
2. No abnormal varus
3. Dial test result for external rotation of the tibia on the femur less than 5 degrees as compared with the uninvolved side tested with the knee at 30 and 90 degrees of flexion

Posterolateral Corner–Posterior Cruciate Ligament Injury Combination

PLC impairment is more frequently associated with multiple ligament injuries, and posterolateral rotatory instability is notably a common condition that occurs secondary to PCL damage. Injury mechanisms include those contributing to isolated PLC injury, hyperextension combined with posterolateral rotatory force, a severe tibial posterolateral rotation force, or a severe varus force.[4,12,45,81] A combined injury may also occur when a flexed knee receives a posterior force on the tibia while externally rotated. In this situation, PCL tension is significantly decreased in comparison to the tension present during neutral tibial rotation because the PLC structures are recruited to resist the applied force.[86] A frank knee dislocation can also produce severe injury to the PLC.[24,81,90]

When a complete PLC injury is combined with a PCL injury, the primary and secondary restraining effects of the PCL are lost at high knee flexion angles. Consequently, there is increased posterolateral rotatory instability, varus displacement, and posterior translation at *all* knee angles.[83] When isolated or combined PLC injury is suspected, stress tests for increased varus displacement and posterolateral rotatory instability should be performed at 30 and 90 degrees and compared with the results in the uninjured knee.[83] An injury to the PLC structures combined with a PCL injury will typically be manifested as follows:

1. Abnormal posterior laxity greater than 20 to 25 mm; tibial step-off is absent and negative
2. Abnormal varus displacement at 30 degrees
3. Abnormal external rotation thigh-foot angle of greater than 10 to 15 degrees in comparison to the normal lower extremity tested at 30 and 90 degrees

Posterolateral Corner–Anterior Cruciate Ligament Injury Combination

Though less well recognized, combined ACL and PLC injury can occur. Collectively, this multiple injury results in increased primary anterior and posterior translation, primary varus laxity, coupled posterolateral rotatory instability, and anterolateral rotatory instability.[82,91] There is disagreement whether the external rotation test at 30 degrees is a reliable method for identifying combined ACL and PLC injury. Although anterolateral rotatory instability is commonly associated with ACL insufficiency, identifying which cases are combined PLC and ACL injuries may require intraoperative assessment. When PLC involvement is suspected, post–ACL reconstruction flexion-rotation drawer and dial tests can verify PLC insufficiency requiring surgical intervention. The data support the clinical observation that cruciate ligament grafts are at risk for failure in knees with untreated posterolateral and anterolateral rotatory instability.[26] Consequently, intraoperative assessment of PLC insufficiency may easily and perhaps should routinely be conducted immediately after postoperative ACL and PCL reconstruction.

DIAGNOSIS AND PHYSICAL EXAMINATION

Because the majority of all PLC injuries occur in conjunction with other ligamentous disruption, they may be overlooked during an initial knee examination.[12,59,75] Patients with PLC injuries typically have diffuse tenderness, ecchymosis, edema, induration and tenderness over the PLC area, and localized tenderness over the fibular head.[3,16] Localized point tenderness at the joint line may indicate a Segond fracture.[45,69,70]

Examination is carried out to ascertain the functional integrity of specific structures, and comparison is made with the uninjured knee. Lesions of the PLC structures are often classified as grade I, II, or III sprains, depending on whether there is minimal, partial, or complete tearing of the ligament.[2,38,43,45] Grade I injuries are not associated with abnormal joint motion, grade II injuries are associated with slight to moderate joint motion, and grade III in injuries are usually associated with markedly abnormal joint motion.[2]

A posterior drawer test should be performed at 30 and 90 degrees.[32] After applying gentle posterolateral rotational force, assess the amount of posterolateral rotation and compare it with the contralateral normal knee. Note that some normal laxity is seen in patients with physiological genu recurvatum. If posterior translation is normal at 90 degrees but is slightly increased at 30 degrees, PLC injury is likely. Not all patients with PCL tears have a positive posterior drawer test on physical examination.[28] Although the PCL is commonly evaluated by performing the posterior drawer test at 90 degrees,[23,25,27,59] it can also be assessed by other methods, including the dynamic posterior shift test,[15] the quadriceps active test, the posterior sag sign, the prone posterior drawer test, and the reverse pivot-shift test.[35] The reverse pivot-shift test has the largest variability of all motion tests (with positive results occurring in 35% of normal knees examined under anesthesia).[11] The knee is flexed to 45 degrees, the foot is externally rotated, and the knee is then extended.

During assessment of patients with known PCL tears, diagnosis of potential injury to the PLC should be undertaken with the patient in a supine position.[13] The posterolateral external rotation test[45] is conducted at 30 and 90 degrees, with a combined posterior and external rotation force being applied while palpating for posterolateral subluxation of the tibia. If subluxation occurs at 30 degrees but not at 90 degrees, an isolated injury of the PLC is indicated. If subluxation occurs at both angles, a combined PLC and PCL injury is suggested.

The dial (tibial external rotation) test assesses increased external rotation and may be performed with the patient supine or prone, although it may be easier to visualize side-to-side differences in the latter position.[1,83] The test should be performed at both 30 and 90 degrees because increased external rotation at 30 degrees but not at 90 degrees indicates an isolated injury to the PLC whereas increased external rotation at both angles suggests injury to both the PCL and the PLC. Differences between the results of the 30- and 90-degree dial tests may be so slight that they are not visually detectable. If external rotation of the injured tibia exceeds 10 degrees in a side-to-side comparison with the noninjured tibia, a PLC injury is suggested.[5] The external rotation recurvatum test[29,32] is used to diagnose posterolateral rotatory instability but is usually indicative of a combined injury with the PCL. The test is performed by lifting the patient's extended legs by the great toes and noting any relative difference in hyperextension, tibial external rotation, and varus.

Assessment of the ACL is commonly undertaken with the Lachman test.[80] A combined ACL and PLC injury should be suspected in severe injuries or if the ACL insufficiency is chronic. Either of these circumstances in the presence of a grade II to III Lachman test *combined with* a grade II to III flexion-rotation drawer test is indicative of a combined injury. It should also be suspected if the patient is undergoing a revision ACL reconstruction and there were no signs of injury, noncompliance with physical therapy, or incorrect surgical methodology.

Patients with PLC injuries usually, but not always, demonstrate varus alignment while standing and may learn to adapt to their instability with a flexed knee gait. This abnormal gait pattern is characterized by a varus thrust, or a hyperextension varus thrust may develop during their stance phase.[60,83]

DIAGNOSTIC IMAGING

Standard anterior-posterior radiographs of a knee with posterolateral injury may show abnormal widening of the lateral joint space or a Segond fracture.[16,41,60] Avulsion of the lateral aspect of the capsule from the tibial plateau (Segond fracture—lateral capsular sign) is typically indicative of an ACL lesion. However, an isolated PLC injury may be seen as avulsion of metaphyseal bone from the tibia.[16,68] Although chronic PLC injuries correlate positively with radiographs demonstrating osteoarthritic changes in the lateral or medial compartment or with patellofemoral arthritis,[6,29] these data have limited use in primary PLC diagnosis.

Magnetic resonance imaging (MRI) is useful in diagnosing PLC injury, particularly in severely traumatized, acutely injured knees wherein a complete and accurate clinical diagnosis is not possible.[54,65,77,88] Coronal oblique T2-weighted MRI has been demonstrated in cadaveric and clinical studies to provide improved visualization of PLC structures when compared with standard coronal or sagittal views.[92] In a prospective clinical study, LaPrade et al[42] used a thin-sliced coronal oblique T1-weighted protocol designed to include the entire fibular head and styloid process in their comparison of seven uninjured knees to 20 patients with grade III PLC injuries. They were able to accurately identify PLC structures individually and determine the chronic or acute nature of the lesions with this protocol.

TREATMENT

Nonoperative

Kannus[38] monitored 23 patients with nonoperated grade II and III sprains of the PLC. Eleven patients with grade II sprains had excellent or good result, 9 were asymptomatic, and all had residual laxity. Twelve patients with grade III sprains all had fair to poor results on their standardized scores, and 6 had post-traumatic arthritis.

Surgical Reconstruction

Reconstruction techniques for the PLC include partial and complete tendon transfers, among which are femoral bone block advancement of the arcuate ligament complex, lateral gastrocnemius muscle advancement, biceps tendon tenodesis, and hamstring or patellar tendon reconstruction of the LCL from the fibular head to the isometric point of the femur.[8,31,47,60,61,85] Individual ligament replacement techniques for PLC insufficiency include an LCL anatomic reconstruction using the central segment of the biceps femoris tendon (Fig. 50–2),[7] reconstruction of the tibial attachment of the popliteus tendon and the PFL with a split patellar tendon graft (an Achilles tendon may also

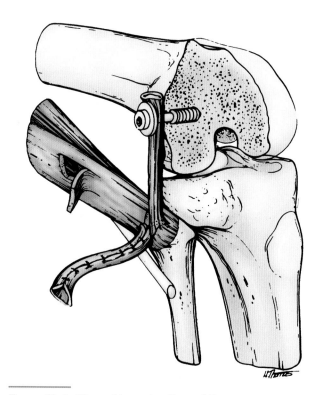

Figure 50–2. View of lateral collateral ligament reconstruction with a central strip of biceps tendon. (From Bowen MK, Warren RF, Cooper DE: Posterior cruciate ligament and related injuries. In Insall J [ed]: Surgery of the Knee, 2nd ed. New York, Churchill Livingstone, 1993.)

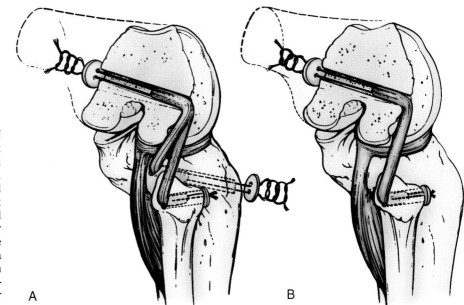

Figure 50–3. **A,** Reconstruction of the popliteus-tibial attachment and popliteofibular ligament with a split patellar ligament graft. Subsequent to proximal femoral tunnel placement, the graft is split and one end placed in the tibial tunnel and the other in the fibular tunnel. **B,** Reconstruction of the popliteofibular ligament with a patellar ligament graft. (From Veltri DM, Warren RF: Posterolateral instability of the knee. Instr Course Lect 44:441-453, 1995.)

A

B

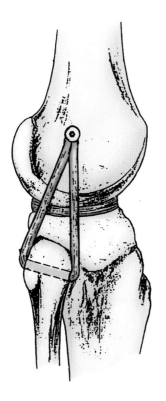

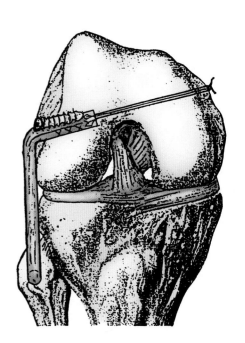

Figure 50–4. Illustration of a lateral collateral ligament and popliteofibular ligament reconstruction with a free semitendinosus tendon graft. (From Fanelli GC, Larson RV, Practical management of posterolateral instability of the knee. Arthroscopy 18(2 Suppl 1):1-8, 2002.)

be used), or isolated reconstruction of the PFL with a graft (Fig. 50–3).[83]

Other reconstruction examples include LCL/PFL substitution with the semitendinosus (Fig. 50–4)[20] and split Achilles (Fig. 50–5),[48] PFL substitution with the semitendinosus without significant varus instability (Fig. 50–6),[20] split biceps tendon transfer (biceps femoris tendon tenodesis),[18] rerouted biceps tendon,[40] and fibular head oblique osteotomy.[64]

Study Results

In 21 patients with combined PLC and cruciate ligament injuries, Noyes and Barber-Westin[61] reported that 13 (61.9%) were fully functional, 6 (28.6%) were partially functional, and 2 (9.5%) were nonfunctional. They used a modified Hughston and Jacobson[30] technique in which the tissue is advanced with the knee in 30 degrees of flexion rather than at 90 degrees. In another combined

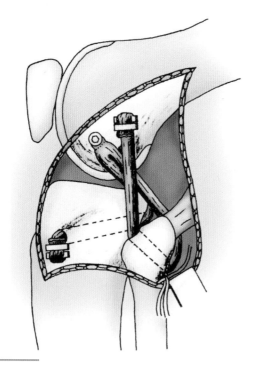

Figure 50–5. Posterolateral reconstruction with a split Achilles tendon allograft. A bone plug is placed in the anteroinferior side tunnel of the femur and secured with a cannulated interference screw. The 6-mm-wide and 7-mm-wide sides of the graft are secured by staples on the femur and tibia, respectively. (From Lee MC, Park YK, Lee SH, et al: Posterolateral reconstruction using split Achilles tendon allograft. Arthroscopy 19:1043-1049, 2003.)

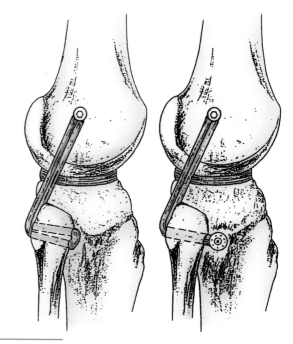

Figure 50–6. Illustration of a semitendinosus free graft used to reconstruct posterolateral corner instability without varus instability and without (**A**) or with (**B**) tibiofibular joint instability. (From Fanelli GC, Larson RV: Practical management of posterolateral instability of the knee. Arthroscopy 18(2 Suppl 1):1-8, 2002.)

PLC and cruciate ligament series involving 39 patients, Clancy and Sutherland[10] performed a tenodesis of the biceps femoris tendon to the lateral femoral epicondyle. They reported that 77% had no restrictions in activities of daily living and 54% were able to return to their previous level of sports competition. In a combined PLC-PCL study by Fanelli et al,[19] all 21 patients had either correction or overcorrection of their posterolateral instability as measured by the tibial external rotation test.

Jacob and Warner[36] suggested that recession of the popliteus tendon and LCL into the lateral femoral condyle can restore tension yet maintain the anatomic attachment sites. This procedure would be appropriate in cases of mild attenuation when the popliteus musculotendinous junction and the PFL are intact. A study by Albright and Brown[1] reported the results of a sling procedure used to approximate reconstruction of the popliteus tendon. This procedure eliminated the reverse pivot shift, hyperextension, and varus laxity in 26 (87%) of the study's 30 patients.

Using a rerouted biceps tendon technique in patients with isolated rotatory instability, Kim et al[40] reported that external rotation was normal in 15 (71%) of the 21 patients at follow-up and loss of correction of more than 5 degrees was found in 3 patients at an average of 1 year postoperatively. Patients were immobilized at 30 degrees for 6 weeks, with partial weightbearing permitted thereafter with passive and active ROM.

Operative Technique

The reconstruction techniques described are all complex and require the rearrangement of normal structures. No matter how carefully done, there is a penalty for moving normal structures to new locations. In an effort to simplify the reconstruction and minimize the associated morbidity of the procedure, we have developed and currently use the following techniques.

ANTEROLATERAL LATERAL AUGMENTATION DESIGNED TO ELIMINATE ANTEROLATERAL ROTATORY INSTABILITY

To minimize donor site morbidity, a semitendinosus or other suitable allograft may be used. However, if allograft tissue is not available, autologous tissue may be substituted. A lateral incision is made through subcutaneous tissue from the lateral femoral epicondyle to Gerdy's tubercle. The fascia lata is divided longitudinally. Gerdy's tubercle is identified along with the site just posterior to the insertion of the LCL on the femur (Fig. 50–7). Slot-eyed Beath pins are then placed in these positions (Fig. 50–8).

Initially, the pins are drilled or tapped a short distance into the bone, and a suitably strong suture material is stretched between these two pins (Fig. 50–9). The knee is then put through full ROM. Tension changes in the suture

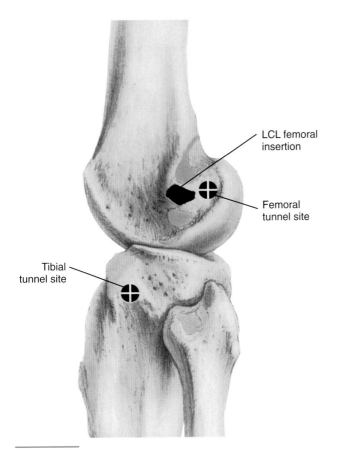

Figure 50–7. The tibial tunnel site is located just anterior to Gerdy's tubercle, and the femoral tunnel site is located just posterior to the insertion of the lateral collateral ligament (LCL) on the femur.

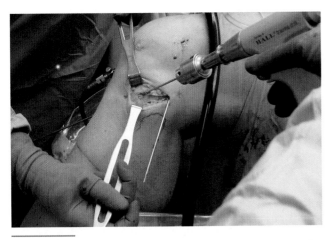

Figure 50–8. Insertion of the slot-eyed Beath pins into the approximated position.

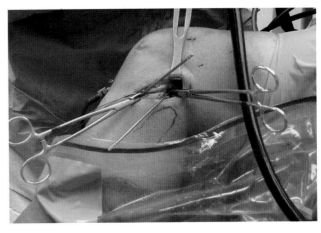

Figure 50–9. Beath pins are wrapped with suture material to determine site-selected isometry of 2-mm or less excursion during range-of-motion testing.

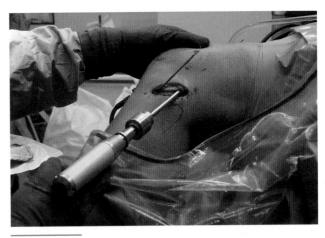

Figure 50–10. Femoral tunnel being overdrilled with a 7-mm reamer to a depth of 25 mm.

so placed should be less than 2 mm. This is a simple, but useful approximation of isometry. If the tension in the suture is inadequate or the suture breaks, which is indicative of a nonisometric position, the pins are reinserted at a more suitable site until satisfactory isometry is established. The work of Sidles et al[71] established that no truly isometric positions exist laterally and extra-articularly.

However, this method produces a useful approximation that will protect the ACL graft in these instances of severe anterolateral rotatory instability.

Once this relatively isometric position is established, the femoral pin is drilled through the femoral cortex with its exit directed medially and sufficiently proximal to avoid the femoral tunnel of the previously reconstructed ACL. The tibial pin is advanced distally and medially to avoid the tibial tunnel and then exits the skin. Once adequate pin position is achieved, a 7-mm cannulated reamer is advanced over the Beath pins, and both tunnels are drilled to a depth of 25 mm (Fig. 50–10). A wire suture is placed at both ends of the graft, which is then advanced into the tunnels with the aid of the slot-eyed Beath pins (Fig. 50–11). With the knee held in 20 degrees of flexion, the graft is tensioned to approximately 5 kg, and direct tendon-to-bone fixation is accomplished with 7×25-mm bioabsorbable interference screws placed over a guide wire (Fig. 50–12). Stability is then checked (Fig. 50–13). The pivot-shift phenomenon should be completely eliminated. The wound is then closed with subcuticular absorbable sutures. Use of this relatively simple extra-articular recon-

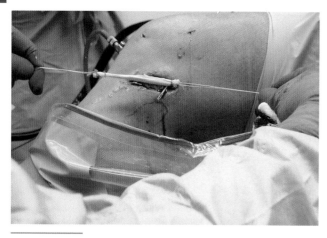

Figure 50–11. Graft shown in preparation for insertion. Note the slot of each Beath pin is positioned to receive the graft wire before placement of the graft ends into their respective tunnels.

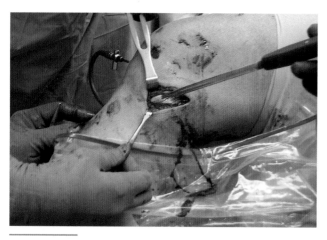

Figure 50–12. Insertion of a 7 × 25-mm headless cannulated bioabsorbable interference screw for direct interference fixation of the tibial side of the graft. Another identical screw is used for femoral side fixation.

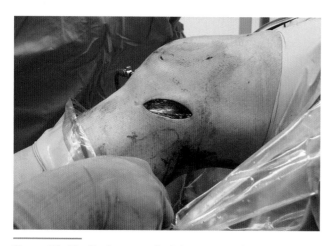

Figure 50–13. Graft secured while awaiting flexion-rotation drawer testing and wound closure with subcuticular absorbable suture.

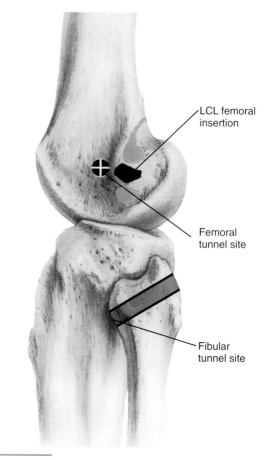

LCL femoral insertion

Femoral tunnel site

Fibular tunnel site

Figure 50–14. The proximal tunnel site is located just anterior to the insertion of the lateral collateral ligament (LCL). The distal tunnel located in the fibular head is drilled obliquely, angling from posterior proximal on the fibular head to anterior distal, and then exits through the skin anteriorly.

struction has significantly improved our success rate in these severely unstable knees.[89]

POSTEROLATERAL LATERAL AUGMENTATION DESIGNED TO ELIMINATE POSTEROLATERAL ROTATORY INSTABILITY

The posterolateral reconstructive surgical technique mirrors that of the anterolateral reconstruction. The only significant difference is the location of the distal and proximal tunnels. To establish the proximal tunnel, a site just anterior to the LCL is identified (Fig. 50–14), and a guide wire is placed in this position. The guide wire and subsequent tunnel should be oriented in a proximal medial direction so that it avoids the femoral tunnel of an ACL reconstruction (Fig. 50–15). The foot is then internally rotated, thereby exposing the head of the fibula. To establish the distal tunnel, a guide wire is drilled obliquely, angling from posterior proximal on the fibular head to anterior distal, and then exits through the skin anteriorly. Like the anterolateral reconstruction, isometry is evaluated with a suture. The final tunnels are drilled, and with

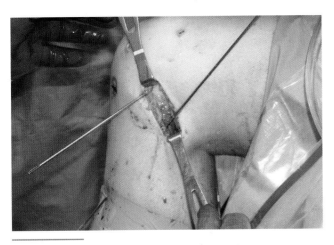

Figure 50–15. Insertion of the slot-eyed Beath pins into their respective approximated positions.

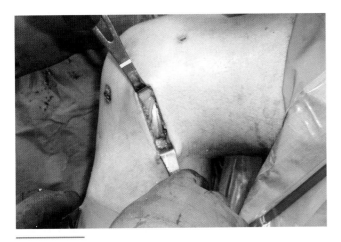

Figure 50–16. Graft secured while awaiting the dial test and wound closure with subcuticular absorbable suture.

the knee in approximately 90 degrees of flexion, direct tendon-to-bone fixation is accomplished with bioabsorbable interference screws. Under tension, the femoral insertion is fixed first, followed by the fibular insertion (Fig. 50–16).[53]

Rehabilitation

The postoperative program is similar to the program after an isolated ACL reconstruction. Postoperative pain may be greater after lateral reconstruction, and therefore proper pain management is crucial so that early rehabilitation can be initiated. Rehabilitation emphasizes ROM, quadriceps strengthening, and patellofemoral joint protection. Patients are allowed weightbearing as tolerated, with the majority returning to full weightbearing by the seventh postoperative day. The postoperative ROM protocol includes continuous passive motion and heel slides, with the goal of full ROM by the sixth postoperative week.

Cold therapy is used to reduce postoperative pain and swelling.

The postoperative exercise program emphasizes quadriceps strengthening and avoids all flexion and extension against resistance. Immediately after surgery all patients begin a strengthening program that consists initially of straight-leg raises. Patients progress to nonimpact sliding/gliding exercises as tolerated. Specifically, patients begin a program consisting of swimming, Nordic track, and stationary bicycling usually beginning by the end of the second postoperative week. If any activity produces pain, patients are instructed to discontinue or limit the extent of that exercise.

DISCUSSION

PLC instability can be anterior, posterior, or both. The instability can be isolated or exist in conjunction with other ligamentous injuries. The possibility of PLC injury should be considered when examining any injured knee for ligamentous injury. However, PLC instability may be best confirmed intraoperatively after completion of ACL or PCL reconstruction. This injury pattern is easily diagnosed, and a MRI study may be helpful in borderline cases.

It has been suggested that all grade I and most moderate grade II injuries of the PLC structures can be treated nonoperatively, but residual laxity may remain, especially in knees with grade II injuries.[13] Mild grade II injuries can probably and occasionally be treated nonoperatively; however, differentiation between grade I and II injury is often complicated by concomitant multiple ligament injuries. Additionally, a poorly reconstructed ACL can mimic injury to the PLC. If the tibial tunnel is placed so posterior that the position of the ACL graft is too vertically oriented, the resulting rotational instability can mimic a PLC injury.

Acute grade III isolated or combined injury of the PLC is best treated early, by direct repair if possible, or else by augmentation or reconstruction of all injured ligaments. Chronic PLC injury, whether isolated or combined, is probably best treated by reconstruction of the PLC along with reconstruction of any coexisting cruciate ligament injury.

Clinical outcomes of PCL reconstruction have not been as successful as those achieved after ACL reconstruction.[9,21,33,49,60,89] The commonly associated PLC injury, if left unattended in PCL disruptions, may contribute to unsuccessful PCL reconstruction. However, there seems to be a greater percentage of posterolateral rotatory instability among PCL-deficient patients than anterolateral rotatory instability among ACL-deficient patients. This may be due to a higher percentage of severe trauma associated with the PCL group. Biomechanical data support the clinical observation that cruciate ligament grafts are at risk for failure in knees with untreated anterolateral or posterolateral rotatory instability.[26] Failure to diagnose and treat a PLC injury in a patient who has a known tear of the ACL or PCL can result in failure of the reconstructed cruciate ligament.

References

1. Albright JP, Brown AW: Management of chronic posterolateral rotatory instability of the knee: Surgical technique for the posterolateral corner sling procedure. Instr Course Lect 47:369-378, 1998.
2. American Medical Association, Committee on the Medical Aspects of Sports: Standard nomenclature of athletic injuries. Prepared by the Subcommittee on Classification of Sports Injuries. Chicago, American Medical Association, 1966.
3. Baker CL Jr, Norwood LA, Hughston JC: Acute posterolateral rotatory instability of the knee. J Bone Joint Surg Am 65:614-618, 1983.
4. Baker CL Jr, Norwood LA, Hughston JC: Acute combined posterior cruciate and posterolateral instability of the knee. Am J Sports Med 12:204-208, 1984.
5. Bleday RM, Fanelli GC, Giannotti BF, et al: Instrumented measurement of the posterolateral corner. Arthroscopy 14:489-494, 1998.
6. Bowen MK, Nuber GW: Management of associated posterolateral instability in posterior cruciate ligament surgery. Op Tech Sports Med 1:148-153, 1993.
7. Bowen MK, Warren RF, Cooper DE: Posterior cruciate ligament and related injuries. In Insall J (ed): Surgery of the Knee, 2nd ed. New York, Churchill Livingstone, 1993.
8. Clancy WG: Posterolateral reconstruction for rotatory instability of the knee. Video J Orthop 7:3, 1992.
9. Clancy WG, Shelbourne KD, Zoellner GB, et al: Treatment of knee joint instability secondary to rupture of the posterior cruciate ligament. Report of a new procedure. J Bone Joint Surg Am 65:310-322, 1983.
10. Clancy WG Jr, Sutherland TB: Combined posterior cruciate ligament injuries. Clin Sports Med 13:629-647, 1994.
11. Cooper DE: Tests for posterolateral instability of the knee in normal subjects. J Bone Joint Surg Am 73:30-36, 1991.
12. Cooper DE, Warren RF, Warner JJP: The posterior cruciate ligament and posterolateral structures of the knee: Anatomy, function, and patterns of injury. Instr Course Lect 40:249-270, 1991.
13. Covey DC: Current concepts review. Injuries of the posterolateral corner of the knee. J Bone Joint Surg Am 83:106-118, 2001.
14. Covey DC, Sapega AA: Anatomy and function of the posterior cruciate ligament. Clin Sports Med 13:509-518, 1994.
15. Covey DC, Sapega AA, Sherman GM: Testing for isometry during reconstruction of the posterior cruciate ligament. Anatomic and biomechanical considerations. Am J Sports Med 24:740-746, 1996.
16. DeLee JC, Riley MB, Rockwood CA Jr: Acute posterolateral rotatory instability of the knee. Am J Sports Med 11:199-207, 1983.
17. Fabricianni C, Oranski M, Zoppi U: Il musculo popliteo, studio anatomico. Arch Ital Anat 87:203-217, 1982.
18. Fanelli CG, Edson CJ: Management of the combined anterior cruciate ligament/posterior cruciate ligament injuries of the knee. In Chow JCY (ed): Advanced Arthroscopy. New York, Springer-Verlag 1999, pp 533-557.
19. Fanelli GC, Giannotti BF, Edson CJ: Arthroscopically assisted combined posterior cruciate ligament/posterior lateral complex reconstruction. Arthroscopy 12:521-530, 1996.
20. Fanelli GC, Larson RV: Practical management of posterolateral instability of the knee. Arthroscopy 18(2 Suppl 1):1-8, 2002.
21. Fleming RE Jr, Blatz DJ, McCarroll JR: Posterior problems in the knee. Posterior cruciate insufficiency and posterolateral rotatory insufficiency. Am J Sports Med 9:107-113, 1981.
22. Frank CB, Jackson WJ: Current concepts review: The science of reconstruction of the anterior cruciate ligament. J Bone Joint Surg Am 79:1556-1576, 1997.
23. Gollehon DL, Torzilli PA, Warren RF: The role of the posterolateral and cruciate ligaments in the stability of the human knee. A biomechanical study. J Bone Joint Surg Am 69:233-242, 1987.
24. Grana WA, Janssen T: Lateral ligament injury of the knee. Orthopedics 10:1039-1044, 1987.
25. Grood ES, Stowers SF, Noyes FR: Limits of movement in the human knee. Effect of sectioning the posterior cruciate ligament and posterolateral structures. J Bone Joint Surg Am 70:88-97, 1988.
26. Harner CD, Vogrin TM, Hoher J, et al: Biomechanical analysis of a posterior cruciate ligament reconstruction. Deficiency of the posterolateral structures as a cause of graft failure. Am J Sports Med 28:32-39, 2000.
27. Henry MH, Berend ME, Feagin JA Jr: Clinical diagnosis of acute knee ligament injuries. Ann Chir Gynaecol 80:120-126, 1991.
28. Hughston JC: The absent posterior drawer test in some acute posterior cruciate ligament tears of the knee. Am J Sports Med 16:39-43, 1988.
29. Hughston JC, Andrews JR, Cross MJ, Moschi A: Classification of knee ligament injuries. Part II. The lateral compartment. J Bone Joint Surg Am 58:173-179, 1976.
30. Hughston JC, Bowden JA, Andrews JR, Norwood LA: Acute tears of the posterior cruciate ligament. Results of operative treatment. J Bone Joint Surg Am 62:438-450, 1980.
31. Hughston JC, Jacobson KE: Chronic posterolateral rotatory instability of the knee. J Bone Joint Surg Am 67:351-359, 1985.
32. Hughston JL, Norwood LA: The posterolateral drawer test and external rotation recurvatum test for posterolateral rotatory instability of the knee. Clin Orthop 147:82-87, 1980.
33. Insall JN, Hood RW: Bone-block transfer of the medial head of the gastrocnemius for posterior cruciate insufficiency. J Bone Joint Surg Am 64:691-699, 1982.
34. Jacobson KE: Technical pitfalls of collateral ligament surgery. Clin Sports Med 18:847-882, 1999.
35. Jakob RP, Hassler H, Stäubli HU: Observations on rotatory instability of the lateral compartment of the knee: Experimental studies on the functional anatomy and pathomechanism of the true and reverse pivot shift sign. Acta Orthop Scand Suppl 191:1-32, 1981.
36. Jakob RP, Warner JP: Lateral and posterolateral rotatory instability of the knee. In Jakob RP, Stäubli HU (eds): The Knee and the Cruciate Ligaments: Anatomy, Biomechanics, Clinical Aspects, Reconstruction, Complications, Rehabilitation. New York, Springer, 1992, pp 463-494.
37. Johansson H: Role of knee ligaments in proprioception and regulation of muscle stiffness. J Electromyogr Kinesiol 1:158-179, 1991.
38. Kannus P: Nonoperative treatment of grade II and III sprains of the lateral ligament compartment of the knee. Am J Sports Med 17:83-88, 1989.
39. Kennedy JC, Alexander IJ, Hayes KC: Nerve supply of the human knee and its functional importance. Am J Sports Med 10:329-335, 1982.
40. Kim SJ, Shin, SJ, Jeong JH: Posterolateral rotatory instability treated by a modified biceps rerouting technique: Technical considerations and results in cases with and without posterior cruciate ligament insufficiency. Arthroscopy 19:493-499, 2003.
41. Krukhaug Y, Molster A, Rodt A, Strand T: Lateral ligament injuries of the knee. Knee Surg Sports Traumatol Arthrosc 6:21-25, 1998.
42. LaPrade RF, Gilbert TJ, Bollom TS, et al: The magnetic resonance imaging appearance of individual structures of the posterolateral knee. A prospective study of normal knees and knees with surgically verified grade III injuries. Am J Sports Med 28:191-199, 2000.
43. LaPrade RF, Hamilton CD, Engebretsen L: Treatment of acute and chronic combined anterior cruciate ligament and posterolateral knee injuries. Sports Med Arthrosc Rev 5:91-99, 1997.
44. LaPrade RF, Resig S, Wentorf F, Lewis JL: The effects of grade III posterolateral knee complex injuries on anterior cruciate ligament graft force. A biomechanical analysis. Am J Sports Med 27:469-475, 1999.
45. LaPrade RF, Terry GC: Injuries to the posterolateral aspect of the knee. Association of anatomic injury patterns with clinical instability. Am J Sports Med 25:433-438, 1997.
46. Last RJ: The popliteus muscle and lateral meniscus. With a note on the attachment of the medial meniscus. J Bone Joint Surg Br 32:93-99, 1950.
47. Latimer HA, Tibone JE, El Attrache NS, et al: Reconstruction of the lateral collateral ligament of the knee with patellar tendon allograft. Report of a new technique in combined ligament injuries. Am J Sports Med 26:656-662, 1998.
48. Lee MC, Park YK, Lee SH, et al: Posterolateral reconstruction using split Achilles tendon allograft. Arthroscopy 19:1043-1049, 2003.
49. Lipscomb AB, Anderson AF, Norwig ED, et al: Isolated posterior cruciate ligament reconstruction. Long-term results. Am J Sports Med 21:490-496, 1993.
50. Markolf KL, Wascher DC, Finerman GAM: Direct in vitro measurement of forces in the cruciate ligaments. Part II: The effect of section of the posterolateral structures. J Bone Joint Surg Am 75:387-394, 1993.
51. Maynard MJ, Deng X, Wickiewicz TL, Warren RF: The popliteofibular ligament. Rediscovery of a key element in posterolateral stability. Am J Sports Med 24:311-316, 1996.
52. McGuire DA, Wolchok JC: Extra-articular lateral reconstruction technique. Arthroscopy 16:553-557, 2000.

53. McGuire DA, Wolchok JW: Posterolateral corner reconstruction. Arthroscopy 19:790-793, 2003.
54. Miller TT, Gladden P, Staron RB, et al: Posterolateral stabilizers of the knee: Anatomy and injuries assessed with MR imaging. AJR Am J Roentgenol 169:1641-1647, 1997.
55. Nielsen S, Helmig P: The static stabilizing function of the popliteal tendon in the knee. An experimental study. Arch Orthop Trauma Surg 104:357-362, 1986.
56. Nielsen S, Helmig P: Posterior instability of the knee joint. An experimental study. Arch Orthop Trauma Surg 105:121-125, 1986.
57. Nielsen S, Ovesen J, Rasmussen O: The posterior cruciate ligament and rotatory knee instability. An experimental study. Arch Orthop Trauma Surg 104:53-56, 1985.
58. Nielsen S, Rasmussen O, Ovesen J, Andersen K: Rotatory instability of cadaver knees after transection of collateral ligaments and capsule. Arch Orthop Trauma Surg 103:165-169, 1984.
59. Noyes FR: PCL & posterolateral complex injuries. Overview. Am J Knee Surg 9:171, 1996.
60. Noyes FR, Barber-Westin SD: Surgical reconstruction of severe chronic posterolateral complex injuries of the knee using allograft tissues. Am J Sports Med 23:2-12, 1995.
61. Noyes FR, Barber-Westin SD: Surgical restoration to treat chronic deficiency of the posterolateral complex and cruciate ligaments of the knee joint. Am J Sports Med 24:415-426, 1996.
62. Noyes FR, Grood ES, Torzilli PA: Current concepts review. The definitions of terms for motion and position of the knee and injuries of the ligaments. J Bone Joint Surg Am 71:465-472, 1989.
63. Noyes FR, Stowers SF, Grood ES, et al: Posterior subluxations of the medial and lateral tibiofemoral compartments. An in vitro sectioning study in cadaveric knees. Am J Sports Med 21:407-414, 1993.
64. Pavlovich RI, Nafarrate EB: Trivalent reconstruction for posterolateral and lateral knee instability. Arthroscopy 18:E1, 2002.
65. Ross G, Chapman AW, Newberg AR, Scheller AD Jr: Magnetic resonance imaging for the evaluation of acute posterolateral complex injuries of the knee. Am J Sports Med 25:444-448, 1997.
66. Sapega AA, Covey DC: The biomechanics of femoral and tibial posterior cruciate ligament graft placement. Clin Sports Med 13:553-559, 1994.
67. Scapinelli R: Studies on the vasculature of the human knee joint. Acta Anat 70:305-331, 1968.
68. Seebacher JR, Inglis AE, Marshall JL, et al: The structure of the posterolateral aspect of the knee. J Bone Joint Surg Am 64:536-541, 1982.
69. Segond P: Pathologie externe. Recherches cliniques et expérimentales sur les épanchemants sanguins du genou par entorse. Progres Med (Paris) 7:297-299, 1879.
70. Shindell R, Walsh WM, Connolly JF: Avulsion fracture of the fibula: "The arcuate sign" of posterolateral knee instability. Nebr Med J 69:369-371, 1984.
71. Sidles JA, Larson RV, Garbini JL, et al: Ligament length relationships in the moving knee. J Orthop Surg 6:593-610, 1988.
72. Skyhar MJ, Warren RF, Ortiz GJ, et al: The effects of sectioning of the posterior cruciate ligament and the posterolateral complex on the articular contact pressures within the knee. J Bone Joint Surg Am 75:694-699, 1993.
73. Smith BA, Livesay GA, Woo SL-Y: Biology and biomechanics of the anterior cruciate ligament. Clin Sports Med 12:637-670, 1993.
74. Staubli HU, Birrer S: The popliteus tendon and its fascicles at the popliteal hiatus: Gross anatomy and functional arthroscopic evaluation with and without anterior cruciate ligament deficiency. Arthroscopy 6:209-220, 1990.
75. Strand T, Molster AO, Engesaeter LB, et al: Primary repair in posterior cruciate ligament injuries. Acta Orthop Scand 55:545-547, 1984.
76. Sudasna S, Harnsiriwattanagit K: The ligamentous structures of the posterolateral aspect of the knee. Bull Hosp Jt Dis Orthop Inst 50:35-40, 1990.
77. Tardieu M, Lazennec JY, Christel P, et al: [Normal and pathological MRI aspects of the posterolateral corner of the knee.] J Radiol 76:605-609, 1995.
78. Terry GC, LaPrade RF: The posterolateral aspect of the knee. Anatomy and surgical approach. Am J Sports Med 24:732-739, 1996.
79. Terry GC, Norwood LA, Hughston JC, Caldwell KM: How iliotibial tract injuries of the knee combine with acute anterior cruciate ligament tears to influence abnormal anterior tibial displacement. Am J Sports Med 21:55-60, 1993.
80. Torg JS, Conrad W, Kalen V: Clinical diagnosis of anterior cruciate ligament instability in the athlete. Am J Sports Med 4:84-93, 1976.
81. Towne LC, Blazina ME, Marmor L, Lawrence JF: Lateral compartment syndrome of the knee. Clin Orthop 76:160-168, 1971.
82. Veltri DM, Deng XH, Torzilli PA, et al: The role of the cruciate and posterolateral ligaments in stability of the knee. A biomechanical study. Am J Sports Med 23:436-443, 1995.
83. Veltri DM, Warren RF: Posterolateral instability of the knee. Instr Course Lect 44:441-453, 1995.
84. Vladimirov B: Arterial sources of blood supply of the knee-joint in man. Nauchni Tr Vissh Med Inst Sofiia 47:1-10, 1968.
85. Wascher DC, Grauer JD, Markoff KL: Biceps tendon tenodesis for posterolateral instability of the knee. An in vitro study. Am J Sports Med 21:400-406, 1993.
86. Wascher DC, Markolf KL, Shapiro MS, Finerman GA: Direct in vitro measurement of forces in the cruciate ligaments. Part I: The effect of multiplane loading in the intact knee. J Bone Joint Surg Am 75:377-386, 1993.
87. Watanabe Y, Moriya H, Takahashi K, et al: Functional anatomy of the posterolateral structures of the knee. Arthroscopy 9:57-62, 1993.
88. Westrich GH, Hannafin JA, Potter HG: Isolated rupture and repair of the popliteus tendon. Arthroscopy 11:628-632, 1995.
89. Wirth CJ, Jager M: Dynamic double tendon replacement of the posterior cruciate ligament. Am J Sports Med 12:39-43, 1984.
90. Wright DG, Covey DC, Born CT, Sadasivan KK: Open dislocation of the knee. J Orthop Trauma 9:135-140, 1995.
91. Wroble RR, Grood ES, Cummings JS, et al: The role of the lateral extraarticular restraints in the anterior cruciate ligament–deficient knee. Am J Sports Med 21:257-262, 1993.
92. Yu JS, Salonen DC, Hodler J, et al: Posterolateral aspect of the knee: Improved MR imaging with a coronal oblique technique. Radiology 198:199-204, 1996.
93. Zimny ML: Mechanoreceptors in articular tissues. Am J Anat 182:16-32, 1988.

CHAPTER 51

Functional Knee Tests and Outcome Scales

Robert S. Gotlin • Joseph E. Herrera

The ability to measure the integrity and stability of a knee after ligament reconstruction is essential for determining the success of surgical intervention and providing a guide for further postsurgical management and rehabilitation. A series of tests have been developed to measure ligament integrity, muscle strength, endurance, and overall functional efficiency of the knee. Commonly used tools that measure these parameters include arthrometry, isokinetic testing, functional hop testing, and outcome scales.

ARTHROMETRY

Standard clinical tests such as the Lachman, sag, and drawer tests have been used to evaluate the integrity of ligaments in the knee, but they are limited because of their subjective nature. The knee ligament arthrometer is a device that provides an objective measure of ligament laxity. It quantifies anterior-posterior translation of the tibia relative to the femur.[22,87] Arthrometry has been used to evaluate side-to-side differences in normal knees,[22,83] in those with acute and chronic ligament disruption,[25,75] and in knees that have undergone ligament reconstruction.[57] The KT-1000/2000 arthrometer (MEDmetric Corp., San Diego, CA), Genucom Knee Analysis System (Faro Medical Technologies, Lake Mary, FL), and Knee Signature System (CA-4000, Orthopedic Systems, Inc., Hayward, CA) are commercially available arthrometers that have been compared and evaluated for reliability.[42,43,62,74,76,94,95] Queale et al compared these three arthrometers and reported the KT-2000 to be the most reliable tool for measuring laxity when used by a single examiner.[74] In our clinic we use the KT-2000.

Instrumentation

The KT-2000 arthrometer (Fig. 49–1) is a device that contains both an arthrometer that measures anterior-posterior translation of the tibia with respect to the femur and a plotter graph that records these translation distances. When evaluating normal patients and those with cruciate ligament disruption, the patient is first placed supine on the examination table. The distal part of the thigh is then placed on a bolster whose inferior aspect is positioned cephalad to the superior aspect of the patella (Fig. 49–2). The bolster allows the knee to be flexed approximately 30 degrees, which helps isolate the anterior cruciate ligament (ACL) and posterior cruciate ligament (PCL) for

evaluation. After aligning the thigh on the bolster, the arthrometer is secured to the anterior aspect of the leg. It is held in place with two Velcro straps. Once secured, the arthrometer is activated by engaging the handle plunger and then pushing the arthrometer handle away from the examiner, toward the examining table. When an audible beep is heard, the device is ready to perform the test, which is accomplished by pulling the handle (with the plunger engaged) toward the examiner to assess the integrity of the ACL and pushing the handle away from the examiner to assess the integrity of the PCL. With each activation of the arthrometer handle, a series of beeps are audible, three for anterior excursion and one for posterior excursion. The three anterior beeps correspond to standardized force readings of 15 lb (67 N), 20 lb (89 N), and 30 lb (134 N), whereas the posterior beep corresponds to 20 lb (89 N) of force. It is at these predetermined levels that we make side-to-side comparisons of excursion distance. We average several trials measuring anterior and posterior excursion of the tibia with respect to the femur at these specific force levels. Measurements (millimeters) of posterior excursion distance at 20 lb (89 N) and anterior excursion distance at 30 lb (134 N) are typically tracked by clinicians. An attached plotter graph displays a force-displacement curve (Fig. 51–3) that allows the examiner to visualize and measure the millimeters of tibial excursion.

Evaluation of a PCL injury with an arthrometer requires an additional step. Because a ruptured PCL may allow the tibia to rest in a relatively posterior position relative to the femur, we must account for this distance before using the arthrometer; otherwise, our recordings may reveal factitious exaggerated measurements for ACL laxity and reduced measurements for PCL laxity. To account for this, we perform the quadriceps active test. First, we must identify the knee's quadriceps neutral angle on the uninvolved limb, or the flexion angle at which there is minimal tibial motion when the quadriceps contracts. The arthrometer is secured to the flexed knee and a gentle quadriceps contraction is performed. The degree of knee flexion when the arthrometer needle moves neither anterior nor posterior on the active quadriceps contraction is the quadriceps neutral angle. After establishing the quadriceps neutral angle, the injured limb is flexed to the degree of knee flexion that established the quadriceps neutral angle on the uninjured knee. The quadriceps is then contracted and the degree of tibial displacement recorded. This value represents the distance (millimeters) that the femur is resting posterior as a result of the ruptured PCL. It is the "correction" that must be made for posterior lay of the resting tibia as a result of the stretched/ruptured PCL. The

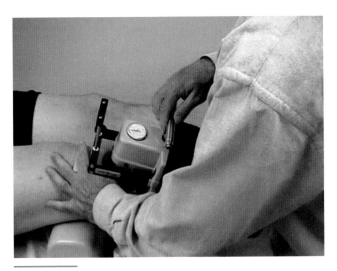

Figure 51–1. KT-2000 arthrometer.

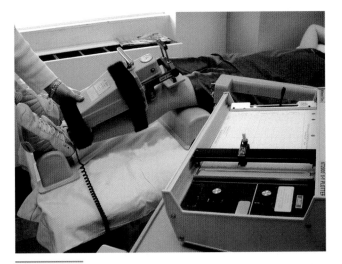

Figure 51–2. Positioning of the inferior aspect of the bolster pad in line with the superior aspect of the patella.

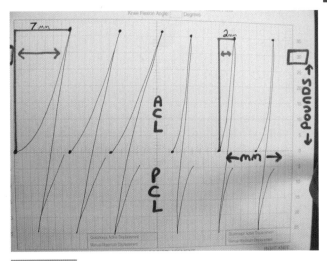

Figure 51–3. Force-displacement graphs of the KT-2000. Millimeters of anterior tibial excursion are noted along the x axis, whereas the force (in foot-pounds) of anterior displacement is noted along the y axis. ACL, anterior cruciate ligament; PCL, posterior cruciate ligament.

millimeters of anterior excursion on quadriceps neutral active testing represents the numeric value to be "added" to the PCL arthrometer results and subtracted from the ACL results. The test is completed by performing KT arthrometry for both the ACL and PCL and correcting for the posterior resting tibia on the side of the PCL tear.[23,24]

Normal Population

In the normal population there is no significant difference in ligament laxity between age and sex groups.[22,23,41,83,93,95] Daniel et al supported this finding by performing arthrometry on 338 normal patients and 33 cadavers.[22] Several studies have also investigated the effect of hormone concentration (during the menstrual cycle) on ligament laxity.[27,50,79,84,88,92] This was prompted by the finding that the incidence of ACL injuries in female athletes is significantly higher than that in males.[63,79] Karageanes,[50] Belanger,[14] and Van Lunen[88] and their colleagues reported

no significant difference in ligament laxity with arthrometry testing during different times of the menstrual cycle. We, in unpublished data, confirmed similar findings (30 patients with <1-mm alteration in side-to-side arthrometry values at different times of the menstrual cycle). Although no significant difference was found between sex and age, arthrometry testing has revealed a difference in laxity when comparing normal knees in the same individual. These studies found a side-to-side difference in laxity of 3 mm or less in 95% of subjects tested with uninjured knees.[22,23,41,65,83,93,95]

Ligament Disruption

Numerous studies have investigated the reliability and validity of quantifying acute and chronic ligament disruption with the use of an arthrometer. These studies have shown that a side-to-side difference in anterior tibial displacement of 3 mm or greater is indicative of ACL disruption.[22,23,41,75,83,93] Rangger et al performed arthrometry with the KT-1000 on 105 patients with acute unilateral ACL disruption and 159 patients with chronic ACL deficiencies.[75] They found that 95% of patients with acute ACL disruptions and 99% with chronic ACL disruptions had a right-to-left difference of 3 mm or greater, thus confirming the results of previous studies.[75] When testing the integrity of the ligaments in the knee, the amount of anterior force used has been the subject of a few studies. Earlier studies used an anterior displacement force of 20 lb (89 N) to evaluate ACL disruptions.[22,25,75,83] Highgenboten et al investigated the reliability of the KT arthrometer when using 15, 20, and 30 lb of anterior force in conscious and unconscious patients. Their findings advocated the use of 30 lb of force when evaluating ACL injuries.[41] In our clinic we track excursions of the tibia relative to the femur at 30 lb of anterior force. One word of caution, because of the varying calf girth of different patients, false recordings may be registered in those with larger calves. In this instance, we use the "manual max" test. For this, the KT arthrometer is attached to the flexed lower extremity, and rather than using the arthrometer handle to move the tibia anterior and posterior, the examiner places one hand on the arthrometer guide and the other hand under the calf. From this position, a manual Lachman maneuver is performed while recording the tibial excursion on the plotter graph.

Although use of an arthrometer is effective and reliable in diagnosing complete ACL disruption, several studies investigated its effectiveness in detecting partial ACL tears.[38,40,44,53,55] Most studies reveal that arthrometry testing is not reliable in detecting partial tears. Hole et al found that only 11% of examiners were able to accurately diagnose partial ACL tears when measuring anterior tibial excursion.[44] The majority of studies used anterior tibial displacement measurements, but according to Liu et al, the compliance index, stiffness, and rate of change in stiffness of anterior force displacement were found to be better at predicting partial ACL rupture in a knee model.[55] Further studies are needed to evaluate the reliability of using these parameters to diagnose partial ligament tears.

As described earlier, evaluation of the PCL requires the use of the quadriceps active test with the knee placed in the quadriceps neutral position. The KT-1000 arthrometer was found to be a moderately reliable tool for measurement of tibial translation in patients with PCL tears when using the aforementioned techniques.[45] Daniel et al studied PCL-deficient knees and found that 41 of 42 knees had an average anterior tibial translation measuring 6 mm in chronic and 4.2 mm in acute PCL disruptions during quadriceps contraction.[24] Although arthrometry testing is effective in quantifying laxity, the amount of knee instability in a PCL-deficient knee as determined by the KT arthrometer was related neither to the patient's return to sports nor to knee satisfaction.[33,73]

Ligament Reconstruction

Even though the KT arthrometer has demonstrated its diagnostic ability for ligament tears, its greatest utility may be in the postoperative setting. Commonly, KT testing is performed approximately 6 months after surgery. The results obtained guide rehabilitation and help determine criteria for return to sports. Although arthrometry serves as a tool to measure laxity in the reconstructed knee, it should not be used in isolation to determine the success or failure of surgery.[85,87] Arthrometry serves an integral role in determining functional success when used in concert with other interventions, including isokinetic testing, hop testing, and outcome scales. Arthrometry has been used to evaluate the integrity of isolated and combined ACL and PCL reconstruction.[5,7,20,30,31,57,64,70,71,87] It has also been used to compare ligament integrity in those undergoing surgery via different operative techniques and as a comparator for various grafts, including patellar tendon autograft, patellar tendon allograft, Achilles

tendon allograft, and semitendinosus/gracilis autograft.[7,20,31,57,64,70,87] Malcolm et al performed arthrometry testing on 43 patients with four different ACL reconstruction grafts and found the four reconstruction types to be equally effective in the immediate restoration of normal laxity in ACL-deficient knees. They advocated use of the arthrometer in the operating room to confirm that ligament integrity was reestablished.[57] When measuring ligament laxity after reconstruction, a side-to-side difference of 5 mm or less has been used as the general criterion for surgical success and a measurement greater than 5 mm is deemed a failure.[3,7,37] Of note, we have found excellent subjective functional results even in some with side-to-side differences greater than 5 mm. Most of these have been in patients who have undergone ACL reconstruction after chronic ACL tears. We find that those with reconstruction of chronic tears may have an excellent functional outcome even with a slightly exaggerated KT finding postoperatively.

As a general guideline, a side-to-side difference in anterior tibial excursion of 4 to 5 mm or less at 30 lb of anterior force would indicate adequate ligament stability to return to previous activity.[37] An anterior tibial excursion difference of 6 mm or greater, after reconstruction, may correlate with a positive pivot-shift test,[10,11,19] which according to many is suggestive of ACL deficiency. Increased laxity found on arthrometry is a concern because of altered contact loading of the articular surfaces and possible inferior structural properties of the graft.[15,19] In our clinic, patients with increased laxity are advised to wear a brace for competitive activities. It must be emphasized that increased laxity alone as found on arthrometric studies should not be the sole criterion to determine return to sports.[87]

Several long-term studies ranging from 2 years to 10 years after reconstruction have been performed to assess the integrity of the graft.* These studies investigated the correlation of increased laxity and the type of rehabilitation performed. A classic review compared those who underwent accelerated rehabilitation, which resulted in return to play 3 to 6 months after surgery,[4,10,72,82] with those who underwent a more "traditional" nonaccelerated protocol, which would delay return to play for 8 to 12 months after surgery.[6,10,35] These studies evaluated data a minimum of 2 years after surgery. There was an increase in laxity with a side-to-side difference of 3 mm or greater in 11% to 52% of those who participated in the accelerated program and 8% to 39% of those in the nonaccelerated programs. Currently, the majority of rehabilitation programs follow the accelerated track.

Barber-Westin et al studied the effect of rehabilitation after reconstruction in 142 patients and found that 2 years postoperatively, 85% had normal displacement of less than 3-mm side-to-side difference at 134 N (10% had a 3.0- to 5.5-mm difference, and 5% had more than a 5.5-mm difference). The researcher's concluded that the increase in laxity was not due to the type of rehabilitation, but postulated that other factors may cause the increase. First, a few millimeters of graft slippage can occur from slight

---

*References 4, 6, 7, 10, 11, 15, 19, 29, 30, 35, 64, 70-72, 82, 87.

shifting of the tibial or femoral bone fixation. Second, elongation of the graft may occur during the healing and maturation period. Third, portions of the graft may have been replaced with collagen tissue of low stiffness because of a delay in maturation and the presence of a large number of small-diameter collagen fibrils.[10]

Confounding Variables

When performing arthrometry, factors that affect accurate measurement of anterior tibial displacement include positioning,[32] knee effusion,[93] muscle relaxation,[22] and tester experience.[39] Fiebert et al conducted a study on 50 subjects in which arthrometry was performed with the lower limb in neutral, internal rotation, and external rotation. They found that internal rotation significantly decreased anterior translation when compared with external rotation and neutral. They concluded that internal rotation of the tibia should be avoided when performing arthrometry.[32] Wright and Luhmann advocated aspirating the knee, if an effusion is present, before arthrometry measurements because of the high incidence of false-positive results. They found that the source of inaccuracy is an inability to stabilize the patella in the trochlear groove because of anterior displacement, which results in incorrect readings on the arthrometer.[93] The most common cause of erroneous measurements is the subject's inability to relax. It has been suggested that monitoring the level of relaxation with electromyography may be the solution for a patient who has difficulty relaxing.[22,32] We find that gently supporting the limb to be tested with the examiner's hands while gently oscillating it to and fro often leads to good relaxation of the limb. The level of experience of the tester has also affected the accuracy of measurements. It has been recommended that a tester have at least 1 month of experience before data collection.[39]

ISOKINETIC TESTING

The return of muscular strength after ligament reconstruction has been shown to be an integral component for successful return to functional and athletic activities.[8,9,37,68] Clinically, muscle strength is evaluated by performing a manual muscle test. Unfortunately, manual muscle testing is faulty because of its subjective nature and its inability to offer information regarding muscular performance. Isokinetic testing provides the physician with a valid, objective, and reliable method to measure muscular performance.[17,26,89-91] Although there is much controversy regarding the reliability of an isokinetic functional testing paradigm because our functional world is largely one of isotonic and not isokinetic activities, we still find isokinetic testing useful as a standardized testing regimen since it gives reliable side-to-side comparisons.

Isokinetic systems such as the Biodex Dynamometer (Biodex Medical Systems, Inc., Shirley, NY), Cybex Dynamometer (Cybex International Inc. Medway MA), and Con-Trex Dynamometer (Con-Trex, Inc., Dueben-

dorf, Switzerland) measure muscle performance during isokinetic muscle loading. Testing involves the use of fixed speeds of movement and variable resistance so that that maximal muscle loading can be achieved throughout the entire range of motion. Testing speed can be adjusted from 0 degrees of movement per second to 450 deg/s to allow the examiner to measure performance at different velocities. We routinely test our patients at a speed of 60 and 180 deg/s. Testing of the uninvolved limb is usually done within the first week of the rehabilitation program to obtain baseline values. Postoperative testing of both the involved and uninvolved limb typically occurs 4 to 6 months after reconstruction.

Instrumentation

After a 10- to 15-minute warm-up (i.e., an exercise bike), the patient is seated on the isokinetic testing device (Fig. 51-4) with the hip flexed 80 to 90 degrees and the thigh and pelvis fixed to the isokinetic device with a Velcro strap. Care is taken to align the knee joint axis with the axis shaft of the dynamometer. Once alignment is accomplished, the leg is then secured with another Velcro strap. After the parameters and testing speed are established, the patient is instructed to extend and flex the knee through a few practice cycles. Then, each lower limb is tested by asking the patient to perform three consecutive sets of maximal knee extension and flexion. The uninvolved extremity is tested first. By doing so, patients are allowed to familiarize themselves with the device and thus reduce hesitancy when testing the involved limb.

Absolute and Relative Contraindications

Isokinetic testing devices are considered to be very safe because testees should never meet more resistance than they can produce. As with every testing device, there are

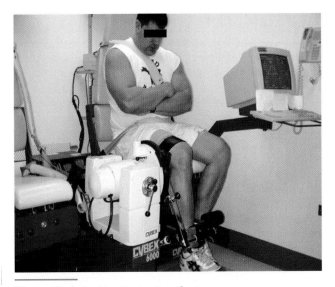

Figure 51-4. Isokinetic testing device.

certain contraindications that must be considered. Absolute contraindications include soft-tissue healing constraints, severe pain, extremely limited range of motion, severe effusion, unstable joint or bone, and acute strains. Some relative contraindications include pain, limited range of motion, and subacute sprain.[26]

Data Interpretation

The data collected include torque, acceleration, force decay rate, range of motion, and muscular performance parameters. Although numerous values may be attained from isokinetic testing, the parameters that have received significant attention with regard to performance include peak torque percentage,[18,19,36,51] percent deficit,[18,34,37] and the agonist-antagonist ratio of the involved limb.[1,18,19,34,37]

Peak torque is the highest torque value developed throughout the range of motion. The peak torque percentage is the ratio of the peak torque of the involved limb to the peak torque of the uninvolved limb multiplied by 100 (involved torque/uninvolved torque × 100). Peak torque measurements (approximately 6 months after ACL reconstruction) reveal quadriceps peak torque of the operated limb to range from 59.5% to 90%.[18,36] The normal quadriceps peak torque ratio is considered to be 90% or greater; however, athletes who have demonstrated a quadriceps ratio of 70% to 75% have been allowed to return to play.[19] The peak torque ratio for hamstrings is also measured with isokinetic testing. This measurement has proved to be useful, especially when the hamstrings are harvested and used as a graft for ACL reconstruction. There was concern that hamstring grafts would adversely affect hamstring strength after reconstruction. Several studies compared the use of hamstring grafts with other grafts after ACL reconstruction.[2,18,54,96] The majority of these studies suggested no significant deficit in the hamstring peak torque ratio with use of the hamstring graft.

Percent deficit is the peak torque percentage subtracted from 100 (100 − peak torque percent). Generally, a deficit of 10% to 15% or greater for the hamstrings and 20% or greater for the quadriceps indicates side-to-side imbalance. Based on combined results with arthrometry measurements, patients with abnormal deficit percentages are advised to use a brace or undergo further rehabilitation.

The agonist-antagonist ratio for the knee compares the peak torque ratio of the hamstrings with that of the quadriceps. Normal values of the ratio are dependent on the speed setting of the isokinetic testing device. For example, the expected ratio for a normal knee tested at a setting of 60 deg/s ranges from 60% to 69%, whereas a knee tested at 180 deg/s will have quadriceps-hamstring ratios ranging from 70% to 79%. In a knee with ACL deficiency, the ratio is usually 10% higher than that on the contralateral side (because of relative quadriceps weakness). Those with PCL injuries will have a ratio that is 10% lower.[26,90] Agonist-antagonist ratios have been used to guide rehabilitation for patients with ligament disruptions. For example, Kannus et al performed isokinetic

testing on 37 patients with ACL disruption and found deficits in hamstring strength; accordingly, an emphasis on knee flexion exercises was recommended in this population.[48] Another variable we monitor is peak torque–percent body weight. The peak torque for both the quadriceps and hamstrings as compared with one's body weight (pounds) is measured. For the quadriceps, females are expected to produce a ratio greater than 70% and males greater than 80%. For the hamstrings, females should produce a ratio greater than 30% and males greater than 40%. Our guidelines for deficits are 10% maximum for the hamstrings and 20% maximum for the quadriceps.

Validity, Reliability, and Limitations

Several studies have investigated the reliability and validity of isokinetic testing for muscular performance.[17,21,26,48,49,89-91] To prove reliability and validity, Wilk and Johnson performed isokinetic testing on 24 subjects for knee flexion and extension at varying velocities. After multiple trials they found a Pearson correlation coefficient indicating that isokinetic testing is reliable when measuring peak torque, peak torque to body weight, and several other parameters.[91] Other investigators have subsequently supported their findings.*

The reliability of isokinetic testing has been questioned when investigating the difference in positioning and inter-machine differences. Currier found a significant difference in knee extensor force with different angles of hip flexion. He advocated the use of an adjustable back stabilization unit in order to perform the test at consistent hip flexion angles.[21] Recently, Bardis et al compared the Con-Trex Dynamometer and the Cybex Dynamometer and found that the reliability of each device used separately was acceptable but that intermachine reliability was suspect.[13] These findings suggest that it is important to perform isokinetic testing in the same position and that all follow-up test should be performed on the same machine.

A few limitations have been noted with isokinetic testing, including the cost of the machine, availability of the machine, availability of personnel trained in data interpretation, inaccurate results because of pathology in the uninvolved leg, and the lack of eccentric loading measurements in some devices.[26] Eccentric contraction of muscles surrounding the knee is an important component during decelerating movements and motion control[46] that must be kept in mind during interpretation of data. It has been shown that when used in combination with hop testing, arthrometry, and outcome scales, isokinetic testing serves a vital role.[17]

FUNCTIONAL HOP TESTING

Return to functionally demanding activities such as running, stair climbing, jumping, and hopping requires

*References 1, 2, 17, 18, 26, 34, 36, 51, 54, 90, 91, 96.

the ability to produce force and to absorb force adequately.[46] Arthrometry and isokinetic testing evaluate ligament integrity and concentric strength of the limb after surgery, but both fail to correlate with functional ability.[66,81] A battery of tests such as the single hop, Noyes hop, figure-of-eight, stair hop, side hop, hop and stop, and shuttle run tests have been developed to evaluate the functional competence of a knee. These tests all have varying levels of reliability.[46,52,68,77,78] We use the Noyes hop test and the hop and stop test.

Noyes Hop Test

The Noyes hop test consists of four components (Fig. 51–5). The test includes a single hop for distance, a timed hop for 6 m, a triple hop for distance, and a crossover hop for distance. The affected and unaffected limbs are tested to formulate a bilateral symmetry score.[67,68] Noyes et al studied normal uninjured subjects and found that a limb symmetry index of 85% or greater was normal for both males and females regardless of dominance and sports activity level.[69] They also performed studies on patients with ACL rupture and found the four tests to be specific for knee pathology.[68] Bolgla and Keskula found the Noyes hop test to be reliable in testing 5 male and 15 female volunteers and calculated an interclass correlation coefficient of 95% to 96% for all four activities.[16]

A few limitations of the Noyes hop test have been noted. First, there are no movement standards that can be followed while testing. For example, limb symmetry scores can be misleading if a subject uses compensatory motion such as an arm swing, which causes the interlimb ratio to appear symmetric.[46] Second, the Noyes hop test measures force production but does not make a distinction for force absorption measurements. As reported in the literature, deceleration parameters such as eccentric contraction and force absorption have a strong correlation with functional performance.[61]

HOP AND STOP TEST

The hop and stop test, as described by Juris et al,[46] consists of two components, a maximal hop for distance and a maximal controlled leap (Fig. 51–6). This test addresses the issues of standard movement and measurement of force absorption. Often, testing paradigms do not account for coordination and force absorption skill. The hop and stop test assesses not only force production ability but also force absorption. The maximal hop for distance is used to measure force production. The subject is instructed to use the same leg for takeoff and landing when performing this test. The maximal controlled leap evaluates force absorption. When performing the leap, the subject uses one leg for takeoff and lands on the other leg, which is the leg being tested. Both these tests require subjects to start with their hands on their hips and the hip and knee flexed to 90 degrees. This requirement eliminates compensatory motion such as arm swing and standardizes motion parameters while testing.

Once the data are collected, the performance variables that are created include hop percent height, hop symmetry, stop symmetry, and hop-to-stop ratio. The hop percent height normalizes the hop distance to the subject's stature. Juris and colleagues found that hop symmetry and stop symmetry had no significant difference in their ability to detect normal or dysfunctional knees. They also found the hop and stop test to be reliable and accurate in assessing the functional performance of the knee because it takes into account force absorption.

OUTCOME SCALES

Arthrometry, isokinetic testing, and functional hop testing provide objective findings to evaluate the lower limb. Subjective reporting of knee stability and function through outcome scales plays an important role in assessing the success of surgical reconstruction, rehabilitation, and

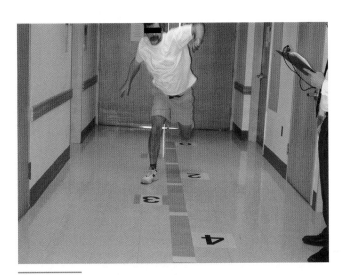

Figure 51–5. Noyes hop testing. A 6-m hop grid is used to evaluate functional hopping.

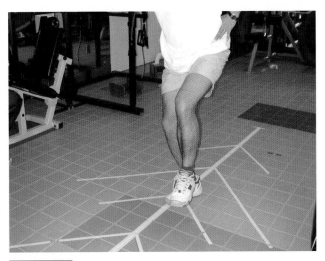

Figure 51–6. Hop and stop testing.

determination of return to unrestricted activities. Several knee rating systems are available to evaluate a patient's symptoms, perception of knee condition, daily functional limitations, and current sports and occupational activity levels. Several studies have examined the reliability, validity, and responsiveness of these scales.[28,58-60,69,86] The most commonly used scales include the Noyes' Cincinnati knee rating questionnaire and the Lyshom scale. In our clinic we use the Cincinnati knee rating questionnaire.

The Cincinnati knee questionnaire is part of the Cincinnati Knee Rating System that was developed by Noyes in 1983; it also includes physical examination, instrumental testing, and radiographic evidence. The questionnaire uses a 100-point rating system that evaluates symptoms such as pain, swelling, and giving way. Patients rate activities such as walking, stair climbing, running, jumping, and twisting. The scale also assesses the patient's overall function. Barber-Westin et al studied 100 subjects and found the questions to be highly responsive in detecting changes between evaluations.[12] This questionnaire has been found to be reliable, valid, and responsive.[12,59]

The Lysholm questionnaire was introduced by Lysholm and Gilquist in 1982.[56] This scale, similar to the Cincinnati questionnaire, is also based on a 100-point rating scale. It assesses symptoms by asking questions about pain, swelling, and instability. The Lysholm scale assigns more points to symptoms than the Cincinnati questionnaire does. Function is gauged by rating activities such as stair climbing and squatting. Other values that are rated in the Lysholm scale include the patient's perception of limp, support, and thigh atrophy. This, like the Cincinnati scale, has been shown to be reliable, valid, and responsive. Marx et al administered this questionnaire to 133 patients and found the intraclass correlation coefficient to be 0.95.[58]

SUMMARY

Each component of functional testing such as arthrometry, isokinetic testing, functional hop testing, and outcome scales has been found to be a reliable and valid measure of limb stability, strength, function, and satisfaction. These tests have been used either individually or cumulatively to assess the success of surgical intervention, rehabilitation, functional ability, and patient satisfaction. It has been shown that the data collected from all the tests cumulatively can accurately guide return to unrestricted activities.[8,11,17] Individually, each test provides limited, but useful information. Although functional testing has been shown to be valid and reliable, a recent survey conducted by Francis et al suggested that only a small percentage of surgeons use these tools to measure outcomes or guide return to unrestricted activity.[33a] This survey highlights the need to standardize outcome measurements postoperatively.[56]

References

1. Aagaard P, Simonsen EB, Magnusson SP, et al: A new concept for isokinetic hamstring: quadriceps muscle strength ratio. Am J Sports Med 26:231-237, 1998.
2. Adachi N, Ochi M, Uchio Y, et al: Harvesting hamstring tendons for ACL reconstruction influences postoperative hamstring muscle performance. Arch Orthop Traumatol Surg 123:460-465, 2003.
3. Aglietti P, Buzzi R, Menchetti PM, Giron F: Arthroscopically assisted semitendinosus and gracilis tendon graft in reconstruction for acute anterior cruciate ligament injuries in athletes. Am J Sports Med 24:726-731, 1996.
4. Aglietti P, Zaccherotti G, Menchetti PPM, et al: A comparison of clinical and radiological parameters with two arthroscopic techniques for anterior cruciate ligament reconstruction. Knee Surg Sports Traumatol Arthrosc 3:2-8, 1995.
5. Anderson AF, Lipscomb AB: Preoperative instrumented testing of anterior and posterior knee laxity. Am J Sports Med 17:387-392, 1989.
6. Bach BR Jr, Jones GT, Sweet FA, et al: Arthroscopy-assisted anterior cruciate ligament reconstruction using patellar tendon substitution. Two- to four-year follow-up results. Am J Sports Med 22:758-767, 1994.
7. Bach BR Jr, Levy ME, Bojchuk J, et al: Single-incision endoscopic anterior cruciate ligament reconstruction using patellar tendon autograft. Minimum two-year follow-up evaluation. Am J Sports Med 26:30-40, 1998.
8. Barber SD, Noyes FR, Mangine R, DeMaio M: Rehabilitation after ACL reconstruction: Function testing. Orthopedics 15:969-974, 1992.
9. Barber SD, Noyes FR, Mangine RE, et al: Quantitative assessment of functional limitations in normal and anterior cruciate ligament–deficient knees. Clin Orthop 255:204-214, 1990.
10. Barber-Westin SD, Noyes FR: The effect of rehabilitation and return to activity on anterior-posterior knee displacements after anterior cruciate ligament reconstruction. Am J Sports Med 21:264-270, 1993.
11. Barber-Westin SD, Noyes FR, Heckmann TP, Shaffer BL: The effect of exercise and rehabilitation on anterior-posterior knee displacements after anterior cruciate ligament autograft reconstruction. Am J Sports Med 27:84-93, 1999.
12. Barber-Westin SD, Noyes FR, McCloskey JW: Rigorous statistical reliability, validity, and responsiveness testing of the Cincinnati knee rating system in 350 subjects with uninjured, injured, or anterior cruciate ligament–reconstructed knees. Am J Sports Med 27:402-416, 1999.
13. Bardis C, Kalamara E, Loucaides G, et al: Intramachine and intermachine reproducibility of concentric performance: A study of the Con-Trex MJ and the Cybex Norm dynamometers. Isokinet Exerc Sci 12:91-97, 2004.
14. Belanger MJ, Moore DC, Crisco JJ 3rd, et al: Knee laxity does not vary with the menstrual cycle, before or after exercise. Am J Sports Med 32:1150-1157, 2004.
15. Beynnon BD, Johnson RJ, Fleming BC: The science of anterior cruciate ligament rehabilitation. Clin Orthop 402:9-20, 2002.
16. Bolgla LA, Keskula DR: Reliability of lower extremity functional performance tests. J Orthop Sports Phys Ther 26:138-142, 1997.
17. Brosky JA Jr, Nitz AJ, Malone TR, et al: Intrarater reliability of selected clinical outcome measures following anterior cruciate ligament reconstruction. J Orthop Sports Phys Ther 29:39-48, 1999.
18. Carter TR: Isokinetic evaluation of anterior cruciate ligament reconstruction: Hamstring versus patellar tendon. Arthroscopy 15:169-172, 1999.
19. Cascio BM, Culp L, Cosgarea AJ: Return to play after anterior cruciate ligament reconstruction. Clin Sports Med 23:395-408, 2004.
20. Chang SK, Egami DK, Shaieb MD, et al: Anterior cruciate ligament reconstruction: Allograft versus autograft. Arthroscopy 19:453-462, 2003.
21. Currier DP: Positioning for knee strengthening exercises. Phys Ther 57:148-152, 1977.
22. Daniel DM, Malcom LL, Losse G, et al: Instrumented measure of anterior laxity of the knee. J Bone Joint Surg Am 67:720-726, 1985.
23. Daniel DM, Stone ML: KT-1000 anterior posterior displacement measurements. In Daniel DM, Akeson WH, O'Connor JJ (eds): Knee Ligaments: Structure, Function, Injury and Repair. New York, Raven Press, 1990, pp 427-447.
24. Daniel DM, Stone ML, Barnett P, Sachs R: Use of the quadriceps active test to diagnose posterior cruciate ligament disruption and measure posterior laxity of the knee. J Bone Joint Surg Am 70:386-391, 1988.

25. Daniel DM, Stone ML, Sachs R, Malcom L: Instrumented measurement of anterior knee laxity in patients with acute anterior cruciate ligament disruption. Am J Sports Med 13:401-407, 1985.
26. Davies GJ: Isokinetic testing. In Davies GJ (ed): A Compendium of Isokinetics in Clinical Usage and Rehabilitation Techniques. Onalaska, WI, S & S Publishers, 1987 pp 19-37.
27. Deie M, Sakamaki Y, Sumen Y, et al: Anterior knee laxity in young women varies with their menstrual cycle. Int Orthop 26:154-156, 2002.
28. Demirdjian AM, Petrie SG, Guanche CA, Thomas KA: The outcomes of two knee scoring questionnaires in a normal population. Am Sports Med 26:46-51, 1998.
29. Fanelli GC, Edson CJ: Arthroscopically assisted combined anterior and posterior cruciate ligament reconstruction in the multiple ligament injured knee: 2- to 10-year follow-up. Arthroscopy 18:703-714, 2002.
30. Fanelli GC, Edson CJ: Combined posterior cruciate ligament–posterolateral reconstructions with Achilles tendon allograft and biceps femoris tendon tenodesis: 2- to 10-year follow-up. Arthroscopy 20:339-345, 2004.
31. Feller JA, Cooper R, Webster KE: Current Australian trends in rehabilitation following anterior cruciate ligament reconstruction. Knee 9:121-126, 2002.
32. Fiebert I, Gresley J, Hoffman S, Kunkel K: Comparative measurements of anterior tibial translation using the KT-1000 knee arthrometer with the leg in neutral, internal rotation, and external rotation. J Orthop Sports Phys Ther 19:331-334, 1994.
33. Fowler PJ, Messieh SS: Isolated posterior cruciate ligament injuries in athletes. Am J Sports Med 15:553-557, 1987.
33a. Francis A, Thomas RD, McGregor A: Anterior cruciate ligament rupture: Reconstruction surgery and rehabilitation. A nationwide survey of current practice. Knee 3(1):13-18, 2001.
34. Gerodimos V, Mandou V, Zafeiridis A, et al: Isokinetic peak torque and hamstring/quadriceps ratios in young basketball players. Effects of age, velocity, and contraction mode. J Sports Med Phys Fitness 43:444-452, 2003.
35. Glasgow SG, Gabriel JP, Sapega AA, et al: The effect of early versus late return to vigorous activities on the outcome of anterior cruciate ligament reconstruction. Am J Sports Med 21:243-248, 1993.
36. Gokeler A, Schmalz T, Knopf E, et al: The relationship between isokinetic quadriceps strength and laxity on gait analysis parameters in anterior cruciate ligament reconstructed knees. Knee Surg Sports Traumatol Arthrosc 11:372-378, 2003.
37. Gotlin RS: Lower extremity. In Scuderi GR, McCann PD, Bruno PJ (eds): Sports Medicine: Principles of Primary Care. New York, CV Mosby, 1997, pp 463-506.
38. Gross SM, Carcia CR, Gansneder BM, Shultz SJ: Rate of force application during knee arthrometer testing affects stiffness but not displacement measurements. J Orthop Sports Phys Ther 34:132-139, 2004.
39. Hanten WP, Pace MB: Reliability of measuring anterior laxity of the knee joint using a knee ligament arthrometer. Phys Ther 67:357-359, 1987.
40. Hewett TE, Noyes FR, Lee MD: Diagnosis of complete and partial posterior cruciate ligament ruptures. Stress radiography compared with KT-1000 arthrometer and posterior drawer testing. Am J Sports Med 25:648-655, 1997.
41. Highgenboten CL, Jackson AW, Jansson KA, Meske NB: KT-1000 arthrometer: Conscious and unconscious test results using 15, 20, and 30 pounds of force. Am J Sports Med 20:450-454, 1992.
42. Highgenboten CL, Jackson A, Meske NB: Genucom, KT-1000, and Stryker knee laxity measuring device comparison: Device reproducibility and interdevice comparison in asymptomatic subjects. Am J Sports Med 17:743-746, 1989.
43. Highgenboten CL, Jackson A, Meske NB: Genucom knee analysis system: Reproducibility and database development. Med Sci Sports Exerc 21:713-717, 1990.
44. Hole RL, Lintner DM, Kamaric E, Moseley JB: Increased tibial translation after partial sectioning of the anterior cruciate ligament. The posterolateral bundle. Am J Sports Med 24:556-560, 1996.
45. Huber FE, Irrgang JJ, Harner C, Lephart S: Intratester and intertester reliability of the KT-1000 arthrometer in the assessment of posterior laxity of the knee. Am J Sports Med 25:479-485, 1997.
46. Juris PM, Phillips EM, Dalpe C, et al: A dynamic test of lower extremity function following anterior cruciate ligament reconstruction and rehabilitation. J Orthop Sports Phys Ther 26:184-191, 1997.
47. Kannus P: Normality, variability and predictability of work, power and torque acceleration energy with respect to peak torque in isokinetic muscle testing. Int J Sports Med 13:249-256, 1992.
48. Kannus P, Jarvinen M, Johnson R, et al: Function of the quadriceps and hamstrings muscles in knees with chronic partial deficiency of the anterior cruciate ligament. Isometric and isokinetic evaluation. Am J Sports Med 20:162-168, 1992.
49. Kannus P, Yasuda K: Value of isokinetic angle–specific torque measurements in normal and injured knees. Med Sci Sports Exerc 24:292-297, 1992.
50. Karageanes SJ, Blackburn K, Vangelos ZA: The association of the menstrual cycle with the laxity of the anterior cruciate ligament in adolescent female athletes. Clin J Sport Med 10:162-168, 2000.
51. Kobayashi A, Higuchi H, Terauchi M, et al: Muscle performance after anterior cruciate ligament reconstruction. Int Orthop 28:48-51, 2004.
52. Lephert SM, Perrin DH, Fu FH, Minger K: Functional performance tests for anterior cruciate ligament insufficient athlete. Athl Train 26:44-50, 1991.
53. Lintner DM, Kamaric E, Moseley JB, Noble PC: Partial tears of the anterior cruciate ligament. Are they clinically detectable? Am J Sports Med 23:111-118, 1995.
54. Lipscomb AB, Johnston RK, Snyder RB, et al: Evaluation of hamstring strength following use of semitendinosus and gracilis tendons to reconstruct the anterior cruciate ligament. Am J Sports Med 10:340-342, 1982.
55. Liu W, Maitland ME, Bell GD: A modeling study of partial ACL injury: Simulated KT-2000 arthrometer tests. J Biomech Eng 124:294-301, 2002.
56. Lysholm J, Gillquist J: Evaluation of knee ligament surgery results with special emphasis on use of a scoring scale. Am J Sports Med 10:150-154, 1982.
57. Malcom LL, Daniel DM, Stone ML, Sachs R: The measurement of anterior knee laxity after ACL reconstructive surgery. Clin Orthop 196:35-41, 1985.
58. Marx RG: Knee rating scales. Arthroscopy 19:1103-1108, 2003.
59. Marx RG, Jones EC, Allen AA, et al: Reliability, validity, and responsiveness of four knee outcome scales for athletic patients. J Bone Joint Surg Am 83:1459-1469, 2001.
60. Marx RG, Stump TJ, Jones EC, et al: Development and evaluation of an activity rating scale for disorders of the knee. Am J Sports Med 29:213-218, 2001.
61. McNair PJ, Marshall RN: Landing characteristics in subjects with normal and anterior cruciate ligament deficient knee joints. Arch Phys Med Rehabil 75:584-589, 1994.
62. McQuade KJ, Sidles JA, Larson RV: Reliability of the Genucom Knee Analysis System. A pilot study. Clin Orthop 245:216-219, 1989.
63. Medrano D Jr, Smith D: A comparison of knee joint laxity among male and female collegiate soccer players and non-athletes. Sports Biomech 2:203-212, 2003.
64. Muren O, Dahlstedt L, Dalen N: Reconstruction of acute anterior cruciate ligament injuries: A prospective, randomised study of 40 patients with 7-year follow-up. No advantage of synthetic augmentation compared to a traditional patellar tendon graft. Arch Orthop Trauma Surg 123:144-147, 2003.
65. Myrer JW, Schulthies SS, Fellingham GW: Relative and absolute reliability of the KT-2000 arthrometer for uninjured knees. Testing at 67, 89, 134, and 178 N and manual maximum forces. Am J Sports Med 24:104-108, 1996.
66. Neeb TB, Aufdemkampe G, Wagener JH, Mastenbroek L: Assessing anterior cruciate ligament injuries: The association and differential value of questionnaires, clinical tests, and functional tests. J Orthop Sports Phys Ther 26:324-331, 1997.
67. Noyes FR: The Noyes Knee Rating System. An International Publication of Cincinnati Sports Medicine Research and Education Foundation, Cincinnati, OH, 1990.
68. Noyes FR, Barber SD, Mangine RE: Abnormal lower limb symmetry determined by function hop tests after anterior cruciate ligament rupture. Am J Sports Med 19:513-518, 1991.
69. Noyes FR, Barber SD, Mooar LA: A rationale for assessing sports activity levels and limitations in knee disorders. Clin Orthop 246:238-249, 1989.

70. Nyland J, Caborn DN, Rothbauer J, et al: Two-year outcomes following ACL reconstruction with allograft tibialis anterior tendons: A retrospective study. Knee Surg Sports Traumatol Arthrosc 11:212-218, 2003.

71. Nyland J, Hester P, Caborn DN: Double-bundle posterior cruciate ligament reconstruction with allograft tissue: 2-year postoperative outcomes. Knee Surg Sports Traumatol Arthrosc 10:274-279, 2002.

72. O'Neill DB: Arthroscopically assisted reconstruction of the anterior cruciate ligament. A prospective randomized analysis of three techniques. J Bone Joint Surg Am 78:803-813, 1996.

73. Parolie JM, Bergfeld JA: Long-term results of nonoperative treatment of isolated posterior cruciate ligament injuries in the athlete. Am J Sports Med 14:35-38, 1986.

74. Queale WS, Mackler LS, Handling KA, Richards JG: Instrumented examination of knee laxity in patients with anterior cruciate deficiency: A comparison of the KT-2000, Knee Signature System, and Genucom. J Orthop Sports Phys Ther 19:345-351, 1994.

75. Rangger C, Daniel DM, Stone ML, Kaufman K: Diagnosis of an ACL disruption with KT-1000 arthrometer measurements. Knee Surg Sports Traumatol Arthrosc 1:60-66, 1993.

76. Riederman R, Wroble RR, Grood ES, et al: Reproducibility of the knee signature system. Am J Sports Med 19:660-664, 1991.

77. Risberg MA, Ekeland A: Assessment of functional tests after anterior cruciate ligament surgery. J Orthop Sports Phys Ther 19:212-217, 1994.

78. Risberg MA, Holm I, Ekeland A: Reliability of functional knee tests in normal athletes. Scand J Med Sci Sports 5:24-28, 1995.

79. Romani W, Patrie J, Curl LA, Flaws JA: The correlations between estradiol, estrone, estriol, progesterone, and sex hormone–binding globulin and anterior cruciate ligament stiffness in healthy, active females. J Womens Health 12:287-298, 2003.

80. Sernert N, Kartus JT Jr, Ejerhed L, Karlsson J: Right and left knee laxity measurements: A prospective study of patients with anterior cruciate ligament injuries and normal control subjects. Arthroscopy 20:564-571, 2004.

81. Sernert N, Kartus J, Kohler K, et al: Analysis of subjective, objective, and functional examination tests after anterior cruciate ligament reconstruction. Knee Surg Sports Traumatol Arthrosc 7:160-165, 1999.

82. Shelbourne KD, Gray T: Anterior cruciate ligament reconstruction with autogenous patellar tendon graft followed by accelerated rehabilitation. A two- to nine-year followup. Am J Sports Med 25:786-795, 1997.

83. Sherman OH, Markolf KL, Ferkel RD: Measurements of anterior laxity in normal and anterior cruciate absent knees with two instrumented test devices. Clin Orthop 215:156-161, 1987.

84. Slauterbeck JR, Fuzie SF, Smith MP, et al: The menstrual cycle, sex hormones, and anterior cruciate ligament injury. J Athl Train 37:275-278, 2002.

85. Snyder-Mackler L, Fitzgerald GK, Bartolozzi AR 3rd, Ciccotti MG: The relationship between passive joint laxity and functional outcome after anterior cruciate ligament injury. Am J Sports Med 25:191-195, 1997.

86. Tegner Y, Lysholm J: Rating systems in the evaluation of knee ligament injuries. Clin Orthop 198:43-49, 1985.

87. Tyler TF, McHugh MP, Gleim GW, Nicholas SJ: Association of KT-1000 measurements with clinical tests of knee stability 1 year following anterior cruciate ligament reconstruction. J Orthop Sports Phys Ther 29:540-545, 1999.

88. Van Lunen BL, Roberts J, Branch JD, Dowling EA: Association of menstrual-cycle hormone changes with anterior cruciate ligament laxity measurements. J Athl Train 38:298-303, 2003.

89. Wilk KE: Dynamic muscle strength testing. In Amundsen LR (ed): Muscle Strength Testing: Instrumented and Non-Instrumented Systems. New York, Churchill Livingstone, 1990, p 123.

90. Wilk KE: Isokinetic testing: Goals, standards, and knee test interpretation. In Isokinetic Source Book. Shirley, NY, Biodex Medical, 1997, pp 5-14.

91. Wilk KE, Johnson RE: The reliability of Biodex B-2000. Phys Ther 68:792, 1988.

92. Wojtys EM, Huston LJ, Boynton MD, et al: The effect of the menstrual cycle on anterior cruciate ligament injuries in women as determined by hormone levels. Am J Sports Med 30:182-188, 2002.

93. Wright RW, Luhmann SJ: The effect of knee effusions on KT-1000 arthrometry. A cadaver study. Am J Sports Med 26:571-574, 1998.

94. Wroble RR, Grood ES, Noyes FR, Schmitt DJ: Reproducibility of Genucom knee analysis system testing. Am J Sports Med 18:387-395, 1990.

95. Wroble RR, Van Ginkel LA, Grood ES, et al: Repeatability of the KT-1000 arthrometer in a normal population. Am J Sports Med 18:396-399, 1990.

96. Yasuda K, Tsujino J, Ohkoshi Y, et al: Graft site morbidity with autogenous semitendinosus and gracilis tendons. Am J Sports Med 23:706-714, 1995.

CHAPTER 52

Disorders of the Proximal
Tibiofibular Joint

David R. Whiddon • Todd A. Parker • John E. Kuhn • Jon K. Sekiya

Instability of the proximal tibiofibular joint is a rare injury. Initially described by Dubreuil in 1848,[9] the largest case series is attributable to Ogden,[26,27] who reported on 43 patients with this disorder. Turco and Spinella[38] described an additional 17 patients with instability and suggested that the disorder may be more common than reported. The varied presentation of instability may occur as an isolated idiopathic subluxation of the joint or as a higher energy injury with associated long bone and ankle fractures. Injury most commonly occurs in young men as a result of sports-related activities where violent twisting motions of the flexed knee occur, such as wrestling, basketball, soccer, gymnastics, parachute jumping, skiing, judo, rugby, football, track, baseball, racquetball, roller skating, and jet skiing.[9,17,24,26,27,37,38] A thorough understanding of the anatomy and biomechanics of the proximal tibiofibular joint, the mechanisms leading to instability, and the symptoms and associated conditions are essential to making this difficult diagnosis.

ANATOMY

The adult proximal tibiofibular joint is a diarthrodial joint consisting of a synovial membrane–lined, hyaline cartilage articulation between the lateral condyle of the tibia and the fibular head. A communication with the knee joint is present in approximately 10% of adults,[10,25,30] although an MRI study showed a communication in 9 of 14 (64%) fresh cadaveric specimens.[4] The joint capsule stabilizes the articulation with ligamentous attachments that are thicker and stronger anteriorly (Fig. 52–1). The anterior portion of the joint is stabilized by two or three broad bands of the anterior tibiofibular ligament, which pass obliquely upward from the fibular head and insert on the anterior aspect of the lateral tibial condyle, and an extension of the deep layer of the biceps femoris tendon, which blends with the anterior proximal tibiofibular ligament and inserts on Gerdy's tubercle.[4,20] Posteriorly the joint is stabilized by two thick bands of the posterior proximal tibiofibular ligament passing obliquely upward from the fibular head and attaching to the posterior aspect of the lateral tibial condyle and covered and reinforced by the popliteus tendon.[4,10,25,30] The joint also may be stabilized by the posterolateral structures of the knee, including the arcuate ligament, the fabellofibular ligament, the popliteofibular ligament, the popliteus muscle, and the fibular collateral ligament.[31,36] Anterior movement of the fibular

head is stabilized by the biceps femoris tendon, which inserts on the styloid process and upper surface of the head of the fibula, and the fibular collateral ligament, which extends from the lateral aspect of the fibular head just anterior to the styloid and attaches to the posterior aspect of the lateral femoral condyle.[10,20,30,31,36] The flexion angle of the knee plays an important role in the injury mechanism.[26] The lateral collateral ligament is tight from approximately 0 to 30 degrees of knee flexion. At higher flexion angles, the lateral collateral ligament and the biceps femoris tendon relax, allowing the proximal fibula to migrate anteriorly. With knee extension, the proximal fibula is pulled posteriorly as these same structures tighten. This anterior-posterior motion is more prominent in children and gradually decreases in adults.[25] This laxity in the joint capsule with knee flexion predisposes the proximal tibiofibular joint to injury primarily in the flexed position.

In addition to the soft-tissue restraints present in the proximal tibiofibular joint, the bony anatomy deserves special consideration. Ogden[25,26] described two variants based on observations from 43 cases of instability that he treated and anatomic dissections of 84 specimens. He divided the specimens into two subgroups based on the horizontal inclination of the joint, with the division chosen arbitrarily as 20 degrees. The first group, described as the horizontal variant, has less than 20 degrees of joint inclination relative to the horizontal plane (Fig. 50–2A); this results in the fibular head being seated in a groove behind a prominent lateral tibial ridge that enhances stability against anterior dislocation. The surface area of the horizontal variant is planar, circular, and relatively large, averaging 26 mm^2. The second group, the oblique variant, has a joint angle of inclination greater than 20 degrees and is highly variable in surface area, ranging from 10 to 40 mm^2 (average 17 mm^2) (Fig. 50–2B). The fibular articular surface configuration can be planar, concave, or convex with an inclination that is highly variable and can reach 76 degrees. The decreased surface area and increased angle of inclination are thought to predispose the oblique variant to greater instability, with 70% of the injuries described by Ogden occurring in oblique joints.[25,26]

The proximal tibiofibular joint acts in concert with the ankle joint to allow external rotation of the fibula with ankle dorsiflexion.[3] As the ankle is dorsiflexed, the lateral plane of the talus rotates. In a stable ankle, the fibula rotates externally about its longitudinal axis effectively to widen the mortise. The oblique variant is more con-

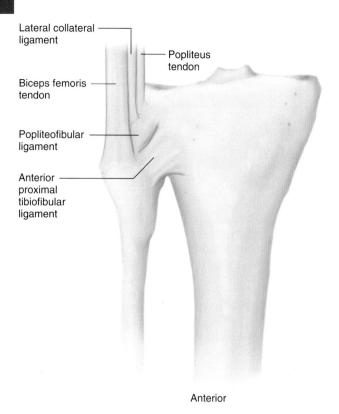

Lateral collateral
ligament

Popliteus
tendon

Biceps femoris
tendon

Popliteofibular
ligament

Anterior
proximal
tibiofibular
ligament

Anterior

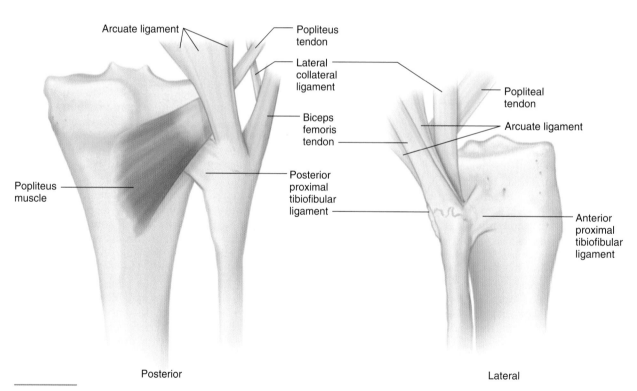

Arcuate ligament

Popliteus
tendon

Lateral
collateral
ligament

Biceps
femoris
tendon

Posterior
proximal
tibiofibular
ligament

Popliteus
muscle

Posterior

Popliteal
tendon

Arcuate ligament

Anterior
proximal
tibiofibular
ligament

Lateral

Figure 52–1. Anatomy of the proximal tibiofibular joint.

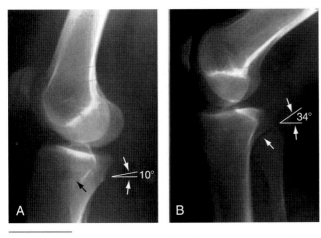

Figure 52–2. Lateral radiographs show anatomic variation of the proximal tibiofibular joint. Increased slope of the articulation is associated with the development of instability. **A,** Horizontal orientation(<20 degrees). (The black arrow points to the joint.) **B,** Oblique orientation (>20 degrees) is more likely to develop instability. (The white arrow points to the joint.) (Copyright 2003 American Academy of Orthopaedic Surgeons. From Sekiya JK, Kuhn JE: Instability of the proximal tibiofibular joint. J Am Acad Orthop Surg 11:120-128, 2003, with permission.)

strained in rotational mobility, and forced ankle dorsiflexion may increase torsional loads on the oblique joint, predisposing to a higher risk of fibular dislocation or fracture.[25]

CLASSIFICATION OF INSTABILITY AND INJURY

Ogden[26] proposed a classification system to describe proximal tibiofibular joint instability. The four types are based on direction of instability: atraumatic subluxation, anterolateral dislocation, posteromedial dislocation, and the rare superior dislocation. In his review of 43 patients, Ogden[26] noted 10 with subluxation, 29 with anterolateral dislocations, 3 with posteromedial dislocations, and 1 with superior dislocation. Four cases of inferior dislocation also have been reported.[12]

Idiopathic subluxation is an atraumatic condition involving excessive symptomatic anterior-posterior motion without actual dislocation of the joint. The condition may occur bilaterally, and patients typically have no history of inciting trauma. Laxity of the capsular ligaments is thought to contribute to subluxation. This disorder tends to be reported in younger individuals and individuals with generalized ligamentous laxity, Ehlers-Danlos syndrome, and other conditions of hypermobility.[7,26,27] In 10 cases of atraumatic subluxation in Ogden's series,[26] only 4 occurred in adults; however, 3 of these cases were associated with peroneal nerve symptoms.

Anterolateral dislocation is the most frequent type of dislocation, involving injury to the anterior and posterior capsular ligaments (Fig. 52–3A). This injury usually results from a fall on a hyperflexed knee with the foot

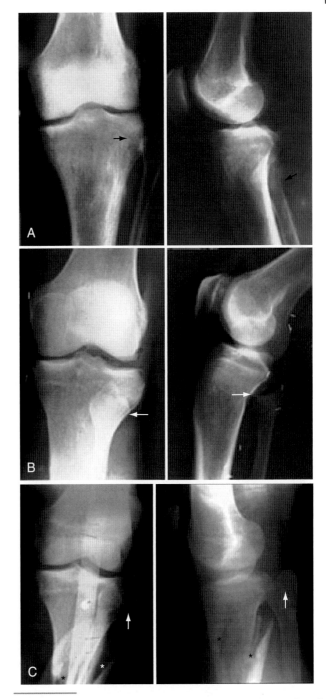

Figure 52–3. **A,** Anteroposterior and lateral radiographs of an anterolateral dislocation of the proximal tibiofibular joint. (The arrows demonstrate the lateral and anterior displacement of the fibula.) **B,** Anteroposterior and lateral radiographs of a posteromedial dislocation of the proximal tibiofibular joint. (The arrows demonstrate the medial and posterior displacement of the fibula.) **C,** Anteroposterior and lateral radiographs of a superior dislocation; note the associated tibia fracture *(asterisks)* with this high-energy injury. (The arrows demonstrate the superior placement of the fibula.) (Copyright 2003 American Academy of Orthopaedic Surgeons. From Sekiya JK, Kuhn JE: Instability of the proximal tibiofibular joint. J Am Acad Orthop Surg 11:120-128, 2003, with permission.)

inverted and plantar flexed, such as landing on a foot caught under the body with a flexed knee.[26,27,38] Higher flexion angles result in relaxation of the lateral collateral ligament and biceps femoris tendon, with twisting of the body creating a torque that moves the fibular head laterally to the edge of the bone buttress of the lateral tibial metaphysis. The ankle inversion and forced plantar flexion cause a reflex contracture of the peroneal, extensor hallucis longus, and extensor digitorum longus muscles, pulling the now laterally displaced fibular head anteriorly. When dislocated in the anterolateral position, the fibular head is stable resulting from the intact pull of the fibular collateral ligament.[26,27,38]

Posteromedial dislocations appear much less frequently in the literature.[1,19,26,27,41] This injury has been reported to result from a direct blow to the knee or from a twisting injury that tears the supporting ligaments. The fibular head is displaced posteriorly and medially along the posterolateral tibial metaphysis by the intact biceps femoris tendon (Fig. 52–3B). This type of dislocation often is associated with a common peroneal nerve injury.

Superior dislocations are essentially a dislocation of the entire fibula (Fig. 52–3C). Usually resulting from a high-energy ankle or leg injury, superior migration of the fibula disrupts the entire tibiofibular interosseous membrane and is associated with lateral malleolar injuries and tibial fractures.[19,26] Atraumatic superior dislocation of the proximal tibiofibular joint also has been associated with congenital dislocation of the knee.[26]

CLINICAL PRESENTATION

The presentation can be subtle, and other etiologies of lateral knee pain must be considered.[33] The differential diagnosis includes biceps femoris tendinitis, meniscal pathology, and posterolateral instability.[32] A thorough physical examination with particular attention to the proximal tibiofibular joint should isolate the location of the pathology. Because of the association with peroneal nerve injuries, and the possibility of longitudinal instability of the fibula, it is important to assess the integrity and functionality of the ankle and peroneal nerve. When the patient presents after high-energy trauma, associated injuries may include fractures of the tibial plateau or shaft, ipsilateral proximal femur, distal femoral epiphysis, ankle fractures, or knee dislocations.[26] When other traumatic injuries such as these are present, the proximal tibiofibular dislocation may be missed initially.

With isolated proximal tibiofibular joint injury, effusions are rarely present. With anterolateral dislocations, there is likely to be a prominent lateral mass, with tenderness to palpation over this mass.[26] The fibular head may be mobile with the knee flexed, but may be relatively fixed with the knee in extension. Examination of the biceps tendon reveals a tense, curved cord, which may be tender to palpation. Pain also may be accentuated by having the patient actively dorsiflex and evert the foot and by extending the flexed knee.

In the absence of acute trauma, when chronic instability or atraumatic subluxation is under consideration, the knee should be flexed to 90 degrees (relaxing the lateral collateral ligament and biceps femoris tendon) and the fibular head palpated for tenderness. Anterior-to-posterior mobility should be assessed by grasping the fibular head between the thumb and index finger, and the patient should be asked if this motion reproduces the symptoms or causes any apprehension.[2] The Radulescu sign, which is performed by having the patient lie prone with the knee flexed to 90 degrees, also may be helpful.[35] One hand stabilizes the thigh, while the other internally rotates the lower leg to see if the fibular head can be subluxated or dislocated anteriorly.

Recurrent or chronic dislocation of the proximal tibiofibular joint is associated with a wide range of symptoms that may mimic other knee conditions.[33] Although patients usually have no problems with activities of daily living, symptoms may be present during activities requiring sudden changes in direction, such as sports movement. Patients may complain of a sensation of instability or of the knee giving way. Stair climbing may aggravate symptoms.[35]

Patients with symptomatic proximal tibiofibular joint ganglia may complain of a sensation of fullness in the lateral knee.[6,22,23] Peroneal nerve symptoms are common, with dysesthesia present in 54% of patients and footdrop in 30%.[22] Anterior compartment syndrome has been reported in association with a proximal tibiofibular joint cyst.[43] Ganglion cysts of the proximal tibiofibular joint may be a sign of degenerative changes involving this articulation.

IMAGING STUDIES

Plain radiographs should be obtained of the knee in true anteroposterior and lateral views with comparison views obtained from the other knee or previous radiographs if possible.[30,39,41] On the anteroposterior view, the medial aspect of the fibular head crosses the lateral border of the tibia. On the lateral view, the fibular head overlies the posteromedial border of the tibia. Resnick and colleagues[30] described a line that follows the lateral tibial spine distally along the posterior aspect of the tibia and defines the most posteromedial portion of the lateral tibial condyle (Fig. 50–4). In a normal knee, this line is found over the midpoint of the fibular head. In anterolateral dislocations, the fibular head is anterior to this line; in contrast, in posteromedial dislocations, all or most of the fibular head is posterior to this line. Although some investigators have disputed the value of oblique radiographs, an oblique view with the knee in 45 to 60 degrees of internal rotation, which places the proximal tibiofibular joint in profile, allows visualization of the width of the articular space and appearance of the subchondral bone.[16,30,41] Although not necessary in all cases, axial CT has been shown to be a reliable and accurate imaging modality to identify injury to the proximal tibiofibular joint.[16,42] It may be most useful when the diagnosis is suspected but not clearly established on plain radiographs, and other etiologies have been eliminated.

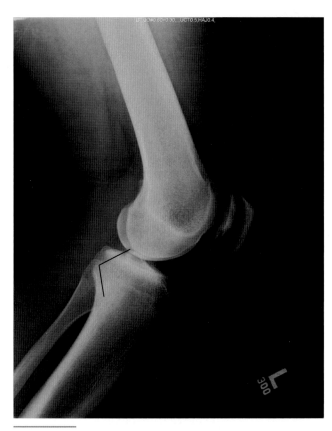

Figure 52–4. Lateral radiograph of a normal knee depicting Resnick's line *(solid line)* for identifying instability of the proximal tibiofibular joint. This line defines the posterior border of the tibia and should intersect near the midpoint of the fibular head.

TREATMENT METHODS

Symptomatic atraumatic subluxation of the proximal tibiofibular joint frequently can be managed nonsurgically.[7,26,27] In immature patients with generalized ligamentous laxity, symptoms generally are self-limiting and resolve with skeletal maturity. Activity modification is important with avoidance of knee hyperflexion.[14,17] A short period (2 to 3 weeks) of cast immobilization for patients with substantial pain may relieve symptoms. For persistent symptoms of instability, a supportive strap similar to a patellar tendon strap, placed 1 cm below the fibular head, combined with exercises to strengthen the hamstring and gastrocnemius muscles, may provide some benefit.[38] The strap should not be placed too tightly to avoid peroneal nerve palsy and should be worn only during activities that produce symptoms.

The acute proximal tibiofibular joint dislocation should be managed initially with closed reduction under either local anesthesia or intravenous sedation.[19,26,38] Closed reduction is best performed by placing the knee in 80 to 110 degrees of flexion, relaxing the lateral collateral ligament and biceps femoris tendon, then applying direct pressure to the fibular head in the appropriate direction. Some authors contend that the foot should be externally rotated, everted, and dorsiflexed while performing the reduction, which relaxes the peroneal, extensor hallucis longus, and extensor digitorum longus muscles, theoretically aiding the reduction.[14,26,37] An audible "pop" may occur as the fibula is reduced, at which point the knee is extended and the lateral collateral ligament assessed for integrity. Reductions without concomitant ligamentous injury are usually stable.

After reduction, some authors advocate a soft dressing, no immobilization, and crutch-assisted weightbearing progressing to full weightbearing over 6 weeks.[28,38] Others advocate immobilization for 3 weeks, with the knee in the neutral to slightly flexed position.[37,41] Ogden[26] reported, however, that 57% of patients who were immobilized after closed reduction later required surgical intervention for continuing symptoms.

Open reduction is required when closed reduction fails.[1,5,11,18,28,38] Failure of closed reduction may occur when the proximal fibula is caught anteriorly on the lateral tibial ridge with an intact, taut fibular collateral ligament. Surgical intervention also is recommended for acute posteromedial dislocations because of poor outcomes from closed reduction.[26] Surgery usually is required after superior dislocation, owing to the high rate of associated tibia and ankle fractures.[19,26,41] Veth and colleagues[41] reported spontaneous reduction of a dislocation after fixation of the associated tibial fracture. After open reduction, the joint should be stabilized using temporary screw or Kirschner wire fixation, combined with a primary repair of the torn capsule and injured ligaments.[1,5,26,29] Postsurgical management usually consists of immobilization of the knee and ankle joints for 6 weeks in a non-weightbearing status. Removal of the screws or Kirschner wires is recommended between 6 and 12 weeks, with a gradual return to full weightbearing status and initiation of muscle-strengthening and range-of-motion exercises.[1,28,38]

Chronic proximal tibiofibular joint instability, missed dislocations, and malreductions may lead to degenerative changes in the joint.[27,41] Ganglion cysts of the proximal tibiofibular joint can be associated with degeneration of the joint or arise de novo.[15,22] Additionally, peroneal nerve symptoms may appear late in cases of recurrent subluxation.[26,27,38] Numerous procedures have been described to address these symptoms, including arthrodesis, fibular head resection, and ligamentous reconstructions.

Arthrodesis of the joint was described by Dennis and Rutledge[7] for the treatment of bilateral atraumatic dislocations. They placed screws well below the level of the joint, however, and the screws eventually worked loose and required removal. Ogden[27] attempted arthrodesis in four patients, one of whom experienced hardware failure. The remaining three went on to bony fusion, but complained of ankle pain and instability at long-term follow-up. Miskovsky and coworkers[22] found arthrodesis to be a useful option in a series of patients with symptomatic proximal tibiofibular ganglia. They noted a high rate of cyst recurrence with primary and secondary excision, but found no recurrence after arthrodesis. Although arthrodesis is useful to relieve pain symptoms, the procedure restricts rotation of the fibula, transferring rotational forces to the ankle.[3] This transfer predisposes the ankle joint to increased pain and instability. Arthrodesis is performed by isolating and protecting the peroneal nerve, after which the articular surfaces of the joint are denuded to bleeding subchondral bone. The joint is reduced and stabilized with one or two cancellous lag screws. Immobilization is recommended for 5 weeks, with progression to full weightbearing after 8 weeks.[2] Because of the constraint of normal fibular rotation at the ankle, arthrodesis is not recommended in athletes and children.[13,26,27] To allow rotation of the distal fibula, several authors recommend resecting 1.5 cm of the fibula at the junction of the proximal and middle third, perhaps reducing the stress at the ankle joint.[14,26]

Ogden[26,27] proposed fibular head resection as an alternative to arthrodesis, which he believed overconstrained normal fibular rotation. This procedure may be indicated when peroneal nerve symptoms or palsy associated with proximal tibiofibular subluxation or dislocation is present.[7,26,27] This procedure involves excision of the head and neck of the fibula, while preserving the fibular styloid process and the attached lateral collateral ligament, which is secured to the underlying tibia.[26,27] Neurolysis should be performed if there are adhesions in proximity to the peroneal nerve. Although this procedure is useful at relieving pain symptoms, especially in a degenerative joint, it also is associated with chronic ankle pain and knee instability.[8,14] Fibular head resection is contraindicated in athletes because of the risk of posterolateral instability and in children because their physes are at risk for injury.

For patients in whom symptoms of recurrent instability predominate, reconstruction of ligamentous structures supporting the proximal tibiofibular joint has shown promise in limited studies.[13,21,34] Giachino[13] reported two cases of ligamentous reconstruction with good results, no recurrent pain or instability, and a return to previous activity levels. He described using a 10-cm rolled strip of deep fascia of the anterolateral compartment of the leg still attached proximally to the fibular head and half of a posterior strip of biceps femoris tendon still attached distally to the fibular head. With the common peroneal nerve isolated and protected, the posterior surface of the proximal tibia is exposed. A hole is drilled from anterior to posterior in the tibia, and the two new ligaments are wrapped around the head of the fibula with the proximal tibiofibular joint held reduced. The grafts are passed through the tibial drill hole from posterior to anterior and anchored to the fascia anteriorly. The knee is immobilized for 6 weeks with subsequent progressive weightbearing. Shapiro and colleagues[34] reported using a distally based 20 × 2 cm strip of iliotibial band, which is tubularized and passed through a drill hole in the tibia at a level just proximal to Gerdy's tubercle. The graft is passed through the posterior capsule and arcuate complex, then through a drill hole from posterior to anterior in the reduced fibula at the fibular head/neck junction. The graft is placed deep to the lateral collateral ligament from anterior to posterior and tightened, then secured to itself and the posterior capsule. Weightbearing as tolerated was allowed, and by 4 months postoperatively, the patient had fully recovered range of motion with no instability.

AUTHORS' PREFERRED TREATMENT

Acute proximal tibiofibular joint dislocations should be managed with closed reduction, under general anesthesia if necessary. Postreduction immobilization is generally unnecessary because most reductions are inherently stable. For dislocations that remain unstable and for posteromedial dislocations, open reduction and temporary internal fixation is required with exploration and repair of the injured anterior and posterior proximal tibiofibular ligaments and capsule. Posterolateral structures should be assessed at the time of surgery and repaired. Protected weightbearing is necessary for 6 weeks or until hardware removal, at which time weightbearing should be advanced and progressive muscle strengthening begins.

Chronic instability should be treated conservatively when possible. A CT-guided injection of the joint may provide useful information regarding the proportion of pain resulting from joint degeneration versus instability. For cases of proximal tibiofibular joint instability, we advocate reconstruction of the proximal tibiofibular joint with the method described by Giachino[13] after failure of conservative management. For the arthritic joint, which initially may respond favorably to injection but then recur, we perform a proximal tibiofibular joint fusion. Surgeons should exercise caution when considering fusion of the unstable joint because the effect of limiting rotation of the fibula seems detrimental to the ankle. In such cases in which proximal tibiofibular joint fusion is performed, a small section of fibula should be resected at its midportion to allow more normal ankle kinematics. There are limited indications for proximal fibular head resection given the importance of the posterolateral knee structures attached to the proximal fibula and the significant risk of posterolateral knee instability after excision.

References

1. Anderson K: Dislocation of the superior tibiofibular joint. Injury 16:494-498, 1985.
2. Baciu CC, Tudor A, Olaru I: Recurrent luxation of the superior tibiofibular joint in the adult. Acta Orthop Scand 45:772-777, 1974.
3. Barnett CH, Napier JR: The axis of rotation at the ankle joint in man: Its influence upon form of the talus and the mobility of the fibula. J Anat 86:1-9, 1952.
4. Bozkurt M, Yilmaz E, Atlihan D, et al: The proximal tibiofibular joint: An anatomic study. Clin Orthop 406:136-140, 2003.
5. Crothers OD, Johnson JT: Isolated acute dislocation of the proximal tibiofibular joint: Case report. J Bone Joint Surg Am 55:181-183, 1973.
6. Damron TA, Rock MG: Unusual manifestations of proximal tibiofibular joint synovial cysts. Orthopedics 20:225-230, 1997.
7. Dennis JB, Rutledge BA: Bilateral recurrent dislocations of the superior tibio-fibular joint with peroneal nerve palsy: A case summary. J Bone Joint Surg Am 40:1146-1148, 1958.
8. Draganich LF, Nicholas RW, Schuster JK, et al: The effects of resection of the proximal part of the fibula on stability of the knee and on gait. J Bone Joint Surg Am 73:575-583, 1991.
9. Dubreuil JM: J Chir 214, 1848. In Pitha, Bilroth (eds): Handbuch der Allgemeinen und Speziellen Chirurgie. Stuttgart, Ferdinand Enke, 1882, p 262.
10. Eichenblat M, Nathan H: The proximal tibio-fibular joint: An anatomical study with clinical and pathological considerations. Int Orthop 7:31-39, 1983.

11. Fallon P, Virani NS, Bell D, et al: Delayed presentation: Dislocation of the proximal tibiofibular joint after knee dislocation. J Orthop Trauma;8:350-353, 1994.

12. Gabrion A: Inferior dislocation of the proximal tibiofibular joint: A report on four cases. Acta Orthop Belg 69:522-527, 2003.

13. Giachino AA: Recurrent dislocations of the proximal tibiofibular joint: Report of two cases. J Bone Joint Surg Am 68:1104-1106, 1986.

14. Halbrecht JL, Jackson DW: Recurrent dislocation of the proximal tibiofibular joint. Orthop Rev 20:957-960, 1991.

15. Ilhali OA, Younas SA, Labbe MR, et al: Prevalence of ganglion cysts originating from the proximal tibiofibular joint: A magnetic resonance imaging study. Arthroscopy 19:150-153, 2003.

16. Keogh P, Masterson E, Murphy B, et al: The role of radiography and computed tomography in the diagnosis of acute dislocation of the proximal tibiofibular joint. Br J Radiol 66:108-111, 1993.

17. Lord CD, Coutts JW: A study of typical parachute injuries occurring in two hundred and fifty thousand jumps at the parachute school. J Bone Joint Surg 26:547-557, 1944.

18. Love JN: Isolated anterolateral proximal fibular head dislocation. Ann Emerg Med 21:757-759, 1992.

19. Lyle HHM: Traumatic luxation of the head of the fibula. Ann Surg 82:635-639, 1925.

20. Marshall JL, Girgis FG, Zelko RR: The biceps femoris tendon and its functional significance. J Bone Joint Surg Am 54:1444-1450, 1972.

21. Mena H, Brautigan B, Johnson DL: Split biceps femoris tendon reconstruction for proximal tibiofibular joint instability. Arthroscopy 17:668-671, 2001.

22. Miskovsky S, Kaeding C, Weis L: Proximal tibiofibular joint ganglion cysts: Excision, recurrence, and joint arthrodesis. Am J Sports Med 32:1022-1028, 2004.

23. Muckart RD: Compression of the common peroneal nerve by intramuscular ganglion from the superior tibio-fibular joint. J Bone Joint Surg Br 58:241-244, 1976.

24. Ogden JA: Dislocation of the proximal fibula. Radiology 105:547-549, 1972.

25. Ogden JA: The anatomy and function of the proximal tibiofibular joint. Clin Orthop 101:186-191, 1974.

26. Ogden JA: Subluxation and dislocation of the proximal tibiofibular joint. J Bone Joint Surg Am 56:145-154, 1974.

27. Ogden JA: Subluxation of the proximal tibiofibular joint. Clin Orthop 101:192-197, 1974.

28. Parkes JC II, Zelko RR: Isolated acute dislocation of the proximal tibiofibular joint: Case report. J Bone Joint Surg Am 55:177-183, 1973.

29. Rajkumar P: A new surgical treatment of an acute dislocation of the proximal tibiofibular joint. Int J Clin Pract 56:556-557, 2002.

30. Resnick D, Newell JD, Guerra J Jr, et al: Proximal tibiofibular joint: Anatomic-pathologic-radiographic correlation. AJR Am J Roentgenol 131:133-138, 1978.

31. Seebacher JR, Inglis AE, Marshall JL, Warren RF: The structure of the posterolateral aspect of the knee. J Bone Joint Surg Am 64:536-541, 1982.

32. Sekiya JK, Kuhn JE: Instability of the proximal tibiofibular joint. J Am Acad Orthop Surg 11:120-128, 2003.

33. Semonian RH, Denlinger PM, Duggan RJ: Proximal tibiofibular subluxation relationship to lateral knee pain: A review of proximal tibiofibular joint pathologies. J Orthop Sports Phys Ther 21:248-257, 1995.

34. Shapiro GS, Fanton GS, Dillingham MF: Reconstruction for recurrent dislocation of the proximal tibiofibular joint: A new technique. Orthop Rev 22:1229-1232, 1993.

35. Sijbrandij S: Instability of the proximal tibiofibular joint. Acta Orthop Scand 49:621-626, 1978.

36. Terry GC, LaPrade RF: The posterolateral aspect of the knee: Anatomy and surgical approach. Am J Sports Med 24:732-739, 1996.

37. Thomason PA, Linson MA: Isolated dislocation of the proximal tibiofibular joint. J Trauma 26:192-195, 1986.

38. Turco VJ, Spinella AJ: Anterolateral dislocation of the head of the fibula in sports. Am J Sports Med 13:209-215, 1985.

39. Veltri DM, Warren RF: Treatment of acute and chronic injuries to the posterolateral and lateral knee. Oper Tech Sports Med 4:174-181, 1996.

40. Veth RP, Kingma LM, Nielsen HK: The abnormal proximal tibiofibular joint. Arch Orthop Trauma Surg 102:167-171, 1984.

41. Veth RP, Klasen HJ, Kingma LM: Traumatic instability of the proximal tibiofibular joint. Injury 13:159-164, 1981.

42. Voglino JA, Denton JR: Acute traumatic proximal tibiofibular joint dislocation confirmed by computed tomography. Orthopedics 22:255-258, 1999.

43. Ward WG, Eckardt DL: Ganglion cyst of the proximal tibiofibular joint causing anterior compartment syndrome: A case report and anatomic study. J Bone Joint Surg Am 76:1561-1564, 1994.

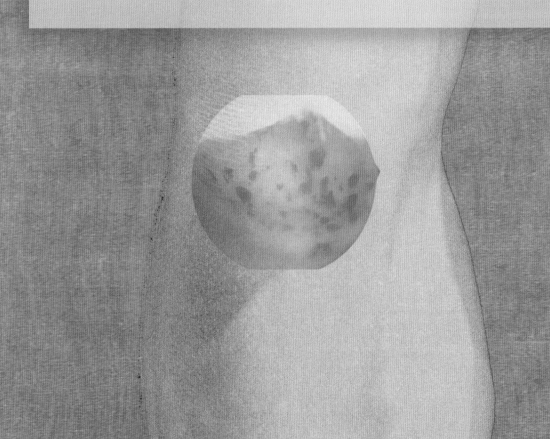

SECTION VI

Patellar and Extensor Mechanism Disorders

CHAPTER 53

Disorders of the Patellofemoral Joint

Paolo Aglietti • Francesco Giron • Pierluigi Cuomo

ANATOMY OF THE PATELLOFEMORAL JOINT

Patella

The patella is roughly an oval bone with a rounded point inferiorly and a transverse diameter slightly longer than its longitudinal diameter. The anterior surface is convex in both the proximodistal and mediolateral directions. The upper two-thirds, the triangular base, receives the insertion of the quadriceps tendon. The V-shaped lower third receives the insertion of the patellar tendon. An anatomic study of 21 fresh patellar specimens revealed the following average dimensions: height of the anterior surface, 4.5 cm (range, 3.8 to 5.3 cm); width, 4.7 cm (range, 4.0 to 5.5 cm); height of the articular surface, 3.5 cm (range, 3.0 to 3.9 cm); and thickness, 2.3 cm (range, 1.9 to 2.6 cm).[325] Our group reported similar measurements.[8] We removed 80 patellae and studied their dimensions by radiographic methods, with the following results: total height, 4.0 cm; total width, 4.1 cm; height of the articular surface, 2.9 cm; width of the articular surface, 3.8 cm; and thickness at the level of the ridge, 2.0 cm.

The posterior surface of the patella can be divided into two portions: the articular superior three-fourths and the nonarticular inferior fourth. The articular surface is oval, with the longest diameter in the transverse plane. It is divided into medial and lateral facets by the central ridge. The respective sizes of the medial and lateral facets vary. Wiberg,[400] in an extensive radiographic study of the patellofemoral joint, classified patellae into three different types, and a fourth type was added by Baumgartl[24]; these four types are shown in Figure 53–1. According to an anatomic study,[325] type II occurs most frequently (57%), followed by type I (24%) and type III (19%). It can be seen that there is an increasing prevalence of the lateral facet over the medial facet when moving from type I to type IV. If it is assumed that the final patellar shape is determined by the stress imposed on it, types III and IV should be the result of lateralized gliding of the patella into the sulcus, whereas type I should develop when the medial and lateral facets are loaded symmetrically.

Wiberg[400] was unable to confirm a relationship between chondromalacia and the morphology of the patella. Nevertheless, patellae showing lateral tracking (as in recurrent subluxation or dislocation) tend to have a predominant lateral facet. An experimental confirmation of this concept[325] showed a correlation between the Wiberg type III shape and the width of the lateral patellofemoral ligament, thus suggesting that a thicker lateral retinaculum causes lateral patellar tracking and hence a patellar shape with lateral predominance. In the experimental study reported here,[325] the dimensions of the patella—height, width, and thickness—were not directly interrelated but tended to vary independently as a result of the pull of the surrounding soft-tissue structures. This concept is confirmed clinically by the small size of the patella in children with a congenital dislocation that was not reduced surgically.

Goodfellow and colleagues[156] described the presence of a secondary ridge on the medial facet that delineates an "odd" facet near the medial border of the patella. This area has been shown to contact the medial femoral condyle with the knee in full flexion. Because this ridge is usually pure cartilage, it cannot be observed in specimens of dried bone.[131] It should be remembered that the shape of the articular surface is determined by the profile of the subchondral bone and the thickness of the cartilage. The articular cartilage is thicker at the level of the central ridge—in fact, it is the thickest cartilage in the human body (up to 5 mm). This thickness perhaps explains why patellar cartilage is diseased more often than trochlear cartilage.

In some cases, a transverse ridge divides the patellar articular surface into a larger superior and a smaller inferior part. This transverse ridge was present in 15 of 21 anatomic specimens (71%).[325]

Grelsamer et al[163] analyzed the shape of the patella in the sagittal plane as visualized on a lateral radiograph. They drew attention to the fact that the relationship between the length of the patella and the length of the articular surface is not constant. In other words, the length of the distal nonarticular portion of the patella varies. Patellar shape was analyzed by computing the ratio of patellar length to length of the articular surface (morphology ratio). A preliminary analysis of 200 knees revealed that the mean morphology ratio was 1.4 ± 0.1. Based on these results, patellae were classified type I if the morphology ratio was between 1.2 and 1.5. Type II patellae were those with a morphology ratio greater than 1 SD above the mean (>1.5)—that is, with a long inferior pole (the long-nosed, or Cyrano, appearance). Type III patellae had a morphology ratio more than 1 SD below the mean (<1.2)—that is, with a short inferior pole (Fig. 53–2). In a group of 235 patients with no evidence of patellofemoral symptoms, there were 94% type I patellae, 4% type II patellae, and 2% type III patellae. In a second group of 202 knees with patellofemoral problems, 76% of the patellae were type I, 17% were type II, and 7% were type III. The group of knees with patellofemoral problems had a sig-

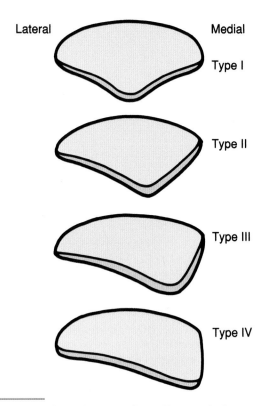

Lateral   Medial

Type I

Type II

Type III

Type IV

Figure 53–1. Classification of patella morphology according to Wiberg and Baumgartl. Type I has medial and lateral facets of roughly the same size, both gently concave. Type II has a medial facet smaller than the lateral facet, and it is flat or slightly convex. Type III has a markedly reduced medial facet compared with the lateral facet, and it is convex and almost vertical. Type IV was described by Baumgartl as the "Jaegerhut" shape, without a central ridge or medial facet.

nificantly higher proportion of type II and type III patellae, with abnormally long or short inferior poles, respectively. Therefore, it appears that patellar shape contributes to pain, although exactly how it does so is unclear.

Femoral Trochlea

The articular portion of the anterior surface of the femur consists of a sulcus with lateral and medial facets. The sulcus continues distally with the intercondylar notch. The medial and lateral facets are in continuity with the femoral condyles. The junction between the trochlear and condylar surfaces is usually marked by a shallow groove, which is determined by contact with the meniscus in the fully extended knee. The two grooves are asymmetric; the lateral groove is more clearly evident. The medial and lateral facets of the femoral trochlea are also asymmetric in that the lateral facet is a few millimeters more prominent than the medial facet in a normal knee. The greater height of the lateral facet and the congruence between the trochlear sulcus and the central ridge of the patella are contributing factors in stabilization of the patella (osseous stabilizers). The sulcus is significantly flatter in knees with

patellar instability, so the stabilizing function of the osseous surfaces is lost to a variable extent.

The lateral trochlear facet extends proximally more than the medial facet. A ridge may be present between the upper margin of the trochlea and the anterior surface of the femur, and the ridge is often more pronounced medially.[309] Until recently, it was widely thought that a conflict between this ridge and the articular surface of the medial patellar facet was a cause of chondromalacia. This hypothesis has now been refuted on the basis of our knowledge that the patella enters the sulcus from the lateral side.

At the lateral margin of the upper trochlea, an area of thickened fibrotic synovium is present as a fibrocartilaginous extension of the lateral facet.[131] This site is where the patella contacts the femur with the knee in full extension and quadriceps contraction.

Passive Soft-Tissue Stabilizers

The patella is effectively anchored to the knee by four structures in a cruciform arrangement as shown in Figure 53–3. These structures guide the patella in its tracking during flexion and extension and are considered to be passive stabilizers.

Patellar Tendon

The patellar tendon, which varies in length, determines the proximodistal (vertical) position of the patella in relation to the joint line—that is, the height of the patella.[204] It is a flat structure that connects the apex of the patella to the tibial tuberosity. It is slightly wider proximally than distally, and its width at the central third varies between 24 and 33 mm in most subjects. Its thickness varies between 3 and 5 mm. The average length of the patellar tendon is 4.6 cm (range, 3.5 to 5.5 cm).[325] It is slightly oblique distally and laterally, thus contributing to the overall valgus alignment of the extensor apparatus. This tendency may be increased in knees with recurrent patellar instability as a result of lateral placement of the tibial tubercle.

Lateral Retinaculum

The anatomy of the lateral retinaculum has been described by Fulkerson and Gossling.[130] It is composed of two layers of fibers: the superficial layer and the deep layer. The superficial layer (the superficial oblique retinaculum) (Fig. 53–4) is composed of oblique fibers running in a distal and anterior direction from the anterior border of the iliotibial band to the lateral margin of the patella and to the lateral aspect of the patellar tendon. The deep layer is composed of three distinct structures (Fig. 53–5). The midportion runs transversely from the deep surface of the iliotibial band to the lateral border of the patella (deep transverse retinaculum). Superior to this portion is the epicondylopatellar band, described by Kaplan,[218] which connects the lateral epicondyle to the superolateral aspect

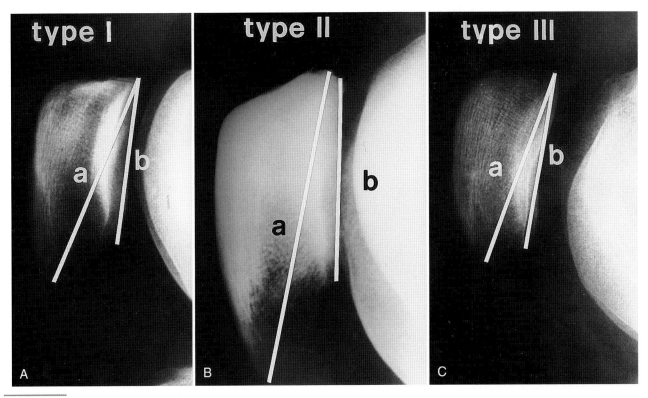

Figure 53–2. Different shapes of the patella in the sagittal plane according to Grelsamer et al.[163] Patellar shape is described by the morphology ratio—that is, the ratio of patellar length to length of the articular surface. **A**, A normal type I patella has a morphology ratio between 1.2 and 1.5. **B**, Type II patella, with a morphology ratio over 1.5—that is, with a long inferior pole (Cyrano appearance). **C**, Type III patella with a morphology ratio below 1.2—that is, with a short inferior pole.

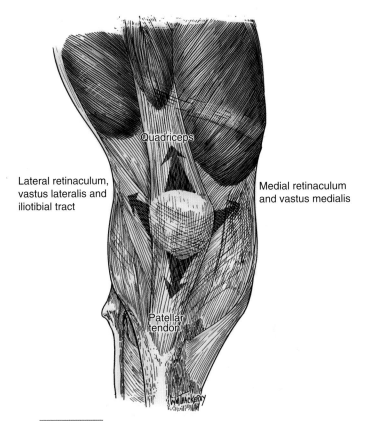

Figure 53–3. The patella is anchored and stabilized to the knee by four structures in a cruciform fashion: the patellar tendon inferiorly, the quadriceps tendon superiorly, and the retinacula medially and laterally.

of the patella. It does not seem to be constant because an anatomic study[325] has confirmed its presence in only 13 of 20 specimens (65%). Inferior to the midportion, the patellotibial band connects the tibia, near Gerdy's tubercle, to the inferolateral aspect of the patella. This portion is also called the patellomeniscal ligament.

The bulk of the lateral retinaculum runs from the lateral margin of the patella and patellar tendon to the anterior aspect of the iliotibial band. With increasing flexion, the iliotibial band is displaced posteriorly, thereby increasing the lateral pull of the patella. If this acts against weakened medial stabilizers, patellar tilt or subluxation may result.

Medial Retinaculum

The medial patellar retinaculum inserts into the upper two-thirds of the medial margin of the patella. Two distinct condensations of fibers are classically described: the medial patellofemoral ligament, which inserts into the medial femoral epicondyle, and the medial patellotibial ligament, which inserts into the medial meniscus and tibia (Fig. 53–6). The medial patellofemoral ligament is less constant than the corresponding lateral ligament. It was present in only 7 of 20 (35%) anatomic specimens.[325] An interesting negative relationship was found between the length of the patellar tendon and the width of the medial patellofemoral ligament[325]: because a high-riding patella is frequently associated with lateral subluxation, it is not

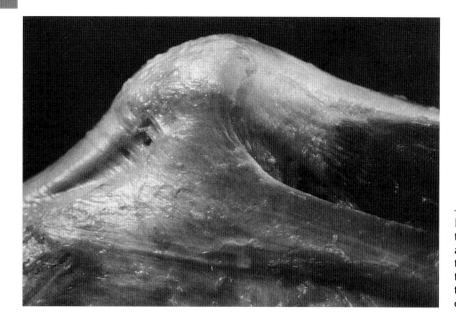

Figure 53–4. The superficial fibers of the lateral retinaculum run from the anterior border of the iliotibial band to the lateral margin of the patella and the patellar tendon in an oblique direction distally and anteriorly (superficial oblique retinaculum).

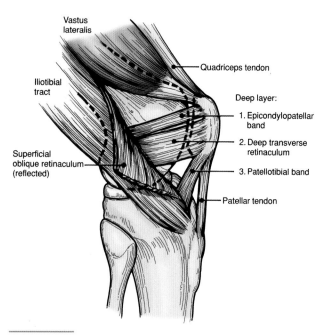

Figure 53–5. Deep to the superficial layer of the lateral retinaculum, the deep layer is composed of three distinct structures, proximally to distally: the epicondylopatellar band, the deep transverse retinaculum, and the patellotibial band. (Modified from Fulkerson JP, Gossling HR: Anatomy of the knee joint lateral retinaculum. Clin Orthop 153:183, 1980.)

surprising to find that the longer the patellar tendon, the weaker the medial stabilizers.

The importance of the medial retinacular structures in restraining lateral displacement of the patella has been re-evaluated.[78] Eight specimens were dissected to better define the local anatomy, and 25 specimens were subjected to mechanical testing. The origin of the vastus medialis obliquus was from the medial intermuscular septum and the adductor magnus tendon proximal to the adductor tubercle (average, 3.3 cm proximal to the tubercle; range, 0.5 to 6 cm). The insertion of the vastus medialis obliquus was on the superomedial and medial margin of the patella. The medial patellofemoral ligament originated at the adductor tubercle and was in the same tissue layer as the medial collateral ligament. The ligament fibers proceed anteriorly toward the undersurface of the vastus medialis obliquus proximally and toward the lateral patellar margin distally. The width of the medial patellofemoral ligament ranged from 0.8 to 2.5 cm (average, 1.3 cm).

In two of the eight specimens that were dissected, no distinct fibers of the medial patellofemoral ligament could be identified. Biomechanical testing showed that the medial patellofemoral ligament was the major soft-tissue restraint to lateral patellar displacement and provided 53% of the restraining force. However, in seven knees, this ligament contributed less than 39% of the restraining force. Four of these seven knees had a wispy or nonpalpable ligament. The medial patellomeniscal ligament was found to be the next important stabilizing structure, and it provided 22% of the restraining force to lateral displacement of the patella. The fibers of the medial retinaculum anterior to the medial collateral ligament provided only 11% of the restraining force; the medial patellotibial ligament provided even less, 5% on average. In conclusion, the medial patellofemoral ligament and the patellomeniscal ligament together accounted for 75% of the restraining force.

A pathoanatomic study[338] of 16 acute patellar dislocations correlates well with the anatomic and biomechanical data reported here. Open surgical exploration revealed tears of the medial patellofemoral ligament off the femur in 15 of 16 cases (94%).

Muscular Active Stabilizers: Quadriceps Tendon

The four components of the quadriceps muscle join distally into the quadriceps tendon. Three muscles—the

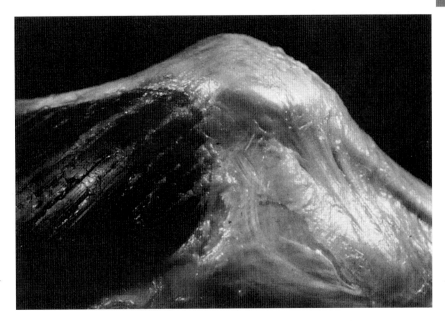

Figure 53–6. The vastus medialis obliquus becomes tendinous just a few millimeters proximal to the patella. Because of the oblique direction of its fibers, it is best suited to resist lateral displacement of the patella. The patellotibial ligament is visible as a distinct structure medial to the patellar tendon.

vastus medialis, vastus lateralis, and vastus intermedius—are monoarticular muscles; the fourth, the rectus femoris, is biarticular and spans both the hip joint and the knee joint. The quadriceps tendon is composed of three layers. The most superficial fibers of the rectus femoris run over the patella and join the patellar tendon, whereas its deeper fibers insert into the base of the patella. The vastus medialis and vastus lateralis unite to form the middle layer of the quadriceps tendon, which inserts into the base of the patella. These muscles also send fibers that blend with the corresponding patellar retinacula. The vastus intermedius inserts into the base of the patella through the third deepest part of the quadriceps tendon.

The vastus medialis muscle has been described as consisting of two portions, the vastus medialis obliquus and the vastus medialis longus.[248] The fibers of the vastus medialis obliquus have a more oblique direction distally and laterally and are therefore better suited to limit lateral displacement of the patella. The angle at which the vastus medialis obliquus fibers approach the patella has been reported to range from 55 to 70 degrees relative to the long axis of the quadriceps tendon.[325] The vastus medialis obliquus fibers become tendinous just a few millimeters proximal to the insertion on the superior third or half of the medial margin of the patella (see Fig. 53–6). The insertion of the vastus medialis obliquus varies, however. Knees with patellar dislocation often have a less well developed vastus medialis obliquus that inserts more proximally on the patella. This fact has been confirmed by a magnetic resonance imaging (MRI) study that compared normal subjects and patients with patellar dislocation.[229] A more proximal insertion of the vastus medialis obliquus renders its medial pull less effective. This observation may lend support to adding vastus medialis advancement to other realignment procedures in these patients.

The fibers of the vastus lateralis approach the patella at a more acute angle in relation to the long axis of the quadriceps tendon than do those of the vastus medialis obliquus, with the angle averaging 31 degrees (range,

22 to 45 degrees). Furthermore, the muscle fibers become tendinous at an average of 2.8 cm (range, 0.5 to 4.5 cm) proximal to the superolateral corner of the patella. Attention has been drawn to the most distal part of the vastus lateralis, which was found to be anatomically distinct and was named the *vastus lateralis obliquus*.[168] These fibers originate from the lateral intermuscular septum and are therefore best suited to application of a lateral displacing force on the patella.

It has been suggested that these fibers can be resected at the time of lateral release without transection of the main tendon of the vastus lateralis to avoid over-release, possible medial instability, and weakening of the quadriceps.[168]

Patellar Dysplasia

Complete absence of the patella (patellar aplasia), a small patella (patellar hypoplasia), and a large patella (patella magna) have been reported in small series[26,33] but are rarely encountered in clinical practice. Patellar duplication has also been reported in a few cases, usually in association with multiple epiphyseal dysplasia. The duplication may be present in the frontal plane (one patella anterior to the other), in the horizontal plane (one superior and one inferior), or in the sagittal plane (one medial and one lateral).[145]

BIPARTITE PATELLA

The most frequent form of patellar dysplasia is patella bipartita. It generally involves the superolateral corner of the patella, but it may be present at the lateral margin, at the apex,[359] or at the superomedial pole. More rarely, the patella may be tripartite or multipartite. The pathogenesis of this disturbance is probably attributable to excessive traction from the surrounding soft tissues on the patella ossification nucleus during the critical phase of ossification. This hypothesis agrees well with the macroscopic and histological characteristics of the junction between the two fragments, which resembles pseudarthrosis with fibrous or cartilaginous tissue filling the gap. According to this hypothesis, the most common superolateral fragment develops under the traction applied by the vastus lateralis. The less common straight lateral fragment is sometimes observed in subluxing patellae, and it is probably due to traction from a shortened lateral retinaculum (Fig. 53–7).

A bipartite patella is most often discovered accidentally during radiographic examination for another disorder of the knee. Some problems may arise in knees that have sustained a direct blow because fractures of the lateral margin and the superolateral corner are sometimes encountered. An accurate radiographic examination, including axial views, may reveal the sharply irregular margins of the fragment and thus allow diagnosis of a recent fracture and lead to appropriate treatment. On the other hand, the junction between the patella and the bipartite fragment is occasionally disrupted and rendered symptomatic by the trauma because of disruption of the nonosseous union. In these cases, if conservative treatment fails, removal of the fragment cures the symptoms. If the fragment involves a significant portion of the articular surface, it should instead be fixed with one or two 4-mm cancellous lag screws.

An alternative approach was described in 1995.[292] In a series of 16 knees with painful bipartite patellae, a modified lateral release was performed wherein a strip of lateral retinaculum was excised that extended proximally around the patella to the proximal attachment of the bipartite fragment. Preoperatively, 11 of 16 knees (69%) also experienced patellofemoral pain. Fifteen of the 16 knees showed evidence of bony union within 8 months after surgery.

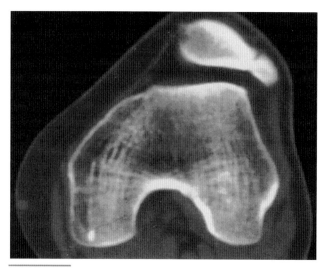

Figure 53–7. Computed tomography scan of a patient with recurrent patellar dislocation. A fragment has separated from the lateral margin of the patella. It probably develops during the ossification period because of traction from a shortened lateral retinaculum, which is visible as a thickened structure.

Tenderness over the separated fragment disappeared in all patients postoperatively, but tenderness about the medial patellofemoral joint persisted in seven knees. We think that this treatment should be reserved for patients with symptomatic bipartite patellae and lateral patella compression syndrome. The extension of the release, which includes the tendon of the vastus lateralis, also raises some concern.

BIOMECHANICS OF THE PATELLOFEMORAL JOINT

Today, there is wide agreement that the most important function of the patella is to improve quadriceps efficiency by increasing the lever arm of the extensor mechanism.[132] The thickness of the patella displaces the patellar tendon away from the femorotibial contact point throughout the range of motion, thereby increasing the patellar tendon moment arm. In an experimental study involving cadaver knees, Wendt and Johnson[397] found that patellectomy decreased quadriceps torque between 0 and 70 degrees, the greatest decrease—almost 40%—occurring between 10 and 30 degrees.

The patella is necessary to centralize the divergent forces from the four heads of the quadriceps and transmit tension around the femur, in a frictionless way, to the patellar tendon and tibial tuberosity. The thick articular cartilage of the patella, the thickest in the human body, is well suited to resist high compressive force with minimal friction, although this may create nutritional problems. Finally, the patella acts as a shield to protect the distal end of the femur and improves the cosmetic appearance of the knee. This can readily be appreciated by observing the squared appearance of the flexed knee in patients who have undergone patellectomy.

It has often been suggested that degeneration of the articular surface of the patella can be attributed to failure to withstand the high compressive loads imposed on it during daily living and sports activities. Therefore, much work has been devoted to calculation of the compressive force experienced by the patella during various activities (the patellofemoral joint reaction force). With knowledge of the patellofemoral joint reaction force and the patellofemoral contact area at a given degree of flexion, one can calculate patellofemoral pressure (load per unit area).

Patellofemoral Joint Reaction Force

The patellofemoral joint reaction force is the result of tension developing in the quadriceps and patellar tendons because of contraction of the quadriceps. It is represented by the resultant vector of the quadriceps tendon force (M1) and the patellar tendon force (M2). The forces M1 and M2 have traditionally been supposed to be equal if the patella works as a frictionless pulley. However, more recent investigations have shown that the ratio M1/M2 is not equal to 1 through most of the range of motion and that the ratio M1/M2 increases with flexion to values up to 1.5.[11,53,188] However, for a rough estimate of patellofemoral joint reaction force, the quadriceps and patellar tendon forces M1 and M2 can be considered equal.

With knowledge of the quadriceps force Fq (and supposing it to be equal to M1 and M2) and the angle between M1 and M2, the patellofemoral joint reaction force (PFJRF) can be calculated (Fig. 53–8) with the following equation.[194]

$$PFJRF = 2Fq \cos J/2.$$

The quadriceps force Fq has been calculated according to static principles. Any flexion moment is balanced by a corresponding extension moment to reach equilibrium. These calculations have been performed by Bandi[22] and by several other authors.[188,270,327] A free-body diagram can be constructed to balance the flexion and extension moments (Fig. 53–9).[194] This diagram reflects the forces encountered in the static position, and the inertial forces of the dynamic situation are ignored. The estimated quadriceps force may therefore be lower than that experienced during in vivo activities. Fq can be expressed by the following equation:

$$Fq = Fwt(f \sin \alpha + t \sin \beta)1/r$$

According to the two equations in this discussion, it appears that in a given person of constant weight who is performing a squat as in Figure 53–9, the patellofemoral joint reaction force varies according to the degree of

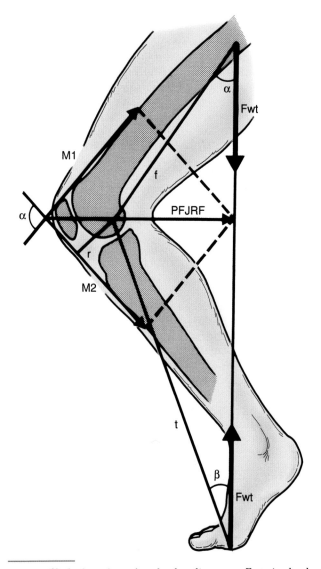

Figure 53–9. Standing free-body diagram. Fwt is body weight; r is the moment arm of the patellar tendon, that is, the perpendicular distance from the center of rotation of the knee to the tendon itself; f is the effective length of the femur from the knee to the intersection with a vertical line passing through the center of gravity of the body; t is the distance from the knee to the point of contact between the foot and the floor; α is the femoral angle with the vertical; and β is the tibial angle with the vertical. If the quadriceps force Fq is supposed to be equal to the quadriceps tendon force M1 and the patellar tendon force M2, Fq can be calculated (see text for equation). (Adapted from Hungerford DS, Barry N: Biomechanics of the patellofemoral joint. Clin Orthop 144:9, 1979.)

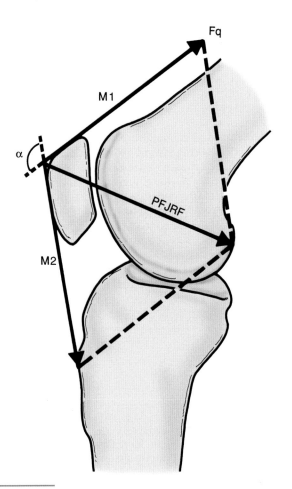

Figure 53–8. Schematic representation of quadriceps force (Fq), quadriceps tendon force (M1), and patellar tendon force (M2). If it is supposed that Fq = M1 = M2 as in a frictionless system, the patellofemoral joint reaction force (PFJRF) can be calculated (see text for equation). (From Hungerford DS, Barry N: Biomechanics of the patellofemoral joint. Clin Orthop 144:9, 1979.)

flexion of the knee. An increase in flexion of the knee increases the angles α and β and therefore the flexion arm of the body weight. Maintenance of a static position requires more quadriceps force. Furthermore, the angle between M1 and M2 decreases with increasing flexion, and the resultant vector of the patellofemoral joint reaction force becomes correspondingly greater.

The extension moment arm r is also variable through the range of motion. The length of the moment arm of the extensor mechanism has been calculated experimentally in cadaver knees by Grood and coworkers.[164] It was maximal at approximately 20 degrees, where it measured 39.6 mm on average. The moment arm decreased rapidly to approximately 20 mm on average when proceeding toward extension and toward 90 degrees of flexion.

The situation represented in Figure 53–9 is useful to obtain a rough estimate of the patellofemoral joint reaction force in the static position, but other factors must be taken into account in daily living activities. One such factor is the inertia of dynamic accelerations and decelerations. In addition, the center of gravity of the body can be displaced forward or backward and can therefore decrease or increase the flexion moment of the body weight. Thus, it appears that several factors, beyond the knee flexion angle, are capable of influencing the magnitude of the patellofemoral joint reaction force.

Regardless of the method used to determine the patellofemoral joint reaction force, high values have been reported by several authors. Reilly and Martens[327] calculated a patellofemoral joint reaction force of 0.5 times body weight at 9 degrees of flexion for level walking, 3.3 times body weight at 60 degrees of flexion during stair climbing or descending, and up to 7.8 times body weight at 130 degrees during deep knee bends. Matthews and coworkers[270] calculated the patellofemoral joint reaction force during the same activities and obtained similar results. Huberti and Hayes[187] calculated a maximum contact force of 4600 N at 90 degrees of flexion during maximum isometric quadriceps contraction, or approximately 6.5 times body weight.

The biomechanics of the knee extension exercise has been also investigated, and the results have clinical relevance. The situation can be described with a free-body diagram (Fig. 53–10). In this position, the flexion moment arm increases steadily during extension and is maximal at full extension. This is different from the standing position shown in Figure 53–9, wherein the moment arm of the body weight increases with increasing flexion. Reilly and Martens[327] calculated a peak patellofemoral joint reaction force of 120 kg at 36 degrees of flexion during the extension exercise with a 3-kg boot.

An experimental study of the knee extension exercise in cadaver knees was performed by Grood and colleagues.[164] They found that the ratio of quadriceps force to leg weight increased from 90 to 50 degrees, remained constant between 50 and 20 degrees, and increased abruptly between 20 degrees and full extension. The relatively constant force required to extend the knee between 50 and 20 degrees was explained by the increasing length of the moment arm of the extensor mechanism in the same arc of motion, which produced the improved quadriceps efficiency necessary to overcome the increasing flexion moment arm. However, in the last 20 degrees of extension, the extensor moment arm decreases rapidly; in fact, a strong quadriceps force is required to reach full extension.

It appears that the extension exercise against resistance is somehow not physiological for the knee because the quadriceps force required increases toward extension. On the contrary, during the more physiological act of squatting from the standing position, the quadriceps demands increase with flexion. Because the patellofemoral contact area increases in flexion, as is described in the next discussion, the knee is likely to experience excessive patellofemoral contact pressure during the knee extension exercise while working toward extension. Hungerford and Barry[194] calculated that the knee extension exercise with a 9-kg boot exceeds the physiological patellofemoral compression force of the squatting exercise at around 50 degrees of flexion. When compared with the squatting exercise, patellofemoral contact pressure during the knee extension exercise was almost six times higher at 30 degrees of flexion.

Clinical experience is consistent with these observations. Patients with patellofemoral symptoms can hardly tolerate the knee extension exercise against resistance or

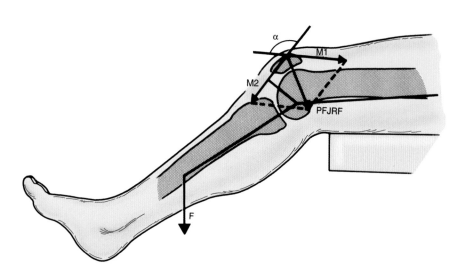

Figure 53–10. Free-body diagram of the extension exercise. The flexion moment increases toward extension, and increasing quadriceps force is required to reach full extension. This is the converse of the squatting exercise reported in Figure 53-8, wherein increasing quadriceps force is required with further flexion. PFJRF, patellofemoral joint reaction force. (Adapted from Hungerford DS, Barry N: Biomechanics of the patellofemoral joint. Clin Orthop 144:9, 1979.)

isokinetic training at low angular speeds in terminal extension. Deep knee bends are equally deleterious. Straight-leg raising or short-arc isotonic exercises are more suitable alternatives to rehabilitate the quadriceps in such patients without increasing symptoms.

Patellofemoral Contact Areas

Patellofemoral contact areas have been studied by several authors using different techniques.[8,155,156,187] Similar results have been achieved for the location and extent of contact areas through the range of motion, which can be summarized as follows (Fig. 53–11).

The articular surface of the patella contacts the upper part of the femoral trochlea at around 20 degrees of flexion. The initial contact may occur earlier or later, according to the length of the patellar tendon. The contact area on the patellar surface is shaped like a horizontal band and extends from the medial facet, near the secondary ridge, to the lateral facet. It is located in the inferior, middle, and superior third of the patella at 30, 60, and 90 degrees, respectively. Therefore, the contact area moves proximally with increasing flexion of the knee. Furthermore, its surface area increases steadily with increasing flexion.

Huberti and Hayes[187] measured contact area with pressure-sensitive film and found that it increased, on average, from 2.6 cm[2] at 20 degrees to 4.1 cm[2] at 90 degrees. This value corresponds to approximately a fifth of the total patellar cartilage area at 20 degrees and a third at 90 degrees. The increase in contact area was mainly due to an increase in the vertical dimensions of the area itself, which increased from 0.6 cm at 20 degrees to 1 cm at 90 degrees of flexion. The contact area reached the most proximal part of the patellar articular surface only at 120 degrees.[187] At this flexion angle, the contact area was dome shaped along the proximal edge of the patellar cartilage and still continuous from the medial to the lateral facet in seven of eight knees.

We reported on two separate contact areas at 120 degrees of flexion.[8] At 120 degrees of flexion, the quadriceps tendon comes in contact with the femoral trochlea, and the tendofemoral contact area was 3.4 cm[2] on average, which represented approximately 75% of the corresponding patellofemoral contact area at the same angle of flexion of the knee.

At 135 degrees of flexion, the contact area on the patella assumes a completely different configuration. The medial facet is free of contact and faces the intercondylar notch. Medially, contact is established between the "odd" facet and the lateral border of the medial femoral condyle. The lateral facet contacts the lateral femoral condyle.

In summary, the contact area on the patella shifts proximally with increasing knee flexion. The contact area increases steadily up to 90 degrees, which helps lower patellofemoral contact pressure. After 90 degrees of flexion, the quadriceps tendon contacts the femur and a tendofemoral contact area is developed to further resist the increasing patellofemoral joint reaction force and therefore lower patellofemoral pressure. The patellar contact area is a continuous band, from the medial to the lateral facet, up to 90 degrees[8,156] or up to 120 degrees, according to other workers.[187] Afterward, separate contact areas on the lateral and medial or odd facet are present.

Patellofemoral Contact Pressure

Patellofemoral contact pressure is probably the most important factor in the biomechanics of the patellofemoral joint. More important than the absolute value of the patellofemoral joint reaction force is the ratio of the patellofemoral joint reaction force to the contact area—that is, contact pressure. Both contact area and contact force vary significantly throughout the range of motion. As we have pointed out, both increase in flexion during the act of squatting. Increasing the contact area in flexion partially compensates for the increasing patellofemoral joint reaction force.

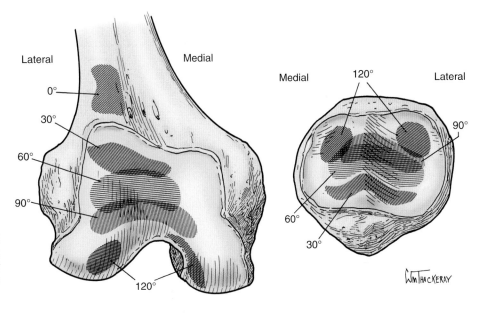

Figure 53–11. Patellofemoral contact zones. (From Aglietti P, Insall JN, Walker PS, et al: A new patella prosthesis. Clin Orthop 107:175, 1975.)

Patellofemoral contact pressure has been measured in eight cadaver knees with pressure-sensitive film.[187] Resultant knee moments, corresponding to a third of the values reported in the literature for maximum isometric voluntary quadriceps contraction, were applied at 20, 30, 60, and 90 degrees of flexion and were 23.6, 30.7, 47.2, and 35 N, respectively. Based on two-thirds of the reported maximum moments, 47.2 N was applied at 120 degrees of flexion. Contact pressure was remarkably uniform over the entire contact area (±0.25 MPa), being approximately the same on both the medial and the lateral facets. The average patellofemoral contact pressure was 2.0 MPa at 20 degrees, 2.4 MPa at 30 degrees, 4.1 MPa at 60 degrees, and 4.4 MPa at 90 degrees. The highest increase was recorded between 30 and 60 degrees. The average patellofemoral contact pressure decreased to 3.5 MPa at 120 degrees. In five knees, patellofemoral pressure was relatively uniform over the contact area, and two knees exhibited higher pressure on the medial facet (medial-lateral ratio, 2.3). The last knee had higher pressure on the lateral facet (3.7 MPa) than on the medial facet (1.7 MPa). At 120 degrees, a definite area of tendofemoral contact was present proximal to the patella. The average tendofemoral contact pressure was about 50% of the patellofemoral contact pressure (1.6 MPa) at the same angle of flexion.

In summary, despite the complex anatomy of the patellofemoral joint and the valgus vector of the extensor mechanism, it appears that patellofemoral contact pressure is uniformly spread over the contact areas. Peak pressure is therefore avoided in the cartilage. Patellofemoral pressure is highest between 60 and 90 degrees of flexion. If the data are extrapolated for a maximum quadriceps contraction, a pressure of 12 MPa can be anticipated. At flexion angles greater than 90 degrees, tendofemoral contact plays an important role in reducing patellofemoral contact pressure.

HISTORY

Regardless of cause, and there are many, the symptoms of patellar dysfunction tend to be the same. In themselves, these symptoms are not distinctive and include pain and instability. Catching or locking is also sometimes reported. Moreover, all these symptoms are produced by other internal derangements. However, the pattern of complaints in patients with patellar disorders is sufficiently specific to focus attention on the patellofemoral joint. Unfortunately, the menisci are usually assumed to be the major cause of mechanical derangement in the knee, and the patella is often ignored.

The onset of symptoms varies and should be carefully investigated. The symptoms can sometimes be attributed to a direct traumatic event involving high-energy force. The typical example is a car accident with a dashboard injury. Indirect force can also cause patellofemoral symptoms. An example is the typical valgus–external rotation injury that causes lateral patellar subluxation or dislocation. Often, the history of patients with patellofemoral pain does not reveal a definite traumatic event. In these cases, pain may result from overuse. Pain occurs when the load imposed on a joint exceeds the joint's ability to sustain the increased demands and adapt. The typical example is a running athlete, but overuse can be also a daily living or work-related problem.

Pain

Typically, patients with patellar complaints have an aching pain situated behind the patella, often on the medial side of the joint and sometimes posteriorly located in the popliteal fossa. The pain is aggravated by activities that require a strong quadriceps contraction, such as squatting, stair climbing, skiing, or riding a bike uphill. Descending stairs requires a strong eccentric quadriceps contraction to proceed to the next step smoothly. This is often more painful than ascending stairs, which requires a concentric quadriceps contraction. Prolonged periods with the knee flexed are usually painful (the movie sign). The reason for this phenomenon is not completely understood but may involve increased tension in the soft tissues or increased compression on the articular surfaces.

Pain may be bilateral, and the onset of symptoms is usually gradual and unrelated to any significant traumatic episode. At times, however, a bout of strenuous activity or a minor injury may seem to have initiated the complaint, although questioning generally demonstrates that such events merely served to worsen a preexisting disorder. Bilaterality and insidious onset are most characteristic of patellar pain.

The origin of pain may be from both the soft tissues and bone. Soft tissues include the retinacula, synovium, tendons, and nerves. Bone and subchondral bone are also richly innervated. Articular cartilage, however, is not so innervated.

The location of the pain can also produce diagnostic errors; the most common site is the anteromedial side of the knee, the same location of pain from a meniscal disorder, a fact that has contributed to the removal of many normal menisci. Less frequently, posterolateral pain may be felt, and when there is local tenderness in this region as well, the diagnosis of bicipital or popliteal tendinitis may be entertained. Popliteal pain is a frequent symptom of patellofemoral arthritis; when an associated popliteal cyst is present, it might be assumed that the cyst is causing the pain, whereas in fact both are secondary to patellar arthritis.

The characteristics and location of pain have been investigated with the use of knee pain diagrams in a group of 109 knees with patellofemoral pain. Patient-drawn diagrams illustrate their perception of pain.[322] A similar diagram was used by a physician to illustrate areas of tenderness. The diagrams were divided into nine zones, including two prepatellar zones, the patellar tendon, upper and lower medial peripatellar zones, upper and lower lateral peripatellar zones, and the medial and lateral joint lines. Pain was usually intermittent (69%) and aggravated by stair climbing (88%) and squatting (85%). The prepatellar area was the most frequently painful area (close to 70%), followed by the medial parapatellar areas (50% to 60%) and the lateral parapatellar areas. The joint line areas were painful in 20% to 30% of cases. Comparison between patient-drawn and physician-drawn diagrams revealed that each patient marked an average of 4.2 zones as compared with 2.6 zones for physicians. Overall, good correlation was found between pain location as perceived by the patient and tenderness localized by physical examination, with complete or some overlap in 88% of cases. Pain diagrams were thought to be a useful adjunct in these patients.

Instability

Instability is the second major symptom of patellar dysfunction. Sometimes, instability represents an episode of dislocation or subluxation that can be documented by examination (objective instability), but on occasion, exactly similar episodes occur in patients in whom it is impossible, even under anesthesia, to displace the patella passively from the femoral sulcus (subjective instability). For this reason, the boundaries between subjective instability, subluxation, and dislocation should not be too fine because other patients with passively dislocatable patellae will not complain of clinical instability. Instability of patellar origin may mimic the buckling caused by meniscal injury or ligamentous insufficiency, but most often it is a different sensation. Although the instability may occur on pivoting or twisting movements, such as when "cutting" in sports, the patient is usually aware that it is the kneecap that has slipped. Otherwise, when the patient does not recognize the nature of the buckling, the event is described in such terms as the knee having "collapsed" or "went forward." There is not the sensation of the joint "coming apart" or of "one bone sliding on the other" that is so typical of ligament insufficiency. Episodes of patellar instability may or may not be followed by pain and swelling lasting for a few days to several weeks.

Locking

A grating sensation, particularly when the patellofemoral joint is loaded as in stair climbing or arising from a chair, is a fairly common complaint and may sometimes be audible. Momentary "catching" may also be experienced, and interruption of smooth patellar gliding may precipitate buckling or giving way. Actual locking of the knee sometimes happens, and curiously, patellar locking is not always transient but may give the impression of a true mechanical block. The mechanism of persistent locking is obscure. Hamstring spasm and secondary contracture of the posterior capsule may contribute to prolonged locking.

Swelling

Many patients with patellofemoral disease complain of swelling. Sometimes this is a subjective sensation because on examination, an effusion is not found and circumfer-

ential measurement of the joint does not show an increase when compared with the opposite side. Synovitis with distention by synovial fluid or blood occurs after an episode of patellar subluxation and sometimes with chondromalacia or arthritis. Cartilaginous or osteocartilaginous loose bodies may be generated from the articular surfaces and contribute to giving way and transient locking, although the patient is usually aware of a free body within the joint that may also be directly felt in the suprapatellar pouch.

PHYSICAL EXAMINATION

During the physical examination, the patient should be sequentially examined while standing, walking, sitting, supine, and prone.

The examination begins with the patient standing with the feet together. Genu varum or valgum can readily be observed, as well as rotatory malalignment such as infacing or "squinting" of the patellae in patients with an increased quadriceps (Q) angle and hip anteversion (Fig. 53–12). Quadriceps tone and development can be appreciated in the standing position or during a half-squat. Hypoplasia of the vastus medialis obliquus should be noted. Normally, the vastus medialis inserts on the upper third or half of the medial border of the patella. In knees with patellofemoral dysplasia, the muscle belly may end a

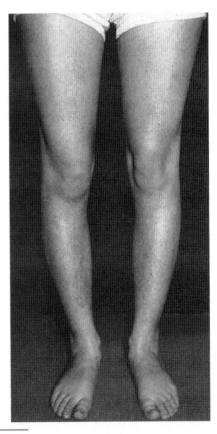

Figure 53–12. Squinting of the patellae caused by rotational malalignment of the limb. The phenomenon is accompanied by an increase in the Q angle.

few centimeters short of the superior patellar margin. The presence of quadriceps atrophy implies decreased dynamic muscle control on the patella.

The position of the foot also deserves attention. Eversion at the subtalar joint is accompanied by compensatory internal tibial torsion, which increases the Q angle and consequently stress on the patellofemoral joint. The subtalar joint is a single-axis joint that acts like a hinge connecting the talus to the calcaneus. The axis of the subtalar joint deviates an average of 23 degrees medially and anteriorly to the long axis of the foot and 41 degrees inferiorly and posteriorly in relation to the horizontal plane. Therefore, internal rotation of the leg causes eversion of the heel and depression of the medial side of the foot. External rotation of the leg produces the opposite effect.[75] Subtalar joint eversion may be either primary or secondary, as in knees with varus alignment or tibia vara, wherein compensatory subtalar joint eversion is required to produce a plantigrade foot. This phenomenon is probably more important in long-distance runners.[210] Eversion of the heel (heel valgus) is readily appreciated by looking at the patient in the standing position from the backside. Abduction of the forefoot is evaluated in the standing position by palpation of the talar head on the anterior aspect of the ankle. The neutral position is defined when the head of the talus can be equally palpated on the medial and lateral sides. During weightbearing, a normal foot is in mild pronation and additional pronation should still be possible.[55]

Gait is observed, and younger patients are asked to squat and hold the halfway position briefly because pain in this position is usually patellar in origin (half-squat test). Whenever possible, both stair climbing and descending should be observed because this activity also provokes patellar symptoms.

With the patient seated on the examining table, the position of the patella is first checked. Normally, it sinks between the femoral condyles with the knee at 90 degrees of flexion. If patella alta is present, its anterior surface points to the ceiling with the knee in the same 90-degree position. Active extension is observed, and the presence of patellar crepitus and painful catching is recorded, as well as abnormal patellar tracking.

Ficat and Hungerford[116] stress the importance of observing the entrance and exit of the patella into and out of the sulcus between 10 and 30 degrees of flexion. They describe four common abnormalities in patellar tracking. Normal patellar tracking is present when the patella glides smoothly into the sulcus, and only minimal lateral displacement may be appreciated in the final extension when the patella exits the trochlear groove. We define more marked lateral displacement as lateralization, whereas greater degrees of pathological tracking are defined as subluxation or dislocation. This finding is also called the J sign because the path resembles an upside-down J. Furthermore, evaluation of the tilt of the patella should be attempted. In normal knees, the medial border of the patella should be at the same level as the lateral border, with a minor lateral tilt in full extension. It should be noted that most of the abnormalities in patellar tracking involve lateral displacement and lateral tilt of the patella in extension, which reduces in flexion. Therefore, we find

it useful to roughly estimate patellar subluxation and tilt during the physical examination (Fig. 53–13) and verify this later with radiographic axial views or computed tomography (CT). Other abnormalities in patellar tracking may be encountered more rarely, including medial dislocation or subluxation of the patella in flexion (after over-release of the lateral structures and excessive medial displacement of the tibial tuberosity) or lateral dislocation in flexion (as in habitual or permanent dislocation).

Patellar crepitation is appreciated during active extension and recorded as absent, mild, moderate, or severe. It should be evaluated in the sitting position, and it is enhanced by the application of manual resistance on the lower part of leg. Because crepitation beyond 90 degrees of flexion cannot be evaluated in the sitting position, it is better assessed during a full squat.

Hughston and Walsh[193] described a lateral position of the patella in the flexed knee for which they coined the term *frog-eye* patella. This seems to be associated with patella alta, which can be suspected clinically when the fat pad is unusually prominent. In fact, the fat pad may, on inspection, be mistaken for the patella because it occupies

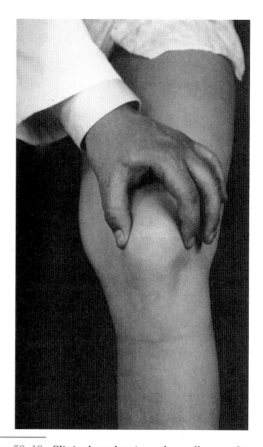

Figure 53–13. Clinical evaluation of patellar tracking. The patient is sitting on a firm examining table with the knee flexed at 90 degrees. The examiner places his hand on the knee so that the medial and lateral borders of the patella are palpated with the index finger and thumb. The patient is asked to actively extend the knee. An effort is made to detect the presence of lateral subluxation (displacement) or lateral tilt (lateral border of the patella lower than the medial border) during tracking.

the femoral sulcus with the knee in extension while the patella is situated in the supracondylar pouch.

With the patient supine on the examining table, tenderness around the patella is evaluated systematically. Tenderness and swelling in the prepatellar area may be indicative of prepatellar bursitis. Evaluation of tenderness around the patella includes assessment of the medial and lateral retinacula, quadriceps, and patellar tendons, including their insertions. Joint line tenderness should also be evaluated. Patellar tenderness can be elicited by the following maneuvers.

Direct Palpation of the Patellar Facets When the Patella Is Displaced Medially or Laterally. This method has a disadvantage in that synovium and capsule are necessarily intervening between the finger and the articular surface. Some authors,[125] in fact, have suggested that the primary source of pain may be in the lateral retinaculum itself and have proposed that it should be selectively palpated by displacing the patella laterally so that the lateral retinaculum is put under tension (Fig. 53–14).

Compressing the Patella against the Femoral Sulcus. The knee must be flexed approximately 30 degrees to bring the patella from its resting and largely supracondylar position into the sulcus. The patella is then pushed medially (Fig. 53–15) and laterally (Fig. 53–16) and compressed into the femoral sulcus. The patient may experience pain and/or apprehension. Pain during medial displacement is common in those with patellar pain syndromes. Apprehension during the medial glide test can be evoked in the presence of medial instability caused by excessive lateral release. Lateral displacement induces the apprehension sign in patients with recurrent patellar subluxation or dislocation. Reflex quadriceps contraction is provoked in an attempt to prevent the dislocation. At the same time, the patient may attempt to push the examiner's hands away.[109]

Direct posterior compression of the patella in the trochlea has been also suggested to elicit pain from cartilage lesions.[321] The pain produced by this test comes from subchondral bone if the examiner is careful to avoid compression of the soft tissues. Compression at variable degrees of knee flexion may be helpful in localizing cartilage lesions.

Pushing Distally on the Patella in a Fully Extended Knee and Asking the Patient to Contract the Quadriceps. Unfortunately, in some knees, especially those with patella alta, this maneuver entraps the synovium of the suprapatellar pouch and produces exquisite pain, even when the patella itself is normal. Because of the frequency of false-positive results, this method is not recommended.

The Q angle is measured by drawing an imaginary line connecting the center of the patella and the anterior superior iliac spine to produce a surface marking that approximates the line of pull of the quadriceps tendon (Fig. 53–17). The direction of the ligamentum patellae is indicated by a second line drawn from the center of the patella to the center of the tibial tubercle. The intersection of these two imaginary lines forms the Q angle. Because this measurement is affected by rotation of the hip, an effort is made to note the position of the medial border of the patient's foot during walking and reproduce this position during the measurement.

Active pronation or supination of the foot should be avoided because these movements are associated with

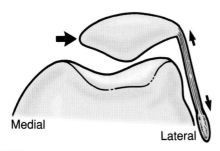

Figure 53–14. Palpation of the lateral retinaculum with the knee in extension. The patella is displaced laterally to place the lateral retinaculum under tension so that tenderness of this structure can be more selectively assessed. (Modified from Fulkerson JP: Awareness of the retinaculum in evaluating patellofemoral pain. Am J Sports Med 10:147, 1982.)

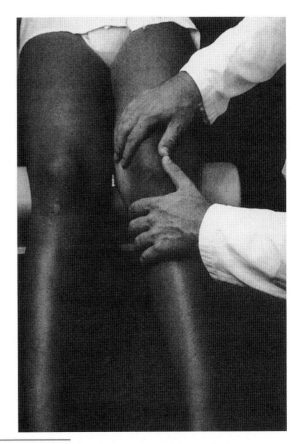

Figure 53–15. Patellar compression test. With the knee resting on a thigh support to flex it at 25 degrees and bringing the patella into the sulcus, the patella is pushed medially. This usually causes marked pain in knees with patellar pain syndromes. We have found it most convenient to use the KT-1000 arthrometer thigh support (MEDmetric Corp., San Diego, CA), which allows optimal relaxation of the thigh muscles.

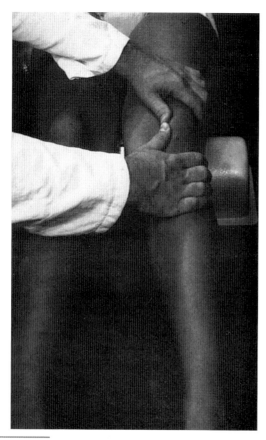

Figure 53–16. Apprehension test. In the same position as described in Figure 53-14, the patella is pushed laterally. In cases of recurrent patella dislocation or subluxation, the patient experiences apprehension, contracts the quadriceps, and attempts to remove the examiner's hands from the knee.

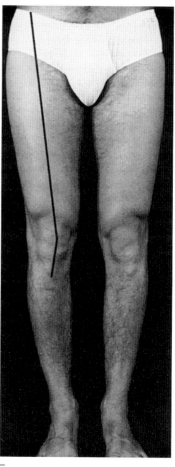

Figure 53–17. The quadriceps angle is measured by drawing two lines from the center of the patella. The first line is drawn up to the anterior superior iliac spine and represents the line of pull of the quadriceps muscle. The second line is drawn down to the tibial tubercle and indicates the line of the patellar tendon.

internal and external rotation of the leg, respectively,[307] and consequently increase and decrease the Q angle.

We measured the Q angle in 150 normal subjects and found it to be 15 degrees (range, 6 to 27 degrees; SD, 3 degrees) (Table 53–1).[7] It was lower in men (14 degrees; SD, 3 degrees) than in women (17 degrees; SD, 3 degrees), and the difference was significant ($p = 0.001$). Only 11 subjects, all women, had Q angles greater than 20 degrees (7%). Therefore, it seems that a Q angle greater than 20 degrees may reasonably be considered abnormal. The Q angle was also measured in a group of pathological knees, including 53 patients with patellar pain and 37 with recurrent subluxation or dislocation. In the knees with patellar pain, the Q angle was significantly increased to 20 degrees; this was true for both men and women. In contrast, the Q angle was not significantly different from normal in knees with recurrent subluxation or dislocation (average, 15 degrees), and the same applied to both men and women. In patients with patellar subluxation or dislocation, the Q angle is usually underestimated for at least two reasons: First, the patella is displaced laterally in extension; second, the quadriceps tendon frequently lies more lateral than predicted when the superior iliac spine is used as the surface marking (Fig. 53–18).

To overcome the problem of lateral patellar displacement and consequent underestimation of the Q angle, Fithian et al[119] measured the Q angle with the knee in 30 degrees of flexion. They simultaneously applied a posteriorly directed force so that the patella symmetrically contacted the trochlea. With this method, the Q angle was 12 degrees in control subjects (11.2 degrees in men and 13.4 degrees in women). A significantly higher value was found in a group of knees with patellar dislocation (average, 19.2 degrees). The contralateral knee of patients suffering from patellar dislocation also showed an increased value of the Q angle (average, 18.4 degrees).

It is debated whether the Q angle is better measured in the supine or the standing position. Woodland and Francis[408] measured the Q angle in the supine and standing position in a large number of normal men[276] and women.[264] The average values in the supine position were 12.7 degrees for men and 15.8 degrees for women. Changing to the standing position increased the Q angle 0.9 degree in men and 1.2 degrees in women. The difference was statistically significant but is probably less significant

Table 53–1. Measurement of Quadriceps Angle and Radiographic Measurements of Patellar Height and Patellofemoral Congruence

	NO. OF SUBJECTS	Q ANGLE	T/P RATIO*	A/B RATIO†	SULCUS ANGLE	CONGRUENCE ANGLE
Normal knees‡	150	15° (3°)	1.04 (0.11)	0.95 (0.13)	137° (6°)	−8° (6°)
Males	75	14°	1.01	0.97	137°	−6°
Females	75	17° (p < 0.001)	1.06 (p < 0.05)	0.94 (NS)	137° (NS)	10° (p < 0.001)
Patella	37	15° (NS)	1.23 (p < 0.001)	1.08 (p < 0.001)	147° (p < 0.001)	16° (p < 0.001)
subluxation						
Males	16	13° (NS)	1.23 (p < 0.001)	1.07 (NS)	149° (p < 0.001)	15° (p < 0.001)
Females	21	16° (NS)	1.22 (p < 0.005)	1.08 (p < 0.001)	146° (p < 0.001)	17° (p < 0.001)
Patellar pain	53	20° (p < 0.001)	1.08 (p < 0.01)	1.91 (NS)	139° (p < 0.01)	−2° (p < 0.001)
Males	18	20° (p < 0.001)	1.11 (p < 0.001)	0.93 (NS)	140° (p < 0.005)	−1° (p < 0.005)
Females	35	19° (p < 0.001)	1.07 (NS)	0.90 (NS)	139° (NS)	−2° (p < 0.001)

The values of statistical significance reported in normal knees refer to the difference between males and females. The values reported in the pathological groups (patellar pain and patellar subluxation) refer to the difference from normal knees.
*T/P ratio: tendon-patella ratio of Insall and Salvati[204] (see text).
†A/B ratio: Blackburne and Peel[38] ratio (see text).
‡Numbers in parentheses indicate standard deviation.
NS, not significant.
Data from Aglietti P, Insall JN, Cerulli G: Patellar pain and incongruence. I: Measurements of incongruence. Clin Orthop 176:217, 1983.

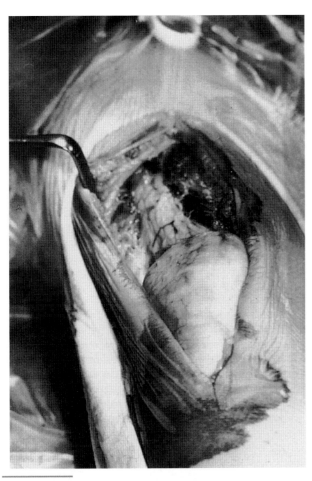

Figure 53–18. The quadriceps tendon often lies more laterally than the surface marking of the Q angle predicts.

tibial rotation[366] because this position would give a more reliable measurement of the maximal valgus vector imposed on the patella. However, the difficulty in achieving standardized knee flexion and hip rotation make the reproducibility of this measurement less reliable. It has also been suggested that the Q angle be measured at 90 degrees of knee flexion,[227] when the patella is centered in the sulcus. The direction of the patellar tendon is measured in relation to the transepicondylar line. Values greater than 10 degrees are considered pathological. However, consistent identification of the transepicondylar line is not easy, especially in obese patients.

In the supine position and with the knee in extension, the patient is asked to contract the quadriceps, and upward movement of the patella is noted (lateral pull test). In a normal knee, the patella is pulled predominantly upward with an associated minor lateral displacement. The lateral pull test result is considered abnormal if lateral displacement is excessive.[227]

Patellar mobility should be evaluated with the knee in full extension and at 30 degrees of flexion. With the knee in extension, the patella is out of the trochlear groove and may be easily displaced medially and laterally. Gross hypermobility, as in patients with patella alta and a dysplastic extensor apparatus, is easily detected in this position. With the knee flexed 20 to 30 degrees, the patella is normally drawn into the trochlear groove and stabilized. Excessive displacement in the lateral direction indicates laxity of the medial retinaculum and vice versa. On the other hand, reduced medial mobility indicates the presence of a tight lateral retinaculum. Kolowich and colleagues[227] suggested that patellar mobility is best evaluated by dividing the patella into longitudinal quadrants (Fig. 53–19). With the knee at 20 to 30 degrees of flexion, mobility in the medial or lateral direction should not exceed two quadrants. A medial glide of one quadrant or less suggests a tight lateral retinaculum, which may also be investigated by trying to lift the lateral border of the patella with the knee in extension (passive patellar tilt) (Fig. 53–20). If the transverse axis of the patella cannot

clinically. It is relevant to note that the values determined by Woodland and Francis[408] are close to those detected by Aglietti et al.[7]

It has been suggested that the Q angle be measured at 30 degrees of knee flexion and with maximum external

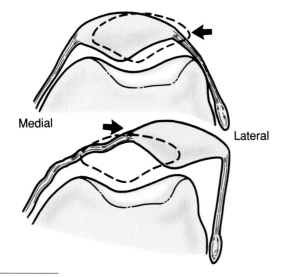

Figure 53–19. The mobility of the patella is best evaluated with the knee flexed to 20 to 30 degrees to engage the patella into the femoral sulcus. Displacement of the patella in the medial or lateral direction is best recorded in quadrants. Displacement in the medial direction of one quadrant or less indicates a tight lateral retinaculum. Displacement in the lateral direction over two quadrants indicates weakened medial stabilizers. (From Kolowich PA, Paulos LE, Rosenberg TD, Farnsworth S: Lateral release of the patella: Indications and contraindications. Am J Sports Med 18:359, 1990.)

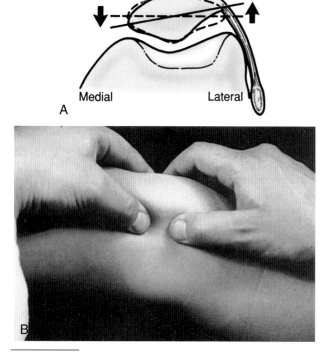

Figure 53–20. **A** and **B**, Passive patellar tilt test. In a normal knee in full extension, it is possible to lift the transverse axis of the patella beyond the horizontal. An inability to perform this maneuver indicates a tight lateral retinaculum. (From Kolowich PA, Paulos LE, Rosenberg TD, Farnsworth S: Lateral release of the patella: Indications and contraindications. Am J Sports Med 18:359, 1990.)

be elevated beyond the horizontal plane, a tight lateral retinaculum is demonstrated.[227]

Medial and lateral displacement of the patella has been measured with a displacement transducer[119] or axial radiographs.[382] Fithian et al[119] used a displacement sensor to record motion in the coronal plane with the knees bent at 30 degrees. Forces of 2.5 and 5 lb were applied with a hand-held force applicator with a load cell. Under a 5-lb force, medial patellar displacement averaged 9.2 ± 3.5 mm and lateral displacement was 7.7 ± 2.6 mm in a group of 188 normal knees. In a group of 22 patients with symptomatic lateral patellar dislocation, medial displacement at 5 lb was 8.3 ± 4.5 mm and lateral displacement was 11.5 ± 4.7 mm. Using the lateral minus medial displacement index, control knees had an average value of -2.1 ± 2.8 mm. Symptomatic knees had a lateral minus medial displacement of 3.2 ± 3.4 mm. The difference was statistically significant. In summary, the total mediolateral displacement of the patella in normal knees under a 5-lb force was close to 17 mm in normal knees and almost 20 mm in knees with patellar instability. The lateral minus medial displacement was useful for differentiating between normal and unstable patellae. Medial displacement was larger than lateral displacement in 81% of control subjects. In unstable patellae, lateral displacement was larger than medial displacement. The asymptomatic knees in patients with unilateral patellar dislocation could not be used as controls because they showed abnormal patellar mobility similar to the symptomatic knees. The authors offered the concept of balance between medial and lateral structures. A normal knee should have greater medial than lateral displacement. If lateral displacement exceeds medial displacement, the restraining structures are unbalanced.

Teitge et al[382] evaluated medial and lateral patellar mobility with an axial radiograph at 30 to 40 degrees of flexion and a spring-loaded scale to apply a 16-lb force (7.3 kg). In a group of 20 asymptomatic knees, medial displacement averaged 11.1 ± 3.6 mm and lateral displacement was 11.6 ± 8.1 mm. The values are higher than those reported in the study by Fithian et al,[119] but the displacing force was also greater (16 lb versus 5 lb). In a group of knees with lateral instability, medial displacement was comparable (11.6 mm on average), whereas lateral displacement was highly increased to 21.9 mm on average.

Torsional abnormalities of the femur and tibia have been described as a possible factor leading to patellar pain or instability. The pattern would involve increased femoral neck anteversion so that the trochlear groove faces inward, the Q angle is increased, and the patellae are squinting. Compensatory external tibial torsion is required to produce a foot aligned in the sagittal plane.

Turner and Smillie[388] measured tibial torsion in 836 patients with a tropometer. They found an average lateral tibial torsion of 19 degrees in control knees, which was increased to 24.5 degrees in knees with patellofemoral instability and to 24 degrees in those with chondromalacia. Because increased tibial rotation was also found in Osgood-Schlatter disease, the finding does not seem to be specific for patellofemoral joint disorders.

The amount of femoral neck anteversion has often been indirectly estimated by measuring the proportion of internal to external rotation of the hips in extension

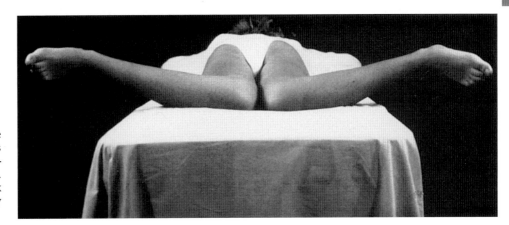

Figure 53–21. Excessive internal rotation of the hips in a patient with recurrent patellar dislocation. Increased femoral neck anteversion is usually present in these cases.

(Fig. 53–21), which would be its major determinant.[15,369,370] Carson and colleagues[55] suggested that if internal rotation of the hip in extension exceeds external rotation by more than 30 degrees, femoral neck anteversion is increased. Insall and colleagues[203] suggested that increased femoral neck anteversion may be present in knees with patellofemoral malalignment. Hvid and Andersen[195] measured the Q angle and internal rotation of the hip in 29 patients with patellofemoral complaints. They found that both the Q angle and internal hip rotation were higher in women than in men. There was a significant correlation between the Q angle and hip rotation, thus suggesting that the Q angle is in fact increased because of excessive femoral neck anteversion. Other authors,[110] however, have failed to identify any significant difference in Q angle, genu valgum, and anteversion of the femoral neck between normal adolescents and adolescents or adults with anterior knee pain. They concluded that because those affected by knee pain are also those most interested in sports activities, the probable cause is chronic overloading rather than faulty mechanics.

More recently, Dejour et al[91] reported CT measurements of femoral anteversion and tibial torsion in normal controls and knees with instability of the patella. They found that femoral neck anteversion was increased in knees with patellofemoral instability (15.6 degrees) as compared with controls (10.8 degrees). Tibial torsion was a less important factor. It was 33 degrees in the control group and 35 degrees in the knees with patellar instability.

In light of the data reported in the literature and our own clinical experience, we think that torsional abnormalities of the lower limb, including femoral neck anteversion and, less significantly, external tibial torsion, may contribute to and play a role in patellofemoral disorders by increasing lateral pull on the patella. However, because these deformities are often less marked and remote from the knee, their importance is minor from the therapeutic and surgical points of view.

In conclusion, we emphasize that there is not a single symptom or sign that is in itself diagnostic of patellar pain or instability. The diagnosis is usually straightforward in recurrent patellar dislocation but may require much more effort in cases of subtle patellar pain with minor anatomic abnormalities. Furthermore, an increased Q angle or a tight lateral retinaculum may be present in a painful knee,

but this does not imply that the patellofemoral joint is in fact causing the problem. The correct diagnosis should therefore rest on accurate interpretation of the symptoms, physical examination, and imaging of the patellofemoral joint.

IMAGING OF THE PATELLOFEMORAL JOINT

Standard radiographic evaluation, including anteroposterior, lateral, and axial views, should be obtained in each patient with patellofemoral disorders to assess the height and congruence of the patella and exclude other bone disorders. CT has been widely used to study the patellofemoral joint in the first 20 degrees of flexion, where it cannot be investigated by traditional radiographic techniques. MRI has also been used to investigate the patellofemoral relationship in extension and early flexion, as well as to detect cartilage lesions. Bone scans can be used to visualize loss of osseous homeostasis.

Radiography

ANTEROPOSTERIOR VIEW

The anteroposterior view is not of much value, although arthrosis of the tibiofemoral joint and varus or valgus malalignment can be observed. For this purpose a 30 × 40-cm weightbearing film is appropriate. In addition, because the outline of the patella is visible, abnormalities such as patella magna or parva, bipartite patellae, and fractures can be seen. Marked lateral subluxation of the patella can also be detected in the anteroposterior view.

LATERAL VIEW

The lateral view is taken with the knee in at least 30 degrees of flexion to place the patellar tendon under tension and demonstrate the functional relationship between the patella and the femur. Excessive rotation should be avoided because it may obscure some of the bony landmarks, such as the tibial tubercle, and make interpretation difficult. The patella is not visualized in the lateral view in rare cases of congenital absence and when it is completely displaced laterally, as in habitual dislocation. In children younger than 5 years, the ossific nucleus has not yet appeared and thus the patella is invisible.

Patellar position is related to the length of the patellar ligament. Patella alta, in particular, is associated with patellar instability, dislocation, and abnormalities of the trochlear groove. Several methods of measurement have been described, including those reported by Blumensaat,[41] Insall and Salvati,[204] Blackburne and Peel,[38] Caton and the Lyon School,[62] Rünow,[335] and Grelsamer and Meadows.[162]

Blumensaat's Line

Blumensaat[41] states that in a lateral radiograph with the knee flexed 30 degrees, the lower pole of the patella should be on a line projected anteriorly from the intercondylar notch (Blumensaat's line). It is difficult to obtain routine radiographs with the knee flexed exactly the required degree, and this limits the usefulness of the method. The Blumensaat method is also inaccurate. Of 44 radiographs of the knee that were flexed exactly 30 degrees, in no case did the lower pole of the patella lie on Blumensaat's line; rather, the patella was positioned above this line.

Insall-Salvati Method

Insall and Salvati[204] sought a method that would fit the following requirements: (1) simple and practical, as well as accurate; (2) applicable to the range of knee positions during routine radiography, which in the lateral view is usually 20 to 70 degrees of flexion; and (3) independent of the size of joint and the degree of magnification of the radiograph. Because the ligamentum patellae is not elastic, its length determines the position of the patella, provided that the point of insertion into the tibial tubercle is constant.

Insall and Salvati[204] describe an expression for normal patellar height in terms of the length of the patellar tendon. Measurements were made on 114 knees in which the diagnosis of a torn meniscus was clearly established by clinical history and examination, by positive arthrographic results, and by the finding of a meniscal tear at arthrotomy. Any case in which the slightest doubt existed was excluded, and it was assumed that the joints examined were structurally normal before a traumatic episode produced a torn meniscus. All patients were adults, and none showed radiological evidence of osteoarthritis. The following measurements were made (Fig. 53–22):

1. T (length of tendon). The length of the patellar tendon was measured on its deep or posterior surface from its origin on the lower pole of the patella to its insertion into the tibial tubercle. The point of insertion is usually represented on the radiograph by a clearly defined notch.
2. P (length of patella). The greatest diagonal length of the patella was measured.

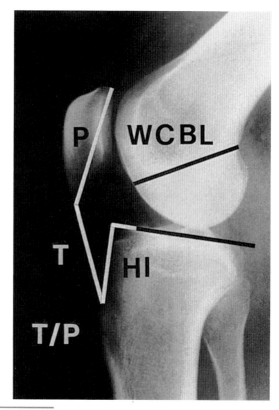

Figure 53–22. Insall-Salvati measurements to determine the height of the patella. T, length of the tendon measured on its deep posterior surface; P, greatest diagonal length of the patella; WCBL, width of the femoral condyles at Blumensaat's line; HI, height of insertion, or the perpendicular distance between the joint line and the insertion of the patellar tendon. (From Insall JN, Salvati E: Patella position in the normal knee joint. Radiology 101:101, 1971.)

3. WCBL (width of the femoral condyles at Blumensaat's line). Both condyles were measured at the level of Blumensaat's line and an average was obtained. This measurement determined whether there was great variation in patellar size. Patellar size was considered to be acceptably constant.
4. HI (height of insertion). The perpendicular distance from the level of the tibial condylar surface to the point of insertion of the patellar tendon was measured to determine whether there was a constant relationship between the level of the tibial tubercle and the tibial plateau. A great variation in tendon insertion would have invalidated the measurements, but the insertion appeared to be acceptably constant. This measurement, therefore, may be disregarded for clinical evaluation.

The length of the patellar tendon (T) was found to be approximately equal to patellar length (P), and this was expressed as a ratio (because of variations in the size of individual knee joints and their projection on radiographs). The average value of the ratio T/P was 1.02, with a mean SD of 0.13. It was concluded that in a normal knee, the length of the patellar tendon should not differ from that of the patella by more than 20%.

The measurements were repeated on bilateral knee radiographs in 50 asymptomatic volunteers by Jacobsen and Bertheussen,[209] who confirmed a similar degree of accuracy. We also measured patellar height according to the Insall-Salvati method in a group of 150 normal knees[7] (see Table 53–1). The T/P ratio was found to be 1.04 on average (range, 0.8 to 1.38; SD, 0.11). The patella was significantly higher in women (1.06) than in men (1.01). In the same group of knees, the distance from the plateau level to the tibial tuberosity and the diagonal length of the patella varied only with sex, with larger values in men than in women. In 53 knees with patellar pain, the patella was slightly but significantly higher than in normal knees, with an average T/P ratio of 1.08 (range, 0.88 to 1.29; SD, 0.09). In a group of 37 knees with recurrent subluxation, the average T/P ratio was clearly increased to an average of 1.23 (range, 0.78 to 1.60; SD, 0.18). In conclusion, using the Insall-Salvati method, an index over 1.2 indicates patella alta, whereas an index below 0.8 indicates a low patella.

Blackburne-Peel Ratio

Blackburne and Peel[38] criticized the T/P ratio on the basis of two observations:

1. The radiographic marking on the tibial tubercle may be indistinct or even unrecognizable when the tibial tuberosity has been affected by Osgood-Schlatter disease.
2. The nonarticular portion of the lower pole of the patella varies considerably in size, and it is instead the position of the articular surface that is of greatest clinical significance.

To overcome these difficulties, they suggested a ratio between the perpendicular distance from the lowest articular margin of the patella to the tibial plateau (A) and the length of the articular surface of the patella (B) as measured on a lateral view of the knee in at least 30 degrees of flexion (Fig. 53–23). The A/B ratio in 171 normal knees was 0.80 (SD, 0.14). There was no difference between the sexes.

We measured the A/B ratio in a group of 150 normal knees[7] and found a slightly higher value than the original authors did: an A/B ratio of 0.95 on average (range, 0.65 to 1.38; SD, 0.13), with an insignificant difference between men and women (see Table 53–1). In a group of patients with anterior knee pain, the A/B ratio was 0.91, an insignificant difference from the ratio in control knees. On the other hand, the A/B ratio was significantly increased in knees with recurrent subluxation (average, 1.08; range, 0.76 to 1.89; SD, 0.19).

Lyon School

The Lyon school[62] criticized the previously existing methods of measuring the height of the patella. They found it difficult to define the insertion of the patellar tendon into the tibial tuberosity in knees with previous transposition of the tuberosity. They further observed that the use of a tangent to the tibial plateaus in the Blackburne and Peel method[38] may be a source of significant error.

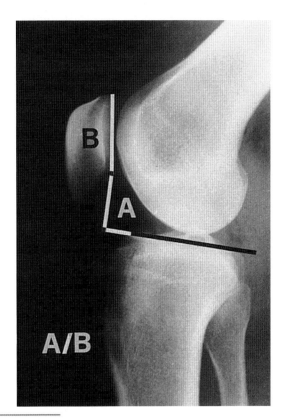

Figure 53–23. Blackburne and Peel method of measuring patellar height. The height is expressed as the ratio between A (perpendicular distance between the lowest part of the articular surface and the joint line level) and B (length of the articular surface of the patella). (From Blackburne JS, Peel TE: A new method of measuring patella height. J Bone Joint Surg Br 59:241, 1977.)

Perfect superimposition of the tibial plateaus is necessary to draw the line. The posterior slope of the tibial plateaus is not constant and may vary within 15 degrees or more in subjects who have undergone anterior tibial epiphysiodesis. To overcome these difficulties, they tried to develop an easy method that could be used on lateral radiographs in flexion between 10 and 80 degrees and that was not influenced by radiographic magnification, by previous transposition of the tibial tuberosity, or by fractures of the tip of the patella. In this method, a ratio is calculated between the distance AT from the inferior point of the articular surface of the patella to the anterosuperior edge of the tibia and the length AP of the articular surface of the patella (Fig. 51–24). The AT/AP ratio was calculated in 141 normal subjects and found to be 0.960[13] in 80 men and 0.990[12] in 61 women. Based on these findings, the authors considered the patella to be infra with a ratio of 0.6 or less and alta if 1.3 or more.

Norman Index

Norman and coworkers[300] observed that the Insall-Salvati method does not describe the relationship between the patella and the femoral sulcus and that proximal or distal transposition of the tibial tuberosity may be performed without affecting the T/P ratio. To overcome these diffi-

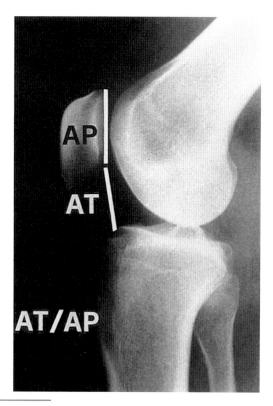

Figure 53–24. Caton's method to measure the height of the patella. The height is expressed as the ratio between the distance (AT) from the lowest point of the articular facet to the most prominent part of the tibial plateau and the length (AP) of the articular facet of the patella. See text for discussion of the ratio AT/AP. (From Caton G, Deschamps G, Chambat P, et al: Les routules basses: Á propos de 128 observations. Rev Chir Orthop 68:317, 1982.)

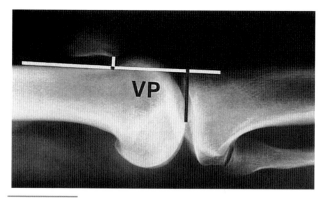

Figure 53–25. Norman's method to measure the height of the patella. A lateral radiograph is obtained with perfect superimposition of the femoral condyles, the knee hyperextended, and the quadriceps contracted to straighten the patellar tendon. A line is drawn tangential to the distal third of the anterior femoral cortex. Two perpendicular lines are then drawn that pass through the femoral-tibial contact point and through the inferior point of the articular facet. The distance between the two perpendicular lines is defined as the vertical position (VP) of the patella, and it is related to the height of the patient in centimeters. The Norman index is expressed as follows: Vertical position of the patella (mm)/Body height (cm). In a normal knee, its average value is 0.21. (From Norman O, Egund N, Ekelund L, Rünow A: The vertical position of the patella. Acta Orthop Scand 54:908, 1983.)

culties, Norman et al described a method wherein a lateral radiograph is obtained with the knee in full extension (hyperextension) and quadriceps contraction to straighten the patellar tendon. The film-focus distance should be kept constant (1 m) and the cassette placed in contact with the lateral aspect of the knee. Various parameters were measured in this radiograph, including the length of the tendon, patella, and articular facet and the vertical position of the patella—that is, the distance from the lowest point of the articular facet to the joint line. These measurements were related to the height of the patient, and it was found that the vertical position of the patella was constant without sex-related differences (Fig. 53–25). The Norman index, defined as the ratio between the vertical position of the patella (in millimeters) and body length (in centimeters), is 0.21 in a normal knee (SD, 0.02). In patients with recurrent dislocation without associated generalized laxity, the index was 0.23 on average; in patients with associated generalized laxity, it was 0.25.

Modified Insall-Salvati Ratio

Grelsamer and Meadows[162] observed that the Insall-Salvati index does not account for the shape of the patella. They found that patients with patella alta and a long distal nose

may have a falsely normal Insall-Salvati index. The presence of patella alta in these patients can be easily verified by indices that use the patellar articular surface and the upper part of the tibia as landmarks (the Blackburne and Peel or the Caton ratio). The variable relationship between the length of the patella and the length of the articular surface as expressed by the morphology index[163] has been presented in the section on anatomy (see Fig. 53–2).

To overcome the problem of variable morphology of the patella, the Insall-Salvati ratio was modified. It was suggested that the ratio of the distance between the inferior articular facet of the patella and the tibial tuberosity and the length of the articular surface be used (Fig. 53–26). In other words, this method uses the same distal reference point as the Insall-Salvati method (the tibial tuberosity) and the same proximal reference point as the Caton method. In a group of 100 control knees, the modified Insall-Salvati ratio was 1.5 on average (range, 1.2 to 2.1) Ninety-seven percent of control knees had a ratio less than 2.0. Therefore, for practical purposes, a ratio of 2 or more can be used as an index of patella alta.

MRI Method

Biedert et al[36] proposed a different method to evaluate patellar height based on MRI scans in extension. The measurements are taken in the central or just lateral sagittal slice where the articular cartilage is thicker. Patellar articular cartilage is projected on trochlear cartilage, and the height of its projection is calculated. The ratio between trochlear articular cartilage height and patellar articular

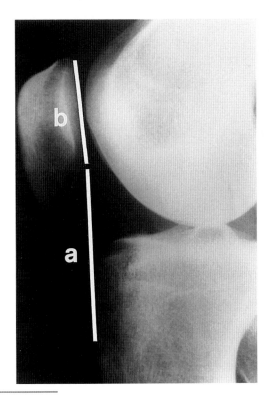

Figure 53–26. The modified Insall-Salvati method as described by Grelsamer and Meadows.[162] The distance between the lowest point of the articular surface of the patella and the tibial tuberosity (distance a) is divided by the length of the articular facet (distance b). A value of 2 or more indicates patella alta.

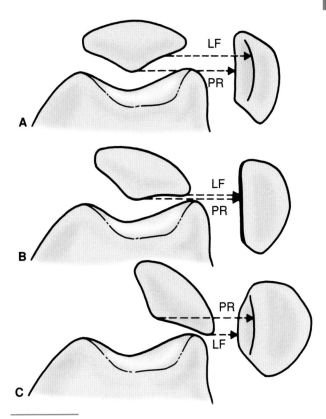

Figure 53–27. Patellar shape on a lateral view with the knee flexed 10 to 15 degrees and good superimposition of the femoral condyles. **A,** In a normal knee, the posterior profile of the patella is represented by two lines: the most posterior one is the patellar ridge (PR); the anterior one is the lateral facet (LF). **B,** If the patella is slightly tilted laterally, the two lines superimpose. **C,** If the patella is severely tilted, the lateral facet overhangs the ridge line posteriorly and the anteroposterior diameter of the patella is increased. (**A,** Modified from Maldague B, Malghem J: Apport du cliché de profil du genou dans le dépistage des instabilites rotuliennes: Rapport préliminaire. Rev Chir Orthop 71[Suppl 2]:5, 1985.)

cartilage height is deemed the patellar index. Normal values are 12.5% to 50%. An index less than 12.5% signifies patella alta, whereas an index higher than 50% indicates patella baja. The main advantage of this method is that it takes into consideration only the articular cartilage very precisely and is not affected by the patellar tendon.

Conclusions

Various methods of measuring the height of the patella have been described. In our opinion, the Insall-Salvati T/P ratio remains a reliable and reproducible method. It does not require perfect alignment of the knee in the lateral view and does not need correction for magnification. Values greater than 1.2 or, more importantly, greater than 1.3 are diagnostic of patella alta. The method may be not be applicable in knees with previous Osgood-Schlatter disease, and the method is not suitable to evaluate patellar position after distal transfer of the tibial tuberosity. For this purpose, we use the Blackburne and Peel or the Caton method, which measure the height of the patella in relation to the tibial plateau and joint line. The main drawback of the Blackburne and Peel method is that it requires a lateral view with superimposition of the femoral condyles to accurately identify the joint line. An image amplifier is required to consistently obtain this degree of accuracy. The same problem is encountered with the Norman technique, which has the additional dif-

ficulty of requiring an effective quadriceps contraction. Furthermore, the film-focus distance (1 m) must be kept constant and the patient's height must be known. In presence of abnormal patellar morphology with a long or short distal pole, the modified Insall-Salvati method should be used.

Attention has been drawn to evaluation of the anatomy of the trochlea and subluxation of the patella as seen on the lateral view. Maldague and Malghem[258] first described the radiographic appearance of the patella and trochlea femoralis in lateral views of normal knees and knees with patellar instability. It is necessary to obtain lateral views with satisfactory superimposition of the posterior and distal femoral condyles, which requires the use of an image amplifier. In the lateral view of a normal knee, the posterior aspect of the patella is represented by two lines: the most posterior one is the patellar ridge, the other is the lateral facet (Figs. 53–27 and 53–28). In knees with mild lateral tilt of the patella, the two lines superimpose. When the patella is more markedly tilted, the lateral facet

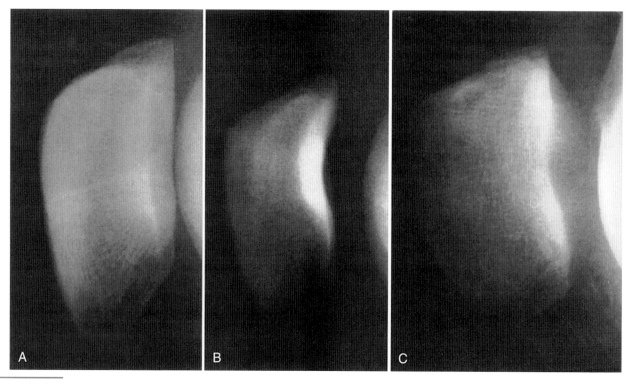

Figure 53–28. Lateral views. **A,** The patella in a normal knee. **B,** A knee with a mildly tilted patella. **C,** A knee with a markedly tilted patella.

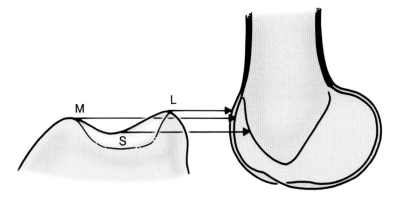

Figure 53–29. Morphology of the trochlea in a lateral radiograph with superimposition of the femoral condyles. The two anterior lines are the projection of the medial (M) and lateral (L) facets of the trochlea. The posterior line is in continuation with the intercondylar roof line and corresponds to the deepest part of the sulcus (S). (Modified from Maldague B, Malghem J: Apport du cliché de profil du genou dans le dépistage des instabilites rotuliennes: Rapport préliminaire. Rev Chir Orthop 71[Suppl 2]:5, 1985.)

overhangs the patellar ridge line posteriorly, and the anteroposterior diameter of the patella is greatly increased. The normal trochlea is composed of three lines: the two anterior lines are projections of the top of the medial and lateral facets of the trochlea; the posterior line, in continuation with the intercondylar roof line, represents the deepest point of the sulcus (Fig. 53–29). The distance between the two anterior lines and the posterior line represents the depth of the sulcus. Maldague and Malghem observed that its depth is normally greater than 1 cm as measured 1 cm distal to the upper part of the trochlea. In knees with patellar instability, the depth of the trochlea is reduced either throughout the length of the sulcus (total deficient sulcus) or only in its upper part (focally deficient sulcus). The authors emphasized the importance of the lateral view in patients with clinically suspected patellar instability and axial views showing negative results.

Because axial views are often obtained in more than 30 degrees of flexion, a lateral view taken at 15 degrees of flexion allows exploration of the patellofemoral congruence at a degree of flexion that cannot be visualized with conventional axial views.

These concepts have been carried a step further by the Lyon school.[91] They examined the lateral views of 143 knees with recurrent or acute dislocation of the patella and compared these with the radiographs of 190 control knees. They studied two quantitative measurements, trochlear bump and trochlear depth, and one qualitative sign, the crossing sign.

On a lateral view with superimposition of the femoral condyles, a line is drawn tangent to the last 10 cm of the anterior cortex of the femur. The line of the femoral sulcus may end in front of (positive value), over, or behind (negative value) the line of the anterior cortex. The distance

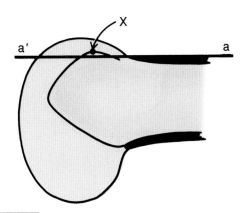

Figure 53–30. Quantification of the trochlear bump. A line (a'-a) is drawn tangential to the last 10 cm of the anterior femoral cortex. The line of the sulcus at its most anterior point X may pass in front (positive value) or behind (negative value) the tangent line. The bump is measured as the distance between the femoral cortex line and the sulcus line in millimeters.

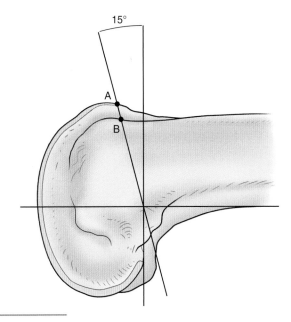

Figure 53–31. Quantification of trochlear depth. It is the distance A-B measured in millimeters along a line subtended 15 degrees from the perpendicular to the posterior femoral cortex line and crossing a line tangential to the posterior femoral condyles and perpendicular to the posterior cortex line.

between the anterior cortex line and the sulcus (saille or bump) is measured in millimeters (Fig. 53–30). The bump of the sulcus line in relation to the anterior femoral cortex was found to be highly useful in differentiating between knees with instability (average, +3.2 mm) and normal knees (average, −0.8 mm). A pathological threshold value for measurement of trochlear bump was identified: 3 mm. Sixty-six percent of knees with patellar instability had anterior trochlear translation of 3 mm or more as compared with only 6.5% of control knees.

The depth of the trochlea was measured as the distance between the floor of the trochlea and the most anterior condylar contour line. First, a line tangent to the posterior cortex of the femur was drawn. A second line was drawn perpendicular to the posterior femoral cortex line and tangent to the posterior aspect of the femoral condyles. A third line was finally drawn that subtended an angle of 15 degrees with the second line and passed through the intersection of the first and the second lines. Trochlear depth was measured along this third line (Fig. 53–31). Trochlear depth was 7.8 mm in the control group and 2.3 mm in knees with patellar instability. A trochlear depth of 4 mm or less was considered pathological. This value was found in 85% of knees with patellar instability and in only 3% of controls.

Dysplasia of the trochlea can be divided into three types according to the point at which the sulcus line crosses the lines of the condyles (the croisement, or crossing, sign) The crossing sign is a simple qualitative criterion defined as the crossing between the floor line and the lateral condylar line. At that level, the trochlea is considered flat (Figs. 53–32 and 53–33).[92]

Type I dysplasia: This form is the mildest. The lines of the condyles are symmetric, and they are crossed at the same point in the proximal part of the trochlea by the floor line. Only the very proximal part of the trochlea is flat.

Type II dysplasia: The lines of the condyles are not superimposed; the line of the sulcus crosses the

medial condyle line first, and the lateral one crosses at a higher level. Separate crossing of the medial and lateral condyle lines is characteristic of this type.

Type III dysplasia: This form is the most severe. The condyle lines are superimposed, but they are crossed low on the trochlea by the sulcus line. Most of the trochlea is therefore flat.

Two types of normal trochlea were identified:

Type A (50%): The sulcus line is posterior to the condyle lines throughout its length (Fig. 53–34).

Type B (50%): The sulcus line joins the line of the medial condyle, but only in the highest part of the trochlea.

Dysplasia of the femoral sulcus, as evidenced by the crossing sign, was present in the majority of knees with patella instability (96%) (Fig. 51–35); the same was true in only 3% of control knees. In light of this study, the authors concluded that in trochlear dysplasia, the trochlea is flat in a zone of variable length and has a shallow groove more distally. According to the authors, trochlear dysplasia is better evaluated on a lateral radiograph than on CT. Such dysplasia is best recognized with the crossing sign, a qualitative factor, which was present in 96% of knees with patellar instability. Two other quantitative measurements, trochlear bump (positive when ≥3 mm) and trochlear depth (positive when ≤4 mm), were both positive in 85% of cases.

More recently, the Lyon School[381] modified this classification and introduced new radiographic signs. The supratrochlear spur is located in the proximal aspect of the lateral trochlea in an attempt to keep the patella in the groove. The double-shape sign has been described as a vertical line of sclerosis that is the projection of the medial

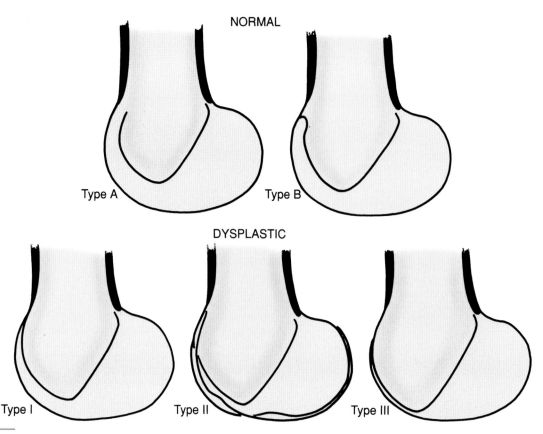

Figure 53–32. The croisement (crossing sign). In normal knees, the sulcus line either is posterior to the condyle lines throughout its length (type A) or joins the medial condyle line only in the upper part of the trochlea (type B). Therefore, there is no crossing between the sulcus line and the condyle line in normal knees. The presence of the crossing sign indicates dysplasia of the femoral trochlea. See text for further discussion. (From Dejour H, Walch G, Neyret P, Adeleine P: La dysplasie de la trochlee femorale. Rev Chir Orthop 76:45, 1990.)

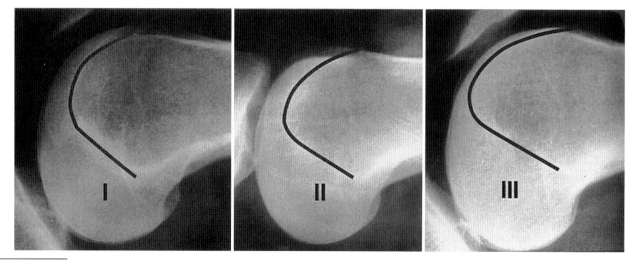

Figure 53–33. Trochlear dysplasia, types I, II, and III. See text for explanation. (From Dejour H, Walch G, Neyret P, Adeleine P: La dysplasie de la trochlee femorale. Rev Chir Orthop 76:45, 1990.)

trochlea. Based on these new signs, trochlear dysplasia has been described as follows:

Grade A: crossing sign (symmetric but less deep trochlea)

Grade B: crossing sign and trochlear spur (flat or convex trochlea)

Grade C: crossing and double-shape signs (asymmetric trochlea, laterally convex and medially hypoplastic)

Grade D: crossing and double-shape signs, trochlear spur (asymmetric trochlea with rapid mediolateral change)

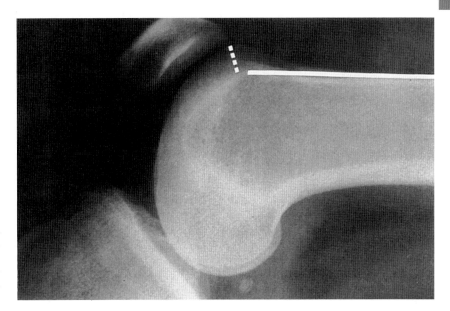

Figure 53–34. Lateral radiograph of a normal knee. The sulcus line is flush with the anterior femoral cortex line, the sulcus depth in its upper part is 8 mm, and there is no crossing between the sulcus and condyle lines.

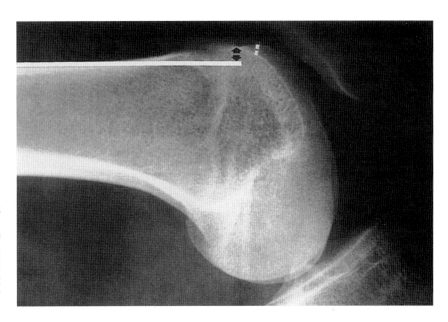

Figure 53–35. Lateral radiograph of a knee with recurrent patellar instability. The sulcus line is anterior to the femoral cortex line (bump of +4 mm), the sulcus depth is only 3 mm, and there is a crossing sign between the sulcus and condyle lines (type I dysplasia).

It is suggested that treatment of instability of the patella be based on the recognized anatomic abnormalities. Recreation of a sulcus of normal depth is theoretically desirable to improve the stability of the patella. This may be achieved by elevating the lateral femoral condyle[12] or by depressing the central part of the trochlea.[269] Elevation of the lateral condyle is a logical approach if the saille of the sulcus is normal; it is contraindicated in knees with a positive saille. Deepening of the sulcus (trochleoplasty) seems to be more logical because it re-creates normal anatomy. However, the procedure is technically more demanding and involves violation of the articular cartilage.

AXIAL VIEWS

An axial view of the patellofemoral joint adds considerably to our knowledge when performed in a correctly standardized manner. Unfortunately, all too often this portion of the examination is either omitted or performed haphazardly, so much useful information is lost. Various techniques are available.

In the method attributed to Settegast,[352] the patient lies prone with the knees acutely flexed. The x-ray plate is placed beneath the knees with the tube directed above so that the beam is at a right angle. This is an easy examination for the technician to perform. Unfortunately, it is also uninformative because if the angle of flexion is poorly controlled, the image of the patella is often distorted and the patella lies on the femoral condyles rather than in the sulcus, which is the most important and functional position.

Hughston and Walsh[193] advocate a modification of the Jaroschy technique.[211] The patient is placed prone with the cassette beneath the knees. The knees are flexed 55 degrees and rest on the tube, which is angled at about 45 degrees. The disadvantages of this method are that images are distorted because the beam strikes the plate at an angle and the knees are flexed more than desirable.

Ficat and Hungerford[116] describe a technique in which the patient's knees are flexed over the end of the x-ray table. The tube is placed at the patient's feet and the cassette is held proximally against the anterior of the thigh. In this position, it is perpendicular to the beam. Flexion views at 30, 60, and 90 degrees can be obtained. The technique is widely used in Europe but seems less popular in the United States, probably because of technical difficulties in obtaining good views.

Merchant and colleagues[284] describe a technique whereby the patient is positioned supine with the knees flexed 45 degrees over the end of the table. The knees are elevated slightly to keep the femora horizontal and parallel with the table surface. The x-ray tube is kept proximally over the patient's head and angled down 30 degrees from the horizontal. The film cassette is placed about 30 cm below the knees, resting on the shins and perpendicular to the x-ray beam (Fig. 53–36). The legs are strapped together at about calf level to control rotation, and both knees are exposed simultaneously. It is important for the quadriceps muscle to be relaxed. The position of 45 degrees of knee flexion was selected as the position of least flexion with which satisfactory results could be obtained.

Two angles are measured on the Merchant view: the sulcus angle and the congruence angle (Fig. 53–37). The congruence angle measures the relationship of the patella to the intercondylar sulcus. For this measurement, the sulcus angle is bisected to establish a zero reference line. A second line is then projected from the apex of the sulcus angle to the lowest point on the articular ridge of the patella. The angle measured between these two lines is the congruence angle. If the apex of the patellar articular ridge is lateral to the zero line, the congruence angle is designated positive. If it is medial, the congruence angle is negative. In a group of 100 normal knees, 50 males and 50

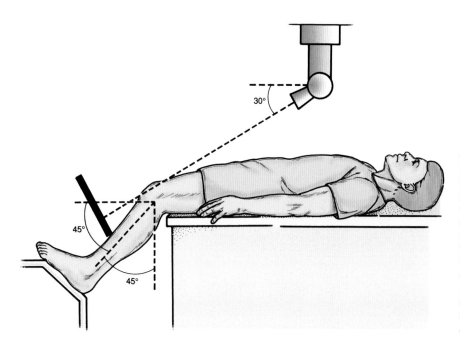

Figure 53–36. Merchant's technique to obtain axial views of the patella. The patient is supine with the knees flexed 45 degrees over the edge of the table and resting on a support. The cassette rests on the shins about 30 cm below the knees. It is struck at a right angle by the x-ray beam, which is angled 30 degrees down from the horizontal. (From Merchant AC, Mercer RL, Jacobsen RH, et al: Roentgenographic analysis of patello-femoral congruence. J Bone Joint Surg Am 56:1391, 1974.)

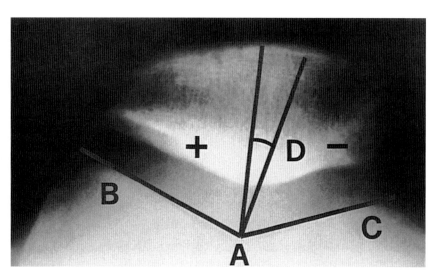

Figure 53–37. Measurement of the sulcus angle and the congruence angle on a Merchant view. The sulcus angle (BAC) is bisected by the reference line. A second line (AD) is then drawn from the sulcus to the patellar ridge. If the apex of the patellar ridge is lateral to the reference line, the value of the angle is positive; if it is medial, the value of the angle is negative. (From Merchant AC, Mercer RL, Jacobsen RH, et al: Roentgenographic analysis of patello-femoral congruence. J Bone Joint Surg Am 56:1391, 1974.)

females, Merchant and colleagues[284] measured an average sulcus angle of 138 degrees (SD, 6 degrees) and an average congruence angle of −6 degrees (SD, 11 degrees). Based on these data, it was suggested that any sulcus angle greater than 150 degrees and congruence angle greater than 16 degrees is abnormal at the 95th percentile. In a group of patients with recurrent patellar dislocation (number not specified), the average congruence angle was +23 degrees, which is well beyond the 95th percentile of normal subjects.

We have repeated the measurements proposed by Merchant et al in normal and pathological knees.[7] In a group of 150 normal knees, the average sulcus angle was 137 degrees (SD, 6 degrees), with no differences between males and females. This is very close to the results of Merchant and associates. On the other hand, we measured an average congruence angle of −8 degrees (SD, 6 degrees), thus suggesting a lower upper limit in normal knees (+4 degrees) than that proposed by Merchant (+16). In 53 knees with anterior knee pain, the sulcus angle was similar to that of controls (average, 139; SD, 4 degrees) and the congruence angle was slightly increased (average, −2; SD, 9 degrees). In 37 knees with recurrent dislocation, the sulcus angle (average, 147 degrees; SD, 7 degrees) and the congruence angle (average, −16; SD, 13 degrees) were both clearly increased over those of controls (Fig. 53–38).

Laurin and coworkers[243,244] described a similar method in which the x-ray tube is positioned distally between the feet and the cassette is held proximally against the anterior of the thighs (Fig. 53–39). The following details should be observed:

The patient should be seated with the feet at the very edge of the table. The x-ray beam is directed parallel to the anterior border of the tibia and the longitudinal axis of the patella. The x-ray beam is thus parallel to the specific proximal segment of the patellofemoral joint that must be visualized.

The knees must be in a position of 20 degrees of knee flexion, and the quadriceps must be relaxed. A special adjustable support under the knees is recommended to maintain the position.

The x-ray plate is held by the patient such that it is at 90 degrees to the long axis of the tibia and x-ray beam; it must not be laid flat against the thighs, nor should it be at 90 degrees to the table top. The patient must forcibly press the lower edge of the plate against the thighs. Otherwise, especially in muscular or obese patients, only the patella appears at the bottom of the x-ray film and the femoral trochlea is not included. Under such circumstances, the radiographs must be repeated and the technique modified either by pushing on the x-ray plate more forcibly or by holding the x-ray plate more proximal on the thighs. The knees must not be flexed more than 20 degrees.

In a correctly obtained Laurin view, the patellofemoral compartment is clearly visualized. The lateral prominence of the trochlea has a rounded contour, whereas the medial prominence is sharp. The lateral patellofemoral angle (Fig. 53–40) can be measured by drawing a line tangent to the top of the medial and lateral femoral condyles and a second line tangent to the lateral facet of the patella.[244] The lateral facet of the patella was chosen as reference because given the wide variations in patellar morphology described by Wiberg[400] and Baumgartl,[24] it retains a relatively constant shape. In a group of 100 normal knees, the lateral patellofemoral angle was open laterally in the great majority (97%), whereas the lines were parallel in only 3%. In 30 knees with patellar subluxation, the lines were parallel in 60% and open medially in 40% (Fig. 53–41). The lateral patellofemoral angle was of no assistance in the evaluation of knees with patellar pain because it was normal (open laterally) in 90% and the lines were parallel in the remainder. In an effort to individuate a radiographic measurement diagnostic of chondromalacia, Laurin and coworkers[243] proposed the patellofemoral index (Fig. 53–42). The basic abnormality underlying patellar subluxation and patellar pain is the same, but it

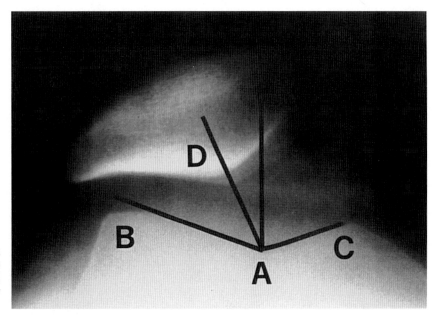

Figure 53–38. Merchant's axial view in a patient with recurrent dislocation of the patella. Both the sulcus angle (BAC) and the congruence angle (CAD) were clearly increased over normal values.

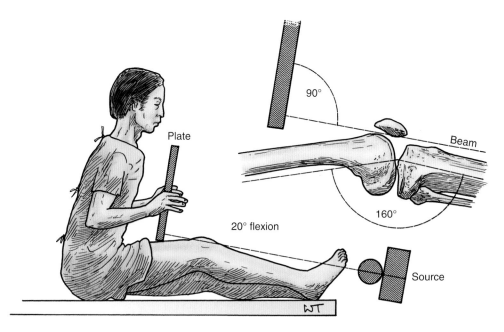

Figure 53–39. Laurin's method to obtain axial views of the patella. The patient is seated on the examining table with the feet near the edge. The x-ray beam is parallel to the anterior border of the tibia, and the knees are flexed 20 degrees. The cassette is held by the patient against the thighs and at 90 degrees to the beam. See text for further discussion. (From Laurin CA, Levesque HP, Dussault R, et al: The abnormal lateral patellofemoral angle: A diagnostic roentgenographic sign of recurrent patellar subluxation. J Bone Joint Surg Am 60:55, 1978.)

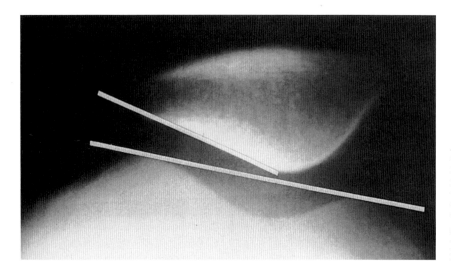

Figure 53–40. Measurement of the lateral patellofemoral angle (LPFA) on a Laurin view. The LPFA is measured by drawing a line tangential to the top of the medial and lateral condyle and a second line tangential to the lateral patellar facet. It is open laterally in normal knees.

is less severe in the second condition. The lateral patellofemoral angle is therefore not altered, whereas the patellofemoral index may show a "minitilt" of the patella. The patellofemoral index is the ratio of the thickness of the medial to the lateral patellofemoral interspace. In normal knees, the medial interspace was equal or slightly wider than the lateral and the patellofemoral index was 1.6 or less. In contrast, the patellofemoral index was higher than 1.6 in 97% of knees with patellar pain. An increased patellofemoral index with widening of the medial interspace indicates a minitilt of the patella.

Malghem and Maldague[259] suggested that axial views be obtained at 30 degrees of flexion and external tibial rotation. This method takes advantage of the lateral pull of the patellar tendon to detect subluxability of the patella.

Lateral rotation is produced manually by external rotation of the forefoot. Counterpressure on the lateral side of the thigh is necessary to keep the knee within the beam axis. The examination is performed sequentially for both knees. The tube is positioned between the feet of the patient, and the cassette rests against the thighs. In 27 knees that underwent surgery for patellar instability, the congruence angle was measured according to the method of Merchant and colleagues,[284] and a value greater than 16 degrees was considered evidence of subluxation. Subluxation was evident in 26% of cases by the 45-degree axial view and in 100% by the 30-degree lateral rotation view. Of these 27 knees, 13 had a centered patella in the 45-degree axial view and showed subluxation in the 30-degree lateral rotation view. In these knees, a 30-degree axial view

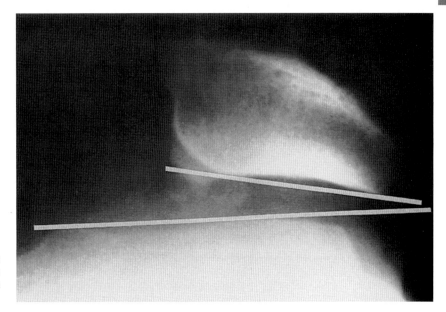

Figure 53–41. Laurin's view in a knee affected by recurrent dislocation of the patella. The lateral patellofemoral angle is open medially.

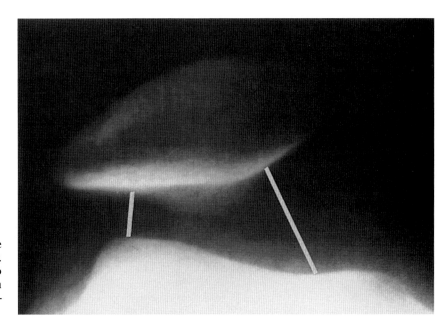

Figure 53–42. Measurement of the patellofemoral index on a Laurin view. The ratio of the medial interspace to the lateral interspace is up to 1.6 in normal knees. In this case, the measurement is clearly pathological.

without external rotation was added. This modification yielded a result (average congruence angle, +10.3 degrees) that was intermediate between the 45-degree (average congruence angle, +1.5 degrees) and the 30-degree (average congruence angle, +26.7 degrees) views with external rotation.

Toft[386] suggested that axial radiographs of the patella in the weightbearing position can detect narrowing of the patellofemoral joint line.

An alternative method to measure tilt of the patella was described by Grelsamer et al.[161] They elected to use a line connecting the two edges of the patella (the corner-to-corner line) instead of the more usual line tangent to the subchondral bone of the lateral facet as recommended by Laurin and associates.[244] They reasoned that the corner-to-corner line is independent of patellar morphology, it is easy to draw, and it corresponds more closely to clinical

evaluation of the tilt. Patellar tilt was evaluated in relation to a horizontal line (Fig. 53–43) and not to a line tangent to the medial and lateral edges of the trochlea. Using a horizontal line as a reference has a drawback because it requires consistent rotational control of the leg and alignment of the cassette parallel to the ground. Rotational alignment of the leg was judged from the foot, which had to point directly upward. The rationale of using a horizontal line is to be independent of the morphology of the anterior trochlea, which is highly variable and may induce underestimation or overestimation of a tilt.

A second alternative is to use a line tangent to the posterior condyles, but this requires a CT scan. Axial views were obtained at 30 degrees of flexion via a Merchant technique. In a group of 100 knees with patellar malalignment, the average tilt angle was 12 ± 6 degrees, and 85% of cases had a tilt greater than 5 degrees. In a control group of 100

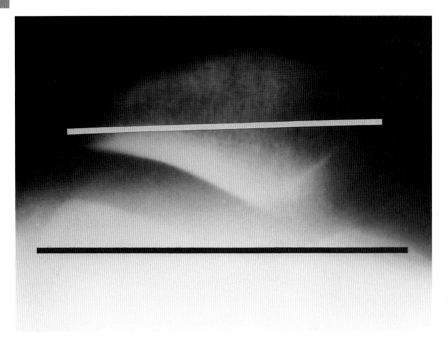

Figure 53–43. Tilt of the patella evaluated according to Grelsamer et al.[161] The tilt is the angle joining the edges of the patella and the horizontal. The axial view is obtained with the knee flexed 30 degrees and careful control of rotation of the leg with the foot pointing directly upward and the lower border of the film parallel to the ground.

knees, the average tilt angle was 2 ± 1 degree ($p < 0.01$), and 92% of cases had a tilt of 5 degrees or less. Patellar tilt greater than 5 degrees is therefore 85% sensitive, 92% specific, and 89% accurate in the diagnosis of patellofemoral malalignment. This method of measuring patella tilt may thus be advantageous if a dedicated radiologist is available to accurately position the patient and the cassette.

In conclusion, we think that standard anteroposterior and lateral radiographs with a Merchant axial view can reasonably be accepted as a first step in the diagnosis of patellofemoral disorders. A lateral view with perfect superimposition of the femoral condyles is necessary to evaluate the morphology of the trochlea for any evidence of dysplasia (flat trochlea). According to our data (see Table 53–1),[7] a normal knee has, on average, a Q angle of 15 degrees, an Insall-Salvati T/P ratio of 1.04, a Blackburne and Peel A/B ratio of 0.95, a sulcus angle of 137 degrees, and a congruence angle of −8 degrees. Slightly, but statistically significantly higher values for the Q angle and T/P ratio have been found in females. For clinical purposes, we consider the following values to be pathological: a Q angle greater than 20 degrees, a T/P ratio greater than 1.2 and certainly greater than 1.3, an A/B ratio greater than 1.2, a sulcus angle greater than 150 degrees, and a congruence angle greater than +4 degrees. Knees with patellar pain showed a clearly increased Q angle (average, 20 degrees), with minor and clinically insignificant differences in the T/P ratio, A/B ratio, and sulcus angle, as well as minor lateralization of the patella (average congruence angle, −2 degrees). Knees with recurrent subluxation or dislocation of the patella showed a high-riding patella with an average T/P ratio of 1.23 and an average A/B ratio of 1.08, a more open femoral sulcus (average sulcus angle, 147 degrees), and gross lateral displacement of the patella (average congruence angle, +16 degrees) (Fig. 53–44). In view of the clear anatomic abnormalities in knees with recurrent dislocation of the patella, these simple radiographic measurements are diagnostic in most cases.

Conversely, patients with anterior knee pain frequently have normal height of the patella and normal-appearing axial views at 45 degrees. In these cases, it is worthwhile to request an axial view at 20 degrees[244] or a CT scan of the patellofemoral joint to detect minor abnormalities in the first 30 degrees of flexion.

Stress axial views of the patellofemoral joint have been used to diagnose medial, lateral, or multidirectional instability.[382] The axial radiographs were of the Merchant type obtained with the knee at 35 degrees of flexion. The examiner applies pressure on the medial and lateral aspect of the patella successively. A 16-lb pressure (7.3 kg) is applied with a spring-loaded scale that has a curved rubber pad. Quadriceps relaxation is essential. Displacement is measured on the axial view with the technique described by Laurin et al[244] as the distance between the medial and lateral edges of the trochlea and the corresponding margin of the patella. Four groups of patients were studied, including 20 volunteers, 27 patients with lateral patellar subluxation, 26 patients with medial instability (after lateral release), and 17 patients with multidirectional instability (after lateral release). The average lateral displacement in control patients was 11.6 mm and 10.3 mm in the two knees. The average lateral displacement in the symptomatic and asymptomatic knees of patients with lateral patellar instability was 21.9 mm and 14.4 mm, respectively; in the knees with medial instability, 13.2 and 13.7 mm; and in those with multidirectional instability, 20.9 and 11.4 mm. The average medial displacement of the patella in control patients was 11.1 mm and 9.9 mm. The average medial displacement in the symptomatic and asymptomatic knees of patients with lateral instability was 11.6 mm and 11.8 mm, respectively; in knees with medial instability, 20.7 mm and 10.4 mm; and in knees with multidirectional instability, 22.1 mm and 11.5 mm.

To summarize, the average medial and lateral displacement in normal knees was close to 10 mm, although the range of variability was large (1 to 32 mm). The side-to-

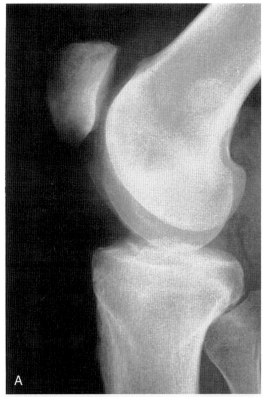

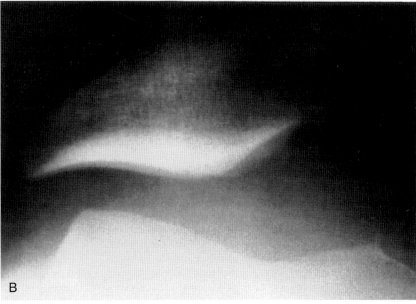

Figure 53–44. Lateral (**A**) and Merchant axial (**B**) views of a knee with recurrent dislocation of the patella. Clear anatomic abnormalities are evident, including a high-riding patella, a flat sulcus, and a positive congruence angle.

side differences were, on average, close to 1 mm. The group of knees with lateral instability were all previously untreated. In these knees, medial displacement was comparable to that in control knees, but lateral displacement was increased to more than 20 mm with a side-to-side difference of 7.5 mm. This finding indicates incompetence of the medial structures. The knees with medial instability all underwent lateral retinacular release without having any evidence of lateral instability, with subsequent worsening of symptoms. This is therefore iatrogenic instability. Lateral displacement was normal, but medial displace-

ment was increased to more than 20 mm on average, with a side-to-side difference greater than 10 mm, indicative of insufficiency of the lateral structures. The knees with multidirectional instability underwent lateral release for the treatment of lateral instability. The apprehension test result was positive in both directions. Medial and lateral displacements were both increased to over 20 mm with side-to-side differences close to 10 mm. We think that stress views are occasionally required to confirm the direction and entity of displacement, especially in patients with iatrogenic instability.

Computed Tomography

The introduction of CT in orthopedics has made it possible to investigate the patellofemoral relationships in the arc between full extension and 30 degrees of flexion. Traditional axial views can be obtained in 20 degrees of flexion according to the method of Laurin and colleagues,[244] but the technique is not easy. Obese or muscular patients render the examination more difficult, and a skilled technician is required to obtain consistent results. Furthermore, the use of CT avoids image overlapping and distortion. For these reasons, CT has gained increasing popularity in the evaluation of patellofemoral disorders.

Delgado-Martins[93] first used CT to evaluate the patellofemoral joints of 12 normal subjects with the knee in extension and compared these images with traditional axial views at 30, 60, and 90 degrees. The patella was considered to be centered when the median crest fit exactly in the intercondylar groove. The author reported that the patella was centered in the groove in 96% of cases at 90 degrees, 63% at 60 degrees, 29% at 30 degrees, 13% in full extension with the quadriceps relaxed, and 4% in full extension with the quadriceps contracted. Although the images reported by Delgado-Martins suggest that some of these patients may suffer from subluxation of the patella, it is well emphasized that evaluation in the first degrees of flexion is far more informative than at 60 or 90 degrees.

Martinez and coworkers[267] made the same observation; they used CT to evaluate 10 normal volunteers and 5 patients with recurrent subluxation. The images were obtained at 0, 20, and 45 degrees of flexion with a special device used to position the knee.[266] The authors measured the sulcus angle and used a line tangent to the posterior condyles as a reference to evaluate the patellar tilt angle, height of the lateral condyle, and centralization of the patella. In extension, 95% of the normal patellae were centralized with the quadriceps relaxed, but this percentage decreased to 85% with quadriceps contraction. Centralization of the patella was maintained in most control subjects at 20 and 45 degrees of knee flexion. The patellar tilt angle was positive (open laterally) in all the normal knees in extension (average, 11 degrees) and did not change with flexion. The sulcus angle was 143 degrees in extension and decreased with flexion. In the five knees with subluxation, the patella was clearly displaced laterally in extension but tended to reduce in flexion. The patellar tilt angle was negative (open medially) in extension but tended to reverse to a positive value (decreased patellar tilt) with flexion. The height of the lateral femoral condyle was decreased and the sulcus angle increased when compared with these values in controls. Martinez and colleagues concluded that axial or CT images at 20 and 45 degrees of flexion can falsely indicate a normal patellofemoral joint.

Sasaki and Yagi[342] used CT to investigate the patellofemoral joint with the knee in extension. They studied 24 knees with patellar subluxation and 24 controls. Lines tangent to the medial and lateral prominences of the trochlea and the transverse axis of the patella were used to measure tilt of the patella. Lateral shift of the patella was measured in relation to the most prominent aspect of the lateral femoral condyle. The results were compared with conventional axial views at 30 degrees of flexion. The mean patellar tilt angles in normal knees with the quadriceps relaxed and contracted were 15 degrees and 14 degrees, respectively. The same values in knees with patellar subluxation were 31 and 40 degrees, respectively. The lateral shift of the patella measured in relation to the transverse diameter was 14% with the quadriceps relaxed and 28% with muscle contraction in the normal knees. These values increased to 31% and 59%, respectively, in knees with subluxation. The values of patellar tilt and shift were significantly higher in patients with subluxation than in controls, and the differences were more evident with the quadriceps contracted. The values of patellar tilt and shift in the knees with subluxation were higher on CT images in full extension than on axial views at 30 degrees. In the 46 knees that underwent extensor mechanism realignment (either proximal or distal), the values of patellar tilt and shift returned to nearly normal on postoperative CT scans. The 35 knees with satisfactory postoperative results showed more improvement in patellar shift (14%) than did the 5 knees with unsatisfactory results (4.3%).

Fulkerson and colleagues have further progressed in CT evaluation of the patellofemoral joint by obtaining images at various degrees of flexion between 0 and 30 degrees and by emphasizing the importance of accurate and standardized scanning. They recommend the use of midtransverse patellar sections and a line tangent to the posterior condyles as reference for the measurements.[140,347,348] Care should be taken to position the patient in the gantry so that normal standing alignment is reproduced and to obtain the cuts through the same point of the patella. Fulkerson and coworkers use the Merchant method to measure the sulcus angle and the congruence angle,[284] tilt of the lateral patellar facet with respect to a line tangent to the posterior condyles (patellar tilt angle), and the height of the lateral condyle from the deepest point of the sulcus.[347] These authors reported the measurement of 10 normal knees and 54 symptomatic knees, including 49 suffering from patellar pain and 5 from patellar dislocation. Evaluation of the congruence angle in the normal knees revealed that the patellae were slightly lateralized in extension (average congruence angle, +2.5 degrees); by 10 degrees of flexion, however, all were centered or slightly medial. Therefore, a patella can be considered subluxated if the congruence angle remains positive beyond 10 degrees of flexion. The patellar tilt angle of control knees was always positive (open laterally) in the first 30 degrees of flexion. None of the normal knees had a patellar tilt angle of less than 8 degrees in the first 30 degrees of flexion. Therefore, a patella was considered tilted if it showed a tilt of less than 8 degrees in any position between 0 and 30 degrees of flexion.

It should be remarked that the congruence angle and the patellar tilt angle are both necessary to describe an abnormal position of the patella. An abnormal congruence angle indicates lateral displacement of the patella (or lateral subluxation), whereas an abnormal patellar tilt angle indicates that the patella is tilted. These changes may occur independently. Based on measurements in normal knees, it was established that a normal patella should be centered by 10 degrees of flexion (congruence angle, 0 degrees or less) and the patellar tilt angle should be open laterally at least 8 degrees in the arc of motion between 0 and 30 degrees.

According to these criteria, three categories of abnormal patellar position were defined: subluxated, tilted, and tilted and subluxated (Fig. 53–45). Knees with subluxation showed a high congruence angle (average, +23 degrees) in extension, which progressively reduced (average, +8 degrees) at 30 degrees of flexion. Knees with

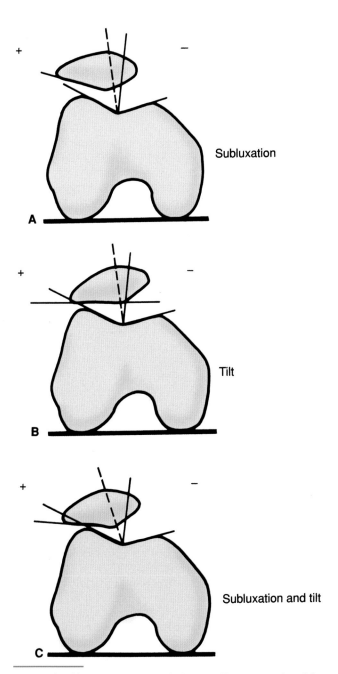

Figure 53–45. The position of the patella as visualized by computed tomography may present the following abnormalities: **A**, Subluxation with a positive congruence angle persisting beyond 10 degrees of flexion. **B**, Tilt with a lateral patellofemoral angle of less than 8 degrees in the first 30 degrees of flexion. **C**, Subluxation and tilt when both abnormalities are present.

subluxation could be further divided into those with an associated tilt and those without. The first group had a patellar tilt near 0 degrees throughout the range of motion, which is significantly different from controls. A third group included knees with an isolated patellar tilt. In these cases, the patellar tilt angle was slightly decreased in extension (10 degrees versus 18 degrees in controls) and decreased further with flexion at 30 degrees (when it was 2 degrees as compared with 16 degrees in controls).

Inoue and colleagues[197] examined 50 knees with patella subluxation and 30 controls with CT in full extension and with traditional axial views at 30 and 45 degrees of flexion (using the technique of Ficat and Hungerford[116]) and at 45 degrees (using the Merchant technique[284]). The position of the patella was described in reference to the lateral patellofemoral angle.[244] The lateral patellofemoral angle was positive (open laterally) throughout the 0- to 45-degree arc of motion in normal knees, increased from 7 degrees in full extension to 11 degrees at 30 degrees of flexion, and finally increased to 12 degrees at 45 degrees of flexion. In knees with subluxation, the lateral patellofemoral angle was open medially in full extension (−17 degrees), decreased to 0 degrees at 30 degrees of flexion, and reversed to positive (+4 degrees) at 45 degrees of flexion. The differences in the lateral patellofemoral angle between normal knees and subluxated knees were more evident in full extension (24 degrees) than at 30 degrees (11 degrees) or at 45 degrees of flexion (8 degrees). The borderline lateral patellofemoral angle was defined as 0 degrees with CT and as 8 degrees with axial views using the Ficat technique.

With these criteria, sensitivity and specificity were calculated for CT in full extension (96% and 90%, respectively) and for axial views using the Ficat technique at 30 degrees (88% and 80%, respectively) and at 45 degrees (80% and 80%, respectively). The congruence angle on the Merchant view was the least sensitive test (30%) when the borderline value of Merchant (+16 degrees) was used. This study confirms that both normal and subluxing patellae tilt laterally when the knee approaches full extension and that the lateral tilt of subluxing patellae is more pronounced with the knee in extension. The use of CT is recommended in patients with persistent knee symptoms and normal-appearing axial radiographic views at 30 and 45 degrees.

The use of CT has allowed exploration of the patellofemoral relationship in the first 30 degrees of flexion. The results from different centers seem to confirm that a normal patella is slightly displaced laterally in full extension (with a positive congruence angle), but that it reduces early in flexion, by 10 or 15 degrees of flexion. The patellar tilt angle measured as the angle between the lateral patellar facet and either the tangent to the posterior condyles[140] or the tangent to the medial and lateral trochlear facets[197] should be open laterally throughout the same arc of motion in normal knees. Knees affected by patellar subluxation or dislocation show excessive lateral displacement and lateral patellar tilt, which are more evident in extension but tend to reduce in flexion.

The importance of quadriceps contraction during CT for evaluation of patellofemoral malalignment has been emphasized[167] in a series of 37 adolescents examined with or without quadriceps contraction with the knee flexed at 15 degrees. Increased lateralization and tilting were noted in 41% of knees with quadriceps contraction. In 11% of these knees, quadriceps contraction changed the type of malalignment. The authors suggested more extensive use of quadriceps contraction during CT of the patellofemoral joint.

In 1978, Goutallier and Bernageau[157] described the method of radiological measurement (with 30-degree axial views) of the distance between the apex of the tibial tuberosity and the deepest point of the trochlear groove. The tibial tuberosity–sulcus femoralis (TT-SF) distance gives a measure of the valgus vector that is imposed on the extensor mechanism at a given degree of flexion. Because the tibial tuberosity lies lateral to the sulcus femoralis, the greater the TT-SF distance, the higher the valgus vector. The TT-SF distance gives a true measure of the Q angle because it is independent of the position of the patella. It is well known that the clinical Q angle in extension is normal in knees with recurrent subluxation or dislocation. This is due to the lateral displacement of the patella, which leads to an underestimate of the true Q angle. Goutallier and Bernageau[157] reported that the average value in a group of 16 normal knees was 13 mm (range, 7 to 17 mm). This distance was increased in most knees with patellofemoral osteoarthritis or recurrent subluxation of the patella. The introduction of CT offered the possibility of measuring the TT-SF distance in full extension by obtaining a first cut through the proximal part of the femoral sulcus and a second cut through the tibial tuberosity. Both should be perpendicular to the long axis of the bones. Dejour et al[91] reported that the average TT-SF distance in normal knees in extension is 12.7 mm whereas in knees with patellar instability, it is 19.8 mm. When 20 mm was used as the borderline value, the distance was greater than this value in 3% of the control knees; the same was true in 56% of the knees with patellar instability. The reproducibility of the measurement was fair, within 4 mm.

A lateralized position of the tibial tubercle in females with patellofemoral pain has been shown by Muneta et al.[294] However, the difference from controls was only 2.5 degrees on average. Their method of measurement is somewhat more complicated because it uses the central point of the intercondylar notch as a reference point and not the deepest point of the trochlea as suggested by Dejour and coworkers.[91]

We have used axial views according to Merchant and colleagues[284] and Laurin and colleagues[244] and CT in 20 and 30 degrees of flexion to evaluate patellofemoral congruence in a group of 86 knees.[9] We included 20 controls, 25 knees with patellar instability, and 41 knees with patellar pain. The results of this study are reported in Table 51–2. In the patellar instability group, the height of the patella was significantly increased in comparison to controls when using both the Insall-Salvati and the Blackburne and Peel methods, whereas the group with patellar pain did not significantly differ from controls. In the Merchant view, the sulcus angle and the congruence angle of the patellar pain group were not significantly different from controls, whereas both values were significantly increased in the instability group. In the Laurin view, the

lateral patellofemoral angle and the patellofemoral index were significantly increased in the instability group but not in the pain group. In the CT scan at 30 degrees, values of the sulcus angle, congruence angle, patellar tilt angle, and sulcus depth were significantly different in the instability group, with a shallower sulcus, a subluxated and tilted patella, and a reduced height of the lateral femoral condyle. The patellar pain group showed a significant difference (at the lowest level) from the control group in only the congruence angle and sulcus depth. The average TT-SF distance was 8.7 mm in controls, 10.2 mm in the pain group, and 14.7 mm in the instability group. The difference between controls and the instability group was significant. Measurements of these parameters on scans with the knee at 20 degrees of flexion did not significantly differ from those at 30 degrees.

We continue to use CT in the evaluation of knees with patellofemoral disorders and have expanded their use to include three degrees of flexion: 0, 15, and 30 degrees. At each angle of flexion, two cuts are made, through the tibia and through the patellofemoral joint. The tibial cut is made through the tibial tuberosity and at 90 degrees to the tibial axis (Fig. 51–46). The femoral cut is oriented to pass through the middle of the patella and the posterior femoral condyles. Because the apex of the patella is a nonarticular surface, a cut passing through the middle of the patellar height actually passes through the lower third of the articular surface. This is the part that contacts the femoral trochlea in the first 30 degrees of flexion. The femoral cut should pass posteriorly through the most posterior aspect of the femoral condyles so that a reference line tangent to the condyles can be reliably identified. On the femoral cut, we measure the sulcus angle and congruence angle,[284] the patellar tilt angle,[347] and the sulcus depth.[347] Furthermore, by superimposing the femoral and tibial cuts, the TT-SF distance can be measured (Fig. 53–47). Examples of CT at 0, 15, and 30 degrees of flexion in a knee with recurrent dislocation and patellar pain are given in Figures 53–48 and 53–49, respectively.

The use of CT images for exploration of the patellofemoral relationship has allowed a better understanding of the dynamics of this joint in normal and pathological knees, and its usefulness for scientific purposes is widely accepted. However, in knees with recurrent episodes of patellar dislocation, the degree of anatomic abnormality is such that it is promptly appreciated on a traditional axial view. If distal realignment is being considered, knowledge of the TT-SF distance may allow more anatomic reconstruction of the joint and thus avoid overcorrection of the transposition itself in knees with a normal TT-SF distance. The usefulness of CT images is probably greatest in knees with patellofemoral disturbances and normal-appearing axial views if some abnormality can be disclosed in a more extended position.

Arthrography

Evaluation of the patellofemoral joint enhanced by the injection of contrast material is not frequently performed

Table 53–2. Radiographic and Computed Tomographic Measurements of the Patellofemoral Joint in Normal and Pathological Knees

	NORMAL KNEES (20)	PATELLAR PAIN (41)	PATELLAR INSTABILITY (25)
Lateral View			
Insall-Salvati (T/P)	$1.06° \pm 0.13°$	$1.09° \pm 0.16°$ NS	$1.30° \pm 0.17°$ $p < 0.001$
Blackburne-Peel (A/B)	$0.96° \pm 0.15°$	$0.95° \pm 0.14°$ NS	$1.20° \pm 0.22°$ $p < 0.001$
Merchant View			
Sulcus angle	$138.6° \pm 6.3°$	$138.2° \pm 6.3°$ NS	$153.6° \pm 10.4°$ $p < 0.001$
Congruence angle	$-6.7° \pm 8.3°$	$-9.2° \pm 9.9°$ NS	$+16.6° \pm 21.4°$ $p < 0.001$
Laurin View			
Lateral patellofemoral angle open laterally	20	39	3
Parallel or open medially	—	2 NS	22 $p < 0.001$
Patellofemoral index	1.41 ± 0.14	1.41 ± 0.42 NS	3.22 ± 3.1 $p < 0.005$
CT at 30°			
Sulcus angle	$137° \pm 7.6°$	$139° \pm 9.7°$ NS	$160° \pm 10.4°$ $p < 0.001$
Congruence angle	$-13.2° \pm 5°$	$-5.7° \pm 11.9°$ $p < 0.05$	$+4.2° \pm 17°$ $p < 0.001$
Patella tilt angle	$+15.4° \pm 5°$	$+14.3° \pm 4.6°$ NS	$+4.85° \pm 5.4°$ $p < 0.001$
Depth of the sulcus	9 ± 1.4 mm	8 ± 1.5 mm $p < 0.05$	4.7 ± 2 mm $p < 0.001$
TT-SF distance	8.7 ± 2.5 mm	10.2 ± 3.1 mm NS	14.7 ± 5.2 mm $p < 0.001$

NS, not significant; TT-SF, tibial tuberosity–sulcus femoralis.
Data from Aglietti P, Pisaneschi A, Allegra M, Villari N: Dolore di rotula: Uno studio con la radiologia convenzionale e con la TAC. Ital J Sports Traumat 10:7, 1988.

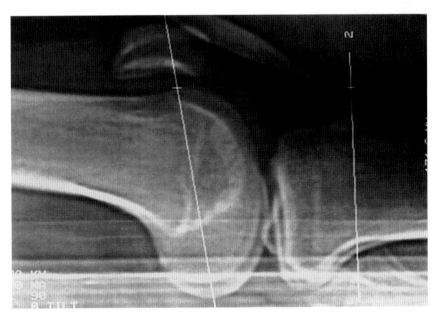

Figure 53–46. Orientation of the femoral cut passing through the middle of the patella, which corresponds to the lower third of the articular surface, and through the posterior aspect of the femoral condyles. Orientation of the tibial cut through the tibial tuberosity and at 90 degrees to the tibial axis.

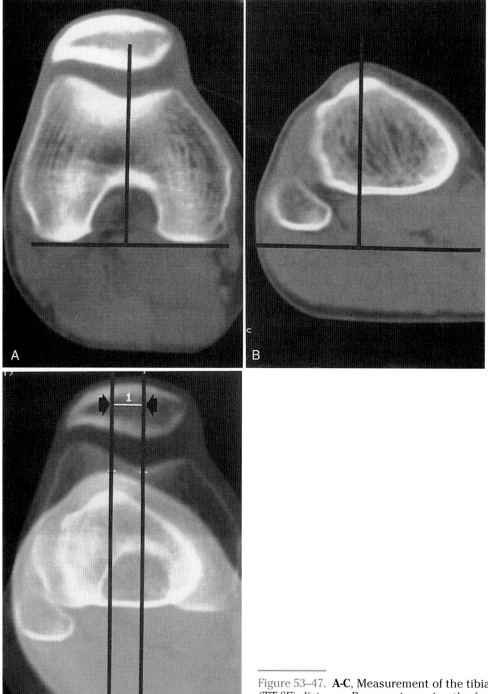

Figure 53–47. **A-C,** Measurement of the tibial tuberosity–sulcus femoralis (TT-SF) distance. By superimposing the femoral and tibial cuts, the distance between the deepest point of the sulcus and the tibial tuberosity can be measured. Values greater than 20 mm with the knee in extension are considered pathological.

because of the inconvenience and low acceptance of the examination. Ficat and Phillippe[118] recommended axial views after single-contrast arthrography to study chondromalacia. Arthrography and axial views have the disadvantage that accurate alignment of the radiograph is required if superimposition is to be avoided. CT avoids this problem. Double-contrast arthrography and CT have been used to study patellar cartilage. Boven and col-

leagues[43,44] proposed a score based on regularity, congruity, and inhibition of cartilage. The results of CT were compared with the macroscopic aspect of cartilage at arthroscopy or arthrotomy or with the clinical diagnosis when it was reasonably certain. In 18 knees with clinically proven chondromalacia, CT-arthrography predicted certain chondromalacia in 78% and probable chondromalacia in 17%. In 29 knees with clinically absent chondro-

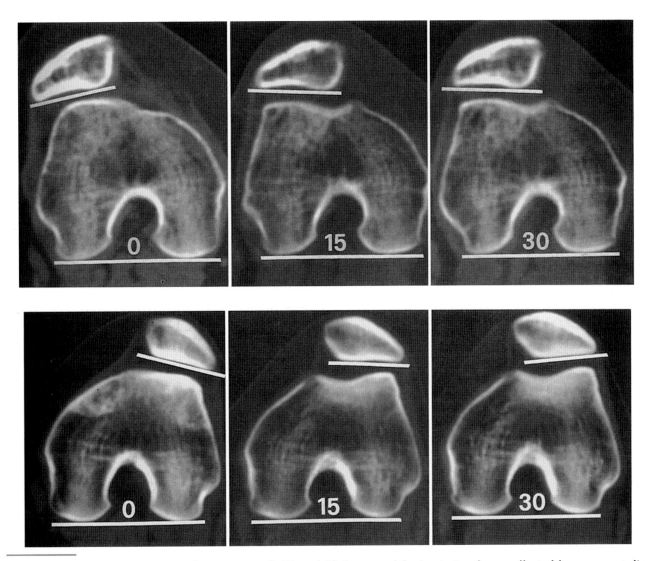

Figure 53–48. Computed tomography images at 0, 15, and 30 degrees of flexion in two knees affected by recurrent dislocation of the patella. Proceeding from extension to flexion, the congruence angle, the sulcus angle, and the patellar tilt angle are reduced, mainly between 0 and 15 degrees of flexion.

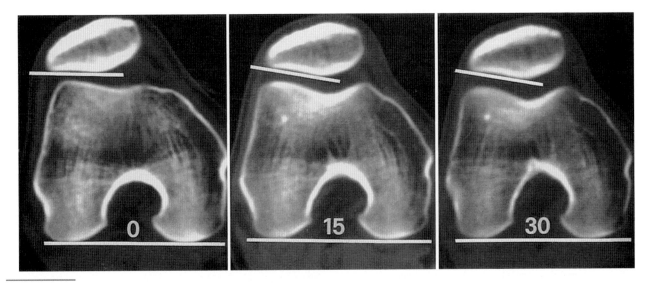

Figure 53–49. Computed tomography images of a knee affected by patellar pain. The patella is tilted laterally in extension, but almost normal congruence is restored by 15 degrees of flexion.

malacia, CT-arthrography predicted no chondromalacia in 65% and probably no chondromalacia in 27%.

The value of double-contrast arthrography and CT has been emphasized by Ihara,[196] who studied 53 normal and 47 pathological knees. The results were compared with the findings at arthrotomy or arthroscopy in 70 knees. Furthermore, chondral lesions were experimentally produced in cadaver knees by using drill bits of different sizes between 0.7 and 5 mm, and the knees were examined with arthrography and CT. When the x-ray beam was focused, 1-mm holes could be detected. Even if the beam deviated from the hole, 1.5-mm holes were visible. In 53 knees with normal cartilage, the cartilage was observed to be thicker at the median ridge, at the secondary ridge, and at the center of the lateral facet. In the 47 pathological knees, it was noted that the use of contrast material was necessary to diagnose fissures, fibrillation, and ulcers. When compared with the arthroscopic findings, the diagnosis was correct in 97% of cases.

It is emphasized that the correct amount of contrast material and air should be used to obtain the greatest accuracy. The x-ray beam should be perpendicular to the cartilage if meaningful data on the thickness of the cartilage are needed. Ihara preferred CT-arthrography to arthroscopy for the assessment of patellar cartilage because it allows more direct visualization of cartilage thinning and extension of ulcers in the deeper layers. However, he admitted difficulty in diagnosing cartilage softening on CT-arthrography. It is our impression that after the introduction of MRI, the reasons for performing CT-arthrography for the evaluation of patellofemoral cartilage are decreased.

Magnetic Resonance Imaging

MRI is a new diagnostic modality for the knee.[207,289,367] It has been reported to be an accurate diagnostic tool for meniscal and cruciate ligament lesions. Because both osseous and soft-tissue structures are visualized, it may be used to assess patellar tracking in the 0- to 30-degree arc of motion, as well as to evaluate lesions in patellar cartilage.

Kujala and coworkers[235] used MRI to evaluate patellar tracking in the 0- to 30-degree arc of motion in 20 normal subjects (10 males and 10 females). Axial midpatellar images were obtained. They found that the sulcus angle became progressively sharper from full extension to 30 degrees of flexion and decreased 13 degrees on average. The lateral patellofemoral angle[244] increased an average of 6 ± 5 degrees during flexion, and lateral patellar displacement[243] decreased an average of 4 ± 3 mm with flexion. The congruence angle[284] shifted 31 degrees (± 13 degrees) medially during flexion. In extension, the congruence angle was positive (open laterally) in all the knees except in one male. At 30 degrees of flexion, the congruence angle was negative (open medially) in all the knees except in one male and one female, where it was zero. Citing these data, Kujala and colleagues concluded that a normal knee (whether male or female) should be congruent (congruence angle, 0 degrees or negative) by 30 degrees of

flexion (but not necessarily in a lesser degree of flexion). Females were found to have significantly more laterally displaced patellae at 10 and 20 degrees of flexion, but the other differences were not significant.

Kujala and coworkers[236] compared the measurements obtained from normal knees and knees affected by recurrent patellar dislocation. For this study, 10 normal women and 11 women with recurrent subluxation were selected. Midpatellar sagittal and axial images were used to measure patellar length, patellar tendon length, Insall-Salvati ratio (T/P), sulcus angle, congruence angle, lateral patellofemoral angle, lateral patellar displacement, and depth of the femoral sulcus. Knees with recurrent patellar dislocation showed higher values for the sulcus angle, lateral patellar displacement, and congruence angle and lower values for the lateral patellofemoral angle, which indicates that dislocating patellae were more lateralized and tilted laterally. The differences were more evident in extension and gradually reduced when proceeding toward flexion. Statistical analysis showed that the two groups were most clearly differentiated by the sulcus angle at 10 degrees and by the lateral patellofemoral angle at 0 degrees. Kujala and colleagues concluded that in patients with recurrent dislocation, tilt and lateralization of the patella are more evident in early flexion. All control patellae were congruent at 30 degrees, but the same was true for most (77%) of the dislocating patellae. Therefore, differences between normal and dislocating patellae are most evident at the beginning of flexion (0 to 10 degrees).

MRI has been used to investigate patellar cartilage. Yulish and colleagues[412] compared the results of 23 MRI examinations with the findings at arthroscopy: 3 patients were asymptomatic volunteers and 20 had patellar symptoms. Normal patellar cartilage appears uniformly smooth on both axial and sagittal MRI views with a signal intensity that is intermediate between that of cortical and cancellous bone. MRI alterations in patellar cartilage were classified as follows:

Stage 1: areas of swelling with decreased signal intensity

Stage 2: irregularity of the articular surface with focal thinning

Stage 3: absence of cartilage with exposure of subchondral bone or synovial fluid extending through the ulcer to subchondral bone

MRI correctly predicted the arthroscopic findings in 20 of 22 knees (91%). It missed a knee with softening of the patella and diagnosed a chondral fracture that was not confirmed by arthroscopy. The presence of joint fluid visible on T2-weighted images was useful to detect the presence of cartilage ulcers, through which fluid leaked to subchondral bone.

An experimental study[170] has compared the accuracy of CT-arthrography and MRI in detecting patellar cartilage lesions. Drill holes ranging from 0.8 to 5 mm in diameter and from 1 to 2 mm in depth were produced in cadaver knees. Double-contrast CT-arthrography easily detected 3- and 5-mm holes, but 50% of the 1.5- and 2-mm lesions were missed. The 0.8-mm holes were not recognized at all. On the contrary, MRI detected the smallest 0.8-mm lesions because they were precisely delineated by intra-articular fluid, which appears bright on T2-weighted images.

In a clinical study, 54 knees were examined by MRI, and evidence of a cartilage lesion was found in 44 cases. At arthroscopy, however, the corresponding lesion was found in only 34 knees (77%), whereas there was no chondral lesion or softening in the remaining 10 knees. When compared with arthroscopy, MRI had 81.5% accuracy, 100% sensitivity, and 50% specificity. As far as staging of the lesion, it was correctly predicted by MRI in 76% of cases, overrated in 5.8%, and underrated in 17.6%. Using these data, Handelberg and colleagues[170] proposed an MRI classification of chondral lesions. It is recognized that MRI yields a discrete incidence of false-positive results, possibly because of detection of early lesions in the deep layers of cartilage that are not visualized at arthroscopy. They are evident as linear, dark areas in the gray signal of cartilage. Further studies are needed to confirm whether these findings represent early lesions or are a variation of normal anatomy.

Stage I lesions, described as softening at arthroscopy, are usually visible as round areas of low signal intensity on "proton density" and T2-weighted images.

Stage II lesions correspond to fissures that appear as zones of low signal surrounding the high signal of fluid leaking into the cleft.

Stage III lesions correspond to superficial or deep defects, which appear as bright images because of the synovial fluid that fills them.

Stage IV lesions involve thinning and irregularity of cartilage as found in degenerative arthritis.

In conclusion, we think that MRI is an attractive diagnostic modality for the patellofemoral joint. It does not involve the use of ionizing radiation or contrast material and allows evaluation of both patellar tracking and cartilage lesions. However, the reduced availability and increased cost of MRI as compared with CT limit the use of MRI.

Radionuclide Imaging

The use of bone scans as an adjunctive procedure to obtain information regarding the osseous metabolic activity of the patellofemoral joint has been investigated by Dye and Boll.[101] They first determined the scintigraphic activity of the patellofemoral joint in a series of patients undergoing technetium Tc 99m methylene diphosphonate (^{99m}Tc-MDP) bone scans for reasons other than lower extremity symptoms. The lateral view was far more informative than the anteroposterior view in providing data on the patellofemoral joint. From the data acquired from this series of control knees, it appeared that the scintigraphic activity of the patella was roughly equal to that of the ipsilateral femoral diaphysis in 96% of cases. Of the control patellae, 4% exhibited a definite increase in activity over the reference region of the femur. ^{99m}Tc-MDP bone scans were obtained in 113 patients complaining of patellofemoral symptoms without previous knee surgery or evidence of osseous abnormalities. Of these symptomatic knees, 49% showed increased uptake of the isotope. When this group was divided into knees exhibiting patellar symptoms and knees with peripatellar symptoms, a high (54%) incidence of positive bone scans was found in the first group (patellar) versus a lower incidence (16%) in the second group (peripatellar). The difference between normal knees (4%) and knees with patellar symptoms (54%) was significant. Knees with increased uptake of the isotope were found to have two different patterns: diffuse (73%) or focal (27%). Increased uptake in the femoral trochlea was found in only 11% of cases, and it was associated with increased patellar uptake in all the cases except two.

Two or more sequential bone scans were obtained in 56 patients after different therapeutic modalities. At follow-up evaluation, 89% of knees with persistent symptoms exhibited positive patellar uptake, including 10 knees with an initially normal-appearing bone scan. After an average period of 6 months (range, 3 to 14 months), 17 knees showed remission of symptoms and normalization of patellar uptake. The knees with focal uptake showed favorable resolution more frequently than did those with diffuse uptake. Despite resolution of the symptoms, 12 knees demonstrated persistent positive patellar uptake.

In conclusion, Dye and Boll believed that increased patellar uptake represents an alteration in osseous homeostasis consisting of increased blood flow and increased bone turnover. The two processes occur simultaneously and somewhat dependently. Bone scans provide information limited to the osseous component of the patellofemoral joint. Therefore, a scan showing positive results is not an indicator of chondromalacia; nearly half the patients in whom a bone scan showed positive results in fact had normal cartilage. The primary indication for obtaining a bone scan in a patient with prolonged symptoms is a doubtful diagnosis, especially in cases with medicolegal or workers' compensation implications. A positive bone scan result confirms the presence of altered osseous metabolism. On the other hand, soft-tissue problems will go undetected. A positive bone scan result may reverse to a negative one with adequate treatment, but the process is prolonged, probably because of the high repetitive force withstood by the patellofemoral joint. The best prognosis for improvement is found in cases with focal uptake in the patella. In contrast, increased uptake in both the patella and femoral trochlea indicates a poor prognosis. Very few of these cases resolved completely, and they may represent a preradiographic stage of osteoarthritis.

Arthroscopy

The role of arthroscopy in evaluation of the patellofemoral joint has been recognized for a long time.[60] It allows direct visualization of both patellar tracking and cartilage abnormalities.

PATELLAR TRACKING

Patellar tracking has been evaluated with the arthroscope inserted through an inferior or a superior portal. Grana and colleagues[158] did not record any significant difference in observing patellar tracking from the standard antero-lateral, anteromedial, or superior portals. They consider the tracking abnormal if the patellar ridge does not seat in the trochlear groove by 45 degrees of flexion. Metcalf[285] popularized the use of the superolateral approach to observe patellar tracking. He considered typical signs of lateral tracking of the patella to be the presence of an "empty sulcus" and "overhang" of the lateral facet beyond the lateral femoral condyle. Lindberg and colleagues[249] proposed the use of the transpatellar tendon approach and the 70-degree arthroscope to visualize the patellofemoral joint.

In a comparative study,[249] two surgeons independently evaluated the patellofemoral joint of 20 knees, one through the suprapatellar and the other through the transpatellar approach. Both techniques gave similar results, but there was a slight difference in the assessment of tracking because three knees with subluxation of the patella were considered normal when visualized through the suprapatellar approach. Overall, the authors concluded that the transpatellar approach allowed better visualization throughout the range of motion. Patellar tracking was considered normal if the ridge of the patella reduced into the sulcus by 10 degrees of knee flexion. Reduction between 10 and 30 degrees was considered first-degree subluxation. Reduction beyond 30 degrees of flexion was classified as second-degree subluxation. The authors also investigated the effects of intra-articular pressure on the position of the patella and found that subluxation could not be increased or reduced by raising intra-articular pressure. This finding is in fact logical because the patella floats up symmetrically with rising pressure.

Lindberg and colleagues,[250] using the criteria just discussed, isolated a group of 122 knees with lateral subluxation of the patella as visualized at arthroscopy. Most of these patients suffered from anterior knee pain (72%). A second group of 50 knees displayed a congruent, but chondromalacic patella at arthroscopy. Symptoms of anterior knee pain were present in only 32% of these patients, a significant difference from the subluxation group. Associated lesions were rare (35%) and mostly traumatic in the subluxation group, but in the group with congruent and chondromalacic patellae, associated lesions were more common (82%) and mostly degenerative. These data seem to support the hypothesis that patellar maltracking and patellar pain syndromes are intimately linked. In contrast, degenerative changes of the patellar cartilage in knees with congruent patella are often associated with degenerative joint disease.

Patellar tracking, including the dynamic effect of the quadriceps muscle, has been evaluated arthroscopically under local anesthesia by Sojbjerg and colleagues.[366] The arthroscope was inserted through the anteromedial portal. Patellar tracking was examined while the knee was passively flexed through a 0- to 90-degree arc of motion. The quadriceps influence was evaluated by asking the patient to contract the quadriceps at 45 degrees of flexion with the tibia in neutral and external rotation. Three groups of knees were examined, including 17 controls, 13 knees with patellar instability, and 20 knees with patellar pain. In normal knees, the lateral facet, median ridge, and

medial facet contacted the femur at average flexion angles of 20, 35, and 50 degrees, respectively. The same values in the group with patellar instability were 30, 55, and 85 degrees, respectively. The difference from the control group was significant for the ridge and medial facet. In the patellar pain group, the average angles at which the lateral facet, ridge, and medial facet contacted the femur were 20, 35, and 50 degrees, respectively. These values were the same as those of controls, but dispersion of the values was much increased. All the control patients were able to bring the medial facet in contact with the femur by contracting the quadriceps while the knee was in neutral or external rotation. The same was true of all the knees with patellar pain except one case. On the other hand, most of the patients with patellar instability were unable to bring the medial facet in contact with the femur by quadriceps contraction with the tibia in external rotation.

We prefer to use the superolateral approach to examine the patellofemoral joint. In our opinion it allows better visualization of the joint because the arthroscope is more mobile and at a greater distance from the patella (Fig. 53–50). The inferior portals are available if the cartilage is to be shaved. Centralization of the patellar ridge in the sulcus (Fig. 53–51) and overhang of the lateral patellar facet (Fig. 53–52) are routinely visible. Because of these data, we think that patellar tracking with centralization of the ridge in the sulcus within 30 degrees of flexion can safely be considered normal. Normal tracking, defined as centralization within 10 degrees,[249] is probably too restrictive. Centralization between 30 and 50 degrees is borderline, whereas beyond 50 degrees it is definitely abnormal. In borderline cases, if the patient is under local anesthesia, it may be useful to note whether centralization is obtained with quadriceps contraction. The patella may also be pushed medially and laterally while one observes the displacement with the arthroscope. Failure to glide medially over one quadrant of its width indicates a tight lateral retinaculum. Excessive lateral gliding (over two quadrants) and possibly patellar dislocation (Fig. 53–53) indicate laxity of the medial stabilizers.

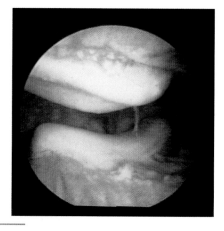

Figure 53–50. Good visualization of the patellofemoral joint can be obtained easily with the arthroscope inserted into the superolateral portal.

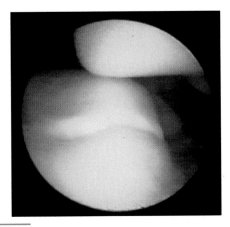

Figure 53–51. Patellofemoral joint of a knee with recurrent dislocation of the patella. The arthroscope is placed in the superolateral portal. With the knee flexed 30 degrees, the patellar ridge contacts the lateral trochlear facet and the sulcus is empty (empty sulcus sign).

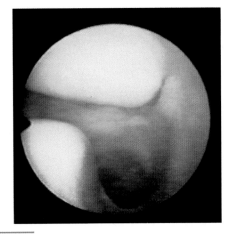

Figure 53–52. Same knee as in Figure 53-51. The lateral patellar facet overhangs the trochlea laterally.

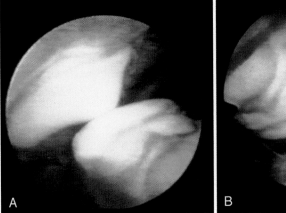

Figure 53–53. Knee affected by recurrent dislocation of the patella. The patellofemoral joint is visualized from the superolateral portal. **A,** With the knee flexed 30 degrees, the patella is markedly lateralized and the sulcus appears flat. **B,** The patella can be easily dislocated.

CARTILAGE ABNORMALITIES

Cartilage lesions can be accurately documented at the time of arthroscopy. Several methods of classification of articular cartilage lesions have been developed. Most of them have the disadvantage of combining depth and size of the lesion in the grading system. In agreement with Casscells,[61] we think that depth, size, and location of the lesion should be recorded separately. We routinely classify the depth of the lesion into five grades:
Grade I: softening (Fig. 53–54)
Grade II: fissuring
Grade III: superficial fibrillation
Grade IV: deep fibrillation (Fig. 53–55)
Grade V: erosion down to subchondral bone
   The size of the lesion is recorded by means of the two greatest perpendicular diameters. The location is best recorded on a sketch of the articular surface of the patella. The three different factors—depth, size, and location—may later be combined in any grading system that is shown to correlate best with the clinical results.
   It is clear from this classification that arthroscopic examination of the patella cannot be considered complete unless a probe has been used to palpate the articular cartilage. Softening may otherwise go undetected. It should be remembered that articular cartilage is thicker on the central ridge, which is therefore more resilient. Some experience is necessary to avoid overestimation of this normal finding.

CLASSIFICATION OF PATELLOFEMORAL DISORDERS

Several attempts have been made to classify patellofemoral disorders, but the greatest progress has followed appreciation of the subsequent two points. First, the term *chondromalacia*, introduced by Aleman,[13] should be used to describe a lesion of the articular cartilage of the patella as observed at arthrotomy or arthroscopy or suspected clinically in the presence of clear patellofemoral crepitation during active extension of the knee. It is now widely accepted that chondromalacia is mostly secondary to patellofemoral overload or malalignment or, more rarely, direct trauma. The term *idiopathic chondromalacia* should

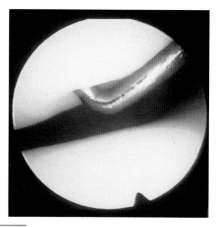

Figure 53–54. Softening of the patellar cartilage. These lesions may be missed unless the articular cartilage is palpated with the probe.

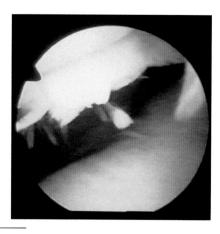

Figure 53–55. Deep fibrillation of the articular cartilage of the patella (grade IV chondromalacia).

be restricted to the infrequent patient with proven damage to articular cartilage without any evidence of mechanical imbalance or history of trauma.

The second important fact is recognition of a group of disorders with variable expression, which can be called *patellofemoral malalignment* or *dysplasia*. These disorders include, to a variable degree, an increased Q angle, a high-riding patella, a shallow femoral sulcus, lateralized tracking of the patella, hypoplasia of the vastus medialis obliquus, increased femoral anteversion, and compensatory external tibial rotation. The most profitable way of thinking of these disorders is as a developmental dysplasia with a continuum of anatomic deficiencies. The analogies with congenital dysplasia of the hip are evident.

It has been disputed which of the anatomic abnormalities are genetically determined and which are adaptive changes. From an embryological point of view, the patella has medial and lateral facets that are initially equal in size. However, by the sixth month of gestation, the dimensions of the lateral patellar facets exceed those of the medial facets, as is found in adults.[394] The definite adult form of

Box 53-1. Insall's Classification of Patellofemoral Disorders

Presence of Cartilage Damage
Chondromalacia
Osteoarthritis
Osteochondral fractures
Osteochondritis dissecans

Variable Cartilage Damage
Malalignment syndromes
Synovial plicae

Usually Normal Cartilage
Peripatellar causes: bursitis, tendinitis
Overuse syndromes
Reflex sympathetic dystrophy
Patellar abnormalities

Data from Insall JN: Disorders of the patella. In Insall JN (ed): Surgery of the Knee. New York, Churchill Livingstone, 1984, p 191.

the trochlea is achieved very early in fetal life.[238,394] According to these data, recurrent dislocation of the patella has been described as a hereditary disease with autosomal dominant transmission.[287] On the other hand, it is well known that patellar dislocation may result from multiple injections in the vastus lateralis with quadriceps fibrosis.[166,184,253] It therefore seems that both genetically determined and acquired forms exist and manifest themselves with lateral tracking of the patella.

Insall's Classification

Insall[200] devised a classification of patellofemoral disorders based on the presence of articular cartilage damage (Box 53–1), which can be present, variable, or absent. In the group with variable cartilage damage, he described malalignment syndromes, which include different clinical afflictions ranging from patellar pain to patellar subluxation and dislocation.

Merchant's Classification

We have found the classification of patellofemoral disorders published by Merchant[282] in 1988 to be useful and practical (Box 53–2). Patellofemoral disorders are classified into five categories: (1) post-traumatic conditions, (2) patellofemoral dysplasia, (3) idiopathic chondromalacia, (4) osteochondritis dissecans, and (5) synovial plicae.

POST-TRAUMATIC CONDITIONS

The post-traumatic category includes three subgroups: acute trauma, repetitive trauma, and late effects of trauma.

Box 53-2. Merchant's Classification of Patellofemoral Disorders

I. Trauma (conditions caused by trauma in an otherwise normal knee)
  A. Acute trauma
    1. Contusion
    2. Fracture
      a. Patella
      b. Femoral trochlea
      c. Proximal tibial epiphysis (tubercle)
    3. Dislocation (rare in a normal knee)
    4. Rupture
      a. Quadriceps tendon
      b. Patellar tendon
  B. Repetitive trauma (overuse syndromes)
    1. Patellar tendinitis ("jumper's knee")
    2. Quadriceps tendinitis
    3. Peripatellar tendinitis (e.g., anterior knee pain in an adolescent as a result of hamstring contracture)
    4. Prepatellar bursitis ("housemaid's knee")
    5. Apophysitis
      a. Osgood-Schlatter disease
      b. Sinding-Larsen-Johansson disease
  C. Late effects of trauma
    1. Post-traumatic chondromalacia patellae
    2. Post-traumatic patellofemoral arthritis
    3. Anterior fat pad syndrome (post-traumatic fibrosis)
    4. Reflex sympathetic dystrophy of the patella
    5. Patellar osseous dystrophy
    6. Acquired patella infra
    7. Acquired quadriceps fibrosis
II. Patellofemoral dysplasia
  A. Lateral patellar compression syndrome
    1. Secondary chondromalacia patellae
    2. Secondary patellofemoral arthritis
  B. Chronic subluxation of the patella
    1. Secondary chondromalacia patellae
    2. Secondary patellofemoral arthritis
  C. Recurrent dislocation of the patella
    1. Associated fractures
      a. Osteochondral (intra-articular)
      b. Avulsion (extra-articular)
    2. Secondary chondromalacia patellae
    3. Secondary patellofemoral arthritis
  D. Chronic dislocation of the patella
    1. Congenital
    2. Acquired
III. Idiopathic chondromalacia patellae
IV. Osteochondritis dissecans
  A. Patella
  B. Femoral trochlea
V. Synovial plicae (anatomic variant made symptomatic by acute or repetitive trauma)
  A. Medial patellar ("shelf")
  B. Suprapatellar
  C. Lateral patellar

From Merchant AC: Classification of patellofemoral disorders. Arthroscopy 4:235, 1988.

Acute Trauma

The sequelae of acute trauma to the patellofemoral joint are commonly encountered in every emergency department: contusions, fractures of the patella, and rupture of the patellar or quadriceps tendon. It is theoretically possible that a direct blow on the medial aspect of the patella can dislocate it laterally. However, clinical experience confirms that patients who suffer patellar dislocation almost invariably have signs of patellofemoral dysplasia, and trauma is not a major cause.[335]

Repetitive Trauma

The consequences of repetitive trauma (overuse syndromes)—patellar tendinitis, quadriceps tendinitis, Osgood-Schlatter disease, Sinding-Larsen-Johansson disease, and prepatellar bursitis—are well-known clinical entities that do not usually constitute a diagnostic problem.

Late Effects of Trauma

Late effects of trauma include, among others, post-traumatic chondromalacia of the patella. This diagnosis should be strictly limited to knees that have sustained major trauma during sports or vehicular accidents (as with a dashboard injury) without evidence of associated patellofemoral malalignment. Reflex sympathetic dystrophy and acquired patella infra (or knee arthrofibrosis) are included among the late consequences of trauma, although some individual predisposition is necessary for these conditions to develop. Acquired quadriceps fibrosis secondary to multiple injections during the neonatal period is a well-described clinical entity that can lead to stiffness of the knee or habitual dislocation of the patella.

PATELLOFEMORAL DYSPLASIA

The category of the various degrees of patellofemoral dysplasia or malalignment (the terms *dysplasia* and *malalignment* are used with the same meaning in this chapter) includes most of the young patients with patellofemoral problems seen in orthopedic practice. From a clinical point of view, the patients may complain of pain, instability, or both.

Lateral Patellar Compression Syndrome

The lateral patellar compression syndrome includes knees with patellar pain aggravated by flexion activities without episodes of true instability. Nevertheless, some patients may refer to the subjective feeling of giving way, probably related to momentary quadriceps inhibition as a result of pain and not to true objective patellar instability. The Q angle has been found to be increased (average, 20 degrees) in these knees, whereas the congruence angle in 45-degree axial views and patellar height show only minor abnormalities.[7] More subtle tracking abnormalities with lateral tilt of the patella may be detected with CT in the 0- to 30-degree arc of motion.[348] In these knees, the pathogenetic mechanism seems to involve increased lateralization force on the patella, which remains stable in the sulcus. Therefore, the term *lateral patellar compression syndrome* seems appropriate.

Chronic Subluxation of the Patella

In many patients who complain mainly of pain, the patella is subluxated laterally in the axial view at 30 or 45 degrees. It is essential to emphasize that the main symptom is pain and that the diagnosis of chronic subluxation of the patella is based on an increased congruence angle (subluxation) on axial views. For practical purposes, a congruence angle of 5 degrees or greater on the Merchant axial view may be considered abnormal at the 95th percentile.[7] The same group of patients has been recognized by Dejour et al,[91] who reported that they constitute about 20% of cases of patellar pain. He named them *instabilities rotuliennes potentielles* (potential instabilities of the patella).

A continuum of abnormalities exists between lateral patellar compression syndrome and chronic subluxation of the patella. The routine use of CT or MRI to evaluate patella tracking in the first 30 degrees of flexion may detect tracking abnormalities in more cases and thus increase the frequency of diagnosis of chronic subluxation of the patella at the expense of diagnosis of lateral patellar compression syndrome. It should be remembered that subluxation of the patella may be present in otherwise asymptomatic knees or in knees evaluated for another disorder (meniscal or ligamentous injuries). Interpretation of the radiographic findings always requires confirmation by an adequate history and physical examination.

Recurrent Dislocation of the Patella

Patients who suffer from recurrent dislocation of the patella have recurrent episodes of patellar instability. As has been pointed out previously, patients with lateral patellar compression syndrome may experience episodes of sudden collapse or giving way of the knee as a result of quadriceps inhibition secondary to pain. They should be differentiated from true episodes of patellar instability. Patients with recurrent dislocation of the patella have a clear "apprehension sign" while attempting to displace the patella laterally with the knee at 20 to 30 degrees of flexion. They usually show lateral tracking (most often

lateral subluxation and tilt) of the patella, which is evident both clinically and on axial views. Furthermore, it should be possible to displace the patella out of its sulcus with the patient under anesthesia. We also think that the term *dislocation*—not subluxation—should be used to describe cases of recurrent instability. Strictly speaking, the term dislocation should be applied in a patient who after a twisting maneuver suddenly falls and notes that the patella lies on the lateral aspect of the knee, with relocation obtained by extending the knee. It is not unusual for the same patient to experience similar episodes later and have a feeling of lateral displacement of the patella but without actually seeing it out of the sulcus. We think that both episodes are probably dislocations, the only difference being the time that the patella is allowed to remain out of the sulcus. For these reasons, the term subluxation should not be used to describe a clinical situation, and perhaps these patients should better be considered as having recurrent instability.

This classification accounts for the fact that chondromalacia or osteoarthritis may follow patellofemoral malalignment and should be recognized as a secondary phenomenon. Nevertheless, patellofemoral arthritis is manifested in many older patients without a previous history of patellar pain or instability and is often associated with variable degrees of medial or lateral tibiofemoral joint arthrosis. It should therefore be recognized that not all the cases of patellofemoral arthritis are necessarily the consequence of patellofemoral dysplasia.

Chronic Dislocation of the Patella

Chronic dislocation of the patella includes knees with a patella permanently dislocated out of its sulcus. A difference can be detected between cases wherein the patella is dislocated both in extension and in flexion (permanent dislocation) and wherein it dislocates each time that the knee is flexed (habitual dislocation). This condition may be congenital or acquired as a result of multiple intramuscular injections.

OTHER CATEGORIES

The diagnosis of idiopathic chondromalacia patellae should be restricted, as previously pointed out, to the few patients with proven cartilage damage and without clinical or radiological evidence of malalignment. Finally, the categories osteochondritis dissecans and synovial plicae complete Merchant's classification. Other infections and tumors are rarely observed and have not been included.

LATERAL PATELLAR COMPRESSION SYNDROME

Lateral patellar compression syndrome is characterized clinically by pain and radiographically by a patella that is centered in the sulcus.

Symptoms

The basic symptoms were described earlier. Pain is characteristically dull, poorly localized, and increased by activities that overload the patellofemoral joint—for example, stair climbing, squatting, and prolonged sitting with the knee flexed. The onset of symptoms may follow trauma, either a direct blow to the patella or a twisting injury. However, the entity of trauma is more often disproportionate to the effects. On the other hand, malalignment of the lower limb seems to be the common denominator of this group of patients, including an increased Q angle and a tight lateral retinaculum. Swelling is often reported by these patients, but effusion is not frequently found at examination. Effusion becomes more common in the presence of chondromalacic changes because cartilage debris causes synovial inflammation. Patients sometimes report catching or momentary locking. These conditions may be caused by momentary quadriceps inhibition secondary to pain or by some cartilage irregularity that locks the smooth gliding movement of the patella during extension. Careful inquiry usually differentiates these episodes from the giving way of ligamentous laxity, from a meniscal tear, or from an episode of true patellar instability.

The diagnosis of chronic anterior cruciate ligament deficiency may be readily excluded through the confirmation of normal anterior tibial translation with a firm endpoint in the Lachman test and a negative pivot-shift test. Differentiating the diagnosis from a meniscal injury is often trickier because medial joint line tenderness is usually positive in patellar pain syndromes. It helps to remember that tibial rotation tests (the Steinmann and McMurray tests) do not increase pain in patients with lateral patellar compression syndrome. Thigh atrophy is a frequent finding in meniscal disorder but is usually absent in knees with lateral patellar compression syndrome.

The most difficult task is probably differentiation between patients suffering from lateral patellar compression syndrome with episodes of buckling or locking and patients with true patellar instability. However, buckling in knees with lateral patellar compression syndrome is usually a secondary complaint. True episodes of patellar instability, followed by considerable swelling that persists for a few days, are lacking. The apprehension test result is negative, and only minor tracking abnormalities of the patella are present.

Physical Examination

The patient is observed while standing. Squinting of the patellae is easily appreciated. A mild varus knee may be present. The axes of the femur and tibia are parallel and connected by an oblique patellar tendon, which slopes downward and laterally (bayonet deformity). The patient is then observed while walking. The presence of associated pronation of the foot is checked. If pronation is present, it is corrected and the effects on alignment of the extensor apparatus (Q angle) are noted. The patient is asked to perform a half-squat and to hold the position for a short time, which usually evokes pain. The full-squat position, or sitting on the heels with the quadriceps relaxed, is usually less painful.

With the patient sitting, the knee is actively extended and tracking of the patella is noted. The physician should concentrate on two factors. The first is lateral subluxation of the patella. The most frequent abnormality is mild lateral displacement in full extension and early flexion that reduces with further flexion. The second factor to note is the tilt of the patella. The transverse axis of the patella, passing through the medial and lateral edges, is normally horizontal or has up to 5 degrees of slope downward and laterally. The presence of a medial border of the patella clearly higher than the lateral border should be considered normal. Crepitus of the patellofemoral joint is also noted during active extension against resistance and classified as mild, moderate, or severe. It is our experience that moderate to severe crepitation is always associated with damage to the patellofemoral cartilage.

Finally, the patient is examined in the supine position. The Q angle is often increased in patients with lateral patellar compression syndrome. Values over 20 degrees are considered definitely abnormal. Alignment of the patellar tendon is again checked with the knee at 90 degrees of flexion. Because derotation of the tibia occurs with flexion of the knee, the extensor mechanism is straighter in flexion than in extension. More than 10 degrees of lateral and downward slope of the patellar tendon with the knee at 90 degrees of flexion, in relation to the transepicondylar line, should be considered pathological.[227]

Assessment of tightness of the lateral retinaculum is critical in the diagnosis of lateral patellar compression syndrome. The examiner should be able to lift the lateral border of the patella until the transverse axis is tilted above the horizontal (passive patellar tilt test). With the knee at 20 to 30 degrees of flexion, it should be possible to push the patella medially more than a quarter of the patellar width. If these test results are positive, a tight lateral retinaculum is diagnosed.

Tenderness of the patellofemoral joint and surrounding structures is checked. Because many structures may be tender, it is essential to proceed in an orderly fashion. We begin with palpation of the medial and lateral retinacula and their insertion into the patellar margins. It has been suggested that the patella be pushed laterally to put the lateral retinaculum under tension and facilitate palpation of it.[125]

In a prospective clinical examination of 78 knees with patellofemoral pain, Fulkerson[126] found that some portion of the lateral retinaculum was tender in 90% of cases, more often at or near the retinaculopatellar junction. Pain in the medial retinaculum was ill defined, less clearly retinacular in nature, and possibly arising from the medial facet. Isolated pain in the medial patellofemoral joint was present in only 10% of knees. Eight patients received a corticosteroid injection in the painful portion of the retinaculum. All the knees experienced pain relief, but finally pain returned in all cases. Our experience contrasts with these findings because tenderness of the medial patellofemoral joint (including the retinaculum and the medial patellar facet) seems to be more frequent than tenderness of the lateral retinaculum.

The examination proceeds with the patellar compression test. With the knee flexed 20 to 30 degrees to engage the patella into the femoral sulcus, the patella is compressed against the trochlea by pushing it medially and laterally. In this way, effective tenderness of the patellar facets may be elicited with less irritation of the surrounding soft-tissue structures. Medial compression of the patella usually evokes pain in knees with lateral patellar compression syndrome, whereas lateral displacement causes less or no pain and no apprehension.

The examination is completed with palpation of the quadriceps tendon and its insertion on the base of the patella, palpation of the patellar tendon and its insertions on the tibial tubercle and the apex of the patella, and palpation of the joint lines. It should be remembered that medial joint line tenderness is often marked in lateral patellar compression syndrome, possibly more marked than tenderness of the medial retinaculum. It has been supposed that this could be mediated by inflammation of the synovium in this zone, but macroscopic or histological evidence of synovitis has not been found.[203] Another possible explanation is tension in the medial patellomeniscal ligament when the patella is tilted laterally. Nevertheless, the examiner should not be deceived by this finding and too easily diagnose a torn medial meniscus.

Radiographic Examination

Routine anteroposterior, lateral, and axial views at 45 degrees of flexion[284] are not very informative in knees with patellar pain and lateral patellar compression syndrome. In a group of 53 patients with patellar pain, we found only minor differences from controls, including a slightly more open sulcus angle (139 degrees versus 137 degrees) and a slightly decreased congruence angle (−2 degrees versus −8 degrees).[7]

Using axial views in a more extended position (20 degrees), Laurin and colleagues[243] reported that the lateral patellofemoral angle was not helpful in the diagnosis of patellar pain syndromes because it was open laterally in 90% of cases, similar to what is found in normal knees (97%). For this reason, the patellofemoral index was developed—that is, the ratio of the thickness of the medial to the lateral patellofemoral joint line. This value was up to 1.6 in normal knees, whereas it was greater than 1.6 in 97% of knees with patellar pain. Laurin and coworkers interpreted this finding as the existence of a minor tracking abnormality of the patella (minitilt).

Our experience using the Laurin view has been less encouraging.[9] In a group of 41 knees with patellar pain, the lateral patellofemoral angle and the patellofemoral index did not significantly differ from these values in controls. The same was true of the average value of the congruence and sulcus angles on the Merchant views. In a group of 20 controls examined in the same study, the following values were considered abnormal: congruence angle greater than 9 degrees, lateral patellofemoral angle open medially, and patellofemoral index greater than 1.7. When these criteria were used in the group of 41 knees with lateral patellar compression syndrome, the congru-

ence angle was abnormal in 5%, the lateral patellofemoral angle in 5%, and the patellofemoral index in 24%. Thus, the patellofemoral index was the most frequently abnormal value, but it was so in only a fourth of cases. Therefore, its diagnostic value in our experience[9] has been less clear than reported by Laurin and colleagues.[243]

The lateral view usually fails to show a significant degree of patella alta in knees with lateral patellar compression syndrome. A high patella (Insall-Salvati index >1.2) was found in only 6% of 53 knees affected by lateral patellar compression syndrome.[7]

Changes in the osseous structure of the patella may occur in lateral patellar compression syndrome in response to excessive loading of the lateral facet and hypopressure on the medial facet as a manifestation of Wolff's law.[406] The subchondral plate of the lateral facet shows increased density, whereas there is a corresponding decrease in density of the subchondral plate of the medial facet. The cancellous trabeculae of the patella may show the same changes. Furthermore, the orientation of the trabeculae, which is normally 90 degrees to the transverse axis of the patella, shifts to the lateral side to become perpendicular to the lateral facet.

Other changes visible on the radiograph may be interpreted as secondary to excessive lateral traction. A thickened lateral retinaculum may be visible on an underpenetrated radiograph, and traction by it may produce an osteophyte on the lateral border of the patella. The same forces, increased lateral pressure and traction from the lateral retinaculum, influence both development of the patella during growth and its final shape. Because the patella and the trochlea ossify rather late, these adaptive modifications represent only the consequence of the Heuter-Volkman law[181,392]: compression retards epiphyseal growth, whereas traction stimulates it. In response to these forces during growth, the final shape of the patella may show a marked predominance of the lateral facet (Wiberg type III), and the prominence of the lateral femoral condyle may be reduced as has been confirmed by CT.[347] Traction from a thickened and shortened lateral retinaculum also seems to be responsible for some bipartite patellae. In these cases, the accessory fragment is located straight on the lateral margin of the patella and not, as usual, at the superolateral corner, where the vastus lateralis tendon inserts. A bipartite patella could represent the end result of a stress fracture of the original ossification center under the influence of excessive traction.

More recently, the introduction of CT has offered the possibility of studying the patellofemoral joint in full extension and early flexion—that is, in the most informative part of the arc of motion, which cannot be explored with conventional axial views. Furthermore, the use of a well-defined reference line tangent to the posterior femoral condyles and avoidance of overlapping of the bones allow detection of more subtle abnormalities. Schutzer and colleagues,[347] using transverse midpatellar sections at 0, 10, 20, and 30 degrees, found that the patella in normal subjects becomes centered in the sulcus by 10 degrees of flexion. Moreover, the angle between the tangent to the posterior femoral condyles and the tangent to the lateral patellar facet (patellar tilt angle) was always open laterally and never less than 8 degrees. Based on these data, it was possible to classify a patella as subluxated if the congruence angle was still positive beyond 10 degrees of flexion and tilted if the patellar tilt angle was less than 8 degrees in the first 30 degrees of flexion.

Using a similar CT technique in knees with patellofemoral disorders, Fulkerson et al[133,140,347] identified a group of knees with tilt but without subluxation. In these knees, the patellar tilt angle was slightly decreased in extension (10 degrees versus 18 degrees in controls) and further decreased in flexion at 30 degrees (2 degrees versus 16 degrees in controls). This has been attributed to a shortened lateral retinaculum. If the situation is allowed to persist, chronic hyperpression of the lateral facet and hypopression of the medial facet may lead to degenerative changes in the patellar cartilage and to patellofemoral arthritis as described by Ficat and colleagues.[115]

We performed CT at 20 and 30 degrees of flexion to investigate a group of 41 knees with patellar pain.[9] In light of the measurements obtained with similar technique in 20 normal knees, we considered the following conditions abnormal: a positive congruence angle, a patellar tilt angle less than 6 degrees, and a TT-SF distance greater than 14 mm. According to these criteria, a pathological congruence angle was the most frequent finding (19%), followed by the TT-SF distance (15%) and the patellar tilt angle, which was pathological in only 5% of knees.

We think that many of the discrepancies on radiographic and CT measurements cited in the literature will be solved if more precise criteria are used. Introduction of the concept of lateral patellar compression syndrome seems to be a significant step forward in this direction. A similar pathological condition was described by Ficat et al,[115] who named it *syndrome d'hyperpression externe*, and more recently by Fulkerson and Hungerford,[134] who named it *excessive lateral pressure syndrome*. To be included in this group, patients should have a well-defined patellar pain syndrome and show clinical evidence of an increased valgus vector of the extensor apparatus, including an increased Q angle and a shortened lateral retinaculum. The axial views or CT should not show subluxation of the patella, but a lateral tilt may be present and the TT-SF distance may be increased. It should be remembered that it is not unusual to find patients who complain of knee pain without any clinical sign of patellar instability but whose axial radiographs reveal lateral subluxation of the patella. Dejour and colleagues[91] stated that these patients constitute about 20% of their patellar pain cases and named them *instabilities rotuliennes potentielles*. Merchant[282] has considered these knees separately as chronic subluxation of the patella. We agree that there are valid reasons to keep these knees separate from the lateral patellar compression syndrome group.

Etiology of Patellofemoral Pain

Several hypotheses have been proposed throughout the years to explain the presence of pain in malalignment syndromes. Because chondromalacia was the most striking finding, it was assumed that pain was coming from the damaged articular surface, and thus patellar pain and chondromalacia became synonymous. This hypothesis has progressively been challenged because (1) cartilage is not innervated and it is therefore insensitive and (2) it has been found that patellar pain may exist with apparently intact articular cartilage. Today, it is widely accepted that chondromalacia in malalignment syndromes is a secondary phenomenon. Two hypotheses are proposed to explain the pathogenesis of pain in malalignment syndromes: (1) abnormal lateral loading of the bony patellar surface and (2) excessive lateral ligament tension.

Insall[199,200] suggested that lateral loading of the patellar ridge is increased in malalignment syndromes. This sometimes causes chondromalacia of the articular surface but does not necessarily mean that chondromalacia is the cause of the pain. In fact, the preoperative severity of pain correlated poorly with the severity and extent of patellar chondromalacia found at surgery. The worst examples of chondromalacia were found in patients with recurrent dislocation who had little or no pain between the episodes of dislocations. It therefore seems likely that pain can occur independently of articular damage and that cartilage failure in patients with "chondromalacia" syndrome may be either coincidental or due to other causes (e.g., patellar malalignment) without itself being responsible for pain.

The pain associated with malalignment is probably explained by the unique anatomy of the patella, which in the region of the vertical crest possesses a convex bony surface covered by a thick layer of relatively soft articular cartilage. A soft convex surface is particularly sensitive to sideways loading, such as would occur in patellar tracking abnormalities. The effect can be visualized by considering the analogy of an eraser on the end of an ordinary pencil. Repetitive sideways loading soon causes the eraser to shear from its attachment to the pencil, whereas direct compression with much greater force has little effect. In the same manner, deformation of the convex articular cartilage of the patella produces abnormal shear loading on subchondral bone even when the cartilaginous surface is intact (Fig. 53–56). Repeated deformation of the vertical crest would also explain the softened and fissured areas that may be found in exactly this region (Fig. 53–57), as well as tangential fissures within the substance of the cartilage itself. According to this hypothesis, the pain threshold in subchondral bone can be exceeded even if the cartilage is intact (1) when excessive stress or force is exerted (e.g., athletics or direct trauma) or (2) when normal stress is applied in an abnormal direction (e.g., lateral loading). Thus, the current view of malalignment is that lateral tracking and lateral loading of the patella are the primary source of pain but may incidentally be the cause of chondromalacia as well.

Fulkerson and Gossling[130] have detailed the anatomy of the lateral retinaculum and emphasized its role in the cause of patellar pain. They substantiated the hypothesis with the following clinical, histological, and surgical observations.

From a clinical point of view, the lateral retinaculum in knees with lateral patellar compression syndrome can be palpated as thickened, indurated, and shortened. The decreased medial mobility and passive patellar tilt demonstrate this fact. The examiner should be alert to the fact

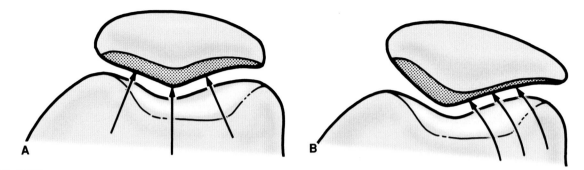

Figure 53–56. **A,** In normal balance, forces across the patellofemoral joint are evenly distributed. **B,** In cases of excessive lateral loading, the articular cartilage in the region of the crest is deformed and excessive loads are transmitted to the subchondral bone.

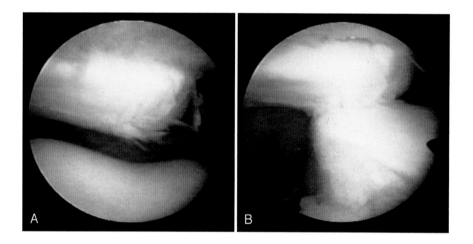

Figure 53–57. Pathogenesis of cartilage lesions. **A,** A knee with patellofemoral malalignment exhibits fissures and fibrillation in the area of the central ridge. **B,** Pushing the patella laterally allows visualization because the ridge is subjected to abnormal shear stress in the region with chondromalacia changes.

that tightness of the lateral retinaculum may be less evident in extension but increases with flexion. In fact, the posterior border of the lateral retinaculum inserts into the iliotibial band. As the knee is flexed, the patella sinks into the sulcus while the fascia lata is displaced posteriorly. This increases tension in the retinaculum. Fulkerson[126] prospectively examined a group of 78 knees in young patients with patellar pain and found that the lateral retinaculum was tender in 90% of cases.

From a histological point of view, Fulkerson and colleagues[141] analyzed 18 biopsy specimens of the lateral retinaculum obtained from knees with patellar pain at the time of lateral release. These specimens were stained with hematoxylin-eosin and with the modified Gomori trichrome stain to better visualize the myelin and connective tissue of the nerves. The results were compared with those in specimens obtained from 3 knees with anterior cruciate ligament insufficiency and 13 cadaver knees. Five knees with patellar pain showed evidence of moderate to severe degenerative neuropathy with slightly increased perineural fibrosis and mild to moderate loss of myelinated fibers. In the cadaver specimens, 23 nerves were identified, 22 of which were normal. Of the three knees with anterior cruciate ligament insufficiency, one showed evidence of minimal nerve injury, and this was attributed to the chronic instability. The findings in the knees with patellar pain were comparable to those present in Morton's neuroma. This affliction is supposed to be

caused by repeated nerve compression leading to nerve edema and perineural fibrosis. A similar irritative mechanism, chronic stretching, causes degeneration of the nerves in the lateral retinaculum. Because there was virtually no evidence of inflammation in the lateral retinaculum of these knees, the presence of degenerative neuropathy was interpreted as the source of pain.

Sanchis-Alfonso et al[341] evaluated 16 lateral retinacula excised at the time of surgery in patients with symptomatic patellofemoral malalignment and described a relationship between the clinical and histological findings. An increase in the proportion of innervated tissue was correlated with anterior knee pain. The more severe the pain, the larger the nerves (24% of nerve fibers surpassing 25 µm in diameter); in addition, these nerves exhibited a zonal disposition in which there were groups of nerve fibers in some fields and no nerve fibers in others. The group with moderate pain had an increase in medium and small nerve fibers (mean diameter, 18 µm), predominantly of tiny perivascular fibers. The same group of researchers in a subsequent study[340] performed an immunohistochemical analysis for neural markers in 13 lateral retinacula excised from symptomatic patients at the time of surgery. The presence of S-100 protein was interpreted as demonstrating a rich perivascular innervation made of tiny fibers in a necklace fashion. Vascular innervation was increased in the lateral retinacula of patients with patellofemoral malalignment as compared with those with other abnormalities and with innervation in the medial retinacula. Richer innervation was evident in patients in whom pain was the main symptom than in patients whose main symptom was instability. The presence of substance P receptors was studied to determine the amount of nociceptive fibers among the proliferated nerves. They found that not all the tiny perivascular or interstitial nerves were nociceptive and that the number of these nociceptive fibers was higher in those suffering from pain as the predominant symptom.

From a surgical point of view, a thick and fibrotic lateral retinaculum is readily evident at the time of open lateral release in knees with lateral patellar compression syndromes. After incision, the two borders of the retinaculum separate promptly. With the knee in 90 degrees of flexion, more than 2 cm of separation is not uncommon. The presence of excessive tension in the lateral retinaculum may be confirmed with the "stitch test." One or two catgut sutures are placed close to the lateral retinaculum in extension. The knee is then flexed to 90 degrees. If excessive tension is present, the sutures will break.[115] The importance of the lateral retinaculum as a source of pain seems to be confirmed by the observation of a small number of patients with residual pain after lateral release. In these knees, a tight lateral band could be appreciated by palpation. The symptoms were relieved by a localized injection of 1% lidocaine. Residual pain was therefore interpreted as being due to incomplete lateral release.[134]

We think that both abnormal lateral loading of the patellar surface and excessive lateral ligamentous tension may contribute to pain in lateral patellar compression syndrome. Nevertheless, we are impressed by the fact that patients with this disorder are usually able to flex and extend the knee throughout the range of motion without much pain. If a load or resistance is added, however, as in the act of squatting, the maneuver becomes very painful. It seems that the main difference between the two situations is the load on the patellofemoral joint. For this reason, we think that abnormal load transmission in the patellofemoral joint with overload of subchondral bone is probably the most important source of pain in lateral patellar compression syndrome.

Treatment

CONSERVATIVE TREATMENT

Appropriate conservative treatment is based on thorough appreciation of the mechanics of the patellofemoral joint and its disturbance, which leads to pain. Conservative treatment traditionally includes rest, quadriceps exercises, knee braces, and anti-inflammatory drugs.

Rest

Rest is initially necessary when the syndrome has an acute onset with severe pain and joint effusion. A large effusion should be aspirated for diagnostic reasons and to make the patient more comfortable. On the other hand, the use of casts or splints for prolonged periods should be discouraged as a treatment of patellofemoral problems because it increases quadriceps atrophy.

Restriction of Activity

Restriction of activity may be a reasonable alternative for some patients. There is the case of a middle-aged woman who complains of anterior knee pain and swelling after prolonged skiing but who is otherwise asymptomatic. She will probably agree to reduce her activity level in that specific sport and avoid prolonged physical therapy or surgery. Unfortunately, most of the patients complaining of pain are young teenagers who want to be active in sports[110] and more often in activities that involve a lot of jumping, such as volleyball or basketball. These patients may not accept modified activity. The same problem arises with a patient who is complaining of pain in activities of daily living, including stair climbing and prolonged sitting. Such patients may well be unable to modify their lifestyle for professional reasons. Nevertheless, a change to less stressful activities remains a reasonable alternative in some patients.

Quadriceps Training

Quadriceps training is probably the most essential component of nonoperative treatment. If the pathogenetic mechanism of pain in lateral patellar compression syndrome is lateral tracking of the patella, strengthening of the quadriceps and, specifically, the vastus medialis obliquus may result in improvement. Isometric and progressive resistive quadriceps strengthening with the knee in extension (straight-leg raises) is probably the most widely used modality. When performed 100 to 200 times a day in sets of 10 to 20 repetitions, such exercises are usually effective and rarely painful. When some increase in quadriceps strength has been built, short-arc isotonic exercises in the last 30 degrees of extension can be introduced in many patients without adverse effects. On the other hand, the knee extension exercise from 90 degrees to full extension with weights on the ankle is often painful and contraindicated.[180] The same applies to isokinetic exercises that impose high loads on the patellofemoral joint.[223]

Knee braces with a patellar cutout and appropriate padding on the lateral aspect of the patella are of some help to patients. The obvious shortcoming is that they can be worn only for limited periods during athletic activities.

Nonsteroidal Anti-inflammatory Drugs

Oral nonsteroidal anti-inflammatory medications can be used to lessen pain and swelling. It has been suggested that they protect articular cartilage by reducing the synthesis of prostaglandins from arachidonic acid.[68] Their usefulness in lateral patellar compression syndrome is limited because lifelong protection against the adverse effects of hyperpressure on cartilage cannot be recommended.

McConnell's Rehabilitation Program

A more refined rehabilitation program has been proposed by McConnell,[272] and we have used it with success in several patients. It is based on precise appreciation of the alterations in the lower limb in the individual patient. First of all, muscle tightness, including the rectus femoris, iliotibial band, hamstrings, and gastrocnemius, should be identified and corrected. A tight iliotibial band increases lateral pull on the patella during flexion of the knee. The traditional stretches of the iliotibial band in the side-lying position seem to affect the proximal part of the muscle, with little effect on its distal attachment. Therefore, tight lateral structures are better stretched by using a strong medial glide or medial tilt of the patella. Stretching of the lateral retinaculum allows the patella to be reduced by the pull of the vastus medialis obliquus. Tight hamstring muscles increase midstance flexion of the knee during running and therefore the loads on the extensor apparatus. Furthermore, increased flexion of the knee requires increased dorsiflexion of the ankle to produce a planti-grade foot. If these cannot be accommodated at the ankle joint, the movement may be transferred to the subtalar joint and result in increased pronation.

A tight gastrocnemius muscle should also be corrected because it limits dorsiflexion at the ankle. Once again, the movement is translated to the subtalar joint, thereby increasing pronation of the foot. Pronation at the subtalar joint is accompanied by internal tibial rotation, which increases the Q angle and lateral tracking of the patella

(Fig. 53–58). McConnell found that in adolescents, sub-talar pronation and not the Q angle was the single most significant factor associated with patellofemoral pain. If pronation is diagnosed, supination exercises are pre-scribed to increase the awareness of foot position. Orthotics to improve foot posture are also useful, espe-cially in runners.

The role of the vastus medialis obliquus is recognized as crucial to centralize the patella after adequate stretch-ing of the lateral structures has been achieved. Some aspects concerning activation of the vastus medialis obliquus are emphasized. Training of the quadriceps muscle with the femur in internal rotation involves con-traction of the tensor fascia lata, which assists extension through the iliotibial band. This increases lateral pull on the patella and therefore decreases the effectiveness of the vastus medialis obliquus. External rotation of the femur is preferable. Most of the fibers of the vastus medialis obliquus originate from the tendon of the adductor magnus. Consequently, contraction of the adductors during knee extension facilitates vastus medialis obliquus activity. Pain during exercises should be avoided because it has an inhibitory effect on muscle contraction and results in muscle atrophy.

Training of a muscle should be specific to mimic the work that the muscle usually performs. The effects of training are specific for limb position, angle of knee flexion, velocity of the movement, and type of contraction (concentric or eccentric). It is therefore unlikely that

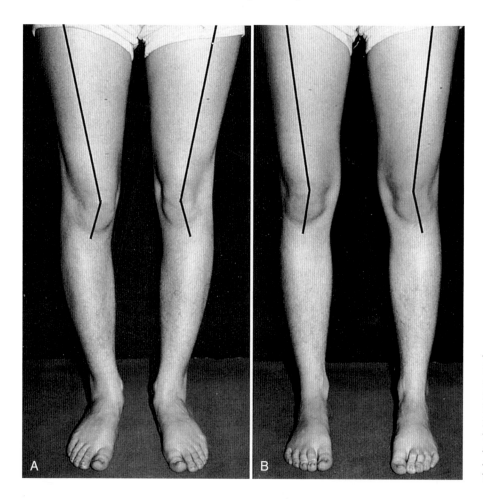

Figure 53–58. Alignment of the extensor apparatus with the foot in pronation and supination. **A,** Pronation at the subtalar joint is accompanied by internal tibial torsion, which increases the Q angle. **B,** Supination reduces the Q angle through external rotation of the tibia.

training with straight-leg raises will cause significant improvement in strength to relieve pain during an eccentric activity such as descending stairs. The "feed-forward" mechanism of muscle contraction, wherein the muscle is set in advance for a particular activity, should be specifically trained. The "feedback" mechanism is too slow to fine-tune patellar tracking because it involves considerably more time to receive the information. When this information is received, the joint is already in a new position.

A new test has been developed to better identify patients who might benefit from this program. Isometric quadriceps contraction is performed at 120, 90, 60, and 30 degrees, and contraction is held for at least 10 seconds. If quadriceps contraction in some of these positions elicits pain, the contraction is repeated after the patella has been pushed medially with both thumbs. McConnell has reported that if pain is reduced or abolished, a favorable outcome with this program can be predicted.

As stated previously, the program is specifically tailored to the findings of the examination in an individual patient. In a series of 35 patients with patellofemoral pain, the most frequent anatomic abnormalities were increased subtalar pronation (63%), tight lateral structures at the knee (60%), and squinting patellae (43%).[272] If tight muscles or structures are identified, the patient is first taught to stretch them. This is particularly so with tight lateral structures at the knee. Taping of the patella is used to reduce pain during the exercises and therefore enhance vastus medialis obliquus activity. Most of the patients have lateral displacement (subluxation) of the patella. This can be corrected by firm taping from the lateral aspect of the patella medially. If patellar tilt is also present, it can be decreased by adding another piece of tape from the midline of the patella medially to lower the medial aspect of the patella and lift the lateral border up (Fig. 53–59).

Because most of the work of the quadriceps (and most of the pain) occurs in the standing position, training in the standing position is encouraged. With the affected limb forward and the knee flexed to 30 degrees, the patient is instructed to selectively contract the vastus medialis obliquus and adductors. The position is held for 10 seconds while the patient supinates the foot and slowly returns in pronation, but without reaching the habitual position of excessive pronation (Fig. 53–60). The exercise is repeated with the knee in increasing flexion up to 75 degrees, if this is not prevented by pain. In general, the greater the flexion of the knee, the more likely pain becomes. This exercise is intended to selectively train the vastus medialis obliquus and increase the awareness of foot position while correcting hyperpronation. Eccentric exercises such as stepping down from a step and exercises in the sitting position are also included. Taping of the patella is useful initially to decrease pain but may be reduced and eventually avoided as quadriceps strength and coordination improve.

The effectiveness of the McConnell taping technique to move the patella medially has been studied in 20 healthy men.[241] An axial weightbearing view with the knee at 40 degrees of flexion was obtained before taping, after taping, and after exercise to stress the tape. Measurement of the congruence angle showed that taping was effective in

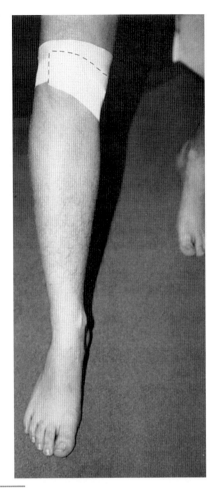

Figure 53–59. Taping of the patella for lateral patellar compression syndrome or subluxation. Lateral displacement of the patella can be corrected by firm taping from the lateral aspect of the patella medially. If lateral tilt is present, a second tape may be added from the midline of the patella medially to lower the medial border of the patella and lift the lateral border.

moving the patella medially, 9 degrees on average. Medial displacement was appreciated in 17 of 20 patellae (85%). Taping was ineffective in only 3 knees (15%). After exercise, no medial movement of the patella could be demonstrated in relation to the baseline situation. However, because the nontaped patella moved laterally an average of 4.6 degrees, taping was effective in preventing this postexercise shift. This study seems to suggest the limitations of taping in centralizing the patella and the need for reapplication of the tape during exercises if it loosens.

Gigante et al[148] performed CT in 16 girls with anterior knee pain related to patellofemoral incongruence to evaluate the effect of taping on patellar mediolateral position and the patellar tilt angle with and without quadriceps contraction. The authors found that taping had no effect on medializing the patella or reducing the tilt angle. On the contrary, Pfeiffer et al performed MRI on 18 healthy girls and found taping effective in reducing lateral patellar tilt.[316]

The clinical effectiveness of patellar taping has been evaluated in a prospective randomized study of 25 patients

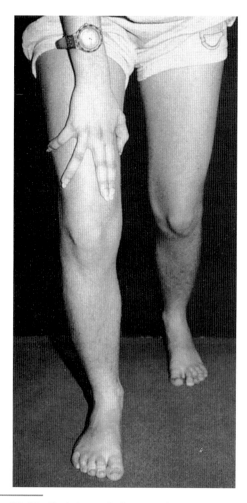

Figure 53–60. Training of the quadriceps muscle (and vastus medialis obliquus) in the standing position. The affected limb is forward, and the knee is flexed to 30 degrees. The patient palpates the vastus medialis obliquus to verify effective contraction of it. The position is maintained while the patient slowly supinates the foot and then returns in pronation, but without reaching the position of usual excessive pronation. The exercise is performed in series of 10 repetitions.

with patellofemoral pain.[230] A standard physical therapy program was used, including stretching exercises and quadriceps muscle strengthening with isometric, isotonic, and isokinetic exercises. Pain, activity, and isokinetic strength improved significantly, but no differences were found between the tape and no-tape groups. Therefore, it is probable that quadriceps strengthening, and not patellar taping, is the major factor in the improvement in such cases.[19]

We have satisfactorily used the program described by McConnell[272] in several patients with patellofemoral pain (lateral patellar compression syndrome) or chronic subluxation. Our success rate of almost 60% was lower than the 96% reported by the originator. It usually takes some time before the patient develops the skill necessary to selectively activate the vastus medialis obliquus and to set it in advance before movement is started. Some patients may never reach this goal. The program seems to give the best results in intelligent and well-motivated patients.

Our impression of conservative treatment of lateral patellar compression syndrome and chronic subluxation of the patella is that it is helpful in over half the patients, but activity modification is an important part of the program itself. It is unusual for a patient with a well-developed clinical syndrome of anterior knee pain to return to unrestricted participation in vigorous sports involving jumping and squatting. Nevertheless, many knees may be improved to the point that daily living and recreational activities can be performed with minor symptoms. A period of conservative treatment is therefore mandatory before surgical treatment. This policy avoids many unnecessary operations. Furthermore, should surgery be needed, the patient will already be aware of the exercises to be performed in the postoperative period.

Whitelaw and colleagues[399] emphasized the importance of reducing activity in the conservative treatment of patients with anterior knee pain. They treated 85 patients with a course of anti-inflammatory drugs, stretching, and quadriceps exercises. After a period of 4 to 6 weeks of treatment, 87% obtained symptomatic improvement. Those who reduced their activity level had a higher success rate (92%) than those who did not (68%). The patients were again reviewed at an average follow-up of 16 months, and the percentage of knees with symptomatic relief decreased (68%). Patients who regularly performed the prescribed home exercise program were more likely to improve knee function (71%) than those who did not (41%).

SURGICAL TREATMENT: LATERAL RETINACULAR RELEASE

Surgical treatment may be undertaken in knees with persistent disabling symptoms that do not improve after a prolonged (at least 6 months) supervised physical therapy course. In knees with pain as a result of lateral patellar compression syndrome, lateral retinacular release has frequently been performed.

Indications

We think that all authors would agree that the primary indication for lateral retinacular release is the demonstration of a tight lateral retinaculum. There is obviously no indication that a lateral release should be performed for a painful, but loose patella, which can be equally displaced medially and laterally. The ideal candidate should show decreased medial glide (one-fourth the patellar width or less) and decreased passive patellar tilt (the transverse axis of the patella cannot be elevated beyond the horizontal). Axial CT views should show patellar tilt with absent or mild subluxation. Fulkerson and Shea[140] think that a knee with an isolated patellar tilt (as shown on CT) but without significant osteoarthritic changes has the greatest likelihood of improving after lateral release.

Anatomic Details

The anatomy of the lateral retinaculum has been described by Fulkerson and Gossling.[130] It consists of two layers. The superficial layer (superficial oblique retinaculum) originates from the anterior border of the iliotibial band, and its fibers are directed anteriorly and distally and insert into the lateral border of the patella and the patellar tendon. If the superficial retinaculum is carefully freed and reflected posteriorly, the deep layer is exposed. It is composed of three different structures. The deep transverse retinaculum consists of fibers running from the lateral border of the patella to the deep aspect of the iliotibial band. The deep transverse retinaculum is less extended in a proximodistal direction than the superficial oblique retinaculum is because the former is present only at the lateral border of the patella whereas the latter extends more distally, along the lateral margin of the patellar tendon. Distal to the deep transverse retinaculum and deep to the superficial oblique retinaculum is a distinct patellotibial ligament that inserts proximally on the lower lateral border of the patella and distally on the lateral meniscus and proximal end of the tibia. Proximal to the deep transverse retinaculum, a second distinct band of fibers can be identified running from the lateral epicondyle and intermuscular septum in a distal and oblique direction to the upper part of the lateral margin of the patella (epicondylopatellar ligament). It seems that these structures are not constantly present and were found with variable frequency in an anatomic study.[325]

Beneath the deep transverse retinaculum is the thin capsulosynovial layer. Posterior to the lateral retinaculum lies the iliotibial tract, which inserts into Gerdy's tubercle distally, whereas proximally it blends with the intermuscular septum.

The anatomy of the vastus lateralis muscle and its junction with the patella has been described by Hallisey and colleagues.[168] Some of the fibers of the vastus lateralis originate from the lateral intermuscular septum and not from the femur (vastus lateralis obliquus). Three different anatomic patterns of insertion of the vastus lateralis obliquus were identified. It has been suggested that sectioning of the lateral retinaculum and vastus lateralis obliquus may be sufficient and save the main tendon of the vastus lateralis.

Open and Arthroscopic Lateral Retinacular Release

Lateral retinacular release can be performed with open or arthroscopic techniques, but the structures to be sectioned are obviously the same. They include the lateral retinaculum in its portion lateral to the patella and the patellar tendon. Proximally, we prefer to limit sectioning to the most distal fibers of the vastus lateralis (vastus lateralis obliquus) (Fig. 53–61). Release of all the tendon of the vastus lateralis has been recommended,[274,285] but this significantly prolongs rehabilitation and carries the risk of over-release (with medial subluxation of the patella) and quadriceps weakness. If the surgeon thinks that additional lateral release is required after sectioning the lateral retinaculum, the release should be extended distally, down to the tibial tubercle, to include the patellotibial and patellomeniscal ligaments. This modification has been shown to increase the effectiveness of lateral release while preserving the vastus lateralis tendon.[268]

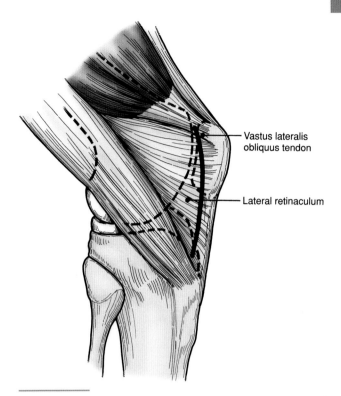

Figure 53–61. Structures to be sectioned at the time of lateral retinacular release (*continuous line*). They include the lateral retinaculum (lateral to the patellar tendon and patellar margin) and the tendon of the vastus lateralis obliquus. The main tendon of the vastus lateralis should be saved.

The lateral restraints to medial glide of the patella with the knee at 30 degrees of flexion have been studied by Johnson[216] at the time of surgery in 38 knees affected by patellar compression syndrome. The vastus lateralis obliquus was the primary restraint to medial glide of the patella in almost half the knees (47.5%), followed by the iliotibial band (16%) and the lateral retinaculum (5%). The three structures contributed equally in the remaining 31.5% of cases. Therefore, sacrifice of the main tendon of the vastus lateralis seems unnecessary.

The superior lateral genicular artery runs deep to the retinaculum along the distal fibers of the vastus lateralis and is sectioned during the procedure. Failure to obtain hemostasis of these vessels results in considerable hematoma formation.

If an open release is planned, it is safer to perform diagnostic arthroscopy first to rule out the possibility of an associated meniscal and ligamentous disorder or the presence of a loose body. After the tibiofemoral compartment is inspected, the arthroscope is placed in the superolateral portal, where tracking of the patella and the presence of cartilage changes are best evaluated. It is our experience that in most cases there is correlation between the clinical, radiographic, and arthroscopic findings. In the presence of normal patellar tracking, normal medial glide of the patella, and no chondromalacia (including no cartilage softening after careful probing), the preoperative diagnosis and the usefulness of a lateral release should be questioned.

After arthroscopic treatment of the associated disorder, lateral release may be safely accomplished through a short 3- to 5-cm lateral incision placed along the upper part of the lateral margin of the patella. After undermining the subcutaneous tissue in a proximal and distal direction (Fig. 53–62), the skin is mobilized to cut the whole retinaculum under direct vision. The superolateral genicular artery is coagulated, and hemostasis is confirmed by releasing the tourniquet before suturing. The capsulosynovial layer is sectioned if the surgeon thinks that it still tethers the patella laterally and if direct inspection of the patella is required. At the end of the procedure, it should be possible to lift up the lateral border and transverse axis of the patella at least 70 degrees from the horizontal axis (Fig. 53–63), and the patella should be free to glide medially over two quadrants with the knee at 30 degrees of flexion. The knee is flexed and extended several times to confirm improved tracking of the patella. If the tracking is still abnormal, as may be the case in knees with recurrent patella dislocation, consideration should be given to imbrication of the medial capsule[193] and possibly transfer of the tibial tubercle, depending on the disorder. Excessive lateral release should not be performed in an attempt to correct persistent lateral tracking.

Lateral retinacular release can also be performed "blindly" or under arthroscopic control. The advantage of this procedure is cosmetic (the skin incision is avoided), but there is a disadvantage in that the superior lateral genicular artery cannot be coagulated unless electrosurgery is used. We have used the technique described by Metcalf[285] in more than 50 cases.

First of all, the joint is thoroughly inspected with the arthroscope in the standard anterolateral portal, and the associated intra-articular disorder is treated. The arthro-

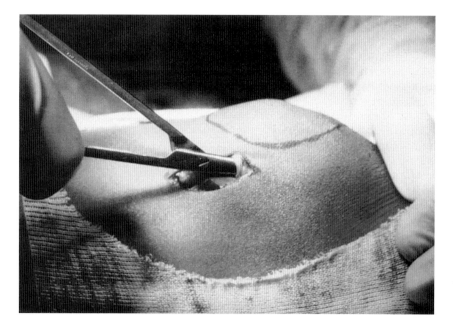

Figure 53–62. Lateral retinacular release can be performed through a short 3- to 5-cm incision placed along the upper part of the lateral border of the patella. After the subcutaneous tissue is undermined in a distal direction, the whole retinaculum can be sectioned under direct vision and the lateral genicular artery can be coagulated.

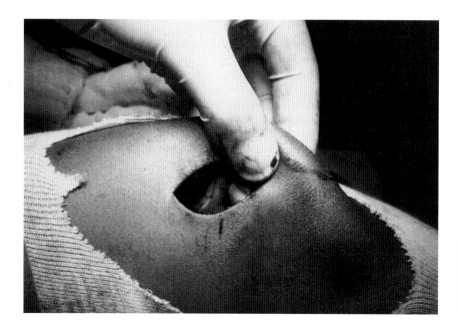

Figure 53–63. After lateral retinacular release, it is necessary to verify that the transverse axis of the patella can be lifted above the horizontal at least 70 degrees (positive turn-up sign).

scope is then inserted in the superolateral portal to better appreciate patellar tracking and the presence of chondromalacia. The articular cartilage can be shaved at this time. The subcutaneous tissue of the lateral parapatellar area is then infiltrated with bupivacaine (Marcaine) plus epinephrine. A subcutaneous tunnel is created from the anterolateral portal proximally toward the superolateral portal and distally toward the tibial tuberosity with Metzenbaum scissors. One blade of the scissors is redirected into the joint from the anterolateral portal, whereas the other stays in the subcutaneous tunnel (Fig. 53–64). The use of scissors with asymmetric blades enhances the operation. The lateral retinaculum is released up to the superolateral portal while staying near the lateral border of the patella.

During this phase, the arthroscope can be left in place or withdrawn to perform the procedure blindly, according to the preference of the surgeon. The direction of the scissors is then reversed and the retinaculum is sectioned from the anterolateral portal down to the tibial tuberosity along the lateral margin of the patellar tendon. The arthroscope is reintroduced in the anterolateral portal, and the proximal part of the sectioned retinaculum is visualized. The release may be extended proximally with 5-mm arthroscopic scissors introduced from an accessory lateral midpatellar portal. As stated earlier, we now do not advise release of the entire tendon of the vastus lateralis from the patella, and we limit the release to the fibers of the vastus lateralis obliquus. This is sufficient to obtain a 70-degree positive "turn-up sign," which should be confirmed at the end of the operation. Improved tracking of the patella can be also visualized by reintroducing the arthroscope from the superolateral portal. The entire procedure is performed under tourniquet control. The tourniquet is not released until a lateral pad and a compressive elastic bandage have been applied (Fig. 53–65). An intra-articular drain is left in the joint for 24 hours.

In recent years, we have used electrosurgery to perform the arthroscopic lateral release to avoid the complication of bleeding and hematoma from the superolateral genicular artery.[355] We perform the procedure with the arthroscope in the superolateral portal, as previously described. The irrigating solution may be changed from saline to distilled water. The release can be performed with a straight blade and the knife introduced in an accessory medial parapatellar portal (Fig. 53–66), or the release can be performed with a hooked blade and the knife introduced from the anterolateral portal. The arthroscope is then shifted to the anterolateral portal, and the release may be extended proximally with scissors introduced from an accessory lateral parapatellar portal. The procedure is performed without a tourniquet so that the bleeding vessels can be identified and soon coagulated.

Postoperative Rehabilitation

After arthroscopic lateral release without coagulation of the superior lateral genicular artery, the patient leaves the operating theater with a lateral compression pad and elastic bandage. If satisfactory hemostasis has been achieved during open surgery or with arthroscopic electrosurgery, a Robert Jones dressing is applied. The drain is removed at 24 hours, and the patient usually leaves the hospital on the first postoperative day.

The importance of starting quadriceps rehabilitation as soon as possible has been widely stressed because the success of the operation depends on the achievement of good quadriceps strength. Straight-leg–raising exercises can be started as soon as the patient recovers from anesthesia. The patient is encouraged to perform 100 repetitions daily in the first days and to increase thereafter. Flexion of the knee is also initiated early, and the patient is expected to reach 90 degrees by the end of the first week. Early recovery of flexion has an important role in preventing the formation of scar tissue across the release because the release opens widely in flexion. Manipulation of the patella with medial glides and lift-up of the lateral border also have a role in preventing scar formation. They

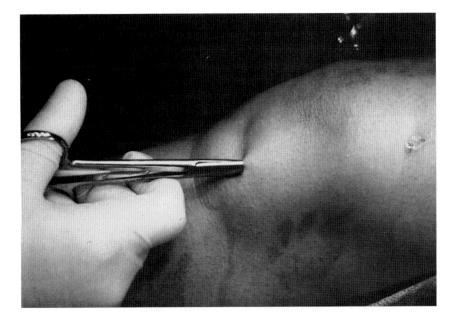

Figure 53–64. Arthroscopic lateral retinacular release according to the Metcalf technique. After diagnostic arthroscopy and treatment of the intra-articular pathology, Metzenbaum scissors with asymmetric blades are introduced from the anterolateral portal to divide the lateral retinaculum toward the superolateral portal.

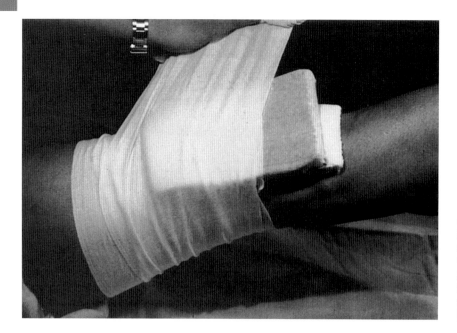

Figure 53–65. After percutaneous or arthroscopic lateral retinacular release without coagulation of the superolateral genicular artery, the tourniquet is not released until a lateral pad and compressive elastic bandage have been applied.

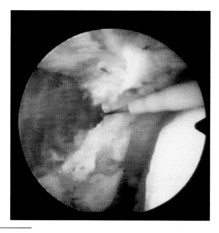

Figure 53–66. Arthroscopic lateral retinacular release using electrosurgery. The arthroscope is inserted into the superolateral portal and the knife into an accessory medial parapatellar portal. The procedure is performed without a tourniquet, and the bleeding vessels are soon coagulated.

can usually be instituted after removal of the dressing 10 days postoperatively. With this rehabilitation course, it does not seem to be necessary to remove a strip of retinaculum to avoid scarring at the release as suggested by Ficat and coworkers.[115]

The patient is allowed to walk with weightbearing as tolerated from the first postoperative day. Most patients prefer to use a cane for a week. Ice must be used liberally. Aspirin and nonsteroidal anti-inflammatory medications are avoided for 2 weeks before and 2 weeks after the procedure because they may increase bleeding.

The dressing is removed at 10 days. If a pressure pad has been applied, the dressing should not be removed earlier to inspect the wound. After 10 days, the stitches are removed and the patient is encouraged to increase flexion beyond 90 degrees and to perform patellar mobi-

lization exercises. The straight-leg–raising exercises are increased in number, and light weights can be added at the ankle. Stretching exercises for the hamstrings and gastrocnemius are added together with exercises for the muscles of the hip. Short-arc quadriceps exercises in the last few degrees of extension can be used if the patient is comfortable and has no patellofemoral crepitation in that arc. A stationary bicycle can be used without resistance and with a high seat.

There is obviously no standard approach to rehabilitation after lateral retinacular release. Progress should be monitored in the individual patient. We think that the most important indicators of improvement are the absence of pain and effusion. If such is the case, rehabilitation can be advanced safely. Ice after the exercises is advised for a long time postoperatively. If the goals of early rehabilitation are successfully met, including recovery of range of motion and sufficient quadriceps strength, more dynamic exercises under weightbearing conditions can be introduced, as explained in the discussion of conservative treatment in this chapter. These exercises are better suited to patients with athletic motivations. Emphasis should be placed on the role of the vastus medialis obliquus and the importance of maintaining its tone. Many patients may prefer to visit a rehabilitation center for some sessions.

Patients should be made aware of the necessity of continuing a home exercise program indefinitely. Recurrence of pain is often associated with low compliance with rehabilitation exercises and insufficient quadriceps tone. It should also be pointed out that some exercises, including the extension exercise with weights on the ankle, deep knee bends, and activities involving squatting and jumping, overload the patellofemoral joint and are likely to cause a relapse of symptoms. They should be limited or, better, avoided. Finally, it should be remembered that although the procedure may seem a minor one, rehabilitation is usually prolonged; most patients require 3 months before they return to recreational activities.

Results of Lateral Retinacular Release for Patellar Pain Syndromes

Evaluation of the results of lateral retinacular release, as well as comparison of publications from different centers, is difficult. Differences between the evaluation methods and rating systems may prevent accurate comparison of the results. Furthermore, there is an additional difficulty with the selection of patients. No classification is used consistently by most authors; therefore, it is not clear whether the cases are comparable. Some authors did not divide the patients suffering from patellar pain from those complaining mainly of instability.[37,180,273,274,283] In other publications, it is clearly stated that patients complained mainly of patellar pain, and these studies are summarized in Table 53–3. It is not clear in most of the series whether only knees with lateral patellar compression syndrome were included—that is, knees with biomechanical abnormalities leading to overload of the lateral facet while the patella remains centered in the sulcus—or there were also knees with chronic subluxation of the patella—that is, knees with subluxation of the patella but in which pain is still the main complaint. Nevertheless, despite the unavoidable differences in the selection of patients, in the methods of clinical and radiographic evaluation, and in the scoring systems, some interesting observations can be made.

Overall, 879 knees treated with open, closed, or arthroscopic lateral retinacular release for patella pain syndromes are included in Table 53–3. They were reviewed with variable follow-ups ranging from 6 to 64 months. The results were satisfactory in 73% of the cases on average. In other words, the results were unsatisfactory in one of four knees.

Unsatisfactory Results. Several authors have attempted to identify factors that correlate with an unsatisfactory result. Micheli and Stanitski[286] found that females had a worse prognosis than males did and that insufficient reduction of the patella on postoperative radiographs and severe chondromalacia were associated with inferior results. Metcalf[285] reported a 12% decrease in the percentage of good and excellent results with follow-up increasing from 1 to 4 years. No deterioration in results was

Table 53–3. Results of Lateral Retinacular Release for Patellar Pain Syndromes

AUTHOR	YEAR	NO. OF KNEES	AVG. FOLLOW-UP (mo)	TYPE OF RELEASE	% SATISFACTORY RESULTS	REMARKS
Ficat & Hungerford[116]	1977	174	6	Open	76	Excessive lateral pressure syndrome
Larson et al[242]	1978	45	18	Open, Z-plasty	82	If the result would be judged satisfactory when pain is absent or mild, only 62% would be in this category
Ceder & Larson[63]	1979	64	15	Open, Z-plasty	81	Patients underwent surgery subsequent to the previous series
Micheli & Stanitski[286]	1981	30	18	Open	76	Males did better (87%) than females (72%); worse results with persistent lateral tracking and severe chondromalacia
Harwin & Stern[174]	1981	25	24–45	Closed	100	No unsatisfactory results using the criteria of Merchant[283]
Metcalf[285]	1982	79	48	Arthroscopic	70	Reported 12% decrease in satisfactory results between 1 and 4 years of follow-up mainly as a result of failure to maintain quadriceps strength in young females
Osborne & Fulford[308]	1982	75	36	Closed	56	Mostly servicemen of the Royal Navy; all cases with advanced chondromalacia unsatisfactory; deterioration of satisfactory results between 1 year (82%) and 3 years (56%) of follow-up
Krompinger & Fulkerson[234]	1983	14	12	Arthroscopic	79	Knees with lateral retinacular pain; worse results in patients with marked malalignment or subluxation
Grana et al[158]	1984	43	30	Arthroscopic	91	Most patients returned to unrestricted vigorous activities (74%)
Ogilvie-Harris & Jackson[304]	1984	56	60	Arthroscopic	66	Good results are maintained at 1-year (88%) and 5-year (85%) follow-up in closed chondromalacia; results deteriorate with time in knees with open chondromalacia or exposed subchondral bone

Table continues

Table 53–3. Results of Lateral Retinacular Release for Patellar Pain Syndromes—Cont'd

AUTHOR	YEAR	NO. OF KNEES	AVG. FOLLOW-UP (mo)	TYPE OF RELEASE	% SATISFACTORY RESULTS	REMARKS
Simpson & Barrett[358]	1984	10	15	Arthroscopic	90	Worse results with age <30 years, hyperlaxity, insufficient release, and poor quadriceps strength
Schonholtz et al[344]	1987	7	48	Closed	14	Worst results reported in the literature
Bray et al[49]	1987	50	27	Arthroscopic	54	Two matched groups according to age and sex, workers' compensation board (WCB) claimant and nonclaimant; subjectively better results in non-WCB claimant group; more subsequent procedures in WCB group
Christensen et al[73]	1988	29	54	Open	76	No deterioration in results between 1-year and 4.5-year follow-up
Johnson[216]	1989	38	64	Open	87	Surgical assessment of primary lateral restraint to medial glide of the patella
Aglietti et al[10]	1989	20	40	Arthroscopic	60	Insufficient pain relief in 40%; vigorous activities in only 55%
Gecha & Torg[146]	1990	44	29	Open	57	Worse results in knees with associated malalignment, patellar hypermobility, and absence of tightness in lateral structures
Dzioba[102]	1990	76	48	Open	83	The following factors correlate with a satisfactory result: preoperative positive Merchant view, intraoperative demonstration of lateral tracking of the patella, thickened retinaculum, and postoperative "reduction" of the patella on the Merchant view

evident in males or in females older than 30 years. Deterioration was more frequent in young females who failed to maintain quadriceps strength with a continuous exercise program. Osborne and Fulford[308] also reported 26% deterioration of results in subsequent follow-up visits at 1 and 3 years postoperatively.

Knees with severe chondromalacia had uniformly unsatisfactory results. Krompinger and Fulkerson[234] reported less satisfactory results when the Q angle was greater than 20 degrees. Ogilvie-Harris and Jackson[304] reported good results in maltracking patellae with closed chondromalacia, with no deterioration between the 1-year (88%) and 5-year (85%) follow-up. Knees with major fasciculation of the patellar cartilage had a satisfactory outcome at 1 year (87%), but the results had deteriorated at 5 years (65%). Knees with exposure of subchondral bone were mostly unsatisfactory, even at the early follow-up visit. Simpson and Barrett[358] obtained less satisfactory results in patients older than 30 years, when the release was insufficient, when the quadriceps was rehabilitated incompletely, or when the patient had generalized ligamentous laxity. We have reported[10] significantly worse results in knees with postoperatively insufficient passive patellar tilt (<20 degrees above the horizontal), which would indicate insufficient release at the time of surgery or scarring across the defect.

Successful Results. Gecha and Torg[146] attempted to define the clinical prognosticators of success in a series of 44 lateral retinacular releases. They reported better results when malalignment and laxity were absent—that is, when there was no increased Q angle; generalized ligamentous laxity; patellar hypermobility; genu varum, valgum, or recurvatum; increased femoral anteversion; external tibial torsion; and abnormal foot pronation. A preoperatively positive Sage sign (medial displacement of the patella less than a fourth of the patellar width), indicating tightness of the lateral structures, also correlated with better results. Dzioba[102] attempted to determine the predictors of a good surgical outcome in a series of 76 knees. Among preoperative factors, the possibility of producing patellar pain by resisted extension of the knee, a positive restriction/apprehension test result, and evidence of patellar subluxation on the Merchant view correlated with better results. Among intraoperative factors, evidence of patellar subluxation at arthroscopy (overhang sign) and a thickened retinaculum at release were important predictors. At follow-up, reduction of the patella on the Merchant view was significantly correlated with a good outcome.

In light of our experience and the publications reported, we think that the following preoperative, intraoperative, and postoperative factors should be considered to be associated with successful results after lateral retinacular release.

Preoperative Factors. Preoperative factors should be carefully evaluated, and such evaluation is part of the patient selection process. The most important factor is probably the demonstration of maltracking of the patella and the presence of an excessively tight lateral retinaculum.[146,227,285] This can best be demonstrated by the presence of decreased medial glide of the patella and decreased lift-off of its lateral border (passive patellar tilt test). Conversely, no advantage can be expected after lateral release in patients with hypermobile patellae and loose joints. Confirmation of patellar maltracking should be obtained on axial views or CT, wherein a lateral patellar tilt, possibly associated with lesser degrees of subluxation, should be present. The presence of a grossly subluxated patella should raise suspicion that a lateral release might be inadequate to reposition the patella. The same is true in the presence of other signs of patellofemoral malalignment, including femoral anteversion, excessive lateral displacement of the tibial tubercle, a flat sulcus, patella alta, and vastus medialis obliquus hypoplasia. The greater their degree, the less likely that correction of a single factor (the retracted lateral retinaculum) may cure the symptoms.

Intraoperative Factors. Intraoperatively, arthroscopic demonstration of patellar maltracking and evidence of a thickened and retracted retinaculum are associated with better results. Incomplete release or scarring at the defect during the healing phase have been reported as causes of unsatisfactory results.[10,358] On the other hand, excessive release or wide release in a knee without underlying malalignment is not without consequences, and medial subluxation may develop.[190,191,382] The importance of associated chondromalacia to the final outcome has been widely debated. It seems that closed chondromalacia or lesser degrees of fibrillation do not affect the result, but diffuse deep fibrillation or exposure of subchondral bone with possible changes in the trochlear surface (early osteoarthritis) has been found to downgrade the result.[286,304,308,358]

Postoperative Factors. Among postoperative factors, most authors have stressed that failure to effectively rehabilitate the quadriceps and vastus medialis obliquus leads to poor results. Dzioba[102] reported that lateral retinacular release failed to center the patella in an axial view obtained a few days after the operation, but that the patella was reduced after 6 weeks of adequate muscular training. Correction of patellar position on postoperative axial views has been reported to correlate with good results.[102,286] Finally, the duration of the follow-up time may influence the rate of success. Some authors did not detect any influence of the follow-up time,[102,180,216,286,344] whereas others have reported decreasing success with longer follow-up intervals.[73,273,285,304,308] It is reasonable to think that some patients do not maintain sufficient quadriceps strength throughout the years and that relapse of symptoms may occur.

Complications

It has been proposed that a simple operation such as lateral retinacular release often helps, but does not harm the patient. This assumption has not proved to be true, and numerous complications have been reported, including hematoma formation, reflex sympathetic dystrophy, deep vein thrombosis, and medial subluxation of the patella.

Hematoma formation has been reported with variable frequency ranging from 1% to 42%.[10,34,63,234,284,344,360] Its incidence is higher after arthroscopic techniques that do not allow coagulation of the superolateral genicular artery. Small[360] reported that among arthroscopic procedures, lateral release had the highest incidence of complications (7.1%) and that 65% of the complications were hemarthrosis. The incidence is lessened by firm application of a pressure pad and elastic bandage, which should not be removed until 10 days after the operation. Aspirin or other anticoagulants should not be administered 2 weeks before and after surgery. More recently, the introduction of electrosurgery has allowed coagulation of bleeding vessels under direct control, thereby reducing this complication.[355] Once significant hemarthrosis has occurred, it can be managed by aspiration and the application of ice with a pressure pad and bandage. Some cases may require coagulation of the bleeding vessels because of recurrent episodes of hemarthrosis.

The significance of hemarthrosis to the final outcome has been interpreted in various ways. There is little doubt that the early rehabilitation phases will be prolonged and recovery delayed. Metcalf[285] thought that after hemarthrosis, there were no consequences for the final outcome except for delayed recovery. Simpson and Barrett[358] thought that hemarthrosis can ultimately lead to poor results, but the data did not substantiate their belief because the incidence of hemarthrosis was similar in the satisfactory and unsatisfactory groups (40% and 44%, respectively).

Medial subluxation of the patella after excessive lateral release or lateral release in a knee without underlying malalignment has been reported.[190,191] Hughston et al[191] reported on 65 knees that underwent surgical treatment to correct medial subluxation of the patella. Fifty-eight of them had undergone lateral release; the remaining cases were due to other surgical or traumatic causes. After exposure of the extensor mechanism, reconstruction of the lateral fascial layers in a side-to-side manner was performed in 39 knees (60%). When the remaining lateral tissue was insufficient, a reconstruction was performed. A 1-cm-wide wide strip of iliotibial band was dissected and left attached to Gerdy's tubercle. The fascia was then inserted into the inferolateral edge of the patella to reconstruct the patellotibial ligaments. This reconstruction was performed in 12 knees (18%). In the remaining 14 knees, iliotibial band tissue was insufficient. A quarter strip of the patellar tendon was detached distally with a piece of bone and reinserted laterally in the region of Gerdy's tubercle. In each case, an effort was made to advance the vastus lateralis distally from its retracted position. The average follow-up was 54 months (minimum, 24 months). Preoperatively, 78% of patients were limited to daily living activities or required external support. At follow-up, only 20% were still at this level. The procedure led to improvement in 75% of patients. Preoperatively, 69% of the knees had severe pain. At follow-up, 77% had no pain or had mild or moderate pain. Six knees required revision because of inadequate or excessive tensioning of the reconstruction. Overall, a good or excellent outcome was achieved in 80% of the knees, and 20% were failures (poor clinical result or revision needed). It appears from these data that these cases are difficult to treat, with many possible complications and a learning curve.

Because treatment of excessive lateral release and medial subluxation (Figs. 53–67 to 53–69) is difficult and the results are often less than optimal, every effort should be made to avoid it. The preoperative diagnosis should be accurate to avoid the risk of performing a lateral release in a knee without malalignment. At the time of release, detachment of the vastus lateralis obliquus is sufficient to allow increased medial glide of the patella.[202] The entire tendon of the vastus lateralis should not be released. If this is not sufficient to reposition the patella, medial plication should be considered with or without transposition of the tibial tuberosity. Over-release of the lateral structures should definitely be avoided. Excessive transposition of the tibial tuberosity in the medial direction is equally dangerous because the normal valgus alignment of the extensor mechanism is converted to varus.

OTHER CAUSES OF PATELLOFEMORAL PAIN

In this discussion, we have grouped several afflictions that although different in pathogenesis, clinical manifestations, and treatment, have a common denominator: The main symptom is peripatellar pain. Before establishing a definite diagnosis of patellar pain as a result of malalignment, it is useful to briefly exclude other causes of peripatellar pain. The diagnosis is usually straightforward in some afflictions such as bursitis or tendinitis but may be trickier in others, as in subtle forms of reflex sympathetic dystrophy. The list is by no means exhaustive because we included the most frequent afflictions only. We consider patellar and quadriceps tendinitis, peripatellar bursitis, reflex sympathetic dystrophy syndrome, osteochondritis dissecans, and synovial plicae. Osgood-Schlatter disease and Sinding-Larsen-Johansson disease are discussed elsewhere in this text.

Overuse Syndromes

Overuse syndromes are caused by repetitive trauma and include tendinitis of the quadriceps and patellar tendon and peripatellar bursitis.

TENDINITIS

Tendinitis is a frequent affliction of the patellar or quadriceps tendon, usually at their insertion on the patella. Tendinitis of the patellar tendon is frequently encountered in young people who play sports that involve a lot of jumping, such as baseball and volleyball (jumper's knee).

However, this affliction is not exclusive to athletes. Quadriceps tendinitis is more common in athletes in their forties. Tendinitis of the patellar tendon is more frequent than tendinitis of the quadriceps tendon.

Pathogenesis

The pathogenesis of the lesion is chronic overload of the tendon itself, which results in microtears within the tendon, fraying of the tendon fibers, and focal degeneration. The lesion is usually more evident in the deep fibers of the patellar tendon near its insertion on the apex of the patella.[82] Histological examination of specimens obtained at surgery has revealed mucoid degeneration and fibrinoid necrosis within the tendon.[265] The inflammatory response further weakens the remaining fibers of the tendon, so progressive weakening of this structure results.

It has been observed[371] that the highest loads are imposed on the tendon during deceleration, as when landing from a jump or when running and suddenly cutting. Curwin and Stanish[82] suggested that the force on the patellar tendon may reach 9000 N during fast running, 8000 N when landing from a jump, and 500 N in level walking. Zernicke and colleagues[413] estimated that 14,500 N was imposed on the patellar tendon of a weightlifter during a 175-kg lift when the tendon ruptured. The rupture took place when the lifter stopped the downward movement of the body (eccentric contraction). The calculated force on the patellar tendon exceeded the body weight of the lifter by more than 17 times. It is in fact during these decelerating activities that a patient suffering from tendinitis experiences the sharpest pain. Therefore, it seems that the tendon is inadequate to match the requests imposed on it during eccentric contractions.

Stress

If the pathogenesis of tendinitis is viewed in light of these considerations, it is not surprising that traditional programs based on rest, casting, and possibly steroid injections yielded a large failure rate. Symptoms subside during the resting period, only to recur as soon as the tendon is loaded again. It is well known that both rest and steroids have a negative effect on the mechanical properties of tendons and ligaments. On the other hand, if progressive stress is imposed on the tendons, tensile strength may be recovered. An extensive review of the effects of stress deprivation on collagen tissue is beyond the scope of this chapter, and the reader is referred to the excellent articles of Amiel and colleagues[16] and Woo et al.[407]

Diagnosis

The diagnosis of patellar or quadriceps tendinitis is usually straightforward and often suggested by the patient, who complains of a sharp localized pain at the upper (quadriceps tendinitis) or lower (patellar tendinitis) pole of the patella that is increased by activities that load the extensor mechanism. The diagnosis can be made through demonstration of tenderness of the affected site. Thickening of the tendon can be appreciated at the same time.

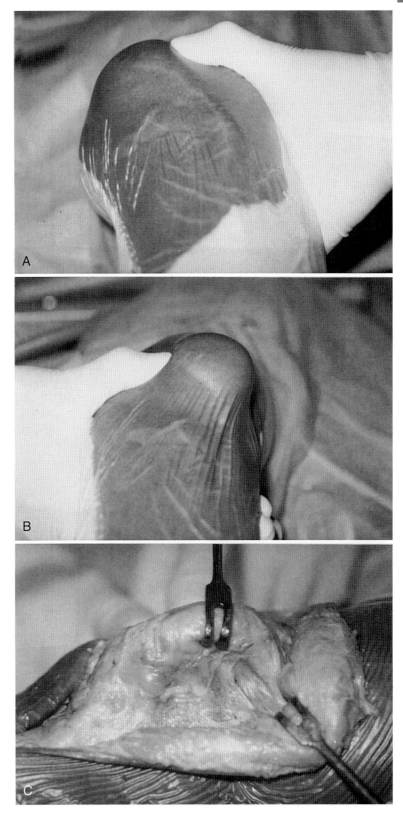

Figure 53–67. Twenty-five-year-old woman with failed reconstruction of the extensor apparatus. She underwent transposition of the tibial tuberosity with wide lateral release and medial plication. At the time of the reoperation, the patella could be abnormally displaced in both the medial (**A**) and lateral (**B**) directions. **C**, At surgery, the lateral retinaculum, the vastus lateralis obliquus, and the vastus lateralis tendons were all absent and substituted by a thin synovial-like tissue.

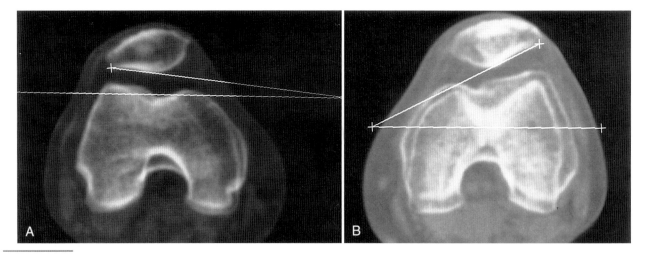

Figure 53–68. Computed tomography (CT) of the patellofemoral joint of a 25-year-old female who underwent proximal realignment (lateral release and medial plication) of both knees for recurrent dislocation of the patella. The first operation, on the right side (**A**), was clinically successful. The second operation, on the left side (**B**), was unsuccessful because of increased pain and feeling of instability. Physical examination showed excessive lateral release and apprehension while the patella was pushed medially. The CT scan shows a wider patellar tilt angle on the left side because of over-release of the lateral structures.

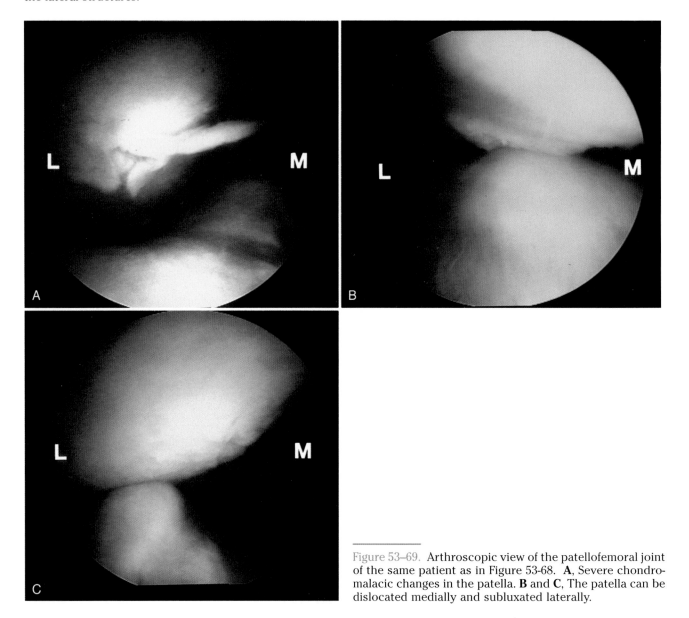

Figure 53–69. Arthroscopic view of the patellofemoral joint of the same patient as in Figure 53-68. **A**, Severe chondromalacic changes in the patella. **B** and **C**, The patella can be dislocated medially and subluxated laterally.

Thorough examination of the knee is mandatory because other causes of knee pain may coexist, especially patellofemoral pain, which often occurs in volleyball or basketball players. Effort should be made in these cases to establish the contribution of each structure to the symptoms of the patient.

Clinical Features

The severity of the lesion is classified clinically according to the severity of pain, the activities that precipitate it, and the duration, as suggested by Blazina and coworkers.[40] According to their classification, four stages are described:

Stage 1: pain only after sports

Stage 2: pain at the beginning of the sport, disappearing with warm-up, and reappearing with fatigue

Stage 3: constant pain at rest and with activity

Stage 4: complete rupture of the patellar tendon

This classification has been modified by Curwin and Stanish[82] and further divided into six stages.

Ultrasonography

We are using ultrasonography with increasing frequency to examine knees with patellar tendinitis. It is useful to confirm the diagnosis in doubtful cases and to monitor the evolution of the disease. Fritschy and De Gautard[124] reported the results of ultrasonographic examination of the patellar tendon in 15 normal subjects and 25 patients with jumper's knee. In normal knees, the average thickness of the tendon is 4 mm, as seen in longitudinal sections, and the average width is 21 mm, as seen in transverse sections. The tendinous fibers are parallel and homogeneous. Hyperechoic and hypoechoic zones alternate regularly in normal tendons. In knees affected by patellar tendinitis, three different aspects can be differentiated:

- Thickening and swelling, which are almost exclusive to the acute forms. The tendon is swollen but still has a homogeneous appearance.
- Heterogeneous structure with hypoechoic zones corresponding to edema and hyperechoic zones corresponding to fibrous scar and intratendinous calcification. This aspect is more frequent in the knees of patients affected for several months.
- Irregularities of the tendinous envelope. The tendinous envelope is thickened and has a poorly defined outline. The tendon has a heterogeneous appearance but is not swollen.

These findings suggest a progression toward the chronic phase, in which inflammation no longer has a major role.

Conservative Treatment

In recent years, we have used the conservative program suggested by Curwin and Stanish[82] with excellent results. As alluded to earlier, the program aims at imposing increasing stress on the patellar tendon so that its strength can be gradually increased. Eccentric exercises are used for this purpose. Furthermore, stretching is an integral part of the program and is used to increase the resting length of the muscle-tendon unit and decrease loads on the tendon. Patients need to exercise every day for at least 6 weeks. Much encouragement is needed because long-standing tendinitis may require 1 month or more before the patient experiences improvement. If improvement is obtained by 6 weeks, the frequency of training sessions may be gradually reduced, but not interrupted. A cooperative patient usually learns the exercises easily, and these exercises can be conveniently performed at home. Half an hour every day is usually sufficient for the average recreational athlete. Sports participation during the 6-week period is allowed, with the exclusion of activities that cause pain at the tendon.

The training program consists of five successive phases.[82]

1. Warm-up for 5 minutes.
2. Stretching of the quadriceps and hamstring muscles, performed in three to five repetitions, 30 seconds each.
3. Eccentric exercises:
   a. The patient begins the exercise in the standing position, suddenly drops to a squatting position, then recoils to the standing position (Fig. 53–70). At the point of reversing direction, some discomfort is usually felt at the affected site.
   b. Three sets of 10 repetitions are used initially and may be increased to five to six sets of 15 to 20 repetitions.
   c. Loads on the tendon can be varied by changing the velocity of the exercise or by adding weights to the shoulders of the patient.
   d. Most recreational athletes start the exercise without weights and increase the speed throughout the week, starting at low speed (days 1 and 2) and then progressing to moderate speed (days 3 to 5) and high speed (days 6 and 7).
   e. If the exercise can be performed without excessive discomfort at the maximum speed, weights can be added to the shoulders, and the sequence is repeated the second week.
   f. In high-level athletes, adding weights to the shoulders may not be convenient because of the excessive loads required.
   g. In selected patients, jumping from increasing heights on the affected limb may be a more reasonable alternative (plyometrics).
4. Stretching of the quadriceps and hamstrings is repeated as indicated in step 2.
5. Crushed ice is applied for 5 to 10 minutes on the affected area.

Using this program, Stanish and colleagues[371] have reported a good success rate in 200 athletes suffering from chronic tendinitis. With an average follow-up of 16 months, 44% had complete pain relief, 43% had a marked decrease in symptoms, 9% were unchanged, and 2% were worse after the program. We have used this program in our patients with quadriceps or patellar tendinitis in recent years. During the same period, only two knees required surgery because of persisting symptoms. It is our

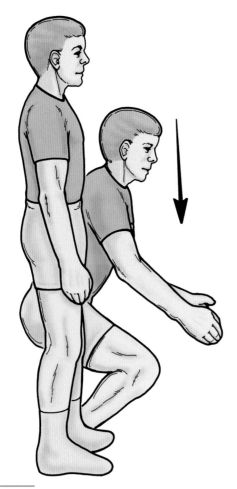

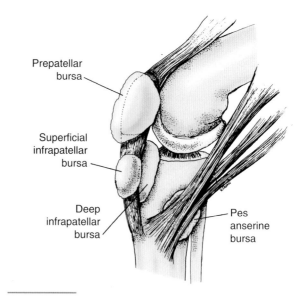

Figure 53–71. Peripatellar bursae. The prepatellar bursa is the most frequent site of inflammation—the so-called housemaid's knee.

Figure 53–70. Eccentric exercise for the treatment of patellar tendinitis. The patient begins the exercise in the standing position and suddenly drops to the squatting position. At the point of reversing the direction of the movement, high loads are imposed on the patellar tendon and some (but not excessive) discomfort should be felt at the affected site. The load on the tendon can be varied by increasing the speed of the exercise or by adding weights on the shoulders. (From Curwin S, Stanish WD: Tendinitis: Its Etiology and Treatment. Lexington, MA, Collamare Press, 1984.)

impression that if the program is diligently followed, only a minority of patients will need surgery.

Surgical Treatment

When surgical treatment is necessary because of failure of conservative regimens, we have used the following operation for patellar tendinitis.[314] The tendon is approached through a short longitudinal, 5-cm skin incision centered over the distal pole of the patella. The tendon is split longitudinally in line with its fibers, in its proximal part up to the apex of the patella. Three or four incisions are usually sufficient to remove the degenerated tissue from within the tendon and to drill the apex of the patella with

a 2-mm Kirschner wire. If severe degenerative changes are noted at the apex, the tendon can be elevated from the apex itself while preserving its continuity with the prepatellar aponeurosis, and the apex is then resected with a rongeur. We have found that this more extensive procedure is rarely necessary.

Postoperatively, the limb is protected in a Robert Jones dressing for 10 days. Partial weightbearing is allowed soon and progresses to full weightbearing by 4 to 6 weeks. Progression in the exercises is dictated by the amount of dissection and detachment of the tendon that has been performed at surgery and by local symptoms. Usually, 3 to 4 months is required before full return to participation in competitive sports.

PERIPATELLAR BURSITIS

Numerous bursae are described around the knee (Fig. 53–71) that under certain circumstances, can become inflamed. The prepatellar bursa is subcutaneous and present in most people. It usually covers the lower half of the patella and the upper half of the patellar ligament. Because it becomes chronically inflamed in those whose occupation involves much kneeling, inflammation of this bursa has been known as "housemaid's knee." It is seldom difficult to recognize. The infrapatellar bursa lies between the lower part of the patellar ligament and the upper part of the tuberosity of the tibia. It is small and separated from the synovial membrane of the knee by the fat pad. The pain, tenderness, and swelling localized in this region are usually distinctive. Pes anserinus bursitis is overdiagnosed; the pain is often attributable to other causes (e.g., medial meniscal tears, degenerative arthritis, or osteonecrosis).

Reflex Sympathetic Dystrophy

Reflex sympathetic dystrophy is a vasomotor disturbance characterized by pain out of proportion to the initial trauma, swelling, stiffness, and discoloration. These are considered the four cardinal findings of reflex sympathetic dystrophy. Secondary findings include osteoporosis, decreased skin temperature, and skin atrophy.[237]

This entity was originally described by Mitchell,[290,291] who described its development after an injury to a major mixed nerve in the extremity. He named it *causalgia*, which literally means "burning pain" in Greek and describes the most evident symptom of this disorder. Because of the original description, several other terms have been used to label this syndrome, including acute atrophy of bone,[377,378] Sudeck's atrophy, reflex dystrophy,[96] minor causalgia,[186] shoulder-hand syndrome, reflex sympathetic dystrophy,[108] and reflex sympathetic imbalance.[237]

Reflex sympathetic dystrophy is the most widely accepted term today to describe this syndrome and is used throughout this chapter. The term in itself has the connotation of a dreadful syndrome that could not be cured until 1930, when the neurosurgeon Spurling reported successful cervicothoracic sympathectomy.[368] Before that time, most patients with a fully developed form of reflex sympathetic dystrophy were doomed to drug abuse and chronic invalidism. Suicide was a possible end result.

The term reflex sympathetic dystrophy underlines the fact that the disorder is mediated by the sympathetic nervous system. The sympathetic nervous system has its cell bodies in the lateral horn of the thoracic and lumbar cord. These send unmyelinated fibers to the sympathetic thoracic and lumbar ganglia. Cell bodies in the sympathetic ganglia send nonmyelinated fibers that join the nerves to reach the periphery of the body. The neurotransmitter of the neurons of the ganglia is norepinephrine, with the exception of the sympathetic fibers to sweat glands, where the neurotransmitter is acetylcholine.

Reflex sympathetic dystrophy has more recently been identified as a definite syndrome of the knee, and recognition of it has allowed understanding of a previously unrecognized source of pain.[79,220,237,305,351,385]

SYMPTOMS

The four cardinal signs of reflex sympathetic dystrophy are pain, stiffness, swelling, and discoloration. Their expression varies among different patients and between the upper and lower extremities. The following discussion is therefore focused on reflex sympathetic dystrophy of the knee.

Pain is an essential symptom for the diagnosis of reflex sympathetic dystrophy. The character of the pain is burning or deeply aching. It is increased by motion and exposure to cold temperatures. The patient is often unable to indicate a specific source of the pain and complains that the knee is diffusely painful on the front, medial, and lateral aspects. Tenderness is equally diffuse.

Stiffness is a common complaint and may consist of the loss of a few degrees of flexion and extension, but it may also be more severe. We have observed patients with fully developed forms of reflex sympathetic dystrophy who had an arc of motion of just a few degrees and walked on a stiff, semiflexed knee. Stiffness is secondary to pain. If it persists for sufficient time, secondary changes in the periarticular soft tissues develop, including capsular fibrosis and proliferation of fibrofatty tissue in the joint.

Swelling is often reported by the patient. At objective examination, induration of the peripatellar tissues is often appreciated. Effusion is a less frequent finding.

Discoloration of the skin around the knee and the skin of the leg and foot is often present with a dusky, cyanotic aspect, which may increase during exposure to cold temperatures.

Secondary changes include osteoporosis, hyperhidrosis, decreased skin temperature, and skin atrophy.

Osteoporosis predominantly involves the patella, but it may spread to the femur and tibia. In more advanced forms, it acquires the typical "patchy" appearance that is suggestive of reflex sympathetic dystrophy (Fig. 51–72).

Hyperhidrosis can be reported by patients in the early stages; such patients tell of changing their socks several times during the day. Decreased skin temperature can be appreciated by palpation or better documented with thermography. Skin atrophy is usually less marked in the knee than in the hand or foot but is sometimes encountered in late stages. Muscle and quadriceps atrophy, however, is present early in the course of the disease.

The evolution of the disease is usually divided into three stages[237,239]: acute, subacute or dystrophic, and chronic or atrophic. The acute stage includes the disease within the first 3 months from onset. Pain, stiffness, increased sweating, and coolness of the limb are characteristic features in this early phase. The subacute stage includes patients with continuing symptoms from 3 months to 1 year. Pain often reaches its maximum intensity during this period and is accompanied by osteoporosis. The limb is pale with dry and fixed skin, and severe quadriceps wasting is noted. The chronic or dystrophic stage includes patients who have had symptoms for a period longer than 1 year. Thickening and fibrosis of the periarticular tissues, osteoporosis, and skin atrophy are the most prominent findings of the late stage.

ETIOLOGY

The accepted pathogenetic theory involves the presence of a painful lesion as a result of trauma or previous surgery. The trauma is often minor. The painful stimulus enters the cord through the afferent sensitive fibers and stimulates an efferent autonomic impulse that produces vasoconstriction, ischemia, and therefore pain. This increases the already-present painful stimulus. A vicious circle is therefore created.[252] Because the painful stimulus is often trivial, it is necessary to postulate a diathesis of patients who would have a hyperactive sympathetic system (Fig. 53–73).

The initial trauma seems to frequently involve the patellofemoral joint. Katz and Hungerford[220] reported that in their series of 36 cases of reflex sympathetic dystrophy of the knee, injuries or operations about the

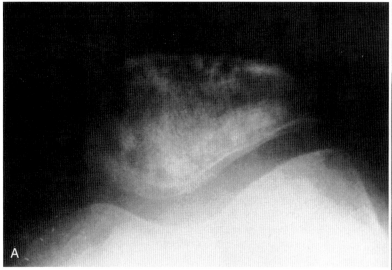
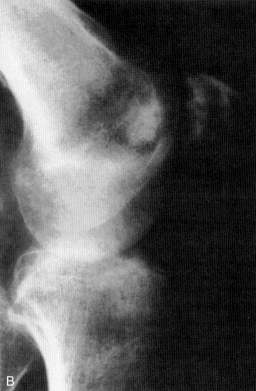

Figure 53–72. Fifty-three-year-old man with a fully developed form of reflex sympathetic dystrophy. The typical patchy osteoporosis is clearly evident in the patella (**A**) but also, to a lesser degree, in the femur and tibia (**B**).

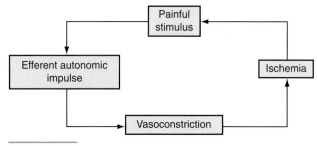

Figure 53–73. The vicious circle of reflex sympathetic dystrophy. A painful stimulus evokes an efferent autonomic impulse, which produces vasoconstriction, ischemia, and therefore pain. (From Livingstone WK: Pain Mechanisms: A Physiologic Interpretation of Causalgia and Its Related States. New York, Macmillan, 1943.)

patellofemoral joint triggered the syndrome in 64% of cases. Surgery on the patellofemoral joint, including chondral shaving and lateral release, was reported in 11 of 14 knees with reflex sympathetic dystrophy by Cooper and colleagues.[79] Injury to a nerve around the knee may also trigger the disease. Poehling and coworkers[319] reported on a group of 35 knees with reflex sympathetic dystrophy. All the patients had evidence of damage to the infrapatellar branch of the saphenous nerve. In their series of 36 cases of reflex sympathetic dystrophy of the knee, Katz and Hungerford[220] found evidence of nerve damage in 6 knees (17%), twice to the peroneal nerve and four times to the infrapatellar branch of the saphenous nerve.

Surgery can trigger reflex sympathetic dystrophy, as has been noted by most authors. In some cases it is not easy to understand whether the syndrome developed after surgery or the symptoms of the disease were present preoperatively and were just worsened by inappropriate surgery. Unfortunate patients undergoing several surgical procedures, with increasing symptoms after each one, are still observed. Repeated arthroscopy to look for some internal derangement that is not found can only cause the symptoms to deteriorate.

Several theories have been proposed to explain the pathogenesis of reflex sympathetic dystrophy. Livingstone,[252] as previously mentioned, suggested that a vicious circle explains this disorder. Chronic irritation of a sensory nerve causes increased afferent input and results in activation of the internuncial neuron pool in the spinal cord, which in turn results in increased sympathetic activity. These concepts have been refined by Melzack and Wall,[280] who described specialized cells located in the substantia gelatinosa of the dorsal horn. These cells would modulate the central transmission of afferent impulses. Small (C) fibers, such as sympathetic fibers, suppress the inhibitory influence of the substantia gelatinosa on afferent impulses and therefore "open the gate," thereby increasing transmission of pain impulses to the brain. In contrast, activation of large (A) fibers stimulates the inhibitory influence of the substantia gelatinosa and therefore "closes the gate." It appears that predominant small-fiber activation results in increased central pain transmission through an open gate (gate theory).

Peripheral mechanisms have been implicated in the genesis of reflex sympathetic dystrophy by Doupe and coworkers.[99] They suggested that in a traumatized nerve, artificial synapses may develop between afferent sensory fibers and sympathetic efferents. Therefore, an afferent stimulus would automatically cause an efferent sympathetic response. This theory fits well in knees with a demonstrable nerve injury but cannot explain cases of reflex sympathetic dystrophy in the absence of a nerve injury. It seems that different mechanisms, both peripheral and central, may cause reflex sympathetic dystrophy. This fact may be of some therapeutic importance.

An apparent contrast exists between increased sympathetic activity in an extremity and the clinical evidence of a swollen, edematous limb with increased blood flow, as shown by plethysmographic studies.[97] This apparent contrast can be explained by the development of arteriovenous shunting at the precapillary level, as suggested by an increased oxygen level in venous blood.[375]

DIAGNOSIS

Clinical Features

The diagnosis of reflex sympathetic dystrophy is primarily clinical, and unless this possibility is remembered, many correct diagnoses will be missed. The main symptom of the syndrome is continuing pain out of proportion to the initial injury. Additional features that may be present to a variable degree include joint stiffness, swelling, discoloration, quadriceps and skin atrophy, decreased skin temperature, and hypersensitivity to touch and cold. Ladd and coworkers[237] proposed the term *reflex sympathetic imbalance* to describe a disorder that does not have all four cardinal signs of reflex sympathetic dystrophy. We think that the key to the diagnosis of reflex sympathetic dystrophy is the coexistence of unduly prolonged pain with vasomotor disturbances and possibly joint stiffness. The correct diagnosis may be difficult to make, especially in patients with previous surgery.

Radiography

Radiographic evaluation is useful to exclude bone lesions and to confirm the presence of osteoporosis primarily involving the patellofemoral joint. Patchy osteoporosis of the patella, though an inconstant finding, is diagnostic of reflex sympathetic dystrophy. Bone scans have been widely used in joints suspected of having this disease.[231,233,256] The usual picture is one of increased uptake in the affected joint. Bone scans have been reported to be highly sensitive (96%) in reflex sympathetic dystrophy of the hand.[256] However, their sensitivity seems to be less at the knee. Increased uptake in knees with this disease has been reported in 61% of cases by Katz and Hungerford,[220] in 88% by Ogilvie-Harris and Roscoe,[305] and in 71% by Cooper and associates.[79] Therefore, a positive bone scan result is not considered essential to diagnosis of the disease in the knee, but it is helpful. Increased uptake of the isotope has often been detected in other asymptomatic joints of the same limb, which is further confirmation of the more diffuse nature of the disease (Fig. 53-74).

Thermography

Thermography has been used to document temperature changes in affected limbs.[389] The expected finding is a skin

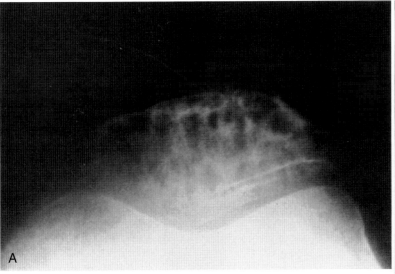
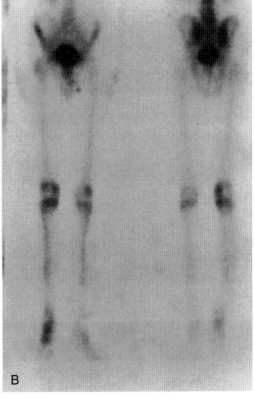

Figure 53-74. Axial radiographic (**A**) and technetium Tc 99m methylene diphosphonate bone scan (**B**) of a 52-year-old man affected by reflex sympathetic dystrophy of the right knee. The typical patchy osteoporosis of the patella is present. Increased uptake of the isotope is evident at the knee, but also at the right ankle, which was asymptomatic at the time of the bone scan.

temperature decreased by 1° or more over the knee,[79,220] but the sensitivity of the examination is not 100%, similar to bone scan examinations. Cold stress testing techniques have also been used to document an abnormal sympathetic response of the limb. The technique of isolated cold stress testing[319] involves placing the feet in a refrigerator unit for 20 minutes (cooling phase) and then at room temperature for another 20 minutes (rewarming phase). Temperature probes taped over the pulp of each digit are used to record temperature changes during the test. In a group of 35 patients affected by reflex sympathetic dystrophy of the knee, the results of isolated cold stress testing correlated with the improvement after vasoactive therapy. The average skin temperature of both limbs was lower in patients who did not experience improvement than in those who benefited from treatment.

Because reflex sympathetic dystrophy and vasomotor instability seem to be a bilateral phenomenon, an average of both limbs was considered. Decreased temperature in nonimproved patients was noted before cooling (23.7° C versus 25.3° C), after cooling (15° C versus 16.4° C), and after rewarming (20.8° C versus 22.2° C). This study suggests that knees with lesser degrees of vasomotor instability (i.e., warmer during the isolated cold stress test) have a better chance of recovery with therapy.

Arthroscopy

Arthroscopy has been performed in knees with reflex sympathetic dystrophy to confirm the absence of a significant intra-articular disorder. Absence of an intra-articular disorder beyond some minor synovitis has been reported in 100% of cases.[305,385] Therefore, the use of arthroscopy in knees with suspected or proven reflex sympathetic dystrophy is not justified and is potentially dangerous because symptoms may become worse afterward. On the other hand, it has been pointed out that an intra-articular disorder may trigger recurrence of the syndrome.[237,301] The safest sequence is to cure reflex sympathetic dystrophy first and then correct the associated—and rarer—intra-articular disorder.

Sympathetic Blockade

Because reflex sympathetic dystrophy is caused by abnormal activation of the sympathetic system, the most direct and effective confirmation of the diagnosis is obtained by sympathetic blockade. This is considered the gold standard in the diagnosis of this disorder.

A sympathetic block is performed by injecting a local anesthetic around the lumbar ganglia of the sympathetic chain. A positive response to the test (or blockade) consists of complete disappearance or relief of most of the pain and an increase in skin temperature of at least 1° C. At the same time, absence of a motor or sensory block should be documented.

Other authors[237] have suggested the use of epidural sympathetic blockade with 0.25% bupivacaine to confirm the diagnosis of reflex sympathetic dystrophy. Spinal blockade has also been suggested as a means of differentiating pain of sympathetic, somatic, and central origin.[351]

With this technique, normal saline is injected first. If relief is obtained, the pain is of psychogenic origin. Otherwise, spinal blockade with a 5% procaine solution is performed. The patient is carefully monitored for pain, pinprick sensation, motor function, skin temperature, and blood pressure to assess sensory, motor, and sympathetic nerve function, respectively. The thickness of the nerve fibers determines their sensitivity to the anesthetic solution. The small preganglionic fibers of the sympathetic system are the most sensitive and therefore recover last. If the patient does not obtain pain relief after introduction of the procaine with an effective sensory and motor block, the pain must be of central origin (psychogenic or malingering). If relief is obtained but pain returns with the pinprick sensation, the pain is of somatic origin because somatic fibers recover faster than sympathetic fibers. On the other hand, if pain relief lasts longer after recovery of sensory and motor function while sympathetic functions are blocked, the pain is presumably of sympathetic origin.

Our preference for the diagnosis of reflex sympathetic dystrophy is direct sympathetic blockade of the lumbar ganglia because the test is easier to interpret.

TREATMENT

It has been suggested that the course of reflex sympathetic dystrophy is self-limited. Unfortunately, many cases persist for years and lead to permanent disability. Poplawski and colleagues[320] examined a series of 126 patients who had post-traumatic dystrophy of the hand and foot with a follow-up longer than 5 years. Nearly all had continuing symptoms. It seems, therefore, that treatment is needed in these patients and early treatment may be especially helpful.[138,346]

Treatment includes physical therapy modalities, sympathetic blockade, regional sympathetic blockade, and sympathectomy.

Physical Therapy

Physical therapy modalities may be sufficient alone in the lightest forms and are used in addition to sympathetic blockade. The goal is to regain function of the atrophied and contracted extremity. Gentle active mobilization of the limb is encouraged. Passive mobilization and manipulation should be avoided because of the potential for deterioration of symptoms. Weightbearing is encouraged as tolerated.

A decrease in edema of the limb is accomplished by frequent elevation above heart level. Elastic stockings are worn if the patient can tolerate them. Distal-to-proximal manual massage is also helpful. Increasing stimulation should be applied to the patient to increase the level of tolerance. This can be achieved by using a whirlpool, hot and cold baths, and massage. The action of desensitization modalities may be related to enhancement of large (A) fiber transmission, which closes the gate to the small, pain fiber input.[346]

Transcutaneous Electrical Nerve Stimulation

Transcutaneous electrical nerve stimulation has often been used for the treatment of reflex sympathetic dystrophy. Melzack[279] suggested that it may work by activating transmission in both large and small fibers. Large fibers would act by "closing the gate" to the afferent input, as noted previously. Small-fiber input also contributes to blocking pain transmission by enhancing the inhibitory areas of the brainstem. Transcutaneous electrical nerve stimulation may be safely added to physical therapy modalities, and complications of this treatment have been reported only sporadically.[346]

Sympathetic Blockade

Sympathetic blockade is the most obvious form of treatment of reflex sympathetic dystrophy because it allows breakage of the vicious circle of pain leading to sympathetic activation leading to ischemia leading to pain. Sympathetic blockade can be achieved by introducing an anesthetic at the level of the lumbar ganglia or in the epidural space. Alternatively, regional sympathectomy of the limb may be achieved by introducing guanethidine or reserpine. Finally, surgical sympathectomy can be performed.

Block of the lumbar ganglia is the most selective modality to obtain sympathetic blockade without motor or sensory blockade. The same procedure can be used as a diagnostic modality, as discussed earlier. The level at which sympathetic blockade should be achieved is an important consideration. Erdemir and associates[106] noted that the upper sympathetic trunks may not be taken into account and lead to incomplete pain relief, as noted in two cases in their series. To establish the correct level, they have suggested sensory epidural anesthesia. The most proximal level at which pain relief is obtained with sensory epidural anesthesia determines the level of sympathetic blockade or surgical sympathectomy.

Pain relief after sympathetic blockade can recur after some time, and the block can be readministered. Up to four or five blocks can be performed. If recurrence of pain is the problem, surgical sympathectomy can be considered.

Cooper and coworkers[79] have suggested the use of an epidural catheter to continuously deliver the anesthetic and obtain prolonged anesthesia. Bupivacaine was used at the beginning in all the patients, and the initial dose was 1 mg of 0.5% solution per kilogram of body weight. After administration of the initial dose, the continuous drip was set at 0.25 to 0.5 mg/kg of body weight per hour, which was tuned to provide complete epidural anesthesia.

During the initial phase, range-of-motion exercises are greatly enhanced by complete sensory anesthesia. Because a motor block is also present, a continuous passive motion machine is used to increase the arc of motion. When the patient has regained motion, usually after 2 to 3 days of bupivacaine, narcotic epidural agents are substituted for the bupivacaine. Morphine, meperidine, or fentanyl is used. They cause a sensory block without a motor block, and the patient can therefore exercise actively and walk. After the pain has been relieved and motion is increased,

the dose of narcotic drugs is progressively decreased and finally interrupted. The epidural catheter is maintained for an average of 4 days. Cooper and colleagues were convinced that epidural blockade has several advantages over sympathetic blockade of the lumbar ganglia. First, complete sympathetic and somatic anesthesia is a desirable factor initially, when aggressive mobilization is required. Second, an epidural block is easier to administer and the procedure is more familiar to most anesthesiologists. Third, the epidural catheter may be left inside for 5 to 7 days to provide continuous pain relief.

O'Brien et al[301] reported a positive experience using sympathetic blockade in a group of 60 patients affected by reflex sympathetic dystrophy of the knee. Forty patients had reflex sympathetic dystrophy as a result of knee surgery. Arthroscopic procedures were the most frequent cause (24 patients), followed by total knee replacement (7 knees). Lumbar sympathetic blockade was performed with 0.5% bupivacaine. Successful blockade was confirmed by a rise in skin temperature of the affected limb and by a concomitant increase in pulse wave plethysmography. The patients underwent sympathetic blockade every other day for 8 days (four sessions) and then one blockade weekly until the patient became asymptomatic. At a 2-year follow-up, 92% of the patients had relief of their reflex sympathetic symptoms with an average of 9 blockades (range, 1 to 30). Sixteen patients underwent additional surgery after the sympathetic blockade as part of the treatment of their reflex sympathetic dystrophy. There was no relationship between the duration of symptoms and the outcome of treatment. The final outcome was significantly related to the presence of an anatomic lesion. Among the 36 patients without a persisting anatomic lesion, 81% were rated good. Among the 24 patients with a persisting anatomic lesion, only 21% were rated good.

Postganglionic regional sympathetic blocks with guanethidine[150,171] or reserpine[31] have been used in limited series. The anesthetic drug is administered according to a modified Bier technique for the induction of local anesthesia. After exsanguination of the extremity with an Esmarch bandage, a pneumatic tourniquet is applied and released after 20 to 30 minutes. Guanethidine accumulates in the intraneuronal storage granules and displaces epinephrine, thereby providing prolonged sympathetic blockade. Reserpine reduces the reuptake of catecholamines.

The sympatholytic effects of intravenous injection of guanethidine and reserpine have been studied in a group of volunteers.[275] Adrenergic (vasomotor) and cholinergic (sweating) sympathetic functions were studied separately. Only guanethidine significantly increased skin temperature after cold stress testing. Neither of the drugs affected cholinergic sympathetic functions. It thus seems that intravenous guanethidine may be especially valuable in the treatment of syndromes wherein vasoconstriction predominates.

Oral sympatholytic drugs may be used in addition to physical therapy in the less severe forms or in conjunction with sympathetic blockade in the more advanced cases. Ca^{2+} channel blockers (usually nifedipine) have also been used to obtain vasodilatation.

Surgical sympathectomy may be indicated if four or five sympathetic blockades fail to achieve consistent pain relief or if the pain relief is incomplete. Alternatively, chemical sympathectomy can be achieved by using alcohol.

Steroids

Systemic steroids have been used in the treatment of reflex sympathetic dystrophy since the original report of Steinbrocker and Argyros.[374] Favorable results have been documented by Christensen and colleagues[74] and Kozin et al.[232,233] The side effects of steroids should not be disregarded, and Glick[149] reported weight increase and moon facies in patients treated with steroids for reflex sympathetic dystrophy. Prednisone has been frequently used at a high dose initially (60 to 80 mg/day in divided doses) and then quickly tapered off.[344] The mechanism of action of corticosteroids has not been elucidated completely. It has been suggested that steroids reduce the chronic perivascular inflammatory infiltrate that has been found in synovial specimens.[232,233] Their stabilizing effect on base membranes can also reduce capillary permeability and therefore decrease the plasma extravasation commonly associated with the early stages of reflex sympathetic dystrophy.[346] Poplawski and colleagues[320] used an intravenous solution of 20 to 30 mL of 1% lidocaine (Xylocaine) without epinephrine and 80 mg of methylprednisolone (Solu-Medrol). The mixture was injected in the previously exsanguinated limb after inflation of the pneumatic tourniquet. The block was maintained for 30 minutes. This treatment was administered to 28 extremities affected by reflex sympathetic dystrophy of the hand or foot. A satisfactory result was obtained in 21 of the 28 cases (75%).

CONCLUSIONS

We think that reflex sympathetic dystrophy of the knee remains an underdiagnosed affliction. It is essential to maintain a high level of suspicion of this disorder in every patient with prolonged, diffuse, and nonspecific pain. Further surgical procedures and the resultant increased disability may be avoided. The gold standard for diagnosing this affliction remains a positive response to sympathetic blockade of the lumbar ganglia. Early treatment (within 6 months) has the highest chance of success.

Synovial Plicae

ANATOMY

The anatomy of synovial folds of the knee joint was first described by Mayeda.[271] Later, in 1939, Jino[214] described the arthroscopic appearance of synovial folds in cadavers. Pipkin[317] first suggested that plicae may be a source of symptoms. Since then, the role of synovial folds as a cause of internal derangement of the knee has remained a matter of controversy. Some authors think that plicae are a fairly

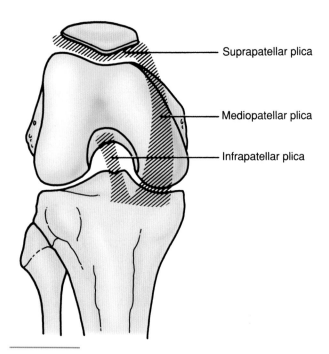

Figure 53–75. The three synovial plicae of the knee joint: suprapatellar, mediopatellar, and infrapatellar.

frequent cause of symptoms that can be cured by resecting the thickened fold, whereas others contend that they are rarely, if ever, symptomatic.

The three synovial plicae of the knee are commonly described as suprapatellar, mediopatellar, and infrapatellar (Fig. 53–75). The suprapatellar plica divides the suprapatellar pouch from the patellofemoral joint. It runs from the anterior surface of the femur to the posterior aspect of the quadriceps tendon in a horizontal plane. The mediopatellar plica lies along the medial wall of the joint. It originates near the suprapatellar plica and runs in the frontal plane down to insert in the fat pad. The infrapatellar plica, or ligamentum mucosum, attaches proximally at the anterior outlet of the intercondylar notch and widens as it runs distally to insert into the fat pad.

DEVELOPMENT

The development of the synovial folds of the knee joint has been the subject of several investigations. It is commonly thought that the knee is initially divided into three compartments, the medial and lateral tibiofemoral compartments and the suprapatellar bursa.[318] The synovial plicae are therefore considered remnants of the original divisions of the joint. A further study of this subject was presented by Ogata and Uthoff,[302] who examined 116 embryos and fetuses. Formation of the joint space was first observed at around 8 weeks of gestation. Multiple small cavitations around the patella and femoral condyles coalesce to form larger cavitations. A single cavity was observed at around 10.5 weeks. However, mesenchymal tissue strands remain at certain sites to form synovial plicae. The presence of residual mesenchymal tissue in the medial patellofemoral joint (mediopatellar plica) is explained by the peculiar anatomy of this region. Contact between the femur and patella is mainly lateral, with a large interval on the medial side and a narrow one on the lateral aspect. Therefore, the amount of mesenchymal tissue is larger on the medial side of the patellofemoral joint. Incomplete resorption of this tissue results in the presence of a mediopatellar plica. The genesis of the other two synovial folds of the knee is different. The suprapatellar plica can be explained as a remnant of the septum between the suprapatellar bursa and the patellofemoral joint. The infrapatellar plica is equally a remnant of the septum between the medial and lateral patellofemoral compartments.

MORPHOLOGY

The frequency and morphology of the synovial folds of the knee have been investigated widely. Sakakibara[337] classified the mediopatellar plica into three types: type A is a cord-like elevation in the synovial wall, type B has a shelf-like appearance but does not cover the femoral condyle, and type C is a shelf-like structure that covers the femoral condyle.

Dandy[84] classified the medial shelf according to its width: absent, ridge, less than 1 cm, less than 2 cm, and more than 2 cm. He also classified the suprapatellar plica according to its width: absent, up to one-fourth of the width of the suprapatellar pouch, between one-fourth and one-third, between one-third and two-thirds, more than two-thirds, and complete and perforated. The anatomy of the suprapatellar and mediopatellar plicae was studied arthroscopically according to these classifications in a series of 500 knees. The suprapatellar plica extended up to one-third of the width of the suprapatellar pouch in 64.2%, between one-third and two-thirds in 4%, and two-thirds or more in 31.6%. The mediopatellar plica was absent or represented by a low ridge in 36%, up to 1 cm wide in 44.8%, and up to 2 cm wide in 12% of the knees. In the remaining knees, the mediopatellar plica was either perforated (1.2%), high (3.8%), or reduplicated (1.6%). There was no correlation between the pattern of the plica and the age of the patient. No association was found between large suprapatellar and large mediopatellar folds, but the mediopatellar shelf was absent significantly more often in knees with a narrow suprapatellar plica.

In patients in whom both knees were examined, the aspect of the plicae was significantly similar between one knee and the other. In conclusion, arthroscopic observation of synovial plicae in a large series of 500 knees indicates that a narrow suprapatellar plica extending up to one-third the width of the suprapatellar pouch was present in about two-thirds of cases whereas a broad suprapatellar plica extending two-thirds or more of the width of the pouch was present in the remaining third. A wide mediopatellar plica, over 2 cm, was rare. One-third of the knees had no plica or just a ridge, almost half had a small plica up to 1 cm, and only 12% had a medium-sized plica, between 1 and 2 cm. There was no relationship between the size of the suprapatellar and the mediopatellar plica, thus suggesting a different developmental mechanism.

PATHOPHYSIOLOGY

The accepted theory of the pathophysiology of the plica syndrome[172] involves an inflammatory process of the fold that alters the extensible qualities of its tissue. Normally, the synovial folds slide gently over the femoral condyle during flexion and extension of the knee. However, a thickened, edematous, and fibrotic fold loses its elasticity and eventually snaps over the condyle during flexion. At this time, further inflammation occurs along with replacement of elastic tissue by fibrous tissue. Friction between the fibrotic fold and articular cartilage can cause degenerative changes in the femoral condyle or patellar cartilage.

SYMPTOMS

The most frequent symptom of plica syndrome is pain.[172,192,208,295,328,391] Previous trauma to the medial aspect of the knee can precede the onset of symptoms. Pain is frequently medial or retropatellar and dull. Swelling, giving way, or snapping is reported by roughly a third of patients. Objective findings include tenderness of the medial side of the patellofemoral joint and possibly palpation of a thickened mediopatellar plica. A snapping sensation may be appreciated during flexion of the knee.

ARTHROSCOPIC SURGERY

A definitive diagnosis of symptomatic mediopatellar or suprapatellar plica syndrome can best be achieved at arthroscopy. Treatment involves sectioning of the plica and removal down to its base with a motorized shaver. Removal of the mediopatellar plica is best accomplished by viewing it from the superolateral approach and working with the instruments through the anteromedial and anterolateral portals.

The results of arthroscopic removal of the mediopatellar plica have been reported to be influenced by the presence of associated disorders. Vaughan-Lane and Dandy[391] reported that the best results were obtained in 26 knees with definite tenderness of the medial shelf; 61% of these results were excellent. On the other hand, in 21 knees with a mediopatellar shelf plus other abnormalities, the result was excellent in only 14%. Similarly, Richmond and McGinty[328] achieved satisfactory results in 86% of knees with an isolated symptomatic mediopatellar plica, whereas the percentage decreased to 69% in knees with associated conditions.

CONCLUSIONS

It is our impression that the diagnosis of plica syndrome should be rare.[226] An associated disorder is frequent and often involves the patellofemoral joint (lateral patellar tracking, chondromalacia). In these cases, the role of a thickened plica remains doubtful. There are certainly cases in which a thickened plica is an isolated finding and arthroscopic resection relieves the symptoms. Nevertheless, such cases are rare in our experience and are encountered probably once or twice a year in the practice of a busy arthroscopist. The placebo effect of arthroscopy should also be accounted for when evaluating the results of this surgery.

Osteochondritis Dissecans

Osteochondritis dissecans of the patella is a rare disease involving the separation of an area of articular cartilage and underlying subchondral bone. The affliction was first described by Rombold.[329] The bone fragment may remain in situ or become detached to form a loose body.

Two theories have been proposed to explain the etiology of osteochondritis dissecans of the patella: interruption of the blood supply (ischemic theory) or mechanical factors (traumatic theory). The trauma may be either a single direct injury or the application of repetitive stress to the patellofemoral joint as a result of sports activities. The presence of a subluxing patella causes tangential stress on the patellar ridge, which has also been reported as a possible cause of osteochondritis dissecans.[316]

Several small series of osteochondritis dissecans of the patella have been reported in the English literature.[95,103,206,312,349,376] A number of common clinical features have been pointed out by various authors. The disease is more common in males than in females, and the second decade of life is the most frequently affected. The most frequent symptom is patellofemoral pain, followed by swelling. Feelings of a loose body, locking, or giving way or episodes of patellar subluxation are reported in roughly a third to a fifth of cases.[349] Bilaterality has been reported in about 20% of cases. The most frequent finding at physical examination is retropatellar crepitus, sometimes accompanied by effusion and retropatellar tenderness. Increased patellar mobility or lateral tracking of the patella can be evident in some cases.

The lesion constitutes a defect of the articular surface of the patella, best visualized on the lateral view. The axial view helps localize the lesion in the medial or lateral facet. CT and MRI studies can be used to better define the site and extension of the lesion. MRI allows determination of the viability of the fragment and the integrity of the overlying articular cartilage when no synovial fluid is identified between the fragment and crater.[316] The lesion may involve virtually every part of the articular surface of the patella, but the distal and medial sites are the most frequently affected. In 77% of the cases of Desai and colleagues[95] and 81% of the cases of Schwartz and coworkers,[349] the lower two-thirds of the central ridge and the medial facet were involved. The upper third of the central ridge and the lateral facet are less frequently affected.

CONSERVATIVE TREATMENT

Conservative treatment is based on restriction of activities and quadriceps strengthening. Although the success rate is not high, such treatment may be worth attempting in younger patients with minor symptoms and the fragment still in situ, without sclerosis of the crater on radiographs or MRI evidence of fluid expression through interrupted cartilage and necrosis of the bone fragment.

SURGICAL TREATMENT

Surgical treatment varies according to the stage of the lesion. In patients complaining mainly of a loose body and locking, arthroscopic removal of the loose body may be all that is needed. If the lesion on the patellar surface is smooth and filled with fibrous tissue, it should be left alone. However, the most frequently encountered situation is a fragment in situ but detached to a variable degree. In these cases, removal of the fragment plus curettage of the defect is performed. The procedure can be performed arthroscopically or through arthrotomy. The first alternative seems preferable because it allows evaluation of the entire joint and assessment of patellar tracking. Other procedures, including lateral retinacular release or realignment, can be added as needed.

The results of surgical treatment of osteochondritis dissecans of the patella, more often removal of the bone fragment and curettage of the crater, have been variably reported. Stougaard[376] and Schwartz and coworkers[349] have reported unsatisfactory results in over half of patients, whereas a better outcome was documented by Edwards and Bentley,[103] Smillie,[362] and Desai and associates.[95] A large lesion is more likely to cause persistent symptoms after removal. In these cases, curettage of the crater and fixation of the bone fragment should be considered, at least in patients with a fragment in situ and no MRI evidence of cartilage interruption or necrosis of the bone fragment. However, it is not yet known whether the results of fixation are superior to simple removal and curettage of the defect.

CONCLUSIONS

Osteochondritis dissecans of the patella is a rare disease that more frequently affects males in their second decade of life. If conservative treatment fails, surgical treatment may offer improvement of symptoms in a number of patients, but the long-term results reported in the literature are not uniformly satisfactory.

Osteochondritis dissecans is even more rarely localized to the femoral trochlea.[251,364] The radiolucent area on the trochlea can easily be missed; this fact probably contributes to the rarity of the lesion. CT are MRI are helpful in better defining these lesions. The principles of treatment previously outlined for osteochondritis dissecans of the patella can also be applied to the trochlear form.

PATELLAR SUBLUXATION AND DISLOCATION

Patellar subluxation and patellar dislocation can be grouped together as patellar instability. The difference is one of degree and not of nature. Subluxation is an alteration in the normal tracking of the patella, but with the patella still within the femoral sulcus. Dislocation means that the patella has been completely displaced out of the sulcus. Therefore, unless the patient has noted the patella lying on the lateral aspect of the knee, it appears that it may be impossible to know whether the patella was subluxated or dislocated during the single episode of instability. Furthermore, the patella may show lateralized tracking without episodes of instability (chronic subluxation of the patella).

From a clinical point of view, the following situations can be encountered and will be described: acute dislocation; chronic subluxation; and recurrent, habitual, and permanent dislocation of the patella.

Acute Dislocation of the Patella

The diagnosis of acute dislocation of the patella is applied to knees seen after the first episode of dislocation.

SYMPTOMS

The patient usually seeks treatment at the emergency department and reports that during a twisting movement of the knee a snap was felt, the knee gave way, and the patient fell down on the ground. The patient may have been able to observe the patella lying on the lateral side of the knee. At this time, the knee is straightened and the patella relocated in the sulcus. Swelling occurs rapidly. Therefore, it is unusual to observe the patella still in the dislocated position in the emergency department.

If the patient has observed abnormal lateral displacement of the patella, the diagnosis is straightforward. Otherwise it can be difficult.[395] The physician is faced with a swollen and tender knee and a nonspecific history of giving way. Aspiration of the joint demonstrates hemarthrosis, and fat droplets may be present if an associated osteochondral fracture has occurred. Careful inquiry about the mechanism of injury often reveals that the patient had the foot fixed on the ground whereas the femur was internally rotated relative to the tibia and the quadriceps was contacted, as in the act of changing direction while running. In this position, the Q angle is increased, and contraction of the quadriceps pulls the patella laterally. This mechanism has also been described in baseball pitchers.[165] More rarely, a direct blow on the medial side of the knee may cause patellar dislocation in a knee with underlying malalignment.

PHYSICAL EXAMINATION

If the knee is grossly swollen, the physical examination is best performed after aspiration of the joint. Tenderness is easily evoked by palpation of the medial retinaculum and medial femoral epicondyle. Attempts to displace the patella laterally are prevented by apprehension. Testing for

ligamentous stability is rendered more difficult by muscle contracture, but with some patience one should be able to confirm the presence of an intact anterior cruciate ligament with a gentle Lachman test.

The differential diagnosis should include anterior cruciate ligament injury and rupture of the quadriceps or patellar tendon. The latter diagnosis can be excluded by asking the patient to perform a straight-leg raise. If the patient is unable to do this exercise and a defect that is proximal or distal to the patella is appreciated, the diagnosis is confirmed.

If an acute patellar dislocation is suspected, it is informative to examine the contralateral knee. Evidence of malalignment or maltracking of the patella may further enhance the correct diagnosis.

PATHOANATOMY AND IMAGING

Routine anteroposterior, lateral, and axial views should be obtained in every patient with a suspected diagnosis of acute patellar dislocation. We have found that a Merchant view[284] can be easily obtained in these patients. Lateral displacement of the patella within the femoral sulcus may be evident, even if less frequently than in knees with recurrent patellar dislocation. In a group of 55 acute dislocations, Vainionpää and colleagues[390] found an abnormal lateral patellofemoral angle on the Laurin view[244] in only 34%. The physician should look for other abnormalities associated with patellar instability, including a high-riding patella and a flat femoral sulcus.

Oblique and notch views may be necessary to exclude the presence of osteochondral fractures (Fig. 53–76) of the medial patellar facet or lateral femoral condyle.[20,331] These fractures are usually produced during relocation of a dislocated patella, when the medial patellar facet strikes against the lateral femoral condyle. The conflict is increased by quadriceps contraction. The frequency of associated osteochondral fractures in knees with acute patellar dislocation has been reported to be around 5%.[330] In 18 knees with this association, the fracture involved the inferomedial aspect of the patella in 14 (78%), the lateral femoral condyle in 2 (11%), and both these structures in 2 (11%). Failure to demonstrate osteochondral fragments on radiography does not imply that there was no damage to the articular surface. In fact, arthroscopic examination of a knee with acute patellar dislocation has often revealed extensive cartilage injury of the patella and/or the lateral femoral condyle. More rarely, a larger portion of the patella is fractured during acute dislocation (Fig. 53–77). In these cases, one should consider fixing the fragment rather than excising it.

A relationship between articular hypermobility and chondral damage after acute patellar dislocation has been suggested.[372] In a series of 30 adolescents with acute patellar dislocation, articular hypermobility was evaluated by using the criteria of Beighton and Horan,[25] including passive thumb apposition to the volar aspect of the forearm, fifth-finger hyperextension, and elbow and knee hyperextension beyond 10 degrees. The patients underwent routine radiography and arthroscopy. Five (33%) of

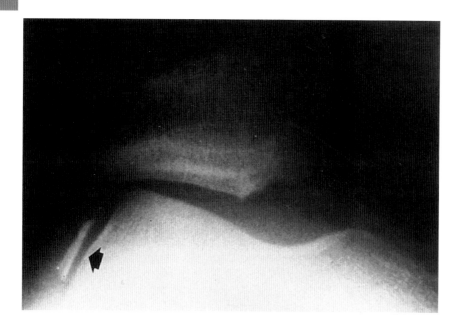

Figure 53–76. An osteochondral fracture occurred during an episode of acute patellar dislocation. The osteochondral fragment is lying in the lateral gutter.

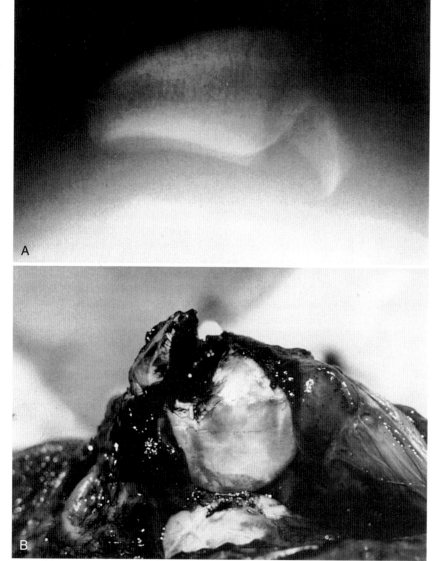

Figure 53–77. Acute patellar dislocation in an 18-year-old boy. A large fragment, involving over 50% of the medial patellar facet, had been detached, as is evident in the axial view (A) and at surgery (B).

the 15 knees with hypermobility had articular injuries as noted at arthroscopy, including 2 displaced and 3 undisplaced osteochondral lesions. Twelve (80%) of the 15 patients without articular hypermobility had evidence of undisplaced (7) or displaced (5) osteochondral injuries. Only 5 (29%) of the 17 osteochondral/chondral lesions were visible on initial radiographs. These data suggest that articular injury is far more common when visualized by arthroscopy than on radiographs. Articular hypermobility is a "protective factor" against chondral damage, with a 2.5 times reduction in the incidence of lesions.

Traction fractures may be revealed by radiographic examination and should be differentiated from osteochondral fractures.[123] They occur on the medial border of the patella (Fig. 53–78), where a small flake of bone may be avulsed by the medial retinaculum put under tension by lateral displacement of the patella.

MRI has been used to investigate knees with acute patellar dislocation.[338] It has allowed a better understanding of the pathoanatomy of this condition. A series of 23 knees were examined with radiographs and MRI, followed by arthroscopy (19 knees) and open exploration of the medial soft tissues (16 knees). Clinically, 83% of the knees exhibited moderate to large effusion and 70% had tenderness over the posteromedial soft tissues and adductor tubercle (Bassett's sign). Radiographs revealed osteochondral fractures of the patella in 21% of cases and fractures of the lateral femoral condyle in 5%. MRI showed moderate to large effusion in all the knees. A tear of the femoral insertion of the medial patellofemoral ligament (at the adductor tubercle) was present in 87% (20 knees). Two knees had a significant sprain of the medial patellofemoral ligament without detachment. One knee had a detachment of the medial retinaculum from the margin of the patella. Variable amounts of retraction of the vastus medi-

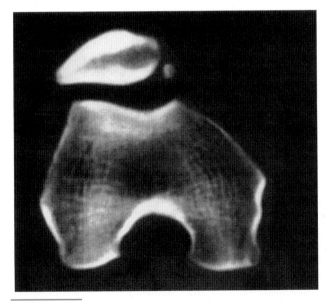

Figure 53–78. A traction fracture of the patella occurred during an episode of acute patellar dislocation. The bone fragments have been detached from the medial margin of the patella by the pull of the medial retinaculum put under tension by lateral displacement of the patella.

alis obliquus and increased signal were present in 78%. Bony injuries were noted in 87% of the lateral femoral condyles, near the sulcus terminalis, and in 30% of the patellae, medially.

Nineteen knees with gross lateral instability underwent arthroscopy and evaluation under anesthesia. Medial soft-tissue tears were not visualized by arthroscopy. Sixteen knees underwent open exploration. The fascia was found to be intact in all cases. After elevation of the vastus medialis, hemorrhage was common in the area of the adductor tubercle. A tear of the femoral insertion of the medial patellofemoral ligament was present in 15 of 16 knees. In some cases, this was a true avulsion. Repair of the torn medial patellofemoral ligament restored stability to the patella. None of the 12 patients with a follow-up of more than 2 years experienced recurrent dislocation, although 4 had episodes of possible subluxation. It appears that detachment of the medial patellofemoral ligament from its insertion into the adductor tubercle is the most frequent lesion in acute dislocation of the patella. This is in agreement with the biomechanical work of Conlan et al,[78] who showed that the medial patellofemoral ligament was the primary restraint to lateral patellar dislocation and provided 53% of the total restraining force, followed by the patellomeniscal ligament, which contributed 22%. Detachment of the vastus medialis obliquus from the adductor tubercle was also evident from MRI and surgical findings.

PROGNOSIS AFTER ACUTE PATELLAR DISLOCATION

Several authors have attempted to define the prognosis after conservative treatment of acute patellar dislocations (Table 53–4). Cofield and Bryan[76] reported a discouraging experience because 52% of their 50 cases were rated as failures. In light of their experience, they recommend selective immediate repair in patients with anatomic variants that would contribute to recurrence in high-level athletes and in knees with displaced intra-articular fractures. Larsen and Lauridsen[240] reviewed 79 acute patellar dislocations. A relevant primary trauma was reported in 41 cases (52%), whereas in 38 (48%), the trauma had been minor or absent. Patella alta and increased passive patellar mobility were more frequent in patients with atraumatic dislocations. The dislocation was more frequently atraumatic in females (57%) than in males (32%). Younger patients had a higher incidence of predisposing factors, which were present in 84% of patients younger than 14 years, in 69% between 15 and 19 years, and in 41% between 20 and 29 years. In agreement with this finding, redislocation was more likely in younger patients (<20 years of age).

Hawkins and colleagues[176] reviewed 27 cases of acute patellar dislocation; 20 of these were treated conservatively with immobilization, whereas 7 underwent immediate surgical stabilization and lateral release. Recurrence of dislocation was encountered in 15% of the conservative group, and a further 20% complained of instability. All three patients with redislocation showed signs of

Table 53–4. Prognosis after Conservative Treatment of Acute Patellar Dislocations

AUTHOR	YEAR	NO. OF KNEES	TREATMENT	AVG. FOLLOW-UP (mo)	REDISLOCATION (%)	REMARKS
Cofield & Bryan[76]	1977	50	Conservative		44	High redislocation rate; 52% of knees were considered unsatisfactory; 27% required further surgery
McManus et al[277]	1979	26	Cast for 6 weeks	31	19	Dislocations in children; 42% complained of instability without dislocation; 38% were asymptomatic
Larsen & Lauridsen[240]	1982	79	Cast or bandage	71	NA	Unable to define factors that may predispose to redislocation except age younger than 20 years
Hawkins et al[176]	1986	20	Arthroscopy (9), cast (11)	40	15	All patients who experienced redislocation had obvious lower limb malalignment; some degree of pain was present in 75% of cases
Cash & Hughston[58]	1988	74	Cast	96	36	Recurrence rate is higher in presence of signs of patellofemoral dysplasia of the opposite knee (43%) than when these are absent (20%); higher redislocation rate in younger patients
Garth et al[144]	1996	39	Functional padded sleeve	46	20	One-third of cases remain unsatisfactory according to subjective and objective criteria
Mäenpää & Lehto[257]	1997	100	Cast (60), splint (17), bandage (23)	156	44	44% redislocation, 19% patellofemoral pain or subluxation; only 37% without complaints

NA, not available.

malalignment of the lower limb. There were no redislocations in the surgical group, but 28% of these patients complained of instability, which was attributed to residual quadriceps atrophy. Residual pain, mostly mild to moderate, was present in 75% of the conservative group and 42% of the surgical group. In light of their data, Hawkins and colleagues recommend surgical treatment of knees that exhibit a combination of predisposing signs, including genu valgum, increased Q angle, patella alta, or abnormal patellar configuration.

Cash and Hughston[58] examined 103 knees with acute dislocation of the patella and divided them into two groups according to the presence or absence of signs of anatomic predisposition to recurrence. These signs were present in 69 knees (67%) and absent in 34 (33%). After conservative treatment, the group with normal anatomy had a low recurrence rate (20%) and a high incidence of satisfactory results (75%); only one patient needed further reconstruction. In contrast, the group with the anatomic abnormalities suffered a higher recurrence rate (43%) and had a lower percentage of satisfactory results (52%); almost a third of these knees needed further surgery. It is noteworthy that in this series of patients with acute dislocation of the patella, 70% were males, contrary to most of the previous series, which reported a female preponderance. Age was a predisposing factor to dislocation. The recurrence rate was highest (60%) in children 14 years or younger; no patient older than 28 years incurred redislocations.

Mäenpää and Lehto[257] reviewed a series of 100 acute patellar dislocations with long-term follow-up (average, 13 years; range, 6 to 26 years). The patients were initially

treated with a cast (60 knees), a splint (17 knees), or a bandage (23 knees), according to the physician's preference. At follow-up, 13% had restricted extension, 21% had restricted flexion, 61% had retropatellar crepitation, and the apprehension test yielded positive results in 52%. Redislocation had occurred in 44% of the knees. The redislocation rate per follow-up year was 0.29 in the patellar bandage group, 0.12 in the cast group, and 0.08 in the splint group. Beyond the 44% incidence of recurrent dislocation, there was a 19% incidence of patellofemoral pain or subluxation. Only 37% of patients had no complaints at the time of follow-up. This series suggests that application of a splint may be preferable to both cast and bandage. However, the duration of the immobilization was different in the three groups. Therefore, redislocation rates are influenced by both the type and the length of the immobilization.

Garth et al[144] reported the results of 39 knees with acute patellar dislocation that were treated functionally. Treatment included immediate straight-leg–raising exercises followed by the application of a laterally padded knee sleeve and immediate mobilization. The average follow-up was 46 months (range, 24 to 71 months). Six patients (15%) experienced recurrent instability. Good or excellent results were achieved in 67% of the knees subjectively and in 69% objectively. This means that the results after functional treatment of acute patella dislocation were not satisfactory in about a third of the knees. These results are similar to those achieved with cast immobilization. However, functional treatment avoids the deleterious effects of immobilization and decreases the convalescence time.

It is tempting to postulate that the greater the anatomic abnormalities, the more likely the patella is to dislocate with a minor injury. Such patients would also experience dislocation at a younger age and are more likely to experience recurrent episodes of instability. Similar concepts have been proposed to interpret recurrent dislocation of the glenohumeral joint. The data reported earlier seem to lend support to this theory, but more research is needed before it can be definitely accepted.

TREATMENT

In view of the incomplete success rate of conservative treatment of acute patellar dislocations, some authors have recommended surgical treatment in the presence of anatomic abnormalities or osteochondral fractures.[42,58,76] The results of surgical treatment of acute patellar dislocations have been summarized in Table 53–5. It appears that the recurrence rate is lower after surgery in the acute phase than after conservative treatment. However, normal knees were not consistently obtained because a significant incidence of retropatellar pain and crepitation is reported. It is interesting to note that in the paper by Dainer and associates,[83] the addition of lateral release to medial reefing worsened the final result by increasing the incidence of recurrence and unsatisfactory results.

Our preferred treatment of acute patella dislocation is conservative. We recognize that nonoperative treatment is doomed to failure in probably a third of cases because of recurrence of the dislocation, but surgery will not produce normal knees in 100% of cases and operative or postoperative complications may occur. Thus, our preferred treatment of the first acute dislocation remains immobilization for around 4 weeks in an "off-the-shelf" immobilizer. Quadriceps strengthening is started soon with straight-leg raises, and partial weightbearing is allowed as tolerated. By 1 month, most patients have sufficient quadriceps strength and decreased tenderness to permit immobilization to be discontinued. Quadriceps strengthening is advised for prolonged periods.

There are exceptions to conservative treatment, the most frequent being the presence of an osteochondral fragment on the radiograph. A large fragment with underlying bone of sufficient thickness should be fixed, but it is an infrequent case. More often, the bone is thin and does not allow firm fixation. In such cases, arthroscopic removal is preferable.

More osteochondral fragments may be found at surgery than identified on preoperative radiographs. Jensen and Roosen[213] performed surgery in a series of 23 acute patella dislocations and removed 5 osteochondral fragments from the medial patella (22%). Only one of these was evident on preoperative radiographs. Similarly, Dainer and coworkers,[83] in a series of 29 arthroscopies for acute dislocations, found 17 defects of the patella (59%) and 13 of the lateral femoral condyle (45%). Radiographs failed to identify 40% of these defects. A similar discrepancy between radiographic and arthroscopic findings has been reported by Stanitski[372]: less than a third of the articular

Table 53–5. Prognosis after Surgical Treatment of Acute Patellar Dislocations

AUTHOR	YEAR	NO. OF KNEES	TREATMENT	AVG. FOLLOW-UP (mo)	REDISLOCATION (%)	REMARKS
Boring & O'Donoghue[42]	1978	17	Modified Hauser (9), medial reefing (8)	98	0	There were no redislocations, but 2 knees had subluxation (12%); 12 knees (70%) were painful, although 8 were so only rarely; all had moderate retropatellar crepitation
Jensen & Roosen[213]	1985	23	Medial reefing (23), lateral release (8)	39	9	Pain with motion was present in 39%, retropatellar crepitus and signs of chondromalacia in 35%; the addition of lateral release did not improve results
Cash & Hughston[58]	1988	16	Medial reefing	97	0	Satisfactory results obtained in 87%
Dainer et al[83]	1988	29	Arthroscopy and cast (14), arthroscopy and lateral release (15)	25	14	All recurrences were in the group treated by lateral release, which had a lower incidence of satisfactory results (73%) than in those treated without lateral release (93%)
Vainionpää et al[390]	1990	55	Medial reefing (55), lateral release (37)	24	9	Satisfactory results in 80%; snapping was reported by 66% and giving way by 20%
Sallay et al[338]	1996	12	Medial patellofemoral ligament suture (12), lateral release (3)	34	0	25% of knees had possible patella subluxation

lesions identified by arthroscopy were visualized on radiographs. Nevertheless, these observations do not justify the routine use of arthroscopy in acute patellar dislocations. Many small fragments may become finally entrapped in the synovium and never become symptomatic loose bodies.

Recent advances in understanding the pathoanatomy of acute patellar dislocation[338] may offer a solution to improve the results over those of conservative treatment. In a series of 12 knees, treatment consisted of suture of the medial patellofemoral ligament. With a minimum follow-up of 2 years, none of the knees had redislocated, although 25% of the patients had episodes compatible with subluxation. If these results are confirmed in larger series, this approach may be the most "conservative" treatment of acute dislocation of the patella.

Chronic Subluxation of the Patella

This category includes knees with patellar pain wherein axial views or CT reveals lateral displacement (subluxation) of the patella. These knees can be interpreted as an intermediate grade of dysplasia of the extensor mechanism, between lateral patellar compression syndrome and recurrent dislocation of the patella: patients complain of pain (as in those affected by lateral patellar compression syndrome), but the patella shows lateralized tracking (as in knees affected by recurrent patellar dislocation). The same group of knees has been described by Dejour et al[91] and was found to account for about 20% of their knees with patellar pain. They named them instabilities rotuliennes potentielles (potential patellar instabilities). These patients may later experience episodes of patellar instability. The symptoms are similar to those described in the discussion of lateral patellar compression syndrome, and initial treatment involves the described nonoperative course. If this fails to relieve the symptoms, lateral retinacular release or other major realignment procedures may be considered, as reported in the next discussion.

Recurrent Dislocation of the Patella

SYMPTOMS

The history is usually self-explanatory and sufficient to make the diagnosis. The patient is generally in the second decade of life. Several authors have reported a female preponderance, but Hughston[189] pointed out that young athletic males are also frequently affected. The patient reports an initial episode of patellar dislocation that was treated conservatively. After the initial episode, the patient suffers one or more similar episodes of instability as a result of trivial injuries. Their severity may vary from lesser forms with just a feeling of insecurity to true dislocations with the patella noted on the outer aspect of the knee. Crosby and Insall[81] have observed that the number of dislocations decreases with increasing age. Patients may learn how to avoid the dislocation; their decreased activity level beyond

the twenties may also contribute to this favorable outcome.

PHYSICAL EXAMINATION

The patient is first observed standing, and the presence of angular deformities (genu varum or valgum) as well as squinting of the patellae is noted. Any excessive degree of pronation of the foot should be recorded.

The patient is asked to sit on the edge of the examining table and straighten the knee while the examiner evaluates patella tracking. A variety of abnormal tracking patterns have been described. In our experience, the most frequent finding is lateral subluxation in extension. The patella is centered in the sulcus with the knee flexed at 90 degrees, but the patella displaces laterally when it exits the sulcus. Subluxation is usually accompanied by lateral tilt of the patella—that is, the lateral border of the patella becomes significantly lower than the medial border while proceeding toward extension. The lateral subluxation (or dislocation) of the patella in the most severe cases may be abrupt and painful to the point at which there is an extension lag.

With the patient lying supine, the Q angle can be measured. With the knee in extension, this angle is normal in most cases because the patella is displaced laterally. An abnormally increased Q angle (and lateral placement of the tibial tuberosity) can better be appreciated with the knee at 90 degrees of flexion because the patella relocates in the sulcus.[227] It has been suggested that obliquity of the patellar tendon greater than 10 degrees from the perpendicular to the transepicondylar line is pathological. We have found it difficult to obtain a precise measurement in degrees because of problems in defining the transepicondylar line. Nevertheless, a qualitative assessment in this position is useful.

Atrophy of the quadriceps and hypoplasia of the vastus medialis obliquus can best be evaluated by asking the patient to contract the quadriceps. The bulk of the vastus medialis obliquus and its insertion on the patella should be noted.[122]

With the knee in extension, mobility of the patella can be grossly estimated. It is better performed by engaging the patella in the femoral sulcus with the knee flexed 30 degrees. The patella is alternately pushed medially and laterally with the quadriceps relaxed. The magnitude of displacement is measured in quadrants. Lateral displacement more than two quadrants (half-width of the patella) indicates laxity of the medial structures. Medial displacement of the patella of one quadrant or less indicates tightness of the lateral structures.[227] This can be also assessed by lifting up the lateral border of the patella with the knee in extension. If the transverse axis of patella cannot be lifted over the horizontal, tightness of the lateral structures is again demonstrated (passive patellar tilt).

Finally, the most informative test is performed, the apprehension test described by Fairbank.[109] With the knee at 20 to 30 degrees of flexion, the patella is pushed laterally. The patient thinks that the patella is going to dislocate and avoids this situation by contracting the quadriceps and displacing the hands of the examiner. The test should be performed gently.

In conclusion, while examining a patient with recurrent dislocation of the patella, the examiner should be aware that several anatomic abnormalities are related to the disease, including soft-tissue and bone abnormalities. Bone abnormalities are best investigated by radiological techniques. Soft-tissue problems are identified by physical examination. Laxity of the medial stabilizers seems to be a prerequisite to allow lateral displacement of the patella. The medial stabilizers include the medial parapatellar retinaculum with the medial patellofemoral ligament,[78] which is a purely passive restraint, and the vastus medialis obliquus, which is an active stabilizer. Conversely, the lateral stabilizers are overdeveloped and include a thick and shortened lateral retinaculum and a well-developed vastus lateralis. Often, hyperlaxity of other joints can be demonstrated (metacarpophalangeal, wrist, knee, and elbow joints). Some patients with recurrent dislocation of the patella also suffer from recurrent dislocation of the glenohumeral joint, more often with bilateral symptoms and without previous trauma. Some of these patients are affected by Ehlers-Danlos syndrome or Marfan's syndrome. It should be remarked that in patients with generalized joint laxity, the lateral structures are not usually tight and the patella can be equally displaced medially and laterally.

The role of the vastus medialis obliquus has been investigated with electromyography by Mariani and Caruso.[264] They examined five normal controls and eight knees with subluxation of the patella. Electromyography of the vastus medialis obliquus and vastus lateralis was performed simultaneously with the patient in the sitting position and actively extending the knee from 90 degrees to full extension against low resistance. Normal subjects showed a comparable high level of activity in the vastus medialis obliquus and vastus lateralis between 30 degrees and full extension. In seven of the eight knees with patellar subluxation, the vastus medialis obliquus showed a decreased level of activity in the whole range, particularly between 30 degrees and full extension. Similar data were obtained by examining the asymptomatic knee of the patients with subluxation. Surgery on the symptomatic knees was performed with the Elmslie-Trillat technique.[387] Electromyograms were obtained again 6 to 12 months after the operation. In all the patients except one, the performance of the vastus medialis obliquus returned to the level of the vastus lateralis. The author interpreted these data as proof that the muscle disorder is secondary to anatomic alterations in the extensor mechanism and can be reversed by correcting these abnormalities.

A different opinion was more recently expressed by Floyd and coworkers.[120] They performed a histochemical and electromyographic study on 12 knees with recurrent dislocation of the patella and 7 normal controls. Muscle biopsies from the controls (vastus lateralis) showed an approximately equal number of type 1 and 2 fibers, with a predominance of type 2A over type 2B. Type 2C fibers are rare in adult muscle. In the knees with patellar subluxation, however, there was a significantly increased number of type 2C fibers and a decrease in type 1. The increase in the percentage of type 2C fibers, which pre-dominate in fetal life, has been interpreted as evidence of a primary myopathy. We think that whether primary or secondary, hypoplasia of the quadriceps and vastus medialis obliquus remains an important factor in recurrent dislocation and should often be addressed at the operation.

RADIOGRAPHIC EVALUATION

Bone abnormalities in recurrent dislocation of the patella can be studied by traditional radiographic and CT techniques. Abnormalities include a high vertical position of the patella, a patella with prevalence of the lateral facet, a flat femoral sulcus, lateral subluxation and tilt of the patella, lateral placement of the tibial tuberosity, and increased femoral anteversion.

Patella alta is not a bone abnormality in itself because it is due to increased length of the patellar tendon. It is best investigated in the lateral view. We have measured the height of the patella with the Insall-Salvati method[204] in 37 knees affected by recurrent subluxation of the patella.[7] The average T/P ratio in this group was 1.23, which is significantly higher than the value (1.04) found in normal knees. The patella was also significantly higher in this group of knees when measured with the A/B ratio of Blackburne and Peel,[38] which was 1.08 versus 0.95 in controls. (See also the section "Imaging of the Patellofemoral Joint," "Lateral View" in this chapter.)

A flat femoral sulcus has been reported by Brattström.[47] Using the Merchant view, we[7] found a significantly shallower sulcus in knees with recurrent instability (average sulcus angle, 147 degrees) than in controls (average sulcus angle, 137 degrees). Furthermore, the patella was subluxated laterally as shown by a positive congruence angle (16 degrees on average as compared with −6 degrees in normal subjects).

Traditional axial views at 30, 45,[284] or 20 degrees[243] of flexion are usually sufficient to show definite abnormalities of the sulcus and patella position in knees with recurrent patella dislocation because of the underlying anatomic dysplasia. Nevertheless, knees with less evident malalignment of the extensor apparatus are better investigated with CT or MRI, which allows visualization of the patellofemoral joint in the range from full extension to 20 degrees of flexion and avoids overlapping of bony contours. Furthermore, these techniques allow identification of the tangent to the posterior condyles, which is used as a reference for measurements of patellar tilt and the height of the lateral femoral condyle. Measurement of the lateral displacement of the tibial tuberosity with respect to the femoral sulcus can be also obtained with CT.

Schutzer and colleagues,[347] using CT in normal knees, pointed out that the patella is slightly lateralized in extension, but that all patellae are reduced by 10 degrees of flexion (congruence angle of 0 degrees or less). The angle between the lateral patellar facet and the tangent to the posterior condyles is always open laterally and never less than 8 degrees. According to these findings in normal knees, three types of abnormal patellar tracking can be identified: subluxation (lateral displacement as indicated by a positive congruence angle beyond 10 degrees of flexion), tilt (a patella tilt angle of <8 degrees), or tilt and subluxation. Subluxation was more evident in extension (average congruence angle, 13 degrees) and tended to reduce with flexion (average congruence angle, 8 degrees). This observation has also been made by Inoue and colleagues.[197] They found that the lateral patellofemoral angle measured on CT images with the knee in full extension was the most sensitive test to differentiate normal knees from knees with patellar subluxation (sensitivity, 96%). Conventional axial views with the knee at 30 and 45 degrees of flexion had lower sensitivity, 88% and 80%, respectively.

MRI has been also used to study the patellofemoral joint in subluxing patellae.[236] Subluxing patellae were more lateralized and tilted than those of normal controls, and the differences were more evident in extension. All the normal patellae were congruent in the sulcus at 30 degrees of flexion, but also at this degree most of the subluxing patellae (77%) had reduced. Thus, it seems that clinical, radiographic, CT, and MRI data concur to demonstrate that the patellae of knees with recurrent dislocation have a more abnormal and lateralized position in extension that reduces in early flexion.

The height of the lateral femoral condyle in reference to the deepest point of the femoral trochlea has been measured on CT images. With the knee at 30 degrees of flexion, we have found that the height of the lateral condyle was 9 mm in normal subjects and 4.7 mm in persons with subluxation, a significant difference.[9] Schutzer and colleagues[348] reported that knees with a subluxated and tilted patella had a significantly reduced height of the lateral femoral condyle when compared with normal knees. Dejour et al[91] observed that in knees with recurrent dislocation, the deepest point of the sulcus is more prominent in relationship to the anterior femoral cortex than it is in normal knees. Therefore, the flat sulcus of knees with recurrent dislocation would be the result of a decreased depth of the trochlea and not a decreased height of the lateral prominence of the trochlea.

Evaluation of the lateral displacement of the tibial tuberosity with reference to the deepest point of the sulcus femoralis has been popularized by Goutallier and Bernageau,[157] who measured it radiographically. This measurement is more informative than the surface Q angle, which is frequently normal in knees with recurrent patellar dislocation because of lateral displacement of the patella in extension. It can be appreciated that if the patella is realigned into the sulcus by tightening the medial structures and releasing the lateral ones, the Q angle and the valgus vector will be increased. Therefore, preoperative measurement of the TT-SF distance would allow the orthopedist to plan a distal realignment in addition to a proximal one. Dejour and coauthors[91] reported that the TT-SF distance of normal knees in extension is 12.7 mm on average whereas it was 19.8 mm in a group of knees with patellar instability. Only 3% of normal knees had a TT-SF distance greater than 20 mm, whereas the same was true of 56% of the knees with unstable patellae. We have measured the TT-SF distance with the knee at 30 degrees of flexion and found an average value of 8.7 mm in normal knees and 14.7 mm in knees with patellar instability, a significant difference.[9]

CLINICAL FACTORS

Bilateral recurrent dislocation of the patella, generalized ligamentous laxity, associated joint dislocations (more often of the shoulder), and a family history of recurrent dislocation of the patella have been reported with variable frequency by several authors.[45,81,90,169,183,287,334]

Rünow[335] clearly recognized that both external and internal factors may contribute to recurrent dislocation. Trauma is an external factor. Anatomic abnormalities of the patellofemoral joint and generalized ligamentous laxity are internal factors. Analyzing a series of 104 patients affected by recurrent patellar dislocation, he tried to identify the interaction of external and internal factors in the genesis of the disease.

An abnormally high Insall-Salvati T/P ratio (>1.3) was chosen as an index of local anatomic abnormality. In Rünow's series, only 2% of the control knees had an Insall-Salvati T/P ratio greater than 1.3, whereas the same was true in 41% of the dislocating knees. Furthermore, bilateral and frequent dislocations (defined as more than two dislocations per year) were three times more common when the patella was alta than when it was normal.

Generalized joint laxity evaluated according to a modified Carter and Wilkinson method[56] was present in 56% of males and 69% of females with recurrent patellar dislocation. Only 10% of the control males and 11% of the control females had generalized ligamentous laxity. Therefore, ligamentous laxity was six times more frequent in knees with recurrent dislocation of the patella. Patients with generalized ligamentous laxity frequently (43%) received orthopedic treatment of other joint disorders, including scoliosis, congenital dysplasia of the hip, flat feet, and equinus feet. This was rare (5%) in patients without associated ligamentous laxity. Of the patients with ligamentous laxity, 33% had relatives with recognized orthopedic abnormalities, but this was true in only 3% of the patients without generalized laxity. In the light of these facts, dislocation of the patella may be viewed as an expression of a systemic disorder of connective tissue.

The importance of trauma was difficult to evaluate, but it appeared that its magnitude was inversely related to joint laxity and anatomic abnormality. Moderate trauma, involving direct force against the patella or indirect force associated with athletics, was present in 55% of cases. In the remaining 45%, the patella dislocated because of a trivial injury (minor trauma).

A classification of patellar instability was based on two independent variables: one local (patella alta according to an Insall-Salvati T/P ratio higher than 1.3) and the other systemic (generalized joint laxity). Four grades were defined: grade I with absence of both factors, grade II with generalized joint laxity and no patella alta, grade III with patella alta and no generalized joint laxity, and grade IV with both factors present. The 104 cases of recurrent patellar dislocation were classified as follows: grade I, 16%; grade II, 35%; grade III, 19%; and grade IV, 30%. This classification seems appropriate if one considers that the age at onset decreased from 19 years in group I to 15 years in groups II and III to 13 years in group IV. The incidence of bilateral dislocation and frequent dislocation (more than twice a year) increased progressively from grade I to grade

IV and was 13%, 19%; 35%, 68%; 13%, 26%; and 60%, 74%, respectively. The incidence of moderate trauma and associated patellar or trochlear fractures decreased from grade I to grade IV and was 76%, 69%; 55%, 26%; 63%, 38%; and 33%, 17%, respectively.

In summary, moderate trauma, defined as the application of direct force on the patella or an indirect twisting mechanism during athletic activities, has a definite role in the absence of predisposing factors, including patella alta and joint laxity. However, grade I knees often had a shallow trochlear groove or a high-riding patella as evaluated with the Norman index.[300] Therefore, trauma is definitely unlikely to produce patellar dislocation in a completely normal knee. A shallow condylar groove was not included in the classification, but Norman thought that it contributed to patellar instability. Generalized ligamentous laxity and patella alta according to the Insall-Salvati index correlated best with the degree of clinical instability of the patella.

It should be remembered that recurrent patellar instability may be part of the clinical picture of Down's syndrome. Dugdale and Renshaw[100] examined 210 institutionalized patients and found an 8% incidence of dislocated or dislocatable patellae. Nevertheless, it appears that this condition interferes with walking capacity in only a minority of patients. Most of them are able to adapt to the problem. Surgery to correct the instability is necessary in only a minority of cases.[91,261]

CONSERVATIVE TREATMENT

Conservative treatment should be attempted in knees with recurrent patellar instability. It is based on strengthening of the quadriceps and vastus medialis obliquus and stretching of the tight lateral structures, as previously described. The frequency of the episodes of instability may be reduced so that surgery is no longer necessary. If disabling symptoms persist, surgical treatment is indicated.

Garth et al[144] reported the results of functional treatment of 30 knees with recurrent dislocation of the patella. Treatment included quadriceps strengthening and a lateral padded knee sleeve. With an average follow-up of 46 months, a satisfactory result was achieved in only 50% of cases, and the recurrence rate was 40%.

SURGICAL TREATMENT

In this section we discuss lateral release and proximal, distal, and combined realignment.

Lateral Retinacular Release

The surgical technique and postoperative treatment of lateral retinacular release have been described earlier in this chapter. The results in knees affected by recurrent patella subluxation and dislocation are reported in Table 53–6. The reported percentage of satisfactory results varies between 30% and 100%. However, the rating systems were not uniformly stringent. We think that any patient with

persistent symptoms of instability cannot be included among satisfactory results. Dandy and Griffiths[86] reported on 41 knees that underwent lateral release for recurrent dislocation. The average follow-up was 4 years. Ninety percent of the knees were classified as satisfactory according to the rating system of Crosby and Insall.[81] However, only 44% of the patellae were stable, 24% were occasionally insecure, and 32% underwent at least one redislocation.

Using an average follow-up of 8 years, Dandy and Desai[85] reviewed 33 knees in which the previous follow-up had been 4 years.[86] The percentage of satisfactory results decreased from 90% at 4 years to 72% at 8 years. Thirty-two percent of the patellae had dislocated at least once before the 4-year follow-up. Twenty-one percent (seven knees) continued to dislocate and underwent tibial tubercle transposition. Subluxation in extension and generalized ligamentous laxity correlated with an increased failure rate. The authors concluded that with these conditions, lateral release does not correct recurrent dislocation.

Our experience with lateral retinacular release for recurrent dislocation of the patella was not completely satisfactory. We reviewed 21 knees.[5] The group included 12 females and 9 males whose age averaged 21 years (range, 12 to 48 years). The operation was performed with the arthroscopic technique described by Metcalf[285] in 18 cases and with an open technique in 3 knees; 20 patients (95%) were reviewed with an average follow-up of 66 months (range, 22 to 101 months). Most of the patients (90%) had no pain or swelling at follow-up, but one knee (5%) had instability during sports activities and six knees (29%) during daily living activities. Therefore, only 66% of the results could be considered satisfactory. On the axial view at 45 degrees of flexion,[284] the congruence angle was 19 degrees preoperatively and decreased to 3 degrees at follow-up, but it was still abnormal in 37% of cases. When satisfactory and unsatisfactory results were compared to identify predictive factors, we found that the prognosis was worse in females ($p = 0.05$) and knees with more than five preoperative dislocations ($p = 0.05$). The persistence of lateral patellar tracking at follow-up as evaluated clinically ($p = 0.02$) and a deficit on the one-leg hop test for distance greater than 15% ($p = 0.05$) correlated with an unsatisfactory result. No correlation was found between the results and generalized joint laxity, passive patellar tilt, congruence angle at follow-up, patellar height, and degree of chondromalacia.

Insall's Proximal Realignment

Proximal realignment is in fact a rearrangement of the muscular attachments to the patella, and its purpose is to alter the line of pull of the quadriceps muscle. The quadriceps angle is not altered, nor is the length of the patellar tendon, but the realignment corrects the adverse effect of patellofemoral incongruence. The method can be applied for both patellar pain and patellar dislocation. It is a major procedure that is indicated only after a protracted period of conservative management.[200,202]

The operation (Figs. 53–79 and 53–80) is performed under tourniquet control after exsanguination of the limb,

Table 53–6. Results of Lateral Retinacular Release for Recurrent Patellar Subluxation and Dislocation

AUTHOR	YEAR	NO. OF KNEES	AVG. FOLLOW-UP (mo)	TYPE OF RELEASE	% SATISFACTORY RESULT	REMARKS
Metcalf[285]	1982	14	48	Arthroscopic	100	No redislocations
Chen & Ramanathan[65]	1984	39	72	Closed	86	Includes 15 acute dislocations, 9 recurrent subluxations, and 15 recurrent dislocations, with similar success rates in the 3 groups
Simpson & Barrett[358]	1984	32	15	Arthroscopic	86	Worse results with age <30 years, incomplete release, quadriceps weakness, and generalized laxity
Ogilvie-Harris & Jackson[304]	1984	46	60	Arthroscopic	44	Results correlate closely with degree of chondromalacia: 100% satisfactory with grade I chondromalacia but only 25% with grade III
Schonholtz et al[344]	1987	15	48	Closed	67	Better results than in pain syndromes
Betz et al[34]	1987	31	48	Closed	74	Knees with subluxation had a higher recurrence rate (64%) than those with dislocation (14%); 1 patient experienced medial subluxation
Sherman et al[355]	1987	45	28	Arthroscopic	75	One recurrence among 15 dislocations (6%); poor results more frequent in dislocators (39%) than in subluxers (15%)
Christensen et al[73]	1988	30	54	Open	30	Deterioration of satisfactory results from the 1-year (73%) to the 4-year (30%) follow-up
Dandy & Griffiths[86]	1989	41	48	Arthroscopic	90	44% of patellae were stable, 24% were occasionally insecure, and 32% had had at least one redislocation; worse results in hyperlaxity and knees with dislocation in flexion
Aglietti et al[10]	1989	20	66	Arthroscopic	65	35% experienced recurrent instability; worse results in females and knees with over 5 preoperative dislocations
Dandy & Desai[85]	1994	33	96	Arthroscopic	72	

either by elevation or with a bandage. A midline skin incision is made that extends proximally from the tibial tubercle for a distance of approximately 6 inches (15 cm). The skin edges are undermined sufficiently to expose the patella and quadriceps expansions; the incision should be sufficiently extensive that the components of the quadriceps muscle are clearly visible. Both the vastus medialis and vastus lateralis must be exposed, as well as the proximal extent of the quadriceps tendon and the insertion of the fibers from rectus femoris. The arthrotomy is performed by making an incision beginning proximally at the apex of the quadriceps tendon and placed within the tendon close to the border of the vastus medialis. The incision is continued distally to the patella and extended across the medial border of this bone and then distally medial to the patellar ligament. The incision described is therefore almost straight. The fibers of the quadriceps expansion medial to the incision are dissected from the bone with a scalpel.

Because of the vertical ridges on the anterior surface of the patella, the incision can be difficult and should be performed with care to preserve the expansion intact without lacerations. This is necessary to obtain secure closure when the quadriceps repair is completed. The fibers of the expansion can easily be separated from the bone if the dissection proceeds from above and below alternately,

thus forming a V and leaving the thinnest central part until last. When the procedure is performed in this manner, the central portion separates from the bone easily and can be fully preserved. Once the medial border of the patella is reached, the synovial lining is incised. Proceeding distally, the fat pad is divided in the line of the capsular incision until the patella can be everted for inspection of the joint.

A second capsular incision is now made on the lateral side beginning proximally in the muscle fibers of the vastus lateralis and extending distally to the tibial tubercle. It is desirable, but not essential to maintain the integrity of the synovium. Sometimes this is not possible because of tight fibrous bands in the substance of the synovium itself. A number of substantial vessels cross to the patella in the lateral retinaculum. There is a group of two or three vessels at the level of the upper pole of the patella that are usually the largest and bleed profusely if not coagulated or ligated. A second group of rather smaller vessels run beneath the retinaculum more distally at the lower pole of the patella, generally one or two in number. These vessels should also be identified and coagulated.

The interior of the knee is thoroughly explored, and selective débridement is performed when necessary. In the malalignment syndrome, regardless of the extent of the patellar lesion, the femoral sulcus is usually normal. (The

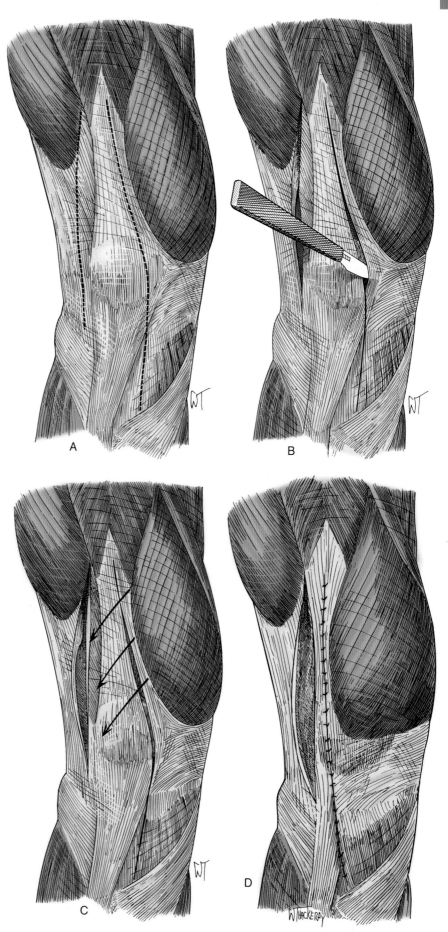

Figure 53–79. Proximal realignment. **A**, After exposure of the quadriceps mechanism, two incisions are made. The first enters the knee joint by a capsular incision placed at the margin of the vastus medialis over the medial quarter of the patella and medial to the patellar tendon. The second is a lateral release extending into the fibers of vastus lateralis. **B**, To preserve continuity of the medial flap, the quadriceps expansion crossing the patella must be carefully preserved and separated by sharp dissection. **C**, Realignment is effected by advancing the medial flap containing the vastus medialis laterally and distally in the line of the fibers of the oblique portion of the vastus medialis. **D**, After suturing, the incision lies in a straight line across the front of the patella, and the lateral release should open widely.

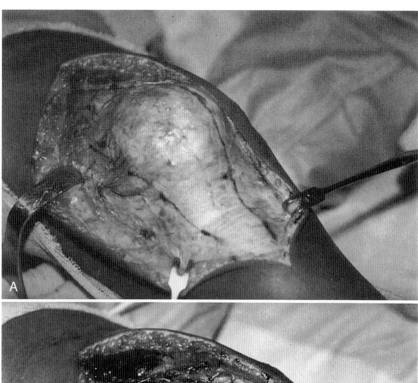
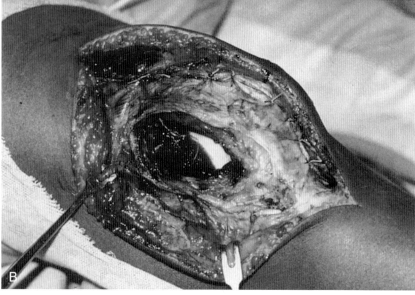

Figure 53–80. Insall's proximal realignment. **A**, After undermining of the subcutaneous tissue to expose the extensor apparatus, the proposed medial capsular incision and the lateral release have been marked with methylene blue. **B**, The medial arthrotomy has been closed with overlapping of the medial flap laterally over the patella. The lateral release opens widely.

exception is occasional evidence of an osteochondral fracture at the lateral border of the femoral sulcus caused by patellar dislocation.)

At this stage of the operation, the tourniquet should be released to enable any bleeding points not previously identified to be coagulated. The tourniquet is reinflated and thorough irrigation performed. The quadriceps must then be reconstructed such that the subsequent line of pull will be in a more medial direction. This is the purpose of the operative procedure, and by altering the direction of quadriceps action, patellar congruence is restored and patellar instability prevented. The first suture is placed so that the most distal part of the vastus medialis is brought laterally and distally to overlap the upper pole of the patella and adjoining quadriceps tendon. Before the overlap is executed, the synovium should be removed from the deep surface of the medial flap, which includes the vastus medialis, the medial part of the quadriceps expansion, and distally the medial capsule of the knee.

The amount of overlap that should be achieved depends on the preoperative laxity of the tissues.

In some knees, the vastus medialis is sutured as far across as the lateral border of the patella, but the more usual amount of overlap is 10 to 15 mm. A second suture is inserted at the lower pole of the patella to bring the medial flap across as tightly as the tissues will allow. The type of suture material may be absorbable or nonabsorbable according to the surgeon's preference. The two initial sutures determine the remainder of the closure, and after they are placed, the knee should flex to 90 degrees without the sutures breaking. The remaining closure is completed distally by suturing the flap as it lies and proximally, with decreasing overlap of the vastus medialis over the quadriceps tendon.

Occasionally in patients with recurrent dislocation and an extreme lateral position of the patella, the medial flap is so stretched that overlapping to the lateral patellar border is still insufficient to hold the patella in the center of the femoral sulcus. In these circumstances, the medial flap, including the vastus medialis, should be everted and the free border rolled back on itself. A series of sutures are inserted so that a tuck is made in the muscle. The reefed vastus medialis and quadriceps expansion are sutured anterior to the patella and quadriceps tendon. The tuck must be sufficient to keep the patella centralized. The resulting bulk of the muscle and capsule lying anterior to the patella may appear aesthetically unpleasant, but the tissue atrophies rapidly so that within a few weeks the enlargement disappears.

Two features of the repair should be emphasized. First, the lateral incision into the vastus lateralis must extend proximally almost as far as the medial incision. The most common error is reluctance to make an adequate division of the vastus lateralis; unless this is done, proximal rearrangement of the quadriceps is not possible. It might be expected that extensive division of the muscle would cause quadriceps weakness, but in practice this has not been observed.

Second, the more distal part of the closure must be snug but not excessively tight. In practice, it is almost impossible to overdo the overlapping in this area because it is prevented by soft-tissue tension and the anatomy of the femoral sulcus. Excessive tightness is revealed through observation of the behavior of the patella when the knee is flexed.

After routine closure of the subcutaneous tissue and skin, a compression dressing is applied.

To partially overcome the cosmetic disadvantage of a 15-cm-long skin incision, the surgical technique can be modified as follows. An 8-cm medial parapatellar skin incision is performed. The subcutaneous tissue is undermined in a proximal and distal direction. A medial capsular incision crossing over the medial third of the patella is performed routinely. After inspection of the joint, lateral retinacular release is performed from within the joint. The technique is the same as that used for total knee replacements. We prefer the multiple-puncture technique to a single incision to avoid the creation of a wide lateral defect. At this point, hemostasis is secured. Suture of the medial capsular incision with overlapping follows as previously described.

The patient is permitted to get out of bed on the second postoperative day and is allowed full weightbearing as tolerated. Crutches are needed only for a few days, and the patient can go home within a week. The compression dressing is left in place for 2 full weeks, at which time the sutures are removed. Straight-leg raises are then begun (if the quadriceps is not working by this time, side raises are performed initially). Flexion is also allowed and encouraged; with normal progress, 90 degrees of flexion is reached 4 to 6 weeks after surgery, by which time gait has returned to normal. For several months, the patient performs 300 straight-leg raises each day. Weights may be avoided because they have not proved necessary to rehabilitate quadriceps strength and may provoke patellar pain if used too vigorously.

The results of Insall's technique have been reported by different centers (Table 53–7). Insall[200] reviewed 75 realignments performed between 1969 and 1979 for patellar pain and instability. Ten operations were bilateral. The procedures were performed in 40 female and 25 male patients, and the average age was 20 years (range, 13 to 32 years). Patients were selected for surgery very carefully. All had dysplasia of the extensor mechanism and serious complaints of pain or instability for a long time, ranging from 1 to 5 years. All had undergone lengthy conservative treatment. The symptoms were always severe enough to interfere with everyday activity, not only with sports. Absence from school was a frequent problem in younger patients.

Of the 75 knees, 36 had an increased quadriceps angle (at least 20 degrees), 21 had a high-riding patella (average T/P ratio, 1.19), and 18 had both conditions (quadriceps angle, over 20 degrees; average T/P ratio, 1.23); a preoperative Merchant view had been obtained in 20 knees, and the findings for the sulcus and congruence angles were in accord with the measurements reported by our group.[7] Thus, the 10 knees with an increased quadriceps angle had an average sulcus angle of 138 degrees and an average congruence angle of 0 degrees. The six knees with a high-riding patella had a sulcus angle averaging 161 degrees and a congruence angle that averaged 25 degrees. The four knees with both variants had an average sulcus angle of 143 degrees and a congruence angle of 19 degrees. The 75

Table 53–7. Results of Proximal Realignment with Insall's Technique

AUTHOR	YEAR	NO. OF KNEES	DIAGNOSIS	AVG. FOLLOW-UP (mo)	% SATISFACTORY RESULT	REMARKS
Insall et al[201]	1983	75	Pain and subluxation	48	91	Better results when the is patella centered in the sulcus after the operation; no correlation with the severity of chondromalacia
Scuderi et al[350]	1988	60	Subluxation and dislocation	42	81	Only one redislocation (1.7%); females and older patients had inferior results; better results with patella centralization
Abraham et al[2]	1989	35	Pain and dislocation	76	62	Less satisfactory results in knees with patellofemoral pain (53%) than in knees with recurrent dislocation (78%)
Aglietti et al[5]	1989	11	Dislocation	102	91	Only 1 case was unsatisfactory because of insufficient quadriceps rehabilitation

knees were divided according to the primary symptoms into 40 knees with patellar pain (32 with an increased quadriceps angle, 3 with a high-riding patella, and 5 with both), 29 knees with subluxation (18 with a high-riding patella, 4 with an increased quadriceps angle, and 7 with both), and 6 knees with both pain and subluxation (all with an increased quadriceps angle and a high-riding patella).

The findings at surgery for patellar surface lesions were normal or grade I in 76%, grade II in 12%, grade III in 4%, and grade IV in 8% of cases. Pain was moderate to severe in 32 of the 57 grade I lesions (56%), in 7 of the 9 grade II lesions (78%), in none of the grade III lesions, and in 4 of the 6 grade IV lesions (67%). At surgery, 14 patellae were shaved, and 7 were shaved and drilled.

The grading system was similar to that described by Bentley.[30] At follow-up ranging from 2 to 10 years with an average of 4 years, the results were as follows: excellent in 37%, good in 54%, fair in 5%, and poor in 4%. Excellent and good results were obtained in 93% of stage I cartilage lesions, 100% of stage II lesions, 33% of stage III lesions, and 83% of stage IV lesions. In the 21 knees in which the patella was shaved or drilled, 86% had satisfactory results. Postoperatively, only 14 patients could not participate in sports.

In 57 knees, a postoperative Merchant view was obtained. In the 52 satisfactory knees, the average congruence angle was −11 degrees; 35 knees had a negative angle, 5 measured 0 degrees, and 12 had a positive congruence angle. Five knees were rated fair or poor, and in these knees the average congruence angle was 0 degrees. (Two knees had a positive congruence angle, two were 0 degrees, and one had a negative angle.) Naturally, one must not put too much store in radiographic measurements of any kind, and some inconsistencies are to be expected. However, these findings suggested a trend in that clinical improvement correlated with correct alignment, whereas no such correlation existed with either the severity of chondromalacia or its treatment by patellar shaving.

The complications of proximal realignment were relatively few and minor. They included superficial phlebitis, hematoma, delayed wound healing, and culture-negative drainage. Five knees (7%) required manipulation under anesthesia to allow better range of motion. One subsequent patellectomy was performed because of persistent patellar pain.

Scuderi and colleagues[350] reported the results of a group of 60 knees with patellar subluxation (34 knees) or dislocation (26 knees) that were treated by Insall's proximal realignment. In this study, 20 knees had undergone previous surgery (33%), including proximal and distal realignment, lateral retinacular release, anterior cruciate ligament surgery, meniscectomy, and removal of loose bodies. Postoperatively, a cast was applied for 1 month. The follow-up period was 3.5 years (range, 2 to 9 years). The results were excellent in 30%, good in 52%, fair in 10%, and poor in 8%. Results were significantly better in males and younger patients. None of the patients younger than 20 years had an unsatisfactory result. The preoperative diagnosis (subluxation or dislocation), the length of follow-up, or the severity of chondromalacia did not correlate with

the result. Knees with a satisfactory result had a greater change in the congruence angle (medial displacement of the patella) than did those with an unsatisfactory grading. The complications were as follows: seven patients (12%) needed postoperative manipulation to increase range of motion, one patient experienced a single episode of recurrent dislocation, three patients underwent arthroscopy for recurrent patellofemoral pain, and one patient underwent bilateral patellectomy for degenerative joint disease. Although the overall results did not correlate with the severity of chondromalacia, it is noteworthy that all the patients who needed a reoperation had severe, degenerative osteoarthritis.

Abraham and colleagues[2] reported the results of Insall's proximal realignment in 15 knees with patellofemoral pain and 9 knees with recurrent dislocation with an average follow-up period of 6.3 years. Satisfactory results in the group of knees with patellofemoral pain decreased from 87% at 2 years to 53% at 5 years. It should be noted that a quarter of these patients had severe grade IV chondromalacia at the operation: none of these knees obtained a satisfactory result. Better results were achieved in knees with recurrent patellar dislocation: 92% were satisfactory at 2 years and 78% remained so at 5 years. Two knees required additional surgery for recurrence of dislocation. An anatomic study in cadaver knees was undertaken to define the innervation of the patella. It was noted that branches of the femoral and lateral femoral cutaneous nerves innervated the patella. All these branches are cut by the skin and subcutaneous incisions and by the medial capsulotomy plus lateral release. In light of these findings, Abraham and coworkers suggested that pain relief may be attributed in part to denervation. No radiographic data were presented to describe the relationship between clinical results and restoration of congruence.

We[5] reported the results of proximal realignment in 11 knees affected by recurrent patella dislocation that were reviewed with a long average follow-up of 102 months. Only one case was considered unsatisfactory because of poor quadriceps rehabilitation. There were no recurrences of dislocation. Eight of these patients (73%) were interested in sports preoperatively, and all returned to their desired sport, including soccer (two), running (three), and aerobics (three). Analysis of the Merchant axial views revealed that preoperatively, the average congruence angle was +16 degrees, with 80% of the knees considered abnormal. At follow-up, only one knee was still abnormal (9%), and the average congruence angle was reduced to −8 degrees. There were no signs of degenerative arthritis during the long period of follow-up.

Arthroscopically Assisted Procedures

Arthroscopically assisted procedures have been described in the literature.[179,361,411] Basically, they include lateral retinacular release and plication of the medial capsule. Plication is achieved percutaneously or through short skin incisions with the use of spinal needles, straight or curved. They are used to deliver sutures into the joint, which are then extracted and tied over the capsule.

These procedures are in fact proximal realignments wherein a simple plication of the medial capsule is performed, without advancement of the vastus medialis obliquus. This technique allows shortening of the medial patellofemoral ligament, which is the primary restraint to lateral displacement of the patella.[78] Distal extension of the plication to the tibial tuberosity (through a short incision) may give additional support by shortening the patellomeniscal and patellotibial ligaments.

We have no experience with arthroscopically assisted procedures. Our concern is that exact tensioning of the medial structures and secure repair may be more difficult to achieve by arthroscopic than by the more traditional open techniques. On the other hand, the cosmetic advantage of arthroscopic surgery cannot be negated, especially in young females. The results of small series of arthroscopically assisted repairs are encouraging.[48,361] However, we think that larger series with longer follow-up are needed.

Distal and Combined Realignment

All the procedures in which the tibial attachment of the patellar ligament or the tibial tubercle is detached and transferred in a medial and possibly distal direction, thereby reducing the Q angle and correcting the height of the patella, are classified as distal or combined realignment. Most of the techniques in use today stem from those originally described by Hauser,[175] Goldthwait,[151,152] and Roux.[332] The procedure known as Goldthwait-Roux is an entirely soft-tissue procedure and involves lateral release, medial plication, and longitudinal splitting of the patellar tendon with transfer of the lateral half medially.[121] The Hauser procedure[175] consists of lateral retinacular release and transfer of the tibial tubercle medially and distally with or without medial plication. Two techniques have been widely used, the Elmslie-Trillat technique in Europe[387] and the Hughston technique[193] in North America.

Elmslie-Trillat Technique. The Elmslie-Trillat operation[80,387] is usually performed through a lateral parapatellar skin incision. A lateral retinacular release is performed and extended proximally as far as needed. The periosteum is elevated from the anteromedial surface of the tibia. An osteotome is inserted in the retropatellar bursa from the lateral aspect and directed distally and medially to osteotomize the tibial tuberosity (Fig. 53–81). A 4- to 6-cm fragment of bone is osteotomized, with care taken to preserve the distal pedicle intact. The tuberosity is then displaced medially, rotated around the distal pedicle, and fixed in the desired position with a screw. A medial arthrotomy may be required to allow inspection of the medial meniscus. Reefing of the medial capsule may be added if the stability of the patella does not appear to be sufficient. In these cases, a strip of the medial retinaculum is resected and the remainder sutured under tension.

Hughston Technique. The Hughston operation[193] involves a lateral curvilinear skin incision, which results in better cosmesis and less interruption of the blood and nerve supply. After extension of the dissection in a medial direction through the prepatellar bursa, release of the lateral retinaculum is performed first (Fig. 53–82). A medial parapatellar arthrotomy is then performed to allow inspection of the joint and correction of the associated

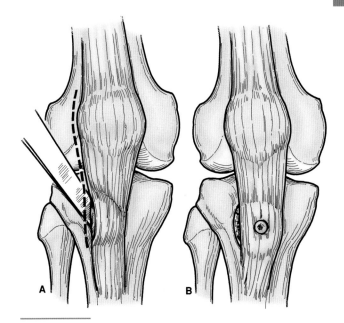

Figure 53–81. The Elmslie-Trillat operation. A lateral retinacular release is performed first. **A**, An osteotome is inserted in the retropatellar bursa from the lateral side and directed distally and medially. Care is taken to create a 4- to 6-cm-long osteotomy and preserve the integrity of the distal pedicle. **B**, The fragment is fixed with a single screw in the desired position. Medial plication may be added if sufficient stability is not restored after the distal transfer.

lesions. In knees with an increased Q angle, distal realignment is recommended. A thin osteotome is inserted into the retropatellar bursa to lift the patellar tendon with a thin wafer of bone. The insertion of the patellar tendon is displaced medially and distally as required and fixed in place with a Stone staple. The tourniquet is deflated at this stage, and hemostasis is achieved. Then the vastus medialis obliquus is advanced in line with its fibers, usually a few millimeters, with the knee flexed at 45 degrees. The muscle is sutured to the patella with nonabsorbable sutures, and motion of the knee is checked every stitch or two. If any abnormal motion is noted, the sutures are removed and the advancement is repeated. Below the vastus medialis obliquus, the capsule is closed without advancement in side-to-side fashion.

Results of Distal Realignment. The results of several series of patients operated on by distal realignment for recurrent dislocation of the patella are summarized in Table 53–8. The results of some early series pointed out that distal realignment according to the Hauser[175] technique was effective in preventing recurrent episodes of patellar dislocation in most cases. However, even when recurrent dislocation was cured, the knees were not normal. McNab[278] reported that whereas 85% of 33 knees with a follow-up of up to 3 years obtained a satisfactory clinical result, none of the 10 knees monitored for a period longer than 8 years could be so defined. Heywood[183] reported a low recurrence rate (6%) in a group of 53 knees monitored for an average of 7 years, but many patients complained of pain and swelling. Bowker and Thompson[45] reported on 26 knees treated surgically by distal realign-

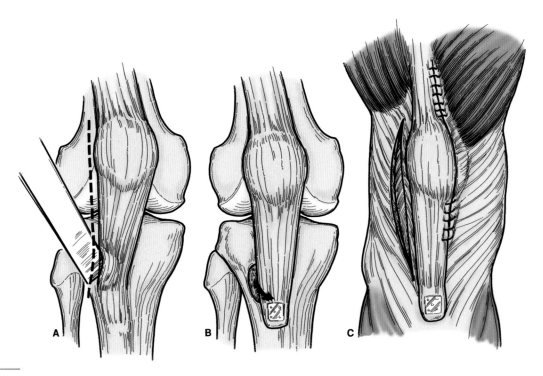

Figure 53–82. Hughston's technique to realign the extensor apparatus. Lateral release is performed first. **A**, In knees with an increased Q angle, the tibial insertion of the patellar tendon is detached with a thin wafer of bone. **B**, The tibial insertion is displaced in a distal and medial direction as required and fixed with a Stone staple. **C**, The vastus medialis obliquus is then advanced in line with its fibers for a few millimeters and fixed in place with nonabsorbable sutures. Smooth movement of the patella is checked every stitch or two; if any abnormality is noted, the stitches are removed and the advancement redone.

ment and monitored for an average of 108 months. The recurrence rate was 12%, but symptoms of patellofemoral arthritis were present in 59% of cases.

During these early years, most authors thought that osteoarthritis was the consequence of many years of maltracking of the patella and that the longer the duration of dislocation, the more likely the development of degenerative changes.[45,183,278] According to this concept, restoration of normal patellar tracking was supposed to stop the progression of degenerative changes.

However, this concept did not hold true. Crosby and Insall[81] reported the results of 81 knees treated surgically for recurrent patellar dislocation by distal realignment according to Hauser's technique (69 knees) or by proximal soft-tissue realignment using Wagner's technique (12 knees). The results were compared with those obtained in 26 knees treated conservatively. The average follow-up was 8 years in the surgical group and 16 years in the conservative one. Further dislocations occurred in 19% of the distal and 25% of the proximal realignments. The frequency of dislocations in nonoperated patients seemed to decrease with increasing age, and there were few dislocations in patients older than 30 years; the patella continued to dislocate more frequently than once a year in only 11% of cases. Satisfactory results were obtained in 59% of the distal realignments, 75% of the proximal realignments, and 65% of the conservative group. Evidence of moderate to severe osteoarthritis was present in 71% of the distal realignments but only 4% of the conservative group. Therefore, osteoarthritis was much less frequent in the

conservative group even if the follow-up period was doubled. It was concluded that medial transfer of the tibial tubercle was responsible for the high incidence of osteoarthritis. This can be explained by the fact that medial displacement of the tibial tubercle according to Hauser's technique[175] is accompanied by posterior displacement because of the triangular shape of the proximal end of the tibia (Fig. 53–83). This displacement in turn decreases the lever arm of the patellar tendon and increases the compressive force on the patellofemoral joint.

It has been calculated experimentally that transfer of the tibial tuberosity 20 mm medially and 15 mm distally implies a posterior displacement of approximately 30% of the sagittal diameter of the tibia. This in turn increases patellofemoral contact force by 20%.[382] An additional factor associated with patellofemoral arthritis may be the external rotation induced in the tibia by the medial transfer, which was noted in some patients who turned the foot out more than they did preoperatively. When compared with distal realignment, proximal soft-tissue procedures had a similar incidence of recurrence, more clinically satisfactory results, and no evidence of osteoarthritis (at least in the three cases in which radiographs were obtained).

A similar disturbing incidence of osteoarthritis was shown by Hampson and Hill,[169] who reviewed 44 knees with an average follow-up period of 16 years after a Hauser distal realignment. At the time of review, 75% of the patients complained of pain and 88% of patellofemoral

Table 53-8. Results of Distal Realignment for Chronic Subluxation, Recurrent Subluxation, or Dislocation of the Patella

AUTHOR	YEAR	NO. OF KNEES	OPERATION	AVG. FOLLOW-UP (mo)	% SATISFACTORY RESULT	REMARKS
McNab[278]	1952	33 10	Hauser Hauser	6-36 96-246	85 0	Encouraging results in the group with short follow-up, but all patients with a long follow-up were disabled by osteoarthritis
Heywood[183]	1961	53	Hauser	84	46	Recurrence rate, 6%
Bowker & Thompson[45]	1964	26	Hauser	108	NA	Recurrence rate, 12%; symptoms of patellofemoral arthritis in 59%
Hampson & Hill[169]	1975	44	Hauser	192	NA	At follow-up, pain was present in 75%, crepitus in 88%, and patellofemoral arthritis in 71%
Crosby & Insall[81]	1976	69	Hauser	96	59	Recurrence rate, 19%; osteoarthritis moderate to severe in 71%
Grana & O'Donoghue[159]	1977	65	Slot-block method	54	83	Recurrence rate, 5%; high postoperative complication rate (26%); progressive patellofemoral arthritis in 9%
Hughston & Walsh[193]	1979	346	Proximal and distal realignment	NA	71	Further proximal or distal realignment in 2.9%
DeCesare[90]	1979	67	Hauser	205	72	Recurrent dislocation, 7%, all in patients with generalized laxity; results deteriorated with increasing follow-up periods; moderate to severe arthritis in 10%
Chrisman et al[72]	1979	47 40	Hauser Roux-Goldthwait	92 92	72 93	Comparative study of the two procedures; higher complication rate after the Hauser (45%) than the Roux-Goldthwait (15%) procedure; the first procedure also showed more redislocations (17% vs. 5%) and less satisfactory results
Deburge & Chambat[89]	1980	114	Elmslie-Trillat	>24	84	Low recurrence rate (1.7%) but higher incidence of pain (19%) and patellofemoral arthritis (16%)
Aglietti et al[6]	1981	30	Putti-Goebbel	156	57	High complication rate with redislocation in 26%, maximum flexion 60°, and patellofemoral arthritis in 23% of knees
Fondren et al[121]	1985	47	Roux-Goldthwait	69	89	Worse results in knees with severe chondromalacia; patellofemoral arthritis developed in these knees
Reigler[326]	1988	42	Elmslie-Trillat	51	81	Muscle strength and endurance were evaluated with a computerized device and correlated with the end result
Cerullo et al[64]	1988	52	Hughston or Elmslie-Trillat	72	88	100% satisfactory results in dislocating patellae, slightly less (82%) in subluxers
Barbari et al[23]	1990	62	Hauser	96	84	High complication rate, including peroneal nerve palsy (3 cases), medial over correction (1), insufficient correction (1), dislocation of the bone block (1), stiffness (2); recurrence rate 10%; pain present in 58%, retropatellar crepitus in 40%; patellofemoral and tibiofemoral arthritis present in 26% and 37%, respectively
Shelbourne et al[354]	1994	45	Elmslie-Trillat	24		Preoperatively, 34 knees had instability and 11 had pain; 0% redislocation rate; 20% postoperative subluxation, which correlated with insufficient correction of congruence angle
Naranja et al[298]	1996	55	Elmslie-Trillat-Maquet procedure	74	60	Main preoperative symptom was pain (17), instability (24), or both (14); better results in knees with pure instability; redislocation rate 16%

NA, not available.

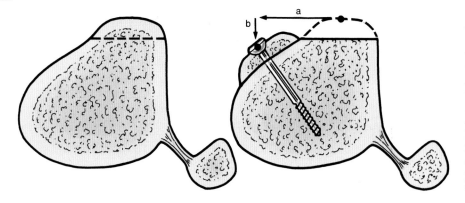

Figure 53–83. Transfer of the tibial tuberosity according to the Hauser technique. Because of the triangular shape of the proximal end of the tibia, medial displacement (a) causes posterior displacement (b) as well. This in turn decreases the lever arm of the patellar tendon and increases the compressive force on the patellofemoral joint, thereby predisposing it to degenerative changes.

crepitation. Patellofemoral arthritis was present in 71% of cases and tibiofemoral arthritis in 48%. The incidence of osteoarthritis increased with longer follow-up periods. Arthritis was present in 50% of the knees with a follow-up of less than 16 years and 90% of those with more than 16 years of observation. In light of these findings, the authors confuted the belief that degeneration can be prevented by Hauser's operation.

Distal and proximal realignment according to the Putti-Goebbel technique resulted in complications similar to those reported in the previous publications[6]: 43 operations were performed; 30 knees in 27 patients were monitored for an average period of 13 years (range, 2 to 18 years). The average age at the time of surgery was 13 years (range, 4 to 33 years). The preoperative diagnosis was recurrent or habitual dislocation of the patella in all the knees.

The Putti-Goebbel technique involves transposition of the tibial tuberosity and soft-tissue realignment. The tuberosity was detached and transposed distally and medially in a window prepared on the medial metaphysis of the tibia. Fixation was obtained with sutures or a single screw. A strip of capsular tissue was then removed from the medial retinaculum and used to fill the defect created after lateral release and closure of the medial arthrotomy. Immobilization in a cast was routinely applied for an average of 6 weeks.

The result was considered satisfactory if pain was absent or minimal, maximum flexion was over 120 degrees, and function was normal for daily living activities. Postoperative complications included one deep infection, which was cured with antibiotics; one case of displacement of the bone block; six cases of hematoma formation; and transient peroneal nerve palsy in two. Manipulation under anesthesia was performed in only two cases. Redislocation occurred in eight knees (27%), which underwent reoperation with further medial displacement of the tuberosity and plication of the medial capsule. None of the knees had redislocated at the time of follow-up.

The final result was satisfactory in 17 cases (57%). Unsatisfactory results were mainly due to stiffness or patellofemoral symptoms. Maximum flexion was less than 60 degrees in seven knees (23%). A recurvatum deformity as a result of growth disturbance of the proximal end of the tibia was present in 23% of cases. The patella was low in 67% of cases, and signs of patellofemoral arthritis were evident in 23%, more frequently in the knees with a low patella.

In summary, the Putti-Goebbel technique, followed by cast immobilization, has shown a high rate of complications consisting of stiffness, residual patellofemoral symptoms, and recurrence of dislocation. Excessive medial displacement with concomitant posterior displacement of the tuberosity and postoperative immobilization have certainly contributed to this unfavorable outcome.

Deburge and Chambat[89] reported the results of 114 Elmslie-Trillat operations performed for recurrent dislocation with a minimum follow-up of 2 years. The recurrence rate was very low (1.7%), but 19% of knees were painful at follow-up. Pain was the main reason for patient dissatisfaction. The results of centralization of the patella in the sulcus femoralis showed that 70% of the patellae were well repositioned and 11% were undercorrected with residual lateralization whereas 18% were overcorrected with medial subluxation. Medial femorotibial arthrosis was found in 28% of knees; previous medial meniscectomy was frequently associated with this condition. Lateral patellofemoral arthritis was present at follow-up in 16% of cases and correlated with the presence of degenerative changes of the patellar cartilage as seen at the operation. As observed by other authors, transfer of the tibial tuberosity in adolescents had an unacceptably high incidence of complications.

A significant incidence of arthritis after Hauser's distal realignment was reported by Barbari and colleagues.[23] They found a 26% and 37% incidence of patellofemoral and tibiofemoral arthritis, respectively, in a group of 62 knees with an average follow-up of 8 years.

The consequences of transfer of the tibial tubercle in a knee with open physes are well known. As a result of the procedure, growth of the tibial plateau is blocked anteriorly and recurvatum ensues. The complication affected a significant percentage of the knees as reported by Heywood[183] (31%), Crosby and Insall,[81] (18%) and DeCesare[90] (60%). In knees with open physes, realignment should therefore be limited to soft-tissue procedures.

A comparative study of the Hauser and Roux-Goldthwait procedures was presented by Chrisman and colleagues.[72] Lateral release and plication of the medial capsule were similarly performed in both series. In the Hauser procedure, the tibial tubercle was transposed medially and distally; in the Roux-Goldthwait procedure, the lateral half of the patellar tendon was freed distally, passed under the remaining medial half, and sutured to the pes anserinus. With an average 7.7-year follow-up, 47

Hauser procedures and 40 Roux-Goldthwait procedures were reviewed. The Hauser procedure showed a higher complication rate (45% versus 15%), a higher redislocation rate (17% versus 5%), and a slightly higher incidence of patellofemoral arthritis (8.5% versus 5%). Excessive medial displacement of the tibial tubercle during the Hauser procedure was thought to lead to patellofemoral degeneration. Overcorrection was more likely to occur in the Hauser than in the Roux-Goldthwait procedure.

An interesting study has been presented by Cerullo and colleagues.[64] They reviewed a series of 94 patients who underwent surgery consisting of extensor mechanism realignment for patellar dislocation (20 knees), subluxation (42 knees), or patellar pain without instability (32 knees). The procedures included the Hughston[193] and the Elmslie-Trillat[387] operations in 70% of cases. In the remaining 30%, only proximal realignment was performed because the Q angle was not increased. The patients were reviewed with an average follow-up of 6 years (range, 3.5 to 11.0 years). All the dislocating patellae achieved a satisfactory subjective and objective result whether they underwent proximal (2 knees) or distal (18 knees) reconstruction. Subluxing patellae incurred 81% subjectively and 97% objectively satisfactory results, without significant differences between proximal (8 knees) and distal (34 knees) realignment. Results were the worst in the group of knees with stable patellae, which were satisfactory in only 50% of cases subjectively and in 59% objectively. In this group, proximal realignment offered better results than distal realignment did, both subjectively (75% satisfactory versus 25%) and objectively (69% versus 50%).

Authors' Experience

We reviewed our experience with surgical treatment of recurrent patellar dislocation.[5] In the years 1979 to 1990, 72 knees underwent surgical treatment of recurrent dislocation of the patella. Only patients with two or more episodes of patella dislocation and age older than 10 years at the first dislocation were included in the study. Sixty-nine knees were available for personal follow-up. Twenty knees underwent lateral release; 14, Insall's proximal realignment; 16, distal realignment; and 19, combined (proximal and distal) realignment. The choice of surgical procedure depended on our attitude toward the treatment of recurrent dislocation of the patella at the time of surgery. In the early 1980s, we used mainly proximal realignment. Later, with the wide diffusion of arthroscopic techniques, lateral retinacular release was performed because in 1984, preoperative CT was used to assess the tuberosity-sulcus distance. When this measurement was abnormal, a distal or combined realignment was performed to reconstruct a more normal anatomy. Distal realignment included lateral retinacular release and medial transposition of the tibial tuberosity according to the Elmslie-Trillat technique. If the patella was high riding, distal displacement was also added. The height of the patella was measured with the Caton index, and values over 1.2 were indicative of a high-riding patella. Combined realignment included lateral release and medial plication according to the Insall technique,

plus transposition of the tibial tuberosity (Figs. 53–84 and 53–85).

Analysis of the preoperative data (Table 53–9) showed that the combined realignment group had, on average, significantly ($p < 0.01$) more preoperative dislocations. Grade III or IV patellar chondromalacia (deep fibrillation or erosion down to subchondral bone) was found at surgery more frequently (57%) in the proximal realignment group.

Preoperative radiographs showed that a flat sulcus (>145 degrees) was present in about half the knees in each group and a positive congruence angle was present in 74% to 94% of cases without significant differences among the four groups. A high-riding patella (Caton's index >1.2) was found more frequently (62%) in the distal realignment group.

The average follow-up was 8 years in both the lateral release and the proximal realignment group, 6 years in the distal realignment group, and 4 years in the combined realignment group.

At follow-up, 40% of knees in the lateral release group had experienced one or more redislocation episodes. The congruence angle remained positive in 40% of these knees. A history of more than five preoperative dislocations correlated with recurrence of dislocation at follow-up.

In the three realignment groups, the incidence of pain at follow-up ranged between 10% and 14%, swelling ranged between 6% and 14%, and recurrent instability ranged between 0% and 7%, without significant differences among the three groups. Patellofemoral crepitation was a frequent finding at follow-up, with a frequency of 26% to 50% in the three groups.

Radiographic analysis at follow-up showed that a positive congruence angle was present in none of the proximal realignments, 25% of the distal ones, and 10.5% of the combined realignments. The average tuberosity-sulcus displacement evaluated with CT scans at follow-up was 19.5 mm on average in proximal realignments, and it was satisfactorily reduced to 12 mm and 10 mm on average in the distal and combined realignment groups, respectively. There was no correlation between tuberosity-sulcus displacement and subjective results.

In conclusion, our experience with isolated lateral release for the treatment of recurrent patella dislocation has been disappointing, with a 40% redislocation rate and a positive congruence angle at follow-up in 40% (see Figs. 51–84 and 51–85). We think that lateral release should be offered only occasionally to patients with recurrent patella dislocation and specifically to those who refuse the larger skin incision required for a formal open realignment. The use of arthroscopically assisted techniques to perform medial plication may help improve the results of isolated lateral release.

Proximal, distal, and combined realignments were effective in preventing recurrent dislocation. However, pain and/or swelling sometimes contributed to an unsatisfactory result. Although redislocation was prevented in most cases, the anatomy of the patellofemoral joint was not returned to normal. Lateral patellar tracking in terminal extension was present in 31% to 57% of cases after realignment. The apprehension test result remained positive in

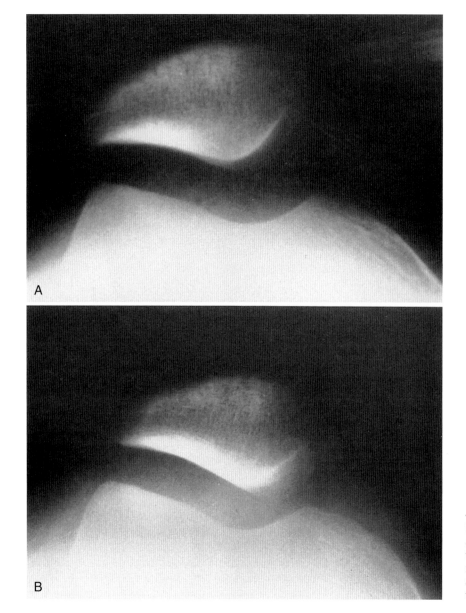

Figure 53–84. Fifteen-year-old girl affected by recurrent dislocation of the patella. After lateral retinacular release with a follow-up of 5 years, the axial Merchant view shows good centralization of the patella.

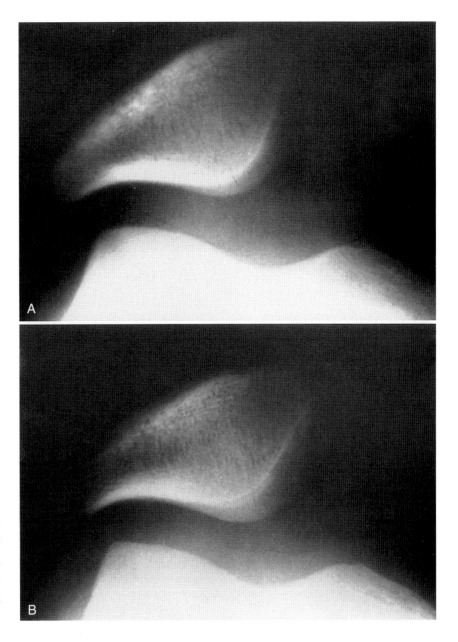

Figure 53–85. Seventeen-year-old male affected by recurrent dislocation of the patella. After lateral retinacular release with a follow-up of 6 years, the axial Merchant view shows insufficient centralization of the patella. This problem was encountered in roughly a third of our patients who were treated by lateral release.

Table 53–9. Comparative Study of Four Different Operations in the Treatment of Recurrent Dislocation of the Patella

	LATERAL RELEASE	PROXIMAL REALIGNMENT	DISTAL REALIGNMENT	COMBINED REALIGNMENT	
Knees	20	14	16	19	
Average age at surgery	21	23	24	20	NS
Females	53%	57%	40%	63%	NS
Preoperative dislocations (average number)	4	6	7	11	$p < 0.01$
Grade III-IV chondromalacia	10%	57%	37%	37%	$p = 0.03$
Preoperative Radiographs					
Sulcus angle > 145°	50%	43%	44%	68%	NS
Congruence angle > 0°	80%	86%	94%	74%	NS
Patella alta, Caton's index > 1.2	10%	43%	62%	37%	$p < 0.01$
Average follow-up (yr)	8	8	6	4	
Symptoms at Follow-up					
Pain	5%	14%	13%	10%	
Swelling	10%	14%	6%	10%	
Instability	40%	7%	6%	0%	
Objective Evaluation at Follow-up					
Abnormal patella tracking	NA	57%	31%	42%	
Moderate to severe patellofemoral crepitus	NA	29%	50%	26%	
Positive apprehension sign		NA	14%	19%	31%
Radiographs at Follow-up					
Congruence angle > 0°	40%	0%	25%	10.5%	NS
Patella alta, Caton's index > 1.2	NA	7%	6%	10.5%	NS
Tuberosity-sulcus displacement	NA	19.5 mm	12.3 mm	10.2 mm	$p = 0.01$

NA, not available; NS, not significant.
Data from Aglietti P, Buzzi R, De Biase P, Giron F: Surgical treatment of recurrent dislocation of the patella. Clin Orthop 308:8, 1994.

14% to 31%. The congruence angle was satisfactorily corrected in all proximal realignments (Fig. 53–86), whereas it was still positive in 25% of the distal and only 10% of the combined group (Fig. 53–87). Therefore, it seems that reefing of the medial soft tissues with proximal realignment plays a major role in centralization of the patella and restoration of a normal congruence angle.

A similar experience with distal realignment was reported by Shelbourne et al.[354] They performed a modified Elmslie-Trillat procedure (lateral release and medial displacement of the tibial tuberosity) on 34 knees affected by patellar instability. With a mean follow-up of 2 years, they saw no recurrence of dislocation, but 20% of patients complained of subluxation. Analysis of the congruence angle in the stable (25) and unstable (9) knees showed that preoperatively, the congruence angle was higher in unstable knees (38 degrees) than in stable knees (20 degrees). Postoperatively, stable knees showed good correction of the congruence angle to an average value of −5.4 degrees. Unstable knees, on the other hand, showed insufficient correction, with an average congruence angle of +17 degrees. The authors observed that correction to at least +15 degrees is necessary to decrease the incidence of postoperative instability.

In a series of 29 anteromedial transfers of the tibial tuberosity studied by Fulkerson,[128] the congruence angle improved from +28 degrees preoperatively to +13 degrees at follow-up, thus achieving incomplete correction. Although no direct correlation between pain relief and congruence angle was observed at follow-up, one patient without improvement in the congruence angle also had no pain relief.

In our opinion, these data support the observation that a major lateral dislocation of the patella cannot be corrected by moving the tibial tuberosity medially unless significant overcorrection is achieved. We think that in these cases, medial plication should be added.

Our current technique of planning and performing a combined realignment will now be described.

A straight midline skin incision extending from 5 cm above the upper pole of the patella to 3 cm distal to the tibial tuberosity is used routinely. A lateral parapatellar incision is equally effective and has a slight cosmetic advantage. Careful preoperative and/or intraoperative planning is necessary to decide on the direction and amount of displacement of the tibial tuberosity.

The height of the patella is measured with the Insall-Salvati,[204] Blackburne and Peel,[38] or Caton[62] methods. The latter two methods, which measure the height of the articular facet of the patella in relation to the tibial plateau, allow postoperative assessment of the correction obtained. The Insall-Salvati method is not affected by distal displacement of the tubercle. The Caton method[62] has the advantage of not requiring perfect superimposition of the

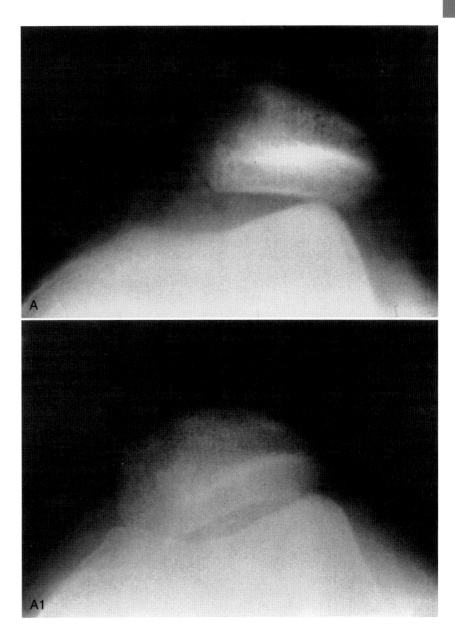

Figure 53–86. Two knees treated surgically with Insall's proximal realignment for recurrent dislocation of the patella. With a long follow-up of over 10 years, the patella shows good centralization on the Merchant axial view. No degenerative changes developed during these years.

(Figure continues)

femoral condyles to draw the joint level line as in the Blackburne and Peel method.[38] We aim at a ratio close to 1.0 with both the Caton and the Blackburne and Peel methods.

If the patella is found to be high, distal transposition is performed. To determine the required amount of distal displacement, the height of the articular facet of the patella is measured (AP in Fig. 53–88). The difference between distance AT and AP, corrected according to the magnification, indicates the amount of distal displacement required to produce an AT/AP ratio of 1.0.

The amount of medial displacement of the tibial tuberosity is assessed by measuring its placement in relation to the deepest point of the sulcus femoralis—that is, the TT-SF distance. This was first measured by Goutallier and Bernageau,[157] who used a radiographic method with a lead marker on the tibial tuberosity. More recently, CT

images have been used. The measure is obtained by superimposing a first cut through the tibial tuberosity on a second one through the upper part of the sulcus. The lateral displacement of the tip of the tuberosity from the deepest point of the sulcus is measured in millimeters. Dejour et al[91] reported that the TT-SF distance in normal knees in extension is around 12 mm and that values over 20 mm are definitely pathological. The reproducibility of the measurement was fair, around 4 mm. We have measured the TT-SF distance with the knee in 30 degrees of flexion and have found an average value of 8.7 ± 2.5 mm in normal knees.[9]

Nevertheless, CT assessment of the TT-SF distance has some disadvantages. First, a dedicated radiologist is necessary. Placement of the femoral and tibial cut with a standardized technique is critical for obtaining meaningful data. The limb of the patient should be fixed to the table

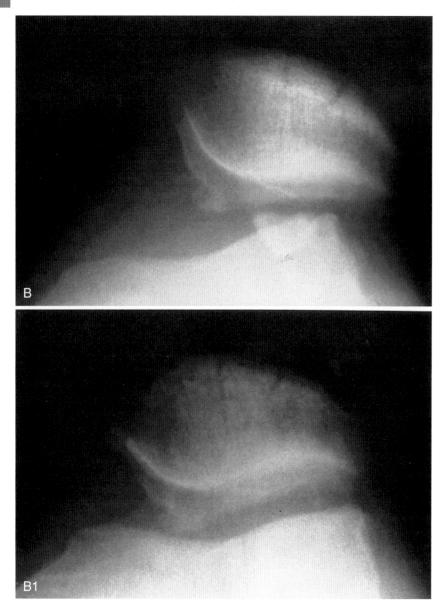

Figure 53–86, cont'd.

with straps to avoid inadvertent movement of the limb between the femoral and the tibial cut. Second, the measurement obtained with CT is in millimeters and does not account for the size of the patient. In other words, the same distance may be pathological in a small knee but within normal limits in a large patient.

To overcome these difficulties, we now prefer to intra-operatively measure the angle between the anterior superior iliac spine (S), the deepest point of the sulcus femoralis (S), and the top of the tibial tuberosity (T), halfway between the medial and lateral margin of the patellar tendon (SST angle) (Fig. 53–89). This measurement can easily be obtained at surgery with a goniometer (Fig. 53–90). The upper limb of the goniometer extends to the anterior superior iliac spine, the probe is in the deepest point of the sulcus femoralis, and the lower limb with the K-wire points to the tibial tuberosity. There are usually no difficulties in locating the iliac spine and tibial tuberosity. However, definition of the deepest point of the sulcus may be difficult or even impossible in knees with severe dysplasia and a flat sulcus. In a preliminary study, we measured the SST angle in normal knees during arthroscopic meniscectomy and have found an average value of 0.16 degree. In knees with recurrent dislocation of the patella, it was increased to an average of 0.25 degree.

There are several advantages of measuring the SST angle at surgery over measuring the TT-SF distance preoperatively with CT. First, the measurement is under direct control of the surgeon. The limb can be positioned in the same rotation as it is during walking. Second, the value obtained is in degrees and therefore independent of the patient's size. Third, the SST angle can be further checked after transposition of the tuberosity and the displacement changed if the alignment is unsatisfactory. We aim at restoration of a normal or slightly decreased SST angle,

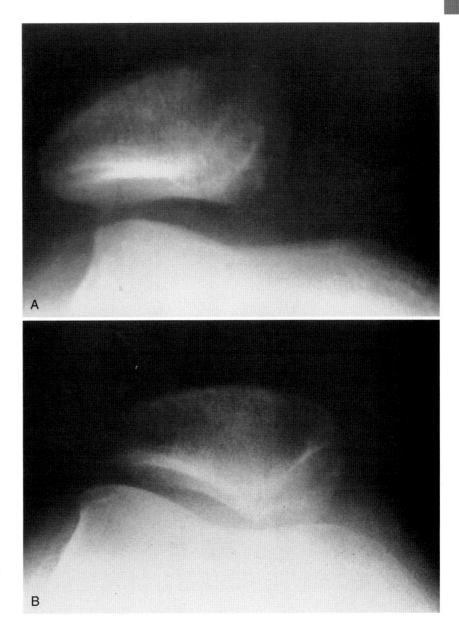

Figure 53–87. Twenty-three-year-old woman affected by recurrent dislocation of the patella. After distal realignment, lateral release, and medial plication (according to Insall's technique) with a follow-up of 4 years, the patella shows good centralization in the sulcus.

but the vector of the extensor apparatus should remain valgus and should not be overcorrected into varus.

After the skin incision, subcutaneous flaps are reflected medially and laterally. Lateral retinacular release is performed first, from the tibial tuberosity to the vastus lateralis obliquus. The tendon of the vastus lateralis is not released. The synovial layer can often be left intact, and doing so helps decrease blood extravasation in the subcutaneous tissue and retain some lateral stability. A wide medial arthrotomy is then performed from the apex of the quadriceps tendon, and the quadriceps expansion is detached from the medial third of the patella and parallel to the medial border of the patellar tendon.[200] The patella is everted, and chondromalacic changes are noted and treated as required. Loose bodies can be removed at this time. The menisci and cruciates are inspected and palpated with an arthroscopic probe.

The tibial tuberosity is defined by entrance into the retropatellar bursa proximally, the muscles are detached laterally, and the periosteum is incised medially. A 5- to 7-cm-long fragment of bone is sculpted after predrilling (two holes) with a 4.5-mm drill bit. The fragment is osteotomized with an oscillating saw. Working from the medial side, the osteotomy should be in the frontal plane or with slight posterior and lateral angulation. This approach ensures that medial displacement is not accompanied by posterior displacement of the tuberosity (Fig. 53–91). We would like to emphasize that a flat cut with the correct orientation can be obtained only when working with the saw or osteotomes from the medial side. The bulky muscles of the anterolateral compartment of the leg prevent working from the lateral side at the proper orientation. The saw blade should be advanced from the medial side until it emerges laterally so that a flat

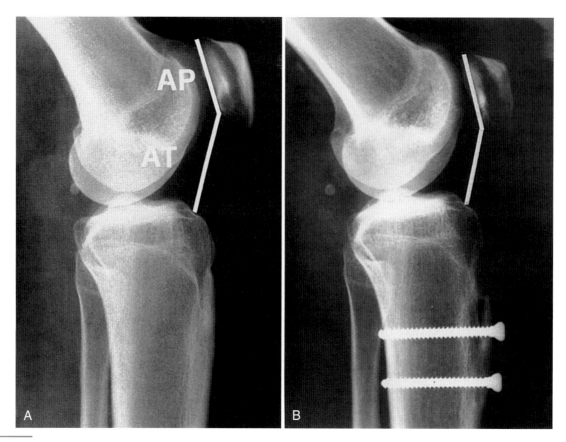

Figure 53–88. Determination of the amount of distal displacement of the tibial tubercle on a lateral radiograph of a knee affected by recurrent dislocation of the patella. The preoperative radiograph shows a high-riding patella with a Caton AT/AP ratio of 1.25. If we aim at obtaining an AT/AP ratio of 0.95, the required millimeters of distal displacement can be calculated as described in the text.

osteotomy is produced. The fragment, 5 to 7 cm long, should be tapered distally. The osteotomy is then completed distally and proximally (Fig. 53–92).

It has often been suggested that the use of an oscillating saw to perform an osteotomy should be avoided because it can cause heat necrosis of bone. We have routinely used an oscillating saw to perform osteotomy of the tibial tubercle and taken the precaution to irrigate the blade with saline. We have not observed any delayed union thus far and continue to use the saw because it allows a more precise cut.

The tuberosity is elevated from its bone bed and displaced medially and distally as planned. For the distal displacement, the distal part of the bone fragment should be resected for a distance equal to the required displacement. Medial displacement is obtained at the proximal part of the bone fragment, whereas the distal part is maintained in alignment with the tibial crest. Medial displacement of more than 12 to 13 mm has not been required in our experience. The tuberosity is temporarily fixed with a 3.2-mm drill bit, and the goniometer is used again to verify that the anatomic Q angle has been corrected satisfactorily. If such is the case, the fragment can be definitively fixed with two cortical lag screws that engage the posterior cortex after countersinking their heads.

The final step is suture of the medial arthrotomy. This is a critical step of the operation. We think that tightening of the lax medial structures according to the Insall technique is the most effective way to reduce lateral subluxation and tilt of the patella. Severe lateral patellar subluxation with tilt cannot be expected to reduce after an isolated lateral retinacular release, which is necessary, but not sufficient to allow medial relocation. Medial displacement of the tibial tuberosity also reduces the valgus vector on the extensor mechanism but cannot be expected to reduce the subluxation in itself unless significant overcorrection is achieved with neutral or varus alignment of the extensor mechanism. Therefore, medial plication should be an integral part of realignment procedure for recurrent patellar dislocation with significant lateral subluxation and tilt of the patella.

On the other hand, we emphasize that overtightening the medial structures is a risk in this procedure. Because the valgus vector of the extensor apparatus is reduced by transfer of the tibial tuberosity, excessive tightening of the medial capsule may lead to medial subluxation of the patella.[190,191] We have noted that overtightening of the medial capsule is more likely if the suturing is performed with the knee in extension. In this position, the patella lies above the sulcus, and medial plication often results in

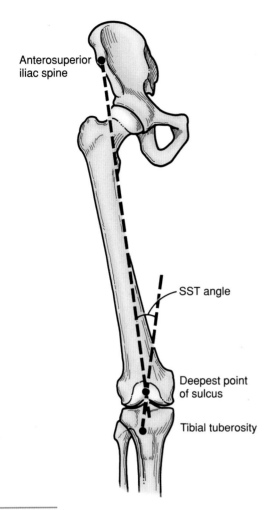

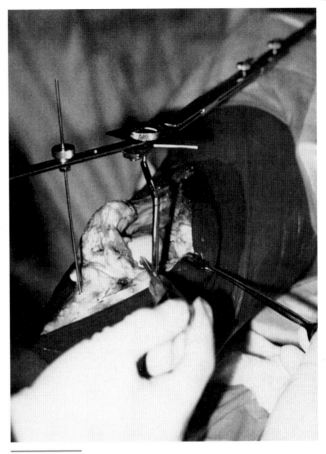

Figure 53–89. Representation of the angle between the anterior superior iliac spine, the deepest point of the sulcus femoralis, and the tibial tuberosity (SST angle). The angle represents a true measure of the valgus vector of the extensor apparatus, and it is not affected by patella position as the surface Q angle is.

Figure 53–90. Measurement of the SST angle at surgery. The upper limb of the goniometer extends to the anterior superior iliac spine, the probe is placed in the deepest point of the sulcus femoralis, and the lower limb of the goniometer with the Kirschner wire points to the tibial tuberosity.

excessive shortening such that the patella dislocates medially when the knee is flexed. To avoid this inconvenience and to fine-tune suturing of the medial arthrotomy, we have found it useful to perform the repair with the knee at 30 degrees of flexion so that the patella is firmly engaged in the sulcus.

Two critical stitches of No. 5 nonabsorbable Ethibond suture are placed at the upper and lower pole of the patella. The needle is passed through the prepatellar tissue, through the medial capsule, and back through the capsule and prepatellar tissue (Fig. 53–93). The amount of overlapping of the medial flap over the patella is determined by the point of penetration through the prepatellar tissue. After these two critical stitches are tightened, tracking of the patella is evaluated in the 0- to 90-degree arc of motion. If it is satisfactory, the remaining part of the arthrotomy is closed with absorbable suture (Vicryl No. 4) without further overlapping. Tracking of the patella is again observed at the end of the suturing, and any obvious abnormality is corrected by adjusting the amount of

overlap of the medial capsule. Lateral mobility of the patella with the knee at 30 degrees is also evaluated and should be less than one quadrant. The wound is closed as is done routinely over suction drainage, and the knee is placed in a bulky Robert Jones bandage. An intraoperative lateral radiograph is useful to check the length of the screws.

In the early postoperative course, the patient is observed carefully. Compartmental syndromes of the leg have been described after the Hauser procedure[401] and attributed to bleeding from the recurrent tibial artery.[393] We have not observed this complication in our series, but this possibility should be known and prompt measures undertaken if there is any suspicion. The dressing is changed on the second postoperative day, and the patient is encouraged to begin active flexion on the bed with the heel sliding on a board. A continuous passive motion device may also be used. Isometric quadriceps contraction is started as soon as possible, but straight-leg raising is not allowed in the first month. The patient is usually discharged on the fifth postoperative day with flexion reaching 60 to 70 degrees. Partial weightbearing is allowed as tolerated, and flexion is progressively increased to 130 degrees by the end of the second month. By the same time,

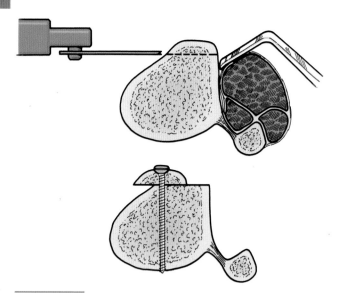

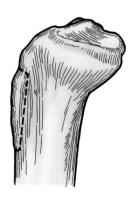

the patient usually walks without crutches and a limp. Quadriceps strengthening is continued for a long time. Isokinetic exercises are not indicated, as is the case in most disorders of the patellofemoral joint. When isometric quadriceps strengthening in extension is well tolerated, short-arc isotonic exercises are introduced without weights on the ankle. If good quadriceps strength and

Figure 53–91. Osteotomy of the tibial tubercle to perform a medial or medial and distal transposition. The osteotomy plane should be horizontal—that is, in the frontal plane—so that no posterior displacement occurs at the time of medial displacement. To allow an approach to the tibia at the correct angle with the saw, the osteotomy is best performed from the medial side to the lateral and with the handle of the saw upward.

Figure 53–92. Osteotomy of the tibial tuberosity to perform a medial or medial and distal transposition. The fragment is tapered distally. The osteotomy is completed distally and proximally to avoid entering the joint.

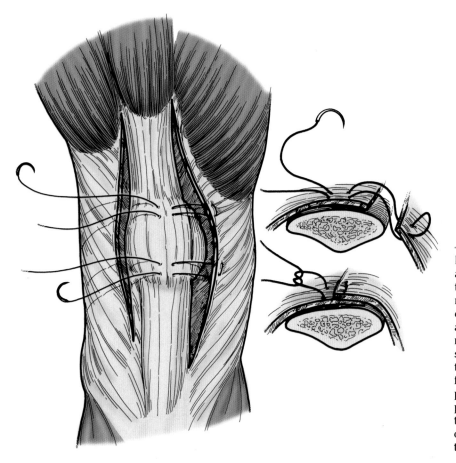

Figure 53–93. Suture of the medial arthrotomy after transposition of the tibial tuberosity in a combined proximal and distal realignment. Two critical stitches are placed at the upper and lower pole of the patella with nonabsorbable No. 5 Ethibond sutures. The suture is passed through the prepatellar tissues, the medial flap, and back through the flap and prepatellar tissues. The point of penetration through the prepatellar tissues determines the amount of overlapping of the medial flap over the patella.

bulk have been achieved and there is no evidence of patellofemoral crepitation on extension of the knee, leg presses with low weights and eccentric exercises can be introduced to the program.

In conclusion, we would like to remark that several anatomic abnormalities have been identified in knees with recurrent dislocation of the patella, including tightness of the lateral and stretching of the medial structures with hypoplasia of the vastus medialis obliquus, lateral placement of the tibial tubercle, a shallow trochlear sulcus, and a patellar shape with prevalence of the lateral facet. The degree of severity of each abnormality varies from knee to knee. From a surgical point of view, one may choose to correct one or more of these factors. If only one factor is going to be corrected, the operation is lateral retinacular release. As noted earlier, the results are unfavorable in more than a third of patients.

If two factors are going to be corrected, we think that the operation should be an Insall proximal realignment, which incorporates lateral release with medial plication. The long-term success of this operation is well documented by ourselves[5] and others,[350] apart from the originator.[200,201] We prefer the medial plication according to Insall's technique over other techniques wherein the vastus medialis obliquus is detached and advanced extra-articularly. With a wide medial arthrotomy and elevation of the quadriceps expansion from the patella, a strong structure is available that can be solidly fixed to allow early motion without fear of dehiscence of the suture line. If only two factors are corrected, it makes much less sense to perform a lateral release and medial transfer of the tibial tuberosity because lateral subluxation of the patella will be reduced incompletely in a number of cases unless excessive medial displacement of the tibial tuberosity is produced.

We would like to repeat that the correct operation to center the patella in the sulcus is Insall's proximal realignment. Medial transposition of the tibial tuberosity is intended to reduce the Q angle and correct excessive lateral placement of the tibial tuberosity, but it cannot be expected to reduce severe lateral subluxation of the patella unless overcorrection is achieved. Hughston[193] and Walsh nicely expressed this concept when they wrote, "Asking a patellar tendon transfer to control the patella is indeed asking the tail to wag the dog." They advocated medial transposition of the tibial tuberosity in selected cases with an increased Q angle.

If three factors are addressed, the operation is lateral release, medial plication of the capsule, and medial and possibly distal transfer of the tibial tuberosity. Medial transfer should be performed only in cases of documented lateral displacement of the tuberosity in relation to the trochlear sulcus, using either CT images or an intraoperative goniometer. The aim should be to correct the valgus vector of the extensor apparatus to values slightly less than normal while avoiding great overcorrections as well as posterior displacement of the tibial transfer. It has been suggested that a fourth factor may require correction.[91] A flat sulcus may be corrected either by elevation of the lateral condyle according to Albee[12] or by depression of the depth of the sulcus as suggested by Masse.[269] We have no experience with these procedures, although we think

that they add to an already complex surgery and possibly increase degenerative changes because of violation of the articular cartilage.

Combined proximal and distal realignment is a more demanding and tricky operation than an isolated Insall proximal operation. We encourage the surgeon to repetitively evaluate patellar tracking during and after the suture phase of the medial arthrotomy. Because the valgus vector of the extensor mechanism is decreased by transposition of the tibial tuberosity, medial subluxation may ensue from an excessively tight medial repair. The final answer regarding the best operation for recurrent dislocation of the patella has not yet been obtained. It will rest on demonstration of better clinical results, low recurrence rates, painless knees, and no degenerative arthritis in the long term. It has yet to be demonstrated that combined realignment, though based on apparently sound mechanical principles, gives results superior to those of proximal realignment. Further studies are needed to elucidate this issue.

Chronic Dislocation of the Patella

The category of chronic dislocation of the patella includes knees with a patella that dislocates laterally each time that the knee is flexed and returns toward the midline with extension of the knee (habitual dislocation). In the most severe cases, the patella is permanently dislocated laterally (permanent dislocation).

Some clinical features allow differentiation from the more common recurrent dislocation of the patella, which usually involves adolescents and wherein patellar tracking shows lateral subluxation with extension and relocation with flexion. Chronic dislocation of the patella is usually detected in children in their first decade of life. The disorder can be classified as congenital or acquired; the acquired form includes cases in which a certain etiological factor has been identified, including multiple injections in the thigh of the infant or, more rarely, trauma. Chronic dislocation of the patella has some relationship to contracture of the quadriceps, which also affects children in their first decade of life. A brief description follows.

Hnevkovsky[184] first reported on 12 children, 8 girls and 4 boys, between 1 and 7 years old who experienced progressive flexion loss of their knees without a history of trauma or inflammation of either the knee or the thigh. Conservative treatment did not improve flexion. The condition was bilateral in four knees. In the affected knee of older children, the patella was higher and more laterally placed than in the normal knee. All the knees underwent surgery. Section of the scarred vastus intermedius allowed improvement in flexion in 10 knees. Histological examination of samples from the quadriceps revealed progressive fibrous degeneration of the vastus intermedius and rectus femoris. Hnevkovsky interpreted the disease as an incompletely developed form of arthrogryposis.

Two cases of quadriceps contracture in identical twins were reported by Fairbank and Barrett.[111] One child underwent surgery; scarring of the vastus intermedius was limiting flexion, with no contribution from the rectus, vastus medialis, or lateralis. Histological examination revealed fibrous and fatty degeneration of the vastus intermedius. Two patients similar to those reported in previous publications were described by Gammie and coworkers.[143] They suggested a similarity between quadriceps contracture and other congenital abnormalities, including clubfoot, Sprengel's shoulder, and congenital wryneck. Karlen[219] reported six cases of quadriceps contracture in Chinese patients, five children between 1 and 9 years old and a 24-year-old man. The best results were obtained after isolated section of the tendon of the vastus intermedius in younger patients. The two older patients, aged 9 and 24 years, obtained less improvement in flexion, possibly because of the changes that occurred in the other structures of the knee, which were due to restriction of flexion over a long period.

Gunn[166] and Lloyd-Roberts and Thomas[253] shed some more light on the etiology of quadriceps contracture in children. Gunn reported on 22 patients with quadriceps contracture. Fifteen of them (68%) had a history of severe illness for which injection therapy into the thigh was almost certainly administered. At surgery, the vastus lateralis and intermedius were involved, alone or in combination, in all the knees. In six cases, the rectus femoris was involved, but only in its lateral half. In only one case did the fibrotic reaction reach the vastus medialis. Contracture of the iliotibial band was common and thought to be secondary to fibrosis of the quadriceps muscle. These data indicate that the quadriceps was affected mainly in its anterior and lateral portion. Some children in this series were affected by chronic dislocation of the patella. If this was prevented by the application of medial pressure on the patella, flexion of the knee was severely limited. Patellar dislocation was therefore interpreted as a way to attain flexion at the expense of patellar stability.

Similar conclusions were reached by Lloyd-Roberts and Thomas,[253] who analyzed the histories of six children with quadriceps contracture. All had received injections or infusions into their thighs soon after birth for serious illnesses. In three patients, the stigmata of injections persisted as skin dimples. The consequences of the intramuscular injections and subcutaneous infusions were related to the local trauma, to the volume of fluid introduced (which can raise intramuscular pressure with subsequent capillary obstruction and muscle ischemia), and to its chemical composition (including pH and osmotic pressure). All these factors lead to intramuscular edema and hemorrhage with widespread ischemic changes in the muscle.

Intramuscular injections seem to be a major cause of quadriceps fibrosis and contracture. In a large series of 2404 cases reported by the Japanese Ministry of Health and Welfare, 76% occurred after injections, 3% were congenital, and 21% were idiopathic.[66] Identification of the original cause of the disease is rendered more difficult by the fact that it may be several months before postinjection stiffness becomes evident. In the series reported by Alvarez and coworkers,[14] the time interval ranged from 3 to 18 months. In five patients with chronic patellar dislocation, the condition was preceded by a period of stiffness of the knee.

Green and Waugh[160] described four cases of congenital lateral dislocation of the patella and emphasized the difficulty in reaching the correct diagnosis in infants. In these patients, the presence of a flexion contracture should alert the physician to the possibility of congenital lateral dislocation of the patella once other causes, including arthrogryposis, have been excluded. In infants, the patella can be palpated with difficulty because it is very small and located on the lateral side. Radiographs are of no help because the patella is not ossified. Green and Waugh described a patient with a strong tendency toward hereditary transmission of the disease. They recommend early treatment of the disease, within the first year of life. A first operation was needed to reach full extension, followed by a second to relocate the patella in the sulcus by means of release of the lateral structures, shortening of the medial capsule, and transfer of the patellar tendon. If the abnormal position of the patella and the flexion contracture are allowed to persist for longer periods, secondary deformities may develop, including genu valgum and external tibial torsion, as a result of the pull of the displaced extensor mechanism.

Williams[404] presented a series of 28 children with quadriceps contracture that led to a stiff knee in 13 cases and to chronic dislocation of the patella in 15. Over half of his patients had a history of intramuscular injections. The children with a stiff knee were initially seen at an average age of 3 years. In some cases kept under observation, the condition proved to be progressive. At surgery, the vastus intermedius contributed to limit flexion in 85% of cases, the vastus lateralis in 54%, and the rectus femoris in 46%. The children with chronic dislocation of the patella were initially evaluated at an average age of 6 years, 3 years older than those with a stiff knee. The patella dislocated laterally each time that the knee was flexed, and flexion did not exceed 30 degrees if dislocation of the patella was prevented by the application of lateral pressure. At surgery, all the components of the quadriceps were involved except the vastus medialis. The vastus lateralis was involved in 73%, the iliotibial band in 53%, and the rectus femoris in 33%. The similarity between a stiff knee with quadriceps contracture and chronic dislocation of the patella was further confirmed by the observation of a boy who had patellar dislocation of one knee and stiffness in the other.

CLINICAL ASPECTS

The congenital form of chronic dislocation of the patella is rarely detected at birth because of the small dimensions of the patella, its lateral placement, and late development of the ossific nucleus, which renders radiographs uninformative in infants. As pointed out by Green and Waugh,[160] the presence of a fixed flexion contracture should remind the physician of the possibility of congenital lateral dislocation of the patella, once arthrogryposis has been excluded. The most frequent clinical situation is when the parents note that the child has difficulty rising from the sitting or squatting position. Even if walking and straight-leg raising are possible, quadriceps power is greatly decreased. The knee at 90 degrees of flexion looks wider than the contralateral normal knee, and the medial femoral condyle can easily be palpated under the skin (Fig. 53–94). If the deformity has persisted for a sufficient period, secondary deformities may develop, including valgus alignment of the knee and fixed external tibial torsion. If dislocation of the patella is prevented, knee flexion will be greatly limited by the tightness of the quadriceps.

The clinical picture in the acquired form is similar. There is often a history of several intramuscular injections in the thighs delivered in the first days of life because of severe illness. Once again, the diagnosis can be missed until the age of 4 or 5 years or even later. Some cases seem to be secondary to trauma. The patient reports that the knee was normal until trauma dislocated the patella laterally. Afterward, lateral dislocation in flexion developed.

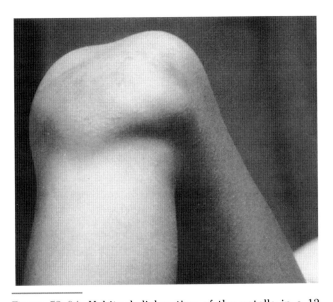

Figure 53–94. Habitual dislocation of the patella in a 12-year-old boy. The knee looks wider than normal, the profile of the medial femoral condyle is well evident medially, and the patella is dislocated laterally.

Because the typical osseous abnormalities of long-standing patellar dislocation (flat sulcus, small patella) are absent in some cases, it seems possible that trauma played a major role.

SURGICAL TREATMENT

The two goals of surgical treatment of chronic patellar dislocation are (1) realignment of the patella and (2) lengthening of the contracted quadriceps. Isolated realignment of the patella may improve tracking of the patella but fails to allow sufficient flexion. Furthermore, the efforts to improve flexion predispose to recurrence of the dislocation.

Williams[404] described a procedure wherein tight lateral bands[212] are first released from the patella (Fig. 53–95) by means of a wide lateral release. Proximal to the patella, the incision parallels the lateral border of the quadriceps tendon, thus releasing the vastus lateralis insertion from the patella and quadriceps tendon. The vastus intermedius is inspected and divided if tight. If the rectus femoris is also tight, it can be lengthened by releasing the vastus medialis from the quadriceps tendon and the rectus femoris at the musculotendinous junction. The knee is flexed, the vastus medialis and lateralis are sutured together, and the quadriceps tendon is lengthened. If the patella still subluxes laterally, medial plication is added, possibly with advancement of the vastus medialis or transfer of the patellar tendon or sartorius. A similar technique has been reported by Fulkerson and Hungerford[135] wherein the quadriceps tendon is lengthened by Z-plasty.

Bergman and Williams[32] reported the results of the Williams operation[404] in a consecutive series of 35 patients (45 knees) with chronic dislocations of the patella. The average age at initial evaluation was 9 years (range, 3 to 15 years). A history of multiple intramuscular injections was present in eight cases (23%). One child had a quadriceps contracture with a stiff knee on the opposite side. There was a family history of patellar dislocation in 10 children (29%). The most common reason for involvement of the orthopedic surgeon was the unusual appear-

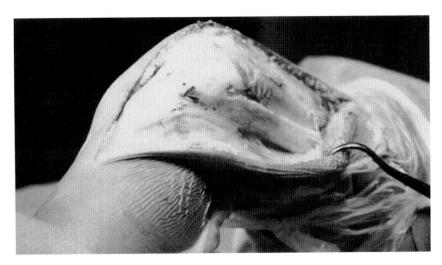

Figure 53–95. Knee affected by habitual dislocation of the patella. An abnormally tight iliotibial band inserts into the lateral border of the patella and tethers it laterally. (From Jeffreys TE: Recurrent dislocation of the patella due to abnormal attachment of the iliotibial tract. J Bone Joint Surg Br 45:740, 1963.)

ance of the knee (43%) as noted by the mother. The abnormality was detected during routine examination of the child in 20% of cases and during examination for unrelated trauma in a further 20%. It is remarkable that the initial symptom was pain in only 11% and inability to run because of instability in 6%. If dislocation of the patella was prevented, the average flexion angle was 35 degrees and never more than 70 degrees. At surgery, the most often contracted structure was the vastus lateralis (72%), followed by the iliotibial band (58%). Contractures involved the rectus femoris in 42% and the vastus intermedius in 16%. The vastus medialis was affected in only one case.

After the operation, the knee was placed in a cast at 90 degrees of flexion for 6 weeks. An extensor lag was present initially in all the knees in which the quadriceps tendon had been lengthened, but it resolved within 1 year on average. The patients were reviewed with an average follow-up of 6 years and 9 months. Patellar redislocation was detected in 12 knees (28%), 10 of which required a repeated quadricepsplasty with a successful final result. At the final follow-up, 34 knees (79%) were normal; of the remaining 9 patients (21%), 6 had a history of occasional giving way and 3 complained of patellofemoral pain.

In France, knees with chronic patellar dislocation are more often treated with a quadricepsplasty according to Judet.[217] After lateral retinacular release, the quadriceps is sharply elevated from the distal to proximal aspects and detached from the lateral intramuscular septum and femoral shaft. If needed, the rectus tendon is detached from the anterior inferior iliac spine. All the quadriceps muscle is therefore allowed to slide distally, and flexion is increased. Additional procedures may be needed to stabilize the patella in the femoral sulcus, including medial plication of the capsule or transfer of the patellar tendon. In a growing child, this is best achieved by medial transposition of the lateral half of the patella tendon (Goldthwait-Roux operation) (Fig. 53–96).

In conclusion, habitual dislocation of the patella is a less frequent, but not less challenging problem than recurrent dislocation. Treatment of it rests on appreciation of the two components of the disease: lateral displacement of the patella and quadriceps shortening. A successful result requires that both be corrected at the same operation.

CHONDROMALACIA PATELLAE AND PATELLOFEMORAL ARTHRITIS

The development and significance of damage to the articular cartilage of the patellofemoral joint have been known and discussed for a long time. As far as known, the first description of chondromalacic cartilage was given by Buedinger.[51,52] He described fissures that he thought were caused by trauma. The term *chondromalacia*, however, was not used by Buedinger himself and is attributed to Aleman.[13] Since the original description, it has been progressively appreciated that the role of trauma is a minor one. Furthermore, a significant incidence of chondromalacic changes has been noted in knees without patellofemoral symptoms at the time of surgery for a meniscal or ligamentous disorder or at autopsy. In this discussion we summarize the current knowledge of chondromalacia patellae. The term should be used strictly to describe changes that occur in the articular cartilage of the patella. Because there is no evidence that chondromalacia of "normal" asymptomatic knees has the same site, characteristics, and evolution of chondromalacia of knees with patellofemoral problems, we have separated the studies describing these two conditions.

Age-Related Changes in Chondromalacia

At autopsy, Owre[311] examined the articular surface of the patella in 124 knees of patients ranging in age from 14 to 80 years. In the five different age groups—14 to 19, 20 to 29, 30 to 39, 40 to 59, and 60 to 80 years—the incidence of "edema" was 28%, 84%, 92%, 94%, and 100%, respec-

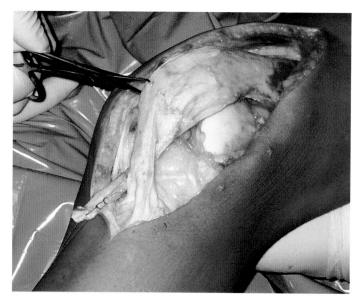

Figure 53–96. Operation for chronic dislocation of the patella, including a wide lateral release, medial plication, and medial transposition of the lateral half of the patella tendon.

tively. In the same groups, the incidence of fissuring was 0%, 56%, 73%, 90%, and 94%, respectively. It seems that fissuring, the more severe change, is rare before the age of 20 years but becomes increasingly common after the second decade of life and affects almost all knees after the fourth decade of life. Owre concluded that "one rarely finds a normal joint after the age of 50 years." However, the extent to which these patellae were involved is not clear.

Wiles and associates[403] reported that chondromalacia was noted in 29% of the knees that underwent meniscectomy at the Middlesex Hospital between 1950 and 1955. Outerbridge[309] also reported the incidence of chondromalacia as observed at the time of meniscectomy. From the second to the seventh decades of life, the reported incidence was 50%, 35%, 44%, 71%, 72%, and 66%, respectively. He noted that the site was almost always the middle of the medial patellar facet or slightly distal to it. In light of this observation, Outerbridge classified chondromalacia into four different grades:

Grade I: softening and swelling
Grade II: fragmentation and fissuring in an area of $^{1}/_{2}$ inch or less
Grade III: area larger than $^{1}/_{2}$ inch
Grade IV: cartilage erosion down to bone

According to his classification, grade I chondromalacia was present in 17%, grade II in 19%, grade III in 10%, and grade IV in 6% of cases. There was no correlation between age at surgery and the severity of chondromalacia. In a subsequent study, Outerbridge[310] reported that in a group of patients undergoing medial meniscectomy, severe (grades III and IV) chondromalacia was more frequent in females (34%; males, 10.4%) and in overweight patients.

Emery and Meachim[104] reported an extensive study of Liverpool necropsies. They found that in young persons, overt fibrillation began at the periphery of the patella, specifically in a limited area of the medial margin of the patella (odd facet). They remarked that this lesion did not progress to fasciculation or bone erosion, even in older subjects. In middle-aged persons, fibrillation appeared in the central medial facet and then spread through the ridge to the lateral facet. Lesions in the central part of the lateral facet first progressed to bony erosion.

Marar and Pillay[263] studied chondromalacia in a series of 100 Chinese cadavers. Both knees were dissected in each cadaver: 30 cadavers had erosion of the articular surface and 21 had fibrillation without erosion of one or both patellae. The age distribution ranged from 32 to 82 years. In the fourth to eighth decades of life, the correlation of age with chondromalacia showed an incidence of 0%, 33%, 39%, 65%, and 57%, respectively. The incidence increased with age, but even after the sixth decade of life the incidence was around 60%, less than that reported by Owre[311] and Wiles and coworkers.[402,403] Chondromalacia involved the medial facet alone in 36 knees, whereas erosion of the lateral facet was present in 16. Therefore, chondromalacia involved the medial facet frequently, but not exclusively. There was no correlation between chondromalacia and the presence of a distinct ridge at the junction between the medial femoral condyle and the anterior surface of the femoral shaft as described by Outerbridge.[309]

Casscells[59] examined the cartilage changes in 300 cadaver knees whose average age was 70 years. Only 8% were younger than 50 years, 39.5% were 50 to 69 years old, 48.5% were 70 to 89 years old, and 4% were older than 90 years. Chondromalacia was classified into four grades according to the severity and extension of the lesion, grade 0 being normal and grade 4 meaning erosion down to subchondral bone in a wide area. Degenerative changes in cartilage were less common in the weightbearing area of the tibiofemoral joint (23%) than in the patellofemoral joint (63%). Chondromalacia was more frequent in females (77%) than in males (60%). The severity of chondromalacia, however, was minor in most cases: 37% of the knees were normal, 25% were grade 1, and 27% were grade 2. Chondromalacia diffused to the entire patellar surface in 51% and was limited to the medial facet in 25%, lateral facet in 12%, and ridge in 12%. Cartilage changes in the trochlea were less frequent than chondromalacia, with 52% of the knees showing absence of changes. Citing these data, Casscells questioned the conclusion of Owre[311] because most of the knees in this group of elderly cadavers had only minor changes in the patellofemoral joint, and these were even rarer in the tibiofemoral joint. Since the introduction of arthroscopy, Casscells[60] observed that chondromalacia is a frequent finding in knees with and without known abnormalities in the patellofemoral joint; he stated, "I am convinced that chondromalacia is rarely the cause of these symptoms."

Abernethy and colleagues[1] studied 100 knees obtained at autopsy from 56 patients ranging in age from 30 to 90 years. The severity of chondromalacia was classified into four grades. The severity of cartilage damage on both the medial and the lateral facets increased with age. Abernethy and coworkers observed that in the less severe grades 1 and 2, changes were almost always located along the periphery of the patella and did not progress. More advanced cartilage damage was observed on the central medial facet, but it did not progress to expose subchondral bone in more than a small minority of cases (4%). The most severe cartilage damage appeared to begin on the lateral facet and could later spread to the medial facet. Overall exposure of subchondral bone was present in only 13% of the lateral facets and 4% of the medial facets. A chronological sequence of the development of chondromalacia was suggested. Early and minor changes usually occur on the medial facet, but with increasing age, changes occur on the lateral facet, where cartilage is more often eroded down to subchondral bone. Based on the high necropsy incidence of cartilage fibrillation of the medial facet (85%), Abernethy and coworkers concluded that this finding is better considered as asymptomatic, age-related, physiological change.

Given the low incidence of patellofemoral disorders in the general population, we think that autopsy studies should reflect the development of chondromalacia in "normal" knees.[1,59,104,263] According to these studies, it seems that fibrillation develops early on the medial facet and at the periphery of the patella. These changes are asymptomatic and mostly nonprogressive. Starting in middle age, changes develop in the lateral facet, and here they are more likely to progress to erosion down to subchondral bone. It is remarkable, however, that progression to severe cartilage damage occurred in only a minority of knees. It seems that cartilage is reasonably well suited to resist the test of time. The arthroscopist should be aware of these facts and avoid overemphasizing the frequent finding of superficial fibrillation of the medial facet. Chondromalacia cannot be assumed to be the cause of pain in itself, and malalignment or another source of pain should be looked for.

Goodfellow and colleagues[155] introduced the term *surface age-dependent degeneration* to describe the sequence of degenerative changes that develop in some part of most human joints as a consequence of aging.[153,154,173] The term seems appropriate because the first changes affect the surface of the cartilage and deeper layers are only secondarily involved. It has been suggested that surface degeneration at the hip, knee, and elbow begins in areas that are seldom used because of human habits. The surgical and autopsy experience of Goodfellow and coworkers suggests that surface degeneration of the patella starts in the "odd" facet. Analysis of the functional anatomy of the patellofemoral joint has confirmed that the odd facet contacts the medial femoral condyle at 135 degrees of knee flexion only. Because this degree of flexion is not habitually reached in occidental people, the concept of disuse is valid. There was no evidence to suggest that surface degeneration of the odd facet is symptomatic, but this is not to say that it is without consequence. Bullough and Goodfellow[54] stressed the unitary nature of cartilage, wherein collagen fibers are arranged to resist tension. Interruption in the transmission of force created by the defect, even in an unloaded area, predisposes the adjacent loaded areas to mechanical breakdown. In other words, the asymptomatic surface degeneration of the odd facet can slowly progress in some patients and spread to the medial and lateral facets, until subchondral bone is exposed. At that time, the process becomes symptomatic and radiography reveals the usual changes of patellofemoral osteoarthritis.

passing transversely across the central area of the patella, with the upper and lower thirds of the articular surface nearly always spared (Fig. 53–97). The medial facet alone was involved in 21% and the lateral facet alone in 7% of cases. They further observed that 9% of the knees that they performed surgery on for patellar pain syndrome in fact had normal patellar cartilage. This finding has also been reported by other authors. Goodfellow and associates[155] found an absence of articular cartilage lesions in 15% of their patients with clinically diagnosed patellar pain. The incidence of knees with patellar pain syndromes that were found to have normal articular cartilage at the time of surgery has been variably reported as being 9% to 69%.[63,102,158,242,274,285,286]

It therefore seems that both pain and cartilage changes may be secondary to a third factor. The mechanisms suggested[200] involve the peculiar anatomy of the patellofemoral joint. The convex central ridge of the patella is covered by a thick layer of cartilage. This layer creates a vertical crest that is subject to lateral shear force. This force is obviously increased in knees with malalignment. Deformation of the thick articular cartilage may produce abnormal loading on subchondral bone and therefore pain, even in the absence of cartilage lesions. On the other hand, repeated deformation of the cartilage around the ridge may well be responsible for cartilage softening, fissuring, and ultimately, degeneration. The effect can be visualized by again considering the analogy of an eraser on the end of an ordinary pencil. Repetitive sideways loading soon causes the eraser to shear from its attachment to the pencil, whereas direct compression with much greater force has little effect.

Goodfellow and colleagues[155] described a different lesion as being responsible for patellofemoral pain in young patients. The lesion involves the deep layer of cartilage, at least in the early phases, and is therefore called *basal degeneration*. In the first stage, the lesion is appreciated as "softening" or as "pitting edema" of the cartilage.

Chondromalacia and Patellofemoral Malalignment

Ficat and colleagues[115] described the excessive lateral pressure syndrome of chondromalacic changes in knees with proven patellofemoral disorders as consisting of a lateral tilt of the patella around the central ridge caused by a shortened lateral retinaculum. According to this pathogenetic mechanism, they defined the critical zone as an area that experiences the highest compression-shear force and consequently has the highest incidence of cartilage degeneration. The critical zone is localized across the ridge of the patella with some extension to the lateral facet. In the craniocaudal direction, the proximal and distal parts of the articular cartilage are often spared, whereas the central part is involved.

Insall and colleagues[203] performed a detailed study on the topographic location of cartilage changes in 105 knees affected by malalignment and patellar pain, including some with recurrent dislocation. They found that the most frequent site of chondromalacia (71%) was in an ellipse

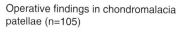

Operative findings in chondromalacia patellae (n=105)

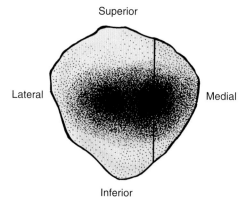

Figure 53–97. Composite of patellar maps made at surgery showing the distribution of chondromalacia in a series of 105 patellae. (From Insall JN, Falvo KA, Wise DW: Chondromalacia patellae: A prospective study. J Bone Joint Surg Am 58:1, 1976.)

The affected area may be sharply separated by the surrounding normal cartilage, and the isolated disk of cartilage may be easily elevated with a small curet. The articular surface of the disk appears glistening and smooth, whereas the deep surface demonstrates thick fascicles of collagen perpendicular to the articular surface. Thus, there seems to be a derangement of the deep layers of cartilage wherein collagen bundles lose cohesion and cartilage is held together by the intact tangential fibers at the articular surface. The lesion may evolve to form a blister, which may successively rupture and originate an area of open chondromalacia.

Goodfellow and colleagues[155] described two preferential sites of this lesion: (1) the secondary ridge between the medial and odd facet and (2) the inferior part of the central ridge, which separates the medial from the lateral facet. The lesion was found in 23 young patients complaining of patellofemoral pain, but it was admitted that not all patients with such pain may be expected to have this lesion. It was not specified whether these knees had associated malalignment. The reason that a basal degeneration lesion causes pain includes the fact that the intermediate layers of cartilage are essential for load transmission to subchondral bone. The nonaligned collagen fibers of the intermediate zone assume a more tangential alignment under load, only to resume their original orientation when the load is removed. The disorganization of the intermediate zone is therefore likely to cause abnormal stress distribution to subchondral bone and hence pain. The development of basal degeneration and its peculiar site was explained by the fact that the secondary ridge is subjected to shear force while the knee is flexed from 90 to 130 degrees, when it glides against the convex surface of the medial femoral condyle.

MACROSCOPIC OBSERVATIONS

Chondromalacia
It seems that regardless of the cause, the development of degeneration of the cartilage of the patella follows a course through a stage of softening and then fissuring, fibrillation, and exposure of subchondral bone.

Cartilage softening (or closed chondromalacia) is the earliest lesion (grade I). Cartilage softening can be demonstrated only with the use of a probe. The cartilage loses its normal resilience to the point that "pitting edema" may be observed after pressure with an instrument. In some cases, a blister is evident on the surface of the patella. Arthroscopic measurement of the stiffness of the cartilage of the medial facet has been performed with a microminiature pressure transducer.[88] Among a group of 50 normal control knees, 51% had softening of the cartilage, whereas 92% of the knees with patellofemoral pain had the same finding. In more than half the knees with patellofemoral pain and cartilage softening, no change was observed in the appearance of the cartilage. This report confirms that softening of patellar cartilage may exist in as many as half the knees without patellofemoral symptoms.

Once the articular surface has been interrupted, the lesion may be classified as open chondromalacia. The second grade is fissuring of the articular surface. Fissures may be superficial or deep down to subchondral bone. Fissuring may proceed to fibrillation (grade III), which can be classified as superficial or deep. Flaps of cartilage may be due to extension of fissures horizontally and tangent to subchondral bone. The last stage is exposure of subchondral bone (grade IV).

The term *chondromalacia* should be limited to disorders that involve articular cartilage only. If the disease has progressed to involve changes in bone (osteophyte formation, subchondral sclerosis, and cysts) and the synovium (synovitis), it is better classified as patellofemoral arthritis. The various stages of chondromalacia can coexist in the same patella. A central area of exposure of subchondral bone may be surrounded by a zone of cartilage fibrillation, which in turn is surrounded by softened cartilage until normal cartilage is encountered.

Patellofemoral Arthritis
Arthritis of the patellofemoral joint predominantly involves the lateral joint line in the great majority of cases. The usual aspect on the axial view includes narrowing of the joint line, osteophytes on the lateral border of the patella and trochlea, subchondral sclerosis of the lateral facet, and possibly cyst formation (Fig. 53–98). The predominant involvement of the lateral joint line in patellofemoral arthritis is explained by the valgus vector of the extensor apparatus.

Patellofemoral arthritis is often associated with tibiofemoral degenerative changes, either in the medial or in the lateral compartment. Valgus alignment is frequently associated with an increased Q angle, which in turn increases the valgus vector of the extensor apparatus. Medial gonarthrosis with varus alignment, on the other hand, may enhance the development of patellofemoral arthritis by releasing breakdown products and lytic enzymes from cartilage.[68]

Arthritis involving predominantly the medial patellofemoral joint line is rare. It is usually iatrogenic and caused by excessive medial displacement of the tibial tuberosity.

HISTOLOGY AND ELECTRON MICROSCOPY

The histological changes of chondromalacia vary according to the stage of the disease.[30,115,136,306] The three components of cartilage—chondrocytes, ground substance, and collagen fibers—are all affected by the disease, and their changes will be described separately in discussions of closed and open chondromalacia.

Closed Chondromalacia
Knees with closed chondromalacia examined by optical microscopy show a continuous surface. The superficial cells often undergo fibrous metaplasia and assume a shape flatter than usual. The deeper layers of cartilage have an apparent increase in the quantity of ground substance, which is described as edema. Ground substance shows a decrease in its staining capacity with Alcian blue, tolui-

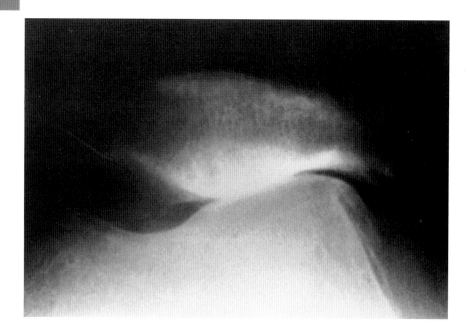

Figure 53–98. Arthritis of the patellofemoral joint. Involvement of the lateral joint line is clearly predominant.

dine blue, and safranin O, which can be correlated with a decrease of the content of glycosaminoglycans. Ohno and colleagues[306] said that loss of glycosaminoglycans is especially centered around the chondrocytes. The chondrocyte number is normal or slightly reduced in the superficial and transitional zone. Ohno and associates described the presence of matrix streaks that were centered on often empty lacunae.

Bony changes have been reported in knees with patellofemoral pain by Darracott and Vernon-Roberts.[87] In 11 patellae, they observed diffuse osteoporosis in 3 cases and isolated foci of osteoporosis in the remaining 8. In some patellae, nodular aggregates of bone on trabeculae were present at the junction of normal and porotic areas.

The findings on electron microscopy are best understood with reference to normal articular cartilage. At the surface of cartilage, electron microscopy reveals a network of collagen fibers oriented parallel to it. The chondrocytes of the superficial zone are flattened (spindle or oval shaped) and have a cytoplasmic structure that is similar to that of fibroblasts, with a Golgi apparatus and rough endoplasmic reticulum, often poorly developed. In the transitional zone is a tridimensional network of collagen fibers within the ground substance. The chondrocytes are more rounded and have a moderately developed rough endoplasmic reticulum.

In knees with closed chondromalacia, electron microscopic examination reveals changes in all three components of cartilage. The collagen fibers of the superficial zone and just beneath it show loss of the usual orientation with a more random distribution, angulation, abrupt change in their direction, and fiber disintegration. The ground substance seems to be increased in volume; this has been correlated with a 9% increase in the water content of osteoarthritic cartilage.[260] Crevices, small fissures, or streaks have been identified in the matrix, more often in the deep superficial or transitional zone. They are centered around cellular lacunae and extend radially from

them. The streaks are obliquely oriented to the surface. They do not reach either the surface or the deep layers of cartilage. The chondrocytes are slightly reduced in number and show signs of both activation (a well-developed Golgi apparatus and rough endoplasmic reticulum) and degeneration (increase in the number of dense bodies, dilatation of the endoplasmic reticulum, and mitochondrial distention). Chondrocytes tend to cluster in the superficial and transitional zones. Necrotic cells or cellular remnants are occasionally visible in early lesions.

Open Chondromalacia

Examination of lesions of open chondromalacia by optical microscopy reveals an obvious fibrillation of the surface. In addition, changes in the constituents of cartilage are more marked and clearly degenerative. Chondrocytes are reduced in number and show obvious clustering. Dead cells are more common. The ground substance is disorganized and stains unevenly.

Bentley[30] described the presence of a greatly increased number of small cells resembling fibroblasts in the superficial layer of areas of open chondromalacia. This was evident in almost half the specimens that he examined. In association with these changes, the cartilage appeared to have repaired and smoothed off. Bentley supplemented the histological examination with an autoradiographic study using SO_4 and tritiated thymidine labeling. In no case was there evidence of SO_4 labeling in the superficial and transitional zones, which indicates extensive cell damage and absence of synthesis of sulfate-containing glycosaminoglycans. Labeling of the nuclei of cells with tritiated thymidine, which indicates impending or recent cell division, was evident in the areas of fibrous metaplasia, in 50% of the clusters of chondrocytes, and sometimes in the deep zone of cartilage. These data have been interpreted as evidence of depletion of glycosaminoglycans from the superficial and middle zone of cartilage. The presence of cell division is attributed to fibrous metaplasia of the superficial layers and to limited attempts at proliferation in the intact cartilage close to the areas of the lesion. This finding contrasts with what has been reported by Lund and Telbag,[255] who failed to show tritiated thymidine labeling in chondromalacic cartilage.

Examination of areas of open chondromalacia with the electron microscope confirms the predominantly degenerative nature of this lesion. Chondrocytes show clear degenerative changes at both the cytoplasmic and nuclear level, and necrotic cells are common; the few remaining chondrocytes are often clustered. Collagen fibers are more dissociated and fragmented. The internal surface of the fissures is lined with amorphous material that appears to merge with the adjacent matrix and is therefore considered matrix in an advanced state of degeneration.

In conclusion, it appears that the earliest changes in chondromalacia affect the transitional zone whereas the surface tangential network of fibers is spared. The cartilage seems to react to the increased loads and demands by an increase in chondrocyte activity. If the demands exceed the potential of the chondrocytes, an increasing number of cells fail. Loss of glycosaminoglycans and an increase in water are noted in the ground substance. Collagen fibrils lose their tridimensional arrangement and become tightly packed in bundles, some of which appear to be interrupted. Matrix streaks have been described around lacunae[306] and interpreted as the earliest sign of matrix failure. The superficial layer increasingly loses the support of the deranged transitional layer, and fissuring of the surface ultimately occurs, either by superficial extension of the matrix streaks or by some other mechanism. The major reparative response that has been observed is fibroblastic metaplasia in the superficial layers, more often at the periphery of the lesion and in contact with the synovium.[306] The significance of the reparative response of the surrounding normal cartilage is less clear.

ETIOLOGY

Chondromalacia

We think that the main cause of chondromalacia patellae in knees with malalignment is the development of high compression force on the lateral facet associated with shear force in the area of the central ridge; such force develops to resist lateral displacement of the patella.[193] In these conditions, the medial facet may also manifest chondromalacic changes as a result of hypopressure, but these changes seem to develop more slowly, probably because the medial facet experiences lower loads. The details of this hypothesis have previously been described. Other conditions have been suspected to cause chondromalacia. Some of these have stood the test of time, whereas others are no longer thought to be true.

In his classic work, Wiberg[400] described three different types of patella morphology. He identified type III as the most dysplastic form, with a marked lateral predominance, a wide lateral facet, and a smaller convex medial facet. Nevertheless, he could not show an association between type III patellae and chondromalacia. The same has been observed by Outerbridge.[309,310] Therefore, it

appears that the shape of the patella cannot be considered an etiological factor of chondromalacia.

Outerbridge[309,310] observed that chondromalacia more frequently involved the medial patellar facet; he suggested that this propensity is related to the presence of an osteochondral ridge between the proximal lip of the trochlea on the medial side and the femoral shaft. He also found a relationship between the height of the ridge and the incidence of chondromalacia. Outerbridge observed that with the knee in extension, the patella lies proximal to the ridge. At the beginning of flexion, the medial facet would impinge against the ridge, thereby leading to chondromalacia. This pathogenetic mechanism has been questioned because of the observation that the patella is lateralized in full extension and enters the sulcus from the lateral side, thus making impingement against the ridge unlikely. In a study of 100 Chinese cadavers, Marar and Pillay[263] found that despite a distinct ridge often visible at this site, it was well covered by the overlying soft tissues and there was no relationship between the ridge and chondromalacia.

Abernethy and colleagues[1] examined 100 cadaver knees and identified a sequence of changes that would occur with increasing age. The earliest changes were observed at the periphery of the patella, then in the central medial facet, and finally in the central lateral facet. Changes in the lateral facet showed the greatest tendency to progress toward the more advanced stages (bone exposure). The presence of chondromalacia was related to the stiffness of the underlying bone, which was indirectly inferred by measurements of bone density. The bone underlying the medial facet was relatively less stiff than the rest of the contact area of the patella. Increased stiffness beneath the lateral facet was associated with more advanced articular damage. There was an abrupt change between relatively compliant bone and stiff bone in the area of the central medial facet. This is the area in which the earliest cartilage damage occurred. The suggested pathogenic mechanism is that the less stiff bone deflects under load more than the stiffer bone does. This causes shear stress in the overlying articular cartilage with consequent degeneration. The objection to this theory is that adjacent areas of the patellar surface do not necessarily experience the same loads. In other words, the differences in bone density may only be a reflection of the different loads that are imposed on the various areas of the patellar surface (Wolff's law). Given the valgus vector of the extensor mechanism, the increased bone density under the lateral patellar facet is not an unexpected finding.

Chondromalacia patellae is a well-known complication that occurs after prolonged immobilization for fractures of the lower limb. In these cases, damage may result from loss of the pumping action that supplies nutrients to the articular cartilage. Patellar cartilage, which is exceptionally thick, may be more vulnerable in this sense. Damage to the cartilage of the trochlea, which is thinner, is less frequent. Furthermore, immobilization of the joint has been shown to cause obliteration of the cavity by proliferation of fibrofatty tissue. Fibrous tissue grows over unapposed articular cartilage, and ulcers develop in apposed cartilage because of prolonged pressure.[107] If the immobilization is of long duration, these changes are not reversible and explain the development of chondromalacia.

Chondromalacia is also known to develop after surgical procedures on the knee joint. Anterior cruciate ligament reconstruction, either open or arthroscopic, has been widely performed, and there is evidence that symptoms of chondromalacia develop in roughly a fourth of cases. Clear patellofemoral crepitation is appreciated in these patients, but fortunately it is painful or causes swelling in only about 5%.

Many factors may contribute to the development of chondromalacia.[4] First, it should be recognized that chondromalacic changes and malalignment may be present (and asymptomatic) preoperatively and become symptomatic postoperatively. Second, trauma to articular cartilage occurs during the operation. Wide medial arthrotomies with detachment of the vastus medialis and subluxation-dislocation of the patella are likely to alter patellar tracking. Healing of the medial retinaculum with some lengthening and atrophy of the vastus medialis increases lateral patellar tracking. An iatrogenic type of hyperpressure syndrome can be created when a strip of iliotibial band is harvested as a graft for intra- or extra-articular reconstruction and the fascia is tightly closed, thereby decreasing the length of the lateral retinaculum. Articular cartilage can be damaged by sharp instruments, but this seems to be more likely in cartilage of the femorotibial compartment during complicated arthroscopic meniscectomy or meniscal repair.

The cartilage of the patellofemoral joint is violated during anterior cruciate ligament reconstruction by removal of the cartilage around the notch (notchplasty). This is a contact area of the patellofemoral joint when the knee is flexed more than 90 degrees. Therefore, excessive and unnecessary removal of cartilage should not be encouraged. The postoperative hemarthrosis has deleterious effects on articular cartilage.[185,373] The consequences of chronic hemarthrosis are evident in hemophilic arthropathy.[373] In this respect, acute hemarthrosis seems to have fewer consequences than the chronic form does.[365]

The postoperative period after anterior cruciate ligament reconstruction is at least as important as the operation itself if changes in articular cartilage are to be prevented. Normal range of motion should be regained while avoiding persistence of a flexion contracture[336] or significant flexion loss.[4] The development of arthrofibrosis with patella infra leads to early degenerative changes in the patellofemoral joint.[313] Prolonged immobilization should be avoided because it increases the likelihood of stiffness and the beneficial effects of early range of motion are negated.[339] On the other hand, it should be recognized that reactive synovitis of variable duration is present after every surgical procedure on the knee. The synthesis of prostaglandins (mediators of inflammation) and aryl sulfatase is increased after meniscal[142] or cartilage injury.[383] The increase in prostaglandins leads to the production of proteolytic enzymes and depletion of cartilage proteoglycans.[129,139] Thus, it seems that the resistance of cartilage may be decreased in the postoperative period and adequate time should be allowed for recovery before heavy exercises are undertaken. The persistence of joint swelling and effusion is probably the most helpful clinical sign, which should discourage the progression to more advanced stages of rehabilitation.[353]

Direct trauma to the cartilage of the patellofemoral joint may result from a dashboard-type injury. Such trauma more often results in an injury to the posterior cruciate ligament because with the knee at 90 degrees of flexion, the tibial tuberosity is the most prominent part of the knee. However, if the knee is bent to 120 degrees, the patella becomes more exposed to direct trauma because it can be driven against the femoral condyles. This may result in an impaction type of injury to the articular cartilage or a chondral or an osteochondral fracture. Degeneration of the articular cartilage of the patella is also frequent after patella fractures or fractures of the femoral condyles, wherein direct trauma to the cartilage and a less than perfect anatomic reduction are the most likely contributing factors. Osteochondral fractures are frequent in knees with recurrent dislocation of the patella. They usually involve the medial patellar facet or the lateral border of the trochlea and seem to occur at the time of reduction of the dislocation.

The biochemical events that lead to chondromalacia and osteoarthritis have been investigated by Chrisman.[68] He thinks that trauma (or repeated microtrauma) may initiate cartilage degeneration by increasing the release of arachidonic acid, a precursor of prostaglandins.[70] Under these circumstances, prostaglandin E_2 is the major product, and through stimulation of cyclic adenosine monophosphate, synthesis of catheptic protease is increased. Catheptic proteases are released in the matrix, where they split the protein bonds to chondroitin sulfates. Loss of matrix and cartilage softening are the end result. The resultant degradation products, especially the protein polysaccharides, can flood the joint and induce chemical synovitis, which is the cause of pain.[69,147] Synovitis also causes the production of a variety of enzymes from the synovial membrane, which again attack the cartilage, thus leading to the development of a vicious circle. Nonsteroidal anti-inflammatory medications can be used to decrease the synthesis of prostaglandins from arachidonic acid and therefore reduce cartilage softening and synovitis.[68,71,303]

This "cascade hypothesis" has been confirmed in the development of osteoarthritis.[68] Shoji and Granda[356] investigated the acid hydrolases and chemical components of the articular cartilage of the patella from normal, chondromalacic, and osteoarthritic patients. They concluded that (1) chondromalacia is a transitional form of osteoarthritis at the pathobiochemical level and (2) degradation of articular cartilage may begin with proteolysis and be further accelerated by depolymerization of glycosaminoglycans. It is attractive to think that some patients with chondromalacia but without evidence of trauma or malalignment have some biochemical derangement of cartilage that makes it susceptible to wear,[67] but this theory has not been proved thus far.

Patellofemoral Arthritis

It is obvious from the foregoing discussion that osteoarthritis defined as loss of articular cartilage is widely regarded as merely the end result of the progression of chondromalacia. As described by Wiles and coworkers,[403] chondromalacic changes become flaky, pieces of cartilage break off, and an ulcer-like lesion develops, at the base of which lies subchondral bone.

Histological and biochemical assays have shown that the residual cartilage located at the margins of this ulcer is indistinguishable from cartilage removed from chondromalacic lesions elsewhere; thus, the concept of chondromalacia progressing through various stages to osteoarthritis is valid. Nevertheless, there are important reasons for regarding patellofemoral arthritis as a separate entity. First, the patients are middle-aged or older and rarely give a long history of pain beginning in adolescence. Rather, these patients usually have symptoms of relatively brief duration before initial evaluation, which typically indicates well-advanced changes of osteoarthritis (loss of cartilage space, sclerosis, and osteophyte formation) at that time. Unquestionably, these advanced findings did not suddenly occur and were preceded by the stages of development observed in autopsy studies by Emery and Meachim.[104]

On the assumption that advanced osteoarthritis takes years, rather than months to develop, the early stages of the process must have taken place without the awareness of the patient (the usual asymptomatic nature of chondromalacic lesions has already been discussed). In established osteoarthritis, similar lesions are nearly always found in the femoral sulcus, unlike the earlier stages, in which this surface is usually normal. In osteoarthritis there is no difficulty explaining the pain mechanism because the sensitive subchondral bony surfaces are in contact with each other. The existence of a pain mechanism, however, does not explain why radiographically similar joints in different patients (or even in the same patient) may be painful in one and not in the other. Similarly, the intensity of symptoms in the same joint varies from time to time even though the radiographic appearance remains unchanged.

Ficat and coworkers[115] are of the opinion that excessive lateral pressure syndrome is the most frequent cause of patellofemoral arthrosis. Certainly in the established picture, cartilage erosion is predominantly lateral and the patella often appears laterally positioned if not laterally subluxated. However, whether this lateralization is a consequence of the loss of cartilage space or whether the cartilage erosion is caused by tight lateral structures remains unclear. Ficat and associates regard excessive lateral pressure syndrome as a separate entity, but others may prefer to regard it merely as a part of a more generalized malalignment of the quadriceps mechanism.[200]

In our experience, it is uncommon for patients with patellofemoral arthrosis to have sustained earlier episodes of patellar dislocation, although this is sometimes the case. In some cases, the arthrosis clearly follows a patellar fracture, other injury, or previous surgery. Medial facet arthrosis is seldom, if ever a primary entity, but it may follow as the late result of tibial tubercle transfer for patellar dislocation.

However, patellofemoral arthrosis usually seems to arise de novo in a structurally normal joint for which no obvious cause can be assigned. Most frequently, there is also associated femorotibial arthrosis. In a series of 600 patients with radiologically established gonarthrosis managed at the knee clinic of the Hospital for Special

Surgery, patellofemoral arthrosis was associated with medial femorotibial narrowing in 65% and with lateral femorotibial narrowing in 20% of cases. The characteristic lateral patellofemoral narrowing and lateral patellar displacement were present in all three types, even when the patellofemoral arthrosis was associated with medial compartment arthrosis and varus angulation. In our opinion, the predominance of lateral facet erosion merely reflects the normal valgus vector of the patellofemoral mechanism.

SURGICAL TREATMENT

It has previously been emphasized that before proceeding to surgery, a full course of conservative treatment is recommended in every case of lateral patellar compression syndrome or recurrent dislocation of the patella. The same is true when dealing with cases of idiopathic chondromalacia or patellofemoral arthritis. When conservative treatment fails, surgery may be indicated.

Operations for patellofemoral chondromalacia or arthritis may be divided into two categories: (1) those that aim at relieving stress on the patellofemoral joint by realignment or improvement of the mechanical advantage of the extensor mechanism and (2) those that directly address the disorder of the articular cartilage. The first category includes operations such as lateral retinacular release, proximal and distal realignment, and elevation of the tibial tubercle. The rationale for performing such operations is the consideration that patellofemoral arthritis or chondromalacia is a secondary phenomenon and correction of the underlying biomechanical abnormality should stop progression of the degenerative changes. The second category of operations includes cartilage shaving, excision, drilling, abrasion of subchondral bone, and spongialization. These operations should be performed as the only surgical act in selected cases in which no underlying biomechanical abnormality is detected (idiopathic chondromalacia). However, these operations are more frequently performed in association with operations that attempt to relieve stress on the patellofemoral cartilage. Finally, patella resurfacing and patellectomy are described.

Patellar Shaving

Interest in patellar shaving has been renewed by the introduction of arthroscopic techniques. Cartilage fibrillation and mobile flaps can conveniently be converted to a smooth surface with a motorized shaver. The aim of the operation is to remove the fronds of cartilage that "catch" during every flexion-extension movement of the knee and cause retropatellar crepitation. The operation is best suited for grade III lesions (fibrillation). The surgeon should resist the temptation to perform aggressive débridement of the cartilage and just try to obtain a smooth surface. Because there is no evidence that cartilage can regenerate to fill partial- or full-thickness defects, the operation should be conservative. We do not advise converting a partial-thickness defect to a full-thickness defect down to subchondral bone. The operation is best performed by using less aggressive shaver tips. The use of aggressive, large-diameter meniscal cutters results in excessive and unnecessary removal of cartilage.

The efficacy of patellar shaving for chondromalacia has varied, and no one has reported uniformly satisfactory results, at least to our knowledge. Bentley[29] compared the results of four different procedures for chondromalacia: patellar shaving, cartilage excision and drilling of subchondral bone, distal realignment with lateral release, and patellectomy. Patellar shaving yielded the worst results, satisfactory in only 25% of cases, regardless of the age and sex of the patient and the grade of chondromalacia.

Ogilvie-Harris and Jackson[304] reported the results of arthroscopic patellar shaving for three different pathologies of the patellofemoral joint. In 33 knees with unstable patellae, shaving and lavage yielded a good result in less than a third of cases. The addition of lateral release to the shaving improved the short-term 1-year results, but there was no improvement by 5 years. Forty-two knees were affected by post-traumatic chondromalacia and were treated by shaving and lavage. The 5-year results in this group varied according to the severity of the involvement of cartilage. The percentage of satisfactory results was 83% in knees with grade I cartilage softening, 73% in those with open chondromalacia, and only 20% in knees with exposed subchondral bone. In a group of 85 knees with idiopathic chondromalacia, satisfactory results were achieved at the 5-year follow-up in only 27% of cases, less frequently (15%) when subchondral bone was exposed. These results suggest that simple lavage plus shaving is not adequate treatment of unstable patellae, for which formal realignment of the extensor mechanism is needed. The results of post-traumatic chondromalacia were strictly linked to the severity of cartilage damage, and it seems that improvement cannot be expected when the disease has progressed to the degree of arthritis. Results in knees with idiopathic chondromalacia were also largely unsatisfactory, as is often the case when one treats the effects without understanding the etiology of the disease.

The results of arthroscopic chondroplasty of the patella in a selected group of 41 knees have been reported by Schonholtz and Ling.[343] Only cases with isolated chondromalacia were included, with exclusion of unstable patellae. Direct trauma was involved in 48% of cases. These cases constituted only 5.8% of a large group of 1083 arthroscopic procedures performed during a 3-year period. With an average follow-up of 40 months, 49% of the knees were satisfactory and 78% of the patients said that they would undergo a similar procedure again if required.

In conclusion, we recommend conservative shaving of open chondromalacic lesions as the only surgical procedure in selected cases of idiopathic or post-traumatic chondromalacia without patellar maltracking or overload secondary to biomechanical abnormalities. Patellar shaving is also recommended as an adjunctive procedure to treat open chondromalacia at the time of realignment procedures for unstable patellae. The effectiveness of the operation seems to be related to the following two factors: (1) unstable flaps of cartilage that can catch and contribute to retropatellar crepitus during flexion and extension of the knee are removed, and (2) the release

of chondral breakdown products, proteoglycans, lytic enzymes, and other inflammatory products is decreased, thus breaking the vicious circle of synovial irritation and further cartilage damage.

Subchondral Bone Drilling, Cortical Abrasion, Spongialization

Subchondral bone drilling, cortical abrasion, and spongialization have been suggested for the treatment of advanced chondromalacia with exposure of subchondral bone. The common rationale for these operations is to encourage fibrous ingrowth of the cartilage defect from the underlying cancellous bone, as originally suggested by Pridie.[323] The cancellous bone can be exposed by drilling through subchondral bone, by removing subchondral bone completely (spongialization),[117] or by abrading it arthroscopically.[215]

Ficat and colleagues[117] have popularized spongialization. The operation is performed through a lateral approach after extensive lateral release with removal of a 1-cm-wide strip of iliotibial band. The cartilage lesion is circumscribed with a knife such that the edge of normal cartilage is left perpendicular to the surface of bone. The subchondral bone is excised completely, either by making a series of drill holes and removing the bridge between them with a rongeur or by using a high-speed drill bit.

Ficat reported the results in 85 patients with a follow-up period ranging from 6 months to 3 years: 79% obtained a satisfactory result. Four knees in this series were re-explored, and tissue specimens were obtained for histological evaluation. The grown tissue was found to be more cellular than normal cartilage and essentially fibrous. Far less satisfactory results have been reported by Bentley.[29] In a series of 20 knees treated by cartilage excision and drilling, only 35% were satisfactory at an average follow-up period of 7 years. Better experience has been reported by Beltran[28] in Saudi Arabian patients, who pose higher demands on the patellofemoral joint because of religious habits that involve kneeling. He operated on 33 knees with patellofemoral arthritis. After entering the joint through a lateral approach, osteophytes were removed, and the entire articular cartilage and subchondral bone of the patella were resected, with a flat surface remaining. One-third to two-fifths of the patellar thickness was resected. At an average follow-up period of 31 months, 60% of the patients were free of pain and 12% had only mild discomfort.

As has previously been pointed out, the surgeon should remember that partial- or full-thickness cartilage defects cannot be filled by regrown hyaline cartilage; at best, they can be filled by fibrous or fibrocartilaginous tissue, whose mechanical properties are inferior to those of cartilage. Therefore, it makes no sense to remove partially damaged cartilage on the assumption that it will regenerate.

It has been observed[177] that early cartilage lesions (grades I and II) at least partially retain the capacity to transfer loads whereas this capacity is lost in advanced (grades III and IV) degenerative areas. Using pressure-sensitive film, Hayes and coworkers[177] demonstrated an even distribution of pressure in the contact areas of normal knees. This was altered in knees with chondromalacia, which showed 53% decreased transmission of pressure over grade I and II lesions and no transmission at all over eroded areas. Peak pressure was observed in the normal cartilage bordering the erosions. In light of these data, it seems unwise to excessively enlarge the margins of the lesion because this will create peak pressure in the surrounding normal cartilage.

Nevertheless, spongialization or abrasion may be the only alternatives to treat limited areas of cartilage erosion. The results of these techniques have been somewhat unpredictable,[198] and we think that improvement is unlikely in the presence of extensive arthritis of the patellofemoral joint. Because these techniques have often been used in association with other procedures that unload the patellofemoral joint (such as the Maquet operation), it is difficult to understand the merits of each procedure.

Lateral Retinacular Release

Open or arthroscopic lateral retinacular release has often been used to relieve stress on the lateral facet in knees with lateral patellar compression syndrome or to improve the congruence in knees with chronic subluxation or recurrent dislocation of the patella. The procedure has also been performed on knees with patellofemoral arthritis. Experimental studies using pressure-sensitive film[177] have shown that plication of the lateral retinaculum in a normal knee increases patellofemoral pressure on the lateral facet, the highest increase occurring at 60 degrees of flexion. Lateral release, on the other hand, did not appreciably influence contact areas or patellofemoral pressure. The pressure changes were highly variable and unpredictable. The authors concluded that with the limitations of the experimental model in normal knees or knees with chondromalacia, lateral retinacular release cannot be expected to reliably unload the lateral facet.

The situation may be different in selected cases with a shortened lateral retinaculum and minimal or absent cartilage changes. Therefore, to maximize satisfactory results, careful preoperative selection of patients is necessary, with demonstration of a tight lateral retinaculum. Fulkerson and Shea[140] have further emphasized this concept by recommending preoperative CT images of the patellofemoral joint. Knees exhibiting lateral patellar tilt without subluxation are the most likely to benefit from a lateral release, provided that extensive degenerative changes of the cartilage have not already occurred.

From a clinical point of view, we have found that 60% of our patients affected by patellar pain syndromes without severe cartilage changes did benefit from the operation.[10] However, only one of six knees with patellofemoral osteoarthritis were improved at an average follow-up of 4 years. Therefore, isolated lateral retinacular release cannot be recommended as treatment of established lateral patellofemoral osteoarthritis.

Elevation of the Tibial Tubercle

Elevation of the tibial tubercle[405] has been recommended by Bandi[22] and Maquet[261,262] as a method to reduce patellofemoral contact pressure. The rationale for this operation was based on analysis of the forces that act on the patellofemoral joint (Fig. 53–99). They can be represented as vectors. M1 is the force of the quadriceps muscle, and M2 is the force of the patellar tendon. The resultant of the forces M1 and M2 is the patellofemoral joint reaction force, which compresses the patella against the femur. The magnitude of the patellofemoral joint reaction force is related to the magnitude of M1 and M2 and to the angle j between the vectors M1 and M2. The angle j increases in extension, therefore decreasing the patellofemoral joint reaction force, whereas it decreases in flexion, where patellofemoral pressure is higher. Based on this biomechanical model, advancement of the tibial tuberosity is expected to decrease patellofemoral pressure by two mechanisms: (1) by increasing the lever arm of the patellar tendon, which is the perpendicular distance between the center of rotation of the knee and the tendon, and (2) by increasing the angle j.

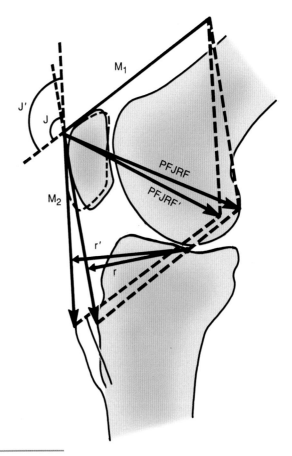

Figure 53–99. Biomechanical effects of advancement of the tibial tuberosity. M1 is the force in the quadriceps tendon, M2 the force in the patellar tendon, and J the angle between M1 and M2. Anterior displacement of the tibial tuberosity causes anterior displacement of the vector M2, which opens the J angle to J′. This in turn causes a reduction in the patellofemoral joint reaction force (PFJRF) to the value of PFJRF′. Furthermore, the lever arm of the patella tendon r is increased to r′, so less force is required in the patellar tendon to produce the same torque.

Maquet[261,262] calculated that a 2-cm advancement of the tibial tuberosity would yield a 50% reduction in patellofemoral compressive force. A 2- to 2.5-cm advancement was the maximum obtainable without severely jeopardizing the skin over the tubercle. Maquet[261] also emphasized that medial displacement of the tuberosity may be required to centralize the patella in the femoral trochlea and redistribute the pressure evenly.

Since the original description of Maquet,[261] further experimental studies have improved our knowledge of the biomechanics of elevation of the tibial tubercle. Ferguson and colleagues[113] used six miniature contact stress sensors to instrument the retropatellar cartilage of cadaver knees subjected to isometric quadriceps extension force. The study demonstrated that elevation of the tubercle relieved contact stress at 0, 45, and 90 degrees of flexion and that the effects were more pronounced at 90 degrees. Contact stress was progressively relieved by increasing elevation of the tubercle, but most of the relief was achieved within the first half inch of elevation. Further elevation to 1.5 inches decreased contact stress only marginally. Furthermore, it was noted that elevation of the tibial tubercle opens the quadriceps tendon–patellar tendon angle and the distal pole of the patella rocks anteriorly. As a consequence of this rocking movement, contact areas are moved more proximally than in a normal knee. Because it was not possible to place the uppermost pair of transducers more proximal on the articular facet of the patella, Ferguson and coworkers suggested that the value recorded may actually represent an underestimation of patellofemoral pressure because the pressure on the most proximal part of the articular surface was not recorded.

Nakamura and associates[297] pointed out that to correctly analyze patellofemoral pressure, two factors must be accounted for: patellofemoral force and contact area. In other words, it is not helpful to reduce patellofemoral force if contract areas are reduced and altered at the same time. Contact area was studied in cadaver knees with casting techniques. The geometry of the knee was studied on lateral radiographs of the knee in the 0- to 110-degree arc of flexion. The tuberosity was elevated 1, 2, or 3 cm with metal wedges. The length of the split down the anterior crest of the tibia was also varied at 5, 10, and 15 cm. Normal subjects were studied to analyze the force at the knee joint during the activity of rising from a chair. The geometric changes occurring in the cadaver knee after advancement of the tuberosity were incorporated in the mathematic model of a "matching" normal subject to study the effects of the operation.

Radiographic analysis showed that the moment arm of the patellar tendon and the angle between the quadriceps and patellar tendon were both increased by the use of progressively thicker wedges but, at least at 90 degrees of flexion, there was not a significant increase in the moment arm between 2 and 3 cm of elevation. Rotation of the patella around a horizontal axis with a floating distal pole was confirmed (Fig. 53–100). The patella is also displaced distally by the elevated tubercle because it moves anteriorly as well as distally. The downward movement of the patella is a function of both the thickness of the wedge and the length of the split. The longer the split, the smaller the downward displacement of the patella (Fig. 53–101).

The analysis of contact area on the femoral side revealed a progressive decrease in the area with increasing thickness of the wedge inserted.

Changes in the contact areas on the patellar side were even more evident. The greater the magnitude of elevation of the tubercle, the larger the decrease in contact area, which tended to displace toward the proximal part of the articular surface. Changes were minimal with a 1-cm elevation but significant with a 2-cm elevation. Analysis of forces at the patellofemoral joint revealed that these were dramatically decreased by the insertion of increasingly thicker wedges at 0, 30, and 60 degrees of flexion, when patellofemoral forces usually are not elevated. However, at 90 and 110 degrees, patellofemoral pressure was reduced by 1-cm elevations but increased by elevations of greater magnitude. The greatest elevation, 3 cm, also increased tibiofemoral compressive force at 110 degrees of flexion and tibiofemoral shear force at 90 and 110 degrees by more than 25%. In light of these results, Nakamura and coworkers[297] concluded that a 1-cm advancement of the tuberosity affords the best compromise between decreasing patellofemoral force and alteration in the contact area.

Ferrandez and associates[114] used an experimental setup consisting of miniature piezoelectric transducers similar to that used by Ferguson and colleagues.[112,113] Their results confirmed that 1-cm displacements afforded the best decrease in patellofemoral pressure. Although larger elevation allowed a greater overall decrease in patellofemoral pressure, other zones of the patella, particularly the proximal and lateral facet, received increasingly higher pressure. A 1-cm elevation, which affords a 50% decompression of the patella, was suggested in most cases.

Hayes and colleagues[177] reported direct measurement of patellofemoral contact area and pressure with the use of pressure-sensitive film in normal knees and after 1.25 and 2.5 cm of elevation of the tibial tubercle. In normal knees, the average patellofemoral contact area increases from 1.8 cm^2 at 30 degrees of flexion to 3.3 cm^2 at 90 degrees, whereas the peak patellofemoral contact pressure increases from 4.2 MPa at 30 degrees to 8.9 MPa at 90 degrees. Peak pressure was 1.39 to 1.58 times the corresponding average pressure. The mean contact area was significantly reduced by 1.25 cm of elevation at 90 degrees of flexion and by 2.5 cm of elevation at both 60 and 90 degrees. There were no significant changes in the contact area at 30 degrees. Cephalad and lateral migration of the contact area followed tubercle elevation, in conjunction with ventral tilting of the inferior pole of the patella. Mean and peak contact pressure did not show significant decreases in comparison to normal knees after tibial tubercle elevation. From their data, Hayes and coworkers concluded that after tibial tubercle elevation patellofemoral contact force can be reduced but, because of the concomitant decrease in contact area, no consistent reduction in patellofemoral peak and average contact pressure can be obtained.

Fulkerson and colleagues[128] evaluated the biomechanical effects of anteromedialization of the tibial tubercle[127] in five cadaver knees with the use of pressure-sensitive film. Before anteromedialization of the tibial tubercle, the load on the lateral facet exceeded that on the medial facet from 0 up to 60 degrees of flexion. At 0 degrees of flexion,

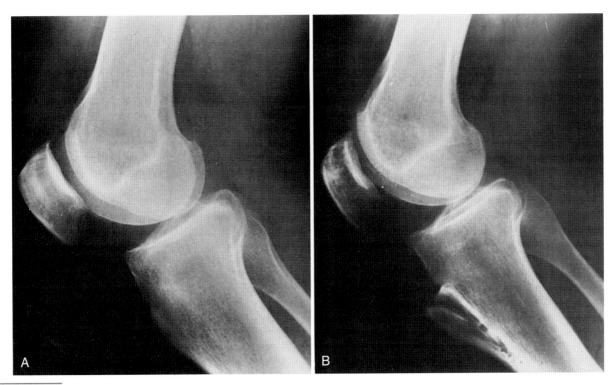

Figure 53–100.   Lateral radiographs before (**A**) and after (**B**) elevation of the tibial tubercle. Note the rotation of the patella with ventral floating of the distal pole.

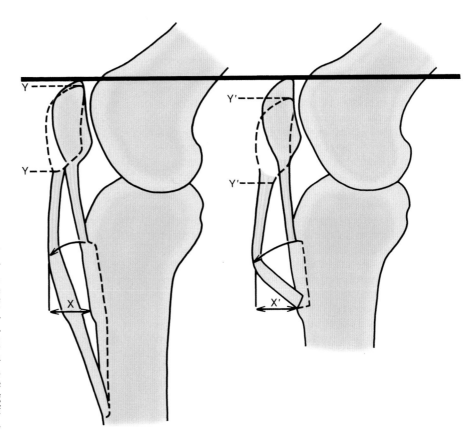

Figure 53–101. Effects of anterior displacement of the tibial tuberosity on the position of the patella. Because of the anterior pull of the patellar tendon, the distal pole of the patella floats anteriorly. Anterior displacement of the tuberosity is accompanied by distal displacement of the patella. For a given anterior displacement X, displacement of the patella in the distal direction is less if a long fragment has been split (Y) than if a shorter one was sculptured (Y).

the average load on the lateral facet was 3.6 MPa as compared with 0.5 MPa on the medial facet, and three of five knees exhibited no load on the medial facet. At 10 degrees of flexion, the patellae remained lateralized, but by 20 degrees of flexion, the patellae were engaged in the trochlea with a significant load on the medial facets. Contact areas varied with flexion and were smallest in extension (0.93 cm²), increased minimally at 10 degrees (1.1 cm²), peaked at 45 degrees (2.3 cm²), and then decreased at 90 degrees (1.8 cm²). Displacement of the tibial tuberosity in an anterior (average, 14.8 mm) and medial (average, 9.2 mm) direction, though causing little difference in the load on the medial facet, greatly decreased the load on the lateral facet between 0 and 30 degrees. Beyond 30 degrees of flexion, patellofemoral pressure was not reduced over preoperative values, although it remained balanced between the medial and lateral facets. The contact area showed a slight proximal migration, but the overall area did not decrease, and decreases on the lateral facet were balanced by increases on the medial facet.

It seems that the experimental work of several authors has allowed considerable progress in understanding the biomechanics of tibial tubercle elevation since the original theories reported by Maquet.[261] Patellofemoral contact force is reduced, but other changes may involve alignment of the patella, such as ventral tilting of its distal pole and possibly distal migration in relation to the joint line. Contact areas may also be reduced and migrate proximally on the patella. Patellofemoral contact pressure is reduced predominantly in early flexion, where it is less elevated. Overall, it seems that the best results can be obtained with elevation of 1 to 1.5 cm.

Technique. A lateral parapatellar skin incision is made and extended distally below the level of the tibial tubercle. The extensor mechanism is exposed, and the joint is entered through a lateral parapatellar approach with division of the lateral retinaculum and the lower fibers of the vastus lateralis (vastus lateralis obliquus). Appropriate débridement of the patellar cartilage and osteophytes is carried out. The tibial tubercle is isolated by a second capsular incision placed medial to the patellar ligament and tubercle. An osteotomy is carried out with osteotomes or an oscillating saw, and the tibial tubercle and adjoining part of tibial crest are split distally for a distance of 10 to 12 cm. Nakamura and colleagues[297] observed that splitting the tubercle and tibial crest for shorter distances produces a comparatively greater lowering effect on the patella in relation to the joint line. Therefore, detachment of a 10-cm bone fragment is recommended. Maquet[261,262] advised that a series of drill holes be made first to outline the osteotomy. The tibial tubercle is levered forward and held by a bone graft taken from the iliac crest (Fig. 53–102). Because the distal cortex is not broken, the fragment of the tibial tuberosity is stable and the bone graft locks in place without internal fixation. The upper margin of the graft should be flush or slightly proximal to the tip of the tubercle (Fig. 53–103) to prevent later fracture of the tubercle itself (Fig. 53–104). Maquet[261] further noted that if medialization of the tuberosity is needed to unload the lateral facet, the fragment of the tuberosity should be displaced forward as well as medi-

ally. The skin is closed with the lateral retinaculum left open. A pressure dressing is applied. The knee is immobilized until wound healing has taken place, after which range-of-motion and rehabilitation exercises are begun. After the first month, weightbearing is permitted as tolerated.

More recently, Fulkerson[127] described a technique that allows anteromedialization of the tibial tuberosity without the need for a bone graft. The author has recommended this operation as a surgical alternative to the Maquet procedure in patients with malalignment and lateral facet arthrosis.[137,140] Fulkerson contended, and we agree, that simple lateral release is insufficient when lateral facet arthrosis is present. In these cases, he suggested anteromedialization of the tuberosity. An anterolateral skin incision is made and extended from the patella to 5 cm distal to the tibial tuberosity. A lateral retinacular release is performed, and the patella is everted to allow shaving of loose cartilage flaps or abrasion of areas of exposed subchondral bone. The muscles of the anterolateral compartment of the tibia are then elevated by subperiosteal dissection from the lateral aspect of the tibia, which is exposed close to its posterolateral corner. It should be remembered that at this level the anterior tibial artery and the deep peroneal nerve run behind the posterolateral corner of the tibia on the anterior surface of the interosseous membrane and should be protected.

The osteotomy plane is outlined with several 3.2-mm drill bits inserted from just medial to the tibial crest to just anterior to the posterolateral corner. The direction of the osteotomy is oblique in a posterior and lateral direction (Fig. 53–105). The osteotomy should taper distally so that

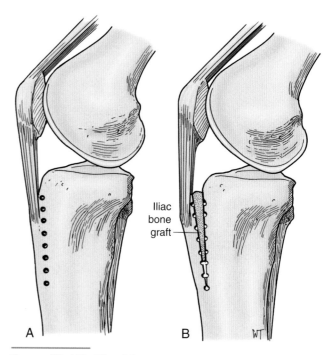

Figure 53–102. The Maquet technique of elevating the tibial tubercle. **A,** A series of holes are drilled first to outline the osteotomy. **B,** The tibial tubercle is then elevated without breaking the distal bridge and held in place by a bone graft taken from the iliac crest.

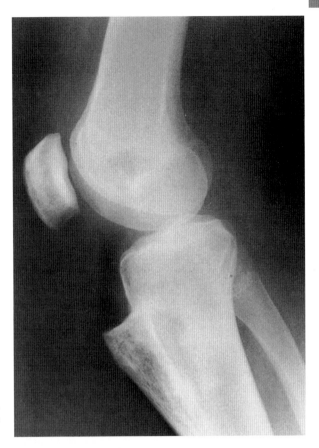

Figure 53-103. Lateral radiograph showing the correct position of the iliac graft, which should be flush with the tip of the elevated tubercle.

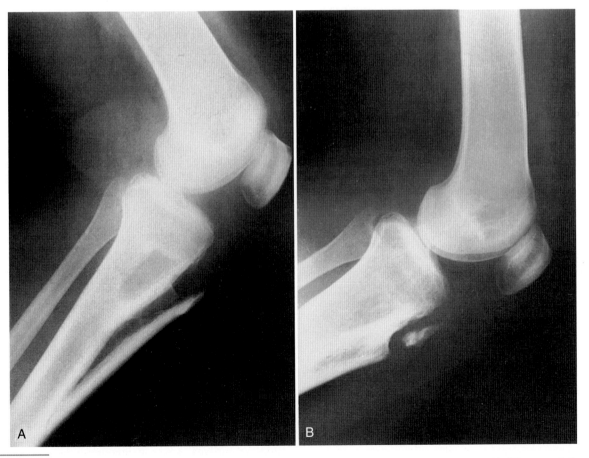

Figure 53–104. **A**, The bone graft was inserted distally to the tip of the elevated tibial tubercle. **B**, The tip of the tibial tubercle fractured, with formation of a separate ossicle.

a 2- to 3-mm bone pedicle is left 5 to 7 cm distal to the tuberosity (Fig. 53–106). The obliquity of the osteotomy can be varied so that the relative amount of anterior and medial displacement can be chosen. Care should also be taken to obtain a perfectly flat osteotomy. The osteotomy can be performed with an osteotome or an oscillating saw. A cut is also made proximally on the lateral aspect of the tibia to avoid proximal extension of the osteotomy into the joint.

Once the osteotomy is completed, the bone fragment is displaced anteromedially along the osteotomy plane by rotation around the intact distal pedicle. Fulkerson and colleagues[128] reported that 12 to 15 mm of anterior displacement of the tibial tuberosity can routinely be achieved with this technique without bone grafts. After patella tracking is observed during the arc of motion, the bone fragment is locked in place with one or two cortical screws engaged in the posterior cortex of the tibia. Early motion can be initiated because fixation is stable. The patient uses a knee immobilizer, which is removed to flex the knee up to 90 degrees. The knee immobilizer is abandoned after 1 month, and progressive weightbearing is allowed. The crutches can be usually discontinued after 6 weeks, when sufficient healing and quadriceps strength have been achieved.

Clinical Results. Good results were reported by Bandi[22] and later by Maquet[261] in his original publication. He reported on 37 knees that underwent isolated elevation of the tibial tubercle and were reviewed with an average follow-up of 4.7 years (range, 1 to 10 years). One patient with multiple scars experienced skin necrosis and required removal of the graft. The remaining 36 knees achieved satisfactory results, but details were not given (Table 53–10).

At the Hospital for Special Surgery, 30 knees were studied after the procedure had been performed according to the Maquet technique.[333] The preoperative diagnosis was chondromalacia in 15 knees and patellofemoral arthrosis in 14 knees; 1 case followed a patellectomy. The average age was 34 years (range, 16 to 38 years). The patients were monitored for 1 to 5 years; 17 knees had undergone various previous procedures, including 5 Hauser procedures and 8 meniscectomies. The initial amount of elevation of the tubercle averaged 1.75 cm, but some settling usually occurred for an average elevation at the time of follow-up of 1.37 cm. The operation was combined with tibial osteotomy in 8 knees, proximal realignment in 6 knees, and patellectomy in 4 knees; in the remaining 12 knees, the tibial tubercle elevation was performed as a solitary procedure.

There were a significant number of complications. Skin necrosis occurred in the region of the tibial tubercle in four knees, which in one case led to a subsequent deep infection, ultimately requiring débridement and skin grafting. A stress fracture through the tibial tubercle proximal to the graft occurred in three knees and resulted in the formation of a separate small ossicle, and in all cases there was some residual tenderness and slight extension weakness. The ossicle was excised in one knee because of local tenderness. A fracture of the proximal end of the tibia occurred in one case, an obese woman who fell 6 weeks

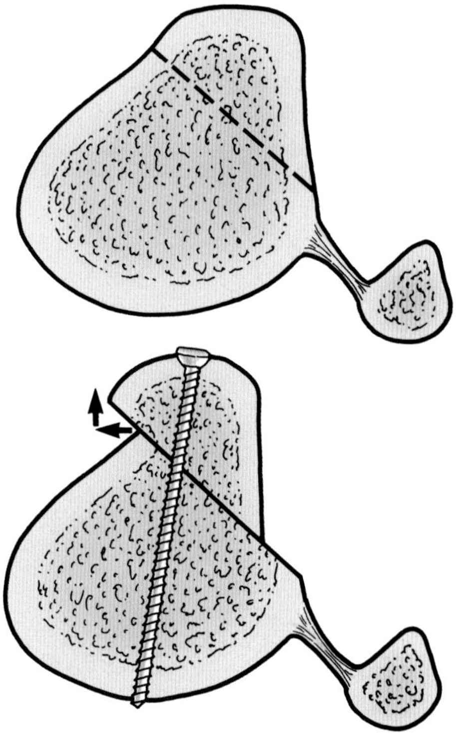

Figure 53–105. Osteotomy of the tibial tubercle according to Fulkerson's technique. The osteotomy plane is oblique in a posterior and lateral direction, so medial displacement is accompanied by anterior displacement. (From Fulkerson JP: Anteromedialization of the tibial tuberosity for patellofemoral malalignment. Clin Orthop 177:176, 1983.)

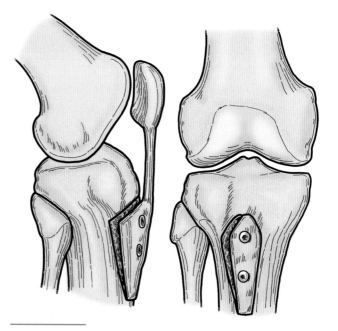

Figure 53–106. Osteotomy of the tibial tubercle according to Fulkerson's technique. The osteotomy is tapered distally, where the thin pedicle is interrupted. An oblique cut is made proximally to avoid entering Gerdy's tubercle and the joint line. (From Fulkerson JP: Anteromedialization of the tibial tuberosity for patellofemoral malalignment. Clin Orthop 177:176, 1983.)

Table 53–10. Results of Elevation of the Tibial Tubercle

AUTHOR	YEAR	NO. OF KNEES	OPERATION	AVG. FOLLOW-UP (mo)	SATISFACTORY RESULT %	REMARKS
Maquet[261]	1976	37	Maquet	55	97	
Rozbruch et al[333]	1979	30	Maquet	12-60	60	Several complications were recorded, including skin necrosis, stress fractures of the tibial tubercle, and 1 fracture of the tibia; better results in knees operated with an isolated Maquet (66% satisfactory) than in those with combined operations (55%)
Ferguson[112]	1982	184	Modified Maquet	24	86	Modified surgical technique with a horizontal skin incision; no skin complications reported
Miller & Larochelle[288]	1986	38	Anteromedialization	30-84	87	Young group of patients (avg. age, 21 years) with intractable patellofemoral pain
Heatley et al[178]	1986	28	Modified Maquet	86	54	Satisfactory results deteriorated from 65% at 3 years to 54% at 6 years
Noll et al[299]	1988	17	Anteromedialization	12-48	86	Heterogeneous group, including patellar pain, subluxation, and previous patellectomies
Engebretsen et al[105]	1989	33	Maquet	65	30	Satisfactory results deteriorated with increasing follow-up from 51% at 2 years to 30% at 5 years
Fulkerson et al[128]	1990	30	Fulkerson	24	89	Satisfactory results in 75% of knees with severe patellofemoral arthritis
Morshuis et al[293]	1990	25	Fulkerson	30	70	Better results in knees with patellofemoral pain without arthritis
Bellemans et al[27]	1997	29	Fulkerson	32	97	Chronic anterior knee pain associated with subluxation-type malalignment

after the operation. The fracture resulted in a nonunion that did not heal despite two bone-grafting procedures. There were two deep infections, one after skin necrosis.

Evaluation of the results was complicated by the varying causes and the additional procedures performed at the same time as the tubercle elevation. However, these variables are also found in other comparable series for which indications for the operation exist.

The major preoperative complaint was pain, and subsidiary complaints in some cases were weakness and buckling. The success or failure of the procedure thus largely depended on relief of pain, with the element of subjectivity that this implies. Complications previously noted were not accounted for except insofar as they affected the end result at the time of the review.

Because of the number of associated procedures, it was decided that the knees be evaluated in two groups: (1) tibial tubercle elevation alone (12 knees), in which the results were good in 8 knees, fair in 2 knees, and poor in 2 knees; and (2) tibial tubercle elevation combined (18 knees), in which the results in this group were good in 10 knees, fair in 7 knees, and poor in 1 knee.

From this it can be seen that about two-thirds of patients gained satisfactory pain relief, whether the Maquet procedure was performed by itself or combined with another operation. The remaining third were not improved, and three knees were actually worse. The poor rating in two knees was directly attributable to a compli-

cation—persistent nonunion of a tibial fracture in one and osteomyelitis after deep infection in the other.

Our conclusion concerning the merits of the operation was that although the procedure did relieve pain in most cases, the significant number of serious complications and the unpredictability of the results must limit the indications to a few severely disabled patients.

Ferguson[112] reported the results of elevation of the tibial tubercle with a modified Maquet technique. He used a horizontal incision with 1.25-cm elevation of the tubercle, which he had previously shown to be sufficient to relieve 57% to 85% of the patellofemoral contact pressure. The graft was harvested from Gerdy's tubercle. The procedure was performed as an isolated operation in all knees. He included 63 patients with chondromalacia, 48 patients with arthritis, 40 with patellar dislocation, 25 with trauma, and 8 with previous patellectomy. The patients were reviewed 2 years after the operation and were classified as either satisfactory or not, depending on return to normal stair climbing and athletic activities. There was no skin sloughing or graft nonunion in this group of patients. Ferguson considered the use of a horizontal incision to be a significant advantage with regard to skin problems. Satisfactory results were obtained in 85% of the overall group, 84% of the chondromalacia group, 92% of the patellofemoral arthritis group, 83% of the recurrent dislocation group, 84% of the post-traumatic group, and 88% of the postpatellectomy group. A prolonged recovery period was needed in most patients to achieve satisfactory pain relief, with 50% of them requiring more than 4 months. The procedure failed to correct the position of the patella in the femoral trochlea, and patellofemoral crepitation persisted during knee motion. The prominence of the tubercle bothered some patients during kneeling.

Miller and Larochelle[288] reported the results of 38 knees treated by anteromedialization of the tibial tuberosity for intractable patellar pain. This was a group of young patients with an average age of 21 years. Malalignment was significant in most of them. A bone fragment that included the tibial tubercle was sculpted from the proximal end of the tibia and displaced medially and anteriorly over the tibial crest. An average anterior elevation of 10 mm was achieved. Satisfactory results were obtained by 87% of patients with a follow-up ranging from 2.5 to 7 years. None was made worse by surgery. There were no skin or soft-tissue problems. The authors stressed the importance of correction of an increased Q angle together with elevation of the tubercle.

Heatley and associates[178] reported the results of anterior displacement of the tibial tubercle in a series of 28 knees with a minimum follow-up of 6 years. This heterogeneous group included patients with patellofemoral arthritis (14 knees), chondromalacia (7 knees), recurrent dislocation (4 knees), and previous surgery (4 knees), mostly treated with a Hauser procedure. Satisfactory results were obtained in 65% at 3 years of follow-up but deteriorated to 54% at 6 years. Satisfactory results varied among the different diagnostic categories and were 43% in those with patellofemoral arthritis, 86% in those with chondromalacia, 25% in those with recurrent dislocation, and 75% in the previous patellar surgery group. There were four postoperative complications, including one deep infection and three stress fractures of the patellar crest. Three of four patients with a postoperative complication achieved a poor end result. A low preoperative clinical score led to an unsatisfactory result in five of six knees with patellofemoral arthritis. In light of this observation, Heatley and coworkers concluded that elevation of the tibial tubercle is likely to be inadequate if the patellar surface is completely worn by the degenerative process.

Engebretsen and associates[105] reported the results of advancement of the tibial tubercle in 33 patients affected by patellar pain. With an average follow-up of more than 5 years, only 10 knees (30%) were improved over their preoperative state. A further seven knees (21%) remained improved as long as 2 years postoperatively, but they were no longer improved 5 years after the operation. In the group that benefited from the operation, eight knees showed involvement of the lateral facet and six had grade III to IV involvement according to Outerbridge. On the other hand, involvement of patellar cartilage was less severe in the knees that were not improved, and only 5 of 23 knees had involvement of the lateral facet. This study failed to report lasting improvement after the Maquet operation in over two-thirds of the knees. More favorable results were reported in knees with advanced chondromalacia and involvement of the lateral facet.

Fulkerson and associates[128] reported the results of the operation that he designed[127] and we described earlier. Simultaneous anterior and medial displacement of the tibial tubercle is achieved without the use of a bone graft; 30 knees were treated surgically for persistent patellofemoral pain with articular cartilage degeneration. They were monitored for more than 2 years, 12 of them for more than 5 years. Good or excellent results were obtained subjectively in 93% of cases and objectively in 89%. The improvement was maintained in all 12 knees monitored more than 5 years. None of the knees with advanced articular cartilage damage (Outerbridge grade III or IV) obtained an excellent result, but 75% were good and all were improved over their preoperative status.

Stiffness was a frequent postoperative complication in the first 25 knees that were immobilized for 1 month postoperatively. Nine of them (36%) required mobilization under anesthesia. After these initial cases, knee motion was started immediately after the operation, and stiffness has no longer been a problem. There were no complications such as skin sloughing, infection, or compartment syndrome. One tibial tubercle fractured through the screw hole, and one avulsed on postoperative day 3 because it was fixed with a single cancellous screw. Both these knees underwent reoperation and healed uneventfully.

The results of Fulkerson's operation have been reported by an independent center.[293] Anteromedialization of the tibial tubercle was performed in a series of 25 knees; they were evaluated with an average follow-up period of 12 months and again at 30 months. Objectively satisfactory results were achieved in 84% and 70% of cases at the first and second follow-ups, respectively. Subjectively satisfactory results decreased from 80% to 65%. Incapacity in kneeling was a problem common to all the knees. The results varied according to the preoperative diagnosis. The best results (100% satisfactory) were obtained in knees with patellar pain and no signs of arthritis. Knees with patellofemoral arthritis and those with lateral subluxation achieved 65% and 60% satisfactory results, respectively.

More recently, Bellemans et al[27] reported the outcome results of Fulkerson procedure in 29 patients treated for chronic anterior knee pain associated with patellar subluxation. Satisfactory subjective and objective results were reported in all patients but one.

Autologous Cartilage Transplantation

Fulkerson's osteotomy provided better results when the chondral damage was located at the distal patellar pole or on the lateral facet. On the contrary, when the chondral damage involved the medial facet or the proximal pole or was pan-patellar, the results were inferior. In these situations cartilage transplantation can be discussed.

Autologous cartilage implantation is a relatively popular procedure generally used to treat large and deep chondral defects, and it aims at replacing the defect with hyaline cartilage[315] after culture of patient's own chondrocytes. It consists of harvesting patients' articular cartilage and implanting it after culture in the laboratory. To the authors' knowledge, no studies that uniquely address cartilage transplantation in the patellofemoral joint have been published. Peterson et al[315] reviewed 61 patients treated with autologous cartilage transplantation of the knee. Seventeen of them had patellar involvement. The mean defect size was 4.4 cm². After 2 years of follow-up, 65% of the patients had a satisfactory result. Minas et al (personal communication) assessed 45 patients at a minimum follow-up of 2 years. Patients were 37 years old on average, and in most of them more than one transplant was performed in the same knee. Patient satisfaction was high, and 87% of the patients said that they would choose the same surgery again.

The main advantage of the technique is that hyaline cartilage is obtained. The main disadvantage is that at least two operations are required. A prerequisite for a satisfactory outcome is that no malalignment or maltracking be present or that they be addressed before or at the same time. In such cases, distal and proximal realignment procedures should be considered, as discussed before. In the case of trochlear involvement with associated dysplasia, a deepening osteotomy should be performed beforehand.

Patellofemoral Resurfacing

McKeever[276] described a cobalt-chromium alloy (Vitallium) prosthesis for resurfacing the patella that was anatomic in shape and had medial and lateral facets. The prosthesis was fixed to the bone with a transfixion screw, and the patella was trimmed to fit the prosthesis. McKeever reported generally good results in 40 knees. Four failures were attributable to infection, but no mechanical failures occurred. DePalma and associates,[94] using McKeever's prosthesis, had a similar experience and reported their results in 17 patients. Eight were rated excellent, six good, two fair, and one poor. However, Levitt[245] found that with longer follow-up, the results in the patients of DePalma and colleagues were not as satisfactory, although some remained pain-free without evidence of progressive arthritis even after many years.

Encouraged by this report of such a satisfactory outcome in some patients, we were led to think that the overall results might be helped by redesigning the shape of the prosthesis and improving fixation with the use of acrylic cement.

In 1973, a new cobalt-chromium patellar prosthesis[8] was designed at the Hospital for Special Surgery; the prosthetic articulating facet had a dome shape, which obviated the need for special rotary alignment. (Binding of the articular surfaces because of incorrect rotary fitting was thought to be a possible source of failure with the anatomic McKeever prosthesis.) The dome prosthesis was available in two sizes, and the anterior surface of the prosthesis had a stud for anchorage to the residual bone of the patella after excision of its articular facets.

Between 1973 and 1976, 31 patellar replacement operations were performed with this prosthesis at the Hospital for Special Surgery.[205] Two patients were lost to follow-up, and the remaining 29 knees (in 28 patients) were studied and reviewed. The diagnosis in 22 knees was patellofemoral osteoarthritis; in 5 knees, chondromalacia patellae after patellar subluxation and realignment by the Hauser technique; and in 2 knees, habitual dislocation with severe osteoarthritis. After a follow-up ranging from 3 to 6 years, the results were excellent in 2 knees, good in 14, fair in 3, and poor in 10. The 10 poor results were all attributable to persistent pain, and in most cases, failure was evident within the first 6 months after surgery. In the osteoarthritic group, the results were better when there

was no femorotibial involvement (67% satisfactory). Surprisingly, because the cartilage of the femoral sulcus was normal, the five knees with patellar chondromalacia did not do better, but perhaps the abnormal patellar mechanics involving the previous tibial tubercle transfer adversely affected the result.

We have not completely given up on this prosthesis and still use it in selected cases. We think that it is indicated for patellofemoral arthritis without evidence of femorotibial narrowing and for young patients after failed patellar surgery. Unfortunately, most patients in this group have undergone a previous Hauser operation and the patellofemoral mechanism has been permanently altered by medial and posterior displacement of the tibial tubercle. Patellar replacement is a type of hemiarthroplasty, and the long-term results are consistent with the results of hemiarthroplasty in other joints. The cases of persistent pain no doubt arise partly from imperfect congruence between the implant and the opposing surface.

Worrell[409] developed an anatomic prosthetic resurfacing of the patella. The cobalt-chromium prosthesis is oval with a vertical ridge that divides the articular surface into a smaller convex medial facet and a larger concave lateral facet. An anchoring stem was added to improve stability. The device is intended for fixation with methylmethacrylate. The author reported results in 15 knees treated surgically with patellar resurfacing for chondromalacia patellae.[410] With a follow-up period ranging from 6 months to 8 years, satisfactory results were achieved in only three knees (20%). Therefore, it does not appear that an anatomic shape of the articular surface improves the end result.

One solution to the problems posed by hemiarthroplasty is to replace the femoral sulcus as well as the patella. Blazina and coworkers[39] reported on such a patellofemoral replacement, and their results seem slightly better than ours with replacement of the patella alone: 78% of 57 patients who underwent patellofemoral replacement were improved by the procedure with an average follow-up of 21 months. However, a large number of their patients (30 of 57, or 53%) underwent secondary or revisionary procedures, and the follow-up time was relatively short (21 months).

The results of 25 patellofemoral arthroplasties have more recently been reported by Arciero and Toomay.[17] Both the patella and the femoral groove were resurfaced. This series differed from that of Blazina and coworkers in that the average age was older (62 years versus 39 years) and the follow-up longer (64 months versus 21 months). Patellofemoral arthritis was present preoperatively in all the knees, whereas malalignment or instability was documented by history in 14 patients. In five knees, tibiofemoral arthritis was also present. Satisfactory results were achieved in 72% of the overall group. The presence of tibiofemoral arthritis, component malposition, and persistent malalignment of the extensor mechanism contributed to the unsatisfactory results.

Patellofemoral arthroplasty has been investigated in France by Cartier et al, who reported their experience[57] in 72 knees with an average follow-up of 4 years (range, 2 to 12 years). They used the Blazina Patella II (64 cases) or the Patella III prosthesis (Richards). The average age in this series was 65 years. Concomitant procedures were frequently performed, including 36 unicompartmental replacements, 34 transfers of the tibial tuberosity, and 27 proximal soft-tissue realignments. This fact renders interpretation of the results more difficult. Nevertheless, 85% of the cases were satisfactory from a subjective and objective point of view: four patients experienced symptomatic degeneration of the medial compartment, one knee had reflex sympathetic dystrophy, and five more cases required revision surgery to achieve a final satisfactory result. Revision surgery included lateral release (one case), transfer of the tibial tuberosity (one case), patellectomy (one case), and exchange of the patellar button (one case). In our opinion, the use of a patellofemoral replacement in conjunction with a femorotibial unicompartmental replacement has no indications given the high success rate of three-compartment prostheses.

With few exceptions,[369,376] the clinical results of patellofemoral arthroplasty have been relatively stable for several decades despite differences in component design and variable indications for surgery.[18,19,42,59,220] The percentage of good and excellent results exceeds 80% in most series. Lonner[254] performed a meta-analysis of 564 patellofemoral arthroplasties and found that only 4 trochlear components (0.7%) and 1 patellar component (0.2%) failed because of loosening. All four reported cases of trochlear component loosening involved uncemented implants. Tibiofemoral degeneration can occur with time, but proper patient selection can delay the onset and reduce the incidence of failure from progressive symptomatic arthritis. In the series with the longest follow-up (15.6 years), Kooijman et al[228] reported that after isolated patellofemoral arthroplasty, 75% of the implants studied were still functioning well into the second decade after implantation. An analysis of failures with particular implant designs is useful. The deep constraining trochlear groove of the Richards I & II (Smith Nephew Richards, Memphis, TN) implants predisposed to subtle maltracking and catching of the patellar component on the trochlear edges, thus prompting secondary surgeries in a relatively high number of cases. de Winter et al[98] reported that 42% of their knees at an average follow-up of 11 years required additional surgery to address patellar maltracking or implant malalignment. The Lubinus patellofemoral arthroplasty has also been associated with a high rate of reoperations for patellofemoral dysfunction. Tauro et al[380] reported a 55% unsatisfactory rate after patellofemoral arthroplasty with the Lubinus implant, including the need for revision in 21 knees (28%) at a mean follow-up of 7.5 years. Fifteen knees were successfully revised for maltracking.

Second-generation implants have been introduced to address maltracking and malalignment. The crucial elements of the trochlear geometry include a proximally and distally prolonged trochlea and a wider sulcus angle. Furthermore, multiple sizes are available. Only early reports on the new implants are available. Lonner[254] used the Avon (Stryker Howmedica Osteonics, Mahwah, NJ) trochlear prosthesis in 22 patients, and the incidence of maltracking was less than 4%. With the same implant, Ackroyd et al[3] reported a 1% incidence of maltracking.

Recently, custom-made trochlear insets have become available. The main advantage of such implants is that they are only 2 mm thick. Bone stock is thus preserved, and in case of failure or progression of tibiofemoral disease, it can be revised to a standard total knee arthroplasty.

A major objection to complete patellofemoral replacement in younger patients is the extreme difficulty of salvage should the operation fail. In case of failure with patellar replacement alone, patellectomy can be performed and the patient is no worse than if patellectomy had been the primary choice. On the other hand, patellectomy does not provide a solution after failure of patellofemoral replacement, and revision is possible only with a total knee prosthesis, clearly an unsatisfactory alternative in younger patients. For this reason, we think that the concept of patellofemoral replacement is debatable; it should not be used in younger patients, and in the elderly, total knee arthroplasty gives better results than either patellofemoral replacement or patellectomy does.

Patellectomy

Patellectomy should be considered the last resort among surgical alternatives for the treatment of disorders. Contrary to what was previously thought,[46,168,182,361] the patella has an important function: displacing the patellar tendon away from the center of rotation of the knee joint and thus lengthening the moment arm of the patellar tendon.

Kaufer[221,222] reported that the knee extension moment arm increases from 3.8 cm at 120 degrees of knee flexion to 5.8 cm in full extension, as determined by mechanical studies in normal cadaver knees. The contribution of the patella to the moment arm increased from 14% at 120 degrees of flexion to 31% in full extension. He assessed that the contribution of the patella to the extensor moment of the knee is produced by two separate mechanisms: (1) it establishes continuity between the quadriceps and patellar tendon, and (2) it displaces the patellar tendon anteriorly, thus increasing the extensor moment arm. In this view, longitudinal repair of the patellar defect is less efficient than transverse repair because the second operation allows direct transfer of tensile force from the quadriceps to the patellar tendon. In longitudinal repair, a significant portion of the tensile force may be transferred to the tibia through the retinacula, which have shorter moment arms. Anterior displacement of the tibial tubercle was found to adequately compensate for the shortening of the extensor moment arm caused by patellectomy.

More recently, Wendt and Johnson[397] examined the relationship between quadriceps excursion and torque in 10 cadaver knees. They found that the mean quadriceps excursion from 0 to 90 degrees of flexion was 66 ± 5 mm and, with the use of 10-degree intervals, that the maximum increment occurred between 30 and 40 degrees (9.5 mm) whereas the minimum occurred between 80 and 90 degrees (5.4 mm). The curve of quadriceps torque correlated closely with the curve of the increments in excursion, with the highest torque occurring at 30 degrees of flexion. Therefore, it was shown that the patella increases quadriceps torque by displacing the tendon away from the axis of rotation of the knee, but that increased quadriceps excursion is required at the same time. Patellectomy decreased quadriceps excursion in the 0- to 90-degree arc of motion from an average value of 66 mm to 51 mm. Quadriceps torque was also decreased by roughly 40% from 0 to 40 degrees of flexion.

Decreased quadriceps strength has been confirmed clinically by Cybex-II isokinetic evaluation of patients with unilateral patellectomy.[396] When compared with the untreated side, the peak quadriceps torque of the knee after patellectomy decreased by an average of 54% at 30 degrees and by 49% at 180 degrees. Quadriceps torque values decreased throughout the range of motion, except near full extension. These data indicate a major deficiency in quadriceps strength and are in perfect agreement with the clinical finding of difficulty rising from a chair or climbing stairs. Furthermore, quadriceps function was also impaired by the inability to rapidly develop quadriceps torque during alternating reciprocal contractions, which contributes to the difficulty that these patients have with running.

Technique. Several techniques have been described for patellectomy. Brooke[50] recommended a transverse incision with enucleation of the patella. Kaufer[221] found that transverse repair was superior to longitudinal repair after patellectomy. An additional 30% of quadriceps force was required to extend the knee after longitudinal repair as compared with only a 15% increase after transverse repair. Because the longitudinal repair was performed without capsular imbrication, it may well be that most of the tensile force was transmitted to the tibia through the parapatellar retinacula.

An additional factor associated with transverse incisions is the need to protect the suture line for longer periods than needed with a longitudinal excision. Longitudinal excision of the patella was recommended by Boyd and Hawkins,[46] along with enucleation of the patella and either side-to-side repair of the capsule or imbrication. The operation can be enhanced by longitudinally dividing the fibers of the quadriceps and patellar tendon and splitting the patella into two halves with an osteotome. During the osteotomy, a retractor is inserted into the joint to protect the trochlear surface. Great care should be taken to preserve the continuity of the prepatellar fibers.

After removal of the patella, the quadriceps, patellar tendon, and prepatellar aponeurosis are sutured with some overlapping, more pronounced in the central portion. The suture line is tested by repeated flexing of the knee up to 90 degrees. Care is taken to verify that the sutured tendon glides in the middle of the trochlea without any tendency toward lateral displacement, especially when the basic disorder was malalignment with patellar dislocation. If this is not the case, lateral retinacular release should be added. The longitudinal approach to patellectomy does not require immobilization. A bulky Robert Jones dressing is applied, and knee flexion and quadriceps strengthening are begun as soon as the wound has healed. Weightbearing is permitted as tolerated.

More recently, Compere and colleagues[77] described a technique by which a tube is created, within which any bone regeneration would be contained. It has been suggested that calcification in the extensor mechanism after patellectomy may be the source of pain; this technique is designed to prevent this problem. Medial and lateral parapatellar incisions are made, and the patella is enucleated.

The medial border of the quadriceps aponeurosis is then brought underneath and sutured to the lateral wound to create a tube. The vastus medialis is then advanced laterally and distally and sutured to the tube. Other techniques of patellectomy that have been described involve Z-plasty,[35] cruciateplasty,[247] realignment,[398] or some form of reinforcement of the patellar defect by turning a flap of the quadriceps or patellar tendon.[296,345,357]

Others have suggested both reinforcement and realignment of the extensor mechanism.[21] However, these procedures are somewhat more complicated and do not seem to have special merit. In our opinion, satisfactory continuity and centralization of the extensor mechanism can be achieved by approximation of a longitudinal incision with some overlapping. An additional lateral retinacular release may be necessary. Regardless of the technique used, the lever arm of the patellar tendon is decreased after patellectomy. To restore the lever arm to normal values, Kaufer[221,222] suggested that a Maquet procedure be used in knees with unsatisfactory quadriceps strength after patellectomy. The procedure has been performed with success in six of nine patellectomized knees by Radin and Leach.[324]

Clinical Results. The clinical results after patellectomy were reviewed in a series of 100 cases at the Hospital for Special Surgery.[224,246] The main indications for the procedure were chondromalacia, patellofemoral arthritis, and comminuted fractures. The average age of the patients was 49, and the average follow-up was 5 years. The group was divided according to the age of the patients, younger or older than 40 years; 22 patellectomies were performed in 19 patients younger than 40 years (average age, 22 years). Chondromalacia and patellar instability were the most frequent diagnoses in this group (16 knees), followed by patellar fractures (5 knees) and patellofemoral arthritis (1 knee). In contrast, the diagnosis in the 78 patients older than 40 years was patellofemoral arthritis in 90% of cases.

An excellent or good result was achieved in 76% of the younger and 70.5% of the older patients. The unsatisfactory results were almost invariably attributable to unrelieved pain with additional complaints of weakness and instability. One poor result in a young patient was attributed to dislocation of the extensor apparatus after patellectomy for patellar instability. The fair and poor results in older patients were often due to associated femorotibial joint disease. Calcification of the patellar tendon did not correlate with pain.[225] No correlation was found between the surgical technique and the end result.

Conclusions. Today there is wide agreement that the patella has an important role in the mechanics of the knee. It increases the lever arm of the patellar tendon and allows the application of quadriceps power around an angle during knee flexion without loss as a result of friction. It protects the femoral trochlea from direct blows and contributes to the normal cosmetic appearance of the knee. These considerations make it clear that patellectomy significantly impairs quadriceps function. Decreased extensor power,[221,222,396] reduced ability to develop quadriceps torque rapidly,[396] decreased stance-phase flexion, and decreased flexion in ascending and descending stairs have all been described.[379] Therefore, we think that the patella should be saved when possible.

We currently recommend patellectomy in the following cases. Severe comminuted fractures of the patella when anatomic reduction is impossible may be treated by partial or total patellectomy. Severe chondromalacia of the patella is usually best treated by realigning the extensor apparatus and shaving or drilling the patellar surface, as required. In the few cases of idiopathic severe chondromalacia with no demonstrable abnormality in patella tracking and in knees with a poor result after realignment, patellectomy may be the only alternative. Severe symptomatic patellofemoral arthritis in a young patient should be treated initially by tibial tubercle elevation, whereas patellectomy should be reserved for knees that did not benefit from the first procedure.

In summary, patellectomy should be considered the last resort in the surgical treatment of patellofemoral disorders. Other alternatives can usually be found. If the surgeon is in doubt, the patella should be saved.

References

1. Abernethy PJ, Townsendt PR, Rose MR, et al: Is chondromalacia patellae a separate clinical entity? J Bone Joint Surg Br 60:205, 1978.
2. Abraham E, Washington E, Huang TL: Insall proximal realignment for disorders of the patella. Clin Orthop 248:61, 1989.
3. Ackroyd CE, Newman JH, Webb JM, Eldridge JD: The Avon patellofemoral arthroplasty. Two to five year results. Presented at a meeting of the American Academy of Orthopaedic Surgeons, 2003, Rosemont, IL, p 607.
4. Aglietti P, Buzzi R, D'Andria S, Zaccherotti G: Patellofemoral problems after intra-articular anterior cruciate ligament reconstruction. Clin Orthop 288:195, 1993.
5. Aglietti P, Buzzi R, De Biase P, Giron F: Surgical treatment of recurrent dislocation of the patella. Clin Orthop 308:8, 1994.
6. Aglietti P, Cantalamessa G, Lucatelli G, et al: Riallineamento distale per lussazione recidivante di rotula. (Risultati a distanza dell'intervento di Putti-Goebbel.) Arch Putti 31:55, 1981.
7. Aglietti P, Insall JN, Cerulli G: Patellar pain and incongruence. I: Measurements of incongruence. Clin Orthop 176:217, 1983.
8. Aglietti P, Insall JN, Walker PS, et al: A new patella prosthesis. Clin Orthop 107:175, 1975.
9. Aglietti P, Pisaneschi A, Allegra M, Villari N: Dolore di rotula: Uno studio con la radiologia convenzionale e con la TAC. Ital J Sports Traumatol 10:7, 1988.
10. Aglietti P, Pisaneschi A, Buzzi R, et al: Arthroscopic lateral release for patellar pain or instability. Arthroscopy 5:176, 1989.
11. Ahmed A, Burke D, Hyder A: Force analysis of the patellar mechanism. J Orthop Res 5:69, 1987.
12. Albee FH: The bone graft wedge in the treatment of habitual dislocation of patella. Med Rec 88:257, 1915.
13. Aleman O: Chondromalacia post-traumatica patellae. Acta Chir Scand 63:149, 1928.
14. Alvarez EV, Munters M, Lavine LS, et al: Quadriceps myofibrosis: A complication of intramuscular injections. J Bone Joint Surg Am 62:58, 1980.
15. Alvik J: Increased anteversion of the femur as the only manifestation of dysplasia of the hip. Clin Orthop 22:16, 1962.
16. Amiel D, von Schroeder H, Akeson WH: The response of ligaments to stress deprivation and stress enhancement: Biochemical studies. In Daniel DM (ed): Knee Ligaments: Structure, Function, Injury and Repair. New York, Raven Press, 1990, p 329.
17. Arciero RA, Toomay HE: Patellofemoral arthroplasty: A three- to nine-year follow-up study. Clin Orthop 236:60, 1988.
18. Argenson JN, Guillaume JM, Aubaniac JM: Is there a place for patellofemoral arthroplasty? Clin Orthop 321:162-167, 1995.
19. Arroll B, Ellis-Pegler E, Edwards A, Sutcliffe G: Patellofemoral pain syndrome: A critical review of the clinical trials on nonoperative therapy. Am J Sports Med 25:207, 1997.
20. Ashtrom JP: Osteochondral fracture in the knee joint associated with hypermobility and dislocation of the patella: Report of eighteen cases. J Bone Joint Surg Am 47:1491, 1965.
21. Baker CL, Hughston JC: Miyakawa patellectomy. J Bone Joint Surg Am 70:1489, 1988.
22. Bandi W: Chondromalacia patellae and femoropatellare arthrose. Helv Chir Acta Suppl 1:3, 1972.
23. Barbari S, Raugstad TS, Lichtenberg N, Refvem D: The Hauser operation for patellar dislocation: 3- to 32-year results in 63 knees. Acta Orthop Scand 65:32, 1990.
24. Baumgartl F: Das Kniegelenk. Berlin, Springer-Verlag, 1944.
25. Beighton P, Horan F: Orthopaedic aspects of the Ehlers-Danlos syndrome. J Bone Joint Surg Br 51:444, 1969.
26. Bell J: Congenital absence of both patellae. J Bone Joint Surg Br 37:352, 1955.
27. Bellemans J, Cauwenberghs F, Witvrouw E, et al: Anteromedial tibial tubercle transfer in patients with chronic anterior knee pain and a subluxation type patellar malalignment. Am J Sports Med 25:375, 1997.
28. Beltran JE: Resection arthroplasty of the patella. J Bone Joint Surg Br 69:604, 1987.
29. Bentley G: The surgical treatment of chondromalacia patellae. J Bone Joint Surg Br 60:74, 1978.
30. Bentley G: Articular cartilage changes in chondromalacia patellae. J Bone Joint Surg Br 67:769, 1985.
31. Benzon HT, Chomka CM, Brunner EA: Treatment of reflex sympathetic dystrophy with regional intravenous reserpine. Anesth Analg 59:500, 1980.
32. Bergman NR, Williams PF: Habitual dislocation of the patella in flexion. J Bone Joint Surg 70:415, 1988.
33. Bernhang AM, Levine SA: Familial absence of the patella. J Bone Joint Surg Am 55:1088, 1973.
34. Betz RR, Magill JT, Lonergan RP: The percutaneous lateral retinacular release. Am J Sports Med 15:477, 1987.
35. Bickel WH, Johnson KA: Z-plasty patellectomy. Surg Gynecol Obstet 132:985, 1971.
36. Biedert R: Patellofemoral disorders. Presented at the ACL Study Group 2004 Congress, Sardinia, Italy.
37. Bigos SJ, McBride GG: The isolated lateral retinacular release in the treatment of patello-femoral disorders. Clin Orthop 186:75, 1984.
38. Blackburne JS, Peel TE: A new method of measuring patella height. J Bone Joint Surg Br 59:241, 1977.
39. Blazina ME, Fox JM, Del Pizzo W, et al: Patellofemoral replacement. Clin Orthop 144:98, 1979.
40. Blazina ME, Kerlan RK, Jobe FW, et al: Jumpers knee. Orthop Clin North Am 4:665, 1973.
41. Blumensaat C: Die Lageabweichungen und Verrenkungen der Kniescheibe. Ergeb Chir Orthop 31:149, 1938.
42. Boring TH, O'Donoghue DH: Acute patellar dislocation: Results of immediate surgery repair. Clin Orthop 136:182, 1978.
43. Boven F, Bellemans MA, Geurts J, Potvliege R: A comparative study of the patello-femoral joint on axial roentgenogram, axial arthrogram and computed tomography following arthrography. Skeletal Radiol 8:179, 1982.
44. Boven F, Bellemans MA, Geurts J, et al: The value of computed tomography scanning in chondromalacia patellae. Skeletal Radiol 8:183, 1982.
45. Bowker JH, Thompson EB: Surgical treatment of recurrent dislocation of the patella. J Bone Joint Surg Am 46:1451, 1964.
46. Boyd HB, Hawkins BL: Patellectomy: A simplified technique. Surg Gynecol Obstet 86:357, 1948.
47. Brattström H: Shape of the intercondylar groove normally and in recurrent dislocation of patella: A clinical and x-ray anatomic investigation. Acta Orthop Scand Suppl 68:134, 1964.
48. Brief LP: Lateral patellar instability: Treatment with a combined open-arthroscopic approach. Arthroscopy 9:617, 1993.
49. Bray RC, Roth JH, Jacobsen RP: Arthroscopic lateral release for anterior knee pain: A study comparing patients who are claiming worker's compensation and those who are not. Arthroscopy 3:237, 1987.
50. Brooke R: The treatment of fractured patella by excision: A study of morphology and function. Br J Surg 24:733, 1937.
51. Buedinger K: Über Ablösung von Gelenkteilen und verwandte Prezesse. Dtsch Z Chir 84:311, 1906.
52. Buedinger K: Über traumatische Knorpelrisse in Kniegelenk. Dtsch Z Chir 92:510, 1908.

53. Buff HU, Jones LC, Hungerford DS: Experimental determination of forces transmitted through the patello-femoral joint. J Biomech 21:17, 1988.

54. Bullough P, Goodfellow J: The significance of the fine structure of articular cartilage. J Bone Joint Surg Br 50:852, 1968.

55. Carson WG, James SL, Larson RL, et al: Patellofemoral disorders: Physical and radiographic evaluation. I: Physical examination. Clin Orthop 185:165, 1984.

56. Carter C, Wilkinson J: Persistent joint laxity and congenital dislocation of the hip. J Bone Joint Surg Br 46:40, 1964.

57. Cartier P, Sanouiller JL, Grelsamer R: Patellofemoral arthroplasty: 2- to 12-year follow-up study. J Arthrop 5:49, 1990.

58. Cash JD, Hughston JC: Treatment of acute patellar dislocation. Am J Sports Med 16:244, 1988.

59. Casscells SW: Gross pathological changes in the knee joint of the aged individual: A study of 300 cases. Clin Orthop 132:225, 1978.

60. Casscells SW: The arthroscope in the diagnosis of disorders of the patello-femoral joint. Clin Orthop 144:45, 1979.

61. Casscells SW: Outerbridge's ridges. Arthroscopy 6:253, 1990.

62. Caton G, Deschamps G, Chambat P, et al: Les routules basses: Á propos de 128 observations. Rev Chir Orthop 68:317, 1982.

63. Ceder LC, Larson RL: Z-plasty lateral retinacular release for the treatment of patellar compression syndrome. Clin Orthop 144:110, 1979.

64. Cerullo G, Puddu G, Conteduca F, et al: Evaluation of the results of extensor mechanism reconstruction. Am J Sports Med 16:93, 1988.

65. Chen SC, Ramanathan EBS: The treatment of patellar instability by lateral release. J Bone Joint Surg Br 66:344, 1984.

66. Chin SS, Mano J, Yukawa YN, et al: Contracture of the quadriceps muscle caused by injection. Acta Orthop Belg 41:306, 1975.

67. Chrisman OD: Biochemical aspects of degenerative joint disease. Clin Orthop 64:77, 1969.

68. Chrisman OD: The role of articular cartilage in patello-femoral pain. Orthop Clin North Am 17:231, 1986.

69. Chrisman OD, Fessel JM, Southwick WO: Experimental production of synovitis and marginal articular exostoses in knee joints of dogs. Yale J Biol Med 37:409, 1965.

70. Chrisman OD, Ladenbauer Bellis IM, Panjabi M: The relationship of mechanical trauma and the early reactions of osteoarthritic cartilage. Clin Orthop 161:265, 1981.

71. Chrisman OD, Snook GA, Wilson TC: The protective effect of aspirin against degeneration of human articular cartilage. Clin Orthop 84:193, 1972.

72. Chrisman OD, Snook GA, Wilson TC: A long-term prospective study of the Hauser and Roux-Goldthwait procedures for recurrent patellar dislocation. Clin Orthop 144:27, 1979.

73. Christensen F, Soballe K, Snerum L: Treatment of chondromalacia patellae by lateral retinacular release of the patella. Clin Orthop 234:145, 1988.

74. Christensen K, Jensen EM, Moer J: The reflex dystrophy syndrome: Response to treatment with systemic cortico-steroids. Acta Chir Scand 148:653, 1982.

75. Close JR, Inman VT: The action of the subtalar joint. Univ Calif Prosthet Devices Res Rep Ser 11, 24, 1953.

76. Cofield R, Bryan R: Acute dislocation of the patella: Results of conservative treatment. J Trauma 17:526, 1977.

77. Compere CL, Hill JA, Levinnek GE, et al: A new method of patellectomy for patellofemoral arthritis. J Bone Joint Surg Am 61:714, 1979.

78. Conlan T, Garth WP, Lemons JE: Evaluations of the medial soft-tissue restraints of the extensor mechanism of the knee. J Bone Joint Surg Am 75:682, 1993.

79. Cooper DE, De Lee J, Ramamurthy S: Reflex sympathetic dystrophy of the knee: Treatment using continuous epidural anaesthesia. J Bone Joint Surg Am 71:365, 1989.

80. Cox JS: Evaluation of the Roux-Elmslie-Trillat procedure for knee extensor realignment. Am J Sports Med 10:303, 1982.

81. Crosby BE, Insall JN: Recurrent dislocation of the patella: Relation of treatment to osteoarthritis. J Bone Joint Surg Am 58:9, 1976.

82. Curwin S, Stanish WD: Tendinitis: Its Etiology and Treatment. Lexington, MA, Collamare Press, 1984.

83. Dainer RD, Barrack RL, Buckley SL, Alexander AH: Arthroscopic treatment of acute patellar dislocation. Arthroscopy 4:267, 1988.

84. Dandy DJ: Anatomy of the medial suprapatellar plica and medial synovial shelf. Arthroscopy 6:79, 1990.

85. Dandy DJ, Desai SS: The results of arthroscopic lateral release of the extensor mechanism for recurrent dislocation of the patella after 8 years. Arthroscopy 10:540, 1994.

86. Dandy DJ, Griffiths D: Lateral release for recurrent dislocation of the patella. J Bone Joint Surg Br 71:121, 1989.

87. Darracott J, Vernon-Roberts B: The bony changes in "chondromalacia patellae." Rheumatol Phys Med 11:175, 1971.

88. Dashefsky JH: Arthroscopic measurement of chondromalacia of the patella cartilage using a microminiature pressure transducer. Arthroscopy 3:80, 1987.

89. Deburge A, Chambat P: La transposition de la tuberosite tibiale anterieure. Rev Chir Orthop 66:218, 1980.

90. DeCesare WF: Late results of Hauser procedure for recurrent dislocation of the patella. Clin Orthop 140:137, 1979.

91. Dejour H, Walch G, Nave-Josserand L, Guier C: Factors of patellar instability: An anatomic radiographic study [invited lecture]. Knee Surg Sports Traumatol Arthrosc 2:19, 1994.

92. Dejour H, Walch G, Neyret P, Adeleine P: La dysplasie de la trochlée femorale. Rev Chir Orthop 76:45, 1990.

93. Delgado-Martins H: A study of the position of the patella using computerized tomography. J Bone Joint Surg Br 61:443, 1979.

94. De Palma AF, Sawier B, Hoffman JD: Reconsideration of lesions affecting the patellofemoral joint. Clin Orthop 18:63, 1960.

95. Desai SS, Patel MR, Michelli LJ, et al: Osteochondritis dissecans of the patella. J Bone Joint Surg Br 69:320, 1987.

96. De Takats G: Reflex dystrophy of the extremities. Arch Surg 34:939, 1937.

97. De Takats G, Miller DS: Post-traumatic dystrophy of the extremities. Arch Surg 46:469, 1943.

98. de Winter WE, Feith R, van Loon CJ: The Richards type II patellofemoral arthroplasty: 26 cases followed for 1-20 years. Acta Orthop Scand 72:487-490, 2001.

99. Doupe J, Cullen CH, Chance GQ: Post-traumatic pain and causalgic syndrome. J Neurol Neurosurg Psychiatry 7:33, 1944.

100. Dugdale TW, Renshaw TS: Instability of the patellofemoral joint in Down syndrome. J Bone Joint Surg Am 68:405, 1986.

101. Dye SF, Boll DA: Radionuclide imaging of the patello-femoral joint in young adults with anterior knee pain. Orthop Clin North Am 17:249, 1986.

102. Dzioba RB: Diagnostic arthroscopy and longitudinal open lateral release: A four year follow-up study to determine predictors of surgical outcome. Am J Sports Med 18:343, 1990.

103. Edwards DH, Bentley G: Osteochondritis dissecans patellae. J Bone Joint Surg Br 59:58, 1977.

104. Emery IH, Meachim G: Surface morphology and topography of patello-femoral cartilage fibrillation in Liverpool necropsies. J Anat 116:103, 1973.

105. Engebretsen L, Svenningsen S, Benum P: Advancement of the tibial tuberosity for patellar pain: A 5-year follow-up. Acta Orthop Scand 60:20, 1989.

106. Erdemir H, Gelman S, Galbraith JG: Prediction of the needed level of sympathectomy for post-traumatic reflex sympathetic dystrophy. Surg Neurol 17:353, 1982.

107. Evans EB, Eggers GW, Butler GK, et al: Experimental immobilization and remobilization of the rat knee joints. J Bone Joint Surg Am 42:737, 1960.

108. Evans JA: Reflex sympathetic dystrophy. Surg Gynecol Obstet 82:36, 1946.

109. Fairbank HA: Internal derangement of the knee in children. Proc R Soc 3:11, 1937.

110. Fairbank JCT, Pynsent PB, Van Poortvliet JA, et al: Mechanical factors in the incidence of knee pain in adolescents and young adults. J Bone Joint Surg Br 66:685, 1984.

111. Fairbank TJ, Barrett AM: Vastus intermedius contracture in early childhood: Case report in identical twins. J Bone Joint Surg Br 43:326, 1961.

112. Ferguson AB: Elevation of the insertion of the patellar ligament for patellofemoral pain. J Bone Joint Surg Am 64:766, 1982.

113. Ferguson AB, Brown TD, Fu FH, Rutkowski R: Relief of patellofemoral contact stress by anterior displacement of the tibial tubercle. J Bone Joint Surg Am 61:159, 1979.

114. Ferrandez L, Usabiaga J, Yubero J, et al: An experimental study of the redistribution of patello-femoral pressures by the anterior displacement of the anterior tuberosity of the tibia. Clin Orthop 238:183, 1989.

115. Ficat P, Ficat C, Bailleux A: Syndrome d'hyperpression externe de la rotule (SHPE): Son interet pour la connaissance de l'arthrose. Rev Chir Orthop 61:39, 1975.

116. Ficat P, Hungerford DS: Disorders of the Patellofemoral Joint. Baltimore, Williams & Wilkins, 1977.

117. Ficat RP, Ficat C, Gedeon P, Toussaint JB: Spongialization: A new treatment for diseased patellae. Clin Orthop 144:74, 1979.

118. Ficat RP, Phillippe J: Contrast Arthrography of the Synovial Joints. New York, Masson, 1981, p 1.

119. Fithian DC, Mishra DK, Balen PF, et al: Instrumented measurement of patellar mobility. Am J Sports Med 23:607, 1995.

120. Floyd A, Phillips P, Khan MRH, et al: Recurrent dislocation of the patella: Histochemical and electromyographic evidence of primary muscle pathology. J Bone Joint Surg Br 69:790, 1987.

121. Fondren FB, Goldner JL, Bassett FH: Recurrent dislocation of the patella treated by the modified Roux-Goldthwait procedure: A prospective study of forty-seven knees. J Bone Joint Surg Am 67:993, 1985.

122. Fox TA: Dysplasia of the quadriceps mechanism. Surg Clin North Am 55:199, 1975.

123. Freiberger RH, Kotzen LM: Fracture of the medial margin of the patella, a finding diagnostic of lateral dislocation. Radiology 88:902, 1967.

124. Fritschy D, De Gautard R: Jumper's knee and ultrasonography. Am J Sports Med 16:637, 1988.

125. Fulkerson JP: Awareness of the retinaculum in evaluating patellofemoral pain. Am J Sports Med 10:147, 1982.

126. Fulkerson JP: The etiology of patello-femoral pain in young active patients: A prospective study. Clin Orthop 179:129, 1983.

127. Fulkerson JP: Anteromedialization of the tibial tuberosity for patellofemoral malalignment. Clin Orthop 177:176, 1983.

128. Fulkerson JP, Becker GJ, Meaney JA, et al: Anteromedial tibial tubercle transfer without bone graft. Am J Sports Med 18:490, 1990.

129. Fulkerson JP, Damiano P: Effect of prostaglandin E$_2$ on adult pig articular cartilage slices in culture. Clin Orthop 179:266, 1983.

130. Fulkerson JP, Gossling HR: Anatomy of the knee joint lateral retinaculum. Clin Orthop 153:183, 1980.

131. Fulkerson JP, Hungerford DS: Normal anatomy. In Disorders of the Patello-Femoral Joint. Baltimore, Williams & Wilkins, 1990, p 1.

132. Fulkerson JP, Hungerford DS: Biomechanics of the patello-femoral joint. In Disorders of the Patello-Femoral Joint. Baltimore, Williams & Wilkins, 1990, p 25.

133. Fulkerson JP, Hungerford DS: Imaging the patellofemoral joint. In Disorders of the Patello-Femoral Joint. Baltimore, Williams & Wilkins, 1990, p 42.

134. Fulkerson JP, Hungerford DS: Patellar tilt compression and the excessive lateral pressure syndrome. In Disorders of the Patello-Femoral Joint. Baltimore, Williams & Wilkins, 1990, p 102.

135. Fulkerson JP, Hungerford DS: Patellar dislocation. In Disorders of the Patello-Femoral Joint. Baltimore, Williams & Wilkins, 1990, p 149.

136. Fulkerson JP, Hungerford DS: Articular cartilage lesions in patello-femoral pain patients. In Disorders of the Patello-Femoral Joint. Baltimore, Williams & Wilkins, 1990, p 176.

137. Fulkerson JP, Hungerford DS: Surgical treatment of patello femoral chondrosis and arthrosis. In Disorders of the Patello-Femoral Joint. Baltimore, Williams & Wilkins, 1990, p 226.

138. Fulkerson JP, Hungerford DS: Reflex sympathetic dystrophy and chronic pain. In Disorders of the Patello-Femoral Joint. Baltimore, Williams & Wilkins, 1990, p 247.

139. Fulkerson JP, Ladenbauer-Bellis JM, Chrisman OD: In vitro hexosamine depletion of intact articular cartilage by E postaglandins. Arthritis Rheum 22:1117, 1979.

140. Fulkerson JP, Shea KP: Disorders of patello-femoral alignment. J Bone Joint Surg Am 72:1424, 1990.

141. Fulkerson JP, Tennaut R, Jaivin JS, Grunnet M: Histological evidence of retinacular nerve injury associated with patello-femoral malalignment. Clin Orthop 197:196, 1985.

142. Galasko CSB, Rushton S, Lacey E: Prostaglandins and the synovitis associated with meniscal lesions. Trans Orthop Res Soc 5:61, 1980.

143. Gammie WFP, Taylor JH, Urich H: Contracture of the vastus intermedius in children: A report of two cases. J Bone Joint Surg Br 45:370, 1963.

144. Garth WP, Pomphrey M, Merrill K: Functional treatment of patellar dislocation in an athletic population. Am J Sports Med 24:785, 1996.

145. Gasco J, Del Pino JM, Gomar-Sancko F: Double patella: A case of duplication of the coronal plane. J Bone Joint Surg Br 69:602, 1987.

146. Gecha SR, Torg JS: Clinical prognosticators for the efficacy of retinacular release surgery to treat patello-femoral pain. Clin Orthop 253:203, 1990.

147. George RC, Chrisman OD: The role of cartilage polysaccharide in osteoarthritis. Clin Orthop 57:259, 1968.

148. Gigante A, Pasquinelli FM, Paladini P, et al: The effects of patellar taping on patellofemoral incongruence. A computed tomography study. Am J Sports Med 29:88-92, 2001.

149. Glick EN: Reflex dystrophy (algoneurodystrophy): Results of treatment by corticosteroids. Rheumatol Rehabil 12:84, 1973.

150. Glynn CJ, Basedow RW, Walsh JA: Pain relief following post-ganglionic sympathetic blockade with I.V. guanethidine. Br J Anaesth 53:1297, 1981.

151. Goldthwait JE: Dislocation of the patella. Trans Am Orthop Assoc 8:237, 1895.

152. Goldthwait JE: Permanent dislocation of the patella: Report of a case of twenty years' duration, successfully treated by transplantation of the patella tendons with the tubercle of the tibia. Am Surg 29:62, 1899.

153. Goodfellow J, Bullough PG: The pattern of ageing of the articular cartilage of the elbow joint. J Bone Joint Surg Br 49:175, 1967.

154. Goodfellow J, Bullough P: Studies on age changes in the human hip joint. J Bone Joint Surg Br 50:222, 1968.

155. Goodfellow J, Hungerford DS, Woods C: Patello-femoral joint mechanics and pathology. 2: Chondromalacia patellae. J Bone Joint Surg Br 59:291, 1976.

156. Goodfellow J, Hungerford DS, Zindel M: Patello-femoral joint mechanics and pathology. 1: Functional anatomy of the patello-femoral joint. J Bone Joint Surg Br 58:287, 1976.

157. Goutallier D, Bernageau J: Mesure de l'écart tubérosité tibiale antérieure-gorge de le trochlée (T.A.-G.T.): Technique résultats intérêt. Rev Chir Orthop 64:423, 1978.

158. Grana WA, Hinkley B, Hollingsworth S: Arthroscopic evaluation and treatment of patellar malalignment. Clin Orthop 186:122, 1984.

159. Grana WA, O'Donoghue DH: Patellar-tendon transfer by the slot-block method for recurrent subluxation and dislocation of the patella. J Bone Joint Surg Am 59:736, 1977.

160. Green JP, Waugh W: Congenital lateral dislocation of the patella. J Bone Joint Surg Br 50:285, 1968.

161. Grelsamer RP, Bazos AN, Proctor CS: Radiographic analysis of patellar tilt. J Bone Joint Surg Br 75:822, 1993.

162. Grelsamer RP, Meadows S: The modified Insall-Salvati ratio for assessment of patellar height. Clin Orthop 282:170, 1992.

163. Grelsamer RP, Proctor CS, Bazos AM: Evaluation of patellar shape in the sagittal plane: A clinical analysis. Am J Sports Med 22:61, 1994.

164. Grood ES, Suntay WJ, Noyes FR, Butler DL: Biomechanics of the knee-extension exercise. J Bone Joint Surg Am 66:725, 1984.

165. Gross RM: Acute dislocation of the patella: The Mudville mystery. J Bone Joint Surg Am 68:780, 1986.

166. Gunn DR: Contracture of the quadriceps muscle: A discussion on the etiology and relationship to recurrent dislocation of the patella. J Bone Joint Surg Br 46:492, 1964.

167. Guzzanti V, Gigante A, Di Lazzaro A, Fabbriciani C: Patellofemoral malalignment in adolescents. Computerized tomographic assessment with or without quadriceps contraction. Am J Sports Med 22:55, 1994.

168. Hallisey M, Doherty N, Bennet W, Fulkerson JP: Anatomy of the junction of the vastus lateralis tendon and the patella. J Bone Joint Surg Am 69:545, 1987.

169. Hampson WGJ, Hill P: Late results of transfer of the tibial tubercle for recurrent dislocation of the patella. J Bone Joint Surg Br 57:209, 1975.

170. Handelberg F, Slahabpour M, Casteleyn PP: Chondral lesions of the patella evaluated with computed tomography, magnetic resonance imaging and arthroscopy. Arthroscopy 6:24, 1990.

171. Hannington-Kiff JG: Relief of Sudeck's atrophy by regional intravenous guanethidine. Lancet 1:1132, 1977.

172. Hardaker WT, Whipple TL, Bassett FH: Diagnosis and treatment of the plica syndrome of the knee. J Bone Joint Surg Am 62:221, 1980.
173. Harrison MH, Schajowicz F, Trueta J: Osteoarthritis of the hip: A study of the nature and evolution of the disease. J Bone Joint Surg Br 35:598, 1953.
174. Harwin SF, Stern RE: Subcutaneous lateral retinacular release for chondromalacia patellae: A preliminary report. Clin Orthop 156:207, 1981.
175. Hauser EDW: Total tendon transplant for slipping patella: A new operation for recurrent dislocation of the patella. Surg Gynecol Obstet 66:199, 1938.
176. Hawkins RJ, Bell RH, Anisette G: Acute patellar dislocation: The natural history. Am J Sports Med 14:117, 1986.
177. Hayes WC, Huberti HH, Lewallen DG, et al: Patellofemoral contact pressures and the effects of surgical reconstructive procedures. In Ewing JW (ed): Articular Cartilage and Knee Joint Function: Basic Science and Arthroscopy. New York, Raven Press, 1990, p 57.
178. Heatley FW, Allen PR, Patrick JH: Tibial tubercle advancement for anterior knee pain: A temporary or permanent solution. Clin Orthop 208:215, 1986.
179. Henry JE, Pflum FA: Arthroscopic proximal patella realignment and stabilization. Arthroscopy 11:424, 1995.
180. Henry JH, Goletz TH, Williamson B: Lateral retinacular release in patello-femoral subluxation: Indication, results, and comparison to open patello-femoral reconstruction. Am J Sports Med 14:121, 1986.
181. Heuter C: Anatomische Studien an den Extremitatengelenken Neugeborener und Erwachsener. Virchows Arch Pathol Anat 25:575, 1862.
182. Hey Groves EW: A note on the extension apparatus of the knee joint. Br J Surg 24:747, 1937.
183. Heywood AWB: Recurrent dislocation of the patella: A study of its pathology and treatment in 106 knees. J Bone Joint Surg Br 43:508, 1961.
184. Hnevkovsky O: Progressive fibrosis of the vastus intermedius muscle in children: A cause of limited knee flexion and elevation of the patella. J Bone Joint Surg Br 43:318, 1961.
185. Hoaglund FT: Experimental hemarthrosis: The response of canine knees to injections of autologous blood. J Bone Joint Surg Am 49:285, 1967.
186. Homans J: Minor causalgia: A hyperesthetic neurovascular syndrome. N Engl J Med 222:870, 1940.
187. Huberti HH, Hayes WC: Patellofemoral contact pressures: The influence of Q-angle and tendofemoral contact. J Bone Joint Surg Am 66:715, 1984.
188. Huberti HH, Hayes WC, Stone JL: Force ratios in the quadriceps tendon and ligamentum patellae. J Orthop Res 2:49, 1984.
189. Hughston JC: Patellar subluxation: A recent history. Clin Sports Med 8:153, 1989.
190. Hughston JC, Deese M: Medial subluxation of the patella as a complication of lateral retinacular release. Am J Sports Med 16:383, 1988.
191. Hughston JC, Flandry F, Brinker MR, et al: Surgical correction of medial subluxation of the patella. Am J Sports Med 24:486, 1996.
192. Hughston JC, Stone M, Andrews JR: The suprapatellar plica: Its role in internal derangement of the knee. J Bone Joint Surg Am 55:1318, 1973.
193. Hughston JC, Walsh WM: Proximal and distal reconstruction of the extensor mechanism for patellar subluxation. Clin Orthop 144:36, 1979.
194. Hungerford DS, Barry N: Biomechanics of the patellofemoral joint. Clin Orthop 144:9, 1979.
195. Hvid J, Andersen LJ: The quadriceps angle and its relation to femoral torsion. Acta Orthop Scand 53:577, 1982.
196. Ihara H: Double-contrast CT arthrography of the cartilage of the patellofemoral joint. Clin Orthop 198:50, 1985.
197. Inoue M, Shino K, Hirose H, et al: Subluxation of the patella: Computerized tomography analysis of patellofemoral congruence. J Bone Joint Surg Am 70:1331, 1988.
198. Insall JN: Intra-articular surgery for degenerative arthritis of the knee: A report of the work of the late K.H. Pridie. J Bone Joint Surg Br 49:211, 1967.
199. Insall JN: Patellar pain. J Bone Joint Surg Am 64:147, 1982.
200. Insall JN: Disorders of the patella. In Surgery of the Knee. New York, Churchill Livingstone, 1984, p 191.
201. Insall JN, Aglietti P, Tria AJ: Patellar pain and incongruence. II: Clinical application. Clin Orthop 176:225, 1983.
202. Insall JN, Bullough PG, Burstein AH: Proximal "tube" realignment of the patella for chondromalacia patellae. Clin Orthop 144:63, 1979.
203. Insall JN, Falvo KA, Wise DW: Chondromalacia patellae: A prospective study. J Bone Joint Surg Am 58:1, 1976.
204. Insall JN, Salvati E: Patella position in the normal knee joint. Radiology 101:101, 1971.
205. Insall JN, Tria AJ, Aglietti P: Resurfacing of the patella. J Bone Joint Surg Am 62:933, 1980.
206. Ireland J, Trickey EL, Leyshon A: Osteochondritis patellae. J Bone Joint Surg Br 63:292, 1981.
207. Jackson DW, Jennings LD, Maywood RM, Berger PE: Magnetic resonance imaging of the knee. Am J Sports Med 16:29, 1988.
208. Jackson RW, Marshall DJ, Fujisawa Y: The pathological medial shelf. Orthop Clin North Am 13:307, 1982.
209. Jacobsen K, Bertheussen K: The vertical location of the patella. Acta Orthop Scand 45:436, 1974.
210. James SL, Bates BT, Ostering LR: Injuries to runners. Am J Sports Med 6:40, 1978.
211. Jaroschy W: Die diagnostische Verwertbarkeit der Patellar-aufnahmen. Fortschr Roentgenstr 31:781, 1924.
212. Jeffreys TE: Recurrent dislocation of the patella due to abnormal attachment of the iliotibial tract. J Bone Joint Surg Br 45:740, 1963.
213. Jensen CM, Roosen JV: Acute traumatic dislocation of the patella. J Trauma 25:160, 1985.
214. Jino S: Normal arthroscopic findings in the knee joint in adult cadavers. J Jpn Orthop Assoc 14:467, 1939.
215. Johnson LL: Arthroscopic abrasion arthroplasty. In Arthroscopic Surgery, Principles and Practice, 3rd ed. St Louis, CV Mosby, 1986.
216. Johnson RP: Lateral facet syndrome of the patella: Lateral restraint analysis and use of lateral resection. Clin Orthop 238:148, 1989.
217. Judet R: Mobilization of the stiff knee. J Bone Joint Surg Br 41:856, 1959.
218. Kaplan E: Some aspects of functional anatomy of the human knee joint. Clin Orthop 23:18, 1962.
219. Karlen A: Congenital fibrosis of the vastus intermedius muscle. J Bone Joint Surg Br 46:488, 1964.
220. Katz MM, Hungerford DS: Reflex sympathetic dystrophy affecting the knee. J Bone Joint Surg Br 69:797, 1987.
221. Kaufer H: Mechanical function of the patella. J Bone Joint Surg Am 53:1551, 1971.
222. Kaufer H: Patellar biomechanics. Clin Orthop 144:51, 1979.
223. Kaufman KR, An K, Litchy WJ, et al: Dynamic joint forces during knee isokinetic exercise. Am J Sports Med 19:305, 1991.
224. Kelly MA, Insall JN: Patellectomy. Orthop Clin North Am 17:289, 1986.
225. Kelly MA, Insall JN: Postpatellectomy extensive ossification of patellar tendon: A case report. Clin Orthop 215:148, 1987.
226. Kinnard P, Levesque RY: The plica syndrome: A syndrome of controversy. Clin Orthop 183:141, 1984.
227. Kolowich PA, Paulos LE, Rosenberg TD, Farnsworth S: Lateral release of the patella: Indications and contraindications. Am J Sports Med 18:359, 1990.
228. Kooijman HJ, Driessen APPM, van Horn JR: Long-term results of patellofemoral arthroplasty. J Bone Joint Surg Br 85:836-840, 2003.
229. Koskinen SK: Patellofemoral relationship and distal insertion of the vastus medialis muscle: A magnetic resonance imaging study in non symptomatic subjects and in patient with patellar dislocation. Arthroscopy 8:465, 1992.
230. Kowall MG, Kolk G, Nuber GW, et al: Patellar taping in the treatment of patellofemoral pain: A prospective randomized study. Am J Sports Med 24:61, 1996.
231. Kozin F, Genant HK, Bekerman C, et al: The reflex sympathetic dystrophy syndrome. II: Roentgenographic and scintigraphic evidence of bilaterality and of periarticular accentuation. Am J Med 60:332, 1976.
232. Kozin F, McCarty DJ, Sims J, et al: The reflex sympathetic dystrophy syndrome. I: Clinical and histological studies: Evidence for bilaterality, response to corticosteroids and articular involvement. Am J Med 60:321, 1976.
233. Kozin F, Ryan LM, Carerra GF, et al: The reflex sympathetic dystrophy syndrome (RSDS). III: Scintigraphic studies, further evi-

dence of the therapeutic efficacy of systemic corticosteroids and proposed diagnostic criteria. Am J Med 70:23, 1981.

234. Krompinger WJ, Fulkerson JP: Lateral retinacular release for intractable lateral retinacular pain. Clin Orthop 179:191, 1983.

235. Kujala UM, Osterman K, Kormano M, et al: Patellar motion analyzed by magnetic resonance imaging. Acta Orthop Scand 60:13, 1989.

236. Kujala UM, Osterman K, Kormano M, et al: Patellofemoral relationship in recurrent patellar dislocation. J Bone Joint Surg Br 71:788, 1989.

237. Ladd AL, De Haven KE, Thanik J, et al: Reflex sympathetic imbalance: Response to epidural blockade. Am J Sports Med 17:660, 1989.

238. Langer M: Uber die Entwicklung des Kniegelenkes. Z Ges Anat 89:83, 1929.

239. Lankford LL, Thompson JE: Reflex sympathetic dystrophy, upper and lower extremity: Diagnosis and management. Instr Course Lect 26, 1977.

240. Larsen E, Lauridsen F: Conservative treatment of patellar dislocations: Influence of evident factors on the tendency to redislocation and the therapeutic result. Clin Orthop 171:131, 1982.

241. Larsen B, Andreasen E, Urfer A, et al: Patellar taping: A radiographic examination of the medial glide technique. Am J Sports Med 23:465, 1995.

242. Larson RL, Cabaud HE, Slocum DD, et al: The patellar compression syndrome: Surgical treatment by lateral retinacular release. Clin Orthop 134:158, 1978.

243. Laurin CA, Dussault R, Levesque HP: The tangential x-ray investigation of the patellofemoral joint: X-ray technique, diagnostic criteria and their interpretation. Clin Orthop 144:16, 1979.

244. Laurin CA, Levesque HP, Dussault R, et al: The abnormal lateral patellofemoral angle: A diagnostic roentgenographic sign of recurrent patellar subluxation. J Bone Joint Surg Am 60:55, 1978.

245. Levitt RL: A long term evaluation of patellar prostheses. Clin Orthop 97:153, 1973.

246. Lewis MM, Fitzgerald PF, Jacobs B, et al: Patellectomy: An analysis of one hundred cases. J Bone Joint Surg Am 58:736, 1976.

247. Lewis RC, Scholz KC: Cruciate repair of the extensor mechanism following patellectomy. In Proceedings of the Western Orthopaedic Association. J Bone Joint Surg Am 48:1221, 1966.

248. Lieb FJ, Perry J: Quadriceps function: An anatomic and mechanical study using amputated limbs. J Bone Joint Surg Am 50:1535, 1968.

249. Lindberg U, Hamberg P, Lysholm J, Gillquist J: Arthroscopic examination of the patellofemoral joint using a central, one portal technique. Orthop Clin North Am 17:263, 1986.

250. Lindberg U, Lysholm J, Gillquist J: The correlation between arthroscopic findings and the patellofemoral pain syndrome. Arthroscopy 2:103, 1986.

251. Linden B: The incidence of osteochondritis dissecans in the condyles of the femur. Acta Orthop Scand 47:664, 1976.

252. Livingstone WK: Pain Mechanisms: A Physiologic Interpretation of Causalgia and Its Related States. New York, Macmillan, 1943.

253. Lloyd-Roberts GC, Thomas TC: The etiology of quadriceps contracture in children. J Bone Joint Surg Br 46:498, 1964.

254. Lonner J: Patellofemoral arthroplasty: Pros, cons, and design considerations. Clin Orthop 428:158, 2004.

255. Lund F, Telbag H: Content and synthesis of nucleic acids in the cartilage in chondromalacia patellae. Acta Orthop Scand 49:535, 1978.

256. MacKinnon SE, Holder LE: The use of three-phase radionuclide bone scanning in the diagnosis of reflex sympathetic dystrophy. J Hand Surg [Am] 9:556, 1984.

257. Mäenpää H, Lehto MU: Patellar dislocation: The long term results of nonoperative management in 100 patients. Am J Sports Med 25:213, 1997.

258. Maldague B, Malghem J: Apport du cliché de profil du genou dans le dépistage des instabilites rotuliennes: Rapport preliminaire. Rev Chir Orthop 71(Suppl 2):5, 1985.

259. Malghem J, Maldague B: Patellofemoral joint: 30° axial radiograph with lateral rotation of the leg. Radiology 170:566, 1989.

260. Mankin H, Thrasher A: Water content and binding in normal and osteoarthrotic human cartilage. J Bone Joint Surg Am 57:76, 1978.

261. Maquet P: Advancement of the tibial tuberosity. Clin Orthop 115:225, 1976.

262. Maquet P: Mechanics and osteoarthritis of the patellofemoral joint. Clin Orthop 144:70, 1979.

263. Marar BC, Pillay VK: Chondromalacia of the patella in the Chinese: A postmortem study. J Bone Joint Surg Am 57:342, 1975.

264. Mariani PP, Caruso C: An electromyographic investigation of subluxation of the patella. J Bone Joint Surg Br 61:169, 1979.

265. Martens M, Wouters P, Burssens A, et al: Patellar tendinitis: Pathology and results of treatment. Acta Orthop Scand 53:445, 1982.

266. Martinez S, Korobkin M, Fondren FB, Goldner JL: A device for computed tomography of the patellofemoral joint. Am J Radiol 140:400, 1983.

267. Martinez S, Korobkin M, Fondren FB, et al: Diagnosis of patellofemoral malalignment by computed tomography. J Comp Assist Tomogr 7:1050, 1983.

268. Marumoto JM, Jordan C, Akins R: A biomechanical comparison of lateral retinacular releases. Am J Sports Med 23:151, 1995.

269. Masse Y: La trochléoplastie: Restauration de la gouttiére trochleenne dans les subluxations et luxations de la rotule. Rev Chir Orthop 64:3, 1978.

270. Matthews LS, Sonstegard DS, Henke JA: Load bearing characteristics of the patello-femoral joint. Acta Orthop Scand 48:511, 1977.

271. Mayeda T: Uber das strangartige Gebilde in der Kniegelenkhole (chorda cavi articularis genu). Mitt Med Fakult Kaiserl Univ Tokyo 21:507, 553, 1918.

272. McConnell J: The management of chondromalacia patellae: A long-term solution. Aust J Physiother 32:215, 1986.

273. McGinty JB: Arthroscopy of the knee. In Insall JN (ed): Surgery of the Knee. New York, Churchill Livingstone, 1984, p 111.

274. McGinty JB, McCarthy JC: Endoscopic lateral retinacular release: A preliminary report. Clin Orthop 158:120, 1981.

275. McKain CW, Urban BJ, Goldner JL: The effects of intravenous regional guanethidine and reserpine: A controlled study. J Bone Joint Surg Am 65:808, 1983.

276. McKeever DC: Patellar prosthesis. J Bone Joint Surg Am 37:1074, 1955.

277. McManus F, Rang M, Heslin DJ: Acute dislocation of the patella in children: The natural history. Clin Orthop 139:88, 1979.

278. McNab J: Recurrent dislocation of the patella. J Bone Joint Surg Am 34:957, 1952.

279. Melzack R: Prolonged relief of pain by brief, intense transcutaneous somatic stimulation. Pain 1:357, 1975.

280. Melzack R, Wall PD: Pain mechanisms: A new theory. Science 150:971, 1965.

281. Mendez AA, Keret D, MacEwen GD: Treatment of patellofemoral instability in Down's syndrome. Clin Orthop 234:148, 1988.

282. Merchant AC: Classification of patellofemoral disorders. Arthroscopy 4:235, 1988.

283. Merchant AC, Mercer RL: Lateral release of the patella: A preliminary report. Clin Orthop 103:40, 1974.

284. Merchant AC, Mercer RL, Jacobsen RH, et al: Roentgenographic analysis of patello-femoral congruence. J Bone Joint Surg Am 56:1391, 1974.

285. Metcalf RW: An arthroscopic method for lateral release of subluxating or dislocating patella. Clin Orthop 167:9, 1982.

286. Micheli LJ, Stanitski CL: Lateral retinacular release. Am J Sports Med 9:330, 1981.

287. Miller GF: Familial recurrent dislocation of the patella. J Bone Joint Surg Br 60:203, 1978.

288. Miller JB, Larochelle PJ: The treatment of patellofemoral pain by combined rotation and elevation of the tibial tubercle. J Bone Joint Surg Am 68:419, 1986.

289. Mink JK, Deutsch AL: Magnetic resonance imaging of the knee. Clin Orthop 244:29, 1989.

290. Mitchell SW: Injuries of Nerves and Their Consequences. Philadelphia, JB Lippincott, 1872.

291. Mitchell SW, Morehouse GR, Keen WW: Gunshot Wounds and Other Injuries of Nerves. Philadelphia, JB Lippincott, 1864.

292. Mori Y, Okumo H, Iketani H, Kuroki Y: Efficacy of lateral retinacular release for painful bipartite patella. Am J Sports Med 23:13, 1995.

293. Morshuis WJ, Pavlov PW, De Rooy KP: Anteromedialization of the tibial tuberosity in the treatment of patellofemoral pain and malalignment. Clin Orthop 255:242, 1990.

294. Muneta T, Yamamoto H, Ishibashi T, et al: Computerized tomographic analysis of tibial tubercle position in the painful female patellofemoral joint. Am J Sports Med 22:67, 1994.

295. Munzinger U, Ruckstuhl J, Scherzer H, Gschwend N: Internal derangement of the knee joint due to pathological synovial folds: The mediopatellar plica syndrome. Clin Orthop 155:59, 1981.
296. Murphy JB: Tuberculosis of the patella. Surg Gynecol Obstet 6:262, 1908.
297. Nakamura N, Ellis M, Seedhom BB: Advancement of the tibial tuberosity: A biomechanical study. J Bone Joint Surg Br 67:255, 1985.
298. Naranja RJ, Reilly PT, Kuhlman JR, et al: Long term evaluation of the Elmslie-Trillat-Maquet procedure for patellofemoral dysfunction. Am J Sports Med 24:779, 1996.
299. Noll BJ, Ben-Itzhak I, Rossouw P: Modified technique for tibial tubercle elevation with realignment for patellofemoral pain. Clin Orthop 234:178, 1988.
300. Norman O, Egund N, Ekelund L, Rünow A: The vertical position of the patella. Acta Orthop Scand 54:908, 1983.
301. O'Brien SJ, Ngeow J, Gibney MA, et al: Reflex sympathetic dystrophy of the knee: Causes, diagnosis and treatment. Am J Sports Med 23:655, 1995.
302. Ogata S, Uhthoff HK: The development of synovial plicae in human knee joints: An embryologic study. Arthroscopy 6:315, 1990.
303. Ogilvie-Harris DJ, Bauer M, Corey P: Prostaglandin inhibition and the rate of recovery after arthroscopic meniscectomy. J Bone Joint Surg Br 67:567, 1985.
304. Ogilvie-Harris DJ, Jackson RW: The arthroscopic treatment of chondromalacia patellae. J Bone Joint Surg Br 66:660, 1984.
305. Ogilvie-Harris DJ, Roscoe M: Reflex sympathetic dystrophy of the knee. J Bone Joint Surg Br 69:804, 1987.
306. Ohno O, Naito Iguchi T, et al: An electron microscopic study of early pathology in chondromalacia of the patella. J Bone Joint Surg Am 70:883, 1988.
307. Olerud C, Berg P: The variation of the Q angle with different positions of the foot. Clin Orthop 191:162, 1984.
308. Osborne AH, Fulford PC: Lateral release for chondromalacia patellae. J Bone Joint Surg Br 64:202, 1982.
309. Outerbridge RE: The etiology of chondromalacia patellae. J Bone Joint Surg Br 43:752, 1961.
310. Outerbridge RE: Further studies on etiology of chondromalacia patellae. J Bone Joint Surg Br 46:179, 1964.
311. Owre A: Chondromalacia patellae. Acta Chir Scand 41(Suppl 77), 1936.
312. Pantazopoulos T, Exarchon E: Osteochondritis dissecans of the patella: Report of four cases. J Bone Joint Surg Am 53:1205, 1971.
313. Paulos LE, Rosenberg TD, Drawbert J, et al: Infrapatellar contracture syndrome: An unrecognized cause of knee stiffness with patella entrapment and patella infera. Am J Sports Med 15:331, 1987.
314. Perugia L, Postacchini F, Ippolito E: I Tendini: Biologia, Patologia, Clinica. Milano, Masson, 1981, p 156.
315. Peterson L, Brittberg M, Kiviranta I, et al: Autologous chondrocyte transplantation. Biomechanics and long-term durability. Am J Sports Med 30:2, 2002.
316. Pfeiffer WH, Gross ML, Seeger LL: Osteochondritis dissecans of the patella: MRI evaluation and a case report. Clin Orthop 271:207, 1991.
317. Pipkin G: Lesions of the suprapatellar plica. J Bone Joint Surg Am 32:363, 1950.
318. Pipkin G: Knee injuries: The role of the suprapatellar plica and suprapatellar bursa in simulating internal derangements. Clin Orthop 74:161, 1971.
319. Poehling GG, Pollock FE, Koman AL: Reflex sympathetic dystrophy of the knee after sensory nerve injury. Arthroscopy 4:31, 1988.
320. Poplawski ZJ, Wiley AM, Murray JF: Post-traumatic dystrophy of the extremities. J Bone Joint Surg Am 65:642, 1983.
321. Post WR: History and physical examination. In Fulkerson JP (ed): Disorders of the Patellofemoral Joint. Baltimore, Williams & Wilkins, 1997, p 39.
322. Post WR, Fulkerson J: Knee pain diagrams: Correlation with physical examination findings in patients with anterior knee pain. Arthroscopy 10:618, 1994.
323. Pridie KH: A method of resurfacing osteoarthritic knee joints. J Bone Joint Surg Br 41:618, 1959.
324. Radin E, Leach R: Anterior displacement of the tibial tubercle for patellofemoral arthrosis. Orthop Trans 3:291, 1979.
325. Reider B, Marshall JL, Koslin B, et al: The anterior aspect of the knee joint. J Bone Joint Surg Am 63:351, 1981.
326. Reigler HF: Recurrent dislocations and subluxations of the patella. Clin Orthop 227:201, 1988.
327. Reilly DT, Martens M: Experimental analysis of the quadriceps muscle force and patello-femoral joint reaction force for various activities. Acta Orthop Scand 43:126, 1972.
328. Richmond JC, McGinty JB: Segmental arthroscopic resection of the hypertrophic mediopatellar plica. Clin Orthop 178:185, 1983.
329. Rombold C: Osteochondritis dissecans of the patella: A case report. J Bone Joint Surg 18:230, 1936.
330. Rorabeck CH, Bobechko WP: Acute dislocation of the patella with osteochondral fracture: A review of eighteen cases. J Bone Joint Surg Br 58:237, 1976.
331. Rosenberg NJ: Osteochondral fractures of the lateral femoral condyle. J Bone Joint Surg Am 46:1013, 1964.
332. Roux C: Recurrent dislocation of the patella: Operative treatment. Clin Orthop 144:4, 1979.
333. Rozbruch JD, Campbell RD, Insall JN: Tibial tubercle elevation (the Maquet operation): A clinical study of 31 cases. Orthop Trans 3:291, 1979.
334. Rubacky GE: Inheritable chondromalacia of the patella. J Bone Joint Surg Am 45:1685, 1963.
335. Rünow A: The dislocating patella: Etiology and prognosis in relation to generalized joint laxity and anatomy of the patellar articulation. Acta Orthop Scand Suppl 201:54, 1983.
336. Sachs RA, Daniel DM, Stone ML, et al: Patellofemoral problems after ACL reconstruction. Am J Sports Med 17:760, 1989.
337. Sakakibara J: Arthroscopic study on Jino's band (plica synovialis mediopatellaris). J Jpn Orthop Assoc 50:513, 1976.
338. Sallay PI, Poggi J, Speer KP, Garrett WE: Acute dislocation of the patella: A correlative pathoanatomic study. Am J Sports Med 24:52, 1996.
339. Salter RB, Simmonds DF, Malcolm BW, et al: The biological effect of continuous passive motion on the healing of full-thickness defects in articular cartilage. J Bone Joint Surg Am 62:1232, 1980.
340. Sanchis-Alfonso V, Rosello-Sastre E: Immunohistochemical analysis for neural markers of the lateral retinaculum in patients with isolated symptomatic patellofemoral malalignment. A neuroanatomic basis for anterior knee pain in the active young patient. Am J Sports Med 28:725, 2000.
341. Sanchis-Alfonso V, Rosello-Sastre E, Monteagudo-Castro C, Esquerdo J: Quantitative analysis of nerve changes in the lateral retinaculum in patients with isolated symptomatic patellofemoral malalignment. A preliminary study. Am J Sports Med 26:703, 1998.
342. Sasaki T, Yagi T: Subluxation of the patella: Investigation by computerized tomography. Int Orthop 10:115, 1986.
343. Schonholtz GJ, Ling B: Arthroscopic chondroplasty of the patella. Arthroscopy 1:92, 1985.
344. Schonholtz GJ, Zahn MG, Magee CM: Lateral retinacular release of the patella. Arthroscopy 3:269, 1987.
345. Schopp AC, Fellhauer CM: Plastic operation in fracture of the patella. J Missouri State Med Assoc 47:179, 1950.
346. Schutzer SF, Gossling HR: The treatment of reflex sympathetic dystrophy syndrome: Current concepts review. J Bone Joint Surg Am 66:625, 1984.
347. Schutzer SF, Ramsby GR, Fulkerson JP: Computer tomographic classification of patellofemoral pain patients. Orthop Clin North Am 17:235, 1986.
348. Schutzer SF, Ramsby GR, Fulkerson JP: The evaluation of patellofemoral pain using computerized tomography: A preliminary study. Clin Orthop 204:286, 1986.
349. Schwartz C, Blazina ME, Sisto DJ, Hirsh LC: The result of operative treatment of osteochondritis dissecans of the patella. Am J Sports Med 16:522, 1988.
350. Scuderi G, Cuomo F, Scott NW: Lateral release and proximal realignment for patellar subluxation and dislocation: A long-term follow-up. J Bone Joint Surg Am 70:856, 1988.
351. Seale KS: Reflex sympathetic dystrophy of the lower extremity. Clin Orthop 243:80, 1989.
352. Settegast A: Typische Roentgenbilder von normalen Menschen. Lehmanns Med Atlanten 5:211, 1921.
353. Shelbourne KD, Nitz P: Accelerated rehabilitation after anterior cruciate ligament reconstruction. Am J Sports Med 18:292, 1990.
354. Shelbourne KD, Porter DA, Rozzi W: Use of a modified Elmslie-Trillat procedure to improve abnormal patellar congruence angle. Am J Sports Med 22:318, 1994.

355. Sherman OH, Fox JM, Sperling H, et al: Patellar instability: Treatment by arthroscopic electrosurgical lateral release. Arthroscopy 3:152, 1987.
356. Shoji H, Granda JL: Acid hydrolases in the articular cartilage of the patella. Clin Orthop 99:293, 1974.
357. Shorbe HB, Dobson CH: Patellectomy: Repair of the extensor mechanism. J Bone Joint Surg Am 40:1281, 1958.
358. Simpson LA, Barrett JP: Factors associated with poor results following arthroscopic subcutaneous lateral retinacular release. Clin Orthop 186:165, 1984.
359. Sinding-Larsen C: A hitherto unknown affection of the patella in children. Acta Radiol 1:171, 1921.
360. Small NC: Complications in arthroscopic surgery performed by experienced arthroscopists. Arthroscopy 4:215, 1988.
361. Small NC, Glogan AI, Berezin MA: Arthroscopically assisted proximal extensor mechanism realignment of the knee. Arthroscopy 9:63, 1993.
362. Smillie IS: Diseases of the Knee Joint, 2nd ed. Edinburgh, Churchill Livingstone, 1980.
363. Smith AM, Peckett WRC, Butler-Manuel PA, et al: Treatment of patellofemoral arthritis using the Lubinus patellofemoral arthroplasty. A retrospective review. Knee 9:27, 2002.
364. Smith JB: Osteochondritis dissecans of the trochlea of the femur. Arthroscopy 6:11, 1990.
365. Soeur R: The synovial membrane of the knee in pathological conditions. J Bone Joint Surg Am 31:317, 1949.
366. Sojbjerg JO, Lauritzen J, Hvid I, Boe S: Arthroscopic determination of patellofemoral malalignment. Clin Orthop 215:243, 1987.
367. Soundry M, Lanir A, Angel D, et al: Anatomy of the normal knee as seen by magnetic resonance imaging. J Bone Joint Surg Br 68:117, 1986.
368. Spurling RG: Causalgia of upper extremity: Treatment by dorsal sympathetic ganglionectomy. Arch Neurol Psychiatry 23:784, 1930.
369. Staheli LT: Medial femoral torsion. Orthop Clin North Am 11:39, 1980.
370. Staheli LT, Lippert F, Denotter P: Femoral anteversion and physical performance in adolescent and adult life. Clin Orthop 129:213, 1977.
371. Stanish WD, Rubinovich RM, Curwin S: Eccentric exercise in chronic tendinitis. Clin Orthop 208:65, 1986.
372. Stanitski CL: Articular hypermobility and chondral injury in patients with acute patellar dislocation. Am J Sports Med 23:146, 1995.
373. Stein H, Duthie RB: The pathogenesis of chronic haemophilic arthropathy. J Bone Joint Surg Br 63:601, 1981.
374. Steinbrocker O, Argyros TG: The shoulder hand syndrome: Present status as a diagnostic and therapeutic entity. Med Clin North Am 42:1533, 1958.
375. Stolte BH, Stolte JB, Leyten JF: Die pathofysiologie von ist shoulder-hand syndrome. Med Tijdschr Geneeskd 114:1208, 1978.
376. Stougaard J: Osteochondritis dissecans of the patella. Acta Orthop Scand 45:111, 1974.
377. Sudeck P: Uber die akute entzundliche Knochenatrophie. Arch Klin Chir 62:147, 1900.
378. Sudeck P: Uber die akute (reflectorische) Knochenatrophie nach Entzundungen und Verletzungen an den Extremitaten und ihre klinische Erscheinungen. Forschr Geb Roentgenstr Nuklearmed 5:277, 1901.
379. Sutton FS, Thompson CH, Lipke J, et al: The effect of patellectomy on knee function. J Bone Joint Surg Am 58:537, 1976.
380. Tauro B, Ackroyd CE, Newman JH, Shah NA: The Lubinus patellofemoral arthroplasty: A five to ten year prospective study. J Bone Joint Surg Br 83:696, 2001.
381. Tavernier T, Dejour D. Knee imaging: What is the best modality? J Radiol 82:387, 407, 2001.
382. Teitge RA, Faerber W, Des Madryl P, Matelic PM: Stress radiographs of the patellofemoral joint. J Bone Joint Surg Am 78:193, 1996.
383. Thompson RC: An experimental study of surface injury to the articular cartilage and enzyme responses within the joint. Clin Orthop 107:239, 1975.
384. Thygesen JEM, Hejgaard N, Tarnhoj J: Is Hauser a harmless procedure? A biomechanical study of the patello-femoral joint related
to the development of secondary chondromalacia. Acta Orthop Belg 48:481, 1982.
385. Tietjen R: Reflex sympathetic dystrophy of the knee. Clin Orthop 209:234, 1986.
386. Toft J: Radiografia sotto carico dell'articolazione femoropatellare. Ital J Orthop Traumatol 7:365, 1981.
387. Trillat A, Dejour H, Couette A: Diagnostic et traitement des subluxations recidivantes de la rotule. Rev Chir Orthop 50:813, 1964.
388. Turner MS, Smillie IS: The effect of tibial torsion on the pathology of the knee. J Bone Joint Surg Br 63:396, 1981.
389. Uematsu S, Hendler N, Hungerford DS, et al: Thermography and electromyography in the differential diagnosis of chronic pain syndromes and reflex sympathetic dystrophy. Electromyogr Clin Neurophysiol 21:165, 1981.
390. Vainionpää S, Laasonen E, Silvennoinen T, et al: Acute dislocation of the patella: A prospective review of operative treatment. J Bone Joint Surg Br 72:366, 1990.
391. Vaughan-Lane T, Dandy DJ: The synovial shelf syndrome. J Bone Joint Surg Br 64:475, 1982.
392. Volkmann R: Chirurgie Erfahrunger über Knochenverbiegungen und Knochenwachstum. Arch Pathol Anat 24:512, 1862.
393. Wall JJ: Compartment syndrome as a complication of the Hauser procedure. J Bone Joint Surg Am 61:185, 1979.
394. Walmsley R: The development of the patella. J Anat 74:360, 1939.
395. Waltson-Jones R: Fractures and Other Bone and Joint Injuries. Baltimore, Williams & Wilkins, 1940.
396. Watkins MP, Harris BA, Wender S, et al: Effect of patellectomy on the function of the quadriceps and hamstrings. J Bone Joint Surg Am 65:390, 1983.
397. Wendt PP, Johnson RP: A study of quadriceps excursion, torque and the effect of patellectomy on cadaver knees. J Bone Joint Surg Am 67:726, 1985.
398. West FE, Soto-Hall R: Recurrent dislocation of the patella in the adult: End results of patellectomy with quadricepsplasty. J Bone Joint Surg Am 40:386, 1958.
399. Whitelaw GP, Rulla DJ, Markowitz HD, et al: A conservative approach to anterior knee pain. Clin Orthop 246:234, 1989.
400. Wiberg G: Roentgenographic and anatomic studies on the patellofemoral joint: With special reference to chondromalacia patellae. Acta Orthop Scand 12:319, 1941.
401. Wiggins HE: The anterior tibial compartment syndrome: A complication of the Hauser procedure. Clin Orthop 113:90, 1975.
402. Wiles P, Andrews PS, Bremner RA: Chondromalacia of the patella: A study of the later results of excision of the articular cartilage. J Bone Joint Surg Br 42:65, 1960.
403. Wiles P, Andrews PS, Devas MB: Chondromalacia of the patella. J Bone Joint Surg Br 38:95, 1956.
404. Williams PF: Quadriceps contracture. J Bone Joint Surg Br 50:278, 1968.
405. Windsor RE: The Maquet procedure. Semin Orthop 5:144, 1990.
406. Wolff J: Uber die innere Architectur der Knochen und ihre Bedeutung fur die Frage von Knochenwachstum. Virchows Arch Pathol Anat 50:389, 1970.
407. Woo SL-Y, Wong CW, Newton PO, Lyons RM: The response of ligaments to stress deprivation and stress enhancement: Biomechanical studies. In Daniel DM (ed): Knee Ligaments: Structure, Function, Injury and Repair. New York, Raven Press, 1990, p 337.
408. Woodland LH, Francis RS: Parameters and comparisons of the quadriceps angle of college-aged men and women in the supine and standing positions. Am J Sports Med 20:208, 1992.
409. Worrel RW: Prosthetic resurfacing of the patella. Clin Orthop 144:91, 1979.
410. Worrel RW: Resurfacing of the patella in young patients. Orthop Clin North Am 17:303, 1986.
411. Yamamoto RK: Arthroscopic repair of the medial retinaculum and capsule in acute patellar dislocations. Arthroscopy 2:125, 1986.
412. Yulish BS, Montanez J, Goodfellow DB, et al: Chondromalacia patellae: Assessment with MR imaging. Radiography 164:763, 1987.
413. Zernicke RF, Garhammer J, Jobe FW: Human patellar tendon rupture. J Bone Joint Surg Am 59:179, 1977.

CHAPTER 54

Surgery of the Patellofemoral Joint: Indications, Effects, Results, and Recommendations*

W. R. Post • John P. Fulkerson

Effective surgical treatment of patellofemoral pain depends on an accurate diagnosis, understanding of the pathophysiology of the condition, and knowledge of the effects of a given surgical treatment on the mechanics and biology of patellofemoral function. Anterior knee pain, often caused by a patellofemoral disorder, is a common disabling complaint in young adults, predominantly women. Fortunately, nonoperative treatment, including quadriceps strengthening, stretching, McConnell taping, and bracing, is usually effective.[4,18,36,60,81,126,140,155] However, when conservative treatment fails and a specific treatable cause of anterior knee pain can be identified after careful physical, radiographic, and in some cases, arthroscopic examination, successful surgical treatment of patellofemoral disorders is likely.

PATHOPHYSIOLOGY OF PATELLOFEMORAL PAIN: IMPLICATIONS FOR TREATMENT

Patients with patellofemoral pain problems typically have various degrees of articular pain, soft-tissue pain from overuse or chronic stretch, and mechanical instability from malalignment or dysplasia of the joint. Quadriceps weakness almost always accompanies anterior knee pain and may be a cause and/or result of knee pain. Restoration of quadriceps strength and flexibility is critical to improving load acceptance. A primary function of the quadriceps is to absorb energy during gait.[195] If the quadriceps is relatively weak and stiff, it can neither generate the desired force concentrically nor absorb the necessary energy eccentrically. In knees with a deficiency of muscular energy absorption as a result of eccentric quadriceps weakness, that energy must be absorbed elsewhere in the extensor mechanism, which may result in painful overload of patellar subchondral bone or excessive stretch of peripatellar soft tissues. Should the peripatellar soft tissues be less compliant and flexible than normal, such loads may be poorly tolerated. Considering the problem as a deficiency in energy absorption, one can imagine that non-operative management must focus on improving strength and flexibility throughout the lower extremities. The rehabilitation regimen must not overload the system. The concept of staying within the "envelope of function" during patellofemoral rehabilitation is especially critical to success.[43] Rehabilitation efforts that attempt to increase strength and function by working the knee as hard as possible are destined to fail in patients with patellofemoral disorders. The prime example is the effect of isokinetic exercise on patients with anterior knee pain. Because isokinetic equipment is designed to produce resistance proportional to the force applied, the joint is forced to work at its upper limits. Already overloaded tissue tolerates this poorly. Instead, emphasize flexibility, strengthening, judicious use of anti-inflammatory medication, and patience to allow the overloaded tissues to heal.

If a dedicated effort at nonoperative management of these patients fails and if malalignment is objectively present, surgery to realign the extensor mechanism and/or decrease patellofemoral joint reaction force may be appropriate. Although our discussion is limited to patellofemoral problems, it is important to remember that anterior knee pain does not necessarily come from patellofemoral disease. Other causes of pain to be considered before planning surgery on the patellofemoral joint itself include symptomatic chondromalacia patellae, patellofemoral arthrosis, plica or fat pad syndrome, iliotibial friction band syndrome, vastus lateralis tendinitis, quadriceps or patellar tendinitis, retinacular strain,[63,166] referred pain,, and chronic effusion from either mechanical (meniscal and/or instability) or inflammatory problems. In addition, one must remember to examine the patient for posterior cruciate ligament deficiency, a condition sometimes associated with anterior knee pain.[106] Anterior cruciate ligament (ACL) deficiency has also been reported to produce anterior knee pain in 20% to 27% of patients with chronic deficiency.[15,23] ACL reconstruction, particularly with the use of a bone–patellar tendon–bone autograft, is well known to activate anterior knee pain in some cases.

Postoperative neuromas or reflex sympathetic dystrophy may further complicate the initial diagnosis. Referred, neoplastic, and nonorganic causes of knee pain must also be excluded.[66] Most diagnoses can be made with the history and physical examination and require only confirmation by radiographic and arthroscopic examination.

*Modified from Post WR, Fulkerson JP: Surgery of the patellofemoral joint: Indications, effects, results, and recommendations. In Scott WN: The Knee, vol 1. St Louis, Mosby–Year Book, 1994, pp 441-468.

Patellofemoral problems, including recurrent dislocation, malalignment causing subluxation and/or tilt, osteoarthrosis, traumatic chondromalacia, and postpatellectomy pain, are at times candidates for surgery. It is imperative to understand the pathophysiology of each diagnosis and whether the goal of surgery should be realignment, soft-tissue débridement, and/or relief of pressure.

Principles of Diagnosis

A rational approach to patellofemoral disorders requires the understanding that various problems have different combinations of articular pain, soft-tissue pain, and lateral instability of the joint. The search for the correct diagnosis will therefore require a search for the cause of the pain and/or instability. Of course, painful stimuli can originate only from tissues that contain pain receptors. Anatomic sources of pain in the patellofemoral joint include retinacular tissue, synovium, and subchondral bone because articular cartilage is devoid of nerve tissue.[44,156] In knees with patellofemoral degenerative disease, afferent pain-transmitting substance P–containing fibers were isolated in the retinaculum, fat pad, periosteum, and subchondral plate of the patella, thus suggesting that anterior knee pain may have multiple origins.[196] Conversely, a deficiency of such fibers has been found in the case of congenital insensitivity to pain.[39]

In contrast, causes of patellar instability are less limited and may include both dynamic and static components. Dynamic (muscular) contributions to lateral instability could result from an increased Q angle or from an unbalanced quadriceps contraction (relative weakness of the vastus medialis obliquus [VMO], delayed VMO firing pattern, or relative hypertrophy of the vastus lateralis muscle). Anteversion of the femoral neck, poor muscular control of external rotation at the hip, pathological tibial torsion, hindfoot pronation, contracture of the retinaculum and/or patellofemoral ligaments, and dysplasia of the patella or trochlea are examples of influences that may increase lateral patellar instability. While performing the history and physical examination on a patient who is suspected to be a surgical candidate, the physician must keep in mind the question of pain versus instability.

History

A thorough history provides important clues to proper diagnosis in many patients. Complaints include components of both pain and instability ranging from recurrent dislocation with minimal pain between episodes to constant pain that is not even related to activity.

ONSET OF THE PAIN

The history of the injury is important. Even in patients who complain primarily of pain, major blunt trauma to a normally aligned and previously asymptomatic patella in a construction worker is a condition very different from the insidious onset of anterior knee pain in an adolescent girl who may have malalignment. Although a patient sustaining a high-energy injury could conceivably have underlying patellofemoral malalignment, it may be present in a patient whose symptoms began after minor trauma, just as a pathological fracture occurs through previously weakened bone.

NATURE OF THE PAIN

Dull, achy, activity-related pain that is increased with climbing, prolonged knee flexion, and squatting is typical in patients with patellofemoral disorders and is helpful in differentiating patients with malalignment from those with other sources of their pain. The increased patellofemoral joint reaction forces involved in such endeavors may cause pain in patients with either soft-tissue or bony origins for their pain. Burning, constant pain, especially in a previously operated knee, suggests the possibility of a painful neuroma or reflex sympathetic dystrophy. Localized constant pain related to a previous surgical incision or site of trauma should lead to suspicion of a neuroma. Pain in the anterior aspect of the thigh may occur when there is a primary hip problem, and pain just above the patella should prompt one to think of referred hip pain, quadriceps tendinitis, or a suprapatellar plica.

GIVING WAY

Unfortunately, this symptom does not seem to be specific for patellar subluxation (transient momentary lateral displacement of the patella from the trochlea) and most often represents pain-mediated quadriceps reflex inhibition. The typical complaint with giving way secondary to quadriceps weakness is giving way into flexion. Intermittent, sharp patellofemoral pain with associated snapping or popping during gait or exercise can at times correlate with a specific anatomic articular flap, plical lesion, or even iliotibial band snapping, but it may also be related to meniscal disease, loose bodies, or ligament instabilities. Sudden giving way also occurs in patients with medial patella subluxation. This is a postoperative problem in the majority of cases and is a new experience, often more debilitating than the original problem for which surgery was performed.

DISLOCATION

An accurate history of true patellar dislocation is important if found and should immediately raise concern that there might be associated articular surface injury. Although some patients report traumatic medial patellar dislocation, in the setting of no previous patellofemoral surgery such reports occur as a result of the patient noticing the prominence of the medial femoral condyle when the patella is dislocated laterally. If the patient then pushes the medial condyle laterally, the laterally displaced patella is thereby reduced. A history of preexisting symptoms suggestive of patellar instability and/or anterior knee pain may be given by some patients and should naturally be considered when selecting a treatment plan for an acute or recurrent dislocator.

Patient-drawn pain diagrams form a useful bridge between the history and physical examination. Patients are asked to illustrate on a simple diagram where their knees hurt (Fig. 54–1). Research has shown that 86% of negative zones accurately predicted no tenderness.[154] Such diagrams can also provide important clues regarding radiculopathy (reflected as a dermatomal pattern or symptom magnification and possibly evidenced by, e.g., stars, exclamation points). Although pain diagrams are certainly not foolproof, they provide an inexpensive insight into areas of pain and tenderness.

Physical Examination

Careful examination is indispensable to proper diagnosis of patellofemoral disorders. The diagnosis of patellofemoral pain is dependent on the physician's ability to reproduce the patient's complaints by physical examination. The search for specific clues, such as an underlying malalignment pattern, abnormally tight soft-tissue structures, generalized ligamentous laxity, and patterns of tenderness, is critical in understanding the pathophysiology of each individual.

Examine the patient while standing and ambulating for evidence of an increased Q angle, torsional deformities of the femur or tibia, knee varus/valgus, pronation of the hindfoot, leg length discrepancy, ankle deformity, scars, and other factors that may affect patellar alignment. Have the patient perform a single-leg knee bend as you watch from the front to see whether the knee rolls inward, thus suggesting weakness of external rotation at the hip. Quadriceps atrophy should also be noted, although we do not believe that apparent "isolated" VMO atrophy is a true finding but rather that it is the superficial reflection of generalized quadriceps atrophy, as suggested by Lieb and Perry.[118,119]

The Q angle is classically measured in extension from the anterior superior iliac spine to the midpoint of the patella and onward to the tibial tuberosity (Fig. 54–2). An increased Q angle should be considered to potentially increase the lateral vector of quadriceps force, possibly causing at least a theoretic tendency to lateral patellar translation (subluxation). Although the Q angle has always been part of the traditional evaluation of the patellofemoral joint, careful review of the available literature reveals that Q angle measurements have not been well standardized. Measurements of the Q angle have been made while the patient is supine and standing. We favor the standing measurement because it includes physiological loading. Unfortunately, the Q angle also has not been proved to correlate with either the incidence of pain or the results of treatment.[152] Normal populations have been measured, and the results are summarized in Table 54–1.[8,10] Although the importance of understanding the lateral extensor moment and its potential effects on patellar alignment is undeniable, we cannot say that the

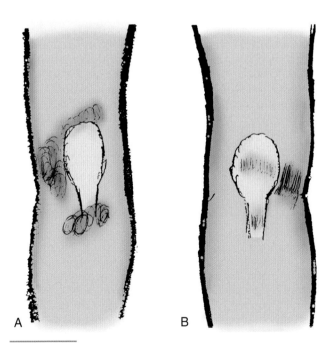

Figure 54–1. Patient-drawn pain diagrams often predict areas of tenderness and help focus the clinical examination. (From Post WR, Fulkerson JP: Knee pain diagrams: Correlation with physical examination findings in patients with anterior knee pain. Arthroscopy 10:486, 1994.)

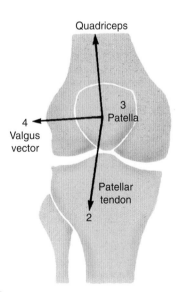

Figure 54–2. The Q angle. Lateralization of either the proximal part of the quadriceps or the tibial tuberosity will increase the resultant valgus vector. (From Fulkerson JP: Disorders of the Patellofemoral Joint. Baltimore, Williams & Wilkins, 1990, p 36.)

Table 54–1. Normal Population Q Angle Review

	SUPINE			STANDING	
Author	Q Angle (Degrees)	No. Knees/Age	Author	Q Angle (Degrees)	No. Knees/Age
Insall et al[1]	14	50/not specified	Woodland[4]	♀ 17.0 ± .072 ♂ 13.6 ± .072	57/20.0 69/22.3
Aglietti et al[2]	♀ 17 ± 3 ♂ 14 ± 3	75/23 75/23	Fairbank[5]	♀ 23 ± 1.2 ♂ 20 ± 1.2	150/14.8 ± 0.1 160/14.6 ± 0.1
Hsu et al[3]	♀ 18.8 ± 4.7 ♂ 15.6 ± 3.5	60/not specified 60/not specified	Horton[6]	♀ 15.8 ± 4.5 ♂ 11.2 ± 3.0	
Woodland et al[4]	♀ 15.8 ± .072 ♂ 12.7 ± .072	57/20.0 69/22.3			

[1]Insall J, Falvo KA, Wise DW: Chondromalacia patellae: A prospective study. J Bone Joint Surg Am 58:1, 1976.
[2]Aglietti P, Insall JN, Cerulli G: Patellar pain and incongruence. Clin Orthop 122:217, 1983.
[3]Hsu RWW, Himeno S, Coventry MB, et al: Normal axial alignment of the lower extremity and load-bearing distribution at the knee. Clin Orthop 255:215, 1990.
[4]Woodland LH, Francis RS: Parameters and comparisons of the quadriceps angle of college-aged men and women in the supine and standing positions. Am J Sports Med 20:208, 1992.
[5]Fairbank JCT, Pynsent PB, van Poortvliet JA, et al: Mechanical factors in the incidence of knee pain in adolescents and young adults. J Bone Joint Surg 66:685, 1984.
[6]Horton MG, Hall TI: Quadriceps femoris muscle angle: Normal values and relationships with gender and selected skeletal measures. Phys Ther 69:897, 1989.
From Fulkerson JP: Disorders of the Patellofemoral Joint. Baltimore, Williams & Wilkins, 1997.

actual measurement of the Q angle has proved clinically useful.

At 90 degrees of flexion, the tuberosity is normally directly inferior to the patella. Lateral deviation of the tubercle can be measured in this position and recorded as the tubercle-sulcus angle.[108] Observation of these relationships allows the clinician to estimate the degree of valgus in the knee, as well as the position of the tibial tuberosity, which may be laterally displaced out of proportion to the tibiofemoral valgus. Lateral displacement of the tibial tubercle is more common in patients with patellofemoral pain and arthrosis and can be detected by physical examination and documented with computed tomography (CT).[101,137,138] The Q angle, as measured clinically, does not directly correlate with patellofemoral pain, and although it is related to patellofemoral mechanics, it is only one of the many factors that influence patellar balance. However, once nonoperative management maximizes dynamic factors, static alignment, including tubercle position relative to the trochlear groove, should be considered. Patellar tracking must be considered as well. Normally, the patella lies superior and lateral to the trochlea on the supratrochlear fat pad in full extension. One may recognize patella alta on examination by the abnormally proximal position of the patella, but it is more accurately diagnosed radiographically. The patella enters the trochlea smoothly from its superolateral position at 10 degrees of flexion and, with increasing flexion, is centered and drawn into the trochlea. If during early flexion the patella tracks laterally and then suddenly shifts medially into the trochlea with active or passive flexion, the J sign is positive. In a review of 210 symptomatic adults, Johnson and van Dyk[99] found no subject with a positive J sign. Also keep in mind the reverse J sign, in which the patella of a patient with medial patella subluxation slides in a medial-to-lateral direction on knee flexion—clearly an abnormal pattern, but often very subtle. As with all tests of alignment, comparison to the other side is important.

PROVOCATIVE TESTS

Strong compression of the patella resulting in pain and crepitus while flexing and extending the knee is helpful in determining whether the patient's pain syndrome has a significant patellofemoral component. Another method of provocative testing is isometric contraction of the quadriceps at different angles of flexion.[126] Isometric contractions, which should be sustained for 10 seconds, have the advantage of avoiding direct palpation in patients who are particularly apprehensive. If one or both of these methods reproduce the patient's complaint, it is likely that they are patellofemoral in origin. These techniques of examination do not, however, distinguish between soft-tissue and articular sources of pain because there is soft-tissue stretch as well as articular compression when the knee is moved or the quadriceps is fired during these examinations.

In an attempt to confirm whether a patient has medial patella subluxation, hold the patella slightly medial with one finger, knee in extension. Then abruptly flex the knee. If this maneuver reproduces the symptom, the patient probably has a problem with medial subluxation, most commonly in the clinical setting of previous lateral release.

PALPATION

The subcutaneous position of the patellofemoral joint makes it uniquely available to careful examination. Palpation of the patellofemoral joint has two goals: (1) to differentiate between soft-tissue and bony pain and (2) to precisely localize the soft-tissue or articular area that reproduces the patient's complaint. Firm compression of the patella directly into the trochlea while the knee is held in various angles of flexion, combined with the knowledge that articulation starts distal on the patella and moves proximally with increasing flexion, can provide information to localize the articular disease. This can be accomplished by direct compression (being careful to not compress adjacent soft-tissue structures). Meaningful specific palpation of either the medial or lateral patellar facets seems anatomically unlikely given the interposition of innervated synovium and retinacular tissue. The degree of crepitus is more significant when absent or asymmetric with the contralateral knee. When evaluating the presence or absence of crepitus, remember that Johnson and van Dyk[99] found 94% of asymptomatic women to have crepitus. It is more important to note whether articular compression reproduces the patient's pain. Also, the character of the crepitus is helpful. Harsh sustained grinding is different from the faint click that is common on flexion and extension of a normal knee.

Soft-tissue palpation should systematically include the retinacular structures, the insertions of the quadriceps tendons into the superior pole of the patella, and the patellar tendon. Structures are generally best palpated in a position that places them on stretch and allows gentle palpation to achieve relative isolation from the underlying structures. This strategy allows discovery of specific points prone to overuse-type injury. We have previously described in detail thorough anatomically and functionally oriented soft-tissue examination, and the reader is encouraged to practice and master these techniques.[56,58,152] Points of intersection between structures, such as the junction of the medial patellar tendon, the inferior pole of the patella, and the medial retinaculum, seem particularly prone to tenderness, perhaps because of the stress concentration at locations where two or more different structures under load meet. These locations are frequently tender in patients with excessive lateral patellar tilt. Cautious search for such locations will often uncover the origin of a patient's soft-tissue pain.

Such differentiation between soft-tissue and articular pain helps surgical planning. Stress-relieving anteriorization should be considered in patients with predominantly articular-based complaints and normal alignment. In contrast, coronal (medial/lateral) realignment may be adequate in cases of malalignment when the articular surface has not degenerated. With severe articular degeneration, the patella may not tolerate even the relatively lower loads present after a procedure that corrects alignment.

STABILITY TESTING

Just as examination for ACL deficiency includes evaluation of the static stability of a joint in several planes, examination of the patellofemoral joint is not complete without evaluation of the static constraints in both the sagittal (tilt) and coronal (medial/lateral) planes. Evaluation of patellar tilt and medial-to-lateral restraints provides important information.

The passive patellar tilt test is performed with the knee in full extension. While the patella is held in the center of the trochlea, the examiner attempts to correct the patellar tilt to neutral or beyond, if possible (Fig. 54–3). We agree with Kolowich and Paulos[108] that normally the tilt should correct at least to neutral, although normal patellae often tilt up to 10 degrees or more past neutral. It is also possible to gain an impression of the nature of the resilience of

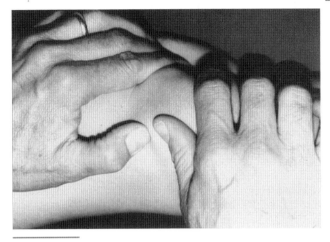

Figure 54–3. Physical examination for patellar tilt. Tilt should correct to neutral. (From Scott WN: The Knee, vol 1. St Louis, Mosby–Year Book, 1994, p 445.)

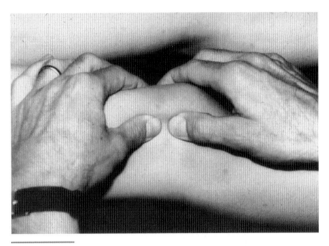

Figure 54–4. Physical examination for patellar glide. Medially directed force is applied to the lateral aspect of the patella. (From Scott WN: The Knee, vol 1. St Louis, Mosby–Year Book, 1994, p 445.)

the lateral retinaculum. Some patients seem to have a springy endpoint, whereas others have a very stiff and unyielding restraint. Comparison with the opposite knee often reveals relatively limited correction of lateral patellar tilt on the symptomatic side. Because the iliotibial band fibers contribute to the lateral retinacular tissue, poor iliotibial band flexibility frequently accompanies abnormal lateral tilt.

Medial and lateral patellar glide testing has also been well described by both McConnell[126] and Kolowich and Paulos.[108] It is similar to the passive hypermobility test described by Hughston.[87] We believe that these tests should be performed with the patella in neutral tilt if possible to compare the medial/lateral restraints consistently. As described, medial patellar glide is tested with medially directed pressure on the patella and the knee in 20 to 30 degrees of flexion to effectively engage the patella in the trochlea (Fig. 54–4). This test is also effective with the knee in extension and earlier degrees of flexion. Near full extension, the ligamentous and muscular restraints may be more isolated because of less bony constraint before engagement of the patella in the trochlea. By testing of lateral glide with the knee in extension it is possible to palpate an endpoint to lateral translation similar to that palpable with the Lachman test. Absence of such an endpoint together with increased translation is highly suggestive of medial patellofemoral ligament (MPFL) deficiency. Any abnormal tightness found in the retinaculum at these lesser angles of flexion can affect the direction of patellar entry into the trochlea. Medial patellar glide is judged abnormal if medial translation is less than one quadrant as described by Kolowich and Paulos. Laterally directed pressure on the neutral patella that results in displacement of three quadrants or more is consistent with an abnormally lax medial restraint. Ligamentous laxity itself, as might be measured by quadrant displacement, should not be confused with actual subluxation and, if found, should generate caution if a realignment procedure is contemplated. Evidence of systemic ligamentous laxity should be sought in such patients before reaching any conclusions regarding specific isolated incompetence of peripatellar restraints or malalignment. In hypermobile patients, the dynamic muscular control of patellar position is even more critical. Place emphasis on active muscular control and be patient. Involuntary quadriceps contraction during positive lateral glide testing or the classic apprehension reaction to the perception of imminent dislocation is strong evidence of clinically relevant patellar instability.

Several tests have been developed to assist in the diagnosis of medial patellar instability, a condition that almost always occurs as a complication of patellar realignment. In patients with symptomatic medial patellar instability, one can displace the patella medially and then passively flex the knee, and the symptoms will be reproduced as the patella moves laterally from the subluxated position into the trochlea.[152] Although the patella is moving laterally, it is moving from a subluxated position into the trochlea, essentially a "reverse apprehension" test. Another helpful test in the setting of potential medial instability is the gravity subluxation test.[142] This test requires that the patient be placed in the lateral decubitus position. The patella is then manually displaced medially. Because of previous operative transection of the vastus lateralis, the patient cannot actively reduce the trochlea. Although provocative testing for medial patellar instability is not routinely necessary, these tests should be regularly included in the evaluation of patients after failed patellofemoral realignment.

FLEXIBILITY

Systematic evaluation of the quadriceps, hamstring, iliotibial band, and gastrocnemius/soleus muscle groups is important because each can contribute to anterior knee pain. Quadriceps tightness is often associated with patellar tendinitis and "failed" postoperative patellar pain patients. Quadriceps tightness is best tested with the patient prone, thereby stabilizing the pelvis. Hamstring contracture may result in abnormally increased knee

flexion during the stance phase and, therefore, increased patellofemoral joint reaction force. Iliotibial band tightness has a more direct effect through its insertion into the lateral retinaculum and, consequently, abnormally increases posterolateral pull with increasing flexion. Increased hindfoot pronation is a result of gastrocnemius and/or soleus contracture in some patients. This causes the subtalar joint to compensate for the relative lack of tibiotalar dorsiflexion with increased hindfoot pronation. The increased subtalar pronation results in increased internal rotation of the tibia and femur and contributes to patellofemoral malalignment. When diminished flexibility is detected, nonoperative management must include stretching.

Radiological Evaluation

Once a complete history and physical examination have been performed, radiological studies are frequently indicated to confirm and document the clinical impression. Standing anteroposterior and lateral x-ray films are important to search for associated conditions and patella alta. A normal ratio of patellar ligament length to patellar length of less than 1.2 has been described by Insall and Salvati.[93] Blackburne and Peel[12] described the ratio of the articular length of the patella to the height of the lower pole of the patellar articular cartilage above the tibial articular surface (normal, <1.0). These ratios can be used to quantify patella alta if desired.

Axial tangential views of the patellofemoral joint such as those described by Merchant and Mercer[131] and Laurin and Dussault[114] may be used as screening tests for malalignment but can be difficult to interpret because of image overlap (unless the image is precisely tangential to the joint). The congruence angle of Merchant and Mercer and the lateral patellofemoral angle of Laurin and Dussault are estimations of lateral subluxation and tilt, respectively. The symmetry of subchondral sclerosis of the patellar facets should also be evaluated for signs of localized sclerosis (indicating unbalanced stress). Both authors and their colleagues recognized the importance of imaging the patella early in flexion in the less constrained proximal femoral sulcus. Kujala and Kormano[111] emphasized imaging the patellofemoral joint in early flexion. They found greater magnetic resonance image (MRI) differences in tilt and lateral subluxation on views with less than 30 degrees of flexion in a group of patients with recurrent patellar dislocations than in a normal control group. CT scans, first suggested by Delgado-Martins[37] in 1979, offer a significant advantage by imaging earlier degrees of flexion with absolutely no image overlap. Advanced imaging studies such as CT scans assist in confirming the diagnosis and should be considered only in the evaluation of an unusual patient in whom nonoperative management fails.

Further work on the CT technique, evaluation, and classification of patellofemoral disorders has been done by Schutzer and associates.[171,172] Several significant advantages of CT evaluation are now clear. Use of the posterior femoral condyles as a reference plane for measurement of

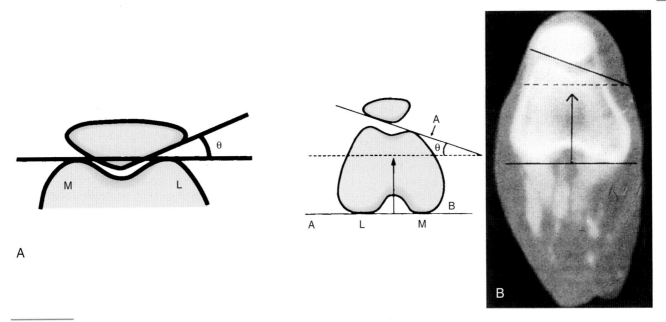

Figure 54-5. **A,** Patellar tilt angle of Laurin measured from an axial radiograph. **B,** Patellar tilt angle measured from a transverse midpatellar computed tomographic scan. (From Fulkerson JP: Disorders of the Patellofemoral Joint. Baltimore, Williams & Wilkins, 1990, pp 50, 60.)

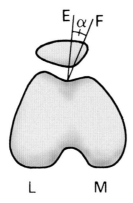

Figure 54-6. Congruence angle as measured on a midtransverse patellar computed tomographic scan. (From Scott WN: The Knee, vol 1. St Louis, Mosby–Year Book, 1994, p 446.)

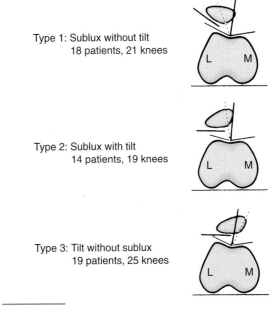

Type 1: Sublux without tilt
18 patients, 21 knees

Type 2: Sublux with tilt
14 patients, 19 knees

Type 3: Tilt without sublux
19 patients, 25 knees

Figure 54-7. Computed tomographic scan classification of patellofemoral malalignment. (From Schutzer SF, Ramsby GR: Computed tomographic classification of patellofemoral pain patients. Orthop Clin North Am 17:235, 1986.)

the patellar tilt angle has been proved to be significantly more consistent than the anterior intercondylar line used by Laurin and Dussault. This increases the precision with which tilt can be measured and also eliminates the variable of femoral rotation[61] (Fig. 54–5). Measurement of the congruence angle is also enhanced by the nature of the CT scan "slice" because it ensures that the trochlear and patellar images being measured are, in fact, at the same level and not artifacts of image overlap (Fig. 54–6). Furthermore, a patellofemoral CT scan can be useful in detecting subtle patellar or trochlear dysplasia, such as a shallow trochlear groove in patients with lateral patellar subluxation. Moreover, a limited CT evaluation of the patellofemoral joint can be accomplished quickly and with expense similar to that of multiple conventional x-ray films. Patterns of patellofemoral malalignment are usefully classified with CT images into three types. Type I is lateral

subluxation, type II combines lateral subluxation and lateral tilt, and type III includes lateral tilt without subluxation (Fig. 54–7). Type IV has been defined as radiographically normal alignment.[62] This classification has been very helpful in confirming the clinical impression of specific patellar malalignment patterns (tilt and/or subluxation). Treatment selection is also dependent on accurate classification, as will be appreciated in the later discussion of our recommended surgical approach.

Nonoperative Management

Most patients with patellofemoral disorders improve without surgery. Dye has provided excellent reviews and a theoretic model that he calls the *envelope of load acceptance model* to better understand the mechanisms and reasons for improvement of patients with patellofemoral pain by rest and activity modification.[43] Initial management of patellofemoral disorders should include the goals of normal flexibility and balanced quadriceps strength. One should remember to include the entire extremity in rehabilitation, especially hip strengthening. This program should be directed by specific physical examination findings. Discussion of specific techniques exceeds the scope of this chapter. In addition to reassurance, strengthening, stretching, and taping techniques, antipronation orthotics and patellar braces may be very beneficial in selected patients. Weight loss in obese patients is imperative in controlling patellofemoral pain.

A RATIONAL APPROACH TO SURGICAL TREATMENT

1. Patellofemoral malalignment (with or without articular degeneration)
2. Articular degeneration without malalignment
3. Soft-tissue disorders without malalignment
4. Patellofemoral instability without static malalignment

Such a classification scheme makes surgical selection rational. Selection of the appropriate surgical procedures in each of these instances depends on an understanding of the pathophysiology of the condition and an appreciation of the mechanics, biology, and history of the surgical alternatives. In general, surgical realignment options for patients with documented patellofemoral malalignment may include lateral retinacular release, tibial tubercle transfer, proximal quadricepsplasty, or a combination of these procedures. Pressure-relieving anteriorization of the tibial tubercle is added when indicated by severe articular degeneration.

For patients who have severe symptomatic articular degeneration in a normally aligned patellofemoral joint, the surgical choices are anteriorization, patellectomy, or patellofemoral arthroplasty. Patellofemoral resurfacing and patellectomy are rarely necessary unless there is no adequate articular cartilage remaining. None of these operations restores the knee to "normal," and nonoperative management is often indicated. Frequently in such patients with severe arthrosis after blunt trauma, there are multiple localized foci of soft-tissue inflammation and overload in addition to the pain from articular degeneration. Patient and persistent treatment directed at the soft tissues (stretching, strengthening, activity modification) can often produce satisfactory improvement without surgery.

Soft-tissue disorders without malalignment, such as patellar tendinitis and pathological hypertrophic plicae, must be distinguished from all of the conditions just mentioned and treated directly. In the unusual patient in whom nonoperative treatment does not resolve these disorders, surgical treatment can often be successful. The underlying principle of this strategy and classification is to define the diagnosis carefully. If, and only if, the symptoms are clearly secondary to documented malalignment should a realignment procedure (including lateral release) be performed.

Patients with normal alignment on physical examination and radiographic imaging who have had episodes of lateral patellar dislocation are logically treated by restoring the normal medial ligament function. This kind of thinking is exactly akin to treating lateral ankle, ACL, or shoulder instability by repairing or reconstructing the injured ligaments that allow symptomatic instability. Such patients had normal or nearly normal alignment and have suffered a traumatic injury to the MPFL, which in some cases fails to heal with sufficient integrity to prevent future instability episodes, even after muscular rehabilitation. These patients typically have more problems with recurrent instability symptoms than with chronic pain. In such patients it makes sense to then perform an operation that restores medial ligament function. Such operations include arthroscopic and open medial reefing procedures and MPFL reconstruction procedures. When considering such a procedure, one must be careful to not "overcompensate" and overtighten the static medial restraints, a situation that can lead to excessive medial patellofemoral articular pressure and a painful result.

Arthroscopic Diagnosis of Patellofemoral Malalignment

CLINICAL EXPERIENCE

Casscells,[26] Metcalf,[132] and Grana and Hinkley[67] discussed arthroscopic malalignment (subluxation) as failure of the midpatellar ridge to centralize during the first 45 degrees of knee flexion. Sojbjerg and Lauritzen[181] reported that 17 normal controls under local anesthesia with 75-mm Hg intra-articular pressure had centralization of the ridge into the trochlea at less than 40 degrees of passive knee flexion with a 95% confidence limit. Patients in their study with a preoperative diagnosis of patellar subluxation had reduction of the midpatellar ridge at a median flexion angle of 55 degrees. The 95% confidence limit was 50 degrees for patients with subluxation. Hadjari and McClish[69] found 85% of normal patellae to centralize in the trochlear groove with flexion of less than 40 degrees. Conversely, in 86% of their patients with patellofemoral subluxation or lateral compression syndrome, the patellae failed to centralize by 40 degrees. These studies confirm the initial observations of Cascells, Metcalf, and Grana and Hinkley. Reproducible measurement depends on consistent technique, including consistent intra-articular pressure. It should be remembered that these criteria have not to date been correlated with treatment results.

Although we routinely use arthroscopy to confirm the diagnosis of malalignment, we believe that such a diagnosis must be made preoperatively based on the history, physical examination, and imaging.

TECHNIQUE FOR PATELLOFEMORAL ARTHROSCOPY

We recommend arthroscopy of the patellofemoral joint without a leg holder to allow easy flexion/extension of the knee. The arthroscope may be inserted through a portal 4 cm proximal to the superomedial pole of the patella, as described by Schreiber.[170] The sharp arthroscopic probe is inserted through the quadriceps, and a blunt trocar is exchanged just before entering the suprapatellar pouch to avoid articular cartilage injury. After joint distention with an arthroscopic pump to ensure reproducible distention, a clear view of the patellofemoral articulation is possible. An inferolateral portal is created for instrumentation (Fig. 54–8). Inspect the articular surfaces as well as the medial and lateral gutters and plicae from this portal. Careful palpation of the articular surfaces should confirm the degree and pattern of articular degeneration present. The knee is then flexed and extended while evaluating patellar tracking with and without fluid distention. Subluxation, tilt, and the degree of flexion necessary to centralize the median ridge should be observed and recorded. This generally serves to confirm the physical examination and radiographic findings and is not depended on for development of a treatment plan. Often, the area of chondrosis corresponds well with the area of initial articulation during flexion. To complete the arthroscopic evaluation and rule out concomitant disease, one should visualize the entire knee through the inferolateral portal and any accessory portals created as necessary to ensure a thorough examination and reconfirm any patellofemoral findings noted proximally. One can perform surgical procedures such as patellar débridement, abrasion arthroplasty, or lateral release through the inferolateral portal as desired.

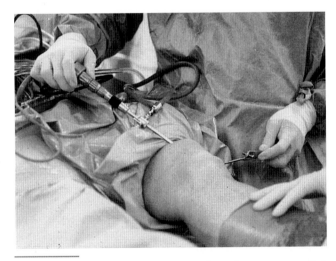

Figure 54–8. A portal 4 cm proximal to the superomedial corner of the patella provides an excellent view of the patellofemoral joint. Palpation of the articular surfaces will help localize areas of chondromalacia. (From Fulkerson JP: Anteromedialization of the tibial tubercle. Master Tech Orthop 1993.)

Procedures for Patellofemoral Malalignment

Once a specific malalignment problem is recognized clinically and nonoperative treatment has failed, a surgical procedure can be selected on the basis of biomechanical theory, the available experimental data from cadaver studies, and previously reported clinical experience. Efforts to decrease the laterally directed component of the quadriceps force can be divided roughly into those primarily involving the quadriceps mechanism proximal to the patella, those distal, and those that are combined. All categories generally include lateral release. Successful realignment of the extensor mechanism requires integration of an accurate clinical diagnosis, the expected biomechanical effect of surgical intervention, careful surgical technique, diligent rehabilitation, and clinical experience.

Proximal Realignment Procedures

LATERAL RELEASE

Theory

Lateral release has been used extensively for the treatment of patellofemoral pain and patellar malalignment. Theoretically, lateral release relieves abnormal posterior and lateral tethering of the patella, which may contribute to lateral tilt and lateral subluxation, respectively. A shortened lateral retinaculum results in excessive pressure on the lateral facet of the patella because as the knee flexes, the iliotibial band is drawn posteriorly. This can cause cartilage degeneration on the overloaded lateral facet. Pathological strain in the lateral retinaculum under these conditions may be the cause of the nerve injury in the lateral retinaculum that has been found histologically in patients with this syndrome.[63] Such neuromatous changes have been shown to be most prominent in patients with the most pain.[166] Surgical release of the lateral retinaculum should ideally relieve excessive articular and soft-tissue strain if the primary malalignment is due to lateral retinacular tightness. In addition, procedures have been developed to medialize the proximal quadriceps vector further by imbrication of the VMO.

Laboratory Data

Measurements of patellofemoral alignment, joint pressure, and joint contact area have failed to show a significant change after lateral release in elderly cadaver knees without documented patellofemoral malalignment.[84,86,116,161] Knees in each of these studies had various degrees of chondrosis but did not necessarily have a tight lateral retinaculum or any malalignment. Desio and Burks[40] found that the lateral retinaculum contributed 10% of the resistance to lateral patellar translation, which could explain why lateral release can make lateral instability worse.

The apparent failure of lateral release to modify normal patellar alignment in the laboratory contrasts with the clinical CT evidence that patellar tilt and, to a lesser extent, lateral subluxation are improved after lateral release.[61] It seems, then, that lateral release will affect patellofemoral mechanics only if malalignment (particularly tilt) is present preoperatively. Unfortunately, the laboratory studies referenced may not have adequately modeled malalignment.

Clinical Data

Evaluation of the many clinical reports of lateral release is muddled by the sometimes unclear indications for surgery. Willner[194] first reported lateral release as successful treatment of recurrent dislocation with a tight lateral retinaculum in 1970. Recurrent patellar subluxation was first considered an indication for lateral release after Merchant and Mercer's study in 1974.[130] Larson and Cabaud[113] later reported their results of lateral release for excessive lateral pressure syndrome. Subsequently, many researchers have presented results of lateral release for various indications from recurrent dislocation to pain without malalignment.* These studies generally report approximately 80% satisfactory results. Unfortunately, many of these reports have follow-up of less than 2 years and do not consistently correlate precise criteria of alignment and articular condition; the results are often based on purely subjective criteria. Follow-up of only 2 years may be of some concern because of reports of deterioration of good results in series of patients with instability. Metcalf's[132] series of arthroscopic lateral release (74% of patients had subluxation on axial radiographs) documented a decline from 86% to 74% good and excellent results between 1 and 4 years postoperatively. A more dramatic drop was found by Betz and Magill[10] in a series of patients (75% with diagnoses of recurrent dislocation/subluxation) whose good/excellent results deteriorated from 82% at 1 year to only 29% at 4 years. Dandy and Desai[34] also found a time-dependent decline in excellent results from 50% to 37% between 4 and 8 years postoperatively. Christensen and Soballe's report[30] of a decline in good results in a group with recurrent subluxation shows a very similar fall from 73% good results at 1.2 years to only 30% good results at 4.6 years. Interestingly, their results showed that lateral release in patients in this same study whose diagnosis was "lateral hypercompression" without symptoms of instability did not deteriorate with time.

The degree of articular degeneration present might logically be expected to correlate with the long-term results. Although this has not been universally found,[27,45,95] it has been a significant factor in most of the studies that specifically studied it. At 3-year follow-up, Osborne and Fulford[146] reported 100% poor results from lateral release in patients with Outerbridge grade III/IV chondrosis. The study of Christensen and Soballe[30] presented only 17% good results in a similar group at 4.6 years. An interesting study by Ogilvie-Harris and Jackson[144] reported 85% good subjective results at 5 years in patients with closed

chondromalacia versus 65% in patients with significant articular fibrillation. Their patients had pain and radiographic evidence of tilt without instability. Of their patients with instability and significant fibrillation, only 33% had good 5-year results. Most recently, Shea and Fulkerson[175] reported only 22% good and excellent results in a group of patients with CT-documented tilt and advanced (Outerbridge III/IV) chondrosis. At an average 3.75-year follow-up, a corresponding group with tilt and minimal articular degeneration enjoyed a 92% good and excellent rating.

Technique of Lateral Release

Both open and arthroscopic techniques of lateral retinacular release have produced successful results. O'Neill[145] compared open and arthroscopic techniques and found similar results. We believe that open release results in satisfactory cosmesis along with the opportunity for meticulous hemostasis and direct observation and palpation of the patella. Arthroscopic techniques for release using scissors, meniscotomes, electrocautery through a lateral parapatellar portal, and laser energy have been described.[55,82,127,174,178,180] The reader is referred to these articles for technical instruction if an arthroscopic technique is desired.

Diagnostic arthroscopy without a tourniquet is performed to confirm the clinical impression of patellar rotational malalignment (tilt) and evaluate the degree of any articular changes. A 2-cm longitudinal incision may be made immediately lateral to the patella with incorporation of the previously placed inferolateral arthroscopy portal, or the release may be performed arthroscopically. The subcutaneous tissues are then spread to reveal the superficial layer of the lateral retinaculum. The lateral retinaculum and synovium are incised midway between the lateral border of the patella and the lateral femoral condyle. A thermal ablator is then used to extend the lateral release proximally in the fatty plane, which can be found between the vastus lateralis and the vastus lateralis obliquus muscles (see Fig. 52–8).[71,153] In most cases, the release will end just at the vastus lateralis obliquus. It is very important to *not* cut the vastus lateralis tendon. Distally, the release may extend to the tibial tubercle, but it usually ends after section of the patellotibial band. Proximally, one must protect the vastus lateralis tendon. Distally, avoid injury to the lateral meniscus. Release is complete when the lateral aspect of the patella can be lifted to allow direct inspection of the articular surfaces (Fig. 52–9). Obtain absolutely meticulous hemostasis. Routine wound irrigation, skin closure, and a light soft dressing precede immediate application of a cooling cuff or ice pack to provide continuous cryotherapy and gentle compression. Patients are encouraged to begin immediate quadriceps exercise and early active and passive range-of-motion exercise. Cryotherapy is used frequently during the first 48 hours and thereafter as necessary during rehabilitation. Clear improvement in patellofemoral pain and stability is generally expected by 1 month but may continue for many months as quadriceps strength improves.

*References 11, 17, 27, 30, 34, 45, 46, 67, 75, 82, 95, 100, 110, 112, 127, 132, 133, 144, 146, 169, 178, 180, 189.

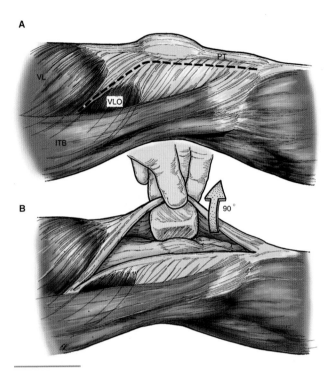

Figure 54–9. **A,** The *dotted line* indicates the extent of lateral release recommended. Note that it extends proximally between the vastus lateralis (VL) and the vastus lateralis obliquus (VLO). PT, patellar tendon. **B,** Lateral release is complete when the patella may be everted 90 degrees to allow direct inspection of the articular surface. (From Scott WN: The Knee, vol 1. St Louis, Mosby–Year Book, 1994, p 451.)

Complications of Lateral Release

The most common acute complication of lateral release is hemarthrosis, which occurs in less than 10% of cases. There are, however, isolated reports of hemarthrosis complicating lateral release in 15% to 42% of cases.[168,169,178] Careful attention to hemostasis, especially the lateral superior geniculate vessels, is important.

Incomplete lateral release or postoperative scarring in the lateral release site may result in persistence or even exacerbation of the preoperative symptoms. Typically, the patient will have had only several months of improvement postoperatively. The residual band becomes the focus of the pathological stress that the lateral release was designed to treat. In a cadaver study that mirrors this clinical scenario, Marumoto and Jordan[125] found that failure to release the patellotibial ligament (i.e., an incomplete lateral release) produced a significant decrease in the ability to translate the patella medially when compared with a lateral release that extended all the way to the tibial tubercle. Careful physical examination is the key to making this diagnosis because pain is typically very well localized to the inferior extent of an incomplete lateral release. Radiographic evaluation, including CT scan of these patients, may be normal. Treatment is release of the residual band.

Medial subluxation has been reported as a complication of lateral release.[88,89,142,177] This unfortunate diagnosis most likely represents the predictable result when a knee

without documented malalignment is treated by lateral release. Radiographic diagnosis of medial subluxation must be cautious because the mean normal congruence angle is considered to be medial to the midpoint of the trochlear sulcus (−8 degrees; standard deviation, 6 degrees).[1] "Apparent" medial subluxation may also be present when lateral patellar tilt results in a medially directed patellar apex—this is a radiographic finding and has nothing to do with true clinical medial patella subluxation.. Clinical examination criteria are best used to establish this diagnosis.[59,88,89,142,152]

Treatment of iatrogenic medial patellar instability must include bracing and eventual repair or reconstruction of the lateral retinacular restraints. Hughston and Flandry[89] described successful use of the lateral third of the patellar tendon and a strip of the iliotibial band to reconstruct the lateral patellotibial ligament in cases in which repair of the release was not possible (Fig. 54–10). Nonweiler and DeLee[142] recommended repair of the lateral release and particularly emphasized the need to repair the vastus lateralis tendon, which was transected in all their cases. It has been our experience that if insufficient tissue is available for repair, reconstruction of the patellotibial ligament with the patellar tendon is a viable option. We have found that in some cases, as described by Nonweiler and DeLee,[151] delayed repair can be successful.[151] When previous realignment included medial tibial tubercle transfer, it may be necessary to transfer the tubercle laterally as well. Additionally, if there is significant medial patellar articular degeneration in the setting of medial subluxation, anterolateralization of the tibial tubercle can be considered. Remember that iatrogenic medial subluxation is best avoided by judicious use of realignment, especially lateral release. To avoid this complication, it is especially important to be certain to spare the vastus lateralis tendon insertion. Surgical treatment, though usually "successful," is frequently a salvage procedure and rarely results in completely normal vigorous knee function.

Lateral Release: Summary

Good short-term results have been achieved in approximately 80% of patients with the use of open and arthroscopic techniques for lateral release. Concern exists over the long-term durability of these results, especially in patients with a history of patellar instability. Further studies that document symptoms, patterns of malalignment, and patterns of chondrosis are necessary to clarify the best indications for lateral release. In our opinion, a good candidate for lateral release has chronic anterior knee pain refractory to at least 3 months of conscientious and well-directed nonoperative management, along with physical examination evidence of tilt, CT scan confirmation of tilt, and arthroscopic confirmation of minimal chondrosis.

LATERAL RELEASE/MEDIAL IMBRICATION PROCEDURES

A number of procedures have been advocated that combine lateral retinacular release with VMO advance-

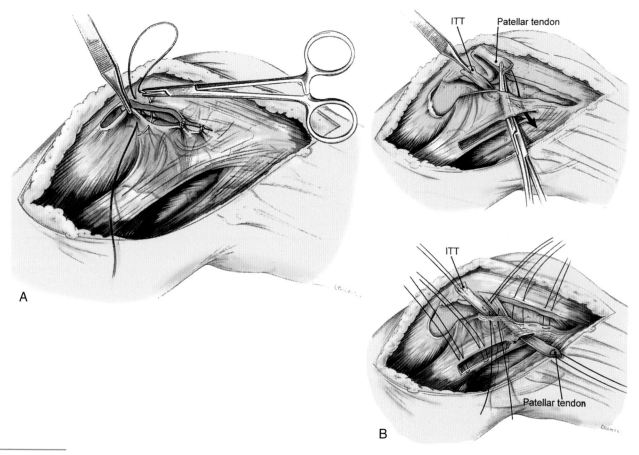

Figure 54–10. **A**, Surgical treatment of iatrogenic medial subluxation. Primary repair of a lateral release defect is possible. **B**, Surgical reconstruction of the lateral retinaculum with the iliotibial tract (ITT) and patellar tendon. (From Hughston JC, Flandry F: Surgical correction of medial subluxation of the patella. Am J Sports Med 24:486, 1996.)

ment. Insall and Falvo[92] reported 81% good to excellent results in 1976 with this procedure for symptoms of recurrent subluxation in 53 knees. In this series, tubercle transfer was chosen for patients with actual dislocations, with a similar percentage of good results. Again, the best results were noted when the articular surfaces were not badly degenerated. In their 1979 study, Insall and Bullough[91] described the proximal "tube" realignment, a procedure that imbricates the medial retinacular structures to lateral tissues after an extensive lateral release that includes the vastus lateralis tendon (Fig. 54–11). A series of lateral release/medial imbrication procedures for subluxation and dislocation was published by Scuderi and Cuomo[173] in 1988, who described good or excellent results in 81% at an average of 3.5 years after surgery (Fig. 54–12). Their outcomes were not affected by the degree of chondromalacia present. Patients who had excellent or good results were those who had the greatest objective improvement in subluxation as measured by the congruence angle on postoperative axial roentgenograms. Hughston and Walsh[90] recommended proximal realignment in patients with symptoms of subluxation when the Q angle was less than 10 degrees and the addition of tibial tubercle medialization with greater Q angles. This strategy resulted in 71% excellent and good results. Overall, lateral release with proximal realignment has produced success rates of

approximately 80%, a rate essentially identical to that for lateral release alone.

Currently, there is considerable interest in mini open proximal realignment. Review of our results (Thomas and Fulkerson—unpublished data) has shown that these procedures are quite effective when there is limited subluxation, no degenerative disease, and no significant medial patellofemoral lesions. Limited-exposure VMO advancement has appeal, particularly since the MPFL interdigitates with the deep VMO and will be tightened with VMO advancement. We strongly recommend examining MPFL open through a 3-cm incision and advancing it, along with the VMO, as a primary stabilizing procedure. This replaces the formal Insall procedure (Fig. 54–11).

MPFL reconstruction has become more popular recently[53] and has an important role in stabilizing the extensor mechanism when there is a dysplastic trochlea or other procedures fail to achieve adequate stability. With this procedure, as with any ligament reconstruction, the critical concern is to place the ligament graft anatomically and avoid overtensioning the reconstruction, which can overload the medial aspect of the patella. Keeping this concern in mind, one must not try to *pull* the patella into an aligned position with a tight medial reconstruction, but rather restore normal resistance to lateral patellar displacement.

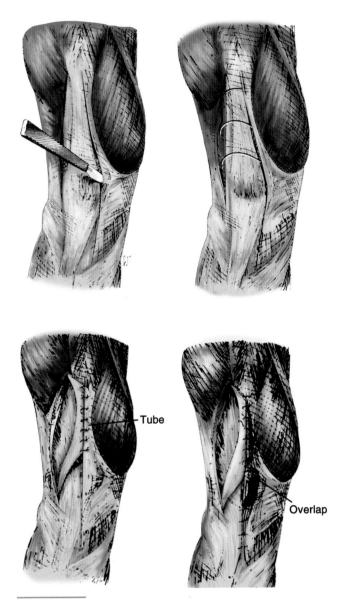

Figure 54–11. Proximal "tube" realignment as described by Insall. (From Insall J, Bullough PG, Burstein AH: Proximal "tube" realignment of the patella for chondromalacia patellae. Clin Orthop 144:63, 1979.) This procedure is not used now in our practices and is replaced by MPFL reconstruction.

Distal Realignment Procedures

THEORY

Distal realignment of the patellofemoral joint by medial transposition of the patellar tendon insertion theoretically decreases the Q angle and thus the laterally directed moment, which tends to cause patellar subluxation with quadriceps contraction. Ideal candidates for distal realignment have laterally displaced tibial tubercles, although this has not been proved to be a prerequisite. Lateral release usually accompanies the various methods of medialization and is important to relieve any lateral tether present. Advancement of the medial structures, alternatively, might potentially create abnormally increased

medial patellar facet pressure. The biomechanics of posterior displacement of the tibial tuberosity dictates an increase in joint reaction force to accomplish the same work, and it should generally be avoided (Fig. 54–13).

CLINICAL DATA

Distal medialization procedures may be divided into two categories: (1) those involving soft tissue only and (2) those involving transfer of the tibial tuberosity. Skeletal immaturity in a patient being considered for distal realignment mandates selection of a procedure that does not violate the proximal tibial physis or the apophysis of the tibial tubercle, a mistake that could cause complications such as genu recurvatum or continued distal migration of the tibial tuberosity with growth.[33,35,52,74,83,120]

SOFT-TISSUE MEDIALIZATION

Historically, options for a skeletally immature patient included the Roux-Goldthwait procedure, in which the lateral half of the patellar tendon is detached distally, passed behind the medial half of the tendon, and sutured to the pes anserinus insertion, and the Galeazzi semitendinosus tenodesis. Each procedure would normally be done with a lateral release. Reports of the Roux-Goldthwait procedure vary from good success rates in two series[29,54] to a high failure rate in another.[16] The mechanics of this operation, however, incurs the risk of inducing undesirable lateral patellar tilt and this procedure is no longer recommended. The Galeazzi tenodesis procedure uses the distally attached semitendinosus tendon to pull the patella distally and medially (Fig. 54–14). Baker and Carroll[5] achieved 81% good and excellent results with only 4% recurrent dislocations when using this technique. In a small series of patients with malalignment reported by Hall and Micheli,[70] 10 of 11 patients had good to excellent results. Perhaps not surprisingly, the authors also reported fair to poor results in 8 of 10 patients when this procedure was performed for dislocation or subluxation caused by ligamentous laxity or a direct blow. They also noted no significant change in their results in patients in whom they combined a Roux-type patellar tendon transfer with the semitendinosus tenodesis. Pes anserinus transposition for lateral patellar instability has been reported by Baksi,[6,7] but we believe that further studies are necessary before widespread use of this technique. These procedures are rarely, if ever necessary. Note that most authors include medial retinacular imbrication/VMO advancement, as well as soft-tissue distal medialization, with each of these procedures. In analysis of these results, it is very difficult to justify distal medialization in skeletally immature patients. Judicious proximal realignment is usually most prudent.

Mini proximal imbrication with MPFL and VMO advancement through a 2-inch incision can be very helpful in many patients and is preferable to alternative procedures when it can restore normal patella tracking. MPFL reconstruction procedures that involve attaching a

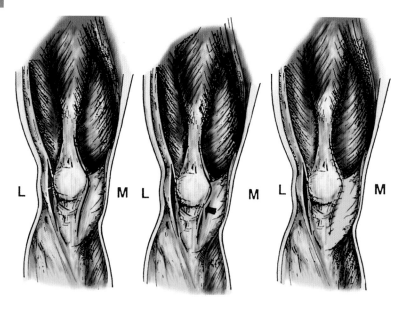

Figure 54–12. Lateral retinacular release with medial imbrication as described by Scuderi. (From Scuderi G, Cuomo F, Scott N: Lateral release and proximal realignment for patellar subluxation and dislocation. J Bone Joint Surg Am 70:856, 1988.) This procedure may be done as a mini-open advancement of the MPFL along with the VMO through a 3-cm incision (Fulkerson).

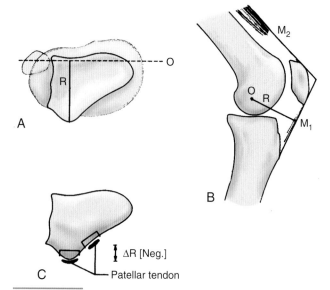

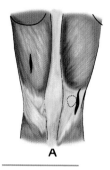

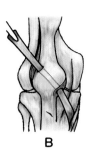

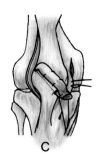

Figure 54–14. Galeazzi semitendinosus tenodesis, an option for soft-tissue distal realignment in the skeletally immature patient. (From Baker RH, Carroll N: The semitendinosus tenodesis for recurrent dislocation of the patella. J Bone Joint Surg Br 54:103, 1972.)

Figure 54–13. **A,** Note the lateral position of the tubercle with respect to the tibial plateau and the posteromedial slope of the anteromedial tibial cortex. Distance R illustrates the lever arm of the quadriceps. **B,** Lateral view illustrating the quadriceps lever R. **C,** Posterior displacement of the tibial tubercle as a result of medial transposition of the tibial tubercle (classic Hauser's procedure). The decreased mechanical advantage of the quadriceps mechanism in this situation results in the need to generate greater quadriceps muscle force to accomplish the same work that results in increased patellofemoral joint reaction force. (From Fulkerson JP: Disorders of the Patellofemoral Joint. Baltimore, Williams & Wilkins, 1990, p 144.)

graft to the region of the medial femoral epicondyle are contraindicated in skeletally immature patients because of the risk of physeal damage. Immediate range of motion is imperative. Another alternative is arthroscopic proximal realignment. Results have been variable with this technique, and the author's (JPF) experience with this technique has been inconsistent when there is more than minimal subluxation. This is probably not an appropriate approach in patients with trochlear dysplasia and more serious subluxation. When arthroscopic realignment is selected, the authors advocate multiple arthroscopic sutures with an emphasis on imbrication of the MPFL. We do not believe that arthroscopic thermal shrinkage has a logical role in patellar realignment.

MPFL reconstruction is best in patients with a dysplastic trochlea and instability that cannot be maintained with less invasive techniques or realignment of the tibial tubercle. This is best accomplished by placing a semitendinosus graft between the saddle region (between the adductor tubercle and medial epicondyle) and the proximal half of the patella to restore normal balance to the extensor mechanism.

TUBEROSITY TRANSFERS

The Hauser procedure, as described in 1938, includes medial and distal transplantation of the tibial tuberosity.[76]

Several authors noted only 67% to 74% rates of good to excellent pain relief and functional improvement after Hauser procedures for diagnoses of chondromalacia resulting from malalignment,[92] recurrent patellar dislocation,[29] and acute and recurrent dislocations.[52] Recurrent dislocation has occurred at similarly steady rates of 17% to 20%.[29,35,102] Generalized ligamentous laxity has been strongly associated with poor results and recurrent dislocation.[35] Furthermore, in some series, a distressingly high percentage of patients (68% to 71%) have had evidence of progression to osteoarthrosis at an average follow-up of 7.3 years,[35] 16 years,[72] and 18 years.[102] Unfortunately, because of the anatomy of the proximal end of the tibia, this procedure resulted in posterior tuberosity displacement (see Fig. 52–13). The high incidence of articular degeneration is consistent with biomechanical theory, which predicts increased stress with distal and posterior transfer of the tuberosity. Posteromedial transfer of the tibial tubercle is rarely, if ever, justified.

Dougherty and Wirth[41] and Grana and O'Donoghue[68] reported modifications of the Hauser procedure in which a slot-block method of fixation of the tibial tuberosity was used for lateral patellar instability. Both had 83% successful results, although Grana and O'Donoghue experienced a 26% rate of significant complications and labeled this procedure technically demanding. Dougherty and Wirth noted worse results in patients with more severe chondromalacia, although specific criteria were not cited. Again, this type of surgery is rarely appropriate and is primarily of historical interest.

Cox[31,32] successfully accomplished distal realignment by medial displacement of the tuberosity while avoiding any posterior displacement with the Roux-Elmslie-Trillat procedure (Fig. 54–15). This technique classically combines lateral release, medial capsular reefing, and medial displacement of the bony insertion of the patellar tendon with distal displacement titrated according to the degree of patella alta measured preoperatively. Excellent and good results were achieved in 77% of 116 patients, with only a 7% recurrence rate. Factors associated with poor outcomes were failure to correct the Q angle or the patella alta adequately, concomitant ACL deficiency, and preexisting patellar degeneration. Using the same procedure, Brown and Alexander[21] found that adequate postoperative correction of the Q angle to 10 degrees or less correlated well with good to excellent results. Shelbourne and Porter[176] also found that postoperative alignment (as measured radiographically by the congruence angle) correlated with the presence of recurrent instability. In their series, 26% (9/34) of patients with preoperative instability had postoperative subluxations. Although the improvement in congruence angle was the same for patients with stable patellae postoperatively, these patients had higher preoperative and postoperative congruence angles. Durable results from tibial tubercle transfer have been reproducible with 10-year minimum follow-up in a number of reports.[28,35,98] No progression of osteoarthrosis was noted, and theoretically one would expect it to be less than with the Hauser procedure, which classically includes posterior tubercle displacement.

In reviewing series of patients treated by distal realignment, one notes that the procedure is often modified in

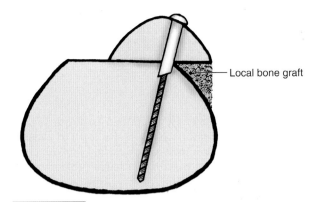

Figure 54–15. Roux-Elmslie-Trillat procedure. Note that this medialization of the tibial tubercle results in no posterior displacement of the tuberosity. (From Cox JS: Evaluation of the Roux-Elmslie-Trillat procedure for knee extensor realignment. Am J Sports Med 10:303, 1982.)

potentially important ways. Tomatsu and Imai[188] compared two groups of similar patients treated with Elmslie-Trillat procedures, but with omission of medial capsulorrhaphy in one group. Results were identical in both groups and very similar to those reported by previous authors. The series of Shelbourne and Porter[176] also omitted medial capsulorrhaphy. Rantanen and Paananen[160] reported on 35 knees treated by medial transfer of the tibial tubercle; they omitted the lateral release in 14 patients. Their results were, again, practically identical to those reported by Cox. Rillmann and Dutly[162] reported yet another modification in which only the medial third of the patellar tendon was transferred and lateral release was included in only 2 of 39 patients. Again, similar outcomes occurred with no redislocations and an 11% rate of postoperative subluxation. Some authors specifically measure patella alta and include distal transfer of the tubercle routinely.[21,31,32,160] Others specifically omit consideration of distal transfer to correct patella alta.[162,176,188] Although the data currently do not allow for definitive guidelines regarding specific operative procedures, we believe that factors such as systemic hypermobility, skeletal alignment, and articular surface condition should be considered when selecting the best procedure to correct instability in any given patient. Patients with severe radiographic malalignment may require medial imbrication, but based on the previous studies it is apparent that many patients do not require medial capsular imbrication.

ANTERIORIZATION

Theory

Anterior elevation of the tibial tuberosity as proposed by Bandi[8] and Maquet[121,122] increases the efficiency of the quadriceps by increasing the lever arm while decreasing the patellofemoral joint reaction force. As illustrated in Figure 54–16, increasing the angle β between the vector of quadriceps pull and the patellar tendon decreases the joint reaction force. The goal is to reduce articular stress by reducing the force and increasing the area of joint contact, thus further decreasing articular stress. Maquet's calculations of patellofemoral compressive force predict an approximately 50% reduction during the stance phase after a 2-cm elevation.

Laboratory Data

This hypothesis is generally confirmed by a progressive reduction in patellofemoral compressive force as cadaver tibial tubercles are advanced. Ferguson and Brown's comparison[50] of six locations on the articular surface of the patella after 1.2-, 2.5-, and 3.7-cm anterior elevation demonstrated significant relief of stress. Overall stress relief with a 1.2-cm advancement at 45 degrees of flexion was 57%. Further elevation to 2.5 and 3.7 cm resulted in additional progressive decreases in average stress of only 30% and 9%, respectively. In a review of these data, Radin[158] noted, however, that the absolute value of total contact stress after 1.2-cm elevation was more than twice that measured after an elevation of 2.5 cm. Ferguson and Brown's study used averaged values obtained from retropatellar sensors and assumed them to be equivalent to the overall average because their model did not permit measurement of contact areas. They concluded that most of the contact stress was relieved with the first 1.2 cm of tendon elevation and that further decreases were believed to represent decreasing returns in exchange for the increasing risk of skin complications. In a similar study using retropatellar piezoelectric transducers, Ferrandez and Usabiaga[51] confirmed close to a 50% decrease in pressure in the first 1 cm, with a more gradual decline with further tubercle elevation.

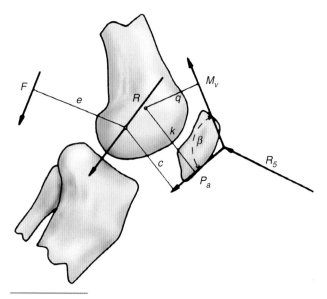

Figure 54–16. Anteriorization of the tibial tubercle decreases the angle β, thereby resulting in decreased patellofemoral joint reaction force. It also tips up the distal patella, thereby unloading distal patellar chondral lesions. (From Maquet P: Mechanics and osteoarthritis of the patellofemoral joint. Clin Orthop 144:70, 1979.)

Lewallen and Riegger[116] used pressure-sensitive film to measure the joint contact force and area after 1.2-cm and 2.5-cm tubercle elevations in eight knees with variable degrees of chondromalacia (Outerbridge grades I to IV). They found significant decreases in joint contact force of 29% and 23% after 1.2-cm elevation at 60 and 90 degrees of flexion, respectively. Contrary to the findings of Ferguson and Brown's study,[50] elevation to 2.5 cm resulted in significant further 60%, 53%, and 55% decreases in force in comparison to "preoperative" values at 30, 60, and 90 degrees. Patellar contact area was observed to shift proximally and laterally with progressive elevation. Interestingly, although force was reduced, joint contact area decreased significantly at 90 degrees of flexion with a 1.2-cm elevation and at 30, 60, and 90 degrees of flexion with 2.5-cm advancement. Similar conclusions were reached by Nakamura and Ellis,[139] who used silicone casting techniques to document progressive decreases in contact area with progressive elevations. Burke and Ahmed,[22] on the other hand, though confirming progressive significant load reduction with progressive advancement to 3 cm, did not find excessive superolateral peak pressures at high degrees of flexion. However, one must keep in mind that these experiments were performed in some normal knees, some with variable amounts of "chondromalacia," and quite possibly some with variable alignment patterns. As regards the suggestions that anteriorization shifts the load proximally, this may occur secondary to the slight distal transfer that occurs as the shingle is rotated forward (and distally).[147] Logically, this effect is increased with shorter shingle length, which produces relatively more distal transfer for the same anteriorization as would a longer shingle. Overall, these findings substantiate the concept of further relief of joint reaction force with increasing elevation even if these particular models do not specifically support or refute Maquet's contention that contact area is increased.

Clinical Experience

Maquet[121] reported on 37 patients with patellar arthrosis and chondromalacia an average of 4.7 years after 2- to 3-cm advancement of the tuberosity; 36 knees were stable with relief of pain and range of motion that approximated preoperative motion. His recommendations included medialization of the tubercle when the patella was subluxated and osteoarthritis was limited to the lateral facet. Medialization was accomplished by notching the graft. Early postoperative motion was possible because of the stable geometry of the iliac graft (Fig. 54–17). In a report by Rozbruch and Campbell[164] at the Hospital for Special Surgery, an additional 16 patients with various diagnoses experienced only 63% good results after Maquet procedures. Radin's[158] 36 patients had successful results from a modified Maquet procedure, including elevation of at least 2 cm, lateral release, and medialization of approximately 1 cm (as necessary to correct subluxation) in 94% with post-traumatic osteoarthrosis, in 88% with chronic patellar subluxation and osteoarthrosis, and in 66% with postpatellectomy pain. Hirsh and Reddy[85] also reported successful results with elevation of 1.7 to 2.5 cm in a small series. Mendes and Soudry,[129] in their series of 27 patients with primarily patellofemoral osteoarthritis, achieved 76% subjective satisfactory results at 5.5 years after a 2.5-cm elevation. Heatley and Allen[78] reported 65% excellent and good results in 29 patients. In a series of 184 patients treated by Ferguson[49] with anterior elevation of 1.25 cm and local bone grafting, satisfactory pain relief plus resumption of lost function was achieved in 92% of patients with "osteoarthrosis" (degree unspecified), 82% of patients with recurrent dislocations, 84% of patients with chondromalacia, 84% of patients with blunt patellar trauma, and 88% of patients with previous patellectomy. Medial transfer of 4 to 5 mm was regularly included in operations for recurrent dislocations and was performed as "desirable" in patients with other diagnoses. Lateral retinacular release was not routinely performed. No internal fixation was used, and patients were placed in a cast for 6 weeks and waited an average of 6 months for symptomatic relief. In general, these reports share a common theme of best results in patients with osteoarthrosis and less consistent results for other diagnoses.

Engebretsen and Svenningsen's results[47] correlated with the pattern of articular degeneration; the best postoperative results were seen in patients with lateral facet degeneration. There was no improvement in 18 of 20 patients with medial facet involvement. At long-term follow-up of 8 to 15 years, anteriorization has been found to be durable; Jenny and Sader[97] reported a 62% success rate. Silvello and Scarponi[179] treated patients with "chondromalacia" and patellofemoral arthritis with somewhat less anteriorization (1.2 to 1.5 cm) than the classic Maquet procedure and achieved only 53% good and excellent results. Conversely, emphasizing the importance of at least 2 cm of anteriorization, Schmid[167] found 80% good/very good results at a mean 16-year follow-up. When considering the use of anteriorization for treatment of anterior knee pain, we believe that it is important to recognize that the severity and pattern of articular degeneration are critical. Distal lateral lesions are probably best suited for relief with this

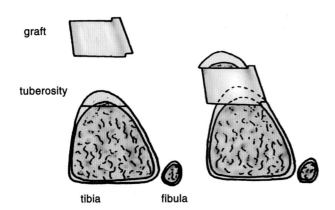

Figure 54–17. Maquet technique. A notched iliac crest graft is used to produce anterior and medial displacement of the tibial tuberosity. This procedure is rarely indicated. (From Maquet P: Advancement of the tibial tuberosity. Clin Orthop 115:225, 1976.)

procedure; however, there are many successes reported in the literature with other lesions. Nonetheless, patients and surgeons must realize that this is generally a salvage procedure and function is rarely truly normal after the procedure. Patients must also understand that the tubercle appears quite prominent after surgery and is usually uncomfortable when kneeling. It is wise preoperatively to show patients photographs of knees after anteriorization to avoid cosmetic dissatisfaction postoperatively.

ANTEROMEDIALIZATION

Although anteriorization procedures have at times included medialization to control subluxation or recurrent dislocation, a number of procedures that routinely combine some degree of anteromedialization have been designed for patients with malalignment. Laboratory evaluation of this concept in a cadaver model with increased lateral facet overload induced by alteration of the proximal vector of the quadriceps showed excellent reduction of lateral facet pressure.[60] This study reported a 30% reduction in lateral facet pressure with anteriorization of 8.8 mm and medialization of 8.4 mm and 65% relief after additional anteromedialization to 14.8/8.4 mm. By 20 to 30 degrees of knee flexion, there was a reduction and equalization of medial and lateral facet pressure with a greater reduction in the more anteriorized group. When compared with previous studies of tubercle anteriorization, a similar slight proximal shift in contact area occurred, although there was no significant undesirable decrease in area as took place with some previous laboratory evaluations of anterior tubercle transfer.[116,139]

Clinical Experience

Anteromedialization of the tibial tuberosity via an oblique osteotomy was introduced by John Fulkerson in 1983 (Fig. 54–18). This procedure allows variable anterior and medial displacement of the tubercle with rigid fixation and early motion while maintaining a broad cancellous surface for primary bone healing.[57] The results of this procedure on 30 knees with patellofemoral pain, moderate articular degeneration, and clinical malalignment indicate excellent/good subjective results in 93%.[60] Objectively, 89% excellent/good results were documented, and the 12 patients monitored for more than 5 years showed no deterioration with time. Mean anteriorization was 10.6 mm. Even 75% of the eight patients with advanced deterioration (Outerbridge grades III to IV) had good results, although excellent results were not achieved in this group. Morshuis and Pavlov[136] described a series of 25 similar osteotomies and reported 84% good and excellent short-term results. Anteriorization was less than 10 mm, and the best results were achieved in patients with mild articular degeneration. Bellemans and Cauwenberghs[9] found consistent clinical improvement and correction of preoperative radiographic pathological tilt and subluxation in 29 patients after anteromedialization by Fulkerson's technique. One noteworthy procedural modification was the

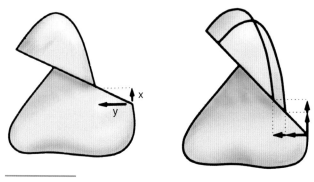

Figure 54–18. An oblique osteotomy allows anterior and medial displacement of the tibial tuberosity without a bone graft. A steeper osteotomy plane will produce more anteriorization along with medialization. (From Fulkerson JP: Anteromedialization of the tibial tuberosity for patellofemoral malalignment. Clin Orthop 177:176, 1983.)

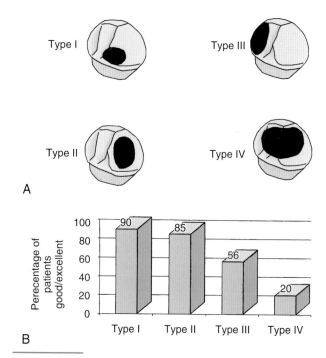

Figure 54–19. **A,** Classification of the location of patellar chondral lesions. **B,** Correlation of good/excellent results after anteromedialization with location of the chondral lesion. (From Pidoriano AJ, Weinstein RN: Correlation of patellar articular lesions with results from anteromedial tibial tubercle transfer. Am J Sports Med 25:533, 1997.)

omission of lateral release in 14 patients with CT-documented normal tilt angles preoperatively.

Pidoriano and Weinstein[149] studied the correlation between the pattern of articular degeneration and the result of anteromedialization and confirmed the theoretic and laboratory findings that distal and lateral lesions should respond best to anteromedialization. Distal lesions and lateral facet lesions, of varying severity, correlated with 87% good to excellent functional results (Fig. 54–19). Conversely, medial facet lesions had just 55% good to excellent functional results. Eight percent of patients with diffuse or proximal patellar lesions did poorly. Patients with severe central trochlear lesions also did poorly. Interestingly, the location of the articular lesion correlated much better with the result than did the absolute degree of articular degeneration, as described by the Outerbridge classification, despite the fact that 28 of 36 patients in the series had grade III/IV articular cartilage degeneration. As predicted by patellofemoral mechanics, the location of the lesion is critical in selecting patients for anteromedialization.

In a later review, Buuck and Fulkerson established effective long-term success of the anteromedial tibial tubercle transfer procedure in a 4- to 12-year follow-up study.[24]

Other techniques of anteromedialization have also been studied. Combined rotation and elevation of the tibial tuberosity with lateral release was reported in 1986 by Miller and LaRochelle.[134] This technique, which uses a wedge-shaped graft rotated medially and fixed with a cortical lag screw, raises the tuberosity 9 to 11 mm and is probably less stable than that described by Fulkerson. Casts were maintained for 4 to 5 weeks postoperatively. Their indications for surgery were refractory patellofemoral pain with normal or increased Q angles. Fifty-five percent of patients had a positive apprehension sign. Pain was decreased in 86% of 38 patients postoperatively, and no patient had residual patellar instability. Another potential problem with this method could be proximal shingle fracture caused by lack of support under the most proximal tip of the shingle.[158] Noll and Ben-Itzhak[141] reported a 1.25-cm elevation with transposition of the tubercle straight medially onto a tapered bony

bed with fixation by a cancellous screw, thereby avoiding the need for bone grafting. Three weeks of cast immobilization followed. Their patients had a variety of diagnoses, primarily patellofemoral pain with an increased Q angle but no patellar instability. Good to excellent relief was obtained in 12 of 14 patients. Naranja et al used a modified Maquet procedure with medialization of the tibial tubercle supported by a local bone graft in 55 knees (80% had preoperative subluxation or dislocation). They found only 53% good/excellent results based on the Fulkerson functional score and 11% recurrent instability in 55 knees. Anteriorization was only 1 cm. The severity of articular cartilage changes was not noted, and some, but not all patients underwent medial reefing and VMO advancement.

In summary, although these series of distal realignment procedures differ in specific details, the results are generally quite good. If the clinician is certain to exhaust nonoperative treatment, document preoperative malalignment, reserve anteromedialization for patients with distal and lateral facet lesions, and avoid technical pitfalls, patient satisfaction is very high.

COMPLICATIONS OF DISTAL REALIGNMENT

Combining six separate reports, potentially disastrous skin necrosis over the tibial tubercle has occurred in 8.8% of 182 reported cases treated by a Maquet procedure with advancement of more than 2 cm.[80,85,121,129,158,164] In contrast, skin necrosis has, to our knowledge, not been reported with lesser advancements and has not been reported or seen by the authors after anteromedial tibial tubercle transfer. Other serious complications are less common but can occur, including acute or stress fractures of the bony shingle, deep venous thrombosis, arthrofibrosis, and compartment syndrome. Acute fracture of the proximal end of the tibia was reported in 6 of 234 patients who were encouraged to initiate immediate full weight-bearing after anteromedialization; accordingly, patients should be advanced to full weightbearing gradually after about 6 weeks with some radiographic evidence of consolidation of the tibial shingle.[184] Compartment syndrome occurred in 12 cases after Hauser procedures,[192] but this procedure is no longer recommended. Emphasis has been placed on strict technique to avoid many of these complications, and indeed, several series have documented a decreased rate of complications as their experience with this procedure increased.[80,158] Radin and Labosky[159] wrote an important article on methods to minimize complications with the Maquet procedure; clinicians planning this procedure would be well advised to study it. Special care should be taken in patients with multiple scars from previous surgery. Avoidance of complications entails careful handling of skin edges, techniques to minimize skin tension, use of suction drains postoperatively, and early motion whenever possible.

FULKERSON'S TECHNIQUE OF ANTEROMEDIALIZATION

After arthroscopic confirmation of the preoperative diagnosis and examination of the medial and lateral joint compartments for associated disease, a straight incision, slightly lateral of midline, is made just lateral to the patellar tendon and tibial crest to a point approximately 5 cm distal to the tibial tuberosity (Fig. 54–20A). It is desirable to make this incision in such a way that a later midline or paramidline incision will be possible if arthroplasty or further surgery becomes necessary. Lateral retinacular release is then performed, including the patellofemoral ligaments (patellotibial and epicondylopatellar bands), synovium, and vastus lateralis obliquus.[71] Proximally, the main tendon of the vastus lateralis is protected. Care is taken distally to avoid injury to the lateral meniscus, which is at the inferior extent of the release. If the release is adequate, 90 degrees of patellar eversion should be possible to allow direct examination and palpation of the articular surfaces (see Fig. 54–9B). Careful observation of the pattern and degree of articular changes and correlation with the patient's symptoms and preoperative evaluation are important in deciding the need for lateral release versus anteromedialization, if the patient has an isolated tilt, or in deciding the degree of anteriorization appropriate for those undergoing anteromedial transfer.

The musculature of the anterior compartment is next sharply released from the tibial crest and elevated atraumatically in a posterior direction to expose the posterolateral corner of the proximal end of the tibia. The anterior tibial artery and the peroneal nerve are at this level (Fig. 54–20B) and must be protected. The medial and lateral borders of the patellar tendon are then defined, with particular care taken to delineate the entire insertion into the tibial tuberosity (Fig. 54–21). Next, a longitudinal incision is made just medial to the tibial crest along the planned osteotomy (closer to the crest for a steeper osteotomy). The osteotomy plane is also tapered distally to create a proximally based pie shape on the medial

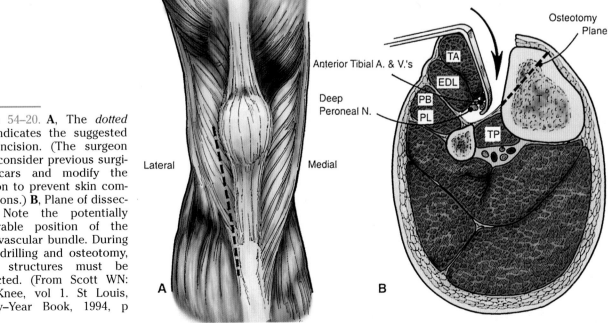

Figure 54–20. **A,** The *dotted line* indicates the suggested skin incision. (The surgeon must consider previous surgical scars and modify the incision to prevent skin complications.) **B,** Plane of dissection. Note the potentially vulnerable position of the neurovascular bundle. During tibial drilling and osteotomy, these structures must be protected. (From Scott WN: The Knee, vol 1. St Louis, Mosby–Year Book, 1994, p 458.)

surface of the tibial narrowing down to a 2- to 3-mm apex 5 to 7 cm distal to the tuberosity (see Fig. 54–21). The periosteum is carefully elevated from the line of the planned osteotomy. While exquisite care is taken to have the posterolateral aspect of the tibia under direct vision at all times, a series of 4.0-mm drill bits may be placed parallel with use of the Hoffmann drill guide or a similar device in a plane from the anteromedial toward the posterolateral aspect of the tibia. Each drill bit should be carefully observed as it penetrates the lateral cortex to avoid injury to the anterior tibial vessels and peroneal nerve. Maintaining bicortical drill bits in the most superior and inferior positions along the drill guide helps place the remaining parallel drill holes accurately, but these bits must be checked frequently to prevent inadvertent and potentially dangerous advancement. A lateral osteotomy must then be made from the superior posterior drill hole to an anterior point proximal to the patellar tendon insertion to prevent propagation of the osteotomy into the proximal end of the tibia (Fig. 54–22). The cortical bone anterior and proximal to the tibial tuberosity is next cut with a $\frac{1}{2}$-inch osteotome while taking care to not injure the tendon (Fig. 54–23). Alternatively, the Tracker AMZ guide (Mitek, Norwood, MA), designed by Jack Farr, may be used to design this osteotomy and make the cut.

The main osteotomy is then completed with an osteotome or saw while using the superior and inferior drill bits as guides to the desired plane (Fig. 54–24). A perfectly flat osteotomy plane is critical to the ultimate apposition of the broad flat cancellous surfaces and the

stability of fixation. Once the osteotomy is complete, the bone pedicle is hinged distally and pushed up the inclined plane. Patellar tracking is then observed, and the optimal amount of medialization is maintained while two countersunk 3.2-mm AO cortical screws are placed into the posterior cortex (Fig. 54–25). Special care is exercised when drilling through the posterior cortex. Anteriorization of 12 to 15 mm is routine without a bone graft, although locally available bone (proximal lateral tibial metaphysis) can be used to neutralize the medialization and add anteriorization in selected rare cases. If pure medialization is desired, the osteotomy is simply modified to eliminate the anterior-to-posterior obliquity. The tourniquet is released and meticulous hemostasis ensured before placement of a suction drain and closure of the subcutaneous and skin layers.

Postoperative Care

A cooling device is placed over light bandages in the operating room to apply continuous cryotherapy and gentle compression. Drains are usually removed in approximately 24 hours when the drainage diminishes. Quadriceps-setting exercises are encouraged the day of surgery, and assuming secure fixation of the shingle, early active and gentle passive motion is begun the next day. Toe-touch weightbearing is allowed with crutches and a knee immobilizer. At 4 to 6 weeks quadriceps strength is improving, bony union has generally occurred, and crutches can be discontinued when the patient can perform a single-leg knee bend without support on the

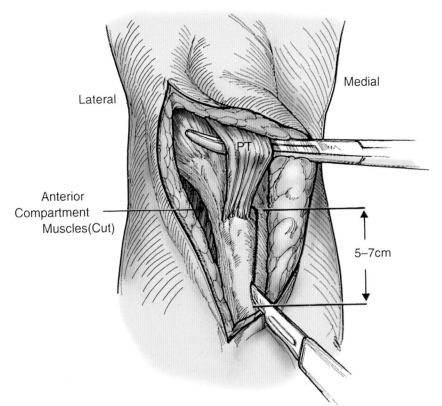

Figure 54–21. The patellar tendon is mobilized. The osteotomy plane is planned. (From Scott WN: The Knee, vol 1. St Louis, Mosby–Year Book, 1994, p 459.)

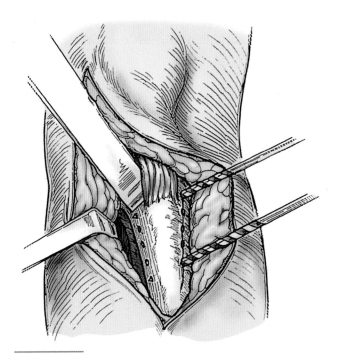

Figure 54–22. Lateral osteotomy frees the superior aspect of the tibial tubercle shingle and prevents propagation of the osteotomy into the proximal end of the tibia. (From Scott WN: The Knee, vol 1. St Louis, Mosby–Year Book, 1994, p 460.)

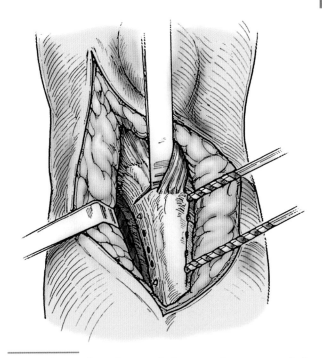

Figure 54–23. Completion of the superior aspect of the osteotomy. (From Scott WN: The Knee, vol 1. St Louis, Mosby–Year Book, 1994, p 460.)

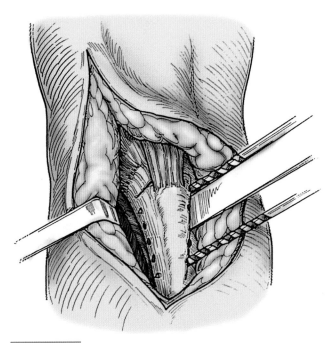

Figure 54–24. A wide osteotome is used to complete the oblique osteotomy along the plane defined by the drill bits previously placed with the parallel drill guide. Care should be taken to make sure that the osteotomy plane is completely flat to ensure good bony apposition. (From Scott WN: The Knee, vol 1. St Louis, Mosby–Year Book, 1994, p 460.)

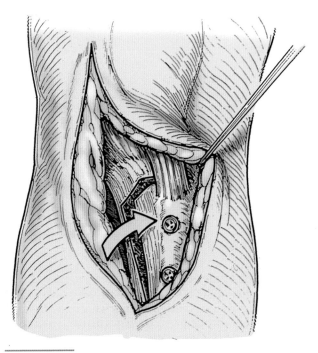

Figure 54–25. The tibial shingle is then pushed anteromedially up the inclined plane and rigidly fixed with two bicortical large-fragment AO cortical lag screws. (From Scott WN: The Knee, vol 1. St Louis, Mosby–Year Book, 1994, p 460.)

operated side. Full recovery is generally achieved between 3 and 4 months.

ARTICULAR DEGENERATION WITHOUT MALALIGNMENT

Theory

If articular degeneration without malalignment is diagnosed, the pathophysiology of the pain is presumed to be subchondral nerve irritation and the inflammatory joint reaction that typically follows the release of proteoglycans from degenerative articular cartilage lesions. Treatment must be directed at decreasing the load on the damaged articular surface, resurfacing, or removing the articular defects. If the defect is eburnated bone, microfracture arthroplasty should be considered to allow potential fibrocartilaginous healing. Anteromedial tibial tubercle transfer is also helpful in unloading areas in which articular cartilage resurfacing has been performed in order to facilitate healing of the transplant.

ARTHROSCOPIC DÉBRIDEMENT

Clinical Experience

Ogilvie-Harris and Jackson[144] reported subjective improvement after arthroscopic débridement, particularly in post-traumatic cases with normal alignment. Federico and Reider[48] reported arthroscopic débridement of loose and fibrillated articular cartilage (without violation of subchondral bone) in 36 patients and found that all but 4 thought that the surgery had a "beneficial effect." Closer scrutiny by more objective measurement with the Fulkerson-Shea joint evaluation score found 58% good to excellent results in patients with traumatic chondromalacia. This apparent paradox illustrates that such patients, though perhaps improved, frequently continue with functional limitations. Nonetheless, this may be satisfactory for some patients and avoids the need for more invasive reconstructive surgery.

ANTERIORIZATION

Clinical Experience

Anteriorization of the tibial tubercle has been reviewed in the previous section. Clinical results with this diagnosis are limited, but encouraging. In articles that reported post-traumatic patients separately, successful results were achieved in at least 84%.[49,157] If a localized articular lesion has been identified, care should be taken that the anteriorization will effectively unload the lesion. It seems likely that the experience reported by Pidoriano and Weinstein[149] would apply equally well to straight anteriorization, with distal lesions being the best candidates for anteriorization. Although average retropatellar pressure is globally decreased after anteriorization, when contemplating this alternative the physician is urged to carefully

consider the data presented previously with regard to the specific local retropatellar effects of tibial tubercle anteriorization.

PATELLECTOMY

Theory/Clinical Experience

Patellar excision as a last resort is certainly a straightforward approach to a painful patella. Of course, one must be certain that the patient's complaints are entirely referable to articular destruction before any consideration of this procedure. The use of this technique as a panacea for patellofemoral problems, including fractures, dislocations, malalignment, and chondromalacia, in the early to mid-20th century arose after a clinical and laboratory report in 1937 by Brooke[19] in which it was concluded that the patella served no important function. Subsequent laboratory investigations[38,77,105,193] and clinical studies[187] have, of course, disproved this opinion. These cadaver and clinical experiences with patellectomy reveal a decrease of as much as 50% in extension power because of the loss of mechanical leverage. Greater percentages of loss of power are to be expected near terminal extension.[105] Animal models of patellectomy have shown consistent evidence of pathological changes in the trochlea.[38,64] Partial patellectomy or "facetectomy" has been suggested as an alternative to sacrifice of the entire patella.[143,165,187] Martens and De Rycke[124] reported lateral release with lateral facetectomy to be satisfactory in 90% of patients with lateral patellar osteophytes. The average age in their series was 60 years with a 2-year follow-up. The results of this procedure for degenerative articular lesions have not been clearly reported, and further studies are necessary before recommending it. Malalignment of the extensor mechanism, if present, must be corrected at the time of patellectomy, if not before.

However, a number of reports do suggest that the results of patellectomy can provide long-term improvement for some patients.[65,107,117,185,186] Such a postpatellectomy knee can probably never be truly "normal" again, but the procedure can allow significant improvement in function if preoperative function is severely limited. Unfortunately, many of these reports combine patients with various diagnoses. Generally, the best results occur in cases in which patellectomy is performed for patella arthrosis when the trochlea is intact. It must, because of the inherent mechanical disadvantage, be viewed as a salvage procedure, and patients should be cautioned against unrealistic expectations.

Technique

Many methods of patellectomy have been advocated. The various techniques represent different strategies for repair of the quadriceps mechanism after removal of the patella. If evidence of patellar malalignment exists, patellectomy must include realignment of the extensor mechanism. Although quadriceps weakness may be minimized by distal advancement of the quadriceps tendon,[105] such advancement may result in limitation of flexion. Side-to-side imbrication and repair have not resulted in extensor lag in our patients. A longitudinal midline incision is selected in the absence of previous surgical scars. Using a scalpel, the patella is then sharply enucleated from the medial and lateral retinaculum. The wound is copiously irrigated. All bone should be meticulously removed. The tourniquet is then released and hemostasis obtained. The quadriceps mechanism is repaired in a side-to-side technique. Clicking and subluxation must be eliminated. Tracking of the repaired quadriceps tendon is carefully evaluated, and the tendon may be imbricated to correct any significant subluxation. Rarely, distal realignment may be necessary. Postoperatively, the patient begins early weightbearing and active and passive range-of-motion exercises. A cooling device is used to provide gentle compression and pain relief postoperatively.

PATELLOFEMORAL ARTHROPLASTY

Theory/Clinical Experience

If an individual patient's pain is purely secondary to isolated patellofemoral articular destruction, resurfacing of the patellofemoral joint could theoretically be considered reasonable. Patellar hemiarthroplasty with an anatomically shaped metallic patellar prosthesis was introduced by McKeever in 1955.[128] Successful arthroplasty in this series was associated with another major intra-articular operation in 39 of 40 patients. Levitt[115] reported satisfactory results in 11 of 20 patients 7 years after implantation of the McKeever prosthesis. Subsequently, Worrell[197,198] reported his results with a modified McKeever-type prosthesis for patellar hemiarthroplasty. His most recent article detailed fair and poor results in 12 of 15 patients younger than 40 years. Pickett and Stoll,[148] however, preferred hemiarthroplasty to patellectomy. Aglietti and Insall[1] and Insall and Tria[94] reported two series of patients treated with a cemented metallic dome-shaped patellar component and found only 67% good results in their patients with isolated patellofemoral arthritis. Using supplemental fixation with bone cement and a McKeever prosthesis for isolated severe patellofemoral arthrosis, Harrington reported 17 of 24 good results at a 5-year follow-up.

Trochlear resurfacing in conjunction with patellar arthroplasty has also been reported.[13,14,25] Patients in each series had often undergone multiple previous procedures. Arciero and Toomey[2] performed 22 cemented patellofemoral arthroplasties and found 85% good results in an older population with isolated patellofemoral arthritis. Krajca-Radcliffe and Coker[109] reported 88% good and excellent results after a 2- to 15-year follow-up. Argenson and Guillaume[3] found the best results in patients after patellar fracture and had a 29% revision rate in those with "primary" patellofemoral arthritis. Outcomes have been satisfactory in many patients, and recent experience by Ackroyd (unpublished) with the Avon prosthesis (Osteonics/Howmedica) has been very promising. In the senior author's (JPF) experience with patellofemoral arthroplasty (22 cases at the time of writing this chapter), this is not a

solved problem by any means. Dysplasia of the trochlea and condyles can cause rotational problems with unicompartmental prostheses, and there are no long-term data with the current designs. Nonetheless, as a salvage procedure in patients with severe isolated patellofemoral arthritis, unicompartmental patellofemoral replacement does have a place because function is better than after patellectomy and the trochlea is resurfaced. In patients with severe trochlea arthritis, we also have limited experience with isolated trochlea resurfacing.

PATELLAR OSTEOTOMY

Osteotomy of the patella has also been suggested as a means to decrease interosseous pressure. Hejgaard and Arnoldi[79] reported that a simple longitudinal osteotomy provided significant pain relief. Longitudinal opening wedge osteotomy with lateral release for severe chondromalacia and normal alignment has also been proposed by Morscher[135] in a preliminary report. Further confirmation of the efficacy of this procedure is necessary before advocating this technique.

ASSORTED SOFT-TISSUE DISORDERS WITHOUT MALALIGNMENT

Patellar Tendinitis

Patellar tendinitis can be diagnosed clinically by the presence of localized tenderness in the patellar tendon, usually at the inferior pole of the patella. Pain is reproduced and well localized with quadriceps contraction. Limited quadriceps flexibility is often noticed during prone testing. If desired, diagnostic confirmation is possible with ultrasound or MRI examination. If a thorough nonoperative program, including relative rest, quadriceps stretching, eccentric strengthening, nonsteroidal anti-inflammatory medication, ultrasound, and iontophoresis, fails, surgery can be successful.[182,183]

Surgical procedures for patellar tendinitis generally involve excision of the abnormal intratendinous tissue with or without repair of the tendon to the inferior pole of the patella.[80,99,100,123] A variable amount of the distal nonarticular patella is sometimes resected.[8,141] We prefer simple excision of the degenerative tendon through a longitudinal incision in the tendon. Karlsson and Lundin[104] presented a similar approach that produced 91% excellent/good results in athletes. Verheyden and Geens[191] found that 26 of 31 knees had very good results with excision of the tendinosis. Popp and Yu[150] found that excision of the pathological angiofibroblastic tissue resulted in excellent outcomes in 7 of 11 knees. The severity of the lesion, as imaged by ultrasonography, was also found to correlate with the success of nonoperative treatment in patients with partial rupture of the tendon; hypoechogenic lesions greater than 20 mm require surgical treatment in 38.5% of cases.[103] If the area of degeneration is adjacent to the inferior pole of the patella, the bony surface is exposed to facilitate a healing response. Similar to the harvest of a patellar tendon graft for other procedures, formal repair of the patellar tendon to the patella is probably not necessary if no more than the central third of the patellar tendon origin is disturbed. Postoperatively, rapid mobilization is encouraged. Cautious and limited arthroscopic débridement of the area of tendinosis and the inferior pole of the patella may be possible.

Pathological Hypertrophic Plica Syndrome

During development of the fetal knee, separate suprapatellar, medial, and lateral compartments are divided by synovial septa. These septa usually recede by the third month of development, with synovial folds called plicae left behind.[42] Suprapatellar plicae and medial patellar plicae are common. Lateral patellar plicae are rare. The pathogenesis of pathological plical hypertrophy is thought to involve blunt or repetitive trauma, which results in scarring, loss of elasticity, and bowstringing. The thickened, stiffened plica can become interposed in the patellofemoral joint or rub over the medial femoral condyle with flexion. This can result in snapping and pain with flexion and cause irritation of surrounding synovium and abrasion of the articular surface. The pathological medial patellar plica can usually be diagnosed by physical examination as a tender palpable cord between the medial patellar border and the medial femoral condyle. The patient's complaints of pain and snapping can often be reproduced and palpated on examination.

Nonoperative management directed at improvement in flexibility and mobilization of the scarred tissue should be attempted. Rovere and Adair[163] showed that injection of a long-acting anesthetic agent and steroid into the medial patellar plica region resulted in full return to activity in 73% of patients. Arthroscopic evaluation and palpation of the pathological plica should show a thickened fibrotic structure. There will usually be surrounding inflammatory synovitis. Superficial fibrillation of the medial femoral condyle may also be present from the repeated friction of the plica over the condyle. If the preoperative complaint, physical examination, and arthroscopic examination correlate, arthroscopic thermal ablation or resection of the pathological plica is indicated.[20,73,96,190] Postoperatively, early motion and return to function are emphasized. In appropriately chosen patients, relief can be dramatic.

Postpatellectomy Pain

One must consider the diagnoses of tendon subluxation versus stress overload to select appropriate intervention in this condition. If the pain is not related to residual soft-tissue malalignment, anteriorization of the tibial tubercle by 1.25 cm has had good results in a total of 13 of 17 patients according to Ferguson,[49] Radin,[157] and Mendes and Soudry.[129] Anteriorization in this situation also might theoretically increase extensor power by increasing the lever arm of the quadriceps mechanism, thus narrowing the mechanical deficit inherent in patellectomy. This has not, however, been clinically proved. If malalignment

exists, appropriate correction, perhaps in conjunction with anteriorization, would be indicated.

Our Recommended Treatment Approach

PATELLOFEMORAL MALALIGNMENT

Patients with patellofemoral pain who have failed nonoperative management may have various degrees of articular pain, soft-tissue pain, and instability. The preoperative history and physical examination supplemented by x-ray film and, when necessary, CT evaluation are used to assess the degree of articular degeneration and the degree of tilt and subluxation present. An appropriate procedure can then be selected to address all components of the problem.

Tilt

Recognized on physical examination and confirmed with x-ray film or more reliably with CT, when isolated (no lateral subluxation or significant articular degeneration), tilt can result in disabling soft-tissue pain. A tight contracted lateral retinaculum draws the patella into increasing lateral tilt with knee flexion as a result of progressive posterior displacement of the iliotibial band (to which a strong portion of the retinaculum is anchored). Soft-tissue pain can result from neuromatous degeneration in the lateral retinaculum under these conditions or from tension overload in the medial tissues. Excessive pressure on the articular surface of the lateral facet is also possible and may conceivably result in progressive degeneration if not corrected in a symptomatic patient. Patients with pure tilt probably represent a subgroup of those labeled as having "chondromalacia" without subluxation in many series. Nonoperative management includes quadriceps strengthening, stretching of the tight lateral retinaculum and iliotibial band, McConnell taping, and bracing and may be supplemented by nonsteroidal anti-inflammatory medication. Lateral release is our procedure of choice in this situation when surgery is necessary and has resulted in 92% excellent or good results in patients with CT-documented tilt and mild cartilage degeneration (Outerbridge grade II chondromalacia or less).[175] CT evaluation of tilt in patients with preoperative tilt and no lateral facet collapse showed consistent improvement to within the normal range 3 to 4 months after lateral release.[61] Medial imbrication has not been necessary to achieve this correction.

Subluxation and Tilt

Patients whose knees fall into this category based on the history, physical examination, and radiographic studies respond less consistently to lateral release alone after failure of conservative care, which should include the use of a brace that can limit instability such as the Trupull (DJ Orthopedics, Vista, CA). Coronal malalignment related to the quadriceps vector and tibial tubercle position is not consistently improved by lateral release, as noted by unchanged postoperative Q angles[110] and by unchanged CT.[61] Medialization of the tibial tubercle helps decrease the Q angle, thus reducing the laterally directed component of the extensor force, which has been shown to contribute significantly to patellar subluxation. Thus, medialization of the tibial tubercle in conjunction with lateral release should be the appropriate procedure in the absence of significant articular damage. We have not found imbrication of the VMO to be routinely necessary.[188] This may be a clinical reflection of the findings of Mariani and Caruso,[123] who found electromyographic evidence of improved VMO function after lateral release and distal realignment.

Patients with a history of traumatic instability and evidence of increased lateral translation on examination under anesthesia would logically be treated with a procedure that restores medial ligament integrity. This could be done with various techniques ranging from arthroscopic imbrication (with or without lateral release) to mini open proximal realignment with advancement of the VMO (which has attachments to the MPFL) to MPFL reconstruction with graft placement. At the present time, the literature does not provide a definitive answer to which procedure is most reliable in specific circumstances. The authors have had experience and success with each of these procedures. Arthroscopic proximal realignment has been helpful in patients with mild subluxation, but we have already seen failures of this technique in patients with more severe subluxation. Careful evaluation of patellar tracking and patellar stability intraoperatively are needed with each technique. More severe cases of subluxation may require a combination of procedures, possibly including tibial tubercle transfer. Documentation of a laterally displaced tubercle by CT scan can help with this decision. We emphasize the importance of examining the MPFL *open* through a small incision as it is usually intact but elongates and may be advanced as needed.

Subluxation and Tilt with Articular Disease

In this situation, one must consider adding pressure relief to the procedure by including anteriorization to the lateral release and medialization. In making this decision, one should recall the characteristic proximal and medial load transfer of anteromedialization in the cadaver models and not transfer increased loads onto damaged proximal articular surfaces. One must also remember that progressive elevation of the tubercle brings increasing relief of force but also increases the risk for complications. Anteriorization of up to 17 mm may be obtained by using Fulkerson's technique of anteromedialization without the addition of an iliac graft. Advantages of the oblique osteotomy as described by John Fulkerson over other techniques with similar goals include a broad flat surface for cancellous healing, rigid internal fixation allowing immediate motion, early functional recovery, and avoidance of skin complications.

Subluxation

Without articular changes greater than Outerbridge I to II and in the absence of tilt, medialization is the primary goal. In milder cases, mini-MPFL advancement alone is satisfactory. When necessary in a *skeletally mature* individual with severe subluxation, our preferred method is a Trillat-type procedure with medial rotation of a flat osteotomy, rigidly fixed, and concomitant lateral release supplemented by MPFL advancement. Avoidance of posterior transposition of the tubercle is imperative to avoid increasing patellofemoral joint contact forces and the resultant high risk for osteoarthrosis.

In children with open proximal tibial growth plates, we perform a lateral release and supplement it with imbrication of the medial patellofemoral ligament (MPFL) if necessary to correct tracking adequately. In patients with mild symptomatic subluxation, arthroscopic medial imbrication may suffice. The Roux-Goldthwait procedure is avoided because of the theoretic potential of inducing iatrogenic lateral tilt.

Another group of patients who have been problematic consists of those with generalized laxity and nondescript anterior knee pain. The author (JPF) believes that there is an analogy to patients with multidirectional shoulder instability such that an imbricating procedure may reduce excessive motion and thereby reduce pain, although definitive proof is as yet lacking in this population.

Patella Alta

Fortunately, distal transfer of the tuberosity occurs with any distally based rotation of a shingle whether the rotation is straight medial, anterior, or somewhere in between. With a longer tibial shingle, less distal displacement occurs. Thus, the degree of patella alta present can be a consideration in selecting the length of the tibial shingle. In patients with severe patella alta in the setting of patellar instability, one may want to be certain that the tubercle osteotomy allows adequate distal transfer for correction.

ARTICULAR DEGENERATION WITH NORMAL ALIGNMENT

In patients who have not undergone previous surgery, sometimes arthroscopic débridement of unstable fragments can bring some relief and is often worth a try. Otherwise, relief of pressure is the goal in this pattern, which may include osteochondral injury or post-traumatic chondromalacia. If articular lesions are not end stage (eburnated bone), the medial trochlea is relatively intact, and the pattern of degeneration or injury spares appropriate areas to make proximal transfer of patellar load an attractive idea, straight anteriorization of the tibial tubercle is appropriate. This type of surgery may be combined with articular cartilage resurfacing. Otherwise, patellectomy and patellofemoral arthroplasty are the remaining surgical options. Our preferred method of anteriorization is to use a steep, oblique osteotomy to achieve anteriorization. Local bone graft may be added if necessary (Fig. 54–26). Another way to this end is a sagittal-plane osteotomy with a lateral back cut to allow straight anteriorization of the tibial tubercle. Rigid fixation with bicortical lag screws

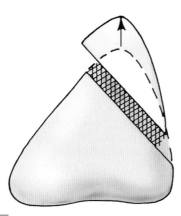

Figure 54–26. An oblique osteotomy with the use of a locally available proximal tibial bone graft results in straight anteriorization without an iliac crest graft. (From Fulkerson JP: Operative management of patellofemoral pain. Ann Chir Gynecol 80:224, 1991.)

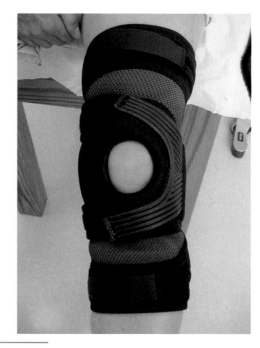

Figure 54–27. Trupull patellofemoral brace (DJ Ortho, Vista, CA).

allows early motion, as with anteromedialization of the tibial tubercle. If pain continues after an attempt at anteriorization, one has not burned any bridges and may still resort to patellectomy or arthroplasty.

THE FAILED PATELLOFEMORAL SURGERY PATIENT

First, rethink the initial diagnosis. Was there trauma? Was there pain? Was there documented instability (dislocation)? Have the complaints changed now? Was there radiographic evidence of malalignment? What was the condition of the articular surfaces at surgery? Was the correct operation performed? Are there any apparent complications of the surgical technique? Was the rehabilitation appropriate and patient enough? Be particularly careful in recommending more surgery to patients who are severely deconditioned with gross strength and flexibility deficits unless a discrete and surgically correctable condition is obvious. A gentle but persistent stretching and strengthening program within the limits of comfort is frequently needed. Beware of reflex sympathetic dysfunction in patients in whom the clinical picture does not make sense and pain appears to be out of proportion. Not always are the classic (skin, temperature, vascular) signs of reflex sympathetic dysfunction present. Diagnosis and management by an aggressive pain clinic can sometimes have dramatically positive effects.

If the previous surgery was lateral release, was the extent of release adequate? If so, patellar tilt should correct at least to neutral on physical examination. If not, one may find poor mobility and a focus of tenderness at the distal extent of the incomplete release. If the preoperative indications were correct for lateral release (pain, no instability, mild articular changes, documented tilt), completing the release may be all that is necessary. If the previous release included the vastus lateralis (determined by palpation and the operative records) and/or one suspects that there was not any preexisting malalignment, be sus-

picious of iatrogenic medial subluxation.[59] Typically, the patient feels the patella slipping laterally—which can be confusing. The event is often sudden and debilitating, worse than what the patient experienced before surgery. This is an iatrogenic complication. The examiner should remember that the patella is slipping from too far medial laterally into the central trochlea! This diagnosis, as described earlier in this chapter, is made best by physical examination. It is surprisingly common after patellofemoral surgery and is often missed! If suspected, we apply a brace capable of providing improved patellar stability, such as the Trupull (Fig. 54–27), to pull the patella laterally and then send the patient home to see whether this brace controls the problem. Reconstruction of the lateral retinaculum (undoing the last operation) is part of the solution, but one must remember to try to determine and treat the initial prelateral release complaint as well. If the patellar articular surface had areas of grade III/IV articular change, especially on the medial facet, medial release and/or anterolateralization will be indicated to unload the patella while realigning a previously overzealous medializing procedure.

Finally, if the patient had a clear preoperative diagnosis of recurrent lateral dislocation and has failed to improve after lateral release, medialization of the tibial tubercle (with anteriorization, depending on the degree of articular changes) is indicated.

Occasionally, a patient will have persistent pain after patellofemoral surgery, which can also be secondary to a neuroma. Physical examination with subsequent confirmatory diagnostic injection of local anesthetic is invaluable to confirm this diagnosis. Physical examination may also reveal foci of tendinosis in the patellar or quadriceps tendons that can respond very well to prone quadriceps stretches because prone quadriceps flexibility is often remarkably deficient in such patients. Severe articular degeneration may be manifested as gross crepitus, pain with direct compression of the patella into the trochlea, and bone scan uptake localized to the patella. Failing patient and complete nonoperative treatment, one might logically consider anteriorization (particularly if the lesion is distal), arthroplasty (particularly if the patient is elderly or inactive), or patellectomy (assuming that the patient understands the expected weakness that accompanies the pain relief). Patients who have failed previous patellofemoral surgeries often present challenging diagnostic dilemmas. Often, it seems that the best answer is no more surgery. However, when patients have symptoms consistent with objective findings, gratifying results frequently occur from surgical intervention. It is most important to listen to these patients and carefully and accurately determine the true cause of the disability.

SUMMARY

Most patients with patellofemoral disorders do not require surgery. Careful attention to the basics of restoring strength and flexibility and correcting instigating factors in the patient's history are often all it takes to treat these problems successfully. When surgery is necessary, meticulous history and physical examination are invaluable. Diagnoses of malalignment should be documented radiographically before surgical realignment. Be patient during rehabilitation of deconditioned patients after patellofemoral surgery. As long as the clinician is careful to precisely define the indications for patellofemoral surgery, accurately perform the surgery, and rehabilitate the patient, successful results are possible in the majority of cases.

References

1. Aglietti P, Insall JN: A new patella prosthesis: Design and application. Clin Orthop 107:175, 1975.
2. Arciero RA, Toomey HE: Patellofemoral arthroplasty: A three- to nine-year follow-up study. Clin Orthop 236:60, 1988.
3. Argenson JN, Guillaume JM: Is there a place for patellofemoral arthroplasty? Clin Orthop 321:162, 1995.
4. Arroll B, Ellis-Pegler E: Patellofemoral pain syndrome: A critical review of the clinical trials on nonoperative therapy. Am J Sports Med 25:207, 1997.
5. Baker RH, Carroll N: The semitendinosus tenodesis for recurrent dislocation of the patella. J Bone Joint Surg Br 54:103, 1972.
6. Baksi DP: Restoration of dynamic stability of the patella by pes anserinus transposition: A new approach. J Bone Joint Surg Br 63:399, 1981.
7. Baksi DP: Pes anserinus transposition for patellar dislocations: Long-term follow-up results. J Bone Joint Surg Br 75:305, 1993.
8. Bandi W: [Chondromalacia patellae and femoro-patellar arthrosis, etiology, clinical aspects and therapy.] Helv Chir Acta 39:1, 1972.
9. Bellemans J, Cauwenberghs F: Anteromedial tibial tubercle transfer in patients with chronic anterior knee pain and a subluxation-type patellar malalignment. Am J Sports Med 25:375, 1997.
10. Betz RR, Magill JTD: The percutaneous lateral retinacular release. Am J Sports Med 15:477, 1987.
11. Bigos SJ, McBride GG: The isolated lateral retinacular release in the treatment of patellofemoral disorders. Clin Orthop 186:75, 1984.
12. Blackburne JS, Peel TE: A new method of measuring patellar height. J Bone Joint Surg Br 59:241, 1977.
13. Blazina ME: Patellofemoral replacement utilizing a customized femoral groove replacement. Tech Orthop 5:53, 1990.
14. Blazina ME, Fox JM: Patellofemoral replacement. Clin Orthop 144:98, 1979.
15. Bonamo JJ, Fay C: The conservative treatment of the anterior cruciate deficient knee. Am J Sports Med 18:618, 1990.
16. Bowker JH, Thompson EB: Surgical management of recurrent dislocation of the patella. J Bone Joint Surg Am 46:1451, 1964.
17. Bray RC, Roth JH: Arthroscopic lateral release for anterior knee pain: A study comparing patients who are claiming worker's compensation with those who are not. Arthroscopy 3:237, 1987.
18. Brody LT, Thein JM: Nonoperative treatment for patellofemoral pain. J Orthop Sports Phys Ther 28:336, 1998.
19. Brooke R: The treatment of fractured patella by excision: A study of morphology and function. Br J Surg 24:733, 1937.
20. Broom MJ, Fulkerson JP: The plica syndrome: A new perspective. Orthop Clin North Am 17:279, 1986.
21. Brown DE, Alexander AH: The Elmslie-Trillat procedure: Evaluation in patellar dislocation and subluxation. Am J Sports Med 12:104, 1984.
22. Burke DL, Ahmed AM: The effect of tibial tubercle elevation on patello-femoral loading. Trans Orthop Res Soc 5:162, 1980.
23. Buss DD, Min R: Nonoperative treatment of acute anterior cruciate ligament injuries in a selected group of patients. Am J Sports Med 23:160, 1995.
24. Buuck D, Fulkerson J: Anteromedialization of the tibial tubercle: A 4-12 year follow up. Op Tech Sports Med 8:131, 2000.
25. Cartier P, Sanouiller JL: Patellofemoral arthroplasty: Two 12-year follow-up studies. J Arthroplasty 5:49, 1990.
26. Casscells SW: The arthroscope in the diagnosis of disorders of the patellofemoral joint. Clin Orthop 144:45, 1979.
27. Ceder LC, Larson RL: Z-plasty lateral retinacular release for the treatment of patellar compression syndrome. Clin Orthop 144:110, 1979.
28. Chambat P, Dejour H: [Transpositions of the anterior tibial tuberosity with a follow-up for more than 10 years.] Rev Chir Orthop Reparatrice Appar Mot 66:222, 1980.
29. Chrisman OD, Snook GA: A long-term prospective study of the Hauser and Roux-Goldthwait procedures for recurrent patellar dislocation. Clin Orthop 144:27, 1979.
30. Christensen F, Soballe K: Treatment of chondromalacia patellae by lateral retinacular release of the patella. Clin Orthop 234:145, 1988.
31. Cox JS: An evaluation of the Elmslie-Trillat procedure for management of patellar dislocations and subluxations: A preliminary report. Am J Sports Med 4:72, 1976.
32. Cox JS: Evaluation of the Roux-Elmslie-Trillat procedure for knee extensor realignment. Am J Sports Med 10:303, 1982.
33. Crosby EB, Insall J: Recurrent dislocation of the patella: Relation of treatment to osteoarthritis. J Bone Joint Surg Am 58:9, 1976.
34. Dandy DJ, Desai SS: The results of arthroscopic lateral release of the extensor mechanism for recurrent dislocation of the patella after 8 years. Arthroscopy 10:540, 1994.
35. DeCesare WF: Late results of Hauser procedure for recurrent dislocation of the patella. Clin Orthop 140:137, 1979.
36. Dehaven KE, Dolan WA: Chondromalacia patellae in athletes: Clinical presentation and conservative management. Am J Sports Med 7:5, 1979.
37. Delgado-Martins H: A study of the position of the patella using computerized tomography. J Bone Joint Surg Br 61:443, 1979.
38. Depalma AF, Flynn JJ: Joint changes following experimental partial and total patellectomy. J Bone Joint Surg Am 40:395, 1958.
39. Derwin KA, Glover RA: Nociceptive role of substance-P in the knee joint of a patient with congenital insensitivity to pain. J Pediatr Orthop 14:258, 1994.
40. Desio SM, Burks RT: Soft tissue restraints to lateral patellar translation in the human knee. Am J Sports Med 26:59, 1998.
41. Dougherty J, Wirth CR: Management of patellar subluxation: A modification of Hauser's technique. Clin Orthop 115:204, 1976.
42. Dupont JY: Synovial plicae of the knee: Controversies and review. Clin Sports Med 16:87, 1997.
43. Dye SF: The knee as a biologic transmission with an envelope of function: A theory. Clin Orthop 325:10, 1996.
44. Dye SF, Vaupel GL: Conscious neurosensory mapping of the internal structures of the human knee without intraarticular anesthesia. Am J Sports Med 26:773, 1998.

45. Dzioba RB: Diagnostic arthroscopy and longitudinal open lateral release: A four-year follow-up study to determine predictors of surgical outcome. Am J Sports Med 18:343, 1990.

46. Dzioba RB, Strokon A: Diagnostic arthroscopy and longitudinal open lateral release: A safe and effective treatment for "chondromalacia patellae." Arthroscopy 1:131, 1985.

47. Engebretsen L, Svenningsen S: Advancement of the tibial tuberosity for patellar pain: A 5-year follow-up. Acta Orthop Scand 60:20, 1989.

48. Federico DJ, Reider B: Results of isolated patellar debridement for patellofemoral pain in patients with normal patellar alignment. Am J Sports Med 25:663, 1997.

49. Ferguson AB Jr: Elevation of the insertion of the patellar ligament for patellofemoral pain. J Bone Joint Surg Am 64:766, 1982.

50. Ferguson AB Jr, Brown TD: Relief of patellofemoral contact stress by anterior displacement of the tibial tubercle. J Bone Joint Surg Am 61:159, 1979.

51. Ferrandez L, Usabiaga J: An experimental study of the redistribution of patellofemoral pressures by the anterior displacement of the anterior tuberosity of the tibia. Clin Orthop 238:183, 1989.

52. Fielding JW, Liebler WA: Tibial tubercle transfer: A long-range follow-up study. Clin Orthop 144:43, 1979.

53. Fithian D, Meier S: The case for advancement and repair of the MPFL in patients with recurrent patella instability. Op Tech Sports Med 7:81, 1999.

54. Fondren FB, Goldner JL: Recurrent dislocation of the patella treated by the modified Roux-Goldthwait procedure: A prospective study of forty-seven knees. J Bone Joint Surg Am 67:993, 1985.

55. Ford DH, Post WR: Open or arthroscopic lateral release: Indications, techniques, and rehabilitation. Clin Sports Med 16:29, 1997.

56. Fulkerson JP: Awareness of the retinaculum in evaluating patellofemoral pain. Am J Sports Med 10:147, 1982.

57. Fulkerson JP: Anteromedialization of the tibial tuberosity for patellofemoral malalignment. Clin Orthop 177:176, 1983.

58. Fulkerson JP: Evaluation of the peripatellar soft tissues and retinaculum in patients with patellofemoral pain. Clin Sports Med 8:197, 1989.

59. Fulkerson JP: A clinical test for medial patella tracking (medial subluxation). Tech Orthop 12:144, 1997.

60. Fulkerson JP, Becker GJ: Anteromedial tibial tubercle transfer without bone graft. Am J Sports Med 18:490, discussion, 496, 1990.

61. Fulkerson JP, Schutzer SF: Computerized tomography of the patellofemoral joint before and after lateral release or realignment. Arthroscopy 3:19, 1987.

62. Fulkerson JP, Shea KP: Disorders of patellofemoral alignment. J Bone Joint Surg Am 72:1424, 1990.

63. Fulkerson JP, Tennant R: Histologic evidence of retinacular nerve injury associated with patellofemoral malalignment. Clin Orthop 197:196, 1985.

64. Garr EL, Moskowitz RW: Degenerative changes following experimental patellectomy in the rabbit. Clin Orthop 92:296, 1973.

65. Geckeler EO, Quarantam AV: Patellectomy for degenerative arthritis of the knee. J Bone Joint Surg Am 44:1109, 1962.

66. Goodman M, Steinberg M: Primary undifferentiated sarcoma of the patella. Orthop Rev 11:85, 1982.

67. Grana WA, Hinkley B: Arthroscopic evaluation and treatment of patellar malalignment. Clin Orthop 186:122, 1984.

68. Grana WA, O'Donoghue DH: Patellar-tendon transfer by the slot-block method for recurrent subluxation and dislocation of the patella. J Bone Joint Surg Am 59:736, 1977.

69. Hadjari MH, McClish LR: Arthroscopic measurement of the patellofemoral articulation angle. Arthroscopy 7:326, 1991.

70. Hall JE, Micheli LJ: Semitendinosus tenodesis for recurrent subluxation or dislocation of the patella. Clin Orthop 144:31, 1979.

71. Hallisey MJ, Doherty N: Anatomy of the junction of the vastus lateralis tendon and the patella. J Bone Joint Surg Am 69:545, 1987.

72. Hampson WGJ, Hill P: Late results of transfer of the tibial tubercle for recurrent dislocation of the patella. J Bone Joint Surg Am 57:209, 1975.

73. Hardaker WT, Whipple TL: Diagnosis and treatment of the plica syndrome of the knee. J Bone Joint Surg Am 62:221, 1980.

74. Harrison MHM: The results of a realignment operation for recurrent dislocation of the patella. J Bone Joint Surg Br 37:559, 1955.

75. Harwin SF, Stern RE: Subcutaneous lateral retinacular release for chondromalacia patellae: A preliminary report. Clin Orthop 156:207, 1981.

76. Hauser EW: Total tendon transplant for slipping patella. Surg Gynecol Obstet 66:199, 1938.

77. Haxton H: The function of the patella and the effects of its excision. Surg Gynecol Obstet 80:389, 1945.

78. Heatley FW, Allen PR: Tibial tubercle advancement for anterior knee pain: A temporary or permanent solution. Clin Orthop 208:215, 1986.

79. Hejgaard N, Arnoldi CC: Osteotomy of the patella in the patellofemoral pain syndrome: The significance of increased intraosseous pressure during sustained knee flexion. Int Orthop 8:189, 1984.

80. Heller L, Hadjipavlou A: Chondromalacia of the patella treated by the Maquet tibial osteotomy. J Bone Joint Surg Br 64:262, 1982.

81. Henry JH, Crosland JW: Conservative treatment of patellofemoral subluxation. Am J Sports Med 7:12, 1979.

82. Henry JH, Goletz TH: Lateral retinacular release in patellofemoral subluxation: Indications, results, and comparison to open patellofemoral reconstruction. Am J Sports Med 14:121, 1986.

83. Heywood AWB: Recurrent dislocation of the patella. J Bone Joint Surg Br 43:508, 1961.

84. Hille E, Schulitz KP: Pressure and contact-surface measurements within the femoropatellar joint and their variations following lateral release. Arch Orthop Trauma Surg 104:275, 1985.

85. Hirsh DM, Reddy DK: Experience with Maquet anterior tibial tubercle advancement for patellofemoral arthralgia. Clin Orthop 148:136, 1980.

86. Huberti HH, Hayes WC: Contact pressures in chondromalacia patellae and the effects of capsular reconstructive procedures. J Orthop Res 6:499, 1988.

87. Hughston J: Patellar Subluxation and Dislocation. Philadelphia, WB Saunders, 1984.

88. Hughston JC, Deese M: Medial subluxation of the patella as a complication of lateral retinacular release. Am J Sports Med 16:383, 1988.

89. Hughston JC, Flandry F: Surgical correction of medial subluxation of the patella. Am J Sports Med 24:486, 1996.

90. Hughston JC, Walsh WM: Proximal and distal reconstruction of the extensor mechanism for patellar subluxation. Clin Orthop 144:36, 1979.

91. Insall J, Bullough PG: Proximal "tube" realignment of the patella for chondromalacia patellae. Clin Orthop 144:63, 1979.

92. Insall J, Falvo KA: Chondromalacia patellae: A prospective study. J Bone Joint Surg Am 58:1, 1976.

93. Insall J, Salvati E: Patella position in the normal knee joint. Radiology 101:101, 1971.

94. Insall J, Tria AJ: Resurfacing of the patella. J Bone Joint Surg Am 62:933, 1980.

95. Jackson RW, Kunkel SS: Lateral retinacular release for patellofemoral pain in the older patient. Arthroscopy 7:283, 1991.

96. Jackson RW, Marshall DJ: The pathologic medical shelf. Orthop Clin North Am 13:307, 1982.

97. Jenny JY, Sader Z: Elevation of the tibial tubercle for patellofemoral pain syndrome: An 8- to 15-year follow-up. Knee Surg Sports Traumatol Arthrosc 4:92, 1996.

98. Jerre T, Knutsson B: Late results of transposition of the tibial tubercle in recurrent dislocation of the patella. Acta Orthop Scand 27:141, 1956.

99. Johnson LL, van Dyk GE: Clinical assessment of asymptomatic knees: Comparison of men and women. Arthroscopy 14:347, 1998.

100. Johnson RP: Lateral facet syndrome of the patella. Lateral restraint analysis and use of lateral resection. Clin Orthop 238:148, 1989.

101. Jones RB, Barlett EC: CT determination of tibial tubercle lateralization in patients presenting with anterior knee pain. Skeletal Radiol 24:505, 1995.

102. Juliusson R, Markhede G: A modified Hauser procedure for recurrent dislocation of the patella: A long-term follow-up study with special reference to osteoarthritis. Arch Orthop Trauma Surg 103:42, 1984.

103. Karlsson J, Kalebo P: Partial rupture of the patellar ligament. Am J Sports Med 20:390, 1992.

104. Karlsson J, Lundin O: Partial rupture of the patellar ligament. Results after operative treatment. Am J Sports Med 19:403, 1991.

105. Kaufer H: Mechanical function of the patella. J Bone Joint Surg Am 53:1551, 1971.

106. Keller PM, Shelbourne KD: Nonoperatively treated isolated posterior cruciate ligament injuries. Am J Sports Med 21:132, 1993.

107. Kelly MA, Insall JN: Patellectomy. Orthop Clin North Am 17:289, 1986.

108. Kolowich PA, Paulos LE: Lateral release of the patella: Indications and contraindications. Am J Sports Med 18:359, 1990.

109. Krajca-Radcliffe JB, Coker TP: Patellofemoral arthroplasty: A 2- to 18-year followup study. Clin Orthop 330:143, 1996.

110. Krompinger WJ, Fulkerson JP: Lateral retinacular release for intractable lateral retinacular pain. Clin Orthop 179:191, 1983.

111. Kujala UM, Kormano OK: Patellofemoral relationships in recurrent patellar dislocation. J Bone Joint Surg Br 71:788, 1979.

112. Lankenner PA Jr, Micheli LJ: Arthroscopic percutaneous lateral patellar retinacular release. Am J Sports Med 14:267, 1986.

113. Larson RL, Cabaud HE: The patellar compression syndrome: Surgical treatment by lateral retinacular release. Clin Orthop 134:158, 1978.

114. Laurin CA, Dussault R: The tangential x-ray investigation of the patellofemoral joint: X-ray technique, diagnostic criteria and their interpretation. Clin Orthop 144:16, 1979.

115. Levitt RL: A long-term evaluation of patellar prostheses. Clin Orthop 97:153, 1973.

116. Lewallen DG, Riegger CL: Effects of retinacular release and tibial tubercle elevation in patellofemoral degenerative joint disease. J Orthop Res 8:856, 1990.

117. Lewis MM, Fitzgerald PF: Patellectomy: An analysis of one hundred cases. J Bone Joint Surg Am 58:736, 1976.

118. Lieb FJ, Perry J: Quadriceps function. An anatomical and mechanical study using amputated limbs. J Bone Joint Surg Am 50:1535, 1968.

119. Lieb FJ, Perry J: Quadriceps function. An electromyographic study under isometric conditions. J Bone Joint Surg Am 53:749, 1971.

120. Macnab I: Recurrent dislocation of the patella. J Bone Joint Surg Am 34:957, 1952.

121. Maquet P: Advancement of the tibial tuberosity. Clin Orthop 115:225, 1976.

122. Maquet P: Mechanics and osteoarthritis of the patellofemoral joint. Clin Orthop 144:70, 1979.

123. Mariani PP, Caruso I: An electromyographic investigation of subluxation of the patella. J Bone Joint Surg Br 61:169, 1979.

124. Martens M, De Rycke J: Facetectomy of the patella in patellofemoral osteoarthritis. Acta Orthop Belg 56:563, 1990.

125. Marumoto JM, Jordan C: A biomechanical comparison of lateral retinacular releases. Am J Sports Med 23:151, 1995.

126. McConnell J: The management of chondromalacia patellae: A long-term solution. Aust J Phys 32:215, 1986.

127. McGinty JB, McCarthy JC: Endoscopic lateral retinacular release: A preliminary report. Clin Orthop 158:120, 1981.

128. McKeever DC: Patellar prosthesis. J Bone Joint Surg Am 37:1074, 1955.

129. Mendes DG, Soudry M: Clinical assessment of Maquet tibial tuberosity advancement. Clin Orthop 222:228, 1987.

130. Merchant AC, Mercer RL: Lateral release of the patella: A preliminary report. Clin Orthop 103:40, 1974.

131. Merchant AC, Mercer RL: Roentgenographic analysis of patellofemoral congruence. J Bone Joint Surg Am 56:1391, 1974.

132. Metcalf RW: An arthroscopic method for lateral release of subluxating or dislocating patella. Clin Orthop 167:9, 1982.

133. Micheli LJ, Stanitski CL: Lateral patellar retinacular release. Am J Sports Med 9:330, 1981.

134. Miller BJ, LaRochelle PJ: The treatment of patellofemoral pain by combined rotation and elevation of the tibial tubercle. J Bone Joint Surg Am 68:419, 1986.

135. Morscher E: Osteotomy of the patella in chondromalacia: Preliminary report. Arch Orthop Trauma Surg 92:139, 1978.

136. Morshuis WJ, Pavlov PW: Anteromedialization of the tibial tuberosity in the treatment of patellofemoral pain and malalignment. Clin Orthop 255:242, 1990.

137. Muneta T, Yamamoto H: Computerized tomographic analysis of tibial tubercle position in the painful female patellofemoral joint. Am J Sports Med 22:67, 1994.

138. Nagamine R, Miura H: Malposition of the tibial tubercle during flexion in knees with patellofemoral arthritis. Skeletal Radiol 26:597, 1997.

139. Nakamura N, Ellis M: Advancement of the tibial tuberosity: A biomechanical study. J Bone Joint Surg Br 67:255, 1985.

140. Natri A, Kannus P: Which factors predict the long-term outcome in chronic patellofemoral pain syndrome? A 7-year prospective follow-up study. Med Sci Sports Exerc 30:1572, 1998.

141. Noll BJ, Ben-Itzhak I: Modified technique for tibial tubercle elevation with realignment for patellofemoral pain. A preliminary report. Clin Orthop 234:178, 1988.

142. Nonweiler DE, DeLee JC: The diagnosis and treatment of medial subluxation of the patella after lateral retinacular release. Am J Sports Med 22:680, 1994.

143. O'Donaghue DH: Facetectomy. South Med J 65:642, 1972.

144. Ogilvie-Harris DJ, Jackson RW: The arthroscopic treatment of chondromalacia patellae. J Bone Joint Surg Br 66:660, 1984.

145. O'Neill DB: Open lateral retinacular lengthening compared with arthroscopic release: A prospective, randomized outcome study. J Bone Joint Surg Am 79:1759, 1997.

146. Osborne AH, Fulford PC: Lateral release for chondromalacia patellae. J Bone Joint Surg Br 64:202, 1982.

147. Pan HQ, Kish V: The Maquet procedure: Effect of tibial shingle length on patellofemoral pressures. J Orthop Res 11:199, 1993.

148. Pickett JC, Stoll DA: Patellaplasty or patellectomy? Clin Orthop 144:103, 1979.

149. Pidoriano AJ, Weinstein RN: Correlation of patellar articular lesions with results from anteromedial tibial tubercle transfer. Am J Sports Med 25:533, 1997.

150. Popp JE, Yu JS: Recalcitrant patellar tendinitis: Magnetic resonance imaging, histologic evaluation, and surgical treatment. Am J Sports Med 25:218, 1997.

151. Post WR: Diagnosis and treatment of patients after failed patellofemoral surgery. In Marder R, Zarins B (eds): Revision of Failed Arthroscopic and Ligament Surgery. Boston, Blackwell Scientific, 1988.

152. Post WR: History and physical examination of patients with patellofemoral disorders. In Fulkerson JP (ed): Disorders of the Patellofemoral Joint. Baltimore, Williams & Wilkins, 1997.

153. Post WR: Lateral retinacular release: Arthroscopic and open techniques. Tech Orthop 12:145, 1997.

154. Post WR, Fulkerson J: Knee pain diagrams: Correlation with physical examination findings in patients with anterior knee pain. Arthroscopy 10:618, 1994.

155. Powers CM: Rehabilitation of patellofemoral joint disorders: A critical review. J Orthop Sports Phys Ther 28:345, 1998.

156. Radin EL: A rational approach to the treatment of patellofemoral pain. Clin Orthop 144:107, 1979.

157. Radin EL: The Maquet procedure—anterior displacement of the tibial tubercle: Indications, contraindications, and precautions. Clin Orthop 213:241, 1986.

158. Radin EL: Anterior tibial tubercle elevation in the young adult. Orthop Clin North Am 17:297, 1986.

159. Radin EL, Labosky D: Avoiding complications with the Maquet procedure. Complications Orthop 48, 1987.

160. Rantanen J, Paananen M: Modified Hauser operation for patellar instability: Immediate mobilization of 35 knees: A 5-8-year follow-up study. Acta Orthop Scand 67:455, 1996.

161. Reider B, Marshall JL: Patellar tracking. Clin Orthop 157:143, 1981.

162. Rillmann P, Dutly A: Modified Elmslie-Trillat procedure for instability of the patella. Knee Surg Sports Traumatol Arthrosc 6:31, 1998.

163. Rovere GD, Adair DM: Medial synovial shelf plica syndrome: Treatment by intraplical steroid injection. Am J Sports Med 13: 382, 1985.

164. Rozbruch JD, Campbell RD: Tibial tubercle elevation (the Maquet operation). Orthop Trans 3:291, 1979.

165. Sacks S: Semipatellectomy: An operation for chondromalacia of the knee joint. S Afr Med J 36:518, 1962.

166. Sanchis-Alfonso V, Rosello-Sastre E: Quantitative analysis of nerve changes in the lateral retinaculum in patients with isolated symptomatic patellofemoral malalignment: A preliminary study. Am J Sports Med 26:703, 1998.

167. Schmid F: The Maquet procedure in the treatment of patellofemoral osteoarthrosis: Long-term results. Clin Orthop 294:254, 1993.

168. Schneider T, Fink B: Hemarthrosis as a major complication after arthroscopic subcutaneous lateral retinacular release: A prospective study. Am J Knee Surg 11:95, 1998.

169. Schonholtz GJ, Zahn MG: Lateral retinacular release of the patella. Arthroscopy 3:269, 1987.

170. Schreiber SN: Proximal superomedial portal in arthroscopy of the knee. Arthroscopy 7:246, 1991.

171. Schutzer SF, Ramsby GR: Computed tomographic classification of patellofemoral pain patients. Orthop Clin North Am 17:235, 1986.

172. Schutzer SF, Ramsby GR: The evaluation of patellofemoral pain using computerized tomography: A preliminary study. Clin Orthop 204:286, 1986.

173. Scuderi G, Cuomo F: Lateral release and proximal realignment for patellar subluxation and dislocation: A long-term follow-up. J Bone Joint Surg Am 70:856, 1988.

174. Shapiro GS, Fanton GS: Lateral retinacular release: The holmium:YAG laser versus electrocautery. Clin Orthop 310:42, 1995.

175. Shea KP, Fulkerson JP: Preoperative computed tomography scanning and arthroscopy in predicting outcome after lateral retinacular release. Arthroscopy 8:327, 1992.

176. Shelbourne KD, Porter DA: Use of a modified Elmslie-Trillat procedure to improve abnormal patellar congruence angle. Am J Sports Med 22:318, 1994.

177. Shellock FG, Mink JH: Evaluation of patients with persistent symptoms after lateral retinacular release by kinematic magnetic resonance imaging of the patellofemoral joint. Arthroscopy 6:226, 1990.

178. Sherman OH, Fox JM: Patellar instability: Treatment by arthroscopic electrosurgical lateral release. Arthroscopy 3:152, 1987.

179. Silvello L, Scarponi R: Tibial tubercle advancement by the Maquet technique for patellofemoral arthritis or chondromalacia. Ital J Orthop Traumatol 13:37, 1987.

180. Simpson LA, Barrett JP Jr: Factors associated with poor results following arthroscopic subcutaneous lateral retinacular release. Clin Orthop 186:165, 1984.

181. Sojbjerg JO, Lauritzen J: Arthroscopic determination of patellofemoral malalignment. Clin Orthop 215:243, 1987.

182. Stanish WD, Curwin S: Tendinitis: The analysis and treatment for running. Clin Sports Med 4:593, 1985.

183. Stanish WD, Rubinovich RM: Eccentric exercise in chronic tendinitis. Clin Orthop 208:65, 1986.

184. Stetson WB, Friedman MJ: Fracture of the proximal tibia with immediate weightbearing after a Fulkerson osteotomy. Am J Sports Med 25:570, 1997.

185. Steurer PA Jr, Gradisar IA Jr: Patellectomy: A clinical study and biomechanical evaluation. Clin Orthop 144:84, 1979.

186. Stougard J: Patellectomy. Acta Orthop Scand 41:110, 1970.

187. Sutton FS Jr, Thompson CH: The effect of patellectomy on knee function. J Bone Joint Surg Am 58:537, 1976.

188. Tomatsu T, Imai N: Simplification of the Elmslie-Trillat procedure for patellofemoral malalignment: Is medial capsulorrhaphy necessary? Int Orthop 20:211, 1996.

189. Vaatainen U, Kiviranta I: Lateral release in chondromalacia patellae using clinical, radiologic, electromyographic, and muscle force testing evaluation. Arch Phys Med Rehabil 75:1127, 1994.

190. Vaughan-Lane T, Dandy DJ: The synovial shelf syndrome. J Bone Joint Surg Br 64:475, 1982.

191. Verheyden F, Geens G: Jumper's knee: Results of surgical treatment. Acta Orthop Belg 63:102, 1997.

192. Wall JJ: Neurovascular complications of the Hauser procedure. Orthop Trans 3:291, 1979.

193. Wendt PP, Johnson RP: A study of quadriceps excursion, torque, and the effect of patellectomy on cadaver knees. J Bone Joint Surg Am 67:726, 1985.

194. Willner P: Recurrent dislocation of the patella. Clin Orthop 69:23, 1970.

195. Winter DA: Energy generation and absorption at the ankle and knee during fast, natural, and slow cadences. Clin Orthop 175:147, 1983.

196. Wojtys EM, Beaman DN: Innervation of the human knee joint by substance-P fibers. Arthroscopy 6:254, 1990.

197. Worrell RV: Prosthetic resurfacing of the patella. Clin Orthop 144:91, 1979.

198. Worrell RV: Resurfacing of the patella in young patients. Orthop Clin North Am 17:303, 1986.

CHAPTER 55

Quadriceps and Patellar Tendon Disruption*

Christopher M. Farrell • Giles R. Scuderi • Mark E. Easley

ANATOMY

The extensor mechanism of the knee consists of the quadriceps musculature, the quadriceps tendon, the patella, and the patellar tendon. The quadriceps musculature is composed of the rectus femoris, the vastus medialis, the vastus lateralis, and the vastus intermedius, which coalesce in a trilaminar fashion to form the quadriceps tendon. The direct head of the rectus femoris takes origin from the anterior inferior iliac spine and the indirect head from the anterior hip capsule. These muscle heads unite distally and form the rectus femoris muscle, the most superficial component of the quadriceps musculature. The muscle bodies narrow to a tendon approximately 3 to 5 cm superior to the patella. The fibers of the quadriceps tendon continue over the anterior surface of the patella and into the patellar tendon. The vastus medialis is divided into two groups: the vastus medialis obliquus and the vastus medialis longus. The muscle fibers of the vastus medialis continue toward the superomedial border of the patella and become tendinous a few millimeters before their insertion. The muscle fibers of the vastus lateralis terminate more proximally than those of the vastus medialis and become tendinous approximately 3 cm from the superolateral border of the patella. The vastus intermedius lies deep to the other three muscles, and its tendinous fibers insert directly into the superior border of the patella and blend medially and laterally with the vastus medialis and vastus lateralis. Aponeurotic fibers from both the vastus lateralis and vastus medialis contribute to the lateral and medial retinaculum.

The patellar tendon is primarily derived from the central fibers of the rectus femoris, which extend over the anterior surface of the patella and form a flat tendinous structure that inserts into the tibial tubercle. It continues past the tubercle and blends with the iliotibial band on the anterolateral surface of the tibia. The average length of the patellar tendon is 4.6 cm (range, 3.5 to 5.5).[96]

ETIOLOGY OF EXTENSOR MECHANISM DISRUPTION

Experimental studies have shown that a normal tendon will not rupture when a longitudinal stress is applied, but rather the disruption will occur at the musculotendinous junction, the muscle belly, or the tendinous insertion into the bone. It has been shown that the normal quadriceps tendon may be able to tolerate up to 30 kg/mm of longitudinal stress before failing. Patellar and quadriceps tendon ruptures therefore occur through a pathological area of the tendon. The estimated force required to disrupt the extensor mechanism of the knee is 17.5 times body weight and usually occurs during a sudden eccentric contraction of the extensor mechanism with the foot planted and the knee flexed as the person falls. With this in mind, many pathological conditions can affect the extensor mechanism, including renal disease, diabetes mellitus, hyperparathyroidism, rheumatoid arthritis, systemic lupus erythematosus, gout, osteomalacia, infection, obesity, steroid use,[61,75] and other metabolic diseases. These metabolic diseases cause microscopic damage to the vascular supply to the tendons or alter the architecture of the tendon. Diabetes has been shown to cause arteriosclerotic changes in the tendon vessels, whereas chronic synovitis causes fibrinoid reactions within the tendon. Muscle fiber atrophy secondary to renal disease and uremia will also weaken the tendon. Pathological changes from advancing age include fatty and cystic degeneration, myxoid degeneration, and calcification, all of which alter tendon architecture. Bone resorption and osteopenia can also occur at the osteotendinous junction with advancing age. A report of spontaneous patellar tendon rupture in identical twins further supports the concept that predisposing factors for extensor mechanism rupture exist.[34] Although quadriceps tendon rupture tends to occur in older patients or those with systemic disease or degenerative changes, patellar tendon rupture or avulsion is more common in patients younger than 40 years.[53,107] Most spontaneous ruptures of the quadriceps tendon occur within 2 cm of the patella through the pathological areas mentioned earlier. Numerous cases of bilateral extensor mechanism rupture have been reported. Although the majority of ruptures occur in patients with predisposing conditions such as obesity, systemic illness,*

*Modified from Scuderi GR, Easley: Quadriceps and patellar tendon disruptions. In Insall JN, Scott WN (eds): Surgery of the Knee, vol 1. New York, Churchill Livingstone, 2001, pp 1074-1086.

*References 1, 5, 35, 41, 49, 57, 62, 64, 66, 88, 95, 98, 100, 109, 111.

and use of anabolic steroids,[61] several authors have reported simultaneous bilateral extensor mechanism rupture in healthy patients without predisposing factors.[12,14,34,36,53,66,79,83,106,113] In a retrospective review of bilateral and unilateral quadriceps tendon rupture, Konrath and associates noted a significant correlation between bilateral simultaneous rupture and systemic disease.[51]

Iatrogenic conditions that may alter the local properties of the extensor mechanism include total knee arthroplasty (TKA),[63] lateral retinacular release,[7,23,104] and harvesting of the central third of the patellar tendon for ligament reconstruction.[8,54,67] Local steroid injection has likewise been implicated as a cause of tendon rupture. Rupture of the quadriceps tendon has also been reported after patellar dislocation.[81]

Disruption of the extensor mechanism is a significant disabling injury and should be diagnosed early.[91,103] Patients usually have an acute onset of knee pain, swelling, and loss of function after a stumble or fall. The physical examination generally reveals a palpable defect in the quadriceps tendon with a low-lying patella. When asked to perform a straight-leg raise, the patient may be unable to do so or will demonstrate an extensor lag. A patellar tendon rupture has similar findings; however, the palpable gap is in the patellar tendon with a proximally retracted patella.

Although extensor mechanism disruptions are typically diagnosed from the history and physical examination, imaging studies often prove useful in confirming the diagnosis of quadriceps and patellar tendon tears or differentiating complete from incomplete tears.[90] Radiographs provide supporting information, especially on the lateral view. A low position of the patella and disruption of the quadriceps tendon shadow are associated with quadriceps tendon rupture (Fig. 55–1), whereas a high patella position and disruption of the patellar tendon shadow are associated with patellar tendon rupture.[42,47,80] Despite relatively obvious findings on physical examination and standard radiographs, delay in diagnosis of exten-

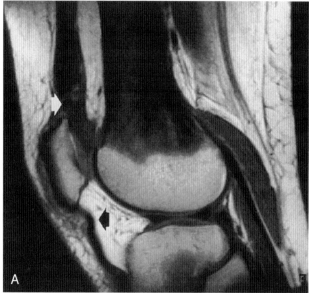

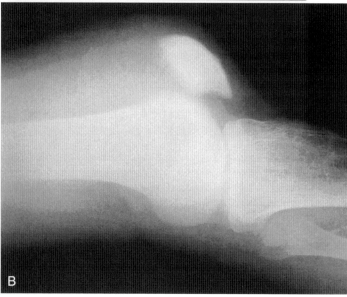

Figure 55–1. **A,** Magnetic resonance image of a torn quadriceps tendon (*white arrow*). Note the laxity of the patella tendon (*black arrow*). **B,** Radiograph showing the low position of the patella associated with quadriceps tendon rupture. This patient has chronic renal failure and hyperparathyroidism. (From Scott WN [ed]: The Knee, vol 1. St Louis, Mosby–Year Book, 1994, p 470.)

sor mechanism rupture still occurs.[60,70,99,107] Several diagnostic imaging modalities may be used in addition to standard radiographs to confirm the diagnosis, including arthrography, ultrasound, and magnetic resonance imaging (MRI). Before the advent of MRI, arthrography was widely used. In the presence of an extensor mechanism tendon rupture, extravasation of radiopaque dye into the defect occurs.[2] Today, however, arthrography has been largely replaced by noninvasive methods such as ultrasound and, more commonly, MRI for evaluation of this problem. High-resolution ultrasonography[6,19,20,59,66,88] may reveal a hypoechogenicity across the entire thickness of the tendon with an acute rupture or tendon thickening and alteration of the normal echo signal with chronic tears. Advantages of ultrasonography include collection of images in real time without exposure to ionizing radiation and relatively limited expense. However, operation of the ultrasound equipment plus interpretation of the images requires the skills of a highly trained and experienced technician and radiologist. Hence, the reliability is highly operator dependent. MRI is the imaging study of choice if the diagnosis cannot be established from the clinical and radiographic examination alone.[8,23,105,108,112] In addition, MRI may be useful to identify other problems within the knee.[116]

QUADRICEPS TENDON RUPTURE

Quadriceps tendon rupture may be complete or incomplete. Whereas incomplete tears may be treated nonoperatively, complete tears are best treated with surgery. These ruptures usually occur at the osteotendinous junction or through an area of degenerative tendon. The rupture originates in the tendon of the rectus femoris, often extending into the vastus intermedius tendon or transversely into the medial and lateral retinacula.

Overview of Surgical Management

Numerous techniques have been described in the literature for repair of acute and chronic rupture of the quadriceps tendon.[18,38,46,55,59,85,89,107] Over the years the repair techniques have progressed from simple suture with catgut or silk[69] to wire-reinforced repairs, suture anchors,[97] autografts,[33] xenografts, allografts, and the use of synthetic material.[31,76] McLaughlin[71-73] has even recommended a two-stage procedure with traction for better approximation of the tendon. With an acute intrasubstance rupture, direct repair may be performed. A straight midline incision will expose the quadriceps tendon rupture, which is then irrigated of hematoma. The tendon edges are débrided and cut fresh to normal-appearing tendon. If there is sufficient tendon proximally and distally, an end-to-end repair is performed with multiple interrupted No. 2 nonabsorbable sutures, and the retinaculum is repaired with multiple interrupted No. 0 absorbable sutures. Once the repair is complete, careful assessment of patellar rotation and tracking should be performed. The knee is then

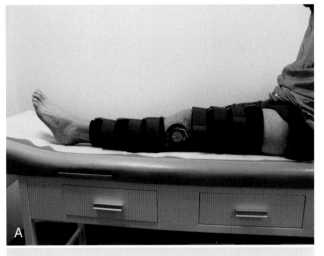
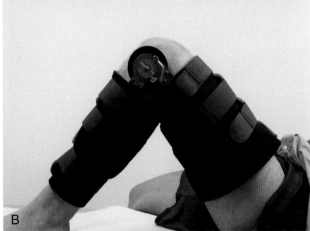

Figure 55–2. A control-dial hinged-knee orthosis with a drop lock to keep the knee in extension (**A**) during early ambulation and allow flexion when exercising (**B**). (Courtesy of Breg, Inc., Vista, CA.)

extended and the repair may be protected with a cerclage wire or nonabsorbable suture. The wound is closed in layers and the leg placed in a cylinder cast for 6 weeks. When the cast is removed, a control-dial hinged-knee orthosis (Fig. 55–2) is used so that flexion can be gradually increased. The brace is discontinued when greater than 90 degrees of flexion has been achieved and quadriceps strength is sufficient to support the limb.

Acute Disruption

When the rupture occurs at the osteotendinous junction, we prefer to repair the tendon with transosseous sutures (Fig. 55–3). The MRI and repair technique is illustrated in the sequence of photos in Figure 55–4. A straight midline incision will expose the quadriceps tendon rupture (Fig. 55–4C). The hematoma is evacuated (Fig. 55–4D), the proximal end of the rectus femoris and vastus intermedius tendon is cut fresh to normal tendon, and the superior pole of the patella is débrided of residual tendon

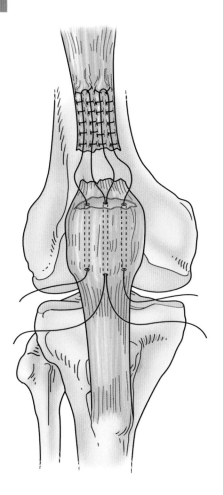

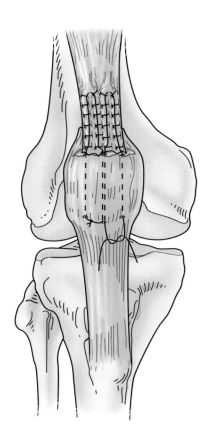

Figure 55–3. Acute repair of the quadriceps tendon into a bony trough. (Redrawn from Scott WN [ed]: The Knee, vol 1. St Louis, Mosby–Year Book, 1994, p 472.)

(Fig. 55–4E). A No. 5 nonabsorbable suture is secured with an interlocking stitch along the lateral portion of the tendon.[52] A second No. 5 nonabsorbable suture is placed in similar fashion along the medial portion of the tendon (Fig. 55–4F). A transverse trough is then made in the superior pole of the patella with a high-speed bur (Fig. 55–4G). To avoid patellar tilt, the trough should be placed as posterior as possible in the patella. Next, three marks are made with a methylene blue pen approximately 1.0 to 1.5 cm apart in the trough (Fig. 55–4H). A Beath pin is used to drill through the medial mark exiting at the inferior pole of the patella (Fig. 55–4I). An anterior cruciate ligament (ACL) drill guide may be used to facilitate precise placement of the drill holes.[84] The medial free end of suture is next placed through the eyelet of the Beath pin and the pin is pulled distally (Fig. 55–4I). The Beath pin is then used to drill and pass the sutures in the central and lateral transosseous patellar tunnels (Fig. 55–4J). The proximal end of the tendon is pulled into the trough and the sutures are held provisionally with a hemostat. The knee is then flexed so that patellar tracking and rotation can be assessed. The repair is completed by tying the No. 5 nonabsorbable suture distally with the knee in full extension (Fig. 55–4K) and repairing the medial and lateral retinacula with multiple interrupted No. 0 absorbable suture (Fig. 55–4L). The repair is then checked to ensure that gapping at the repair site does not occur at 20 to 30 degrees of flexion (Fig. 55–4M). Augmentation is typically not necessary.[51,64,107] However, if the strength

of the repair is in doubt, augmentation may be achieved with wire or Mersilene tape.[72,76] Satisfactory results have also been obtained with suture anchors in lieu of transosseous suture.[97] After closure of the subcutaneous layer and skin, a cylinder cast is applied with the knee in full extension. Postoperatively, the cylinder cast is maintained for 6 weeks and the patient is allowed weightbearing as tolerated with a walker or crutches. Once the cast is removed, a control-dial hinged-knee orthosis is used until 90 degrees of flexion is achieved and quadriceps strength returns. Although we prefer immobilization in the immediate postoperative period, some authors advocate early passive and active assisted range of motion of the knee after quadriceps tendon repair.[59]

The Scuderi technique[40,41,101,102] for repairing acute rupture of the quadriceps tendon has been popular (Fig. 55–5). Using a midline longitudinal incision, the tendon rupture is exposed and the tendon edges are débrided until solid tendinous material is achieved. The knee is extended and the tendon edges are pulled with clamps, overlapped, and repaired with interrupted absorbable suture. A triangular flap 2.4 to 3.2 mm thick, 7.5 cm long on each side, and 5.0 cm at the base is fabricated from the anterior surface of the proximal part of the tendon. The base of the flap is left attached about 5.0 cm proximal to the rupture. The flap is folded distally over the rupture and sutured in place. A Bunnell pullout wire is placed along the medial and lateral side of the quadriceps tendon, patella, and patellar tendon. The wound is closed in layers

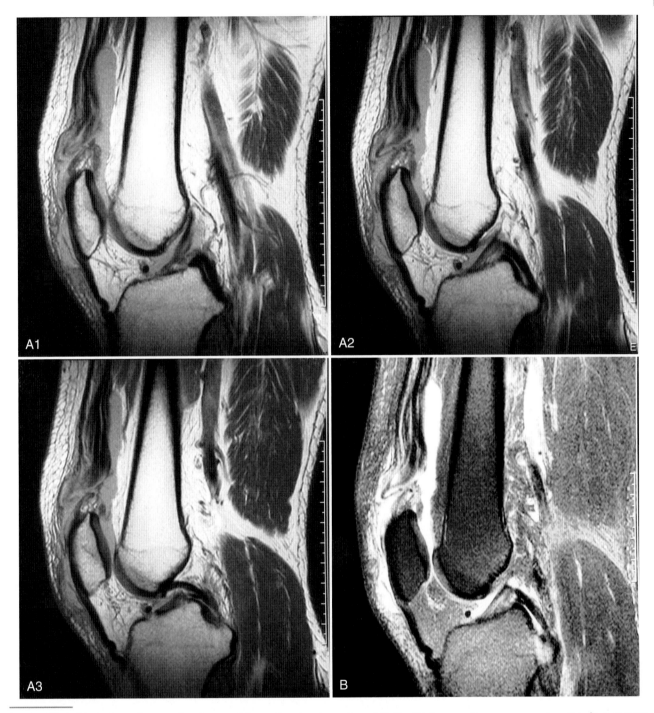

Figure 55–4. Technique for repair of a quadriceps tendon tear. **A** and **B,** Sagittal magnetic resonance images demonstrating a quadriceps tendon tear at the osteotendinous junction.

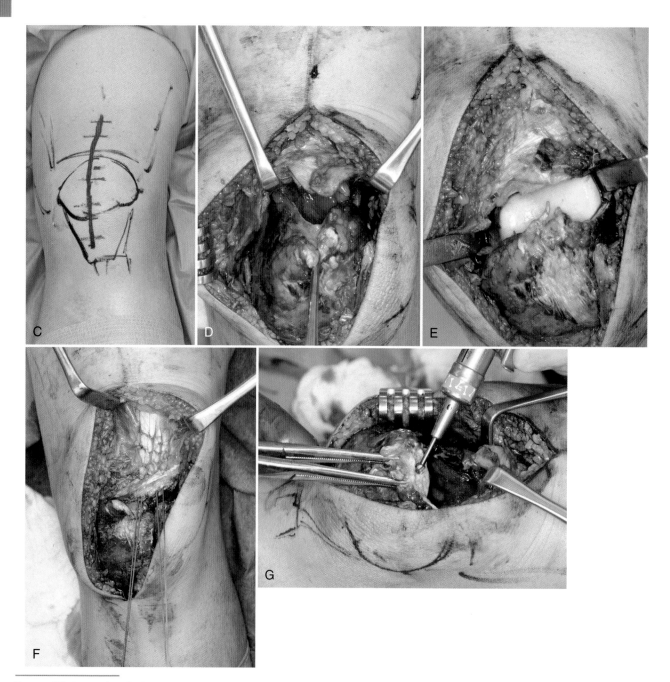

Figure 55–4, cont'd. **C,** Straight midline incision for exposure of the quadriceps tendon rupture. **D,** Hematoma is evacuated and the free tendon ends exposed. **E,** The proximal rectus femoris and vastus intermedius tendon edges are débrided to healthy tendon, and the superior pole of the patella is débrided of residual tendon. **F,** Two No. 5 nonabsorbable sutures are placed along the medial and lateral border of the quadriceps tendon in an interlocking fashion. **G,** A bur is used to create a transverse trough in the superior pole of the patella near the chondral surface.

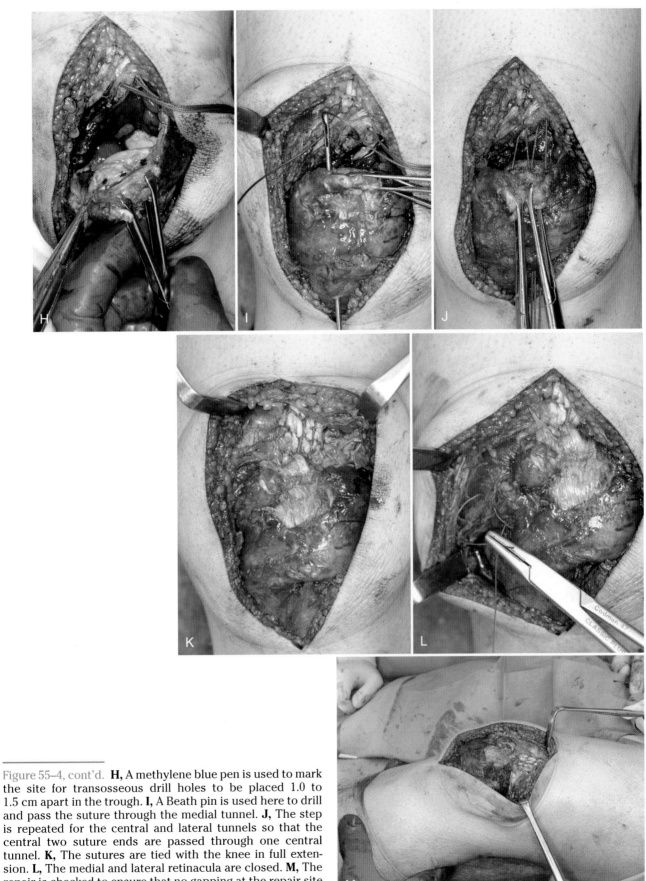

Figure 55–4, cont'd. **H,** A methylene blue pen is used to mark the site for transosseous drill holes to be placed 1.0 to 1.5 cm apart in the trough. **I,** A Beath pin is used here to drill and pass the suture through the medial tunnel. **J,** The step is repeated for the central and lateral tunnels so that the central two suture ends are passed through one central tunnel. **K,** The sutures are tied with the knee in full extension. **L,** The medial and lateral retinacula are closed. **M,** The repair is checked to ensure that no gapping at the repair site occurs with 20 to 30 degrees of flexion.

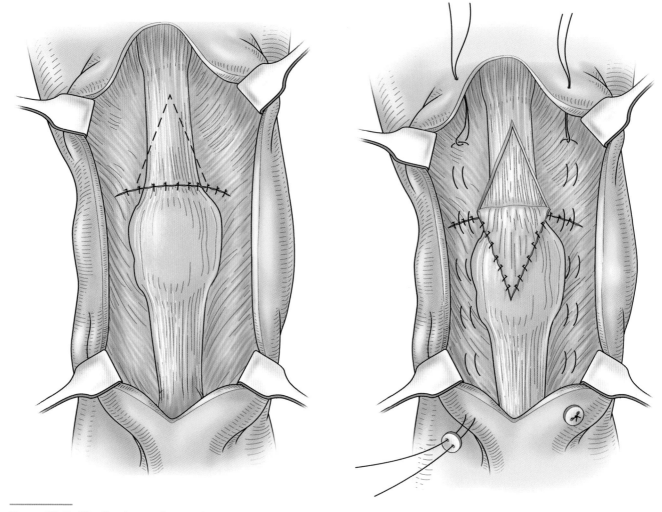

Figure 55–5. The Scuderi technique for repairing acute tears of the quadriceps tendon. (Redrawn from Scuderi GR: Extensor mechanism injuries: Treatment. In Scott WN [ed]: Ligament and Extension Mechanism Injuries of the Knee. St Louis, Mosby–Year Book, 1991, p 190.)

and the leg placed in a cylinder cast with the knee in the extended position. Postoperatively, the cylinder cast is maintained for 6 weeks, and at 3 weeks the pullout wires are removed. When the cast is removed, a control-dial hinged-knee orthosis is used so that flexion can be gradually increased. It is also recommended that the patient undergo physiotherapy, especially a quadriceps-strengthening program.

Chronic (Neglected) Disruption

Neglected or chronic rupture of the quadriceps tendon presents a difficult reconstruction, and the results after repair of such tears are less satisfactory than after treatment of acute tears.[99] A longitudinal midline incision is the preferred approach, and the exposure may reveal a

large gap between the tendon edges. When the tendon edges can be apposed, the ends are débrided and repaired with the Scuderi technique, as described earlier. However, when there is contraction of the tendon and a large gap, a Codivilla tendon-lengthening and repair procedure is recommended (Fig. 55–6). An inverted V is cut through the full thickness of the proximal part of the quadriceps tendon, with the lower margin of the V ending approximately 1.3 cm proximal to the rupture. The tendon ends are apposed and repaired with multiple No. 0 nonabsorbable sutures. The medial and lateral retinacula are also repaired at this time with multiple interrupted No. 0 absorbable sutures. The flap is then brought distally and sutured in place. The open upper portion of the V is closed with interrupted No. 0 absorbable suture. The reconstruction should be protected with a pullout cerclage wire. Postoperative treatment is similar to that after the Scuderi procedure.

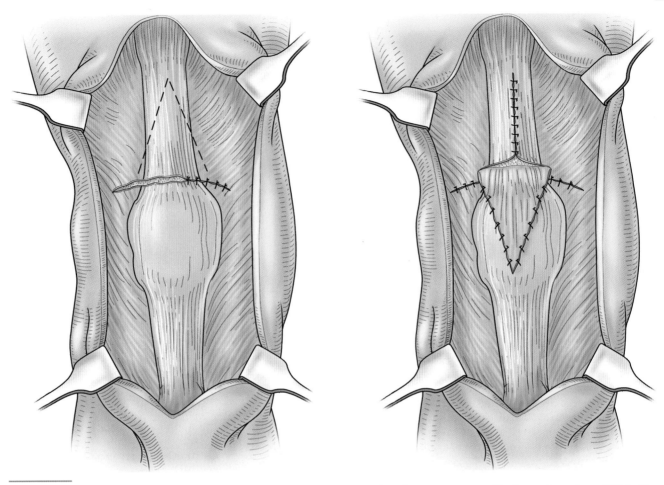

Figure 55–6. The Codivilla quadriceps tendon lengthening and repair for chronic ruptures. (Redrawn from Scott WN [ed]: The Knee, vol 1. St Louis, Mosby–Year Book, 1994, p 473.)

RESULTS OF SURGICAL MANAGEMENT OF QUADRICEPS TENDON RUPTURE

Results of repair and/or reconstruction of acute quadriceps tendon disruptions are generally favorable,[51,91,99] irrespective of the type of repair[59,91,99] or location of the tear[93,99] (avulsion from the patella versus midsubstance tendon disruption). Results are comparable between unilateral and simultaneous bilateral disruption.[51] Although 15% to 53% of patients may have quadriceps tendon deficits based on isokinetic testing postoperatively,[21,51,99] the majority are able to return to their preinjury occupations.[51] However, fewer than half the patients reach their preinjury recreational activity level.[51] Range of motion is typically recovered postoperatively and approaches the motion of the contralateral extremity.[51,99] Although Konrath and colleagues found no detrimental effect of delay in repair, others have shown a delay in surgical repair to be the single most important factor predictive of a poor outcome.[51] Rougraff and colleagues[99] suggested that a

delay of 1 week compromises the outcome of quadriceps tendon repair, with significantly worse functional results and lower satisfaction scores. These findings are supported by Siwek and Rao[107] and Scuderi,[101] who observed worse results with a delay in surgical repair of 2 weeks and 3 days, respectively. In a study of 29 quadriceps tendon repairs, Wenzl and colleagues demonstrated a significantly higher probability of a successful outcome with repairs performed within 2 weeks from the time of injury.[114] Levy and associates also noted the best results in patients managed acutely with a Dacron graft. Surgical débridement of scar tissue plus direct repair of the quadriceps tendon is effective in the management of partial quadriceps rupture.[59] Complications include rerupture and wound compromise. In a series of 53 repairs, Rougraff and colleagues[99] observed two reruptures; in Konrath and coworkers' series[51] of 51 patients, one rerupture was noted. No large series of surgical repair of chronic or neglected quadriceps tendon rupture is available; however, multiple case reports suggest favorable results with several different reconstruction methods.

Quadriceps Tendon Disruption Associated with Total Knee Arthroplasty

Tears of the quadriceps tendon after TKA are quite rare, with a reported incidence ranging from 0.1% to 1.1%.[22,63] Although a traumatic event may result in a quadriceps tendon tear, the contribution of other factors such as systemic disease, local injury, and factors related to the TKA technique may predispose an individual. With only a few series in the literature, these factors may only be speculated on and may include rheumatoid and other inflammatory arthritides, diabetes mellitus, chronic renal failure, hyperthyroidism, and systemic and local steroid use. Possible factors related to the arthroplasty include over-resection of the patella with subsequent quadriceps tendon injury, vascular injury to the tendon resulting from lateral retinacular release,[63] incomplete healing after extensile approaches, and manipulation.[86]

As in the case of the native knee, incomplete tears of the quadriceps tendon in patients with a TKA generally do well with nonoperative treatment. In a series from Dobbs and colleagues,[22] seven partial quadriceps tendon ruptures were treated nonoperatively, all with a satisfactory outcome. One of these seven ruptures was diagnosed 1 year after partial rupture and had no further treatment. This patient had a persistent extensor lag of 10 degrees and a palpable defect in the quadriceps tendon. Sixteen patients with a partial quadriceps tendon rupture underwent primary repair. These patients had a high complication rate (5/16), and 4 ultimately had an unsatisfactory result. This suggests that early diagnosis is imperative and nonoperative management consisting of immobilization of the knee in extension for 4 to 6 weeks with weightbearing as tolerated can yield good results for partial quadriceps tendon tears.

In contrast to the native knee, the results of complete quadriceps tendon tears in patients with a TKA are less predictable. In Dobbs and colleagues' series,[22] 11 patients were identified with a complete quadriceps tendon tear. Ten underwent primary repair and only 4 had a satisfactory result. Complications included four reruptures, two infections, and one patient with symptomatic recurvatum and instability. Likewise, Lynch and colleagues[63] reported unsatisfactory results with direct suture repair for three quadriceps tendon ruptures, with one sustaining a rerupture and the other two demonstrating limited knee flexion and significant extensor lag. Because of the discouraging results of operative treatment by direct suture repair, augmentation with either autogenous graft material such as semitendinosus tendon or graft material such as Marlex mesh should be considered.

PATELLAR TENDON RUPTURE

Overview

Rupture of the patellar tendon is less common than rupture of the quadriceps tendon and generally occurs in patients younger than 40 years.[46,107] Systemic inflammatory diseases, chronic metabolic disorders, anabolic steroid abuse, local steroid injections, and most commonly, progressive degenerative processes of the tendon have all been implicated as potential factors associated with an increased risk for tendon rupture.[15,43,75,78,98] Most of these ruptures occur at the inferior pole of the patella, but they may also take place in the midsubstance of the tendon or rarely at the insertion of the tubercle.[16,65] The patella may be displaced 5 cm proximally as a result of associated retinacular and capsular disruption caused by the strong pull of the quadriceps mechanism. Disruptions through the substance of the patellar tendon can occur spontaneously but, more often, are caused by trauma or laceration. Early diagnosis and treatment provide the best results. Historically, McLaughlin[72,73] recommended that repair of the patellar tendon be reinforced with the use of stainless steel wire anchored to a bolt placed in the tibial tubercle. Hsu and coworkers[39] reported a technique of primary repair reinforced with a neutralization wire. Siwek and Rao[107] also recommended that all immediate repairs of the patellar tendon be reinforced by external devices. Several reports have described reinforcing the repair with various augmentation grafts, including autografts, allografts[24,45] (fascia lata, semitendinosus, gracilis) and synthetic grafts (Mersilene,[76] Dacron,[29,30,59] carbon fiber,[27] and a poly-p-dioxannone cord[50]). In a study by Ravalin and associates,[94] 12 fresh frozen cadaveric specimens were used to compare standard repair with transosseous sutures without augmentation, with augmentation using a No. 5 Ethibond suture, and with augmentation using 2.0 Dall-Miles cable. Gap formation at the repair site was assessed after cycling the knees in a custom knee jig; it was greatest in the repairs without augmentation and the least in the group augmented with the cable. However, recent clinical reports have demonstrated satisfactory results of acute patellar tendon disruption repaired without augmentation. In a series of 15 consecutive patients, Marder and Timmerman published excellent results with primary repair of acute patellar tendon disruption treated by suture repair alone.[65]

Acute Disruption

Complete patellar tendon rupture requires surgical intervention to restore extensor mechanism function. A straight midline incision is made, and small full-thickness medial and lateral subcutaneous skin flaps are developed. The paratenon overlying the patellar tendon is identified and carefully incised longitudinally. The paratenon is elevated medially and laterally and preserved for subsequent repair at the time of closure. Hematoma within the disrupted tendon is evacuated. In situations in which rupture of the patellar tendon occurs at the osteotendinous junction, the free tendon is freshened and a horizontal trough is then made along posterior half of the inferior pole of the patella (Fig. 55–7). Two No. 5 nonabsorbable sutures are then placed along the medial and lateral halves of the patellar tendon with an interlocking (Krackow[52]) stitch such that the four free ends of suture are left emanating from the proximal portion of the tendon. Using a Beath

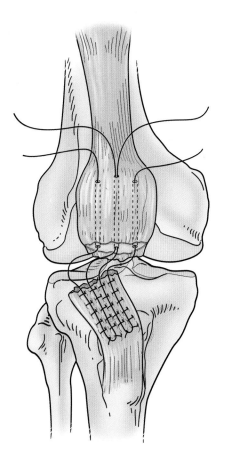

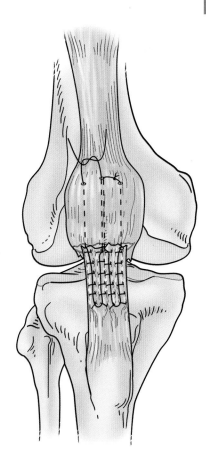

Figure 55–7. Acute repair of the patellar tendon into a bony trough. (Redrawn from Scott WN [ed]: The Knee, vol 1. St Louis, Mosby–Year Book, 1994, p 474.)

pin, a longitudinal drill hole is placed centrally in the patella at the base of the trough with exit at the superior pole of the patella. An ACL drill guide may be used to precisely place the patellar drill holes.[84] The two central free ends of suture are then placed through the eyelet of the Beath pin, and the pin is pulled proximally. The Beath pin is used to drill and pass the sutures on the medial and lateral sides of the patella approximately 1.0 to 1.5 cm apart. The sutures are then pulled taut, and the free end of the patellar tendon should be seated within the trough. The sutures are held provisionally with a hemostat to assess patellar tracking and rotation. It is important to ensure that the repair has not produced patella infra. At 45 degrees of flexion the inferior pole of the patella should be above the roof of the intercondylar notch. A mosquito clamp is then used to pass one of the central sutures medially and the other laterally so that the suture knots may be placed over bone rather than the quadriceps tendon. The medial and lateral retinacula are repaired with No. 0 absorbable suture. In most cases we prefer to tie the sutures with the knee in full extension and augment the repair with Mersilene tape placed circumferentially around the repair through drill holes in the patella and the anterior cortex of the proximal end of the tibia. The wound is then closed in layers, and a cylinder cast with the knee in extension is applied and maintained for 6 weeks. The patient may ambulate with full weightbearing as tolerated with crutches. When the cast is removed, the control-dial hinged-knee orthosis allowing progressive flexion of the knee is used. When the patient has

achieved greater than 90 degrees of flexion and sufficient quadriceps strength to support the limb, the orthosis is discontinued.

Acute ruptures that occur within the substance of the patellar tendon can be repaired with running interlocking sutures of No. 2 nonabsorbable suture material (Fig. 55–8). The distally based tendon is reinforced through longitudinal drill holes in the patella, whereas the proximally based tendon is repaired through a horizontal drill hole in the tibial tubercle. Each flap is repaired side to side with interrupted No. 0 absorbable suture. The medial and lateral retinacula are also repaired with No. 0 absorbable suture at this time. The postoperative course is similar to that described earlier. If secure repair of the patellar tendon cannot be achieved with either of the repairs described previously, augmentation with the semitendinosus or gracilis tendon is recommended (Fig. 55–9).[45,56] Through the original midline incision the insertion sites of the semitendinosus and gracilis are identified. While preserving the distal insertion, a tendon stripper is used to divide the tendon proximally. If only the semitendinosus is used for augmentation, it should be passed through an oblique drill hole at the tibial tubercle in a medial-to-lateral direction. The graft is then pulled superiorly, passing laterally to medially through a transverse drill hole in the inferior aspect of the patella, and then sutured to the origin of the semitendinosus with No. 0 nonabsorbable suture. This technique creates a box around the patellar tendon. The corners of the graft are sutured with nonabsorbable suture to prevent slippage. If

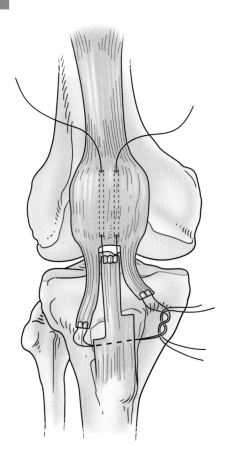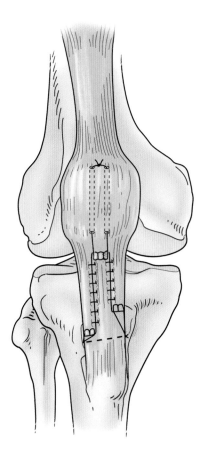

Figure 55–8. Acute repair of intrasubstance tears of the patellar tendon. (Redrawn from Scott WN [ed]: The Knee, vol 1. St Louis, Mosby–Year Book, 1994, p 475.)

the semitendinosus tendon is thin and further augmentation is needed, the gracilis tendon can also be used. The origin of the gracilis tendon is maintained distally, and the tendon is passed in a medial-to-lateral direction through a second horizontal drill hole in the patella; it then circles the patellar tendon and returns in a lateral-to-medial direction through the oblique tibial drill hole. The postoperative course is similar to that described earlier, with 6 weeks of immobilization in a cylinder cast. We prefer a postoperative course of immobilization in a cylinder cast before initiation of a physical therapy program. However, Larson and Simonian[56] have suggested that immediate mobilization with initial passive and active assisted exercises after reconstruction of the patellar tendon with semitendinosus augmentation may be beneficial. Bhargava and coauthors[4] reported on 11 patients treated with primary repair protected by a cerclage wire and early mobilization. All did well; however, patients with history of systemic collagen vascular disorders or previous steroid injection were excluded. Levy and colleagues[59] also recommended immediate postoperative mobilization after reconstruction with a Dacron graft. Marder and Timmerman[65] have used early mobilization in athletes younger than 40 years after primary repair without augmentation.

Fulkerson and Langeland's technique,[32] in which the central quadriceps tendon is harvested with a patellar bone graft for ACL reconstruction, has also been applied to repair/reconstruct patellar tendon disruptions. Williams and colleagues[115] reported success with this technique in three cases of patellar tendon compromise, one acute, one chronic, and one with patella infra. The patellar bone graft is inset into the tibial tubercle, and the quadriceps tendon graft is secured with sutures passed through the patella in a distal-to-proximal direction. In a case report Edwards and associates[25] used this technique to reconstruct an acute patellar tendon disruption associated with bony compromise of the tibial tubercle.

Chronic (Neglected) Disruption

Chronic rupture of the patellar tendon poses a particular problem, especially if there is retraction of the quadriceps tendon with proximal migration of the patella. Previously, a two-stage reconstruction with preoperative traction through a transverse Steinmann pin placed in the patella was described. Presently, mobilization of the patella and quadriceps tendon can be achieved by clearing the medial and lateral gutters into the suprapatellar pouch and subperiosteally elevating the vastus intermedius from the anterior aspect of the femur.[110] A lateral retinacular release is also performed. If necessary, a medial retinacular release can be performed, but this may increase the risk for avascular necrosis of the patella.[103,105] Several techniques have been described for reconstruction of chronic tears of the patellar tendon, including direct repair with augmentation using cerclage wires, autograft, allograft, and synthetic grafts. Direct repair may be performed with transosseous sutures or the more recently described suture anchors.[37] Regardless of the technique performed, it is important that care be taken to maintain normal patellar tracking, rota-

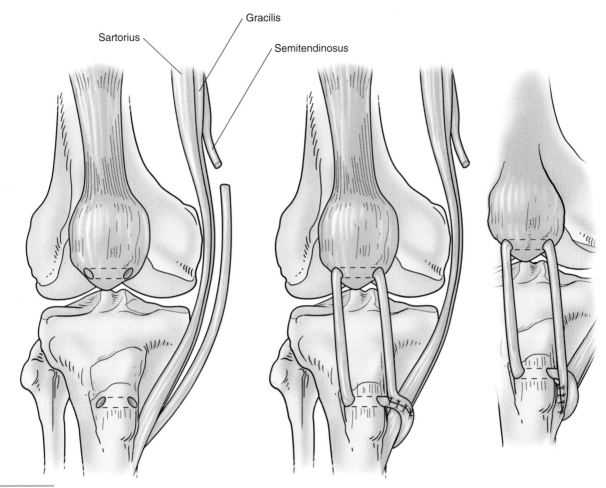

Figure 55–9. Augmentation of a patellar tendon repair with the semitendinosus tendon. (Redrawn from Scuderi GR: Extensor mechanism injuries: Treatment. In Scott WN [ed]: Ligament and Extension Mechanism Injuries of the Knee. St Louis, Mosby–Year Book, 1991, p 191.)

tion, and height. Preoperative planning should include a lateral radiograph of the contralateral knee to determine patellar height. Intraoperatively, the inferior pole of the patella should be above the roof of the intercondylar notch at 45 degrees of flexion. The knee should be able to achieve 90 degrees of flexion, and when in full extension, the patellar tendon should be lax, approximately 1.0 to 1.5 cm.

Reconstruction of chronic patellar tendon rupture is performed through a longitudinal midline incision. The paratenon is incised longitudinally to expose the patellar tendon. If sufficient tendon is available, the ends are cut fresh and sutured as described earlier for the acute repair, but augmentation with a semitendinosus and/or gracilis autograft is typically recommended. A bone tenaculum can be used to pull the patella distally, and the semitendinosus and gracilis are sutured under tension. Recently, Casey and Tietjens[13] reported on their series of four patients with neglected patellar tendon rupture repaired primarily and augmented with three 1.5-mm cerclage wires in a figure-of-eight pattern from the quadriceps tendon to the tibial tubercle. All underwent a supervised therapy program and immediate mobilization in a brace.

Average range of motion was 112 degrees, and no extensor lag was reported. All had the hardware removed between 3 and 13 months postoperatively.

When there is a deficiency of remaining tendon or the remaining tendon is attenuated and scarred, a Z-shortening of the patellar tendon and a Z-lengthening of the quadriceps tendon can be performed (Fig. 55–10). This technique requires intraoperative radiographs to determine appropriate patellar height and position because of the increased tendency for patella infra with this reconstruction. Once the proper position of the patella has been determined, the Z-plasty is reinforced with multiple interrupted No. 0 nonabsorbable sutures. This reconstruction requires augmentation with the semitendinosus and gracilis tendons, which are harvested as two free tendons and sutured end to end. The hamstring tendons pass through a transverse drill hole in the midportion of the patella and then through a transverse hole in the tibial tubercle in a figure-of-eight fashion. The semitendinosus and gracilis grafts are secured to the patellar tendon with absorbable suture. Alternatively, the quadriceps tendon–patellar bone graft technique described earlier may be applied.[32,115] The postoperative course is similar to that described previ-

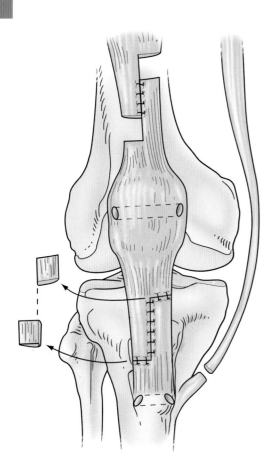
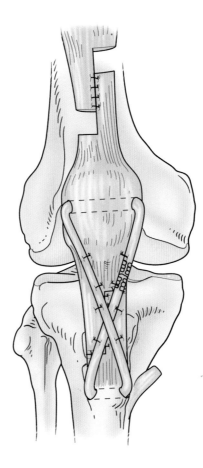

Figure 55–10. Repair of a chronic patellar tendon rupture with a Z-shortening of the patellar tendon and a Z-lengthening of the quadriceps tendon plus augmentation with the semitendinosus and gracilis tendons sutured end to end. (Redrawn from Scott WN [ed]: The Knee, vol 1. St Louis, Mosby–Year Book, 1994, p 476.)

ously. Some authors suggest that a judicious program of immediate postoperative mobilization is possible when the repair is augmented with the semitendinosus tendon or a Dacron graft.[56,59]

Recently, allografts[28,74,87] have been used for reconstruction of neglected patellar tendon rupture (Fig. 55–11). The Achilles tendon with a corticocancellous calcaneal bone block is a convenient allograft. The tibial tubercle is prepared with an oscillating saw or bur to create a trough measuring 2.5 to 3.0 cm long, 1.5 to 2.0 cm wide, and 1.5 cm deep. The bone block is contoured and press-fit into the trough. It is then secured with two 4.0-mm cancellous screws. The Achilles tendon graft is divided into thirds. The central third, which should measure 8 to 9 mm in width, is pulled through a slit in the residual patellar tendon. The graft is then passed through a longitudinal, 8- to 9-mm-wide drill hole in the patella. This drill hole enters the inferior pole of the patella and exits at the superior border proximally, 3 mm posterior to the central portion of the quadriceps tendon. The tendon is then pulled through a vertical slit in the quadriceps tendon. The tendon is sutured at the inferior pole of the patella and at the quadriceps tendon with multiple interrupted No. 0 nonabsorbable sutures. Patella height should be determined at this time. The knee should flex to 90 degrees, and at 45 degrees of flexion the inferior pole of the patella should be superior to the roof of the intercondylar notch. Once the patellar position has been determined to be correct, the medial and lateral flaps are sutured to the medial and lateral retinacula with multiple

No. 0 nonabsorbable sutures. If the paratenon is present, it should be closed over the graft with 2-0 absorbable suture. The wound is closed in layers and a cylinder cast is applied. The cast is worn for 5 weeks and then a control-dial hinged-knee orthosis is worn until 90 degrees of flexion has been achieved and quadriceps strength is sufficient to support the limb during ambulation. Wascher and Summa[112] described a technique in which an Achilles tendon allograft was used to reconstruct a ruptured extensor mechanism after patellectomy that had failed two previous attempts at primary repair.

RESULTS OF SURGICAL REPAIR OF PATELLAR TENDON DISRUPTION

As for quadriceps tendons, the results of patellar tendon repair are favorable, regardless of the location of the rupture or the method of repair.[39,53,56,68,107] Again, delayed repairs have worse outcomes than do repairs performed in the acute setting.[39,68,107] When the patellar tendon is repaired in the acute setting, range of motion approaching that of the contralateral knee is typically regained,[53,68,107] and in athletic individuals, premorbid activity levels and strength can be expected.[53] No large series of neglected patellar tendon ruptures managed with patellar ligament reconstruction are available. Complications include rerupture, wound problems, and patellofemoral symptoms. Rerupture is generally related

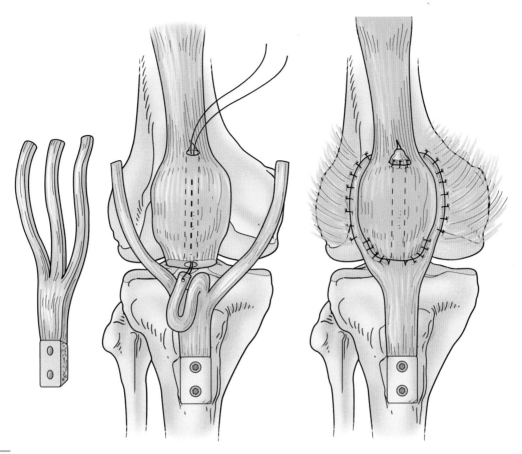

Figure 55–11. Allograft reconstruction for neglected patellar tendon rupture. (Redrawn from Scott WN [ed]: The Knee, vol 1. St Louis, Mosby–Year Book, 1994, p 476.)

to return to rigorous activity before completion of proper physical therapy. Wound complications are more common than with quadriceps tendon disruption because of the thinner skin at the tibial tubercle; therefore, it is recommended that the skin incision be made adjacent to, but not directly over the tubercle. Patellofemoral symptoms have been managed with lateral release.[51] Obtaining an intraoperative radiograph at completion of the patellar tendon repair is prudent to ensure that patella baja has not been created.

Patellar Tendon Disruption Associated with Total Knee Arthroplasty

Rupture of the patellar tendon after TKA is a rare, but devastating complication with a reported prevalence ranging from 0.17% to 2.5%.[63,92] Ruptures may occur intraoperatively, in the immediate postoperative period, or at some time after the postoperative period. Intraoperative ruptures can occur during exposure, especially while trying to evert the patella in a stiff knee. Patients with multiply operated knees are at a significant risk, probably because of soft-tissue scarring, stiffness, and devascularization of tissues. Previous distal alignment procedures,[92] excessive patellar resection,[26] and hinged implants[77] have all been implicated as potential contributors to patellar tendon

rupture after TKA. Postoperatively, rupture can occur during manipulation of a stiff knee, from trauma, or as a delayed complication such as chronic attrition from impingement against the tibial insert[26] or an anteriorly overhanging tibial tray.

Prevention is of paramount importance. Awareness of this potential problem should be raised preoperatively in patients with a stiff or multiply operated knee. Intraoperatively, if difficulty with exposure is encountered, several techniques may aid in safely performing a TKA. Posteromedial dissection from the tibia may help allow external rotation of the tibia, which can markedly relieve tension on the patellar tendon. Incising the lateral patellofemoral ligament in primary TKA and excision of scar tissue in the lateral gutter and beneath the patellar tendon in revision TKA can oftentimes allow the extensor mechanism to sublux laterally more easily. A quadriceps snip should be performed if there is still significant tension. Finally, if none of these measures adequately decrease tension on the patellar tendon, a tibial tubercle osteotomy or quadriceps turndown may be required to safely expose the knee.[86]

Management of patellar tendon rupture after TKA is considerably more difficult than management of rupture arising in the native knee. Patellar tendon avulsions that occur intraoperatively and have an intact periosteal sleeve may be reattached with staples, transosseous sutures,[92] or suture anchors. However, late ruptures are much more difficult to treat. Rand et al[92] reviewed 18 patients with patellar tendon rupture. Nine patients underwent primary suture repair, and in all nine cases the repair failed.

As a result, late rupture of the patellar tendon in patients after TKA generally requires a more extensive reconstruction to restore extensor mechanism function. Options for reconstruction include primary repair augmented with semitendinosus tendon autograft,[11] Achilles tendon allograft,[17] and quadriceps tendon–patella–patellar tendon–tibial tubercle allograft.[9,58,92] Cadambi and Engh[11]

described a technique for primary repair augmented with an autogenous semitendinosus tendon. In this procedure, the semitendinosus tendon is harvested at the musculotendinous junction, with the distal insertion left intact. The tendon is routed medially through a drill hole in the distal pole of the patella and then sutured to itself at its distal insertion. The knee was immobilized for 6 weeks and patients were permitted to bear weight as tolerated. In their series of seven patients, the average extensor lag was 10 degrees with an average flexion of 79 degrees. The

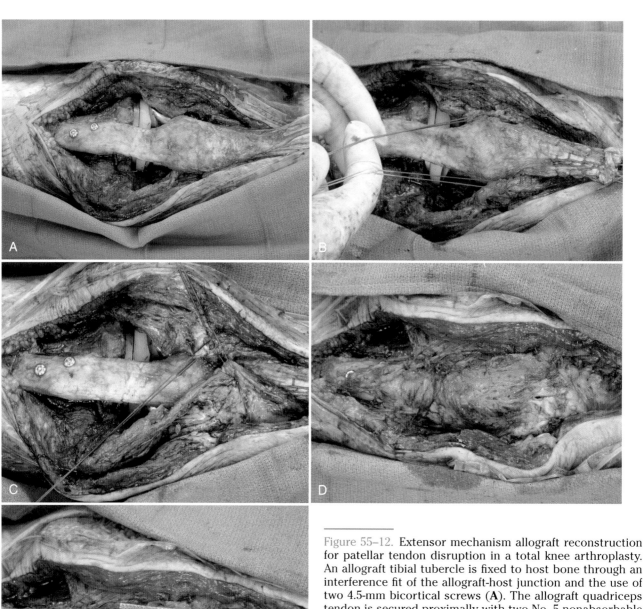

Figure 55–12. Extensor mechanism allograft reconstruction for patellar tendon disruption in a total knee arthroplasty. An allograft tibial tubercle is fixed to host bone through an interference fit of the allograft-host junction and the use of two 4.5-mm bicortical screws (**A**). The allograft quadriceps tendon is secured proximally with two No. 5 nonabsorbable sutures in the Krackow method with the knee in full extension. The length of the allograft is adjusted to ensure that the allograft patella lies in the trochlear groove. Two sutures are then placed in the host retinacular tissue (**B**). The residual host extensor tissue is then sewn over the allograft reconstruction in a pants-over-vest method (**C**) and (**D**). Marlex mesh is used to reinforce the repair (**E**). (Modified from Scuderi GR, Easley ME: Quadriceps and patellar tendon disruptions. In Insall JN, Scott WN [eds]: Surgery of the Knee, vol 1. New York, Churchill Livingstone, 2001, pp 1074-1086.)

authors concluded that the use of autogenous semitendinosus tendon augmentation of primary patellar tendon repairs could restore sufficient quadriceps strength and motion.

Achilles tendon allograft has also been used to reconstruct chronic patellar tendon rupture after TKA. Crossett and colleagues[17] reviewed their experience with fresh frozen Achilles tendon allograft with an attached calcaneal bone graft in nine knees. The calcaneal bone block is cut to match a defect created in the tibia, and the bone block is impacted with an interference fit. The bone block is secured with a screw or wires. The allograft tendon is then sewn to the underlying extensor mechanism with nonabsorbable suture while the knee is in full extension. Postoperatively, the knees were immobilized in extension for 4 weeks, and then progressive flexion was allowed. The average extensor lag improved from 44 degrees preoperatively to 3 degrees postoperatively, and although two grafts had failed, both were repaired successfully.

Emerson and colleagues[26] were the first to describe an allograft reconstruction using the quadriceps tendon, a patella with a cemented prosthesis, the patellar tendon, and the tibial tubercle. In their description, the allograft tubercle is fixed to the host tibia with screws or wire and the patella is placed on the anterior flange of the femoral component. The allograft quadriceps tendon is then sutured to the host tendon with nonabsorbable suture while the extensor mechanism construct is placed under slight tension. There was a high complication rate, with a third of the patients demonstrating an extensor lag of 20 to 40 degrees. Leopold and colleagues[58] reconstructed seven extensor mechanisms with Emerson's technique and rated all seven as failures based on persistent extensor lag of more than 30 degrees.

Nazarian and Booth[82] studied a larger series of 36 patients with chronic extensor mechanism disruption and used a modification of Emerson's technique. In their technique the distal extensor allograft was tensioned with the knee in full extension. The average extensor lag was 13 degrees. Twenty-three had achieved full active extension that equaled passive extension. However, eight knees required a repeat allograft reconstruction. This modification seems to provide improved active knee extension. This finding is supported by Burnett and colleagues,[9] who evaluated 20 extensor mechanism allografts: group I consisted of 7 knees reconstructed with the allograft slightly tensioned, and group II consisted of 13 knees with the allograft tightly tensioned in full extension. The average postoperative extensor lag was 59 degrees in group I and 4.3 degrees in group 2. All 7 reconstructed with the graft slightly tensioned were clinical failures, whereas all 13 reconstructed with the allograft tightly tensioned in full extension were clinical successes.

Other techniques described include a medial gastrocnemius flap,[10] the use of synthetic ligament augmentation,[3] and patellotibial fusion.[48]

The technique for extensor mechanism allograft that we prefer (Fig. 55–12) is similar to that described by Nazarian and Booth. A long midline incision is used to provide wide exposure and preserve as much of the residual extensor mechanism tissue as possible. The host tibia is exposed by subperiosteal dissection. Full passive extension of the knee is achieved. The allograft tibial tubercle is then prepared with a microsagittal saw to fashion a bone block approximately 3 cm long, 1.5 cm wide, and 1 cm deep and an oblique "dovetail" proximal cut.[11] The host tibia is then prepared to create a "lock-and-key fit." The allograft tibia is secured with either screws or wires. Two nonabsorbable No. 5 sutures are then secured to the allograft quadriceps tendon with a locking Krackow stitch. The residual extensor mechanism tendon is sewn over the extensor mechanism allograft construct in a pants-over-vest technique. As emphasized by Nazarian and Booth[82] and Burnett and colleagues,[9] the graft is tensioned with the knee in full extension. Marlex mesh is then used to reinforce the repair. This is but one method to reconstruct the extensor mechanism in TKA. A more comprehensive review of this problem is found elsewhere in these volumes.

References

1. Anderson WE, Habermann ET: Spontaneous bilateral quadriceps tendon rupture in a patient on hemodialysis. Orthop Rev 17:411, 1988.
2. Aprin H, Broukhim B: Early diagnosis of acute rupture of the quadriceps tendon by arthrography. Clin Orthop 195:185, 1985.
3. Aracil J, Salom M, Aroca JE, et al: Extensor apparatus reconstruction with Leeds-Keio ligament in total knee arthroplasty. J Arthroplasty 14:204-208, 1999.
4. Bhargava SP, Hynes MC, Dowell JK: Traumatic patella tendon rupture: Early mobilisation following surgical repair. Injury 35:76, 2004.
5. Bhole R, Johnson JC: Bilateral simultaneous spontaneous rupture of quadriceps tendons in a diabetic patient. South Med J 78:486, 1985.
6. Bianchi S, Zwass A, Abdelwahab IF, et al: Diagnosis of tears of the quadriceps tendon of the knee: Value of sonography. AJR Am J Roentgenol 162:1137, 1994.
7. Blaiser RB, Ciullo JV: Rupture of the quadriceps tendon after arthroscopic lateral release. Arthroscopy 2:262, 1986.
8. Bonamo J, Krinick R, Sporn A: Rupture of the patellar ligament after use of its central third for anterior cruciate ligament reconstruction: A report of two cases. J Bone Joint Surg Am 66:1294, 1984.
9. Burnett RS, Berger RA, Paprosky WG, et al: Extensor mechanism allograft reconstruction after total knee arthroplasty. A comparison of two techniques. J Bone Joint Surg Am 86:2694, 2004.
10. Busfield BT, Huffman GR, Nahai F, et al: Extended medial gastrocnemius rotational flap for treatment of chronic extensor mechanism deficiency in patients with and without total knee arthroplasty. Clin Orthop 428:190, 2004.
11. Cadambi A, Engh GA: Use of a semitendinosus tendon autogenous graft for rupture of the patellar ligament after total knee arthroplasty: A report of seven cases. J Bone Joint Surg Am 74:974, 1992.
12. Calvo E, Ferrer A, Robledo AG, et al: Bilateral simultaneous spontaneous quadriceps tendon rupture: A case report studied by magnetic resonance imaging. Clin Imaging 21:73, 1997.
13. Casey MT Jr, Tietjens BR: Neglected ruptures of the patellar tendon: A case series of four patients. Am J Sports Med 29:457 2001.
14. Chmell SJ: Bilateral spontaneous patellar tendon rupture in the absence of concomitant systemic disease or steroid use. Am J Orthop 24:300, 1995.
15. Clark SC, Jones MW, Choudhury RR, Smith E: Bilateral tendon rupture secondary to repeated local steroid injections. J Accid Emerg Med 12:300, 1995.
16. Cooper ME, Selesnick FH: Partial rupture of the distal insertion of the patellar tendon: A report of two cases in professional athletes. Am J Sports Med 28:402, 2000.
17. Crossett LS, Sinha RK, Sechriest VF, Rubash HE: Reconstruction of a ruptured patellar tendon with Achilles tendon allograft following total knee arthroplasty. J Bone Joint Surg Am 84:1354, 2002.
18. Dabezies EJ, Schutte J: Orthopedic grand rounds: Quadriceps rupture: Case report. Orthopedics 4:357, 1981.

19. Daffner RH, Riemer BL, Lupetin AR, et al: Magnetic resonance imaging in acute tendon ruptures. Skeletal Radiol 15:619, 1986.
20. Davies SG, Baudouin CJ, King JD, et al: Ultrasound, computed tomography and magnetic resonance imaging in patellar tendinitis. Clin Radiol 43:52, 1991.
21. De Baere T, Geulette B, Manche E, Barras L: Functional results after surgical repair of quadriceps tendon rupture. Acta Orthop Belg 68:146, 2002.
22. Dobbs RE, Hanssen AD, Lewallen DG, Pagnano MW: Quadriceps tendon rupture after total knee arthroplasty. Prevalence, complications, and outcomes. J Bone Joint Surg Am 87:37, 2005.
23. Driesen R, Victor J, Fabry G: Quadriceps tendon rupture complicating patellar tendon release. Acta Orthop Belg 59:301, 1993.
24. Ecker ML, Lotke PA, Glazer RM: Late reconstruction of the patellar tendon. J Bone Joint Surg Am 61:884, 1979.
25. Edwards TB, Lewis JE, Guanche CA: Patellar tendon and tibial tubercle reconstruction using quadriceps tendon with patellar bone plug autograft. J Orthop Trauma 11:304, 1997.
26. Emerson RH Jr, Head WC, Malinin TI: Extensor mechanism reconstruction with an allograft after total knee arthroplasty. Clin Orthop 303:79, 1994.
27. Evans PD, Pritchard GA, Jenkins DH: Carbon fibre used in the late reconstruction of rupture of the extensor mechanism of the knee. Injury 18:57, 1987.
28. Falconiero RP, Pallis MP: Chronic rupture of a patellar tendon: A technique for reconstruction with Achilles allograft: A case report. Arthroscopy 12:623, 1996.
29. Frazier CH: Tendon repairs with Dacron vascular graft suture: A followup report. Orthopedics 4:539, 1981.
30. Frazier CH, Clark EM: Major tendon repairs with Dacron vascular graft suture. Orthopedics 3:539, 1981.
31. Fujikawa K, Ohtani T, Matsumoto H, et al: Reconstruction of the extensor apparatus of the knee with the Leeds-Keio ligament. J Bone Joint Surg Br 76:200, 1994.
32. Fulkerson JP, Langeland R: An alternative cruciate reconstruction graft: The central quadriceps tendon. Arthroscopy 11:252, 1995.
33. Gallie WE, LeMesurier AB: The late repair of fractures of the patella and of rupture of the ligamentum patellae and quadriceps tendon. J Bone Joint Surg 9:47, 1927.
34. Goodier D, Flores M, Shedden RG: Patellar tendon rupture in identical twins. J Trauma 38:665, 1995.
35. Goodrich A, Difiore RJ, Tippens JK: Bilateral simultaneous rupture of the infrapatellar tendon: A case report and literature review. Orthopedics 6:1472, 1983.
36. Greenbaum B, Perry J, Lee J: Bilateral spontaneous patellar tendon rupture in the absence of concomitant systemic disease or steroid use. Orthop Rev 23:890, 1994.
37. Ho HM, Lee WK: Traumatic bilateral concurrent patellar tendon rupture: An alternative fixation method. Knee Surg Sports Traumatol Arthrosc 11:105, 2003.
38. Hohl M, Larson RL, Jones DC: Disruption of the extensor mechanism. In Rockwood CA, Green DP (eds): Fractures in Adults. Philadelphia, JB Lippincott, 1984, pp 1429-1591.
39. Hsu KY, Wang KC, Ho WP, et al: Traumatic patellar tendon ruptures: A followup study of primary repair and a neutralization wire. J Trauma 36:658, 1994.
40. Ilan DI, Tejwani N, Keschner M, Leibman M: Quadriceps tendon rupture. J Am Acad Orthop Surg 11:192, 2003.
41. Kamali M: Bilateral traumatic rupture of the infrapatellar tendon. Clin Orthop 142:131, 1979.
42. Kaneko K, DeMouy EH, Brunet ME, et al: Radiographic diagnosis of quadriceps tendon rupture: Analysis of diagnostic failure. J Emerg Med 12:225, 1994.
43. Kannus P, Jozsa L: Histopathological changes preceding spontaneous rupture of a tendon. A controlled study of 891 patients. J Bone Joint Surg Am 73:1507, 1991.
44. Katzman BM, Silberberg S, Caligiuri DA, et al: Delayed repair of a quadriceps tendon. Orthopedics 20:553, 1997.
45. Kelikian H, Riashi E, Gleason J: Restoration of quadriceps function in neglected tear of the patellar tendon. Surg Gynecol Obstet 104:200, 1957.
46. Kelly DW, Carter VS, Jobe FW, et al: Patella and quadriceps tendon ruptures—jumper's knee. Am J Sports Med 12:375, 1984.
47. Kelly DW, Godfrey KD, Johanson PH, et al: Quadriceps rupture in association with the roentgenographic "tooth" sign: A case report. Orthopedics 3:1206, 1980.
48. Kempenaar JW, Cameron JC: Patellotibial fusion for patellar tendon rupture after total knee arthroplasty. J Arthroplasty 14:115, 1999.
49. Keogh P, Shanker SJ, Burke T, et al: Bilateral simultaneous rupture of the quadriceps tendons. Clin Orthop 234:139, 1988.
50. Kinmont JC, Walter E, Curtis MJ: Augmentation of patellar tendon repair with poly-p-dioxanone cord. Injury 33:263, 2002.
51. Konrath GA, Chen D, Lock T, et al: Outcomes following repair of quadriceps tendon ruptures. J Orthop Trauma 12:273, 1998.
52. Krackow KA, Thomas SC, Jones LC: Ligament-tendon fixation: Analysis of a new stitch and comparison with standard techniques. Orthopedics 11:909, 1988.
53. Kuechle DK, Stuart MJ: Isolated rupture of the patellar tendon in athletes. Am J Sports Med 22:692, 1994.
54. Langan P, Fontanetta AP: Rupture of the patella tendon after use of its central third. Orthop Rev 16:317, 1987.
55. Larsen E, Lund PM: Ruptures of the extensor mechanism of the knee joint. Clin Orthop 213:150, 1986.
56. Larson RV, Simonian PT: Semitendinous augmentation of acute patellar tendon repair with immediate mobilization. Am J Sports Med 23:82, 1995.
57. Lavalle C, Aparicio LA, Moreno J, et al: Bilateral avulsion of quadriceps tendons in primary hyperparathyroidism. J Rheumatol 12:596, 1985.
58. Leopold SS, Greidanus N, Paprosky WG, et al: High rate of failure of allograft reconstruction of the extensor mechanism after total knee arthroplasty. J Bone Joint Surg Am 81:1749, 1999.
59. Levy M, Goldstein J, Rosner M: A method of repair for quadriceps tendon or patellar ligament (tendon) ruptures without cast immobilization. Clin Orthop 218:297, 1987.
60. Li PL: Acute bilateral rupture of the quadriceps tendon—an obvious diagnosis? Injury 25:191, 1994.
61. Liow RY, Tavares S: Bilateral rupture of the quadriceps tendon associated with anabolic steroids. Br J Sports Med 29:77, 1995.
62. Lombardi LJ, Cleri DJ, Epstein E: Bilateral spontaneous quadriceps tendon rupture in a patient with renal failure. Orthopedics 18:187, 1995.
63. Lynch AF, Rorabeck CH, Bourne R: Extensor mechanism complications following total knee arthroplasty. J Arthroplasty 2:135, 1987.
64. MacEachern AG, Plewes JL: Bilateral simultaneous spontaneous rupture of the quadriceps tendons: Five case reports and a review of the literature. J Bone Joint Surg Br 66:81, 1984.
65. Marder RA, Timmerman LA: Primary repair of patellar tendon rupture without augmentation. Am J Sports Med 27:304, 1999.
66. Margles SW, Lewis MM: Bilateral spontaneous concurrent rupture of the patellar tendon without apparent associated systemic disease: A case report. Clin Orthop 136:186, 1978.
67. Marumoto JM, Mitsunaga MM, Richardson AB, et al: Late patellar tendon ruptures after removal of the central third for anterior cruciate ligament reconstruction. Am J Sports Med 24:698, 1996.
68. Matava MJ: Patellar tendon ruptures. J Am Acad Orthop Surg 4:287, 1996.
69. McBurney C: Suture of the divided ends of a ruptured quadriceps extensor tendon with perfect recovery. Ann Surg 6:170, 1887.
70. McGrory JE: Disruption of the extensor mechanism of the knee. J Emerg Med 24:163, 2003.
71. McLaughlin HL: Repair of ruptures through the larger tendons by removable staple suture. Arch Surg 52:547, 1946.
72. McLaughlin HL: Repair of major tendon rupture by buried removable suture. Am J Surg 74:758, 1947.
73. McLaughlin HL, Francis KC: Operative repair of injuries to the quadriceps extensor mechanism. Am J Surg 91:651, 1953.
74. McNally PD, Marcelli EA: Achilles allograft reconstruction of a chronic patellar tendon rupture: A case report. Arthroscopy 14:340, 1998.
75. Miles JW, Grana WA, Egle D, et al: The effect of anabolic steroids on the biomechanical and histological properties of rat tendon. J Bone Joint Surg Am 74:411, 1992.
76. Miskew WBW, Pearson RL, Pankowich AM: Mersilene strip suture in repair of disruptions of the quadriceps and patellar tendons. J Trauma 20:867, 1980.
77. Mochizuki RM, Schurman DJ: Patellar complications following total knee arthroplasty. J Bone Joint Surg Am 61:879, 1979.
78. Morgan J, McCarty DJ: Tendon ruptures in patients with systemic lupus erythematosus treated with corticosteroids. Arthritis Rheum 17:1033, 1974.

79. Munshi NI, Mbubaegbu CE: Simultaneous rupture of the quadriceps tendon with contralateral rupture of the patellar tendon in an otherwise healthy athlete. Br J Sports Med 30:177, 1996.

80. Nance EP, Kaye JJ: Injuries of the quadriceps mechanism. Radiology 142:301, 1982.

81. Naver L, Aalberg JR: Rupture of the quadriceps tendon following dislocation of the patella: A case report. J Bone Joint Surg Am 67:324, 1985.

82. Nazarian DG, Booth RE: Extensor mechanism allografts in total knee arthroplasty. Clin Orthop 367:123, 1999.

83. Oladipo OOJ, Whitelaw GP, Shah BP: Bilateral simultaneous rupture of the quadriceps tendon: Case report. Am J Knee Surg 10:89, 1997.

84. Ong BC, Sherman O: Acute patellar tendon rupture: A new surgical technique. Arthroscopy 16:469, 2000.

85. Oni OO, Ahmad SH: The vastus lateralis–derived flap for repair of neglected rupture of the quadriceps femoris tendon. Surg Gynecol Obstet 161:385, 1985.

86. Parker DA, Dunbar MJ, Rorabeck CH: Extensor mechanism failure associated with total knee arthroplasty: Prevention and management. J Am Acad Orthop Surg 11:238, 2003.

87. Phillip BB: Knee injuries. In Crenshaw AH (ed): Campbell's Operative Orthopaedics. St Louis, Mosby–Year Book, 1992, pp 1895-1938.

88. Preston ET: Avulsions of both quadriceps tendons in hyperparathyroidism. JAMA 221:406, 1972.

89. Quenu E, Duval P: Traitement operatoire des ruptures sous-rotuliennes du quadriceps. Rev Chir 31:169, 1905.

90. Raatikainen T, Karpakka J, Orava S: Repair of partial quadriceps tendon rupture: Observations in 28 cases. Acta Orthop Scand 65:154, 1994.

91. Ramsey RH, Muller GE: Quadriceps tendon rupture: A diagnostic trap. Clin Orthop 70:161, 1970.

92. Rand JA, Morrey BF, Bryan RS: Patellar tendon rupture after total knee arthroplasty. Clin Orthop 244:233, 1989.

93. Rasul AT, Fischer DA: Primary repair of quadriceps tendon ruptures: Results of treatment. Clin Orthop 289:205, 1993.

94. Ravalin R, Mazzocca AD, Grady-Benson JC, et al: Biomechanical comparison of patellar tendon repairs in a cadaver model: An evaluation of gap formation at the repair site with cyclic loading. Am J Sports Med 30: 2002.

95. Razzano CD, Wilde AH, Phalen GH: Bilateral rupture of the infrapatellar tendon in rheumatoid arthritis. Clin Orthop 91:158, 1973.

96. Reider B, Marshall JL, Koslin B, et al: The anterior aspect of the knee joint: An anatomic study. J Bone Joint Surg Am 63:351, 1981.

97. Richards, DP, Barber AF: Repair of quadriceps tendon ruptures using suture anchors. Arthroscopy 18:556, 2002.

98. Rose PS, Frassica FJ: Atraumatic bilateral patellar tendon rupture: A case report and review of the literature. J Bone Joint Surg Am 83:1382, 2001.

99. Rougraff BT, Reeck CC, Essenmacher J: Complete quadriceps tendon ruptures. Orthopedics 19:509, 1996.

100. Schwartzberg RS, Csencsitz TA: Bilateral spontaneous patellar tendon rupture. Am J Orthop 25:369, 1996.

101. Scuderi C: Ruptures of the quadriceps tendon: Study of twenty tendon ruptures. Am J Surg 95:626, 1958.

102. Scuderi C, Schrey EL: Ruptures of the quadriceps tendon: Study of fourteen tendon ruptures. Arch Surg 61:42, 1950.

103. Scuderi GR: Extensor mechanism injuries: Treatment. In Scott WN (ed): Ligament and Extensor Mechanism Injuries of the Knee. St Louis, Mosby–Year Book, 1991, pp 183-193.

104. Scuderi GR, Scharf SC, Meltzer LP: The relationship of lateral releases to patella viability in total knee arthroplasty. J Arthroplasty 2:209, 1987.

105. Scuderi GR, Scharf SC, Meltzer L: Evaluation of patella viability after disruption of the arterial circulation. Am J Sports Med 15:490, 1987.

106. Shah M, Jooma N: Simultaneous bilateral quadriceps tendon rupture while playing basketball. Br J Sports Med 36:152, 2002.

107. Siwek CW, Rao JP: Ruptures of the extensor mechanism of the knee joint. J Bone Joint Surg Am 63:932, 1981.

108. Spector ED, Di Marcangelo MT, Jacoby JH: The radiologic diagnosis of quadriceps tendon rupture. NJ Med 92:590, 1995.

109. Stern RE, Harwin SF: Spontaneous and simultaneous rupture of both quadriceps tendons. Clin Orthop 147:188, 1980.

110. Thompson TC: Quadricepsplasty to improve knee function. J Bone Joint Surg Am 36:366, 1944.

111. Walker LG, Glick H: Bilateral spontaneous quadriceps tendon ruptures: A case report and review of the literature. Orthop Rev 18:867, 1989.

112. Wascher DC, Summa CD: Reconstruction of chronic rupture of the extensor mechanism after patellectomy. Clin Orthop 357:135, 1998.

113. Webb LX, Toby EB: Bilateral rupture of the patella tendon in an otherwise healthy male patient following minor trauma. J Trauma 26:1045, 1986.

114. Wenzl ME, Kirchner R, Seide K, et al: Quadriceps tendon ruptures—is there a complete functional restitution. Injury 35:922, 2004.

115. Williams RJ, Brooks DD, Wickiewicz TL: Reconstruction of the patellar tendon using a patella-quadriceps tendon autograft. Orthopedics 20:554, 1997.

116. Yu JS, Petersilge C, Sartoris DJ, et al: MR imaging of injuries of the extensor mechanism of the knee. Radiographics 14:541, 1994.

Index

Note: Page numbers followed by f, t, and b refer to figures, tables, and boxed material, respectively.

A

Abrasion, synovial, in meniscal repair, 487, 487f, 488f
Abrasion chondroplasty
  for chondromalacia, 918-919
  for juvenile osteochondritis dissecans, 1239
  for osteoarthritis, 354-355
  for osteonecrosis, 453
Abrasive wear. *See* Wear.
ACE bandage, in knee denervation surgery, 1088-1089
Acellularized tendon grafts, 668
Acetaminophen, for arthritis, 334, 999, 1641
Achilles tendon allograft
  in ACL reconstruction, 252
    vs. patellar tendon graft, 606, 669-670
  in extensor mechanism reconstruction, 1822-1823
  in LCL reconstruction, 628-630, 630f
    in knee dislocation, 767
  in PCL reconstruction, 245
    in knee dislocation, 767
  in posterolateral corner injuries, 780, 781, 781f, 782f
ACL. *See* Anterior cruciate ligament (ACL).
Acquired immunodeficiency syndrome. *See also* Human immunodeficiency virus infection.
  definition of, 1049
  diseases associated with, 1057-1060
    infectious, 1057-1058
    inflammatory, 1058-1059
    necrotic, 1059-1060
    neoplastic, 1060
    osteoporotic, 1060
  transfusion-related, in hemophiliacs, 1010
Acticoat, 1107
Activity level
  chondral injuries and, 433
  preoperative, as guide for osteotomy, 1325
Activity score, improved, after autologous chondrocyte transplantation, in athletes, 382-383, 383t
Acufex Knee Signature System, 588. *See also* Arthrometry.
Acupuncture, for osteoarthritis, 332-333
Acute normovolemic hemodilution, reduced blood loss with, 1830-1831
Adalimumab, for rheumatoid arthritis, 997
Adductor magnus muscle, anatomy of, 45f, 51
Adductor tubercle, 43f, 1119
Adeno-associated virus, in gene therapy, 318, 319f
Adenovirus, in gene therapy, 318, 319f
Adhesions
  after ACL reconstruction, 642-643
  after PCL reconstruction, 754
Adolescents. *See* Pediatric patients.
Advance PS prosthesis, 1537-1538, 1538f
Aerobic conditioning, for osteoarthritis, 330-331

Age
  gestational, estimation of, 1183
  patient. *See also* Elderly; Pediatric patients.
    in ACL reconstruction, 635
    in bone tumors, 1851, 1852t
    in chondral injury, 433
    in high tibial osteotomy, 1325
    in proprioception, 113
    in unicompartmental arthroplasty, 1423
    in wound healing, 1103
    instability and, 513
Agility drills, after ACL reconstruction, 712
AIDS. *See* Acquired immunodeficiency syndrome.
Alendronate, for reflex sympathetic dystrophy, 1077
Algodystrophy, 1074. *See also* Reflex sympathetic dystrophy.
Alignment. *See also* Malalignment.
  in computer-assisted surgery, optimization of, 1690-1691
  in preoperative osteotomy planning, 1303, 1303t
  in total knee arthroplasty. *See* Total knee arthroplasty, alignment in.
  patellar. *See also* Patellar tracking.
    evaluation of
      in physical examination, 86, 87f
      radiographic, 147-149, 151f
    valgus, in patellar dislocation, 1750
Alignment guide, for total knee arthroplasty, 1478-1479, 1479f
  anatomic method in, 1479-1480, 1480f
  classic method in, 1479, 1479f
Alloantibody inhibitor, in hemophilia, 1036-1037
Allogenic antibody, in hemophilia, 1034-1035
Allograft(s). *See also specific types and procedures.*
  acellularized, 668
  bacterial contamination of, 690-691
  cryopreservation of, 502, 668-670, 687, 688, 1822
  disadvantages of, 252
  donor screening for, 501-502, 688-689
  freeze-dried, 502, 687, 688, 1822, 1882
    vs. fresh-frozen allografts, 1822
  fresh, 687
  fresh-frozen, 687, 688, 1822, 1882
    vs. freeze-dried allografts, 1822
  historical perspective on, 686
  HIV transmission via, 252
  immune response to, 408, 421-422, 500-501, 664-665, 665f, 686
  incorporation of, 687
  infections from, 252, 665-668, 690-691
    prevention of, 406-407, 663-664, 688-691
  insertion of, surgical technique in, 508, 508f, 509f
  lyophilization of, 502
  physiology of, 687
  preparation of, 507-508, 507f, 508f

Allograft(s) *(Continued)*
  processing of, 502, 667-668, 686-687
  procurement of, 501-502
  rejection of, 501
  safety of, 406-407, 663-664, 667-668, 688-691
  sizing of, 503-504
  sterilization and irradiation of, 252, 502, 667-668, 687-688
  storage of, 407-408, 407t, 421
  tissue banking of, 667-668, 688-690
Allograft-prosthetic composite reconstruction, 1877-1885
  advantages of, 1877, 1878f
  composite cementing in, 1878-1879
  extensor mechanism repair in, 1882, 1883f
  extensor mechanism transplant in, 1884-1885
  fixation in, 1878
  graft size in, 1879-1880
  graft-host junction in, 1878, 1879f
  of distal femur, 1884, 1885f
  of tibia, 1880-1882
  overview of, 1877
  principles of, 1878-1880
  soft tissue coverage in, 1880
Allowash technology, 667-668
Alternating current technology, in electromagnetic computer-assisted navigation, 1707
Alumina, in total knee arthroplasty, 267-268
Alveolar soft part sarcoma, 1030
Ambulatory aid, for arthritis, 1642
American Association of Tissue Banks (AATB) guidelines, 406-407, 667, 688
American College of Chest Physicians (ACCP) guidelines, for thromboprophylaxis, 1844
American Orthopaedic Society for Sports Medicine Study Group Knee Score, 563, 564f, 565f
Aminolevulinic acid–dehydratase deficiency porphyria, 578-581, 949-951, 950f
Amoxicillin, prophylactic, in total knee arthroplasty, 1784t
Ampicillin, prophylactic, in total knee arthroplasty, 1784t
Amputation
  for flexion deformity, 1219
  for malignant bone tumors, 1871-1872
  for reflex sympathetic dystrophy, 1078
  salvage, of infected prosthesis, 1789
Anakinra, for rheumatoid arthritis, 997
Analgesia. *See also* Pain *and specific analgesics.*
  for arthritis, 334, 1641
  for osteonecrosis, 452
  for reflex sympathetic dystrophy, 875-876
Anatomic axis, of knee, 86, 87f, 146f, 147
Anderson Knee Stabler, 715-716
Anderson technique, for pediatric ACL reconstruction, 1247, 1250f

Patellofemoral arthroplasty, 1442-1453, 1442f-
1443f
  Autocentric implant in, 1448t, 1449, 1450f
  Avon implant in, 1448t, 1450-1451, 1450f
  Bartlett patella score in, 1445t
  Bristol patella score in, 1445t
  clinical evaluation for, 1444
  clinical results of, 6-8, 1446f, 1448t, 1449-
    1453, 1449f-1452f
  design characteristics in, 1451
  for chondromalacia, 927-928, 959
  for osteoarthritis, 1647-1648
  for patellofemoral arthritis, 927-928
  Fulkerson patellofemoral score in, 1446t
  late failure of, 1452-1453
  Lonner patellofemoral score in, 1447t
  Low Contact Stress implant in, 1447, 1448t,
    1449, 1449f
  Lubinus implant in, 1448t, 1449-1450,
    1450f
  Nexon implant in, 1448t, 1450
  patient selection for, 1443
  postoperative management of, 1444-1445
  postoperative radiographs of, 1451-1452,
    1451f, 1452f
  Richards I, II, and III implants in, 1446-
    1447, 1446f, 1448t
  scoring systems in, 1445, 1445t, 1446t,
    1447t
  surgical technique of, 1444
Patellofemoral bracing, 723-724, 723f, 724f,
  726t, 962, 962f. See also Brace/bracing.
Patellofemoral index, 833-834, 841t
Patellofemoral instability, 817, 1189. See also
  Patellar dislocation; Patellar subluxation;
  Patellofemoral joint, disorders of.
  after patellar resurfacing, 1580, 1581f, 1582
  apprehension test in, 819, 820f, 884-885
  classification of, 886-887
  continuum of, 1206
  in pediatric patients, 1278-1291
    anatomic aspects of, 1278-1281, 1280f,
      1281f
    biomechanics of, 1278-1281
    classification of, 1282-1283, 1282f, 1283t
    developmental aspects of, 1278
    imaging of, 1284-1285, 1285f
    injury history in, 1283
    natural history of, 1283
    nonoperative management of, 1285-1286
    operative management of, 1286-1290
      indications for, 1286
      with medial patellofemoral ligament
        repair, 1286-1289, 1288f, 1289f
      without medial patellofemoral ligament
        repair, 1289-1290
    physical examination in, 1283-1284
    risk fractures for, 1281-1282
  operative management of
    medial patellofemoral repair/
      reconstruction of, 948
    in pediatric patients, 1286-1289
    without medial patellofemoral repair/
      reconstruction of, in pediatric
      patients, 1289-1290
Patellofemoral joint, 807-930
  anatomy of, 807-812, 1278-1281, 1280f,
    1281f
    of femoral trochlea, 808
    of lateral retinaculum, 808-809, 810f
    of medial retinaculum, 809-810, 811f
    of patella, 807-808, 808f
    of patellar tendon, 808
  arthroscopy of, 944-945, 945f

Patellofemoral joint (Continued)
  articulation of, in mobile-bearing prosthesis,
    1566-1567
  biomechanics of, 812-816, 1278-1281
  contact areas in, 815, 815f
  contact pressure in, 815-816
  disorders of
    anatomic aspects of, 807-812
    apprehension test in, 819, 819f, 884-885
    autologous chondrocyte transplantation
      in, 383-388, 384f, 385f, 386t, 387t
    biomechanical aspects of, 812-817
    classification of, 847-850
    femoral neck anteversion in, 822-823
    hip rotation in, 822-823
    history in, 816-817
    imaging in, 823-846. See also
      Patellofemoral joint, imaging of.
    instability in, 817
    locking in, 817
    osteochondral allograft for, 415
    outcome scales for, 578
    pain in, 816-817, 850-878. See also
      Patellofemoral pain.
    patellar compression test in, 819, 819f
    patellar mobility evaluation in, 821-822,
      822f
    patellar tilt test in, 821-822, 822f
    patellar tracking in, assessment of, 818,
      818f
    physical examination in, 817-823
    post-traumatic, 848-849
    Q angle measurement in, 819-821, 820f
    surgical treatment of, 944-963
      failure of, 962-963
      for articular degeneration without
        malalignment, 958-959, 961
      for malalignment, 944-958, 960-961
      for soft-tissue disorders without
        malalignment, 959, 961
    swelling in, 817
    tibial torsion in, 822, 823
    vastus medialis hypoplasia in, 817-818
  embryology of, 848, 1278
  imaging of, 823-846, 841t
    arthrography in, 840-844
    arthroscopy in, 845-846
    computed tomography in, 838-840, 839f-
      841f, 841t
    magnetic resonance imaging in, 844
    normal findings on, 841t
    radiographic, 823-837, 841t
      anteroposterior view in, 823
      axial view in, 831-837, 832f-837f
      Blumensaat's line in, 824
      double-bubble sign in, 829-830
      in patellar height measurement, 823-
        831. See also Patella, height of,
        radiologic evaluation of.
      in sulcus evaluation, 829, 830f, 831f
      in trochlear evaluation, 827-831
      lateral view in, 823-831, 841t
      Laurin view in, 833-834, 834f, 841t
      Merchant view in, 832-833, 832f, 833f,
        841t
      patellar shape on, 827, 827f
      patellar tilt on, 827-828, 828f
      stress, 836-837
      sulcus line on, 828-831, 830f, 831f
    radionuclide imaging in, 845
  lesions of, débridement and microfracture
    of, rehabilitation protocol after, 363
  magnetic resonance imaging of, 173-174,
    174f-176f

Patellofemoral joint (Continued)
  malalignment of, 849
    arthroscopic diagnosis of, 944-945, 945f
    authors' preferred treatment of, 960-961
    chondromalacia and, 853, 912-913, 912f,
      915
    definition of, 848
    distal realignment procedures for, 949-
      958
      complications of, 954-955
      results of, 949-954
    Insall's proximal realignment for, 948,
      949f
    lateral, 850-866. See also Lateral patellar
      compression syndrome.
    lateral release for, 945-947, 947f, 948f
      with medial imbrication, 947-948, 949f
    pain in, 853-855. See also Patellofemoral
      pain.
    patellar dislocation and. See Patellar
      dislocation.
    taping for, 857-858, 857f
    tibial transfer for, 893-897, 893f, 894f,
      895t, 950-951
    tibial tubercle anteriorization for, 919-
      926, 919f, 921f-924f, 925t, 951-953,
      952f, 953f, 958
      complications of, 954-955
      results of, 121t, 924-926, 952-953,
        958
      technique of, 922-926, 922f-924f
    tibial tubercle anteromedialization for,
      384-385, 385f, 953-958, 954f-957f
    tibial tubercle unloading procedures for,
      1441
  palpation of, 89, 940-941, 898f
  stabilizers in
    muscular active, 810-811, 811f
    passive soft-tissue, 808, 809f
Patellofemoral joint reaction force, 812-815,
  813f, 814f
Patellofemoral ligament
  anatomy of, 42, 43f
  medial
    anatomy of, 809-810, 811f
    deficiency of, patellar glide test for, 810
    injury of, in patellar dislocation, 881
    reconstruction of, 948
Patellofemoral osteoarthritis. See
  Patellofemoral arthritis.
Patellofemoral outcome scales, 578. See also
  Knee rating scales.
Patellofemoral pain, 850-878
  after ACL reconstruction, with patellar
    tendon autograft, 643
  after patellectomy, 960
  basal degeneration and, 912-913
  characteristics of, 938
  crepitus and, 940-941
  diagnosis of, 938
  etiology of, 853-855
  flexibility evaluation in, 942
  from malalignment, 944-958. See also
    Patellofemoral joint, malalignment of.
  history in, 938-939
  in articular degeneration without
    malalignment, 958
  in lateral patellar compression syndrome,
    850-866. See also Lateral patellar
    compression syndrome.
  in overuse syndromes, 866-870
  in patellar dislocation, 938-939
  in patellar subluxation, 938, 961
  in peripatellar bursitis, 870

Semitendinosus/gracilis tendon allografts, in ACL reconstruction, 663-664, 664f
in double-bundle technique, 684
Semitendinosus/gracilis tendon autografts, in ACL reconstruction, 647, 648
Sensorimotor system
capsuloligamentous mechanoreceptors in, 99-100, 100f, 100t
histology and structural anatomy of, 99-102
in neuromuscular control, 104, 106-110
balance and posturography and, 110, 110f
dynamic electromyography of, 106-107, 108f
for force perception, 106
for proprioception and kinesthesia, 106, 106f, 107f
Hoffmann reflex and, 108-109, 109f
isokinetic research and, 109-110, 109f
microneurography of, 107, 108f
muscle stiffness and, 110
reflexive muscle activation and, 107, 108f
somatosensory evoked potentials and, 109
twitch interpolation and burst superimposition and, 110
tenomuscular receptors in, 100-102, 101f
Septic arthritis
in HIV/AIDS, 1058
magnetic resonance imaging of, 184-185
synovianalysis in, 1007
Sexual transmission, of HIV, 1052
Sham incision, 1110, 1112f
Shiers prosthesis, 1369, 1371f
Shock absorption, by meniscus, 313, 482-483
Shoe modification, for arthritis, 1642
Short arc quad exercise, 698f, 705
Siderosome, 1008
in cartilage damage, 1037-1038
Silicon sheeting, for scar hypertrophy, 1112, 1113f
Silvadene, for skin loss, 1107
Sinding-Larsen-Johansson disease
magnetic resonance imaging of, 211
radiography of, 156, 156f
Skin
bacterial contamination of, 1106
blistering of, circulatory compromise and, 1105, 1105f
breakdown of, in distal femoral fracture, 1128
closure of, wound healing in, 1104-1105, 1105f
healing of, 1105-1108
compromise of, 1106-1108
surgical preparation of, 1106
Skin graft, for wound complications, 1111-1113, 1112f, 1113f
Skin necrosis, after total knee arthroplasty, 1722, 1722f
Skin tape, 1105
Skyline view, radiographic, 145
Sleeve, for arthritic knee, 724-725, 726t
Sleeve fractures, patellar, 1273-1276, 1275f, 1276f
Sliding hammer, prosthetic component removal with, in revision arthroplasty, 1762, 1764f
Slocum test, 96, 96f, 619-620, 620f
Smillie's approach, 125
Smoking
consent form in, 1101, 1102f
in wound healing, 1101

Snapping knee syndrome, 1228, 1229. See also Meniscus, discoid.
Soccer players, autologous chondrocyte transplantation in, 382-383, 383t
Soft tissue
healing of, 1099-1108. See also Wound healing.
irritation of, from patellar hardware, 1164
local manipulations of, 1110-1111, 1111f
magnetic resonance imaging of, 161-175
radiography of
abnormal findings on, 153-161
normal findings on, 145-147
Soft-tissue expansion, before total knee arthroplasty, 1110-1111, 1112f
Soft-tissue impingement, of patella, 1752-1753, 1752f
Soft-tissue sarcoma, 1908
Soft-tissue tumors, 1903-1908
benign, 1907-1908
calcifications in, 157, 159f
clinical features of, 1903
cystic, 1904-1907
evaluation of, 1903-1904
imaging of, 186-187, 190f, 1904, 1904f
malignant, 1908
Soft-tissue procedure, in ACL reconstruction, computer-assisted, 1666-1667, 1667f
Soleus muscle, anatomy of, 53
Somatosensory evoked potentials, testing of, 109
Spacer block technique, extramedullary, for unicompartmental arthroplasty, 1435, 1437f
Spherocentric prosthesis, 1369, 1371f
loosening rate of, 1731-1732
Spinal anesthesia, 1064-1065. See also Anesthesia.
for reflex sympathetic dystrophy, 875-876
Spinal cord stimulation, for reflex sympathetic dystrophy, 1078
Spinning, in knee kinematics, 228, 229f
Spin-out, catastrophic, of mobile-bearing prosthesis, 1570-1571, 1570f
Splints. See also Brace/bracing.
for MCL injuries, 621
Split biceps tendon graft, in PCL reconstruction, 751, 752f
Split patella approach, Insall's modification of, 122-123, 123f
Spondyloarthropathies, 989-990
magnetic resonance imaging of, 184-185
Spongialization, for chondromalacia, 918-919
Spontaneous osteonecrosis of knee, magnetic resonance imaging of, 183-184, 184f-186f, 218, 219f
Sporting activity
return to. See Return to sports.
transmission of HIV during, 1055
Sports knee osteotomy, 517-530
associated ligament deficiencies and, 523-524
cartilage repair and, 523
complications of, 528-530, 529t
contraindications to, 518-520, 519t
counseling for, 520
for valgus deformity, 528, 529f
for varus deformity, 524-528, 525f-527f
indications for, 517-518, 519f
malalignment with isolated gonarthrosis and, 521-523, 521f, 522f
patient selection for, 517-520
physical examination for, 520
preoperative planning for, 520-524

Sports knee osteotomy (Continued)
radiologic evaluation for, 520-521
results of, 530
surgical techniques of, 524-528
closing wedge, 525-526, 525f-526f
distal femoral closing wedge, 528, 529f
opening wedge, 527-528, 527f
treatment algorithm for, 521-524
Sprains, 549, 550f. See also Ligament(s), injury of.
classification of, 549, 550f
Squinting, patellar, 817, 817f
S-shaped posterior incision, 132, 132f
SST angle, intraoperative measurement of, 902-903, 905f
Stability. See also Instability.
after total knee arthroplasty, with PCL retention/substitution, 1383, 1383f, 1384f
meniscal role in, 483
of mobile-bearing prosthesis, 1564
Standards for Tissue Banking (AATB), 667
Staphylococcal infections, from allografts, 666, 667, 690-691
Stapling, 1104-1105
anterior femoral, for flexion deformity, 1219
for juvenile osteochondritis dissecans, 1239
STAR technique, 683
Steadman Hawkins Clinical Research Database, 364, 364t
Steegast's method, in patellofemoral joint radiography, 831
Steinmann pin, in tibial tubercle fracture fixation, 1749
Steinmann test
first, 90, 91f
second, 90, 90f
Stem, prosthetic. See Prosthesis, stems of.
Stem cells, in gene therapy, 319, 319f
Sterilization
of allografts, 252, 502, 667-668, 687-688
of ultrahigh molecular weight polyethylene components, 265
Stiffness, 99, 110
after knee denervation surgery, 1092
after osteotomy, 1316
after total knee arthroplasty, 1730
in ACL-deficient knee, 112
in chronic patellar dislocation, 908
in quadriceps contracture, 908
in reflex sympathetic dystrophy, 871, 873
Stocking, compression, thromboprophylaxis with, 1841
Storage
of osteochondral allograft, prior to transplantation, 407-408, 407t
of osteochondral bulk allograft, science in, 421
Straight instability, 551-553
Straight-leg raising. See Quadriceps exercises.
Strapping, for proximal tibiofibular dislocation, 801
Strength testing, isokinetic, 791-792, 791f
Strengthening exercises. See Exercises.
Streptococcal infections, from allografts, 666, 667, 690-691
Stress
avoidance of, in PCL-retaining total knee arthroplasty, 1527
in finite element protocol, of polymer insert damage, 279-280
in wound healing, 1104
with PCL-substituting total knee arthroplasty, 1527

Vascular injuries
    after tibial osteotomy, 1315, 1346
    after total knee arthroplasty, 1723, 1723f
    in knee dislocation, 756, 757-758, 757f
    repair of, 762, 763, 765
Vascular response, to meniscal injury, 484-485,
    485f
Vascular theory, of osteonecrosis, 450
Vascularity
    meniscal, 311-312, 312f, 483-484, 483f,
    484f
    patellar, 1576
Vasodilation, in wound healing, 1100
Vastus intermedius muscle, 1148
    anatomy of, 38, 38f, 39f
Vastus lateralis intermedius muscle, anatomy
    of, 810-811, 811f
Vastus lateralis muscle, 1148
    anatomy of, 38, 38f, 39f, 810-811, 811f
Vastus medialis muscle, 1148
Vastus medialis obliquus muscle
    activity of, in neuromuscular control,
    105f
    advancement of, with lateral retinacular
    release, 948, 950f
    anatomy of, 38, 38f, 39f, 40, 41f, 45f, 810-
    811, 811f
    hypoplasia of, 75, 817-818
    in minimally invasive surgery, for total knee
    arthroplasty
        limited midvastus approach to, 1634,
        1634f
        limited subvastus approach to, 1633-
        1634, 1634f
    training of, in lateral patellar compression
    syndrome, 856-857, 858f
Vectors, in gene therapy
    nonviral, 317, 319f
    viral, 318, 319t
Venography, positive, in thromboembolism
    therapy, 1720
Venous thrombosis
    after knee arthroplasty, 1716-1720
    after tibial osteotomy, 1346
    deep
        anesthetic considerations in, 1068
        detection of, 1717-1718
        documented, protocol for, 1720
        incidence of, 1717
        prophylaxis for, 1718-1720, 1718f
            comparative studies of, 1719
        risk of, after knee surgery, 1837
    in calf veins, 1716, 1717f
    prophylaxis for
        ACCP guidelines in, 1844
        duration of, 1842-1844, 1844f
        mechanical, 1841
        pharmacological, 1838-1841, 1838f,
        1839f
        risk of, randomized trials in, 1840t
Vertical transmission, of HIV, 1055
Viability, of chondrocytes
    in osteochondral allografts, 406, 407, 407t
    in osteochondral bulk allografts, 421, 422
Video fluoroscopy, 1592. See also
    Fluoroscopy.
VIGOR trial, of COX inhibitors, 335, 994
Villonodular synovitis, pigmented, 1043-1046,
    1046f. See also Synovitis, pigmented
    villonodular.
Viral infections, from tendon allografts, 666
Viral vectors, in gene therapy, 318, 319t
Visual analog scale, 574, 576f

Vitamin C, in wound healing, 1104
Vitamin E, in wound healing, 1104
Von Willebrand's disease, vs. hemophilia A,
    1034
V-Y quadriceps tendon lengthening, for
    congenital knee dislocation, 1195,
    1197f

W
Wall slides, 697f
Warfarin. See also Anticoagulants.
    ACCP dosing guidelines for, 1844
    action and administration of, 1839t
    dose-adjusted
        anesthetic considerations associated with,
        1069
        efficacy of, 1838
        thromboprophylaxis with, 1718, 1720,
        1838-1839
WasherLoc fixation, of graft, in ACL
    reconstruction, 253
Water, in articular cartilage, 308
Wear
    after total knee arthroplasty, 1746-1748,
    1746f-1749f. See also Total knee
    arthroplasty, component wear in.
    in total knee arthroplasty, 267
    of femoral component, 1746
    of mobile-bearing prosthesis, 1561-1562
    of patellar component, 1747
        metal-backed, 1747, 1761, 1762f
    of polyethylene component, 1746, 1747,
    1748, 1749f
        after PCL-retaining total knee
        arthroplasty, 1383-1384, 1384f
        after PCL-substituting total knee
        arthroplasty, 1551, 1552f-1555f
        ultrahigh-molecular-weight, 265-267,
        266f
    of tibial component, 1746, 1746f
    prosthesis failure due to, 297-298, 297f
Webbing syndromes, flexion deformities in,
    1209-1221. See also Flexion deformity.
Wedge
    metal augmentation. See Metal wedge
    augmentation.
    sizing of, for osteotomy, 1333, 1335
Wedge osteotomy. See also Osteotomy; wedge
    Osteotomy.
    closing wedge proximal valgus
        with internal blade-plate fixation, 1330-
        1331, 1332f
        with internal plate fixation, 1331, 1333,
        1333f-1335f
    in sports knee
        closing wedge, 525-526, 525f-526f
        distal femoral closing, 528, 529f
        opening wedge, 527-528, 527f
    lateral closing tibial, for varus deformity,
    1307-1309, 1310f
    medial closing femoral, for valgus deformity,
    1312-1314, 1313f
    medial opening tibial
        for osteoarthritis, 1644, 1644f
        for varus deformity, 1309-1310, 1311f
    opening tibial
        advantages and disadvantages of, 1335
        by callus distraction (hemicallostasis)
            advantages and disadvantages of, 1338-
            1339
        technique of, 1337-1338, 1339f

Wedge osteotomy (Continued)
    technique of, 1333, 1335f-1337f
        wedge size calculation in, 1333, 1335
    opening vs. closing, 1307t
Weight. See also Obesity.
    influence of, in osteotomy planning, 1326
Weight reduction
    for arthritis, 1641
    for osteoarthritis, 331
Welding, thermal, of meniscal tissue, 489
Western Ontario McMaster Osteoarthritis
    Score (WOMAC), 364-365, 384
Wet-to-dry dressings, 1107
White-white meniscal tear, 485
Wire fixation
    of patellar fracture, tension band. See
    Tension band wiring, of patellar
    fracture.
    of tibial plateau fracture, 1143-1144, 1145f,
    1146f
Women
    ACL injuries in, predisposing factors for,
    610-611, 634, 1242
    ACL reconstruction in, results of, 610-
    611
    arthrometry in, 610-611
Worker's compensation claims, arthrometry
    results and, 610
Wound, coverage options for, 1110-1115
Wound care, 1105-1106, 1107
Wound drainage
    after total knee arthroplasty, 1721-1722,
    1721f
        prolonged, 1786, 1786f
    postoperative management of, 1832-1833
Wound healing, 1099-1108
    age in, 1103
    anemia effects on, 1103
    aspirin in, 1103
    bacterial contamination in, 1106
    cellular elements of, 1100-1101
    chemotherapy in, 1103
    cigarette smoking effects on, 1101, 1102f
    circulatory compromise in, 1105-1106
        blistering from, 1105, 1105f
    complications of
        anticipation of, 1110, 1111f
        fascial flaps for, 1114
        fasciocutaneous flaps for, 1114-1115, 1115f
        free flaps for, 1114-1115, 1115f
        muscle flaps for, 1113-1114, 1113f
        myocutaneous flaps for, 1113-1114
        skin graft for, 1111-1113, 1112f, 1113f
    corticosteroid effect on, 1103
    delayed, after total knee arthroplasty,
    1722
    diabetes mellitus effects on, 1101-1102
    difficulties in, planning for, 1110-1111,
    1111f, 1112f
    dressings for, 1107
    edema in, 1106
    epidermis in, 1106-1107
    factors affecting, 1101-1105
    fibroblastic proliferative phase of, 1100
    growth factors in, 1108
    hematoma in, 1106
    history of, 1099-1100
    hyperbaric oxygenation therapy in, 1101,
    1102f
    infection in, 1106
    inflammatory phase of, 1100
    maturation phase of, 1100
    necrosis in, 1106, 1107